SURGERY OF THE SKIN

PROCEDURAL DERMATOLOGY

PLEASE READ THE FOLLOWING AGREEMENT CAREFULLY BEFORE USING THIS DVD-ROM PRODUCT. THIS DVD-ROM PRODUCT IS LICENSED UNDER THE TERMS CONTAINED IN THIS DVD-ROM LICENSE AGREEMENT ("Agreement"). BY USING THIS DVD-ROM PRODUCT, YOU, AN INDIVIDUAL OR ENTITY INCLUDING EMPLOYEES, AGENTS AND REPRESENTATIVES ("You" or "Your"), ACKNOWLEDGE THAT YOU HAVE READ THIS AGREEMENT, THAT YOU UNDERSTAND IT, AND THAT YOU AGREE TO BE BOUND BY THE TERMS AND CONDITIONS OF THIS AGREEMENT. ELSEVIER INC. ("Elsevier") EXPRESSLY DOES NOT AGREE TO LICENSE THIS DVD-ROM PRODUCT TO YOU UNLESS YOU ASSENT TO THIS AGREEMENT. IF YOU DO NOT AGREE WITH ANY OF THE FOLLOWING TERMS, YOU MAY, WITHIN THIRTY (30) DAYS AFTER YOUR RECEIPT OF THIS DVD-ROM PRODUCT RETURN THE UNUSED, PIN NUMBER PROTECTED, DVD-ROM PRODUCT, ALL ACCOMPANYING DOCUMENTATION TO ELSEVIER FOR A FULL REFUND.

DEFINITIONS As used in this Agreement, these terms shall have the following meanings:

"Proprietary Material" means the valuable and proprietary information content of this DVD-ROM Product including all indexes and graphic materials and software used to access, index, search and retrieve the information content from this DVD-ROM Product developed or licensed by Elsevier and/or its affiliates, suppliers and licensors.

"DVD-ROM Product" means the copy of the Proprietary Material and any other material delivered on DVD-ROM and any other human-readable or machine-readable materials enclosed with this Agreement, including without limitation documentation relating to the same.

OWNERSHIP This DVD-ROM Product has been supplied by and is proprietary to Elsevier and/or its affiliates, suppliers and licensors. The copyright in the DVD-ROM Product belongs to Elsevier and/or its affiliates, suppliers and licensors and is protected by the national and state copyright, trademark, trade secret and other intellectual property laws of the United States and international treaty provisions, including without limitation the Universal Copyright Convention and the Berne Copyright Convention. You have no ownership rights in this DVD-ROM Product. Except as expressly set forth herein, no part of this DVD-ROM Product, including without limitation the Proprietary Material, may be modified, copied or distributed in hardcopy or machine-readable form without prior written consent from Elsevier. All rights not expressly granted to You herein are expressly reserved. Any other use of this DVD-ROM Product by any person or entity is strictly prohibited and a violation of this Agreement.

SCOPE OF RIGHTS LICENSED (PERMITTED USES) Elsevier is granting to You a limited, non-exclusive, non-transferable license to use this DVD-ROM Product in accordance with the terms of this Agreement. You may use or provide access to this DVD-ROM Product on a single computer or terminal physically located at Your premises and in a secure network or move this DVD-ROM Product to and use it on another single computer or terminal at the same location for personal use only, but under no circumstances may You use or provide access to any part or parts of this DVD-ROM Product on more than one computer or terminal simultaneously.

You shall not (a) copy, download, or otherwise reproduce the DVD-ROM Product in any medium, including, without limitation, online transmissions, local area networks, wide area networks, intranets, extranets and the Internet, or in any way, in whole or in part, except for printing out or downloading nonsubstantial portions of the text and images in the DVD-ROM Product for Your own personal use; (b) alter, modify, or adapt the DVD-ROM Product, including but not limited to decompiling, disassembling, reverse engineering, or creating derivative works, without the prior written approval of Elsevier; (c) sell, license or otherwise distribute to third parties the DVD-ROM Product or any part or parts thereof; or (d) alter, remove, obscure or obstruct the display of any copyright, trademark or other proprietary notice on or in the DVD-ROM Product or on any printout or download of portions of the Proprietary Materials.

RESTRICTIONS ON TRANSFER This License is personal to You, and neither Your rights hereunder nor the tangible embodiments of this DVD-ROM Product, including without limitation the Proprietary Material, may be sold, assigned, transferred or sublicensed to any other person, including without limitation by operation of law, without the prior written consent of Elsevier. Any purported sale, assignment, transfer or sublicense without the prior written consent of Elsevier will be void and will automatically terminate the License granted hereunder.

TERM This Agreement will remain in effect until terminated pursuant to the terms of this Agreement. You may terminate this Agreement at any time by removing from Your system and destroying the DVD-ROM Product. Unauthorized copying of the DVD-ROM Product, including without limitat tary Material and documentation, or otherwise failing to con rms and conditions of this Agreement shall result in autom n of this license and will make available to Elsevier legal re termination of this Agreement, the license granted herein and You must immediately destroy the DVD-ROM Product panying documentation. All provisions relating to propriet l survive termination of this Agreement.

LIMITEL Y AND LIMITATION OF LIABILITY NEITHER ELSEVIE CENSORS REPRESENT OR WARRANT THAT THE DVD-ROI WILL MEET YOUR REQUIREMENTS OR THAT ITS OPERATI BE UNINTERRUPTED OR ERROR-FREE. WE EXCLUDE ESSLY DISCLAIM ALL EXPRESS AND IMPLIED WARRAN TATED HEREIN, INCLUDING THE IMPLIED WARRANTIES NTABILITY AND FITNESS FOR A PARTICULAR PURPOSE ON, NEITHER ELSEVIER NOR ITS LICENSORS MAKE ANY TATIONS OR WARRANTIES, EITHER EXPRESS OR IMPLIE ING THE PERFORMANCE OF YOUR NETWORK OR COMPU M WHEN USED IN CONJUNCTION WITH THE DVD-ROM F E SHALL NOT BE LIABLE FOR ANY DAMAGE OR LOSS OF A RISING OUT OF OR RESULTING FROM YOUR POSSESSIO OF THE SOFTWARE PRODUCT CAUSED BY ERRORS OR S, DATA LOSS OR CORRUPTION, ERRORS OR OMISSIONS ROPRIETARY MATERIAL, REGARDLESS OF WHETHER S ITY IS BASED IN TORT, CONTRACT OR OTHERWISE AND I BUT NOT LIMITED TO, ACTUAL, SPECIAL, INDIRECT, INC R CONSEQUENTIAL DAMAGES. IF THE FOREGOING LIMITA LD TO BE UNENFORCEABLE, OUR MAXIMUM LIABILITY TO Y NOT EXCEED THE AMOUNT OF THE LICENSE FEE PAID BY THE SOFTWARE PRODUCT. THE REMEDIES AVAILABLE TO NST US AND THE LICENSORS OF MATERIALS INCLUDED IN T VARE PRODUCT ARE EXCLUSIVE.

If this DVD-ROM s defective, Elsevier will replace it at no charge if the defective D Product is returned to Elsevier within sixty (60) days (or the grea d allowable by applicable law) from the date of shipment.

Elsevier warrants software embodied in this DVD-ROM Product will perform in sub ompliance with the documentation supplied in this DVD-ROM Pro u report a significant defect in performance in writing to Elsevier, ier is not able to correct same within sixty (60) days after its recei r notification, You may return this DVD-ROM Product, including a and documentation, to Elsevier and Elsevier will refund Your mor

YOU UNDERSTAND EXCEPT FOR THE 60-DAY LIMITED WARRANTY RECITED A ELSEVIER, ITS AFFILIATES, LICENSORS, SUPPLIERS AND AG MAKE NO WARRANTIES, EXPRESSED OR IMPLIED, WITH RES O THE DVD-ROM PRODUCT, INCLUDING, WITHOUT LIMITATIO PROPRIETARY MATERIAL, AND SPECIFICALLY DISCLAIM VARRANTY OF MERCHANTABILITY OR FITNESS FOR A PART PURPOSE.

If the information provic this DVD-ROM Product contains medical or health sciences informa is intended for professional use within the medical field. Informati ut medical treatment or drug dosages is intended strictly for pro al use, and because of rapid advances in the medical sciences, ndent verification of diagnosis and drug dosages should be mad

IN NO EVENT WILL ELSE ITS AFFILIATES, LICENSORS, SUPPLIERS OR AGENTS, BE LIABLE YOU FOR ANY DAMAGES, INCLUDING, WITHOUT LIMITATION, A ST PROFITS, LOST SAVINGS OR OTHER INCIDENTAL OR CONSEC IAL DAMAGES, ARISING OUT OF YOUR USE OR INABILITY TO US DVD-ROM PRODUCT REGARDLESS OF WHETHER SUCH DAMAG E FORESEEABLE OR WHETHER SUCH DAMAGES ARE DEEME RESULT FROM THE FAILURE OR INADEQUACY OF ANY EXC E OR OTHER REMEDY.

U.S. GOVERNMENT REST D RIGHTS The DVD-ROM Product and documentation are provide restricted rights. Use, duplication or disclosure by the U.S. Gover t is subject to restrictions as set forth in subparagraphs (a) through f the Commercial Computer Restricted Rights clause at FAR 52.2271 in subparagraph (c)(1)(ii) of the Rights in Technical Data and Compu oftware clause at DFARS 252.2277013, or at 252.2117015, as applica Contractor/Manufacturer is Elsevier Inc., 360 Park Avenue South, New NY 10010 USA.

GOVERNING LAW This Agree t shall be governed by the laws of the State of New York, USA. In any oute arising out of this Agreement, You and Elsevier each consent to th clusive personal jurisdiction and venue in the state and federal courts n New York County, New York, USA.

SURGERY OF THE SKIN

PROCEDURAL DERMATOLOGY

EDITORS

June K Robinson MD
Section Chief of Dermatology
Professor of Medicine
Dartmouth-Hitchcock Medical Center
Lebanon, NH, USA

Roberta D Sengelmann MD
Assistant Professor
Departments of Medicine (Dermatology) and Otolaryngology
Director, Center for Dermatologic and Cosmetic Surgery
Washington University School of Medicine
St Louis, MO, USA

C William Hanke MD MPH
Medical Director
Laser and Skin Surgery Center of Indiana
Clinical Professor of Otolaryngology – Head and Neck Surgery
Indiana University School of Medicine
Indianapolis, IN, USA

Daniel Mark Siegel MD MS (Management and Policy)
Clinical Professor of Dermatology
Director, Procedural Dermatology Fellowship
Department of Dermatology
State University of New York Health Sciences Center at Brooklyn
New York, NY, USA

DVD EDITORS

Ashish C Bhatia MD
Assistant Professor of Clinical Dermatology
Department of Dermatology
Northwestern University, Chicago, IL, USA;
Director of Mohs Micrographic Surgery
Cutaneous Oncology, Laser and Cosmetic Surgery
River North Dermatology – DuPage Medical Group
Naperville, IL, USA

Thomas E Rohrer MD
Clinical Associate Professor of Dermatology
Boston University School of Medicine
SkinCare Physicians of Chestnut Hill
Chestnut Hill, MA, USA

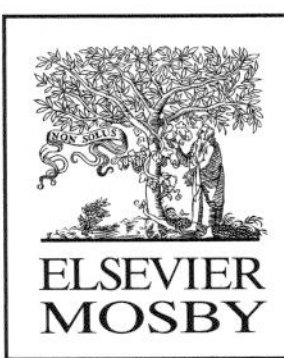

Philadelphia Edinburgh London New York Oxford St Louis Sydney Toronto 2005

ELSEVIER
MOSBY

Mosby is an affiliate of Elsevier Inc.

First published 2005

Notice

Medical knowledge is constantly changing. Standard safety precautions must be followed, but as new research and clinical experience broaden our knowledge, changes in treatment and drug therapy may become necessary or appropriate. Readers are advised to check the most current product information provided by the manufacturer of each drug to be administered to verify the recommended dose, the method and duration of administration, and contraindications. It is the responsibility of the practitioner, relying on experience and knowledge of the patient, to determine dosages and the best treatment for each individual patient. Neither the Publisher nor the editors or contributors assume any liability for any injury and/or damage to persons or property arising from this publication.

The Publisher

ISBN 0-323-02752-0

British Library Cataloguing in Publication Data
A catalogue record for this book is available from the British Library

Library of Congress Cataloging in Publication Data
A catalog record for this book is available from the Library of Congress

Printed in Spain

Last digit is the print number : 9 8 7 6 5 4 3 2 1

The publisher's policy is to use **paper manufactured from sustainable forests**

Commissioning Editor: Sue Hodgson
Project Development Manager: Joanne Scott
Project Manager: Glenys Norquay
Design Managers: Jayne Jones, Andy Chapman
Illustration Manager: Mick Ruddy
Illustrators: Richard Tibbits, Paul Richardson

Contents

*denotes chapters with video footage on the accompanying DVD 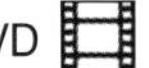

List of Contributors *vii*
Preface *xi*
Acknowledgments *xii*
Dedications *xiii*

PART ONE: Basic Surgical Concepts

1.* Skin Structure and Surgical Anatomy *3*
June K Robinson MD and E Ratcliffe Anderson Jr MD

2. Aseptic Technique *25*
Christie T Ammirati MD

3.* Anesthesia and Analgesia *39*
Teresa T Soriano MD, Gary P Lask MD, and Scott M Dinehart MD

4. Instruments and Materials *59*
Melissa A Bogle MD and Aaron K Joseph MD FAAD

5. Patient Evaluation, Informed Consent, Preoperative Assessment and Care *67*
Howard Fein MD and Allison T Vidimos RPh MD

6. Digital Imaging in Dermatologic Surgery *77*
Rhett J Drugge MD and Mark Naylor MD

7. Wound Healing *97*
Jie Li MD PhD and Robert S Kirsner MD PhD

8.* Dressings and Postoperative Care *117*
May Leveriza-Oh MD and Tania J Phillips MD FRCPC

9. Antibiotics *137*
Ann F Haas MD

10. Large Equipment and Design of the Surgical Suite, Including Monitoring Devices *147*
Brett M Coldiron MD FACP and Mary Maloney MD

11. Dermatology Office Accreditation *159*
W Patrick Davey MD FACP

PART TWO: Essential Surgical Skills

12.* Electrosurgery, Electrocoagulation, Electrofulguration, Electrodesiccation, Electrosection, Electrocautery *177*
Seaver L Soon MD and Carl V Washington Jr MD

13.* Cryosurgery *191*
Gilberto Castro-Ron MD and Paola Pasquali MD

14.* Skin Biopsy Techniques *203*
Carlos Garcia MD

15. Incision, Draining and Exteriorization Techniques *213*
Jeffrey A Squires MD and Frederick S Fish III MD FACP

16.* Suturing Technique and Other Closure Materials *225*
Sarah Weitzul MD and R Stan Taylor MD

17.* Hemostasis *245*
Tri H Nguyen MD

18.* Ellipse, Ellipse Variations and Dog-ear Repairs *259*
Samuel E Book MD, Sumaira Z Aasi MD, and David J Leffell MD

19.* Layered Closures, Complex Closures with Suspension Sutures and Plication of SMAS *273*
Edgar F Fincher MD PhD, Hayes B Gladstone MD, and Ronald L Moy MD

20.* Repair of the Split Earlobe, Ear Piercing and Earlobe Reduction *291*
Sirunya Silapunt MD and Leonard H Goldberg MD

21.* Random Pattern Cutaneous Flaps *311*
Jonathan L Cook MD and Glenn D Goldman MD

22.* Axial Pattern Flaps *345*
Joel Cook MD and John A Zitelli MD

23.* Skin Grafting *365*
Dane R Christensen MD, Christopher J Arpey MD, and Duane C Whitaker MD

24.* Regional Reconstruction: Trunk, Extremities, Hands, Feet, Face (Perioral, Periorbital, Cheek, Nose, Forehead, Ear, Neck, Scalp) *381*
Camille L Mason MD, Christopher J Arpey MD, and Duane C Whitaker MD

25.* Scar Revision *401*
Ken K Lee MD, Annalisa K Gorman MD, and Neil A Swanson MD

PART THREE: Aesthetic Surgical Procedures

26. Psychosocial Issues and the Cosmetic Surgery Patient *413*
Dee Anna Glaser MD and Jason Layman BS

27. Evaluation and Management of the Aging Face *425*
Lisa M Donofrio MD

28.* Soft-tissue Augmentation *437*
Roberta D Sengelmann MD, Stacey Tull MD MPH, and Sheldon V Pollack MD

29.* Chemical Peels *463*
Sue Ellen Cox MD and Kimberly J Butterwick MD

30.* Implants *483*
J Michael Carney MD

31.* Use of Botulinum Toxin Type A in Facial Rejuvenation *501*
Alastair Carruthers MD and Jean Carruthers MD

32.* Liposuction *513*
Naomi Lawrence MD and Janie M Leonhardt MD

33.* Autologous Fat Transfer: Evolving Concepts and Techniques *535*
Kimberly J Butterwick MD

34.* Follicular Unit Hair Transplantation *549*
Robert M Bernstein MD

35. Laser Hair Removal *575*
Sandy S Tsao MD and George J Hruza MD

36.* Microdermabrasion and Dermabrasion *589*
James M Spencer MD MS and Christopher B Harmon MD

37.* Laser Treatment of Tattoos and Pigmented Lesions *599*
Vivek Iyengar MD, Kenneth A Arndt MD, and Thomas E Rohrer MD

38.* Laser Skin Resurfacing: Ablative and Non-ablative *611*
Tina S Alster MD and Elizabeth L Tanzi MD

39.* Laser and Light Treatment of Acquired and Congenital Vascular Lesions *625*
Arielle NB Kauvar MD and Agneta Troilius MD PhD

40.* Endovenous Ablation Techniques with Ambulatory Phlebectomy for Varicose Veins *645*
Mitchel P Goldman MD and Robert A Weiss MD

41.* Minimum Incision Face Lift *657*
Robert C Langdon MD, Gerhard Sattler MD, and C William Hanke MD MPH

42.* Blepharoplasty and Brow Lift *673*
Brent R Moody MD and Paul J Weber MD

43.* Rejuvenation of the Neck Using Liposuction and Other Techniques *691*
Carolyn I Jacob MD and Michael S Kaminer MD

PART FOUR: Special procedures

44. Keloid Management *705*
Hilary Baldwin MD

45.* Nail Surgery *719*
Eckart Haneke MD PhD and Monica Lawry MD

46.* Leg Ulcer Management *743*
Carlos A Charles MD, Anna F Falabella MD, and Adolfo C Fernández-Obregón MD

47.* Benign Subcutaneous Lesions: Cysts and Lipomas *767*
Jessica J Krant MD MPH and John A Carucci MD PhD

48. Mohs Micrographic Surgery and Cutaneous Oncology *777*
Hubert T Greenway MD and Kurt L Maggio MD

49. Skin Cancer in the Organ Transplant Patient *801*
Daniel Berg MD FRCPC and Thomas Stasko MD

50. Management of Dysplastic Nevi and Melanomas *821*
Carol L Huang MD, Ashfaq A Marghoob MD, and Allan C Halpern MD

INDEX *841*

List of Contributors

Sumaira Z Aasi MD
Assistant Professor
Department of Dermatology
Yale School of Medicine
New Haven, CT, USA

Tina S Alster MD
Director, Washington Institute of Dermatologic Laser Surgery
Clinical Professor, Georgetown University Medical Center
Washington, DC, USA

Christie T Ammirati MD
Assistant Professor of Dermatology
Department of Dermatology
Penn State Milton Hershey Medical Center
Hershey, PA, USA

E Ratcliffe Anderson Jr MD
Professor of Medicine
Cardinal Bernardin Cancer Center
Loyola University Stritch School of Medicine
Maywood, IL, USA

Kenneth A Arndt MD
Clinical Professor of Dermatology,
Yale Medical School
New Haven, CT, USA;
Clinical Professor of Dermatology,
Harvard Medical School
Boston, MA, USA;
Adjunct Professor of Medicine (Dermatology),
Dartmouth Medical School
Hanover, NH, USA
Co-Director,
SkinCare Physicians of Chestnut Hill
Chestnut Hill, MA, USA

Christopher J Arpey MD
Associate Professor of Dermatology
Department of Dermatology
University of Iowa Hospitals and Clinics
Iowa City, IA, USA

Hilary Baldwin MD
Associate Professor of Clinical Dermatology
Department of Dermatology
State University of New York - Downstate
Brooklyn, NY, USA

Daniel Berg MD FRCPC
Associate Professor of Dermatology
Director, Dermatologic Surgery
University of Washington
Seattle, WA, USA

Robert M Bernstein MD
Associate Clinical Professor of Dermatology
College of Physicians and Surgeons
Columbia University
New York, NY, USA

Ashish C Bhatia MD
Assistant Professor of Clinical Dermatology
Department of Dermatology
Northwestern University, Chicago, IL, USA;
Director of Mohs Micrographic Surgery
Cutaneous Oncology, Laser and Cosmetic Surgery
River North Dermatology – DuPage Medical Group
Naperville, IL, USA

Melissa A Bogle MD
Laser Surgery Fellow
Skin Care Physicians of Chestnut Hill
Newton, MA, USA

Samuel E Book MD
Clinical Assistant Professor of Dermatology
Section of Dermatologic Surgery and Cutaneous Oncology
Yale School of Medicine
New Haven, CT, USA

Kimberly J Butterwick MD
Dermatology/ Cosmetic Laser Associates of La Jolla
La Jolla, CA, USA

J Michael Carney MD
Assistant Clinical Professor
Department of Dermatology
University of Arkansas for Medical Sciences
Little Rock, AR, USA

Alastair Carruthers MD
Clinical Professor
Division of Dermatology
University of British Columbia
Vancouver, BC, Canada

Jean Carruthers MD
Clinical Professor
Division of Ophthalmology
University of British Columbia
Vancouver, BC, Canada

John A Carucci MD PhD
Chief, Mohs Micrographic and Dermatologic Surgery
Assistant Professor of Dermatology
Weill Medical College of Cornell
New York Presbyterian Hospital
New York, NY, USA

Gilberto Castro-Ron MD
Chief of Dermatology and Cryosurgery
Department of Dermatology
Instituto Oncológico Luis Razetti
Caracas, Venezuela

Carlos A Charles MD
Dermatology Resident
Department of Dermatology and Cutaneous Surgery
University of Miami School of Medicine
Miami, FL, USA

Dane R Christensen MD
Fellow, Dermatologic Surgery
Department of Dermatology
University of Iowa Hospitals and Clinics
Iowa City, IA, USA

Brett M Coldiron MD FACP
Clinical Assistant Professor of Dermatology
University of Cincinnati
Cincinnati, OH, USA

Joel Cook MD
Associate Professor of Dermatology
Department of Dermatology
Medical University of South Carolina
Charleston, SC, USA

Jonathan L Cook MD
Associate Professor of Medicine, Dermatology
Assistant Professor of Surgery
Director of Dermatologic Surgery
Duke University Medical Center
Durham, NC, USA

Sue Ellen Cox MD
Clinical Associate Professor
Department of Dermatology
University of North Carolina
Chapel Hill, NC, USA

W Patrick Davey MD FACP
Clinical Professor of Medicine
Dermatology Associates of Kentucky
Lexington, KY, USA

Scott M Dinehart MD
Clinical Professor
Arkansas Cancer Research Center
University of Arkansas for Medical Sciences
Little Rock, AR, USA

Lisa M Donofrio MD
Associate Clinical Professor of Dermatology
Yale University School of Medicine;
Assistant Clinical Professor of Dermatology
Tulane University School of Medicine
New Haven, CT, USA

Rhett J Drugge MD
Private Practice
Stamford, CT, USA

Anna F Falabella MD CWS
University of Miami School of Medicine
Department of Dermatology and
Cutaneous Surgery
VA Medical Center
Miami, FL, USA

Howard Fein MD
Clinical Fellow
Section of Dermatologic Surgery and
Cutaneous Oncology
Department of Dermatology
The Cleveland Clinic Foundation
Cleveland, OH, USA

Adolfo C Fernández-Obregón MD
Assistant Clinical Professor
Department of Dermatology
New York Medical College
Valhalla, NY, USA

Edgar F Fincher MD PhD
Clinical Instructor
West Los Angeles Veterans Administration
Hospital
Los Angeles, CA, USA

Frederick S Fish III MD FACP
Associate Clinical Professor
Department of Dermatology
University of Minnesota
Minneapolis, MN, USA

Carlos Garcia MD
Assistant Professor
Director of Dermatologic Surgery and
Cutaneous Oncology
Department of Dermatology
Oklahoma University Health Sciences Center
Oklahoma City, OK, USA

Hayes B Gladstone MD
Director, Division of Dermatologic Surgery
Department of Dermatology
Stanford University School of Medicine
Stanford, CA, USA

Dee Anna Glaser MD
Associate Professor and Vice Chairman
Director of Cosmetic Services
Department of Dermatology
St Louis University School of Medicine
St Louis, MO, USA

Leonard H Goldberg MD
Adjunct Professor of Dermatology
MD Anderson Cancer Center
Houston, TX, USA

Glenn D Goldman MD
Associate Professor of Dermatology
Department of Dermatology
Fletcher Allen Health Care
Burlington, VT, USA

Mitchel P Goldman MD
Associate Clinical Professor of
Dermatology/Medicine
La Jolla Spa MD
La Jolla, CA, USA

Annalisa K Gorman MD
Clinical Instructor
Division of Dermatology
University of Washington School of Medicine
Seattle, WA, USA

Hubert T Greenway MD
CEO Scripps Clinic
Director of Cutaneous Oncology
Division of Mohs Surgery
Scripps Clinic
La Jolla, CA, USA

Ann F Haas MD
Senior Dermatologist
Sutter Medical Group;
Assistant Clinical Professor of Dermatology
Department of Dermatology
University of California, Davis
Sacramento, CA, USA

Allan C Halpern MD
Professor of Dermatology
Memorial Sloan-Kettering Cancer Center
New York, NY, USA

Eckart Haneke MD PhD
Professor of Dermatology
Department of Dermatology
University Medical Center St Radboud
Nijmegen, Netherlands

C William Hanke MD MPH
Medical Director
Laser and Skin Surgery Center of Indiana
Clinical Professor of Otolaryngology – Head
and Neck Surgery
Indiana University School of Medicine
Indianapolis, IN, USA

Christopher B Harmon MD
Clinical Instructor
Department of Dermatology
University of Alabama at Birmingham
Birmingham, AL, USA

George J Hruza MD
Clinical Associate Professor
Departments of Dermatology and
Otolaryngology
St Louis University School of Medicine
Medical Director
Laser & Dermatologic Surgery Center
St Louis, MO, USA

Carol L Huang MD
Clinical Instructor of Dermatology
Memorial Sloan-Kettering Cancer Center
New York, NY, USA

Vivek Iyengar MD
Associate Director, Dermasurgery
Section of Dermatology
University of Chicago
Chicago, IL, USA

Carolyn I Jacob MD
Associate Clinical Instructor
Department of Dermatology
Chicago Cosmetic Surgery and Dermatology
Chicago, IL, USA

Aaron K Joseph MD FAAD
Clinical Assistant Professor
Department of Dermatology
University of Texas Medical School
Houston, TX, USA

Michael S Kaminer MD
Assistant Professor of Dermatology
Yale and Dartmouth Medical Schools
SkinCare Physicians of Chestnut Hill
Chestnut Hill, MA, USA

Arielle N B Kauvar MD
Clinical Associate Professor
Department of Dermatology
New York University School of Medicine
New York, NY, USA

Robert S Kirsner MD PhD
Associate Professor of Dermatology
Department of Dermatology
University of Miami School of Medicine
Miami, FL, USA

Jessica J Krant MD MPH
Assistant Clinical Professor of Dermatology
Department of Dermatology
SUNY Health Science Center at Brooklyn
New York, NY, USA

Robert C Langdon MD
Associate Clinical Professor of Dermatology
Yale University School of Medicine
New Haven, CT, USA

Gary P Lask MD
Clinical Professor of Medicine (Dermatology)
Director, UCLA Dermatologic Surgery and
Laser Center
University of California
Los Angeles, CA, USA

Naomi Lawrence MD
Head of Procedural Dermatology
Center for Dermatologic Surgery
Cooper University Hospital
Marlton, NJ, USA

Monica Lawry MD
Assistant Clinical Professor
Department of Dermatology
University of California, Davis
Sacramento, CA, USA

Jason Layman BS
Department of Dermatology
St Louis University School of Medicine
St Louis, MO, USA

Ken K Lee MD
Director of Dermatologic Surgery
Assistant Professor of Dermatology, Surgery,
Otolaryngology/Head and Neck Surgery
Oregon Health & Science University
Portland, OR, USA

David J Leffell MD
Professor of Dermatology and Surgery
Department of Dermatology
Yale School of Medicine
New Haven, CT, USA

Janie M Leonhardt MD
Center for Dermatologic Surgery
Cooper University Hospital
Marlton, NJ, USA

May Leveriza-Oh MD
Dermatology Fellow, Wound Healing
Department of Dermatology
Boston University School of Medicine
Boston, MA, USA

Jie Li MD PhD
Assistant Professor of Dermatology
Department of Dermatology and Cutaneous Surgery
University of Miami School of Medicine
Miami, FL, USA

Kurt L Maggio MD
Director of Mohs Surgery and Cutaneous Oncology
Walter Reed Army Medical Center;
Assistant Clinical Professor of Dermatology
George Washington University
School of Medicine;
Howard University School of Medicine
Washington DC, USA
Uniformed Services University of the Health Sciences
Bethesda, MD, USA

Mary Maloney MD
Chief, Division of Dermatology
University of Massachusetts Medical School
Worcester, MA, USA

Ashfaq A Marghoob MD
Assistant Professor of Dermatology
Department of Dermatology
Memorial Sloan-Kettering Cancer Center
Hauppauge, NY, USA

Camille L Mason MD
Fellow, Dermatologic Surgery
Department of Dermatology
University of Iowa Hospitals and Clinics
Iowa City, IA, USA

Brent R Moody MD
Assistant Professor
Director of Cosmetic Dermatologic Surgery
Vanderbilt University
Nashville, TN, USA

Ronald L Moy MD
Associate Clinical Professor
VA West LA Medical Center
Division of Dermatology
David Geffen UCLA School of Medicine
Los Angeles, CA, USA

Mark Naylor MD
Associate Professor
Department of Dermatology
University of Oklahoma Health Sciences Center
Oklahoma City, OK, USA

Tri H Nguyen MD
Associate Professor, Dermatology and Otolaryngology
Director, Mohs and Dermatologic Surgery
MD Anderson Cancer Center
The University of Texas
Houston, TX, USA

Paola Pasquali MD
Attending Physician and Professor
Department of Dermatology
Instituto Oncológico Luis Razetti
Caracas, Venezuela

Tania J Phillips MD FRCPC
Professor of Dermatology
Department of Dermatology
Boston University School of Medicine
Boston, MA, USA

Sheldon V Pollack MD
Associate Professor of Medicine
Faculty of Medicine
University of Toronto
Toronto, ON, Canada

June K Robinson MD
Section Chief of Dermatology
Professor of Medicine
Dartmouth-Hitchcock Medical Center
Lebanon, NH, USA

Thomas E Rohrer MD
Clinical Associate Professor of Dermatology
Boston University School of Medicine
SkinCare Physicians of Chestnut Hill
Chestnut Hill, MA, USA

Gerhard Sattler MD
Medical Director
Rosenpark Clinic for Aesthetic Operative Dermatology and Plastic Surgery
Darmstadt, Germany

Roberta D Sengelmann MD
Assistant Professor
Departments of Medicine (Dermatology) and Otolaryngology
Director, Center for Dermatologic and Cosmetic Surgery
Washington University School of Medicine
St Louis, MO, USA

Daniel Mark Siegel MD MS (Management and Policy)
Clinical Professor of Dermatology
Director, Procedural Dermatology Fellowship
Department of Dermatology
State University of New York
Health Sciences Center at Brooklyn
New York, NY, USA

Sirunya Silapunt MD
Dermatologist
DermSurgery Associates
Houston, TX, USA

Seaver L Soon MD
Resident in Dermatology
Department of Dermatology
Emory University School of Medicine
Atlanta, GA, USA

Teresa T Soriano MD
Assistant Professor of Medicine (Dermatology)
Co-Director, UCLA Dermatologic Surgery and Laser Center
University of California
Los Angeles, CA, USA

James M Spencer MD MS
Professor of Clinical Dermatology
The Mount Sinai School of Medicine
New York, NY, USA

Jeffrey A Squires MD
Adjunct Associate Professor
Department of Dermatology
University of Minnesota
Minneapolis, MN, USA

Thomas Stasko MD
Associate Professor of Medicine
Department of Dermatology
Vanderbilt University
Nashville, TN, USA

Neil A Swanson MD
Professor and Chairman
Department of Dermatology
Oregon Health & Science University
Portland, OR, USA

Elizabeth L Tanzi MD
Co-director of Laser Surgery
Washington Institute of Dermatologic Laser Surgery
Washington, DC, USA

R Stan Taylor MD
Professor of Dermatology
Department of Dermatology
University of Texas
Southwestern Medical School
Dallas, TX, USA

Agneta Troilius MD PhD
Associate Clinical Professor
Department of Dermatology
University Hospital
Malmo, Sweden

Sandy S Tsao MD
Instructor in Dermatology
Harvard Medical School;
Clinical Director
MGH Dermatology Laser Center
Massachusetts General Hospital
Boston, MA, USA

Stacey Tull MD MPH
Chief Resident
Division of Dermatology
Washington University School of Medicine
St Louis, MO, USA

Allison T Vidimos RPh MD
Section of Dermatologic Surgery and Cutaneous Oncology
Department of Dermatology
Cleveland Clinic Foundation
Cleveland, OH, USA

Carl V Washington Jr MD
Associate Professor
Department of Dermatology
Emory University School of Medicine
Atlanta, GA, USA

Paul J Weber MD
Private Practice
Fort Lauderdale, FL, USA

Robert A Weiss MD
Associate Professor
Department of Dermatology
Johns Hopkins University School of Medicine
Baltimore, MD, USA

Sarah Weitzul MD
Assistant Professor
Department of Dermatology
University of Texas
Southwestern Medical School
Dallas, TX, USA

Duane C Whitaker MD
Professor of Dermatology
Department of Dermatology
University of Iowa Hospitals and Clinics
Iowa City, IA, USA

John A Zitelli MD
Adjunct Associate Professor of Dermatology
and Otolaryngology
University of Pittsburgh
Pittsburgh, PA, USA

Preface

In 2003, several decades of dermatologic surgery evolution was recognized with the designation of fellowships in procedural dermatology. The editors have encouraged the contributing authors to capture the art and practice of dermatologic surgery at the beginning of this century. We use the available technology to present the core curriculum to the learner in a way that promotes those who read the text, view the demonstrations of techniques on the CD and the website to further our understanding of the field in the next decade. The textbook, *Surgery of the Skin: Procedural Dermatology*, is organized into four sections: basic concepts, basic surgical procedures, aesthetic surgical procedures, and special procedures. This format allows the novice to learn sequentially as the book unfolds. Those who have mastered some aspects can move from highly specialized procedures toward the beginning of the book to refresh their knowledge of basic surgical procedures and concepts. The chapters are organized with consistent heading levels throughout the book, which makes thumbing ahead or back an easy task.

Reading can take the learner just so far, but then a point is reached where hands on training is the best way to learn. We learn by watching the movement of the hands of those performing surgery as well as reading the writing of those same hands. The educational methods used in this text allow the reader to watch the hands of those performing the procedures. The operative sequences are taken from the 'surgeon's view' of the operative field. Eventually, the learner simply has to take the plunge and perform the surgery. When the mentor is in the surgical room during performance of the procedure, the experience of the senior physician naturally serves to troubleshoot the novice's first attempt at performing a new procedure. Experience is the best teacher but also the toughest teacher. The experienced teacher allows the student to make small mistakes in order to learn judgment and technique and buffers the patient from large errors from which there is no recovery. At certain points in a procedure, the teacher may need to take over the more difficult or delicate portions of the procedure because only the experienced hands can achieve the result needed. Also, there is a need for the teacher to 'feel the tissue' to evoke their memory and experience. Some teachers have learned to verbalize their tactile skills and teach by both demonstrating and describing what they are doing at the surgical table. Others have learned how to commit those experiences to writing. The editors present the work of these highly skilled teachers to you in their writing and by having you watching them. The future of our specialty rests within these physicians, who represent the art and form of dermatologic surgery. Each author is a treasure of surgical experience learned from the preceding generation of dedicated teachers, developed over the years as each individual daily practices the art of dermatologic surgery, and devotedly teaches their students.

As we apply the knowledge gained from ongoing basic research to solve clinical problems, we will continue to improve the overall quality of patient care. Dermatologists have a tradition of outpatient ambulatory surgery and have expanded the scope of procedures performed in this setting. Historically, dermatology and especially dermatologic surgeons have generously shared their knowledge with other dermatologists and with physicians from other disciplines. This cooperative learning is integral to the successful evolution of dermatologic surgery. The editors wish the website version of this textbook to provide an international forum for interactive learning and discussion. This discourse, which represents the joining of hands in cyberspace, will enhance the evolution of the field.

The hands of the surgeon are the meeting place of mind, matter and spirit. Surgeons' hands become a metaphor for their creative manual and intellectual skills as well as their knowledge and memory. The sense of touch and motion of the hands are necessary to inscribe and recall ordered sequences in performing procedures. Our hands are our messengers to the world of surgery and to our patients. We hold the book in our hands. Physicians' hands are unique because our hands perform procedural dermatology, comfort patients by laying on our hands, and our guiding hands comfort the family. As we care for others with our hands, we demonstrate that we are the handiwork of the creator. May this textbook and its components, the work of our hands, be inspirational to you.

"… the hand is the instrument of instruments."
Aristotle, De Anima, 3.8

June K Robinson MD
C William Hanke MD
Roberta D Sengelmann MD
Daniel Mark Siegel MD
2005

Acknowledgments

The editors are grateful to two groups of amazing people. First, we are indebted to the contributors who expended considerable time and effort in completing their chapters and sharing their experience. Second, the editors and contributors have shifted personal time away from families and friends to complete their work. Hopefully the final product has been worth the sacrifice of all.

Dedications

This book is dedicated to our families, our teachers, our patients, and our students and to the team at Elsevier. All helped us learn the art of skin surgery and how to share our experience with others.

To William T Barker, my husband, whose encouragement and unwavering support help sustain my professional life.
- June K Robinson MD

To my daughters, Sarah and Katherine, my sons, David and Peter, and to my wife, Margaret, whose support, love, and friendship continues to guide my life.
- C *William Hanke MD MPH*

To all the residents and fellows in training whose queries and open-mindedness continue to "keep me on my toes" by stimulating new ideas and novel approaches in clinical practice. I would also like to thank my father, Dr Robert Sengelmann, a plastic and reconstructive surgeon still in practice today at nearly 70 years of age, for imparting his love for surgery and teaching to me. Thanks, Dad.
- Roberta D Sengelmann MD

For my wife, Susan, my friend and companion who has helped me navigate an exciting and ongoing journey.
- Daniel Mark Siegel MD MS

PART 1

Basic Surgical Concepts

1 Skin Structure and Surgical Anatomy

June K Robinson MD and E Ratcliffe Anderson Jr MD

Summary box

- Wound healing and eventual scar formation depends on the anatomical location, structure and function of the skin in the region.
- The cosmetic units of the face and skin tension lines are used to plan a procedure.
- Knowledge of the sensory nerves is necessary for effective regional nerve blocks.
- The depth of the initial incision, the proper level of undermining, and placement of sutures depend on the underlying anatomy.
- Knowledge of the anatomy and drainage of the lymphatic system is vital when treating melanoma, squamous cell carcinoma, and other aggressive cutaneous malignancies.

■ INTRODUCTION

Why begin with anatomy? Mastery of names and locations is the basis for communication and learning. Learning anatomy allows the physician to practice surgery of the skin according to the guiding rule of medicine, 'primum non nocere,' first do no harm! Understanding anatomy supports the planning of surgical procedures by a series of steps that ultimately leads to the rearrangement or restoration of function as well as aesthetics. Each step depends on the physician's familiarity with the regional anatomy of the surgical site.

The decision to perform surgery requires an assessment of the risks and benefits of the procedure to the individual patient. The anticipated wound healing, which is based on the structure and function of the skin, must be considered. The cosmetic units of the face and skin tension lines are used to plan the procedure. Providing safe and sufficient anesthesia requires a knowledge of the sensory nerves to allow for effective regional nerve blocks. The depth of the initial incision requires the ability to anticipate anatomical structures from the surface landmarks to the underlying vital structures. The proper level of undermining, which is used to mobilize tissue, requires an understanding of the horizontal arrangement of the cutaneous, muscular, and fascial soft tissue planes of the head and neck. Suture placement depends on this vertical and horizontal orientation.

It is critically important to understand the drainage pattern of the lymphatic system, which must be examined for cutaneous metastasis of melanoma, squamous cell carcinoma, and other aggressive cutaneous malignancies, which may initially spread to primary echelon nodes. Designing flaps to prevent persistent postoperative lymphedema provides improved outcomes for the patient.

■ TECHNICAL ASPECTS

Skin structure

The skin is the largest organ of the body and the most accessible to the external environment. In the average 75 kg man, the skin weighs 2 kg and covers 1.8 m^2.[1] The large surface area puts the skin at great risk for trauma. The skin's response to injury with its innate ability to control bleeding and infection, are paramount to the survival of the individual. The remarkable healing potential of the skin is determined by its unique structure and physiology. The skin's physiology also determines the appearance of the skin. Healthy appearing skin, especially facial skin, is often associated with emotional well-being and success of the individual.

By its multilayer organization of the epidermis, dermis, and appendages (hair, nails, and sebaceous and other glands), the skin maintains water equilibrium, protects against ultraviolet radiation and invasion by foreign agents, and maintains immunologic surveillance and thermal regulation (Fig. 1.1). The structural elements with relevance to wound healing are particularly relevant to those performing procedures.

Epidermis

The outermost layer of the skin, the epidermis, is a continuous self-regenerating layer of stratified squamous epithelium varying in thickness from 0.04 mm on the eyelids and genitalia to 1.5 mm on the palms and soles. The

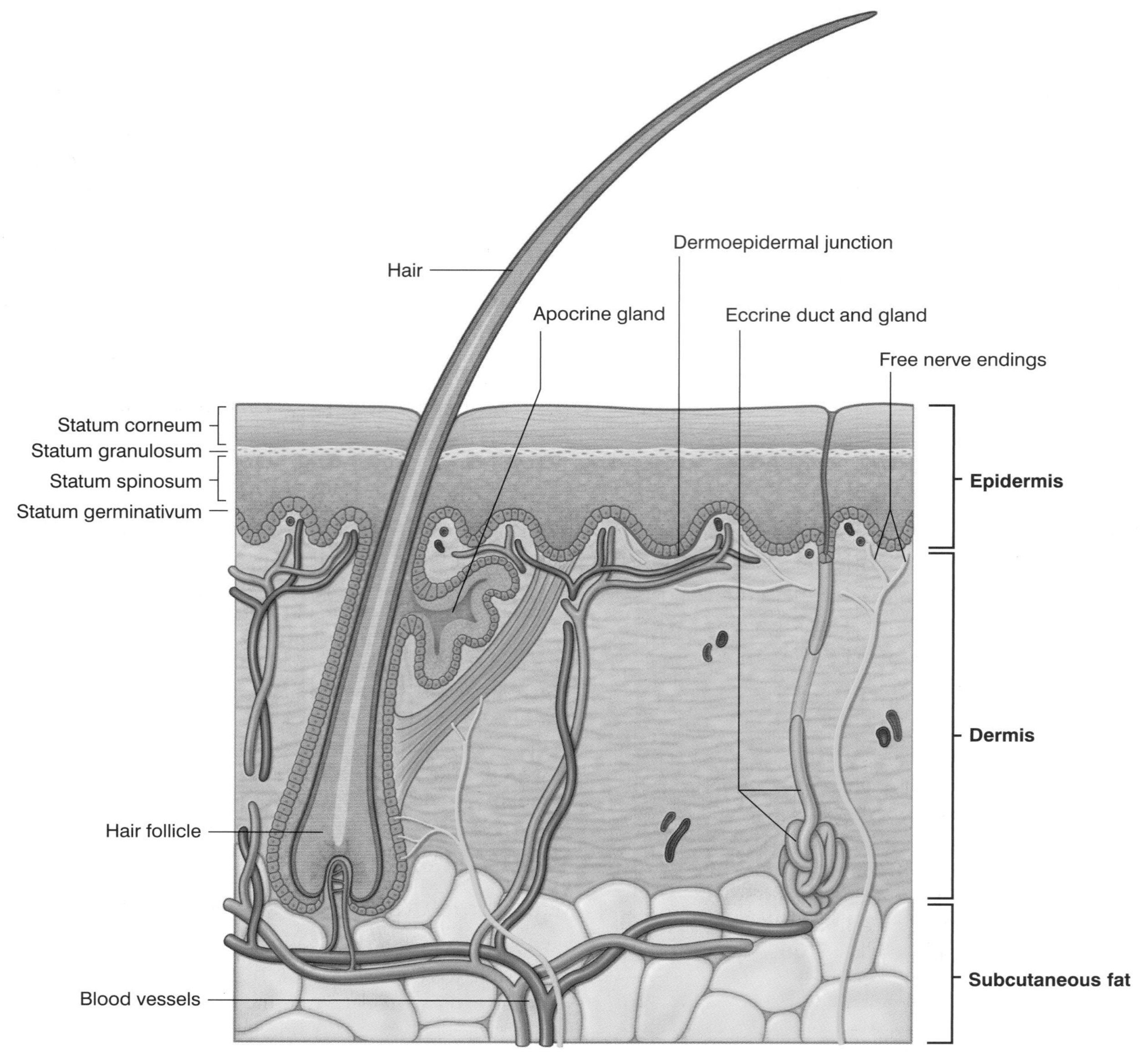

Figure 1.1 Skin consists of three major divisions: epidermis, dermis, and subcutaneous fat. (After White et al. 1996[2] with permission from Saunders.)

individual cells, keratinocytes, are organized into layers based on distinct structural features. These layers from deep to superficial, include the stratum germinativum, stratum spinosum, stratum granulosum, and stratum corneum. Each layer represents a distinct stage of keratinization, which is manifest by progressive flattening of the cellular architecture and an increase in cell size. The end-product of this process is the stratum corneum, the dead outermost layer of skin composed of terminally differentiated keratinocytes, a plasma membrane, filamentous and matrix proteins, and lipids.

The stratum germinativum, or basal cell layer, is composed of a single row of columnar epithelial cells arranged with their long axes perpendicular to the dermoepidermal junction.[2] Basal keratinocytes are the active stem cells that proliferate heterogeneously and maintain homeostasis by balancing proliferation (S phase) and noncycling (G_0, G_1, G_2 phase) cells. Additional noncycling stem cells can be recruited by stimuli such as mitogens, hormones (estrogen, progesterone, epidermal growth factor), wounding, and carcinogens. Only 30–40% of the basal cell layer germinal cells are mitotically active.[3] Cellular synthesis of DNA takes approximately 16 hours and the average germinal cell replicates once every 19 days. Cell cycling time varies between 200 and 400 hours. The actively cycling cells generate committed keratinocytes, which ultimately differentiate into stratum corneum. The normal transit time for a cell to travel between the stratum germinativum and the stratum corneum is 40–56 days, and an additional 14 days are needed for corneocyte desquamation from the stratum corneum. The total epidermal renewal time varies from 58 to 74 days.

Dermoepidermal junction

The dermoepidermal junction is a large, specialized anchoring site, with an ultrastructure that resembles a tongue and groove pattern.[4] The major function of the dermoepidermal junction is to keep the epidermis firmly attached to the dermis. Other functions include support, wound healing, and regulation of permeability.

The attachment function is accomplished through:

- A series of interacting filamentous molecules that exist in the hemidesmosomes of the keratinocyte (bullous pemphigoid antigen 2—referred to as collagen type XVII and integrin)
- The anchoring filaments (kalinin, nicein, and epiligrin, which is referred to as laminin 5).
- The lamina densa (type IV collagen, nidogen/entactin, laminins 1, 6, and 7, and the heparan sulfate proteoglycan perlecan).
- The anchoring fibrils (type VII collagen) that entrap dermal banded collagen fibers (collagen types I, III, and V).
- Other fibrous papillary dermal elements (the beaded microfilaments containing type VI collagen and the elastic microfibrils made of the protein fibrillin).[5]

Type IV collagen, a 400-kD molecule whose monomers resemble hockey sticks, forms a lattice network here that is important in wound healing.

Dermis

The flexible dermal connective tissue wraps around the body and provides much of the structural integrity of the skin and protection against mechanical trauma. The dermis is an intricate connective tissue network of collagen and elastin fibers embedded in a ground substance matrix that accommodates nerve bundles, sensory receptors, lymphatic channels, and vasculature. Beneath the dermoepidermal junction, collagen, especially collagen type I, constitutes 75% of the dermis. Collagen is composed of three alpha helical chains coiled into a triple helix, which are cross-linked and aligned in a staggered parallel manner to form microfibrils.[6] These microfibrils are assembled into bundles to form fibrils, which are organized into collagen fibers. In the adventitial and papillary dermis, collagen fibers are loosely arranged and form a fine meshwork, whereas in the reticular dermis, they are assembled into thick interwoven bundles.

Elastic fibers constitute approximately 3% of the dermis by dry weight, measure 1–3 μm in diameter, and play a major role in skin elasticity and resilience.[7] Elastic fibers are confined to the lower portion of the dermis, where they are arranged parallel to the epidermis.

The third component of the dermis is the ground substance, an amorphous material that fills spaces between the fibrillar and cellular components of the dermis, imparting turgidity and resilience. The ground substance is composed of water, electrolytes, plasma proteins, and mucopolysaccharides. In human skin the dermal matrix consists of glycosaminoglycans (hyaluronic acid and dermatan sulfate) and glycoproteins. Fibronectin, the major filamentous glycoprotein component of the dermal matrix, is produced by fibroblasts. Fibronectin ensheaths collagen and elastin bundles and plays a role in the attachment of keratinocytes to the basal lamina, which is important in wound healing.

Intrinsic elasticity

The intrinsic elasticity of the skin, its 'stretchability', is an important characteristic to understand during wound closure. In areas where the dermis is relatively inflexible and lacks elasticity (back, scalp), even small degrees of tissue rotation may result in protrusion of the pivot point, whereas in areas where the skin possesses significant elasticity (young facial skin), larger angles of rotation are absorbed by tissue compression without causing significant protrusion. Lifting and stretching the skin between the surgeon's index finger and thumb is a helpful means for estimating the elasticity of the skin before wound reconstruction.

Intrinsic tissue elasticity is related to the patient's age, amount of photodamage, and anatomic site. In general, younger patients possess greater tissue elasticity for a given anatomic site than older patients. Skin that demonstrates marked photodamage will possess less elasticity than photoprotected skin. In some anatomic sites, such as the back of the hand or elbow, the skin is easily movable but quite inelastic. In this skin, even a 30° angle of closure may produce a noticeable tissue protrusion.

Biomechanical skin responses

Ultimately its biomechanical properties determine the response of tissue to intraoperative conditions. These properties are measured by stress, elasticity, creep, and stress relaxation. Stress (load) can be defined as force versus cross-sectional area. Strain is the change in length versus original length. The load versus length relationship is the stress–strain curve (Fig. 1.2). During the initial stages of loading, the material deforms in direct proportion to the stress, as seen by the early straight-line relation between

The stress–strain relationship

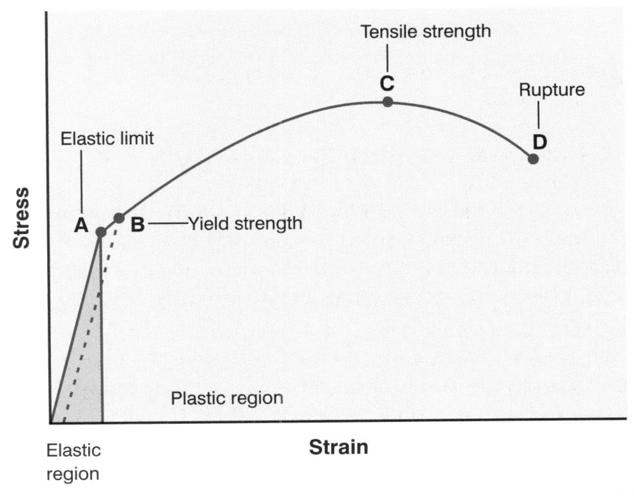

Figure 1.2 The stress–strain relationship. (After Marcus et al. 1990[8] with permission from Journal of the American Academy of Dermatology Inc.)

stress and strain. The slope of this curve up to point A, the elastic region of the stress–strain curve, is Young's modulus or the modulus of elasticity (E).[8,9] The equation of this line, Hooke's law, is $\sigma = Ee$, where σ is defined as stress and e is defined as strain. Materials with larger E values are stiffer or more rigid than those with low E values.

A material loaded with stress beyond point A will not completely return to its original shape on removal of the stress. Point A represents the elastic limit. Loading beyond point A produces permanent deformation; this region of the curve is the plastic region. As the stress is removed, the elastic portion recovers along a line parallel to the original slope (see Fig. 1.2, dashed line), leaving permanent deformation. The limit of usable elastic behavior is defined as point B, the yield strength. As loading continues into the plastic region, the increasing stress does produce increasing strain, but not in a linear fashion (see Fig. 1.2, points B and C). The specimen elongates on continued application of the load until the point is reached at which the specimen is unable to adapt enough to continue to support the load (see Fig. 1.2, point C, tensile strength). After the maximal load is exceeded, the specimen elongates rapidly and rupture occurs (see Fig. 1.2, point D). Obviously, during intraoperative loading of the skin, the surgeon seeks to maximize the stress to produce the greatest strain that can be tolerated by the skin. Thus the region of this curve BC must be used to optimal advantage, but the load should not exceed the tensile strength of the skin or the tissue will slip into the portion of the curve CD that leads to rupture.

Mechanical creep occurs when the skin is stretched at a constant force and eventually contributes to skin deformation. The constant force results in extrusion of tissue fluid from the interstices of the collagen network and stretching of skin beyond its inherent extensibility. The stretching achieved during mechanical creep does not retract and the blood supply is not disturbed. A corollary to mechanical creep is stress relaxation, which occurs when skin is stretched for a given distance and held constant. Intraoperative loading with a constant force is achieved by placing temporary retention sutures for about 15 minutes. Another way of achieving mechanical creep is load cycling, which is performed with strong traction exerted with skin hooks at 3-minute intervals over four cycles. When skin stretched by these two methods is anchored to a fixed point by suspension sutures, the elastic fibers do not revert to their original state.

Head and neck soft tissue anatomy

Several significant variations in the skin of the head and neck and the relationship to underlying adipose tissue, cartilage, and bone occur within dramatically short distances of just a few centimeters of the scalp, eyelids, lips, and chin (Fig. 1.3)

The scalp is classically divided into five layers that are identified by the mnemonic 'SCALP' which describes the layers from superficial to deep as S, Skin; C, subCutaneous tissue; A, Aponeurosis (galea); L, Loose connective tissue; P, Periosteum.[10] The cutaneous nerves and vessels of the scalp are in the dermal skin layer with larger vessels in the subcutaneous fat. There are virtually no vessels in the subgaleal space of loose connective tissue, which makes it the ideal plane to undermine scalp tissue. However, scattered emissary vessels that are transmitted through the skull are occasionally encountered and must be planned for during scalp surgery. All nerves and vessels of the scalp originate below the level of the brow when extended circumferentially around the scalp. No motor nerves are found on the scalp.

Fibrous bands connect the dermis to the aponeurosis or fascia on the face and the body, but these bands are accentuated in the scalp. Thus, during surgery in the subcutaneous fat in this area, there is significant resistance to lateral movement and substantial undermining has to be performed to close even small wounds.[11] The rich vascular supply of the scalp means that undermining in the subcutaneous tissue is routinely associated with heavy bleeding. To mitigate this problem, most dermatologic surgeons carry their incision through the galea. Because the galea is so inelastic, the underside of it may be scored (galeotomy) to enhance its ability to stretch over the periosteum to close the defect. The galea is an aponeurosis connecting the frontalis muscle of the forehead with the occipitalis muscle of the posterior scalp, which is why these are often referred to as one structure, the occipitofrontalis muscle. The galea extends from the superior occipital line to approximately 2 cm below the frontal hairline on the forehead where it interdigitates with the superficial muscular aponeurotic system (SMAS).

The skin of the eyelids, which is the thinnest on the entire body, has a rich vascular supply and no subcutaneous fat. The skin lies directly on the muscle, with a minimal or no fatty layer. Caution is needed when making incisions because even an incision of several millimeters is relative deep here and inadvertent injury to the orbital septum and highly vascular retro-orbital fat must be prevented.

Like the periorbital area, the voluntary muscles of the perioral and chin area insert directly into the skin, which is why dynamic (animation) wrinkles in these areas are so prominent. The muscles are thick and large, especially on the chin, and undermining is often difficult and associated with increased bleeding. Blunt dissection on the chin is often hampered by the presence of the diagonally and vertically inserting muscular fibers and minimal subcutaneous space to dissect within. By contrast, the skin of the lateral cheeks has no direct muscle insertions and blunt undermining in subcutaneous tissue can be carried out with minimal effort.

In the postauricular area, anterior to the mastoid area, the fatty layer is often very thin. The most posterior aspect of the parotid gland is in this area and protects the facial nerve. The gland is grayish tan in color and a bit denser in consistency than adipose tissue and must be avoided.

Cosmetic units of the face

Boundaries or junctions of anatomic units on the face, including the nasolabial fold, the nasofacial sulcus, the mentolabial crease, and the preauricular sulcus form some of the contour lines of the face. Other examples are eyelid margins, philtral columns, nasal contours, the vermilion border, and eyebrows. These junction lines divide the face into cosmetic units.[12,13] (Figs 1.4–1.7). It is important that these boundaries are respected as much as possible during surgery to minimize distortion. Other facial contour lines are wrinkles, which are best delineated in the seated and

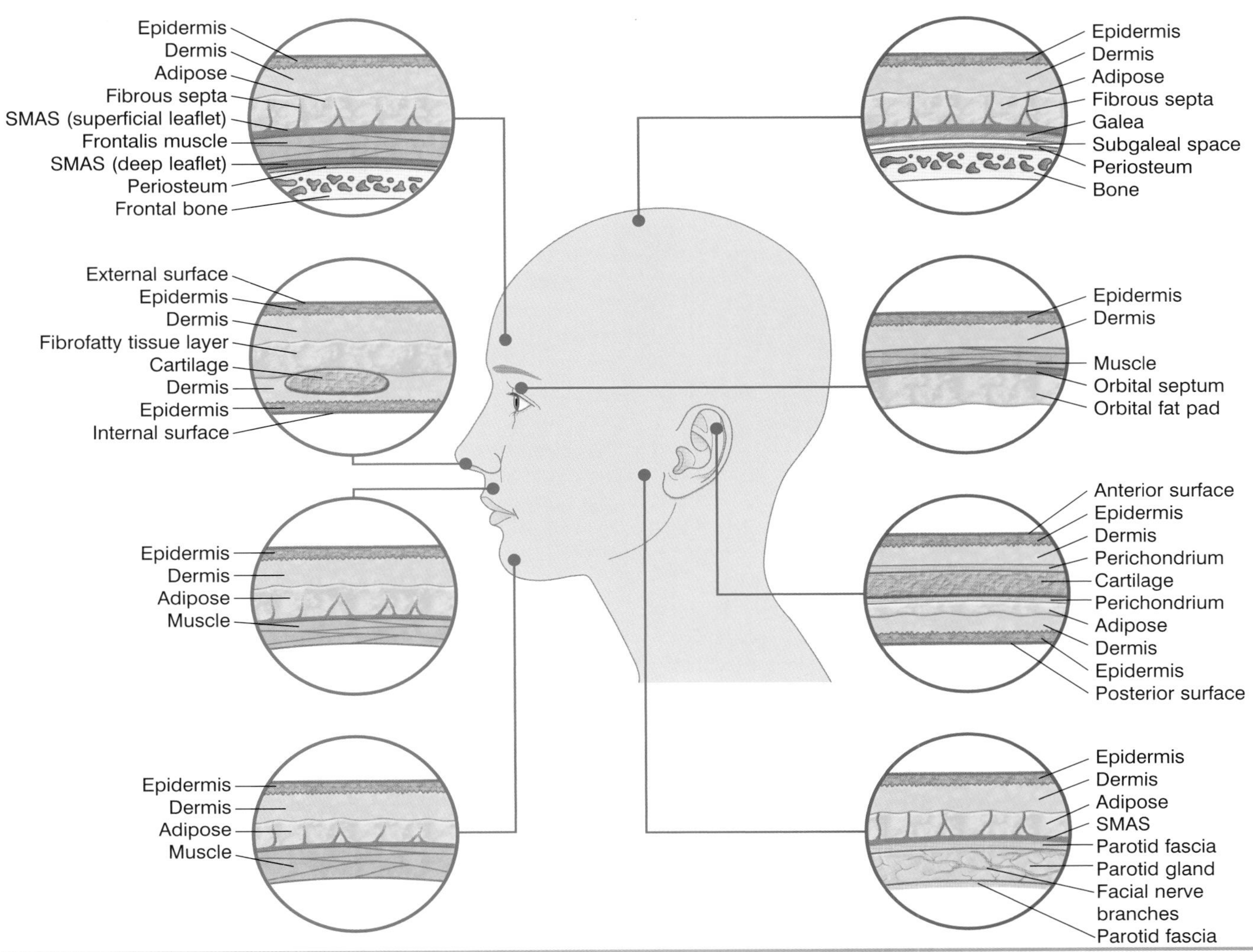

Figure 1.3 Facial skin cross sections showing variations of the skin and its relationship to deeper layers. (Modified with permission from Wheeland RG. Cutaneous Surgery. Philadelphia: WB Saunders; 1994:51.)

animated patient. Age and sun exposure can accentuate the wrinkles that appear along the course of the relaxed skin tension lines. These lines generally occur perpendicular to the long axis of the underlying musculature.

The major aesthetic units of the face (the forehead, nose, eyes, lips, cheeks, and chin) (see Figs 1.4–1.7) are subdivided into units whose skin surface attributes are consistent within the unit. Surface characteristics such as pigmentation, texture, hair quality, pore size, sebaceous quality, and response to blush stimuli are similar within a single unit. Elasticity and mobility of the skin may vary within a unit. The boundaries of these cosmetic units may provide good places to electively situate incisions. For instance, the junction of the nose and medial cheek (the nasofacial sulcus) provides a natural line of definition along which an incision may be camouflaged. These cosmetic units also reflect the surface anatomy.

Skin tension lines

The inherent properties of the dermal collagen and elastic tissue of skin in various regions combined with the tension intermittently exerted on it by the underlying muscles results in linear wrinkles (Figs 1.8–1.10). Over the years stretching of the collagen in the direction of the pull of the muscles produces wrinkles. The elastic tissue is able to maintain the smooth shape of the skin; however, as the skin loses its elasticity with age, the redundant skin ripples into wrinkles and folds. The linear wrinkles on the face form along the attachments of the fibers of the SMAS. When fibrous attachments of the skin to the underlying muscle do not exist, gravitational forces pull the skin into baggy areas. Examples of this include infraorbital festooning, medial cheek jowling, and 'turkey gobbler' neck deformity.

Facial surface anatomy and relation to bony structures of the face

The surface anatomy of the face is best appreciated by referring to the bony landmarks of the frontal, maxillary, zygomatic, and mandibular bones. Each of these bones has distinctive features that contribute to the surface landmarks of the face—the orbital rims, zygomatic arch, the mastoid process, and the mentum.

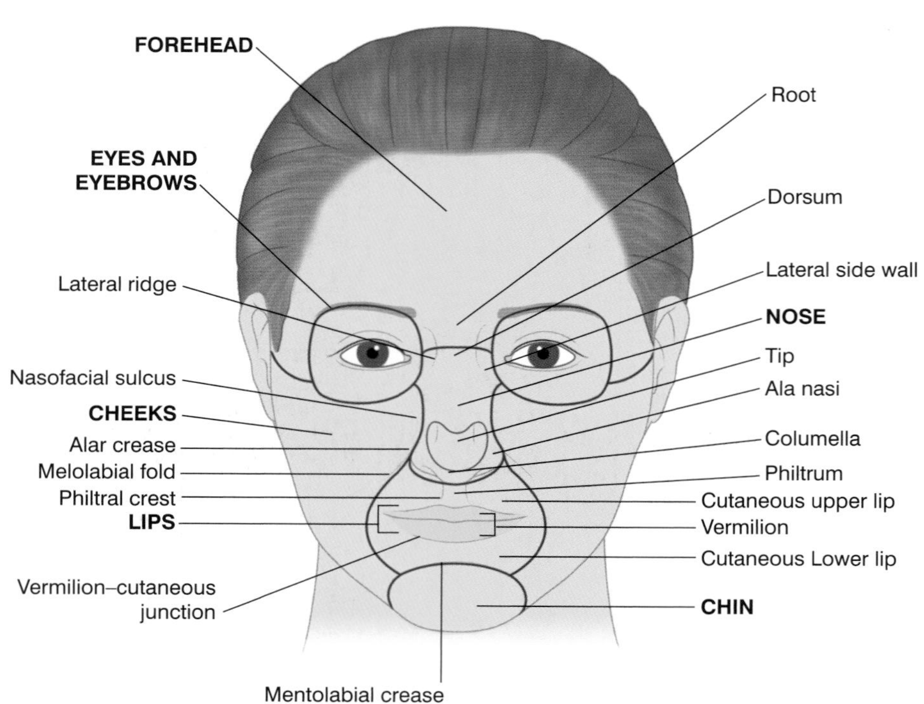

Figure 1.4 The boundaries of the five cosmetic units of the face (forehead, cheeks, eyes, nose, lips, and chin) are defined by the contour lines of the nose, lips, and chin. (After Robinson 1996[12] with permission from Saunders.)

Four components form cosmetic unit of forehead

General forehead
Superior eyebrow
Temporal
Glabellar

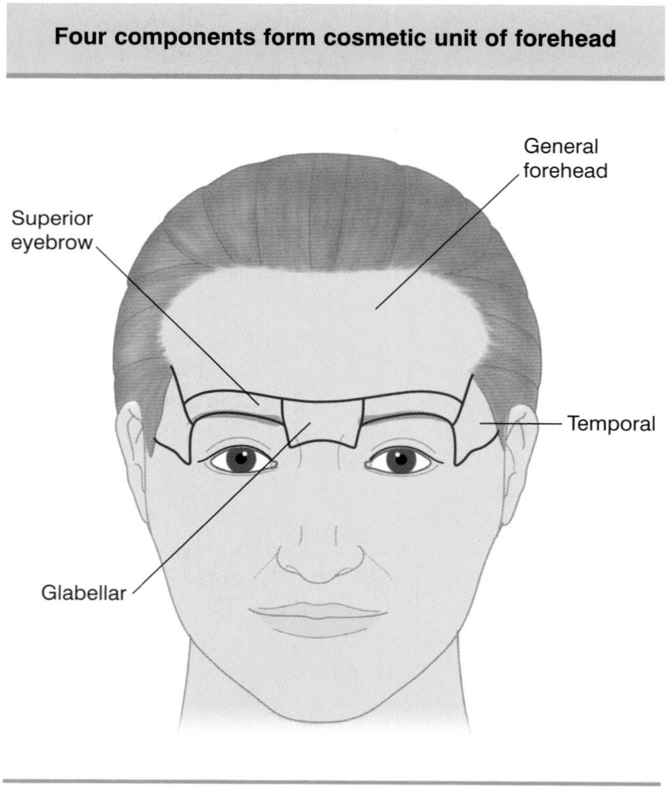

Figure 1.5 Four components of the forehead. (After Robinson 1996[12] with permission from Saunders.)

Five components form cosmetic unit of cheek

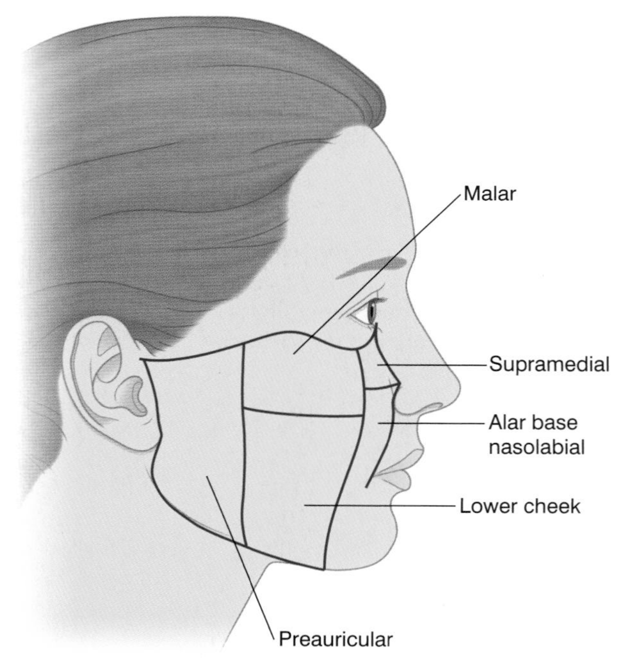

Figure 1.6 Five components of the cheek. (After Robinson 1996[12] with permission from Saunders.)

Topographic landmarks and components of the periorbital region

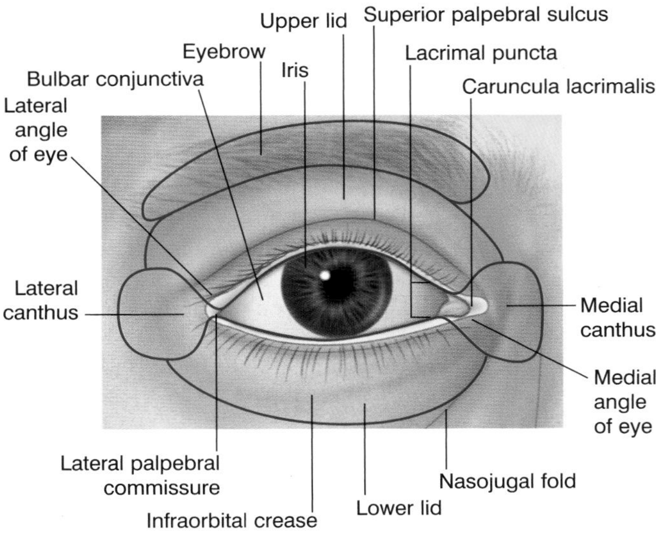

Figure 1.7 Topographic landmarks of the periorbital region. (After Robinson 1996[12] with permission from Saunders.)

Relationship of facial muscles and skin tension lines

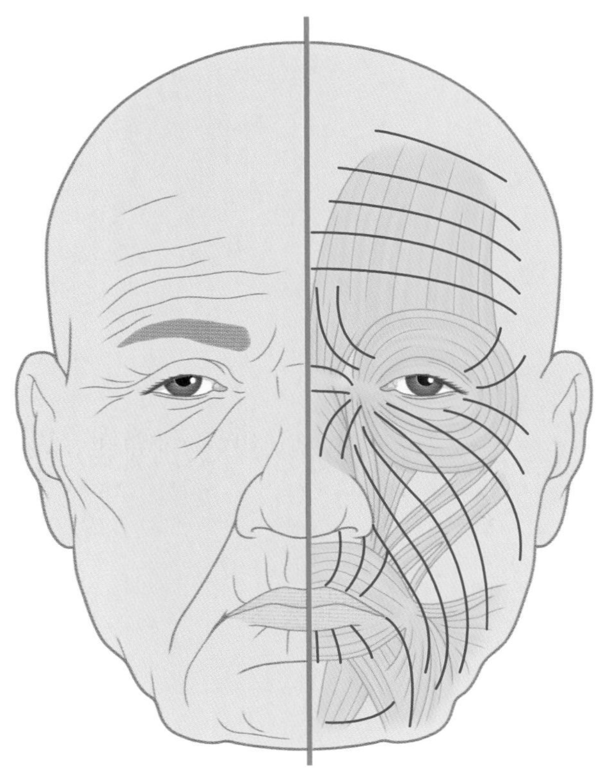

Figure 1.8 Facial skin tension lines and the facial muscles. Over a period of years the pulling of the muscles of facial expression on the skin and lose of elasticity results in the redundant skin forming wrinkles. (After Salasche et al. 1988[13] with permission from The McGraw Hill Companies Inc ©.)

Relaxed skin tension lines of body

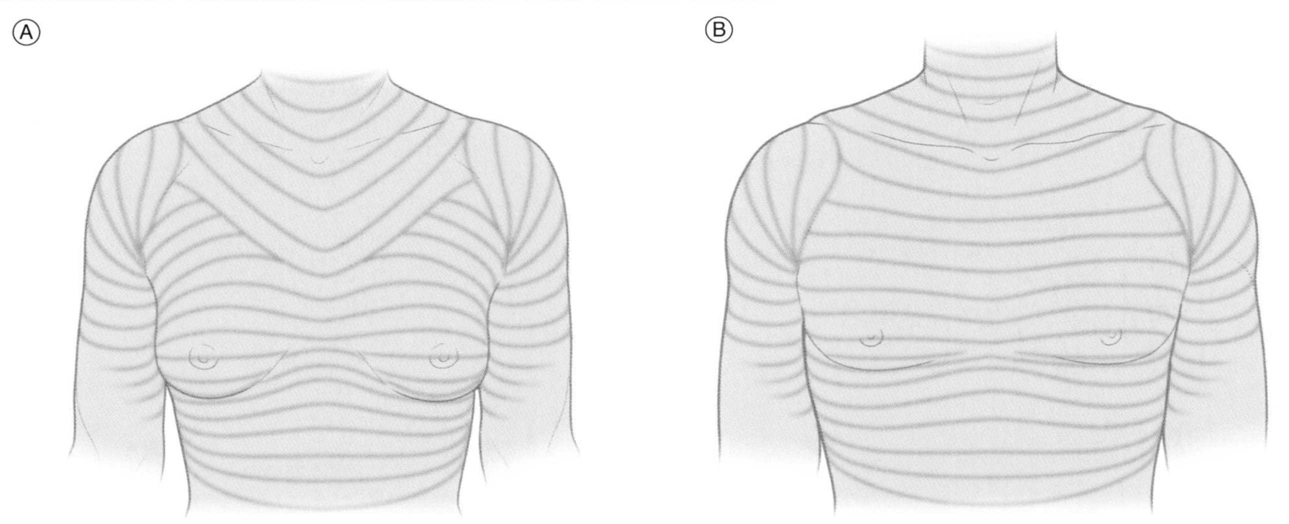

Figure 1.9 Relaxed skin tension lines of the body in (A) a woman; (B) a man. (After Robinson 1996[12] with permission from Saunders.)

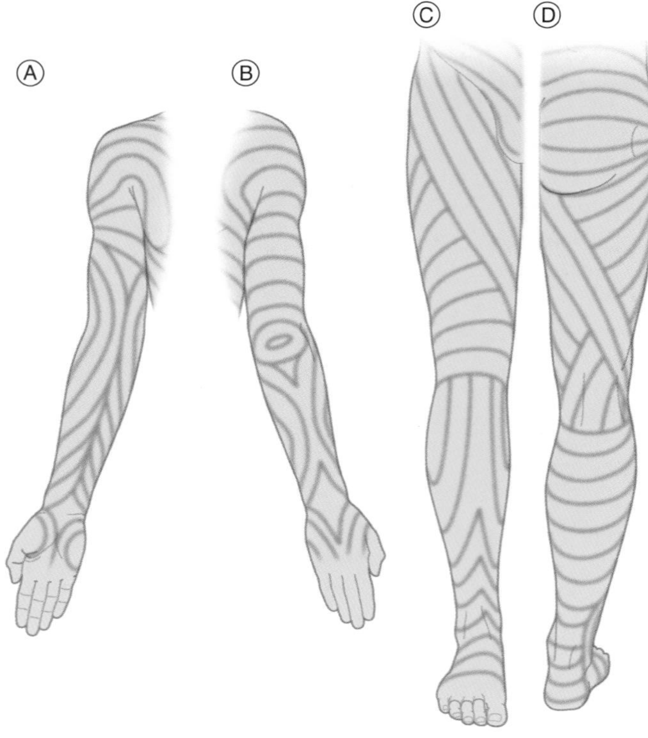

Figure 1.10 Relaxed skin tension lines of the extremities. (A) Upper arm; (B) lower arm; (C) anterior leg; (D) posterior leg. (After Robinson 1996[12] with permission from Saunders.)

The zygomatic arch is the most prominent bone of the lateral cheek. The posterior aspect of the arch helps to define the superior pole of the parotid gland, the superficial temporal artery, and some branches of the facial nerve. The mastoid process is the most inferior portion of the temporal bone and is easily palpated as a rounded projection at the inferior aspect of the postauricular sulcus. It is the landmark for identification of the emergence of the facial nerve trunk. In the adult, the mastoid process protects the facial nerve as it exits the skull through the stylomastoid foramen. The mastoid process is not fully developed until puberty during which time the facial nerve is not fully protected. The mental protuberance of the mandible forms the prominence of the chin. The body of the mandible supports the teeth and presents a sharp inferior margin of the lower face.

The portion of the frontal bone forming the forehead has rounded projections (frontal eminences). The superciliary arches deep to the eyebrows are prominent ridges with a small elevation between the two arches (the glabella). The nasion is formed by the articulation of the paired nasal bones with the frontal bone.

The three important foramina in the facial bones can be identified from the surface (see Practical Applications, page 21). The supraorbital, infraorbital, and mental foramina are found along a vertical line extending from the supraorbital foramen or notch and passing though the center of the pupil (Fig. 1.11). The supraorbital foramen is 2.5 cm or approximately one thumb-breadth from the midline of the nasal root.[13] It can be palpated immediately above the orbit as a notch on the underside of the orbital rim. From this notch the supraorbital artery, vein, and nerve emerge from the skull.

The infraorbital vessels and nerve pass through the infraorbital foramen, which is found in the maxillary bone below the infraorbital rim. In non-obese people, it can usually be palpated as a small opening 1 cm below the infraorbital rim on the backward slope of the maxilla and superolateral to the nasal ala in people. While the mental foramen is not usually palpable, it is typically present at the midportion of the mandible along the same vertical line from the supraorbital foramen (see Fig. 1.11). With age there is a reduction in the height of the mandible; the mental foramen may therefore assume a more superior location. In patients with dentures, the position of the foramen is best located by measuring about 1.0 cm from the inferior margin of the mandible superiorly along the midpupillary line.

Anthropometric landmarks

A series of measures and angles form the points of reference for aesthetic planes, which attempt to codify the ideal parameters of beauty and proportion of the face. Most of these points refer to the depressions and prominences of the profile (Fig. 1.12). Pleasing facial proportions divide the face into relatively equal thirds. The upper face is measured from the trichion (the anterior hairline) to the glabella (which delineates the most prominent projection of the forehead at the eyebrows). The middle third of the face extends from the eyes and nose at the glabella to the subnasale (the inferior aspect of the nose at the junction of the columella and the cutaneous upper lip). The lower third extends from the subnasale to the menton (the lowest point on the chin contour of the mandible).[14]

The face divides vertically into fifths, with each segment being equal to the width of the eye measured from medial to lateral contours. The width of the eye equals the distance between the eyes (inner canthal distance); the distance from the lateral canthus to the outer rim of the helix of the ear in a full frontal view; and the width of the nose from ala to ala (Fig. 1.13). The central facial dimensions are further related by the interpupillary distance (solid line A) being equal to the vertical distance between the medial canthi and the most inferior point of the vermilion of the upper lip (the stomion superius; solid line B).

The ideal brow is defined by two lines; one drawn from the lateral alar rim to the outer canthus of the eye which continues on to the lateral tail of the brow. The other line, drawn obliquely from the lateral alar rim through the medial canthus to the brow defines the highest point of the brow arch. The lips ideally extend from the medial limbus of one eye to the medial limbus of the other. A slanted line connecting the highest point of the upper lip at Cupid's bow with the most lateral aspect of the vermilion border of the upper lip should parallel a line connecting the mid and highest point of the supracanthal fold of the eyelid and the lateralmost border of this fold. These landmarks can be helpful to achieve the most aesthetically pleasing results during facial reconstruction surgery.

Anatomic landmarks of the face

Parotid gland

Before planning a surgical procedure, the important structures that lie below the surface are localized by

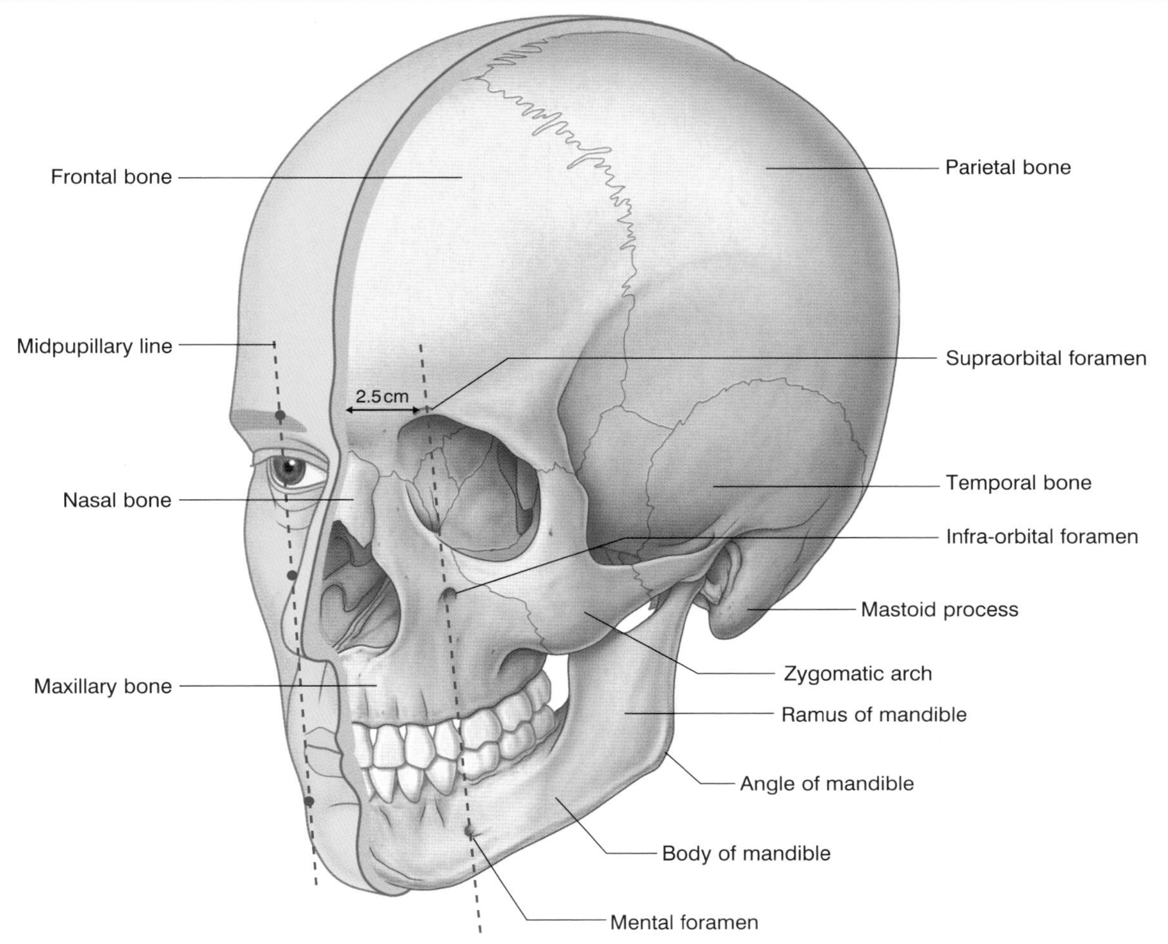

Figure 1.11 A vertical line approximates the location of the supraorbital, infraorbital, and mental foramina 2.5 cm from the midline.

referring to surface landmarks. Asking patients to clench their teeth and jaw and palpating the leading edge of the muscle on the cheek identifies the masseter muscle. The muscle originates on the zygomatic arch and inserts on the ramus, angle, and body of the mandible. The parotid gland is on the posterior half of the masseter muscle and extends from the tragus to just above the angle of the mandible. It has a somewhat triangular shape with the parotid duct (Stensen's duct) emerging from the anterior border of the parotid. The duct drains the secretions of the parotid gland into the interior of the mouth as it enters the mouth opposite to the second molar tooth. The duct courses along the middle third of a line drawn from the notch of the ear above the tragus to a point midway between the oral commissure and the alar rim (Fig. 1.14). This structure can be palpated as it runs across the masseter muscle when the teeth are clenched. At the anterior border of the masseter muscle the duct makes a sharp right angle and passes through the buccinator muscle to enter the buccal mucosa at the position of the second upper molar. Cutting into the parotid gland creates a draining sinus that often heals spontaneously in a few days, but cutting the parotid duct often produces a chronic draining sinus that requires a procedure to repair it.

The facial nerve is associated with the parotid gland. Although the parotid gland protects the fibers of the facial nerve posteriorly, the branches are closer to the surface at the anterior margin of the parotid gland. The branches of the facial nerve exit the superior, anterior, and inferior poles of the parotid gland from its deep aspect and generally lie on the deep fascia of the masseter muscle (see Fig. 1.14). Although relatively deep in this area, the nerve branches are potentially exposed to surgical procedures and injury.

Another structure that can be located by its relationship to the parotid gland is the superficial temporal artery, which traverses the posteroinferior aspect of the parotid gland from infralobular to pretragal and enters the subcutaneous fat at the superior pole of the parotid gland at the zygomatic arch. The pulsation of the artery can be easily palpated pretragally and as it crosses the zygomatic arch and continues into the temple (Figs 1.15, 1.16).

Temporal fossa

The zygomatic arch, the tail of the eyebrow, the coronal suture line, and the temporal hairline delineate the boundaries of the temple. It lies superior to the lateral cheek and above the parotid gland. This area is an important landmark for identification of the most superficial course of

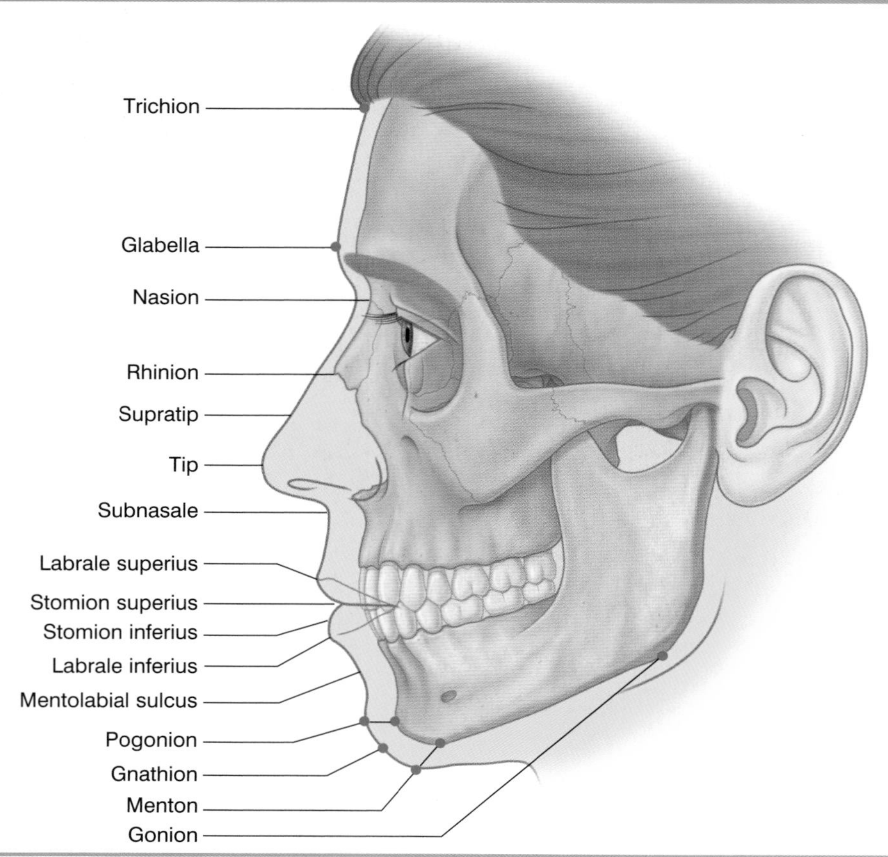

Figure 1.12 Anthropometric landmarks of the profile. (After Salasche et al. 1988[13] with permission of The McGraw Hill Companies Inc ©.)

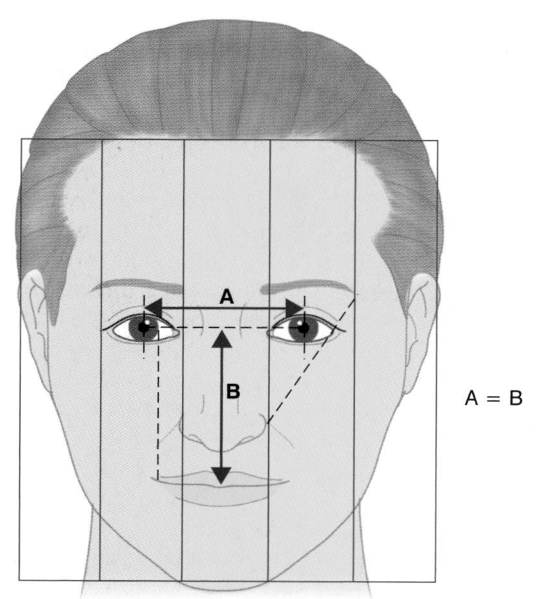

Figure 1.13 Central facial relationships. (After Salasche et al. 1988[13] with permission of The McGraw Hill Companies Inc ©.)

the temporal branch of the facial nerve and is therefore called a danger zone. The lateral margin of the frontalis muscle generally extends to the lateral tip of the eyebrow along the coronal suture line. Medially and superiorly to this point, the branches of the nerve are protected by their location below the muscle; however, lateral to the brow the nerve overlies the SMAS and is only protected from injury by a very thin fatty layer (Fig. 1.17).

Facial artery

The facial artery, a branch of the external carotid artery, is palpated as it crosses the inferior mandibular rim immediately anterior to the insertion of the masseter muscle (Fig. 1.18 and see Practical Applications, page 21). This point is also helpful in locating the course of the mandibular branch of the facial nerve. After crossing the mandibular rim, the facial artery and vein then follow an anterosuperior course in the direction of the oral commissure (Fig. 1.19). Near the angle of the mouth, the inferior labial artery and then the superior labial artery branch off medially. The facial artery then courses along the medial cheek near the nose as the angular artery and enters the orbit immediately above the medial canthal tendon to anastomose with the ophthalmic artery branches (Fig. 1.20).

Sternocleidomastoid muscle

The sternocleidomastoid muscle originates from the sternum and clavicle and extends in a posterior diagonal fashion to insert onto the ipsilateral mastoid process and

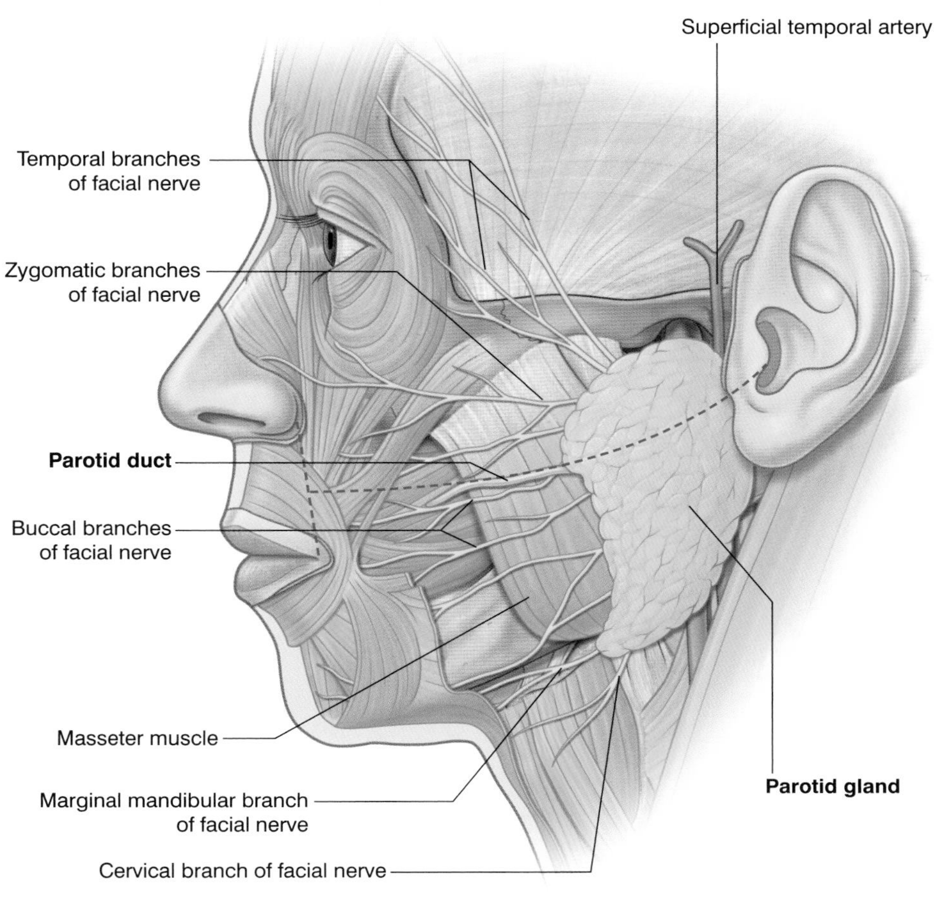

Figure 1.14 Branches of the facial nerve exit the anterior, superior, and inferior poles of the parotid gland. The point where the parotid duct crosses the anterior border of the masseter muscle is plotted along a line connecting the tragus to the middle of the upper lip, the tragolabial line. (After Robinson 1996[12] with permission from Saunders.)

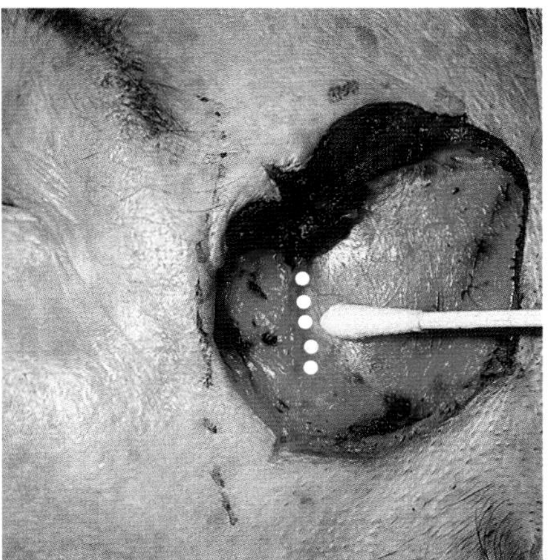

Figure 1.15 Relationship of the temporal artery to the temporal branch of the facial nerve. The frontal branch of the temporal artery lies to the left of the line of white dots pointed to with the cotton-tip applicator. One of the temporal branches of the facial nerve is marked on the skin with Gentian violet. (After Robinson 1996[12] with permission from Saunders.)

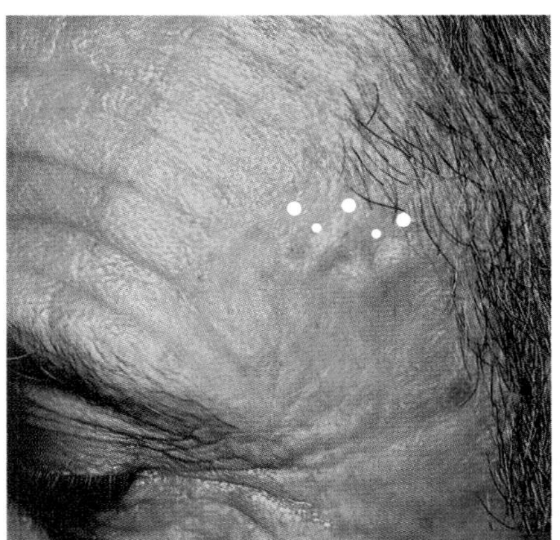

Figure 1.16 The tortuous engorged frontal branch of the temporal artery is visible on the surface of the skin (highlighted by white dots). (After Robinson 1996[12] with permission from Saunders.)

lateral portion of the occipital ridge. The muscles work together to flex the neck and work individually to turn the neck and elevate the chin. With the head rotated away from the observer, the sternocleidomastoid muscle becomes a prominent surface landmark that divides the neck into the anterior and posterior triangles. The muscle and the mastoid process are important landmarks used to identify the spinal accessory nerve at its most exposed location in the posterior triangle (Fig. 1.21)

Facial muscles

Branches of the facial nerve innervate all the muscles of facial expression (Table 1.1). These muscles originate or insert into the skin itself. This is in contrast to the muscles of the body, which originate and insert on the bony structures that they move. The major function of the facial muscles is expression, which is important to nonverbal communication, and mouth and eyelid function. The SMAS represents a continuous layer of fascia which encases and

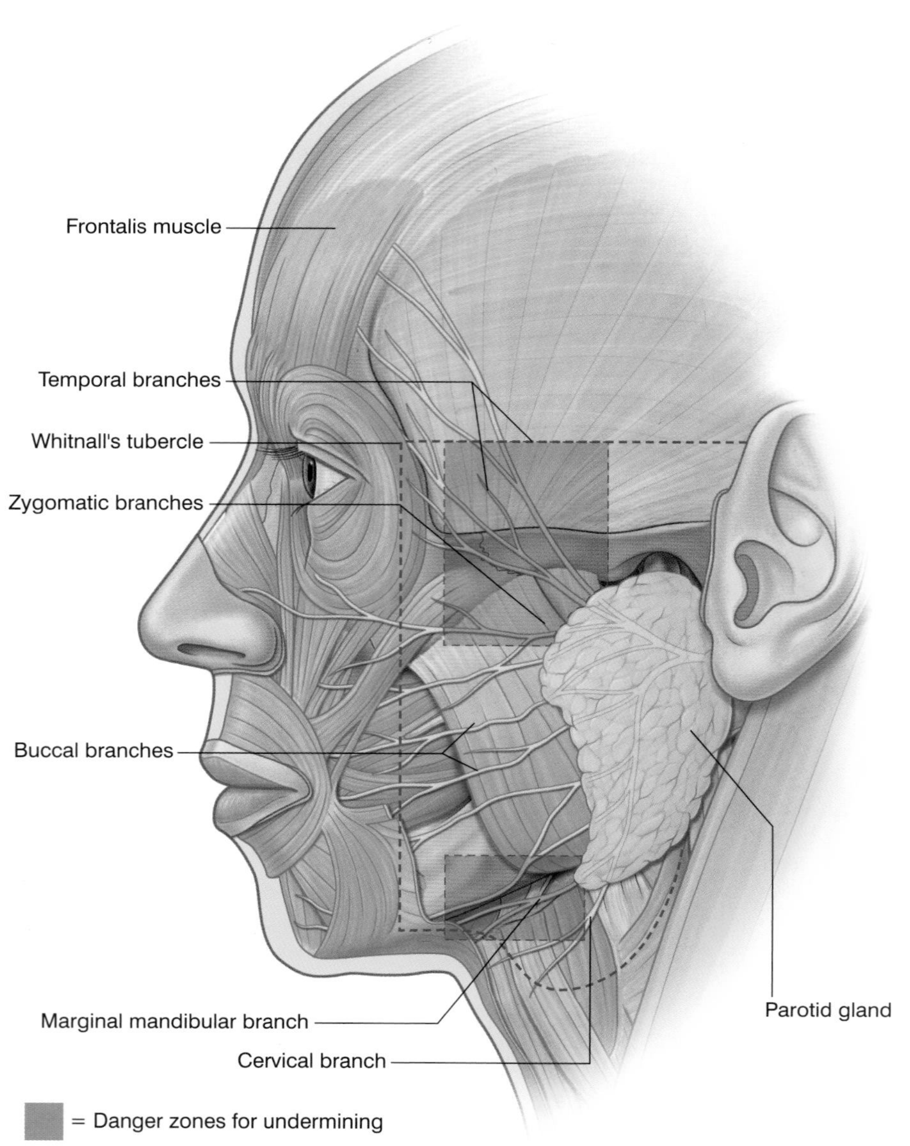

Figure 1.17 Branches of the facial nerve. The shaded area represents the 'nonprotected zone' where branches have emerged from the parotid gland. (After Robinson 1996[12] with permission from Saunders.)

connects all the muscles of facial expression with overlying skin through fibrous bands. It interconnects, integrates, and unifies the action of the facial muscles and creates facial expression. The importance of the facial muscles is obvious in the patient who has lost the function of the facial nerve because of trauma or stroke or as the temporary result of local anesthesia (Fig. 1.22). If, for example, temporal nerve injury causes permanent loss of the ipsilateral frontalis muscle causing loss of horizontal forehead rhytides and descent of the brow on the affected side, the normal side may be temporarily treated by injection of botulinum toxin to block the function of the nerve or a brow-lift may ensue.

The muscles are best thought of by regions of the face, with groups of muscles acting in concert together thanks to the SMAS, rather than as individual muscles (e.g. mouth, nose, eye, and ear). Muscles of the upper face (periorbita) act primarily in the vertical direction, whereas those of the lower face (perioral) work in both vertical and horizontal directions. The frontalis muscles of the upper face normally function as one unit that raises the eyebrows and secondarily, the eyelids. Nerve injury here causes more of a cosmetic than a functional derangement, whereas injury to motor nerves of the lower face causes substantial cosmetic and functional loss as a result of mouth dysfunction.

Periorbital muscles

The major muscle around the eyes is the orbicularis oculi, which has an orbital and a palpebral component. The palpebral muscle is further divided into preseptal and pretarsal components. The muscle only inserts into the bone at the medial canthus. The palpebral portion, which covers the eyelid, acts to gently close the lid. Contracting the orbital portion of the muscle closes the lids more tightly and draws them medially. The orbicularis oculi muscle does

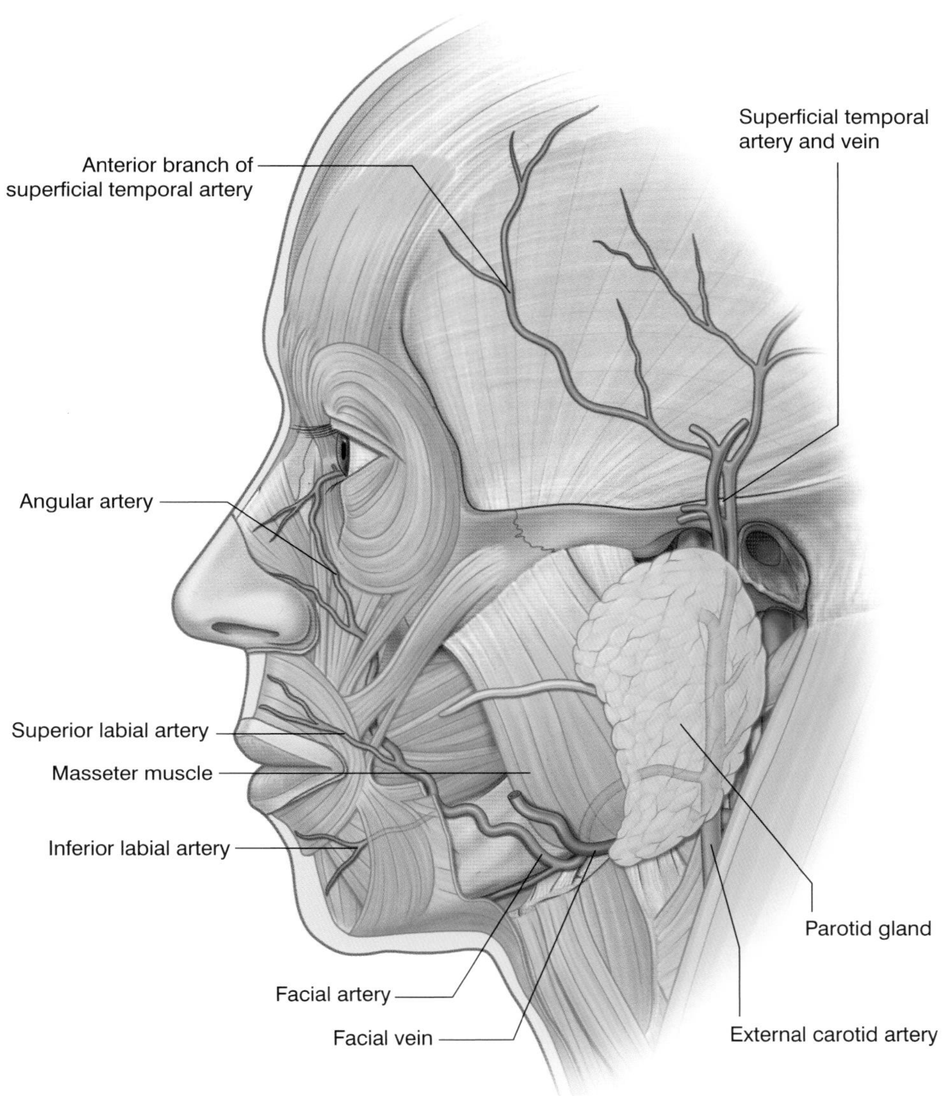

Figure 1.18 Arterial supply of the face in relationship to the masseter muscle and parotid gland. (After Robinson 1996[12] with permission from Saunders.)

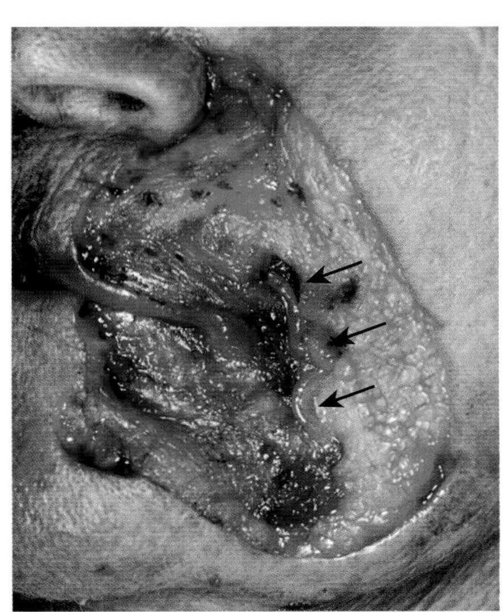

Figure 1.19 The course of the facial artery is shown as it enters the face at the lower border of the jaw, just in front of the anterior border of the masseter muscle. It is possible to palpate the pulsation here. The diagonal path across the face lateral to the oral commissure is shown by the arrows. (After Robinson 1996[12] with permission from Saunders.)

not open the eyelids. The eyelid is opened by the levator palpebrae superioris, which originates within the orbit and is innervated by branches of the third cranial nerve. Thus, loss of function of the orbicularis oculi results in the levator superioris working unopposed so the eyelids do not close. The orbicularis oculi muscle is innervated primarily by the zygomatic branch of the facial nerve, but the upper portion of the muscle is also partially innervated by the temporal branch of the facial nerve (Fig. 1.23). Paralysis of these muscles by nerve loss leads to inability to fully or tightly close the lids and possibly ectropion formation.

The bilateral corrugator supercilii muscles arise from the medial part of the superciliary ridge to insert into the skin of the brow. They draw the brow medially causing 'hooding,' and contribute to the formation of the deep vertical furrow of the glabella.

The procerus muscle is a solitary midline muscle that originates from the superior aspect of the nasal bones

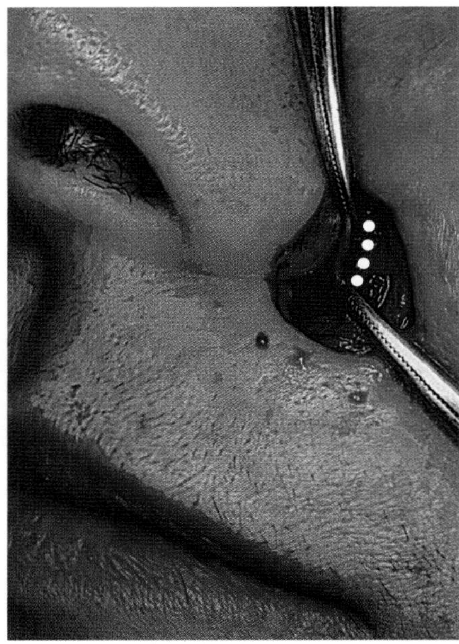

Figure 1.20 The facial artery lies adjacent to the nose as the angular artery. It is to the left of the line of white dots.

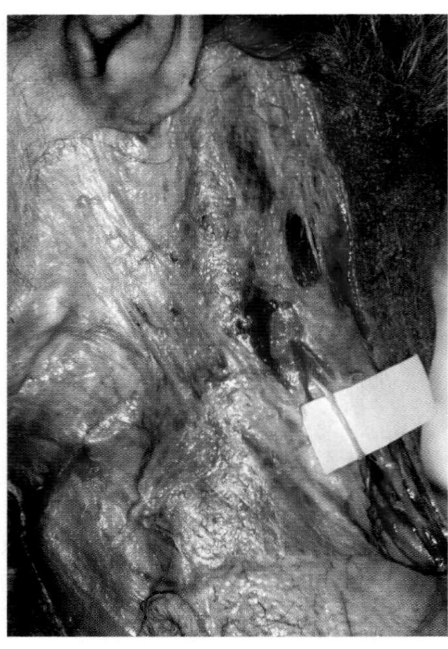

Figure 1.21 The spinal accessory nerve at its most exposed location. (After Robinson 1996[12] with permission from Saunders.)

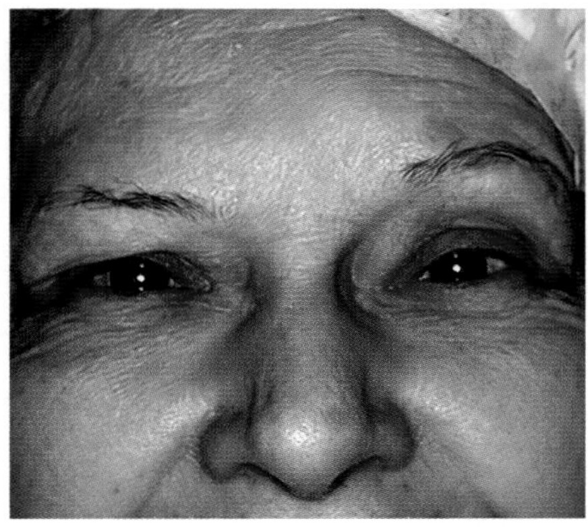

Figure 1.22 Loss of function of the temporal branch of the facial nerve results in a depressed brow. (After Robinson 1996[12] with permission from Saunders.)

Table 1.1 Muscles of facial expression and their functions

Region	Muscle	Actions	Innervation
Forehead and brow	Frontalis	Raises the eyebrows and accentuates the horizontal wrinkles of the forehead, assists opening of the eyelid widely	Temporal branch of the facial nerve
	Corrugator supercilii	Produces scowling by drawing the brow medially and downward	Temporal branches of the facial nerve
	Procerus	Draws the forehead and brows inferiorly to create transverse wrinkles at the nasal root	Zygomatic branch of the facial nerve
Eyelid	Orbicularis oculi	Closes the eye and blinks	Zygomatic branch of the facial nerve
	Levator palpebrae superioris	Opens the upper eyelid	
	Frontalis		
	Procerus		
Mouth	Orbicularis oris	Draws the lips together, pulls the lips against the teeth, and puckers the mouth	Buccal and marginal mandibular branches of the facial nerve
Buccinator	Flattens the cheek against the teeth and assist with whistling	Buccal branches of the facial nerve	
	Levator labii superioris alaeque nasi, levator labii superioris, zygomaticus major, zygomaticus minor	Lip elevators—produce the smile	Zygomatic branch of the facial nerve
	Levator anguli oris, risorius	Lip elevators—produce the smile	Buccal branch of the facial nerve
	Depressor anguli oris, depressor labii inferioris	Lip depressors	Marginal mandibular branch of the facial nerve
	Platysma	Lip depressor	Cervical branch of the facial nerve.
	Mentalis	Lower lip elevation and protrusion	Marginal mandibular branch of the facial nerve

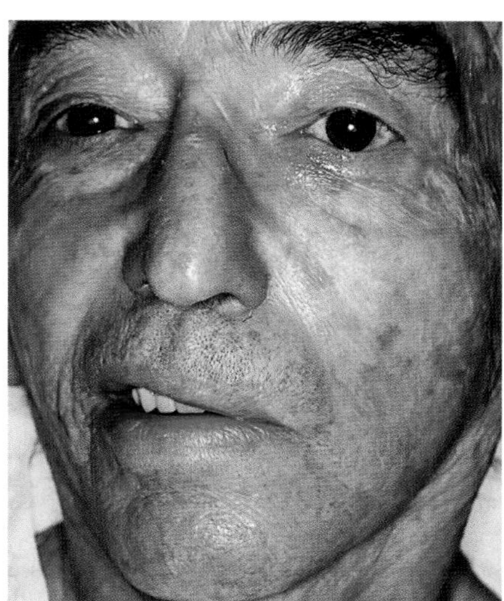

Figure 1.23 While providing anesthesia for the surgical procedure, the buccal and zygomatic branches of the facial nerve are temporarily paralyzed.

to insert into the skin overlying the root of the nose. It pulls the medial aspect of the eyebrows inferiorly and is innervated by the temporal branches of the facial nerve.

Nasal muscle

The muscles of the nose are variable in their development and have little functional importance.

Perioral muscles

Of the muscles of the lower face, those around the mouth are the most important. These can be divided into muscles that elevate, depress, and encircle the lips. The muscles insert directly into the skin. The elevators from medial to lateral as they insert into the lip are the levator labii superioris, levator labii superioris alaeque nasi, zygomaticus major and minor, levator anguli oris, zygomaticus minor, and zygomaticus major muscles. These muscles originate from the upper maxilla in the infraorbital areas, insert into the upper lip and melolabial fold, and as they contract pull the mouth up and out. The levator anguli oris, which originates in the canine fossa of the maxilla, inserts into the angles of the mouth bilaterally, and is the deepest of the elevator muscles.

The mentalis muscle is innervated by the marginal mandibular nerve. It interdigitates with the lip depressors above and platysma below, and contraction causes protrusion of the lip as well as 'apple dumpling' chin (fine pits in the skin where muscle fibers tug on overlying skin).

The depressors of the mouth from medial to lateral according to insertion in the lip include the depressor anguli oris, depressor labii inferioris and the platysma. These three muscles, which are innervated by the marginal mandibular branch of the facial nerve, pull down the lip and angle of the mouth. Injury to this vulnerable nerve results in an unopposed upward and diagonal pull on the lips causing lower lip elevation on this side, which is most prominent when smiling. At worst, this may give the appearance of a sneer. This may also be associated with some loss of function (i.e. drooling).

The orbicularis oris is the sphincter muscle responsible for pursing the lips and tight lip closure. Its muscle fibers are blended with those of many of the elevators and depressors as well as those of the platysma and risorius muscles. The deep buccinator muscle, which is also innervated by the buccal branches of the facial nerve, is the fleshy part of the mid cheek. It helps keep food from accumulating between the gums and the cheek while eating by forcing it back into the path of the teeth.

Lateral movement of the mouth is a function of the superficial platysma and risorius. The risorius is a paper-thin muscle that arises from the parotid fascia and passes anteriorly to insert into the skin and mucosa at the corner of the mouth. It pulls the labial commissure laterally, widening the mouth by making a smirk.[6]

The platysma muscle is important anatomically but has little functional role. It is innervated by the cervical branches of the facial nerve. The muscle originates in the superficial cervical fascia and inserts into the orbicularis oris muscle as well as skin of the lips and chin. It is usually a broad but extremely thin muscular sheet that is responsible for tensing the skin of the neck, which gives vertical banding to the level of the clavicle in exaggerated cases. It covers and attempts to protect the marginal mandibular branch of the facial nerve as well as the facial artery and vein.

Despite the prominence of the temporalis and masseter muscles, these are not muscles of facial expression, but rather muscles of mastication.

Ear muscles

The muscles of the ear are of no functional significance.

Superficial muscular aponeurotic system

The SMAS is composed of muscle and a thin superficial layer of fascia that invests nearly all of the muscles of facial expression, especially those of the lower face, mid-face, and forehead regions. The fascial component of the SMAS arises from the superficial cervical fascial layer, envelops the platysma muscle, sweeps over the mandible, and invests the muscles of the face. Posteriorly, the fascia is tightly attached to the mastoid process of the temporal bone, the fascia over the sternocleidomastoid muscle, the superficial fascia of the parotid gland about 1–2 cm anterior to the tragus, and the zygomatic arch.

Functionally, the SMAS forms a network that binds nearly all of the muscles of facial expression together and ensures that they act in concert. The fascia provides a method of distributing the pull of the muscles evenly over the skin and acts as a deterrent to prevent spread of infection from the superficial to the deep areas of the face.

The axial arteries are found either in the superficial aspect of the SMAS or at the SMAS–subcutaneous fat border. Thus, the sub-SMAS layer is relatively bloodless. All sensory nerves lie above the SMAS whereas all motor muscles lie just deep to the SMAS. Dissection beneath the SMAS on the cheek is only safe when directly over the parotid gland where the nerves are found within the parenchyma of the gland. In the temporal area, dissecting above the SMAS ensures the integrity of the facial nerve. The unique features of the SMAS have resulted in significant innovations in cosmetic surgery, especially neck and face-lift surgery.[15]

Nerve supply of the head and neck

Sensory innervation

The sensory innervation of the face is derived from branches of cranial nerve V (the trigeminal nerve). It has three branches: V_1—the ophthalmic (superior branch); V_2—the maxillary nerve (middle branch), and V_3—the mandibular nerve (lower branch); these exit the skull through the supraorbital foramen, infraorbital foramen, and mental foramen, respectively. All the foramina are located along a vertically-orientated midpupillary line. Effective regional nerve block anesthesia can be achieved by blocking the nerves as they exit the foramina.

Cervical nerves derived from C2 to C4 form a plexus deep to the sternocleidomastoid muscle. The largest nerve to emerge from this plexus is the greater auricular nerve, which exits from behind the posterior border of the muscle and courses upward toward the lobule of the ear lateral to the jugular vein. It supplies the skin of the lateral neck and the skin at the angle of the jaw as well portions of the ear. The lesser occipital nerve also emerges from behind the muscle slightly superior to the exit of the greater auricular nerve and courses upward to innervate the neck and the scalp posterior to the ear. The transverse cervical nerve emerges from behind the muscle several centimeters inferior to the great auricular nerve and crosses the muscle transversely to supply the skin of the anterior neck. This area of emergence of the great auricular, lesser occipital and transverse nerves is Erb's point (see Surgical Anatomy of the Neck, below and Fig. 1.28). The importance of Erb's point is that the spinal accessory nerve (the motor nerve to the trapezius muscle) also emerges in this vicinity.

Motor innervation

The facial nerve innervates all the muscles of facial expression; therefore, it is of unique importance during surgery of the skin. In many instances, the branches of this nerve are superficial and vulnerable to trauma during surgery. When surgery is planned in these areas, patients need to be advised preoperatively of the risk of trauma to the facial nerve and the functional deficits that may result because of it.

The facial nerve has five major branches—temporal, zygomatic, buccal, marginal mandibular, and cervical. In general, the branches of the facial nerve enter the muscles that they innervate at their posterior and deep surfaces. The branches generally travel below SMAS fascia, as opposed to sensory nerves, which run over the SMAS. If a branch is injured anterior to a vertical line drawn from the lateral canthus, the nerve can be expected to regenerate with partial function over the course of several months. Once the facial nerve branches leave the parotid gland they are less well protected and more prone to inadvertent trauma. Hence, this region is called a 'danger zone' (see Fig. 1.17). The danger zone is described within the following boundaries:

- Starting at the ear, a horizontal line 1 cm above the zygoma and ending at Whitnall's tubercle (see Fig. 1.17). The lateral aspect of the brow is a useful landmark for the upper border of the danger zone.
- A vertical line starting at Whitnall's tubercle and ending at the inferior margin of the mandible.
- Starting at the inferior margin of the mandible, a curved line extending 2 cm below the margin of the mandible and ending at the angle of the mandible.

The temporal branch is considered to be one of the most vulnerable branches of the facial nerve (Fig. 1.24). Drawing one line from the earlobe to the lateral tip of the highest forehead crease and a second line from the earlobe to the lateral tip of the brow and then connecting these two end points can identify the course of this nerve. After leaving the upper pole of the parotid gland the nerve, which may be singular or exist as multiple branches, courses upwards to innervate the frontalis muscle, upper portion of the orbicularis oculi muscle, and corrugator supercilii. The nerve is most vulnerable as it crosses the zygomatic arch and temple where it is protected only by skin, subcutaneous fat, and a thin layer of SMAS. In elderly patients in particular, who have little to no subcutaneous layer, this nerve sits only millimeters below the skin surface (Fig. 1.25). The major effect of injuring the nerve is flattening of the forehead with drooping of the eyebrow and inability to close the eye tightly. Descent of the brow into the orbital area may interfere with upward and lateral gaze, which can be repaired with a brow lift.

The other branch of the facial nerve at risk because of its superficial location is the marginal mandibular branch as it exits the inferoanterior pole of the parotid gland at the angle of the mandible and as it courses upwards posterior to the facial artery onto the face just anterior to the masseter muscle to innervate the lip depressors. In these locations, as it crosses the angle of the mandible it is covered only by skin, subcutaneous fat, and the SMAS. Usually, the marginal mandibular nerve remains at or above the lower level of the mandible in its course. However, in 20% of people, this nerve is found to descend 1–2 cm into the neck at the mandibular angle, so caution must be exercised in this area[16] (Fig. 1.26). When the head is hyperextended in the opposite direction to expose the submandibular area for surgery, the nerve may be as much as 2 cm or more below the mandible even in patients in whom this is not usually the case. The platysma muscle is superficial to the marginal mandibular branch and may protect it from trauma. Unfortunately, the platysma muscle is highly variable and not always clearly identifiable. Trauma to the marginal mandibular branch can produce appreciable functional and cosmetic deficits, allowing lateral and upward pull on the mouth. The ipsilateral side tends to be frozen in a persistent grimace because of the lack of opposing downward muscular contraction.

Lymphatics of the head

The vessels of the lymphatic system tend to parallel the venous system and have valves every 2–3 mm. In general the drainage is from superficial to deep, and from medial to lateral, and caudad in a downward diagonal direction. It has been estimated that between 20 and 50% of normal individuals have palpable benign lymph nodes in the neck. These lymph nodes are generally less than 1 cm in size.[17]

The major facial lymph node basins of the head and neck are in the parotid, submandibular, and submental areas. The major lymphatic drainage of the face consists of channels that run posteriorly in a downward diagonal direction. The scalp and posterior aspect of the ear drain to the

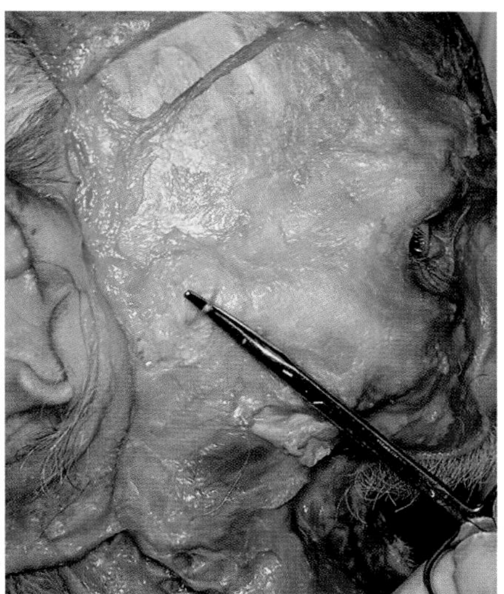

Figure 1.24 Cadaver prosection of the rami of the temporal branch of the facial nerve as it crosses the zygomatic arch. (After Robinson 1996[12] with permission from Saunders.)

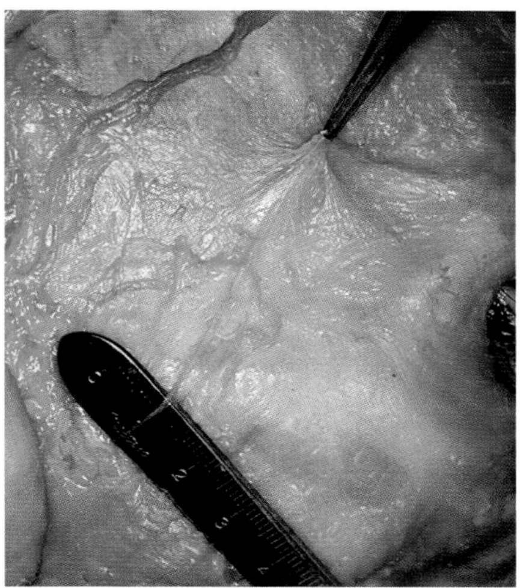

Figure 1.25 Cadaver prosection close-up of the same area seen in Figure 1.24. The scalpel handle is under the temporal branch of the facial nerve, which has been dissected out of the SMAS at the zygomatic arch. On the forehead, about 2 cm above the brow, the forceps picks up the nerve as it is covered with the SMAS. The nerve is clearly visible through the distance between the two surgical instruments. (After Robinson 1996[12] with permission from Saunders.)

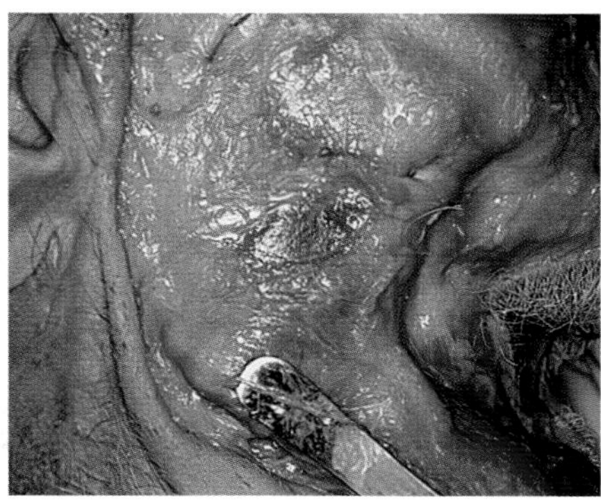

Figure 1.26 Marginal mandibular nerve descends into the neck. The surgical instrument is placed below the nerve to demonstrate the location of the nerve in this cadaver dissection. (After Robinson 1996[12] with permission from Saunders.)

postauricular and occipital nodes, which then drain to the deeper cervical lymph nodes of the spinal accessory, transverse cervical, and internal jugular nodes. Although the parotid nodes are identified as being both preauricular and infra-auricular, they are both within the gland and in the surrounding glandular fascia, and behave as a single unit serving the basin of the lateral cheek, anterior surface of the ear, forehead, and lateral canthal area. The submental nodes drain their respective side of the medial and lower face, the medial eyelid, the lateral aspects of the lip, the nose, the gingivae of the mouth, the soft palate, the anterior two-thirds of the tongue, and the palatine fossa. The submental glands are in the midline and have the potential to drain from either the right or left central facial region of the middle two-thirds of the lip and the chin. The submental and submandibular nodes are surrounded by glandular fascia.

The parotid nodes are examined with the patient seated and directly facing the physician, but the submental and submandibular nodes are best palpated with the chin drawn inferiorly to relax the platysma muscle overlying these areas. This procedure may be further enhanced by a bimanual examination with one finger placed in the floor of the mouth and the fingers of the other hand pressing upward against the submental and submandibular basin. The submental nodes are often palpable in healthy people.

Drainage to the postauricular nodes is from the upper posterior aspect of the ear, and the posterior parietal, mastoid, and temporal areas of the scalp. From here, drainage continues into the nodes beneath the upper portion of the sternocleidomastoid muscle and the superior junction of the internal jugular and spinal accessory node chains. The occipital nodes drain the muscular layers of the neck and posterior aspect of the scalp. They then also drain into the cervical lymph node chain (Fig. 1.27). Ultimately the lymphatic system of the head and neck blend into a solitary trunk that empties into the venous circulation by the thoracic duct on the left and the jugular and subclavian veins on the left.

Surgical anatomy of the neck

The skin of the neck is relatively loose with transverse creases and wrinkles. Elective incisions are easily placed in these lines. Because of the concave shape of the neck, vertical incisions have a tendency toward scar contracture with web formation, which may have functional as well as cosmetic implications.

The superficial landmarks of the neck are the hyoid bone anteriorly and the sternocleidomastoid muscle laterally, which divides the neck into the anterior and posterior triangles. The posterior triangle of the neck is important to identify because the spinal accessory nerve, which innervates the trapezius muscle, emerges from the posterior aspect of the sternocleidomastoid there. The spinal accessory nerve, which is covered only by skin and superficial cervical fascia, is vulnerable to injury during surgery in the posterior triangle. Trauma to the nerve results in loss of function of the trapezius muscle, with winging of the scapula, inability to shrug the shoulder, difficulty abducting the arm, and chronic shoulder pain. Unlike the distal aspects of the facial nerve, when this nerve is transected, it has no ability to regenerate. It exits behind the sternocleidomastoid muscle and travels diagonally in a downward direction across the posterior triangle to innervate the trapezius muscle. The exit of the spinal accessory nerve from the sternocleidomastoid muscle is known as Erb's point (Fig. 1.28).

Erb's point is located by turning the head away and bisecting a horizontal line connecting the angle of the jaw to

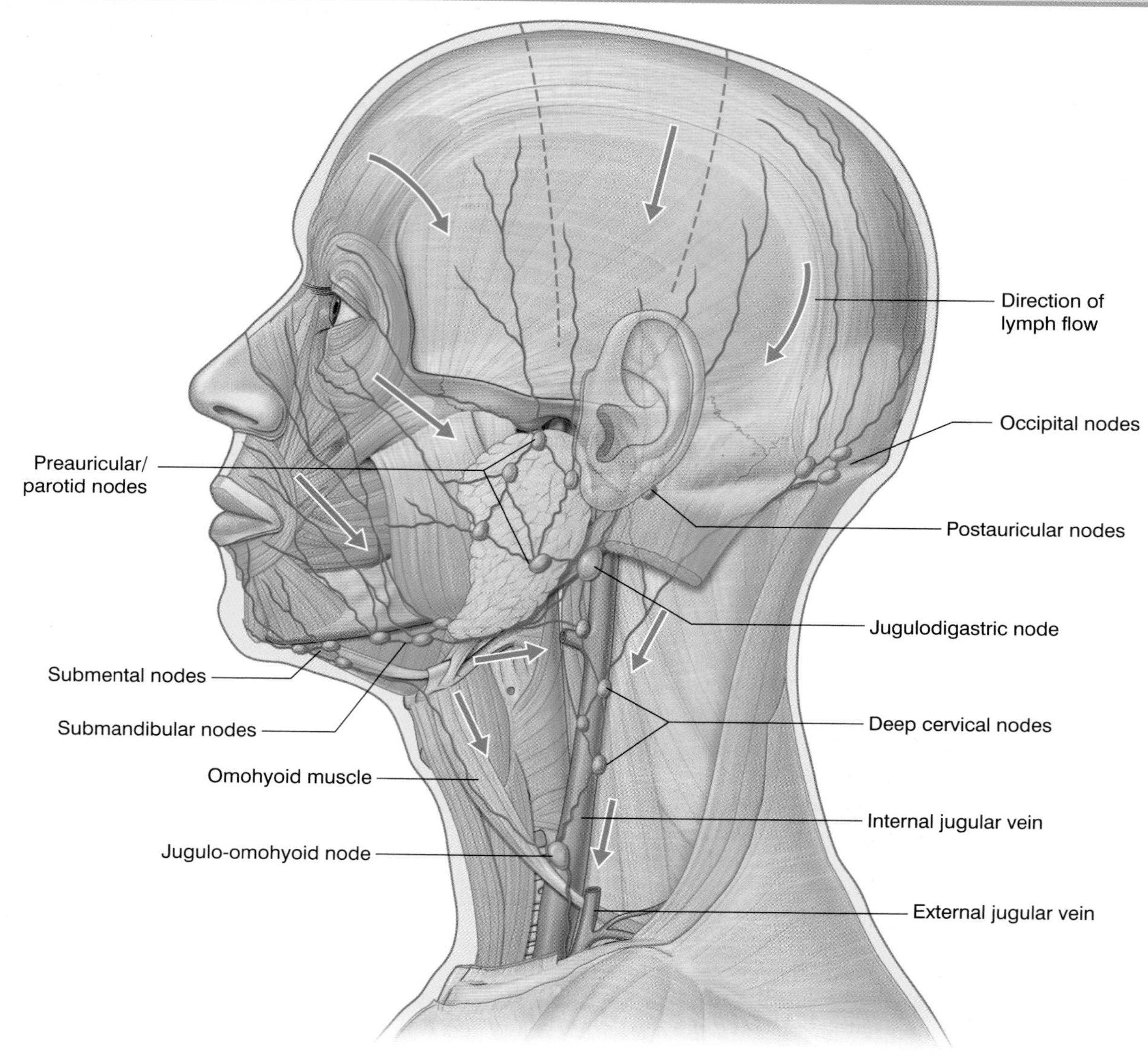

Figure 1.27 Lymphatic system of the head and neck. Dotted lines indicate the borders between the drainage areas and arrows indicate the direction of lymph flow. (After Robinson 1996[12] with permission from Saunders.)

the mastoid process with a vertical line drawn from the midpoint to the posterior border of the sternocleidomastoid muscle. If a vertical line is dropped 6 cm from the midpoint of this line, it will intersect the sternocleidomastoid muscle near to the point of emergence of the nerve.[18] Another way of identifying this area is to draw a horizontal line from the thyroid notch across the neck through the posterior triangle—2 cm above and below the point where this line intersects the posterior margin of the sternocleidomastoid muscle is the approximate site where the spinal accessory nerve traverses the posterior triangle of the neck. Transecting the spinal accessory nerve, which supplies the trapezius muscle, results in difficulty raising the shoulder.

Superficial anatomy of the hand and foot

Dermatologic surgery of the hand and foot is generally limited to surgery of the skin and subcutaneous tissue. In planning a procedure in these areas, every effort must be made to preserve functionality. Vital structures, including nerves, arteries, veins, ligaments, and tendons, sit superficially below a thin layer of skin and fat and are often palpable. The loose dorsal skin and fascia of the hand and foot become tight when in full flexion. Procedures are planned with this in mind, so as to avoid placing undue tension on wound edges that might limit range of motion and cause wound dehiscence and unsightly scarring.

The dorsal surface of the hand is innervated by the sensory branch of the radial nerve, which is vulnerable to injury because of its superficial location, and by the dorsal branch of the ulnar nerve. Palmar skin and fascia are thick and inelastic with flexion creases (Fig. 1.29). The palmar surface is innervated by the radial, median, and ulnar nerves.

Palmar incisions parallel flexion creases or cross high-tension crease areas at an angle of 45° or less. Incisions that cross creases at angles approaching a right angle produce a

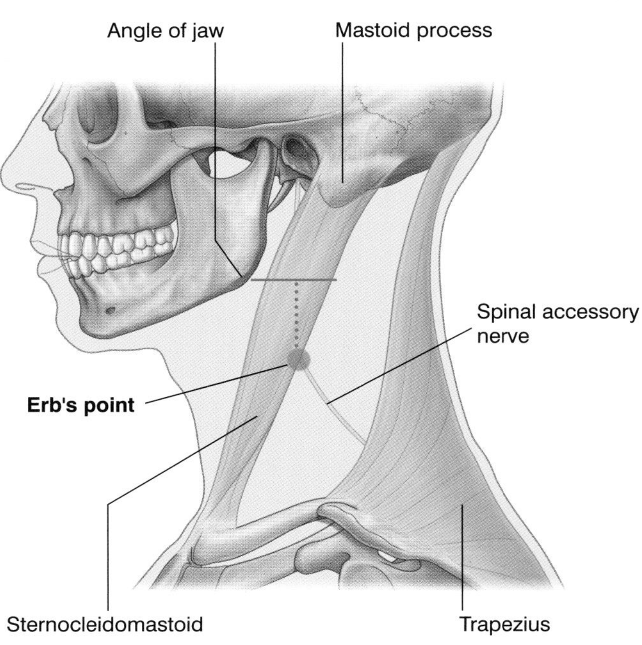

Figure 1.28 Erb's point is located by bisecting a horizontal line connecting the angle of the jaw to the mastoid process with a vertical line drawn from the midpoint to the posterior border of the sternocleidomastoid muscle. Within a short distance of this point, the spinal accessory nerve, lesser occipital nerve, great auricular nerve, and transverse cervical nerves all emerge from the posterior border of the muscle. (After Robinson 1996[12] with permission from Saunders.)

Practical applications of understanding skin structure and surgical anatomy

- Recognize the danger zones for arterial bleeding:
  - the frontal branch of the temporal artery at the temple.
  - the facial artery as it crosses the mandibular rim.
  - the angular artery as it courses near the nose.
- Recognize the danger zones for nerve transection:
  - the temporal branch of the facial nerve.
  - the spinal accessory nerve in the posterior triangle of the neck.
  - the marginal mandibular nerve as it courses in the neck below the mandible.
- Know where to perform nerve blocks:
  - facial nerve blocks at the supraorbital, infraorbital, and mental nerve foramina—all the foramina are located along a vertically oriented midpupillary line.
  - digital blocks in the web space rather than along the digit to decrease the risk of nerve injury by compression with the volume of local anesthesia.
  - ankle block—posterior tibial nerve (see Chapter 3).
- Know where to place sutures:
  - layered closures—place sutures in the muscle, SMAS and deep subcutaneous fat, superficial subcutaneous fat, and deep dermis before the sutures that close the surface.
- Palpation of lymph nodes in head and neck:
  - postauricular nodes drain the upper posterior aspect of the ear, and the posterior parietal, mastoid, and temporal areas of the scalp.
  - parotid nodes drain the lateral cheek, anterior surface of the ear, forehead, and lateral canthal area.
  - submental nodes drain the medial and lower face, the medial eyelid, the lateral aspects of the lip, the nose, the gingivae of the mouth, the soft palate, anterior two-thirds of the tongue and the palatine fossa, and because they are in the midline they have the potential to drain from either the right or left central facial region of the middle two-thirds of the lip and the chin.

scar that may be tender and limit movement (see Chapter 24). Transverse dorsal incisions on the dorsum of the hand are more cosmetically acceptable. Curvilinear lazy 'S' incisions are better over the dorsal surface of the digits to prevent scar contracture from a longitudinal incision that may impair joint mobility. The oblique aspect of the S curve minimizes the risk of injury to longitudinal structures of the digit.

On the dorsal foot it is preferable to make longitudinal incisions that are perpendicular to relaxed skin tension lines to avoid damaging the underlying structures. The plantar foot skin adheres to deeper structures via many fibrous bands, which make for limited tissue movement during surgery. The anatomy of the medial aspect of the foot and ankle is particularly relevant for performing posterior tibial nerve blocks (Fig. 1.30).

SUMMARY

The anatomy of the head and neck is complex. As a great deal of surgery of the skin performed by dermatologic surgeons involves the face and neck, in-depth knowledge of

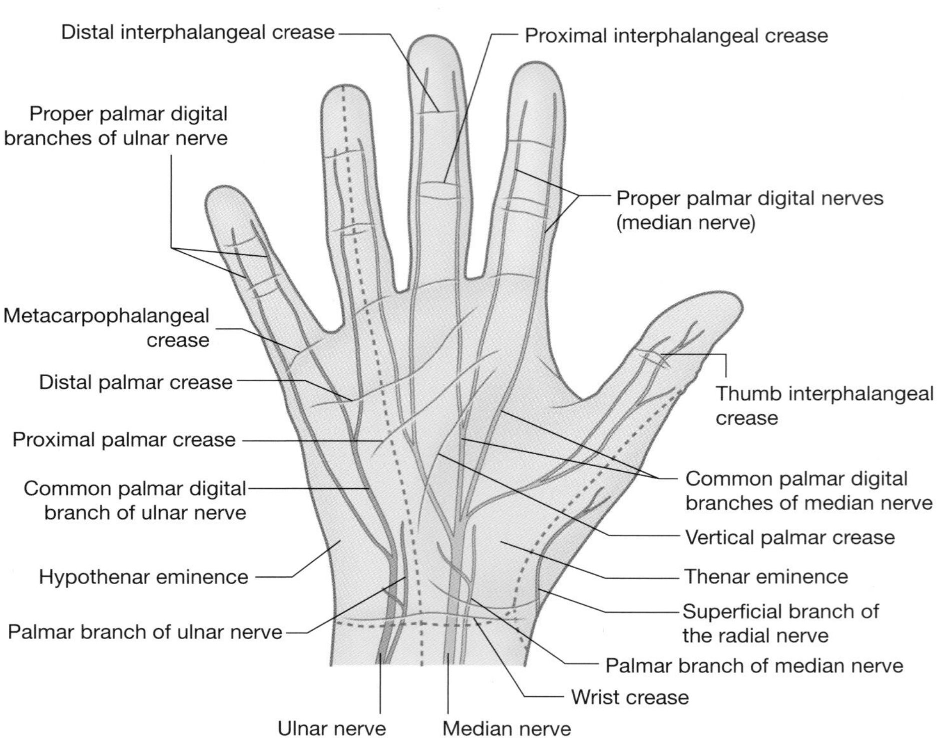

Figure 1.29 Palmar topical landmarks and cutaneous innervation of the hand. Dotted lines indicate boundaries of the innervation of the palmar surface: three and one-half digits by the median nerve, one and one-half digits by the ulnar nerve. (After Robinson 1996[12] with permission from Saunders.)

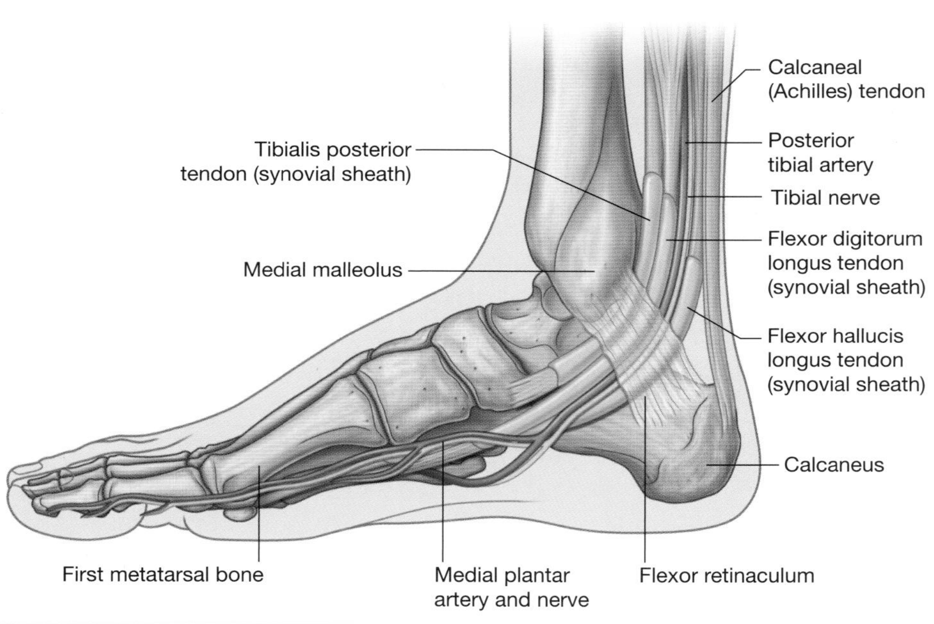

Figure 1.30 Medial surface of the foot and ankle with the underlying tendons and the palpable artery. (After Robinson 1996[12] with permission from Saunders.)

Optimizing facial surgery

- Preserve the cosmetic units of the face. Remove additional tissue to place incisions at the junction of cosmetic units; use suspension sutures to fix advancing tissue to underlying support to prevent distortion of the free margins of the lip and eyelid.
- Place incisions into relaxed skin tension lines. With the patient seated, observe the formation of lines with animation of the face (e.g. grimace, frown, smile, pucker).
- Place suspension sutures into deep supporting structures. The mental crease, nasolabial fold at the junction with the alae, the zygomatic arch, the orbital rim.
- Mobilize tissue. Plan tissue movement to access the lax tissue of the temple, nasolabial fold, paranasal cheek, supraorbital and infraorbital lids glabella, neck; use cycles of intraoperative loading with skin hooks on the skin of the wound edges to produce stress relaxation; temporary retention sutures place constant force on the wound edges.
- Reduce the wound size. Undermine tissue widely in a tissue plane that results in the least amount of bleeding and plicate the SMAS.

Pitfalls and their management

- Facial nerve injury. When facial nerve injury is the result of blunt trauma, inflammation, or heat, the nerve may recover over a period of 2–6 months; if the loss of function does not risk loss of an important function, a period of observation is appropriate.
- Sectioning of the temporal branch of the facial nerve results in brow and lid ptosis and the inability to tightly close the eyes. Dissect above the SMAS at the temple. Botulinum toxin injections of the unaffected forehead on the contralateral side will result in the brows being at the same level. Brow-lift on the side with the brow ptosis may also be performed.
- Sectioning of the zygomatic branch causes paralysis of upper lid resulting in epiphora and exposure keratitis. Short-term management: immediately postoperatively provide a moisture chamber for the eye with lubrication. Long-term management: gold weight implant into the upper eyelid provides closure by gravity with lateral tarsorrhaphy; lateral canthoplasty.
- Sectioning of the marginal mandibular branch results in protrusion of the corner of the lower lip. Botulinum toxin injections of the unaffected side. Suspension of the lid at the commissure or facial nerve graft if the transection is distal may provide relief.
- Spinal accessory nerve injury. When planning surgery, locate Erb's point by turning the head away and bisecting a horizontal line connecting the angle of the jaw to the mastoid process with a vertical line drawn from the midpoint to the posterior border of the sternocleidomastoid muscle. A vertical line is dropped 6 cm from the midpoint of this line and it will intersect the sternocleidomastoid muscle near to the point of emergence of the nerve.
- Arterial bleeding. When approaching areas where there is likely to be arterial bleeding have two hemostats available for each artery in the field; palpate the area to feel the pulsation of the artery at the inferior mandibular rim and the temple; undermine in the plane with the least risk of transecting arteries; on the scalp undermine in the subgaleal space, and on the forehead below the muscle and over the periosteum; undermine the wound edges to see the artery and clamp it before cutting it. Ligate arteries.

these areas is required to optimize outcomes and minimize patient risks. This chapter and accompanying CD-ROM are a source of information that would ideally be augmented and tested in cadaver dissection courses, with accurate anatomic models, and by observing surgical procedures with an experienced surgeon. Anatomy knowledge is essential for sound surgical judgment and advanced surgical skills. This chapter is the tinder that kindles the flame of procedural dermatology.

"The mind is not a vessel to be filled but a fire to be kindled" (Plutarch).

REFERENCES

1. Farmer ER, Hood AF. Pathology of the skin. Norwalk, CT: Appleton & Lange 1990; 3–29.
2. White CR, Bigby M, Sangueza OP. What is normal skin? In: Arndt KA, LeBoit PE, Robinson JK, Wintroub BU, eds. Cutaneous medicine and surgery. Philadelphia: Saunders 1996; 3–41.
3. Briggaman RA, Kelly T. Continuous thymidine labeling studies of normal human skin growth on nude mice: measurement of cycling basal cells. J Invest Dermatol 1982; 78:359.
4. Briggaman RA, Wheeler CE Jr. The epidermal–dermal junction. J Invest Dermatol 1975; 65:71–84.
5. Katz SI. The epidermal basement membrane zone – structure, ontogeny, and role in disease. J Am Acad Dermatol 1984; 11:1025–1037.
6. Eyre DR. Collagen: molecular diversity in the body's protein scaffold. Science 1980; 207:1315–1322.
7. Uitto J, Olsen DR, Fazio MJ. Extracellular matrix of the skin: 50 years of progress. J Invest Dermatol 1989; 92:61S–77S.
8. Marcus J, Horan DB, Robinson JK. Tissue expansion: past, present, and future. J Am Acad Dermatol 1990; 23:813–825.
9. Greener EH, Harcourt JK, Lautenschlager EP. Materials science in dentistry. Baltimore: Williams and Wilkins 1972; 46–52.
10. Chayen D, Nathan H. Anatomical observations on the subgaleotic fascia of the scalp. Acta Anat 1974; 87:427–428.
11. Dzubow LM. Facial flap – biomechanic and regional applications. Norwalk, CT; Appleton & Lange; 1989.
12. Robinson JK. Basic cutaneous surgery concepts. In: Robinson JK, Arndt KA, LeBoit PE, Wintroub BU, eds. Atlas of cutaneous surgery. Philadelphia: Saunders 1996; 1–4.
13. Salasche SJ, Bernstein G, Senkarik M. Surgical anatomy of the skin. Norwalk, CT: Appleton & Lange; 1988.
14. Ellis DAF. Pelausa EO. Cosmetic evaluation of the lower third of the face. Fac Plast Surg 1987; 4:159–164.
15. Owsley JQ Jr. SMAS–platysma face lift. Plast Reconstr Surg 1983; 71:573–576.
16. Dingman RO, Grabb WC. Surgical anatomy of the mandibular ramus of the facial nerve based on the dissection of 100 facial halves. Plast Reconstr Surg 1962; 29; 266–272.
17. Sage H. Palpable cervical lymph nodes. JAMA 1958; 168;496–498.
18. King IJ, Motta G. Iatrogenic spinal accessory nerve palsy. Ann R Coll Surg Engl 1983; 65:35–37.

2 Aseptic Technique

Christie T Ammirati MD

Summary box

- In surgical procedures, there are four potential sources of contamination: the personnel, the surgical environment, the patient, and the instruments, with the patient's normal flora being the most common reservoir.
- Appropriate measures to ensure aseptic technique depend upon the procedure being carried out and the risk of infection, but there are basic precautions that should be adhered to whatever the procedure:
  - hands should be washed before donning surgical gloves and after their removal
  - alcohol-containing preparations are extremely flammable and should be allowed to dry completely before laser or electrocautery are used
  - chlorhexidine gluconate should not be allowed to contact the eye or middle ear
  - povidone-iodine must be left on the skin to be effective
  - hair removal is only indicated if the hair will obscure the surgical field or hinder proper surgical technique.
- Good surgical technique is directly related to the degree of contamination a wound can overcome without becoming infected and includes:
  - atraumatic handling of tissue
  - effective hemostasis without compromising blood supply
  - limiting the amount of implanted material (particularly braided suture).

INTRODUCTION

When it had been shown by the research of Pasteur that the septic property of the atmosphere depended not on the oxygen or any gaseous constituent but on minute organisms suspended in it...it occurred to me that decomposition in the injured part might be avoided...by applying some materials capable of destroying the life of the floating particles. The material which I have employed is carbolic...acid

Lister J. On the antiseptic principle in the practice of surgery. Lancet 1867; 2:353–356.

Before 1860 most surgery was performed reluctantly and with the understanding that the operation was as likely to kill the patient as the disease. This was because regardless of the success of the operation the vast majority of patients died within a few days from overwhelming sepsis. Although less than 150 years ago, this was a time when the prowess of a surgeon was evidenced by the amount of blood encrusted on his coat.[1] If a scalpel became dull during an operation it was promptly sharpened on the sole of an assistant's shoe and then placed back into the wound. Lint and sawdust from the floor were used as hemostatics, surgical sponges were reused without laundering, and it was believed wound infections were generated spontaneously by exposure to air.

The modern era of surgery began in the mid-19th century, with the development of anesthesia. Once the pain from surgery had been conquered, surgeons were free to focus on technique rather than speed. Despite their best efforts, hospital gangrene and death remained dreaded but frequent outcomes of most major operations. This dismal mortality rate remained unchanged until Pasteur introduced the germ theory of disease, which would later form the basis of Joseph Lister's principles of surgical antisepsis. In 1867, Lister deduced that '...the essential cause of suppuration in wounds is decomposition, brought about by the influence of the atmosphere'.[2] Unlike Pasteur, Lister could not boil or 'pasteurize' surgical wounds to remove these particles. Instead he turned to carbolic acid (phenol), which in the form of coal tar was known to remove the odor from municipal sewage and to delay the putrefaction of dead bodies. After initial success with carbolic-soaked bandages on open compound fractures, Lister extended its use to the operating room. His antiseptic surgical technique consisted of washing the surgeon's hands, the instruments, the operating room environment, and the surgical site with carbolic acid. He also devised an atomizer, which produced a continuous mist of carbolic acid into the air during surgery. In 1870, Lister published an article describing the influence of these measures on the deplorable conditions of the surgical wards at the Glasgow Royal Infirmary, the stench of which was notorious. After 9 months of strict antisepsis there was not a single case of hospital gangrene, pyemia, or erysipelas in the entire ward.[3] Unfortunately, these dramatic findings were met with strong opposition from the medical community and it took almost 10 years before surgeons began to adopt this technique universally.

'Listerism,' or antisepsis, markedly decreased the mortality from surgery, but the atmosphere of the surgical suite was laden with carbolic acid, which was toxic to surgeons and other personnel who were chronically exposed to its vapors. It was also somewhat caustic when applied directly to open wounds. This prompted the search for alternative antiseptics with less morbidity, such as iodine and alcohol. Sterilization of instruments and bandages became possible in 1886 when von Bergmann developed a superheated steam system similar to the modern autoclave. Sterilization of the surgeon's hands remained a challenge until Halsted introduced 'boilable' rubber gloves in 1890. Mikulicz added further refinement to aseptic technique when he described the benefits of wearing a gauze mask in 1897, and MacDonald recognized the infection risk posed by 'theatre spectators' gathered around the operating table.[1]

Over the last 100 years aseptic technique has evolved into a set of well-defined practices designed to reduce the risk for surgical site infection. Dermatologic surgeons perform a broad range of procedures in a variety of settings. Appropriate measures to ensure aseptic technique will depend on the invasiveness of the proposed procedure and the risk for infection. These measures range from the use of non-sterile gloves and an alcohol skin wipe for shave biopsies, to full surgical dress and strict asepsis for liposuction. The following chapter outlines the major components of aseptic technique and their applicability to dermatologic surgery.

Normal flora

> For my part I judge, from myself…that all the people living in our United Netherlands are not as many as the living animals that I carry in my own mouth this very day…
>
> *Anthony van Leeuwenhoek (1683) Letter to the Royal Society of London. Cited in: Dobell C. Antony van Leeuwenhoek and his little animals. New York: Russell & Russell Inc; 1958*

The human body is colonized with microorganisms that are collectively known as indigenous or normal flora. The density and composition of these microorganisms vary with the different portions of the body, and on the skin are largely determined by local humidity and lipid content. Skin flora can be divided into two distinct populations, resident flora and transient flora.

Resident flora

Resident flora maintain stable population densities and can be isolated in similar numbers from most individuals. These commensal microorganisms help protect the host from infection by competing with pathogens for substrate and tissue receptors. Resident flora inhabit the surface of the skin, as well as deeper portions such as the pilosebaceous unit. Deeply embedded organisms are resistant to mechanical removal and are beyond the reach of topical antiseptic solutions. Given this inherent limitation, the goal of preoperative skin cleansing is to decrease resident flora to its lowest possible level, with the realization that it cannot be completely eradicated.

The most common resident organisms are the coagulase-negative staphylococci, with *Staphylococcus epidermidis* accounting for more than 90% of resident aerobes.[4] Anaerobic diphtheroids such as *Propionibacterium acnes* are common in lipid-rich locations, such as the pilosebaceous unit. Gram-negative bacteria represent a small portion of the resident flora and are mostly limited to the humid intertriginous areas with *Enterobacter*, *Klebsiella*, *Escherichia coli*, and *Proteus* spp. being the predominant organisms.

Transient flora

Transient flora are acquired through contact with people, objects, or environment. They are loosely attached to the surface of the skin and are amenable to removal by washing. The majority of postoperative wound infections are due to transient microorganisms that contaminate the wound during surgery. In most cases the source is the endogenous flora of the patient's nose, throat, or skin.[5] Exogenous sources of contaminating flora include the surgical personnel, the local environment (including air), surgical instruments, and materials brought into the sterile field during surgery. *Staphylococcus aureus* is the most frequent cause of surgical site infection, followed by coagulase-negative staphylococci, *Enterococcus* spp., *E. coli*, and less commonly group A streptococci and *Pseudomonas aeruginosa*.[6]

Most pathogens are transmitted via one of four basic routes: contact, airborne, vehicle, or vector. For surgical procedures, the contact and airborne routes are the most likely means of contamination. Contact transmission may be indirect where organisms are transferred via fomites (for example, if suture touches contaminated skin and are then placed into the wound) or direct (if contaminated skin of the patient or surgeon touches the wound). During airborne transmission, microorganisms are not suspended freely but carried on desquamated skin cells, aerosolized water droplets, or dust particles.[7] In this way, the gowns, linens, surgical tables, and operating room floors are easily contaminated, particularly with staphylococci and enterococci which are resistant to desiccation.

Surgical site infection

> …I have as yet, scarcely lost a case in true consequence of surgery…yet nearly half of those that I have operated on for hernias have died and more than half after tracheotomy and nearly all after trephining. But these were deaths after operations; not because of them.
>
> *Paget J. Address in surgery. BMJ 1862; 2:157.*

Center for Disease Control definition

The Center for Disease Control (CDC) defines surgical site infection as any surgical wound that produces pus (suppurates) within 30 days of the procedure, even in the absence of a positive culture.[8] An exception to this rule would be a suture abscess, which may suppurate but resolves with the removal of the suture and is not considered to be a wound infection. Inflammation is frequently associated with wound infection but in the absence of suppuration, is not sufficient to classify the wound as infected. A positive culture does not necessarily confirm a wound infection, because chronic wounds may be colonized but not infected. In this case, it is the quantity of bacteria per gram of tissue (usually $>10^5$) that determines whether infection is present.

Categories of risk

The risk for developing a surgical site infection can be categorized by the degree of contamination within the wound.[9] Wounds are defined as clean if they are elective incisions carried out on non-inflamed tissues under strict aseptic technique and if there is no entry into the gastro-intestinal, respiratory or genitourinary tracts. If there are minor breaks in aseptic technique, or entry into the gastro-intestinal, respiratory or genitourinary tracts, the wound is considered to be clean–contaminated. Contaminated wounds include those where major breaks in aseptic technique have occurred, or there is inflammation, but no frank purulence encountered. A dirty wound contains frank purulent fluid such as an abscess. It may also involve the perforation of a viscus or fecal contamination.

In addition to the local condition of the wound, patient and operative characteristics may influence the risk for developing a surgical site infection. A more comprehensive method, such as that proposed by the CDC, takes into account comorbid factors such as the patient's age, malnutrition, obesity, hypothermia, blood transfusions, or use of immunosuppressants (including alcohol).[9] The length of operation is also factored into risk assessment, with long procedures carrying a greater risk of contamination than brief procedures. The inclusion of these additional parameters allows for comparison of rates that are risk-adjusted for specific procedures, and helps identify patients at high risk for surgical site infection.

■ PREOPERATIVE PREPARATION

Preparation of surgical personnel

Surgical hand scrub

The surgeon's hands and forearms, along with those of assisting personnel, are placed in close contact with the surgical wound and represent a significant potential source of contamination. The surgical hand scrub serves to remove transient flora and soil from the fingernails, hands and forearms. Its effectiveness relies on the antiseptic agent chosen and its method of application. If performed correctly, it can reduce the microbial load by 90–99% and maintain this reduction for several hours.[10]

Antiseptic agents

> They and their disciples teach, and almost all modern surgeons follow them, that pus should be generated in wounds. There could be no greater error than this. For it does nothing else but hinder the work of nature, prolong disease, prevent healing and the closing up of wounds....My father used to heal almost every kind of wound with wine alone...'
>
> *Theodoric of Lucca (1210–1298) Bishop of Cervia, Physician and Surgeon. Borgognoni T (Theordoric of Lucca). The Surgery of Theodoric. Translated from the Latin by Campbell E, Colton J. New York: Appleton-Century-Crofts Inc; 1955.*

The ideal antiseptic agent should be broad-spectrum, non-irritating, fast-acting and provide continued antimicrobial action within the moist environment of the surgical glove. There are several commercially available antimicrobial ingredients approved for surgical hand scrubs. Each agent has its own unique characteristics and action spectrum but none is ideal for every situation. A thorough working knowledge of the strengths and limitations of these ingredients is essential to choosing the appropriate agent for each setting (Table 2.1).

In the USA the most common agents are povidone-iodine and chlorhexidine gluconate with and without alcohol.[9] Povidone-iodine is a broad-spectrum antiseptic with well-known skin-staining and fabric-staining qualities. It works within minutes but must be left on the skin to have a persistent effect. It is quickly inactivated in the presence of blood or sputum, and chronic maternal use has been associated with hypothyroidism in newborns.[11]

Chlorhexidine gluconate has a similar antimicrobial spectrum as povidone-iodine but when combined with alcohol has a more rapid onset.[12] Chlorhexidine gluconate binds to the stratum corneum and maintains residual activity in excess of 6 hours, even when wiped from the field. Its action is not affected by the presence of organic matter but it should be used with caution around the eyes as it has been known to cause conjunctivitis and severe corneal ulceration. It may also cause significant ototoxicity if allowed to enter the middle or inner ear through a perforated tympanic membrane.[13]

Alcohol-based preparations, which are the standard of care in Europe, are gaining popularity in the USA.[14] Multiple studies have confirmed their safety, speed, and broad range of antimicrobial activity.[15,16] Alcohol-based solutions do not necessarily have detergent qualities and should only be applied to clean skin and fingernails.[17] For maximum effect, they should be dispensed in sufficient volumes so as to keep the hands wet while rubbing for at least 2 minutes.[14] Alcohol-containing products are highly flammable and should be allowed to dry before electrocautery or a laser is used (Figs 2.1, 2.2). When applied as a single agent, alcohol is rapidly germicidal, but once evaporated it does not have significant residual activity.[17] To address this limitation, alcohol-based preparations are frequently combined with a second agent that has a sustained effect, such as chlorhexidine gluconate. Often the mixture achieves better antisepsis than either agent alone.[15,18]

Parachlorometaxylenol (PCMX), also known as chloroxylenol, has good Gram-positive bacteria coverage but notably poor activity against *P. aeruginosa*. Several PCMX formulations have an added chelator, such as ethylenediaminetetraacetic acid (EDTA), which markedly increases the anti-*Pseudomonas* activity of the mixture.[9] PCMX maintains residual activity for several hours, but this is less than that induced by chlorhexidine gluconate. It is minimally affected by the presence of organic matter and, although it can be absorbed through the skin, adverse reactions are rare.

New agents

The majority of new surgical hand scrub solutions are alcohol-based for speed and ease of application. Triseptin (Healthpoint Ltd, Fort Worth, TX) is a brushless surgical

Table 2.1 Common antiseptic agents*

Agent	Action Spectrum	Rapidity of Onset	Sustained Activity	Cautions
60–95% Alcohols	++++ Gram-positive ++++ Gram-negative +++ *Mycobacterium tuberculosis* +++ Fungi +++ Enveloped viruses	Fastest	Minimal as a single agent	Flammable Poor cleansing agent Use liberal amount and allow to dry
Chlorhexidine gluconate	++++ Gram positive +++ Gram negative + *Mycobacterium tuberculosis* ++ Fungi +++ Enveloped viruses	Fast	Excellent Additive effect with repeated use	Keratitis Ototoxicity
Povidone-iodine	++++ Gram positive +++ Gram negative +++ *Mycobacterium tuberculosis* +++ Fungi +++ Enveloped viruses	Fast	Intermediate to minimal if wiped from the skin	Potential systemic toxicity with neonates or large body surface area Rapidly neutralized by blood, serum proteins or sputum
Para-chloro-meta-xylenol (PCMX)	+++ Gram positive ++ Gram negative† ++ *Mycobacterium tuberculosis* ++ Fungi ++ Enveloped viruses	Intermediate	Intermediate to excellent, depending on formulation	Poor *Pseudomonas* coverage as a single agent

* *Adapted from Wade and Casewell[12] and Parienti et al.[15]*
† *Improved Pseudomonas coverage with addition of chelating agent such as EDTA.*
Spectrum of action: ++++, excellent; +++, good; ++, fair; +, poor.

Figure 2.1 70% isopropyl alcohol pad igniting seconds after contact with electrocautery tip.

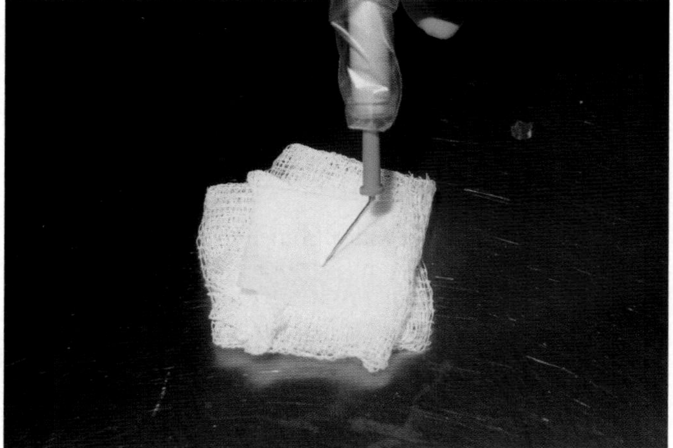

Figure 2.2 Same type of alcohol pad as used in Figure 2.1 but allowed to dry. It does not ignite despite prolonged contact with the electrocautery tip and maximum settings.

hand scrub that contains a combination of 70% ethyl alcohol, zinc pyrithione (to enhance persistence of effect), emollients, and surfactants. It achieves initial and 6-hour persistent hand antisepsis after a 3-minute brushless application and has been shown to be significantly superior to scrub-brush application of either chlorhexidine gluconate for 3 minutes or povidone-iodine for 5 minutes.[16]

N-duopropenide (NDP) is a newly developed cationic antiseptic that belongs to the quaternary ammonium chemical family. It has good Gram-positive and Gram-negative coverage along with activity against fungi and yeasts. It also has reported activity against *Bacillus* and *Clostridium* endospores. Clinical studies have shown that NDP in combination with 60% isopropanol (NewGer-spray, Biogenetic Labs, Madrid, Spain) and emollients provides rapid antisepsis with persistent activity at 3 hours.[19]

Duration and method

Hand scrub solutions can become contaminated and support microbial growth. To limit this risk, they should be stored in closed receptacles and either supplied in single-use containers or dispensed from a foot-operated system.[20] The outer surfaces of a hand pump frequently become contaminated and should, therefore, be replaced with a more hygienic system. Another potential source of contamination is the bacteriological quality of the water used to rinse the skin after completion of the hand scrub. In one modern operating room, plumbing manipulations resulted in water flowing from the surgical sink that was contaminated with Gram-negative bacteria and atypical mycobacterium.[21] This led to an outbreak of surgical infections and illustrates that water supplies should be periodically monitored, particularly after servicing.

Recent studies have refuted the need for the traditional 5–10 minute surgical scrub and suggest that a shorter application time may be just as effective. Combining agents that complement each other can decrease the required duration of the scrub. For example, an initial 1–2-minute scrub with chlorhexidine gluconate, followed by an alcohol-based hand rub, is as effective as a 5-minute scrub with either agent alone.[15,18] While the importance of cleaning under the fingernails remains unchallenged, the need to scrub the skin with a brush has been debated. Several studies have confirmed that rubbing the hands together briskly to generate friction may be as effective as using a scrub brush, particularly if an alcohol-based product is used.[16]

Fingernails should be kept short to facilitate cleaning, and artificial nails—which are known to harbor significantly more microorganisms than natural or polished nails—should not be worn during surgical procedures.[22] There are conflicting data regarding nail polish and its effect on the surgical hand scrub. It is generally agreed that nail polish may be worn as long as it is not chipped or dark in color, potentially obscuring the presence of subungual debris. Jewelry is known to harbor bacteria beneath it and to decrease the effectiveness of the hand scrub, but it is not known whether this sequestration leads to increased risk for surgical site infection.[23] Despite the lack of consensus or scientific data, jewelry and long fingernails (natural or artificial) clearly limit dexterity, and increase the risk for glove perforation, and are therefore best avoided during surgery.

Surgical attire

Surgical attire can be divided into non-sterile and sterile items, each serving different functions. Non-sterile attire is designed to reduce microbial shedding from surgical personnel and subsequent contamination of the surgical environment. It consists of a scrub suit, cover gown, face mask, shoe protection, and hair cover. These items are permeable to moisture and should be changed immediately should they become wet with blood or another body fluid.

Sterile surgical attire, such as impervious surgical gowns and sterile gloves, are designed to maintain a sterile field and protect personnel from exposure to blood-borne pathogens during surgery.

Scrub suits

Scrub suits are made of loosely woven material for comfort, and serve to reduce bacterial shedding from the skin of surgical personnel. The perineum is heavily colonized and the friction generated by walking can liberate bacteria-laden skin cells into the operating room environment.[24] A scrub shirt tucked into pants that are constricted at the waist and ankles is an efficient means of reducing perineal dispersal. Wearing a long-sleeved scrub jacket that snaps closed in the front can decrease bacterial shedding from the forearms (Fig. 2.3). However, there are no scientific data to show that wearing scrub suits rather than street clothes affects

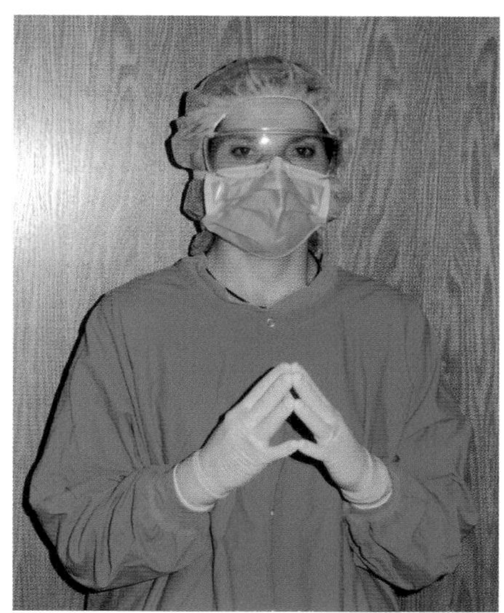

Figure 2.3 Suggested apparel to limit contamination of the sterile field from normal flora of the surgeon. Note that the cuffs of the gloves are pulled over the wristband of the scrub jacket. A bouffant-style hair cover provides maximum containment of the surgeon's hair.

the incidence of surgical site infection.[25] Scrub suits serve as personal protective gear but they are not impermeable to blood or body fluids. While they add to the overall hygiene of the surgical environment, they may be considered optional for minor surgical procedures. For procedures where exposure to body fluids is expected, such as liposuction, their use—along with impermeable gowns—should be strongly considered.

Regardless of the apparel chosen, any item of clothing that becomes soiled during surgery should be changed immediately. At the end of the day all surgical apparel (including scrub suits and lab coats that may appear to be clean) should be placed in a laundry bin—not hung in a locker to be worn the next day. Pathogenic bacteria and fungi can survive for extended periods on fabrics, particularly the polyester/cotton blends that are commonly used for scrub suits and lab coats.[26]

Cover gowns

Cover gowns are non-sterile reusable long-sleeved garments that cover the front of the scrub suit from the neck to the knees and tie in the back. They became popular when it was found that scrub suits, which were protected by cover gowns when worn outside the operating room, had significantly less contamination than those that were not.[27] Despite the potential for contamination there is currently no evidence to link the use of cover gowns with a lower incidence of surgical site infection, and neither the CDC nor the Association of Operating Room Nurses (AORN) guidelines require their use.[9,28]

Face masks

Face masks were originally designed to limit contamination of the surgical site from microorganisms expelled by surgical personnel. The effectiveness of a face mask is defined by its shape, the materials from which it is made, and the way in which it is worn. Loose-fitting masks allow up to 40% of expired air to escape backward past the cheeks and ears, particularly when sneezing or coughing, and must be tied snuggly to be effective.[29] At the end of each surgery, face masks should be discarded promptly and not placed in the pocket for future use, or left dangling around the neck. The inner surface of the mask becomes contaminated with expired microorganisms and, once removed, should be handled only by the ties.

There are conflicting data regarding the ability of face masks to reduce surgical site infection, and their necessity in the operating room has been questioned. Several clinical studies found no difference in bacterial counts or wound infection rates when surgical personnel wore face masks during surgery.[30] It has been suggested that face masks may even increase the risk for contamination by 'wriggling' around on the face and abrading skin cells into the sterile field.[31] Studies have found a clear relationship between bacterial contamination of the surgical field and the volume at which the person speaks.[32] Speaking in a normal tone for up to 30 minutes without a face mask projects relatively few bacteria. Conversely, speaking in a loud tone, even briefly, liberates significantly more bacteria—up to 1 meter away—and coughing or sneezing can propel bacteria up to 3 meters.[33] Given these findings, it is possible that operating in silence without a mask may provide the least risk for surgical site contamination.

However, caution is advised before discontinuing the routine use of face masks because it is not always known if talking will be needed during a procedure, or if an unexpected cough or sneeze will occur. A second consideration is the role that face masks play in universal precautions. They not only protect the surgical wound from airborne contamination but also serve to protect the wearer's mouth and nose from unexpected splashes of blood and body fluids.

Surgical footwear

Footwear worn during surgery should be fluid resistant and have impervious soles. It should be cleaned regularly and restricted to use in the operating room environment. These measures serve to limit contamination of the operating room floor and protect the healthcare worker from body fluid spills. If such footwear is not available, paper booties with elastic at the ankles can be worn over street shoes. These disposable covers protect the shoes from exposure to blood-borne pathogens and add to the overall hygiene of the operating room environment. However, there is little evidence that their use directly affects wound infection rates.[34,35]

Hair covers

The majority of patients and surgical personnel carry bacteria on the surface of their hair, which may be shed during surgery and contaminate the surgical field.[36] Disposable hair covers are a convenient and inexpensive means of reducing this contamination. Of the available varieties, bouffant and hood-style covers provide maximum coverage and are preferred over skullcaps that do not cover the hair over the ears or the nape of the neck (Fig. 2.3).

Surgical gloves

> In the winter of 1889–1890…the nurse in charge of my operating-room complained that the solutions of mercuric chlorid [*sic*] produced a dermatitis of her arms and hands. As she was an unusually efficient woman…I requested the Goodyear Rubber Company to make as an experiment two pair of thin rubber gloves with gauntlets.… Thus the operating in gloves was an evolution rather than inspiration or happy thought, and it is remarkable that during the four or five years when as operator I wore them only occasionally, we could have been so blind as not to have perceived the necessity for wearing them invariably at the operating-table.
>
> *Halsted WS. Surgical papers. Baltimore: The Johns Hopkins Press; 1924.*

Surgical gloves provide a second line of defense against potential contamination from the hand flora of the surgical team. They also protect surgical personnel from exposure to blood-borne pathogens. In dermatologic surgery, gloves become perforated in approximately 11% of procedures, and the wearer recognizes that a perforation has occurred in only 17% of cases.[37] In this fashion, the aseptic barrier between the surgeon's hand and the patient's wound can be unknowingly breached for extended periods. Even in the absence of visible perforation, the hands should always be washed after removing gloves. Occult glove perforations raise significant concern for exposure of the surgeon to the patient's body fluids. This margin of safety may be increased by the use of thicker 'tear-resistant' gloves or double-gloving.

Despite evidence-based data that these measures reduce the risk of exposure, most surgeons find that double-gloving limits their dexterity, and do not use this practice consistently.[38]

Aside from exposure concerns, there is little evidence that occult perforations influence bacterial counts on the surgeon's hands or on the outside of the gloves.[39] These findings should be interpreted with caution, as they were obtained from sterile gloves worn over hands that had undergone a traditional surgical hand scrub using an antiseptic agent with sustained effect. There are no available studies that evaluate the degree of surgical site contamination or wound infection rate from sterile glove perforation without a preceding surgical hand scrub.

Sterile surgical gowns

Sterile surgical gowns are worn as a barrier to fluid and microbial transmission during surgery. They have long sleeves with elastic cuffs and they maintain the sterile barrier between the surgical field and the surgeon's clothes or exposed arms. They are made from either impermeable material or a water-resistant, tightly woven fabric, and have been shown to decrease bacterial counts in the operating room.[40] The effect of contamination via this route, as reflected in the development of surgical site infection, is not known. Sterile surgical gowns are generally not necessary for most dermatologic procedures, but may be considered as protective gear for liposuction or other procedures with expected exposure to body fluids.

Preparation of the patient

> The man who is stretched on the operating table in one of our surgical hospitals is in greater danger of dying, than was the English soldier on the battlefield of Waterloo.
>
> *James Simpson (1811–1870), Scottish surgeon to the soldiers at the Battle of Waterloo. Cited in: Glaser H. The road to modern surgery. New York: EP Dutton & Co; 1962.*

Removal of street clothes

Regardless of the scheduled procedure, most hospital-based operating rooms require that patients remove all of their clothing, including underwear, and put on a cotton gown. This empiric practice is based on the perception that street clothes and shoes may contaminate the operating room environment, but is not supported by scientific data. Patients in street clothes disperse the same amount of bacteria as those dressed in a clean cotton gown, covered with a cotton sheet.[24] Infection rates for same-day surgery are not significantly affected when patients remain fully dressed.[41] Aside from causing embarrassment, removal of underwear and putting on a minimally secured gown allows for increased bacterial shedding from the perineum into the environment. Therefore, unless a gown facilitates exposure of the surgical site, or body fluid spillage is expected, the scientific literature does not support the need for patients to remove their street clothes before dermatologic surgery.

Hair removal

While some surgical rituals may be empiric, and not based on scientific data, they are generally considered sensible, and at best harmless. One exception to this observation would be preoperative shaving on the night before surgery and the erroneous belief that removing hair from the surgical site decreases the risk for infection. Shaving with a razor in particular should be avoided, because it causes abrasions which compromise skin integrity and allow bacteria to flourish. The time lapse between shaving and surgery plays a key role in the risk for infection. Seropian and Reynolds found a wound infection rate of 3.1% in patients shaved immediately before surgery that was significantly higher than the rate of 0.6% that occurred in those who were not shaved.[42] The infection rate rose to 7.1% when shaving was done the day before surgery, and to as much as 20% when performed more than 24 hours before surgery. Cruse and Foord performed a 5-year prospective study of surgical wounds and found a 2.3% infection rate in patients who were shaved, 1.7% in patients who had their hair clipped, and 0.9% in patients whose hair was not removed from the surgical field by any method.[43]

From an infection standpoint, it is generally agreed that hair should be left intact within the surgical field. That being said, the frustration of attempting to suture on the scalp when hair is caught with each throw of the knot is well known to surgeons who work in this area. If care is not taken, the entangled hair can decrease knot security and can increase the risk of a foreign-body reaction. One way to avoid this is to secure the hair away from the field with sterile hair clips, rubber bands, or lubricating gel (Fig. 2.4). If these methods do not prove sufficient, and removal is required, the hair should be judiciously clipped at the skin with a pair of scissors or electric clippers before establishing a sterile field.

Surgical site preparation

The goal of preoperative skin preparation is to lower the risk for surgical site infection by removing skin debris, dirt, and transient microorganisms. Like the surgical hand scrub, it seeks to lower the resident bacterial count as much as possible and limit rebound growth, but with minimal skin irritation. On the night before surgery, a preoperative shower with chlorhexidine gluconate has been shown to decrease wound infection rates, particularly those from *Staphylococcus aureus*, and may be considered for procedures with large surgical fields such as liposuction.[44] The most commonly used agents for surgical site preparation are chlorhexidine gluconate, povidone-iodine, *para*-chlorometaxylenol (PCMX) and alcohol-based products (Table 2.1). Some antiseptic agents are mutually inactivating and if repeated application is expected (such as during multiple stages of Mohs micrographic surgery followed by reconstruction) the same agent should be used for each consecutive application.[41]

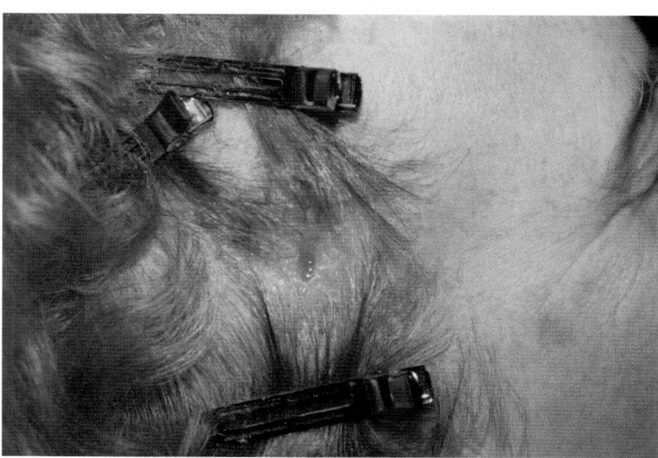

Figure 2.4 Suggested means to limit the need for hair removal. Hair is held away from the sterile field with water-soluble lubricating gel and hair clips.

Draping

Sterile drapes serve to protect the surgical site from microorganisms present on the surrounding non-sterile surfaces. Tightly woven cotton surgical drapes are softer and arguably more comfortable for patients than disposable impermeable drapes, but they may absorb fluid during surgery and 'wick' bacteria into the sterile field.[45] The fabric's weave may loosen with repeated washing and may become perforated by repeated clamping with towel clamps. To limit the risk for contamination, woven drapes should be chemically treated to retard water, inspected frequently for wear, and changed immediately if they should become wet. Alternatives to woven drapes are disposable plastic and plastic-lined paper drapes, which are impermeable to moisture and bacteria. The drawback is that they may be stiff and have a tendency to shift during surgery.

Environmental cleaning

> ...the surgeon's duty under ordinary circumstances is not to find what are the most dangerous sanitary conditions under which he dare operate, it is rather to discover the causes of the pestilence and banish them as far as possible from his field of action. The desiderata to be secured are a pure air, healthy conditions and strict cleanliness...
>
> *From an address by Sir William Scovell Savory (1879) to the British Medical Society. Cited in: Elliot IMZ, Elliott JR. A short history of surgical dressings. London: The Pharmaceutical Press; 1964.*

Microorganisms from both the patient and surgical personnel are continually shed into the operating room environment via desquamated skin cells. Once dispersed, they eventually settle onto horizontal surfaces such as the surgical field, floor, or counter tops. This reservoir can be reaerosolized from the passage of feet across the floor and by the breeze generated from opening the surgical room door.[46,47] To limit potential contamination, doors should be kept closed, the passage of non-essential personnel should be minimized, and cleaning and disinfection of surgical rooms should be performed on a scheduled basis.[48] It also follows that all people involved—the surgeon, patient and surgical assistant—need to reprep if there is a break in sterile technique, or they need to leave the room. Upon resuming surgery, the surgical site must be reprepped and draped, and surgeons must don fresh gloves. At no time should a surgeon leave the surgical suite with contaminated gloves.

Personnel outside of a hospital setting will need to be instructed in the unique cleaning needs of a surgical room and the ways in which they differ from routine office cleaning. There are no current studies that define the frequency and extent to which environmental cleaning should be carried out. For brief surgical procedures without fluid spillage, such as obtaining a Mohs layer, mopping the floor and wiping down counter tops after each patient is impractical and is not supported by the literature or the CDC.[9,49] Most guidelines recommend visible inspection of the room in between procedures, and prompt clean-up of any visible soiling or discarded surgical items that may have fallen onto the floor. Terminal cleaning, including wet vacuuming of the entire floor and disinfection of all environmental surfaces, is recommended at the end of each day of use.

Surgical instrument sterilization

Sterilization refers to a chemical or physical process that completely destroys or removes all forms of viable microorganisms, including spores, from an object. Surgical instruments and materials that come in contact with sterile tissue, cavities, or bloodstream must be unconditionally sterile. Instruments that are sterilized outside of the hospital settings, such as in a physician's office, are not subject to centralized control. It is essential that designated personnel be thoroughly trained in proper sterilization technique, with the ultimate responsibility for ensuring its adequacy resting upon the operating surgeon.[50,51] There are several sterilization methods available and while some systems are amenable to use in a physician's office, others are best suited to a hospital or industrial setting.

Steam under pressure (autoclave)

Most office-based dermatologic surgeons use an autoclave, which is considered the most efficient, economical and easily monitored method for sterilizing instruments.[52,53] Autoclaving generates pressures of 2 Pascals and temperatures of 121 °C that must be maintained for 15–30 minutes depending on the density of the surgical package. This form of sterilization is useful for liquids, glass, metal instruments, paper, and cotton, but should not be used with heat-sensitive plastics or oils.[52] A potential limitation to autoclave sterilization is that repeated exposure to high humidity may dull sharp cutting surfaces, particularly the high-grade carbon steel edges of hair-transplant punches and scalpel blades.

Heated chemical vapor

Sterilization by heated chemical vapor is a low-humidity method that can be used on sharp instruments, with less concern for dulling. It has the added benefits of not requiring a drying phase, and shorter heat-up time than an autoclave. However, instead of heating with distilled water, this method uses alcohol and formaldehyde, which necessitates use of protective gear, adequate ventilation, and safety monitoring.

Dry heat

Dry heat may be used for glass, oils, and instruments that can withstand prolonged exposure to temperatures of 121–204°C. As this method is humidity-free, it does not dull sharp instrument edges, and has no corrosive or rusting effects on instruments. The most common safety hazard with dry heat sterilization is burn injury to personnel, so protective equipment must be available and used consistently.

Gas sterilization

Gas sterilization with ethylene oxide or formaldehyde is an effective method for sterilizing heat-sensitive and moisture-sensitive instruments. A significant drawback is that ethylene oxide and formaldehyde are both toxic if inhaled and known carcinogens. In addition, gas sterilization requires prolonged exposure times and extensive venting systems.[50] The Occupational Health and Safety Administration (OSHA) requires strict monitoring of these highly toxic gases and, given its hazardous potential, gas sterilization is rarely performed outside hospital settings.

Chemical immersion

Sterilization by immersion in solutions such as glutaraldehyde or aqueous formaldehyde may be used for heat-sensitive items. The most frequently used 'cold sterilant' is 2% glutaraldehyde, but it is not reliably sporicidal and may be more accurately termed a 'cold disinfectant'.[53] Both glutaraldehyde and formaldehyde are highly toxic, require immersion for 6–12 hours, and do not have reliable means to ensure sterility. Once instruments are removed from the solution they must be handled aseptically, rinsed in copious amounts of sterile water, and dried on a sterile towel. They cannot be wrapped for storage and must be used immediately or their sterility is compromised.

New methods

Ortho-phthalaldehyde (OPA) is a relatively new chemical sterilant that received approval from the US Food and Drug Administration (FDA) in 1999. When compared to glutaraldehyde and formaldehyde, OPA sterilizes much faster (10–15 minutes) and has superior mycobactericidal and sporicidal activity.[55] It is highly stable, not irritating to the eyes or nasal passages, and does not require exposure monitoring. Disadvantages are that it may stain the skin gray and, as for other immersion methods, instruments cannot be wrapped for storage.

■ TECHNIQUES AND OPTIMIZING OUTCOMES

Surgical hand scrub

For minor or short-lived procedures (such as biopsies or electrodesiccation and curettage), the literature does not support the need for a formal surgical hand scrub, but it is recommended before more lengthy or invasive procedures. Before beginning the hand scrub, any jewelry on the fingers and wrists should be removed. Next, wash the hands and forearms thoroughly with a detergent-based solution to remove visible soiling. Recall that the majority of hand flora is found under and around the fingernails, so a disposable orange stick or nail pick will be needed to remove subungual debris and the fingernails should be kept trimmed. After a thorough cleansing, rinse and apply a liberal amount of an antiseptic solution to all the surfaces of the fingers, hands, and forearms. The effective duration and method of application varies with the solution chosen, but should be at least 2 minutes. The arms should be kept flexed at the elbow and rinsed from the fingertips downward, allowing water to drip from the elbows. Use a sterile or single-use disposable towel for drying. Allow any residual moisture to be air dried before donning surgical gloves. Ideally, the water supply should be controlled by a foot pedal, which removes the need to manually close a contaminated faucet.

Face masks

For maximum effect, crimp the face mask to fit the contour of the nose and tie it firmly at the back of the head, so that it covers nose and mouth. Should it become necessary to cough or sneeze while wearing a face mask, step backwards and face the surgical field rather than turning to one side. Change the face mask immediately if it becomes wet and discard it at the end of each major procedure, regardless of its condition. If a face mask is not worn during surgery, intraoperative talking should be kept to a minimum.

Surgical gloves

Remember that surgical gloves do not replace the need for clean hands and are considered a second line of defense. They should be inspected for tears or imperfections before and during surgery. If they become perforated, they should be changed immediately. Double-gloving provides additional protection from perforation but may limit dexterity and is not 100% effective. A double-glove puncture indication system (Biogel Reveal, Regent Medial, Norcross, GA) that shows punctures as a green color may be considered for high-risk patients or procedures.

Hair Removal

Hair should only be removed if its presence will obscure the surgical field or hinder proper surgical technique. If hair removal is deemed necessary, clip it judiciously at the skin with a pair of scissors or electric clippers before establishing the surgical field. Hair removal should be limited to the immediate peri-incisional area.

Surgical site preparation

For procedures with large surgical fields, such as liposuction, consider having the patient shower the night before surgery with chlorhexidine gluconate. At the time of surgery, place the patient on the table in the position in which surgery will be performed. Remove any visible dirt from the surgical site with a detergent-based solution and friction. Heavily colonized areas such as the umbilicus or nasal vestibule should receive close attention. After a thorough cleansing, blot the skin with a sterile or single-use towel and apply an appropriate antiseptic solution for the location and condition of the surgical site. Paint the solution or gel onto the skin in concentric circles beginning at the proposed incision site and extending several centimeters beyond the expected draped perimeter. It is important to remember that alcohol-containing solutions are flammable and must be allowed to dry before surgery or laser procedures are begun.

Draping

Once the skin has been prepared, the drapes should be gathered or folded in a compact manner. They should be held higher than the surgical table and placed along the perimeter of the sterile field extending into the periphery. Drapes should be placed so that they overlap several centimeters of prepared skin, and once set down they should not be lifted or repositioned. When possible, apply drapes to the patient's head and neck so as to direct the patient's expired air away from the surgical field. Woven drapes are no longer considered sterile if they become wet and should be changed immediately.

Environmental cleaning

At the beginning of each day, equipment, lights, tables, switch plates, and counter tops should be damp-dusted with a clean lint-free cloth and disinfectant. Perform a visible inspection of the room at the end of each procedure and any visible soiling or discarded surgical items that may have fallen onto the floor should be picked up and disposed of.

At the end of the day, the entire floor, including the surfaces underneath equipment, should be cleaned with a wet-vacuum. Alternatively, a two-mop system may be used, where the first mop applies the disinfectant solution and the second mops it up. Only freshly laundered mops should be used because they are easily contaminated and can spread bacteria from another location, such as a bathroom, to the floor of the operating room.

Instrument cleaning and sterilization

It is important to begin with high-grade stainless steel instruments that will withstand repeated use. There should be a formal protocol that designates the person responsible for removing all sharp objects, such as suture needles and scalpel blades, from the surgical tray at the end of each procedure. Once all the sharps have been removed, the instruments are taken to the processing area, completely disassembled, and placed in a presoaking solution to soften any adherent debris. At the end of the day the instruments are either cleaned manually or put in a washer/sterilizer. Cleaning must be meticulous because residual blood, tissue, and other organic matter may shield microorganisms and affect the reliability of sterilization methods.[56] Irregular surfaces, crevices, or hinged mechanisms may require ultrasonic cleaning or special brushes. After cleaning, the instruments are rinsed and inspected for residual organic debris or surface damage. Forceps and hemostat tips should be exactly aligned, and scissor blades should cut tissue paper without resistance. Any defective instrument should be set aside for repair. Instruments with moving parts should be placed into an instrument 'milk' that serves as a water-soluble lubricant and decreases the friction between opposing surfaces.

Instrument packaging and quality assurance

When the processing method permits, place instruments that are to be sterilized into individual pouches that can be opened as needed. Choose a packaging system that assures sterility until opened, permits identification of the contents, and resists tears, punctures or abrasions.[57] Instruments with delicate tips can be protected with special heat-tolerant tip guards (Fig. 2.5). A sterilization process indicator, such as heat-sensitive tape or an insert that turns dark with heat exposure, should be in a visible location on the package. This identifies packages that have been exposed to one or more steps in the sterilization process, but does not verify sterility. The only means of assuring the efficiency of a sterilizer is to perform quality assurance tests with heat-resistant *Bacillus* spp. spores at regular intervals (at least weekly). The spores' lack of viability after passing through the process demonstrates that conditions necessary to achieve sterilization were met during the cycle being monitored.

Maintaining a sterile field

To limit airborne contamination, cover instruments with a sterile drape when they are not in use. Do not allow sharp or heavy objects to drop onto the tray where they may perforate the sterile field. Instead, they should be presented directly to the gloved person. To limit splashing that may compromise the sterile field, dispense solutions by pouring them slowly into a receptacle that is placed on the edge of the surgical tray or held by the scrub person.

All devices that enter the sterile field must be sterile or placed within a sterile barrier. Autoclavable electrocautery hand-pieces are available, but many dermatologic surgeons use non-sterile hand-pieces attached to wall units. Use disinfectant to wipe any non-sterile item to be used during surgery (such as an electrocautery hand-piece) and place it in a sterile covering, such as a proprietary sterile sheath, a Penrose drain, or a sterile surgical glove (Figs 2.6, 2.7), before use.

Surgical technique

Surgical skill does not negate the need for aseptic technique but the competence with which the tissues are handled is closely tied to the degree of contamination a wound can overcome. To assure maximum blood supply to the healing tissue, it must be handled gently with either a skin hook or toothed tissue forceps, and unnecessary tension on the wound edges during closure avoided. Hemostasis should be achieved in a manner that does not compromise blood supply, implant excessive amounts of suture, or induce unnecessary thermal damage. Electrocautery is an indispensable tool but it must be used judiciously. Excessive

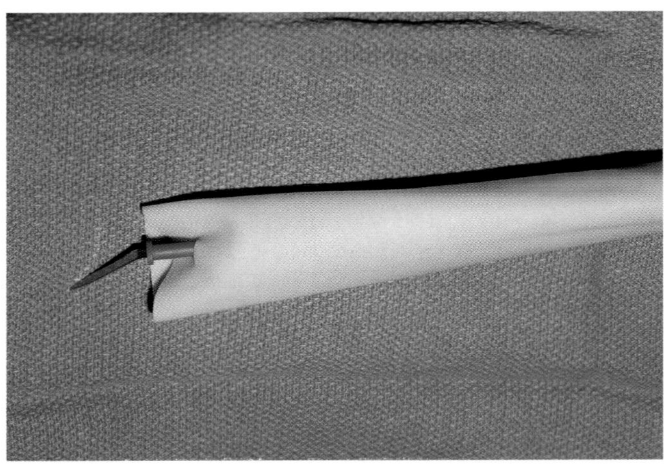

Figure 2.6 A small incision at the edge of the Penrose drain helps secure it around the sterile electrocautery tip and limits exposure of the non-sterile hand-piece.

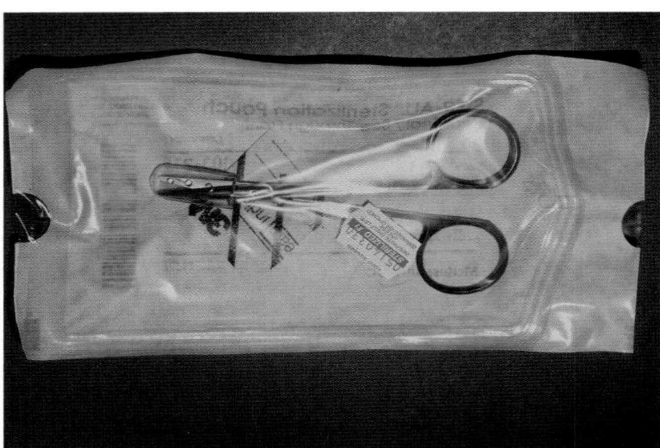

Figure 2.5 Self-sealing sterilization package that allows visualization of the contents. Note the guard placed over the delicate tips of the instrument to protect them during the sterilization process, the clearly identifiable sterilization load number, and the heat-sensitive tape.

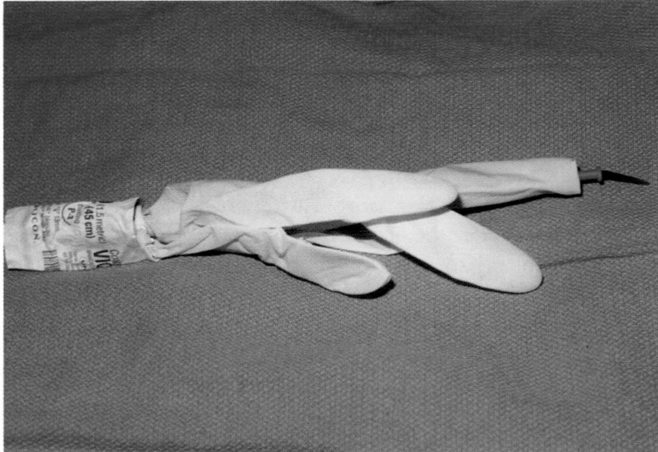

Figure 2.7 Using a sterile foil suture package around the cuff of a sterile glove helps secure it to the non-sterile electrocautery hand-piece.

thermal destruction of tissue is associated with an increased risk for infection.[43] Consider bipolar cautery, which directs current between the tips of the forceps, and produces significantly less tissue necrosis than monopolar cautery at comparable energy settings.[58] Avoid extensive thermal damage by tying off large-diameter vessels or muscular arteries. When possible, use the smallest effective monofilament suture and limit unnecessary suture, particularly braided silk, which enhances the virulence of staphylococci 10 000-fold.[59]

Wound dressings

Wound dressings are an important part of surgical site care. Ideally a bandage should be placed over the wound while the sterile field is still in place. The patient is instructed to leave the dressing undisturbed for at least 48 hours, which allows a degree of epithelialization to take place and seals the wound edges from bacterial contamination.[60] This does not apply to blood-soaked bandages, which may enhance bacterial passage. Saturated bandages should be changed promptly regardless of the timing.

PITFALLS AND THEIR MANAGEMENT

As can be seen in this discussion, the use of aseptic technique is never entirely infallible, particularly in view of the normal flora of human skin and the inability to render it completely sterile. In the postoperative period, patients should be monitored for surgical site infection and appropriate therapy should be instituted. Chapter 9 discusses antibiotic therapy in detail, and Chapters 7, 8 and 15 give further information on wound healing, dressings, and postoperative care, and drainage.

SUMMARY

Most surgical site infections are due to contamination that occurs during surgery. Common and often overlooked sources of contamination are the surgical environment, instruments, and the normal flora of the patient and surgical personnel. The key to considering any of these sources of infection is the nature of the potential pathogens—including the ease with which they are spread from one location to another and their ability to flourish in broken skin. Indeed, the discovery that preoperative shaving is associated with a greater infection rate than leaving the hair intact clearly shows how our knowledge continues to develop. As the variety and complexity of procedures performed by dermatologists expands, so will the need to adopt aseptic measures appropriate to each procedure's risk for wound infection. This will range from minimal ones, like the use of gloves and alcohol skin wipes for a shave biopsy, to full surgical dress and strict asepsis for liposuction.

REFERENCES

1. Glaser H. The road to modern surgery. New York: EP Dutton; 1962.
2. Lister J. On the antiseptic principles in the practice of surgery. Lancet 1867; 2:353–356.
3. Lister J. On the Antiseptic system of treatment upon the salubrity of a surgical hospital. Lancet 1870; 1:194–200.
4. Marples MJ. The normal microbial flora of the skin. Soc Appl Bacteriol Symp Ser 1974; 3:7–12.
5. Altemeier WA, Culbertson WR, Hummel RP. Surgical considerations of endogenous infections—sources, types, and methods of control. Surg Clin North Am 1968; 48:227–240.
6. National Nosocomial Infections Surveillance (NNIS) System Report: Data summary from January 1992 to June 2002, issued August 2002. Am J Infect Control 2002; 30:458–475.
7. Davies RR. Dispersal of bacteria on desquamated skin. Lancet 1962; 2:1295–1297.
8. Horan TC, Gaynes RP, Martone WJ, et al. CDC definitions of nosocomial surgical site infections, 1992: a modification of CDC definitions of surgical wound infections. Am J Infect Control 1992; 20:271–274.
9. Mangram AJ, Horan TC, Pearson ML, et al. Guideline for prevention of surgical site infection, 1999. Centers for Disease Control and Prevention (CDC) Hospital Infection Control Practices Advisory Committee. Am J Infect Control 1999; 27:97–132.
10. Cheng SM, Garcia M, Espin S, et al. Literature review and survey comparing surgical scrub techniques. Assoc Operat Room Nurses J 2001; 74:218;221–224.
11. Danziger Y, Pertzelan A, Mimouni M. Transient congenital hypothyroidism after topical iodine in pregnancy and lactation. Arch Dis Child 1987; 62:295–296.
12. Wade JJ, Casewell MW. The evaluation of residual antimicrobial activity on hands and its clinical relevance. J Hosp Infect 1991; 18(Suppl B):23–28.
13. Perez R, Freeman S, Sohmer H, et al. Vestibular and cochlear ototoxicity of topical antiseptics assessed by evoked potentials. Laryngoscope 2000; 110:1522–1527.
14. Larson EL. APIC guideline for handwashing and hand antisepsis in health care settings. Am J Infect Control 1995; 23:251–269.
15. Parienti JJ, Thibon P, Heller R, et al. Hand-rubbing with an aqueous alcoholic solution vs traditional surgical hand-scrubbing and 30-day surgical site infection rates: a randomized equivalence study. JAMA 2002; 288:722–727.
16. Hobson DW, Woller W, Anderson L, et al. Development and evaluation of a new alcohol-based surgical hand scrub formulation with persistent antimicrobial characteristics and brushless application. Am J Infect Control 1998; 26:507–512.
17. Boyce JM, Pittet D. Center for Disease Control Guideline for Hand Hygiene in Health-Care Settings: Recommendations of the Health-Care Infection Control Practices Advisory Committee and the HICPAC/SHEA/APIC/IDSA Hand Hygiene Task Force. MMWR 2002; 51(RR-16):1–45.
18. Deshmukh N, Kramer JW, Kjellberg SI. A comparison of 5-minute povidone-iodine scrub and 1-minute povidone-iodine scrub followed by alcohol foam. Military Med 1998; 163:145–147.
19. Herruzo-Cabrera R, Vizcaino-Alcaide MJ, Fdez-Acinero MJ Usefulness of an alcohol solution of N-duopropenide for the surgical antisepsis of the hands compared with handwashing with iodine-povidone and chlorhexidine: clinical essay. J Surg Res 2000; 94:6–12.
20. Reybrouck G. Handwashing and hand disinfection. J Hosp Infect 1986; 8:5–23.
21. Dharan S, Pittet D. Environmental controls in operating theatres. J Hosp Infect 2002; 51:79–84.
22. Hedderwick SA, McNeil SA, Lyons MJ, Kauffman CA. Pathogenic organisms associated with artificial fingernails worn by healthcare workers. Infect Control Hosp Epidemiol 2000; 21:505–509.
23. Salisbury DM, Hutfilz P, Treen LM, et al. The effect of rings on microbial load of health care workers' hands. Am J Infect Control 1997; 25:24–27.
24. Bethune DW. Dispersal of *Staphylococcus aureus* by patients and surgical staff. Lancet 1965; 1:480–483.
25. Belkin NL. Use of scrubs and related apparel in health care facilities. Am J Infect Control 1997; 25:401–404.
26. Perry C, Marshall R, Jones E. Bacterial contamination of uniforms. J Hosp Infect 2001; 48:238–241.
27. Copp G, Mailhot CB, Zalar M, et al. Covergowns and the control of operating room contamination. Nurs Res 1986; 35:263–268.
28. Mathias JM. Sacred cow survey. Use of cover gowns, shoe covers falls to new low. OR Manager 2000; 16:1;9–11;13–14;*passim*.
29. Belkin NL. The evolution of the surgical mask: filtering efficiency versus effectiveness. Infect Control Hosp Epidemiol 1997; 18:49–57.
30. Tunevall TG. Postoperative wound infections and surgical face masks: a controlled study. World J Surg 1991; 15:383–388.
31. Schweizer RT. Mask wiggling as a potential cause of wound contamination. Lancet 1976; 2:1129–1130.

32. Schiff FS. The shouting surgeon as a possible source of endophthalmitis. Ophthalmic Surg 1990; 21:438–440.
33. Doust BC, Lyon AB. Face masks in infection of the respiratory tract. J Am Med Assoc 1918; 71:1216–1219.
34. Humphreys H, Marshall RJ, Ricketts VE, et al. Theatre overshoes do not reduce operating theatre floor bacterial counts. J Hosp Infect 1991; 17:117–123.
35. Weightman NC, Banfield KR. Protective overshoes are unnecessary in a day surgery unit. J Hosp Infect 1994; 28:1–3.
36. Recommended practices for surgical attire. Assoc Operat Room Nurses J 1998; 68:1048–1052.
37. Gross DJ, Jamison Y, Martin K, et al. Surgical glove perforation in dermatologic surgery. J Dermatol Surg Oncol 1989; 15:1226–1228.
38. Tanner J, Parkinson H. Double gloving to reduce surgical cross-infection. Cochrane Database Syst Rev 2002; CD003087.
39. Dodds RD, Guy PJ, Peacock AM, et al. Surgical glove perforation. Br J Surg 1988; 75:966–968.
40. Sanzen L, Carlsson AS, Walder M. Air contamination during total hip arthroplasty in an ultraclean air enclosure using different types of staff clothing. J Arthroplast 1990; 5:127–130.
41. Woodhead K, Taylor EW, Bannister G, et al. Behaviours and rituals in the operating theatre. A report from the Hospital Infection Society Working Party on Infection Control in Operating Theatres. J Hosp Infect 2002; 51:241–255.
42. Seropian R, Reynolds BM. Wound infections after preoperative depilatory versus razor preparation. Am J Surg 1971; 121:251–254.
43. Cruse PJ, Foord R. A five-year prospective study of 23 649 surgical wounds. Arch Surg 1973; 107:206–210.
44. Hayek LJ, Emerson JM. Preoperative whole body disinfection—a controlled clinical study. J Hosp Infect 1988; 11(Suppl B):15–19.
45. Blom AW, Gozzard C, Heal J, et al. Bacterial strike-through of re-usable surgical drapes: the effect of different wetting agents. J Hosp Infect 2002; 52:52–55.
46. Ayliffe GA. Role of the environment of the operating suite in surgical wound infection. Rev Infect Dis 1991; 13 Suppl 10:S800–S804.
47. Ritter MA, Eitzen H, French ML, et al. The operating room environment as affected by people and the surgical face mask. Clin Orthop 1975; 111:147–150.
48. Recommended practices for traffic patterns in the perioperative practice setting. Association of periOperative Registered Nurses. Assoc Operat Reg Nurses AORN J 2000; 71:394–396.
49. Weber DO, Gooch JJ, Wood WR, et al. Influence of operating room surface contamination on surgical wounds: a prospective study. Arch Surg 1976; 111:484–488.
50. Sebben JE. Surgical preparation, facilities and monitoring. In: Roenigk RK, Roenigk HH, eds. Roenigk & Roenigk's Dermatologic Surgery. 2nd edn. New York: Marcel Dekker; 1996. pp. 1–24.
51. Allen KW, Humphreys H, Sims-Williams RF. Sterilization of instruments in general practice: what does it entail? Public Health 1997; 111:115–117.
52. Recommended practices for sterilization in perioperative practice settings. Association of periOperative Registered Nurses. AORN J 1999; 70:283–293.
53. Sebben JE. Survey of sterile technique used by dermatologic surgeons. J Am Acad Dermatol 1988; 18(5 Pt 1):1107–1113.
54. Simmonds WL. Sterilization. Cutis 1980; 25:78–80.
55. Rutala WA, Weber DJ. New disinfection and sterilization methods. Emerg Infect Dis 2001; 7:348–353.
56. Recommended practices for cleaning and caring for surgical instruments and powered equipment. AORN J 2002; 75:627–630, 633–636, 638 passim.
57. Recommended practices for selection and use of packaging systems. Association of Operating Room Nurses. AORN J 1996; 63:949–953.
58. Ferguson DJ. Clinical application of experimental relations between technique and wound infection. Surgery 1968; 63:377–381.
59. Edlich RF, Panek PH, Rodeheaver GT, et al. Physical and chemical configuration of sutures in the development of surgical infection. Ann Surg 1973; 177:679–688.
60. Hochberg J, Murray GF. Principles of operative surgery. Antisepsis, technique, sutures and drains. In: Sabiston Jr DC, ed. Textbook of surgery. 14th edn. Philadelphia: WB Saunders; 1991.

Appendix
Online Resources

Association of Operating Room Nurses (AORN)
Recommended Practices
http://www.aorn.org (last accessed June 2004)
http://www.findarticles.com/cf_dls/PI/index.jhtml (last accessed June 2004)

Association for Professionals in Infection Control and Epidemiology (APIC)
APIC guideline for handwashing and hand antisepsis in healthcare settings
http://www.apic.org/pdf/gdhandws.pdf (last accessed June 2004)

Canada Communicable Disease Report (CCDR)
Hand washing, cleaning, disinfection and sterilization in health care
http://www.hc-sc.gc.ca/pphb-dgspsp/publicat/ccdr-rmtc/98pdf/cdr24s8e.pdf (last accessed June 2004)

Center for Disease Control and Prevention (CDC)
http://www.cdc.gov
Guideline for prevention of surgical site infection, 1999
http://www.cdc.gov/ncidod/hip/SSI/SSI_guideline.htm (last accessed June 2004)
Guideline for hand hygiene in health care settings, 2002
http://www.cdc.gov/mmwr/preview/mmwrhtml/rr5116a1.htm (last accessed June 2004)

Food and Drug Administration (FDA)
FDA-cleared sterilants and high level disinfectants
http://www/fda.gov/cdrh/ode/germlab.html (last accessed June 2004)

National Nosocomial Infection Survey (NNIS)
http://www.cdc.gov/epo/mmwr/preview/mmwrhtml/00001772.htm (last accessed June 2004)

Occupational Safety & Health Administration (OSHA)
http://www.osha.gov (last accessed June 2004)

3 Anesthesia and Analgesia

Teresa T Soriano MD, Gary P Lask MD, and Scott M Dinehart MD

Summary box

- Most skin surgery can be performed under local anesthesia, avoiding the risks associated with general anesthesia.
- Local anesthetics reversibly interrupt propagation of nerve impulses by interfering with sodium ion influx into peripheral nerve cells.
- Topical application is particularly effective for mucosal surfaces because of their enhanced absorption.
- For other surfaces, intradermal or subcutaneous infiltration are the most commonly used techniques, the former being more immediate in onset and more prolonged, but also causing more tissue distortion and pain.
- To anesthetize a large area of skin a nerve block may be more appropriate, injecting a small amount at the major cutaneous nerve trunk that supplies the area, therefore avoiding the use of potentially toxic amounts of anesthetic.
- Choice of anesthetic and delivery method depends on the type of surgery planned and patient characteristics.
- Local adverse effects may occur, but allergic reactions are rare.
- Serious systemic adverse effects can result from inadvertent intravascular injection, excess amounts, and abnormal drug metabolism; an awareness of the effects associated with the different anesthetics is important.

INTRODUCTION

The expanding field of dermatologic surgery requires the proper selection and administration of anesthesia to maximize patient safety and comfort. Most cutaneous procedures can be optimally performed under local anesthesia. Because it reliably provides effective anesthesia and avoids the increased risks of morbidity and mortality associated with general anesthesia, local anesthesia is preferred for most cutaneous surgical procedures.

Investigations of local anesthetic agents similar to ones used today began in the late 19th century. In 1860, Neiman isolated cocaine from the shrub of *Erythroxylon coca* and noted its numbing effect on the tongue.[1] In 1880, Von Anrep recognized cocaine's anesthetic properties after injecting it into animals and into his own arm.[1] In 1884, Koller, influenced by Sigmund Freud, introduced cocaine into the clinical arena when he used cocaine as a local anesthetic during surgery for a patient with glaucoma.[1] Soon thereafter, Hall and Halsted performed the first peripheral nerve block using cocaine.[1] However, as the use of cocaine for local anesthesia expanded, reports of its potential toxicity and addictive effects also emerged.[1]

Further developments aiming for safer local anesthetics occurred during the past century. In 1904, Alfred Einhorn synthesized procaine, an ester of para-aminobenzoic acid (PABA).[1] In 1905, Braun reported the successful use of procaine with epinephrine (adrenaline) for local anesthesia.[1] In 1930, a more potent PABA ester, tetracaine was introduced.[2] Although both had utility as anesthetics, they had the tendency to produce allergic reactions. In 1943, Lofgren and Lundqvist synthesized lidocaine, an amide derivative of diethlyaminoacetic acid.[2] Its superior safety and efficacy has led to its widespread use, and lidocaine has become the prototype of local anesthetics. Subsequently, other amide derivatives have been developed.

Several local anesthetics with various methods of delivery are now available for cutaneous surgery. Appropriate, safe, and effective use of these compounds depends on understanding the pharmacological properties, different applications, and proper technique of administration. Proper use of local anesthesia maximizes patient safety, minimizes pain, and allows for the ease of surgical procedures.

Structure and physiology of anesthetics

Most local anesthetic agents have similar chemical structures, consisting of three components: an aromatic portion, an intermediate chain, and an amine portion (Fig. 3.1). Modifications of any of these components can affect the pharmacological properties of the anesthetic agent. The

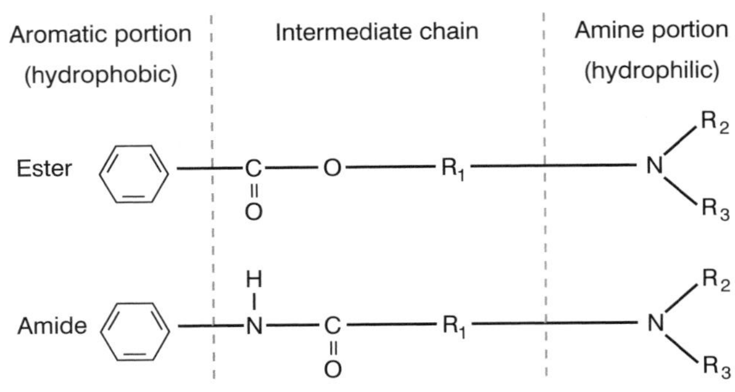

Figure 3.1 Basic structures of ester and amide type local anesthetics.

Table 3.1 Local anesthetics

Type	Generic name	Some trade names
Esters	Procaine	Novocain
	Tetracaine	Pontocaine
	Benzocaine	Hurricane
	Chloroprocaine	Nesacaine
	Cocaine	(None)
Amides	Lidocaine	Xylocaine
	Bupivacaine	Marcaine
	Mepivacaine	Carbocaine
	Prilocaine	Citanest
	Etidocaine	Duranest
	Ropivacaine	Naropin
	Levobupivacaine	Chirocaine

aromatic end provides most of the lipophilic properties of the compound. It facilitates the diffusion of the anesthetic through membranes, which correlates to the potency of the anesthetic.[3] The hydrophilic end, usually consisting of a tertiary amine, is involved in binding within the sodium channel.[4] An intermediate chain, consisting of either an ester or amide, links these two domains. An intermediate chain length between 3 and 7 carbon-equivalents is necessary for local anesthetic activity.[4] Disruption of this chain initiates the drug's metabolism and allows for the reversible nature of the anesthetic.[4]

The differences in the intermediate chain linkage (ester versus amide) classifies local anesthetics into two groups (Table 3.1). They differ in their metabolism and potential for sensitization.[5] Ester-type compounds tend to have a shorter duration of action because they are rapidly hydrolyzed by plasma pseudocholinesterases to form metabolites excreted by the kidneys.[5] Individuals with atypical forms of pseudocholinesterase may be prone to the toxic effects of these agents.[5] PABA is a major metabolic product and is responsible for the higher incidence of allergies with ester-type anesthetics.[6] Amide derivatives are not readily hydrolyzed. They are metabolized by microsomal enzymes in the liver, and excreted by the kidneys.[5] Individuals with compromised liver function are more susceptible to the toxic effects of amide anesthetics.[7]

The pharmacological properties of common ester and amide anesthetics are outlined in Tables 3.2 and 3.3. The molecular structure and dissociation constant (pKa) of local anesthetics affect their potency and toxicity.[8] Changes in the molecule's structure affect lipid solubility and protein binding. In general, lipid solubility determines the potency of the agent while protein binding dictates its duration of action.[8] For example, the addition of a 4-carbon group to procaine creates tetracaine, which is more lipid soluble and potent. Highly protein-bound agents, such as bupivacaine, are tightly associated with the neural membrane, leading to a longer duration of action.[4] The pKa influences the onset of action of local anesthetics.[8] For the most part, the shorter-acting anesthetics tend to have a faster onset of action and less toxicity. However, peak plasma concentrations depend on various factors including the concentration of anesthesia, the duration of infiltration, the site of injection and the rate of metabolism of the agent.[9]

The pKa of local anesthetics and the hydrogen ion concentration (pH) of the solution and tissue influence the pharmacologic activity of local anesthetics.[4] Local anesthetics are weak bases, with a pKa between 7.7 and 9.1. They are usually prepared as solutions of hydrochloride salts with a pH of 5.0–6.0 to enhance their solubility and stability.[4] In tissue, they exist as an uncharged base or as a cation, with their relative proportions determined by the pKa of the anesthetic and the pH of solution.[8] The nonionized base form can readily diffuse across lipid nerve sheaths and cell membranes while the ionized form can diffuse through the extracellular space and intracellular cytoplasm.[8] In general, a lower pKa correlates to a higher concentration of base and a faster onset of action.[4] Alkalinization of the anesthetic solution increases the amount of base and the anesthetic's onset of action.[10] In addition, the pH of the tissue can also affect the action of local anesthetics. Infected tissues tend to be acidic and impair the effectiveness of local anesthetics.[11]

Local anesthetics can cross the placenta by passive diffusion; however, they are generally safe to use during pregnancy.[12] Studies have shown no maternal or teratogenic effects from the administration of lidocaine during the first trimester of pregnancy.[13] Lidocaine, etidocaine, and prilocaine are labeled pregnancy category B. Because of the potential of causing fetal bradycardia, bupivacaine and mepivacaine are labeled category C.[13] Local anesthetics can be excreted in breast milk and result in toxicity to the infant if a large amount of anesthetic is used.[13]

Mechanism of action

Local anesthetics act by reversibly interrupting the propagation of impulses and blocking nerve conduction.[8] In the resting state, the electric potential is negative intracellularly relative to the extracellular space as a result of the ionic gradient of sodium and potassium ions. This gradient is maintained by the cellular membrane, which allows free movement of potassium, and by Na^+/K^+ adenosine triphosphatase (ATPase) pumps. During conduction of an impulse, sodium channels open and allow sodium ions to move across the membrane and generate an impulse or action potential. By interfering with the influx of

Table 3.2 Ester local anesthetics

Anesthetic	Onset (min)	pKa	Duration (min)		Maximal recommended dose (mg/kg) for adults	
			Without epinephrine (adrenaline)	With epinephrine (adrenaline)	Without epinephrine (adrenaline)	With epinephrine (adrenaline)
Procaine	5	8.9	15–30	30–90	10	14
Chloroprocaine	5–6	9.0	30–60	N/A	10	N/A
Tetracaine	7	8.6	120–240	240–480	2	2

See Table 3.11 for pediatric dosage.

Table 3.3 Amide local anesthetics

Anesthetic	Onset (min)	pKa	Duration (min)		Maximal recommended dose (mg/kg) for adults	
			Without epinephrine (adrenaline)	With epinephrine (adrenaline)	Without epinephrine (adrenaline)	With epinephrine (adrenaline)
Lidocaine	<1	7.7	30–120	60–400	5	7
Bupivacaine	2–10	8.1	120–240	240–480	2.5	3
Mepivacaine	3–20	7.6	30–120	60–400	6	8
Prilocaine	5–6	7.7	30–120	60–400	7	10
Etidocaine	3–5	7.7	200	240–360	4.5	6.5
Ropivacaine	1–15	8.2	120–360	Not yet defined	3.5	Not yet defined
Levobupivacaine	2–10	8.1	120–240	Not yet defined	2.1	Not yet defined

See Table 3.11 for pediatric dosage.

sodium ions into the cells, local anesthetics prevent the depolarization of peripheral nerves and subsequent nerve conduction.[8] The exact mechanism of action by which local anesthetics interfere with the movement of sodium ions is unclear. One postulated mechanism involves the local anesthetic binding to receptors in sodium channels and when enough sodium channels within an axon are blocked, conduction is interrupted.[14] The binding site of local anesthetics may be at the channel's pore or within the protein subunits with the channel.[15,16]

Nerve fibers are divided into three main categories (Table 3.4):[6] A, B, and C fibers. A and B fibers are myelinated and C fibers are unmyelinated. The A fibers are the largest and are subdivided into four types: alpha, beta, gamma, and delta. The A-alpha fibers conduct motor impulses whereas A-beta fibers primarily conduct light touch and pressure. A-gamma fibers are responsible for joint proprioception. The A-delta fibers, which are the smallest of the A type fibers, conduct pain and temperature. The B fibers are preganglionic sympathetic fibers. The C type fibers are the smallest and like the A-delta fibers, conduct pain and temperature. In general, smaller myelinated fibers are easier to block than larger myelinated fibers; therefore, pain and temperature sensation may be eliminated before the loss of vibration and pressure.[6] This translates clinically as locally anesthetized patients may not feel pain and temperature, but still feel a pressure sensation during a procedure.[6]

Additions to local anesthetics

Substances are frequently added to local anesthetics to augment analgesia and enhance the ease and safety of the surgery (Table 3.5). Some of these products are commercially available premixed by the manufacturer.

Vasoconstrictors

Most local anesthetics, except for cocaine, promote vasodilatation by relaxation of vascular smooth muscle. This results in increased bleeding at the operative site and increased diffusion of anesthetics away from the site of injection. Vasoconstrictors are commonly added to local anesthetics to decrease bleeding and thereby, facilitate the ease of surgery. In addition, they retard the absorption of anesthetics, which in turn, minimizes the amount of drug injected and decreases systemic toxicity. By localizing the drug to the field injected, vasoconstrictors also prolong the duration of the anesthesia. This added benefit does not seem to hold true for more lipid-soluble, long-acting agents such as bupivacaine and ropivacaine, which are already highly tissue-bound.[8]

Epinephrine (adrenaline) is the most common vasoconstrictor added to local anesthetics to enhance efficacy. Although the anesthetic may have an immediate onset of action, full vasoconstriction with epinephrine typically requires 7–15 minutes.[6] Epinephrine is commercially

Table 3.4 Types and properties of nerve fibers

Type of nerve fiber	Myelinated	Property/innervation
A alpha	Yes	Motor
beta	Yes	Light touch and pressure
gamma	Yes	Proprioception
delta	Yes	Pain and temperature
B	Yes	Preganglionic sympathetic fibers
C	No	Pain and temperature

With permission from Grekin RC, Auletta MJ. Local anesthesia in dermatologic surgery. J Am Acad Dermatol 1988; 19:599–614.[6]

Table 3.5 Additives to local anesthetics

Additive	Dosage	Purpose
Epinephrine (adrenaline)	1 : 100 000 or less	To decrease bleeding, prolong anesthesia, reduce anesthetic toxicity
Hyaluronidase	150 units added to every 30 mL of anesthetic	To facilitate drug diffusion, decrease tissue distortion with infiltration
Sodium bicarbonate (8.5%)	1 mL (1 mEq/mL) for every 10 mL of 1% lidocaine with epinephrine (adrenaline)	To decrease pain with infiltration of acidic solution

available premixed at concentrations of 1 : 100 000 and 1 : 200 000 with lidocaine. The optimal dose of epinephrine has been debated.[17,18] However, for dermatologic surgery concentrations greater than 1 : 200 000 are probably not necessary and concentrations greater than 1 : 100 000 are associated with an increased risk for side-effects.[19] The maximum dose of epinephrine for local anesthesia injected in healthy individuals should generally not exceed 1 mg (100 mL of 1 : 100 000 solution).[6]

Epinephrine (adrenaline) is labeled pregnancy category C. Concerns about the safety of use during pregnancy were raised when epinephrine was shown to reduce uterine blood flow in experimental animals.[12] Decreased placental perfusion can theoretically interfere with fetal organogenesis particularly in the first trimester. Later in the pregnancy, decreased uterine blood flow by epinephrine absorption may induce premature labor. Given these potential risks, it is prudent to postpone non-urgent procedures requiring the use of epinephrine until after pregnancy. Some have advocated the use of dilute concentrations (e.g. 1 : 300 000) of epinephrine in necessary procedures during pregnancy.[20]

To prevent the degradation of epinephrine in an alkaline pH, commercially prepared lidocaine with epinephrine contains acidic preservatives, such as sodium metabisulfite and citric acid.[21] The resulting acidic solution tends to cause more pain on injection.[22] Freshly mixed solutions of lidocaine with epinephrine results in a less acidic solution; therefore, less discomfort with injection.[21] Freshly prepared anesthetic solution having a 1 : 100 000 concentration of epinephrine can be made by adding 0.5 mL of 1 : 1 000 epinephrine to 50 mL of lidocaine. Adding half as much epinephrine in this mix would give a concentration of 1 : 200 000 epinephrine.

Sodium bicarbonate

The addition of sodium bicarbonate to commercially available lidocaine with epinephrine reduces the pain on infiltration.[23] The pH of lidocaine is around 5.0 to 7.0. However, the addition of acidic preservatives lowers the pH of commercially prepared epinephrine and lidocaine solutions to around 3.3–5.5, so causing more discomfort with injection. Buffering with 8.4% sodium bicarbonate in a ratio of 1 sodium bicarbonate to 10 epinephrine 1 : 100 000 or 1 sodium bicarbonate to 15 epinephrine 1 : 200 000 increases the pH, bringing it closer to physiologic pH, and reduces pain.[24]

Adjusting the pH of the solution can affect other pharmacologic properties of these agents. Epinephrine is chemically unstable in anesthetic solutions alkalinized by sodium bicarbonate. Neutralizing lidocaine and bupivicaine solutions containing epinephrine with bicarbonate decreases the activity of epinephrine over 24 hours.[25] In addition, alkalinization of local anesthetics allows for increased amounts of uncharged, lipid-soluble base, which more readily crosses the nerve membrane, leading to a faster onset of action. Clinically, alkalinization of mepivacaine and lidocaine for use in peripheral nerve blocks leads to more rapid nerve blockade.[4]

Hyaluronidase

Hyaluronidase is an enzyme that depolymerizes hyaluronic acid, one of the acid mucopolysaccharides present in intercellular ground substance. It is typically prepared in 150 unit vials. Its addition to local anesthetics facilitates diffusion of injectable solutions through tissue planes, thereby, increasing the area of anesthesia and minimizing tissue distortion by fluid infiltration.[26] It facilitates undermining in the subcutaneous plane by hydrodissection of fatty tissue.[27] Clinically, hyaluronidase may be a useful adjunct in surgery in the periorbital region to minimize the number of anesthetic injection sites and potential ecchymosis. It may also be helpful in harvesting split-thickness skin grafts when wider areas of local anesthesia can be attained with minimal loss of anatomic contour.[28] Uniform dosage recommendations for cutaneous surgery are not available, but 150 units in 20–30 mL of anesthetic have been used.[27]

Hyaluronidase has disadvantages that limit its use in cutaneous surgery. It decreases the duration of anesthesia and potentially increases the risk of anesthetic toxicity as a result of increased absorption.[27,29] Hyaluronidase contains the preservative thimerosal, which is a contact allergen.[28] Because rare allergic reactions have been reported, preoperative skin testing has been recommended.[27] Hyaluronidase is not recommended for tumescent liposuction because it does not augment the degree of anesthesia with the tumescent technique and increases the rate of absorption of lidocaine, and therefore the potential for systemic toxicity.[29]

Other anesthetics

Different local anesthetics are sometimes mixed together to capitalize on the useful properties of each drug. For example, a longer-acting anesthetic with a delayed onset of action, such as bupivacaine, can be mixed with a quicker-onset anesthetic, such as lidocaine.[28] A study that evaluated the efficacy of such a mixed solution found no difference in onset or duration of action than with bupivicaine alone.[30] To date, it has not been shown that mixing anesthetics with different properties together confers an advantage over using either one alone. Although premixing anesthetics may not be advantageous, the addition of a longer-acting anesthetic into an operative site previously anesthetized with a shorter-acting anesthetic may provide more optimal anesthesia when a prolonged procedure is anticipated.[28]

■ TECHNIQUES

Topical anesthesia

Topical application of anesthesia has been particularly effective on mucosal surfaces, but caution must be taken regarding increased systemic absorption leading to toxicity. Some products are particularly formulated for application on mucosal surfaces (Table 3.6). The stratum corneum presents the major barrier to the delivery of topical anesthesia on intact skin.[31] The development of novel delivery systems has allowed for increased penetration and greater efficacy of newer topical agents.[32]

Cryoanesthesia

Applying cold agents to the skin can be useful in reducing the pain associated with minor surgical procedures. The placement of ice cubes on the skin is a rapid, inexpensive, and easy method to minimize the discomfort during needle injections.[33]

Topical freezing agents or vapocoolants rapidly cool the skin and provide enough anesthesia for injections or brief superficial surgical procedures. Held 10–30 cm (4–12 in.) from the skin, the refrigerant is sprayed toward the lesion just until the area turns white. Various topical freezing agents are available (Table 3.7)[34] Care should be taken to protect the eyes and avoid inhalation of vapor when using these agents. Cryoanesthesia has the potential risks of causing pigmentary alterations and scarring. In addition, some vapocoolants, such as ethyl chloride, are flammable.[34,35] The concern about the potential harmful effects of the vapocoolants to the ozone layer led to the ban of production of hard chlorofluorocarbons in 1996, and the development of more ozone-safe hydrofluorocarbons.[34,35]

Various cooling methods to the skin are used with several laser procedures. These include the application of a cooled gel, a cold glass window, and other contact cooling devices to the skin being treated. The delivery of refrigerated air onto the skin has also been used. Some laser devices are equipped with dichlorodifluoromethane and tetrafluoroethane cryogen sprays that deliver transient cooling to the epidermis.[35] These cooling methods provide some anesthesia and protect against laser-induced epidermal thermal injury.

Cocaine

Cocaine (see Table 3.6) is an ester anesthetic that, unlike other local anesthetics, possesses vasoconstrictive properties. Available as a 4% and 10% solution, it is primarily used for intranasal surgery.[36] Anesthesia occurs within 5 minutes of application and lasts up to 30 minutes. The maximum recommended dose is 200 mg/kg. Potential toxicity, including hypertension, tachycardia, and arrhythmias, can result from blocking the reuptake of norepinephrine (noradrenaline). In addition, decreased coronary blood flow can occur, leading to myocardial infarction.[36] Dopamine reuptake blockade results in central nervous system stimulation.[36] The risks of adverse events and the potential for abuse limits cocaine's anesthetic use over safer alternative agents.

Benzocaine

Benzocaine (see Table 3.6) is a topical ester anesthetic available as an aerosol spray, gel, ointment or solution ranging from 5–20%. It is commonly used for achieving rapid anesthesia on mucosal surfaces. Although topical benzocaine can cause contact sensitization, it is still widely used. The 20% gel known as Hurricane gel applied with a dry gauze for 30–60 seconds or Hurricane aerosol spray for less than 2 seconds achieves anesthesia within 15–30 seconds.[37] The anesthetic effect lasts for about 12–15 minutes. Available as a spray and liquid, cetacaine is a mixture of 14 % benzocaine, 2 % butyl aminobenzoate, and 2% tetracaine hydrochloride that produces rapid mucosal anesthesia that lasts for approximately 30–60 minutes.[36] Benzocaine-containing preparations should be avoided in infants because of the risk of methemoglobinemia.[39]

Table 3.6 Common topical anesthetics formulated for mucosal surfaces

Anesthetic	Trade Name	Concentration (%)	Vehicle	Onset of action	Duration of action	Clinical use
Cocaine		4, 10	Solution	1–5 minutes	30–60 minutes	Intranasal
Lidocaine	Xylocaine	2–5	Gel, ointment, topical and viscous solution	1–2 minutes	15–20 minutes	Oral mucosa
Benzocaine	Hurricane	20	Liquid, gel, spray	<5 minutes	15–45 minutes	Oral mucosa
Benzocaine combination	Cetacaine	*	Spray, liquid	30 seconds	30–60 minutes	Oral mucosa
Proparacaine	Alcaine	0.5	Solution	20 seconds	15–20 minutes	Ophthalmic
Tetracaine	Pontocaine	0.5	Solution	20 seconds	12–20 minutes	Ophthalmic

**Cetacaine contains 14% benzocaine, 2% tetracaine and 2% butyl aminobenzoate*

Table 3.7 Examples of vapocoolants used for cutaneous local anesthesia

Vapocoolant	Ingredients
Ethyl chloride*,† (Gebauer Company, Cleveland, OH)	50% dichlorodifluoromethane, 50% trichloromonofluoromethane
Instant Cold Spray† (HL Moore, New Britain, CT)	10% isopentane, 90% butane
Fluoro Ethyl‡ (Gebauer Company, Cleveland, OH)	75% dichlorotetrafluoroethane, 25% ethyl chloride
Fluori-Methane‡ (Gebauer Company, Cleveland, OH)	15% dichlorodifluoromethane, 85% trichloromonofluoromethane
Frigiderm‡ (Delasco, Council Bluffs, IA)	dichlorotetrafluoroethane

**Flammable; †ozone-safe; ‡manufacture discontinued, but still available. With permission from Plotkin S. Clinical comparison of preinjection anesthetics. J Am Podiatr Med Assoc 1998; 88:73–9.*[33]

Table 3.8 Common topical anesthetics useful for cutaneous surfaces

Anesthetic	Ingredients	Vehicle	Onset of action (min)
EMLA*	2.5% lidocaine with 2.5% prilocaine	Oil in water	60–120
ELA-Max (now LMX 4)*,†	4% lidocaine	Liposomal	30–60
ELA-Max 5 (now LMX 5)*,†	5% lidocaine	Liposomal	30–60
Topicaine*,†	4% lidocaine	Microemulsion	30–60
Tetracaine§	4% tetracaine	Lecithin gel	60–90
Betacaine-LA§	Lidocaine, prilocaine, dibucaine	Vaseline ointment	60–90

**FDA approved; †over-the-counter product; §compounded anesthetic*

Lidocaine

Lidocaine, available in a 2–5% gel and topical and viscous solutions, has been used reliably for topical anesthesia on mucosal surfaces. However, these compounds are formulated in conventional vehicles that often do not provide adequate and consistent anesthesia for intact skin surfaces. A lidocaine 5% patch is available that is marketed primarily for postherpetic neuralgia. Over the past 40 years, mixtures of higher concentrations of lidocaine have been specially compounded to achieve topical anesthesia for minor surgical procedures.[37] Topical preparations of 30% lidocaine prepared using Acid Mantle (Doak Pharmacal Co Inc, Westbury, NY) or Velvachol (Novartis, East Hanover, NJ) as a vehicle result in hydrophilic mixtures that hydrate the stratum corneum and facilitate penetration of lidocaine through the stratum corneum.[37] Over the past decade, topical anesthetics in more sophisticated vehicles have become commercially available that allow for better efficacy in reducing pain during superficial cutaneous surgery (Table 3.8).

EMLA

A widely used agent over the past decade, EMLA (a eutectic mixture of local anesthesia) cream, is a 5% eutectic mixture composed of 2.5 mg/mL of lidocaine and 2.5 mg/mL of prilocaine in an oil-in-water emulsion cream. A eutectic mixture is a formulation that melts at a lower temperature than any of its individual components. EMLA's formulation contains emulsifiers that enhance skin penetration and increase the anesthetic concentration to 80% in the oil droplets while maintaining a low overall concentration of 5%, thereby minimizing the risk of systemic toxicity.[37] Several clinical trials have shown its efficacy in alleviating pain during various dermatologic procedures, including laser surgery, chemical peels, harvesting split-thickness skin grafts, skin biopsies, and curettage and electrosurgery.[32,37]

EMLA is available as a cream and a patch. It was temporarily pulled from retail pharmacies, but has since been reintroduced. It has a redesigned child-resistant closure that complies with the Poison Prevention Packaging Act issued by the US Consumer Product Safety Commission requiring products containing over 5 mg of lidocaine in a single package to be child resistant. EMLA is available as a 30 g tube in retail pharmacies and a 5 g tube in the hospital setting for inpatient use. EMLA is also packaged as an anesthetic disc, which contains 1 g of EMLA emulsion, with an active contact surface area approximately 10 cm^2. Generally, a 60-minute application period under an occlusive dressing—Tegaderm (3M Healthcare, St Paul, MN), Saran Wrap (Dow Chemical Company, Midland, Michigan)—before the procedure is necessary to achieve effective anesthesia; however, this may vary depending on the location of the treatment. Effective anesthesia after 25 minutes of EMLA application to the face, and after 5–15 minutes on mucosal surfaces has been reported.[32] Increased duration of application over 2 hours has been shown to correspond to enhanced depth of analgesia. The depth of analgesia after 60 minutes is 3.0 mm and after 120 minutes, 5.0 mm.[37] Because of the risk of methemoglobinemia associated with prilocaine, EMLA should be used with caution in infants.[40] Alkaline injury to the cornea has been seen with EMLA, so the use of EMLA close to the eyes should be avoided.[41]

LMX

LMX (Ferndale, Michigan; originally named ELA-Max) is a more recently developed topical anesthetic containing lidocaine encapsulated in a liposomal delivery system and is available without a prescription. The liposomal vehicle facilitates penetration and provides sustained release of the anesthetic. In addition, liposomes may enhance the anesthetic's duration of action by protecting it from metabolic breakdown.[32] LMX 5% is labeled as an anorectal cream indicated for the temporary relief of local discomfort associated with anorectal disorders. It tends to have a faster onset of action; a 30-minute application time before the procedure is recommended. In studies comparing EMLA and LMX 5% used for dermatologic procedures, both were effective in reducing pain; however, LMX 5% had a longer duration of action.[42] Its has been used, without the need for occlusion, to decrease pain induced during medium-depth chemical peels and laser hair removal.[43,44] Its use on mucosal or conjunctival surfaces is not recommended because of the risk of increased absorption and the potential for irritation of the cornea.[37] In a child weighing less than 20 kg, a single application of LMX should be limited to an area of less than100 cm^2.[32]

Topicaine

Topicaine contains 4% lidocaine in a gel microemulsion vehicle. Released in 1997, it is an over-the-counter product approved for pain relief of intact skin.[32] The recommended application time is 30–60 minutes under occlusion. One study demonstrated its effectiveness in providing anesthesia for laser treatment after 30 minutes of application.[45]

Tetracaine

Tetracaine, a long-acting ester anesthetic, is available in a 0.5% solution and is used most commonly for ophthalmic procedures. It can provide anesthesia to the mucous membranes for up to 45 minutes. A formulation of 0.5% tetracaine, 0.05% epinephrine (adrenaline) 1 : 2000, and 11.8% cocaine in normal saline—termed TAC—has been compounded by pharmacists for over 20 years for anesthesia and vasoconstriction before repairing superficial lacerations, especially in children.[37] Its limited absorption on intact skin limits its utility for other cutaneous procedures. One study found EMLA cream to be superior to TAC solution for anesthesia of lacerations on the extremities.[46]

Concern over the potential systemic absorption of cocaine led to the substitution of 4% lidocaine for cocaine (LAT formulations).[37] More recently, tetracaine 4% gel in a lecithin gel base has been introduced, though studies are still needed regarding its efficacy and safety compared to other available compounds.[32] One study showed its effectiveness in reducing laser-induced pain after a 60-minute occlusion period.[45]

Amethocaine 4% gel, a preparation with 4% tetracaine, currently not approved for use in the US, is marketed in Europe as a topical anesthetic that provides more rapid and longer duration of action than EMLA and can be safely used in children and adults.[32] A study comparing 4% amethocaine and EMLA for pain relief during pulsed dye laser treatments found amethocaine superior to EMLA.[47] Adverse events tend to be transient and include erythema, edema, and pruritus.[32]

Other topical agents

Other mixed formulations have been reported to provide effective topical anesthesia, but further studies are required to determine their clinical benefits over available agents. Betacaine-LA (Medical Center Pharmacy, Tampa, FL) ointment is a specially compounded formulation that contains lidocaine, prilocaine, dibucaine, and a vasoconstrictor.[32] It is not FDA approved and is only available from the manufacturer by a doctor's request. Novel formulations of lidocaine and tetracaine are currently undergoing clinical trials. The S-Caine patch (Ferndale, Michigan) contains a 1 : 1 eutectic mixture of lidocaine and tetracaine coupled with a disposable, oxygen-activated heating element. The drug delivery system aims at utilizing controlled heating to facilitate the anesthetic delivery into the dermis.[32] Similarly, containing a eutectic lidocaine/tetracaine mixture, the S-Caine peel (Johnson and Johnson) is a cream that dries upon exposure to air to form a flexible film that can be easily removed. The S-Caine peel, applied to the face for 20–30 minutes, has been shown to provide rapid, safe, and effective anesthesia for pulsed dye laser treatments on the face.[48] In this study, side-effects were limited to minimal erythema; no edema or skin blanching was reported.

Iontophoresis

Iontophoresis has been used as a method of delivering solutions of lidocaine with epinephrine (adrenaline) into the skin without the pain of needle injections. With this system, an electrical current draws ionically charged drugs into the skin. The dose is dependent on the total electric charge delivered. It has been found useful for cutaneous procedures especially in the pediatric population.[49] A study comparing iontophoresis of lidocaine with EMLA found iontophoresis to be more effective in achieving anesthesia.[50] Disadvantages of iontophoresis include additional equipment and learning curve, difficulty in application to certain regional areas, and limited depths of penetration of the anesthetic.[49,50]

Ophthalmic

Ophthalmic solutions provide safe and effective topical anesthesia to the mucous membranes of the sclera and the conjunctiva. They are often useful when placing corneal eyeshields before periocular surgery and laser procedures. Common topical eye preparations include proparacaine 0.5%, tetracaine 0.5%, and benoxinate 0.25%. Rapid absorption and onset of anesthesia occurs within 30 seconds after placement of one to two drops of anesthesia into the conjunctival sac.[37] A stinging sensation may be felt upon instillation of the anesthetic drops. The anesthetic affect usually lasts 15 minutes or longer. An eyepatch should be placed until the anesthesia resolves to prevent inadvertent trauma to the cornea.[37] One study[51] showed that tetracaine eye drops cause more pain than proparacaine eye drops, and proparacaine provided slightly longer duration of anesthesia than tetracaine (10.7 vs 9.2 minutes). For procedures requiring prolonged anesthesia, instillation of one drop of proparacaine every 10 minutes for 5–7 doses may be used.

Infiltrative techniques

Local infiltration

Local infiltration of anesthesia that involves the injection of the anesthetic into the surgical site is the most commonly used technique in cutaneous surgery. This is administered either intradermally and/or subcutaneously. Intradermal injection results in an immediate onset and prolonged duration of anesthesia compared to deeper injections. However, it tends to cause more tissue distortion and pain. Subcutaneous injection of anesthetics produces less tissue distortion and pain, but has slower onset and duration as a result of diffusion and increased absorption.

Various techniques can diminish the pain and make local infiltration of anesthesia better tolerated (see Optimizing Outcomes).[50] Providing a calm and comfortable environment with the patient reclining and reassuring the patient can diminish fear and anxiety as well as the perception of pain. Patients often feel a 'stick' and 'burning' sensation associated with the entry of the needle into the skin and the infiltration of the anesthesia. The use of small-diameter needles, such as the 30-gauge needles commonly used in cutaneous surgery, minimizes the pain associated with the initial puncture of the skin.[20] The application of topical anesthetics, ice, or other cooling devices before the initial injection may be helpful for children and extremely anxious individuals.[33] Warming lidocaine to body temperature may also help attenuate the pain with infiltration.[39] Providing counter-irritation by pinching the skin around the needle entry point can diffuse the pain stimulus.[20] As multiple needle punctures can be painful, re-entering at previously anesthetized areas can further reduce discomfort, especially when working on larger areas.

Tissue distension with infiltration of the anesthetic produces pain. Injecting slowly and using only the volume necessary to achieve adequate anesthesia can attenuate the pain associated with tissue distension.[20] The use of smaller-diameter needles also lends to a decreased rate of infiltration with slow tissue distension and less pain. More recently, computer-controlled injection devices such as the Wand (Milestone Scientific) have been developed that control the rate of injection, and limit patient discomfort.[52] In addition, various needle-free devices have been investigated.[53] These systems have been marketed primarily for dentistry, and their practical utility in decreasing pain during various cutaneous procedures is yet to be determined.

Field block

Field or ring-block involves the placement of anesthesia circumferentially around the operative site (Fig. 3.2). It is useful when direct infiltration into the surgical field is undesirable. Examples include cyst excisions because injection directly into the cyst can lead to rupture of cystic contents, and working with inflamed or infected tissue when local infiltration may not produce as effective anesthesia in an acidic environment.[5] This technique can also minimize the total amount of anesthetic required, which is beneficial for procedures involving larger areas that would usually require more anesthesia via local infiltration.[20] To obtain optimal anesthesia using ring blocks, the anesthetic should be injected into the superficial and deep planes.[20]

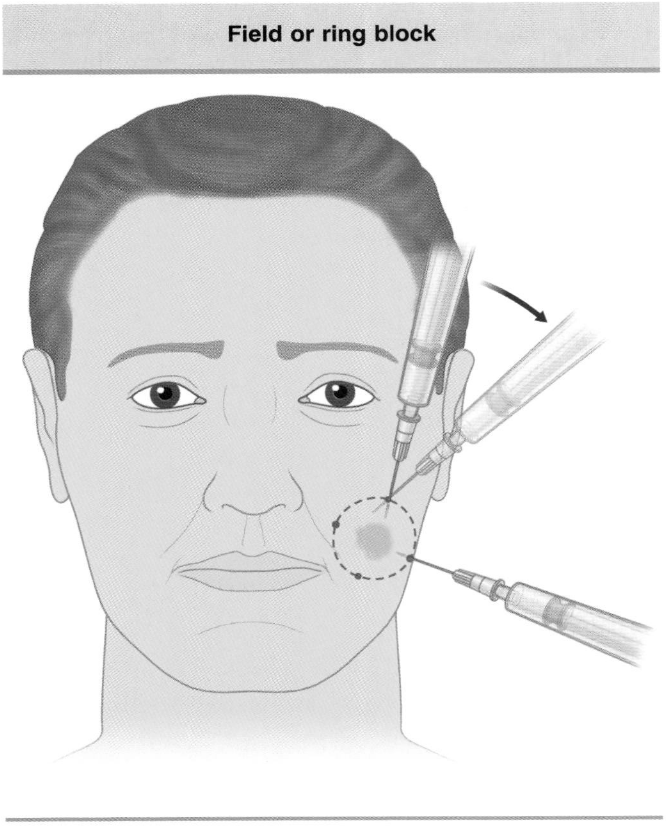

Field or ring block

Figure 3.2 Field or ring block. Anesthetic is injected circumferentially around the surgical site. This approach is useful on any part of the body, especially where a regional nerve block is not an option, and to treat larger areas.

Tumescent anesthesia

The tumescent technique involves the delivery of large volumes of dilute anesthesia (usually 0.05–0.1% lidocaine with 1 : 1 000 000 epinephrine (adrenaline)) into subcutaneous fat until the tissue distends. It has been widely used for liposuction, hence the name tumescent liposuction, in which as much or more dilute anesthesia is administered as fat is removed (see Chapter 32). The anesthetic is typically delivered through 0.5–1.5-mm multiport infiltration cannulas or 18–20-gauge blunt-tipped spinal needles. To administer the large volumes typically necessary for liposuction, special pumping devices aid infiltration.

Although the basic tumescent solution described by Klein contains 0.05% lidocaine, the concentrations of lidocaine and epinephrine can be tailored, depending on the site and nature of the procedure (Table 3.9)[54] The safe upper limit of lidocaine dosage with this technique is estimated to be 55 mg/kg.[55] Warming of the tumescent solution before infiltration to 104 °F (40 °C) and slowing the rate of infiltration have been shown to reduce pain in liposuction patients.[56] The tumescent technique allows procedures to be performed safely with minimal blood loss without the risks of general anesthesia and its prolonged duration of action provides postoperative analgesia.[57,58]

Although best known for use during liposuction (see Chapter 32), the tumescent technique is helpful whenever large areas are to be treated to obtain adequate and safe anesthesia. Examples are endovenous ablation with lasers or radiofrequency devices, ambulatory phlebectomy, and face-lifting.

Nerve blocks

Knowledge of the anatomic distribution of sensory nerves of the head, neck, and hands and feet enables one to anesthetize large areas of skin using a small amount of anesthesia using a nerve block. Injecting at the point of major cutaneous nerve trunks, this method of anesthesia is efficient when dealing with wider anatomic areas where

Table 3.9 Klein's basic tumescent anesthetic solution

Component	Final concentration	Amount added to one liter normal saline
Lidocaine	500 mg/L	50 mL of 1% lidocaine
Epinephrine (adrenaline)	0.5 mg/L	0.5 mL of 1 : 1 000 000 epinephrine (adrenaline)
Sodium bicarbonate	10 mEq/L	10 mL of 8.5% sodium bicarbonate

With permission from Klein, JA. Anesthetic formulation of tumescent solutions. Dermatol Clinics 1999; 17:751–759.[54]

larger amounts of anesthesia would otherwise be needed by local infiltration. The smaller volume of anesthetic required not only reduces the risk for toxicity, but also decreases tissue distortion at the operative site. If wide undermining is planned and hemostasis is needed, a more dilute lidocaine with epinephrine concoction can be infiltrated painlessly in the field following the block. In general, nerve blocks cause less discomfort for the patient given the limited number of injections especially during a mucosal approach. They can also avoid the need for additional sedation or general anesthesia. In dermatologic surgery, nerve blocks are commonly used on the face and digits, but can be used to anesthetize other areas, such as the ears, feet, hands, penis, and lateral thigh.

Because of their usefulness in cutaneous surgery, it is important to carefully learn the proper technique for peripheral nerve blocks to minimize potential adverse effects. For optimal results, administering nerve blocks requires technical skill and knowledge of local neuroanatomy. Once analgesia is obtained, an infiltration of vasoconstrictor at the surgical site is often necessary because nerve blocks do not usually provide sufficient hemostasis. Risks include direct nerve injury leading to dysesthesias and paresis as well as vessel trauma causing ecchymosis and hematoma formation.[52]

Amide-type anesthetics are most commonly used for nerve blocks. As smaller volumes are injected, higher concentrations of anesthetic, such as 2% lidocaine, may be used to enhance diffusion of the anesthetic around the nerve.[52] Vasoconstrictors, such as epinephrine 1 : 200 000, may be added to the anesthetic agent. Epinephrine can have the advantages of slowing absorption of the anesthetic from the injected site, prolonging the duration of anesthesia, decreasing the amount of anesthetic needed, and improving hemostasis.[59] The use of epinephrine in digital blocks has been avoided given the potential risk of vasoconstrictor-induced ischemia; however, some debate this risk as theoretical when a proper technique is employed.[59,60]

Nerve blocks involve injecting anesthesia adjacent to a nerve or within the same fascial compartment as the nerve to be anesthetized. Typically, a 1-inch 30-gauge needle is selected; the smaller-caliber needle tends to be less painful and allows a slower and controlled delivery of anesthesia.[60,61] As vessels tend to travel along sensory nerves, care must be taken to avoid injecting into a vessel by aspirating before injection. Some advocate the use of a 25-gauge needle for nerve blocks because the smaller-caliber needles may be less reliable in aspirating blood during inadvertent intravascular placement.[6] After the needle is placed into the desired area, a small volume of anesthetic is injected and allowed to diffuse around the nerve. Take caution not to inject into the nerve itself, which can cause a neuropraxia resulting in paresthesia in the distribution of the nerve. Rarely this can be permanent.[61] Peripheral nerve blocks require diffusion into larger-sized nerves, and thus require a longer onset of action than local infiltrative anesthesia. Usually the block is effective after 5–10 minutes. The duration of anesthesia depends upon the anesthetic chosen.[6]

Nerve blocks on the face

Cutaneous branches of the trigeminal nerve and the cervical plexus convey sensory innervation from the face (Table 3.10).[61]

The trigeminal nerve has three main branches: the ophthalmic, maxillary, and mandibular. These convey sensation from the face, scalp to the vertex, conjunctiva, oral cavity, and teeth. Bony landmarks on the face help identify the location of the main trunk of the cutaneous branches of the trigeminal nerve (Fig. 3.3). The cervical plexus, a network arising from the anterior rami of the four superior cervical nerves, innervates the angle of the mandible, the submandibular area, and the neck.[60]

Supraorbital and supratrochlear nerve

The supraorbital and supratrochlear nerves are branches of the frontal nerve, which arises from the ophthalmic (V_1) nerve, and innervate the ipsilateral forehead and frontal scalp to the vertex. The supraorbital nerve emerges from the supraorbital foramen or notch, which is on the superior orbital rim in the midpupillary line. The supratrochlear nerve lies along the upper medial corner of the orbit approximately 1.5 cm medial to the supraorbital notch (see Chapter 1). Both nerve blocks can be achieved by entering just lateral to the supraorbital notch in the midpupillary line and injecting 1–2 mL of anesthetic toward the midline.[62]

Table 3.10 Facial nerve blocks useful in dermatologic surgery

Nerve	Distribution of sensory innervation	Location of emergence of nerve
Supraorbital	Forehead, frontal scalp to vertex	Supraorbital notch—at the superior orbital rim at the midpupillary line (approximately 2.5 cm from midline)
Supratrochlear	Mid-forehead, frontal scalp to vertex	Above eyebrow, approximately 1 cm lateral to midline and 1.5 cm medial to supraorbital nerve
External nasal	Dorsum, tip, and columella of nose	At the junction of the upper lateral cartilage and nasal bones
Infraorbital	Lower eyelid, nasal sidewall, upper lip, medial cheek, upper teeth, maxillary gingiva	Infraorbital notch—midpupillary line, approximately 1 cm inferior to the lower orbital rim and superolateral to nasal ala
Mental	Lower lip and chin	Mid-height of the mandible in the mid papillary line, approximately 1 cm inferior to second premolar
Auriculotemporal	Temporal scalp, anterior auricle, lateral temple	Just superior to the temporomandibular joint at zygomatic arch
Greater auricular and transverse cervical	Posterior auricle, angle of mandible, submandibular area	Posterior margin of sternocleidomastoid muscle at its midpoint (Erb's point) (see Chapter 1)

With permission from Eaton JS, Grekin RC. Regional anesthesia of the face. Dermatol Surg 2001; 27:1006–1009.[60]

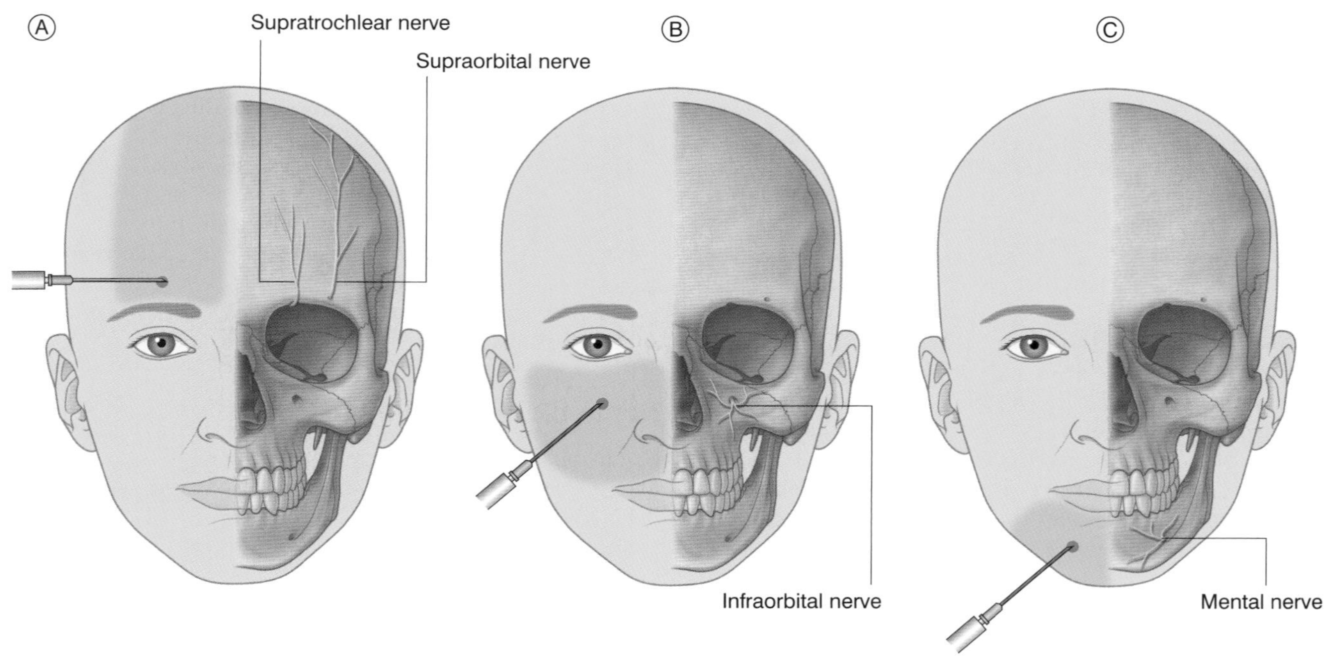

Figure 3.3 Location and sensory distribution for nerve blocks. (A) Supraorbital and supratrochlear nerve block. (B) Infraorbital nerve block. (C) Mental nerve block. (For additional information, see Fig. 1.11.)

External nasal nerve

The external nasal nerve, a branch of the anterior ethmoidal nerve, emerges from between the lower border of the nasal bone and the upper lateral nasal cartilage. Anesthesia to the skin of the ipsilateral nasal dorsum, nasal tip, and columella can be obtained by injecting approximately 1 mL of anesthetic bilaterally just off the midline after palpating for the junction between the mobile lateral cartilage and the firm nasal bones.[60]

Infraorbital nerve

The infraorbital nerve, the largest branch of the maxillary nerve (V_2), emerges from the infraorbital foramen to provide terminal branches that innervate the ipsilateral lower eyelid, nasal sidewall and ala, upper lip, and medial cheek. The infraorbital foramen is just medial to the midpupillary line approximately 0.7–1 cm below the infraorbital rim. Blocking the nerve at its point of emergence can be achieved percutaneously or intraorally. With the intraoral approach, the needle is advanced through the gingival buccal sulcus at the apex of the canine fossa for about 1 cm, at which point 1–2 mL of anesthetic is injected just over periosteum (Fig. 3.4).[60] The intraoral route tends to be less painful and the use of a topical mucosal anesthetic on the mucosal surface before injecting can further decrease the discomfort of the initial needle stick.[6]

Mental nerve

The mental nerve, a terminal branch of the mandibular nerve (V_3), can be blocked as it emerges from its foramen located approximately 2.5 cm lateral to the midline just medial to the midpupillary line and midway along the vertical height of the mandibular bone. The position of the foramen can vary with the age of the patient. Because the mandible atrophies at the alveolar ridge with age, the foramen lies closer to the upper margin of the mandible in older patients (Fig. 3.5).[60]

Blocking the mental nerve provides anesthesia to the ipsilateral chin and lower lip, including its adjacent mucosa and gingiva.[60] Like the infraorbital block, this can be approached by either the percutaneous or intraoral route (see Fig. 3.4). Using the intraoral route, anesthetic is injected into the inferior labial sulcus between the lower first and second premolars and injecting 1–2 mL just over periosteum.[62]

Auriculotemporal nerve

Another branch of the mandibular nerve (V_3), the auriculotemporal nerve, runs deep and posterior to the temporomandibular joint before it emerges superficially to travel with the superficial temporal artery. Blocking this nerve as it passes superiorly across the zygomatic arch provides anesthesia to the ipsilateral anterior auricle, lateral temple, and temporal scalp. This nerve block can be achieved by palpating for the temporomandibular joint with the jaw open and injecting 2–3 mL superior to this joint over periosteum at the zygomatic arch.[60]

Greater auricular and transverse cervical nerves

The greater auricular and the transverse cervical nerves arise from the cervical plexus and emerge near the midpoint of the posterior border of the sternocleidomastoid muscle, also known as Erb's point (Fig. 3.6). The greater auricular nerve passes upward toward the ear along the external jugular vein and innervates the ipsilateral angle of the jaw to the submandibular area and the posterior auricle.[60] Arising approximately 1 cm inferior to the greater auricular nerve,

Intraoral route for blocking infraorbital and mental nerves

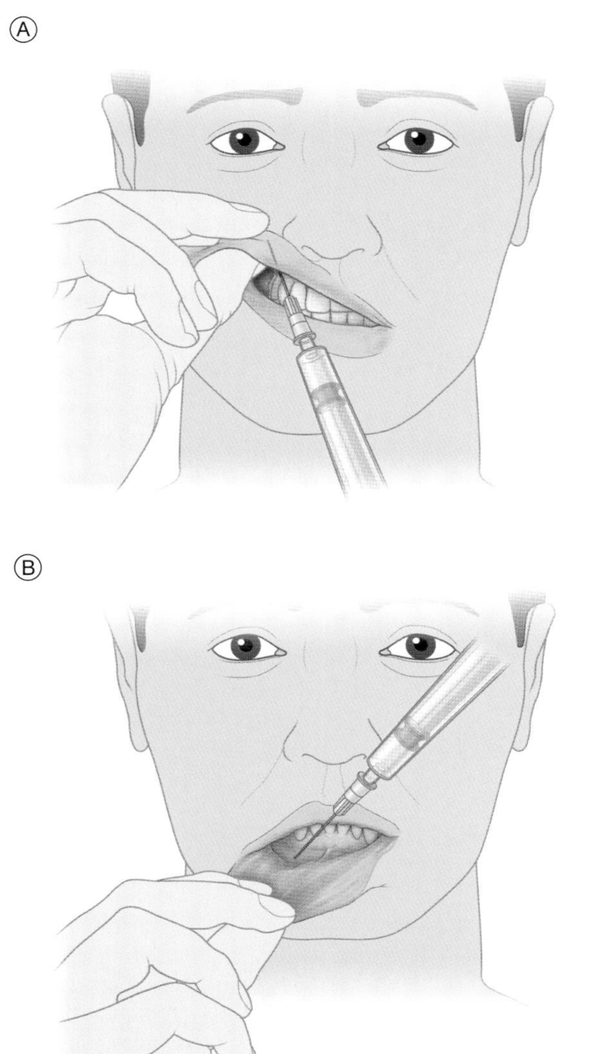

Figure 3.4 Intraoral route for blocking (A) infraorbital and (B) mental nerves.

Changing location of mental foramen with age

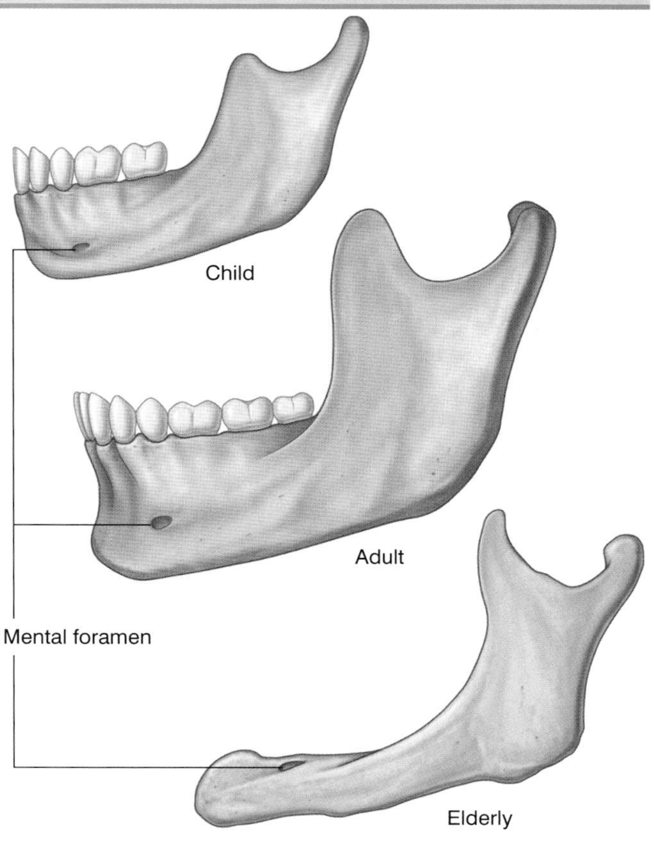

Figure 3.5 Changing location of the mental foramen with age. (For additional information, see Fig. 30.3D.)

the transverse cervical nerve heads in the anterior direction to provide sensory innervation to the ipsilateral inferior central border of the mandible and anterior neck. Turning the head at 45° against resistance to accentuate the landmarks and injecting into Erb's point will block both nerves.[60]

Nerve blocks for the extremities

Nerve blocks are useful for procedures involving the digits and wider surface areas of the palms and soles.

Digital block

Digital nerve blocks are useful for procedures involving the nails and phalanges. Two dorsal and two ventral nerves lie along the lateral aspects of the digits and innervate each digit (Fig. 3.7). Placement of anesthetic around these nerves at the base of the digits anesthetizes the finger. The addition of epinephrine in digital blocks has generally not been recommended because of the risk of vascular compromise. Controllable vasoconstriction to achieve an avascular surgical field can be safely achieved with the proper use of a tourniquet.[28]

The dorsal approach tends to be less painful than entering from the palmar or plantar surface (Fig. 3.7).[28] The needle is placed into the webspace at the dorsolateral aspect of the finger and the anesthetic is slowly deposited. The needle is partially withdrawn and redirected to deliver anesthesia to the dorsoventral aspects of the digit. The procedure is repeated on the opposite side of the digit. A total volume of 1–3 mL of 2% lidocaine typically provides adequate anesthesia.[28]

Although complications from digital blocks are unusual, care must be taken to avoid digital ischemia. Various factors that have been reported to contribute to digital gangrene include epinephrine, ring block technique (circumferential anesthesia), excessive tourniquet pressure, and postoperative burns from hot soaks to anesthetized fingers.[63] Epinephrine should be avoided in patients with severe hypertension, and peripheral vascular and vasospastic disease.[63] The pressure from the injection of excessive volumes (more than 8 mL) of anesthetic can also compromise the vascular circulation.[6] Digital blocks should be avoided in situations that potentially compromise the digital vessels at the base of the proximal phalanx (i.e. trauma or infection).[59]

Greater auricular and transverse cervical nerve

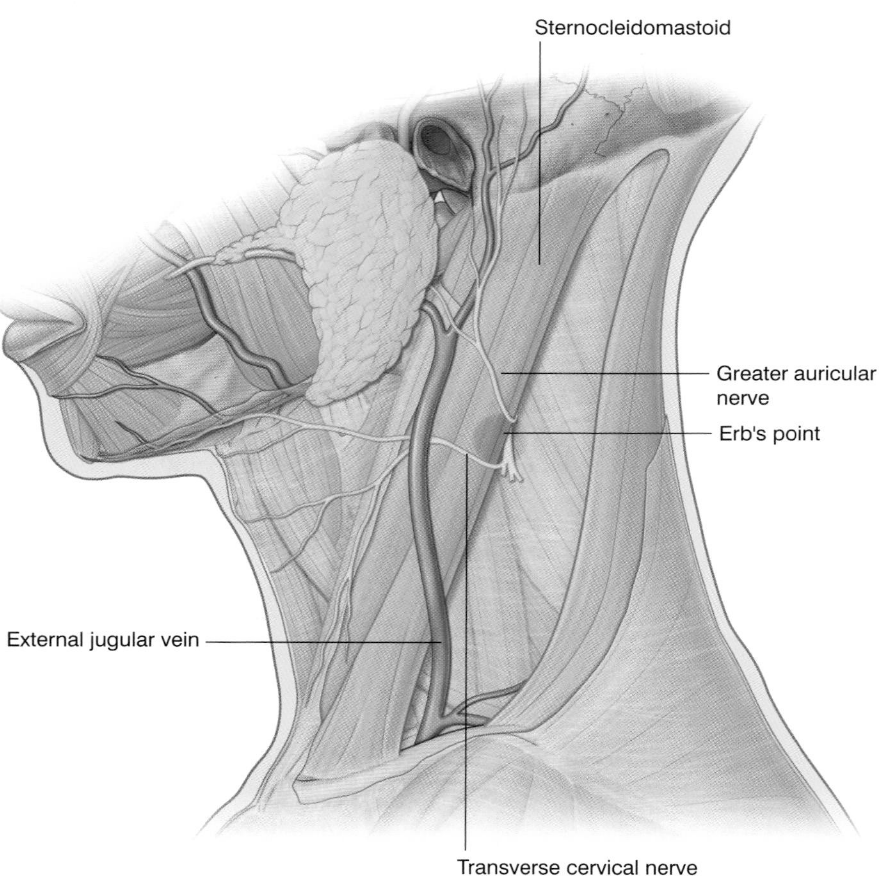

Figure 3.6 Nerve block of greater auricular nerve and transverse cervical nerves as they emerge at the midpoint of the posterior border of the sternocleidomastoid muscle, Erb's point. (For additional information, see Fig. 1.28.)

Digital innervation and nerve block

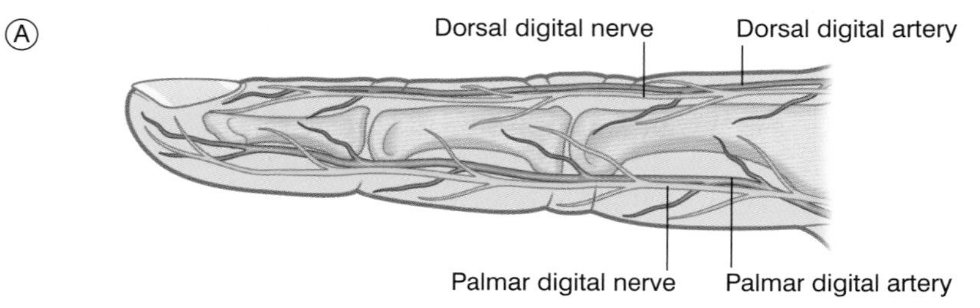

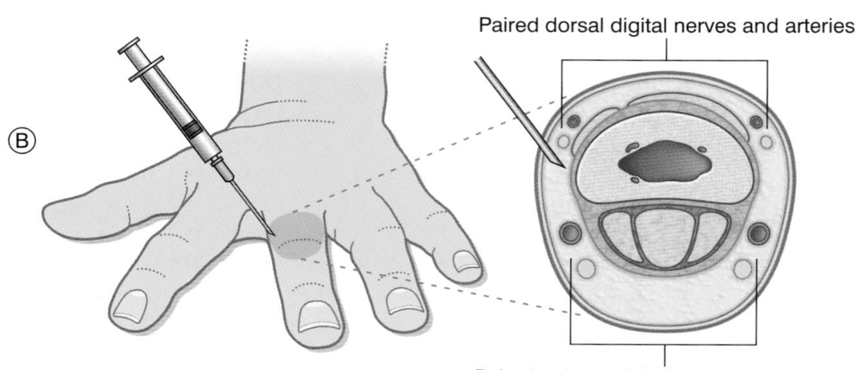

Figure 3.7 The digit. (A) Dorsal and palmar digital arteries and nerves run together. (B) Dorsal approach in administering digital nerve block allows anesthesia of dorsal and palmar bundles with one puncture.

Wrist blocks

Anesthesia to the hand can be achieved by blocking selected nerves at the wrist level. Wrist blocks are particularly useful for dermatologic procedures on the palm when multiple injections can be quite painful. The median and ulnar nerves, and superficial branch of the radial nerve provide sensory innervation to the palm (Fig. 3.8).[64]

The median nerve is located in the midline of the volar side of the wrist between the palmaris longus tendon and the flexor carpi radialis tendon.[65] Having the patient place the thumb and last two digits together accentuates the palmaris longus tendon, which is almost universally present.[62] (Fig. 3.9) Injecting 3–5 mL of anesthetic just to the radial side of the palmaris tendon and under the flexor retinaculum at the proximal crease of the wrist crease will block the median nerve and provide anesthesia to most of the radial side of the palm.[64,65]

The ulnar nerve runs beneath the flexor carpi ulnaris tendon and its insertion into the pisiform bone.[65] Flexing the wrist in a slightly ulnar direction helps identify the flexor carpi ulnaris tendon.[65] Inserting a needle just radial to this tendon on the proximal crease of the wrist at the ulnar styloid process and injecting 3–5 mL of anesthetic in the tissue blocks the ulnar nerve.[63,64]

The radial nerve lies on the lateral border of the radius just dorsal to the radial styloid.[65] Blocking the superficial branch of the radial nerve provides anesthesia to the palmar surface of the thumb.[64] Radial nerve block can be attained by infiltrating 4–6 mL of anesthetic in the area lateral to the radial artery extending toward the dorsum of the wrist.[64] Suboptimal anesthesia in this area may occur as a result of anatomic variation of sensory innervation.[65]

Palmar innervation and wrist nerve block

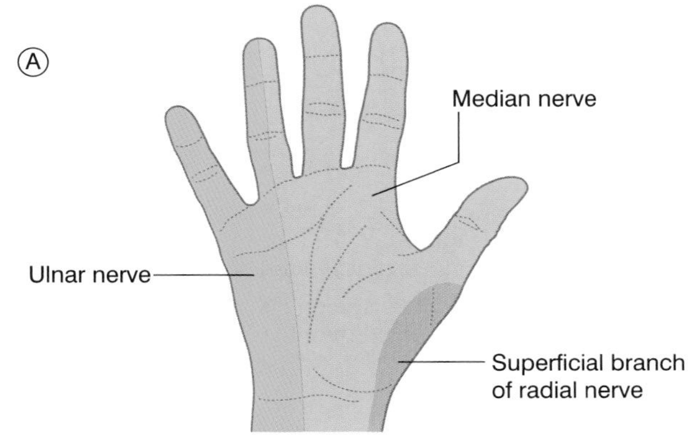

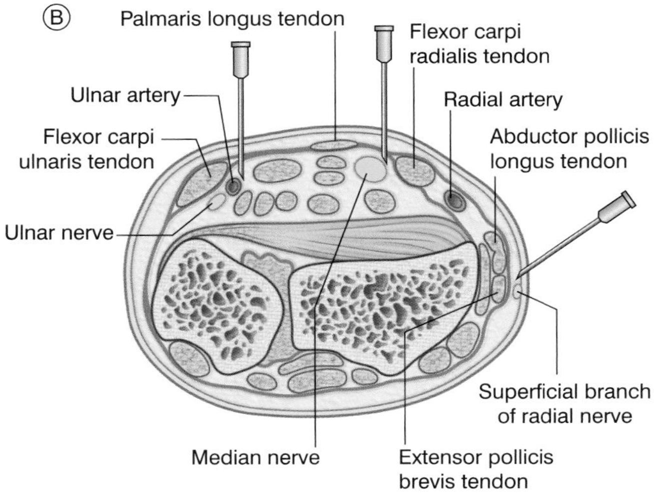

Figure 3.8 The palm. (A) Sensory innervation; (B) Nerve blocks at the wrist.

Ankle blocks

Five nerves provide sensory innervation to the foot: the posterior tibial, sural, saphenous, superficial fibular, and deep fibular (Fig. 3.10).[62] The posterior tibial nerve innervates the plantar surface except for small areas on the lateral and medial aspects, which are supplied by the sural and saphenous nerves, respectively. The superficial fibular, sural, saphenous, and deep fibular nerves innervate the dorsum of the foot. To achieve a peripheral nerve block of the feet requires that the particular nerve trunks be accessed at the level of the ankle. Blocking all five nerves (Fig. 3.11) can be performed with the patient supine and the foot placed on a padded support; however, some prefer to block the posterior tibial and sural nerves with the patient prone.

At the ankle, the posterior tibial nerve passes posterior to the posterior tibial artery between the calcaneal tendon and the medial malleolus and travels distally deep to the flexor reticulatum.[61] The posterior tibial nerve can be accessed with the patient supine and with the foot extended and externally rotated.[64] A needle is placed at the level of the upper half of the medial malleolus, posterior to the posterior tibial artery pulse and anterior to the calcaneal tendon.[61] The needle is advanced toward the posterior tibia, withdrawn slightly, and 3–4 mL of anesthetic is injected.[61]

The sural nerve, arising from branches of the common fibular and tibial nerves, passes more superficially between the Achilles tendon and the lateral malleolus as it travels toward the lateral border of the foot.[61] The sural nerve block is performed with the patient prone.[61] A needle is inserted 1–1.5 cm distal to the tip of the lateral malleolus and 3–5 mL of anesthetic is injected.[66]

The saphenous nerve, a terminal branch of the femoral nerve, runs along the medial surface of the calf, passes subcutaneously anterior to the medial malleolus, and extends toward the medial surface of the foot.[61] Injecting 3–4 mL of anesthetic into the subcutaneous tissue medial to the saphenous vein and anterior to the medial malleolus blocks the saphenous nerve.[61]

The superficial fibular nerve, a branch of the common fibular nerve, travels along the anterolateral border of the calf. It arises subcutaneously above the ankle where it divides into its branches, the intermediate and medial dorsal cutaneous nerves, before entering the foot.[60] Blocking the superficial fibular nerve by injecting 3–4 mL of anesthetic into the subcutaneous tissue midway between the anterior tibial surface and the lateral malleolus provides anesthesia to a major surface of the dorsal foot.[61]

The deep fibular nerve supplies a small portion of the foot, the first webspace. The deep fibular nerve block is rarely necessary in cutaneous surgery because anesthesia to this area can be adequately achieved by local infiltration.

Landmarks for median and ulnar nerve

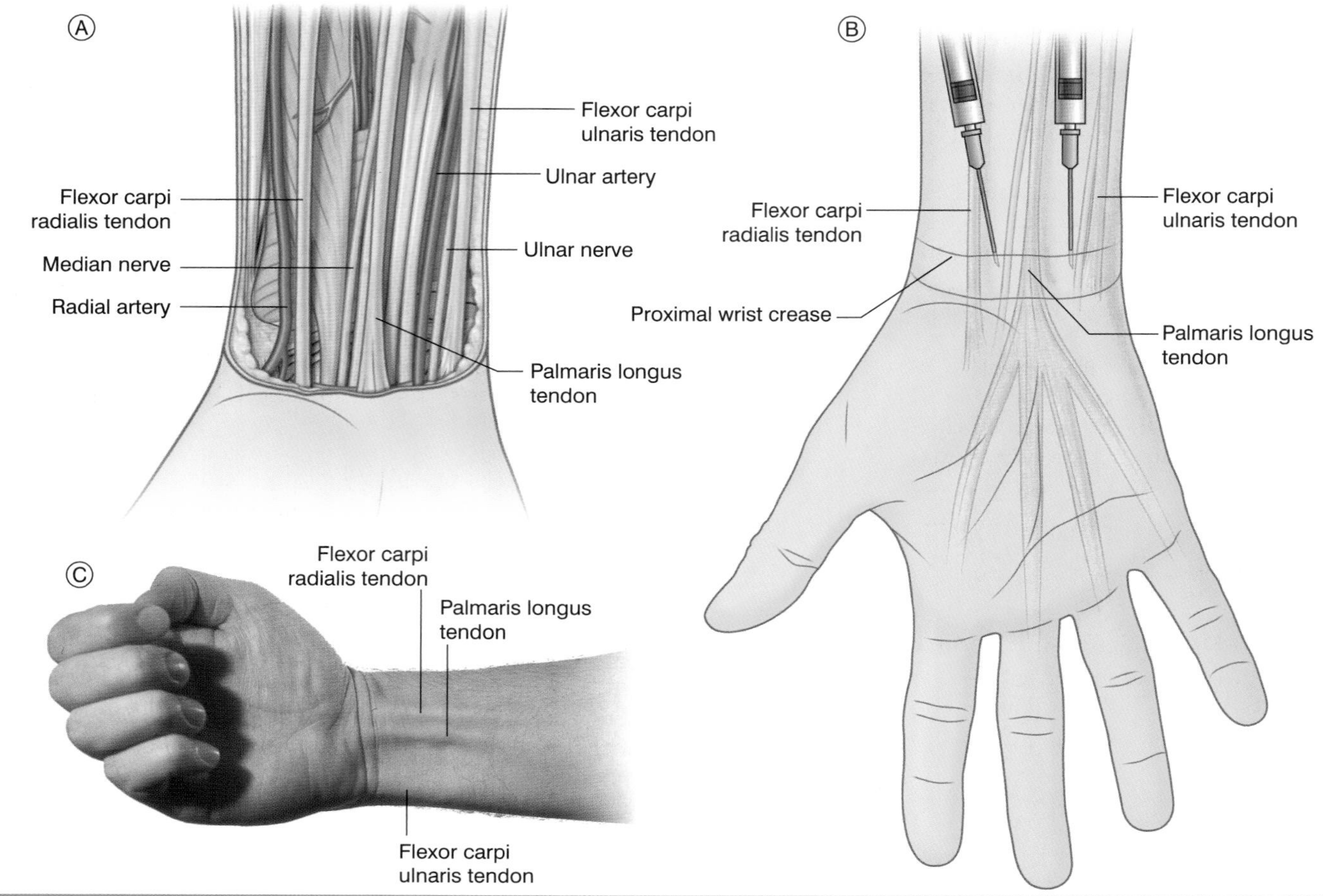

Figure 3.9 Landmarks for median and ulnar nerve blocks. (A) The median nerve lies between the palmaris longus tendon and the flexor carpi radialis tendon. The ulnar nerve runs beneath the flexor carpi ulnaris tendon and its insertion into the pisiform bone. (B) The tendons can be easily visualized and palpated. (C) Nerve blocks are delivered by insertion of needles at the proximal crease of the wrist.

Optimizing outcomes

Techniques to minimize discomfort during the administration of local anesthesia

- Reassure the patient.
- Position the patient with head supported, leaning back in a chair or on the table.
- Use small diameter (30-gauge) needles.
- Minimize patient viewing of needle and injection.
- Add sodium bicarbonate to neutralize premixed epinephrine (adrenaline)-containing solutions (and use within 24 hours to minimize loss of vasoconstrictor effect of epinephrine).
- Warm the anesthetic solution.
- Use counter-irritation of adjacent skin.
- Inject and infiltrate anesthetic slowly, deep to more superficial.
- Use adequate volume of anesthetic only; too much increases risk of toxicity; too little increases patient discomfort and bleeding.
- Minimize the number of skin punctures.
- Reintroduce needle at previously anesthetized areas.
- Consider using topical agents (anesthetics, ice, gentle cryotherapy) before injecting in children and extremely anxious patients.
- Consider using field or nerve blocks for larger areas.
- Avoid injecting into the nerve during nerve blocks.
- When treating a small child it may be comforting to parent and child to enlist the parent's support in stabilizing the patient. Consider conscious sedation or general anesthesia.

Sensory innervation of the foot

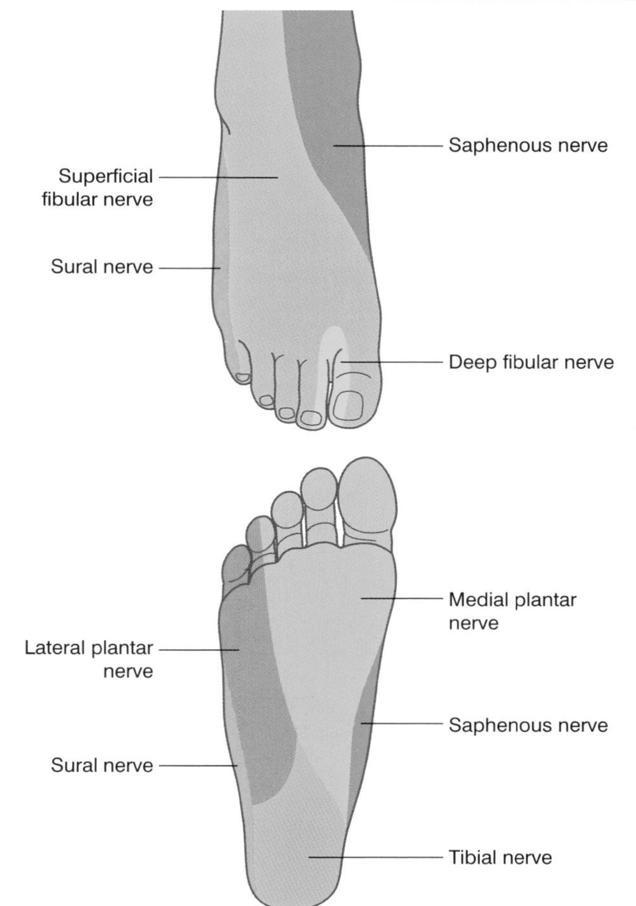

Figure 3.10 Sensory innervation of the foot.

Ankle block

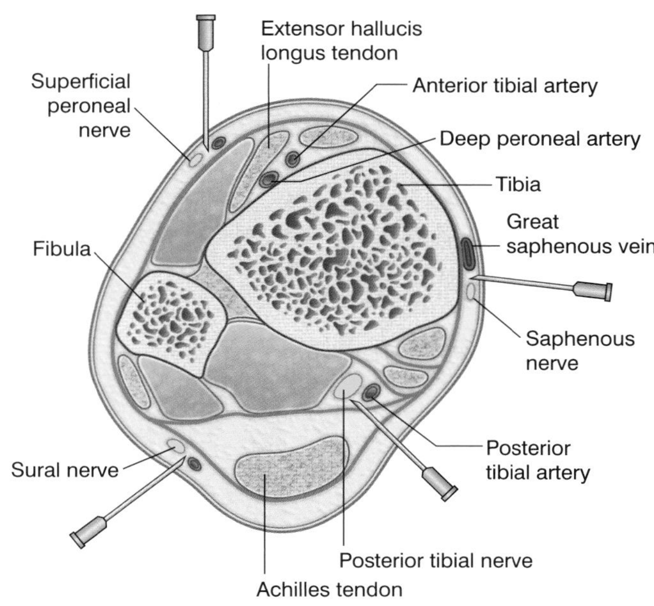

Figure 3.11 The ankle block. Transverse section of right leg above malleoli to show location of the sensory nerves—the sural, superficial fibular, posterior tibial, and saphenous nerves.

PITFALLS AND THEIR MANAGEMENT

Pitfalls and their management

- Prevention of digital injury associated with local anesthesia:
  - avoid the use of epinephrine (adrenaline) especially in patients with peripheral vascular disease
  - use small needles (30-gauge) to avoid vessel injury
  - limit volume of anesthetic used to 1–2 mL
  - avoid circumferential block of the digits
  - block at the level of the metacarpal heads
  - do not use digital block if there is infection or trauma of the proximal phalanx (distal to the injection site)
  - ensure bandages are not too constrictive
  - counsel patients to avoid postoperative hot soaks
- Prevention of allergic reactions to lidocaine:
  - obtain thorough drug, surgical, and past allergy history
  - refer for allergy testing to confirm diagnosis and test for alternative agents
  - use preservative-free solution if paraben allergy present
  - use alternative agents when true lidocaine allergy noted: amide anesthetic, benzyl alcohol, diphenhydramine, or normal saline (the anesthetic effect of 0.9% saline results from tissue distention and pressure on nerve endings as well as the presence of benzyl alcohol preservative)
  - consider using conscious sedation or general anesthesia if concerned local anesthesia may be inadequate
- Prevention of methemoglobinemia associated with local anesthesia:
  - adhere to recommended anesthetic dosages
  - avoid using prilocaine and benzocaine in patients with risk factors:
  - age <3 months
  - hereditary methemoglobinemia
  - glucose-6-phosphate dehydrogenase deficiency
  - concomitant oxidant drugs such as dapsone, nitroglycerin, nitrites, nitrates, phenacetin, primaquine, sulfonamides

Local anesthetics are generally easy and safe to administer; however, they can cause local and systemic adverse reactions. Local reactions can occur regionally around the site of administration. These commonly result from improper technique or the addition of epinephrine. Allergic reactions to local amide anesthetics are rare.[67] Although idiosyncratic systemic toxicity can occur at low plasma levels of local anesthetics, most systemic signs of toxicity are present at increased plasma levels.[67] Systemic toxicity due to local anesthetics primarily affects the central nervous and cardiovascular systems. Methemoglobinemia can occur particularly in predisposed individuals (see pages 43 and 56).

Local adverse effects

Regional reactions associated with local anesthetics are often due to the technique of administration of the agent or the addition of epinephrine. Tenderness, ecchymosis, and hematoma can occur, but are seldom of consequence. Epinephrine, when added to local anesthetics for its vasoconstrictive properties, has been implicated in tissue necrosis, particularly of the digits.[59] Patients with hypertension, peripheral vascular disease, and vasospastic disease are at increased risk.[59,63] For this reason, it is generally recommended to avoid local anesthetic infiltration of epinephrine-containing solutions to the fingers and toes. Digital ischemia can also occur after ring blocks and injection of excessive volumes of anesthesia even without the addition of epinephrine.[63,68] Local injections of phentolamine 0.5 mg/mL and topical application of nitroglycerin have been used to reverse epinephrine-induced digital vasospasm.[59,68] Phentolamine is an α-adrenergic blocker that competitively blocks both presynaptic (α-2) and postsynaptic (α-1) receptors producing vasodilatation and a decrease in peripheral resistance. It is available in a 5-mg powder and can diluted in normal saline.

Paresthesias due to nerve injury can occur, particularly with peripheral nerve blocks. Nerve injury may result from transection of the nerve, pressure-induced ischemic injury with intraneural injection, vascular compromise by injury to local vasculature, or direct toxicity of injected agents.[69] Acute pain or paresthesias on injection of local anesthetic can signify intraneural injection and should be avoided.

Inadvertent thermal and chemical burns have been associated with the use of local anesthetics. To allow for adequate penetration, EMLA is formulated in an alkaline vehicle with a pH of approximately 9.4. Alkaline chemical injuries to the eye have been reported with the use of EMLA near the eyes.[41] These manifest as corneal abrasions and ulcerations and require immediate ophthalmologic evaluation and management.

Accidental thermal burns postoperatively have also been associated with local anesthesia. Although longer duration of anesthetic action provides postoperative analgesia, it also places individuals at risk for accidental thermal burns. Reports of thermal and cigarette burns to anesthetized areas have been reported after digital blocks and tumescent liposuction.[70,71] Counseling patients on the duration of anesthesia before discharge should avoid this potential complication.

Systemic adverse effects

Life-threatening allergic reactions to local anesthetics are rare.[67] Psychogenic attacks and epinephrine reactions should be differentiated from true allergic reactions.[4] Psychogenic attacks, which frequently manifest as vasovagal episodes, occur as a result of patients' response to anxiety, fear of needles and/or pain of injection. Increased parasympathetic tone caused by the stress of injection leads to lightheadedness, diaphoresis, nausea, syncope, bradycardia, and hypotension. Reassurance and positioning the patient in the Trendelenburg position typically relieves the patient's symptoms. Symptoms of flushing, palpitations, and malaise related to the adrenergic effects of epinephrine may be mistaken for an allergic reaction. Although tachycardia is typically present in both an epinephrine reaction and an anaphylactic reaction, blood pressure tends to be elevated with the former and decreased during anaphylaxis.

The addition of epinephrine poses a risk for potential adverse reactions in certain clinical settings. Caution should be taken in using epinephrine in patients taking tricyclic antidepressants and β-blockers. The interaction of tricyclic antidepressants and epinephrine may lead to hypertension, tachycardia, and arrythmias.[12] Injection of epinephrine-containing anesthetic has been reported to cause hypertension followed by bradycardia in patients taking propanolol.[12] This is likely a result of unopposed alpha-adrenergic vasoconstriction. Epinephrine should be avoided in patients with hyperthyroidism, severe hypertension, and pheochromocytoma.

Several reports of allergic reactions, ranging from contact dermatitis to anaphylaxis, have been described.[72] Allergic reactions occur more commonly with ester derivatives than amides. Esters are metabolized to PABA, which is a potential allergen. Cross-reactivity may occur among ester-type anesthetics, paraphenylenediamine hair dyes, sulfonylureas, and thiazides.[12] However, there is no cross-reactivity between esters and amide anesthetics. Methylparaben, an allergen chemically related to PABA, is a preservative added to anesthetics. Reactions to lidocaine may be due to these preservatives and not to the anesthetic itself.[67]

Mild allergic reactions can be treated with antihistamines and corticosteroids. Management of anaphylactic reactions includes the administration of 0.3–0.5-mg epinephrine subcutaneously, basic life support, and transport to an acute care facility.[73]

Although uncommon, delayed-type hypersensitivity from the topical use of ester and amide anesthetics has been reported. Multiple exposures to increasingly popular over-the-counter products containing lidocaine may contribute to topical sensitization to lidocaine.[74]

There are no specific recommendations on the most reliable method of testing for suspected allergy to anesthetics.[72] The possibility of reaction to preservatives should be considered. If there is a clear history of procaine or PABA sensitivity, the use of preservative-free lidocaine is recommended.[72] The use of patch testing and intradermal skin testing with preservative-free lidocaine has been suggested as a rational approach.[72,74] An alternative in dealing with anesthetic allergy is the use of other agents for local anesthesia. Benzyl alcohol 0.9%, diphenhydramine

1%, and 0.9% saline (which contains benzyl alcohol) have been used to provide anesthesia for minor cutaneous procedures.[20,75,76] However, the depth and duration of anesthesia have been shown to be less with diphenhydramine and benzyl alcohol compared to lidocaine.[75,76] In addition, diphenhydramine induced more pain than lidocaine,[75] caused skin necrosis in one patient,[76] and can potentially be sedating. Intradermal tramadol and metoclopramide have also been shown to have local anesthetic properties.[77,78] Intradermal tramadol 5% provided loss of sensation to pinprick, cold, and light touch 30 minutes after intradermal injection.[79] In a study comparing intradermal 5% tramadol to prilocaine, both provided similar local anesthetic effect, but tramadol had significantly increased incidence of local rash at the injection site.[78] Because alternatives to local anesthetics are not ideal, referral for allergy testing to rule out a true allergy or to identify a safe anesthetic is recommended.

Systemic toxicity affecting the central nervous and cardiovascular systems occurs with higher blood levels resulting from inadvertent intravascular injection, administering excess amounts, rapid drug absorption, and abnormal drug metabolism (Table 3.11).[67] Delivering anesthesia to a vascular area results in an increased rate of absorption.[67] Rapid absorption also typically occurs in the mucous membranes. Abnormal drug metabolism can occur in conjunction with liver disease, pseudocholinesterase deficiency, and interactions with other medications.[80,81] Amide-type anesthetics are metabolized by microsomal enzymes in the liver, specifically cytochrome p450–3A4. Concurrent use of medications that inhibit cytochrome p450–3A4 can potentially result in systemic toxicity, especially when larger amounts of anesthetics are used (Table 3.12).[81]

Table 3.11 Maximum lidocaine dosages

	Without epinephrine (adrenaline)	With epinephrine (adrenaline)
Adults	5 mg/kg	7 mg/kg
Children	1.5–2.0 mg/kg	3.0–4.5 mg/kg

Table 3.12 Cytochrome p450-3A4 inhibitors

Amiodarone	Methylprednisolone
Benzodiazepines (midazolam, triazolam)	Metronidazole
Carbamazepine	Miconazole
Cimetidine	Nicardipine
Clarithromycin	Nifedipine
Chloramphenicol	Pentoxifylline
Cyclosporine	Propofol
Danazol	Propranolol
Dexamethasone	Quinidine
Diltiazem	Selective serotonin reuptake inhibitors
Erythromycin	Tetracycline
Fluconazole	Terfenadine
Itraconazole	Thyroxine
Isoniazid	Verapamil
Ketoconazole	Valproic acid
Methadone	Verapamil

Signs of central nervous system toxicity to local anesthetics manifest in a concentration-dependent manner (Table 3.13).[67,72] Early symptoms of lidocaine toxicity include drowsiness and circumoral paresthesia. This can progress to lightheadedness, restlessness, and irritability.[72] At higher concentrations, muscle twitching, nystagmus, blurred vision, and confusion appear; seizures and cardiac toxicity do not usually occur until plasma concentrations approach 10 μg/mL.[67] Increasing blood levels lead to coma and respiratory arrest.[67]

Local anesthetics can affect the cardiovascular system. Transient reactions can occur when using solutions containing epinephrine. These include tachycardia, diaphoresis, tremor, headache, elevated blood pressure, and chest pain. Slow injections and careful aspirations to avoid intravascular injection prevent rapid systemic absorption of epinephrine. In healthy patients, increased blood pressure and arrhythmias do not usually occur if the dose of epinephrine is limited to 0.5 mg (50 mL of 1 : 100 000 dilution).[12] However, patients with underlying systemic diseases, such as hyperthyroidism, cardiac disease, peripheral vascular disease, and pheochromocytoma, as well as those with anxiety disorder may be more sensitive to epinephrine.[6] The maximum epinephrine dose recommended for such patients is 0.2 mg.[12]

Higher toxic blood levels of anesthetics such as lidocaine lead to vasodilatation, hypotension, and bradycardia, which progress to cardiovascular collapse and cardiac arrest. Signs of cardiovascular compromise usually do not manifest until after signs of CNS toxicity.[81] Anesthetic potency directly correlates to the degree of myocardial depression. More potent anesthetics, such as bupivicaine and etidocaine, appear to be more cardiotoxic than other anesthetics.[81] Furthermore, because bupivacaine enters the sodium channel rapidly, but leaves it slowly, it has a greater potential to induce serious re-entrant arrhythmias that may be refractory to treatment.[81] The cardiac toxicity of bupivacaine can be more severe during pregnancy, which may be due to increased progesterone and the adverse effects of pregnancy on venous return during resuscitation.[4]

Early recognition of anesthetic toxicity can lead to proper and timely management. Initial management of allergic and toxic reactions includes halting the delivery of the anesthetic and maintaining ventilation and oxygenation.

Table 3.13 Lidocaine levels and symptoms of toxicity

Lidocaine level (μg/mL)	Symptoms of toxicity
1–6	Subjective toxicity: lightheadedness, euphoria, tongue and circumoral paresthesia, tinnitus, blurred vision
5–9	Objective toxicity: vomiting, tremors, muscular fasciculations
8–12	Seizures, cardiopulmonary depression
12–20	Coma, respiratory and cardiac arrest

With permission from Faccenda KA, Finucane BT. Complications of regional anesthesia. Incidence and prevention. Drug Saf 2001; 24:13–442 and 69[67] and McCaughey W. Adverse effects of local anesthetics. Drug Saf 1992; 7:178–189.[72]

Hypoxia and acidosis decrease the seizure threshold and contribute to the cardiodepressant effects of local anesthetics.[81] Seizures can be treated and potentially prevented with thiopental sodium, diazepam, or propofol.[81] Neuromuscular blocking agents such as succinylcholine may be needed to aid in intubation.[81] Hypotension is treated by the administration of fluids; profound hypotension may require vasopressors, such as epinephrine, ephedrine, or phenylephrine. Bradycardia and decreased myocardial contractility may require inotropic agents, such as epinephrine or ephedrine.[75] Bretyllium is used to treat recalcitrant dysrhythmias. Amrinone can be used when conventional inotropes are ineffective.[81] Amrinone is a phosphodiesterase inhibitor that leads to increased cAMP in the myocardium and enhanced cardiac contractility. Naguib et al[81] describe a detailed algorithm showing the treatment of local anesthetic-induced acute cardiovascular toxicity and seizures.

Methemoglobinemia, the presence of increased hemoglobin in the oxidized state instead of the oxygen-carrying reduced state, can occur following the use of local anesthetics.[82] Benzocaine and prilocaine are local anesthetics most commonly associated with clinically significant methemoglobinemia. Several reported cases have occurred in infants or young children after the topical use of benzocaine to mucosal surfaces, and more recently, after the application of EMLA to the skin.[81] Infants and children are at greater risk than adults because hemoglobin F is more susceptible to oxidation, newborns have lower levels of reductive enzymes, and the dose tends to be greater per kilogram of body weight.[81] Limiting use to recommended dosages tends to avoid problems; however, susceptibility may increase with glucose-6-phosphate dehydrogenase deficiency, rare methemoglobinemia and methemoglobin reductase deficiency, and concomitant administration of other methemoglobin-forming drugs, such as sulfonamides and antimalarials.[73]

Methemoglobinemia presents with a cyanotic appearance in the skin, lips and nail beds at methemoglobin levels of 10–20 %.[73] In addition to the drug history, the presence of cyanosis without cardiorespiratory disease suggests a diagnosis of methemoglobinemia.[82] Symptoms frequently do not occur for 1–3 hours following treatment because methemoglobinemia is caused by metabolites of the anesthetic.[73] Conventional pulse oximeters are usually unreliable in the presence of methemoglobinemia; therefore arterial blood gases and methemoglobin levels are recommended.[80] Management depends on the level of toxicity. Methemoglobinemia with a level below 30% can usually be managed by removal of the causative drug, oxygen, and observation.[73] Higher levels may need intravenous methylene blue 1–2 mg/kg as a 1% solution. Methylene blue is contraindicated in patients with glucose-6-phosphate deficiency. Ascorbic acid 300–1000 mg/day intravenously in three to four doses is recommended in these patients.[82] Hemodialysis may be considered if symptoms persist.[82]

Special precautions should be taken when using local anesthetics in children. Recommended maximum dosages of lidocaine for children over 3 years of age are 1.5–2.0 mg/kg for lidocaine without epinephrine and 3.0–4.5 mg/kg for lidocaine with epinephrine.[38] Because parabens can potentially displace bilirubin by competitively binding to albumin, the use of preservative-free anesthetic solutions has been suggested in jaundiced neonates.[28] Lastly, given the risk of lidocaine toxicity and methemoglobinemia, the quantity of topical anesthetics should be limited to established recommendations (Table 3.14).[38]

■ PRACTICAL APPLICATIONS

Local anesthesia for most cutaneous surgery is generally achieved easily and effectively by local infiltration using 1% lidocaine with or without epinephrine. When longer procedures are anticipated, longer-acting anesthetics, such as bupivacaine and etidocaine, may be mixed to maximize benefit while minimizing risks. Local infiltration is typically delivered using 30-gauge, $\frac{1}{2}$ or 1-inch needles. Larger-diameter needles tend to cause more pain while 32-gauge needles tend to be too flexible and small for easy injection. Infiltration may distort lesional and anatomic borders; therefore, markings on the operative site before infiltration are helpful. Because local anesthetics tend to be less effective in acidic environments, infected areas may require greater amounts of anesthetic to achieve adequate anesthesia.

Field or ring blocks (see Fig 3.2) are practical for cyst excisions and incision and drainage of abscesses. In addition, they are commonly used for procedures in certain anatomic areas, such as the scalp and the pinna of the ear. A scalp block can be performed by injecting anesthetic approximately 4–5 cm apart starting at the mid forehead extending circumferentially toward the occiput and back around to the mid forehead. A ring block around the circumference of the ear provides anesthesia to the ear except for the concha and the external auditory canal. A field block around the nose can also be useful, particularly for rhinophymectomy surgery and other resurfacing procedures.

Nerve blocks are useful for procedures involving large surface areas of the face, scalp, hands, and feet, as well as procedures in particularly sensitive areas, such as lips, palms, soles, and digits. A prerequisite is that regional nerves are available to block, which is not so on most areas

Table 3.14 Recommended use of EMLA

Age and weight	Maximum total dose (g)	Maximum application area (cm^2)	Maximum application time (hours)
0–3 months or <5 kg	1	10	1
3–12 months and >5 kg	2	20	4
1–6 years and >10 kg	10	100	4
7–12 years and >20 kg	20	200	4

With permission from Physicians' Desk Reference. 57th edn. New Jersey: Thompson PDR; 2003.[38]

of the neck, trunk, and extremities. The benefits of nerve blocks include decreased amount of anesthetic, fewer needle injections, and reduced tissue distortion. One obvious disadvantage is the lack of hemostasis that comes with tissue infiltration. The administration of nerve blocks can be especially helpful for the following procedures—surgical excisions in acral and facial areas, ablative laser resurfacing of the face, laser therapy of plantar warts, botulinum toxin injections to the palms and soles, hair transplantation, medium and deep chemical peels of the face, and perioral injection with fillers.[61,64,84]

The tumescent anesthesia technique employs the delivery of large volumes of dilute anesthetic. It allows treatment of larger areas where nerve blocks are not possible (i.e. trunk and limbs) and for higher maximum doses of lidocaine to be delivered without toxicity. It has mainly been used for tumescent liposuction; however, its utility has been expanded to other procedures as well, including laser resurfacing, dermabrasion, face-lifting/neck-lifting, ambulatory phlebectomy, and soft tissue reconstruction.[83–85] The concentration of lidocaine and epinephrine can be varied depending on the clinical requirements. For instance, liposuction of fibrous areas, such as the back, upper abdomen, and breasts, tends to require higher concentrations of lidocaine (1000–1250 mg/dL). As these areas tend to be associated with increased bleeding, they also benefit from higher concentrations of epinephrine (1 mg/dL).[54] In contrast, less fibrous areas, such as the hips and thighs, may not require concentrations beyond 500–700 mg/dL of lidocaine and 0.5–0.65 mg/dL of epinephrine.

In the past, the effective use of topical anesthetics was limited to mucosal surfaces. The development of EMLA and newer topical agents has extended their application to cutaneous surfaces. For optimal results, topical anesthetics should be applied appropriately for the recommended duration before the procedure. Insufficient volume and incorrect application were often found to be the causes of inadequate anesthesia after using EMLA.[39] Topical anesthetics are useful in minimizing the pain associated with superficial surgical procedures, laser procedures, filler injections, and chemical peels. In addition, topical anesthetics are particularly helpful in performing superficial cutaneous procedures in children. They also decrease the pain associated with the introduction of a needle for infiltrative or nerve block administration of anesthesia.

A combination of the above techniques can be employed in cutaneous surgical procedures to achieve optimal anesthesia and obviate the need for general anesthesia. Under certain circumstances, conscious sedation and general anesthesia may be necessary and must be assessed on a case-by-case basis.

■ SUMMARY

The use of local anesthesia is ideal for most cutaneous surgical procedures. Knowledge of the pharmacologic properties, potential adverse effects, and different applications and techniques of administration is crucial to the practice of cutaneous surgery. With proper use, the available anesthetic agents provide safe and effective anesthesia and analgesia. Although local infiltration remains the most commonly used method, other techniques of drug delivery have expanded the use of local anesthetics in the field of dermatologic surgery. The use of nerve blocks, tumescent technique, and topically effective agents, alone or in combination, has provided optimal regional anesthesia without the risks of general anesthesia. As the use of local anesthesia broadens with the emergence of new laser technology and new surgical techniques, the impetus will hopefully be present to develop novel agents and delivery systems with even greater safety, efficacy, and ease of administration profiles.

■ REFERENCES

1. Calatayud J, Gonzalez A. History of the development and evolution of local anesthesia since the coca leaf. Anesthesiology 2003; 98:1503–1508.
2. Wildsmith JA, Strichardtz GR. Local anaesthetic drugs—an historical perspective. Br J Anaesth 1984; 56:937–939.
3. Covino BG. Local anesthesia. N Engl J Med 1972; 286:975–983.
4. Tetzlaff JE. The pharmacology of local anesthetics. Anesthesiol Clin North Am 2000; 18:217–231.
5. Covino BG. Local anesthesia—second of two parts. N Engl J Med 1972; 286:1035–1042.
6. Grekin RC, Auletta MJ. Local anesthesia in dermatologic surgery. J Am Acad Dermatol 1988; 19: 599–614.
7. Selden R, Sasahara AA. Central nervous system toxicity induced by lidocaine: a report of a case in a patient with liver disease. JAMA 1967; 202:908–909.
8. Covino BG. Pharmacology of local anesthetic agents. Br J Anaesth 1986; 58:701–716.
9. Klein JA. Tumescent technique for regional anesthesia permits lidocaine doses of 35 mg/kg for liposuction. J Dermatol Surg Oncol 1990; 16:248–263.
10. Catchlove RFH. The influence of CO_2 and pH on local anaesthetic action. J Pharmacol Exp Ther 1972; 181:298–309.
11. Bieter RN. Applied pharmacology of local anesthetics. Am J Surg 1936; 34:500–510.
12. Lawrence C. Drug management in skin surgery. Drugs 1996; 52:805–817.
13. Richards KA, Stasko T. Dermatologic surgery and the pregnant patient. Dermatol Surg 2002; 28:248–258.
14. Fink BR. The long and short of conduction blockade. Anesth Analg 1989; 68:551–555.
15. Butterworth JF, Strichartz GR. Molecular mechanisms of local anesthesia: a review. Anesthesiology 1990; 72:711–734.
16. Ragsdale DS, McPhee JC, Scheuer T, et al. Molecular determinants of state-dependent block of Na+ channels by local anesthetics. Science 1994; 265:1724–1728.
17. Siegel RJ, Vistnes LM, Iverson, RE. Effective hemostasis with less epinephrine: an experimental and clinical study. Plast Reconstr Surg 1973; 51:129–133.
18. Fante, RG, Elner VM. The use of epinephrine in infiltrative local anesthesia for eyelid reconstruction. Plast Reconst Surg 1998; 102:917.
19. Moore DC, Bridenbaugh DL, Thompson GE, et al. Factors determining dosage of amide-type local anesthetic drugs. Anesthesiology 1997; 47:263–268.
20. Auletta MJ, Grekin RC. Local anesthesia for dermatologic surgery. New York: Churchill Livingstone; 1990.
21. Moore DC. The pH of local anesthetic solutions. Anesth Analg 1981; 60: 833–834.
22. Howe NR, Williams JM. Pain on injection and duration of anesthesia for intradermal infiltration of lidocaine, bupivicaine, and etidonate. J Dermatol Surg Oncol 1994; 20:459–464.
23. McKay W, Morris R, Mushlin P. Sodium bicarbonate attenuates pain on skin infiltration with lidocaine with or without epinephrine. Anesth Analg 1987; 66:572–574.
24. Stewart JH, Cole GW, Klein JA. Neutralized lidocaine with epinephrine for local anesthesia. J Dermatol Surg Oncol 1989; 15:1081–1083.
25. Robinson J, Fernando R, Sun Wai WY, et al. Chemical stability of bupivacaine, lidocaine, and epinephrine in pH-adjusted solutions. Anesthesia 2000; 55:853–858.

26. Lewis-Smith PA, Adjunctive use of hyaluronidase in local anesthesia. Br J Plastic Surg 1986; 39:554–558.
27. Clark LE, Mellette JR. The use of hyaluronidase as an adjunct to surgical procedures. Dermatol Surg 1994; 20:842–844.
28. Dinehart SM. Topical, local, and regional anesthesia. In: Wheeland R, ed. Cutaneous surgery. Philadelphia: WB Saunders; 1994:105–110.
29. Klein, JA. Pharmacology of lidocaine In: Klein JA. Tumescent technique, tumescent anesthesia and microcannular liposuction. St. Louis: Mosby; 2000:127.
30. Galindo A, Witcher T. Mixtures of local anesthetics: bupivacaine–chloroprocaine. Anesth Analg 1980; 59:683–685.
31. Adriani J, Dalili H. Penetration of local anesthetics through epithelial barriers. Anesth Analg 1971: 50:834–841.
32. Friedman PM, Mafong EA, Friedman BS, et al. Topical anesthetics update: EMLA and beyond. Dermatol Surg 2001; 27:1019–1026.
33. Kuwahara RT, Skinner RB. EMLA versus ice as a topical anesthetic. Dermatol Surg 2001; 27:495–496.
34. Plotkin S. Clinical comparison of preinjection anesthetics. J Am Podiatr Med Assoc 1998; 88:73–79.
35. White, J, Siegfried E, Boulden M, et al. Possible hazards of cryogen use with pulsed dye laser. A case report and summary. Dermatol Surg 1999; 25:250–253.
36. Latorre F, Klimek L. Does cocaine still have a role in nasal surgery? Drug Saf 1999; 20:9–13.
37. Huang W, Vidimos A. Topical anesthetics in dermatology. J Am Acad Dermatol 2000; 43:286–298.
38. Physicians' Desk Reference. 57th edn. New Jersey: Thompson PDR; 2003.
39. Chen BK, Eichenfield L. Pediatric anesthesia in dermatologic surgery: when hand-holding is not enough. Dermatol Surg 2001; 27:1010–1018.
40. Rincon E, Baker RL, Iglesias AJ, et al. CNS toxicity after topical application of EMLA cream on a toddler with molluscum contagiosum. Pediatr Emerg Care 2000; 16:252–254.
41. Eaglstein NF. Chemical injury to the eye from EMLA cream during erbium laser resurfacing. Dermatol Surg 1999; 25:591–591.
42. Bucalo BD, Mirikitani EJ, Moy RL. Comparison of skin anesthetic effect of liposomal lidocaine, nonliposomal lidocaine and EMLA using 30-minute application time. Dermatol Surg 1998; 24:537–541.
43. Altman, DA, Gildenberg SR. High-energy pulsed light source hair removal device used to evaluate the onset of action of a new topical anesthetic. Dermatol Surg 1999; 25:816–818.
44. Koppel RA, Coleman KM, Coleman WP. The efficacy of ELMA versus ELA-Mac for pain relief in medium-depth peeling: a clinical and histopathologic evaluation. Dermatol Surg 2000; 26:61–64.
45. Friedman PM, Fogelman JP, Nouri K, et al. Comparative study of the efficacy of four topical anesthetics. Dermatol Surg 1999; 25:950–954.
46. Zempski WT, Karasic RB. EMLA versus TAC for topical anesthesia of extremity wounds in children. Ann Emerg Med 1997;30:163–166.
47. McCafferty DF, Woolfson AD, Handley J, et al. Effect of percutaneous local anesthetics on pain reduction during pulsed dye laser treatment of portwine stain. Br J Anaesth 1997; 78:286–289.
48. Bryan HA, Alter TS. The S-caine peel: a novel topical anesthetic for cutaneous laser surgery. Dermatol Surg 2002; 28:999–1003.
49. Greenbaum SS, Bernstein EF. Comparison of iontophoresis of lidocaine with a eutectic mixture of lidocaine and prilocaine (EMLA) for topically administered local anesthesia. J Dermatol Surg Oncol 1994; 20:579–583.
50. DeCou JM, Abrams RS, Hammond JH, Lowder LR, Gauderer MW. Iontophoresis: a needle-free, electrical system of local anesthesia delivery for pediatric surgical office procedures. J Pediatr Surg. 1999; 34:946–949.
51. Bartfield JM, Holmes TJ, Raccio-Robak N. A comparison of proparacaine and tetracaine eye anesthetics. Acad Emerg Med 1994; 1:364–367.
52. Hawkins, JM, Moore PA. Local anesthesia: advances in agents and techniques. Dent Clin N Am 2002; 46:719–732.
53. True RH, Elliott RM. Microprocessor-controlled local anesthesia versus the conventional syringe technique in hair transplantation. Dermatol Surg 2002; 28:463–468.
54. Klein, JA. Anesthetic formulation of tumescent solutions. Dermatol Clinics 1999; 17:751–759.
55. Ostad A, Kageyama N, Moy RL. Tumescent anesthesia with a lidocaine dose of 55 mg/kg is safe for liposuction. Dermatol Surg 1996; 22:921–927.
56. Kaplan B, Moy RL. Comparison of room temperature and warmed local anesthetic solution for tumescent liposuction. A randomized double-blind study. Dermatol Surg 1996; 22:707–709.
57. Klein J. Tumescent technique. Am J Cosm Surg 1987;4:263–267.
58. Lillis PJ. Liposuction surgery under local anesthesia: limited blood loss and minimal lidocaine absorption. J Dermatol Surg Oncol 1988;14:1145–1148
59. Denkler K. A comprehensive review of epinephrine in the finger: to do or not to do. Plast Reconstr Surg 2001; 108:114–124.
60. Eaton JS, Grekin RC. Regional anesthesia of the face. Dermatol Surg 2001; 27:1006–1009.
61. Cohen SJ, Roenigk RK. Nerve blocks for cutaneous surgery of the foot. J Dermatol Surg Oncol 1991; 17:527–534.
62. Randle HW, Salassa JR, Roenigk. Local anesthesia for cutaneous lesions of the head and neck. Practical applications of peripheral nerve blocks. J Dermatol Surg Oncol 1992; 18:231–235.
63. Wilhelmi BJ, Blackwell SJ, Miller JH, et al. Do not use epinephrine in digital blocks: myth or truth? Plast Reconstr Surg 2001; 107:393.
64. Trindade de Almeida AR, Kadung BV, Martins de Oliveira EM. Improving botulinum toxin therapy for palmar hyperhidrosis: wrist bock and technical considerations. Dermatol Surg 2001; 27:34–36.
65. Earle AS, Blanchard JM. Regional anesthesia in the upper extremity. Clin Plast Surg 1985; 12:97–114.
66. Sarrafian SK, Ibrahim IN, Breihan JH. Ankle-foot peripheral nerve block for mid and forefoot surgery. Foot Ankle 1983; 4:86–90.
67. Faccenda KA, Finucane BT. Complications of regional anesthesia. Incidence and prevention. Drug Saf 2001; 24:413–42.
68. Heard CMB, LaJohn S, Fletcher JE. An accidental ring block of the great toe? Paediatr Anaesth 2001; 11:123.
69. Ben-David B. Complications of peripheral blockade. Anesthesiology Clin N Am 2002; 20:695–707.
70. O'Donnell J, Wilson K, Leonard PA. An avoidable complication of digital nerve block. Emerg Med J 2001: 18:316.
71. Grose DJ. Cigarette burn after tumescent anesthesia and intravenous sedation. Dermatol Surg 2003; 29:433–435.
72. McCaughey W. Adverse effects of local anesthetics. Drug Saf 1992; 7:178–189.
73. Finder RL, Moore PA. Adverse drug reactions to local anesthesia. Dent Clin North Am 2002; 46:747–757.
74. Mackley CL, Marks JG, Anderson BE. Delayed-type hypersensitivity to lidocaine. Arch Dermatol 2003; 139:343–346.
75. Bartfield JM, Jandreau SW, Raccio Robak. Randomized trial of diphenhydramine versus benzyl alcohol with epinephrine as an alternative to lidocaine local anesthesia. Ann Emerg Med 1998; 32:650–654.
76. Dire DJ, Hogan DE. Double-blinded comparison of diphenhydramine vs lidocaine as a local anesthetic. Ann Emerg Med 1993; 22:1419–1422.
77. Pang WW, Mok MS, Chang DP, Huang MH. Local anesthetic effect of tramadol, metoclopramide, and lidocaine following intradermal injection. Reg Anesth Pain Med 1998; 23:580–583.
78. Altunkaya H, Ozer Y, Kargi E, Babuccu O. Comparison of local anaesthetic effects of tramadol with prilocaine for minor surgical procedures. Br J Anaesth 2003; 90:320–322.
79. Pang WW, Mok MS, Chang DP, et al. Intradermal injection of tramadol has local anesthetic effect: a comparison with lidocaine. Acta Anaesthesiol Sin 1998; 36:133–136.
80. Klein JA, Kassarjdian N. Lidocaine toxicity with tumescent liposuction. A case report of probable drug interactions. Dermatol Surg 1997; 23:1169–1174.
81. Naguib M, Magboul MM, Samarkandi AH, et al. Adverse effects and drug interactions associated with local and regional anesthesia. Drug Saf 1998; 184:334–5.
82. Coleman MD, Coleman NA. Drug-induced methaemoglobinaemia. Treatment issues. Drug Saf 1996; 14:394–305.
83. Keel D, Goldman MP. Tumescent anesthesia in ambulatory phlebectomy: addition of epinephrine. Dermatol Surg 1999; 25:371–372.
84. Hanke CW. The tumescent facial block: tumescent local anesthesia and nerve block anesthesia for full-face laser resurfacing. Dermatol Surg 2001; 27:1003–1005.
85. Coleman WP, Klein JA. Use of the tumescent technique for scalp surgery, dermabrasion, and soft tissue reconstruction. J Dermatol Surg Oncol; 1992; 18:130–135.

4 Instruments and Materials

Melissa A Bogle MD and Aaron K Joseph MD

Summary box

- A skilled dermatologic surgeon requires knowledge of basic instrumentation and wound closure materials.
- Any dermatologist performing surgical procedures should invest in the highest quality instruments practical for their needs.
- Proper maintenance will enhance the longevity of surgical instrumentation and protect the surgeon's investment.
- Wound closure materials may be ordered according to the type, size, length, and color of suture material, as well as the type and size of the attached needle.
- Finely tuned surgical excision and repair trays can improve the efficiency and safety of office procedures.
- Proper safety procedures must be followed when working with surgical instrumentation to avoid injury to the patient, surgeon, or surgical personnel.

■ INTRODUCTION

Contemporary dermatology practice incorporates an ever-increasing number of surgical procedures. Knowledge of the best equipment and supplies to carry out particular procedures can make a good dermatologic surgeon even better. Properly organizing the surgical tray can greatly improve the efficiency and safety of everyone within the surgical suite. In addition, thorough instrument care will greatly extend the life of the tools and the investment of the surgeon.

■ TECHNICAL ASPECTS

Instruments

Scalpels, scissors, forceps, skin hooks, hemostats, needle holders, and curettes constitute the basic armamentarium of the dermatologic surgeon. In general, instruments used for dermatologic procedures are small, fine, and lightweight, allowing atraumatic handling of delicate tissues. All instruments are available in various grades of quality, and in general it is a good investment to use the best surgical instruments practical and affordable for a practitioner's needs.

Scalpel handles and blades

A scalpel consists of a blade and a handle. Blades are composed of either carbon steel or stainless steel. Carbon steel blades are sharper but dull fairly quickly with use. Stainless steel blades, on the other hand, are not as sharp but they will maintain their sharpness longer than carbon steel blades.[1] Scalpel blades are also available with Teflon coatings to reduce drag when cutting through tissue.[2]

The two basic types of scalpel handles are the Bard-Parker #3 handle and the Beaver handle (Fig. 4.1). The Bard-Parker #3 handle is flat or rounded, and is available with an etched ruler on the side which is helpful for intraoperative measurements. It is probably the most versatile handle and can hold a variety of scalpel blades including the #10, #11, and #15 Bard-Parker blades (Fig. 4.2). The #10 blade is wide with a sharp, convex belly,

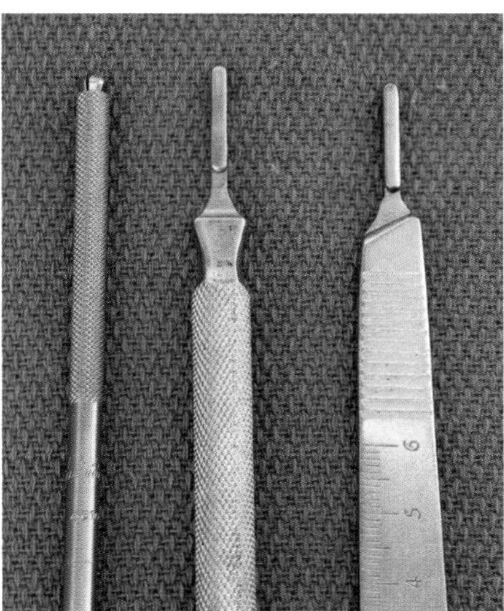

Figure 4.1 Scalpel handles: (left to right) the Beaver round knurled handle, the Bard-Parker round knurled #3 handle, and the Bard-Parker #3 standard handle.

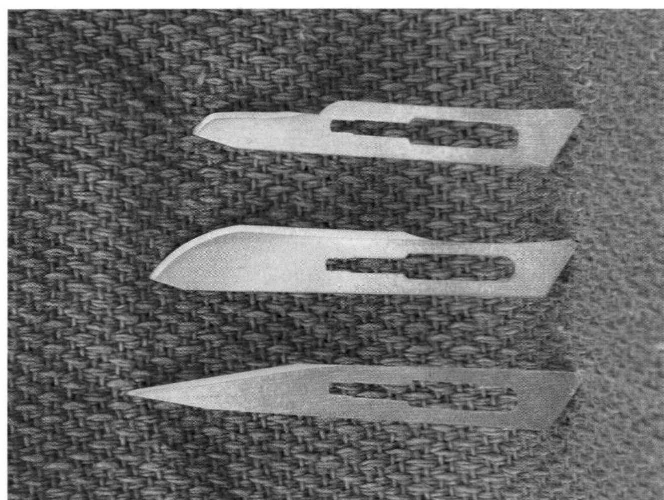

Figure 4.2 Scalpel blades: (top to bottom) the Bard-Parker #15, #10, and #11.

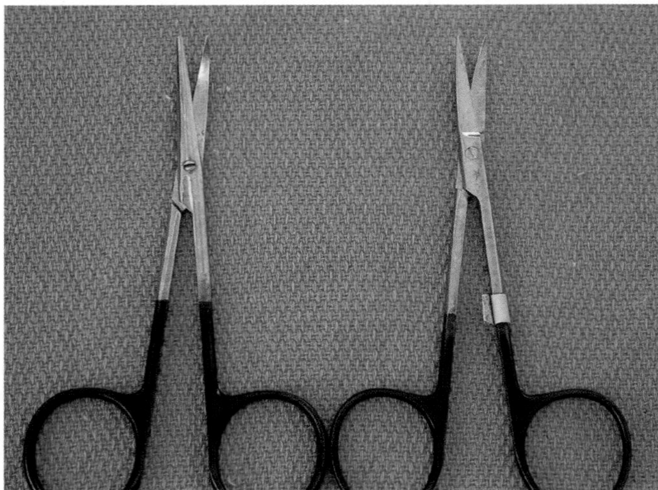

Figure 4.3 Scissors: curved iris scissor with two smooth blades (left), and straight Strabismus scissors with sharp tips (right).

making it ideal for large excisions on thick skin such as the trunk. The #11 blade is tapered to a sharp point and used primarily for incision and drainage or for cutting sharp angles on flaps. The #15 blade is the most commonly used blade in excisional surgery. It is shaped like a smaller version of the #10 blade with the sharpest portion at the tip. A variant of this is the #15c blade which is even smaller; this is used when working in areas of thin, delicate skin such as that around the eye.

The Beaver handle is round or hexagonal, like a pencil, and it holds a smaller, sharper blade (Fig. 4.1). It is the handle of choice for small, delicate work. Standard blades cannot be used with the Beaver-style handle as the blade is fitted between two jaws (a collet) which tighten when the handle is rotated. Like the Bard-Parker #3 handle, a choice of blades works well with the Beaver system. The two most commonly used are the #67 and #64 blades. The #67 Beaver blade is small and curved convexly with a sharp tip similar to the #15c blade. The #64 Beaver blade has a rounded tip with a sharp cutting edge which is useful for working in concavities such as the conchal bowl.

While not used in surgical excisions, a third cutting instrument that should be mentioned is the razor blade. The disposable double-edged razor blade is sharp, economical, and ideal for shave biopsies or removal of lesions on the surface of the skin (such as seborrheic keratoses). The surgeon has a relative degree of control over the depth of the shave according to how much curvature is applied to the blade. The blades are generally used from a clean, non-sterile package, as heat sterilization will dull the blade.[1] Single-edged prep razor blades are also available for removing hair preoperatively. The blades are designed to fit in a razor handle with or without a guard comb for lifting long, thick hair and for increased skin protection.

Scissors

There are many types of scissors available to the dermatologic surgeon. There are choices in the length of the handle (short or long), the blade (straight or curved, smooth or serrated), and the tip (sharp or blunt). Each feature affects the utility of the tool and makes it suited to a particular use. Respect for this knowledge will not only enhance a surgeon's skills but, will protect the scissor blade from dulling and keep the tips in good alignment. In general, short-handled scissors are useful for fine work and are probably the most versatile for delicate dermatologic surgeries on the head and neck. Long-handled scissors are ideal in cases where the surgeon must reach under tissue for a long distance, as occurs in extensive undermining or freeing up large flaps. Curved blades are ideal for blunt dissection and allow easy movement around tumors and cysts. Straight blades are used for gross trimming such as with flaps or grafts and cutting suture. Adding a serrated edge to the blade allows for less slipping of the tissue during cutting, making it particularly useful in areas of thin skin with little subcutaneous tissue. Finally, sharp-tipped scissors are used for dissection, whereas blunt-tipped scissors are better suited to atraumatic undermining and freeing up of flaps such as the island pedicle.

The iris scissor is a sharp-tipped, short-handled scissor most often used for blunt or sharp dissection and cutting on the head and neck. It is available with a straight or curved blade and also with a choice of either two smooth blades or one smooth blade and one serrated blade (Fig. 4.3). The Gradle scissor is similar to the iris except the blades are curved and tapered to a fine pointed tip. This makes it ideal for particularly delicate dissection as, for instance, in the periorbital region. The Westcott scissor is also good for delicate dissection around the eye area due to its sharp, fine, pointed tip. It is unique in that it operates on a spring system where the blades come together as the handle arc is squeezed. The Mayo scissor has an almost 1 to 1 handle to blade ratio and is used for coarse dissection (Fig. 4.4). The Metzenbaum scissor is a long-handled scissor that comes in varying lengths, making it ideal for blunt or sharp dissection in areas that require long reach. It also comes with either a straight or curved blade and a sharp or blunt tip (Fig. 4.4). The LaGrange scissor is a longer-handled scissor with a strongly curved tip and a reverse curve on the handle shank. It is used primarily to harvest hair transplant donor grafts but is also ideal for removing punch biopsy specimens.

Supercut scissors are a relatively new addition to the dermatologic surgeon's armamentarium. They are made with a special sharpening technique such that one of the

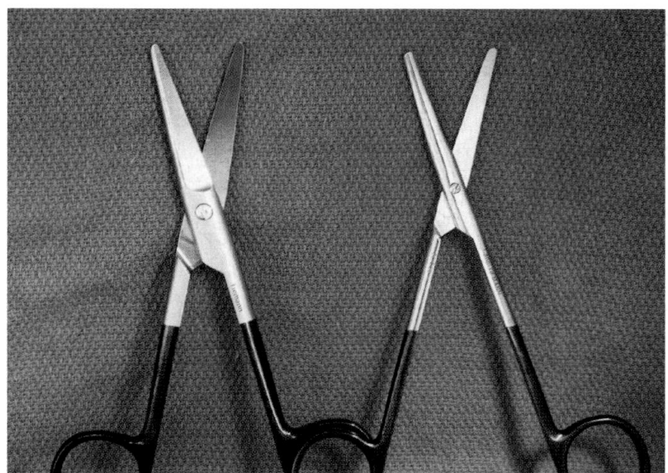

Figure 4.4 Scissors: the curved Mayo scissor (left), and the straight Metzenbaum scissor with blunted tips (right).

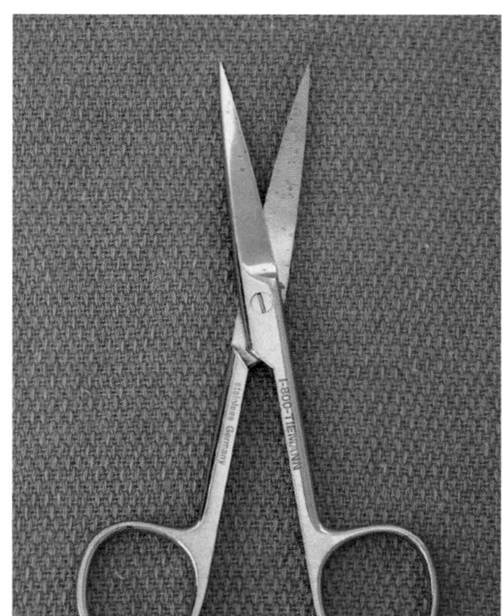

Figure 4.5 Scissors: general operating scissors for suture cutting.

blades has a razor edge. They are available as an option for most of the scissor models discussed above.

Finally, a short discussion of suture-cutting scissors is warranted (Fig. 4.5). While it is not crucial to buy separate scissors only for cutting suture, scissors that are used for cutting tissue will dull much faster if used to cut suture as well. As a general rule, fine, sharp, cutting instruments such as iris, Gradle, or Westcott scissors should never be used to cut suture. Distinct suture cutting scissors such as the Northbent scissor are available with a curved blade and a notch near the tip of one blade that particularly suits the purpose.

Forceps

Like the majority of instruments used in dermatologic surgery, forceps tend to be fine and lightweight. Their tips vary from smooth, to serrated, to toothed. The advantage of serrated forceps is that they allow firm grasp of tissue. However, they can easily cause crush injury in delicate areas, which may hinder optimal wound healing and cosmesis. Toothed forceps were developed to allow a firm grasp of tissue with reduced crush injury (Fig. 4.6).

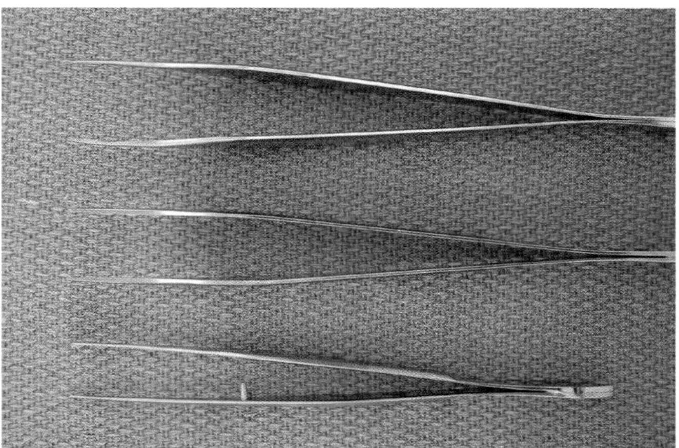

Figure 4.6 Forceps: (top to bottom) heavy, smooth, straight forceps, heavy 1 × 2 toothed straight forceps, and delicate 1 × 2 toothed straight forceps.

Adson forceps are the most versatile forceps. They have a relatively broad handle that tapers to a long, narrow tip. They come in both serrated and toothed models. Brown–Adson forceps are similar, but have a row of eight or nine tiny teeth along the length of the tips for enhanced tissue grasping. Bishop–Harmon forceps are small and delicate with fine tips, either with or without teeth. They are designed with three holes on each side of the handle, making them particularly lightweight and good for delicate work. Jeweler's (splinter) forceps are also small and delicate with an extremely fine and sharp tip. They are best used for grasping small vessels or retrieving suture fragments. Both the DeJardin and Graefe cartilage forceps have wide jaws with teeth used for grasping cartilage.

Skin hooks

Some surgeons prefer the use of skin hooks when manipulating tissue that is to be sutured or to simulate flap movements because hooks are far less traumatic to the epidermis. Skin hooks come in a variety of models, with single or multiple prongs, of varying length, sharpness, and curvature. Single-pronged and double-pronged skin hooks are used most commonly for stabilizing tissue that is to be sutured, and for executing flaps and grafts. They may also be used for planning and removing dog-ear defects and to retract the wound to give tension when placing buried or running sutures.

Hemostats

Hemostats are used for hemostasis of bleeding vessels. Their main use is in clamping off vessels either for electrocoagulation or ligation with suture. Like most instruments, those used in dermatologic surgery should be fine and lightweight. Probably the best-suited hemostat for cutaneous surgery is the Jacobsen hemostat because its fine tip is easily able to grasp small vessels. It is available in both curved and straight models.

Needle holders

There are a great variety of needle holders from which to choose. A general rule is to use a small needle holder with small needles and a large needle holder with large needles

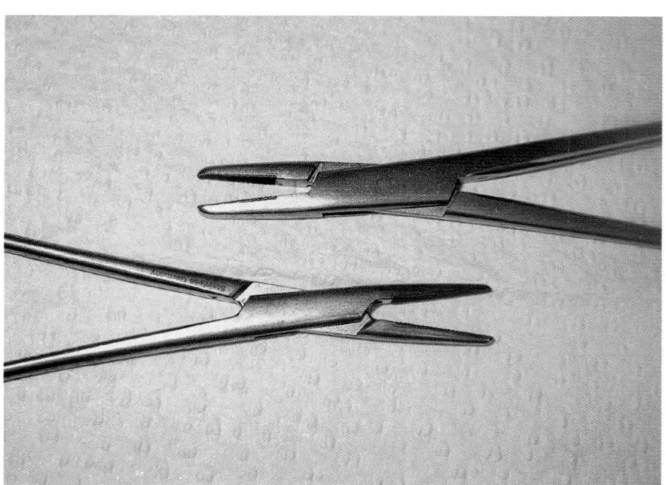

Figure 4.7 Needle holders: smooth (top) and fine-toothed (bottom) variants.

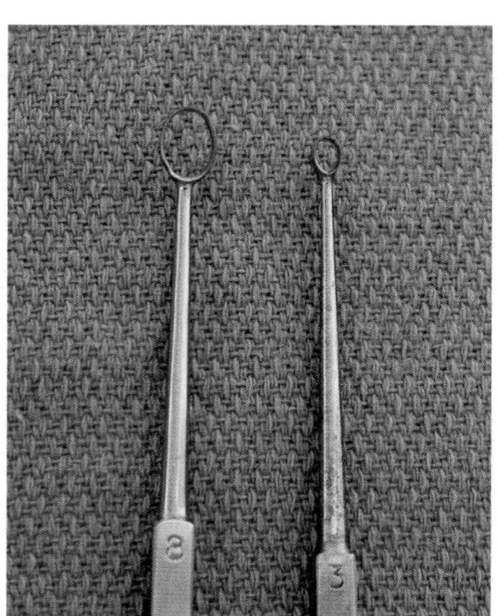

Figure 4.8 Curettes: large (left) and small (right) variants with oval heads.

to avoid needle slippage and damage to both the needle and the instrument. Apart from size, the jaws of needle holders also vary; they can be smooth or fine toothed (Fig. 4.7). Smooth jaws are less damaging to the fine needles and suture used in delicate procedures. In addition, high-end instruments often have metal alloy inserts on the working surface of the jaws, both for protection of the instrument and for secure grasping of the needle.

Crile–Wood needle holders are long with gently tapered, blunt tips. They are used primary when working with larger suture material (5-0 and larger) in areas such as the back or scalp. Neuro-smooth needle holders are similar but have narrow, parallel tips making them ideal for finer suture material (5-0 and smaller). The Webster needle holder is short with narrow jaws so that it is suitable for fine suture work in small, deep areas. The Castroviejo needle holder has a detachable spring handle similar to that of the Westcott scissor and is used for extremely delicate procedures such as those on the eyelid.

Curettes

Curettes are used primarily for the treatment of benign or low-grade malignant tumors and for debulking tumors prior to Mohs micrographic surgery. They come in many handle styles with either round or oval heads of varying sizes from 1 mm to 9 mm (Fig. 4.8). The choice of curette is largely personal preference, but smaller heads should be used for finer procedures. Furthermore, as with any instrument, care must be taken not to dull the sharp edge of the curette. A dull curette will create excessive tissue trauma and a suboptimal outcome.

Miscellaneous instruments

Other instruments that are useful in a dermatologic surgery suite include: towel clamps, periosteal elevators, bone chisels, and nail splitters. Towel clips come in conventional or cross-action models of varying sizes. They are useful for securing towels during lengthy procedures and for anchoring the electrocautery handle within the surgical field. They may also be used for holding skin under tension, as with large scalp wounds. Periosteal elevators and bone chisels are useful when working on the head and neck for sampling periosteum or bone thought to be invaded by tumor. In addition, elevators can be used to aid in nail avulsion procedures.

Wound closure materials

A thorough understanding of suture materials and needles is essential in dermatologic surgery.[3,4] The choice of materials is dictated by the procedure and the personal preference of the surgeon. Sutures may be ordered according to the type, size, length, and color of suture material as well as the type and size of attached needle. Like suture, needle selection depends upon the type and location of wound closure as well as the size of the associated suture material.

Suture

The choice of suture material (Table 4.1) requires an understanding of certain descriptive terms. Tensile strength is analogous to the strength of the suture and is calculated by dividing the weight necessary to break the suture by its cross-sectional area. Sutures with larger diameters generally have greater tensile strengths, however the type and configuration of suture material also contributes. Smaller 5-0 and 6-0 sutures are used on the face and neck, while 3-0 and 4-0 sutures are used on the trunk and extremities. Wounds with a great deal of tension will require 3-0 or 4-0 sutures.

Suture configuration refers to whether it is composed of a single strand (monofilament) or multiple strands (polyfilament). Polyfilament sutures can be braided to increase the ease of handling but have a higher incidence of wound infection.[3] This occurs because the braided configuration has crevices that may harbor bacteria in a wound and a high capillarity that may 'wick' bacteria into a wound.

Elasticity refers to a suture material's ability to stretch (e.g. with wound edema) and then return to its original form. Plasticity, on the other hand, refers to a suture material's ability to stretch and maintain its new length. Memory defines the stiffness of the suture and its inherent ability to return to its original shape after deformation. Sutures with high memory are generally more difficult to handle and tie. Knot strength is the force required to cause knot slippage and it depends on the smoothness and

Table 4.1 Sutures used in skin surgery

Absorbability	Suture (Trade Name)	Configuration	Uses
Absorbable	Surgical gut	Virtually monofilament	Rarely used but good for skin graft closure, tying off superficial vessels, wound closure in children
	Polyglycolic acid (Dexon)	Polyfilament	Buried sutures
	Polyglactin 910 (Vicryl)	Polyfilament	Subcutaneous closure, vessel ligature
	Polydioxanone (PDS)	Monofilament	Where infection would cause significant discomfort, e.g. cartilage
	Polyglyconate (Maxon)	Monofilament	Subcutaneous closure in high-tension areas
Non-absorbable	Silk	Polyfilament	Mucosal surfaces, around eyelids, intertriginous areas
	Nylon: Ethilon, Dermalon	Monofilament	Skin closure
	Nylon: Surgilon, Nurolon	Polyfilament	Skin closure
	Polypropylene: Prolene, Surgilene	Monofilament	Subcuticular running intradermal sutures
	Polyester: Mersilene, Dacron, Ethibond	Polyfilament	Mucosal surfaces
	Polybutester: Novafil	Monofilament	Subcuticular running; elasticity responds well to wound edema
	Stainless steel	Monofilament and polyfilament	Tendon repair

memory of the suture. Finally, tissue reactivity refers to the body's inflammatory response to a given suture material. In general, monofilament and synthetic sutures have less tissue reactivity than polyfilament and natural sutures.[3]

The broadest distinction in suture materials is between absorbable and non-absorbable sutures. Absorbable suture, by definition, loses most of its tensile strength within 60 days of placement through either enzymatic digestion or tissue hydrolysis. Absorbable sutures are used mainly for buried stitches to close the dermis and decrease epidermal wound tension. Commonly used absorbable sutures include surgical gut, polyglycolic acid (Dexon; Davis and Geck Inc, Tyco Healthcare Group LP, Mansfield, MA), polyglactin 910 (Vicryl; Ethicon Inc, Johnson and Johnson Co, Somerville, NJ), and polydioxanone (PDS (Ethicon)) and polyglyconate (Maxon (Davis and Geck)).

Surgical gut is a natural suture made from animal collagen. It is available plain or treated with chromium salts for increased strength and decreased tissue reactivity. Both varieties come packaged in alcohol and will break easily if allowed to dry out. Surgical gut is rapidly degraded in 4–5 days making it useful for epidermal approximation of skin grafts, for tying off superficial blood vessels, or closure of wounds in children where it may be challenging to remove sutures at a later date. A fast-absorbing variant also exists which is heat-treated so that it absorbs completely in 2–4 weeks. The disadvantages of surgical gut include poor tensile strength, high tissue reactivity, and poor knot stability. The body's significant inflammatory response occurs because the suture is broken down by lysosomal proteolytic enzymes as opposed to hydrolysis.

Absorbable polyfilament sutures include polyglycolic acid (Dexon) and polyglactin 910 (Vicryl). Polyglycolic acid (Dexon) is a braided synthetic polymer of glycolic acid and loses approximately 50% of its strength at 2–3 weeks. It is broken down by tissue hydrolysis that decreases tissue reactivity and inflammation. Its main use is for buried sutures, however it should be avoided in contaminated wounds due to its braided configuration and higher incidence of infection. If placed too superficially, the sutures may be transepidermally eliminated ('spit') before they have a chance to be completely absorbed. Polyglycolic acid is available in either a clear or green color, and can be either coated (Dexon Plus) or uncoated (Dexon-S). The coated variety allows the suture to pass more easily through tissue. Polyglactin 910 (Vicryl) is a braided synthetic copolymer of lactide and glycolide which is similar to polyglycolic acid but with a lubricant coating of polyglactin 370 and calcium stearate for easier pull through tissue. It has a high tensile strength, minimal tissue reactivity, and is available in either a white or violet color. The violet color should be avoided in areas of thin skin where it may be visible through the closed wound.

Absorbable monofilament sutures include polydioxanone (PDS) and polyglyconate (Maxon). Polydioxanone (PDS) is a synthetic polymer of *p*-dioxanone with a very high tensile strength and minimal tissue reactivity. It is absorbed much more slowly than Dexon or Vicryl suture, retaining approximately 74% of its strength at 2 weeks and not completely dissolving until 180 days. It is ideal for suturing areas such as cartilage, where tissue inflammation would cause significant discomfort, and it is a better choice for wounds that may be contaminated because of its monofilament configuration. The main disadvantage of polydioxanone is that it can be stiff and difficult to work with and tie. Polyglyconate (Maxon) is composed of glycolic acid and trimethylene carbonate and is similar to polydioxanone in terms of tensile strength. Its main advantage is that it is not as stiff as polydioxanone so that it has greater knot stability and easier handling.

Non-absorbable sutures are resistant to degradation and will maintain most of their tensile strength at 60 days after placement. The most common are silk, nylon, polypropylene (Prolene, Surgilene), polyester, and stainless steel.

Silk is a natural braided fiber that handles very well and is easy to tie. It is unlikely to tear tissue and can lie flat in areas such as mucosal surfaces, around eyelids, and in intertriginous areas. It has a relatively low tensile strength compared to the other non-absorbable sutures, retaining only 0–50% of its original strength at 1 year. The disadvantages of silk are its high tissue reactivity and increased potential for wound infection due to the braided configuration.

Nylon is a synthetic polyamide polymer with low tissue reactivity, excellent elasticity, and high tensile strength. It is available in a variety of configurations including monofilamentous (Ethilon (Ethicon) and Dermalon (Davis and Geck)) or polyfilamentous (Surgilon (Ethicon) and Nurolon (Ethicon)). The monofilament variety comes in black, green and clear colors. Its major disadvantage is high memory, causing more difficult handling and knot tying capabilities. The braided polyfilament variant is easier to handle.

Polypropylene (Prolene (Ethicon), Surgilene (Davis and Geck)) is a flexible synthetic monofilament of linear hydrocarbon polymers. It has good tensile strength, little tissue reactivity, and a smooth surface allowing it to pull easily through tissue. This is useful for subcuticular running intradermal sutures. Its plasticity allows it to accommodate tissue swelling, however it does not retract once the swelling subsides which can lead to poor wound approximation. The disadvantages of polypropylene are that its memory and smoothness can compromise knot security.

Polyester suture is a braided synthetic polyfilament of polyethylene terephthalate. It has minimal tissue reactivity and an extremely high tensile strength, remaining in tissue indefinitely. It is available in either a green or white color, and either uncoated (Mersilene (Ethicon) and Dacron (Davis and Geck)) or coated with polybutilate (Ethibond (Ethicon)) to allow for easier pull through tissue. The braided configuration gives it better handling and knot tying capabilities than nylon or polypropylene, and it has less risk for infection than silk because it is synthetic. Polybutester (Novafil (Davis and Geck)) is a monofilamentous suture composed of polyglycol terephthalate and polybutylene terephthalate. It combines the high tensile strength, low tissue reactivity, and easy handling capabilities of polyester with the plasticity and smoothness of polypropylene.

Stainless steel suture is extremely strong and maintains its strength indefinitely. It is available in monofilament or polyfilament (twisted or braided) varieties. It is difficult to tie without breaking and has a tendency to cut through tissue. Although rarely used in dermatologic surgery, it is a good choice for tendon repair.

Needles

Needles are designed to carry suture material through the skin with minimal tissue trauma. The needle itself is divided into the shank that connects to the suture, the body, and sharp point. The body of the needle comes in round, triangular or flattened varieties. Round bodies will gradually taper to a point and triangular bodies have cutting edges on three sides. Flattened bodies are designed to eliminate needle twisting during procedures. Some needles will have ridges along the body to aid in securing the needle in the needle holder. The curvature of the needle arc varies, but the most commonly used in dermatologic surgery are from $\frac{3}{8}$ to $\frac{1}{2}$ circle.

The needle point is available in three variants: conventional cutting, reverse cutting, and round with a tapered point (Fig. 4.9). Conventional cutting points are triangular in cross-section with a cutting edge on the inside of the needle arc. Reverse cutting points have a cutting edge on the outside of the needle arc to minimize the risk of tearing through tissue when placing a stitch. Round point needles have no cutting edges and are less likely to tear tissue. They are used primarily for suturing fascia, muscle, and aponeuroses.

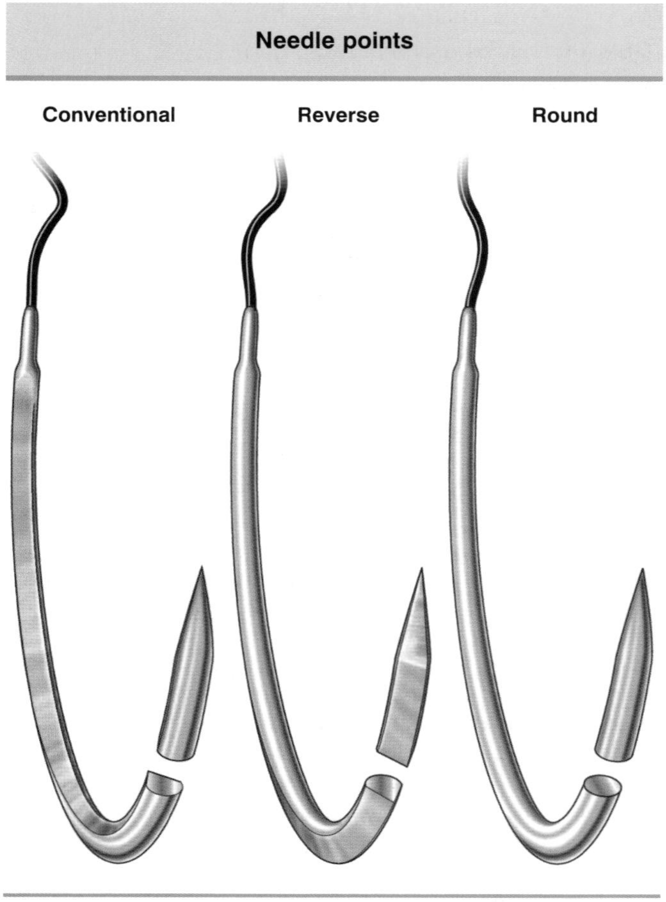

Figure 4.9 Needle points: (left to right) conventional cutting, reverse cutting, and round.

Different manufacturers have different nomenclature for needles and identification is not standardized. The most commonly used series in dermatologic surgery are those made by Ethicon and Davis and Geck. Ethicon manufactures the for skin (FS), plastic skin (PS), precision point (P), and precision cosmetic (PC) needles. The FS is a large, inexpensive, reverse cutting needle with a triangular body for use on thick skin or for buried sutures. The PS is also a reverse cutting needle, however it is sharper than the FS and good for cosmetic procedures. The P is similar to the PS but smaller and even sharper for fine cosmetic work. The PS and P styles both have an oval body that is flattened on the sides. The PC is a sharp, conventional cutting needle with a flattened body for less tissue trauma in delicate cosmetic work.

Davis and Geck manufactures the cutting (CE), plastic reverse (PRE), skin closure (SC), and slim blade (SBE) needles. The E designates a $\frac{3}{8}$ circle needle. The CE is a reverse cutting needle comparable to the Ethicon FS needle. The PRE is a sharp, reverse cutting needle which is ideal for fine cosmetic work similar to the Ethicon PS and P needles. The SC is a conventional cutting needle, and the SBE is a reverse cutting needle with a very thin body. Also available is the diamond point (DP) needle which has a more precise tip.

■ OPTIMIZING OUTCOMES

It is important to properly care for surgical instruments to get the maximum longevity and function out of each tool. As previously stressed, instruments are geared for a particular use, so using a tool to perform a function outside of that use may damage the instrument and shorten its lifespan. Instruments must also be properly cleaned after use.[5]

Ideally, all instruments should be placed in a solution with warm water and a commercially available instrument detergent promptly after use. After soaking, the instruments are gently scrubbed with a plastic brush to remove foreign matter and organic debris. An ultrasonic cleaner may be used to dislodge particulate matter that is not otherwise removed, but adds to instrument wear and tear.[6] The instruments are then rinsed with water to remove detergent and allowed to dry completely. If the instruments are not allowed to dry completely before sterilization they can become stained from water spots.[5] This is also a good time to inspect the instruments for signs of disrepair. Scissor blades should be inspected to make sure they do not have nicks or malapproximation at the tips. Forceps, hemostats, and needle holders should also be checked to make sure the tips meet properly and they are in good working order. If needed, instruments can be lubricated at the hinge with a water- and steam-soluble solution such as instrument milk. Oils or grease should never be used for lubrication as they will turn hard during the sterilization process and cause the joint to become stiff.[5]

There are four main types of instrument sterilization. Dry-heat sterilization is advantageous because it will not corrode the instruments, however the instruments cannot be placed in the standard paper or plastic packages due to the high temperatures during sterilization. This creates a problem when storing the instruments in a sterile fashion for later use. This type of sterilization is most commonly used for rapid sterilization of a contaminated instrument needed for a particular procedure.[6] Steam sterilization is the most popular office method of sterilization. This type of autoclave uses high temperature and pressure to destroy microorganisms. One drawback is that steam autoclaves may dull sharp instruments because of the humidity.[2] The chemical autoclave is similar but uses formaldehyde and alcohol instead of distilled water so there is less dulling of the instruments. The final type of sterilization is ethylene oxide gas sterilization. The setup for this type of sterilization is impractical in an office-based setting, but it is useful for devices that would be otherwise destroyed by heat or moisture, such as dermabrasion handpieces, electrosurgical handles, or wiring. Cold sterilization is not considered adequate for invasive surgical procedures.[6]

■ PITFALLS AND THEIR MANAGEMENT

Any chapter on surgical instrumentation should include a discussion on preventing injury to the surgeon, the patient, or one of the surgical personnel. The first recommendation when using sharps is to always work away from the surgeon's own hand or an assistant's hand that may be in the field.[7] Furthermore, tissue should be handled strictly with instruments such as forceps or skin hooks to avoid unnecessarily exposing hands to the field. Likewise sharp objects such as needles or scalpel blades should be handled with another instrument such as a needle holder or forceps. If a hand must enter the surgical field when a sharp instrument is present, for example for blotting tissue, only one hand should be in the field and the sharp instrument should not be moving at the same time. All parties should wear properly fitted gloves, as loose gloves may obscure the field and make it difficult to hold sharp instruments properly.[7] The surgical tray should be kept clean at all times and all instruments should point in the same direction, away from the surgeon's hand. Needles or sharp instruments should not be obscured by gauze pads or unnecessary items like discarded needle sleeves. Needle recapping should be avoided.

Avoidance of pitfalls

- Keep surgical trays, and the area in which surgery is performed, well organized and tidy to avoid injury from instruments.
- Handle instruments correctly to avoid injury.
- Use fitted gloves both for precision and so that the field of view is not obscured.

■ PRACTICAL APPLICATIONS

Surgical instruments can be set up on a Mayo surgical stand with a removable stainless steel tray. The Mayo stand comes in two styles: an easily maneuverable four-wheeled version and a two-wheeled version. The stand may be adjusted to the desired height. Trays should be kept neat and all instruments should be placed so that needle-stick injuries are minimized. Two trays can be prepared and sterilized for use: an excision tray and a repair tray.

The organization of the excision tray is important for safety and efficiency (Fig. 4.10). At the very least it should contain a scalpel handle, a ruler, a curette for debulking tumors, tissue scissors, forceps, and either a marking pen or a cup containing Gentian violet to delineate tumor margins for Mohs micrographic surgery or excision. The excision

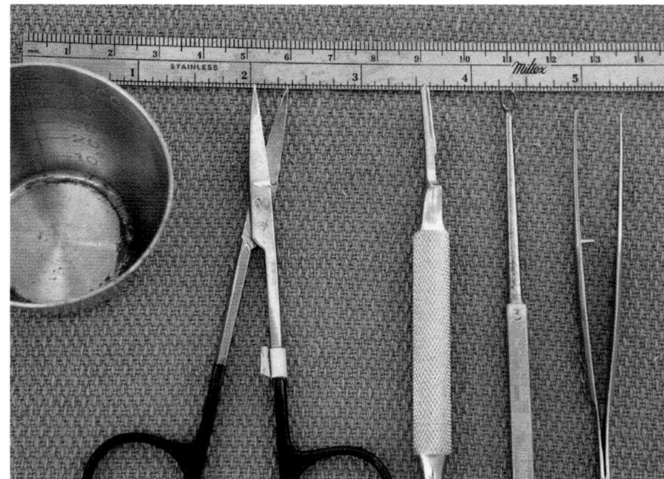

Figure 4.10 Mohs layer/excision tray containing a ruler, stainless steel cup, tissue scissors, scalpel handle, curette and forceps.

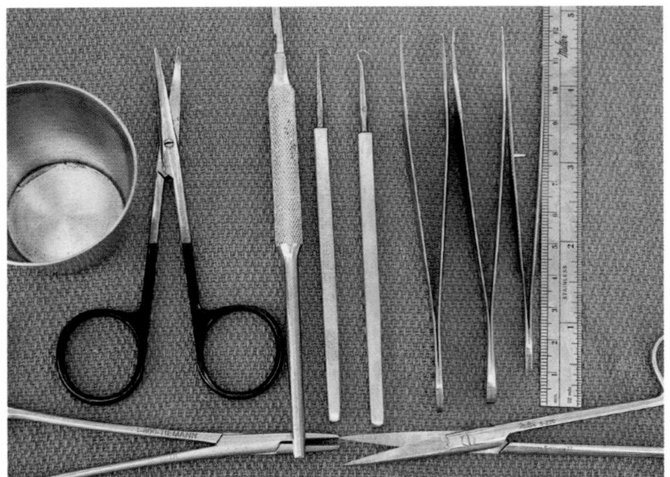

Figure 4.11 Repair tray containing tissue and suture scissors, a scalpel, skin hooks, a variety of forceps, a needle holder, ruler and a stainless steel cup.

tray should also contain towel clamps for holding sterile drapes if the drapes are not self-adhering. Sterile gauze, scalpel blades, and Telfa (Tyco Healthcare Group LP, Mansfield, MA) pads to transport surgical specimens to the laboratory should be added when the tray is opened. Cotton-tipped applicators are also useful for hemostasis and the stick can be used for marking with Gentian violet.

The repair tray should contain roughly the same items as the excision tray, plus additional specific instruments (Fig. 4.11). The repair tray may also include a needle holder, undermining and suture-cutting scissors, a variety of forceps, skin hooks, and a cup with sterile saline for storing skin grafts. Sterile gauze, cotton-tipped applicators, scalpel blades, and suture should be added when the tray is opened.

■ SUMMARY

Knowledge of surgical instruments and wound closure materials is important to the dermatologic surgeon. The surgeon should invest in the highest quality tools available and should take care to maintain the instruments properly, to optimize their effectiveness and durability. Likewise, well-planned surgical excision and repair trays will improve the efficiency and overall safety of surgical procedures.

■ REFERENCES

1. Neuberg M. Instrumentation in dermatologic surgery. Semin Dermatol 1994; 13:10–19.
2. Weber LA. The surgical tray. Dermatol Clin 1998; 16:17–24.
3. Ratner D, Nelson BR, Johnson TM. Basic suture materials and suturing techniques. Semin Dermatol 1994; 13:20–6.
4. Campbell JR, Marks A. Suture materials and suturing techniques. In Practice 1985; 7:72–5.
5. Sebben JE. Sterilization and care of surgical instruments and supplies. J Am Acad Dermatol 1984; 11:381–92.
6. Geisse JK. The dermatologic surgical suite. Semin Dermatol 1994; 13:2–9.
7. Trizna Z, Wagner RF. Preventing self-inflicted injuries to the dermatologic surgeon. J Am Acad Dermatol 2001, 44:520–522.

5 Patient Evaluation, Informed Consent, Preoperative Assessment and Care

Howard Fein MD and Allison T Vidimos RPh MD

Summary box

- Preoperative consultation should include the following elements: medical, surgical and social history, list of current medications, thorough physical examination, and explanation of any proposed procedure.
- Medical conditions may impact outcomes of cutaneous surgery, including pregnancy, hypertension, and cardiovascular disease.
- The potential risks, benefits, and alternatives of the proposed surgical procedure must be adequately discussed in order to obtain informed consent.

INTRODUCTION

The preoperative surgical evaluation is often the initial and perhaps most important encounter between a surgeon and prospective patient. It is during this critical time that the physician can adequately assess the patient's particular medical problem, and determine suitability for a particular procedure, as well as discuss relevant underlying health problems. Preoperative evaluations additionally allow physicians ample opportunity to make appropriate changes to the patient's medications and to explain the various risks, benefits, and alternatives to the proposed surgical procedure. Patients benefit in many ways: they have the opportunity to gain a thorough understanding of the proposed treatment, to have questions or concerns addressed, and they have an opportunity to consider possible treatment alternatives. Lastly, preoperative evaluations can help enhance the physician–patient relationship by creating an open, two-way dialogue.

The consultation area

In general, a clean well-lit area will suffice for most purposes. Consider replacing the standard bulbs in fluorescent ceiling light fixtures with full-spectrum bulbs which more accurately replicate the wavelengths of natural sunlight and better reveal skin tones. Full-spectrum light bulbs are relatively inexpensive and are readily available from retailers (including Lowe's and Home Depot in the USA). A portable overhead light, or simply a flashlight, is useful for illuminating localized areas of skin that cause concern.

All consultation rooms should be equipped with a sink, along with a supply of clean towels and non-irritating facial cleanser because patients may need to remove their make-up to allow for adequate cutaneous examination. Mirrors, both hand-held and wall-mounted, are essential for allowing patients to point out particular areas of concern.

A powered examination table is desirable and allows for comfortable and safe positioning of patients during the physical examination (Chapter 10). Although the cost of these tables can be significant, certain discounts and tax deductions may be available when purchasing at a professional society exhibit, or under the Americans with Disabilities Act; interested physicians should consult their tax professional. In addition, all rooms should be equipped with comfortable chairs in which patients and their significant other(s) can wait before the consultation.

Consider placing pamphlets detailing the various procedures performed in your office on wall-mounted racks. If patients will be spending considerable time waiting in the room a supply of current magazines is also a nice diversion.

During the initial preoperative consultation it is important for the physician to respect and maintain the patient's privacy. We have found that using an opaque, retractable curtain in all rooms for patients to change behind is an invaluable fixture. The consulting physician should attempt to give their complete attention to the patient during the visit. Unnecessary distractions, whether from incoming phone calls, pagers, or office staff interruptions, should be kept to a minimum.

Components of the preoperative consultation

The primary goals of the preoperative consultation are to evaluate, to educate, and to obtain informed consent. While the exact details of the initial consultation may vary depending on such factors as whether or not the patient is new to the practice, the patient's prior medical knowledge, and particular medical problem, the overall components of the preoperative consultation remain unchanged. The following six elements should be included in every preoperative consultation:

- medical history
- surgical history with an emphasis on past dermatologic and/or cosmetic procedures
- complete medication list including use of over-the-counter (OTC) drugs, vitamins and nutritional supplements
- problem-focused physical examination (Fig. 5.1)
- social history
- detailed explanation of the proposed procedure, treatment alternatives, and informed consent.

Medical history

The basic components of a medical history include a detailed accounting of current and past medical conditions, possible drug or latex allergies, as well as current drug and nutritional supplement use. Obtaining a medical history can be facilitated through the use of preprinted patient questionnaires, which can be completed at the time of the preoperative evaluation. A sample questionnaire, as shown in Figure 5.2, can be further modified to meet the needs of each practice.

Medical conditions affecting cutaneous surgery

The underlying health status of each patient should be carefully considered before any surgical procedure. In fact, several medical conditions can be identified that may effect the intraoperative and postoperative success of a given procedure.

Pregnancy

Pregnancy should always be considered as a possibility in women of childbearing age. Screening questions for occult pregnancy should be included in the medical history questionnaire. Since medications such as local anesthetics and antibiotics—commonly used in the perioperative setting—may act as potential teratogens, each should be considered carefully. Non-emergent surgical procedures should be delayed until the postpartum period; however exceptions will arise. The US Food and Drug Administration (FDA) has categorized the teratogenic risk of medications using an A to X rating scale.[1] In general, category A and category B medications can be used safely used during pregnancy, while medications belonging to categories C, D, and X cannot.

Local anesthetics can cross the placental barrier and may accumulate preferentially in the fetus.[2] Potential complications from use of local anesthetic during pregnancy include both fetal bradycardia and central nervous system toxicity. Lidocaine and prilocaine are listed as pregnancy category B agents and are the preferred anesthetics for use during pregnancy. Furthermore, several studies examining the use of lidocaine during pregnancy have shown no increase in adverse fetal events or teratogenicity.[3–5] A similar safety profile is not seen with other amide anesthetics, as intrauterine exposure to both bupivicaine and mepivacaine has been associated with an increased risk for fetal bradycardia.[6] Epinephrine (noradrenaline), which is frequently combined with local anesthetics such as lidocaine, is pregnancy category C and should be used cautiously.

Pregnant patients may require antibiotics in the perioperative setting. Appropriate pregnancy class B antibiotics include penicillin and cephalexin. In penicillin-allergic patients, erythromycin base, and azithromycin are both pregnancy category B, and are acceptable alternatives. Category D antibiotics that are contraindicated in pregnancy include erythromycin estolate, tetracycline, doxycycline, and minocycline. Erythomycin estolate has been associated with hepatotoxicity when taken during pregnancy.[7] Intrapartum use of tetracycline may result in staining of fetal dental enamel and must be avoided.[8]

Hypertension

Blood pressure should be checked during the preoperative consultation. Elevated blood pressure may be associated with increased intraoperative and postoperative bleeding and can complicate the process of wound reconstruction. The use of epinephrine-containing local anesthetics may lead to vasoconstriction, which can further elevate blood pressure. The increased bleeding risk associated with uncontrolled hypertension is perhaps most apparent when working on highly vascular structures such as the nose and scalp.

Patients with persistently elevated blood pressure, who have not previously been diagnosed with hypertension, should be referred to their primary care physician for further evaluation. In our practice, hypertensive patients with a systolic pressure of greater than 170 mmHg and/or a diastolic pressure greater than 100 mmHg are routinely excluded from surgical procedures until their blood pressure can be further lowered. Beyond bleeding risk, exacerbation of hypertension perioperatively may lead to stroke.

Cardiovascular disease

Patients with underlying cardiac disease may have an increased complication risk during surgical procedures and should be identified during the preoperative consultation. Special attention must be given to patients with a history of coronary artery disease, cardiomyopathy, and cardiac valve disease.

Epinephrine (adrenaline) is commonly added to local anesthetic solutions. It is an α-adrenergic agonist and as such has both cardiostimulatory and vasoconstrictive effects which could tax the heart in a person with cardiac disease.[9] Studies performed in patients with advanced cardiac disease, however, showed that small volumes of epinephrine-containing anesthetics could be given safely without significant adverse consequences.[10] Judicious use of epinephrine (adrenaline) is nevertheless advisable in these patients and can be accomplished through use of highly dilute solutions, such as 1 : 200 000, 1 : 500 000, or even 1 : 1 000 000.

Various cardiac conditions are associated with an increased risk for developing bacterial endocarditis following a surgical procedure.[11] The risk associated with each condition has been stratified into high, moderate, and low or negligible categories by the American Heart Association (AHA) (Chapter 9).[11] High-risk categories include patients

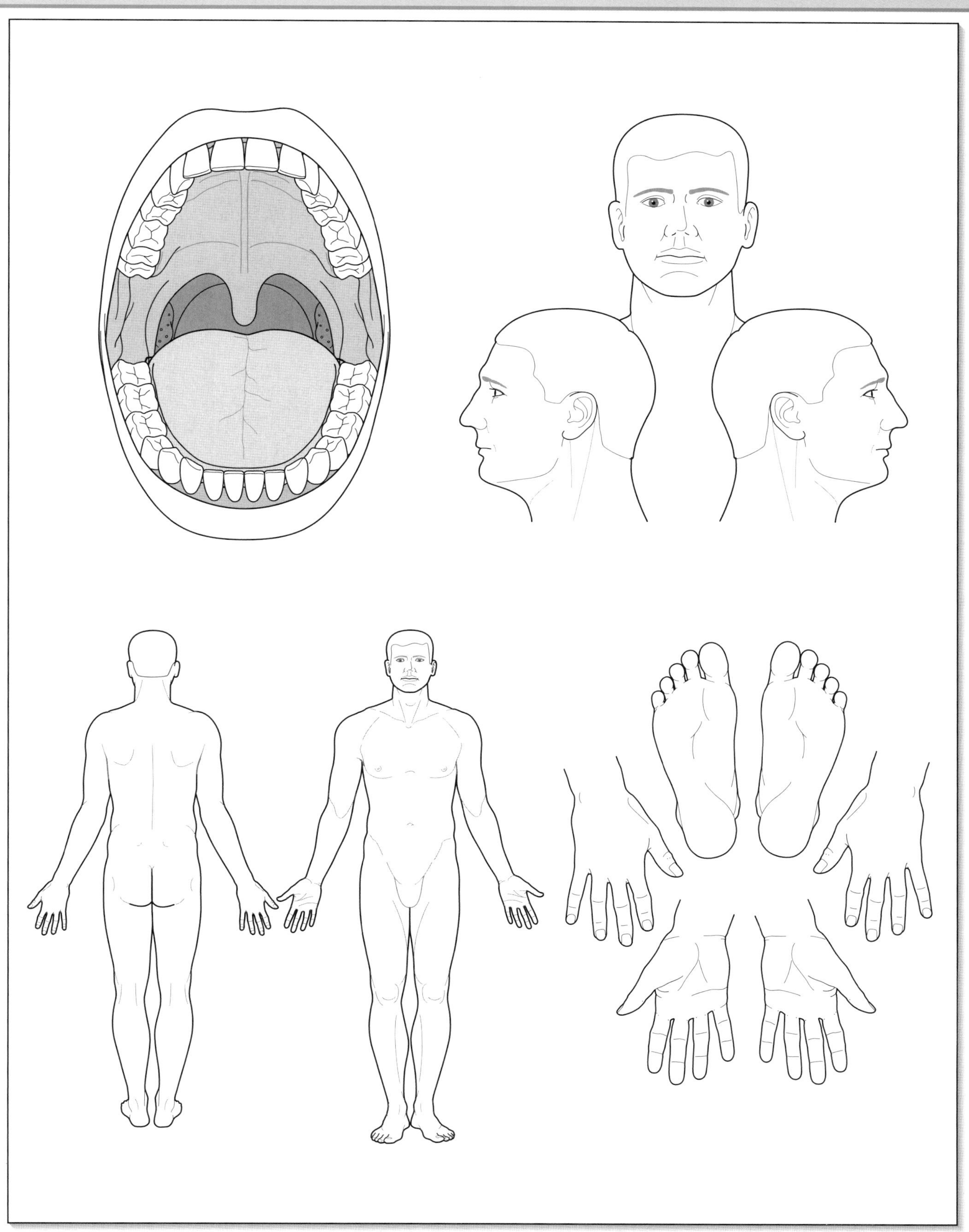

Figure 5.1 Problem-focused physical examination.

Dermatology health questionnaire

HEALTH QUESTIONNAIRE

1

IMPRINT/LABEL

Age: ....

Occupation: .... Name of referring doctor: ....

Why are you seeing the dermatologist today? ....

Prior treatments used for it? ....

What part(s) of your body is(are) affected? .... Have you had it before? ....

How long have you had the problem? .... Does it bleed? ....

Does it itch? .... Does it hurt? .... Has it formed an open wound? ....

Has it been infected? ....

List all current medications (including non-prescription and vitamins): **If none, check here** ❒

Name of Drug	Dosage	Route	Frequency

List all medication allergies: **If none, check here** ❒

Drug ....

....

List hospitalizations for major illnesses and surgeries: ....

....

....

....

Figure 5.2 A patient health questionnaire.

Dermatology health questionnaire (continued)

2

Past personal skin problems:

- ❐ Abnormal moles
- ❐ Melanoma
- ❐ Skin cancer
- ❐ Thick scars or keloid
- ❐ Eczema or Dermatitis
- ❐ Other – specify..
- ❐ Psoriasis
- ❐ Acne

Family history of skin disease:

- ❐ Eczema or Dermatitis
- ❐ Skin cancer
- ❐ Keloids
- ❐ Abnormal moles
- ❐ Melanoma
- ❐ Other – specify..
- ❐ Psoriasis
- ❐ Cancer (*not skin*)

Do you need to take antibiotics before routine dental cleaning? ❐ Yes ❐ No

If yes, why?..

Habits:

Alcohol (amount per week)..

Tobacco (amount per day)..

Aspirin (number per day)..

Do you have any of the following conditions? if yes, place a check:

- ❐ Pacemaker
- ❐ Hepatitis
- ❐ Anemia
- ❐ Gout
- ❐ Artificial heart valve
- ❐ High blood pressure
- ❐ Asthma
- ❐ Diabetes
- ❐ AIDS or HIV infection
- ❐ Thyroid problems
- ❐ Heart murmur
- ❐ Artificial joint
- ❐ Arthritis
- ❐ Cancer (*not skin cancer*)
- ❐ None of the above
- ❐ Other – specify:..

Women only:

Are you pregnant? ❐ Yes ❐ No ❐ Not sure

Are you trying to become pregnant? ❐ Yes ❐ No

Are your menstrual periods regular? ❐ Yes ❐ No

Date of last menstrual period:..

Birth Control method:..

Signature:.. Date:............../............../..............

Reviewed by:.. Beeper#:..

Figure 5.2, continued

with prosthetic valves, a previous history of endocarditis, complex congenital cyanotic heart disease, and surgically constructed systemic–pulmonary shunts or conduits. Moderate-risk patients include those with hypertrophic cardiomyopathy and mitral valve prolapse with regurgitation. Low- or negligible-risk categories include people with implanted cardiac pacemakers and defibrillators, with physiologic heart murmurs, surgically repaired atrial or ventral septal defects. Coronary artery stenting is an increasingly popular cardiovascular procedure and is fairly common among patients undergoing dermatologic surgery. Although no formal AHA guidelines exist regarding the use of prophylactic antibiotics in these patients, some authors have advocated antibiotic prophylaxis for periods ranging from one to six months after stent implantation.[12] The rationale behind these recommendations is presumably to allow for complete re-epithelialization of the implanted stent device. In summary, the exact antibiotic prophylaxis recommendations for dermatologic surgery are unclear as official skin-specific guidelines do not exist, leaving physicians to adapt regimens intended for 'dental, oral, respiratory tract, or esophageal procedures.'

In most cases, a single dose of 2 g of amoxicillin given 1 hour preoperatively is the preferred prophylactic regimen for bacterial endocarditis.[11] In penicillin-allergic patients, alternatives include cephalexin 2 g, azithromycin 500 mg, or clindamycin 600 mg given 1 hour preoperatively.[11] Patients who are unable to take medications orally can be given prophylaxis with either 600 mg of clindamycin or 1 g cefazolin, intravenously or intramuscularly, 30 minutes preoperatively.[11]

Although the risk of bacterial endocarditis for patients undergoing dermatologic surgery is exceedingly low, there are some exceptions. Procedures involving infected or eroded skin are associated with a significantly higher infection risk and warrant the use of prophylactic antibiotics. This is particularly important in both the AHA high-risk and moderate-risk patients.[13] Appropriate antibiotic regimens should typically provide coverage against *Staphylococcus aureus*, a likely pathogen, and include dicloxacillin, cephalexin, and clindamycin.[13]

Patients with implanted cardiac pacemakers and defibrillators must be identified during the preoperative evaluation. Electrical currents generated by electrosurgical units may adversely affect the function of implanted cardiac devices[14] (Chapter 12). In most circumstances, heat electrocautery (which avoids transfer of current to the patient) is the preferred method for achieving hemostasis. Disposable electrocautery 'pen' units are inexpensive and widely available. Bipolar coagulation (in which small forceps are used to grasp bleeding vessels) minimizes current transfer to the patient and has also been advocated.[15] In patients with automatic internal cardiac defibrillators (AICDs) it is also recommended that a magnet is used to inactivate the device just before coagulation. This can be done relatively easily in the outpatient setting. We recommend that contact be made with the patient's cardiologist if that person has an AICD. Often the manufacturer of the defibrillator will send a technician to educate and assist the novice at doing this. After doing it a few times the simple technique becomes routine, but Advanced Cardiac Life Support (ACLS) training for physicians taking care of these patients cannot be overemphasized.

Hepatitis and HIV infection

To minimize exposure risk, all patients treated should be regarded as potentially infectious and universal precautions should be practiced. In addition to surgical gloves, appropriate eyewear and protective garments are needed. Offices can minimize the risk of 'sharps' injury by using a scalpel blade remover or disposable scalpels, placing sharp objects in designated areas on surgical trays, readily disposing of all sharps when finished with them, and using double-layered surgical gloves. Inadvertent fluid exposure to areas such as the eyes and mouth can be prevented through the use of splash-resistant surgical masks and safety eyewear.

Organ Transplantation

Because of the immunosuppressive regimens required to prevent allograft rejection, these patients may be at increased of postoperative wound infection and delayed wound healing.[13] Some patients may be instructed by their transplant physicians and internists to take prophylactic antibiotics before dental or surgical procedures; in these cases, the guidelines of the AHA for endocarditis prophylaxis should suffice.[11]

While not formally supported by AHA guidelines, in our practice we routinely prescribe prophylactic antibiotics for patients undergoing prolonged surgical procedures (Mohs micrographic surgery, liposuction, laser resurfacing) as well as those involving infected or ulcerated skin. Commonly used prophylactic antibiotic regimens in our practice include cephalexin 1 g, dicloxacillin 1 g, or azithromycin 500 mg given orally 1 hour before the procedure.

Other prosthetic devices

No specific antibiotic prophylaxis guidelines exist for dermatologic surgery in patients with non-cardiac prosthetic devices (Chapter 9). Such implanted devices include various orthopedic prostheses, indwelling catheters, ventricular shunts, as well as penile and breast implants. A comprehensive discussion of the role of antibiotic prophylaxis for patients with these devices has been carefully examined by Haas and Grekin.[13] In general, the physician responsible for implanting a prosthetic device should be consulted in advance of a proposed surgical procedure. In instances where antibiotic prophylaxis is warranted, it would be reasonable to follow the AHA guidelines for endocarditis prophylaxis.

Herpes simplex virus infection

A prior history of herpes simplex virus (HSV) infection should be assessed during the preoperative evaluation. This is especially important in people undergoing medium-depth chemical peels, facial laser resurfacing, and potentially for those undergoing imiquimod treatment around the mouth. Similar precautions should be taken in patients undergoing extensive genital procedures who have a history of herpes genitalis.

Various factors experienced during the course of a surgical procedure, such as tissue trauma and psychological stress, can precipitate an acute herpetic flare. For high-risk procedures such as skin resurfacing, appropriate antiviral prophylaxis is indicated regardless of the historical HSV infection status. Common regimens for patients undergoing facial resurfacing procedures include acyclovir 400 mg three times daily, valacyclovir 500 mg twice daily, and famciclovir 250 mg twice daily. Typically, these medications are begun within 48 hours preoperatively and continued until reepithelialization is complete, generally in 7–10 days.

Inherited bleeding disorders

Patients with inherited bleeding disorders such as hemophilia A, hemophilia B, and von Willebrand's disease are at higher risk for significant perioperative bleeding.[16] Consequently, people with a known or suspected bleeding disorder should be referred to a hematologist for appropriate preoperative evaluation and management. Depending on the disorder, various clotting factors may be given intravenously shortly before a planned surgical procedure. In addition to clotting factor replacement, meticulous attention to hemostasis is essential. Where available, physicians should consider using a carbon dioxide laser in cutting mode to further reduce the possibility of bleeding.[17]

Implanted deep-brain stimulators

Deep-brain stimulators are electrical devices implanted into the thalamus or subthalamus for the treatment of movement disorders such as essential tremor and Parkinson's disease.[18] Electrical currents generated by electrosurgical devices including electrodesiccators and electrocoagulators have the potential to interfere with and adversely affect the function of these devices.[19] Electrocautery, which transfers no current to the patient, is therefore the preferred method of achieving hemostasis in these patients.[19] Alternatively, the deep-brain stimulator can be safely inactivated externally by the patient's neurologist shortly before the surgical procedure. This will, however, result in the immediate recrudescence of tremors in a previously nontremulous patient, which might interfere with the planned procedure. In our experience, inactivation of the deep-brain stimulator has never been necessary as effective hemostasis of skin and soft tissue defects commonly encountered in dermatologic surgery can be readily achieved with electrocautery.

Medications

A comprehensive inventory of both prescription and non-prescription medication use is an essential component of the preoperative evaluation. Information derived from the medication list may reveal undisclosed medical problems, possible drug interactions, and avoid potential perioperative complications.

Anticoagulants

Traditional anticoagulants include aspirin, various non-steroidal anti-inflammatory drugs (NSAIDs), coumadin, heparin, and dipyridamole. Recently, however, several newer derivatives have been introduced including the family of low-molecular-weight heparins (LMWHs) such as Fragmin (dalteparin sodium) (Pfizer Inc, New York, NY), Lovenox (enoxaparin sodium) (Aventis Pharmaceuticals Inc, Bridgewater, NJ), Normiflo (ardeparin sodium) (Wyeth-Ayerst Laboratories, St Davids, PA), and Orgaran (danaparoid sodium) (Organon, Roseland, NJ).[20–23] LMWHs are indicated for the treatment of deep venous thrombosis, pulmonary embolism, and postsurgical anticoagulation.[20–23] These medications offer heparin-like anticoagulation but with the convenience of subcutaneous dosing. Plavix (clopidogrel) (Bristol-Myers Squibb, New York, NY) and Ticlid (ticlopidine) (Roche Pharmaceuticals, Nutley, NJ) are adenosine diphosphate (ADP) receptor antagonists with powerful antiplatelet effects.[24,25] Clopidogrel is approved for preventing thrombotic events in patients with recent myocardial infarction, stroke, acute coronary syndrome, and peripheral arterial disease.[24] The anticoagulant effect of clopidogrel can be enhanced by the addition of aspirin and the two are frequently combined in anticoagulant regimens.[24] Aggrenox (Boehringer Ingelheim, Ridgefield, CT), which contains a combination of aspirin and extended-release dipyridamole, has been recently approved for reducing the risk of subsequent stroke in people with a history of transient ischemic attacks or thrombotic, ischemic stroke.[26]

Multiple nutritional supplements have also been shown to have anticoagulant effects, although their impact on dermatologic surgery is unknown. Perhaps most notable is vitamin E, or α-tocopherol, which is often overlooked by both patients and physicians as a potential anticoagulant. Other common nutritional supplements with anticoagulant properties include garlic, ginseng, ginger, gingko, St John's Wort, feverfew, and numerous others. For a more comprehensive review see the article by Collins and Dufresne.[27] Alcohol has also been shown to interfere with platelet aggregation *in vitro*, which may result an increase in bleeding potential.[28]

Clearly, increased bleeding during the perioperative period can significantly prolong the course of a surgical procedure, and increase the risk of postoperative complications interfering with healthy wound repair. Ideally, use of anticoagulant medication would be discontinued before initiating a surgical procedure. However, more recent studies examining the effect of continued anticoagulant use on the incidence of postoperative bleeding in patients undergoing dermatologic surgery have failed to show an increased rate of significant adverse effects.[29,30] In fact, in one study of patients undergoing cardiac surgery, pretreatment with coumadin not only failed to increase the risk for bleeding complications, but also was actually associated with decreased intraoperative blood loss.[31] More importantly, however, are multiple reports which show that discontinuation of anticoagulant before dermatologic surgery in patients at risk for thrombotic events has resulted in an increased rate of perioperative stroke, blindness, pulmonary embolism, and even death.[32,33]

Based on the above findings, our general recommendations for anticoagulant discontinuation before surgery are as follows:

- Only patients taking aspirin for 'preventive' purposes, without a history of coronary or cerebrovascular disease, or without explicit instructions from their physician, are instructed to discontinue use 7 days before their surgical procedure.
- Patients taking NSAIDs for pain relief are asked to discontinue use 7 days before a surgical procedure and to use non-aspirin or non-NSAID pain relievers instead (like acetaminophen or cyclooxygenase COX-2 inhibitors).
- All nutritional supplements, including multivitamins, are to be discontinued 7 days before the surgical procedure.

- Alcoholic beverages are to be avoided for 2 days before the surgical procedure. All other anticoagulant regimens, including coumadin, clopidogrel, dipyridamole and aspirin-anticoagulant combinations, are routinely continued without explicit instructions from the patient's internist.

Nonselective β-blockers

The potential for disastrous complications resulting from the use of epinephrine-containing local anesthetics in patients taking non-selective β-blockers is often overlooked. Through inhibition of vasodilatory β2-adrenergic receptors, non-selective β-blockers such as propranolol may actually potentiate the alpha-adrenergic vasoconstrictive effects of epinephrine leading to malignant hypertension, profound reflexive bradycardia, and even death, when combined with epinephrine (adrenaline).[34] In such instances, treatment with intravenous vasodilators such as hydralazine or chlorpromazine may be appropriate.[35] Similar cardiac effects however are not observed with the selective β1-blocker, metoprolol. Despite this, we suspect there are many patients taking non-selective β-blockers who receive epinephrine-containing anesthetics in the course of dermatologic procedures without any adverse effect. The ultimate significance of this potential interaction in dermatologic surgery is therefore unknown and—as some speculate—idiosyncratic.[36] In the event that a medication change is desired, consultation with the patient's primary care physician is essential first.

Allergies

A list of medication allergies should be included in the preoperative evaluation. In particular, dermatologic surgeons should pay special attention to patients with possible allergy to local anesthetics, antibiotics, pain medications, latex, or surgical wound dressings.

Local anesthetics

True allergy to ester anesthetics is not uncommon and necessitated the development of less allergenic compounds, the amide anesthetics. True allergy to newer amide local anesthetic is generally rare and can be documented through skin testing.[37] In many cases of suspected amide anesthetic allergy, the 'allergen' is actually not the anesthetic itself, but rather the preservatives such as *para*-aminobenzoic acid (PABA), parabens, or metabisulfite, which are commonly added to the solutions.[37,38] In most instances of suspected anesthetic allergy, the solution is simply to substitute an anesthetic belonging to a different class, such as an ester (procaine) for an amide (lidocaine), as cross-reactivity is not observed. For patients with documented allergy to parabens, paraben-free anesthetics are widely available.

Antibiotics

Patients with allergies to oral antibiotics should be treated with appropriate alternatives. Cephalosporin antibiotics can usually be safely given to penicillin-allergic patients who do not exhibit an anaphylactic response to penicillin.[39,40] Other alternatives in penicillin-allergic patients include macrolides such as azithromycin, clarithromycin, and erythromycin.

Antibiotic allergy may also occur with topically applied agents. Although most reactions are typically due to neomycin, an aminoglycoside antibiotic, bacitracin allergy has recently been reported with increased frequency.[41] In patients with suspected topical antibiotic allergy, wounds should be dressed with petrolatum or Aquaphor ointment (Beiersdorf, Wilton, CT). Alternatively, Bactroban (mupirocin) ointment (GlaxoSmithKline, Research Triangle Park, NC), if medically indicated, can be safely used in patients with either bacitracin or neomycin allergy.

Latex

Latex allergy is common in medical settings, affecting approximately 12% of all healthcare workers.[42] Symptoms may range from localized urticaria to anaphylaxis.[43] Common sources for allergens include disposable exam gloves, elastic dressings, and surgical tubing.

Examination glove allergy is generally caused by hypersensitivity to the natural rubber latex molecule. The 'powder' present in latex examination gloves has been shown to be an important vehicle for environmental aerosolization. However, true allergy to the absorptive agents such as cornstarch and talc, which are used in powdered examination gloves, is exceedingly rare.

Screening questions for latex allergy should be included in the preoperative evaluation. Extra pairs of vinyl or nitrile gloves should be kept in examination rooms for latex-sensitive patients. Environmental aerosolization of latex allergens may be further minimized through the use of powder-free latex gloves. Many medical centers have taken a preemptive approach by eliminating latex-containing products from patient-care areas.

Surgical history

Targeted questions can be used to identify patients at high risk for perioperative complications. Questions relating to the patient's previous experience with surgical and dental procedures can help to elucidate these issues. Examples include:

- Have you ever had problems with excessive bleeding?
- Have you ever had problems with scar or keloid formation?
- Have you ever had difficulty with wound healing?
- Have you ever had a wound infection?
- Have you ever had problems with local or general anesthesia?
- Do you have any other concerns you would like to tell me before scheduling surgery?

Once identified, patients at risk for particular surgical complications can be counseled appropriately.

Social history

Social factors play an important role in determining the ultimate success of a surgical procedure and should not be overlooked. In particular, physicians should try to assess the suitability of a particular patient for a given procedure. Is the patient likely or able to comply with the postoperative care instructions? Is a caretaker, such as a spouse or relative, available to assist with wound care? Additionally, patients who drive considerable distances to an office for a procedure may require assistance returning home afterwards. All of these issues should be considered during the preoperative evaluation, and plans made accordingly.

Smoking

Tobacco use may adversely effect dermatologic surgery by enhancing cutaneous vasoconstriction, impairing wound healing, and increasing wound infection risk.[44–46] Prospective patients should be informed of these possibilities during the preoperative evaluation and strongly encouraged to discontinue or minimize their perioperative tobacco use. Ideally, the patient will discontinue tobacco use 1–2 weeks before and after surgery. It is often useful if the patient contacts and meets with their internist to discuss medications useful during this process and to establish a support system that may foster continued abstinence. Not infrequently, patients are able to cease smoking if they receive ample support before surgery. These people are helped in a way that may be ultimately even more beneficial than the surgery performed.

Informed consent

Informed consent is the process by which patients become fully informed about the potential risks, benefits, and alternatives of a proposed medical procedure. It is through the process of informed consent that patients are given the ability to decide their medical fate. However, in order for patients to provide truly informed consent, first they must be mentally competent, and capable of making their own decisions.

In general, the process of informed consent should include the following basic elements:

- a description of the proposed medical procedure in layman's terms
- a reasonable explanation of any treatment alternatives
- information about the relative risks and benefits of the proposed treatment
- a general assessment of patient's comprehension and decision-making ability
- a verifiable acceptance by the patient to undergo a particular procedure.

The exact standard for what constitutes 'informed consent' varies from state to state and country to country. Interested physicians should contact their State Medical Board for further information.

Optimizing outcomes

- Build a relationship with the patient and the patient's family.
- Make sure that more than one person reviews the patient's medical history.
- Check with the patient on the day of surgery whether conditions have changed (e.g. new medications) since the initial consultation.

Pitfalls

- Failure to obtain an adequate medical history, which adversely impacts the surgical outcome.
- Failure to obtain an adequate medication history, which results in an adverse drug reaction.
- Failure to obtain informed consent by not adequately explaining the proposed procedure.
- Failure to consider occult pregnancy in a female of childbearing potential.

REFERENCES

1. http://www.perinatology.com/exposures/Drugs/FDACategories.htm. Retrieved August 6, 2003.
2. Philipson EH, Kuhnert BR, Syracuse CD. Maternal, fetal, and neonatal lidocaine levels following local perineural infiltration. Am J Obstet Gynecol 1984; 149:403–407.
3. Heinonen OP, Sloane D, Shapiro S, eds. Birth defects and drugs in pregnancy. Littleton, CO: Publishing Sciences Group, 1977.
4. Fujinaga M, Maxxe RI. Reproductive and teratogenic effects of lidocaine in Sprague-Dawley rats. Anesthesiology 1986; 65:626–632.
5. Gormley DE. Cutaneous surgery and the pregnant patient. J Am Acad Dermatol 1990; 23:269–279.
6. Moore PA. Selecting drugs for the pregnant patient. J Am Dent Assoc 1998; 129:1281–1286.
7. McCormack WM, George H, Donner A, et al. Hepatotoxicity of erythromycin estolate during pregnancy. Antimicrob Agents Chemother 1977; 12:630–635.
8. Richards KA, Stasko T. Dermatologic surgery in the pregnant patient. Dermatol Surg 2002; 28:248–256.
9. Rainer TH, Robertson CE. Adrenaline, cardiac arrest, and evidence based medicine. J Accid Emerg Med 1996; 13:234–237.
10. Niwa H, Sugimura M, Satoh Y, Tanimoto A. Cardiovascular response to epinephrine-containing local anesthetics in patients with cardiovascular disease. Oral Surg Oral Med Oral Pathol Oral Radiol Endod 2001; 92:610–616.
11. Adnan S. Dajani. Prevention of bacterial endocarditis. Circulation 1997; 96:358–366.
12. Roberts HW, Redding SW. Coronary artery stents: review and patient-management recommendations. J am Dent Assoc 2000; 131:797–801.
13. Haas AF, Grekin RC. Antibiotic prophylaxis in dermatologic surgery. J Am Acad Dermatol 1995; 32:155–76.
14. LeVasseur JG, Kennard CD, Finley EM, Muse RK. Dermatologic electrosurgery in patients with implantable cardioverter-defibrillators and pacemakers. Dermatol Surg 1998; 24:233–240.
15. El-Gamal HM, Dufresne RG, Saddler K. Electrosurgery, pacemakers and ICDs: a survey of precautions and complications experienced by cutaneous surgeons. Dermatol Surg 2001; 27:385–390.
16. Peterson SR, Joseph AK. Inherited bleeding disorders in dermatologic surgery. Dermatol Surg 2001; 27:885–889.
17. Santos-Dias A. CO_2 laser surgery in hemophilia treatment. J Clin Laser Med Surg 1992; 10:297–301.
18. Starr PA, Vitek JL, Bakay RA. Deep brain stimulation for movement disorders. Neurosurg Clin N Am 1998; 9:381–402.
19. Weaver J, Kim SJ, Lee MH, Torres A. Cutaneous electrosurgery in a patient with a deep brain stimulator. Dermatol Surg 1999; 25:415–417.
20. http://www.lovenox.com (last accessed June 2004).
21. http://www.nlm.nih.gov/medlineplus/druginfo/medmaster/a696006.html (last accessed June 2004).
22. http://www.nlm.nih.gov/medlineplus/druginfo/uspdi/203494.html (last accessed June 2004).
23. http://www.orgaran.com (last accessed August 2003)
24. http://www.plavix.com (last accessed June 2004).
25. http://www.nlm.nih.gov/medlineplus/druginfo/medmaster/a696006.html (last accessed June 2004).
26. http://www.aggrenox.com (last accessed June 2004).
27. Collins SC, Dufresne RG Jr. Dietary supplements in the setting of Mohs surgery. Dermatol Surg 2002; 28:447–452.

28. Rand ML, Packham MA, Kinlough-Rathbone RL, Fraser Mustard J. Effects of ethanol on pathways of platelet aggregation in vitro. Thromb Haemost 1988 16; 59:383–387.
29. Kovich O, Otley CC. Perioperative management of anticoagulants and platelet inhibitors for cutaneous surgery: a survey of current practice. Dermatol Surg 2002; 28:513–517.
30. Billingsley EM, Maloney ME. Intraoperative and postoperative bleeding problems in patients taking warfarin, aspirin, and nonsteroidal antiinflammatory agents. A prospective study. Dermatol Surg 1997; 235:381–383.
31. Dietrich W, Dilthey G, Spannagl M, Richter JA. Warfarin pretreatment does not lead to increased bleeding tendency during cardiac surgery. J Cardiothorac Vasc Anesth 1995; 9:250–254.
32. Alam M, Goldberg LH. Serious adverse vascular events associated with perioperative interruption of antiplatelet and anticoagulant therapy. Dermatol Surg 2002; 28:992–998.
33. Kovich O, Otley CC. Thrombotic complications related to discontinuation of warfarin and aspirin therapy perioperatively for cutaneous operation. J Am Acad Dermatol 2003; 48:233–237.
34. Foster CA, Aston SJ. Propranolol–epinephrine interaction: a potential disaster. Plast Reconstr Surg 1983; 72:74–78.
35. McGillis ST, Stanton-Hicks U. The preoperative patient evaluation: preparing for surgery. Dermatol Clin 1998; 16:1–15.
36. Dzubow LM. The interaction between propranolol and epinephrine as observed in patients undergoing Mohs surgery. J Am Acad Dermatol 1986; 15:71–75.
37. Glinert RJ, Zachary CB. Local anesthetic allergy: Its recognition and avoidance. J Dermatol Surg Oncol 1991; 17:491–496.
38. Campbell JR, Maestrello CL, Campbell RL. Allergic response to metabisulfite in lidocaine anesthetic solution. Anesth Prog 2001; 48:21–26.
39. Goodman EJ, Morgan MJ, Johnson PA, Nichols BA, Denk N, Gold BB. Cephalosporins can be given to penicillin-allergic patients who do not exhibit an anaphylactic response. J Clin Anesth 2001; 13:561–564.
40. Anne S, Reisman RE. Risk of administering cephalosporin antibiotics to patients with histories of penicillin allergy. Ann Allergy Asthma Immunol 1995; 74:167–170.
41. Katz BE, Fisher AA. Bacitracin: a unique topical antibiotic sensitizer. J Am Acad Dermatol 1987; 17:1016–1024.
42. Liss GM, Sussman GL, Deal K, et al. Latex allergy: epidemiological study of 1351 hospital workers. Occup Environ Med 1997; 54:335–342.
43. Woods JA, Lambert S, Platts-Mills TA, Drake DB, Edlich RF. Natural rubber latex allergy: spectrum, diagnostic approach, and therapy. J Emerg Med 1997; 15:71–85.
44. Sorensen LT, Karlsmark T, Gottrup F. Abstinence from smoking reduces incisional wound infection: a randomized controlled trial. Ann Surg. 2003; 238:1–5.
45. Lind J, Kramhoft M, Bodtker S. The influence of smoking on complications after primary amputations of the lower extremity. Clin Orthop 1991; 267:211–217.
46. Yaffe B, Cushin BJ, Strauch B. Effect of cigarette smoking on experimental microvascular anastomoses. Microsurgery 1984; 5:70–72.

6 Digital Imaging in Dermatologic Surgery

Rhett J Drugge MD and Mark Naylor MD

Summary box

- Digital imaging is cost-effective and facilitates efficient storage, retrieval and analysis of dermatologic images.
- Analogue cameras capture more information than the human eye can perceive or the digital camera can capture, therefore, if digital images are to be clinically useful and easily used, an understanding of the nature of digital images and their production is important when setting technical standards and selecting a digital system.
- Sophisticated storage and cataloguing systems are available for digital images.
- Users can perform image analyses that are impractical with analogue images, but are of benefit in clinical practice (e.g. in melanoma detection).
- Digital files can be easily copied and exchanged so patient privacy and consent issues must be well understood by technicians and healthcare professionals.

INTRODUCTION

Digital imaging enhances surgical dermatology. Photography is now open to instant machine analysis, dramatically closing the gap between data acquisition and interpretation. Not only do digital cameras allow images to be readily organized within and reported from an electronic medical record, but the synthesis of image capture with analytic computing allows for a powerful synapse that was unthinkable in the era of film photography. The digital camera is efficient and cost-effective and is the portal to a new era of quantitative dermatology.

Dermatologic digital cameras cover a broad range of scales, from photomicroscopy ($1\ m^{-6}$ per visual field) to total body photography ($1.5\ m^2$ per visual field). Mapping consistently across the boundaries of scale (microscope to skin) has been successfully carried out in pigmented skin lesion tracking and micrographic surgery.[1]

The paramount difference between traditional film cameras and digital cameras is the capture medium. Elimination of film, with its inherent expenses and problems accounts for much of the advantage of digital photography. Film is costly to purchase and develop, and is time consuming to handle. Photograph quality may not be assessed until the film is developed, sometimes days or weeks removed from the actual patient encounter. Digital technology has considerable advantages over film photography because of its low cost and because it allows instant feedback, easy editing, easy sharing, inexpensive storage, perfect archives, phenomenal portability, accessible documentation and rapid printing (Table 6.1).

TECHNICAL ASPECTS

Hardware for digital image capture

Optical sensors

The optical parts of a digital camera are analogous to their film counterparts, but the silicon image capture device sets digital apart from film technology. In most digital cameras this initial image capture device is either a charge couple device (CCD) or complementary metal oxide semiconductor (CMOS) chip. The initial image is formed in a screen buffer by the capture device and can be viewed on a preview screen. The image is stored in removable storage media (see below) before being transferred to a computer for further processing and long-term archiving.

CCD and CMOS image capture devices

The heart of most digital cameras today is either a CCD or, increasingly, a CMOS sensor, which forms the initial digital image. On the surface of each of these square centimeter-size ranged silicon chips is a grid containing hundreds of thousands or millions of photosensitive diodes called photo elements (or pixels). Each single pixel captures a set of information with a place in the matrix of the photo image. CMOS sensors are currently not as popular as CCD devices, but are being used for an increasing number of professional quality cameras.

Table 6.1 Advantages of digital technology over film photography

Advantage	Reasons
Low cost	A perfectly adequate single camera set-up can cost less than US$500 and allows for a virtually unlimited number of shots
Instant feedback	Most digital cameras display the picture immediately on the color liquid crystal display (LCD) screen, which is usually on the back of the camera
Easy editing	Once transferred to a computer, amazing transformations can take place. With inexpensive photo editing software, lesion details emerge from dark shadows, patient identities are masked, and dull colors become bright
Easy sharing	Electronic mail allows images to be shared with an online dermatology community, such as RxDerm—a powerful ally in solving challenging clinical problems
Inexpensive storage	Digital photographs can be archived on long-term storage media such as DVD, which can easily hold 40 000 images in a compressed format (assuming 120 KB per image) or 400 images in an uncompressed format (assuming an 8 × 10 magazine print quality, large format image of 12 MB). On pricewatch.com prices on 10 May 2004 were: DVD-R—$35 for 100 4.7 GB disks, or 7 cents per gigabyte; and CD-R—$17 for 100 700 MB disks, or 23 cents per gigabyte
Perfect archives	Digital photos, because they are expressed as binary information, do not change with time because of loss of physical media as long as the information is transferred before media degradation occurs. Film images, with color slides being the most long-lived example, eventually deteriorate because they are based on a constantly degrading physical medium rather than a logical data set archived in an electronic medium
Phenomenal portability	A career's worth of compressed clinical images may be held on a small memory chip barely larger than a silver dollar
Accessible documentation	Digital images may be recalled through patient record identification using manual data entry, and now increasingly by computer recognition of voice, face, or other features.
Rapid printing	Digital photos are printed in a matter of minutes

A CMOS sensor is a more complex type of image capture device, which was difficult to fabricate in the early days of digital technology, but as techniques for chip fabrication have advanced, CMOS chips are rivaling, and perhaps exceeding, in some ways the more mature CCD technology. CMOS offers more processing on the chip itself, but there are trade-offs arising from technical issues such as nonuniformity of pixel processing and somewhat less sensitivity per unit area. CMOS sensors typically have lower power consumption than the typical CCD device. Current technology has advanced to the point that either device can function well in a camera designed to take advantage of the strengths of the capture device while minimizing its weaknesses. Picking a camera with favorable features and characteristics is probably more important than the particular imaging technology used by a manufacturer at this point in time.

Image resolution

Resolution on a digital camera is determined by the size and pixel density of the image capture medium. In the vernacular of digital cameras, a million pixels is a megapixel (1000 × 1000 pixels). CMOS and CCD sensors range from a low-end of 1 megapixel to a high-end of 75 megapixels. Resolutions comparable to 35 mm film have been achieved and surpassed. A sharply focused color slide photograph may contain of the order of 15–20 megapixels of information expressed in digital terms. Most digital cameras have CCDs that capture much less. There is a practical limit to the resolution that can be perceived by the human eye; within that limit, more resolution is not helpful. Color slides have data in them that is difficult to access. A slide made from a 2-megapixel digital photograph and a color slide made from color slide film look identical to the human eye when projected on a typical computer monitor.

Most modern digital cameras exceed the minimum resolution requirements for providing diagnostic dermatology images.[3] In one study diagnostic dermatology image displays established that there is no significant difference in the useful information delivery between digital images (574 × 489 pixels full color resolution) and slide images.[4] In another study, side-by-side comparison using projected slides verified that 768 × 512 pixels full color resolution is sufficient for viewing dermatology images.[5]

Too many high-resolution photos can make a PowerPoint (Microsoft Corporation, Redmond, WA) presentation so unwieldy that it crashes computer systems. High-resolution images can put a strain on removable storage media, camera-to-computer transfer time, random access memory (RAM), hard drive space, processing power, print time, printing ink, and network transmission bandwidth.

These problems have been lessened by the introduction of more affordable processing power, memory, and bandwidth. Software is available to reduce image size and resolution to eliminate awkward image management problems. PowerPoint for Windows XP and above now includes a compression utility that will bring the images down to the maximum screen viewable or projectable output with only a few keystrokes

Disparity in print and display resolutions

Image printing requires four times as many dots per inch (DPI) for the same quality of image as a screen display; print resolutions may vary from 150 to 1200 DPI, whereas normal screen resolution is from 75 to 96 DPI. Digital cameras that produce images greater than 2 megapixels exceed the display capacity of most computer monitors; therefore, the utility of these cameras is limited to improving print quality or magnifying sections of the image. The disparity between the requirements for digital image print and display is reinforced by the growing popularity of flat screen monitors, which use lower display resolutions than older cathode ray tube (CRT) monitors.

Camera memory systems

Digital cameras employ a temporary digital storage medium that captures the images after they are obtained from the image sensor. A variety of storage media are available on different digital camera models. Commonly found media are presented in Table 6.2.

The digital pictures are usually moved from temporary storage media to a computer hard drive. Computer hard drives are not considered a stable environment for permanent medical record keeping. For such archiving, a 'read only memory' (ROM) should be placed on a compact disk (CD) or digital video disk (DVD). Some cameras write directly to a CD as the initial storage medium. Long-term usability of digital images is achieved by migrating data to future technology generations, adhering to standard image file-header formats, and monitoring for media degradation.[6]

Camera liquid crystal displays

LCD screens are valuable for image composition and initial image checking. However, sharpness of focus may not be appreciated at the resolutions allowed by the LCD. These images are shown on the preview LCD for a user-determined number of seconds or a manufacturer preset time. Because of the awkward positioning sometimes imposed by anatomic photography, the ability to rotate the LCD screen is a useful camera characteristic pioneered by Nikon. Digital cameras can be switched to a display mode to review the images using the camera LCD.

Selecting a digital camera

The more important considerations in selecting a digital camera are resolution, macro capabilities, and the camera's acceptance of dermatologic adapters. Other issues include ergonomic comfort factors, size, cost, and the type of storage media. Cameras at the current low-end of the consumer market create a higher resolution picture than most computer monitors can display; 1 megapixel is sufficient for display through a typical LCD, though such cameras are disappearing from the marketplace as they are being displaced by larger format cameras. Paradoxically, the older, bulkier technology, the CRT monitors, may display up to 5 megapixels of information, justifying the use of the current crop of higher resolution cameras. Ultimately, the pixel requirement depends on the product of the required resolution and size of the area imaged.

The term 'interpolated' resolution can be confusing. Interpolation makes the image larger and slightly fuzzy and allows the manufacturer to claim a larger resolution than there are optical pixels. This technique does not improve the quality of the image.

One feature that deserves consideration in this context is the shutter lag (time between shutter press and image capture). Shutter lag is not normally published in the technical specifications of a camera, and varies with flash recharging time. The camera cycle time is also slowed by increasing resolution. A 35 mm single lens reflex (SLR) camera can take action shots at rates unmatched by digital cameras.

A strong macro focus is an essential for close-up views of lesions. Some digital cameras can focus within several centimeters, although to accomplish this, external lighting may be required. An optical zoom enhances macro imaging because it increases the pixel density while a 'digital' zoom adds no new information but simply crops an image without providing additional pixels.

Ultra compact cameras excel in portability and may produce an image quality comparable to bulkier cameras (Table 6.3). A variety of sources exist online for digital camera reviews and among the most useful are http://www.steves-digicams.com/ and http://www.dpreview.com/

Digital camera integration with other devices

Incorporating the digital camera with personal digital assistants (PDAs) and cell phones permits new horizons in image usage. One such example is the Sony CLIE PEG-NZ90 (www.sony.com), a PDA that integrates a 2-megapixel camera (1600 × 1200) with video, sound, pen, and keyboard capture. Although it lacks an optical zoom, it can focus as close as 10 cm and generates screen filling images at 240 × 320 pixels. The PDA easily integrates with wireless networks through an 802.11b card, 128 MB of memory, and sound recording, which allows for text, sound, and video annotation of images in a network environment. Such devices, because of their portability and their integration of other forms of documentation have a valuable role in the electronic medical record. The on-board computing capability of PDAs allows for digital image analysis. The PDA is the likely winner in the coming convergence of phone, camera, and computer.

Table 6.2 Digital camera removable storage media

Media	Abbreviation	Maximum	Comments	US$/128 MB
Compact Flash	**CF**	2 GB	3.3 mm thick, most common	20
Smart Media	**SM**	128 MB	Kodak, Olympus	20
Memory Stick	**MS**	1 GB	Sony	28
Memory Stick Pro	**MS Pro**	2 GB	May not be compatible MS slots	Not available
Compact Flash Type II	**CF/2**	1 GB	5 mm thick	Not available
3½ in floppy diskette	**Floppy**	1.44 MB	Older Sony Mavicas	Not available
Multi Media Card	**MMC**	128 MB	Kodak	49
xD Picture Card	**XD**	128 MB	Olympus	56
8 cm CD disk	**CD-R/CD-RW**	156 MB	Sony Mavicas, Mini CD disks add to the bulk of the device	14
Secure Digital	**SD**	1 GB	Fuji	44
IBM Hitachi Microdrive (Compact Flash II compatible)		5 GB	Most CF/2 compatible	Not available

MB, megabyte; GB, gigabyte

Table 6.3 Select ultra compact digital cameras

	Pentax OptioS (www.pentax.com)	Canon S400 (www.canon.com)	Coolpix SQ (www.nikon.com)	Olympus Stylus 400 (www.olympus.com)
Effective pixels (megapixels)	3.14	**4.0**	3.1	**4.0**
Optical zoom	**3×**	**3×**	**3×**	**3×**
Macro (mm)	58	**7.4**	37	196
Width (inches)	3.3	3.4	**3.2**	3.9
Height (inches)	**2.0**	2.2	3.2	2.2
Depth (inches)	**0.8**	1.1	1.0	1.3
Weight (ounces)	**4.1**	6.5	6.3	5.8
Media	**Secure Digital/Multi Media Card (SD/MMC)**	**Compact Flash type 1**	**Compact Flash type 1**	**xD-Picture Card**
Batteries	**Rechargeable lithium ion Battery**	**Rechargeable lithium ion battery**	**Rechargeable lithium ion battery**	**Rechargeable lithium ion battery**

Best features in **bold**.

Other digital camera features

Lenses

The lens options and requirements are similar in conventional and digital cameras. Many low-cost cameras with fixed lens systems can be modified by lens adapters. Newer models increasingly use retractable lenses that do not allow lens adapters or filters. Interchangeable lenses are restricted to the high-end digital SLR cameras targeted primarily for the professional photography market. Digital SLR cameras use the same lenses as their film camera counterparts, but their focal length may differ from their labeled one because of differences in the size of the film they were intended for and the size of the chip in the camera. Newer high-end digital cameras have sensor chips that are 36 mm × 24 mm, the same as a frame of 35 mm film, eliminating the need for recalculating focal length.

Adapters

The range of digital cameras may be extended with adapters. However, some of these adapters are available only for a select number of digital cameras. Adapter manufacturers generally document the compatibility. Table 6.4 outlines digital camera adapters used in dermatology.

Table 6.4 Digital camera adapters used in dermatology

Adapter	Some manufacturers
Dermoscopy	3Gen (www.3Gen11c.com)
Slide copying adapter	Canfield Imaging (www.canfieldsci.com)
Endoscope adapter	Canfield Imaging
Close-up scale	Canfield Imaging
Microscope	Various
Ring flash	Various

Digital imaging techniques

Basic digital photography

The optical processes of film and digital cameras are equivalent; thus, considerations such as focus, focal length, exposure, shutter speed, and aperture are all still relevant. With adequate computer skills, experienced film camera photographers soon learn to appreciate the speed and simplicity of digital cameras.

Prerequisite computer skills

To use a digital camera effectively it is necessary to have knowledge of a commonly used operating system, file management, computer printing, memory card use, picture quality options, image compression, image editing, and slide show software.

Proper exposure

Automatic exposure settings greatly simplify image capture on most digital cameras. Techniques that help minimize overexposed photos are to maximize the flash-to-subject distance, to increase background luminosity, and to override the auto exposure settings.

Most overexposure results from specular reflection. It results from a sharply defined beam reflecting off a smooth surface directly back into the camera, causing local overexposure of the CCD. Such pixels are subjected to intense reflection resulting in no contrast or differences in surrounding pixels. Methods to minimize specular reflection (areas of white reflection) include cross-polarizing the light source, suspending the highly reflective stratum corneum in a liquid covered with glass, making the light source tangential to the subject, and maximizing the subject-to-flash distance. This can be done with flashes mounted on brackets off camera or using studio lighting.[7]

Sharpness (focus)

Sharply focused photographs reveal a rich level of detail. Methods to enhance sharpness include providing a label at the plane of focus to minimize auto focus failure on unmarked skin (Fig. 6.1), lighting the subject adequately, and avoiding camera movement. If auto focus is a problem, take a series of manually focused images.

Macro photography

The minimum focusing distance limits the resolution with which small objects may be photographed. Digital cameras vary substantially in their minimum focusing distance. The addition of a macro lens can markedly enhance the capacity to take good macro shots. Some adapters provide lens systems that are the equivalent of a skin surface microscope. These macro lenses are available for some

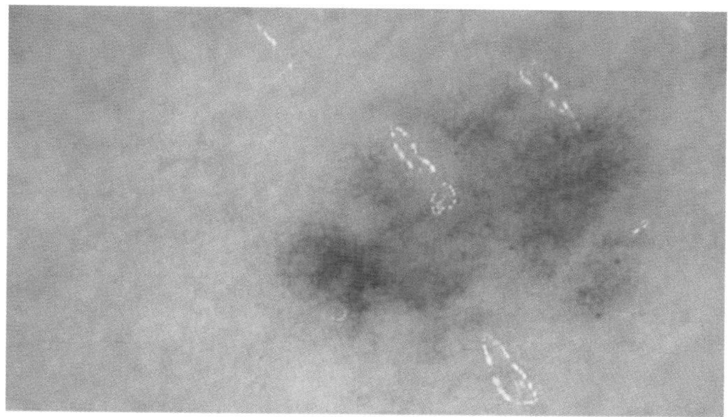

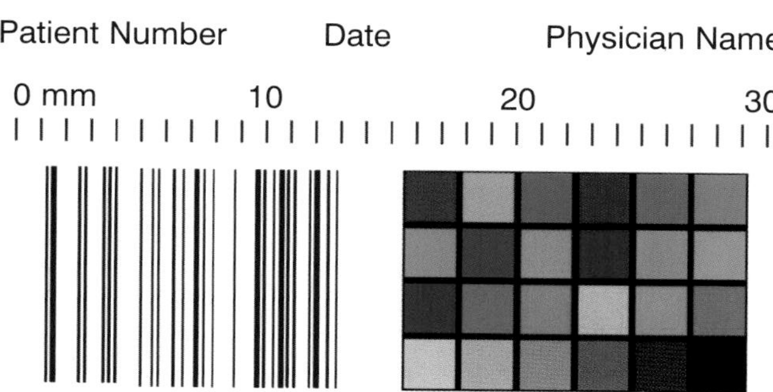

Figure 6.1 A label at the plane of focus to minimize auto focus failure on unmarked skin. This sample label incorporates an absolute color reference chart, patient identification, a metric scale, a bar code for automated identification, date, and physician identification.

lower end digital cameras and have the additional capability of shooting with cross-polarized light or oil immersion to minimize specular reflection.

View finders

In indoor lighting conditions, the LCD monitor provides a view finder superior to the optical view finder. In outdoor settings with high ambient light, the LCD monitor washes out and may force the use of the optical view finder. For practitioners making the conversion to digital media from film, the LCD usually becomes the preferred way to compose photographs. Additionally, the LCD shows the true image to be captured while optical viewfinders may not give accurate composition information for macro photographs because of parallax errors.

Image labels

Image labels within each image are a valuable adjunct to proper image identification. Such labels can sometimes be printed out from the patient schedule on a daily basis and attached to the patient chart. Labels also act as a high-contrast target for focusing. Standardized image labels may incorporate an absolute color reference chart, patient identification, a metric scale, a bar code for automated identification, date, and physician identification (see Fig. 6.1).

Color imaging

Color imaging must be considered in two contexts: human and machine vision. Human vision is dependent on the complementary aspects of scene perception,[8] which limits the value of true color reproduction, whereas machine vision is sensitive to true color.

Bit depth

Each pixel of a digital color image contains a series of color information units (bits). With a 24-bit depth, 8 bits are dedicated to each of the three additive primary colors—red, green, and blue. This bit depth is also called true color because it can produce the one million colors potentially discernible to the human eye, while a 16-bit display is only capable of producing 65 536 colors. No studies have been done on bit depth requirements for diagnostic dermatology imaging.

Red–green–blue (RGB) imaging

Most CCD devices currently on the market utilize the RGB principle. An RGB image has four default channels—red, green, blue, and composite, the latter to display all the color information. Digital cameras use physical RGB color filters on the individual pixels. Chip-specific software filters further modify the color from silicon capture media. The color profile information along with the camera and exposure data are stored in the Journalist Photo Experts Group (JPEG) file header.

Another confounding element of true color analysis of images is that different spectral distributions can result in the same encoded signals being sent to the brain and hence cause the perception of the 'same' color. This phenomenon is called metamerism. Combinations of different frequencies striking the cone cells of the retina cause the sensation of different colors (e.g. the sensation of purple can be created by simultaneously stimulating the eye with color intensities in both the red and blue spectral regions and thus a pixel with equal intensities of R and B and nil of G will appear purple).

Multispectral imaging

Multispectral imaging[9] eliminates the variations in reproduction of colors caused by metamerism. Furthermore, precision color sensing in the near infrared can discriminate the exact temperature of the skin. Digital infrared photography also sends a strong temperature-dependent signal for surgical wound evaluation and provides insight about flap viability and wound infection. Blood and melanin signals have been modeled for melanoma diagnosis.[10] In many cases, multispectral medical imaging may replace invasive diagnosis.

Ultraviolet (UV) photography

UV photography was first applied in dermatology in 1983.[11] Today it is used clinically to detect sun damage in adults[12] and in children.[13] An inexpensive method for UV photography using a digital CCD camera and image processing has recently been documented.[14]

Photodynamic fluorescent photography

Photodynamic fluorescent photography involves the application of aminolevulinic acid (ALA) followed by an incubation period of several hours in contact with the skin. Exposure of the ALA to enzymatic receptors in the rapidly proliferating epidermis converts the ALA to protoporphyrin. Basal cell carcinoma reacts with a bright signal, best emitted with 400 nm light.[15] Unfortunately, in the heavily sun damaged skin, inflammatory and neoplastic changes are easily come by and the test suffers from a lack of discrimination as a result of false-positive signals (personal communication, RJD).

Color balance

In medical photography, absolute color can be an issue. For example, the intensity of shades of red (erythema) is an important clinical measure. Color correction can be achieved by including a color card containing standardized gray scale and color swatches within the image for an absolute color reference. Digital cameras and image editing software typically provide useful color filters to account for lighting sources such as fluorescent light, sunlight, and incandescent light. Check the camera's manual to optimize these settings.

Storing, retrieving, and processing digital images

Storage and retrieval software

Reviews of many software systems for storing and retrieving digital photographs are available at sites like www.dpreview.com. These programs are most commonly called photo album software. Reviews and demonstration copies can be found on the Internet at sites such as www.download.com and www.photographyreview.com. A 2003 search of the phrase 'photo album software' run on Google yielded over 64 900 hits! Image storage and display solutions are being built into operating systems such as Windows XP and Mac OS X. Dermatology-specific solutions have added features which address the special needs of dermatologists.

Diagnostic indexing of patient images

Significant progress has been made in the past several years in lexicography for disease categorization and image labeling for dermatology, so that now dermatologists can take advantage of several different disease-oriented language systems. The Image Library Manager is such a system derived from the Lexicon of the British Association of Dermatologists. Led by Robert Chalmers, the program takes advantage of recent advances in both data storage technology and dermatological disease classification. Designed specifically for dermatologists and dermatopathologists, it uses the strongest available dermatologic language tool to facilitate the tasks of filing images and of creating and storing image sets for research, lectures, and other educational purposes. The project software is available online at http://www.data-soft.co.uk/index.html. In the US, The National Library of Medicine recently awarded a grant for a dermatology lexicon to researchers at the University of Rochester. That project's goal is the creation of a universally accepted and comprehensive dermatology terminology that should produce a good labeling standard for dermatology photographs. Information on the project is available at the Center for Future Health—http://www.futurehealth.rochester.edu/dlp/. Archival software using a dermatology language system may require considerable time and expertise in entering new photographs.

Alternative patient image labeling conventions

Patient images may be stored in JPEG format, archived by folders, according to the date of service on CDs or DVDs. The file names of the images include as a suffix the name given to the image by the digital camera, preceded by the first two letters of the last name, followed by the first letter of the first name, and then followed by the date of birth in six digit format (Table 6.5). These would then be labeled along with the photographs taken of other people on that day and saved with a transcriptionist's dictation in a text file.

This approach has several advantages—it is inexpensive, independent of a software developer, has a universal format, is searchable by patient initials, images are noted by date, and basic displaying and rotating of photos can be done through programs such as IrfanView from www.irfanview.com, Cumulus from www.canto.com, or ACDSee from www.acdsystems.com.

Total immersion photography

An instrument invented by one author (RJD) uses a fluorescently lit stage with 24 digital cameras to automate the process of total body photography. This system is called Total Immersion Photography. Patients position themselves for front and back views under the supervision of a technician who fires the system. The file names are automatically generated as follows: chart number—anatomic position—date—time.jpg. Patient images are stored in a directory named by their chart number. In the automated Total Immersion Photography system, software performs all of these labeling and file transfer procedures on two separate computers once the patient's chart number has been entered and the imaging session is triggered. Images are automatically archived by mirroring the complete contents of each new session on the reciprocal computer. Alphanumeric sorting of images then produces an array of photographs according to the patient, location, date, and time (Table 6.6), which may be reviewed by any slide show software, such as is embedded in current operating systems or downloadable from the web.

The advantages of this approach are that there is no photographic skill requirement and that it achieves total body photography with reproducible lighting, reproducible positioning, private image booth, minimal operator training (novice computer users), and minimal operator time (2 minutes). The obvious downsides are the dedication of office space and the initial outlay of money for such a system. Yet there is the obvious benefit of comprehensive, reproducible automated skin image documentation.

Table 6.5 Alternative patient image labeling conventions

Folder name	Patient initials	DOB label	Camera assigned suffix	Relative file address
Date of service	First two letters of the last name followed by the first letter of the first name	Date of birth in six digit format	Suffix the name given to the image by the camera operating system	.../011503/NAM110954 DSCN7453.JPG

Table 6.6 Total immersion photography

Folder name	Chart number	Position label	Date mmddyyyy	Time hhmmss	File extension	Relative file address
000001	000001	B2	08182003	081839	.jpg	…/000001/000001-B2-08182003-081839.jpg

Table 6.7 Dermatology-specific software featuring image storage, retrieval, and processing

Software genre	Product name	Web address
Esthetic simulation software	Mirror Suite	http://www.canfieldsci.com/software/suite.shtml
	CosMax	http://www.derma.co.at/cosmax/english/english1.htm
Body mapping software	DermaGraphix	http://www.canfieldsci.com/products/dermagraphix.html
	MoleMax	http://www.derma.co.at/molemax1/molemax1.htm
	BodyScan	http://www.fotofinder.de/neu/english/index.htm
Image management software	Image Library Manager*	http://www.data-soft.co.uk/index.html
	FOTOsoft	http://www.dermlite.com/fotosoft.html
Pigmented skin lesion expert system	MoleAnalyzer	http://www.moleanalyzer.com/engl/frameset.htm

* *Image Library Manager incorporates the British Association of Dermatologists' Diagnostic Index*

Diverse types of dermatology software

Many practice genre-specific needs are addressed by dermatology software, which features storage, retrieval, and image processing. Table 6.7 gives examples of such products.

File formats

A dizzying array of file formats is available for digital images. The most popular are represented in Table 6.8. The most standard form of file format is the bitmap (BMP) image. BMP is a standard Windows image format found on DOS and Windows compatible computers. JPEG and TIFF are common file formats produced by digital cameras. The compressed file format used most commonly in dermatology is JPEG, which may allow for compression ratios of 30 : 1 on certain clinical images.

Table 6.8 Popular image file formats

File extension	Web?	Compression?	Format name
RAW	No*	No	Raw Image File
JPEG	Yes	Yes	Journalist Photo Experts Group
BMP	No*	No	Bit Map
GIF	Yes	Yes	Graphic Interchange Format
EXIF	No*	No	Exchangeable Image File Format
TIFF	No*	No, commonly	Tagged Image File Format

* *May be opened within a web browser, but only with the aid of an external program*

File compression

Digital photography creates potentially large files; even a low resolution 640 × 480 pixels image may occupy a megabyte or more of storage space. Digital cameras use compression to ease image storage and transmission. However, most of these algorithms, such as the popular JPEG format, involve data loss. The loss is usually not clinically meaningful at capture, but editing and resaving with further compression may severely degrade an image. Most software allows the user to turn off further compression to minimize this effect. Most digital cameras allow the user to set compression levels at fine (minimal compression), normal (default), or basic (high compression), though the precise descriptors vary by vendor.

Reliable archival storage

Dermatology images fall under medical record storage requirements. As such, a hard copy must be kept for at least 7 years. The most common and cost-effective strategy for archival purposes is to transfer electronic medical records to read only digital media such as the CD read only memory (CD-ROM) or DVD read only memory (DVD-ROM). Such hard copy archives should be created on a frequent basis to avoid information loss. Hard disk or digital tape back-up systems should be in place and used on a near constant basis. Hard disks can be made to mirror each other's contents to provide near instantaneous back-up, ensuring minimal risk to the integrity of electronic medical records.

CD-ROMs and DVD-ROMs are the most reliable media on which to store photos; once written to, the photos will be retrievable for at least several decades. The major limitation to storage time with these media is the optical clarity of the plastic, which will eventually become unreadable to the laser head as the plastic coating of the CD oxidizes with time. The better quality media has a 30–50-year life. If a CD becomes unreadable because the optical face gets too scratched, there are services that will restore the media to a readable condition. Failed hard drives and other defective media may also be recovered in whole or in part.

Methods to secure medical records are mirror hard drives, keeping a second hard copy off-site to avoid fire, flood, or other natural disasters, and a CD and/or a DVD burner to handle long-term storage needs.

Image editing

The full details of image editing are beyond the scope of this chapter, but they need to be acknowledged as a tool for refining and extracting digital photographic information. The most commonly used image editing tools are cropping and resizing. Although many different programs exist for photo editing, by far the most powerful (although not necessarily the easiest to learn to use) is Adobe Corporation's Photoshop. Diverse photo editing software is widely available. IrfanView, a package mentioned above, is both powerful and stable and excellent for basic editing. It is important that the user turns off software compression when editing an image. If the image is recompressed each time it is saved, detail may be lost rapidly due to the algorithms used by JPEG compression.

Exposure correction

Exposure correction is used when an image is too dark or light. Although it is always better to get a good photograph that is properly exposed, mild exposure problems can be handled by digital manipulation. One of the easiest problems to resolve is a photograph that is slightly dark. Additional details can sometimes be reclaimed from shadowy areas in a slightly underexposed image by increasing the brightness and contrast settings with image enhancement software. Within our specialty, differing levels of editing may be acceptable. Adjustment of an image that demonstrates tumor size, location, ablation, and repair frequently need far less proof of legitimacy than images demonstrating subtle anti-aging changes (i.e. cosmetic improvements can result from differences in photographic technique or, potentially, digital image tampering). For the latter, significant adjustment may bring into question whether the image demonstrates the effects of the dermatologic procedure or the capabilities of the editing software and user. For circumstances where precise comparisons are needed, the user optimally captures images that need no adjustment.

Color correction

Digital cameras usually impose camera-specific color filters on their output, which may be organized automatically by a built-in light meter or imposed manually by a choice of lighting source. Once captured and processed by the camera, the colors of an image may be corrected to bring out desired features of the image or to normalize the colors with standardized colors included within the image to provide a reference. The final output of an image may be color corrected by comparing the output to a second color swatch.

Image resizing

Digital cameras capture and store images in a variety of resolutions. Occasionally, an image must be resized (e.g. before sending an image through email because of the potential bulk of the digital file). Two elements—image dimensions and compression—may be adjusted. Photo editing programs enable image cropping or shrinking to control image dimensions. Compression is usually performed in a JPEG format. Excessive resizing or compression may degrade the clinical value of the photograph; the resulting image may not retain sufficient quality to make a fair representation. For JPEG clinical images, reducing the size to less than 25 KB in a 72 DPI 800 × 600 pixel image jeopardizes quality, whereas image sizes greater than 60 KB are excessively large files. Image resizing options include reducing the height and width of the image proportionally, reducing the resolution, compressing the image, and cropping the image.

Annotation

Images may be annotated with voice through many cameras or by text with several text annotation programs. Many still digital cameras include video subsystems, and many digital video cameras include still digital capture. Thus still images may be annotated by video capture within the same capture instrument. Another potential form of annotation is derived from image analysis algorithms, which highlight skin lesions; for instance, a changed pigmented skin lesion may be annotated by a color code. Highlighting techniques are discussed below.

Prints, presentations, email, and telemedicine

Prints

A color laser printer is a fast and effective way to print photographs. High-quality photographs can also be produced with relatively inexpensive inkjet printers. Although black and white laser printers are faster than color, and they are as effective for mapping lesions, they fail to convey comparable diagnostic information. For many applications high-quality black and white images are acceptable, and serve as an accurate map of the size and locations of lesions (such as atypical nevi). Resolution requirements for printing are presented in Table 6.9.

Presentations

Slide shows may be generated directly from a series of properly sorted digital photographs. Most photo album and dermatology-specific software facilitate such presentations.

Table 6.9 Relationship of image resolution and print size

Print size—single (inches)	Megapixels	Image resolution pixels
Wallet (2 × 3)	0.3	640 × 480
4 × 5	0.4	768 × 512
5 × 7	0.8	1152 × 768
8 × 10	1.6	1536 × 1024
16 × 20	3.1	2048 × 1536
20 × 30	5	2560 × 1920

However, Microsoft's presentation software PowerPoint dominates dermatology meetings, both live and virtual; PowerPoint presentations may be offered on the internet with minimal effort. Digital cameras enable slides, photographs, radiographs, and textbook images to be digitized in seconds with adequate quality for most common clinical and educational applications.[16]

Email

Digital images may be readily attached to email messages. This property of email has revolutionized dermatology communications with diagnostic visuals. Many language-specific dermatology email groups have been able to effect cross-cultural case exchanges, greatly enhancing the range of exposure of participating dermatologists to foreign-acquired diseases in an increasingly global community. Rapid communication of challenging or rare diseases has thrust digital image enhanced email to the forefront of dermatology clinical practice and continuing education. Armed with digital cameras and email networks, the dermatology community can rapidly define emerging epidemics.

Image databases

Eloquently described compilations of digital images of the skin are freely available through the internet. One need only perform an image search on Google for a condition such as pemphigus to uncover hundreds of relevant images. Properly organized and indexed digital image collections are excellent teaching tools. The patient population derives tremendous insight through this process. As digital cameras have become ubiquitous, so has accompanying disease imagery. Well-known resources that have flourished over the past few years include the Atlas of Dermatology at http://www.dermis.net and the Dermatology Image Atlas—Johns Hopkins University at http://dermatlas.med.jhmi.edu/derm/.

Teledermatology

Advances in digital cameras initiated the era of store and forward teledermatology in the closing decade of the 20th century. Review of patient images and histories is an effective and efficient modality for the evaluation and management process of dermatology consultations.[17] Parallel studies in teledermatopathology reveal comparable reliability to traditional histologic slide evaluation.[18] With the advent of megapixel cameras and ubiquitous computer networks, teledermatology and telepathology have gained widespread acceptance as a health service for initial dermatology consultations in remote clinical sites.

Acceptance of store and forward teledermatology is limited by several factors: the difficulty of reimbursement (only in special case settings), the expertise required for point and shoot photography, and the labor of history taking. Photographic skills for the non-dermatologists are not trivial. Courses have been run for non-dermatologists to learn dermatologic photography, yet after several days of lessons one primary care physician related feeling daunted by the task of dermatologic photography (C Sneiderman, National Library of Medicine, personal communication). Commercial application service providers such as TeledermSolutions at http://www.teledermsolutions.com have been pioneers in the field.

Management of medical imaging services

Consent and privacy

Networked environments present new challenges to medical record privacy. Patient consent and privacy are key issues in the current era of data protection legislation, for example compliance with the Health Insurance Portability and Accountability Act (HIPAA) in the US.

Patient photography may make a physician liable for invasion of privacy. US courts have imposed liability, primarily when the provider has exploited the patient for commercial benefit. However, courts have also imposed liability when the patient's name or likeness was used for non-commercial purposes, finding that even taking a picture without the patient's expressed consent was an invasion of privacy.[19]

Dermatologists may be liable for publishing photographs under the type of invasion of privacy known as public disclosure of embarrassing private facts. In one case, the court ruled that a physician had invaded a patient's privacy by using 'before' and 'after' photographs of her face to demonstrate the effects of a face lift. The use of the photographs publicized the fact the patient had a face lift, which she found embarrassing and distressing.[19] The American Health Information Management Association has developed a valuable practice brief entitled *Patient Photography, Videotaping, and Other Imaging.*[20] A photographic consent form is accessible online through a variety of online sources.[21] Guidelines for a dermatology office setting are as follows:

- Imaging technicians and health care professionals understand computer security before participating in image management.
- Image databases require users to log in with a username and password.
- Improper username and password combinations are locked out of workstations.
- Medical records workstations automatically log out after a short idle time.
- Systems are set up to inhibit the display of any other patients' information or images.
- Standard operating procedures are in place for patient images and signed by key employees.

Personnel

A dermatology imaging technician may be hired as a key employee in dermatology practices intent on maximizing digital imagery. This employee should be trained to perform full and partial body photography of patients and contribute to a smooth, efficient patient flow. The person must be able to manage patient records in a private and confidential manner within a selected database/application, and also needs to manage and support the dermatology imaging systems and its users. Depending on the network topology, a working knowledge of Windows 2000 or XP or Mac OS X and relational databases is required. The ability to run queries, configure the workstation to communicate within the network, and ensure all equipment is appropriately connected to the workstation (e.g. cables, cameras, and other accessories) is critical. Problem solving and troubleshooting skills and a familiarity with photographic equipment and principles are also necessary. In small practices, the most computer-literate employee usually assumes this role.

Office space for imaging

Optimally, an entire room, or a large part of it, should be permanently reserved for obtaining reproducible sets of images of the face and neck[22] and the whole body. Fixed staging creates the most consistent lighting, pose, and reproducible information for cancer and cosmetic conditions alike. Placing high-resolution cameras with mounting arms in communication with PCs in the clinics may be useful, but eliminates the portability of compact digital cameras and the reproducible structure of staged imaging.

Specific internet resources for digital cameras

Internet websites and consumer magazines are good places to find professional and semi-professional reviews of camera features and include *The Imaging Resource* (http://www.imaging-resource.com/), *Digital Photography Review* (http://www.dpreview.com/), and *Steve's Digicams* (http://www.steves-digicams.com/).

■ PRACTICAL APPLICATIONS

Image processing techniques with special relevance to dermatology

Digital images can be considered data sets susceptible to the mathematical constructs of addition, subtraction, and multiplication as well as more esoteric operations. Image analysis algorithms used in dermatology include the following.

Affine plane transforms

Four points define an affine plane necessary for digital image morphing (warping) between two planar images. If multiple planes are involved, each plane must be defined by an additional four points. The points of reference are known as control points. The affine plane transformation is useful in skin change analysis.

Pigmented lesion area matching

For high-risk patients, photographic records are invaluable; time lapse comparison of digital images may be clarified by using pigmented lesions as control points in an image registration algorithm. Several equations have been demonstrated to accomplish this feat.[23,24]

Edge detection

Edge detection algorithms analyze images for curvilinear color gradients, which are interpreted as edges. Anatomic structures present edges for automatic feature recognition.

Segmentation

Segmentation algorithms are defined to extract regions of interest from skin images. The concept of skin lesion and region of interest become synonymous; this area is now available for further analysis. Segmentation is used extensively in pigmented skin lesion analysis.

Area measurements

Many skin diseases present as well-circumscribed areas (segments) in a background of normal skin. Machine vision is capable of rapid objective measurement of such diseased areas, whereas the human visual cortex fails to perform these precise measurements. Time-lapse evaluations of areas of involvement are critical for accurate evaluations of therapeutic efficacy.[25]

Melanoma analysis algorithms

Once segmented, pigmented skin lesions may be classified by a variety of algorithms for their likelihood of being a melanoma.[26]

Morphing

In image morphing, a variety of algorithms allow two or more images to dissolve or mesh into a single image. In view morphing, one or many images are transformed to provide a fresh, virtual perspective. In dermatology a common application is in assessment of patient cosmetic facial improvement through morphing between images before and after procedures.

Image difference highlighting techniques

Visual appreciation of changes in dermatologic conditions may be accentuated through the use of the image processes described below.

Flicker

If the time-lapse patient images are well aligned, the images may be flickered at 0.5-second intervals to accentuate changes.

Color coding

Areas of interest, such as image changes from one study to another, may be highlighted with color codes.

Side by side

With this process, comparison of images is facilitated by close apposition.

Standardized photography

For optimum results, maximum efficiency, and ease of comparing photographs taken over time, standardizing images is invaluable. The subject's position should be fixed in the same location and pose with identical camera distances and angles to optimize visualization. With respect to serial clinical images, this means that the patient position for imagery must be reproducible.

Specific procedural imaging

Oral photography

Intraoral photography may be difficult with the equipment typically used for cutaneous imaging. Difficulties include poor response to auto focus systems as well as limited magnification and lighting restrictions.[27] A ring flash and dental lip retractors are useful for photographing this area.

Facial photography for surgical procedures

According to the Clinical Photography Committee of the Plastic Surgery Education Foundation, the same camera, lens, setting, lighting, and patient positioning should be used for each photograph to ensure reproducibility. First, full face views are taken of the patient in the frontal position, both oblique positions, and both lateral positions. Orienting the camera horizontally, the patient is photographed from the front with eyes open, from the front with eyes closed, and with a frontal gaze upward. The patient is photographed in both oblique positions, both lateral positions, and from a basal view with the tip of the nose aligned with the upper eyelid crease (Fig. 6.2).[28]

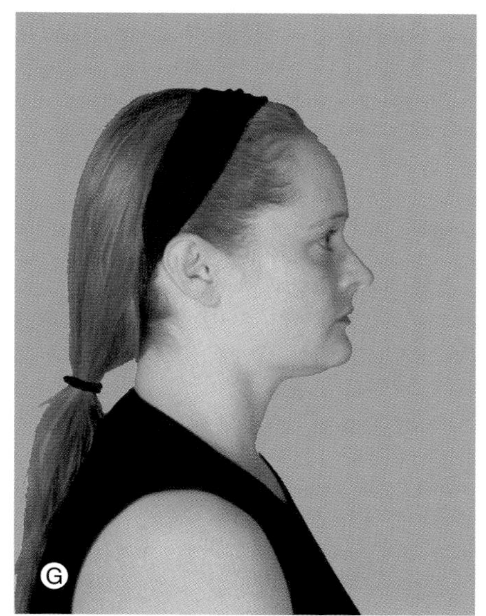

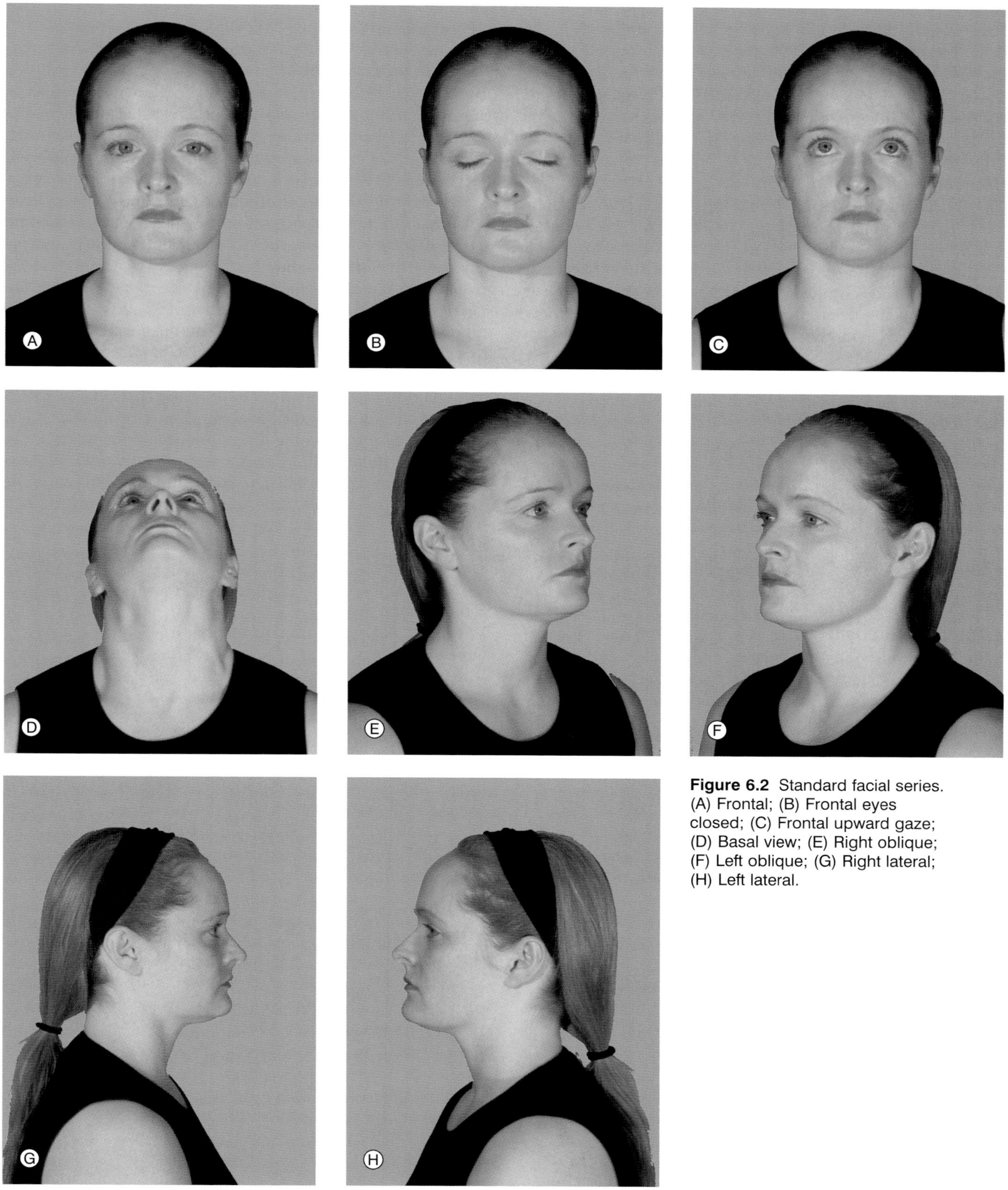

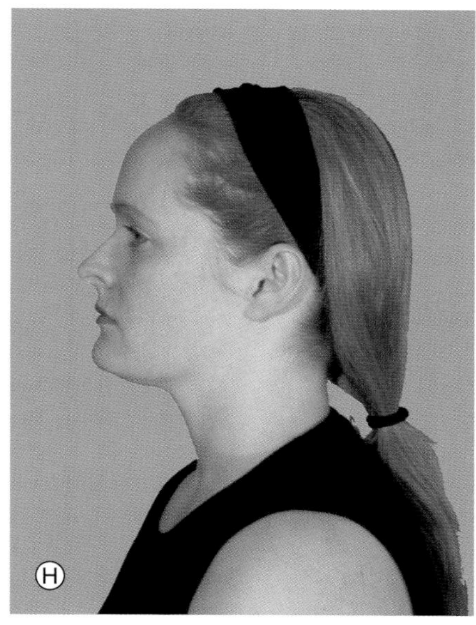

Figure 6.2 Standard facial series. (A) Frontal; (B) Frontal eyes closed; (C) Frontal upward gaze; (D) Basal view; (E) Right oblique; (F) Left oblique; (G) Right lateral; (H) Left lateral.

Blepharoplasty

Imaging the eyes for blepharoplasty[29] requires a series of close-up views, differentiating it from the standard facial cosmetic surgical series (Fig. 6.3).

Hair restoration

Surgical and medical hair evaluations are enhanced by systematic photography. Methods for computer image analysis of hair were introduced in 1986 (Fig. 6.4).[30]

Botox documentation

Photographs are taken both at rest and during muscle contraction to highlight the wrinkles that are being treated. Follow-up photographs are taken 1–4 weeks after treatment to allow for the best comparison (Figures 6.5–6.7).[31]

Chin augmentation

The chin should be imaged with standard facial photographs (see Fig. 6.2). The usual views, full face, oblique, lateral, and base, are generally adequate for this evaluation. From the lateral view, the zero degree meridian and other types of analysis can be employed to determine the grade of retrusion and the desired augmentation.[32] The lateral view is emphasized, but the full face view is mandatory to evaluate chin width. Photographs should be taken with the patient smiling and in repose. These will provide additional information and documentation of labial competence (Fig. 6.8).

Brow lift

The patient must be prompted to contract the brow to create this image series (Fig. 6.9).

Surgical specimen tracking

Digital imagery has been deployed for surgical specimen tracking. In this process the lesion areas are imaged in a sequence of steps to enhance the clinicopathologic correlation—the first image is obtained *in vivo*, the second at the level of gross pathology, and the third at the level of microscopy. Careful specimen mapping and marking is also employed in the Mohs micrographic surgery technique.[33] The marking map is composed directly on the image of the postexcision defects.

Total body photography

The probability of cure of skin cancers depends in part on the time lapse between onset and removal. Digital cameras permit screening protocols that improve productivity and lead to early surgical removal of skin cancers in the at-risk population. The presurgical diagnosis of melanoma currently only occurs by the visualization of the skin of susceptible individuals, but digital detection provides another pathway. Early detection of potentially metastatic skin cancers, especially melanomas, may be facilitated by the detection of pigmented lesion changes.[34,35] Detection and surgical treatment of the early stages of this malignancy are usually curative. In contrast, treatment of advanced melanoma continues to yield dismal results (see Chapter 50).

Patients who are at high risk for melanoma followed up with periodic surveillance have been proven to have significantly thinner and less invasive melanomas than patients whose tumors are diagnosed at first encounter.[36] It has been postulated that small tumors might otherwise be overlooked in the absence of baseline photography.[37] In general, small diameter tumors are more likely to be thinner

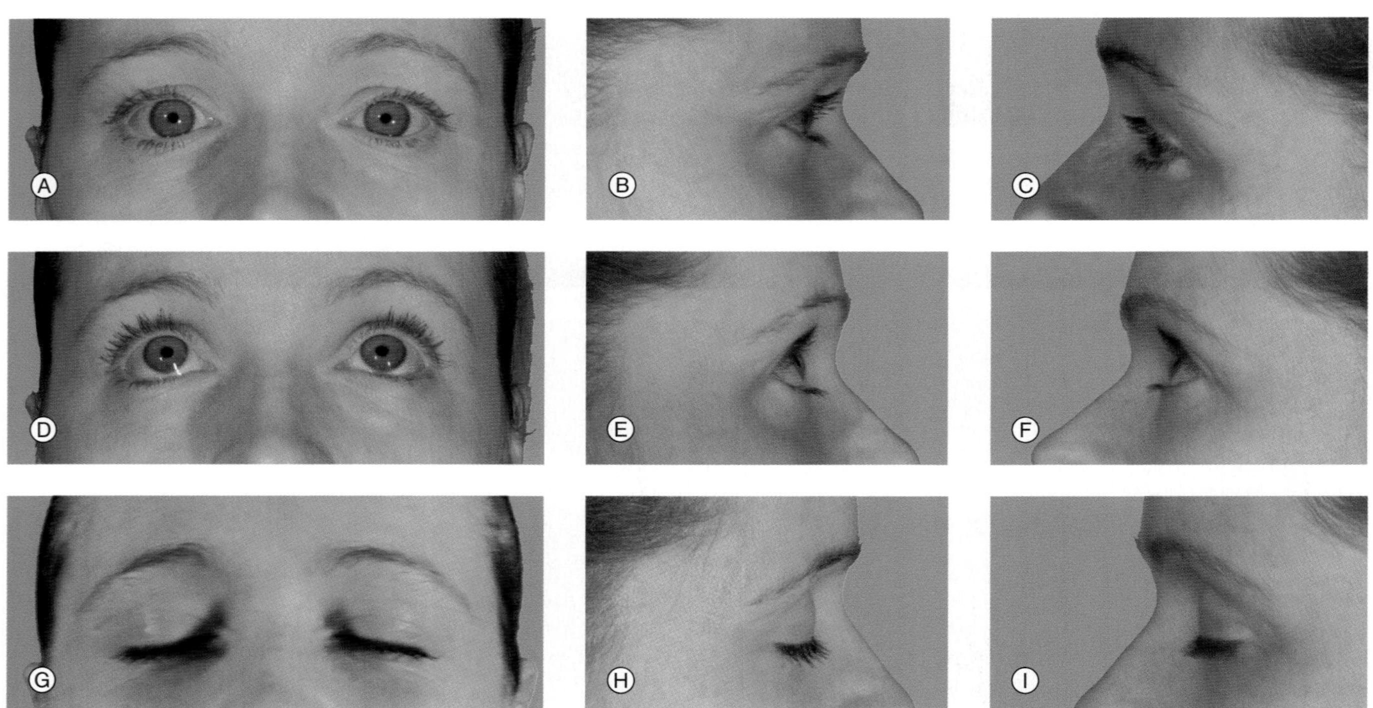

Figure 6.3 Blepharoplasty series. (A) Frontal; (B) Right lateral; (C) Left lateral; (D) Frontal upward gaze; (E) Right lateral upward gaze; (F) Left lateral upward gaze; (G) Frontal eyes closed; (H) Right lateral eyes closed; (I) Left lateral eyes closed.

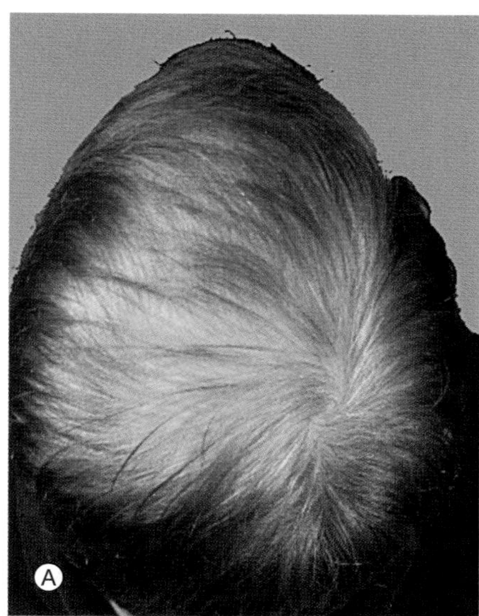

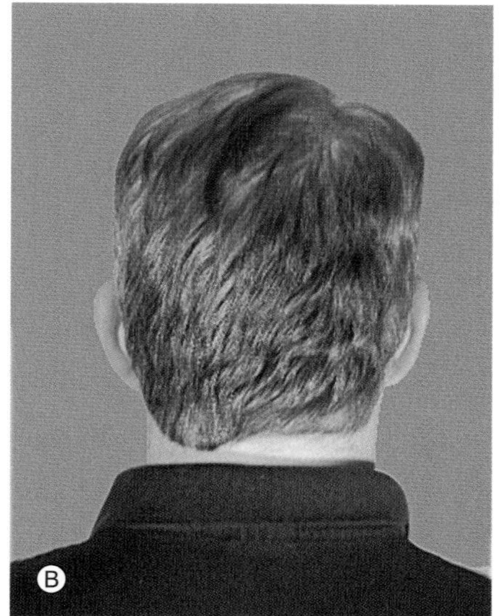

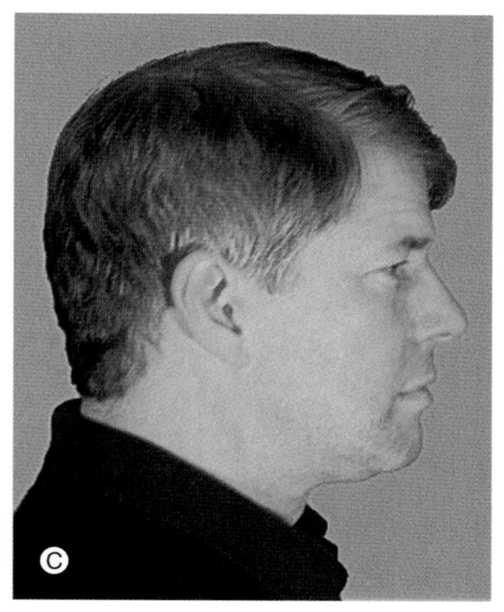

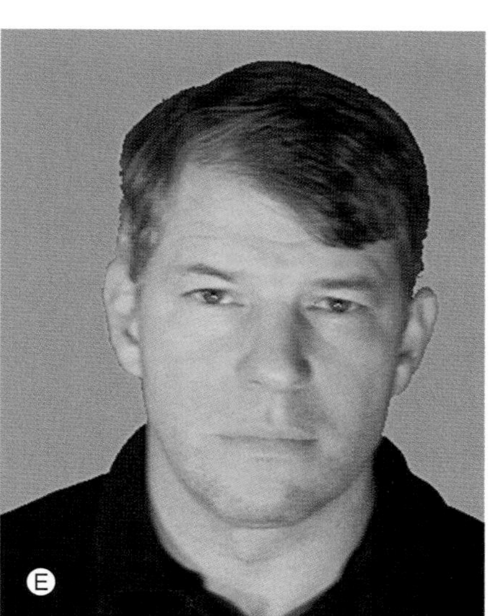

Figure 6.4 Hair restoration series. (A) Crown; (B) Occiput; (C) Right lateral; (D) Left lateral; (E) Frontal.

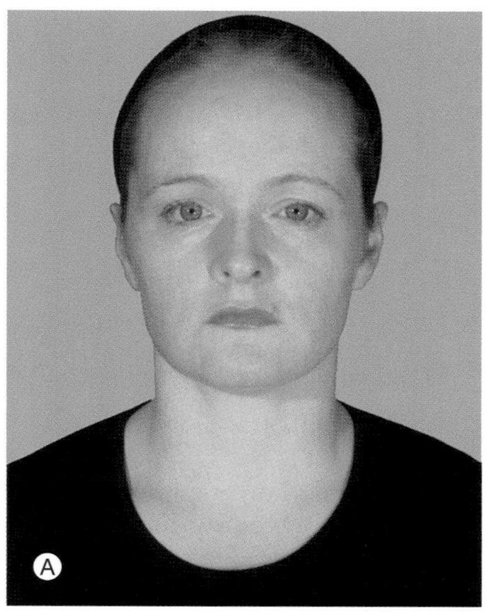

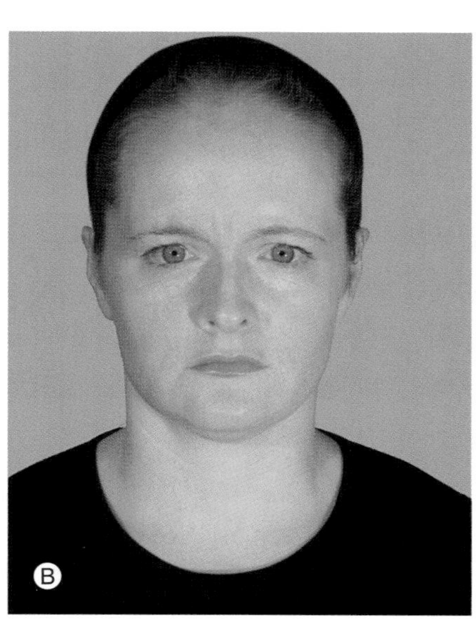

Figure 6.5 Botox glabella series. (A) Frontal face (at rest); (B) Frontal face with contraction of the procerus and corrugator muscles.

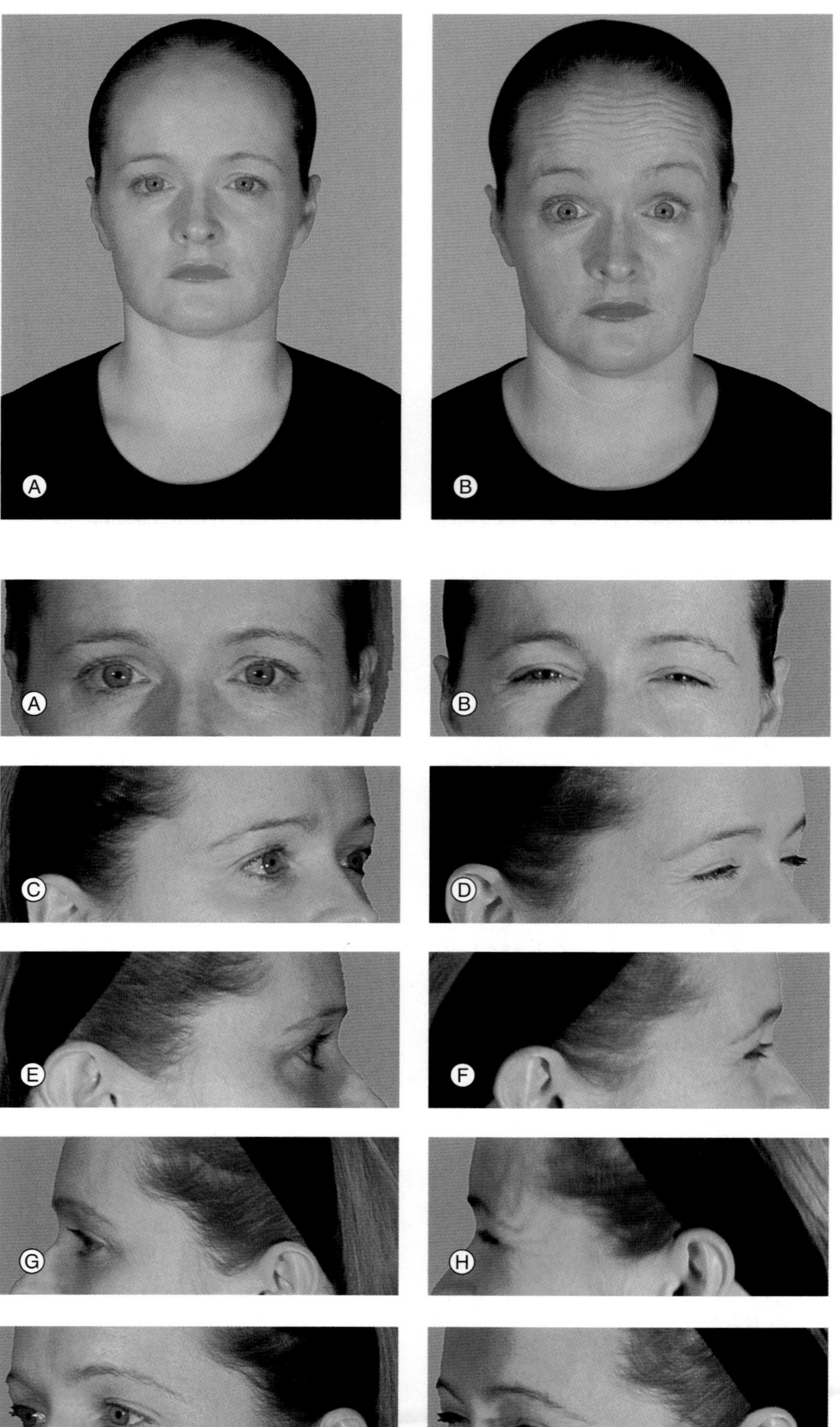

Figure 6.6 Botox frontalis series. (A) Frontal face (at rest); (B) Frontal face with brow fully contracted.

Figure 6.7 Botox series for lateral fibers of the orbicularis oculi. (A) Frontal, relaxed; (B) Frontal, squint; (C) Right oblique, relaxed; (D) Right oblique, squint; (E) Right lateral, relaxed; (F) Right lateral, squint; (G) Left lateral, relaxed; (H) Left lateral, squint; (I) Left oblique, relaxed; (J) Left oblique, squint.

or *in situ* compared with larger diameter skin cancers.[38–40] Photographic changes provide evidence of growth and have been used to advantage in combination with dermoscopic features to classify pigmented skin lesions for malignancy.[41]

Dermatologists are encountering an ever increasing number of people with multiple atypical nevi that are at elevated risk for melanoma. Monitoring these individuals for changes is difficult, but digital photographic techniques have the potential for making the job easier. In the US and elsewhere, total body photography may face two significant and related obstacles: lack of appropriate reimbursement for the procedure; and the inordinate amount of time consumed with this endeavor. Although it is not likely to be a lucrative or time-efficient procedure, total body

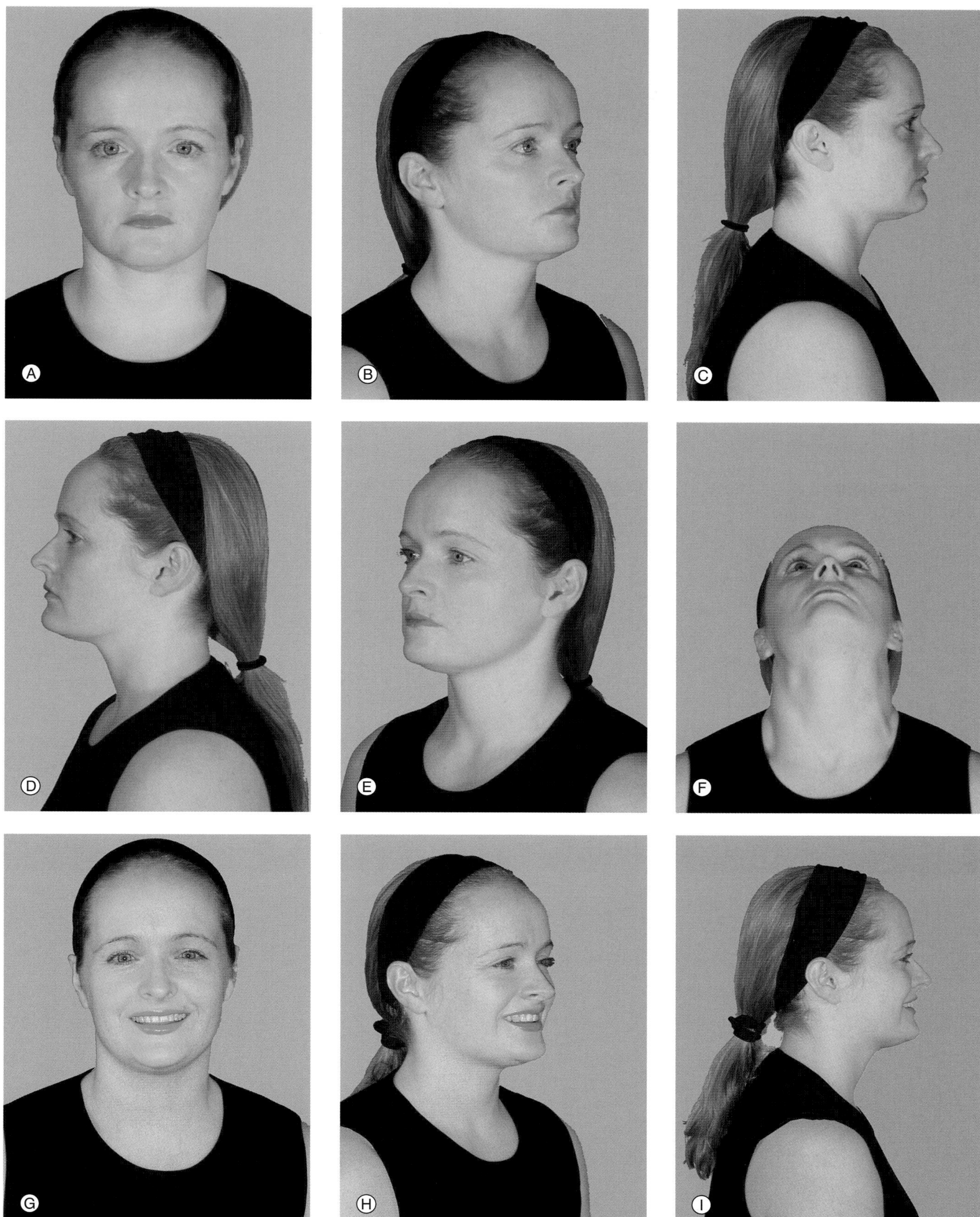

Figure 6.8 Chin augmentation series. (A) Frontal; (B) Right oblique; (C) Right lateral; (D) Left lateral; (E) Left oblique; (F) Basal view; (G) Frontal smile; (H) Right oblique smile; (I) Right lateral smile.

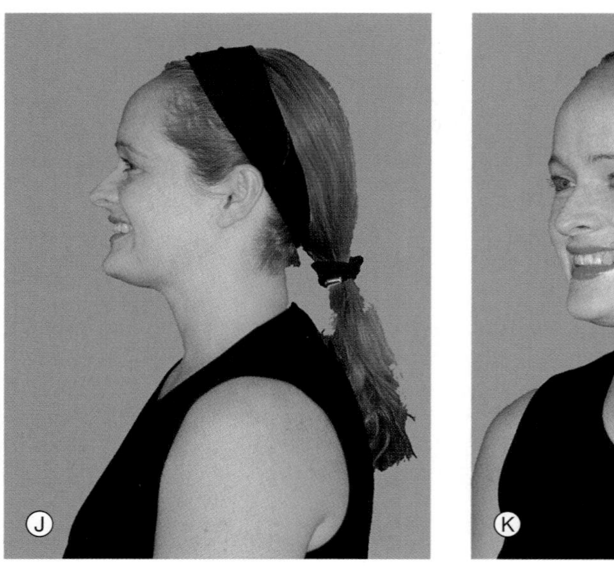
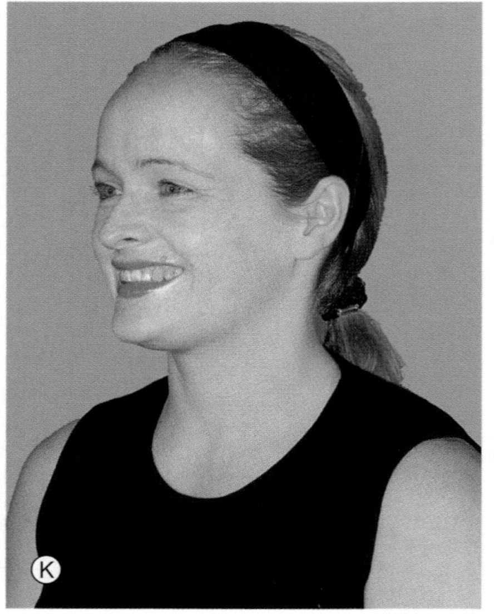
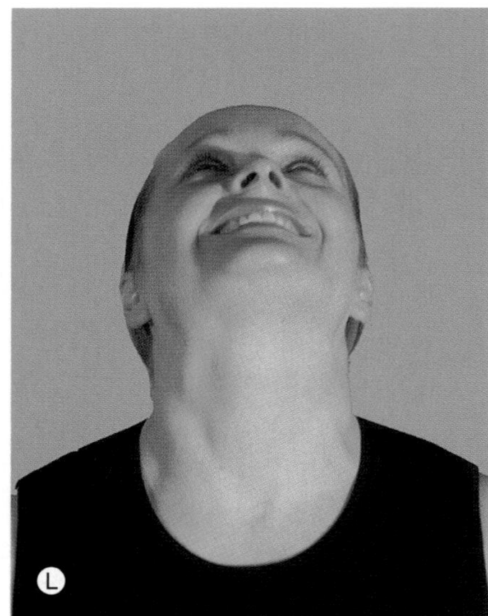

Figure 6.8, continued. (J) Left lateral smile; (K) Left oblique smile; (L) Basal view smile.

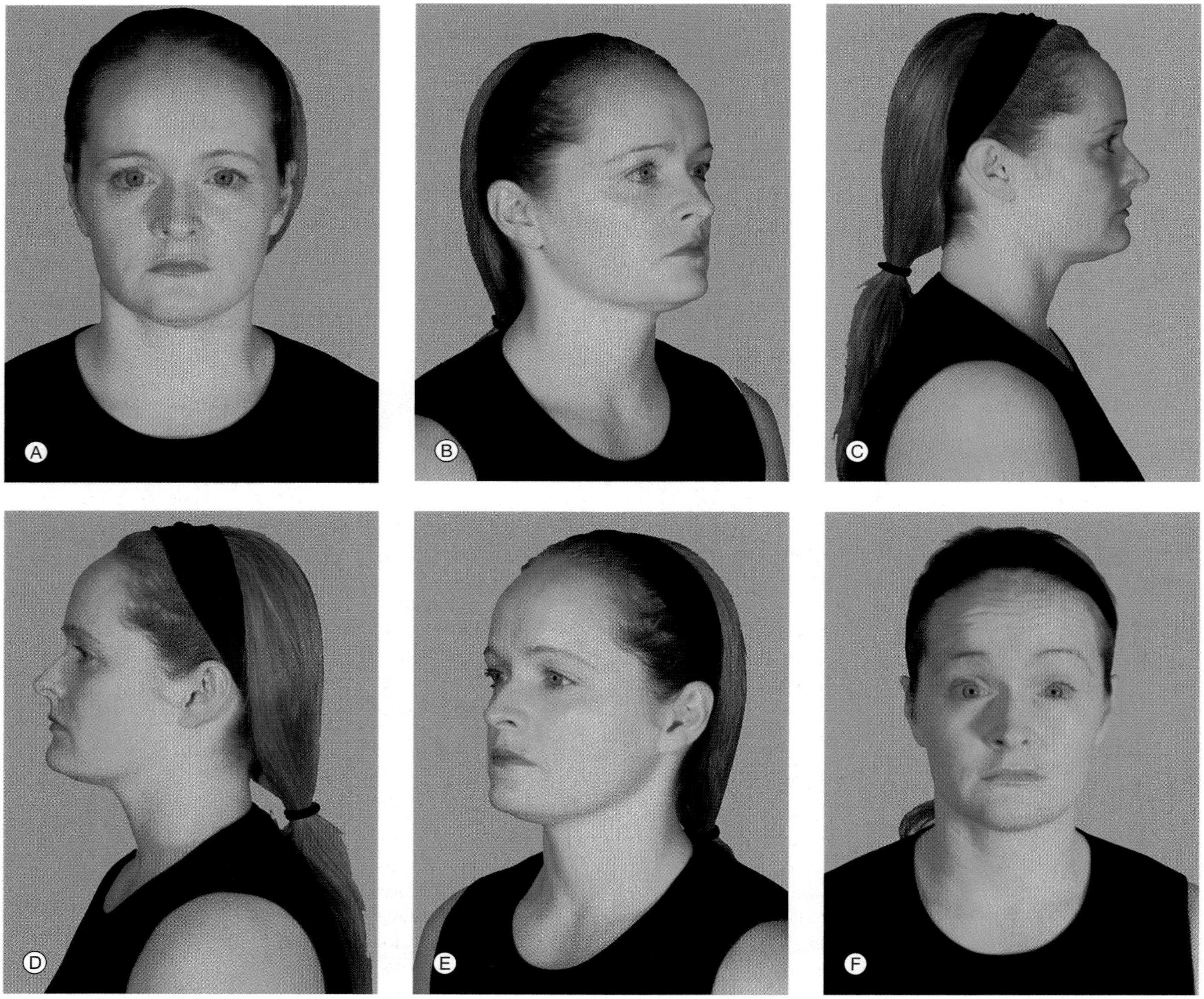

Figure 6.9 Brow lift series. (A) Frontal; (B) Right oblique; (C) Right lateral; (D) Left lateral; (E) Left oblique; (F) Frontalis contracted.

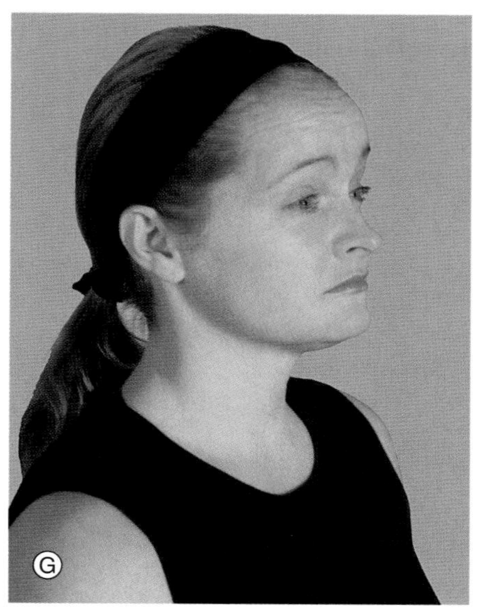

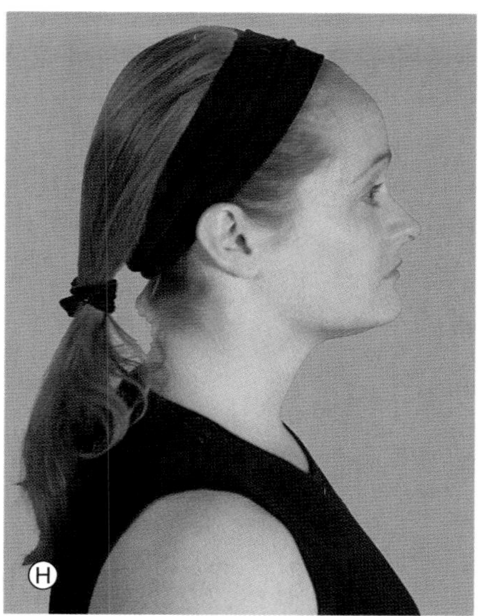

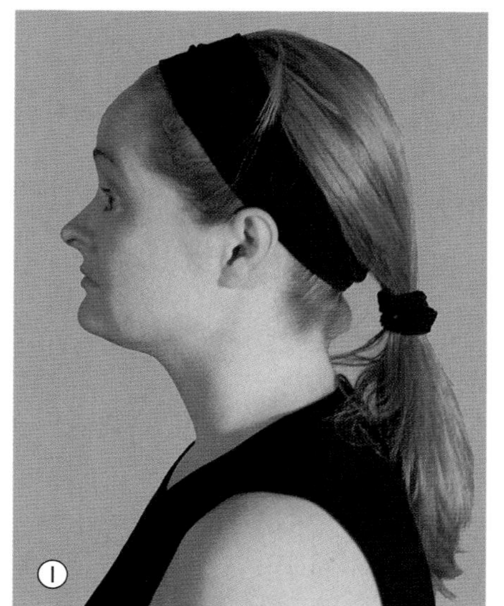

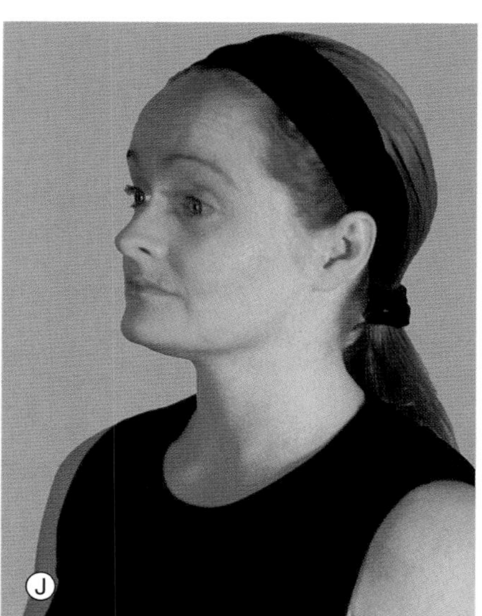

Figure 6.9, continued. (G) Right oblique frontalis contracted; (H); Right lateral frontalis contracted; (I) Left lateral frontalis contracted; (J) Left oblique frontalis contracted.

photography with conventional digital techniques can be a useful tool in the management of such people.

One technique can be carried out by a trained nurse in approximately 10 minutes. The various views utilized are shown in Figure 6.10. A recommended procedure when carrying this out is to take at least two shots of each view to improve image quality. The major goal of photographs of this type is usually to provide a baseline against which future changes can be judged. These photographs can be repeated every few years to provide a more recent baseline, but more frequent imaging other than for following individual lesions is not currently cost-effective. This is not really intended as a tool for the physician to monitor changes, which would consume an impractical amount of time; it is intended to be used with traditional methods for following these individuals, namely, follow-up visits at appropriate intervals to go over history and repeated direct physical examination to look for individual lesions that are suspicious based on instantaneous gross or dermatoscopic morphology. Because these photographs are not intended for close scrutiny by the physician, a useful thing to do is to print a back and/or torso shot and give this to the people photographed so that they (or their partners) can use it for comparison to detect new or changing lesions.

In the future, computerized systems may make it feasible for professionals to directly search digital images and actually use them to monitor for the earliest clues to changing lesions, but for the present this remains beyond the realm of practicality for most private practices. Fotofinder (discussed further below) is a system that includes some computerized comparison capabilities, and such systems may be an early indication of even more sophisticated and practical systems in the not too distant future.

An automated approach invented by one of the authors (RD) for monitoring the skin employs a large, 28-digital camera network surrounding a well-lit stage. Patients undergo Total Immersion Photography in this fluorescent lit booth where images of exposed skin are automatically captured and labeled. Mirror software then synchronizes the contents of the image directories between the two operating computers, ensuring secure back-up. The study takes less than 2 minutes to perform and is instantly available for analysis.

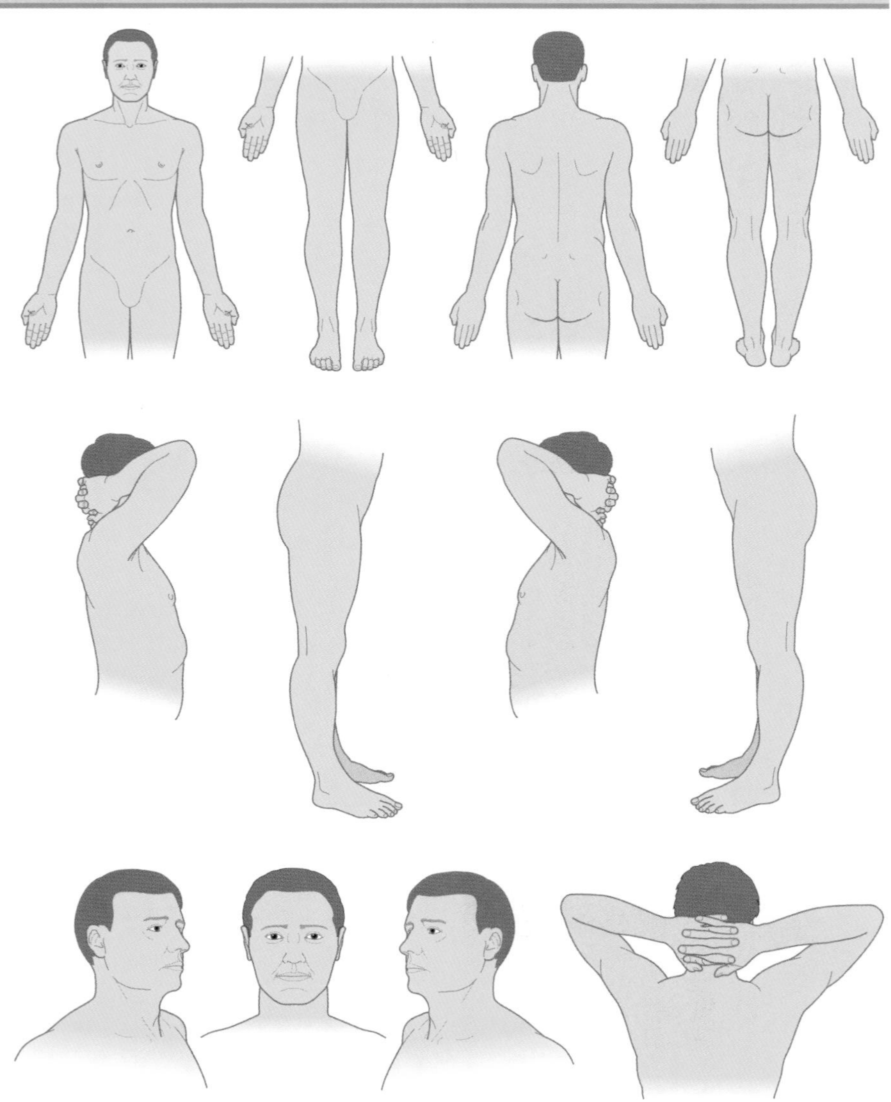

Figure 6.10 Twelve poses for rapid photographic mapping.

In the MoleMax (http://www.molemaxii.com/) system, skin surface microscopy is used to image, archive, and link each suspicious lesion to its precise location on the body. These images are of epiluminescence microscopy (ELM) and a magnification of 30 times. A third image is also taken, which is comprised of a high-resolution image of the lesion as it appears to the naked eye. Through the comparison of all three images over time MoleMax is able to identify new and changing moles and thus detect melanoma early. All images are diagnosed and reported on by dermatologists qualified in the art of ELM before being permanently archived on the computer system for future comparisons.

Fotofinder (http://www.fotofinder.de/neu/english/index.htm) is an interesting competitor to the MoleMax system. The MoleMax system may be preferred over the Fotofinder system with its self-contained database of dermoscopy and gross photographs, but the Fotofinder has certain advantages. It interoperates with any digital camera, resulting in the potential for high-quality images. Fotofinder is slow compared to the MoleMax system. However, the camera provided with Fotofinder enables comparison between two different photographs of the same subject and provides a computerized algorithm to find differences.

Skin surface microscopic photography (photographic dermoscopy)

Dermaphot (http://heineopto.com) is an oil immersion system that has a very limited field of view (about 2.0 cm across, which includes 12.6 cm^2 of surface area), but other than these limitations, works very well. These are made for the most popular types of SLR cameras. The DermLiteFOTO (http://www.dermlite.com/index.html) has the advantage of being able to shoot with (or without) a glass plate or just using cross-polarized light instead of oil/glass (i.e. works just like a DermLite (www.dermlite.com) as opposed to a traditional dermatoscope [Heine, http://www.heineweb.com/]). This camera system has a much larger field of view, about 4 cm across (or about

50 cm^2)—considerably more area than the traditional oil/glass Dermaphot. This is a device that works with most popular digital cameras. The Dermaphot and DermLite FOTO are both units that allow photodermoscopy at a reasonable cost. Live video units allow for direct patient education about their pigmented skin lesions, although this may be inordinately time consuming. Such systems create low-resolution screen capture photographs inferior to those of a low priced digital still camera. Dermoscopy photography documentation may be delegated to properly trained staff, leaving the dermatologist to interpret the results.

Two step method: digital total body photography and digital dermoscopy

There is a growing consensus within dermatology that screening for melanoma should employ the use of digital total body photography followed by dermoscopy. In this case, the patient is imaged, the images are reviewed by the dermatologist, and dermoscopy is performed.[42]

Greater integration of digital imaging and computers can automate much of the melanoma detection process. With incremental refinements in our health service model, the demonstrated benefits of skin cancer detection within digital images will lower the barriers to early diagnosis.

Biometrics

An intense recent focus on security techniques based on body surface scanning has created an enormous wealth of opportunity for dermatologists in pursuit of further knowledge because these biometric analytics have enormous potential value in diagnostic screening as well as patient identification and privacy (Table 6.10). Unfortunately, as biometric security technology improves, ever more sophisticated ways to bypass the technology are developed.[43]

Networked environments

As photography is a tool of communication, optimal usage of digital imagery in dermatology practice may be enhanced by a network of computers that facilitate image sharing. Images may be shared within an office, hospital, or network of allied health facilities. Cases may be shared by email with consultants.[44]

Table 6.10 Biometric digital imaging studies in dermatology

Biometric test	Potential application
Fingerprint scanning	Alterations in dermatoglyphics
Facial recognition	Skin cancer, facial aging, inflammatory diseases
Hand geometry	Skin cancer, inflammatory hand diseases
Subcutaneous hand scan	Vascular disease, panniculitis, arthritis, aging, tumor
Vein verification	Vascular disease, tumors
Ear shape comparison	Cancer, inflammatory diseases
Nail bed identification	Systemic and local diseases
Thermal facial scan	Inflammatory facial diseases

■ SUMMARY

Digital imaging has the potential to expand the usefulness of dermatology. By extending our range of vision, digital cameras alter dermatology; the changes will occur as imaging abandons the role of passive documentation and evolves into an instrument of intelligent signal processing.[45] Better use of these technologies needs to be explored carefully because integration of new technologies into the outpatient dermatologic surgery environment may depress productivity. Bottlenecks and benefits in the application of digital imaging need to be sought out, understood, and refined. Ahead is a long journey upon which we have just recently embarked.

■ REFERENCES

1. Taylor RS, Lin BB. Digital photography for mapping Mohs micrographic surgery sections. Dermatol Surg 2001; 27:411–414.
2. Huntley AC, Smith JG. New communication between dermatologists in the age of the Internet. Semin Cutan Med Surg 2002; 21:202–204.
3. Siegel DM. Resolution in digital imaging: enough already? Semin Cutan Med Surg 2002; 21:209–215.
4. Perednia DA, Gaines JA, Butruille TW. Comparison of the clinical informativeness of photographs and digital imaging media with multiple-choice receiver operating characteristic analysis. Arch Dermatol 1995; 131:292–297.
5. Bittorf A, Fartasch M, Schuler G, Diepgen TL. Resolution requirements for digital images in dermatology. J Am Acad Derm 1997; 37:195–198.
6. Erlandsson A. Electronic medical records, a literature review. Online. Available: ICA Studies/Études CIA 10: http://www.ica.org/biblio/cer/litrev.rtf Apr 1996
7. Gilmore J, Miller W. Clinical photography utilizing office staff: methods to achieve consistency and reproducibility. J Dermatol Surg Oncol 1988; 14:281–286.
8. Foster DH. Does colour constancy exist? Trends Cogn Sci 2003; 7:439–443.
9. Multispectral consists of tens of bands, and bandwidth of 0.1 microns; hyperspectral consists of hundreds of bands and bandwidth of 0.01 microns; ultraspectral consists of thousands of bands and bandwidth of 0.001 microns. Sensors Volume, New World Vistas – Air and Space Power for the 21st Century. USAAF Advisory Board, December 1995:156.
10. Hojjatoleslami A, Claridge E, Montcrieff M. Accuracy of the skin model in quantifying blood and epidermal melanin. In: Arridge S, Todd-Pokropek A, eds. Medical image understanding and analysis 2000. 2000:53–56. http://www.cs.bham.ac.uk/~exc/Research/Papers/miua00_skin.pdf
11. Kikuchi I, Inoue S, Idemori M, Uchimura H. Reflection ultraviolet photography as surface photography proof of the skin. J Dermatol 1983; 10:551–559.
12. Fulton JE. Utilizing the ultraviolet camera to enhance the appearance of photodamage and other skin conditions. Dermatol Surg 1997; 23:163–169.
13. Pagoni A, Kligman AM. UV photography to identify early photodamage in young children. Br J Dermatol 1997; 137:321–322.
14. Niamtu J. Digitally processed ultraviolet images: a convenient, affordable, reproducible means of illustrating ultraviolet clinical examination. Dermatol Surg 2001; 27:1039–1042.
15. Ericson MB, Sandberg C, Gudmundson F, Rosén A, Larkö O, Wennberg A. Fluorescence contrast and threshold limit: implications for photodynamic diagnosis of basal cell carcinoma. J Photochem Photobiol B: Biology 2003; 69:121–127.
16. Niamtu J. Techno pearls for digital image management. Dermatologic Surg 2002; 28:946–950.
17. Whited JD, Hall RP, Simel DL, et al. Reliability and accuracy of dermatologists' clinic-based and digital image consultations. J Am Acad Dermatol 1999; 41:693–702.
18. Piccolo D, Soyer HP, Burgdorf W, Talamini R, Peris K, Bugatti L. Concordance between telepathologic diagnosis and conventional histopathologic diagnosis: a multiobserver store-and-forward study on 20 skin specimens. Arch Dermatol 2002; 138:53–58.
19. Roach WH Jr, Conner C, Younger P, Cartwright KK. Medical records and the law. Gaithersburg, MD: Aspen Publishers, Inc; 1994:207–208.

20. Hjort B. Patient photography, videotaping, and other imaging (updated) (AHIMA Practice Brief). J AHIMA 2001; 72:64M-Q. Online. Available: http://library.ahima.org/xpedio/groups/public/documents/ahima/pub_bok2_000585.html.
21. Drugge RJ. Photographic teledermatology consent form. Stamford, CT: Internet Dermatology Society; 1995. Online. Available: http://www.telemedicine.org/consent.htm.
22. Meneghini F. Clinical facial photography in a small office: lighting equipment and technique. Aesth Plast Surg 2001; 25:299–306.
23. White RG, Perednia DA. Automatic derivation of initial match points for paired digital images of skin. Comput Med Imaging Graph 1992; 16:217–225.
24. Macgregor B. Automated registration of lesions of pigmented skin lesions. Pattern Recognition 1998; 31:805–817.
25. Edwards C. Techniques of image enhancement and analysis for area and severity assessments of skin disease. J Eur Acad Dermatol Venereol 1997; 9:S109–S110.
26. Rosado B, Menzies S, Harbauer A, et al. Accuracy of computer diagnosis of melanoma: a quantitative meta-analysis. Arch Dermatol 2003; 139:361–367; discussion 366.
27. Lynch D. Oral examination. Online. Available: http://www.emedicine.com/derm/topic836.htm#section~pictures 16 Nov 2001.
28. Schwartz MS, Tardy ME Jr. Standardized photodocumentation in facial plastic surgery. Facial Plast Surg 1990; 7:1–12.
29. Clark JM, Cook TA. Preblepharoplasty facial analysis. Online. Available: http://www.emedicine.com/ent/topic618.htm 2 Nov 2001.
30. Gibbons RD, Fiedler-Weiss VC, West DP, Lapin G. Quantification of scalp hair—a computer-aided methodology. J Invest Dermatol Volume 1986; 86:78–82.
31. Malhotra P, Dahaney D. Botox injections for hyperfunctional facial lines. Online. Available: http://www.emedicine.com/ent/topic134.htm July 2002.
32. Doud Galli, SK, Miller, PJ. Chin implants. Online. Available: http://www.emedicine.com/ent/topic628.htm May 2002.
33. Taylor RS, Lin BB. Digital Photography for mapping Mohs micrographic surgery sections. Dermatol Surg 2001; 27:411–414.
34. Menzies SW, Gutenev A, Avramidis M, Batrac A, McCarthy WH. Short-term digital surface microscopic monitoring of atypical or changing melanocytic lesions. Arch Dermatol 2001; 137:1583–1589.
35. Kittler H, Binder M. Risks and benefits of sequential imaging of melanocytic skin lesions in patients with multiple atypical nevi. Arch Dermatol 2001; 137:1590–1595.
36. Richert SM, D'Amico F, Rhodes AR. Cutaneous melanoma: patient surveillance and tumor progression [abstract]. J Invest Dermatol 1997; 108:36.
37. Rhodes AR. Intervention strategy to prevent lethal cutaneous melanoma: use of dermatologic photography to aid surveillance of high-risk persons. J Am Acad Dermatol 1998; 39:262–267.
38. Carli P, Borgognomi L, Reali UM, Giannotti B. Clinicopathological features of small diameter malignant melanoma. Eur J Dermatol 1994; 4:440–442.
39. Shaw HM, McCarthy WH. Small-diameter malignant melanoma: a common diagnosis in New South Wales, Australia. J Am Acad Dermatol 1992; 27:679–682. (Comment. J Am Acad Dermatol 1993; 29:1060–1061.
40. Kopf AW, Rodriguez-Sains RS, Rigel DS, et al. 'Small' melanomas: relation of prognostic variables to diameter of primary superficial spreading melanomas. J Dermatol Surg Oncol 1982; 8:765–770.
41. Lucas CR, Sanders LL, Murray JC, Myers SA, Hall RP, Grichnik JM. Early melanoma detection: nonuniform dermoscopic features and growth. J Am Acad Dermatol 2003; 48:663–671.
42. Malvehy J, Puig S. Follow-up of melanocytic skin lesions with digital total-body photography and digital dermoscopy: a two-step method. Clin Dermatol 2002; 20:297–304.
43. Tsutomu Matsumoto, Hiroyuki Matsumoto, Koji Yamada, Satoshi Hoshino. Impact of artificial 'gummy' fingers on fingerprint systems. Datenschutz und Datensicherheit 2002; 26.
44. van den Akker TW, Reker CH, Knol A, Post J, Wilbrink J, van der Veen JP. Teledermatology as a tool for communication between general practitioners and dermatologists. J Telemed Telecare 2001; 7:193–198.
45. Ennett J. The impact of emerging technologies on future air capabilities. DSTO Aeronautical and Maritime Research Laboratory, Melbourne, Australia, section, 4.15.6. Online. Available: http://www.dsto.defence.gov.au/corporate/reports/DSTO-GD-0186.pdf. Dec 1999.

7 Wound Healing

Jie Li MD PhD and Robert S Kirsner MD PhD

Summary box

- Wound healing occurs in overlapping phases—the inflammatory, the proliferative, and the remodeling phase.
- The depth of the wound determines the degree of contraction and the source of keratinocytes used for re-epithelialization.
- Sharp wounds created by scalpels heal faster than wounds created by destructive or ablative methods.
- Platelets are the first cell to appear in the healing process, and macrophages are the most important cell in the healing process; they both mediate their actions through cytokines or growth factors.
- Wound healing is a complex event that is highly regulated by signals from both serum and the surrounding extracellular matrix environment.
- Physicians can speed wound healing by a variety of mechanisms; by avoiding toxic substances being placed on the wound, by keeping the wound free of necrotic tissue, and by using occlusive dressings appropriately.

INTRODUCTION

Dermatologists and dermatologic surgeons create and care for more wounds than all other specialties combined. Therefore knowledge of wound healing is critical. Wound healing is a dynamic process and involves the complex interaction of many cell types, their cytokines or chemical mediators, and the extracellular matrix. Vascular responses, cellular and chemotactic activity, and the effects of chemical mediators within wounded tissues form the interrelated components of healing. Understanding the processes involved in wound repair is exquisitely important for a specialty that devotes a significant amount of time to create wounds with either diagnostic or therapeutic procedures.

Wound repair is an orderly, continuous process and can be divided into three phases—the inflammatory, the proliferative, and the remodeling phases (Fig. 7.1). However, the process is not a simple linear one because the phases overlap. Therefore, the conceptual distinction between phases serves only as an outline to facilitate the discussions about events occurring during wound repair. The point when wound healing begins and ends often has been based on macroscopic examination. Though not seen clinically, injury and repair of the skin occurring at a microscopic or a molecular level likely occur with even greater frequency. Although not yet quite clear, our understanding of events that occur during wound repair may be invaluable for enhancing our knowledge of wound repair, and for improving healing, leading to the restoration of both anatomic and functional integrity of the wounded tissue.

TYPES OF WOUNDS

Acute versus chronic wounds

Wounds can be conveniently classified as acute or chronic, whereby the healing process proceeds in a timely or an untimely (slow) fashion, respectively. Determining the exact time taken to heal and whether a wound is designated

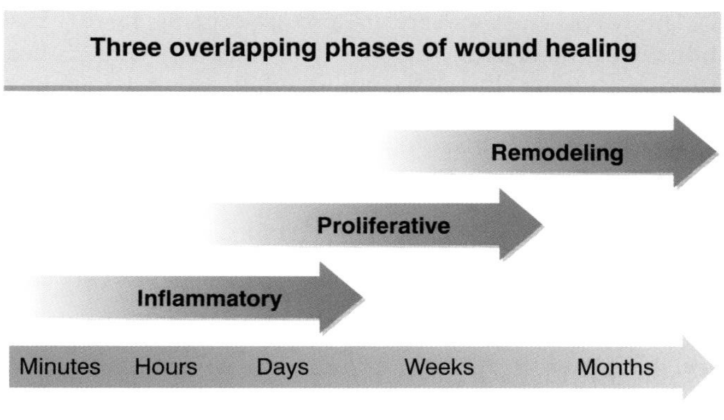

Figure 7.1 Three overlapping phases of wound healing.

acute or chronic remains arbitrary; such decisions are based on several factors that include location, shape, and cause of the wound, as well as the age and physical condition of the patient. For example, an elliptical wound on the face of a healthy child will heal faster than a circular burn wound on an elderly infirm person, even though both might heal in a timely fashion given the circumstances.

Partial-thickness versus full-thickness wounds

Injury to only the epidermis differs from injury involving the underlying dermis. If an injury is limited to the epidermis, the epidermis restores itself to a structure similar to the preinjury state. In contrast, if injury is deeper to the dermis, regeneration does not normally occur, but rather repair occurs and the wound heals with scaring. In certain situations after dermal injury regeneration occurs. This occurs in early fetal skin wounds, where higher concentrations of type III collagen and glycosaminoglycans and decreased amounts of transforming growth factor β1 (TGF-β1) as well as reduced inflammatory response are likely important in mediating regeneration as opposed to repair.[1]

Skin wounds can be categorized depending on their depth as erosion, partial-thickness or full-thickness wounds. If only the epidermis is lost, this is called an erosion. When the wound involves structures deep to the dermis, it is termed an ulcer. Ulcers that involve the epidermis and varying parts of the dermis are termed partial-thickness wounds, while those that involve all of the dermis and deeper structures are called full-thickness wounds (Fig. 7.2). Chronic wounds are also categorized by the thickness of the wound, for example staging of pressure ulcers depends upon wound depth[2] (Fig. 7.3).

For acute wounds there is the added importance of differentiating partial-thickness wounds from full-thickness wounds in that they epithelialize by different mechanisms (Table 7.1). In partial-thickness wounds, since the deep dermis has not been lost or destroyed, skin appendages remain. These structures serve as a reservoir of epithelium to repopulate the epidermis. Keratinocytes from these structures, as well as from the wound edge, migrate across the wound surface, forming new epidermis that covers the wound (Fig. 7.4). In full-thickness wounds, on the other hand, adnexal structures have been destroyed and keratinocytes can, therefore, only migrate from the wound edge. In addition, the wound repair will not regenerate these appendages but replace them with scar.

The depth of wound is also a critical factor that influences the healing outcome. Full-thickness wounds heal to some extent by contraction, while there is minimal contraction in partial-thickness wounds[3] (Fig. 7.5). During contraction, the wound area is decreased and involves movement of pre-existing tissue centripetally. Clinically, contraction of the wound may result in cosmetically disfiguring contractures.

Primary versus second intention healing

When an acute wound is left to heal on its own, it is termed second intention healing. Primary intention healing occurs when a surgeon directs closure of the wound by approximating the wound edges. There are three major methods a

Comparison of erosion, partial thickness and full thickness wounds

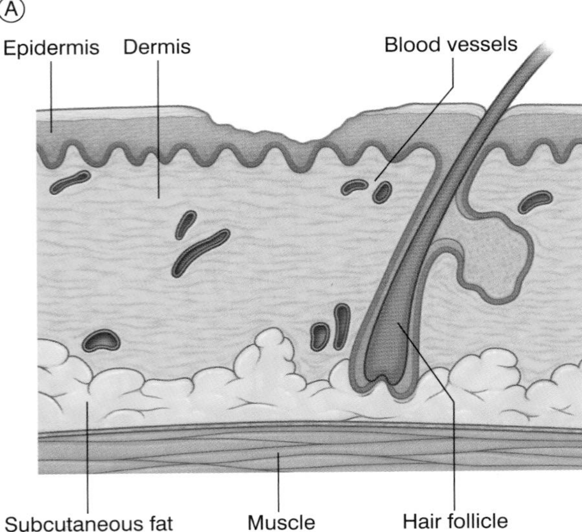

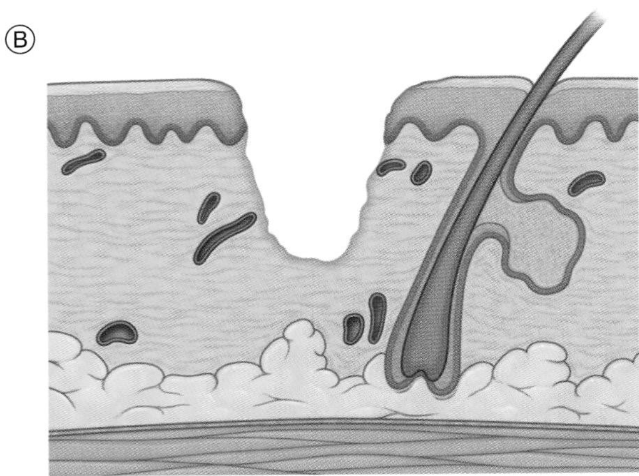

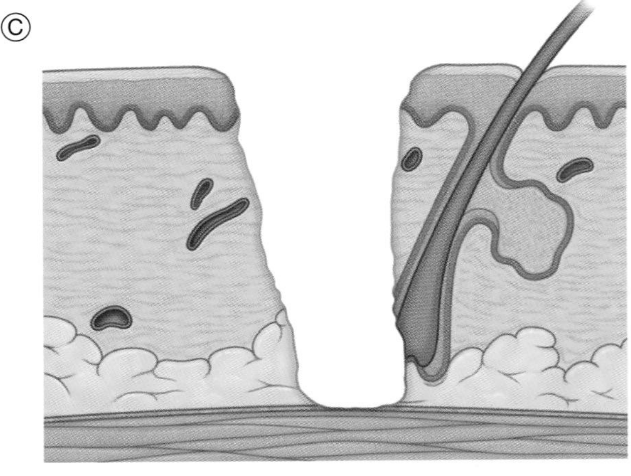

Figure 7.2 Comparison of erosion, partial-thickness and full-thickness wounds. (A) Erosion: only the epidermis is lost. (B) Partial-thickness wound: the epidermis and part of the dermis are missing but some adnexal structures remain. (C) Full-thickness wound: all of the epidermis and dermis along with adnexal structures are missing. The full-thickness skin loss involves the subcutaneous fat tissue and may extend down to, but not through, the underlying fascia.

surgeon may use to repair a wound defect—including direct closure, flap and graft—depending on the size, shape and location of the wound. Direct closure is through a direct side-to-side closure, where the two sides of the wound are sutured or stapled together. The flap method involves moving adjacent tissue into the wound defect to close the wound (flap), where the blood supply is provided by a pedicle. The graft method utilizes skin tissue from a distant location (graft). By definition, a graft has been separated from its own blood supply and therefore its blood supply is provided by the wound bed on which it is placed. Even if the wound edges are approximated using a primary intention method the wound still needs to proceed through the three phases of healing.

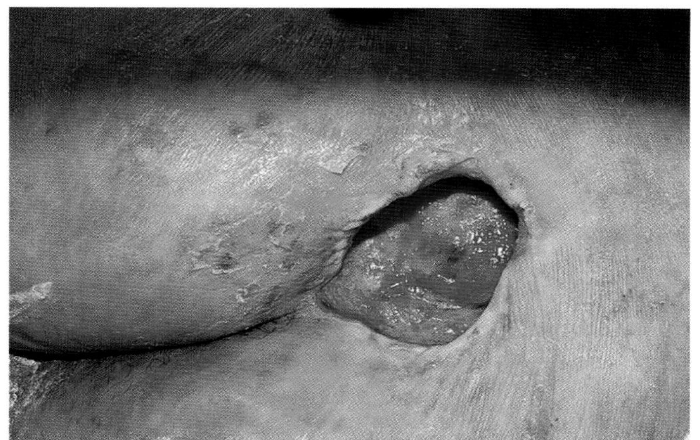

Figure 7.3 Sacral pressure ulcer in nursing-home patient.

Methods of creating acute wounds

The method by which wounds are created may also influence their healing. Acute wounds may be created in a variety of ways. For example, a surgeon may utilize a scalpel (steel), laser (heat), liquid nitrogen (cold), or chemicals (acid) to create a wound. Alternatively, a patient may develop an acute wound in various ways, through burns or traumatic accidents. Depending upon how the wound was created, wounds heal differently and at different rates. In general, wounds created by sharp steel, such as surgical incisions, heal faster than other methods of wounding. Burn wounds have a lag period prior to healing.[4] Healing of traumatic wounds may be slowed due to foreign substances inoculated into the wound, causing prolongation of the inflammatory phase.

■ PHASES OF WOUND HEALING

Inflammatory phase

The initial reaction to wounding can be subdivided into a vascular and cellular response, and in total is manifest as the inflammatory response (Fig. 7.6). Early in the wounding process local vasodilatation, blood and fluid leakage into the extravascular space, and blocking of lymphatic drainage can produce the cardinal signs of inflammation, including rubor (redness), tumor (swelling), and calor (heat). This acute inflammatory response usually lasts 24–48 hours and may be misinterpreted as an infectious process of pathogenic infection. Although usually lasting 1–2 days, it may persist for up to 2 weeks in some cases and proceed into chronic inflammation.

Tissue injury causes blood vessel disruption and bleeding. Platelets, the first cells to appear after wounding, not only

Table 7.1 Wound depth and repair types

Wound Type	Dermis Involvement	Reepithelialization	Main Repair Type
Erosion	None	From wound edge and appendages	Regeneration
Partial thickness	Partial	From wound edge and appendages	Repair with scar
Full thickness	All	From wound edge	Scar and contraction

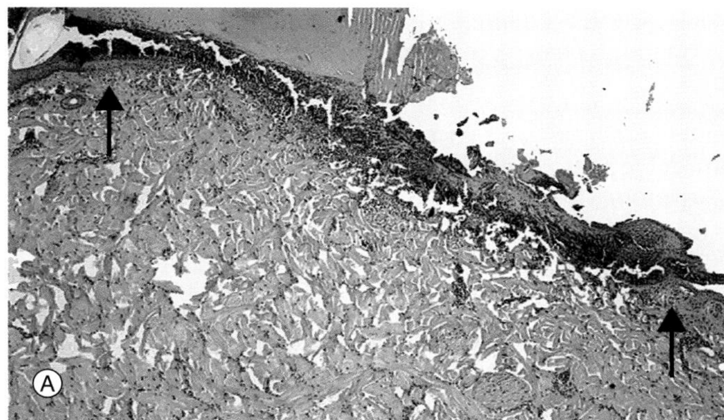

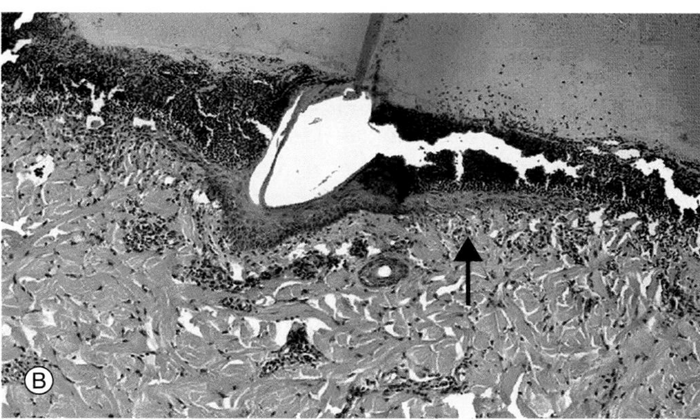

Figure 7.4 Re-epithelialization of a partial-thickness wound in a pig. After partial-thickness wounding, microscopic adnexal structures remain as a source of keratinocytes. (A) Two days after wounding, keratinocytes migrate from both the wound edges and hair follicles (arrows). Magnification × 50. (B) Higher magnification of (A) (× 100) showing that keratinocytes migrate from hair follicle (arrow).

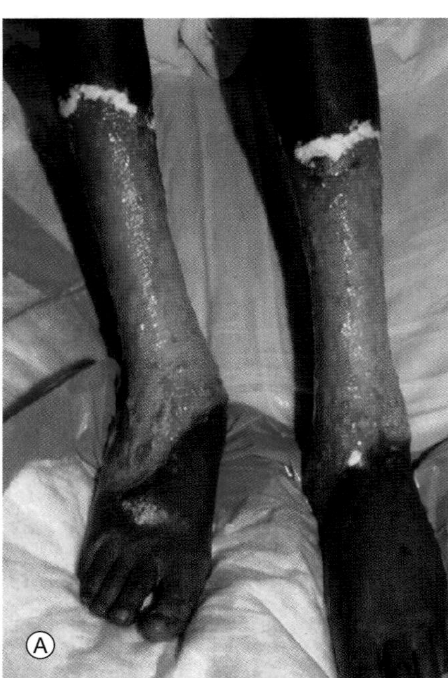

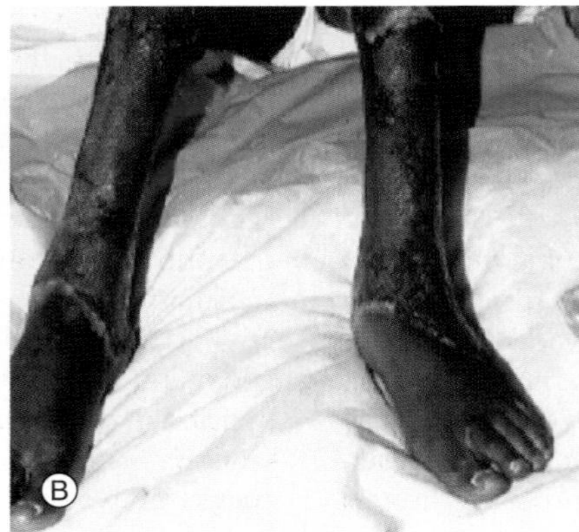

Figure 7.5 Leg ulcer secondary to sickle cell anemia. (A) Wound prior to split-thickness skin graft. (B) Several days after placement of split-thickness skin graft.

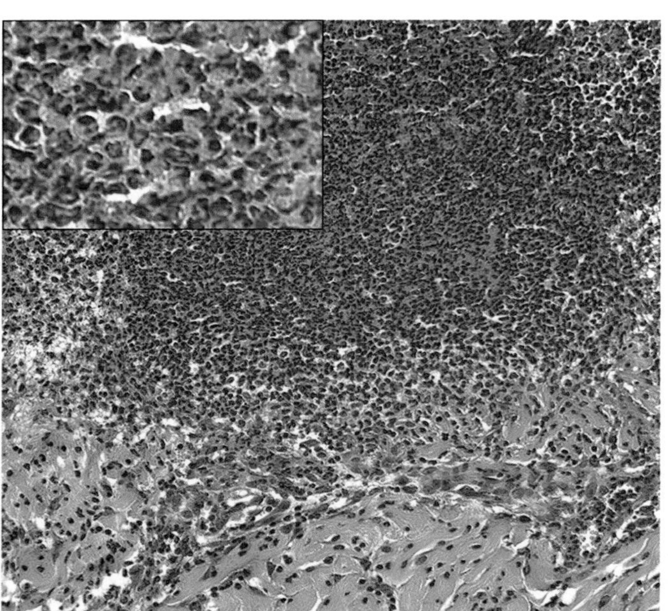

Figure 7.6 Acute inflammatory response. Photo of a 2-day-old partial-thickness wound in a pig, showing leukocyte infiltration in the wound area and emigration from surrounding blood vessels (× 200). Insert: infiltration with neutrophils predominant (× 600).

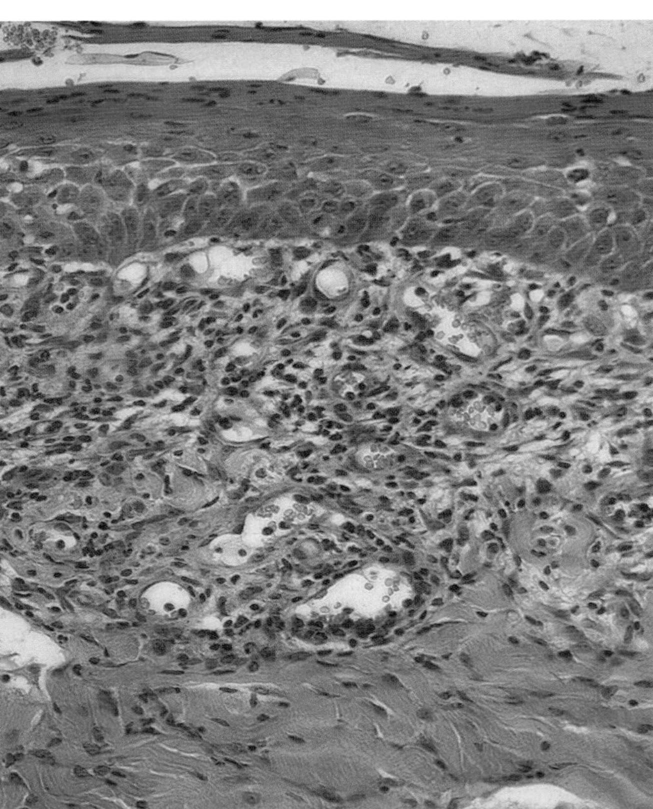

Figure 7.7 Formation of granulation tissue. Photo of a 5-day-old partial-thickness wound in a pig, showing that, underneath newly formed epidermis, the granulation tissue characterizes the proliferative phase with angiogenesis and fibroplasia (× 320).

aid in hemostasis but also initiate the healing cascade via release of important mediators including chemoattractants and growth factors such as platelet-derived growth factor (PDGF).[5] Some authors have defined healing as occurring in four stages, with the first stage being hemostasis, highlighting the importance of platelets in the healing process. In response to chemoattractants and cytokines, leukocytes (including neutrophils and macrophages) infiltrate the wounded area and clear damaged tissue debris and foreign particles. Other infiltrating cells such as mast cells, basophils and eosinophils participate in the inflammation by releasing chemicals or proteases. In the tissue, monocytes become activated and transform into macrophages. In addition to the phagocytosis, macrophages produce several growth factors and cytokines important for the initiation of formation of granulation tissue (Fig. 7.7).

Vascular response

Initial vasoconstriction causes injured small vessels to be pressed together. This induces a stickiness within the endothelial lining that is capable of occluding vessels. Shortly thereafter, histamine is released into the area from mast cells, basophils, and platelets, which causes vasodilatation and blood leakage and an increase in permeability of the endothelial wall.

A surgical incisional wound is the most common acute wound. Using this wound as a conceptual model, one can easily envision that there is concomitant bleeding due to the disruption of blood vessels and extravasation of blood components. Therefore, the first immediate step of wound healing is hemostasis.[6] Hemostasis can be divided into two parts—development of a fibrin clot, and coagulation (Table 7.2). Platelets are the first cells to appear after injury. With injury to endothelial cells and blood vessels, collagens and other extracellular matrix proteins are exposed. Platelets are activated at the site of blood vessel injury by locally generated thrombin, in addition to exposed extracellular matrix, especially fibrillar collagen, and undergo adhesion and aggregation. Upon activation, they release many mediators from their granules including serotonin, adenosine diphosphate (ADP), thromboxane A_2, fibrinogen, fibronectin, thrombospondin, and von Willebrand factor VIII. Induced by these chemicals, other passing platelets adhere to the exposed extracellular matrix of the endothelial wall, resulting in a relatively unstable platelet plug that may temporarily occlude injured small vessels. Concomitantly, endothelial cells produce prostacyclin, which inhibits platelet aggregation and thus limits the extent of platelet aggregation. Platelet-derived fibrinogens are converted by thrombin to fibrins, which are deposited into and about the platelet plug and form the core of the fibrin clot (that is more stable than the platelet aggregation plug) that slows or stops bleeding. This fibrin clot also acts as a scaffold matrix[7] (called provisional matrix) for the migration of leukocytes, fibroblasts, and endothelial cells, and serves as a reservoir of growth factors. In addition, platelets influence leukocyte infiltration by releasing chemotactic factors. Platelets also promote new tissue regeneration by releasing some growth factors implicated in wound repair. These include transforming growth factor TGF-α, TGF-β and PDGF. They have strong effects on promoting cell migration and proliferation and formation of granulation tissue. These functions mean that platelets are not only important in hemostasis, but also significantly contribute to re-epithelialization, fibroplasia, and angiogenesis.

The second part of hemostasis is coagulation, which can be customarily divided into intrinsic and extrinsic pathways, both of which converge at the point where factor X is activated. Damaged tissue releases a lipoprotein known as tissue factor, which activates the extrinsic coagulation pathway. The activated monocytes and endothelial cells also express this tissue factor on their surface and participate in the coagulation. Platelet aggregation triggers a specific enzyme in blood known as Hageman factor XII to initiate the cascade of intrinsic coagulation with a series of converting proenzymes to activated enzymes, culminating in the transformation of prothrombin into thrombin. This in turn converts soluble fibrinogen to insoluble fibrous fibrin. In addition to coagulation, thrombin has multiple effects on platelets, macrophages, fibroblasts, and endothelial cells.

Cellular response

Leukocytes

The inflammatory phase of wound healing derives its name from the influx of white blood cells into the area of injury. Almost immediately after injury, leukocytes (polymorphonuclear leukocytes) begin to adhere to the sticky endothelium of venules. Within 1 hour of the onset of inflammation the entire endothelial margin of the venules may be covered with neutrophils (this is termed

Table 7.2 Hemostasis in wound healing

Activities/Substances	Effects
Development of Platelet Fibrin Clot Substances of platelet granule	
ADP	Platelet aggregation
Fibrinogen	Platelet aggregation
Fibronectin	Platelet aggregation
Thrombospondin	Platelet aggregation
Von Willebrand factor VIII	Platelet activation and adhesion to fibrillar collagen
PDGF, TGF	Leukocyte recruitment, extracellular matrix synthesis
Serotonin	Vasoconstriction, fibroblast proliferation, collagen cross-linking
Chemoattractants	Leukocyte recruitment
Products during fibrin clot development	
Thrombin	Platelet activation, conversion of fibrinogen to fibrin
Platelet aggregation	Core of fibrin clot
Fibrin	Core of fibrin clot
Fibrin clot	Hemostatic plug, provisional matrix for cell migration, reservoir of growth factor
Coagulation	
Hageman factor fragments	Initiate intrinsic coagulation, increased vasopermeability
Bradykinin	Vasodilatation, increased vasopermeability
Complement activation	Leukocyte recruitment, increased vasopermeability
Thrombin	Leukocyte recruitment, conversion of fibrinogen to fibrin, fibroblast proliferation

ADP, adenosine diphosphate; PDGF, platelet-derived growth factor; TGF, transforming growth factor.

margination). Soon after, polymorphonuclear leukocytes begin amoeboid activity by inserting narrow projections into the junctions between endothelial cells, and they release chemotactic factors. In the early inflammatory state, neutrophils (with a survival time in the circulation of only a few hours) and monocytes are the predominant cells at the site of injury (Fig. 7.6). Later in inflammation, the number of neutrophils declines and macrophages (tissue-derived monocytes) predominate.

Neutrophils, the first white blood cells to arrive, and monocytes are recruited to the wound by chemotactic factors released from mast cells (Table 7.3) or produced by the coagulation cascade. Substances released by mast cells, such as tumor necrosis factor (TNF), histamine, proteases, and some other substances such as leukotrienes and cytokines (interleukins), represent chemotactic signals for the recruitment of leukocytes. Growth factors of PDGF and TGF-β are also potent chemotactic factors for leukocytes. The chemotactic factors from the coagulation process (kallikrein, fibrinopeptides released from fibrinogen, and fibrin degradation products) also serve to upregulate the expression of important intercellular adhesion molecules. Upregulated adhesion molecules allow cell–cell interactions, which facilitate diapedesis of neutrophils. Endothelial cells that were previously thought to be bystanders in inflammatory processes are now believed to play an active role in facilitating leukocyte migration. Neutrophils release elastase and collagenase, which likely enhance their passage through the blood vessel basement membrane. Once in the wound site, integrin receptors found on the surface of neutrophils enhance cell–matrix interactions. This allows neutrophils to perform their functions of killing and phagocytosing bacteria and damaged matrix proteins within the wound bed. The neutrophil infiltration normally lasts only a few days. The presence of wound contamination prolongs the neutrophilic presence within the wound. The eosinophil also has low capacity for phagocytosis, but the basophil does not. Basophils contain histamine, which is released locally following injury, to contribute to the early increased vascular permeability (Table 7.3).

Monocytes migrate from the capillary into the tissue spaces; once in the tissue they are activated and transformed into larger phagocytic cells—the macrophages. Monocytes and their tissue counterparts, macrophages, soon become the dominant figures in inflammation. Monocytes are initially attracted to the wound site by some of the same chemoattractants that attract neutrophils, and their recruitment continues through signals released by monocyte-specific chemoattractants, such as monocyte chemoattractant protein-1 (MCP-1)[8] and macrophage inflammatory protein-1 (MIP).[9] Extracellular matrix degradation products—collagen fragments, fibronectin fragments, and thrombin—are also chemoattractant specific for monocytes.[10] Macrophages are critical to repair and are considered the most important regulatory cells in the inflammatory reaction during wound healing (Table 7.4). Macrophages phagocytize, digest, and kill pathogenic organisms, scavenge tissue debris, and destroy any remaining neutrophils. After binding to the extracellular membrane, bacterial, cellular, and tissue phagocytosis and subsequent destruction are accomplished through release of

Table 7.3 Inflammatory cells and their major proteases/chemicals

Cell type	Protease/Chemicals	Major Effects or Substrates
Mast cell	Histamine	Vasopermeability, vasodilatation, EC proliferation
	Heparin	Anticoagulation, fibrinolysis
	Serotonin	Vasoconstriction
		Fibroblast proliferation, collagen cross-linking
	tPA	Plasminogen
	PAF	Platelet activating and aggregation
	Protease-3	Trypsin-like effect
	MMP-9	Gelatin, collagen IV and V
	Tryptase	ProMMP-3, uPA
	Chymase	ProMMP-1, -3
	Leukotrienes	Chemotactic for granulocytes
Neutrophil	Elastase	Elastin, proteoglycans, collagen III, V
	MMP-8	Collagens I, III, VII, and X
	MMP-9	As above
	MT1-MMP	ProMMP-2, -13, collagen I, III, fibronectin
	Heparanase	Heparan sulfate proteoglycans
Eosinophil	MMP-1	Collagens I, III, VII, and X
	MMP-9	As above
	β-glucuronidase	Proteoglycans
Basophil	Histamine	As above
Monocyte/macrophage	MMP-9	As above
	MMP-12	Elastin, collagen IV, laminin, fibronectin
	MT1-MMP	As above
	tPA	As above
	PDGF, IGF-1, FGF, TGF-β, VEGF	See Table 7.5
T lymphocyte	MMP-2	Gelatin, collagen VI, V and I, laminin, fibronectin, proMMP-9, -13
	MMP-9	As above

EC, endothelial cell; FGF, fibroblast growth factor; IGF, insulin-like growth factor; MMP, matrix metalloproteinase; PAF, platelet-activating factor; PDGF, platelet-derived growth factor; TGF, transforming growth factor; tPA, tissue plasminogen activator; VEGF, vascular endothelial growth factor.

Table 7.4 Macrophages in wound repair

Activities	Effects
Recruitment and maturation	Transformation from monocyte to tissue macrophages
Chemoattractant release	Leukocyte recruitment
Phagocytosis of bacteria	Wound decontamination
Phagocytosis of tissue debris	Wound debridement
Phagocytosis of extravasated granulocytes	Resolution of inflammation
MMP release	Matrix degradation (collagen, elastin), granulation tissue formation and remodeling
Growth factor release (FGF, IGF-1, PDGF, TGF-α, TGF-β, VEGF)	Regulation of fibroplasias, angiogenesis, tissue remodeling

FGF, fibroblast growth factor; IGF, insulin-like growth factor; PDGF, platelet-derived growth factor; TGF, transforming growth factor; tPA, tissue plasminogen activator; VEGF, vascular endothelial growth factor.

biologically active oxygen intermediates and enzymatic proteins. These all-important processes performed by the monocyte/macrophage allow for induction of angiogenesis and formation of granulation tissue.[11]

Macrophages tolerate severe hypoxia well. This may explain why they are usually present in the chronic inflammation. In addition, macrophages release chemotactic factors (for example, fibronectin) which attract fibroblasts to the wound and play a role in localizing inflammation and in adhesion of fibroblasts to fibrin during the transition between the inflammatory and proliferative phases of wound repair. In this regard, macrophages may enhance collagen deposition because their depletion markedly decreases deposition of collagen in the wound.[11] In the absence of macrophages, fibroblasts migrate to the site of injury in considerably reduced numbers, and when found they are somewhat immature. The angiogenic potential of macrophages has also been demonstrated by inducing neovascularization in the cornea using a rat model with macrophage-derived growth factor. New blood vessel growth follows a gradient of angiogenic factor produced by hypoxic macrophages, as macrophages do not produce this angiogenic factor when either fully oxygenated or anoxic. If macrophages are removed from the tissue spaces, angiogenesis and wound debridement may be temporarily or permanently inhibited.[12] In total, macrophages can be considered factories for production of growth factors, for synthesizing and secreting PDGF, fibroblast growth factor (FGF), vascular endothelial growth factor (VEGF), TGF-β, and TGF-α.[13] These cytokines are important in inducing cell migration and proliferation, as well as in matrix production. Thus, macrophages appear to play a pivotal role in the transition between inflammation and repair.

Mast cells

In more recent years mast cells have acquired increasing attention in the wound healing field.[14] Studies have found that skin mast cells, which are usually located near vessels and nerves in the dermis, are activated directly by immunological signals and stimuli of nerve origin, as well as by numerous stimuli of physical, chemical or mechanical nature. Once stimulated by direct tissue injury, mast cells are immediately activated by degranulation and release mediators (Table 7.3), such as histamine and TNF, which are essential for triggering the inflammatory response and influencing the local endothelial cells, causing vasodilatation and increased vascular permeability. Mast cells actively participate in the regulation of hemostasis by release of substances such as platelet-activating factor (PAF), heparin, tryptase, chymase and t-plasminogen activator (tPA). In addition, TNF, histamine, proteases and other substances such as leukotrienes and cytokines (interleukins) serve as chemotactic signals for the recruitment of leukocytes. Further, the histamine, heparin, cytokines and growth factors released from mast cells (such as PDGF, VEGF, TGF and FGF) also mediate the processes of angiogenesis, extracellular matrix deposition and remodeling.

Chemical mediators of inflammation

A number of chemical substances are involved in the initiation and control of inflammation. These chemicals work in concert; some are protagonists and others are antagonists of inflammation. The actions of some of these substances may be synergistic, while for many their precise role has not been clearly elucidated.

Histamine

One of many substances released from mast cell granules is histamine. Mast cells are the major source of histamine production, which is also found in blood platelets and basophils. Histamine acts on the type 1 histamine receptor (H1) and causes dilatation of arterioles and increased permeability of venules. When mast cells are depleted of histamine, or H1 receptors are blocked, the early increase in vascular permeability is prevented. In addition to histamine, mast cell granules, released at the time of injury, contain a number of active materials including serotonin and heparin, which lead in part to the initial short-lived increase in permeability of venules. Heparin, an anticoagulant, serves to prevent coagulation of the excess tissue fluid and blood components during the early phase of the inflammatory response.

Serotonin

Serotonin, or 5-hydroxytryptamine (5-HT), is released from platelets and mast cells and is a potent vasoconstrictor, though it is unlikely that it has a significant effect on vascular permeability in humans. However, serotonin appears to be involved in other activities related to the later phases of wound healing, such as fibroblast proliferation and the cross-linking of collagen molecules. Cross-linking of collagen molecules not only affects the tensile strength of newly formed desirable scar tissue, but also accounts for certain negative effects of scarring such as toughness, and the lack of resilience of unwanted fibrous adhesions.

Kinins

The kinins are biologically active and nearly indistinguishable peptides that are found in areas of tissue destruction. The most familiar kinin, bradykinin, is a potent inflammatory substance released from plasma proteins in injured tissue by the plasma enzyme, kallikrein. The action of the kinins on the microvasculature is similar to that of histamine, that is, potent vasodilatation. Kinins are rapidly destroyed by tissue proteases, suggesting their importance is limited to the early inflammatory stage of wound healing.

Prostaglandins

Prostaglandins (PG) are extremely potent biologic substances and are produced by nearly all cells of the body in response to cell membrane injury. When cellular membranes are altered, their phospholipid content is degraded by the enzyme phospholipases that result in the formation of arachidonic acid. Oxidation of arachidonic acid by the enzyme lipoxygenase forms a series of potent compounds, the leukotrienes. Several types of leukotrienes combine to form slow-reacting substance of anaphylaxis (SRS-A) which alters capillary permeability during the inflammatory reaction.

Subsequently a cascade effect occurs, as arachidonic acid is converted by cyclooxygenases to thromboxanes and several prostaglandins. Specific classes of prostaglandin appear to control or perpetuate the local inflammatory response. Prostaglandin E2 (PGE2) may increase vascular permeability by antagonizing vasoconstriction, and its chemotactic activity may attract leukocytes to the locally inflamed area. Some prostaglandins are pro-inflammatory (for example, PGE2) and synergize with other inflammatory substances such as bradykinin. Proinflammatory prostaglandins are thought to be responsible for sensitizing pain receptors, causing a state of hyperalgesia associated with the inflammatory reaction, while other classes of prostaglandin act as inhibitors. Together, these opposing effects of various prostaglandins lead to a tightly controlled response. Prostaglandins may also regulate the repair processes during the early phases of healing by contributing to the synthesis of mucopolysaccharides.

One action of corticosteroids such as prednisone and non-steroidal anti-inflammatory drugs (NSAIDs) such as aspirin is inhibition of prostaglandin synthesis via inhibition of cyclooxygenase activity. Suppressing the inflammatory response and its associated pain may be appropriate treatment for chronic inflammation but is usually not indicated for the normal acute inflammatory response.

Complement system

The complement system collectively describes a system of about 11 principal proteins, many of them enzyme precursors. All of these proteins may be present among the plasma proteins that leak from capillaries into the tissue spaces. When antibody binds antigen, the same antibody also binds with a specific protein molecule of the complement system. This triggers a cascade of sequential reactions that produce multiple end-products which help prevent damage by the invading organism or toxin. With regard to wound healing, some of the end-products activate phagocytosis by both neutrophils and macrophages, whereas others enhance lysis and agglutination of invading organisms. Still others activate mast cells and basophils to release histamine.

Growth factors

Numerous terms are used to designate growth factors, including cytokines, interleukins, and colony-stimulating factors.[13] This fact, coupled with the fact that the name of a growth factor does not in reality identify its only or its primary biologic role, has made the nomenclature for growth factors quite confusing. For instance, platelet-derived growth factor (PDGF) is found in platelets but is also found in keratinocytes and other cells.[5] Growth factors work through cell surface receptors and may bind to single or multiple receptors. Growth factors can have an effect on the cells of origin (autocrine mode), on neighboring cells (paracrine mode), or on distant cells (exocrine mode). Growth factors have been shown to play multiple and critical roles in wound repair processes (Table 7.5). Many growth factors secreted by macrophages are pleiotropic and influence cell proliferation, angiogenesis, and extracellular matrix synthesis. For example, TGF-α plays an important role in wound re-epithelialization, TGF-β1, -β2, and -β3 strongly promote the migration of fibroblasts and endothelial cells, and deposition of extracellular matrix by fibroblasts during formation of granulation tissue. While increased TGF-β1 promotes scar formation, TGF-β3 exhibits an antiscarring effect.[1] PDGF is chemotactic and mitogenic for fibroblasts and smooth muscle cells in vitro.[5] PDGF is also chemotactic for monocytes, macrophages,[15] and neutrophils[16] and thrombin-activated platelets possess angiogenic activity.[17]

Chronic inflammation

Most of the symptoms associated with the acute inflammatory response last approximately 2 weeks. However, if inflammation persists for months or years, it is called chronic inflammation. Chronic inflammation associated with wounds often occurs when a wound is habitually sealed by necrotic tissue, is contaminated with pathogens, or contains foreign material that cannot be phagocytized or solubilized during the acute inflammatory phase. Granulocytes disappear through lysis and migration with the resolution of the acute inflammatory phase, while mononuclear cells—specifically lymphocytes, monocytes,

Table 7.5 Growth factors in cutaneous wound healing

Growth Factors	Effects
EGF	Epidermal keratinocyte migration, proliferation, differentiation, re-epithelialization
FGF-1, -2	Fibroblast and keratinocyte proliferation; endothelial cell proliferation, migration, survival, angiogenesis
IGF	Cell proliferation
KGF/FGF-7	Keratinocyte proliferation
PDGF	Fibroblast chemotaxis, proliferation, contraction
TGF-α	Similar to EGF
TGF-β1, -β2, -β3	Fibroblast chemotaxis, promote extracellular matrix deposition, inhibition of cell proliferation, inhibition of protease inhibitor secretion; endothelial cell migration, survival, angiogenesis
VEGF	Endothelial cell proliferation, migration, survival, increases vasopermeability, angiogenesis

EGF, epidermal growth factor; FGF, fibroblast growth factor; FGF-7, keratinocyte growth factor (also known as FGF-7); IGF, insulin-like growth factor; KGF, keratinocyte growth factor; PDGF, platelet-derived growth factor; TGF, transforming growth factor; tPA, tissue plasminogen activator; VEGF, vascular endothelial growth factor.

and macrophages—persist at the site of inflammation. The chronic inflammatory response may not be characterized by the cardinal signs of inflammation. At times, the body responds to the presence of persistent foreign material and/or infection by local proliferation of mononuclear cells. In particular, macrophages that have ingested foreign particulate material will remain in the tissue if they are unable to solubilize the material. Macrophages attract fibroblasts, and over time may produce increased quantities of collagen, leading to a slowly forming encapsulated mass of fibrous tissue—a granuloma—and this is considered to be the body's last defense against a foreign material that cannot be phagocytized or solubilized.

Proliferative phase

The initial inflammatory responses to injury provide the necessary framework for the production of a new functional barrier. In this phase of healing, cellular activity predominates. Proliferation requires the creation of a permeability barrier (re-epithelialization) but part of this process is the establishment of an appropriate blood supply (neovascularization) and reinforcement of the injured tissue (fibroplasia).

Re-epithelialization

Re-epithelialization is the process responsible for restoring an intact epidermis following cutaneous injury. In general, re-epithelialization involves several processes: the migration of epidermal keratinocytes from wound edges; the proliferation of keratinocytes that are used to supplement the advancing and migrating epithelial tongue; differentiation of the neo-epithelium into stratified epidermis; restoration of an intact basement membrane zone that connects the epidermis and underlying dermis; and the repopulation of specialized cells that direct sensory function (Merkel's cells), pigmentation (melanocytes), and immune functions (Langerhans cells).

Keratinocyte migration

Keratinocyte migration is an early event in wound re-epithelialization. Epidermal keratinocytes initially respond to an epidermal defect by migrating from the free edges of the wound within 24 hours. The keratinocyte migration in partial-thickness wounds also occurs from remaining skin appendages, including the hair follicle (Fig. 7.4). Epidermal stem cells from the hair follicle are now thought to originate from the hair bulge, which is believed to be the germinative portion of the hair.[18] A change in the activity of keratinocytes is required for re-epithelialization to occur. In the unwounded stable state, cuboid-shaped basal keratinocytes interact with each other by a desmosomal intercellular bridge, and are connected to their own basement membrane zone by hemidesmosomes. Approximately 12 hours after wounding, epidermal cells become somewhat flattened and elongated, develop pseudopod-like projections named lamellipodia, lose their cell–cell and cell–matrix attachments, retract their intracellular tonofilaments, and form actin filaments at the edge of the cell cytoplasm. While epidermal cells are migrating, their proliferative potential is inhibited. The migrating basal cells are thought to differ from normal basal cells and may express selective cell surface markers such as CD44, as well as some markers usually expressed by squamous cells.[18]

The mechanisms of wound re-epithelialization have been debated for a long time but remain unclear. The migration of keratinocytes over the wound surface may occur in several ways. Currently, a 'leap frog' theory is the more commonly accepted model[19] whereby epidermal cells migrate two or three cell lengths from their initial position and slide or roll over epidermal cells previously implanted in the wound. The migrating cells become fixed, and other epidermal cells successively migrate over these cells. The epidermal layer progressively advances and closes the epithelial defect.

Keratinocytes use their surface integrin receptors to interact with fibronectin from fibronectin-rich provisional matrix for their migration. The direction of migration is also regulated by the binding of keratinocytes through integrin to the newly formed collagen molecules in the wound bed. Subsequent dissociation of the bindings allows the keratinocytes to move forward. An early provisional matrix formed by fibrin, fibronectin, and type V collagen enables keratinocytes to migrate and dissect under eschar and debris covering the wound.[20] Keratinocytes dissect under eschar because a moist environment is necessary for their migration, and this may be one reason for the success of occlusive dressings in speeding wound healing. Fibronectin produced from plasma initially, and from plasma and fibroblasts later, may also be derived from the migrating keratinocytes themselves. This suggests that the migrating tongue of epithelial cells may provide its own lattice for continued migration. Among the stimuli for re-epithelialization thought to be important are TGF-β, keratinocyte growth factor (KGF), and epidermal growth factor (EGF).

Migrating keratinocytes produce matrix metalloproteases (MMPs) to degrade damaged matrix. An example of the active role of basal keratinocytes in cell migration is their secretion of MMP-1 (collagenase-1) when in contact with fibrillar collagens, but not while on intact basement membrane.[21] MMP-1 disrupts any attachment to fibrillar collagen and allows for continued migration of keratinocytes. Once the wound is epithelialized, keratinocytes bind to α2, β1 integrin, and production of MMP-1 stops. The specificity described above with regard to MMP-1 impacts not solely on the outcome of epithelial migration but also on the maintenance of the directionality of the migrating tongue of epithelium.

Keratinocyte proliferation and differentiation

Re-epithelialization also involves increased proliferation of the keratinocytes located behind the migrating cells at the tongue front, thus ensuring an adequate supply of cells to migrate and cover the wound. When migration ceases, possibly due to contact inhibition, keratinocytes reattach themselves to the underlying substratum, reconstitute the basement membrane, and then resume the process of terminal differentiation to generate a new, stratified epidermis. One can observe that towards the wound center there are single-layered keratinocytes, while near the wound edges there are multiple-layered or stratified keratinocytes. Near the wound margin, the differentiation of the neo-epidermis (keratins 1/10, filaggrin, and loricrin) and regeneration of the dermoepidermal junction (laminin 5 and collagen IV) are more advanced than toward the wound center, where the proliferative index is found to be significantly increased.[19]

Restoration of the basement membrane zone

The formation of intact basement membrane zone (BMZ), which is normally located between epidermis and dermis, is essential for re-establishing the integrity and function of the skin. Within 7–9 days of the re-formation of the epidermis, the BMZ returns to normal. The BMZ forms an adhesion structure, the upper part of which serves as an attachment site for basal keratinocytes through the formation of a hemidesmosome-anchoring filament complex; the lower portion stabilizes the attachment to the underlying dermis by anchoring fibrils (Fig. 7.8). The importance of individual BMZ proteins is evidenced by a group of inherited blistering diseases known as epidermolysis bullosa (EB). These include the mutations of hemidesmosome component collagen XVII as in atrophic epidermolysis bullosa, the defects of laminin 5 of major anchoring filaments as in junctional epidermolysis bullosa, and the deficiency of collagen VII anchoring fibrils as in dystrophic EB.[22]

Collagens

The BMZ of the skin consists of many extracellular matrix proteins, with collagens and laminins as the major components. Collagen IV, collagen VII and collagen XVII are the major collagens in the BMZ, while collagen IV is the most abundant. Collagen IV forms a three-dimensional lattice network within the lamina densa of skin BMZ. In addition, collagen IV is also the predominant collagen in the BMZ of dermal blood vessels. Collagen VII proteins, also called anchoring fibrils, span from the lamina densa to the upper papillary dermis where they form a structure known as anchoring plaque that also contains collagen IV. Anchoring fibril loops are also associated with interstitial collagens of primarily types I and III. Collagen XVII, also known as bullous pemphigoid antigen (BPAG-2 or BP180), is a 180-kDa transmembrane protein located on the hemidesmosome complex of basal keratinocytes. Collagen XVII has a short *N*-terminus inside the cell and a long triple helix collagenous extracellular domains at its C-terminus that associates with anchoring filaments at the lamina lucida of the cutaneous BMZ.[22]

Laminins

Laminins are the major non-collagenous extracellular matrix components in a wide range of BMZ within human tissues. All laminins are large heterotrimeric glycoproteins, each composed of an α, β and γ chain, forming an asymmetric cross-shaped structure (Fig. 7.9). Several laminins have been reported to be present in the BMZ of the dermal–epidermal junction.[23] Laminin 1 was the first laminin identified in the lamina densa. Three $\alpha3$-chain-containing laminins, laminin 5 ($\alpha3\beta3\gamma2$; previously named kalinin, epiligrin, nicein, BM600), laminin 6 ($\alpha3\beta1\gamma1$; previously called k-laminin) and laminin 7 ($\alpha3\beta2\gamma1$) are the integral components of the anchoring filaments, traversing from the hemidesmosome across the lamina lucida to the lamina densa.[24] There is evidence that laminins are also actively involved in wound repair. In response to wounding, the leading keratinocytes in the migrating front edge deposit laminin 5, which serves as a track that migrating keratinocytes can follow to spread.[25] More recently, a new laminin member, laminin 10 ($\alpha5\beta1\gamma1$), has been located within the lamina densa.[26] It has also been found to be a major laminin of dermal microvascular blood vessels.[27] Laminin 10 showed strong promoting effects on human keratinocyte attachment. The skin of laminin 10-knockout mice exhibited discontinuity in the lamina densa of BMZ and causes a defect in hair development.[28]

Dermal–epidermal basement membrane zone

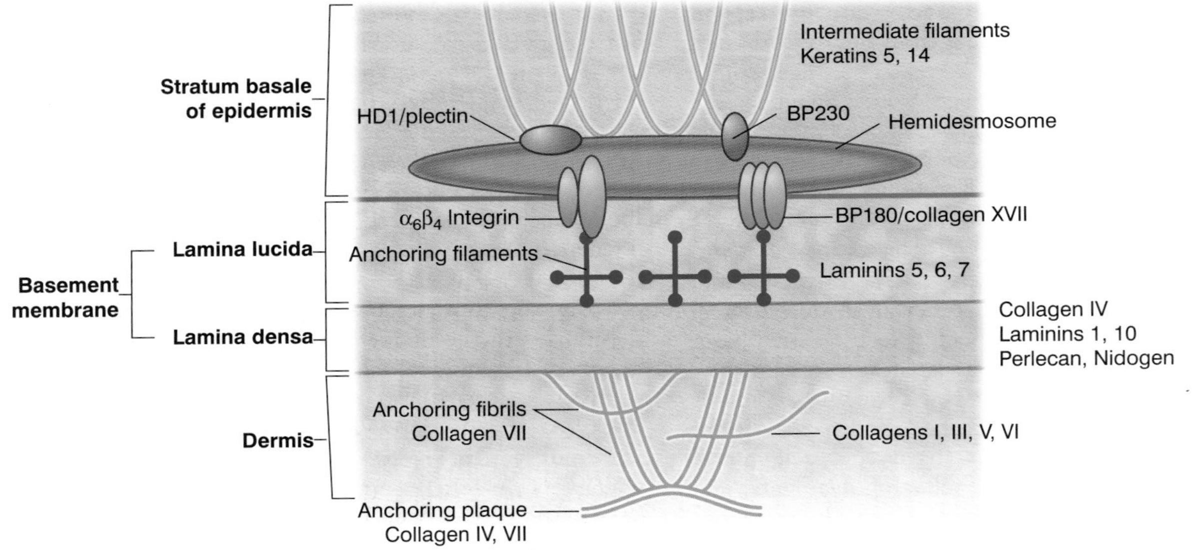

Figure 7.8 Schematic structure of dermal–epidermal basement membrane zone.

Reconstitution of the dermis

Granulation tissue, a sign of progression of healing, begins to form within 3–4 days of injury. The provisional extracellular matrix, fibrin clot, which is rich in fibronectin, promotes formation of granulation tissue by providing scaffolding and contact guidance for cells to migrate into the wound space, and for angiogenesis and fibroplasia to occur to replace the wounded dermal tissue.

Fibroplasia

Granulation tissue consists of new vessels that migrate into the wound as well as the accumulation of fibroblasts and ground substances (Fig. 7.7). Fibroplasia is used to describe a process of fibroblast proliferation, migration into the wound's fibrin clot, and production of new collagens and other matrix proteins, as well as cytokine regulation; this process contributes to the formation of granulation tissue during wound repair. As an early response to injury, fibroblasts in the wound edges begin to proliferate, and at about day 4 they start to migrate into the provisional matrix of the wound clot where they lay down collagen-rich matrix.[29] Fibroblasts perform several functions and may undergo phenotypic changes over a period of time in order to accomplish these different functions.[30] However, it is possible that certain subpopulations of these cells exist (similar to lymphocytes) and these individual subpopulations may perform different roles during wound healing.

First, fibroblasts migrate and later produce large amounts of matrix materials, including collagen, proteoglycans, and elastin.[31] Once the fibroblasts have migrated into the wound, they gradually switch their major function to protein synthesis and change to profibrotic phenotype, which is characterized by abundant rough endoplasmic reticulum and Golgi apparatus filled with new matrix proteins. As was the case for fibroblast proliferation, optimal conditions for fibroblasts to produce matrix proteins consist of an acidic, low-oxygen environment. Fibroblasts are also modulated into the phenotype of myofibroblasts and participate in wound contraction.[3]

Fibroblastic chemotactic factors are complex but are, in part, derived from macrophages already present in the wound. Both PDGF and TGF-β can stimulate fibroblast migration and upregulate the expression of integrin receptors.[32] EGF, and FGF, among others modulate fibroblast proliferation and migration.[33,34] Fibroblast proliferation is also stimulated by low oxygen conditions found in the center of the wound. As angiogenesis proceeds with the formation of new vessels and increased oxygen carrying capacity, this stimulus diminishes.

Structural molecules of the early extracellular matrix, such as fibronectin and collagen, also contribute to the formation of granulation tissue by providing a scaffold for contact guidance and a reservoir for cytokines and growth factors. Fibronectin, a glycoprotein, is a major component of the gel-like cellular substance initially secreted and provides for enhanced fibroblast activity. Thrombin and EGF stimulate fibronectin synthesis and secretion. Fibronectin allows fibroblasts to bind to the extracellular matrix and provides an adherent base for cell migrations, allowing fibroblasts to attach to collagen, fibrin, and hyaluronic acid.[35] The fibronectin matrix provides a scaffold for collagen fibrils and mediates wound contraction. The vectors of fibroblast migration into the wound are directed by the molecular and gross fibrillar structure of fibronectin and, therefore, play a critical role in the speed and direction of dermal repair. Fibroblasts migrate by pulling themselves along a fibronectin matrix, which occurs by contraction of intracellular microfilaments.

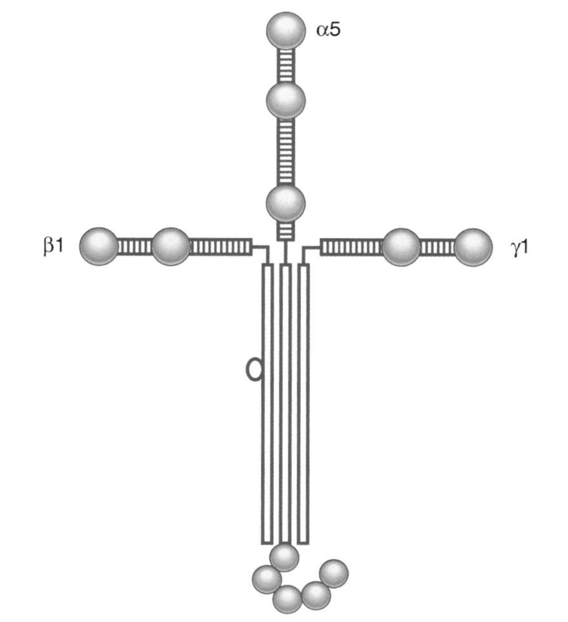

Figure 7.9 Schematic structure of laminin 10.

Integrin receptors in wound healing

Extracellular matrix binds cells through specific cell surface receptors, of which integrins are the major receptors for extracellular matrix. The sequence Arg-Gly-Asp (RGD) has been found frequently to be the major recognition sequence for integrin receptors. Integrins are a family of heterodimeric transmembrane proteins, each consisting of one α chain and one β chain. Integrins mediate the cell–cell and cell–matrix interactions, and transduce the signals between them (Fig. 7.10). Many signaling pathways activated by integrin activation are also activated following growth factor stimulation, suggesting that cellular responses mediated by integrins and growth factors may act synergistically or coordinate cellular biochemical changes.[36,37]

Integrin receptors are involved in all phases of wound repair. Immediately after injury, integrin αIIbβ3 conducts the interaction of platelet with extracellular matrix, including fibrin, fibronectin and thrombospondin, for stable clot formation. During later phases of wound healing, migration of cells including leukocytes, keratinocytes, fibroblasts and endothelial cells into the wound requires rapid binding and dissociation with extracellular molecules to permit cell movement. After fibroblasts cease migration and begin wound contraction, they need to bind tightly to collagens and fibronectin and organize a contractile cytoskeleton. Integrins may play central roles in these processes. Cells might express and use different integrins

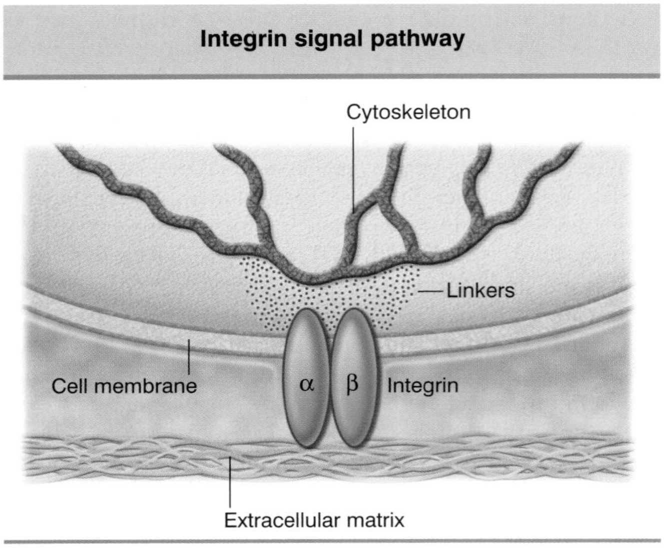

Figure 7.10 Schematic model of integrin signal pathway.

for their migration and attachment. For example, in normal epidermis, $\alpha3\beta1$ integrins mediate the interactions between keratinocytes, and $\alpha6\beta4$ integrins connect basal keratinocytes to the BMZ laminins. $\alpha2\beta1$ and $\alpha5\beta1$ integrins mediate keratinocyte migration on collagen and fibronectin during wound repair.[38,39]

Mechanism of wound contraction

The degree of wound contraction varies with the depth of the wound. For full-thickness wounds, contraction begins soon after wounding and peaks at 2 weeks. In these wounds contraction is an important part of wound healing, accounting for up to a 40% decrease in the size of the wound. In partial-thickness wounds, parts of the adnexa remain and allow epithelialization to occur from within the wound. Therefore, partial-thickness wounds contract less than full-thickness wounds and in direct proportion to their depth. Myofibroblasts are the predominant mediator of this contractile process because of their ability to extend and retract.

During formation of granulation tissue, fibroblasts are gradually modulated into myofibroblasts.[40] By day 7, abundant extracellular matrix has accumulated in the granulation tissue and fibroblasts begin to change into myofibroblast phenotype, which is characterized by actin microfilaments bundles, similar to those seen in smooth muscle cells, along their plasma membrane. The normal skin fibroblasts generally contain β and γ cytoplasmic actins that are organized in a network (not in bundles). A study of electron microscopy and immunohistochemical staining identified a gradual increase of the expression of α-smooth muscle actin, smooth muscle myosin, and desmin, which are markers for smooth muscle differentiation, in wound granulation tissue. This started on day 6 and reached a maximum at day 15, when 70% of fibroblasts showed positivity for these markers. Then there was a progressive regression.[41]

Myofibroblasts probably contain higher concentrations of actinomyosin than any other cell. The cells within the wound align themselves along the lines of contraction—unlike other cells. This muscle-like contraction of the myofibroblasts is mediated by prostaglandin F1, 5-hydroxytryptamine, angiotensin, vasopressin, bradykinins, epinephrine (adrenaline) and norepinephrine (noradrenaline). This contraction is unified and requires cell–cell and cell–matrix communication.[42] Fibronectin not only provides the multiple functions described previously but also assists in wound contraction.[43] Myofibroblast pseudopodia extend, its cytoplasmic actin binds to extracellular fibronectin, attaches to collagen fibers and retracts, drawing the collagen fibers to the cell, thereby producing wound contraction. The rate of contraction is proportional to the number of cells and is inversely proportional to the collagen concentration of the lattice.[44]

Contraction of the wound occurs in predictable directions, via so called 'skin tension lines.' Surgeons often place incisions in the direction of the skin tension lines to direct the contracture. They may also place a full-thickness graft or an acellular dermal equivalent into a full-thickness wound to inhibit wound contraction and subsequent contracture.[45]

Wound angiogenesis

Angiogenesis refers to new vessel growth or neovascularization by sprouting of pre-existing vessels. New capillary buds extend to the wound from blood vessels adjacent to the wound. Newly formed blood vessels participate in formation of granulation tissue and provide nutrition and oxygen to growing tissues. In addition, inflammatory cells require interaction with and transmigration through the blood vessel to enter the site of injury. During angiogenesis, endothelial cells also produce and secrete biologically active substances or cytokines. Neovascularization involves a phenotypic alteration of endothelial cells, directed migration, and various mitogenic stimuli. Cytokines released by cells such as macrophages stimulate angiogenesis during wound healing, as do low oxygen tension and lactic acid, and biogenic amines can potentiate angiogenesis.[46]

As in most normal adult tissues, the dermal blood vasculature remains quiescent. In response to injury, the microvascular endothelial cells initiate an angiogenic process consisting of activation of endothelial cells, local degradation of their basement membrane, sprouting into the wound clot, cell proliferation, formation of a tubule structure, reconstruction of basement membrane and stabilization, and eventually regression and involution of the newly formed vasculature as tissue remodeling (Fig. 7.11).[47] Similar to the migrating tongue of epithelium, endothelial cells at the tips of capillaries migrate into the wound, but do not undergo active proliferation.[48] Cytoplasmic pseudopodia extend from endothelial cells on the second wound day, collagenase is secreted, and there is migration into the perivascular space.[49] On the other hand, proliferation of endothelial cells has been postulated to be a secondary effect to cell migration. Therefore fibronectin, heparin, and platelet factors that are known to stimulate endothelial cell migration into the wound also directly or indirectly stimulate endothelial cell proliferation.

Angiogenic growth factors

Several growth factors have shown to play critical roles in wound angiogenesis including VEGF, angiopoietin, FGF and TGF-β. The cooperative expression of these angiogenic

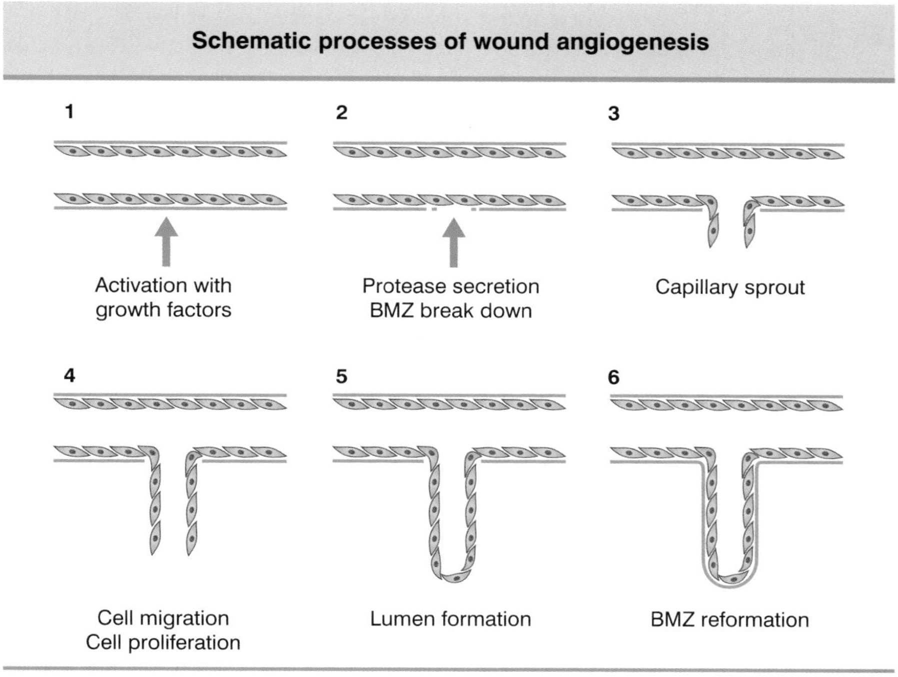

Figure 7.11 Schematic processes of wound angiogenesis. It is initiated when blood vessel endothelial cells in the wound edge are activated by growth factors (activation) to produce and release proteases that degrade the basement membrane zone (BMZ).

Table 7.6 Growth factor regulation of EC in wound angiogenesis

	VEGF	Ang-1	FGF-1, -2	TGFβ
Proliferation	+	±	+	–
Migration	+	+	+	+
Tubule formation	+	+	+	+
Survival	+	+	±	±
EC-specific receptors	Yes	Yes	No	No
Upregulation of integrin, ECM	+	±	+	+
Vasopermeability	+	–	±	–
Vessel wall integrity	–	+	±	+

Ang-1, angiopoietin 1; EC, endothelial cell; ECM, extracellular matrix; FGF, fibroblast growth factor; TGF, transforming growth factor; VEGF, vascular endothelial growth factor.
Note: +, positive effect; –, negative effect; ±, no established effect.

growth factors is essential in wound angiogenesis (Table 7.6).

VEGF exerts its biological activity predominantly on endothelial cells. It is a key mediator of angiogenesis, which performs multiple functions on endothelial cells through two specific receptors, VEGFR-1 or Flt-1 and VEGFR-2 or Flk-1/KDR. VEGF is known also as vascular permeability factor (VPF), due to its potent vasopermeability actions. VEGF is a potent mitogen for endothelial cells and induces endothelial cell migration and sprouting by upregulation of several integrin receptors including αvβ3, α1β1 and α2β1.[50] VEGF acts as a survival factor for endothelial cells through induction of the expression of the antiapoptotic protein Bcl-2.[51] Many different cell types, such as keratinocytes, fibroblasts and endothelial cells, are able to produce VEGF. VEGF is expressed at low levels in normal human skin, but its expression is highly upregulated during wound healing. Low oxygen tension, as occurs in tissue hypoxia during tissue injury, is a major inducer of this growth factor.[52]

Extracellular matrix in wound angiogenesis

Migration of endothelial cells and development of new capillary tubule structure is dependent upon not only the cells and cytokines present but also the production and organization of extracellular matrix components, including fibronectin, collagen, vitronectin and laminin, both in granulation tissue and in endothelial basement membrane. The extracellular matrix is critical for blood vessel growth and maintenance, by acting as both scaffold support, through which endothelial cells may migrate, and reservoir and modulator for growth factors, such as FGF-2 and TGF-β, to mediate intercellular signals.[53]

As a good example, when grown in two-dimensional collagen matrix gel, endothelial cells migrate, proliferate and express PDGF receptors, a situation that mimics the cell population of an active, migrating and proliferating tip of an angiogenic sprout. In this case, deposition of basement membrane proteins of laminin and collagen IV is irregular and discontinuous. When grown in a three-dimensional system, cell proliferation is inhibited and cells form a capillary-like tubule structure, and lose expression of PDGF receptors. This pattern simulates the quiescent, differentiating cell population away from the angiogenic sprout tip and close to the parental vessel, where laminin and collagen IV are deposited in a continuous pattern.[47] Once again, depending on the model system, differential effects may be observed. One measure of the significance of the extracellular matrix is that pharmacological agents aimed at affecting angiogenesis by interfering with the structure and function of the extracellular matrix have been studied.[54]

Remodeling phase

Remodeling, the third phase of wound repair, consists of the deposition of matrix materials and their subsequent change over time (Fig. 7.12). In fact the remodeling occurs through the whole process of wound repair, from the provisional

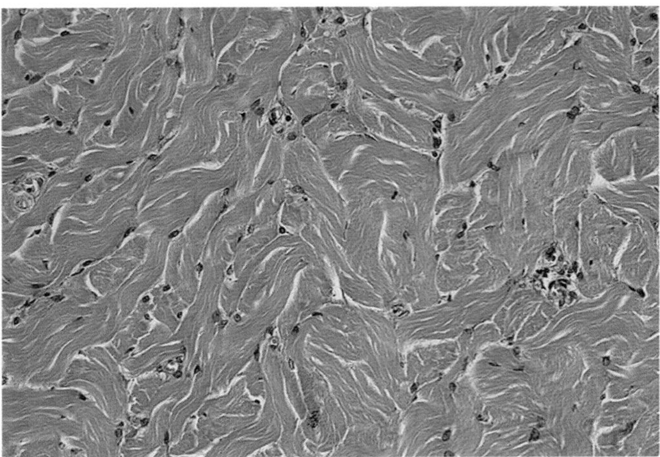

Figure 7.12 The remodeling phase of wound healing. Photo of a 3-week-old partial-thickness wound in a pig, showing some fibroblasts among abundant collagen fibers in the dermis with a new blood vessel supply (× 200).

matrix of the fibrin clot that contains much fibronectin, to the granulation tissue that is rich in type III collagen and blood vessels, and to the mature scar that is collagen I predominant with less blood supply.

Long after the skin's epidermal barrier is restored, events continue to occur that are related to wound injury and repair. The total amount of collagen increases early in repair, reaching a maximum between 2 and 3 weeks after injury. Tensile strength, a functional assessment of collagen, increases to 40% of strength prior to injury at 1 month, and may continue to increase for up to a year. Even at its greatest, the tensile strength of the healed wound is never greater than 80% of its preinjury strength.[55]

Type III collagen, as mentioned above, is the major collagen synthesized by fibroblasts in granulation tissue. Over the period of a year or more, the dermis returns to the stable pre-injury phenotype, consisting largely of type I collagen. In addition, the composition of other extracellular material within the wound changes as the water content and glycosaminoglycan level decrease. The process of this conversion of the dermis is accomplished through tightly controlled synthesis of new collagen and lysis of old. Collagen lysis is accomplished through the actions of collagenases. This leads to a change in the orientation of scar tissue.

Extracellular matrix

Connective tissues are composed of three elements: cells, fibers, and amorphous ground substance. Fibers and ground substances collectively are referred to as extracellular matrix, in part made up by glycosaminoglycans and proteoglycans. Ground substance is an amorphous viscous gel secreted by fibroblasts, which occupies the spaces between the cells and fibers of connective tissue. It helps determine compliance, flexibility, and integrity of the dermis and also provides strength, support, and density to tissue; reduces friction between connective tissue fibers during tissue stress or strain; and protects tissue from invasion by microorganisms. Ground substance allows tissue fluid, which contain nutrients for the cells as well as waste products, to diffuse among cells and capillaries. It also transports many soluble substances and stores electrolytes and water. Substrates of ground substance are water, salts, and glycosaminoglycans. Most glycosaminoglycans are linked covalently to protein and, thus, are termed proteoglycans.

Hyaluronic acid is non-sulfated glycosaminoglycan, and is found in the highest amounts in the first 4–5 days of healing wound.[16] Hyaluronic acid serves as a stimulus for fibroblast proliferation and migration[56] and can absorb large amounts of water, producing tissue edema. This swelling provides additional space for migration of fibroblasts into the wound. Hyaluronidase enzymatically degrades hyaluronic acid.

Sulfated glycosaminoglycans are proteoglycans. They provide a stable and resilient matrix that inhibits cell migration and proliferation. The sulfated glycosaminoglycans chondroitin-4-sulfate and dermatan sulfate eventually replace hyaluronic acid as the major glycosaminoglycan on days 5–7. Saccharide chains in the chondroitin sulfate–protein complex cross-link with collagenous fibers. There are proportional differences in the glycosaminoglycan content of human skin, with a progressive decrease from fetal development to maturity in non-weight-bearing skin. In contrast, weight-bearing skin, such as the plantar aspect of the foot, demonstrates minimal change in glycosaminoglycan composition with aging. Constituents of glycosaminoglycans, particularly chondroitin sulfate, increase proportionally in pathologic states of altered skin, such as Dupuytren's contracture or hypertrophic scarring. Proteoglycans regulate collagen fibrillogenesis and accelerate polymerization of collagen monomers. Heparan sulfate, a proteoglycan which is absent initially after wounding, controls cell division and inhibits the growth of smooth muscle cells. The synthesis of these matrix proteins occurs concomitantly with the production of new collagen.

Collagen

Collagen fibers constitute approximately 80% of dry weight of the dermis in human skin and are the principal proteins providing structure, strength, and stiffness to dermal tissue.[57] In normal adults, type I collagen accounts for approximately 80% of collagen, and type III collagen constitutes 10% of collagen in the dermis. In addition to their structural scaffold roles, collagens promote cell attachment and migration. Collagen varies genetically and structurally. All collagens possess triple-helix structures but differ in the primary structure of their polypeptide chains (α-1 and α-2). Biochemically, collagen is composed of three polypeptide alpha chains. Type I collagen is formed by two α-1 (type I) and one α-2 chains, whereas type III collagen consists of three α-1 (type III) chains. The three α chains are arranged in a triple helix. Several helices are cross-linked to form collagen fibrils that are subsequently entwined to form collagen fibers. The fibers align in directions that accommodate applied stress, thereby allowing the skin to stretch.[57]

Type III collagen presents in large quantities in fetal dermis and is a minority component of normal adult collagen, but during early wound healing it is the predominant collagen synthesized. Type III collagen first appears after 48–72 hours and is maximally secreted after 5–7 days. With wound closure, a gradual turnover of collagen occurs, as type III collagen undergoes degradation and type I collagen synthesis increases. Stimulus for this conversion may be the biomechanical stress and strain placed across a closed wound. As in wound repair, type III collagen is gradually replaced by type I collagen with aging. Stress and strain also may direct realignment of connective tissue fibers. Collagen fibers under tension appear to be resistant to the action of collagenase. In contrast, random fibers not under tension are susceptible to lysis by collagenase. The amount of stress on the wound is responsible for how much scar tissue forms. For example, more scar tissue is necessary in wounds that are on mobile extremities than over a less mobile area such as the abdomen.

Biosynthesis of collagen

Collagen synthesis begins with transcription from DNA to messenger RNA within fibroblast nucleus (Fig. 7.13). Protein translation occurs in endoplasmic reticulum. Both magnesium and zinc trace minerals are needed for translation to occur. Following the synthesis, polypeptide chains undergo several enzymatic modifications, including hydroxylation of proline and lysine which requires oxygen, ferrous iron, and ascorbic acid (vitamin C). Following hydroxylation, the polypeptide chains aggregate into a triple-helix molecule, procollagen, which is released from the fibroblast. Once extracellular, the terminal propeptides are removed by peptidases, and tropocollagen is formed. Tropocollagen, then, aligns in a quarter-staggered array reflected as a helix. The tropocollagen molecules are initially united by hydrogen bonding then stable covalent cross-links, both intramolecularly and intermolecularly, are formed. This creates collagenous fibrils. The intermolecular cross-links are likely to be responsible for tensile strength.

The regulation of collagen synthesis is controlled at several levels. A number of growth factors including TGFβs and FGFs have strong effects on collagen gene expression. TGF-β stimulates both type I and III collagens. Excess TGF-β1 has been found in the dermis of chronic venous ulcers and may play a role in fibrosis.[58] Oxygen and trace minerals also play critical roles in collagen synthesis. Collagen deposition and remodeling is also controlled by various proteinases that degrade collagens (Fig. 7.13).

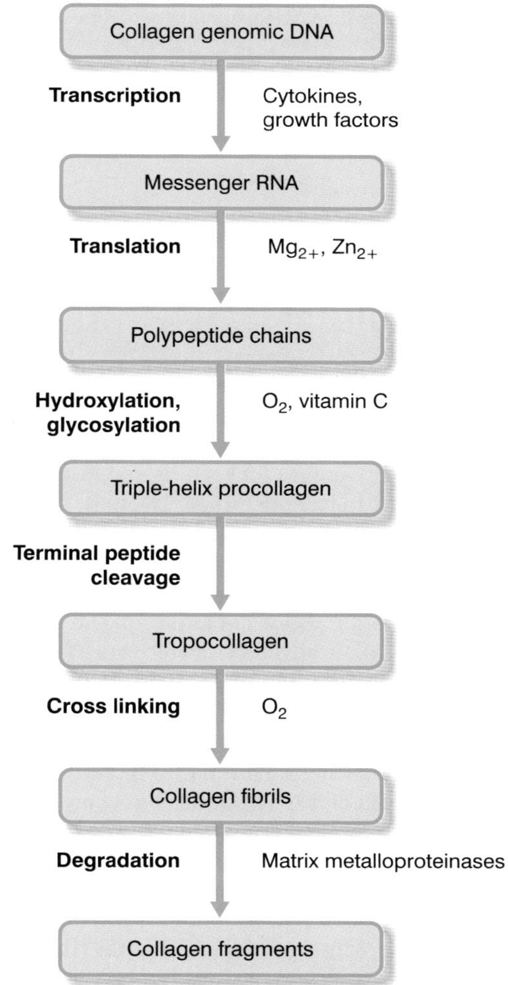

Figure 7.13 Collagen synthesis, degradation, and regulation in wound repair.

Elastic fibers

Elastic fibers are long, thin, and highly retractile. Elastin, as its name implies, provides elasticity and extensibility to the dermis and assists in recovery from deformation.[59] Elastin is a highly hydrophobic structural protein making up only 2% of the total protein in the dermis.[59] Elastin, lipids, and glycoproteins bind to form microfibrils that serve as the scaffolding or as a foundation for fiber orientation. The microfibrils are infiltrated and surrounded by elastin and fuse to form solid elastic fibers. The characteristically wavy elastic fibers are entwined among collagenous fibers. The orientation of elastin varies from a horizontal arrangement in the deep dermis to a more vertical arrangement closer to the epidermis. With aging, the number of microfibrils declines; however, the amount of the amorphous component, elastin, increases.

Proteinases and tissue remodeling

Tissue remodeling is characterized by high levels of extracellular proteolytic activities. The degradation of collagens and other extracellular components is controlled by a group of proteinase enzymes released from inflammatory cells, keratinocytes and fibroblasts under appropriate stimulation. The most important proteinases are matrix metalloproteinases (MMPs).[60] MMPs can be divided into several groups, including the collagenases, the stromelysins, and the gelatinases (Table 7.7). The best characterized subgroup of MMPs are tissue collagenases, which cleave the triple helix of native fibrillar collagens (types I, II and III) in a site-specific fashion.[21] Thus the actions of these enzymes are the rate-limiting step in the turnover of the major extracellular matrix in the dermis, type I and type III collagens. After this cleavage, at body temperature, collagen will be denatured (turn into gelatin) and become susceptible to further degradation by the gelatinases.

With a few exceptions (matrilysin produced in eccrine glands; gelatinase A stored but not produced), MMPs are not detectable or are at very low levels in healthy resting tissue, but are induced in physiologic (repair, remodeling, proliferation) or pathologic states (inflammation, tumor growth) in response to cytokines, growth factors, and cell contact with extracellular matrix. The catalytic activity of

Table 7.7 Major human matrix metalloproteinases (MMPS)

Groups	MMP Type	Major Substrates
Collagenases		
Collagenase-1 (interstitial collagenase)	MMP-1	Fibrillar collagens (types I, II, III VII, X), proMMP-2, -9
Collagenase-2 (neutrophil collagenase)	MMP-8	Fibrillar collagens
Collagenase-3	MMP-13	Fibrillar collagens
Gelatinases		
Gelatinase-A	MMP-2	Gelatin, types IV, V collagen, laminin, fibronectin, proMMP-9, -13
Gelatinase-B	MMP-9	Gelatin, types IV, V collagen
Stromelysins		
Stromelysin-1	MMP-3	Non-fibrillar collagen, gelatin, laminin, fibronectin, proMMP1, -9, -13
Stromelysin-2	MMP-10	Non-fibrillar collagen, gelatin, laminin, fibronectin
Stromelysin-3	MMP-11	Weak activity with non-fibrillar collagen, gelatin, laminin, fibronectin
Matrilysins		
Matrilysin-1	MMP-7	Non-fibrillar collagen, gelatin, laminin, fibronectin, proMMP-1, -9
Matrilysin-2 (endometase)	MMP-26	ProMMP-9, fibronectin, vitronectin
Membrane-type MMPs		
MT1-MMP	MMP-14	ProMMP-2, -13, fibrillar collagens, gelatin, fibrin, laminin, fibronectin
MT2-MMP	MMP-15	ProMMP-2, gelatin, laminin, fibronectin
MT3-MMP	MMP-16	ProMMP-2, collagen III, gelatin, laminin, fibronectin
MT4-MMP	MMP-17	Gelatin, fibronectin, fibrinogen
MT5-MMP	MMP-24	ProMMP-2, gelatin, fibronectin
MT6-MMP	MMP-25	ProMMP-2, collagen IV, gelatin, fibrin, fibrinogin, fibronectin
Others		
Macrophage MMP (metalloelastase)	MMP-12	Elastin

MMPs is also controlled, in part, by a family of tissue inhibitors of metalloproteinases (TIMP-1, TIMP-2, TIMP-3, TIMP-4), which specifically bind MMPs and are natural inhibitors to MMPs. The balance between the activities of MMPs and TIMPs is critical to the wound repair process and remodeling.[60]

■ FACTORS AFFECTING WOUND HEALING

Wound healing can be delayed by various systemic and local factors. Systemic factors that may be detrimental to wound healing include malnutrition, protein deprivation, and deficiencies of vitamin A and vitamin C. Medications such as corticosteroids, penicillamine, nicotine, non-steroidal anti-inflammatory drugs, and antineoplastic agents may interfere with the wound healing at various stages. Chronic debilitating illness, endocrine disorders, systemic vascular disorders, and connective tissue disease often have adverse effects on wound healing. In addition, advancing age contributes to poor wound healing, possibly through impaired expression of metalloproteinases.[61]

Local factors that adversely affect wound healing include poor surgical techniques (excessive tension or excess devitalized tissue); vascular disorders (arteriosclerosis or venous insufficiency); tissue ischemia; infectious processes;[62] certain topically applied medications;[63–65] extravasation of antineoplastic drugs; hemostatic agents such as aluminum chloride or ferric subsulfate; foreign body reactions; or an adverse wound microenvironment (such as the use of dry versus occlusive dressings). Pressure, neuropathy, and chronic radiation injury all adversely affect wound healing.

Lack of cellular oxygen impedes wound healing. Hypoxia that occurs without neovascularization reduces energy production. In addition, tissue oxygen tension is important in collagen synthesis and for the tensile strength of wounds.[66] Wound environments that are anoxic inhibit collagen cross-linking as oxygen is a necessary cofactor. Some elements that may hinder wound healing include medications such as antineoplastic agents and antibiotics. Penicillin, for example, decreases cross-linking of collagen and, therefore, impairs the strength of the wound. Ascorbic acid (vitamin C) is also a cofactor for the collagen cross-linking.[67] Lack of available ascorbic acid (e.g. vitamin C deficiency or scurvy) impedes the hydroxylation and, consequently, the collagen fails to aggregate into fibers. Vitamin A also potentiates epithelial repair and collagen synthesis by enhancing inflammatory reactions, particularly macrophage availability.[68] Minerals also may affect healing; zinc deficiency reduces the rate of epithelialization and retards cellular proliferation and collagen synthesis.[69]

A direct relationship exists between available macrophages and fibroblast production. In fact, if the initial inflammatory process is blocked by the use of systemic steroids during the first 3 days after wounding, healing time is retarded with a resultant loss of skin turgor. Furthermore, the mitotic activity of fibroblasts are suppressed by steroids. The suppression of wound healing caused by corticosteroids has been shown to be ameliorated with administration of local and systemic vitamin A,[68] and a single injection of TGF-β.[70]

OPTIMIZING OUTCOMES

In acute wounds, wound edges may be brought together by direct closure. The apposition of the edges of the wound decreases the distance that cells need to migrate and the size of granulation tissue that must be produced. Aseptic surgical technique minimizes the risk of bacterial contamination which can prolong healing. Prevention of hematoma formation through proper hemostasis and elimination of necrotic tissue also decreases the chance for infection. Therefore, surgical techniques involving steel instruments—as opposed to electrosurgery or cryosurgery—limit the risk for infection because less necrotic tissue is produced, and speed healing as well. Elimination of dead space through the appropriate use of buried deep sutures also lessens the risk for hematoma and subsequent infection. However, wounds closed too tightly with sutures may become ischemic and subsequently necrotic at the edges, and healing may be delayed.

The intelligent use of occlusive dressings can be most effective in speeding wound healing (Fig. 7.14). Stemming from observations in which blisters that remained roofed healed faster than those that had their roof removed, it was found that wounds covered with an occlusive dressing healed up to 40% faster than those left air-exposed. There are many ways in which occlusive dressings might function, including enhancement of keratinocyte migration by maintaining a moist environment, prevention of infection, establishment of an electromagnetic current, or containment of wound fluid and the growth factors present within it.[71]

The choice of occlusive dressings in acute wounds is generally dictated by the clinical setting. Film dressings are commonly used on the face and other cosmetically important areas. Hydrocolloid dressings are recommended in unusually exudative wounds, as they absorb wound fluid as well as provide protection in areas susceptible to trauma. Foam dressings are also absorbent and are extremely effective in reducing the pain associated with some wounds. It is recommended that these dressings be left on the wound until the build-up of exudate causes the fluid to leak from the sides. Because early removal of adherent occlusive dressings can strip away newly formed epithelium, the misuse of occlusive dressings can lead to the prolongation of healing.

Several growth factors including PDGF, growth hormone, EGF, and FGF have been shown to speed the healing of acute wounds in various settings. The use of autologous and allogeneic grafts speed healing of acute wounds as well.

SUMMARY

Wound healing is a complex process, and an understanding of its underlying mechanisms is vital for practitioners of a discipline in which wound creation and repair are fundamental. Advances in immunology and molecular biology have greatly increased our knowledge of the events that take place in inflammation, proliferation and remodeling—the three overlapping phases of healing.

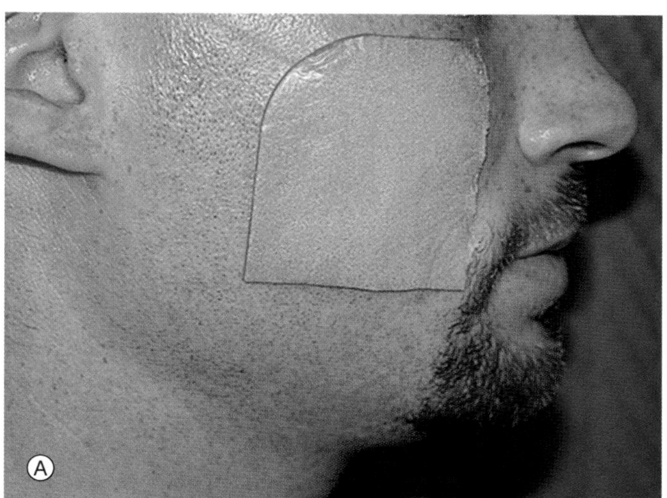

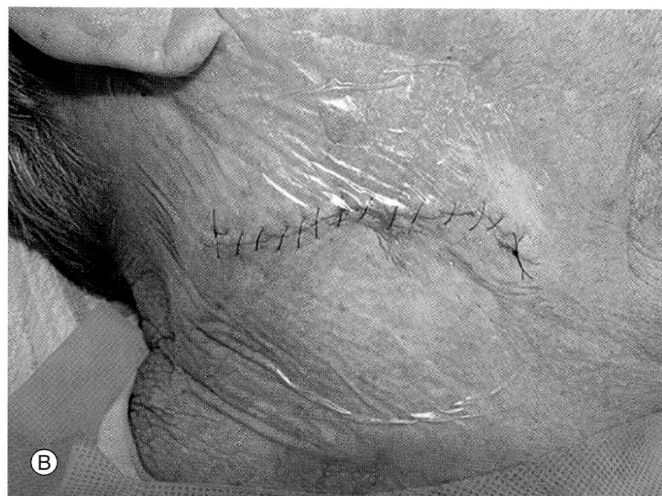

Figure 7.14 Use of occlusive dressings on acute wounds speeds healing and improves cosmesis even over primarily closed wounds. (A) Hydrocolloid dressing on the right cheek. (B) Polyurethane film dressing covering a sutured wound.

■ REFERENCES

1. Scheid A, Wenger RH, Schaffer L, et al. Physiologically low oxygen concentrations in fetal skin regulate hypoxia-inducible factor 1 and transforming growth factor-β3. FASEB J 2002; 16:411–413.
2. Kanj LF, Wilking SV, Phillips TJ. Pressure ulcers. J Am Acad Dermatol 1998; 38:517–536.
3. Welch MP, Odland GF, Clark RA. Temporal relationships of F-actin bundle formation, collagen and fibronectin matrix assembly, and fibronectin receptor expression to wound contraction. J Cell Biol 1990; 110:133–145.
4. Hell E, Lawrence JC. The initiation of epidermal wound healing in cuts and burns. Br J Exp Pathol 1979; 60:171–179.
5. Katz MH, Alvarez AF, Kirsner RS, et al. Human wound fluid from acute wounds stimulates fibroblast and endothelial cell growth. J Am Acad Dermatol 1991; 25:1054–1058.
6. Kirsner RS, Eaglstein WH. The wound healing process. Dermatol Clin 993; 11:629–640.
7. Grinnell F, Billingham RE, Burgess L. Distribution of fibronectin during wound healing in vivo. J Invest Dermatol 1981; 76:181–189.
8. Kunkel SL, Standiford T, Kasahara K, Strieter RM. Stimulus specific induction of monocyte chemotactic protein-1 (MCP-1) gene expression. Adv Exp Med Biol 1991; 305:65–71.
9. Sherry B, Tekamp-Olson P, Gallegos C, et al. Resolution of the two components of macrophage inflammatory protein 1, and cloning and characterization of one of those components, macrophage inflammatory protein 1 beta. J Exp Med 1988; 168:2251–2259.
10. Postlethwaite AE, Kang AH. Collagen- and collagen peptide-induced chemotaxis of human blood monocytes. J Exp Med 1976; 143:1299–1307.
11. Lewis JS, Lee JA, Underwood JC, et al. Macrophage responses to hypoxia: relevance to disease mechanisms. J Leukoc Biol 1999; 66:889–900.
12. Simpson DM, Ross R. The neutrophilic leukocyte in wound repair: a study with antineutrophil serum. J Clin Invest 1972; 51:2009–2023.
13. Falanga V. Growth factors and wound healing. J Dermatol Surg Oncol 1993; 19:711–714.
14. Noli C, Miolo A. The mast cell in wound healing. Vet Dermatol 2001; 12:303–313.
15. Hosgood G. Wound healing. The role of platelet-derived growth factor and transforming growth factor beta. Vet Surg 1993; 22:490–495.
16. Deuel TF, Senior RM, Huang JS, Griffin GL. Chemotaxis of monocytes and neutrophils to platelet-derived growth factor. J Clin Invest 1982; 69:1046–1049.
17. Knighton DR, Hunt TK, Thakral KK, Goodson WH. Role of platelets and fibrin in the healing sequence: an in vivo study of angiogenesis and collagen synthesis. Ann Surg 1982; 196:379–388.
18. Sun TT, Cotsarelis G, Lavker RM. Hair follicular stem cells: the bulge-activation hypothesis. J Invest Dermatol 1991; 96:77S–78S.
19. Laplante AF, Germain L, Auger FA, Moulin V. Mechanisms of wound re-epithelialization: hints from a tissue-engineered reconstructed skin to long-standing questions. FASEB J 2001; 15:2377–2389.
20. Grove GL. Age-related differences in healing of superficial skin wounds in humans. Arch Dermatol Res 1982; 272:381–385.
21. Parks WC. Matrix metalloproteinases in repair. Wound Repair Regen 1999; 7:423–432.
22. Uitto J, Pulkkinen L, McLean WH. Epidermolysis bullosa: a spectrum of clinical phenotypes explained by molecular heterogeneity. Mol Med Today 1997; 3:457–465.
23. McGowan KA, Marinkovich MP. Laminins and human disease. Microsc Res Tech 2000; 51:262–279.
24. Carter WG, Kaur P, Gil SG, et al. Distinct functions for integrins alpha 3 beta 1 in focal adhesions and alpha 6 beta 4/bullous pemphigoid antigen in a new stable anchoring contact (SAC) of keratinocytes: relation to hemidesmosomes. J Cell Biol 1990; 111:3141–3154.
25. Nguyen BP, Ryan MC, Gil SG, Carter WG. Deposition of laminin 5 in epidermal wounds regulates integrin signaling and adhesion. Curr Opin Cell Biol 2000; 12:554–562.
26. Miner JH, Cunningham J, Sanes JR. Roles for laminin in embryogenesis: exencephaly, syndactyly, and placentopathy in mice lacking the laminin alpha5 chain. J Cell Biol 1998; 143:1713–1723.
27. Li J, Zhang YP, Kirsner RS. Angiogenesis in wound repair: angiogenic growth factors and the extracellular matrix. Microsc Res Tech 2003; 60:107–114.
28. Li J, Tzu J, Chen Y, et al. Laminin 10 is crucial for hair morphogenesis. EMBO J 2003; 22:2400–2410.
29. Kurkinen M, Vaheri A, Roberts PJ, Stenman S. Sequential appearance of fibronectin and collagen In experimental granulation tissue. Lab Invest 1980; 43:47–51.
30. Clark RA. Basics of cutaneous wound repair. J Dermatol Surg Oncol 1993; 19:693–706.
31. Woodley DT, O'Keefe EJ, Prunieras M. Cutaneous wound healing: a model for cell–matrix interactions. J Am Acad Dermatol 1985; 12:420–433.
32. Gailit J, Xu J, Bueller H, Clark RA. Platelet-derived growth factor and inflammatory cytokines have differential effects on the expression of integrins alpha 1 beta 1 and alpha 5 beta 1 by human dermal fibroblasts in vitro. J Cell Physiol 1996; 169:281–289.
33. Roberts AB, Sporn MB. Transforming growth factor-beta: potential common mechanisms mediating its effects on embryogenesis, inflammation-repair, and carcinogenesis. Int J Rad Appl Instrum B 1987; 14:435–439.
34. Ross R, Bowen-Pope DF, Raines EW. Platelet-derived growth factor: its potential roles in wound healing, atherosclerosis, neoplasia, and growth and development. Ciba Found Symp 1985; 116:98–112.
35. Pearlstein E. Plasma membrane glycoprotein which mediates adhesion of fibroblasts to collagen. Nature 1976; 262:497–500.
36. Giancotti FG, Ruoslahti E. Integrin signaling. Science 1999; 285:1028–1032.
37. Sepp NT, Li LJ, Lee KH, et al. Basic fibroblast growth factor increases expression of the alpha v beta 3 integrin complex on human microvascular endothelial cells. J Invest Dermatol 1994; 103:295–299.
38. Kim JP, Zhang K, Chen JD, et al. Mechanism of human keratinocyte migration on fibronectin: unique roles of RGD site and integrins. J Cell Physiol 1992; 151:443–450.
39. Mercurio AM. Lessons from the alpha 2 integrin knockout mouse. Am J Pathol 2002; 161:3–6.
40. Majno G. The story of the myofibroblasts. Am J Surg Pathol 1979; 3:535–542.
41. Darby I, Skalli O, Gabbiani G. Alpha-smooth muscle actin is transiently expressed by myofibroblasts during experimental wound healing. Lab Invest 1990; 63:21–29.
42. Mudera V, Eastwood M, McFarland C, Brown RA. Evidence for sequential utilization of fibronectin, vitronectin, and collagen during fibroblast-mediated collagen contraction. Wound Repair Regen 2002; 10:397–408.
43. Singer II, Kawka DW, Kazazis DM, Clark RA. In vivo co-distribution of fibronectin and actin fibers in granulation tissue: immunofluorescence and electron microscope studies of the fibronexus at the myofibroblast surface. J Cell Biol 1984; 98:2091–2106.
44. Bell E, Ehrlich HP, Buttle DJ, Nakatsuji T. Living tissue formed in vitro and accepted as skin-equivalent tissue of full thickness. Science 1981; 211:1052–1054.
45. Yannas IV. Studies on the biological activity of the dermal regeneration template. Wound Repair Regen 1998; 6:518–523.
46. Remensnyder JP, Majno G. Oxygen gradients in healing wounds. Am J Pathol 1968; 52:301–323.
47. Marx M, Perlmutter RA, Madri JA. Modulation of platelet-derived growth factor receptor expression in microvascular endothelial cells during in vitro angiogenesis. J Clin Invest 1994; 93:131–139.
48. Folkman J. Angiogenesis: initiation and control. Ann N Y Acad Sci 1982; 401:212–227.
49. Kalebic T, Garbisa S, Glaser B, Liotta LA. Basement membrane collagen: degradation by migrating endothelial cells. Science 1983; 221:281–283.
50. Senger DR, Claffey KP, Benes JE, et al. Angiogenesis promoted by vascular endothelial growth factor: regulation through alpha1beta1 and alpha2 beta1 integrins. Proc Natl Acad Sci USA 1997; 94:13612–13617.
51. Gerber HP, Dixit V, Ferrara N. Vascular endothelial growth factor induces expression of the antiapoptotic proteins Bcl-2 and A1 in vascular endothelial cells. J Biol Chem 1998; 273:13313–13316.
52. Detmar M, Brown LF, Berse B, et al. Hypoxia regulates the expression of vascular permeability factor/vascular endothelial growth factor (VPF/VEGF) and its receptors in human skin. J Invest Dermatol 1997; 108:263–268.
53. Feng X, Clark RA, Galanakis D, Tonnesen MG. Fibrin and collagen differentially regulate human dermal microvascular endothelial cell integrins: stabilization of alpha v/beta 3 mRNA by fibrin 1. J Invest Dermatol 1999; 113:913–919.
54. Ingber DE, Folkman J. How does extracellular matrix control capillary morphogenesis? Cell 1989; 58:803–805.

55. Abercrombie M, Flint MH, James DW. Wound contraction in relation to collagen formation in scorbutic guinea pigs. J Embryol Exp Morph 1956; 4:167–175.

56. Toole BP, Gross J. The extracellular matrix of the regenerating newt limb: synthesis and removal of hyaluronate prior to differentiation. Dev Biol 1971; 25:57–77.

57. Booth BA, Polak KL, Uitto J. Collagen biosynthesis by human skin fibroblasts. I. Optimization of the culture conditions for synthesis of type I and type III procollagens. Biochim Biophys Acta 1980; 607:145–160.

58. Shah M, Foreman DM, Ferguson MW. Neutralisation of TGF-beta 1 and TGF-beta 2 or exogenous addition of TGF-beta 3 to cutaneous rat wounds reduces scarring. J Cell Sci 1995; 108:985–1002.

59. Braverman IM, Fonferko E. Studies in cutaneous aging: I. The elastic fiber network. J Invest Dermatol 1982; 78:434–443.

60. Visse R, Nagase H. Matrix metalloproteinases and tissue inhibitors of metalloproteinases: structure, function, and biochemistry. Circ Res 2003; 92:827–839.

61. Ashcroft GS, Herrick SE, Tarnuzzer RW, et al. Human ageing impairs injury-induced in vivo expression of tissue inhibitor of matrix metalloproteinases (TIMP)-1 and -2 proteins and mRNA. J Pathol 1997; 183:169–176.

62. Leyden JJ. Effect of bacteria on healing of superficial wounds. Clin Dermatol 1984; 2:81–85.

63. Corball M, O'Dwyer P, Brady MP. The interaction of vitamin A and corticosteroids on wound healing. Ir J Med Sci 1985; 154:306–310.

64. Eaglstein WH, Mertz PM. 'Inert' vehicles do affect wound healing. J Invest Dermatol 1980; 74:90–91.

65. Geronemus RG, Mertz PM, Eaglstein WH. Wound healing. The effects of topical antimicrobial agents. Arch Dermatol 1979; 115:1311–1314.

66. Jonsson K, Jensen JA, Goodson WH, et al. Tissue oxygenation, anemia, and perfusion in relation to wound healing in surgical patients. Ann Surg 1991; 214:605–613.

67. Geesin JC, Darr D, Kaufman R, et al. Ascorbic acid specifically increases type I and type III procollagen messenger RNA levels in human skin fibroblast. J Invest Dermatol 1988; 90:420–424.

68. Hunt TK. Vitamin A and wound healing. J Am Acad Dermatol 1986; 15:817–821.

69. Agren MS, Franzen L. Influence of zinc deficiency on breaking strength of 3-week-old skin incisions in the rat. Acta Chir Scand 1990; 156:667–670.

70. Beck LS, DeGuzman L, Lee WP, et al. One systemic administration of transforming growth factor-beta 1 reverses age- or glucocorticoid-impaired wound healing. J Clin Invest 1993; 92:2841–2849.

71. Eaglstein WH. Experiences with biosynthetic dressings. J Am Acad Dermatol 1985; 12:434–440.

8 Dressings and Postoperative Care

May Leveriza-Oh MD and Tania J Phillips MD FRCPC

Summary box

- Dressings function to cover the wound, absorb drainage, apply pressure, and provide a moist environment.
- Dressings should be selected to keep the wound moist, but not too wet nor too dry.
- Moist wound healing enhances epithelial migration, stimulates angiogenesis, helps in retention of growth factors, facilitates autolytic debridement and fibrinolysis, protects against exogenous organisms, and maintains voltage gradients.
- Healing in a moist environment accelerates the healing of acute wounds. In chronic wounds, moist dressings can relieve pain, promote autolytic debridement, and decrease the frequency of dressing changes.
- Various types of occlusive dressings, as well as skin grafts and skin substitutes, are currently available as dressing options.

DRESSINGS

INTRODUCTION

A dressing is defined as a covering applied to a lesion. This simple definition belies the importance of dressings in wound healing and the complexities of choosing the correct dressing for a particular lesion. At present, there is a myriad of categories, subcategories, and types of dressings with different functions, structural compositions, and physical and chemical characteristics, some common and some very unique.

HISTORICAL PERSPECTIVE

Even during ancient times, the Egyptians had a keen interest in wound healing. They formulated homemade concoctions of lint, grease, and honey as topical therapy for wounds, or would soak strips of bandage material in oils and resins and use them as dressings. They even recommended the use of raw, fresh meat to cover wounds during the first day of healing.[1]

In 1867, the first antiseptic dressings were introduced by Lister who soaked lint and gauze in phenol and then applied them to wounds. In general, before the 20th century, it was believed that wounds healed best when left open (to allow them to breathe) and dry (to keep them 'germ-free') as advocated by Pasteur.[2] This view began to change in 1958 when Odland observed that a blister healed faster when left unbroken.[3] This was further supported by Winter's landmark study on swine in 1962, which showed that superficial wounds kept moist by covering them with a film healed twice as fast as those exposed to the air.[4] Hinman and Maibach repeated Winter's study using humans and found a similar increase in epithelialization rate for occluded wounds.[5]

These studies revolutionized the approach to wound care by demonstrating the importance of moist wound healing. Since then, a multitude of more sophisticated occlusive dressings made of newer materials and agents have been formulated, studied, and become commercially available.

FUNCTIONS OF DRESSINGS

Dressings serve several basic functions (Table 8.1).

Acute wounds vs chronic wounds

Acute wounds

Acute wounds are wounds with no underlying healing defect that proceed to heal in an orderly and timely fashion, passing through well-defined phases of an inflammatory response, granulation tissue formation, and remodeling.[6] In acute wounds, the function of dressings in maintaining a moist environment is critical in facilitating healing. In fact, acute wounds have been shown to heal 40% faster in a moist environment than when air-exposed.[7] The specific effects of a moist environment and occlusion on wound healing are well-established in this wound type.

Table 8.1 Basic functions of wound dressings

Function	Benefit
Cover wound	Protection from trauma and contamination from bacteria and foreign materials Minimize fluid and heat loss
Absorb wound drainage	Keep wound moist, but not wet Minimize maceration
Compression	Increase hemostasis Minimize edema and hematoma formation Prevent dehiscence
Provide moist environment	Facilitate healing of acute wounds Reduce pain in chronic wounds

Enhancement of epithelial migration

Rovee established that in moist wound healing of acute wounds, wound resurfacing occurs more rapidly because keratinocytes begin to migrate sooner, and not because of a higher rate of mitosis.[8]

Stimulation of angiogenesis

Moist wound healing promotes a greater rate of vascularization. The accumulation of angiogenesis-stimulating factors, such as tumor necrosis factor and heparin, under the dressing partly accounts for this.[3] In addition, because hypoxia often stimulates angiogenesis, the dressing establishes a steep oxygen gradient, which stimulates capillary growth toward the more hypoxic center.[9]

Retention of growth factors

Acute wound fluid beneath occlusive dressings has been shown to stimulate proliferation of fibroblasts, keratinocytes, and endothelial cells.[10] The growth factors involved in this were platelet-derived growth factor (PDGF), basic fibroblast growth factor (bFGF), transforming growth factor (TGF)-beta, epidermal growth factor (EGF), and interleukin (IL)-1.[3] PDGF is a powerful mitogenic, chemotactic, and angiogenic factor. EGF is an important player in epidermal cell growth, survival, and differentiation. TGF-beta induces angiogenesis, fibrosis, differentiation, and proliferation.[11]

Facilitation of autolytic debridement

Retained water and proteolytic enzymes interact and achieve painless wound debridement of necrotic tissue.

Protection against exogenous organisms

Although the bacterial count is higher in occlusive dressings than nonocclusive dressings, this does not predispose to infection.[12] Overall infection rate is 2.6% for occlusive dressings versus 7.1% for nonocclusive dressings.[13] As well as acting as a physical barrier, occlusive dressings allow neutrophils to infiltrate easily and function more actively. Occlusion is also associated with the presence of higher levels of lysozymes and globulins.[3] Lastly, occlusion maintains a mildly acidic pH, which is inhibitory to the growth of some bacteria, especially *Pseudomonas* and *Staphylococcus* spp.[14]

Maintenance of voltage gradients

Moist wound healing helps in the maintenance of an electric field, which is essential in keratinocyte migration. Also, an increase in the synthesis of growth factors by human fibroblasts has been demonstrated during in-vitro electrical stimulation.[7]

Chronic wounds

Chronic wounds are wounds in which the normal process of healing has been disrupted at one or more points in the phases of hemostasis, inflammation, proliferation, and remodeling.[6] In this wound type, there is usually an underlying pathology, which produces a delay in the healing process.[15] The effect of occlusion in these wound types is not as well established because there is a dearth of randomized controlled trial data for chronic wounds.

In contrast to acute wound fluid, chronic wound fluid was found to be inhibitory to epithelialization, and to contain degradation products of vitronectin and fibronectin, which inhibit keratinocyte migration.[16] Further, when chronic wound fluid is added to cultures of keratinocytes, fibroblasts, or endothelial cells, it fails to stimulate DNA synthesis directly, contrasting the DNA-synthesizing ability of acute wound fluid.[17,18] Another important biochemical difference in chronic wounds is that they exhibit considerably higher protease activity than acute wounds.[19]

A study on occluded versus nonoccluded venous ulcers showed that the difference in the number of wounds healed at the end of 12 weeks was not statistically significant; however, the rate of healing was more rapid in the occlusive dressing group.[20] For patients with chronic wounds, moisture-retentive dressings do offer the advantages of pain relief, painless wound debridement, containment of wound exudates, reduction in the incidence of complications, and improved quality of life.[3]

■ TYPES OF DRESSINGS

Dressings may be classified based on their clinical functions as well as their physical appearance and composition (Table 8.2).

Nonadherent fabrics

Nonadherent fabrics are derived from a combination of fine mesh gauze and tulle gras, commonly impregnated with chemicals to potentiate the dressing's occlusive or nonadherent characteristics, its ability to facilitate healing, or its antimicrobial properties.[21] They may be subdivided into hydrophobic and hydrophilic types. Hydrophobic fabrics have greater occlusive capability, but hinder fluid drainage through them. These include Vaseline gauze (The Kendall Co, Mansfield, MA), Xeroform (The Kendall Company, Mansfield, MA), and Telfa (The Kendall Co, Mansfield, MA). In contrast, the hydrophilic dressings are less occlusive, but have the ability to readily facilitate the drainage of fluids and exudates into overlying dressings. Examples are Xeroflo (The Kendall Company, Mansfield, MA), Mepitel (Molnlycke Health Care, Gotenberg, Sweden), Adaptic (Johnson & Johnson Medical, Arlington, TX), and N-Terface (Winfield Laboratories, Dallas, TX).

Table 8.2 Types of dressings
Nonadherent fabrics
Absorptive Gauze Foams Alginates
Occlusive/moisture-retentive dressings
Nonbiologic—traditional Foams Films Hydrocolloids Hydrogels Alginates
Nonbiologic—new Hydrofiber dressings Collagen dressings Hyaluronic acid dressings
Biologic—grafts Split-thickness skin grafts (STSG) Full-thickness skin grafts (FTSG) Composite grafts
Biologic/biosynthetic—skin substitutes Cultured epidermal grafts Dermal replacements Composite skin substitutes
Antimicrobial dressings

Absorptive dressings

Gauze is one of the most commonly used absorptive dressings. It is excellent at drawing fluids and exudates away from the wound surface, but loses its efficacy when saturated. It is usually used to cover nonocclusive, nonadhering fabric dressing materials and absorbs discharges, which drain through them. It may also be used, however, over occlusive dressings as a secondary dressing to keep them in place. Wide mesh gauze is usually not placed in direct contact with wounds because it adheres to the surface of the wound, resulting in pain on removal. The only occasions this is done on purpose is when mechanical debridement is desired.[21]

Foam dressings and alginates are classified as both absorptive and occlusive/moisture-retentive dressings.

Occlusive/moisture-retentive

A moist wound environment is provided by a dressing that transmits moisture vapor at a rate lower than that at which a wound loses moisture. This is measured as moisture vapor transmission rate (MVTR) through the dressing when it is left in place for 24 hours. MVTR of intact normal skin is about 200 $g/m^2/day$, while that of wounded skin is 40 times higher. Dressings with an MVTR of less than 35 $g/m^2/hr$ are defined as occlusive or moisture-retentive.[22]

Nonbiologic occlusive dressings

Traditional occlusive dressings are classified into five basic categories (Table 8.3).

Table 8.3 Types and characteristics of occlusive/moisture-retentive wound dressings

Type	Advantages	Disadvantages	Indications	Examples
Foams	Absorbent, conform to body contours	Opaque, require secondary dressing	Partial-thickness wounds, moderately to heavily exudative wounds, pressure relief	Allevyn Flexzan Hydrasorb Lyofoam Vigifoam
Films	Transparent, create bacterial barrier, adhesive without secondary dressing	May adhere to wounds, can cause fluid collection	Donor sites, superficial burns and ulcers, partial-thickness wounds with minimal exudates	Tegaderm Bioclusive Blisterfilm Omniderm Transeal
Hydrocolloids	(+) autolytic debridement, enhance angiogenesis, absorbent, create bacterial and physical barrier	Opaque, gel has unpleasant smell, expensive	Partial- or full-thickness wounds, mildly to moderately exudative wounds, pressure ulcers, venous ulcers, donor sites, acute surgical wounds	Duoderm NuDerm Comfeel Cutinova Replicare
Hydrogels	Semitransparent, soothing, do not adhere to wounds, hydrating	Require secondary dressing, frequent dressing changes	Painful wounds, partial-thickness wounds, wounds after laser, dermabrasion, or chemical peel, donor sites	Vigilon Tegagel Curagel, Clearsite Curafil Elasto-Gel Solosite wound gel 2nd Skin
Alginates	Highly absorbent, hemostatic, do not adhere to wounds, fewer dressing changes	Require secondary dressing, gel has unpleasant smell	Highly exudative wounds, partial- or full-thickness wounds, after surgery	Algiderm Algisite Algisorb Kaltostat Curasorb Polymen SeaSorb Sorbsan

Foams

Foam dressings are composed of hydrophobic, polyurethane foam sheets and are characteristically soft, highly absorbent, and opaque (Fig. 8.1). They are available in varying forms and may be adhesive or nonadhesive, and thick or thin. They have the unique ability of being able to expand to conform to the size and shape of the wound to be dressed.

Some commercially available foam dressings are Allevyn (Smith & Nephew United, Largo, FL), Biopatch (Johnson & Johnson Medical, Arlington, TX), Curafoam (The Kendall Company, Mansfield, MA), Flexzan (Dow B. Hickam, Inc, Sugarland, TX), Hydrasorb (Tyco Health Care/The Kendall Company, Mansfield, MA), Lyofoam (ConvaTec, Princeton, NJ), Mepilex (Molnlycke Health Care, Gotenberg, Sweden), Polymen (Ferris Corp, Burr Ridge, IL), and Vigifoam (Bard, Murray Hill, NJ).

The primary advantages of foam dressings are that they can be used on wounds with unusual configurations and are highly absorptive. Other advantages are that they do not stick to the wound surface and can thus be easily removed for cleaning, and that they may be utilized for pressure relief, such as in cushioning bony prominences.[23]

Because they are opaque, foam dressings allow limited inspection. Their high absorptive properties may also be a disadvantage in that they may dry up the wound bed. Foams often require a secondary dressing.

Foams are used on moderately to heavily exudative wounds as well as infected wounds. Foams themselves may be used as secondary dressings when additional absorption is needed. Because of their dehydrating capabilities, they are not to be used on dry wounds.

Technique

During application, a 2 cm margin is left around the wound edges. The nonadhesive foam is kept in place with tape or gauze rolled around it. Foam dressings are relatively easy to remove. If the dressing has dried up, it has to be soaked first with saline solution before removal to prevent damage to the epithelium.[23]

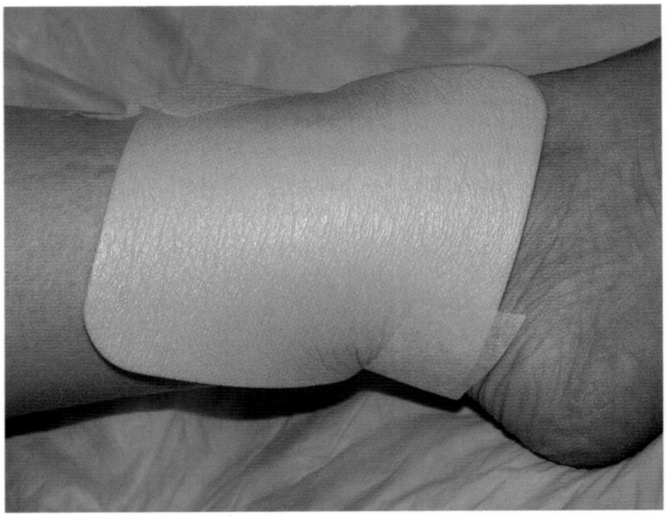

Films

Films are generally made of clear polyurethane membranes with acrylic adhesive on one side for adherence. They are thin, transparent sheets that are permeable to oxygen, carbon dioxide, and water, and impermeable to fluids and bacteria. The specific type of product determines the degree of permeability. Examples are Tegaderm (3M Healthcare, St Paul, MN), Bioclusive (Johnson & Johnson Medical, Arlington, TX), Blisterfilm (The Kendall Company, Mansfield, MA), Omniderm (Omikron Scientific Ltd., Renovot, Israel), Polyskin II (Kendall Healthcare, Mansfield, MA), Proclude (ConvaTec, Princeton, NJ), Mefilm (Molnlycke Health Care, Gotenberg, Sweden), Carrafilm (Carrington Lab, Irving, TX), and Transeal (DeRoyal, Powell, TN).

Because this type of dressing is relatively transparent, it has the distinct advantage of permitting easy visualization of the underlying wound for observation and monitoring purposes (Fig. 8.2). In addition, because they are thin and self-adhesive, they generally do not require a secondary dressing, minimizing their interference with the patient's normal function. This type of dressing can also stay in place for several days and decrease pain.

The biggest disadvantage of film dressings is that because they are nonabsorptive, there is a tendency for fluid to collect under them and eventually leak out. This breaks the antibacterial seal created by the dressing's adhesive and necessitates frequent dressing changes.[21] It also requires intact periwound skin for dressing adherence because there is the possibility that it could adhere to the wound itself, and thereby strip away newly formed epidermis on removal. Minor disadvantages of films are their tendency to wrinkle easily, making them hard to handle, and occasional contact dermatitis from adhesives.

Film dressings are ideally used for mildly exuding wounds, including lacerations, superficial surgical and burn wounds, donor sites, superficial ulcers, and arterial and venous catheter sites. They may also be used as secondary dressings over alginates, foams, and hydrogels. They are not

Figure 8.1 A foam dressing on a lesion medial aspect of the lower leg.

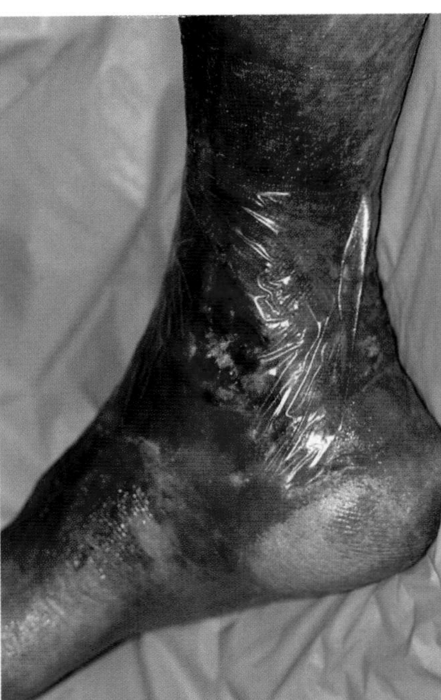

Figure 8.2 A film dressing covering an ulcer on the medial malleolus.

to be used as primary dressings of moderately to heavily exuding or infected wounds, sinus tracts, or cavities. They are also not recommended for patients with fragile skin, such as the elderly.

Technique

The area surrounding the wound should be clean and dry. The recommended margin is 3–4 cm around the wound.[23] The best way to apply the film is to gradually peel off the backing while simultaneously pressing the dressing onto the skin. The uninitiated should be forewarned that the film sticks to latex gloves and to itself very easily.

During removal, film dressings should be peeled off with care. Stretching the film with light pressure disrupts the continuity of the adhesive and makes it easier to remove. The accumulation of a pocket of fluid within the dressing signals that it is time for a dressing change.[23]

Hydrocolloids

Hydrocolloid dressings are a family of dressings containing a hydrocolloid matrix consisting of materials such as gelatin, pectin, and carboxymethylcellulose (Fig. 8.3). They are opaque, absorbent, adhesive waterproof wafers that contain hydrophilic colloidal particles in a hydrophobic polymer. Upon contact with wound exudates, the hydrophilic particles absorb water, swell, and liquefy to form a gel over the wound, which enhances autolytic debridement. Hydrocolloids are impermeable to water vapor, oxygen, and carbon dioxide. They come in preparations of varying thickness and are even available as powders and pastes.

Examples of hydrocolloid dressings are Duoderm (ConvaTec, Princeton, NJ), NuDerm (Johnson & Johnson Medical, Arlington, TX), Comfeel (Coloplast Sween, Inc, Marietta, GA), Hydrocol (Dow Hickman, Sugar Land, TX), Cutinova (Smith & Nephew, Largo, FL), Tegasorb (3M, New York, NY), Replicare (Smith & Nephew United, Largo, FL), and Restore (Hollister, Libertyville, IL).

The advantage of using hydrocolloids is that the autolytic debridement enhances angiogenesis, granulation tissue formation, and healing.[23] Hydrocolloid dressings are slightly bulkier than other dressings such as films, providing more physical protection for the wound. In practical terms, their impermeability to water allows patients to bathe and swim freely.

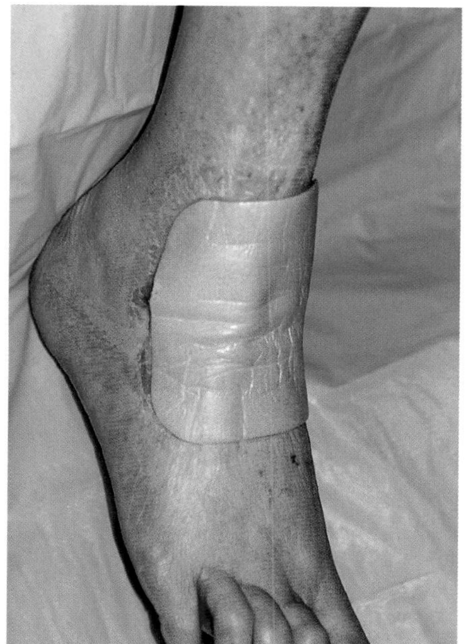

Figure 8.3 A hydrocolloid dressing covering a lesion on the anterior aspect of the ankle.

One of the disadvantages of hydrocolloids is that due to their debriding abilities, they may initially cause the size of the wound to increase. Occasionally the skin surrounding the wound macerates.[24] Hydrocolloids are also associated with the formation of a yellow gel, which has a characteristic unpleasant odor and can be easily confused with infection of the wound.

Indications for the use of hydrocolloids are abrasions, postoperative wounds, pressure and venous ulcers, burn wounds, and donor sites. They are not to be used in third-degree burns or actively infected ulcers.

Technique

The periwound area is cleansed and dried for maximum adherence. Ideally, the dressing is cut extending 2 cm beyond the wound margins. Using scissors to round the corners will minimize rolling up of the hydrocolloid dressing. The backing is peeled off carefully while pressing the pad gently on the skin. The warmth of the hand can be used to help seal the dressing. At the start of treatment, the dressing usually needs to be changed frequently, sometimes daily. However, as the amount of material draining from the wound decreases, the frequency of changing the dressing is likewise decreased, eventually becoming every 3–7 days. Zinc oxide applied to the wound margins can be used to minimize the maceration, irritation, or inflammatory responses of the periwound area.[23]

For removal, hydrocolloids are peeled off the overlying skin with minimal trauma. Remnants of the hydrocolloid left sticking on the intact skin are removed easily using mineral oil. The wound bed is subsequently cleaned with saline to make sure there is no hydrocolloid left on the bed. Patients and caregivers should be advised that removing the dressing prematurely can injure newly formed epidermis.

Hydrogels

Hydrogel dressings consist of a hydrophilic polymer, usually a starch polymer such as polyethylene oxide, and up to 80% water.[21] They are available as gels, sheets, or impregnated gauze, which are absorbent, nonadherent, semitransparent, and semipermeable to water vapor and gases. Their high water content gives them the ability to rehydrate dry wounds, giving them a soothing and cooling effect.[25] Hydrogels also act on necrotic tissue by autolytic debridement, thereby facilitating granulation tissue formation.[23]

Trade names are Vigilon (CR Bard, Murray Hill, NJ), Nu-gel (Johnson & Johnson Medical, Arlington, TX), Tegagel (3M, New York, NY), FlexiGel (Smith & Nephew, Largo, FL), Curagel (The Kendall Company, Mansfield, MA), Flexderm (Dow B. Hickam, Inc, Sugarland, TX), Clearsite (Conmed Corp, Utica, NY), Curafil (The Kendall Company, Mansfield, MA), Curasol (The Kendall Company, Mansfield, MA), Carrasyn (Carrington Laboratories, Irving, TX), Elasto-Gel (SW Technologies, North Kansas City, MO), Hypergel (Scott Health Care, Philadelphia, PA), Normgel (SCA Hygiene Products, Eddy Stone, PA), Solosite wound gel (Smith & Nephew, Largo, FL), 2nd Skin (Spenco Medical, Ltd, Waco, TX), and Transigel (Smith & Nephew, Largo, FL).

Because they are semi-transparent, hydrogels allow some degree of wound inspection. Refrigeration augments their cooling and soothing effects on the wound. As hydrogels are nonadherent, they require a secondary dressing or tape to hold them in place. They also have very little absorptive ability.

Wounds that respond best to hydrogels are dry and mildly exuding wounds, after-procedures such as dermabrasion and chemical peeling wounds, superficial burns, and blisters and ulcers with a necrotic bed. Heavily exuding wounds should not be dressed with hydrogels.

Technique

The hydrogel sheet must first be cut to the appropriate size in relation to the size and configuration of the wound. These sheets are manufactured with a protective covering on both sides. The covering on one side of the sheet is removed to expose the hydrogel (Fig. 8.4), and the exposed side is then placed on the wound. Tape is then used to secure it. The gel form of this type of dressing can be squeezed into the wound cavity. A secondary dressing such as film, foam, or hydrocolloid is used as a protective cover.

To prevent the hydrogel from adhering to the wound bed, the sheets should not be allowed to dry out. They are usually changed every 3 days for necrotic wounds, and every 7 days on granulating wounds.[23] They must be removed very gently to avoid damage to the forming granulation tissue. The gel form is irrigated with saline to facilitate removal.

Alginates

Alginate dressings consist of the soft nonwoven fibers of a cellulose-like polysaccharide derived from the calcium salts of seaweed.[26] They are biodegradable, hydrophilic, non-adherent, and highly absorbent. When the insoluble calcium alginate of this type of dressing comes into contact with wound exudate, a soluble sodium salt is produced, and a hydrophilic gel is formed as a byproduct in the process. Alginates are commercially available as pads (Fig. 8.5), ropes, or ribbons.

Examples are Algiderm (Bard, Murray Hill, NJ), Algisite (Smith & Nephew, Largo, FL), Algisorb (Calgon-Vestal, St Louis, MS), Algosteril (Johnson & Johnson Medical, Arlington, TX), Kaltostat (ConvaTec, Princeton, NJ), Curasorb (The Kendall Company, Mansfield, MA), Carasorb (Carrington Lab, Irving, TX), Dermacea (Sherwood Medical Co, St. Louis, MO), Melgisorb (Molnlycke Health Care, Gotenberg, Sweden), SeaSorb (Coloplast, Holtedam, Denmark), Kalginate (DeRoyal, Powell, TN), and Sorbsan (Dow B. Hickam, Inc, Sugarland, TX).

Because of their exceptional absorptive qualities, alginates are primarily used for heavily exuding wounds.[21] They can also be utilized for deep wounds, sinuses, and cavities. The rope and ribbon forms can be used for packing narrow wounds and sinuses. They are to be avoided in dry or mildly exuding wounds because they may dry out these types of wounds. Their use in deep narrow sinuses is also contraindicated because removal may be difficult.[27]

As well as their absorptive ability, alginates also have hemostatic properties. This sometimes lessens the number of dressing changes needed. Their disadvantages are that the gel formed may be foul-smelling or misleadingly appear purulent, and because they are nonadherent, a secondary dressing is needed.

Technique

Before the application of an alginate dressing, the wound is cleaned with saline and left wet while the surrounding skin is dried. The alginate is applied in a dry condition to the wound surface with a margin of at least 2 mm around the wound edges.[23] When ribbons or ropes are to be used, they are wound in a loose spiral fashion into the wound, doubling back on themselves until the entire wound is covered. A secondary dressing is placed over the dressing.

For removal, the gel formed by the alginate is simply lifted carefully from the wound surface. Irrigation with

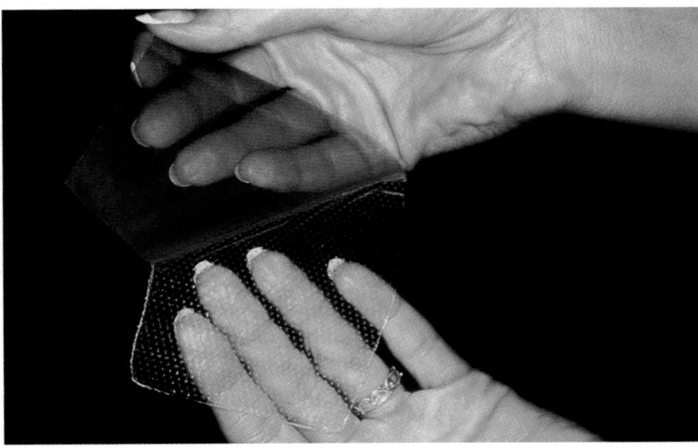

Figure 8.4 A hydrogel dressing being peeled carefully from its backing.

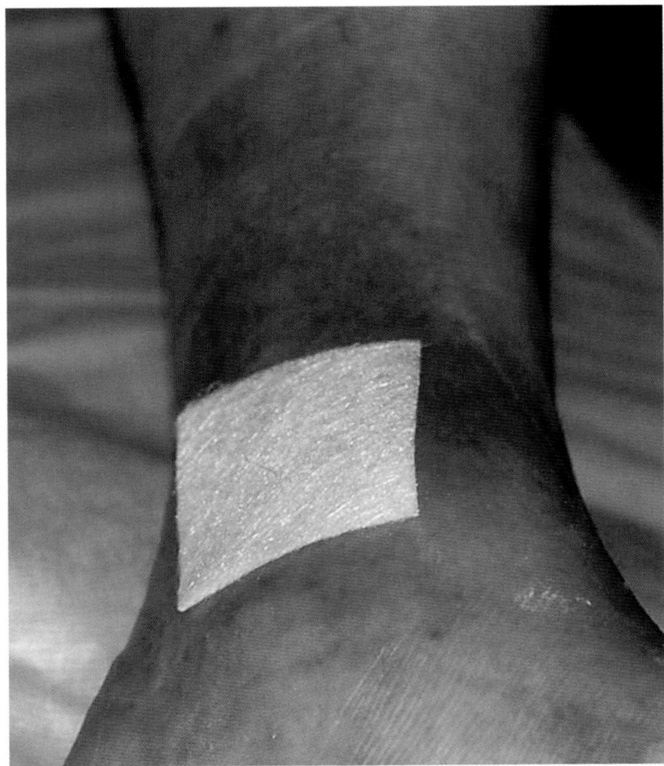

Figure 8.5 An alginate dressing on a lesion on the medial malleolus.

saline solution and the use of forceps after moistening may remove any components of the dressing left behind after lifting.

Hydrofibers

Hydrofiber dressings are composed of soft, absorbent carboxymethyl cellulose fibers that interact with wound exudates to form a soft gel. They are available as nonwoven pads or ribbons under the trade name Aquacel.

They are especially useful for moderately to heavily exuding wounds (Fig. 8.6) and wounds that are prone to bleeding because they are almost three times more absorbent than alginates.[23] They are indicated for abrasions, lacerations, after excision wounds, pressure or leg ulcers, burns, and donor sites. Hydrofiber ribbons may also be used for packing wound cavities.

Technique

Hydrofibers are applied to the wound site and reinforced with a secondary dressing. In removing the dressing, it may be necessary to irrigate the wound with saline solution to remove the gel and prevent stripping of the granulating tissue.

Collagen dressings

Collagen dressings are derived from cowhide and consist of type 1 bovine collagen. They are available as particles, sheets, or gels, and are used for moderately exudative wounds and recalcitrant ulcers.[23] They act by providing a collagen matrix for cellular migration. Examples are Fibracol (Johnson & Johnson, Skillman, NJ), Medifil (Biocore Medical Technologies, Inc, Silver Spring, MD), and Nugel collagen wound gel (Johnson & Johnson Medical, Arlington, TX). They have been known to occasionally cause irritation or increased drainage on initial use.

Technique

First clean the wound, then apply the collagen dressing directly, followed by a secondary dressing. Carefully remove the secondary dressing, then moisten with saline solution.

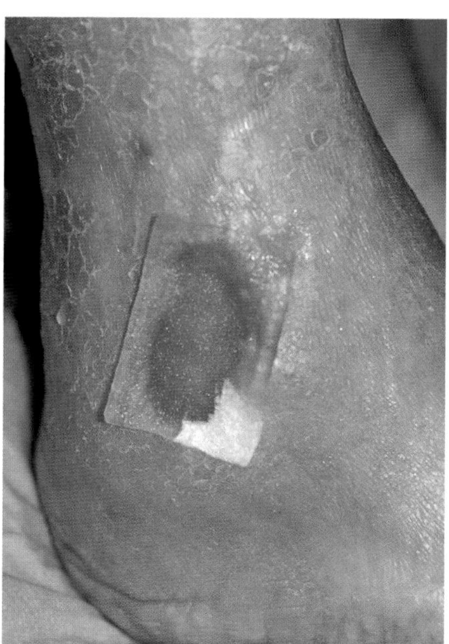

Figure 8.6 A hydrofiber dressing on a moderately exudative lesion on the lateral malleolus.

Hyaluronic acid dressings

Hyaluronic acid dressings are biodegradable, absorbent biopolymers that form a hydrophilic gel with the serum or exudates of the wound. Topical application accelerates granulation tissue formation and re-epithelialization. An example is Hyalofil (ConvaTec, Princeton, NJ).

Biologic/biosynthetic dressings

Grafts

Grafts are pieces of skin that have been separated completely from their local blood supply and transferred to other locations so that they are wholly dependent on the development of a new blood supply from the recipient bed.[28] They may be classified according to the source of donor tissue. A xenograft is a graft transplanted between different species. In humans, the most common xenografts used are derived from pig skin.[21] They are temporary dressings in the sense that they are eventually rejected and replaced by host epithelium.[29]

Autografts are grafts taken from the patient, meaning skin in one area of a patient harvested and transplanted to another area. Allografts are taken from donors of the same species. This could mean cadaveric skin or skin from other living humans. Technological advances have resulted in cultured dermal and epidermal components *in vitro*, which have been used individually or combined as biologic wound dressings, commonly referred to as skin substitutes.

Skin grafts can be categorized based on their thickness or composition. Partial or split-thickness skin grafts (STSGs) contain epidermis and a portion of the dermis while full-thickness skin grafts (FTSG) contain the entire thickness of the epidermis, dermis, and various amounts of subcutaneous tissue.[30] Table 8.4 compares STSGs and FTSGs. Composite grafts are composed of at least two different types of tissues, most frequently skin and cartilage. They are very useful for the repair of full-thickness nasal alar rim defects. (See also Chapter 23.)

Skin substitutes

The quest for developing a widely available product with structural and functional properties as close as possible to those of natural skin continues. Currently, a variety of skin substitutes are available for clinical use and many more are undergoing testing or are pending FDA approval.

Skin substitutes act as a scaffold for tissue regeneration *in vivo*, or as tissue replacement, providing matrix material and cells when grown *in vitro*. They can be temporary or permanent; synthetic, biosynthetic, or biologic.

Based on their components, skin substitutes can be classified into three categories—epidermal grafts, dermal replacements, or composite grafts consisting of both epidermal and dermal components (Table 8.5).

Cultured epidermal grafts

Cultured epidermal autografts Cultured epidermal autografts are grown from the patient's own skin. The technique currently in use for the culturing of epidermal grafts was designed in 1975 by Rheinwald and Green. By serial subculture of human keratinocytes, they were able to grow large epidermal sheets from a small sample in vitro.[32]

Ideally, epidermal cultured autografts need to be sutured or stapled onto the recipient's tissues to prevent separation from the wound bed. At least two other layers of dressings

Table 8.4 Split-thickness versus full-thickness skin grafts

	STSG	FTSG
Composition	Epidermis plus part of the dermis	Epidermis plus dermis plus various amounts of fat
Survival	Greater, because requires less revascularization after transfer	Less chance of survival
Resistance to trauma	Less resistant	More resistant
Cosmetic appearance	Poor cosmetic appearance owing to poor color and texture match; does not prevent contraction	Superior cosmetic appearance; it is thicker, preventing wound contraction or distortion.
Indications	Temporarily or permanently after removal of skin cancer with a high chance of recurrence If a flap is not viable, in areas with limited vascular supply	When aesthetic outcome is essential (e.g. facial defects)
Common uses	Chronic lower leg ulcers (e.g. venous, irradiated tissues; exposed periosteum, cartilage, or tendon) Surgically induced large defects (e.g. for birthmarks, nevi)	Facial defects—nasal tip, dorsum, ala or sidewall, lower eyelid, ear
Donor site tissue	Anteromedial thigh Others—buttock, abdomen, inner or outer aspect of arm, inner forearm	Nearby site, with similar color or texture to skin surrounding the defect (e.g. preauricular and postauricular, supraclavicular, clavicular, neck, nasolabial folds, inner arms)
Disadvantages	Poor cosmetic appearance (e.g. color and texture mismatch, greater chance of distortion or contraction)	Greater risk of failure If not closed primarily, the donor wound site has a prolonged healing time and a greater risk of distortion and hypertrophic scar formation

Adapted from Valencia IC, Falabella AF, Eaglestein WH. Skin grafting. Dermatol Clin 2000; 18:521–532.[28]

Table 8.5 Advantages, disadvantages, and indications for skin substitutes

Type	Advantages	Disadvantages	Indications
EPIDERMAL			
Cultured keratinocyte autograft	Coverage of large area from small skin biopsy Permanent wound coverage Acceptable cosmetic results	3-weeks for graft cultivation Graft fragility, blistering Susceptibility to infection Unstable without dermal substitute Expensive	Burns Leg ulcers
Cultured keratinocyte allografts (Epicel—Genzyme Tissue Repair Co, Cambridge, MA)	No biopsy necessary Immediate availability Cryopreservation and banking	Possibility of disease transmission Expensive Not commercially available	Acute and chronic wounds
DERMAL			
Human cryopreserved allograft skin	Immediate availability Good base for cultured keratinocytes (when de-epidermized)	Temporary coverage Possible disease transmission	Burns
Human allograft skin treated by decellularization, matrix stabilization, and freeze drying (Alloderm)	Immediate availability Immunologically inert Allows ultrathin STSG	Allograft procurement Virus screening	Surgical wounds
Bovine collagen and chondroitin sulfate over silastic (Integra)	Immediate availability Allows ultrathin STSG, less scarring than STSG alone	Susceptibility to infection Complete wound excision before application	Excised burn wounds
Fibroblasts in bioabsorbable mesh (Dermagraft)	Immediate availability	Expensive Multiple applications	Burns (Transcyte) Diabetic foot ulcers (Dermagraft)
COMPOSITE			
Bilayered skin equivalent: bovine collagen, fibroblasts, and keratinocytes (Apligraf)	Immediate availability Easy handling Does not require subsequent skin grafting	Limited viability Expensive	Venous ulcers Diabetic ulcers

Adapted from Bello YM, Phillips TJ. Recent advances in wound healing. JAMA 2000; 283:716-718.[31]

are needed to protect the autograft. A secondary dressing, usually a mesh gauze, is used to cover the graft and is left in place for 7–10 days. Another more outer dressing is then placed over the secondary dressing.[33] This functions to absorb wound exudates, and is changed every or every other day depending on the amount of drainage from the wound.

Cultured keratinocyte autografts were initially used in the 1980s to treat severely burned patients.[34] At present, they are utilized for burns, chronic leg ulcers, epidermolysis bullosa wounds, scar revision, wounds resulting from excision of giant congenital nevi, and vitiligo.[35]

One of the major disadvantages of cultured autografts is that they require a 2–3-week period for growth of an adequate amount of epithelial sheets. Other disadvantages include the difficulty of handling fragile keratinocyte sheets, the lack of a dermal component, and the short-term stability of the graft.

Cultured epidermal allografts For cultured epidermal allografts, the skin is obtained from allogeneic tissue, such as newborn foreskin. Cadaver skin was first used as the source of cultured allografts; however, because of the many problems associated with their use, such as the potential for transmitting disease, limited supply, and variable quality, its use as donor tissue has been reduced.[36–38] Neonatal skin is now the tissue source of choice for cultured epidermal allografts owing to its increased sensitivity and responsiveness to incorporated mitogens, and its own release of growth-stimulating factors and mediators, such as epidermal-derived thymocyte activating factor, interleukins, fibronectin, and TGF-beta.[39]

Cultured allografts were originally thought to act directly as a skin replacement. However, recent studies have shown that allografts are progressively replaced by the patient's own skin. Some investigators suggest that cultured epidermal allografts function by stimulating migration and multiplication of the recipient's keratinocytes,[40] probably by way of growth factors rather than by permanent take of the allograft itself.[41] Others theorize that allografts provide a potent stimulus for wound healing simply by the production of a biologic dressing that prevents dehydration.[42] Although they do not survive permanently on the wound bed, cultured allografts provide efficient pain relief within hours after grafting in addition to their protective functions.

Cultured epidermal allografts have been used to treat donor sites, partial-thickness burns, chronic leg ulcers, epidermolysis bullosa, and wounds resulting from tattoo removal.[28] Many investigators have reported the acceleration of healing of STSG donor sites and partial-thickness burns, resulting in re-epithelialization in 4–7 days.[43]

Cultured epidermal allografts have the significant advantage of avoiding the creation of a donor wound site. In addition, they are readily available, and do not require the 2–3 week growth interval of cultured epidermal autografts.

Cultured epidermal allografts are not commercially available in the US. They are available in only some centers, are expensive, and require a tissue culture facility.

Dermal replacements A variety of products are available as dermal replacements. These are synthetic, biosynthetic, or biological materials with functional or structural similarities to the dermis. The dermis is composed of cellular (fibroblasts) and extracellular components (collagen, matrix proteins) and plays a vital role in the healing of skin by influencing epithelial migration and differentiation, dermoepidermal junction formation, wound contraction, and scar formation.

Skin substitutes functioning as dermal replacements include cadaveric allograft skin, BioBrane (Dow B. Hickam, Inc, Sugarland, TX), EZ Derm (Brennen Medical Inc, St. Paul, MN), Oasis (Cook Inc, Bloomington, IN), Transcyte (Smith and Nephew, Largo, FL), and Dermagraft (Advanced Tissue Sciences Inc, La Joya, CA).

In cadaveric dermal replacements, human cadaver skin is chemically treated to remove its antigenic components, which are usually found as cellular elements. This results in an immunologically inert complex made up of an acellular collagen dermal matrix and an intact basement membrane. This can be used alone or in combination with other grafts or skin substitutes. AlloDerm (Life Cell Co, Woodlands, TX), a human cryopreserved, acellular cadaveric de-epidermalized dermis has been successfully used in combination with STSGs to treat burn wounds and dermal defects, and for periodontal, plastic, and reconstructive surgery.[35]

Biosynthetic dressings were initially introduced for the coverage of burns and donor sites. Biobrane consists of a bilaminate biosynthetic material made up of silicone film and nylon fabric containing porcine collagen peptides as the biological component.[35] When used on donor sites, Biobrane proved superior to Scarlet Red (The Kendall Company, Mansfield, MA) in pain relief, healing time, and absorption of exudates.[44]

Another biosynthetic porcine-derived dermal substitute is EZ Derm in which the porcine collagen is chemically cross-linked using an aldehyde. There are perforated and nonperforated types and it comes attached to a gauze liner, which is detached before grafting. It is used for temporary coverage of partial-thickness skin loss injuries, including burns and ulcers. It has the advantages of immediate availability, a long shelf life, and the absence of human communicable disease.[34] Limited clinical studies have been carried out.

Oasis is a biologic dressing derived from porcine small intestinal submucosa that has been processed to exclude the serosa, smooth muscle, and mucosa layers, producing a collagenous, acellular matrix rich in cytokines and cell adhesion molecules. Because it is packaged dry and then rehydrated, Oasis has the advantage of a longer shelf life than other porcine heterografts. It is also relatively easy to apply and reapply.[35] One of its primary disadvantages is that because it is very thin, it is easily traumatized, so requiring a secondary dressing for additional protection and to prevent it from drying up.

Integra (Integra LifeSciences Corp, Plainsboro, NJ) is a biosynthetic, temporary, bilaminated skin substitute consisting of a matrix of bovine collagen and chondroitin-6-sulfate covered by a synthetic silicone elastomer (Silastic). It is FDA-approved for the treatment of burns. In a 2-year study, Integra was successfully used in the reconstruction of burn scars of the upper extremities, and was shown to be a good alternative for patients with severe burns in whom there is insufficient available skin for a full-thickness skin graft.[45] The dermal component is designed to be slowly biodegradable while the silicone layer is removed and covered with an autograft. This allows for harvesting of thinner epidermal autografts compared to conventional autografts. Thinner autografts enable donor sites to heal faster, allowing earlier reharvesting and less hypertrophic scarring of the donor site.[35] The FDA requires clinicians to complete a company-sponsored training program before using Integra. Its application procedure is complex, and there is an increased susceptibility to infection in comparison to autografts.[35]

Refinements of the matrix concept led to the development of Transcyte (formerly known as Dermagraft-TC). This is a live, metabolically dynamic, immunologically inert human dermis made up of a matrix synthesized by the proliferation of allogeneic human neonatal fibroblasts on a nylon bioabsorbable mesh and an outer silicone polymer layer. The fibroblasts are capable of undergoing cell division and secreting growth factors. Transcyte provides a temporary covering that helps protect the wound from desiccation and contamination. It has been successfully used for temporary wound coverage of partial-thickness burns. It was shown to be superior to silver sulfadiazine in achieving faster re-epithelialization in partial-thickness burns.[46]

Dermagraft evolved as a modified version of Transcyte. It consists of neonatal fibroblasts seeded on a three-dimensional polyglactin bioabsorbable mesh with no outer silicone membrane, so allowing for a single-step procedure (Figs 8.7, 8.8). This skin substitute stimulates the formation of granulation tissue, re-epithelialization, and angiogenesis.[35] The fibroblasts produce fibronectin, glycosaminoglycans, collagens, and growth factors. Dermagraft was designed as a skin substitute for full-thickness wounds. It has the advantages of avoidance of nonhuman tissue, ready availability, less chance of wound contracture and scarring, and mesh absorption in 60–90 days.

In the treatment of chronic diabetic ulcers, Dermagraft was shown to be of significant clinical benefit in achieving wound closure within 12 weeks compared to conventional therapy alone (30 vs 18.3%, P = 0.023).[47] It has also been shown to be more cost-effective,[48] and currently has FDA approval for this indication. Clinical trials are underway to assess its efficacy in the treatment of venous ulcers.

Composite skin substitutes Composite skin substitutes contain both epidermal and dermal components. The first true composite skin equivalent consisting of both epidermal and dermal elements, each with living cells, approved for use by the FDA is Apligraf (Organogenesis, Canton, MA; also known as Graftskin). This is a biosynthetic, bilayered living construct made up of cultured human neonatal foreskin keratinocytes overlying fibroblasts cultured on a dermal matrix of bovine type I collagen (Figs 8.9, 8.10). It is metabolically, morphologically, and biochemically similar to human skin,[28] but lacks appendages, nerves, and blood vessels, and is immunologically inert. Because it lacks macrophages, lymphocytes, and Langerhans' cells,[21] there appears to be no host antibody or cell-mediated response or clinical rejection.

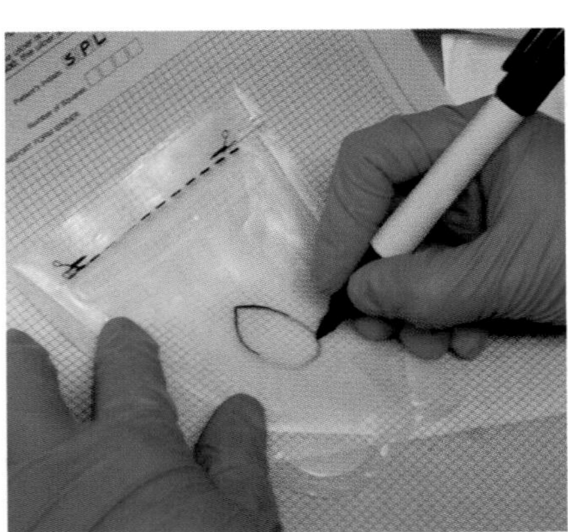

Figure 8.7 Preparation for applying Dermagraft. The configuration of the ulcer is traced on the transparent protective covering of the Dermagraft.

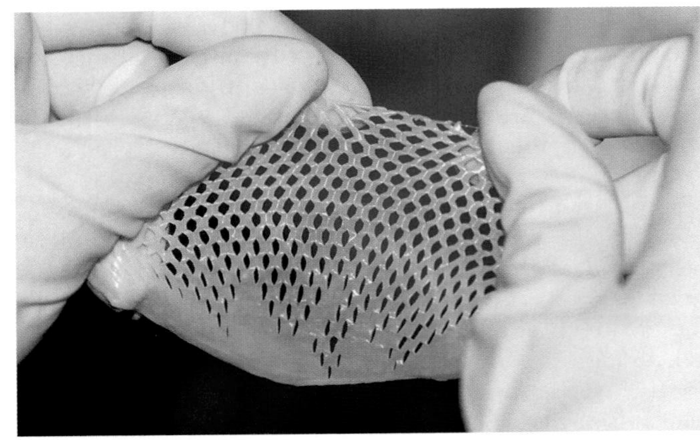

Figure 8.9 The meshed-type Apligraf before application.

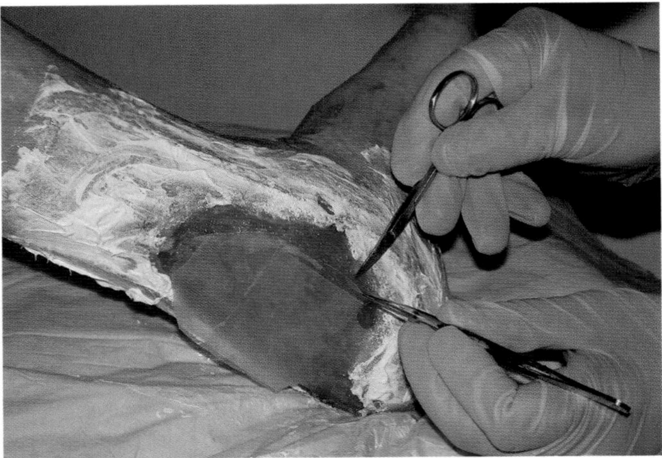

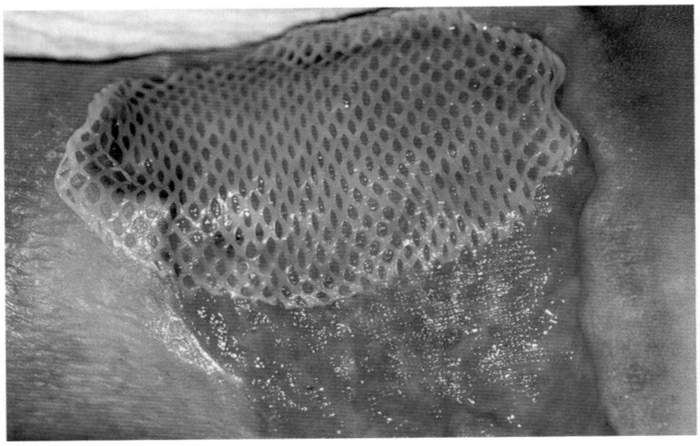

Figure 8.8 Dermagraft being applied to an ulcer.

Figure 8.10 A close-up of the meshed-type Apligraf overlying an ulcer.

Apligraf is a useful adjuvant to standard ulcer therapy for patients with venous leg ulcers or neuropathic diabetic foot ulcers that do not respond to conventional ulcer therapy,[49,50] and is FDA approved for these indications. In a multicenter study of 293 patients with nonhealing venous ulcers, treatment with Apligraf in conjunction with standard compression was shown to be more effective than compression therapy alone in achieving wound closure within 6 months (63 vs 49%; P = 0.02), and to be superior in healing larger (>1000 mm^2, P = 0.02) and deeper ulcers (P = 0.003), and ulcers of more than 6 months' duration (P = 0.001). Median time to complete wound closure was also significantly shortened in the Apligraf-treated group (61 vs 181 days; P = 0.003).[51] In a multicenter study of 208 patients with diabetic foot ulcers comparing Apligraf treatment with saline-moistened gauze (both with standard adjunctive therapy including debridement and foot off-loading), Apligraf resulted in complete wound closure in 56% of patients versus 38% in the control group (P = 0.0042) at the end of 12 weeks. Median closure time was also shorter (65 vs 90 days; P = 0.0026).[52]

Apligraf was a suitable and clinically effective treatment for excised burn wounds when applied over meshed autografts. Furthermore, cosmetic and functional advantages were demonstrated over standard therapy.[53]

Bilayered cellular matrix (BCM) or OrCel (Ortec International Inc, New York, NY) consists of a porous collagen sponge containing cultured keratinocytes and fibroblasts derived from allogeneic cells harvested from neonatal foreskins. This has been FDA approved for use in treatment of split-thickness donor sites of burn patients and patients with recessive dystrophic epidermolysis bullosa. Clinical trials for its use in the treatment of burns, diabetic ulcers, and venous ulcers are underway.

Antimicrobial dressings

Silver-impregnated dressings are becoming popular antimicrobial dressings. They are bactericidal without antibiotics while maintaining a moist environment to facilitate wound healing.[54] Silver has broad-spectrum action on bacteria, including against vancomycin-resistant enterococci and methicillin-resistant *Staphylococcus aureus*. It acts on bacterial cell wall synthesis, ribosome activity, and transcription. It also exhibits activity against fungi and yeast. Commercially available examples of silver-containing dressings include Aquacel Ag (ConvaTec, Princeton, NJ), Contreet (Coloplast Sween, Inc, Marietta, GA), Arglaes (Medline Industries, Mundeline, IL), Acticoat (Smith & Nephew, London, UK), Silveron (Silveron Consumer Products, Mundeline, IL), and AcryDerm Silver (AcryMed, Inc, Portland, OR). In a matched pair randomized study on burns, silver-coated Acticoat dressings resulted in less pain and decreased sepsis compared to the application of silver nitrate.[55]

Cadexomer iodine, a slow-release formulation of iodine, is composed of starch microspheres cross-linked with ether bridges and iodine. It slowly absorbs moisture while releasing iodine in low concentrations, which are antibacterial yet not cytotoxic.[3] Cadexomer iodine provides broad-spectrum antibiotic coverage, and can significantly decrease the bacterial load on the wound surface. It resulted in a significant reduction in *S. aureus* (P < 0.001), beta-hemolytic streptococci, proteus, and klebsiella in a randomized control trial on venous ulcers.[56] Iodosorb, a cadexomer iodine ointment, is antibacterial and an effective debriding agent in pressure, venous, and diabetic ulcers.[57]

■ POSTOPERATIVE CARE AND WOUND CARE

Acute wounds

Postoperative wound management involves caring for patients from the conclusion of their surgical procedure (which may take hours) through the early remodeling phase of the surgical site (which may take weeks to months).[54] The importance of postoperative management in obtaining satisfactory results cannot be overemphasized.

The desired end-result is the most cosmetically acceptable healed wound in the least amount of time.[53] This involves the absence of scarring, infection, and contact dermatitis from topical medications used; and can be achieved by good postoperative care techniques including the proper choice of dressings.

Excisional surgery is one of the most common procedures carried out by dermatologists. After excision, wounds may heal by primary or second intention. In primary intention closure, there is direct apposition of wound edges by suturing. In contrast, in second intention healing, the wound is left open after the surgery and allowed to epithelialize from its edges.[28]

Postexcision wounds healing by primary intention

Wounds sutured closed after excisional surgery, in most instances, do not require special dressings because normal immunity from phagocytes ingesting and killing bacteria is often sufficient to prevent infection.[59] A simple low- or nonadherent gauze dressing secured with tape, or a semipermeable film will usually suffice. For postexcision sites that are still actively bleeding, a thicker more absorbent dressing is needed. Despite the low infection rate, some clinicians still opt to include an antibiotic or aquaphor ointment in the contact layer, if only to make the patient more comfortable.

Wounds healing by primary intention rarely require cleansing.[60] In fact, disturbance of the dressing should be minimized to prevent bacterial contamination as well as removal of re-forming epithelium. When needed, cleansing is usually done with care using saline. Changes of dressing are likewise carried out as needed.

It takes approximately 1 week for sutured wounds to re-epithelialize. The correct time for suture removal depends on several factors, and therefore the practitioner can only follow general guidelines: 4–6 days for the head and neck, 7 days for the upper limbs, 10 days for the trunk and abdomen, and 14 days for the lower limbs.[60] Some problems that may be encountered in sutured wounds are dehiscence, hematoma formation, and suture reactions.[58]

Postexcision wounds healing by second intention

'Shave' or tangential removal of skin is usually performed by dermatologists for biopsy, transverse excision of lesions such as moles, or for Mohs surgery layers.[54] (See also Chapter 48.) It results in an open wound, which is left to heal by second intention and will generally take longer to heal than a sutured wound.

The traditional approach to this type of wound is to apply an ointment followed by two or more layers of dressing. Many dermatologists prefer Polysporin (Pfizer, Inc, New York, NY) or Bacitracin (Fougera and Co, Melville, NY) ointments, and avoid neomycin-containing ointments because of their well-established increased potential for causing contact dermatitis.[61] However, randomized controlled trials have shown that white petrolatum is as safe and effective as Bacitracin with less risk for inducing allergy.[62]

After the ointment layer, the contact layer, which directly touches the wound, is applied. It is usually composed of nonadherent pads such as Telfa and Adaptic, which do not disturb forming granulation tissue. An absorptive layer consisting of gauze pads can be used for draining wounds.

The last layer is the binding or securing layer, which keeps the dressing in place and may also function in compression and immobilization, if needed. Adhesive tape is most commonly used; however, tubular gauze, elastic bandages, and gauze rolls may be added. To increase the holding property of tape, especially when working on a mobile or sebaceous region, the area can be degreased with acetone or alcohol and prepped with liquid adhesive (Mastisol—Ferndale Labs, Ferndale, MI).[63] Hairy areas on which tape is to be applied should be shaved, except for the eyebrows.

The dressing is to be left undisturbed for 48–72 hours after surgery, mainly to reduce the risk of incidental trauma and contamination to the fresh wound.[58] This also allows the patient physical and psychological relief at the time the wounds are most likely to cause pain and discomfort. However, if the dressing becomes soaked with blood or wound exudate before then, a change of dressing is necessary.

At home, gentle cleansing is carried out once or twice a day using soap and water, saline solution, or half-strength hydrogen peroxide. There is some controversy about the use of hydrogen peroxide because it has been shown to have an inhibitory effect on fibroblasts and the microcirculation,[64] and might therefore actually retard healing. However, its effervescence is excellent in removing dried-up debris and crusts on wounds, and the few minutes of contact with it has been deemed more helpful than harmful.[58] Saline is the most commonly used irrigation solution for the removal of inflammatory contents from the wound surface.[57]

In removing the initial dressing, the patient is instructed to wash or wet the dressing first to reduce pain and prevent damage to the granulating wound bed. Cleansing the wounds with normal saline delivered at $8 lb/in^2$ (35-ml syringe and 19-gauge angiocatheter) is usually enough to dislodge debris from the wound bed.[23] A sterile cotton-tipped applicator may also be used to carefully remove debris from more superficial wounds. For deeper wounds, the cleansing solution can be poured over the surface then blotted with sterile gauze. The layered dressing is then reapplied. This is continued until complete re-epithelialization has occurred (several weeks or more for open wounds). Usually, if no complications occur, changes of dressing become less frequent as the wound site gradually re-epithelializes and exudes less fluid.

Another alternative for postexcision wounds is the use of occlusive dressings with or without a secondary dressing. This gives adequate protection from trauma, desiccation, contaminants, and bacteria while providing a moist environment, which facilitates wound re-epithelialization.[21] For the more superficial wounds with minimal exudation, films may be used. For the deeper wounds, hydrogels or hydrocolloids may be used. If the wound is highly exudative, foams and alginates are preferred. There are no hard-and-fast rules about how long this type of dressing should stay on the wound, but it is recommended that the dressing is changed before leakage occurs.

For superficial wounds on the face, one of the more practical options is to simply apply an antibacterial ointment. Its main advantage is that it is a one-step procedure, and interferes minimally with function and appearance.[21] Its main disadvantage is that the ointment can be easily wiped off unintentionally, so providing limited protection and absorption.

Postoperative care in laser resurfacing

After laser resurfacing, there is swelling, pain, burning, and stinging for the first few days. During the first 1–2 days, there is oozing of exudate, with some sloughing of thermally denatured collagen, crusting, and erythema. Bleeding rarely occurs because of the hemostatic action of the laser.[25] During this period, the application of ice packs is recommended to reduce pain, swelling, and discomfort.

Two techniques commonly employed postoperatively are the open and closed techniques (Table 8.6). In the open technique, frequent soaks with dilute acetic acid, saline solution, or cool water are performed to reduce the oozing and crusting. Ointment such as petrolatum or aquaphor is used over the wounded area to protect it and prevent it

Table 8.6 Postoperative care in laser resurfacing

Technique	Advantages	Disadvantages
Closed	Decreased pain Decreased pruritus Less erythema Less crust formation Comfortable Promotes moist healing environment Decreased exudative phase of wound healing Faster re-epithelialization Decreased scarring	Difficult to keep in place on motile areas (perioral) Not tolerated for long period of time (>2 days) Risk of infection if left in place >72 hours Expensive Time consuming Cosmetically unattractive Patient discomfort, claustrophobia
Open	Inexpensive Easy to use Less time consuming for doctors	Hypersensitivity reactions Crusting, desiccation Prolonged erythema Trauma when sleeping (sticking to the pillows) Wound care relies on patient compliance Frequent application of the ointment (every 2 hours) More intense erythema Milia and acne from overuse

Adapted from Lopez AP, Phillips TJ. Wound healing. In: Fitzpatrick RE, Goldman MP, eds. Cosmetic laser surgery. St. Louis: Mosby; 2000.[25]

from drying up. Topical antibiotics are avoided because of their potential for sensitization.[65]

In the closed technique, an occlusive or semiocclusive dressing, such as Flexan (Dow B Hickam, Inc, Sugarland, TX), 2nd Skin, N-Terface, and Omniderm, is used after initially cleansing the resurfaced area. These are generally changed once or twice a day because of the copious exudate.

The disadvantages of the closed technique are difficult visualization and inspection, an increased potential for infection, and patient discomfort. Patients generally do not tolerate having the face covered for more than 48 hours.[25] However, in studies comparing the open and closed technique, the closed technique showed more rapid epithelialization[66] and was associated with less pain. Some authors recommend a combination of the two approaches with the closed technique being used for the first 48 hours, then followed by the open technique.[67]

Uncomplicated partial-thickness and full-thickness wounds

An approach applicable for both partial- and full-thickness wounds is the use of the moisture-retentive occlusive dressings. The moist environment provides the optimal conditions to facilitate healing and relieve pain. The choice of dressing depends on the type of wound and its characteristics.

Options for the treatment of partial- and full-thickness burns are biologic and biosynthetic skin grafts and skin substitutes such as STSGs, FTSGs, cultured epidermal autografts,[34] Alloderm,[35] Integra,[45] Transcyte,[46] and Apligraf.[53]

Chronic wounds

For chronic wounds, it is essential to define and treat the underlying cause. The most common causes such as venous insufficiency, arterial insufficiency, diabetic neuropathy, and pressure necrosis are considered first.[54] When these are ruled out or unlikely, less common causes such as vasculitis, pyoderma gangrenosum, malignancy, and infection are to be taken into account. Determining the etiology of the wound is a key component in deciding how to approach treatment of the wound as well as the underlying condition. Treatment of the most common types of chronic wounds is briefly discussed below.

Venous ulcers

Venous ulcers are the most common form of leg ulcers.[60] The cornerstone of treatment comprises compression, edema reduction, and improvement of venous return. This can be achieved by bed rest, leg elevation, and the use of compression devices, such elastic support stockings, elastic bandages, nonelastic bandages such as Unna's boots, and pneumatic compression pumps.

To improve abnormal venous return, patients are advised to elevate the affected leg 18 cm above the level of the heart or 'toes higher than the nose' for 2–4 hours during the day as well as the night.[68] Before compression is applied to the limb, occlusive arterial disease should be ruled out, and the ulcer base should be clean and uninfected. Compression should be applied on arising from bed and removed at bedtime. The recommended ankle pressure in patients with venous ulcers of the leg is 30–40 mm Hg.[68] The most effective way of delivering compression remains controversial. The advantages and disadvantages of different compression systems are shown in Table 8.7.

Table 8.7 Types of compression therapy

Type	Advantages	Disadvantages
Elastic wrap	Inexpensive, can be reused	Often applied incorrectly by the patient, tends to unravel, does not maintain sustained compression, loses elasticity after washing
Self-adherent wraps	Self-adherent, maintains compression	Expensive, cannot be reused
Unna boot	Comfortable, protects against trauma, full maintenance of ambulatory outpatient status, minimal interference with regular activities, substitute for a failing pump	Pressure changes over time, needs to be applied by trained physician or nurse, does not accommodate highly exudative wounds
Four-layer bandage	Comfortable, can be left in place for 7 days, protects against trauma, maintains a constant pressure for 7 days due to the overlap and elasticity of the bandages, used for highly exudative wounds	Needs to be applied by well-trained physician or nurse
Graduated compression stocking	Reduces the ambulatory venous pressure, increases the venous refilling time, improves calf pump function, different types of stocking accommodate different types of leg, dressings underneath can be changed frequently	Often cannot monitor patient compliance, difficult to put on
Orthotic device	Adjustable compression, sustained pressure, easily put on and removed, comfortable	Expensive, bulky appearance
Compression pump	Augments venous return, improves hemodynamics and microvascular functions, enhances fibrinolytic activity, prevents postoperative thromboembolic complications in high-risk patients	Expensive, requires immobility for a few hours/day

Adapted with permission from Blackwell Publishing Ltd from Phillips TJ. Current approaches to venous ulcers and compression. Dermatol Surg 2001; 27:611–621.[68]

Compression stockings

Some patients find it difficult to put on compression stockings, especially those who are elderly and have arthritis. Some types have silk liners, which allow them to slide onto the leg more easily, while others have a zipper to make them easier to put on and remove.

Compression bandages

Elastic bandages

Various types of elastic bandages are available. One of the more familiar ones is the ACE type, which has the advantage of being reusable. Its primary disadvantage is that because it is not self-adherent, it often unravels. Also if improperly applied by the patient, it does not achieve the correct level of compression.

Compression bandages

Compression bandages should be applied evenly from right above the toes to just below the knee. A useful guide for instructing caregivers about how to apply the appropriate tension to elastic compression bandages is to use a bandage with a rectangle drawn on it—Setopress (Conva Tec Professional Services, Princeton, NJ) or Surepress (ConvaTec, Princeton, NJ). This rectangle turns into a square when the bandage is stretched to the correct tension. It should be applied in a spiral with 50% overlap between turns to produce a double-layer bandaging effect and provide sustained pressures.[68]

Unna boot

The Unna boot is a semirigid paste bandage that is applied by a physician or nurse with the foot at a 90° angle (Fig. 8.11). It should be replaced weekly, or more frequently if heavy drainage is present. Some physicians theorize that the rigid compression is beneficial in that it makes the calf muscles press against the rigid bandage when the patient walks, ensuring the pumping effect of the calf muscles. Other physicians feel that the rigidity is disadvantageous in that the bandage fails to accommodate changing leg volume during fluctuations in edema. The Unna boot can also cause an unpleasant odor, which develops from the wound exudates and has the potential for causing contact dermatitis.

Four-layer bandage

The four-layer compression bandage has been proposed to be the optimal device for achieving compression. It is more flexible and absorbent than the Unna boot, and is capable of maintaining evenly distributed pressure throughout the affected limb for long periods of time. From innermost to outermost, its four layers consist of an orthopedic wool layer, a crepe layer, an elastic layer applied in a figure of eight pattern, and an elastic layer applied in a spiral pattern.

Orthotic device

A legging orthosis with Velcro tape is an adjustable device that can be loosened and tightened as needed to adjust to changes in leg circumference (Fig. 8.12). It is useful in patients who cannot tolerate other compression modalities or who require frequent dressing changes.

Pneumatic compression

For patients who are unresponsive to conventional compression bandages or stockings, home compression pumps may be used. They were developed for the prophylaxis of deep venous thrombosis, and should be considered when a venous ulcer does not respond to standard compression therapy. They can be rented or bought for outpatient use. They are contraindicated in patients with uncontrolled congestive heart failure, during episodes of inflammatory phlebitis, or when increased venous or lymphatic return is undesirable.

Wound dressings

Moisture retentive dressings combined with compression therapy may produce more rapid healing rates initially, but long-term follow-up has failed to demonstrate any statistically significant advantage over compression therapy alone.[20] However, these dressings are beneficial in that they relieve pain, reduce the infection rate, and enhance autolytic debridement and granulation tissue formation.[69]

Larger venous ulcers may require the use of skin grafts or skin substitutes. Meshing of STSGs is helpful for venous ulcers because it allows drainage of wound fluid without disturbing the adherence of the graft to the wound bed. Another treatment option for persistent venous ulcers is

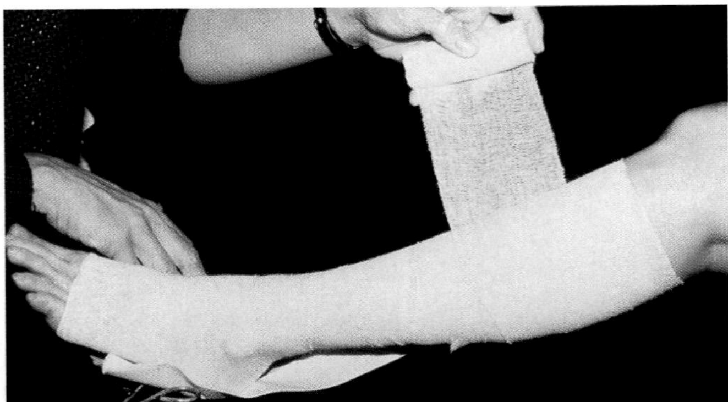

Figure 8.11 Unna Boot application. The boot is applied with the foot at a 90° angle, starting just above the toes, in a figure-of-eight manner around the ankle, and up to the knee in a spiral fashion with 50% overlap. A layer of self-adherent elastic bandage is frequently wrapped around it.

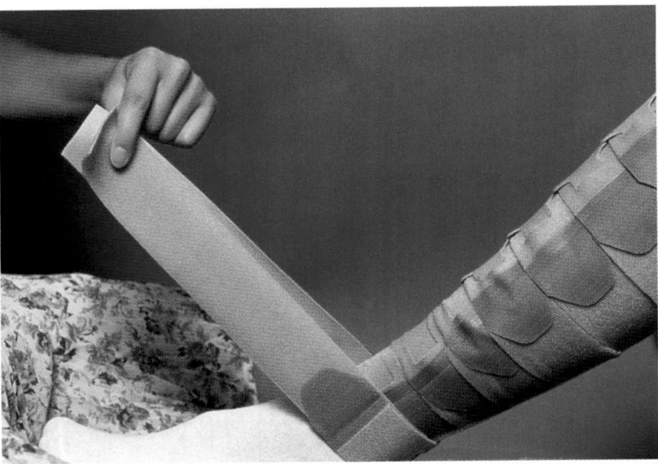

Figure 8.12 A legging orthosis using Velcro tape.

shave therapy. This involves the excision of ulcers with the surrounding lipodermatosclerotic tissue and covering the wounds with meshed split skin grafts. Healing rates of 79% of 59 patients after 3 months, and 88% of 18 patients after an average of 2 years after shave therapy were observed.[70]

Apligraf is FDA-approved for the treatment of venous ulcers, and in combination with compression therapy has been shown to be significantly better at healing ulcers secondary to venous insufficiency compared to compression alone. It is especially helpful in treating venous ulcers of greater than 6 months duration.[50]

Arterial ulcers

Management of arterial ulcers requires surgical re-establishment of an adequate vascular supply whenever possible. Diabetes mellitus, cigarette smoking, hypertension, and hyperlipidemia should be controlled. Moderate exercise may promote development of collateral circulation, and elevation of the head of the bed 10–15 cm (4–6 in) improves gravity-dependent arterial flow.[71] Limbs should be kept warm. Patients should observe good foot care. General principles for proper wound care as well as choice of dressings are observed for arterial ulcers.

Diabetic foot ulcers

Good diabetic foot ulcer care starts with a thorough assessment of the ulcer, including determining whether neuropathy or peripheral vascular disease is present. The principles of good wound care include use of proper footwear and the correct antibiotics when needed, avoidance of weightbearing, pressure-relieving aids, debridement as necessary, aggressive revascularization, and control of the serum glucose levels.[72]

There is a remarkable lack of consensus over dressing choice for the diabetic foot ulcer.[73] The principle of moist healing does still apply, but it has been questioned whether this philosophy applies to all diabetic wounds.[74] The ideal dressing should protect the wound space from secondary contamination, maintain a moist environment, remove exudates, be able to be removed without trauma to the wound, and resist the stresses of standing and walking.

Topical antibiotics keep the surface bacterial colony count low while providing a moist environment in which healing may occur. Saline-moistened gauze also provides a moist wound environment. Occlusive dressings such as hydrogels, hydrocolloids, and polymers play a big role in the treatment of diabetic ulcers.[72] In addition to the traditional occlusive dressings, the latest state-of-the-art biosynthetic dressings Dermagraft[47] and Apligraf[50] have likewise been shown to be effective in the treatment of these ulcers, and have been approved for this use by the FDA. Bilayered Cellular Matrix (BCM; Ortec International Inc, New York, NY) has also shown promise in the treatment of diabetic ulcers, but is not yet FDA approved for this indication.[75]

The total contact cast is commonly used in the US, but requires skilled application and close follow-up.[73]

Pressure ulcers

The most important aspect of treatment of pressure ulcers is tissue load management.[76] This refers to specific interventions designed to decrease the magnitude of pressure, friction, and shear on the tissue. The goal is to create an environment that enhances soft tissue viability and promotes healing of the pressure ulcers, and can be met through vigilant use of proper positioning techniques and support surfaces, whether the individual is in bed or sitting on a chair.[76]

Management also involves addressing factors such as nutrition, immobility, and comorbid disease, and protection from fecal or urine soiling.[77] Nutrition is very important in preventing and healing pressure ulcers, especially an adequate protein content in the diet. Incontinence contributes significantly to the development of pressure sores because constant exposure of skin to urine and stool leads to maceration, weakening of the tissue, and eventual breakdown. Containment devices and skin-protective barriers are useful in counteracting moisture from incontinence.

Wound care of the pressure ulcer involves debridement of devitalized tissue, wound cleansing, application of dressings, and possible adjunctive therapy with electrical stimulation for Stage III and IV unresponsive ulcers. These are full-thickness ulcers that may extend to the subcutaneous tissue (Stage III) or to muscle and bone (Stage IV).[76] Normal saline is the preferred cleansing agent. In the selection of dressings, the cardinal rule is to choose a dressing that will keep the ulcer tissue moist and the surrounding intact skin dry.[76] Studies comparing different types of moist wound dressings showed no differences in pressure ulcer healing outcomes;[76] however, sequential dressing therapy using alginates followed by hydrocolloids showed significantly faster healing ($P < 0.001$) in Stage III and IV ulcers compared to hydrocolloid alone.[78] Foams or wound fillers may be adjunctively used to eliminate dead space in deep ulcers.[77] Dressings applied near the anus should be given special attention because they are difficult to keep intact. Picture-framing or taping the edges of the dressing may reduce this problem.[76]

PITFALLS AND THEIR MANAGEMENT

It is always easier to avoid complications than to treat them.

Pitfalls in postoperative care and the use of dressings and their management

- Infection—use topical and systemic antibiotics as needed, practice clean or aseptic techniques for dressing wounds, irrigate under pressure or debride to remove necrotic tissue (Fig. 8.16).
- Contact dermatitis (Fig. 8.17)—switch to another type of dressing, adhesive, or topical ointment or antibiotic, apply zinc oxide or other lubricating protectants to periwound area, apply low-potency topical corticosteroids.
- Seroma formation—aspirate with a large-bore needle, puncture with a lancet.
- Excessive pressure from dressing—loosen dressing.
- Excessive granulation tissue—apply pressure, change dressing type, pare with curette, cautery with silver nitrate.
- Pigmentary alteration—may be left alone (improves with time).
- Milia or suture granuloma—usually resolve spontaneously, may be left alone.

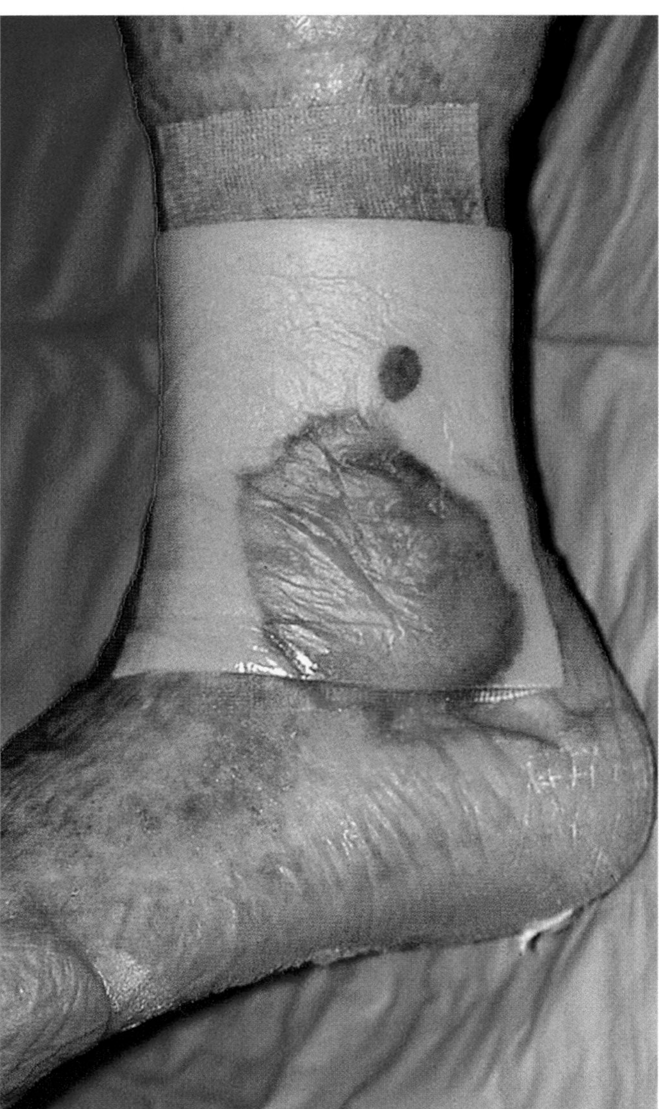

Figure 8.13 Leakage through a foam dressing applied on the ankle occurs because of an inadequate inferior margin.

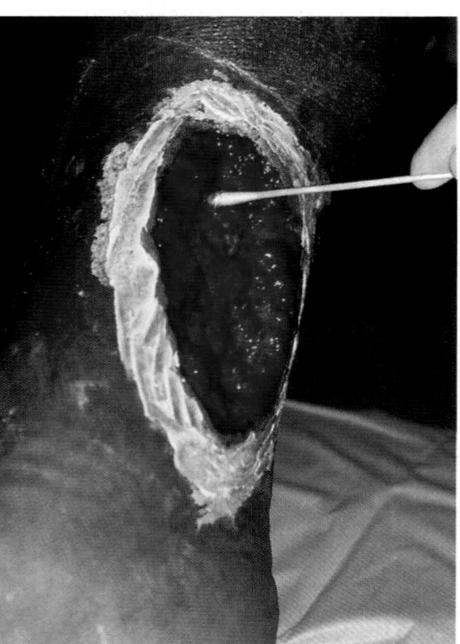

Figure 8.14 Zinc oxide paste is applied on the periwound area to function as a protectant and minimize maceration.

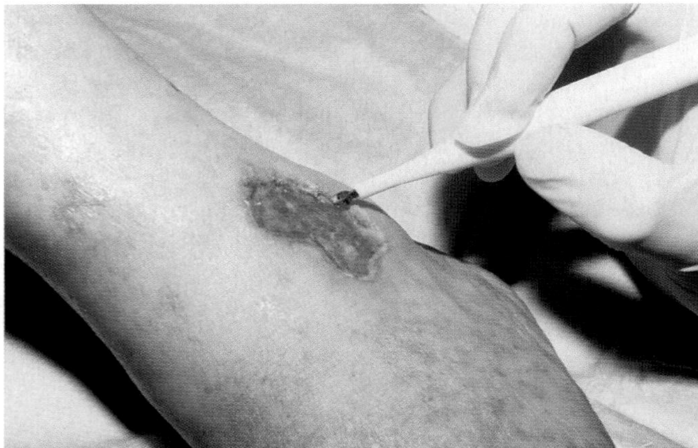

Figure 8.15 Surgical debridement using a curette to remove necrotic tissue and debris from the ulcer bed.

OPTIMIZING OUTCOMES

Ways to optimize results in wound care

- Avoid leakage—provide adequate margins of dressing around wound edges (Fig. 8.13), vary frequency of dressing changes as needed, increase thickness of absorptive layer, select proper dressing (e.g. alginates and foams for heavily exuding wounds).
- Control pain—avoid trauma to site, use moisture-retentive dressings (especially hydrogels), oral analgesics (e.g. acetaminophen), apply EMLA (Astra-Zeneca Pharmaceuticals, Wilmington, DE) for 30–45 minutes before debridement.
- Prevent maceration—apply zinc oxide paste on the periwound area (Fig. 8.14), do not leave on dressings for prolonged periods of time.
- Minimize odor—apply Metrogel (Galderma Laboratories, Inc, Fort Worth, TX), use odor-absorbing dressings—e.g. Actisorb Plus (Johnson & Johnson Medical, Arlington, TX), Lyofoam C (ConvaTec, Princeton, NJ), Carboflex (ConvaTec, Princeton, NJ).
- Remove necrotic tissue—perform debridement: mechanical (Fig. 8.15), autolytic, enzymatic, or biologic; irrigate under pressure during cleansing.
- Ensure patient compliance—instruct the patient and caregiver thoroughly, regular follow-up visits.
- Check intrinsic factors—address any underlying systemic conditions (e.g. venous or arterial disease, hypertension, psychological stress, debility, immunocompromised state), ensure proper nutrition (especially protein).
- Keep wound moist, but not wet—use dressings of appropriate absorbency (e.g. alginates for highly exuding wounds).

PRACTICAL APPLICATIONS

In general, once the underlying cause of a wound has been addressed along with any conditions that may impair healing, wounds have relatively straightforward requirements. Specific needs may be determined by the physical characteristics of the wound including its size, shape, location, depth, phase of healing, tissue type and quantity, condition of the skin surrounding it, and bacterial and

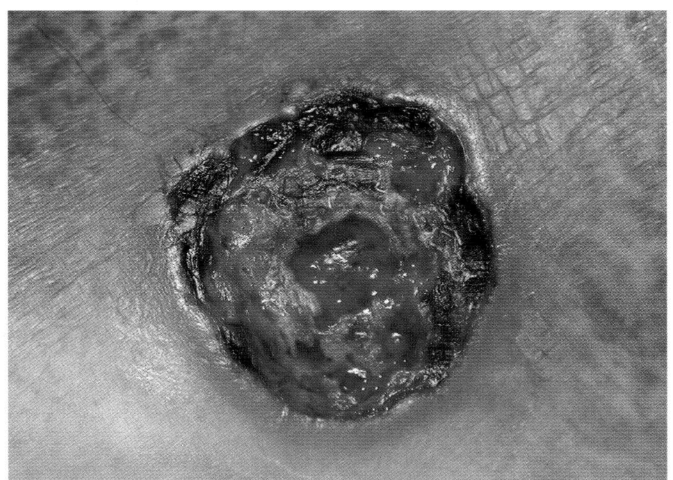

Figure 8.16 Necrotic tissue such as eschar is an optimal substrate for microbial growth which may lead to local and systemic infection.

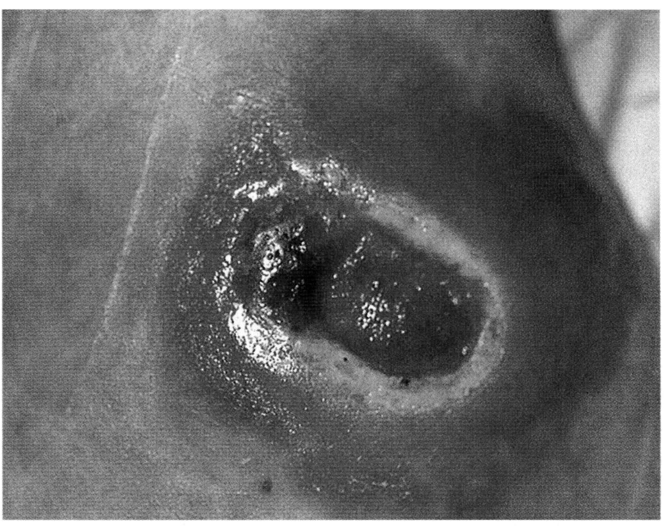

Figure 8.17 Typical appearance of contact dermatitis on the periwound area. Note the erythema.

Table 8.8 Dressing materials and relative performance

Dressing material	Absorption level	Adhesive quality	Conformability	Hydration/ debridement ability	Odor control ability	Clinical applications
Film	None	Fully adhesive	Conformable to surface anatomy	Will hydrate slowly	None	Superficial, lightly exuding wounds, as a secondary dressing
Hydrogel	Low	Nonadhesive or adhesive borders	Conformable to surface anatomy	Will hydrate moderately	None	Superficial, light to moderately exuding wounds, painful wounds
Hydrocolloid	Low to moderate	Fully adhesive surface	Conformable to surface anatomy	Will hydrate moderately to quickly depending on water content	May exacerbate odor (without ill effect)	Superficial light to moderately exuding wounds
Foam	High	Nonadhesive, fully adhesive surface, adhesive borders	Some versions conformable to cavities	Not hydrating	Slight, due to absorption only, some versions contain charcoal for active control	Superficial to deep, moderately to heavily exuding wounds
Alginate	High	Nonadhesive	Conformable to cavities	Not hydrating	Anecdotal evidence for minor effect, charcoal version exists	Superficial to deep, moderately to highly exuding wounds
Contact layer	None	Nonadhesive	Conformable to surface anatomy	Slightly hydrating, depending on cover dressing	None	Superficial wounds of any exudate level

Adapted from Ovington LG. Wound dressings: their evolution and use. In: Falanga V, ed. Cutaneous wound healing. London: Martin Dunitz Ltd; 2001.[79]

exudate levels. Dressing functions to be considered are absorptive capacity, hydrating capacity, adhesive quality, debriding capabilities, conformability, and odor control ability (Table 8.8).[79]

No single dressing can provide all things to all wounds, especially because most wounds have a variety of needs. This leaves clinicians to weigh the pros and cons of possible dressing choices, and to make the decision about which they think is the most appropriate. As the patient's wound progresses, several different categories of dressing may be necessary during the wound-healing process to address the changing wound parameters.

Cost versus cost-effectiveness

A prevalent misconception is that the use of occlusive dressings is too costly in comparison to traditional materials like gauze. However, the cost of wound care is not simply the cost of the dressing material, but the labor cost (especially if a healthcare professional is required), the indirect costs of ancillary supplies (e.g. gloves, biohazardous waste disposal), and the duration of care.[79] Some studies have shown that a more expensive dressing that requires less frequent changes is actually less expensive to use than a cheaper dressing that requires more frequent changes.[79] Not only do occlusive dressings require fewer changes, they also shorten the healing time and provide superior protection, so shortening the total duration of treatment and reducing expenses from possible complications such as infection.

■ SUMMARY

This chapter presents an extensive discussion of the different types of dressings currently available, including their advantages, disadvantages, and indications. From simple gauze dressings, advances in technology have led to the development of complex biosynthetic dressings, which closely approximate the structure and function of natural skin. From the belief that wounds heal best when kept dry and exposed to air, it has been established that acute wounds undoubtedly heal best in a moist environment and why.

This chapter also reviews the technical aspects for applying some types of dressings as well as specific dressings for venous ulcers and techniques for postlaser resurfacing care. The importance of postoperative care cannot be stressed enough. It may make the difference between patient and doctor satisfaction and dissatisfaction. Once the surgical procedure is completed, a careful selection of dressings, close monitoring of the phases of healing, and prompt and correct management of complications all come into play. It is useful to remember that postoperative complications are always easier to prevent than to treat.

■ REFERENCES

1. Majino G. The healing hand: man and wound in the ancient world. Cambridge, MA: Harvard University Press; 1975.
2. Bradley M, Cullum N, Nelson EA, et al. Systemic reviews of wound care management: (2) Dressings and topical agents used in the healing of chronic wounds. Health Technol Assess 1999; 3:1–18.
3. Choucair MM, Bello YM, Phillips TJ. Wound dressings. In: Freedberg IM, Eisen AZ, Wolff K, et al, eds. Fitzpatrick's dermatology in general medicine, 6th edn. New York: McGraw-Hill; 2003.
4. Winter, GD. Formation of scab and the rate of epithelialization of superficial wounds in the skin of the young domestic pig. Nature 1962; 193:293–294.
5. Hinman CD, Maibach HI. Effect of air exposure and occlusion on experimental human skin wounds. Nature 1963; 200:377–378.
6. Lazarus GS, Cooper DM, Knighton DR, et al. Definitions and guidelines for assessment of wounds and evaluation of healing. Wound Rep Reg 1994; 2:165–170.
7. Eaglstein WH. Experiences with biosynthetic dressings. J Am Acad Dermatol 1985; 12:434–440.
8. Rovee DT. Effect of local wound environment of epidermal healing. In: Maibach HI, Rovee DT, eds. Epidermal wound healing. Chicago: Mosby; 1972.
9. Field CK, Kerstein MD. Overview of wound healing in a moist environment. Am J Surg 1994; 167:2S–6S.
10. Katz M, Alvarez A, Krisner R, et al. Human fluid from acute wounds stimulates fibroblast and endothelial cell growth. J Am Acad Dermatol 1991; 25:1054–1058.
11. Falanga V, Shen J. Growth factors, signal transduction and cellular responses. In: Falanga V, ed. Cutaneous wound healing. London: Martin Dunitz Ltd; 2001.
12. Hutchinson, JJ, McGuckin M. Occlusive dressings: a microbiologic and clinical review. Am J Infect Control 1990; 18:257–268.
13. Hutchinson JJ. Prevalence of wound infection under occlusive dressings: a collective survey of reported research. Wounds 1989; 1:123–133.
14. Lilly HA. *Pseudomonas aeruginosa* under occlusive dressings. In: Alexander JW, Thomson PD, Hutchinson JJ, eds. International forum on wound microbiology, Barcelona, Spain. London: Excerpta Medica; 1990.
15. Eaglstein WH, Falanga V. Chronic wounds. Surg Clin North Am 1997; 77:689–700.
16. Grinnell F, Ho CH, Wysocki A. Degradation of fibronectin and vitronectin in chronic wound fluid: analysis by cell blotting, immunoblotting, and cell adhesion assays. J Invest Dermatol 1992; 98:410–416.
17. Harris IR, Yee KC, Walters CE, et al. Cytokine and protease levels in healing and non-healing chronic venous leg ulcers. Exp Dermatol 1995; 4:342–349.
18. Bucalo B, Eaglestein WH, Falanga V. Inhibition of cell proliferation by chronic wound fluid. Wound Repair Regen 1993; 1:181–186.
19. Enoch S, Harding K. Wound bed preparation: the science behind the removal of barriers to healing. Wounds 2003; 15:213–229.
20. Cordts PR, Hanrahan LM, Rodriguez AA, et al. A prospective, randomized trial of Unna's boot versus DuoDERM CGF hydroactive dressing plus compression in the management of venous leg ulcers. J Vasc Surg 1992; 15:480–486.
21. Lionelli GT, Lawrence WT. Wound dressings. Surg Clin North Am 2003; 83:639–658.
22. Bolton L, Pirone L, Chen J, et al. Dressings' effects of wound healing. Wounds 1990; 2:126–134.
23. Bello YM, Phillips TJ. The practical aspects of dressing therapy. Dermatol Therapy 1999; 9:69–77.
24. Phillips TJ, Dover JS. Leg ulcers. J Am Acad Dermatol 1991; 25:965–987.
25. Lopez AP, Phillips TJ. Wound healing. In: Fitzpatrick RE, Goldman MP, eds. Cosmetic laser surgery. St. Louis: Mosby; 2000.
26. Piacquadio D, Nelson DB. Alginates: a 'new' dressing alternative. J Dermatol Surg Oncol 1992; 18:990–998
27. Choucair M, Phillips TJ. A review of wound healing and dressing materials. Wounds 1996; 8:165–172.
28. Valencia IC, Falabella AF, Eaglestein WH. Skin grafting. Dermatol Clin 2000; 18:521–532
29. Eaglestein WH, Falanga V. Tissue engineering and the development of Apligraf, a human skin equivalent. Cutis 1998; 62S:1–8.
30. Johnson TM, Ratner D, Nelson BR. Soft tissue reconstruction with skin grafting. J Am Acad Dermatolol 1992; 27:151–165.
31. Bello YM, Phillips TJ. Recent advances in wound healing. JAMA 2000; 283:716–718.
32. Rheinwald JG, Green H. Serial cultivation of strains of human epidermal keratinocytes: The formation of keratinizing colonies from single cells. Cell 1975; 6:331–334.
33. Ongenae KC, Phillips TJ. Cultured epidermal grafts. In: Robinson JK, Arndt KA, LeBoit PE, et al, eds. Atlas of cutaneous surgery. Philadelphia: WB Saunders; 1996.
34. O'Conner NE, Mulliken JB, Banks-Schlegel S, et al. Grafting of burns with cultured epithelium prepared from autologous epidermal cells. Lancet 1981; 1:75–78.
35. Bello YM, Falabella AF. Use of skin substitutes in dermatology. Dermatol Clin 2001; 19:555–561.
36. May SR, DeClement FA. Skin banking: Part I. Procurement of transplantable cadaveric allograft skin for burn wound coverage. J Burn Care Rehabil 1981; 2:7–23.
37. May SR, DeClement FA. Skin banking: Part II. Low contamination of cadaveric dermal allograft for temporary burn-wound coverage. J Burn Care Rehabil 1981; 2:64–76.
38. May SR, DeClement FA. Skin banking: Part III. Cadaveric allograft skin viability. J Burn Care Rehabil 1981; 2:128–141.
39. Hefton JM, Amberson JB, Biozes DG, et al. Loss of HLA-DR expression of human epidermal cells after growth in culture. J Invest Dermatol 1984; 83:48–50.
40. Leigh, IM, Purkis P, Navsaria H, et al. Treatment of chronic venous ulcers with sheets of cultured allogeneic keratinocytes. Br J Dermatol 1987; 117:591–597.
41. Kirsner RS, Falanga V, Kerdel FA, et al. Skin grafts as pharmacological agents: pre-wounding of the the donor site. Br J Dermatol 1996; 135:292–296.

42. Phillips, TJ. Cultured skin grafts: Past, present and future. Arch Dermatol 1988; 124:1035–1038.
43. Madden JR, Finkelstein JL, Staiano-Coco L, et al. Grafting of cultured allogeneic epidermis on second and third degree burn wounds in 26 patients. J Trauma 1986; 26:955–960.
44. Zapata-Sirvent R, Hansborough JF, Carroll W, et al. Comparison of Biobrane and Scarlet Red dressings for treatment of donor site wounds. Arch Surg 1985; 120:743–745.
45. Chou TD, Chen SL, et al. Reconstruction of burn scar of the upper extremities with artificial skin. Plast Reconstr Surg 2001; 108:378–384.
46. Noordenbos J, Dore C, Hansborough JF. Safety and efficacy of TransCyte for the treatment of partial-thickness burns. J Burn Care Rehabil 1999; 20:275–278.
47. Marston WA, Hanft J, Norwood P, et al. The efficacy and safety of Dermagraft in improving healing of chronic diabetic foot ulcers: results of prospective trial. Diabetes Care 2003; 26:1701–1705.
48. Allenet B, Paree F, Lebrun, et al. Cost-effectiveness modeling of Dermagraft for the treatment of diabetic foot ulcers in the French context. Diabetes Metab 2000; 26:125–132.
49. Falanga V, Margolis D, Alvarez O, et al. Randomized trial comparing cryopreserved cultured epidermal allografts with hydrocolloid dressings in healing chronic venous ulcers. J Am Acad Dermatol 1993; 29:982–988
50. Curran MP, Plosder GL. Bilayered bioengineered skin substitute (Apligraf): a review of its use in the treatment of venous leg ulcers and diabetic foot ulcers. BioDrugs 2002; 16:439–455
51. Falanga V, Margolis D, Alvarez O, et al. Rapid healing of venous ulcers and lack of clinical rejection with an allogeneic cultured human skin equivalent. Arch Dermatol 1998; 134:293–300.
52. Veves A, Falanga V, Armstrong DG, et al. Graftskin, a human skin equivalent, is effective in the management of noninfected neuropathic diabetic foot ulcers: a prospective randomized multicenter clinical trial. Diabetes Care 2001; 24:290–295.
53. Waymack, P, Duff RG, Sabolinski M. The effect of a tissue engineered bilayered living skin analog, over meshed split-thickness autografts on the healing of excised burn wounds. The Apligraf Burn Study Group. Burns 2000; 26:609–619.
54. Mostow EN. Wound healing: a multidisciplinary approach for dermatologists. Dermatol Clin 2003; 21:371–387.
55. Tredget EE, Shankowsky HA, Groeneveld A, et al. A matched-pair randomized study evaluating the efficacy and safety of Acticoat silver-coated dressings for the treatment of burn wounds. J Burn Care Rehab 1998; 19:531–537.
56. Skog E, Arnesjo B, Troeng T, et al. A randomized trial comparing cadexomer iodine and standard treatment in the out-patient management of chronic venous ulcers. Br J Dermatol 1983; 109:77–83
57. Browne A, Dow G, Sibbald RG. Infected wounds: definitions and controversies. In: Falanga V, ed. Cutaneous wound healing. London: Martin Dunitz Ltd; 2001.
58. Arpey CJ, Whitaker DC. Postsurgical wound management. Dermatol Clin 2001; 19:787–797.
59. Cho M, Hung TK. The overall clinical approach to wounds. In: Falanga V, ed. Cutaneous wound healing. London: Martin Dunitz Ltd; 2001.
60. Dibyeshwar B, Jones V, Harding KG. The overall clinical approach to chronic wounds. In: Falanga V, ed. Cutaneous wound healing. London: Martin Dunitz Ltd; 2001.
61. Kaye ET. Topical antibacterial agents. Infect Dis Clin N Am 2000; 14:321–339.
62. Smack DP, Harrington AC, Dunn C, et al. Infection and allergy incidence in ambulatory surgery patients using white petrolatum vs bacitracin ointment. A randomized controlled trial. JAMA 1996; 276:972–977.
63. Grabski WJ, Giandoni MB. Surgical wound dressing. In: Robinson JK, Arndt KA, LeBoit PE, Wintroub BU, eds. Atlas of cutaneous surgery. Philadelphia: WB Saunders; 1996.
64. Vessey NK, Lee KH, Blacker KL. Characterization of the oxidative stress initiated in cultured human keratinocytes by treatment with peroxides. J Invest Dermatol 1992; 99:859–863.
65. Gette MT, Marks JG Jr, Maloney ME. Frequency of postoperative allergic contact dermatitis to topical antibiotics. Arch Dermatol 1992; 128:365–367.
66. Collawn SS. Occlusion following laser resurfacing promotes reepithelialization and wound healing. Plast Reconstr Surg 2000; 105:2180–2189.
67. Newman PJ, Koch J, Goode R. Closed dressings after laser skin resurfacing. Arch Otorhinolaryngol 1998; 124:751–757.
68. Phillips TJ. Current approaches to venous ulcers and compression. Dermatol Surg 2001; 27:611–621
69. Rojas AI, Phillips TJ. Venous ulcers and their management. In: Falanga V, ed. Cutaneous wound healing. London: Martin Dunitz Ltd; 2001.
70. Schmeller W, Gaber Y, Gehl HB. Shave therapy is a simple, effective treatment for persistent venous ulcers. J Am Acad Dermatol 1998: 39:232–238.
71. Phillips TJ. Successful methods of treating leg ulcers. Postgrad Med 1999; 105:159–180
72. Steed DL. Foundations of good ulcer care. Am J Surg 1998; 176:20S–25S.
73. Vowden P, Vowden KR. The management of diabetic foot ulcers. In: Falanga V, ed. Cutaneous Wound healing. London: Martin Dunitz Ltd; 2001.
74. Fisken RA, Digby M. Which dressing for diabetic foot ulcers? J Br Pod Med 1997; 52:20–22.
75. Lipken S, Chaikof E, Isseroff Z, et al. Effectiveness of bilayered cellular matrix in healing of neuropathic diabetic foot ulcers: results of a multicenter pilot trial. Wounds 2003; 15:230–236.
76. Bergstrom, N, Bennett MA, Carlson CE, et al. Treatment of pressure ulcers. Clinical Practice Guideline, No. 15. Rockville, MD: US Department of Health and Human Services. Public Health Service, Agency for Health Care Policy and Research. AHCPR Publication No. 95-0652. December 1994.
77. Wooten MK. Long-term care in geriatrics. Clin Fam Pract 2001; 3:599–626.
78. Belmin J, Meaume S, Rabus MT, et al. Sequential treatment with calcium alginate dressing and hydrocolloid dressings accelerates ulcer healing in older subjects: a multicenter randomized trial of sequential versus nonsequential treatment with hydrocolloid dressings alone. J Am Geriatr Soc 2000; 50:269–274.
79. Ovington LG. Wound dressings: their evolution and use. In: Falanga V, ed. Cutaneous Wound healing. London: Martin Dunitz Ltd; 2001.

9 Antibiotics

Ann F Haas MD

Summary box

- Routine use of antibiotics to prevent wound infection and endocarditis is discouraged because antibiotic-resistant organisms are becoming more common.
- Patient factors, local wound factors, preparation of surgical personnel, and surgical technique are all potential contributory factors to the development of surgical wound infections.
- Antibiotics to prevent wound infection are selected for procedures that have high infection rates or involve implanted prosthetic material or where the consequences of infection are especially serious.
- The choice of antibiotic is based on the most likely infecting organism.
- If used prophylactically, antibiotics need to be in the tissue before the time of wounding and contamination (i.e. there must be a preoperative dose).
- The medical literature and the new American Heart Association (AHA) guidelines recommend both a decrease in dosing (usually only a preoperative dose) and a limit on the situations in which antibiotics are even recommended.

INTRODUCTION

With increasing attention to antisepsis and aseptic technique, dermatologic surgeons, like our general surgical colleagues, have emphasized both the prevention of surgical site infections (SSIs) and appropriate treatment when they occur. The routine use of prophylactic antibiotics to prevent wound infection or endocarditis has fallen into disfavor, especially because of the recent prevalence of antibiotic-resistant organisms. This chapter examines factors involved in the development of SSIs and the controversy surrounding the development of endocarditis, and suggests reasonable guidelines for the use of antibiotics in dermatologic surgery.

Antibiotic resistance

Most antibiotic resistance develops inside hospitals, but the major development outside hospitals has been an increase in the prevalence of β-lactamase-producing bacteria, rendering penicillins less effective. The most important resistance problems facing dermatologists involve *Staphylococcus aureus*, coagulase-negative staphylococci, streptococci, and *Propionibacterium acnes* (with resistance of *Enterobacteriaceae* and *Pseudomonas aeruginosa* primarily involving in-hospital immunocompromised patients).[1] Recently, the major resistance problem has been caused by methicillin-resistant *S. aureus* (MRSA), with the frequency in hospital acquired infections often upwards of 50%. The coagulase-negative staphylococci, which often cause infections in immunocompromised patients, are also showing resistance to methicillin and other antibiotics.

We have also recently seen hospital infections with vancomycin-resistant enterococci, which, although normally not particularly pathogenic, might be able to transfer their vancomycin resistance genes to *S. aureus* (vancomycin resistance in *S. aureus* is already being reported). Resistance of *S. aureus* to erythromycin, tetracycline, fusidic acid, and quinolones is now being reported. Coagulase-negative staphylococci can apparently become resistant for some drugs (penicillin and methicillin) based on the same genes as for *S. aureus*. Clearly, physicians have contributed to the emergence of resistant organisms by their extensive use of antibiotics.

As the best established infection control practice has been thought to be handwashing, and antimicrobial use is the major determinant in the development of resistance, it is conceivable that paying more attention to aseptic technique and less to overprescribing antibiotics can help reduce the risk of resistant organisms developing (see Chapter 2).

Factors involved in the potential development of wound infection

Contamination of surgical wounds by microorganisms set the stage for the potential development of SSIs. Essentially, the dose of the bacterial contamination combined with the virulence of the microorganism exceeds the resistance of the host patient and so increases the risk of SSI.

According to the National Nosocomial Infections Surveillance (NNIS) published by the Centers for Disease Control and Prevention (CDC), the profile of pathogens seen in SSIs has not changed over the past decade.[2] The most frequently isolated pathogens were *S. aureus*, coagulase-negative staphylococci, *Enterococcus* spp., and *Escherichia coli*. The increase in SSIs caused by MRSA, *Candida albicans*, and fungal infections over the time period was also noted and attributed to both the increasing numbers of very ill and immunocompromised patients as well as the frequent use of broad-spectrum antibiotics.

The CDC has estimated that approximately 75% of all operations performed in the US are carried out in an 'ambulatory, or outpatient setting.'[2] Most studies evaluating the development of SSIs comes from hospital operating rooms, so may not therefore be directly applicable to outpatient dermatologic surgery. Additionally, many of the specific factors evaluated have not been examined 'in isolation' apart from other potential confounding factors. However, examination of some of these issues is still of benefit to the dermatologic surgeon and they may be at least partially applicable to the outpatient or office ambulatory surgery setting.

Patient factors

Many pre-existing, sometimes coexistent, conditions have been identified in the literature as risk factors for SSIs, including diabetes mellitus, obesity, smoking, corticosteroid use, malnutrition, and renal failure.[2,3] In addition, certain kinds of operations combined with patient characteristics have also been implicated in the development of SSIs, so making it difficult to attribute SSI development to any one specific factor in isolation. For instance, factors which have been shown to be of predictive risk for development of sternal SSIs in patients receiving coronary artery bypass grafts include diabetes, obesity, COPD, postoperative tracheotomy and total time on cardiopulmonary bypass.

Distant focus of infection

Usually a distant focus of infection is a respiratory, urinary, or skin infection that seeds the operative site.[2,3] One study demonstrated that surgical incision or antibiotic prophylaxis of a skin abscess the night before surgery did not change the rate of postoperative wound infection; however, treating the skin abscess more than 24 hours before surgery reduced the rate of wound infection so that it was close to the rate for patients who did not have a remote infection.[4] Remote skin infection may be a consideration in those with severe acne, actively inflamed epidermal inclusion cysts, or significant atopic dermatitis, and can be a significant problem for those undergoing implantation of a prosthetic device.

Diabetes mellitus

Diabetes mellitus has been associated with defects in leukocyte mobilization and other immune system abnormalities, many of which can be corrected by normalizing blood glucose. Although some studies have associated both increasing levels of HbA_{1c} or elevated glucose levels in the immediate postoperative period with increasing SSI rates, this phenomenon has not been studied in a strictly controlled fashion, in the absence of other potentially contributing factors.[2] The incidence of SSI development in people with diabetes mellitus is variable, depending on the study quoted. It has been shown that people with well-controlled diabetes mellitus do not seem to have an increased infection rate compared with people who do not have diabetes mellitus, so it may be well worth the effort to achieve good control of diabetes mellitus preoperatively.[3]

Smoking

Nicotine use delays primary wound healing and has been noted in studies as an important SSI risk factor. However, the contribution of smoking as an independent variable has not been strictly analyzed in the absence of other potential contributing variables.[2]

Malnutrition

It would seem reasonable that a low serum albumin would be a causal factor in wound healing problems, but it has not been explicitly implicated as a single predictive variable in SSIs. Although nutritional support is routinely given to patients undergoing general surgery and to those undergoing prolonged intubation after trauma, there are many reasons for this and it is not specifically aimed at preventing SSIs.

Age

Advanced age is a variable that is probably additive in contributing to the potential risk of SSI. Older patients have a higher tendency to have multiple medical problems, which can cause malnutrition and hypoxia, for example. Additionally, elderly patients may be on a significant number of medications, which can adversely effect wound healing and so potentially increase the risk of development of SSI.

Intranasal colonization with Staphylococcus aureus

The CDC reports a large study indicating that treating nasal carriage of *S. aureus* effectively reduced SSI development in cardiac surgery.[2] The use of prophylactic mupirocin for those with intranasal colonization is discussed later in this chapter. If a patient repeatedly seems to develop superficial staphylococcal infections without any obvious underlying immunodeficiency consideration might be given to intranasal cultures.

Altered immune response

Many studies have equated immunosuppressant medications and immunosuppressant states (leukemia, Chediak-Higashi syndrome, Job's syndrome) with difficulties in wound healing. Whether this extrapolates to the development of SSIs, specifically, is clearly controversial. For example, corticosteroid use suppresses wound healing by a number of mechanisms, but the relationship between corticosteroid use and SSI risk has not been definitively proven. It has been suggested that stopping corticosteroids a couple of days preoperatively, might positively influence wound healing. Whether this is possible for most patients and whether this would affect the rate of SSIs remains uncertain.[3]

The use of prophylactic antibiotics in patients receiving cytotoxic drugs is also controversial. *The Medical Letter* consultants have recommended prophylactic oral antimicrobial agents in those receiving cytotoxic drugs when their granulocyte counts are below 1 000/mm^3; or when the insult of the surgical procedure will result in significant bacterial contamination; or when the patient's host defenses are inadequate to resist a bacterial insult of any size.[5] However, it is also possible that this may increase colonization of the patient with organisms resistant to these antimicrobial agents.[6] If the dermatologic surgeon is planning a surgical procedure on a patient on immunosuppressant medication, it would be prudent to contact the hematologic specialist to discuss the potential risk of bacteremia in light of the patient's overall immune status, before making a decision about prophylactic antibiotics.

HIV infection and AIDS

Because of the variable clinical features of HIV infection and AIDS, it is difficult to make global assessments of the risk of SSI development for this group of patients. According to studies of patients with HIV infection undergoing emergency surgery reviewed by Burns and Pieper,[7] morbidity and mortality rates appeared to be not directly related to HIV infection. Instead, most of the SSIs in patients with HIV infection undergoing exploratory laparotomy were related to the presence of intra-abdominal malignancy, and perioperative $CD4^+$ counts did not predict postoperative outcomes. Although these outcomes may vary with the type of surgical procedure, it appears that, as an isolated variable, HIV infection does not, in itself, predispose to SSI.

Heavy microbial colonization

It has been shown that if a surgical site is contaminated with more than 10^5 microorganisms per gram of tissue, the risk of SSI is markedly increased (but the dose of microorganisms to induce infection may actually be less if foreign material is present in the wound).[2] For most SSIs the source of pathogens is the endogenous flora of the patient's skin or mucous membranes. The organisms are usually aerobic Gram-positive cocci (staphylococci), but can include anaerobic bacterial and Gram-negative aerobes if the surgical site is close to the perineum or groin. For dermatologists, patients in this category might include those with extensive atopic dermatitis, psoriasis, or other dermatitis. Although preoperative showers can reduce the skin's microbial count, they have not been directly correlated with a reduction in SSI development.

■ PREOPERATIVE PREPARATION

Preparation of personnel and the surgical site

Hair

It has been shown that shaving a preoperative site the night before surgery is associated with much higher SSI rates than with using a depilatory or not removing the hair at all.[2] The higher rates of SSI with shaving are thought to be due to the resultant microscopic nicks in the skin, which can serve as nidi for the development of subsequent skin infection. It has been shown that, if it can be managed, not removing hair at the surgical site is preferable in reducing the potential for SSI. If hair must be removed, clipping the hair immediately before the procedure is associated with a lower risk of SSI than having the patient shave or clip the hair the night before the procedure.[2]

Surgical site

No studies have been conclusive when comparing effects of the commonly available iodophors, alcohol-containing products, and chlorhexidine gluconate on the risk of developing SSIs. Iodophors can be inactivated by blood, but exert an effect as long as they are on the skin. Chlorhexidine gluconate causes greater reductions in microbial counts and greater residual activity after one application and is not inactivated by blood (see Chapter 2). Alcohol is probably the most effective and rapid-acting skin antiseptic, and is quite popular as a skin preparation in Europe (see Chapter 2). Alcohol is inexpensive, effective, and rapid-acting, and is active against bacteria, fungi, and viruses, but not against spores. However, alcohol is flammable, potentially limiting its use around certain lasers or in the standard operating room, depending on the equipment being used. Before applying the antiseptic agent, the skin needs to be cleansed of gross contaminants (including foreign body particles) and the preparation carried out in an enlarging circular fashion, large enough to extend the prepared area several centimeters past where the drapes will be placed. It may not make a significant difference which agent is used, as long as the skin is first cleansed of gross contamination, and then the surgical preparation is applied correctly.

Finally, an interesting study demonstrated a statistically significant decrease in wound infection when benzoyl peroxide was applied prophylactically for 7 days before skin surgery in seborrheic areas with a high density of sebaceous glands.[8] Further studies of risks and potential gains are needed before this can be advised as a practice tool.

Surgical personnel

Handwashing

Although no clinical trials have evaluated the impact of scrub agent choice on SSI risk, handwashing, particularly in between patients has been shown to decrease the SSI risk (see Chapter 2). Many antiseptic agents are available (see Chapter 2); with alcohol-based products becoming more popular in Europe.[2,9] There is no 'gold standard' handwashing technique that has proven to be superior over others. It is interesting that examination of the standard 'surgical scrub' carried out by operating room personnel has shown that scrubbing for at least 2 minutes was as effective as the 10-minute scrub in reducing hand bacterial colony counts.[2] The wearing of artificial nails is increasingly being banned in standard operating rooms because of their risk of carrying Gram-negative organisms[2] (see Chapter 2). The literature is less clear about the risks of nail polish and the transmission of potentially pathogenic organisms (see Chapter 2).

Gloves

The use of gloves to reduce the incidence of SSIs has not been demonstrated. Transfer of skin bacteria from the surgical team to the patient through perforated gloves has also not been demonstrated.[10] Therefore, the routine use of clean, nonsterile or sterile gloves for certain minor procedures could be up to the surgeon's discretion. Glove use is important in protecting the surgeon from contamination by blood-borne pathogens and may help alleviate the risk of development of SSIs.

Masks, gowns, and drapes

The use of masks and gowns are also not conclusively linked to a decreased risk of SSI.[2] Occupational Safety and Health Administration (OSHA) regulations require masks and protective eyewear to protect the surgeon against splash, spray, or spatter. A mask would protect both surgeon and patient in the event that one or the other may have an upper respiratory tract infection. Sterile surgical gowns and drapes provide a potential barrier between the operative site and sources of bacteria. Once again, these barrier devices also serve to protect the surgeon from blood-borne pathogens encountered via total saturation, or 'strike through' of wet gowns, splash, or plume. Certain types of fabrics are more fluid impermeable than others, and any protective clothing or drape material, if it becomes saturated, ceases to act as a protective barrier. As such, wet cloth drapes and garments should be changed immediately during an operation. More details on surgical attire are given in Chapter 2.

Issues specific to surgical personnel

Surgical personnel with active infections or colonized with certain microorganisms have been linked to the development of SSIs.[2] Certainly personnel who are ill should minimize patient contact, and the use of masks is prudent for those personnel with upper respiratory infections. A recent study also documented that surgeons who sweat may be more likely to contaminate the surgical field than the non-sweating surgeon.[11] This is particularly important during more physically demanding procedures, such as tumescent liposuction, where surgeons must take care to protect patients from secretions, and this may mean changing their surgical gown a few times during each procedure.

PRACTICAL APPLICATIONS

Wound classification

Surgical wound classification has long been used in general surgery to attempt to define potential intraoperative microbial contamination, and therefore provide guidelines for the decision to give antibiotic prophylaxis based on a surgical wound class for a given operation. This has been extrapolated to dermatologic surgery (Table 9.1), where most of the wounds encountered are either Class I or Class II wounds, with relatively low infection rates.[3] Antibiotic prophylaxis is not indicated for Class IV wounds; rather, antibiotics are given therapeutically for established infections.

Antibiotics to prevent wound infection

Generally, antibiotic prophylaxis is considered to prevent potential wound infection, endocarditis, and infection of implanted prosthetic devices. The risk–benefit ratio for providing prophylactic antibiotics must be weighed against the risk of toxic or allergic reactions, bacterial resistance, drug interactions, and superinfection. The medical literature continues to suggest giving prophylactic antibiotics only for procedures with high infection rates, for those involving the implantation of prosthetic material, and for procedures in which the consequences of infection are especially serious.[2,3,12]

In surgery of the skin the incidence of wound infection is very low. The reported incidence of bacteremia following dermatologic surgical procedures is also low, and although surgical implantation of prosthetic material is becoming more common in dermatology, it is still relatively infrequent.[3,13] *The Medical Letter* consultants have concluded, 'The small number of wound infections that would be prevented by antimicrobial prophylaxis make it unwarranted for ... varicose vein surgery, most dermatologic and plastic surgery ... repair of simple lacerations, outpatient treatment of burns .....'[11]

Nonetheless, there may be situations where the dermatologic surgeon feels antibiotic prophylaxis is warranted. There are some anatomic areas traditionally considered 'dirty' such as the axilla, groin, external genitalia, and feet, where wounds might be at higher risk of infection.[14] Certain patients might be heavily colonized with *S. aureus* (especially those with extensive atopic dermatitis or psoriasis), and might have additional other factors predisposing them to the development of SSI. Mohs surgery procedures, which result in having a large open wound for several hours, especially in a 'dirty' area, might also be considered for prophylaxis.

There are situations where dermatologists may routinely use prophylaxis in which it may not be necessary. One example of such controversy involves surgery of the ear, particularly when cartilage is exposed. One article discussing second intention healing of auricular defects after Mohs surgery recommended that prophylactic antibiotics were not used routinely even when cartilage is exposed, whereas others consider that antibiotics may be appropriate.[13,15] There may be some geographic areas where a hot, humid, or tropical climate tends to predispose to the development of pseudomonas infection postoperatively in the ear. Perhaps substituting a dilute acetic acid wash (quarter strength white vinegar in the USA would be 1.25%) to the postoperative ear wound daily rather than administration of prophylactic antibiotics might control potential pseudomonal growth at this anatomic site, especially if pseudomonal infection is not an endemic problem in the geographic area.

A limited study of incision and drainage of acute abscesses in 50 afebrile patients in the emergency room demonstrated no associated bacteremia,[16] suggesting that the routine use of antibiotics may not be necessary before incision and drainage.

Table 9.1 Classification of surgical wounds and antibiotic prophylaxis

Class	Infection rate (%)	Consider antibiotic prophylaxis for dermatologic surgery
I. Clean—noncontaminated skin, sterile technique	5	No
II. Clean-contaminated—wounds in: oral cavity, respiratory tract, axilla/perineum	10	Controversial; case-by-case basis
III. Contaminated—trauma, acute, non-purulent inflammation, major breaks in aseptic technique	20–30	Yes
IV. Infected—foreign body contamination, devitalized tissue	30–40	Antibiotics therapeutic, not prophylactic

Choice of antibiotic

The choice of antibiotic is made with consideration of the most likely infecting organism. The likely pathogens encountered in dermatology are *S. aureus*, *S. viridans* (oral cavity), *E. coli* (gastrointestinal tract [GIT]), and rarely, enterococcus (perineal skin). Occasionally, although *Staphylococcus epidermidis* is not a common pathogen in wound infections, *S. epidermidis* wound infections have been reported in the sternal incisions of patients who have cardiothoracic surgery.

The incidence of infection following skin surgery is so low that standard medical publications describing guidelines for antimicrobial prophylaxis in surgery do not even list cutaneous surgery as a category for consideration.[12] 'Head and Neck surgery' is usually listed, with the stipulation that the specific procedures considered for antimicrobial prophylaxis usually involve some type of incisional procedures through the oral or pharyngeal mucosa.

Most articles suggest that an early generation cephalosporin is considered when prophylaxis is needed for skin surgery because they are active against many Gram-positive and Gram-negative organisms.[2,3,12,17] For those allergic to penicillin, an alternative for Gram-positive coverage would be clindamycin. Vancomycin, which must be given intravenously, is not recommended as first-line prophylaxis for any surgery, except for patients suspected of having MRSA. Erythromycin is no longer considered an optimal choice because of the emergence of resistance and its side-effect profile. Amoxicillin and clindamycin are alternatives for the oral cavity, and trimethoprim–sulfamethoxazole and ciprofloxacin are alternatives for *E. coli* coverage in the perineal area. The agent used to cover enterococcus, which is not a common wound pathogen and is difficult to treat, is vancomycin (Table 9.2). Vancomycin is also considered the drug of choice in situations where *S. epidermidis* is considered a pathogen, for MRSA, and for patients with 'early' prosthetic cardiac valves (those < 60 days old). Vancomycin is a difficult drug to use in the outpatient setting because it must be given intravenously. Transient or permanent ototoxicity has been reported. Problems with too rapid an infusion of vancomycin can include exaggerated hypotension and, rarely, cardiac arrest. Vancomycin should be used with caution in patients with renal insufficiency, because the risk of vancomycin nephrotoxicity is increased by high, prolonged blood concentrations.

Timing and dosing of antibiotics

The timing of prophylactic antibiotic administration has been well documented, and needs to reach adequate tissue concentrations before the time of wounding and contamination. This allows the drug to be incorporated into the wound coagulum, which normally develops within the first couple of hours after wounding, and can protect trapped bacteria from systemic antibiotics if they are given after the coagulum develops.[2,3]

Most of the general surgical literature recommends single preoperative dosing only in most circumstances, and this dosing strategy has carried through to dermatologic surgery.[2,3,12] Most dermatologic surgery cases are of short duration, and the single preoperative dose should be adequate. Once the wound is closed, there is generally no further contamination. Even wounds that are created by electrodesiccation and curettage (ED and C), a surgical technique unique to dermatology, tend not to become infected. It has been noted that wound colonization with normal skin flora does not influence wound healing, light colonization with pathogenic bacteria may not interfere, but infection will inhibit wound healing.[18] Wound infection of wounds healing by second intention is 'rare' if the wounds are properly cared for.[19] Finally, it is conceivable that a rare, prolonged dermatologic procedure would require a second dose of antibiotics 6 hours postoperatively to maintain tissue levels of antibiotic.

Role of topical and incisional antibiotics

Topical antibiotics are traditionally used in dermatologic surgery to cover wounds left to heal by second intention. However, sutured wounds would not be expected to become contaminated after closure, so the postoperative application of topical antimicrobials would not seem to decrease the risk of SSI. A study comparing applications of bacitracin and white petrolatum after dermatologic procedures demonstrated no significant difference in overall infection rate between the two groups.[20] The dermatologic procedures

Table 9.2 SSI prevention: antibiotic guidelines

Area	Potential pathogen	Antibiotic choices	1-hour-preoperative dose*
Skin	*S. aureus*	First-generation cephalosporin	1 g orally
		Dicloxicillin	1 g orally
		Clindamycin	300 mg orally
		Vancomycin†	500 mg intravenously
Oral	*S. viridans*	First-generation cephalosporin	1 g orally
		Amoxicillin	1 g orally
		Clindamycin	300 mg orally
Gastrointestinal/genitourinary	*E. coli*	First-generation cephalosporin	1 g orally
		TMP–SMX—double strength‡	1 tablet orally
		Ciprofloxacin	500 mg orally

**Single preoperative dose in most cases; if second dose is necessary, reduce the dose by half at 6 hours. Exceptions are prolonged cases in 'contaminated area' if risk of SSI is high; liposuction; possibly full-face laser resurfacing (see text); 12-hour dosing interval with TMP–SMX and ciprofloxicin; implantation of prosthetic materials (e.g. expanded polytetrafluoroethylene [ePTFE])*

†For methicillin-resistant S. aureus, *or if suspect* S. epidermidis *is pathogen, not contaminant*

‡TMP–SMX, trimethoprim–sulfamethoxazole

included in the study were shave and punch biopsy, curettage and electrodesiccation, excision, Mohs micrographic surgery with simple and complicated repairs (flaps and grafts) and dermabrasion. The infections that occurred in the bacitracin group (also the group with the higher incidence of contact dermatitis) were caused by Gram-negative bacilli, requiring systemic antibiotic coverage that was more costly than the antibiotics needed to treat the *S. aureus* infections occurring in those in the petrolatum group.[20]

The use of intraincisional antibiotics has also been described in dermatologic surgery, both by direct administration into the wound, or mixed with lidocaine, and injected at the time of local anesthetic administration.[21,22] Side-effects have been demonstrated, and although the antibiotic–lidocaine mix did reduce the (low) infection rate in the study further, it is unclear whether this is necessary, given the known low incidence of wound infection for dermatologic surgery.

Mupirocin is the most effective narrow-spectrum antistaphylococcal topical antibiotic, and has been used both for the treatment of infected wounds and to eliminate nasal carriage of *S. aureus* (for prophylaxis against incisional wound infections in patients with recurrent staphylococcal skin infections). Additionally, regimens of both oral clindamycin and topical mupirocin have significantly decreased episodes of infections in those with recurrent staphylococcal skin infections.[17] Because there is now some staphylococcal resistance with mupirocin, it has been recommended that nasal mupirocin should not be used in patients with culture-proven staphylococcal skin infections unless these patients also demonstrate nasal culture-positive *S. aureus*.[17,23]

Special situations in dermatology

Laser resurfacing

There is considerable controversy about antibiotic prophylaxis to prevent SSIs following full-face laser resurfacing.[24–26] Many of the studies are small and poorly designed, and infection rates were compared with and without antibiotics without controlling for the type and duration of application of occlusive dressings. Interestingly, some of the wound infections were delayed in onset; one case of atypical mycobacterial infection occurred 1 month after resurfacing, and another study reported infections developing 3–5 weeks after the procedure.[27,28] What may be more important in these patients is close follow-up after laser resurfacing for an extended period of time, with meticulous patient guidance about postprocedure wound care.

Tumescent liposuction

Tumescent liposuction appears to be associated with a low risk of postoperative infection. One expert attributes this to a variety of factors, including in-vivo bacteriostatic and bactericidal effects of buffered lidocaine with epinephrine (adrenaline), the low incidence of hematomas and seromas, less surgical trauma when carried out as a single surgical procedure, and the careful selection of healthy patients.[29]

Many liposuction surgeons routinely recommend prophylactic antibiotics, extending several days after the procedure, during the period of time that insertion sites are left open to drain residual tumescent fluid or a foreign body drain is employed.[30] Given the cosmetic nature of the procedure and that numerous stab incisions are created to pass cannulas through, the lengthiness of the procedure, and the large surface areas that might be involved, this seems prudent. The most common pathologic organism causing infection is *S. aureus*, but rapidly growing atypical mycobacteria and fatal necrotizing fasciitis (caused by *Streptococcus pyogenes*) following liposuction have been reported.[31–33] Technique-related factors that may minimize the potential for infection after liposuction include extensive tumescent infiltration, open drainage (elimination of sutures that can predispose to foreign body reaction, wound inflammation, and incision site infections), adequate compression (to eliminate the possibility of seromas and hematomas that could predispose to infection), awake patients (which permits early diagnosis of inadvertent visceral penetration by the cannula), cleaning the patient's skin after the procedure, and removing surgical drains as soon as possible.[30]

Management of postoperative surgical site infection

Patients who develop a postoperative SSI usually present between postoperative days 4 and 10 with swollen, tender, erythematous wounds that may be draining malodorous, purulent material. In a sterile setting under local anesthesia, some or all sutures are removed and, after a wound culture is sent, the wound is lavaged to remove debris. The wound can then either be packed with sterile gauze or allowed to remain open to heal by second intention. In cases of purulent drainage, the latter is indicated. Empirical antibiotics are commenced, based on the presumed causal pathogen and can be adjusted based on the culture susceptibility profile.

Careful wound care instructions and close follow-up are mandatory (especially of those patients with higher risk factors, as has been discussed) to guard against the progression of the infection or unusual complications, such as necrotizing fasciitis. Scars can always be revised at a later date, but generally these wounds will demonstrate acceptable wound healing, depending on location.

Antibiotics for prophylaxis of endocarditis

The two types of endocarditis are infective endocarditis (IE) and prosthetic valve endocarditis (PVE). Infective endocarditis refers to infection of the endocardial surface of the heart, usually the heart valves (most often the mitral valve), but may also involve septal defects, mural endocardium, arteriovenous and arterioatrial shunts, and coarctation of the aorta. Certain strains of bacteria appear to adhere more selectively to platelets or fibrin. The most common microorganisms implicated in IE are streptococci and staphylococci.

Prosthetic valve endocarditis (PVE) is associated with valve replacement surgery and can be a cause of significant morbidity and death. The 'early' form of PVE is usually the result of a hospital-acquired microorganism and occurs within the first 60 days of valve placement. The most common cause of early PVE is *S. epidermidis*, although aerobic Gram-negative bacilli and fungi can also be causal. During this tenuous period it is recommended that intravenous vancomycin is given prophylactically for surgical procedures. The 'late' form of PVE occurs after the first

60 days of valve placement and most often involves the aortic valve. The most common cause of late PVE is non-group D streptococci. As the microbial cause of late PVE closely resembles native valve endocarditis, the potential pathogenesis has been postulated to be similar.

The traditional approach to endocarditis prophylaxis has been based on several controversial, and some unproven, considerations. First, the assumption was made that individuals with some types of either acquired or congenital cardiac disease may have an increased risk for developing endocarditis. Next, it was assumed that most cases of endocarditis are caused by streptococci that have predictable antibiotic susceptibility patterns. Additionally, it was thought that the risk of endocarditis increases after traumatic procedures to mucosal surfaces that are likely to produce bacteremia. Finally, it was assumed that giving antimicrobial therapy against streptococci to people 'at risk' for endocarditis undergoing these types of procedures can decrease their risk. None of these assumptions have been established by controlled trials.[34]

The recommendations by the AHA were revised in 1997 to deal in part with the criticism surrounding some of these considerations.[35] The AHA acknowledges that bacteremia may be common after many invasive procedures, but only certain bacteria commonly cause endocarditis, and it is not always possible to predict which patients will develop endocarditis or which procedure may be responsible. Because of the lack of susceptibility of certain causative agents, the lack of recognized predisposing factors in many patients, and the high incidence of daily transient bacteremias, one author calculated that fewer than 10% of cases of endocarditis are theoretically preventable.[36] The AHA also acknowledges that there are no randomized human trials to determine whether antibiotic prophylaxis really protects against the development of endocarditis during bacteremia-producing procedures, and they acknowledge that most cases of endocarditis are not attributable to an invasive procedure.[37]

Bacteremia in dermatology

It has been clearly demonstrated that bacteremias occur frequently after normal activities of daily living such as brushing teeth or eating hard candy. Endocarditis prophylaxis ideally would be used against significant bacteremias caused by organisms associated with endocarditis, and attributable to identifiable procedures. Manipulation of clinically infected skin is associated with a high incidence (>35%) of bacteremia with organisms known to cause endocarditis.[3] Although few studies have investigated bacteremia associated with dermatologic surgery procedures, those that do exist seem to indicate that the incidence of bacteremia following dermatologic surgery is low, and the bacteremia, generally occurring within the first 15 minutes of the procedure is short-lived.[3] In one small study where blood cultures were obtained from patients 30 minutes after undergoing excision or ED and C of eroded, noninfected or intact skin lesions, all blood cultures were negative.[38] In another study of a small number of patients undergoing a variety of dermatologic surgery procedures, blood cultures obtained from three patients were positive at 15 minutes, but grew organisms not commonly causing endocarditis.[39] The fact that transient bacteremia from other surgical and dental procedures involving mucosal surfaces or contaminated tissue also rarely persists for more than 15 minutes, has also been recognized by the AHA.

New Guidelines from the American Heart Association

The AHA defines certain 'high risk' cardiac conditions associated with endocarditis more often than others, and recommends prophylaxis in people with higher risk than the general population and for those in whom endocardial infection is associated with high morbidity and mortality rates. Those conditions that the AHA deems at 'high risk' for the development of endocarditis include those with prosthetic cardiac valves, a history of previous bacterial endocarditis, complex cyanotic congenital heart disease (i.e. single ventricle, transposition of the great vessels, tetralogy of Fallot), and those with surgically constructed systemic pulmonary shunts or conduits. Conditions considered by the AHA to fall into the 'moderate risk' category include acquired valve dysfunction (as in rheumatic heart disease), hypertrophic cardiomyopathy, mitral valve prolapse (MVP) with valvular regurgitation and/or thickened leaflets, and other congenital cardiac malformations, excluding those considered at high risk and those considered a negligible risk. The conditions that the AHA considers to be 'negligible risk' include isolated secundum atrial septal defects, surgical repair of atrial septal defect, ventricular septal defect or patent ductus arteriosus (without residua beyond 6 months), MVP without valvular regurgitation, physiologic 'innocent' heart murmurs, previous Kawasaki disease without valvular dysfunction, and previous rheumatic fever without valvular dysfunction.

The AHA spent considerable time re-evaluating recommendations about patients with mitral valve prolapse (MVP). They recommend prophylaxis for patients with a murmur from mitral regurgitation, and recommend that if the status of the patient's degree of mitral regurgitation is not known, that they either be referred for evaluation (which would potentially consist of echocardiogram and/or Doppler studies) or if there is an immediate need for the procedure in question, that the patient be given prophylaxis. Children also need to be considered because MVP is an important underlying diagnosis associated with pediatric endocarditis.

The AHA has recognized the short duration of transient bacteremia following procedures and some types of instrumentation (which is certainly consistent with what is experienced in dermatologic surgery), and has dropped its previous recommendation for a postprocedure dose of antibiotics for endocarditis prophylaxis.

Perhaps the most significant declaration in the new guidelines (which still do not address dermatologic surgical procedures specifically), is the statement that 'invasive procedures performed through surgically scrubbed skin are not likely to produce (such) bacteremias' ... (the significant bacteremias caused by organisms commonly associated with endocarditis). The AHA does mention 'incision or biopsy of surgically scrubbed skin,' but includes it under the category of procedures for which it does not recommend prophylaxis. The only procedure listed that has specific relevance for dermatology is incision and drainage of infected tissues. The AHA recommends that for individuals at moderate and high risk for endocarditis it would be advisable to give antibiotic prophylaxis for incision and drainage or other procedures involving infected tissues.

The previous AHA recommendations have included erythromycin as an alternative for penicillin-allergic patients. The current guidelines no longer include erythromycin.

Guidelines for endocarditis prophylaxis

It would seem that the risk–benefit ratio for dermatologic surgery suggests that endocarditis prophylaxis is only necessary for those patients the AHA considers 'high' or 'moderate' risk, when dealing with infected tissues. Whether or not to give endocarditis prophylaxis when working on eroded or inflamed, but noninfected tissue, in 'high' or 'moderate' risk patients is much less clear; but given the fact that dermatologic surgery procedures do tend to be performed through 'surgically scrubbed skin,' and that the incidence of bacteremia is not high for dermatologic surgery procedures, there certainly would be justification for not giving prophylactic antibiotics in these cases. The decision in the situation of a 'high' or 'moderate' risk patient before surgery of inflamed but noninfected tissue is probably best handled on a case-by-case basis, perhaps in consultation with the patient's cardiologist.

The guidelines for endocarditis prophylaxis for adults, based on the specific recommendations of the AHA, are listed in Table 9.3.[11] It is important to note that the 'contaminated skin' category is no longer included in the table by the AHA in their revised recommendations; however, it was a part of their previous recommendation. Undoubtedly, the reason for this is that the AHA does not consider that there is much of a bacteremic risk for dermatologic surgery procedures, especially when operating through intact, surgically scrubbed skin. There is discussion in the revised AHA guidelines about 'procedures involving infected tissues,' and the recommendation given is to use prophylaxis directed against the most likely pathogen causing the infection, for those in the 'high' and 'moderate' cardiac risk categories.

Because it is occasionally the case that 'contaminated' or 'infected' skin issues are relevant to the dermatologic surgeon who might also be encountering a 'high' risk cardiac patient, the AHA's recommendations regarding non-oral soft tissue infections are placed into Table 9.3 with changes in drug dosing to reflect the AHA's dosing for the same antibiotic regimens for dental and upper respiratory procedures. In addition, not all of the parenteral options for endocarditis prophylaxis for dental and upper respiratory procedures are included in Table 9.3 for the sake of simplicity because this route of antibiotic administration would not be routinely selected by the dermatologic surgeon in the outpatient setting. Other specific changes reflected in the revised guidelines include reduction in the amoxicillin dose, removal of erythromycin as an option, and the removal of the 6-hour postoperative dose.

Prophylaxis for indwelling devices

The AHA has included 'cardiac pacemakers and implanted defibrillators' on the list of entities for which endocarditis prophylaxis is not recommended. The issue occasionally arises about the use of prophylactic antibiotics to prevent infection of a previously implanted prosthetic device (usually prosthetic joints and vascular grafts). Most of these devices become infected at the time of actual implantation.[3,17] Occasionally, this type of implanted device can become infected as a result of an infection at some other remote site. Antibiotic prophylaxis for patients with an orthopedic prosthesis who undergo an invasive procedure that could be a potential source of bacteremia is controversial, and for the same reasons this issue is controversial in the potential development of endocarditis. The orthopedic literature suggests that after joint arthroplasty patients may be 'at risk' for the first 2 years post procedure. As a general rule, elective procedures potentially causing bacteremia,

Table 9.3 Endocarditis prophylaxis for moderate-to-high risk cardiac patients—infected or abscessed skin, presence of remote skin infection. Based on AHA guidelines.

Area	Potential pathogen	Antibiotic choices	1-hour-preoperative dose*
Contaminated skin	*S. aureus*	First-generation cephalosporin	2 g orally
		Dicloxicillin	2 g orally
		Clindamycin	600 mg orally
		Vancomycin†	1 g intravenously
Gastrointestinal/genitourinary	Enterococcus		
	Low risk	Amoxicillin	2 g orally
	High risk	Ampicillin + gentamicin (+ amoxicillin or ampicillin 6 hours later)	2 g + 1.5 mg/kg intramuscularly/intravenously (+1 g amoxicillin orally or 1 g ampicillin intramuscularly/intravenously 6 hours later)
		Alternatively: vancomycin + gentamicin‡	1 g intravenously + 1.5 mg/kg intravenously/intramuscularly
Oral	*S. viridans*	Amoxicillin	2 g orally
		Clindamycin	600 mg orally
		First-generation cephalosporin	2 g orally
		Azithromycin	500 mg orally
		Clarithromycin	500 mg orally

**As most dermatologic surgery procedures are short duration (15 minutes of bacteremia), the 6-hour postoperative dose is rarely necessary. If given, the 6-hour postoperative dose is generally half the preoperative dose.*

†For pathogenic S. epidermidis*, MRSA, or patients with newly implanted prosthetic cardiac valves*

‡Can repeat in 8 hours, if indicated

according to one source, should be avoided if possible for at least the first 6 months postoperatively, if not longer. The prophylaxis regimen suggested is for 'high risk' dental procedures, for 'high risk' patients.[37] The dental literature lists orthopedic joint prosthesis and orthopedic pins and screws under the category where prophylaxis is not recommended for dental procedures.[40] Considering that dental procedures, as a rule, have a far higher incidence of bacteremia than dermatologic procedures, it should also not be necessary to provide routine antibiotic prophylaxis for patients with orthopedic joint prostheses, pins and screws who are undergoing dermatologic surgery.

There may be a 'protective time element' as well, following the implantation of vascular grafts. The development of pseudointima of the graft surface during the month after graft placement appears to provide protection from bacteremic graft infections in the animal model. It is probably the case that the incidence of bacteremia following most dermatologic surgery procedures would not warrant antibiotic prophylaxis to prevent infection of these types of prostheses. Again, the dental literature includes arterial grafts in the category of situations where prophylaxis is not recommended for their procedures.[40]

Just as with the implantation of other prostheses, the introduction of soft tissue prostheses such as malar or chin implants, acellular human collagen sheets (Alloderm-Lifecell Inc), expanded polytetrafluoroethylene (ePTFE) implants, and others, are prone to implantation infection. Dermatologic surgeons are generally familiar with the ePTFE implants, which are medically inert and have been used for many other medical applications, such as vascular grafts and reinforcement for hernia repairs. These products come in various shapes (sheets, solid or hollow strands, threads, three-dimensional shapes for bony landmark augmentation) and sizes. The most common cosmetic uses for these devices are for the augmentation of nasolabial folds, oral commissures, the vermilion border, acne scars, and the glabellar furrow. These devices are to be implanted subdermally (see Chapter 28). As the ePTFE devices are frequently implanted into the lips or close to the oral cavity, it may be prudent to use antibiotic prophylaxis at the time of implantation. Once in place, these prostheses are then overgrown and surrounded by fibroblasts, which may be protective, in much the same manner as with the vascular grafts. It would probably not be necessary to use antibiotic prophylaxis to cover previously implanted ePTFE devices, unless surgery is being carried out on an inflamed or infected lesion close to the implanted device.

■ OPTIMIZING OUTCOMES AND POSTOPERATIVE CARE

Optimizing outcomes

- Good surgical technique, including meticulous hemostasis, reduces the risk of SSI.
- Minimize the entry of foreign bodies during wound closure and use sutures that have minimal potential for infection development (monofilament sutures).
- Use occlusive wound dressings with antibiotic ointment.
- Educate patients about postoperative wound care.

Surgical technique

Good surgical technique is critical in the prevention of SSIs.[2] Hematomas have long been associated with the development of postoperative wound infection. Maintaining good hemostasis and eliminating 'dead space' with the appropriate use of sutures are significant surgical considerations in minimizing postoperative morbidity. The use of pressure dressings designed to cover areas where there has been extensive undermining or 'bolster' dressings over grafts to minimize shearing forces and prevent fluid loculation also help negate the risk of hematoma. Gentle handling of tissues, including the use of hooks or delicate teethed forceps on the wound margins, helps to prevent ischemia. Well-designed flaps and grafts will maximize blood supply and minimize ischemia, which can lead to the development of devitalized tissue and the potential for wound infection. Removal of devitalized tissue while at the same time maintaining good blood supply is essential, and should be the endpoint of careful and meticulous electrocautery. Minimizing foreign bodies during wound closure can minimize inflammation at the surgical site and decrease the possibility of SSI. Suture material is a commonly used foreign body, with monofilament sutures seeming to have the lowest potential for the development of infection.[2] Finally, wound dressings that include an occlusive contact layer (antibiotic ointment) that is least conducive to the development of contact allergy followed by sterile Telfa (Kendall, Mansfield, MA) and tape (with or without pressure to encourage hemostasis as previously discussed) are important in preventing wound infection. Patient education for appropriate wound management that is carefully detailed verbally and in writing is a valuable component of good surgical technique.

■ SUMMARY

Many factors can contribute to the development of SSIs, and rarely is any one factor the single cause. Reducing infectious complications involves knowing the patient and understanding the significance of patient risk factors, preparation of the surgical site, and maintaining good surgical and aseptic technique. As the incidence of SSIs in dermatologic surgery is low, it is not necessary to provide antibiotic prophylaxis to prevent wound infections or endocarditis in the vast majority of dermatologic surgery (excisional cases). Where necessary, antibiotics are selected to cover the probable pathogenic organism and are best given as a single preoperative dose. Extensive and prolonged surgery, such as tumescent liposuction and laser resurfacing may not conform to these general guidelines and more frequently require antibiotic prophylaxis, especially because wounds are left open as part of the normal healing process. In these cases a postoperative course of antibiotics and close follow-up until the wounds are healed may be prudent. When in doubt, it is advisable for the dermatologic surgeon to consult with the patient's primary care physician to discuss the potential risks and benefits of prophylaxis. Hopefully dermatologic surgery can be a specialty that truly minimizes overuse of 'routine' antibiotics, so helping to minimize the development of bacterial resistance.

REFERENCES

1. Shapiro DB. Postoperative infection in hand surgery. Hand Clin 1998; 14:669–681.

2. Mangram AJ, Horan TC, Pearson M, et al. Guideline for prevention of surgical site infection, 1999. Am J Infect Control 1999; 27:97–134.
3. Haas AF, Grekin RC. Antibiotic prophylaxis in dermatologic surgery. J Am Acad Dermatol 1995: 32:155–179.
4. Valentine RJ, Weigett JA, Dryer D, et al. Effect of remote infections on clean wound infection rates. Am J Infect Control 1986; 14:64–67.
5. Antimicrobial prophylaxis and treatment in patients with granulocytopenia. Med Lett Drugs Ther 1981; 23:55–56.
6. Peterson LJ. Antibiotic prophylaxis against wound infections in oral and maxillofacial surgery. J Oral Maxillofac Surg 1990; 48:617–620.
7. Burns J, Pieper B. HIV/AIDS: impact on healing. Ostomy Wound Manage 2000; 46:30–40.
8. Bencini PL, Galimerti M, Signorini M. Utility of topical benzoyl peroxide for prevention of surgical skin wound infection. J Dermatol Surg Oncol 1994; 20:538–540.
9. Parenti JJ, Thibon P, Heller R, et al. Hand-rubbing with an aqueous alcoholic solution vs traditional surgical hand-scrubbing and 30-day surgical site infection rates. JAMA 2002; 288:722–727.
10. Whyte W, Hambraeus A, Laurell G, et al. The relative importance of routes and sources of wound contamination during general surgery. I. Non-airborne. J Hosp Infect 1991; 18:93–107.
11. Mills SJC, Holland DJ, Hardy AE. Operative field contamination by the sweating surgeon. Aust NZ J Surg 2000; 70:837–839.
12. Antimicrobial prophylaxis in surgery. Med Lett Drugs Ther 1999; 41:75–80.
13. Futoryan T, Grande D. Postoperative wound infection rates in dermatologic surgery. Dermatol Surg 1995; 21:509–514.
14. Brooks RA, Hollinghurst D, Ribbans WJ, et al. Bacterial recolonization during foot surgery: a prospective randomized study of toe preparation techniques. Foot Ankle Int 2001; 22:347–350.
15. Levin BC, Adams LA, Becker GD. Healing by secondary intention of auricular defects after Mohs surgery. Arch Otolaryngol Head Neck Surg 1996; 122:59–66.
16. Bobrow BJ, Pollack CV, Gamble S, et al. Incision and drainage of cutaneous abscesses is not associated with bacteremia in afebrile adults. Ann Emerg Med 1997; 29:404–408.
17. Hirschmann JV. Antimicrobial prophylaxis in dermatology. Semin Cut Med Surg 2000; 19:2–9.
18. Falanga V, Zitelli JA, Eaglestein WH. Wound healing. J Am Acad Dermatol 1988; 19:559–562.
19. Zitelli JA. Secondary intention healing. Clin Dermatol 1984; 2:92–106.
20. Smack DP, Harrington AC, Dunn C, et al. Infection and allergy incidence in ambulatory surgery patients using white petrolatum vs bacitracin ointment. A randomized controlled trial. JAMA 1996; 276:972–977.
21. Bencini PL, Galimberti M, Signorini M, et al. Antibiotic prophylaxis of wound infections in skin surgery. Arch Dermatol 1991; 127:1357–1360.
22. Griego RD, Zitelli JA. Intraincisional prophylactic antibiotics for dermatologic surgery. Arch Dermatol 1998; 134:688–692.
23. Kluytmans J, vanBelkum A, Verbrugh H. Nasal carriage of *Staphylococcus aureus*: epidemiology, underlying mechanisms and associated risks. Clin Microbiol Rev 1997; 10:505–520.
24. Alster TS, Lupton JR. Prevention and treatment of side effects and complications of cutaneous laser resurfacing. Plast Reconstr Surg 2001; 109:308–316.
25. Walia A, Alster TS. Cutaneous CO_2 laser resurfacing infection rate with and without prophylactic antibiotics. Dermatol Surg 1999; 25:857–861.
26. Goldman MP, Roberts TL, Skover G, et al. Optimizing wound healing in the face after laser abrasion. J Am Acad Dermatol 2002; 46:399–407.
27. Christian MM, Vehroozan DS, Moy RL. Delayed infections following full-face CO_2 laser resurfacing and occlusive dressing use. Dermatol Surg 2000; 26:32–36.
28. Rao J, Golden TA, Fitzpatrick RE. Atypical mycobacterial infection following blepharoplasty and full face skin resurfacing with CO_2 laser. Dermatol Surg 2002; 28:768–771.
29. Klein JA. Tumescent technique; tumescent anesthesia and microcannular liposuction. St. Louis: Mosby 2000; 129.
30. Klein JA. Tumescent technique; tumescent anesthesia and microcannular liposuction. St. Louis: Mosby 2000; 88–89.
31. Murillo J, Torres J, Bofill L, et al. Skin and wound infection by rapidly growing mycobacteria; an unexpected complication of liposuction and liposculpture. Arch Derm 2000; 136:1347–1352.
32. Behroozan DS, Christian MM, Moy RL. *Mycobacterium fortuitum* infection following neck liposuction: a case report. Dermatol Surg 2000; 26:588–590.
33. Heitmann C, Czermak C, Germann G. Rapidly fatal necrotizing fasciitis after aesthetic liposuction. Aesth Plast Surg 2000; 24:344–347.
34. Durack DT. Prevention of bacterial endocarditis during dentistry: time to scale back. Ann Intern Med 1998; 129:829–831.
35. Dajani AS, Taubert KA, Wilson W, et al. Prevention of bacterial endocarditis: recommendations by the American Heart Association. Circulation 1997; 96:358–366.
36. Kaye D, ed. Prophylaxis against bacterial endocarditis: a dilemma. American Heart Association (Monograph No. 52) 1977; 67–69.
37. Hanssen AD, Osmon DR. The use of prophylactic antimicrobial agents during and after hip arthroplasty. Clin Orthop 1999; 369:124–138.
38. Zack L, Remlinger K, Thompson K, et al. The incidence of bacteremia after skin surgery. J Infect Dis 1989; 159:148–150.
39. Halpern AC, Leyden JJ, Dzubow LM, et al. The incidence of bacteremia in skin surgery of the head and neck. J Am Acad Dermatol 1988; 19:112–116.
40. Epstein JB. Infective endocarditis: dental implications and new guidelines for antibiotic prophylaxis. J Can Dent Assoc 1998; 64:281–291.

10 Large Equipment and Design of the Surgical Suite, Including Monitoring Devices

Brett M Coldiron MD FACP and Mary Maloney MD

Summary box

- Take time in design.
- Bigger is better.
- Ensure walls and floors are washable.
- Ensure privacy.
- Aim to have plenty of storage.
- Equip with power tables.
- Plan plenty of light.
- Consider used equipment.
- Be prepared for emergencies.

INTRODUCTION

Well-designed surgical office space is critical for surgeon, staff, and patient comfort, as well as office efficiency. Identifying the proper space for your practice and building it requires a significant investment, not only in time and money, but also emotionally. The outcome of the project will be experienced by many for years to come. As such, it is important to seek expert advice in space planning, architecture, and internal design early because fixing a problem later can be far more expensive. Another tremendous resource is provided by our colleagues who have gone before us in building or redesigning a surgical suite. Touring their offices and getting their feedback in advance of proceeding will be exceedingly helpful.

TECHNICAL ASPECTS AND PRACTICAL APPLICATIONS

Surgical suite

As much as we would all love to have one or more oversized operating suites, the reality is that often we are constrained by space availability and overall building configuration. It is important to get professional advice to meet local codes and provide maximal utilization of space. The design should include features to allow for the easy movement of patients (ambulatory or not), patient safety, and comfort. The appearance of the operating room has the ability to reassure patients, or to frighten them.

Design of the office space is key, and the process should not be rushed. Use the plans shown in Figures 10.1 and 10.2 as a starting point and modify as needed. A professional medical architect can be very helpful. Be comfortable with your plans before construction begins because changes may be very expensive. Note that your personal office, unless used for consultations, is the least important room in the building because it generates no income.[1]

Patient privacy should be a major concern, especially with the new Health Insurance Portability and Accountability Act of 1996 (HIPPA) guidelines. Special acoustic insulation can be installed in the walls and on top of the ceiling tiles so that conversations are private. Curtained areas for privacy while changing can be installed in almost any examination room.

Sample office surgery layout

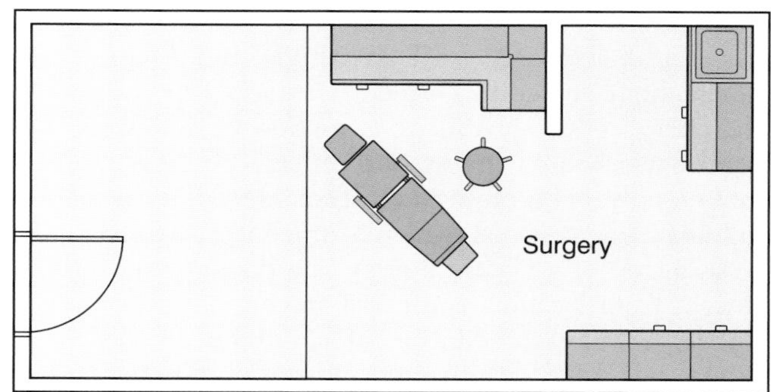

Figure 10.1 Sample office layout with a surgical suite. Note the extensive cabinet space. (Courtesy of Midmark Corporation, Versailles, OH.)

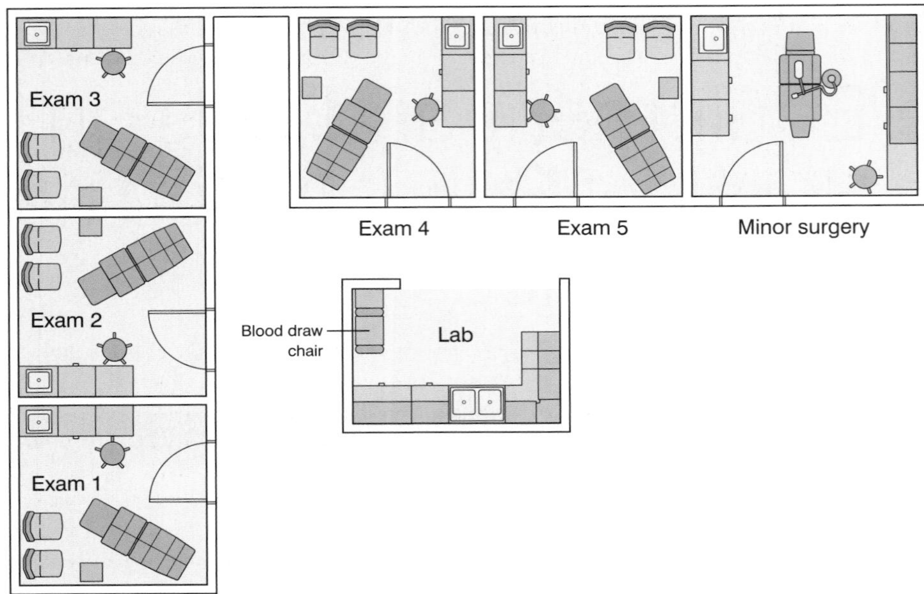

Figure 10.2 Dermatology office floor plan. This is a smaller surgical suite than in Fig. 10.1. Note that the suite is at the end of the corridor. There is a separate laboratory room for cleaning and sterilization of instruments. It may be wise to plan a wall in the laboratory room to separate the 'clean' and 'dirty' to avoid cross-contamination. (Courtesy of Midmark Corporation, Versailles, OH.)

Designing a facility for approval as an ambulatory surgery center (ASC) is beyond the scope of this chapter, but information can usually be obtained from your state board of health and the fire safety codebook. Specific requirements for ASCs vary greatly from state to state. If you are designing an office from scratch, however, you may want to consider in your design the possibility of building such a facility in the future.

Many of the general specifications for ASCs require extensive preplanning and may not be feasible in some office sites. Some of these requirements include a separate entrance, a separate waiting room, a dedicated recovery room, automatically activated fireproof doors, and a sprinkler system ceiling. Some other ASC design features include at least 1-hour fire breaks in the walls, 2-hour firebreaks in the floor, and a back-up power source for key equipment (generator or battery power). Sinks are not allowed in the operating room of an ASC, but are allowed in the recovery room.

There are several exceptions in the fire safety code for offices that use only local anesthesia, but Medicare and independent accrediting agencies usually require that the fire safety code for ASC construction be followed. Most local zoning boards, states, and office accrediting agencies, only require that a physician's office meets the commercial building code standard, which is much less expensive.

Note that office accreditation is a distinct and different process from building and certifying an ASC. Contrary to popular belief, accreditation of an office doesn't usually require difficult-to-meet physical plant requirements. Most of the requirements are centered on the establishment of protocols for governance, charting, record keeping, and quality assurance. Many office surgeons consider that office accreditation is a good route to take, if for no other reason than for public relations. Office accreditation is discussed in detail in Chapter 11.

A word needs to be said about consultants. Always interview three people and collect three bids. The disparities may be astounding. In general, the architect should be knowledgeable enough in this area to walk you through the design and construction of an office or an ASC. You should not have to pay much more than $150 per square foot for construction (unless you are in a chic location in a major urban area), and the architect should settle for 6–10% of the construction cost. Some consultants will take you through the entire process, but are quite expensive. On the other hand, an argument can be made that a consultant can easily save you whatever they cost. In any case, particularly if building an ASC or getting an office accredited, you should not expect to remain remote from the process. You will have to become intimately familiar with all the rules and regulations because their ultimate enforcement will rest with you.

Size

More is better was never truer than in the office operatory. The generally accepted minimum size is 12 × 12 feet (3.7 m × 3.7 m), but 20 × 20 feet (6 m × 6 m) would offer a range of advantages. Cabinetry, table, and equipment will take up a large amount of space. Windows are desirable and supply additional light, but must be secured shut to comply with aseptic technique. Often it is helpful to have windows tinted to protect patient privacy, depending on how accessible they are to the world outside (see Chapter 2). The room must be well-ventilated and temperature control is essential because the lights can produce extensive 'waste' heat.

Plumbing and wiring

Multiple outlets are essential, especially if one intends to use the room for a variety of surgical procedures such as reconstruction, electrosurgery, lasers, intense pulsed light, and liposuction. One block of sockets should be available on each wall, at a minimum. Even if not currently utilizing lasers, wire one socket in some of the surgical rooms for 220 volts to be prepared for the addition of laser or other special equipment in the future. Each room should be plumbed for a sink unless the room is an ASC. Sinks can come built into the cabinets and can be fitted with foot controls, allowing 'scrubbing' before a case. They require additional piping and drainage in each room.

In anticipation of a centrally placed power table, an outlet can be wired into the floor, eliminating power cords running across the floor to the wall socket. Some tables come with additional outlets built into them, which can be helpful when using electrical accessories such as dermatomes or Wood's lamp. Make sure the floor outlet is placed out of the walkway to avoid anyone tripping over it, and designed with an elevated lip to prevent cleaning solutions or water from causing a short during mopping.

Also consider installing ceiling sprinklers. These are expensive, but a safety feature that may qualify the office for decreased insurance rates.

When wiring the office, consider hardwiring fire detectors that will connect to a security system. Other wiring considerations include security elements (motion detectors) in each room to deter break-ins, camera cables for visual monitors, phone lines, and computer wiring.

Plan for as much general lighting in the operating and examination rooms as possible. The value of lighting cannot be overemphasized, particularly in dermatologic surgery. Install as many banks of fluorescent lights as possible. These can be fitted with special reflectors to create a shadowless light. You may also want additional lights focused on the examination table. Fluorescent floodlights can be installed in these to decrease heat production. Articulating lights with adjustable focal lengths are worth the added expense.

Emergency exit lights, and illuminated exit signs, separately powered, are required to pass fire code for any publicly accessed building.

Walls

The wall needs to be bright in color yet washable. A washable off-white or beige latex is an alternative to the sterile white color of most operating rooms. A washable vinyl wall covering is another option. Some decorators advise that a light blue or pastel color can be reassuring while others say blue is cold and pastel unprofessional. Trust your own instincts about your patients and remember that you and your staff will be in the rooms most often, so please yourself. Plan on repainting and recovering every few years.

Floors

It is inevitable that blood, chemicals, and marking dye will be spilled in the operating room. Recent evidence shows that carpeting does not increase the risk of bacterial contamination, and may in fact decrease dust particles in the air.[2,3] Carpet can, however, be stained or soiled, and can be very difficult to clean, giving the room a 'dirty' appearance and creating a biohazard. Considering this, carpet cannot be recommended for flooring in the surgery suite.

Linoleum costs more than carpet, particularly if installed as a single sheet lapping up the wall. However, it lends itself to being easily and thoroughly cleaned.

Ceramic tile can also be used, but the grout lines between tiles can be difficult to clean. Although ceramic tiles are attractive, they can also be slippery when wet. Ceramic tiles and grout are also less durable than linoleum over time, requiring more frequent maintenance.

Doors

The door to the room must be wide enough to allow the entrance of wheelchairs and stretchers. A 48-inch (1.222 m) door offers the greatest access although 44 inches (1.12m) is the minimum. Hallways need to be wide enough to allow stretchers to turn. Unfortunately this takes space away from the examination and operating rooms. It can be difficult to achieve this width when remodeling an existing building in which hallways have been notoriously tight. Ideally, during suite design, doorways from entry to office to at least one operating room are in a straight line without a need to turn.

Ceilings

Nine-foot (2.74 m) ceilings offer the advantage of compatibility with most of the better commercial lighting fixtures that are designed to be suspended from this ceiling height. Once again, it can be difficult to find a pre-existing older office space with ceilings this high. Ceilings in ASCs should be washable, but this is not required in a non ASC office operating room. Suspended ceilings are acceptable but require more maintenance to replace soiled or stained tiles.

Large equipment

Large equipment includes, but is not limited to, surgical tables, lights, cabinets, carts, sinks, suction machines, waste receptacles, Mayo stands, intravenous drip poles, crash carts, electrical cautery units, lasers, light sources, radiofrequency units, liposuction apparatus, and monitoring equipment.

On a general note be aware that much equipment is available used, and this is generally a valuable option. For example, hydraulic power tables will last many years. They may only need upholstering and minor servicing for improved longevity. Replacement bulbs can be found for almost any light. Stainless steel cabinets and sinks rarely wear out, or can be repaired. Suction machines can wear out, but because of infrequent use, have a long life. Great savings can be made with prudent shopping. If buying new, be aware that discounts of 10% or greater can be obtained at conventions, and that these same discounts may be extended at other times if requested. For sample costs see Table 10.1, and see Appendix for a list of equipment suppliers.

It is important to consider which and how many pieces of large equipment you may need over time so that you can design your suite with this growth in mind. If you are planning to own and operate a full scope laser center think about

Item	Cost new (US$)	Cost used (US$)
Power table	7000–14 000	3000–5000
Double overhead lights	3400–7500	1000–2000
Matching cabinets with sink	4000–10 000	500–1000
Suction machine	3000–3500	1500–2000
Pulse oximeter	700–7000	300–2000

Table 10.1 Estimated costs of new and used large equipment

storage and outlets well in advance. Similarly, crash carts come in many shapes and sizes, but most are fairly bulky. It is wise to determine which device you will purchase and where this will be strategically placed between operating suites in advance and designing this space in your plans rather then waiting to find that you do not have the room to place one juxtaposed to the surgical area.

Operating room tables

The operating table is important. The surgeon must be able to get close to the operative field, and the patient needs to be both comfortable and at ease. Tables with thin padding (frequently the less expensive tables) will become uncomfortable during prolonged procedures. You may want to evaluate a table yourself by lying on it in the surgical position for 10–15 minutes. Additionally, talk to other physicians from related specialties to determine how satisfied their patients are with different tables.

There are basically two types of tables, the hydraulic and the electric-powered nylon screw. Hydraulic tables are powered by a hydraulic pump, which forces hydraulic fluid (mineral oil) through hydraulic pistons (Fig. 10.3). A central rotating nylon screw powers the other tables. Hydraulic tables will last a long time, but they are somewhat slow to move. The nylon screw tables can be moved much faster, but the screw eventually wears out. There are multiple options for each kind of table, ranging from essential to elective options. Some of these are discussed below.

The number of mobile joints or 'break' points is important for patient positioning. The options include back, foot, and table elevation as well as tilt and head articulation (which is usually manual). The back elevation allows the patient to recline while foot elevation allows a patient to be in a sitting position with the lower leg (below knees) either up (at same level as the pelvis and thighs) or down. Some tables come with a permanent foot elevation, making table access difficult for some patients.

Another important feature is how low the table can descend toward the floor to allow easy access, especially for handicapped patients and transfers from wheelchairs. This prevents having to hoist or lift patients up from the standing position onto the surgical table. The table itself should adjust to the desired work level of the surgeons using it and provide a comfortable working position for any particular procedure.

Lastly, the tilt adjustment angles the table back, allowing the patient to be put in the Trendelenburg position, which is especially helpful in managing a vasovagal reaction to stress. For this reason alone, all surgical tables should allow the patient to be put in the Trendelenburg position with the head below the heart. Additionally, patients find the 'tilt' position very comfortable because they do not get the sensation that they are sliding off the table.

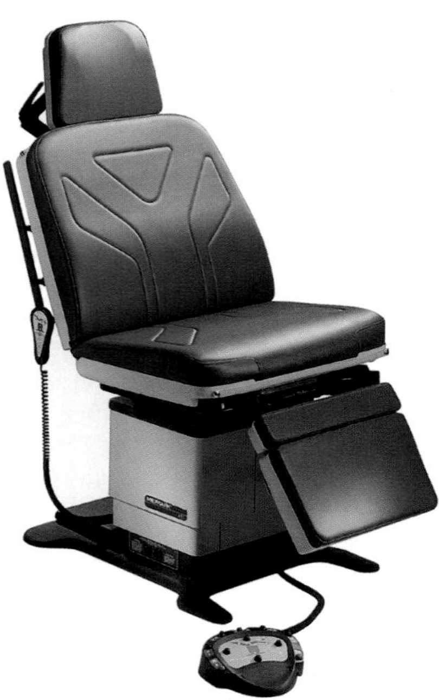

Figure 10.3 Rotating power table with three break points, and programmable hand and foot controls. (Courtesy Midmark Corporation, Versailles, OH.)

Variations of these positions allow flexibility in patient positioning and comfort according to individual needs. The programmable control feature available on many newer models allows the table to be placed in the exact same position accurately on demand. This feature is useful, and because surgical sites are never in the exact same location and patients are never exactly the same size, minor additional table adjustments can be easily made. Although foot controls 'clutter' the floor, they enable the operating surgeon to adjust the patient's position once a sterile surgical environment has been prepared and the case is underway.

The ability to convert to a full flat table position is essential for placing patients in the prone position. In these cases, it is useful to have a table with a large enough headrest that patients feel supported and can even position their hands around their head if more comfortable. Some tables come with a smaller headrest, as compared with table diameter. This can be a useful option for cases where the surgeon needs to get close to the head and neck, such as during head and neck cancer resection and reconstruction, as well as aesthetic rhytidectomy surgery. On the other hand, some surgeons prefer a larger headrest because it provides an area to brace the arms while working. These are clearly personal preferences, which should be explored before making an investment.

An adjustable arm board for procedures on the arm and hand is a useful option.

Tables that rotate can be useful in smaller suites or when operating on a site distant from the cautery unit or light, such as the leg.

Adjustable operating stools with foot or hand pedals can usually be obtained at a discounted rate if purchased with a table. Added features for these stools include back support and arm rests, which some find helpful for delicate facial surgery. Some surgeons stand, some sit. But even if you prefer to stand while operating, it is useful to be able to sit down at the same level of the patient preoperatively to review treatment options and risks. The stool can then be rolled out of the way into a corner or under a writing surface in the room.

Operating room lights

From the surgeon's perspective, the most important purchase for an operative suite besides the instruments is the lighting. Poor lighting is a point of aggravation for any surgeon. Lights must be reliable, have adequate candlepower, and not drift out of position. Less expensive lights tend to have greater drift than more expensive lights. Be wary of the salesman who tells you an inexpensive light will not drift. The mobile operating room light on a stand takes up valuable floor space and has been the least reliable light source for an operating room. Probably the only role for the mobile light is that of ancillary lighting in emergency situations.

Ceiling mounted lights are the gold standard. They are easily adjustable and provide adequate illumination, even in moderately deep cavities. Costs vary widely, as does quality and candlepower. There are a few common design types. The first has multiple lights set in a concave 'head'. Each of the smaller inset lights has a slightly different angle, to provide a widely lighted area with minimal shadows. The second type of light has a single central bulb with a reflective concave surface providing a field of light. A third option is that of smaller lights that are dual mounted to give illumination, and limit shadows (Fig. 10.4).

Lights need to be adjustable during the procedure. This may be accomplished by sterile disposable handle covers, or with autoclavable handles that can be screwed on just before the case. These are generally purchased separately.

Cabinets and storage

There can never be too many cabinets or too much storage (Fig. 10.5). Surgical rooms need an adequate amount of storage so that equipment and supplies are always at hand. This prevents staff from coming and going to supply a procedure and prevents delays in getting urgently needed instruments or equipment. Glass front cabinets are tremendously useful to showcase supplies for ready access.

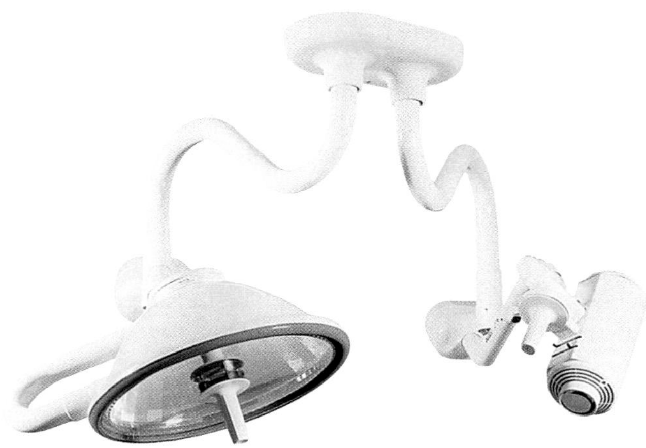

Figure 10.4 Double-headed light—one back illuminated, one spot. (Courtesy of Midmark Corporation, Versailles, OH.)

Any carpenter can design cabinets for you, but custom cabinets may be more expensive than those that are prebuilt. Many of the medical suppliers also supply matching modular cabinets, which are adequate, and some of the vendors will also help with office design.

Carts

Metal carts can be obtained very inexpensively from hardware suppliers and can be adapted for a variety of uses. The top can be used as a supply tray or surgical tray, and equipment such as cautery units and blood pressure cuffs can be mounted on the sides (Fig. 10.6). The additional shelves can be used to store frequently-used supplies. One great feature of such carts is that they can be moved to sites distant from the head and neck, such as the legs, bringing the cautery and supplies to the patient.

Surgical sink

A surgical sink with the water being operated by foot pedals is important for handwashing. This may be positioned in the hall, which is a requirement for an ASC, otherwise it may be more convenient if it is actually within the surgery room itself.

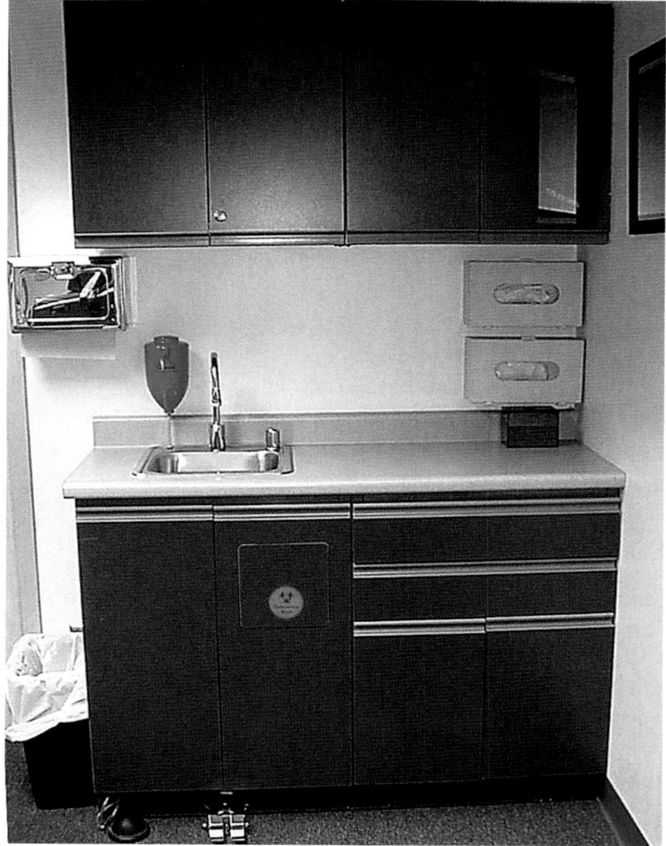

Figure 10.5 Matching cabinets (casework) with built-in sink, which is a useful feature. Note the water is foot operated, as is the soap dispenser. The glove dispenser, paper towel dispenser, and trashcan are all located nearby. There is also a mirror for patients to use when taking off their make-up and organizing when dressing.

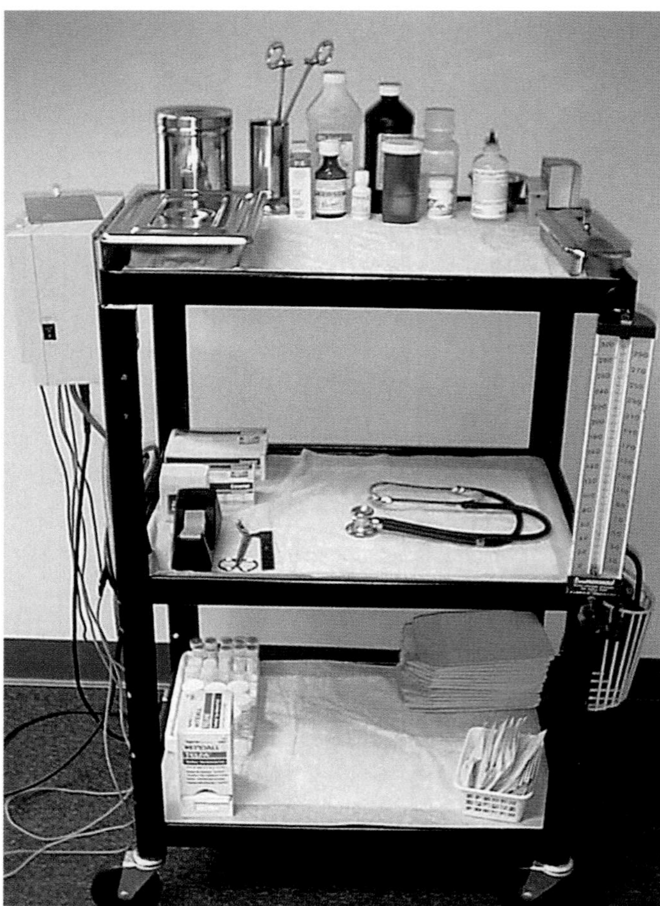

Figure 10.6 A 'customized' metal cart with wheels. Note that the cautery and manometer are mounted. There is room for supplies and small equipment and the cart can move around to distant operative sites.

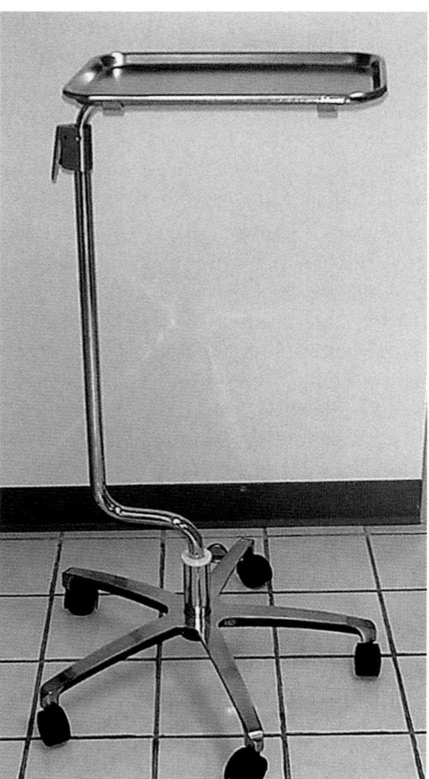

Figure 10.7 Mayo stand with wheels. These devices should last forever.

A sink depth of 18–24 inches (46–61 cm) decreases splash and allows a good stream of water while scrubbing. The foot pedals prevent recontamination of the hands when turning off water controls. Foot-operated soap dispensers work in a similar fashion. These sinks are available through surgical suppliers.

Suction

Suction is useful during surgeries in which difficulty maintaining hemostasis intraoperatively might impair field visualization and surgical outcome. Although some dermatologic surgeons never use suction, it is invaluable when operating in deep cavities or in those with a coagulopathy while trying to preserve adjacent vital neurovascular and anatomic structures. It improves visualization during the procedure to reveal vital structures before they are severed.

Out of the hospital setting, wall suction may be difficult to come by because it is very expensive to install and maintain. Portable units, however, are adequate. Many brands and models are available. There are both small tabletop units as well as rolling units, with the size and configuration of the surgical suite dictating the best unit purchased for any particular practice. Disposable supplies for suction units include presterilized suction tubing and tips. The suction tips include commercially available cannulas or sterile eyedroppers, which are small enough to get into almost any location.

Waste disposal

Waste cans are important in every surgical suite. Standard garbage cans with a footlift top are not appropriate to handle contaminated waste. Kick buckets are stainless steel short waste receptacles on wheels that are easily juxtaposed to the surgeon for ready access and disposal of contaminated waste. At least one such unit should be available in each surgical suite and placed directly under or near the Mayo stand or instrument table.

Mayo stand

Mayo stands are the working surface of the surgical suite, permitting easy access to surgical instruments or any other equipment need at the surgical field (Fig. 10.7). The variety of differences in stands includes size, movement of the platform, mechanism for raising and lowering the platform, the 'legs' or base of the stand, and lastly, its rolling mechanism. Choices between the various options are largely personal preference. A stand with a circular base for support is useful in that a kick bucket can fit within it for space efficiency.

Arrangement of equipment

Access to equipment is as important as space to maneuver around the suite. The operating table should be positioned in such a way that there is free movement around the room and full access to the surgical suites, with the table fully extended. All the equipment should be mobile or portable (i.e. placed on a Mayo stand) so that it can be moved into position where and when it is needed. Fixed equipment is limited because surgical sites may be anywhere on the body. Equally important, equipment that is mobile can also be pushed out of the way along the wall when not needed.

Room maintenance

For equipment maintenance all surfaces should be cleaned and free of debris after a procedure. Surfaces in contact with patient care materials, such as instruments and dressings, should be cleaned between patients. As this cleaning is not sterilization, a multitude of cleaners can be used. Glutaraldehyde acts as a disinfectant. Alcohol and 4% chlorhexidine gluconate are also effective. A 10% bleach solution has gained popularity because it can kill numerous organisms, including the human immunodeficiency virus (HIV). However, it will pit and corrode instruments and should therefore never be used in instrument cleaning. Other commercial medical cleaners are also acceptable (see Chapter 2).

General room cleaning should be carried out daily, paying attention to floors and fixtures. A regularly scheduled cleaning of walls should be performed monthly and as needed for gross contamination.

The best method of decreasing colonization of the surgical suite is to keep known 'dirty' cases out of the room. Abscesses should be drained in another room, never in the designated operating room, and care should be taken not to transfer materials or equipment back to the surgical suite before they have been fully cleaned.

Monitoring equipment

A pulse oximeter is useful in elderly and fragile patients with respiratory disease and is essential if conscious sedation is to be used in the office. The pulse oximeter has revolutionized anesthesia, and makes any procedure using a central nervous system depressant much safer. Automatic blood pressure cuffs may be an adjunct, but are not a substitute because they will detect an adverse event much later than a pulse oximeter.

Pulse oximeters work on the principal of Beer's law, determining the concentration of a given solute in a solvent based on the amount of light that is absorbed at a specific wavelength.[4] Unbound hemoglobin has an absorption peak at 660 nm, whereas hemoglobin with bound oxygen absorbs at 940 nm. The pulse oximeter uses two light emitting diodes and a light sensor, allowing the oximeter to calculate the saturation of oxygen via a computer algorithm. The oximeter also has a plethysmographic function, which provides for timed measurements during arterial pulsations and subtraction of the background venous blood saturation.[5]

The oximeter is usually clipped on the ear or fingertip and can display cardiac rhythm, as well as oxygen saturation. Newer units display respirations, body temperature, and blood pressure as well as end-tidal carbon dioxide levels when the appropriate cuffs and probes are attached (Fig. 10.8).

Pulse oximeters have automatic alarms to indicate critical values. Despite the annoying 'beeping' that is so characteristic of them, disabling the automatic alarm mitigates their ability to alert you to prevent a tragic outcome.

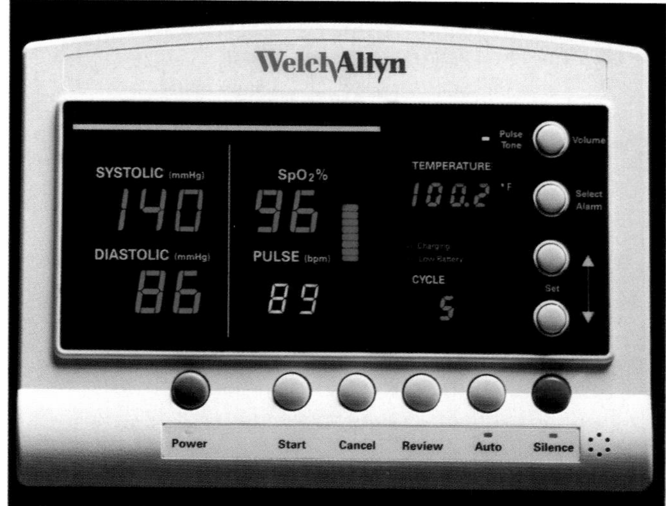

Figure 10.8 Pulse oximeter. These units cost from $1000–7000 depending on how elaborate they are. (Courtesy of Welch-Allyn, Skaneateles Falls, NY.)

It should be noted that a pulse oximeter may not work if the patient is hypovolemic, has serious tricuspid regurgitation, cannot hold the finger still, and while electrocautery is in use.

There are a number of manufacturers of pulse oximeters. A used machine may be acceptable if verified to be in proper working order. The manufacturers usually recommend a once-a-year inspection by their technicians.

A printer unit is optional, and should be obtained if considering office accreditation or ASC status. Regular printouts for quality control will be important to you. If you are planning to use conscious sedation you should probably also plan for office accreditation. Office accreditation may be mandatory for the use of intravenous sedation in the office setting in the future.

Resuscitative equipment

Physicians carrying out large, complex surgeries, with or without conscious sedation, should have resuscitative equipment available. This equipment should include an ambulatory ventilation bag, oxygen, a defibrillator, and the appropriate medications to handle any complication. Physicians performing these advanced procedures should maintain basic and advanced cardiac life support certification, especially if using conscious sedation. The emergency kit shown in Fig. 10.9 is the bare minimum for any office. It includes equipment and medications for anaphylactic reactions and other common emergencies.

Physicians should consider purchasing an automatic external defibrillator (AED). These units are simple to operate, and instruction in their use is now part of basic life support training. These devices are available in airports and restaurants, and should be available in physician's offices. According to the American Red Cross each minute that defibrillation is delayed reduces the chance of survival by 10%.[6]

Monitoring is not required for procedures carried out with local anesthesia. Monitoring is also usually not required for cases carried out with minimal sedation (oral or sublingual medications), in addition to local anesthesia.

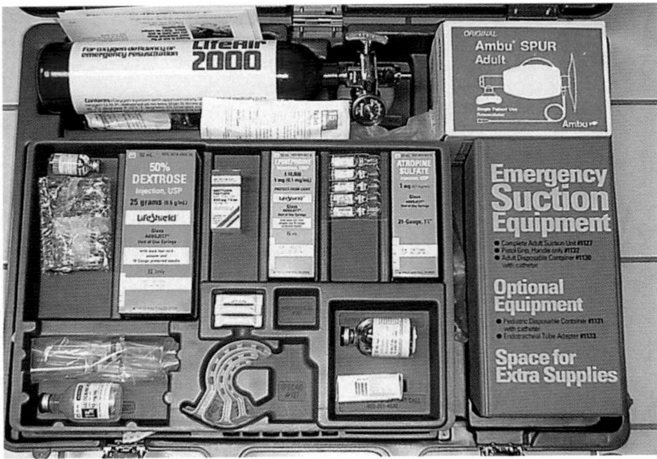

Figure 10.9 Office emergency kit. The bare minimum for offices not using conscious sedation.

Optimizing outcomes

- Include design features to allow easy movement of patients (ambulatory or not), patient safety, and comfort.
- Ensure at least one block of sockets on each wall.
- Ensure the floor outlet is placed out of the walkway.
- Plan for as much general lighting as possible—lights must be reliable, have adequate candlepower, and not drift out of position; ceiling mounted lights are the gold standard and lights need to be adjustable during the procedure.
- Emergency exit lights and illuminated exit signage, separately powered, are required to pass fire code for any publicly accessed building.
- Linoleum flooring can be easily and thoroughly cleaned.
- The door to the room must be wide enough to allow the entrance of wheelchairs and stretchers; hallways need to be wide enough to allow stretchers to turn.
- All surgical tables should allow patients to be put in the Trendelenburg position with the head below the heart.
- There can never be too many cabinets or too much storage (see Fig. 10.5).
- Standard garbage cans with a footlift top are not appropriate to handle contaminated waste.
- All equipment should be mobile or portable.
- A pulse oximeter is essential if conscious sedation is to be used in the office.
- Physicians carrying out large, complex surgeries with or without conscious sedation should have resuscitative equipment available and should maintain basic and advanced cardiac life support certification, especially if using conscious sedation.

PITFALLS AND THEIR MANAGEMENT

Pitfalls

- Not enough space, particularly in the operating room and storage.
- Not visualizing and planning for future expansion.
- Overpaying for equipment and consultants.
- Not compiling a budget before beginning.
- Not obtaining adequate financing in advance.
- Proceeding before adequate planning and consultation.

Seek expert advice in space planning, architecture, and internal design from experts and colleagues who have already built or redesigned a surgical suite. Touring their offices and getting their feedback in advance of proceeding will be exceedingly helpful.

A consultant can easily save whatever they cost. But always interview three people and collect three bids. The disparities may be astounding.

Get professional advice to both meet local codes and provide maximal utilization of space.

Great savings can be realized with prudent shopping. If buying new, be aware that discounts of 10% or greater can be obtained at conventions, and these same discounts may be extended at other times if requested

SUMMARY

When planning a surgical suite seek expert advice in space planning, architecture, and internal design before proceeding too far along because fixing a problem later can be far more expensive than approaching the issue correctly at the start. Bigger is better—the generally accepted minimum size is 12 × 12 feet (3.7 m × 3.7 m)—to accommodate cabinetry, table, and equipment. All walls and floors need to be washable, and all equipment should be mobile or portable. Ensure privacy for patients, plan plenty of storage, sockets, outlets and light, and be prepared for emergencies.

This chapter has been adapted from Maloney M. The surgical suite. In: Grekin RC, ed. The dermatologic suite: design and materials, 1st edition. New York: Churchill Livingstone; 1991: 1–16.

REFERENCES

1. Tobin HA. Office surgery: the surgical suite. J Dermatol Surg Oncol 1998; 14:247–255.
2. Rutala WA, Weber DJ. Surface disinfection: should we do it? J Hosp Infect 2001; 48(suppl A):S64–S68.
3. Skoutelis AT, Westenfelder GO, Beckerdite M, Phair JP. Hospital carpeting and epidemiology of *Clostridium difficile*. Am J Infect Control. 1994; 22:212–217.
4. Maloney M. The surgical suite. In: Grekin RC, ed. The dermatologic surgical suite, design and materials, 1st edn. New York: Churchill Livingstone; 1991.
5. Wilson WC, Shapiro B. Perioperative hypoxia, the clinical spectrum and current oxygen monitoring methodology. Anesth Clin North Am 2001; 19:769–812.
6. American Red Cross. First aid/CPR/AED program. 2001:52.

Appendix
Equipment Suppliers

In the US

Adjustable Fixture Co.
3726 North Booth Street
Milwaukee, WI 53212
Phone: (414) 964-2626; Fax: (414) 964-2944; Toll free: 800-558-2628
Examination lamps, lights

Ameda Medical Technologies
50 Hammerstone Cres.
Thornhill, Ontario
Canada L4J 8B4
Phone: (905) 731-2991; Fax: (905) 731-3298
Ambulatory blood pressure, defibrillators

Ancom Business Products
2831 Center Road
PO Box 150
Brunswick, OH 44212-0150
Phone: (330) 225-1510; Fax: (330) 225-3434; Toll free: 800-845-9010
www.ancom-filing.com
Medical cabinets

BCI, Inc.
N7 W22025 Johnson Road
Waukesha, WI 53186
Phone: (262) 542-3100; Fax: (262) 542-0718; Toll free: 800-558-2345
www.smiths-bci.com;
email: info@smiths-bci.com
Blood pressure monitoring, capnometers, medical monitoring systems, pulse oximeters, vital signs monitors

Burton Medical Products
21100 Lassen Street
Chatsworth, CA 91311
Phone: (818) 701-8700; Fax: (818) 701-8725; Toll free: 800-444-9909
www.burtonmedical.com
Examination lamps

Cardioline USA, Inc.
3200 Dutton Avenue
Santa Rosa, CA 95407
Phone: (707) 547-1740; Fax: (707) 547-1742; Toll free: 800-942-0442
Defibrillators

Criticare Systems, Inc.
20925 Crossroads Circle
Waukesha, WI 53186
Phone: (262) 798-8282; Fax: (262) 789-8290; Toll free: 800-458-4615
Tech. support: 800-458-2697
www.csiusa.com
Blood pressure monitoring, capnometers, carbon dioxide monitors, defibrillators, medical monitoring systems, pulse oximeters

Datex Ohmeda, Inc.
1315 W. Century Drive
Louisville, CO 80027
Phone: (303) 666-7001; Fax: (303) 665-9175; Toll free: 800-652-2469
www.datexohmeda.com
Capnometers, pulse oximeters

ENOCHS Examining Room Furniture
PO Box 50559
Indianapolis, IN 46250
Phone: (317) 842-6255; Fax: (317) 842-6569; Toll free: (800) 428-2305
Tech. support: (800) 322-6416
www.enochsmed.com;
email: enochs@enochsmed.com
Medical cabinets, examination room furniture, stools

Hausmann Industries, Inc.
130 Union Street
Northvale, NJ 07647
Phone: (201) 767-0255;
Fax: (201) 767-1369;
Toll free: 888-HAUSMANN
Custom medical products, examination room furniture, homecare products, office furniture/examination tables, physical therapy

Hewlett-Packard Corporation
Cardiology Business Unit
204 Andover Street
Andover, MA 01810
Toll free: 800-228-4636
Tech. support: 800-548-8833
Defibrillators

Hill Laboratories Company
PO Box 2028, 3 Bacton Hill Road
Frazer, PA 19355
Phone: (610) 644-2867;
Fax: (610) 647-6297
www.hilllabs.com;
email: info@hilllabs.com
Power tables, examination tables, office furniture/examination tables, stools

Marquette Electronics, Inc.
8200 West Tower Avenue
Milwaukee, WI 53223
Phone: (414) 355-5000;
Fax: (414) 355-3790;
Toll free: 800-558-5120
Defibrillators

Med-Electronics, Inc.
9723 Baltimore Avenue
Suite 5 College Park, MD 20740
Phone: 301-345-8826;
Fax: 301-345-5686;
Toll free: 888-321-1300
www.med-electronics.com
email: sales@med-electronics.com
Defibrillators, examination room furniture, examination lights, examination tables, pulse oximeters, automatic blood pressure cuffs.

Medtronic Physio-Control
11811 Willows Road, NE Redmond, WA 98052
Phone: 425-867-4000
Fax: 425-867-4416
Toll free: 800-442-1142
Defibrillators

Midmark Corporation
60 Vista Drive, PO Box 286
Versailles, OH 45380
Phone: (937) 526-3662;
Fax: (937) 526-4604;
Toll free: 1-800-MIDMARK
www.midmark.com
Medical cabinets, examination lamps, examination room furniture, lights, office furniture/examination tables, stools

MRL, Inc.
1000 Asbury Drive
Buffalo Grove, IL 60089
Phone: 847-520-0300; Fax: 847-520-0303; Toll free: 800-462-0777
www.mrlinc.com; www.aedsolutions.com
Defibrillators, vital signs monitors

Multiplex Display Fixture Co.
1555 Larkin Williams Road
Fenton, MO 63026
Phone: 800-325-3350; Fax: (314) 326-1716
Office furniture, examination tables

Nasiff Associates, Inc.
9422 LeBean Lane
Brewerton, NY 13029
Phone: (315) 676-2346; Fax: (315) 676-4711; Toll free: 866-627-4331
www.nasiff.com
email: nasales@nasiff.com
Blood pressure monitoring, pulse oximeters, vital signs

Nevin Laboratories, Inc.
5000 S. Halsted Street
Chicago, IL 60609
Phone: (312) 624-4330; Fax: (312) 624-7337; Toll free: 800-428-2253
Cabinetry, examination tables, stools

Nonin Medical Inc.
2605 Fernbrook Lane
North Plymouth, MN 55447-4755
Phone: (763) 553-9968; Fax: (763) 553-7807; Toll free: 800-356-8874
www.nonin.com
email: info@nonin.com
Pulse oximeters

Pace Tech Inc.
510 N. Garden Avenue
Clearwater, FL 34615
Phone: (813) 442-8118; Fax: (813) 443-7257; Tech. Support: 800-722-3024
Noninvasive blood pressure (automatic) monitors, patient monitors, pulse oximeters, vital sign monitors

Palco Labs
8030 Soquel Avenue, Ste. #100
Santa Cruz, CA 95062
Phone: (831) 476-3151; Fax: (831) 476-0790; Toll free: 800-346-4488
Tech. support: 800-472-3200
www.palcolabs.com
email: info@palcolabs.com
Pulse oximeters

Physio Control International Corp
11811 Willows Road
Redmond, WA 98072
Phone: (425) 867-4452; Fax: (425) 867-4252; Toll free: 800-442-1142
Blood pressure monitoring, defibrillators, pulse oximeters, vital signs monitor

QRS Diagnostic, LLC
14755 27th Avenue
North Plymouth, MN 55447
Phone: (763) 559-8492; Fax: (763) 559-2961; Toll free: 800-465-8408
www.QRSdiagnostic.com;
email: sales@QRSdiagnostic.com
Medical monitoring systems, pulse oximeters, cabinetry, modular, manual exam/treatment tables, power procedure/examination treatment tables

Skytron
5000 36th Street, SE
Grand Rapids, MI 49512
Phone: (616) 957-0500; Fax: (616) 957-5053; Toll free: 800-SKYTRON (759-8766)
Lights

Spacelabs Medical, Burdick Products
500 Burdick Parkway
Deerfield, WI 53531
Phone: (608) 764-1919; Fax: (608) 764-2394; Toll free: (800) 777-1777
Tech. support: (800) 333-7770
www.spacelabs.com;
email: burdickproducts@slmd.com
Defibrillators, pulse oximeters

United Metal Fabricators
1316 Eisenhower Blvd
Johnstown, PA 15904
Phone: (814) 266-8726; Fax: (814) 266-1870; Toll free: 800-638-5322
www.umf-exam.com

In the UK

Actamed Ltd
Calder Island Way, Wakefield
W. Yorkshire WF2 7AW
Tel: +44 (0)1924 200550; Fax: +44 (0)1924 200518
www.actamed.co.uk

Amazon Medical Ltd
Carringtom Business Park, Carrington
Manchester, M13 4XL
Tel: +44 (0)161 7764336; Fax: +44 (0)161 7764339
www.amazonmedical.co.uk/layout.html

Albert Waeschle
PO Box 19,
123–125 Old Christchurch Rd,
Bournemouth, Dorset, BH1 1EX
Tel: +44 (0)1202 204803; Fax: +44 (0)1202 204800
www.albertwaeschle.com/aboutAW.html

Beaver Medical Products Ltd
BMP House, 21 Mansion Close,
Moulton Park, Northampton NN3 6RU
Tel: +44 (0)1604 499427; Fax: +44 (0)1604 492212
www.beavermedical.com/products_home.htm

Berchtold UK Ltd
Hartham Park,
Corsham SN13 0RP
Tel: +44 (0)1249 700770; Fax: 01249 700001

Brandon Medical Limited
Holme Well Road
Leeds, W. Yorkshire LS10 4TQ
Tel: +44 (0)113 277 7393; Fax: +44 (0)113 272 8844
www.brandon-medical.co.uk/products.php

Cory Bros
6 Bittacy Business Centre, Bittacy Hill
London, NW7 1BA
Tel: +44 (0)208 349 1081; Fax: +44 (0)208 349 1962
www.corybros.co.uk/

Caterham Surgical Supplies
Caterham House
89a Gloucester Road
Croydon CR0 2DN
Tel: +44 (0)208 683 1103/4; Fax: +44 (0)208 683 1105
www.caterhamsurgical.co.uk/

Erbe Medical (UK) Ltd
The Antler Complex,
2 Bruntcliffe Way
Morley, Leeds LS27 0JG
Tel: +44 (0)113 2530333; Fax: +44 (0)113 2532733
www.erbe-uk.com/

Eschmann Equipment
Peter Road,
Lancing, West Sussex BN15 6TJ
Tel: +44 (0)1903 753322; Fax: +44 (0)1903 766793
www.eschmann.co.uk

Henleys Medical Supplies Ltd
Brownfields
Welwyn Garden City, Herts AL7 1AN
www.henleysmed.com/shop/enter.html

Heraeus Med
8 Calbeck Rd, Croft Business Park
Bromborough, Wirral CH 62 3PL
Tel: +44 (0)1513 430545; Fax: +44 (0)1513 439883
www.heraeusmed.com/about.htm

Landmark Surgical Ltd
21 Woodland Road, Rock Ferry
Merseyside CH42 4NT
Tel: +44 (0)151 643 1323; Fax: +44 (0)151 643 9312
www.landmark-surgical.co.uk/pages/aboutlandmark.html

Luxo UK Ltd
4 Barmeston Road
London SE6 3 BN
Tel: +44 (0)20 8698 7238; Fax: +44 (0)20 8265 1093
www.luxo.com

Medix Instruments
Monitor House, Hitchin Street
Baldock, Herts SG7 6AE
Tel: +44 (0)1462 635 333; Fax: +44 (0)1462 635 444
www.medixuk.demon.co.uk/

Medtronic Physio-Control (UK) Ltd
Leamington Court, Andover Road
Newfound, Basingstoke, RG23 7HE
Tel: +44 (0)1256 782727; Fax: +44 (0)1256 782728
www.medtronicphysiocontrol.com/

Navrish Ltd
17 Bishops Close, Mays Lane,
Arkley, Barnet, Herts, EN5 QH
Tel: +44 (0)181 3648363; Fax: +44 (0)181 4416813
www.navrish.co.uk/html/about_us.html

Proact Medical Ltd
Cobden Street,
Kettering, Northampton NN16 8ER
Tel: +44 (0)1536 416816; Fax: +44 (0)1536 416716
www.proactmedical.co.uk/page01.html

Radiometer Ltd
Manor Court,
Manor Royal
Crawley, West Sussex RH10 2PY
Tel: +44 (0)1293 517599;
Fax: +44 (0)1293 531579
www.radiometer.com

Response Medical Equipment Ltd
Rourke's Drift House,
Station Road
Chipping Campden,
Glos. GL5 6HY
www.response-medical.co.uk

Seward Ltd
98 Great North Road
London N2 0GN
Tel: +44 (0)20 8365 4100;
Fax: +44 (0)20 8365 3999
www.seward.co.uk/news.htm

Siemens Medical Engineering
Oldbury
Bracknell, Berks RG12 8FZ
Tel: +44 (0)1344 396321;
Fax: +44 (0)1344 396337
www.medical.siemens.com

Steris Ltd
Cornbury Park,
Charlbury, Oxon OX7 3EH
Tel: +44 (0)800 252609;
Fax: +44 (0)1608 811854
www.steris.com

Stryker UK Ltd
Stryker House,
Hambridge Road
Newbury, Berks RG14 5EG
Tel: +44 (0)1635 262400;
Fax: +44 (0)1635 580300
www.stryker.co.uk

Tyco Healthcare Ltd
154 Fareham Road
Gosport, Hants PO13 0AS
Tel: +44 (0)1329 224114;
Fax: +44 (0)1329 224390
www.tycohealthcare.com

Vicarey Davidson & Co
Unit 10 30A, Cumberland Street
Glasgow G5 9QJ
Tel: +44 (0)141 420 1778;
Fax: +44 (0)141 429 3273
www.vicareydavidson.com/

Zoll Medical (UK) Ltd
Unit 13 Empress Business Centre
380 Chester Road, Old Trafford,
Manchester M16 9EB
Tel: +44 (0)161 8772883;
Fax: +44 (0)161 8772884
www.zoll.com/contact.htm

11 Dermatology Office Accreditation

W Patrick Davey MD FACP

Summary box

- Accreditation focuses on the quality of patient care provided, while Medicare standards tend to focus on the physical aspects of healthcare facility and environment.
- An accreditation survey reviews every aspect of the healthcare facility and confirms that the facility does what it says it is doing.
- A year-long preparation for an accreditation survey is usually necessary.
- A consultant can provide helpful guidance regarding state licensure and certificate of need; healthcare legislation and regulation for ambulatory service centers (ASCs) varies between states.
- Pitfalls in achieving accreditation include outdated and irrelevant policies and procedures, inaccurate and incomplete patient care documentation, credentialing and privileging, and inadequate quality improvement and risk management activities.
- Patient safety in office-based facilities is enhanced by accreditation.

INTRODUCTION

The concept of accreditation started with hospitals, but now it has moved into dermatology offices. The focus of accreditation is the quality of patient care provided by the organization. The process is designed to verify that the organization meets specific criteria indicative of quality patient care, and it helps an office to deliver high-quality patient care. Accreditation is the highest form of public recognition a healthcare organization can receive. Achieving accreditation helps an organization find new ways to improve the care and services offered, increase efficiency and reduce costs, develop better risk management programs, lower liability insurance premiums, motivate staff by instilling pride and loyalty, strengthen public relations and marketing efforts, and to recruit and retain qualified professional staff members. Office-based accreditation can be obtained through accreditation organizations such as the Accreditation Association for Ambulatory Health Care (AAAHC) (see Tables 11.1, 11.2), the Joint Commission on Accreditation of Healthcare Organizations (JCAHO) and the American Association for Accreditation of Ambulatory Surgical Facilities (AAAASF). Accreditation through these non-governmental organizations is viewed by the state regulatory agencies as a private means to provide quality oversight. The private accrediting organizations enforce minimal standards and improve patient safety, thereby reducing the burden of government bodies with respect to regulation of the quality of patient care.

TECHNICAL ASPECTS

The accreditation survey process

An outline of the accreditation survey process is given in Figure 11.1.

Table 11.1 AAAHC member organizations[2]

American Academy of Cosmetic Surgery (AACS)
American Academy of Dental Group Practice (AADGP)
American Academy of Dermatology (AAD)
American Academy of Facial Plastic and Reconstructive Surgery (AAFPRS)
American Academy of Family Physicians (AAFP)
American Association of Oral and Maxillofacial Surgeons (AAOMS)
American College Health Association (ACHA)
American College of Obstetricians and Gynecologists (ACOG)
American College of Occupational and Environmental Medicine (ACOEM)
American Gastroenterological Association (AGA)
American Society for Dermatologic Surgery (ASDS)
American Society of Anesthesiologists (ASA)
Federated Ambulatory Surgery Association (FASA)
Medical Group Management Association (MGMA)
Outpatient Ophthalmic Surgery Society (OOSS)
Society for Ambulatory Anesthesia (SAMBA)

Table 11.2 Healthcare organizations with AAAHC accreditation (in descending frequency)

Ambulatory surgery centers
Office-based surgery organizations
Student or Indian health centers
Endoscopy centers
Group practices or Health Maintenance Organizations (HMOs)

The accreditation process

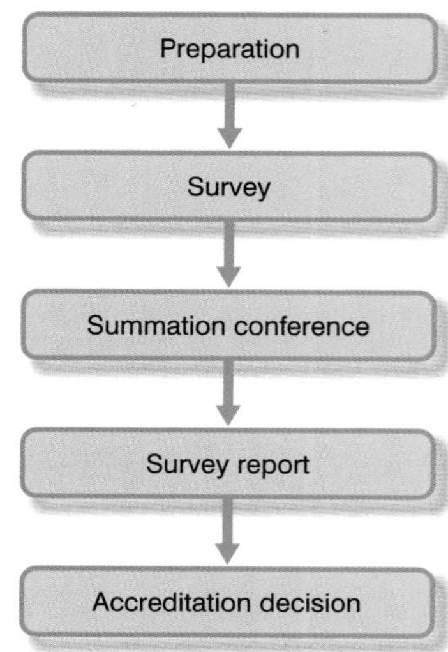

Figure 11.1 The accreditation process.

Preparation

The surveyed organization may need a year to prepare for an accreditation survey. In order for the surveyors to carry out the accreditation survey, a wealth of information must be provided (Table 11.3). Information is reviewed about the patients themselves and patient services, including patient satisfaction, clinical records, patient handouts, marketing materials, and statements of patient rights and responsibilities. Items needed about the physician and other staff members include continuing education schedules and personnel records. Other details must be supplied regarding emergency drills, maintenance, laboratory statistics, committee and governing body meetings, credentialing and privileging policies, audit and balance sheets, Medicare reports, and quality improvement.

A mock survey is invaluable. Some healthcare organizations hire a consultant to help with the preparation for an accreditation survey, although such consultants are not allowed to actively participate in the survey.

In recognition of the need for quality consultative guidance, the AAAHC established Healthcare Consultants International to provide office-based policy and procedure manuals, telephone consultation, and on-site training. Private consulting organizations provide similar services.

Table 11.3 Items reviewed during an accreditation survey

Statement of patient rights and responsibilities
Governing body and committee meeting minutes
Personnel records for physician and non-physician staff
Credentialing and privileging policies
Patient satisfaction surveys
Clinical records
Recent audit and balance sheets
Emergency drill records
Patient handouts and marketing materials
Laboratory statistical reports
Maintenance logs
Reports of Medicare, local or state surveys
Continuing education schedules for physicians and non-physicians
Peer-based quality improvement program
Risk management program

Accreditation survey

An accreditation survey is an educational and consultative procedure and should not be seen as punitive. The survey reviews every aspect of the healthcare facility, not just the physical environment (Fig. 11.2), and surveyors will take time to check a number of policies and procedures, including those listed in Table 11.3. The purpose of this review is to make sure the surveyed organization is doing what they say they are doing. Similar to the clinical record, if it is not written down, it did not happen.

The surveyor inspects the facilities and the environment during an initial orientation tour, and again while watching a typical surgical procedure. All medical equipment must have maintenance tags to show that it is in proper working condition. All medications and materials in the crash cart and surgical areas must be up-to-date. There should be a safe procedure for handling narcotics. A surgical procedure is observed to ensure that proper sterile technique is followed, to assess surgical skill, and to follow postoperative recovery.

The accreditation survey is usually performed by one or two surveyors over a day, or a day and a half, depending on the size and scope of the organization. In this time, surveyors may speak with the staff informally, or during formal interviews, to gain an understanding of the general climate of the organization. Personnel may be asked questions about several issues, thus:

- What do you think is good about the organization and what should be changed?
- Would you bring family members to the facility to be seen as patients?
- Are you happy with your employment?
- Are you aware of the policy or procedure for a particular activity?
- Are you involved in quality improvement?
- How is information shared within the organization?
- What are you most proud of in the organization?

Personnel should answer these questions honestly and should avoid fabricating their answers. If they are unable to answer a question they should say 'I do not know the answer but I know where I can find the answer.' The

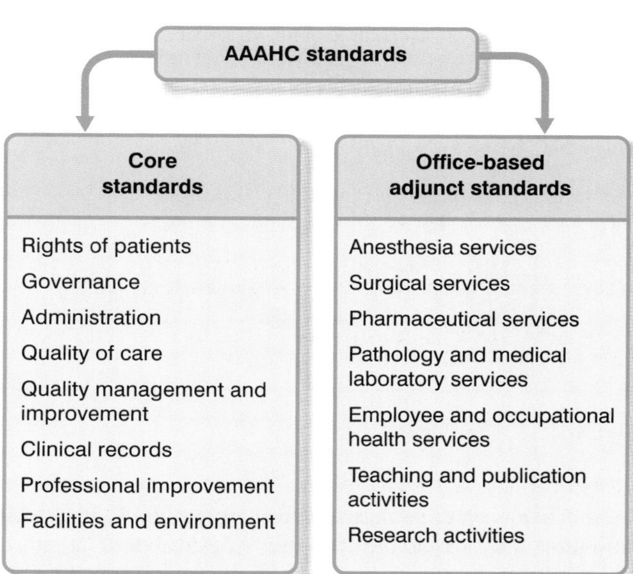

Figure 11.2 AAAHC standards.[2]

personnel should be reassured by the surveyed organization that their comments will not be the cause of a failure to achieve accreditation.

Documented policies, procedures, credentialing, privileging, quality improvement, and risk management activities are points of emphasis by the surveyors.

Summation conference

Unless the survey is for a Medicare Certificate, an accreditation decision will not be given for several months. The surveyors report the findings to the healthcare organization at a summation conference, which involves a dialogue between the surveyors and the principals of the organization.

Survey report and accreditation decision

After the summation conference a survey report is submitted to an accreditation committee, which decides whether or not accreditation is granted. The whole process takes time, and so it may take several months for final notification to come through. The AAAHC gives various accreditation decisions based upon compliance with the standards, and these are:

- 3-year, 1-year or 6-month accreditation terms
- a deferred accreditation decision
- a denial of accreditation.

Of course, the healthcare organization has the right to appeal the decision.

Ongoing changes in the accreditation process for office-based surgery

Because of the explosive growth in office-based surgery, an estimated 82% of surgical cases will be carried out in the outpatient setting by 2006. These figures have had a profound impact on the private accreditation organizations and on the government. In September 2001, the AAAHC established an Office-Based Surgery Accreditation program in an attempt to streamline the accreditation process. This program utilizes a single surveyor for a 1-day survey, using a special AAAHC handbook which emphasizes and explains the standards specifically required of small offices. The program is designed for an organization with no more than four surgeons or dentists and with no more than two operating rooms.[1]

In the various states of the USA an inconsistent patchwork of regulations is being promulgated regarding office-based physicians. Uniform federal involvement is not likely.

Credentialing and privileging

Both credentialing and privileging are time limited, and they must be renewed every 2–3 years. As regards the survey, both processes consist of three stages, and all of these must be completed for accreditation.

Credentialing involves reviewing documentation that shows an individual meets specific criteria for working within an organization. These documents include diplomas, current licenses, board certification, and Drug Enforcement Administrative (DEA) certificates. Thus the three stages of credentialing are:

- to establish that minimum training, experience and other requirements are appropriate
- to establish a process to review, assess and validate an individual's qualifications
- to carry out the review, assessment, and validation independently.[2]

It should be noted that an organization cannot rely upon another entity, such as a hospital, to verify credentials.

Privileging determines the specific procedures and treatments that a healthcare professional can perform. For example, a physician might be able to carry out specific activities, such as admitting a patient, or performing surgery. The three stages of privileging are:

- to determine which clinical procedures and treatments are offered to patients
- to determine the qualifications related to training and experience required to obtain each privilege
- to establish a process to evaluate the applicant's qualifications.[2]

National standards do not exist for credentialing and privileging, so each organization must have in place its own processes and standards. The credentials and privileges of the individual practitioners will have been reviewed by the appropriate medical staff committee and the governing body.

A dermatologist who provides satisfactory evidence of completion of an appropriate training course for specific surgical procedures should be credentialed and privileged to perform those procedures. Dermatology organizations should carry out an independent evaluation process to confirm clinical competency.

It is rare that dermatologists are represented on hospital medical staff credentialing committees, because they work primarily in the outpatient setting. Of course, hospitals compete economically with ASCs and office-based facilities, meaning that any legislative, regulatory, or administrative requirements mandating that dermatologists obtain hospital credentialing and privileging to perform outpatient procedures will limit patient choice and increase the cost of care.[3] The standards of the AAAASF require that a physician should have hospital privileges in order to perform procedures in the outpatient setting, and the JCAHO has established a standard that whereby physicians must perform a minimum number of procedures in the hospital each year to retain privileges in the outpatient setting.

Several states are developing alternative credentialing and privileging programs for outpatient surgical procedures. These are usually administered through the state medical licensing board. Dermatologists need to be involved in the development of these legislative, regulatory and administrative requirements.

Quality assurance and improvement

To obtain accreditation, a healthcare organization must develop a quality assurance and improvement program that links quality improvement activities, peer review, and risk management in an organized and systematic manner. The organization under investigation should be able to produce a document which outlines the structure and design of the quality assurance and improvement program. The plan should be simple and understandable, and must be accomplishable in the office setting. Samples of such plans have been published.[4,5]

Quality assurance and improvement studies should be carried out using the scientific method, whereby a question is clearly identified, the data are collected, a hypothesis is developed and tested, and a theory is established. This method relies on logic, data, and commonsense.

Quality improvement techniques

Quality improvement techniques analyze processes that increase efficiency and productivity. We know that 85% of medical errors result from faults in a process and 15% result from human error.

The process to be improved—the problem—must be identified. It must be relevant to the physician's office. Suitable targets for analysis might include clinical problems, administrative functions, cost of care issues, and ultimately patient outcomes.[5,6] Remember that problems which occurred only once should have been fixed already and should not, therefore, be made the subject of a quality assurance and improvement study. Patient satisfaction surveys can indicate problem areas and can be a starting point for a quality assurance and improvement study.

One or more methods to improve the process are selected. The new process is then tested and improvement is verified over time, following the Deming circle (Fig. 11.3), which summarizes the problem analysis process in terms of planning, doing, checking and acting. On completion of the quality assurance and improvement study, the results are reported to the governing body.

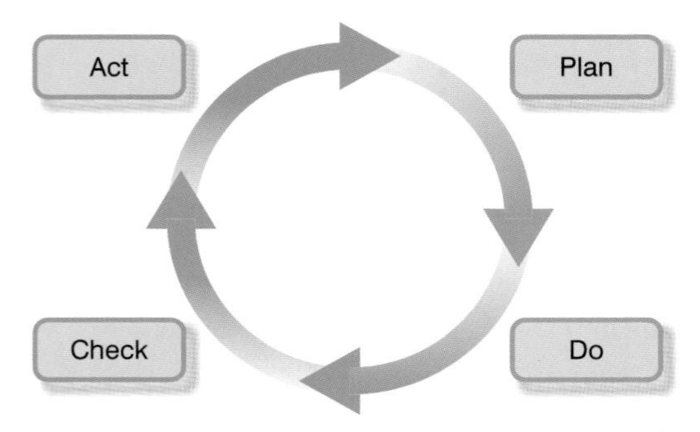

Figure 11.3 The Deming circle.

Another way to look at improving quality is by 'closing the loop,' as advocated by the AAAHC and shown in Figure 11.4. In this scheme, a problem is identified, the process is evaluated, corrective actions are implemented, the process is reevaluated, and the results are reported to the governing body. Ideally, to provide peer-based review, at least two physicians should be actively involved in quality improvement activities. 'Peer-based' means that physicians evaluate physicians, nurses evaluate nurses, and administrators evaluate administrators.

In solo dermatology practices, peer-based review can involve exchanging patient charts, pathology slides, or Mohs sections with another physician—preferably a dermatologist. These physicians are involved in the development of criteria to judge the quality of dermatologic care provided by the participants. If a dermatology office has few employees, the quality assurance and quality improvement committee can be small, but it should not be a committee of one.

Quality improvement activities require written documentation, just like the clinical record. The results of all the activities, even in a solo practice, need to be reported to the governing body. The results should also be communicated to

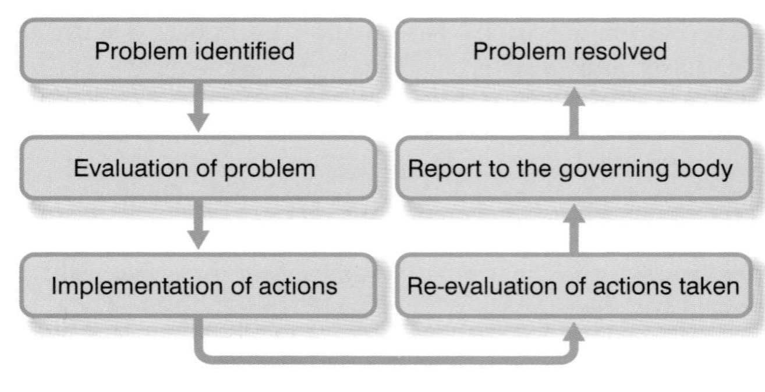

Figure 11.4 Closing the quality improvement loop.

other personnel, and presented during educational sessions such as staff meetings.

Accrediting bodies such as the AAAHC and the JCAHO require accredited healthcare organizations to compare themselves to similar organizations. This comparison is called benchmarking, and it compares key indicators, performance or outcome measures. A healthcare organization can benchmark against itself, or against the medical literature, or it can join a national study. These national studies are carried out by:

- the Institute for Quality Improvement (IQI), a non-profit subsidiary of AAAHC
- the Federated Ambulatory Surgery Association (FASA).

Dermatologists need to be actively involved in developing these comparisons.

Medicare certification and reimbursement

Medicare certification must be obtained in order to receive a facility fee from Medicare. The surgeons' fees are usually reduced when billed with a facility fee, but the net effect is increased reimbursement.

Achieving Medicare certification involves three main steps:

- operate according to the Medicare Conditions of Coverage standards—which can be obtained from the Centers for Medicare and Medicaid Services (CMS)
- obtain a Medicare survey
- obtain a Medicare provider number.[7]

Medicare standards tend to focus on the healthcare facility and environment rather than the quality of care. There are nine national standards and state-by-state Medicare standards.

Medicare surveys may be carried out by a state agency or an accreditation body with deemed status. Three national accrediting bodies, the AAAHC, JCAHO and AAAASF, have been deemed (approved) by the CMS to determine whether a healthcare facility meets the Medicare Conditions of Coverage (standards). During a deemed status survey, the additional Medicare standards are applied. Medicare surveys are always carried out on an 'unannounced' basis.

Office of Inspector General

The Office of Inspector General (OIG) enforces the Medicare certification process through unannounced inspections. The mission of the OIG is 'to protect the integrity of the Department of Health and Human Services programs as well as the health and welfare of beneficiaries served by them. This statutory mission is carried out through a nationwide program of audits, investigations, inspections, sanctions, and fraud alerts.'[8]

The problem is that OIG inspectors have no accountability. They interpret the Medicare Conditions of Coverage according to their own bias and prejudice. Their mission is to find fault with an ASC.

After an OIG inspection the ASC must offer a Plan of Correction, usually within 10 days, or else they risk losing Medicare certification and the resulting facility fees. The Plan of Correction is a detailed point-by-point response to the deficiencies in the Medicare Conditions of Coverage as documented by the OIG.

State licensing and certificate of need

Early in the development of an ASC two questions need to be answered:

- Is licensure of ASCs required in your state?
- Is a certificate of need (CON) required?

State licensing requirements vary from those that are non-existent to those involving many pages of specifications. Procedures that may be performed can be limited by state regulations. Some states offer exemptions from all or some of the requirements for ASCs in physicians' offices, smaller facilities, and single specialty facilities. Exemptions can be obtained on an individual basis.

In more than half of the states, CON laws regulate the building, opening, expansion, services provided, and sales of ASCs (see Tables 11.4, 11.5, 11.6). Exemptions may be obtained for office-based surgery, for new projects costing less than a specific dollar amount, for relocations, expansions or renovations, and for change of ownership.

Ambulatory surgery centers in office-based practices may be exempt from the CON regulations in many states if certain conditions are met. Such factors include the following:

- the ASC will not be Medicare certified
- only physicians in the practice will use the facility
- the number of operating rooms does not exceed a specified number
- the dollar amount spent on the facility and equipment does not exceed a specified amount.

However, payers may refuse to pay facility fees by arguing that the facility is a physician practice and not an ASC.

Most states require that a letter of intent be filed before a CON application. This letter may need to provide detailed information about the location, the number of operating rooms, the area served, the types of services provided, and the source of financing. It informs not only the respective state agency about the intent to file a CON, but also any group that may oppose the development of an ASC. Typically the opponents will be hospitals or other ASCs that do not want competition. The CON may be contested by hospitals or other ASCs through an administrative appeal, or by legal action.

States may use objective numeric criteria or subjective criteria to judge whether or not to approve a CON. The objective criteria may be based on population per operating room, number of cases per operating room, or similar factors, in the area served by the CON applicant.

Throughout the CON application and the hearing process three or four key arguments in favor of granting the CON should be developed. For example, one argument is that the ASC can provide lower costs for patients and payers than local hospitals. This can be demonstrated when comparing the explanation of benefits (EOBs) and co-payments for Medicare patients from local hospitals against those for an ASC. Letters from prominent individuals, payers, and community groups should confirm that the ASC should result in a higher quality of patient care and lower costs than hospitals.

Table 11.4 States with CON laws applying to ASCs	
Alabama	Mississippi
Alaska	Missouri
Connecticut	Montana
Delaware	Nevada
District of Columbia	New Hampshire
Georgia	New York
Hawaii	North Carolina
Illinois	Rhode Island
Iowa	South Carolina
Kentucky	Tennessee
Maine	Vermont
Maryland	Virginia
Massachusetts	Washington
Michigan	West Virginia

Table 11.5 States with CON laws that do not apply to ASCs	
Arkansas	Ohio
Florida	Oklahoma
Louisiana	Oregon
Nebraska	Wisconsin
New Jersey	

Table 11.6 States with no CON laws	
Arizona	New Mexico
California	North Dakota
Colorado	Pennsylvania
Idaho	South Dakota
Indiana	Texas
Kansas	Utah
Minnesota	Wyoming

A second argument might be developed if it can be shown that patients have to wait for surgery because community operating rooms are busy. This is an easy argument if 950 or 1000 cases per year are carried out in each operating room. If the operating rooms are being used for less than 700 or 800 cases per year it is difficult to demonstrate overuse. Alternatively, operating room capacity can be estimated by dividing the total number of hours that an operating room is open by the average number of hours spent on each case. As inpatient cases generally take longer than outpatient cases, it is important to distinguish between inpatient and outpatient operating rooms.

A third argument may focus on the preferred way for the community to expand services. Factors to take into account include the cost of reconfiguring a hospital, and the relative cost of outpatient surgery in a hospital, in an ASC, and in an office.

Of critical importance is to define the CON planning area in a way that is favorable to the project. This is the equivalent of gerrymandering a political district.

State legislation and regulation

Office-based surgery has been regulated primarily by one of two methods:

- individual states have laws and regulations and the penalty for non-compliance is a disciplinary proceeding against the physician's or dentist's license, or a fine (Table 11.7)
- a few states have voluntary guidelines or position statements, which may be used to establish standards in cases of medical malpractice.

Typically, the requirements address the duration of surgery, the level of anesthesia, emergency protocols, the training and qualifications of the surgeon and other personnel, the necessary equipment, and the reporting of adverse outcomes.

The regulatory process begins with passing a law (statute) which is enforced through regulations developed by the appropriate state agency. Many states have regulated office-based surgery through state boards of medicine. The following examples illustrate the varied approaches taken by the states:

The political climate changed in September 1994 with the regulation of office-based medicine by California legislation under AB 595.[9] These regulations apply to facilities using anesthesia (excluding local anesthesia and nerve blocks). The current Californian definition includes conscious sedation. The legislation requires offices to obtain:

- a state license
- Medicare certification or accreditation by an approved organization
- a written transfer agreement with a hospital, physician staff privileges at a hospital, or a plan for handling medical emergencies.

The law was revised in 1999 to require a minimum level of liability insurance coverage, the reporting of complications, and prominent display of the accreditation certificate.

In Florida from 1999 to 2000, the board of medicine adopted a set of rules which require that the following are mandatory:

- hospital privileges for offices using 'level 3' anesthesia (general anesthesia, spinal anesthesia, major intravenous anesthesia)
- hospital transfer agreements
- reporting of adverse incidents in medical offices.

State societies representing dermatology, plastic surgery, and cosmetic surgery sued for injunctive relief and won in a lower court only to have it reversed by the Court of Appeals. The New York State Department of Health developed guidelines in consultation with dermatologic surgeons. The guidelines were overturned by the New York Supreme Court, which said that the department did not have the authority to promulgate guidelines or regulations. Several bills to require regulations have been defeated in the New York state legislature. The state of New Jersey developed regulations in 1999 that required hospital privileges for 'surgery' in medical offices or 'alternative' credentialing by the board of medicine. The final program is still in the development stage.

In a process which began in 2001, the Ohio Board of Medicine deliberated for over 2 years about regulations for

Table 11.7 Office-based surgery statute or rule (revised 22 October 2003)

Current Laws and Regulations			
State Statute or Rule	**Entity**	**Agency**	**Description**
Arizona			
Az. Rev. Stat., Sect. 36–402(3)	Physician offices	Dept of Health Services, Divn of Assurance and Licensure Services	The department accepts accreditation reports from recognized entities such as AAAHC in lieu of licensing inspections for health care institutions. Physician offices and clinics are exempt from the licensing requirements applicable to healthcare institutions unless patients are kept overnight as bed patients or treated otherwise under general anesthesia, except where treatment by general anesthesia is regulated under the dentistry statutes.
California			
Health Safety Code, Ch. A.3, Section 1248; Bus. & Prof. Code, Sect. 216.1, 2216.2, 2240	Outpatient facilities	Medical Board of California	Licensure, Medicare certification, or accreditation is required for all outpatient settings where anesthesia is used (excluding local or peripheral nerve blocks). The Division of Licensing has approved AAAHC, JCAHO, AAAASF and IMQ as state-recognized accreditation agencies. The legislation also contains a number of other requirements such as those relating to liability insurance coverage, reporting complications, adequate personnel, and written discharge criteria. Facilities must be state licensed, Medicare-certified, or accredited by an accrediting agency approved by the medical board in order to charge and collect a facility fee for use of the emergency room or operating room of the facility for services provided to injured employees under the state's workers' compensation laws. Liposuction extraction and postoperative care standards for outpatient settings went into effect on February 20, 2003. Procedures performed under general anesthesia or intravenous sedation, or which result in the extraction of 5000 or more cubic centimeters of total aspirate, must be performed in a hospital or an outpatient setting that is licensed, or accredited by one of the approved entities listed above.
Colorado			
Policy Statement 40–12	Office-based surgery and anesthesia	Board of Medical Examiners	In November 2001 the board adopted a policy statement regarding the provision of surgical and anesthesia services in office settings. Overnight patient stays are not recommended unless the facility is accredited as a 'Class B or C facility' by the AAAHC, JCAHO, AAAASF, or Colorado Dept of Public Health and the Environment.
Connecticut			
Conn. Gen. Stats Sect. 19a-691; SB 1148 (signed into law on June 26, 2003)	Offices where certain types of anesthesia are administered	Dept of Public Health	Any office or unlicensed facility at which moderate sedation/analgesia, deep sedation/analgesia, or general anesthesia is administered must be accredited by AAAHC, JCAHO or AAAASF, or be Medicare-certified, within 18 months of administering such sedation or anesthesia, or by December 31, 2002, whichever is later. Legislation enacted in 2003 impacts physician offices in which moderate or deep sedation or general anesthesia is performed. The law places a 1-year moratorium, until July 1, 2004, on development of such new outpatient surgical centers unless they submit to the CON process. The law also establishes an advisory committee to review CON and its potential impact on outpatient

Table 11.7 Office-based surgery statute or rule—cont'd

Current Laws and Regulations			
State Statute or Rule	**Entity**	**Agency**	**Description**
			surgical centers, as well as requiring the department to develop a system of licensure for outpatient surgical centers by 2007.
District of Columbia			
	Office-based surgery	Board of Medicine	The Board issued an advisory in 2000 that it will follow ASA guidelines in determining the acceptable standard of care in cases involving office-based anesthesia.
Florida			
Fla. Stats. Sect. 458.309(1), (3); 458.351(6); 455.681 Fla. Admin. Code Rules 64B-9.009, 9.0091, 9.0092	Office surgery performed in facility not regulated by AHCA or the Dept of Health	Board of Medicine Dept of Health	Florida law requires Dept of Health inspections for physician office facilities where certain levels of surgery are performed, unless a nationally recognized accrediting agency or another accrediting organization subsequently approved by the Board of Medicine accredits the offices. Physicians performing certain levels of surgery in an office are required to register with the board and indicate whether their office is accredited or subject to a state inspection. The rules recognize AAAHC, JCAHO, AAAASF and the Florida Academy of Cosmetic Surgery as approved accrediting agencies. The rules also require compliance with a number of state standards for office-based surgery. *In Aug. 2000, the board imposed a 90-day moratorium on Level III surgery performed in physician offices that are not licensed as ASCs. Level III surgery is defined as surgery that involves, or reasonably should require, the use of a general anesthesia or major conduction anesthesia and preoperative sedation. The moratorium expired in November 2000, but in July 2001 the board imposed new restrictions on surgery performed on certain high-risk patients, limited volume removal for liposuction performed in combination with other procedures, adopted ASAs standards for basic anesthetic monitoring and required a risk management program.*
Illinois			
Rules for the Administration of the Medical Practice Act of 1987, Sect. 1285.340; added at 26 Ill. Reg. 7243	Office-based anesthesia	Dept of Professional Regulation	The department has established minimum CME and ACLS certification requirements for operating physicians, anesthesiologists and CRNAs who administer certain levels of anesthesia in physician offices. The requirements are phased in beginning on December 31, 2002.
Kansas			
	Office-based surgery	Kansas Medical Society	The society adopted guidelines for surgical and special procedures performed in offices and other unregulated clinical locations, involving anesthesia levels greater than minimal sedation. The guidelines encourage accreditation, especially for locations where procedures are performed that require general anesthesia.
Massachusetts			
Massachusetts Medical Society Guidelines for Office-Based Surgery; S. 639 (introduced in 2003)	Office-based surgery	Mass. Medical Society Board of Registration in Medicine	In December 2002, the Board endorsed the medical society's guidelines, which are based on the level of anesthesia and the complexity of the procedures performed. In addition to other requirements, the recommendations provide that offices where surgery other than minor procedures are performed should be

Table 11.7 Office-based surgery statute or rule—cont'd

Current Laws and Regulations			
State Statute or Rule	**Entity**	**Agency**	**Description**
			accredited by AAAHC, JCAHO, AAAASF, AOA, AAOMS Office Anesthesia Evaluation program, or any other agency approved by the Board. S. 639 was introduced to require licensure and a determination of need for any entity that provides ambulatory surgery. The legislation's sponsor indicated that he will amend the bill to exempt accredited entities.
Mississippi			
Mississippi State Board of Medical Licensure, Rules and Regulations, Article XXIV	Office-based surgery	State Board of Medical Licensure	Depending on the level of surgery performed, the board's requirements address surgeon registration, surgical logs and records, reporting of adverse incidents, equipment, supplies, and training of surgeons. The board provides an alternative credentialing mechanism for procedures outside a physician's core curriculum. Strong recommendations are included for amount of fat to be removed using tumescent liposuction.
New Jersey			
NJAC 13:35–4A.12; 17; A. 2758 (pending)	Office-based surgery and anesthesia	Board of Medical Examiners	Regulations govern the administration of office-based anesthesia, including standards for training, credentialing, staffing, equipment, and reporting. In December 2002 the Board issued the final rule detailing the alternative privileging mechanism for office-based physicians who do not hold hospital privileges. Certain documentation of competence, training, and clinical experience are required to obtain privileges for performing surgery or special procedures, performing or supervising general and regional anesthesia or conscious sedation, or utilizing lasers. The privileging requirement is not imposed for 'minor surgery' although certain procedures, such as liposuction and breast augmentation, are not considered minor. Privileges are granted for 2 years. Initial applications should have been submitted by 16 December 2003. Physicians who submit an application for alternative privileging may continue to provide services until the Board acts on their application. With the adoption of the rule, the Board has begun developing the list of acceptable in-office procedures, the alternative privileging application forms, and criteria for selecting entities to review the documentation submitted along with application. In September 2002, A. 2758 was introduced proposing that the department regulates and inspects unlicensed surgical offices of physicians who are not accredited, who do not participate in Medicare or HMO provider networks, and do not have hospital privileges.
New York			
A 5017, S 4235, S 4724 (introduced in 2003)	Office-based surgery	State Department of Health	In 2000, the department adopted a committee report recommending voluntary clinical guidelines for office-based surgery to serve as an appropriate standard of care, excluding minor procedures. The guidelines contain recommendations for qualification of practitioners and staff, equipment, facilities and policies and procedures for patient assessment and monitoring. The report recommends that office-based practices strongly consider the use of outside accrediting agencies to help assure

Table 11.7 Office-based surgery statute or rule—cont'd

		Current Laws and Regulations	
State Statute or Rule	**Entity**	**Agency**	**Description**
			the public that they are providing care and services in a safe environment and adhering to the highest standards of quality and professionalism. The report describes AAAHC, JCAHO, AAAASF and AMAP as accrediting organizations. A state court ruled that the department did not have legal authority to adopt and may not enforce the guidelines. Legislation was introduced in 2003 to establish enforceable office-based surgery standards and require reporting of incidents.
North Carolina			
Position Statement on Office-based Procedures	Office-based surgery	North Carolina Medical Board	On 23 January 2003, the board approved a position statement of standards of practice. By January 2004 any physician performing level II or III procedures in an office should be able to demonstrate substantial compliance with the guidelines, or obtain accreditation by a nationally recognized agency such as AAAHC, JCAHO, AAAASF, HFAP, or other board-approved agency. Other guidelines address physician credentialing, including an alternative privileging option, emergencies, performance improvement, medical records, patient selection, equipment and supplies, and personnel. Failure to comply creates the risk of disciplinary action by the board.
Ohio			
Administrative Code Sect. 4731–25–01 to 07	Office-based surgery	State of Ohio Medical Board	The Medical Board approved regulations requiring accreditation of offices where physicians or podiatrists perform surgery using moderate sedation or higher anesthesia. The rule took effect on 1 January 2004. Application is required within 18 months of that date and accreditation must be obtained within 3 years of that date. AAAHC, JCAHO, AAAASF, HFAP, and any other board-approved agencies are recognized. The rules also contain education, training and experience requirements for surgery and anesthesia, and limits on liposuction.
Oklahoma			
	Office-based surgery	State Board of Medicine	The Board adopted guidelines for physicians who perform procedures that require anesthesia or sedation in an office setting.
Oregon			
Oregon Admin. Rules Sect. 818-012-0005	Office-based surgery	Oregon Medical Assoc.	The medical association has developed standards for accreditation of facilities where minor procedures or those requiring conscious sedation are performed in an office setting. The association is considering revisions, including possible use of accreditation by outside entities.
Pennsylvania			
Pa. Rules and Regulations, Title 28, Part IV, Subpart F, Ch. 551–571 Pa. Rules and Regulations, Title 28, Part I, Ch. 9	Ambulatory surgery facilities (includes physician offices with a distinct part used solely for surgery on a regular and organized basis) HMOs	Dept of Health	For class A, limited to local or topical anesthesia, ASFs must register and obtain accreditation from AAAHC, JCAHO or AAAASF. For higher classes, B and C, licensure is required, although the rules allow the department. to delegate the survey function to nationally recognized accreditation agencies. At this time, the department does not recognize accreditation for class B or C licensure but

Table 11.7 Office-based surgery statute or rule—cont'd

	Current Laws and Regulations		
State Statute or Rule	**Entity**	**Agency**	**Description**
			conducts its own licensure surveys. External quality review is required for licensure of HMOs. AAAHC accreditation has been recognized as meeting this requirement. The department revised its regulations and is expected to issue RFPs to approve external quality reviews organizations.
Rhode Island			
RI Stats., Ch. 23–17 Dept of Health Rules and Regulations, R23–17-POSPST	Office-based surgery	Dept of Health	The department issued regulations requiring licensure for offices in which surgery other than minor procedures is performed, along with other requirements. Physicians who provide such services must be licensed. Application for accreditation by AAAHC, JCAHO or AAAASF is required within 9 months from initial licensure, with accreditation required within 2 years after licensure. Accreditation must be maintained as a condition of licensure thereafter. In June 2002 the enabling law was amended to specifically include office-based podiatry.
South Carolina			
	Office-based surgery	Board of Medical Examiners	The board approved guidelines for office-based surgery, requiring accreditation by an approved agency, including AAAHC, JCAHO, AAAASF, and AOA for offices in which level II and III procedures are performed, in addition to certain other requirements. The guidelines are recommended as an appropriate standard of care.
Texas			
22 TAC Sect. 192.1–192.6 22 TAC Sect. 221.1–221.17	Outpatient surgical settings that are not part of a licensed hospital or ASC	State Board of Medical Examiners State Board of Nursing Examiners	The two boards adopted regulations governing physicians and CRNAs providing or administering general or regional anesthesia, or monitored anesthesia, in outpatient settings. The regulations exempt licensed ASCs and outpatient settings accredited by AAAHC, JCAHO, and AAAASF.
Virginia			
18 VAC 85-20-310 to 390 (Emergency Regulations effective until 17 November 2003)	ASCs and office-based surgery	Board of Medicine	The board issued emergency regulations governing office-based anesthesia to be effective from 18 November 2002 to 17 November 2003. The regulations cover non-hospital settings where moderate sedation or higher levels are administered, and include reporting and other requirements. Legislation required the board to adopt regulations by 7 January 2003, but it could not complete the regulatory process by that date, thus necessitating emergency regulations until the adoption of a final rule.
Washington			
	Office-based surgery	Washington State Medical Assoc.	The state medical assn. adopted guidelines for office-based anesthesia that include accreditation by AAAHC, JCAHO, AAAASF or Medicare of offices that conduct conscious or deep sedation, or general anesthesia. The Medical Quality Assurance Commission has begun a process to draft regulations for oversight of office-based surgery. Four public workshops were held in 2003.

Table 11.7 Office-based surgery statute or rule—cont'd

Regulations in Developmental or Drafting Stage†			
Statute or Rule	**Entity**	**Agency**	**Description**
Alabama			
Ch. 540-X-10, Rules of the Alabama Board of Medical Examiners	Office-based surgery	Alabama Board of Medical Examiners	In conjunction with an ad hoc multispecialty committee, the board proposed regulations for office-based surgery procedures. As revised on 20 August 2003 the proposed regulations encourage accreditation surveys for facilities where deep sedation/analgesia or general anesthesia is provided.
Arizona			
	Office-based surgery	Arizona Board of Medical Examiners	A board-appointed committee is drafting guidelines.
Iowa			
HB 256 (introduced in February 2003)	Office-based surgery	Dept of Inspections and Appeals	Legislation was introduced to provide for licensing and regulation of office-based surgical sites.
Louisiana			
Proposed Administrative Code Title 46, Ch. 73	Office-based surgery	State Board of Medical Examiners	In October 2003 the board published a notice of intent to adopt rules to regulate office procedures requiring deep sedation or general anesthesia. Exemptions include offices accredited by AAAHC, JCAHO, or AAAASF, and procedures performed by an oral and maxillofacial surgeon within the dentistry scope of practice. The rules will take effect in 2005 and include reports of adverse incidents. The board accepted public comments until November 21 2003.
Tennessee			
Proposed Rule 0880-2-21	Office-based surgery	Tennessee Board of Medical Examiners	The board has proposed detailed regulations that include administration, quality of care, clinical, credentialing, anesthesia, liposuction, and laser surgery limits and requirements. A surgeon would not be allowed to keep patients past midnight unless the office where the procedure is performed is accredited by AAAHC or AAAASF. The board is considering another draft that would require accreditation of certain offices.

**For office-based surgery procedures meeting certain thresholds, Connecticut, Ohio, Pennsylvania, and Rhode Island require accreditation. California and Florida require state certification or accreditation. North Carolina and Texas exempt accredited settings from surgery/anesthesia standards. Illinois, Mississippi, New Jersey, and Virginia adopted office anesthesia or surgery regulations. Colorado, District of Columbia, Kansas, Massachusetts, New York, North Carolina, Oklahoma, and South Carolina adopted voluntary guidelines or policy statements. Oregon and Washington adopted guidelines through their state medical association. Arizona prohibits treatment under general anesthesia in unlicensed physician offices.*

†This information was compiled from a variety of sources, including NCSL, AMA, medical specialty societies, regulators, and accreditation organizations. AAAHC cannot guarantee its complete accuracy, and continues to research state statutes and rules governing ambulatory health care.

AAAASF, American Association for Accreditation of Ambulatory Surgical Facilities; AAAHC, Accreditation Association for Ambulatory Health Care; AMA, American Medical Association; AOA, American Osteopathic Association; ASC, ambulatory surgical center; CME, continuing medical education; CON, Certificate of Need; CRNA, Certified Registered Nurse Anesthetist; HFAP, Healthcare Facilities Accreditation Program; HMO, health maintenance organization; JCAHO, Joint Commission on Accreditation of Healthcare Organizations; NCSL, National Conference of State Legislatures; OIG, Office of Inspector General; RFP, request for proposal.

Table 11.8 Useful website addresses

American Academy of Dermatology (AAD)	www.aad.org
Accreditation Association for Ambulatory Health Care (AAAHC)	http://www.aaahc.org (last accessed June 2004)
American Association for Accreditation of Ambulatory Surgical Facilities (AAAASF)	http://www.aaaasf.org (last accessed June 2004)
Centers for Medicare and Medicaid Services (CMS)	http://www.cms.gov (last accessed June 2004)
Federated Ambulatory Surgery Association (FASA)	http://www.fasa.org (last accessed June 2004)
Joint Commission on Accreditation of Healthcare Organizations (JCAHO)	http://www.jcaho.org (last accessed June 2004)
Office of Inspector General (OIG)	http://www.oig.hhs.gov/

office-based surgery. The very restrictive language used in the initial regulations proposed by the board was modified following aggressive lobbying by the state dermatology society. In Texas, the state dermatology society has been very active and effective in lobbying the board of medicine to develop fair, appropriate and reasonable regulations.

These examples show that laws and regulations can be modified at many points in the process, including the legislature where the law is passed, the state agency or board of medicine where the regulations are formulated, and in the courts where the whole process can be overturned. It is extremely important to have an active state dermatology society, working in the legislative, executive, and judicial branches.

In a position statement on office-based medicine posted on its website (Table 11.8) The American Academy of Dermatology (AAD) supported the following:

- mandatory reporting of adverse incidents in a non-judgmental manner to the appropriate state agency—the way in which the basic information is reported and made available to appropriate researchers should not, however, subject the practitioner to malpractice challenges
- the use of general anesthesia in accredited facilities only
- 'reasonable, appropriate and fair' physician credentialing by state medical boards
- emergency transfer protocols for medical offices where surgical procedures are performed.

The AAD opposed the requirement for mandatory hospital staff privileges, hospital admitting privileges, and hospital transfer agreements for office-based surgery.

PITFALLS AND THEIR MANAGEMENT

Outdated and irrelevant policies and procedures

Dermatologic offices may have problems obtaining accreditation if they present outdated, irrelevant policies and procedures that were developed for another healthcare organization or written for the surveyor.[10] The policies and procedures must match what is really occurring in the office. Ideally the policies and procedures should be developed by the staff that follow them. If an organization uses a consultant's manual, or hospital or ASC policies and procedures as a model, it needs to modify them to fit its practice. Simply filling in the blanks and replacing the hospital's name is not appropriate.

Optimizing outcomes

- Expect preparation to take 1 year—a mock survey is invaluable, and a consultant can help in preparation.
- Update all documented policies and procedures.
- Make sure that all patient documentation is accurate and complete.
- Make sure that all credentialing and privileging is in order.
- Review and improve if necessary quality assurance/improvement and risk management activities.
- Check that all medications and materials in the crash cart and surgical areas are all up-to-date.
- Check that there is a safe procedure for handling narcotics.
- Check that all medical equipment has maintenance tags and is in excellent working condition.
- Ensure that all surgical procedures are carried out with proper sterile technique, appropriate surgical skill and postoperative recovery.

Inaccurate and incomplete documentation, credentialing and privileging

Incomplete or illegible medical charts can lead to failure of an accreditation survey. Common problems include failure to document the presence or absence of allergies, incomplete forms, or missing signatures. Medical charts need to be able to be read by the office staff.

A healthcare organization may fail an accreditation survey if credentialing is not completed, or if the information provided on, for example, diplomas, current licenses, board certification, and DEA certificates, is not independently verified. The organization should go directly to the source, whether medical school, state board or federal government agency, to verify the information. It is not sufficient to rely on the hospital or ASC for credentialing. A credentials verification organization (CVO) can perform this task for a nominal fee.

Another problem area is that of privileging. Privileges need to be site specific, reflecting the competence of the surgeon in that setting. For example, a surgeon may be able to perform cardiac transplantation in a hospital but not in an office-based facility.

Inadequate quality improvement program and safety plans

The organization should have a peer-based quality improvement program, which includes risk management. Organizations may also make mistakes in executing the program. The quality improvement studies should be simple, and frequently a one-page summary is adequate. It should address such topics as clinical issues, administrative problems, cost of care, and patient outcomes.

A one-time audit of charts is not a study—for example, operative reports are missing in 20% of patient charts. Changes in processes need to be made and followed over time, perhaps over 1, 3, 6, 9 or even 12 months. Safety plans should be active, with at least four fire and emergency drills performed each year. These drills should include response to a fire in the facility, and patient evacuation in response to a bomb threat or tornado, earthquake, or other natural disaster. Documentation should cover procedures that are carried out correctly and things that go wrong.

Inadequate government inspections

In March 2000 the OIG released a comprehensive evaluation of the accreditation survey process. It found that while private accreditation organizations were providing a good service, government inspections were inadequate.[8] In their report *Quality Oversight of ASCs: A System in Neglect*, the OIG assessed how state agencies and accreditation organizations oversee ASCs and their accountability to the CMS.

The evaluation was carried out by OIG personnel trained as surveyors who accompanied state agency and other surveyors on ASC surveys. The OIG report found that:

- regulation of ASCs has become increasingly important because the number of Medicare ASCs doubled between 1990 and 2000 and the number of major procedures increased from 12 000 to 101 000 per year
- almost one-third of ASCs certified by state agencies have not been re-certified in 5 years or more, whereas the private accreditation organizations survey every 3 years
- the approach of private accreditation organizations is more consultative and educational, rather than just a check on compliance
- the CMS does not hold the state agencies accountable to Medicare or the public

The OIG report goes on to recommend that:

- the CMS should determine a minimum cycle for surveying ASCs certified by state agencies
- the Medicare Conditions of Coverage used to determine compliance with Medicare standards should add sections on patient's rights and continuous quality improvement and should be adjusted to reflect the level of surgery (local anesthesia to general anesthesia) carried out by different ASCs
- the CMS should ensure that state agency certification and accreditation have the appropriate balance between compliance and continuous quality improvement
- the state agencies should be accountable to the Medicare program and the public for their performance in regulating ASCs.

PRACTICAL APPLICATIONS

Practical benefits for the dermatology office

The process of obtaining accreditation helps a dermatology office to:

- improve the care and services offered
- increase efficiency and reduce costs
- develop better risk management programs
- lower liability insurance premiums
- motivate personnel by instilling pride and loyalty
- strengthen public relations and marketing efforts
- recruit and retain qualified professional personnel.

Enhanced patient safety

Patient safety is a prime concern for all medical personnel and in office-based facilities this can be enhanced by accreditation, as documented by chart review[11] and questionnaire[12] studies.

A chart review study of 3615 patient charts with a 30-day follow-up period revealed no deaths, ventilator requirements, deep venous thromboses, or pulmonary emboli among those who had multiple procedures (24.3% of charts) though two patients (0.05%) had unplanned hospital admissions within 24 hours.[11]

A questionnaire study covered 400 675 operative procedures in 418 accredited office surgical facilities over a 5-year period.[12] The death rate was 1 in 57 000 (0.0017%) and the rate for significant complications (hematoma, hypertensive episode, wound infection, sepsis, or hypotension) was 1 in 213 cases. These rates are comparable to those of hospital and ambulatory surgery centers (ASCs).

One study demonstrated no difference in patient deaths between accredited and non-accredited facilities, but it did not state the total number of surgical procedures reviewed.[13] Patient deaths seem to be associated with general anesthesia and with prolonged combined procedures such as liposuction and abdominoplasty or face lift.

Using information collected by state agencies on the safety of office-based surgery, it has been concluded that 'mandatory reporting of adverse outcomes from office-based surgery is warranted to identify modifiable risk factors and reduce the risk of adverse outcomes.'[2]

To this end, more comprehensive studies of the perioperative risk for patients receiving office-based surgical care are needed.

SUMMARY

Dermatology office accreditation is important to improve the quality of medical, surgical, and cosmetic dermatologic care provided. Patient safety in office-based facilities can be enhanced by accreditation,[11,12] and this is a key healthcare issue. Accreditation can also be protective by reducing the imposition of government-mandated guidelines, regulations, and rules.

REFERENCES

1. Accreditation Association for Ambulatory Health Care. AAAHC Guidebook for Office Based Surgery Accreditation. 2003.
2. Balkrishnan R. No smoking gun: Findings from a national survey of office-based cosmetic surgery adverse event reporting. Dermatol Surg 2003; 29:1093–1099.
3. Accreditation Association for Ambulatory Health Care. Accreditation Handbook for Ambulatory Health Care. 2003; 23–25.

4. Davey WP. Quality improvement and management in a dermatology office. Arch Dermatol 1997; 133:1385–1387.
5. Kesheimer K, Davey WP. Continuous quality improvement in a dermatologic surgery office. Arch Dermatol 2000; 136:1400–1403.
6. American Academy of Dermatology Quality of Care Committee. Quality Assurance/Quality Improvement Self-Assessment Program. Schaumberg, IL: American Academy of Dermatology; 2001.
7. Becker S, Downing S, Moran M. Protecting Your ASC: A Legal Handbook. Alexandria, VA: Federated Ambulatory Surgery Association; 2002
8. Office of Inspector General. Quality oversight of ASCs: A system in neglect. OEI-01-00-00450. Boston: OEI.
9. Private communication from Larry Lanier, American Academy of Dermatology.
10. Taylor D, Iqbal Y. How to clear accreditation. Outpatient Surg Mag 2001: 2: 32–39.
11. Bitar G, Mullis W, Jacobs W, et al. Safety and efficacy of office-based surgery with monitored anesthesia care/sedition in 4778 consecutive plastic surgery procedures. Plast Reconstr Surg 2003; 111:150–156.
12. Morello DC, Colon GA, Fredericks S, et al. Patient safety in accredited office surgical facilities. Plast Reconstr Surg 1997; 99:1496–1500.
13. Coldiron B. Office surgical incidents: 19 months of Florida data. Dermatol Surg 2002; 28:710–712.

PART 2

Essential Surgical Skills

12 Electrosurgery, Electrocoagulation, Electrofulguration, Electrodesiccation, Electrosection, Electrocautery

Seaver L Soon MD and Carl V Washington Jr MD

Summary box

- Electrosurgery refers to thermal tissue damage as a result of tissue resistance to the passage of high-frequency, alternating electric current. It includes electrofulguration, electrodesiccation, electrocoagulation, and electrosection. Electrocautery is not a true form of electrosurgery as no current flows through the patient.
- The precise effect of electric current on tissue—whether superficial tissue dehydration, deep coagulation, or pure cutting—depends on current density, voltage, and electromagnetic waveform.
- Electrosurgery may be indicated for a variety of benign and superficially invasive malignant neoplasms.
- Electrodesiccation and curettage generally provide high cure rates for superficial and nodular basal cell carcinoma (BCC), although these rates depend significantly on lesion size, histologic subtype, and anatomic location.
- Randomized controlled studies suggest that modern electrosection units provide superior speed, hemostasis, cosmetic outcome, and less postoperative pain compared to conventional scalpel surgery, with comparable postoperative wound healing and infection rates.
- Adverse events associated with electrosurgery include electrical burns, electric shock, infection transmission, eye injury, and cardiac pacemaker and implantable cardioverter–defibrillator (ICD) malfunction. The actual risk of pacemaker and ICD malfunction is extremely low.

INTRODUCTION

Electrosurgery refers to the use of electricity to cause thermal tissue destruction, most commonly in the form of tissue dehydration, coagulation or vaporization. Electrosurgical procedures may be divided into four types based on their mechanism of tissue damage.

- Electrolysis—in which direct current induces tissue damage through a chemical reaction at the electrode tip.
- Coblation— in which high-frequency alternating current ionizes an electrically conductive medium, usually isotonic saline solution, which transmits heat to cause superficial epidermal and dermal damage with minimal collateral tissue destruction. Coblation is used for facial rejuvenation.
- High-frequency electrosurgery— in which tissue resistance to the passage of high-frequency alternating current converts electrical energy to heat, resulting in thermal tissue damage. Heat generation occurs within the tissue, while the treatment electrode remains 'cold'. This method includes electrodesiccation, electrofulguration, electrocoagulation, and electrosection.
- Electrocautery— in which direct or high-frequency alternating current heats an element, which causes thermal injury by direct heat transference. Unlike electrosurgery, the element in electrocautery is hot.

This chapter addresses high-frequency electrosurgery and electrocautery. Readers interested in electrolysis are referred elsewhere.[1] It is important that dermatologic surgeons using these techniques are familiar with fundamental concepts in the physics of electricity—such as current, resistance, voltage, power, and electrosurgical waveform output—as well as their effects on the skin. Sound knowledge in this area may optimize preoperative planning, choice of therapy, and postoperative results, and minimize the risk of electrical injury to both patient and physician.

Principles of electricity

Current, resistance, voltage, power, and electrosurgical waveform output are of clinical relevance because they determine the quality and extent of tissue damage. Electrical current refers to the net flow of electrons through a conductor per second, and is measured in amperes (where

1 ampere = 6.242 × 10^{18} electrons per second). An important concept regarding electricity in medicine is that the amount of current (defined as the number of electrons moving past a point per second) is the same for all cross-sections of a given conductor. This quantity refers to current density, defined as the amount of current per cross-sectional area (mathematically, $j = i/A$, where j is current density, i is current, and A is the cross-sectional area of the conductor). Thus, the thinner the electrosurgical tip (i.e. decreasing the cross-sectional area of the conductor, A), the greater the current density, j, at the point of electrode contact. High current density results in greater tissue injury, and is the basis of surgical diathermy (Fig. 12.1). Similarly, increasing the cross-sectional area of the electrode by a sufficient amount may decrease current density to a level of nondestructive tissue warming. This warming effect is the basis of medical diathermy (Fig. 12.2).[2,3]

The body acts as a conductor for electrical current as a result of the electrolyte composition of its cells. In living tissue, current flow consists of the transfer of charged ions within cells. There are two main types of current: direct and alternating. Direct current refers to electron flow in one direction, and is usually produced by a battery. When applied to living tissue, direct current depolarizes cell membranes and leads to neuromuscular excitation. Should this current be sustained for a period of time sufficient to prevent cell repolarization, the cells enter a refractory period wherein neuromuscular activity ceases. If the molecular reorientation induced by the direct current persists beyond this refractory period, cell death occurs. Therapeutic uses of direct current include electrolysis, iontophoresis, and, sometimes, electrocautery. To maintain cell viability, direct current may be applied in intermittent pulses to allow for cell membrane repolarization.[2,4]

Unlike direct current, alternating current continuously switches direction. It is produced in power generators and is available at electrical outlets. In the US, the average electrical outlet carries an alternating current with a frequency of 60 Hz (1 Hz = 1 cycle per second). When this type of current is applied to tissue, cellular ions are alternately pulled to and fro, resulting in rapid cellular depolarization, followed by repolarization as the current changes direction. Because cell membranes are rapidly depolarized and then repolarized, alternating current causes tetanic neuro-

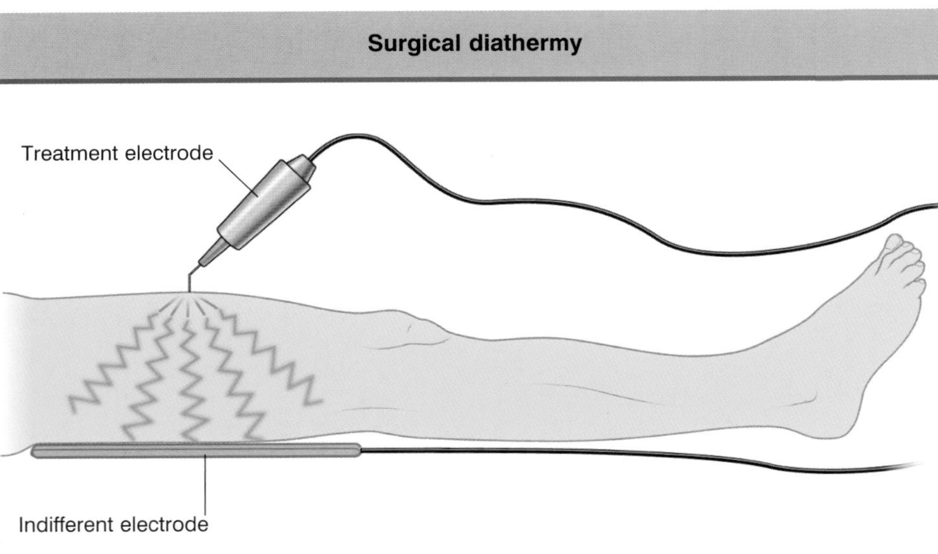

Figure 12.1 Decreasing the surface area of the treatment electrode increases current density.

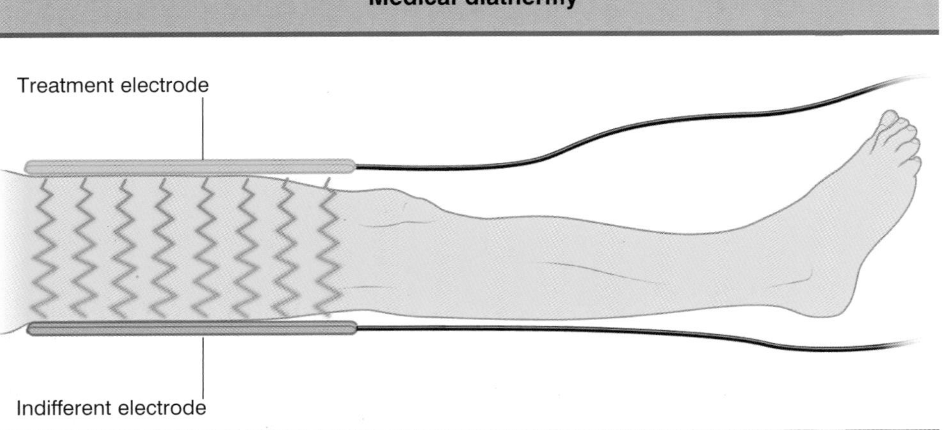

Figure 12.2 Increasing the surface area of the treatment electrode decreases current density.

muscular contraction with frequencies less than 1 kHz (kilohertz). This adverse effect decreases as frequency increases above 1 kHz, and becomes negligible at frequencies of 100 kHz or more. At these high frequencies, current reversal is so rapid that cellular ion position change is essentially nil, and depolarization fails to occur. Instead, electrical energy is converted to heat as a result of ionic collision. High-frequency alternating current thus makes it possible to exploit the heating effects of electricity while avoiding the undesirable neuromuscular effects. Electrosurgical units for electrosurgery and electrocautery utilize frequencies of 500–2000 kHz.[4,5]

Important concepts related to current include resistance and voltage. Resistance refers to the ability of a conductor to impede the passage of an electric current, and is measured in ohms (Ω). The resistance of a substance correlates with its length and cross-sectional area, as well as its resistivity (mathematically, $R = \rho \times l/A$, where R is resistance, ρ is resistivity, l is length, and A is cross-sectional area). Resistance is proportional to the length of the substance, and inversely proportional to its cross-sectional area. A material's resistivity refers to its inherent capacity to resist electric current. The human body is not a homogeneous electrical conducting medium, but consists of different tissues of varying resistivity. Fat has high resistivity, whereas muscle has low resistivity. Skin has variable resistivity depending on whether it is wet or dry: the resistivity of dry skin is colossal at 100 000 Ω, whereas that of wet skin is much lower at 200 Ω.

Voltage refers to the electrical force that induces electron flow when it is applied to a conductor, and is measured in volts (V). This so-called 'electromotive' force is generated by an electrical potential difference between the two ends of the conductor: one end is considered the negative pole (having a high concentration of negatively-charged electrons), while the other is considered the positive pole (having a low concentration of negatively charged electrons). Electric current always flows from a region of high electron concentration to one of low electron concentration. Ohm's law captures the relationship between voltage, current, and resistance mathematically as $V = iR$ (where V is voltage, i is current, and R is resistance). It is clear that for a given resistance, R, increasing the voltage increases current flow through a conductor, whereas decreasing the voltage decreases this flow. In the US, the average voltage available at electrical outlets is 110 V.[6]

The concept of power encompasses how current, voltage, and resistance interact to produce heat in tissue. Power is defined as the rate at which work is done ($P = W/t$, where W is work, and t is time) and is measured in watts (joules/second). This equation states that a given amount of work can be done in less time with increasing power. Work is defined as the product of force by the distance over which the force is applied ($W = F \times d$, where F is force and d is distance), and is measured in joules. In electricity, the work done refers to current flow over a specific distance as a result of a voltage difference. Tissue resistance to the passage of this current results in heat production. Power thus refers to the rate of heat energy produced as a result of tissue resistance to the passage of current induced by a voltage potential. Mathematically, $P = iV$ (where P is power, i is current, and V is voltage). By substituting Ohm's law ($V = iR$, or $i = V/R$), it is apparent that $P = i^2R$, or $P = V^2/R$. That is, power or heat produced is proportional to the product of the square of the current and tissue resistance, or the square of the voltage divided by tissue resistance. Thus power will increase with increments in both current and voltage; however, because resistance is constant, power increases more significantly with an increase in current rather than voltage. Most electrosurgical units operate using between 15 and 150 watts of power, which confers enough heat energy to vaporize water.[2,6]

'Ohmic heating,' or heat production as a result of tissue resistance to electric current, depends on factors such as resistance (and hence the resistivity and the length of the conductor), current density, and the duration of current application. For a given current density, heat production is greater in fat than muscle because of its higher resistivity. As resistance is proportional to conductor length, increasing the distance between a treatment and an indifferent electrode on the body similarly yields greater heat. Minimal heat is generated in substances of little resistance; a clinical example is the inefficacy of electrosurgery in the presence of blood, an electrolyte conductor. Increasing the current density or the duration of current application also results in greater thermal injury.[2,4]

As mentioned, standard electrical outlets in the US provide an alternating current of 60 Hz and 110 V. Electrosurgical procedures, however, require much higher frequencies (because low frequencies cause tetany), a range of voltage, and current intensities, as well as different waveforms to provide the appropriate level of destruction for the clinical indication. These ends are achieved through current modification by the electrosurgical unit.

Electrosurgical units and waveforms

An electrosurgical unit is essentially a high-frequency current generator consisting of three components: a transformer, which modifies the voltage; an oscillating circuit, which increases the frequency; and the patient circuit, which comprises the handpiece, the patient, and, in certain cases, the indifferent electrode.

A transformer is a device that uses alternating current in one circuit to produce a voltage and current in a second circuit, and consists of two wire coils placed adjacent to one another. Available current from the electrical outlet flowing through the first or primary coil induces current flow in the secondary coil as a result of electromagnetic induction. The voltage of the induced current is directly proportional to the number of windings in the secondary coil relative to the primary coil. For example, if the number of windings in the secondary coil is ten times that of the primary coil, then the voltage of induced current is increased tenfold. This type of transformer is termed a 'step-up' transformer to reflect this voltage amplification. The voltage of the induced current may be similarly decreased should the secondary coil have fewer windings than the primary coil. This type of transformer is termed a 'step-down' transformer. Whereas a 'step-up' transformer is used in the spark gap electrosurgical unit, and typically increases the available electrical voltage from 120 V to 550–> 2000 V, both 'step-up' and 'step-down' transformers are used in the vacuum tube electrosurgical unit (Fig. 12.3).[7]

Following voltage transformation, current from the secondary coil enters an oscillating circuit, which increases

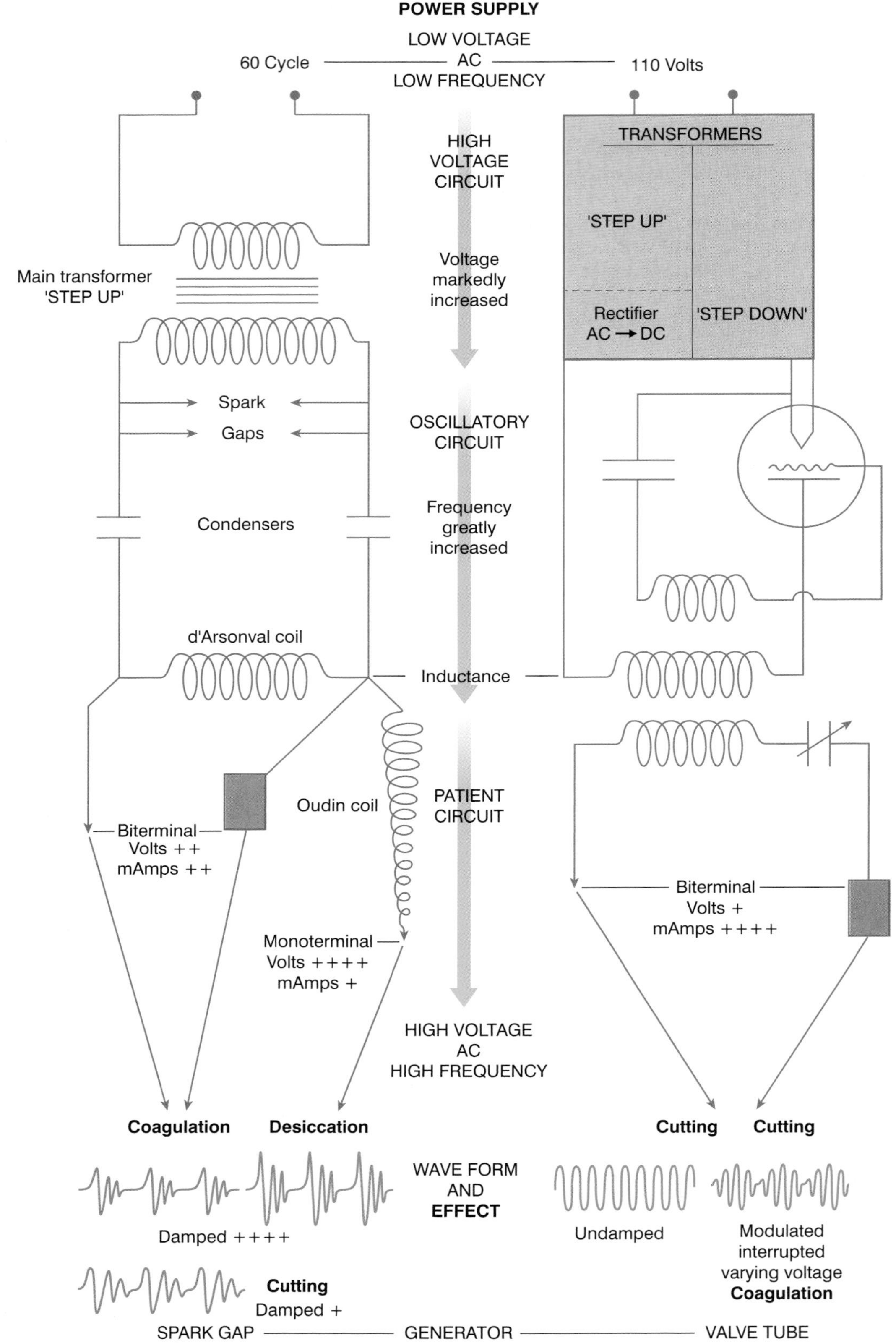

Figure 12.3 Spark-gap units produce damped waveforms. Vacuum-tube units produce undamped as well as blended waveforms. (Adapted from Crumay HM. Electrosurgery, cryosurgery, and hyperbaric oxygen therapy. In: Moschella SL, Hurley HJ. Dermatology. Philadelphia: WB Saunders; 1985.)

the frequency from the available 60 Hz to over 200 kHz. Two types of oscillatory circuits exist based on the component that produces the oscillation: the spark-gap unit and the vacuum-tube unit. Both consist of a condensor (or a capacitator, which stores electric charge), a coil of wire (termed a solenoid), and a small air gap—a spark gap in the case of the spark-gap type, or a thermionic tube in the case of the vacuum-tube unit. The air gap in the spark-gap apparatus resists electric current, whereas that in the vacuum-tube type may include a rectifier, which decreases or even neutralizes this resistance. A third type of oscillating circuit, the solid-state transistor, produces waveforms similar to vacuum-tube units, but allows for smaller, more reliable units by using transistors to control the current.[7,8]

The output waveform determines the precise effect of current on tissue. High-frequency, alternating current generates electromagnetic fields consistent with medium-frequency, sinusoidal radio waves. The term 'waveform' refers to the shape of these waves, specifically, whether they are undamped or damped, and continuous or discontinuous (Fig. 12.4). An undamped wave refers to a pure sine wave of electromagnetic energy that causes pure tissue separation with minimal hemostasis. As the wave dampens, oscillations exhibit amplitude surges that progressively decrease, resulting in marked tissue destructive effects.

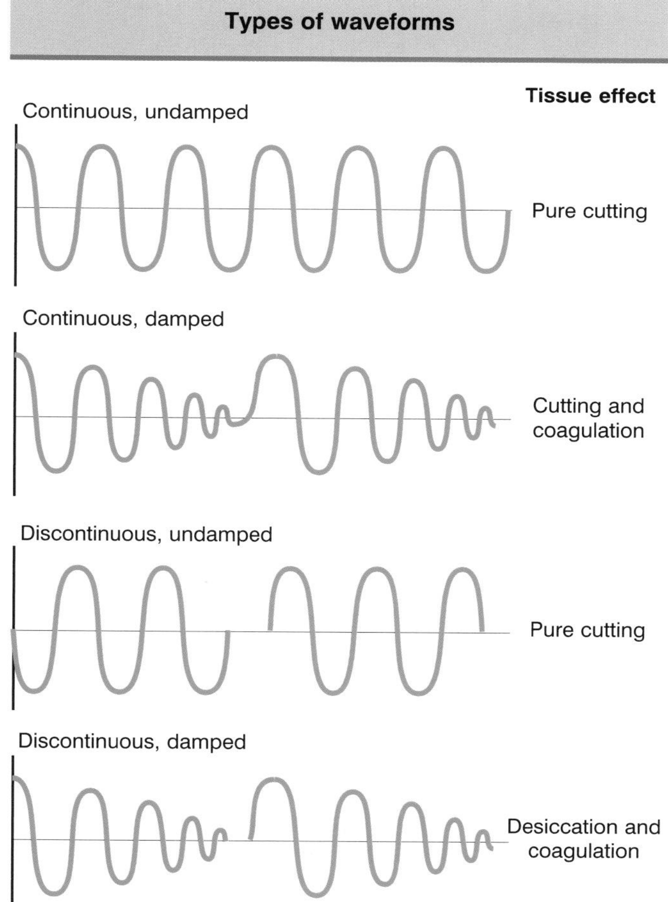

Figure 12.4 Specific waveforms yield specific tissue effects. Adapted from Sebben JE. Electrosurgery principles: cutting current and cutaneous surgery – part 1. J Dermatol Surg Oncol 1988; 14:29–31.

Greater damping leads to increased tissue damage and hemostasis, whereas lesser damping leads to less hemostasis but better healing.

Uninterrupted waveforms are continuous, whereas interrupted waveforms are discontinuous. Continuous wavetrains result in greater tissue heating because the current flows for a longer period of time.[2,9]

Spark-gap units produce damped waveforms because the resistance offered by the spark-gap causes successive wave amplitudes to gradually decrease to zero. Vacuum-tube units, by contrast, produce undamped waveforms because the thermionic tube neutralizes the internal resistance within the circuit, and allows the waveform to continue unchanged (see Fig. 12.3). Changing the characteristics of the oscillating unit, however, modifies the output waveforms in both units. In the spark-gap unit, widening the spark gap requires a greater voltage to jump the gap and produces highly damped waves with the potential for great tissue destruction and hemostasis. Narrowing the spark gap decreases the voltage necessary to jump the gap, and causes the wavetrains to be less damp and to occur closer together. Because this waveform more closely resembles a sine wave, it has less potential for tissue damage and hemostasis. Spark-gap units may thus be used for damped, as well as relatively undamped, output.

A vacuum-tube unit may produce waveforms that are partially rectified, fully rectified, or filtered and fully rectified, depending on the components in its oscillating unit. Partial rectification yields moderately damped waveforms, whereas full rectification yields slightly damped waveforms. Full, filtered rectification yields a completely undamped sine wave. Markedly damped waveforms are used in electrofulguration and electrodesiccation; moderately damped waveforms in electrocoagulation; and undamped waveforms in electrosection (Table 12.1). Similar to spark-gap units, vacuum-tube units may produce a spectrum of waveforms, from moderately damped to purely undamped, depending on the components of their oscillating unit. As they profoundly influence the quality and extent of tissue injury, intelligent use of such electrical concepts as current density, resistance, voltage, power and waveform output may optimize therapy and minimize adverse events during electrosurgery.[4,7,9]

■ PREOPERATIVE PREPARATION

Preoperative care should attempt to minimize risks specific to electrosurgery. History and physical examination should characterize risk factors for excessive blood loss, such as bleeding diathesis, or poor healing, such as vasculopathy, malnutrition, diabetes mellitus, or poor general medical condition. Patients with cardiac pacemakers or implantable cardiodefibrillators must also be identified because these devices may malfunction in the presence of electromagnetic radiation. Patients should remove all jewelry, and avoid contact with grounded metal objects to minimize the risk of electric burns. A nonalcohol-containing prep solution, such as chlorhexidine or povidone-iodine, should be used because alcohol may ignite when exposed to spark or heat. In the perianal region, moist packing should be placed over the anus to prevent ignition of methane.[8,10,11]

Table 12.1 Types of electrosurgical procedures[2,3,32]

Type of procedure	Circuit	Tissue contact with active electrode	Voltage	Amperage	Air-gap output	Tube output	Histology
Electrofulguration	Monoterminal	No	High	Low	Markedly damped	—	Tissue desiccation: cell outlines preserved, but shrunken. Nuclei elongated. Some vessel thrombosis
Electrodesiccation	Monoterminal	Yes	High	Low	Markedly damped	—	Tissue desiccation: cell outlines preserved, but shrunken. Nuclei elongated. Some vessel thrombosis
Electrocoagulation	Biterminal	Yes	Low	High	Moderately damped	Partially rectified	Tissue coagulation: cell outlines lost from massive protein denaturation. Homogeneous hyalinized appearance. Vessel thrombosis
Electrosection with coagulation	Biterminal	Yes	Low	High	Slightly damped	Fully rectified	Cell disintegration forming approximately 0.1 mm incision; adjacent cellular outline elongation and mild coagulation effect
Electrosection	Biterminal	Yes	Low	High	Undamped	Filtered, filtered, fully rectified	Cell disintegration forming approximately 0.1 mm incision; minimal coagulation effect
Electrocautery	None (hot wire)	Yes	Low	High	N/A	N/A	Amorphous tissue with charred foci and formation of steam spaces

■ TECHNIQUES AND PRACTICAL APPLICATIONS

Before considering various types of electrosurgical procedures, clarification of four, often misused, terms is necessary. These terms are monopolar, bipolar, monoterminal, and biterminal.

Monopolar versus bipolar

In electrosurgery, alternating current variably enters and exits the tissue through the treatment electrode. As a result, the treatment electrode is not a true positive or negative pole. Use of the terms monopolar and bipolar to describe any procedure using alternating current is therefore incorrect. Only electrosurgery based on direct current, such as electrolysis, is truly polar in that the treatment electrode functions as a negative pole that transmits unidirectional current. The terms 'monoterminal' and 'biterminal' are technically more correct when referring to electrosurgical procedures.[12]

Monoterminal versus biterminal

The prefix 'mono-' and 'bi-' terminal refers to the number of treatment electrodes used in electrosurgery. Monoterminal indicates that only one electrode delivers current to the patient, whereas biterminal indicates that two electrodes are used for this purpose. The second electrode is often an indifferent electrode, serving to complete an electrical circuit that begins in the electrosurgical unit, flows through the patient, and then returns to the unit. Procedures not using an indifferent electrode, such as electrodesiccation and electrofulguration, are monoterminal, whereas procedures employing an indifferent electrode, such as electrocoagulation or electrosection, are biterminal. In monoterminal procedures, electrons are dispersed randomly to the environment.[2,7]

Electrosurgical procedures

Electrosurgical procedures (see Table 12.1) may be classified according to the degree of tissue destruction produced: superficial tissue destruction (produced by electrodesiccation and electrofulguration), deeper tissue destruction (resulting from electrocoagulation), and tissue cutting (produced by electrosection).

Electrofulguration and electrodesiccation

Electrofulguration and electrodesiccation use markedly damped, high-voltage, low-amperage current in a monoterminal fashion to produce superficial tissue destruction. The absence of an indifferent electrode implies that current accumulates within the patient; as a result, high voltage is required to sustain current flow. Low amperage allows for nominal tissue damage. In electrodesiccation, the electrode contacts the skin and superficial skin dehydration occurs as a result of Ohmic heating (Fig. 12.5). Most damage is epidermal and there is minimal risk of scarring with lower power settings. Higher power settings, however, may be associated with increasing dermal coagulation, superficial scarring, and hypopigmentation.

Electrofulguration represents a variation of electrodesiccation in which the electrode is held 1–2 mm from the skin surface, and causes tissue dehydration by sparks (Fig. 12.6). High voltage allows the current to overcome the resistance of the air gap between the tissue and the electrode tip, producing electrical sparks, which cause superficial epidermal carbonization. This carbon layer has an insulating effect and minimizes further damage to the underlying dermis. As a result, lesions treated by electrofulguration usually heal rapidly with minimal scarring. Because of their low amperage, electrodesiccation and electrofulguration are best suited for superficial and relatively avascular lesions, such as verrucae and seborrheic keratosis. Treatment of highly vascular lesions often results in a bloody operative field, which quickly dissipates the heat produced by these low-amperage modalities.[3,8,9]

Electrocoagulation

Electrocoagulation uses low-voltage, moderately damped or partially rectified, high-amperage current in a biterminal fashion to cause deeper tissue destruction and hemostasis with minimal carbonization (Fig. 12.7). Low voltage is sufficient to establish current flow because the indifferent electrode prevents current accumulation in the patient, which would impede current flow by decreasing the voltage gradient between electrode and patient. High amperage causes deep tissue destruction and hemostasis. In electrocoagulation, one applies and slowly moves the electrode across the lesion until slightly pink to pale coagulation occurs. A curette may then be used to remove the coagulum. One should avoid damaging tissue to the extent that a friable, charred coagulum results because this eschar may easily dislodge and result in delayed bleeding. Coagulated tissue has greater resistance to electrical current than normal skin, and limits the amount of damage. The deep destruction provided by electrocoagulation results in scarring, and this should be noted when discussing therapeutic alternatives with the patient.[3,8,9]

One may achieve hemostasis by touching the electrode directly to the bleeding vessel, or by using biterminal forceps. With either method, the heat generated seals the vessel by fusion of its collagen and elastic fibers, and the operative field must be dry for maximal efficacy. The hemostatic and destructive capacity of electrocoagulation makes it ideal for the treatment of deeper and more vascular lesions (e.g. pyogenic granuloma).[3,8,9]

Electrosection

Electrosection uses undamped or slightly damped, low-voltage, high-amperage current in a biterminal fashion to vaporize tissue with minimal peripheral heat damage. Undamped current yields cutting without coagulation, whereas slightly damped current provides some coagulation. The

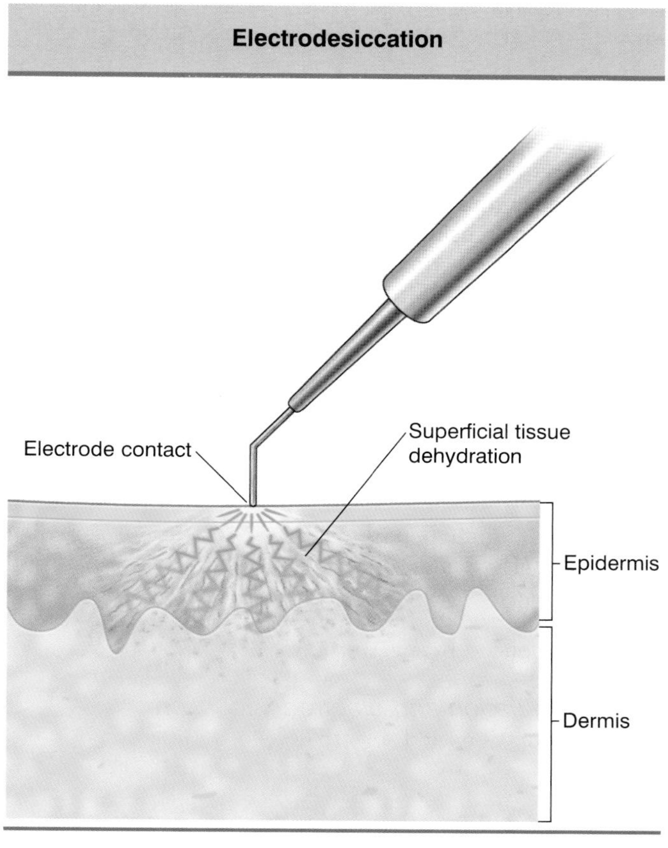

Electrodesiccation

Electrode contact

Superficial tissue dehydration

Epidermis

Dermis

Figure 12.5 Electrodesiccation results in superficial tissue dehydration. Adapted from Sebben JE. Electrosurgery. In: Ratz JL, ed. Textbook of Dermatologic Surgery. Philadelphia: Lippincott-Raven; 1998.

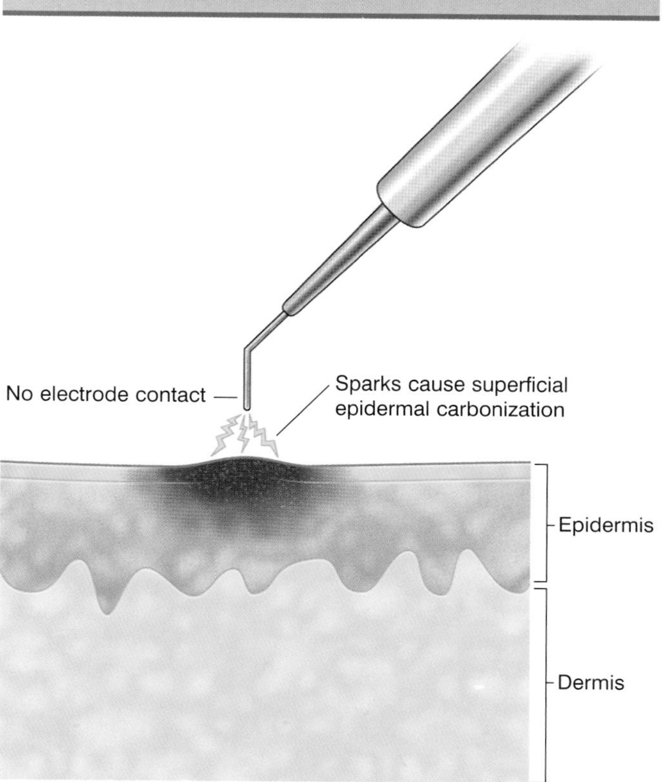

Figure 12.6 Electrofulguration results in superficial tissue carbonization. Adapted from Sebben JE. Electrosurgery. In: Ratz JL, ed. Textbook of Dermatologic Surgery. Philadelphia: Lippincott-Raven; 1998.

Electrocoagulation

Electrode contact

Deeper tissue coagulation

Epidermis

Dermis

Indifferent electrode

Figure 12.7 Electrocoagulation results in deeper tissue coagulation. Adapted from Sebben JE. Electrosurgery. In: Ratz JL, ed. Textbook of Dermatologic Surgery. Philadelphia: Lippincott-Raven; 1998.

presence of an indifferent electrode permits high current flow at a relatively low voltage, while the high amperage allows for highly focused tissue destruction. The precise mechanism by which continuous sinusoidal waveforms cut tissue is unclear, but it may relate to the formation of explosive microbubbles of steam within tissue cells, or to direct mechanical cell disruption by electromagnetic wavetrains. As most of the energy dissipates during tissue vaporization, minimal collateral tissue damage occurs.

As pure sine waves cut without coagulating, electrosection using pure sine waves provides no benefit over conventional scalpel surgery. Currents therefore commonly 'blend' damped and undamped wavetrains to cause simultaneous cutting and coagulation. Increasing the voltage increases coagulation by increasing waveform amplitude variability.

A variety of electrode tips are available when applying cutting current, most commonly including thin wire electrodes, wire loops, and spatulas. When performed correctly, electrosection requires almost no manual pressure from the operator because the electrode glides through tissue with minimal resistance. If sparking occurs, the power setting is likely too high. If the electrode drags, the power setting is likely too low. Advantages of electrosection are its speed and its ability to simultaneously cut and seal bleeding vessels, for instance, in the excision of large, relatively

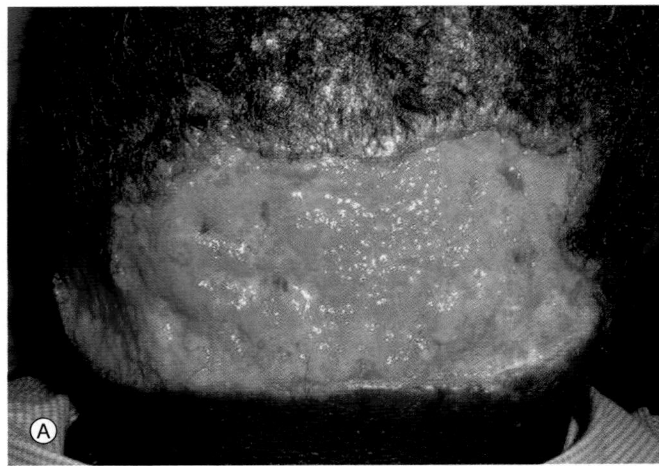

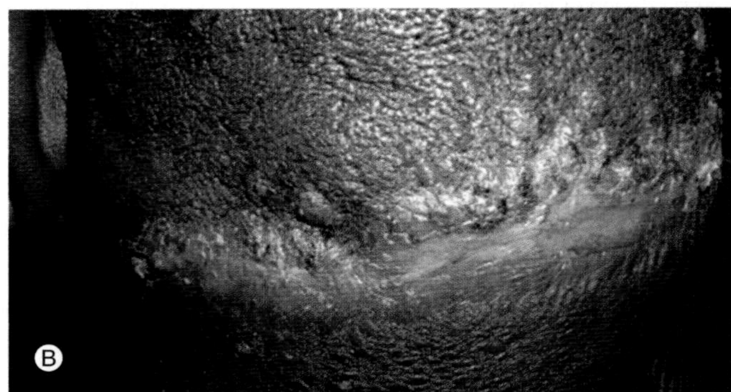

Figure 12.8 (A) Patient 6 weeks after electrosurgical removal of acne keloidalis nuchae. (B) At 4.5 months after surgery the wound is closed by contraction and granulation tissue formation.

vascular lesions, such as acne keloidalis nuchae and rhinophyma. Surgical defects may be allowed to heal by second intention (Fig. 12.8).[2,3,7,10,13]

Electrocautery

Electrocautery uses low-voltage, high-amperage, direct or alternating current to heat a surgical tip to cause tissue desiccation, coagulation, or necrosis by direct heat transference to tissue. Electrocautery is excellent for pinpoint hemostasis and is compatible with patients who may not tolerate current flow (e.g. pacemaker patients). Most destruction with electrocautery occurs close to the heating element, and is thus more readily seen and controlled compared to electrosurgery. The Shaw scalpel is a variation of electrocautery, and consists of a heated sharp scalpel that simultaneously cuts and coagulates bleeding vessels.[2,3]

■ OPTIMIZING OUTCOMES

Electrosurgical procedures may be used to treat a diversity of benign and superficially invasive, malignant neoplasms. Appropriate choice of electrosurgical procedure requires an understanding of the nature of the destructive modality, lesional histology, and anticipated consequences, including pigmentary change and scarring (Table 12.2).

A general therapeutic principle is to use the minimum power setting necessary to achieve the desired effect. Excessive power causes disproportionate tissue damage, and is associated with complications such as increased fibrosis,

Table 12.2 Potential indications for electrosurgery[8,10,15,26]

Type of lesion	Technique
Benign lesions	
Acne keloidalis nuchae	S
Acrochordon	D. F, S
Angioma, cherry	C, D, F
Angioma, spider	C
Condyloma acuminatum	D
Dermatosis papulosis nigra	D, F
Molluscum contagiosum	D, F
Mucous cyst	D, F
Nevi	S
Oral fibroma	D, F
Papilloma	D, F
Pyogenic granuloma	S, C
Rhinophyma	S
Seborrheic keratosis	D, F
Sebaceous hyperplasia	C
Syringoma	D
Telangiectasia	C
Verruca vulgaris	D
Verruca plana	D, F
Premalignant lesions	
In-situ squamous cell carcinoma without extensive follicular involvement	D, F
Actinic keratosis	D, F
Malignant lesions	
Nodular basal cell carcinoma	S, D, F
Superficial basal cell carcinoma	

C, electrocoagulation; D, electrodesiccation; F, electrofulguration; S, electrosection. This list is not comprehensive and electrosurgery may not be the treatment of choice for each lesion

susceptibility to wound infection, and delayed wound healing. The treatment electrode should always be clean of carbonized tissue, which decreases current density and insulates against current flow, thereby reducing cutting and coagulation effect. If carbon build-up seems rapid and excessive, the power setting may be too high, or the procedure rate too slow. It is often useful to combine routine electrosurgery with other surgical modalities (e.g. use of a scalpel, curette or scissors to remove the bulk of a large lesion before use of electrosurgery to treat the base). Combination therapy provides superior control of the depth of destruction, as well as a specimen for histological examination.[4,7,9,13,14]

Clinical outcomes in electrosurgery may include such patient-important outcomes as cure and recurrence rates, postoperative infection rates, severity of postoperative pain, and the cosmetic acceptability of the surgical scar. Although outcomes important to patients are, by definition, important to physicians, other outcomes may also be important to the busy dermatologic surgeon, including speed of surgery and amount of blood loss.

Electrodesiccation and curettage

Electrodesiccation and curettage (ED&C) is a procedure well-known to dermatologists for the treatment of benign and superficially invasive neoplasms (Table 12.2). It involves a sequence of curettage followed by electrodesiccation applied in two to three repetitions to the lesion. Considerations in the decision to perform ED&C include assessment of the depth and histology of the lesion, the thickness of the underlying dermis, and the presence of deep-seated hair follicles. Broad, superficial lesions in areas with thick underlying dermis, such as the trunk and extremities, are ideal candidates for ED&C. Lesions in these locations are often clinically well-defined and easily removed by curettage following desiccation, yielding rapid healing and high cure rates. If one reaches subcutaneous fat during ED&C, the procedure should be abandoned and excision performed because ED&C is less effective for deeper malignancies. ED&C should be used with caution in lesions with the potential for deep follicular extension because there is a higher risk of recurrence.[15]

Basal cell carcinoma

Perhaps the most common and significant indication of electrosurgery is ED&C for the treatment of BCC. The success rate of ED&C is highly operator-dependent because adequate treatment requires that the clinician possess the skill to detect subclinical tumor extension by its physical consistency using the curette. ED&C may be used to treat nodular and superficial BCC, whereas recurrent and micronodular/morpheaform BCCs should be excised because of their penchant for deep dermal infiltration. Case series involving over 1000 BCCs report cure rates ranging from 88 to 99%, although these figures may overestimate benefit as a result of referral bias and insufficient follow up. Studies that report the highest cure rates destroy a substantial peripheral margin around the initial curettage, ranging from 2 to 8 mm. Undermined epidermis at the periphery of the curettage site may be trimmed using scissors.[15] One study summarized all studies of BCC treated by ED&C since 1947 and reported a weighted average 5-year recurrence rate of approximately 8%.[16]

Another study reported determinants of 5-year recurrence rates of 2314 primary BCCs treated by ED&C between 1955 and 1982. Multivariate regression analysis established that patient age, sex, and lesion duration before treatment were not significant determinants of 5-year recurrence. Increasing lesion diameter and occurrence in a high- or middle-risk anatomic site, however, were independent determinants of 5-year recurrence ($P < 0.001$). High-risk sites include the nose, paranasal, nasolabial fold, ear, chin, mandibular, perioral, and periocular areas; middle-risk sites include the scalp, forehead, pre- and postauricular, and malar areas; low-risk sites include the neck, trunk, and extremities (Fig. 12.9).

Basal cell carcinoma in low-risk sites demonstrated an acceptable 5-year recurrence rate of 3% after ED&C, irrespective of lesion diameter. By contrast, middle-risk sites demonstrated a 5-year recurrence of 5% for lesions < 10 mm in diameter, whereas lesions ≥ 10 mm in diameter demonstrated almost five times this recurrence rate, at 23%. In high-risk sites, lesions < 5 mm in diameter demonstrated an acceptable 5-year recurrence of 5%, whereas those ≥ 6 mm in diameter exhibited almost triple the recurrence rate, at 18%. These differences were statistically significant ($P < 0.05$). This study suggests that all lesions occurring in low-risk sites, as well as any lesion

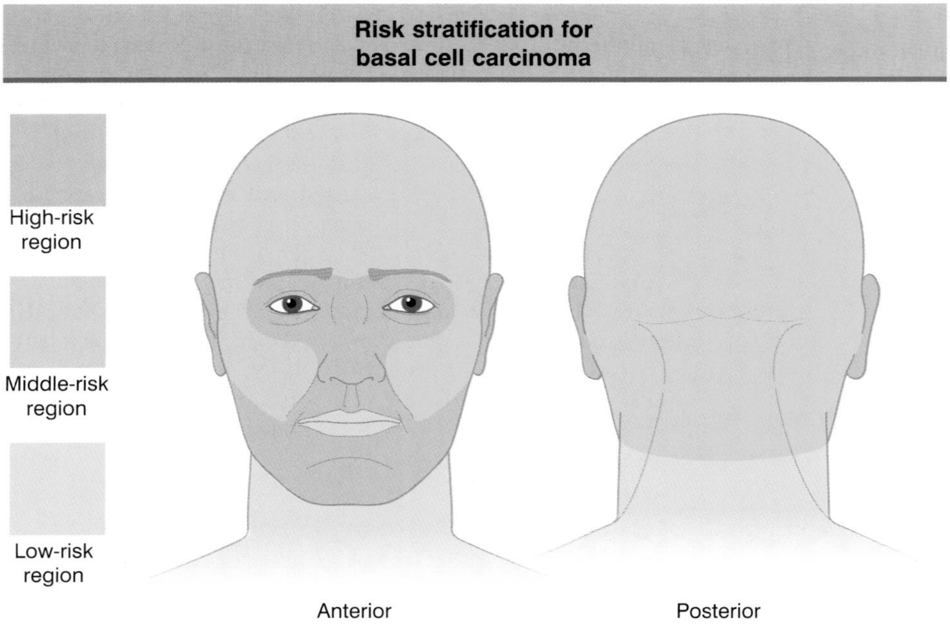

Figure 12.9 Risk of recurrence of BCC treated by electrodesiccation and curettage is significantly dependent on tumor location. Lesions developing on the central face, ears, and mandibular region have the highest risk.

< 5 mm in diameter (regardless of anatomic site) may be treated with ED&C with a high probability of cure at 5 years follow-up. Lesions ≥ 10 mm in diameter in middle-risk and those ≥ 6 mm in diameter in high-risk sites, however, exhibit unacceptably high recurrence rates after ED&C. Excision or Mohs micrographic surgery may achieve superior outcomes in these cases.[17]

Cosmetic outcome following ED&C is site dependent. On the trunk and extremities, ED&C generally results in flat white macules or patches, but may occasionally lead to atrophic, hypertrophic, or even keloidal scars. Several months usually elapse before the scar attains its final appearance, and, until this time, may remain pink, pruritic, and hypertrophic. On the face, ED&C heals with a fine white macule or patch, but may be depressed or produce an indurated, circular scar from wound contraction. Surgical excision often leads to a better cosmetic outcome on the face compared to ED&C. In the study of BCC recurrence following ED&C, 76% patients (1285/1691) rated their ED&C scar as 'good–excellent' in terms of cosmesis 1 year after treatment. ED&C thus provides excellent treatment and cosmetic outcomes for superficial and nodular BCC, although these depend significantly on anatomic location and lesion size.[15,17]

Electrocoagulation

Outcomes relevant to electrocoagulation include hemostasis and, rarely, surgical incision. Hemostasis should be reserved for vessels < 1 mm in diameter; larger vessels or arterioles have a greater chance of delayed bleeding and should be ligated with a dissolvable suture. To optimize hemostasis, the operative field should be dry because current flowing from the electrode is diffused by blood. Care should be taken to apply the minimum amount of time and power, as well as to clamp only the minimum amount of tissue necessary to seal the vessel. Lack of restraint in any of these areas may lead to excess vessel damage, and increased risk of postoperative bleeding. Another problem during electrocoagulation is an apparently sudden decrease in power. Instead of increasing the power setting, confirm good contact between the indifferent electrode and the patient to ensure adequate current drain-off, and that the electrosurgical tip is clean. Incisions made with electrocoagulation should be avoided because animal studies demonstrate that they are associated with higher postoperative infection rates than incisions made with a scalpel or with electrosection.[7,18]

Electrosection

Relevant outcomes include optimizing cutting capacity, as well as incisional speed, postoperative pain and infection, wound healing, and scar cosmesis. The most effective cutting occurs with high current density, which increases as the radius of the electrode decreases. Thus, a needle electrode often provides the most precise cutting effect. Larger electrodes, such as blades and loops, require greater electrical energy to produce the same cutting effect, causing greater peripheral tissue destruction, which may impair wound healing. For debulking procedures, such as rhinophyma excision, however, wire loop electrodes may be used to remove tissue efficiently. Electrosection results in more collateral tissue damage than scalpel surgery, with some histologic distortion of surgical margins. For specimens requiring histopathologic analysis, a filtered, fully rectified current should be used (cutting without coagulation) to prevent significant electrosurgical artifact.[10,13]

As electrosection may often serve as an alternative to conventional scalpel surgery, it may be important to compare these modalities with respect to outcomes such as incisional speed, postoperative pain and infection, wound healing, and scar cosmesis. Reports of impaired wound healing and increased postoperative infection rates associated with early model electrosection units have discouraged the widespread use of electrosection for skin incision.

Several randomized controlled trials (RCTs) from the surgical literature now compare electrosection against other incisional modalities in terms of these outcomes. One RCT compared carbon dioxide (CO_2) laser, conventional scalpel, and electrosection in 88 cholecystectomy patients in terms of incisional time, incisional blood loss, postoperative pain, and wound healing. As expected, incisional time and blood loss were significantly less for electrosection compared to other modalities ($P < 0.05$). No statistically significant difference was observed in the degree of postoperative pain, the number of wound seromas/infections, and wound healing.[19] It is of interest, however, that animal studies consistently demonstrate slower wound healing with electrosection compared to scalpel surgery.[20,21]

Another RCT compared electrosection to scalpel surgery in 84 patients undergoing inguinal herniorrhaphy or cholecystectomy in terms of incisional time, cosmetic outcome, postoperative pain, and wound complications. Incisions by electrosection were significantly faster and were associated with superior cosmetic outcome relative to scalpel incision ($P < 0.01$), whereas no significant difference was observed between groups for postoperative pain and wound complications.

A final RCT compared electrosection versus scalpel incision for elective midline laparotomy in 100 patients in terms of incisional time, incisional blood loss, total intraoperative blood loss, postoperative wound pain, and number of wound complications. Electrosection was associated with significantly quicker incision and less blood loss relative to scalpel surgery (0.8 mL/cm^2 versus 1.7 mL/cm^2, respectively; $P = 0.002$). Electrosection was further associated with significantly lower postoperative pain scores 48 hours after operation, as well as lower total morphine requirements 5 days after operation relative to scalpel surgery (66 mL versus 92 mL, respectively; $P < 0.05$). Wound infection rates were comparable between groups at discharge and at 1 month follow-up.[22] The results of these RCTs suggest that modern electrosection units provide superior speed, hemostasis, cosmetic outcome, and decreased postoperative pain than conventional scalpel surgery, while providing comparable postoperative wound healing and infection rates.

■ POSTOPERATIVE CARE

Immediate postoperative care

Superficial electrosurgical wounds heal well by second intention with basic wound care principles—specifically, cleansing with hydrogen peroxide or saline daily followed by application of an antibiotic ointment and protective dressing. Wounds created by cutting currents may be sutured because minimal tissue damage occurs along the lines of incision. These wounds do not develop tensile strength as rapidly as scalpel wounds: they are weaker for 21 days postoperatively, and thereafter exhibit tensile strength equal to scalpel wounds. A bulky pressure dressing is advisable because some postoperative bleeding is expected, normally within 3 days after surgery. A nonadherent dressing should be placed on the wound surface to minimize vessel irritation when the dressing is removed 1 or 2 days postoperatively.[13,14]

Long-term postoperative care

Hypertrophic scarring may complicate healing in a proportion of electrosurgical wounds. These lesions may be managed conservatively using massage, and, when appropriate, intralesional corticosteroid injection.

■ PITFALLS AND THEIR MANAGEMENT

Pitfalls and their management[2,23–26]

- Burns
  - use non-flammable cleanser such as chlorhexidine or povidone-iodine
  - avoid alcohol cleanser, ethyl chloride anesthesia, or use of flowing oxygen
  - ensure that the indifferent electrode has broad contact with skin, and is not placed over a bony prominence, scar tissue, or implanted metal
  - ensure patient is not touching grounded metal objects
  - consider the risk of current 'channeling'
- Electric shock
  - use a three-pronged receptacle that is not overloaded
  - do not use treatment table outlet
  - surgeon should not make or break contact with patient during current delivery
- Transmission of infection
  - use smoke evacuator with intake nozzle 2 cm from operative site
  - wear surgical mask and eye protection when working with human papillomavirus-related lesions
- Eye injury
  - avoid using treatment electrode close to eye, if possible
  - use corneal shields
- Cardiac pacemaker and defibrillator malfunction

  preoperative:
  - consider preoperative cardiology consult
  - consider alternative therapy in patients that are medically unstable, pacemaker or defibrillator-dependent, or with an external pacemaker
  - consider changing pacemakers to fixed-rate mode
  - consider magnetically deactivating ICD during electrosurgery
  - avoid cutting current outside the hospital setting

  operative:
  - consider using electrocautery, Shaw scalpel (no current flow through patient) or biterminal forceps (minimizes current leakage in patient)
  - choose a site far from the heart and pacemaker for grounding and ensure that the heart does not lie directly in the path between the treatment and indifferent electrodes; do not work near the heart or pacemaker
  - check peripheral pulse and level of consciousness during electrosurgery
  - keep electrosurgical current bursts < 5 seconds

  postoperative:
  - consult cardiology to check or reset device

Although generally safe, electrosurgery is not without risks. These include electrical burns, electric shocks, infection transmission, eye injury, and cardiac pacemaker or defibrillator malfunction.

Electrical burns

Electrical burns reflect concentrated tissue damage when high current density flows through a small surface area. This scenario arises principally from faulty application of the indifferent electrode, failure to isolate the patient from metal surfaces during current application, or from current 'channeling' to a site distant from the treatment area. Faulty application of the indifferent electrode may include placement over a bony prominence, scar tissue, or metal implants, or such that only a small surface area contacts the patient. Current becomes concentrated in this small surface area, resulting in high current density. If this application continues for a sufficient period of time, an electrical burn ensues. If the patient is conscious, he or she usually complains of pain in the area before the burn occurs; however, complaints of pain are impossible under general anesthesia, resulting in increased risk.

Burns may also occur if the patient touches a grounded metal object, particularly if the indifferent electrode is in poor contact or is broken. In this case, the current seeks any alternative low-resistance pathway from the patient to the ground; a burn results from current concentration through a small surface area in contact with the metal object. Common hazards include an electrocardiogram needle or plate, intravenous pole, rectal temperature probe, or photocell ear plethysmograph.

Finally, current may concentrate as it flows through a small area, a phenomenon known as current 'channeling'. This problem occurs when current is applied to a mass with a narrow stalk or base, leading to current concentration when it traverses this narrowed region. Current flowing through a large papilloma with a thin stalk may concentrate and cause a burn at its base. Channeling may also occur when current contacts tissue, such as nerve or a vessel, which is more conductive than the surrounding tissue. The resultant distant coagulation occurring in a nerve or a vessel may have grave consequences when it occurs in an isolated region, such as the finger or the penis. Current channeling has been reported on the scrotum with subsequent necrosis (Fig. 12.10).[2,4]

Reports of burns during electrosurgery are uncommon in dermatology, and most of the experience with this adverse event stems from the surgical literature. Certain precautionary measures may nonetheless minimize the risk of electrical burns. Because inadvertent activation of the treatment electrode may cause burns, the active electrode should never be left on the patient while not in use. An attempt should be made to ensure approximately 20 square inches of surface contact area for the indifferent electrode because this is usually sufficient for current dispersion. Use of modern, indifferent electrodes that are sufficiently flexible to conform to the body as well as the use of a protective interface gel may minimize the risk of faulty application. The indifferent electrode should not be cut to the desired size or bent because this decreases the dispersion area and may create sharp points where current concentration may occur. The surgical staff should ensure

Channeling of electrosurgical current

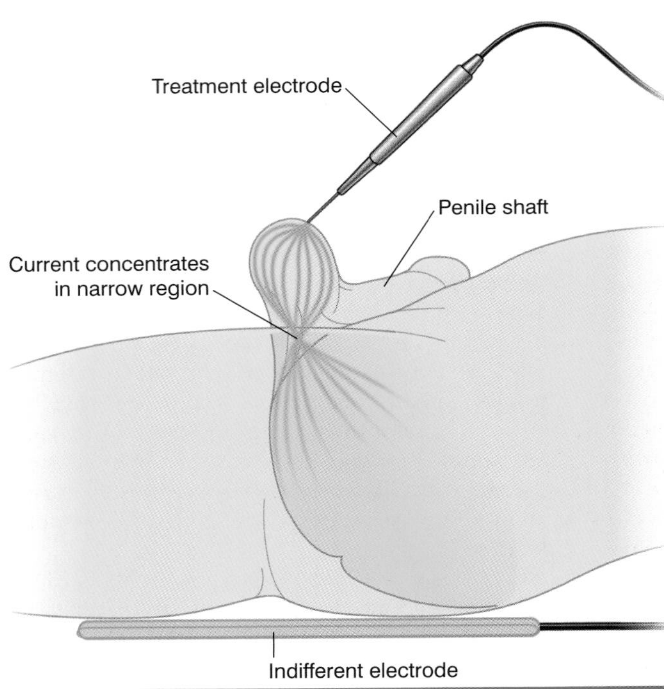

Figure 12.10 Current channeling leads to current concentration in narrowed regions, such as the base of the scrotum. The increased current density may result in electric burns and tissue necrosis.

that the patient is not in contact with any grounded metal object. Current channeling is rare at normal power settings. The risk may be further minimized by using bipolar forceps, an indifferent electrode, or by increasing the cross-sectional area of current flow, for example, by wrapping a saline-soaked sponge (an electrolyte conductor) around the narrow base of the mass being treated.[2,4,23]

Electrocution and electric shocks

Electrocution results from electrically-induced ventricular fibrillation, and is most likely when a low-resistance path directly delivers current to the heart. The risk of electrocution with modern electrosurgical units is minimal because transformers separate the treatment electrodes from the power source, and, in the event of unit malfunction, a three-pronged grounding plug diverts any current leakage to ground.

In cases where no indifferent electrode is used, the patient becomes a receptacle for static electricity and may deliver painful electric shocks to nearby grounded persons. To minimize the risk of electric shock, the staff should not make or break contact with the patient during current application.[14]

Infection transmission

Some physicians believe that the heat induced by electrosurgery sterilizes the electrode tip. Although this statement is true for electrocautery, it does not apply to electrosurgery, where heat production occurs only in tissue. Electrosurgery thus carries the potential of transferring surface bacteria and viruses to the surgical wound. In experimental settings, electrodesiccation has been associated with transmission of hepatitis B virus, human papillomavirus (HPV), and *Staphylococcus aureus*, although reported wound infection rates remain low. HPV may become aerosolized in blood microdroplets and in electrosurgical smoke, with potential transmission to the patient and the surgical staff. To minimize these risks, disposable or sterilized treatment electrodes and protective covers for electrode handles should be used for each procedure. A smoke evacuator, facial masks, and protective eyewear should be used whenever treatment involves HPV-related lesions or creates a smoke plume.[27–29]

Eye injury

When electrosurgery is performed in the periorbital region, sparks may arc towards the globe and result in corneal damage and scarring. When possible, one should avoid electrosurgery in this area, or apply special corneal shields to protect the eyes.[14]

Cardiac pacemaker or defibrillator malfunction

High-frequency electrosurgery may interfere with cardiac pacemaker and ICD function, with the potential for patient fatality. Pacemakers may be classified as either fixed rate (in which the pacemaker fires at a predetermined rate irrespective of intrinsic cardiac rhythm) or demand type (in which the pacemaker fires at a predetermined rate in the absence of intrinsic cardiac rhythm). Demand-type pacemakers are further classified as either 'ventricular-inhibited' or 'ventricular-triggered'. The most common pacemaker in the US is the ventricular-inhibited, demand-type pacemaker. Pacemaker types and potential complications are summarized in Table 12.3.

Fixed-rate pacemakers have no sensing circuitry, and thus resist interference from extraneous electrical signals. All demand pacemakers have sensing circuitry, and are thus susceptible to this type of interference. A ventricular-inhibited, demand pacemaker does not fire in the presence of sensed ventricular contraction. In the absence of sensed ventricular depolarization, it generates an impulse to stimulate ventricular contraction, thus preventing bradycardia or asystole. Ventricular-triggered units, by contrast, stimulate ventricular contraction with each sensed ventricular depolarization. Because the ventricles have already depolarized, no signal capture and no effect on the heart occurs. In the absence of sensed ventricular depolarization, it generates an impulse to stimulate ventricular contraction, thus preventing bradycardia or asystole.[24,30]

In the context of electrosurgery, the sensing circuitry of demand pacemakers may misread the electromagnetic output of electrosurgery as spontaneous ventricular contraction. The cardiac sequelae of this misinterpretation depend on whether the pacemaker is of the ventricular-inhibited, or ventricular-triggered type. In the former, the unit misreads the electrosurgical signal as a spontaneous heartbeat, and erroneously enters standby mode. In patients who are pacemaker-dependent, this malfunction may result in profound bradycardia or asystole, with syncope, seizures, and death. In the latter, the unit misreads the electrosurgical signal as a spontaneous heartbeat, which triggers it to erroneously stimulate ventricular contraction. This output may result in extrasystole, or in life-threatening tachyarrhythmias or ventricular fibrillation should it occur during the vulnerable cardiac repolarization period. Risk of arrhythmia is low in healthy individuals, but increases with myocardial anoxia, electrolyte imbalance, or drug toxicity. Electrosection poses the greatest risk for pacemaker-related complications, but these may occur with all electrosurgical procedures.[25,30]

Table 12.3 Effect of electrosurgical interference on pacemaker function[24]

Pacemaker type	Function	Consequence of electrosurgical interference
Fixed rate	Fires at predetermined rate irrespective of intrinsic cardiac rhythm	No effect
Demand:		
1. Ventricular-inhibited	Fires when intrinsic cardiac rhythm is slower than preset rate	Bradycardia, asystole
2. Ventricular-triggered	Fires with each spontaneous heart beat; in the absence of intrinsic rhythm, fires at predetermined rate	Extrasystole, tachyarrhythmia, ventricular fibrillation

An ICD is a device that sends a defibrillatory shock to the heart when it senses ventricular fibrillation or tachyarrhythmia. It is indicated for refractory ventricular tachyarrhythmias, and consists of a sensing circuit and current generator inserted in an abdominal or infraclavicular subcutaneous pocket. The sensing circuit of the ICD may misinterpret electrosurgical output as a tachyarrhythmia or as ventricular fibrillation. As a result, it may erroneously deliver a defibrillating shock to the heart, which may in turn induce true tachyarrhythmia. Permanent ICD damage may also result if the interference is sufficient.[25]

Given the potential severity of these complications, the question of their frequency becomes a pressing issue. A survey of 166 Mohs surgeons with a total of 1959 years of experience determined the number and type of complications as a result of electrosurgery in the dermatologic setting. This study reported an exceedingly low incidence of interference (1.6 cases/100 years of surgical practice) and of clinical adverse events (0.8 cases/100 years of surgical practice), with no significant morbidity or death rate. Twenty-five cases of interference were reported, consisting of skipped beats (8 patients), pacemaker reprogramming (6 patients), ICD firing (4 patients), asystole (3 patients), bradycardia (2 patients), shortened battery life (1 patient), and tachyarrhythmia (1 patient). Of these 25 cases, 18 patients experienced a clinical adverse outcome—syncope (6 patients), altered sensorium (5 patients), palpitations (3 patients), outpatient cardiology consult (3 patients), and hemodynamic instability (1 patient). The most common electrosurgical procedures associated with interference, in order of increasing frequency, were electrofulguration, electrosection, electrocoagulation, and electrodesiccation. The safety record of electrosurgery in the dermatologic setting thus appears to be excellent, with no significant reports of morbidity or deaths.[31]

Fortunately, pacemaker technology has kept pace with the potential for interference with electrosurgical devices. Most modern pacemakers are designed with metallic covers and filters that minimize the risk of pacemaker malfunction by effectively rejecting extraneous electrical interference. Several authors have also recommended precautionary measures when approaching a pacemaker or ICD patient as a candidate for electrosurgery (see Pitfalls and their management, above). Although these guidelines are excellent, the low incidence of complications in the dermatologic setting suggests that they should not be followed categorically, but tailored to the clinical scenario.

■ SUMMARY

Electrosurgery refers to a procedural class that uses tissue resistance to the passage of high-frequency alternating current to generate thermal tissue damage. These treatments range from superficial tissue dehydration (as in electrodesiccation and electrofulguration), deep tissue coagulation (as in electrocoagulation), to tissue cutting (as in electrosection). Electrocautery is not a true form of electrosurgery as no current flows through the patient. The precise effect of electrical current on tissue depends on such electrical concepts as current density, resistance, voltage, power, and waveform output. Electrosurgical units increase the amperage and frequency of the available current, and modify its waveform to that appropriate for the clinical indication. Spark-gap units are most commonly used for electrodesiccation, electrofulguration, and electrocoagulation, whereas vacuum-tube units are used for electrosection. The waveform output of both, however, may be modified by adjusting their oscillating units.

Electrosurgery may be indicated for a variety of benign and superficially invasive malignant neoplasms. ED&C is one of the most effective treatments for superficial and nodular BCC, although cure rates depend significantly on the lesion size, histology, and anatomic location. Recent RCTs from the surgical literature suggest that modern electrosection units provide superior speed, hemostasis, cosmetic outcome, and postoperative pain compared to conventional scalpel surgery, while providing similar postoperative wound healing and infection rates.

Potential adverse events associated with electrosurgery include electrical burns, electric shock, infection transmission, eye injury, and pacemaker and ICD malfunction. The incidence of these adverse events, however, is relatively low.

In the correct clinical context, electrosurgery provides a rapid, efficacious means of treating benign and superficially invasive malignant neoplasms with minimal blood loss, and represents an important procedure for dermatologic surgery.

■ REFERENCES

1. Wagner R, Tomich J, Grande D. Electrolysis and thermolysis for permanent hair removal. J Am Acad Dermatol 1985; 12:441–449.
2. Bennett R. Electrosurgery. In: Bennett R, ed. Fundamentals of cutaneous surgery. St Louis: The CV Mosby Company; 1988; 553–590.
3. Boughton R, Spencer S. Electrosurgical fundamentals. J Am Acad Dermatol 1987; 16:862–867.
4. Schellhammer P. Electrosurgery: principles, hazards, and precautions. Urology 1974; 3:261–268.
5. McCarthy J. Electrosurgery. In: McAinsh T, ed. Physics in medicine and biology encyclopedia. New York: Pergamon Press; 1986; 319–323.
6. Jensen T. Physics for the health professions. 3rd edn. New York: John Wiley & Sons; 1982.
7. Pollack S, Grekin R. Electrosurgery and electroepilation. In: Roenigk R, Roenigk H, eds. Dermatologic surgery: principles and practice. New York: Marcel Dekker, Inc.; 1989; 187–203.
8. Zalla M. Basic cutaneous surgery. Cutis 1994; 53:172–186.
9. Sebben J. Electrosurgery: high-frequency modalities. J Dermatol Surg Oncol 1988; 14:367–371.
10. Sebben J. Electrosurgery principles: cutting current and cutaneous surgery—part I. J Dermatol Surg Oncol 1988; 14:29–31.
11. Stone S. Electrodesiccation and fulguration of lesions of the skin. J Fam Pract 1979; 8:171–174.
12. Sebben J. Monopolar and bipolar treatment. J Dermatol Surg Oncol 1989; 15:364–366.
13. Sebben J. Electrosurgery principles: cutting current and cutaneous surgery—part II. J Dermatol Surg Oncol 1988; 14:29–31.
14. Sebben J. Electrosurgery. In: Ratz J, ed. Textbook of dermatologic surgery. Philadelphia: Lippincott-Raven Publishers; 1998:457–472.
15. Goldmann G. The current status of curettage and electrodesiccation. Dermatol Clin 2002; 20:569–578.
16. Rowe D, Carroll R, Day C. Long term recurrence rates in previously untreated (primary) basal cell carcinoma: implications for patient follow-up. J Dermatol Surg Oncol 1989; 15:315–328.
17. Silverman M, Kopf A, Grin C, Bart R, Levenstein M. Recurrence rates of treated basal cell carcinomas. Part 2: curettage–electrodesiccation. J Dermatol Surg Oncol 1991; 17:720–726.
18. Kim H, Brunner E, Ritter E, Thompson D, Devereux D. Relevance of methods of skin incision technique on development of wound infection. Am Surg 1991; 57:129–130.
19. Pearlman N, Stiegmann G, Vance V, et al. A prospective study of incisional time, blood loss, pain and healing with carbon dioxide laser, scalpel and electrosurgery. Arch Surg 1991; 126:1018–1020.
20. Hambley R, Hebda P, Abell E, Cohen B, Jegasothy B. Wound healing of skin incisions produced by ultrasonically vibrating knife, scalpel, electrosurgery, and carbon dioxide laser. J Dermatol Surg Oncol 1988; 13:1213–1217.
21. Fry T, Gerbe R, Botros S, Fischer N. Effects of laser, scalpel, and electrosurgical excision on wound contracture and graft 'take'. Plast Reconstr Surg 1980; 65.
22. Kearns S, Connolly E, McNally S, McNamara D, Deasy J. Randomized clinical trial of diathermy versus scalpel incision in elective midline laparotomy. Br J Surg 2001; 88:41–44.
23. Aigner N, Fialka C, Fritz A, Wruhs O, Zoch G. Complications in the use of diathermy. Burns 1997; 23:256–264.
24. Sebben J. Electrosurgery and cardiac pacemakers. J Am Acad Dermatol 1983; 9:457–463.
25. LeVasseur J, Kennard C, Finley E, Muse R. Dermatologic electrosurgery in patients with implantable cardioverter-defibrillators and pacemakers. Dermatol Surg 1998; 24:233–240.
26. Hainer B, Usatine R. Electrosurgery of the skin. Am Fam Physician 2002; 66:1259–1266.
27. Bennett R, Kraffert C. Bacterial transference during electrodesiccation and electrocoagulation. Arch Dermatol 1990; 126:751–755.
28. Sherertz E, Davis G, Rice R, Harris B, Franzini D. Transfer of hepatitis B virus by contaminated reusable needle electrodes after electrodesiccation in simulated use. J Am Acad Dermatol 1986; 15:1242–1246.
29. Feutherer J, Colver G. Herpes simplex virus dispersal by Hyfrecator electrodes. Br J Dermatol 1987; 117:627–629.
30. Krull E, Pickard S, Hall J. Effects of electrosurgery on cardiac pacemakers. J Derm Surg 1975; 1:43–45.
31. El-Gamal H, Dufrersne R, Saddler K. Electrosurgery, pacemakers, and ICDs: a survey of precautions and complications experienced by cutaneous surgeons. Dermatol Surg 2001; 27:385–390.
32. Roenigk R, Roenigk H. Current surgical management of skin cancer in dermatology. J Dermatol Surg Oncol 1990; 16:136–151.

13 Cryosurgery

Gilberto Castro-Ron MD and Paola Pasquali MD

Summary box

- Treatment option for benign and malignant lesions and for palliation.
- Less preoperative and operative time than other techniques.
- Many lesions can be treated at one time.
- Treatment can be carried out in conventional and nonconventional surgical settings.
- Easy, faster to learn, and low-cost technique.

INTRODUCTION

Cryosurgery is the surgical method where very low temperatures are applied to a lesion to cause local destruction. It is an extremely valuable alternative when having to choose between different surgical options because of its cost-effectiveness, efficacy, and excellent aesthetic results. With proper training, its easy delivery allows treatment of common skin diseases in a variety of settings, e.g. nursing homes.

The basic cryosurgery principle is to freeze with subzero temperature and allow a later sloughing of the damaged tissue. The depth of damage depends on the technique and the freezing time.

From a biological point of view, the use of subzero temperatures for therapeutic goals will cause structural changes, as a result of heat loss from the living cell. The goal is to achieve a certain final low temperature by freezing the tissue at a constant velocity with an initial low temperature. Thermodynamically, a temperature flow occurs from hot to cold resulting in death.

An important consideration is conductivity. Air is a poor thermal conductor, while water is a better one; some metals are ideal thermal conductors (especially copper). Ice is a better conductor than water. Therefore, freezing using metal as a conductor will result in lower temperatures than freezing by spraying the cooling substance in the air.

When a living system is exposed to subzero temperatures, ice crystal formation will begin in the extracellular system. As a result of osmosis, water will tend to leave the cell, with a resulting intracellular dehydration; water that has left the inside of the cell will eventually freeze. During high freezing velocity, osmotic water movement will be slower allowing internal crystallization. At this point, the process of cell membrane shrinkage will inevitably begin. Crystallization will begin to form inside the cell, which will expand and break the cell membrane.

When freezing temperature is not optimal—which occurs with low freezing velocity—there will only be ice formation in the extracellular system, which can cause distortion and damage to the cell, but tends to be sublethal. This is in contrast to fast freezing velocity, which will cause intracellular ice formation (because water gets trapped inside the cell) and cell destruction.[1–4]

Ice crystals damage organelles and membranes. Slow thawing will extend the time the tissue is kept at low subzero temperatures, increasing the probability of intracellular ice formation and solute damage.[1] All this explains the direct cellular damage. The indirect damage results from freezing the vessels surrounding the frozen tissue that act as feeding vessels. Experimentally, the vascular-mediated injury is responsible for most injury at the edge of the frozen region of microvascular perfused tissue.[2]

Another important concept in cryosurgery relates to the interface. In physics, the surface is the common limit between two bodies. In cryosurgery, it is the contact area between the heat extractor and the final target lesion. The larger the surface or interface, the poorer the conductance. Thick tumors with large amounts of keratin have a large interface and will not allow a uniform adherence of the probe to the surface, in addition to the fact that keratin is a poor conductant. Therefore, it is important to remove this upper surface to allow proper adherence of the probe to the lesion surface.

Concepts such as total freeze time (which can vary from 30 to 60 seconds), halo thaw time, and total thaw time are useful indicators for measuring the adequacy of freeze. Ideally, total freeze time should be shorter than total thaw time to ensure the golden cryosurgery rule: freeze fast, thaw slowly. In addition, when a freeze/thaw cycle is repeated, the cell is damaged further because ice formation is faster. A single freeze/thaw cycle is reserved for benign flat lesions; repeated cycles are used for bulky benign or malignant lesions.

■ HISTORICAL VIGNETTE

Cold has been used for medical purposes since ancient times. It was first applied as a local anesthetic, to reduce body temperature by simple transfer and to diminish malignant tumor pain and size.

The first substance tried as a cryogen was ice, and then salt and water solutions were mixed with crushed ice. By 1885, the observation that atmospheric gases warm up when compressed and cool down when expanded, led to the use of liquefied oxygen, hydrogen, and nitrogen as cryogens.

Reports from the early 20th century show the use of cold to treat dermatological lesions with different methods and cryogens, among them, carbon dioxide (dry ice) and liquid nitrogen-soaked cotton applicators, with variable results. In the 1960s, Zacarian and Adham increased the depth of destruction by using copper disks immersed in liquid nitrogen, taking advantage of copper's excellent thermal conductance properties. The breakthrough in cryosurgery came in 1961 when Cooper and Lee introduced an automated apparatus that used liquid nitrogen in a closed system. Heat could now be extracted from tissue in a controlled manner.

Dermatologists soon took control of this technique with Torre, Zacarian, Adham, and Garamy formally introducing cryosurgery into the dermatologist office. In 1968, Michael Bryne developed the first commercially available handheld cryosurgical device. Papers followed in clinical and research publications by Gage, Graham, Lubritz, Kuflik, the Spillers, and Rubinsky,[5] among others. Worldwide, growth of the field involved people such as Castro-Ron, Turjansky, and Stolar in Latin America; Dawber, Shepperd, and Sonnex in Great Britain; Sohonen in Finland; Goncalves in Portugal; and Korpan in Austria.[6]

■ PREOPERATIVE PREPARATION

Preoperative care is minimal when compared to that for other surgical techniques. This makes cryosurgery particularly useful and practical for the treatment of older patients, who have difficulties lying down on the examination table or who come into the office in a wheelchair or cannot leave their homes or nursing homes. Cryosurgery is a surgical technique that can be carried out in a wide variety of settings.

Another versatile aspect of cryosurgery is the fact that it can be safely applied to patients with underlying medical conditions, such as bleeding problems, heart conditions, and metabolic diseases. Large malignant lesions can be safely treated without having to expose a debilitated patient to a risk of major bleeding.

Diagnostic tests should include skin biopsy to confirm the diagnosis and the type of lesion, and to determine the required freezing depth. Laboratory data may also be required when the history suggests cryoglobulinemia. Other tests may include ultrasound, radiography, magnetic resonance angiogram with contrast enhancement (particularly useful in vascular tumors), and computed tomography scans.

Preoperative protection of vital areas should avoid metal devices, which are excellent cold conductors and adhere to the protected area. Use plastic or wood retractors, goggles, and cotton for ear or nose canals.

Instruments and supplies we have available are curette, scissors, punch, blade, electrosurgical unit, hemostatic agents, suture material, basic surgical pack and gauze. For patients with a known blood-transmittable disease (such as hepatitis or HIV) use the cryospray technique or the closed method with a proper cover for the probe (such as a latex sleeve obtained from a finger of a latex glove). This allows safe treatment of these patients and reduces the contamination risk to both surgeons and nurses.

For very anxious patients, anxiolytic medication may be prescribed the night before and a pain reliever just before the procedure.

Cold tolerance is variable from person to person and difficult to assess until exposed to cold. When treating multiple lesions, apply cold first to one or two areas and see how tolerant the patient is to cold. For multiple superficial lesions, patients who tolerate subzero temperatures might feel less pain if the treatment is carried out without local anesthesia. Multiple lidocaine injections can be more painful than local tissue freezing because cold is slightly anesthetic.

The painful part of the cryosurgical treatment is usually the thawing time more than the freezing time. Curiously, thawing pain is not necessarily reduced by using anesthesia, while freezing pain is. Topical anesthesia is time consuming in its application and has unpredictable results, but it can be an alternative for large treatment areas.

For actinic keratosis, preoperative topical treatment with 5-fluorouracil (5-FU) and/or retinoids will expose the affected areas and reduce the amount of local keratin, so increasing cold conductance. Debulking the lesion is useful for thick and elevated lesions. For verrucae, previous treatment with salicylic acid preparation 10 or 15 days earlier will reduce the amount of keratin and the cryosurgical procedure will be more effective and shorter. Reducing a thick tumor by shaving or curettage, although ideal, might not always be possible, especially when treating patients with coagulopathies, blood-borne diseases (e.g. HIV infection, hepatitis), or anemia.

For children with hemangiomas, the caregiver is asked not to feed the child for at least 3 hours previous to the procedure. The child is sedated with a preparation of oral chloral hydrate, and local anesthesia is applied at the base of the lesion, so allowing treatment of a peaceful patient. The baby is fed immediately after the procedure—food is the best postoperative anesthesia!

■ TECHNIQUES AND TECHNICAL ASPECTS

Cryosurgery can be applied with three different techniques: the open (or spray) technique; the chamber technique; and the closed (contact or probe) technique.

Open technique

In the open technique the cryogen is released from the unit through tips of different diameters—A (the largest), B, C, or D (the smallest) or with numbers 1, 2, 3, 4—through a needle or using a cannula. The tip diameter, intermittent use of the cryogen, and the distance from tip to target are important factors in determining the amount of cold applied to an individual lesion. It is therefore extremely difficult to establish duration of treatments because many factors are involved. Duration of treatment will always be approximate.

Other aspects of treatment that will also influence the result are skin type and thickness of lesion. Type I and II skins tend to be more sensitive to cold. The surgeon should always be more conservative when applying cold to them to avoid overtreatment and severe secondary effects. As far as thickness is concerned, a thicker, more keratinized lesion should be treated for a longer time than a thinner one because keratin is a poor cold conductor.

Cones are available in different sizes and are made of rubber, neoprene, or plastic. They are used to contain the sprayed liquid nitrogen within a defined area, allowing monitoring of the advance of the freeze front through the outside of the cone walls.

Chamber technique

The chamber technique is a variation of the open technique. Chambers are commercially available in different diameters (Fig. 13.1). The spray is released thought an orifice into an open chamber, which is applied with pressure to the skin. The result is that liquid nitrogen comes out of the unit and is trapped within this chamber where it begins a turbulent movement, which tends to lower the temperature of the cryogen further. Chambers have to be used with extreme care because the final temperature is obtained faster and tends to be lower than with the open technique and even with probes. We limit its use to malignancies, such as squamous cell carcinomas, and for palliative cryosurgery. It can work very well for keratoacanthomas because of the large amount of keratin that has to be destroyed.

Closed technique

The closed technique implies the use of probes. Liquid nitrogen leaves the unit through a conduit line that maintains it in a closed system. Probes are built up with metal, usually copper, which is an excellent thermal conductor, and they come in different shapes (Fig. 13.2).

Ideally, the probe should be chosen to best fit the shape of the target lesion. That is why the best equipment for a cryosurgeon has the largest number of probe shapes. If at the time of the procedure, the cryosurgeon does not have the right size of probe available, a valuable rule of thumb is to choose one that is smaller than required rather than a larger one. Using a smaller probe allows the surgeon to let a larger visible freezing front develop and avoids overtreatment of hidden areas.

Many probes are built with Teflon on the outer surface to avoid undesirable sticking to the area, which will pose a risk of inadvertently breaking the tissue with a sudden movement of the unit. When not teflonized, one can avoid adherence to the surface by previously freezing the probe before contacting the surface. This tip is very useful when treating hemangiomas or mucosal lesions. If a probe adheres to the surface and needs to be removed to avoid further freezing, allow warm water or solution to run fast and freely over the area until total thawing is obtained and the probe detaches.

Probes, chambers, and cones of the most diverse shapes and sizes have been developed to adapt to the numerous lesions treated with cryosurgery. Manufacturers are also willing to build probes of different shapes on demand, to comply with the cryosurgeon's needs.

Technical aspects

Sticking can occur, even when performed by a careful operator. The best advice is to be patient and allow complete thawing before attempting to remove the probe otherwise the frozen tissue can be fractured, with probable profuse bleeding when the tissue thaws.

It is not recommended to use cotton swabs for cryosurgery. It is an obsolete method and temperature control is completely lost. Cotton swabs have a poor thermal capacity and there is a real risk of working with suboptimal temperatures. Contrary to spray or probe cryosurgery, where the temperature is known and maintained during the entire procedure, with cotton swabs dipped in liquid nitrogen, the initial temperature of swab immersed in nitrogen will rapidly increase as the surgeon moves the cotton tip from the container toward the patient lesion. Moreover, cotton swabs are inadequate probes, particularly when surgeons apply 'pressure' over the lesion to imitate the probe technique. These improvised techniques tend to cause all the undesirable effects of cold and few of the desired ones and are responsible for many of the failures unjustly attributed to cryosurgery. Furthermore, studies carried out with cryogens other than liquid nitrogen have shown an increased risk of infections.[7]

As far as equipment is concerned, cryosurgery uses cryogens as freezing substances. Cryogens need to be not only safely stored, but also applied to the target lesion in a safe, practical, relatively simple way. Many different substances have been tried as cryogens, including nitrous oxide, helium, freons, fluorocarbonated sprays, liquid

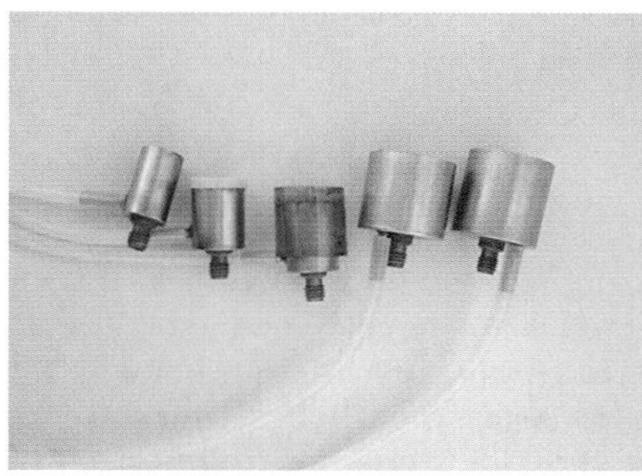

Figure 13.1 Different types of chambers.

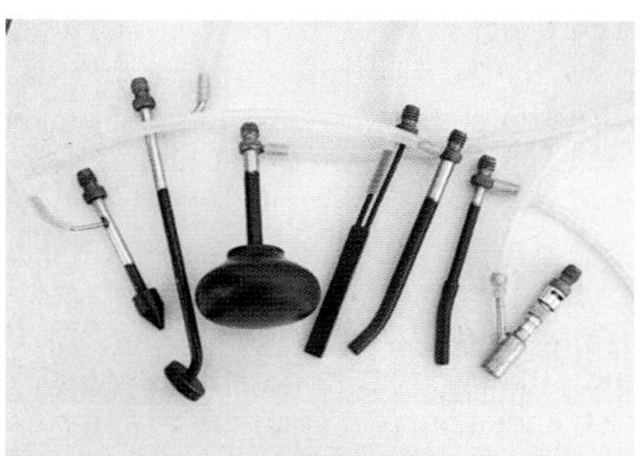

Figure 13.2 Different types of probes.

nitrogen, and solid carbon dioxide. Solid carbon dioxide achieved a certain popularity and was widely used in the early 1900s, but does not achieve temperatures below –79 °C. Over the years, liquid nitrogen has been widely accepted as an ideal cryogen because of its safety in transportation, its low cost, and ease of storage, and its low temperature (–196 °C), which allows for the ideal freezing temperatures needed to destroy malignancies. The goal of treatment is to obtain temperatures of –50 °C to –60 °C at the periphery of the ice ball. From this point on in this chapter the cryogen or freezing substance described will be exclusively liquid nitrogen.

Storage tanks for liquid nitrogen are commercially available in capacities of 4, 5, 10, 25, 30, 35 and 50 liters. They are constructed with insulated material and covers to provide long holding times (Fig. 13.3). Different gadgets, such as gloves, tank stands, and withdrawal devices are also available to facilitate manipulation of the cryogen. Over the years, cryosurgical units have developed from heavy, difficult-to-handle bottles to the low-cost, highly efficient, low-weight, handheld, and easy-to-use format of today. Even the smaller units have enough cryogen capacity to allow freezing of many small lesions or a few large ones from one single fill.

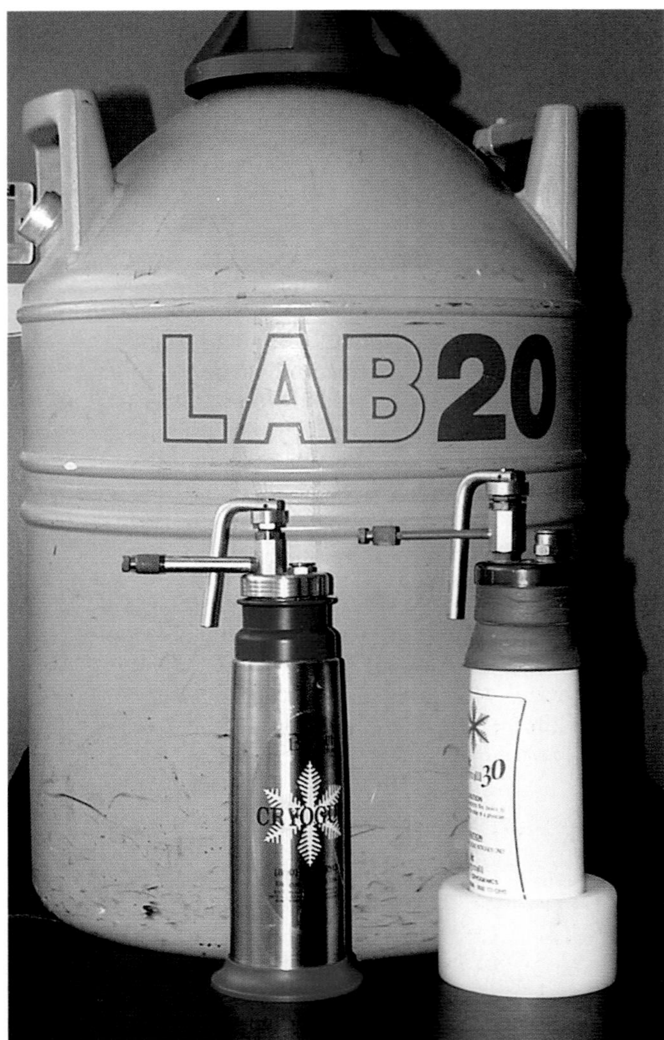

Figure 13.3 Storing tank and handheld units.

Tissue temperature can be monitored using thermocouple needles, which are connected at one end to a temperature monitor and are inserted into the tissue on the other end. Over time, these monitors have been supplanted by clinical experience including halo thaw measurements and now are mostly of academic interest.

Before starting a procedure, the surgeon must decide which technique will be more appropriate to treat the patient's lesion—the open, chamber, or closed technique. If the decision is to use the closed technique, the probe has to be carefully selected. Different probes have to be tried over the target lesion until the one that fits best is found. The general criterion is to choose a probe that fits the lesion's size as closely as possible. The second best option is the next smaller probe. With larger probes than ideal it is not possible to check the advance of the freezing front correctly, so there is a risk of overtreatment.

For very large lesions, it is best to divide the lesion into working areas and to treat each one separately, making sure to slightly overlap the contiguous freezing fronts to ensure a complete treatment. This technique will reduce the risk of leaving untreated areas between one working area and the next. When treating lesions with highly irregular surfaces, it is recommended that excess keratin is eliminated by curettage until a fairly flat surface is obtained, and then a probe is chosen to match this surface. Irregular surfaces will cause a larger interphase and as a consequence lower thermal conductivity.

Once the surface is flattened, it is necessary to have a bloodless area. Hemostatic substances, such as aluminum chloride, work well in stopping bleeding. This is extremely important because blood rapidly increases the local temperature—an effect to be avoided. Trichloroacetic acid, although an excellent hemostatic, should not be used because it leaves a white halo as a result of protein precipitation. The halo may be confused with the advancing freezing front.

The second choice for irregular surfaces is cryospray. This is the correct alternative for lesions that bleed easily, for patients with coagulopathies, for elderly patients needing shorter operative times, and for patients with blood-borne infections, such as HIV infection and hepatitis, where avoiding bleeding is preferred.[8]

■ PRACTICAL APPLICATIONS

Many diseases can be treated with cryosurgery (Table 13.1).[9] As a surgical technique, cryosurgery can be used whenever it is necessary to eliminate tissue; proper training and experience will allow the surgeon to decide when cryosurgery is the best choice of treatment.

The most common conditions treated with cryosurgery and some for which cryosurgery can be considered as a first choice option are described below.

Papillomavirus Infection

For verrucas[29,30] the first consideration that should be taken into account when the decision has been taken to treat with cryosurgery is that keratin is a poor cold conductor. Therefore, it is advisable to either reduce the lesion with keratolytic substances (lactic and salicylic acid) a few weeks earlier or shave off the excess keratin prior to treating with

Table 13.1 Diseases that can be treated with cryosurgery

Benign lesions	Infectious diseases: warts, molluscum contagiosum, larva migrans, leishmaniasis,[10–12] chromomycosis[13] Seborrheic keratosis Pigmentary lesions: lentigines, lentigo simplex, solar lentigo, ephelides Cystic acne, rosacea Hypertrophic lichen planus, lichen sclerosus et atrophicus[14] Keloids Prurigo nodularis[15] Dermatofibroma,[16] chondrodermatitis nodularis helicis chronica Mucocele, myxoid cyst[17] Vascular lesions: hemangiomas, vascular malformations, venous lake,[18] angiokeratoma, cherry and spider angiomas, angiolymphoid hyperplasia, pyogenic granuloma Alopecia areata[19] Sebaceous hyperplasia, steatocystoma multiplex, syringomas, xanthelasma[20] Granuloma annulare[21] Lymphocytoma cutis[22] Trigeminal neuralgia[23] Pearly penile papules[24]
Premalignant lesions	Leukoplakia, actinic cheilitis[25] Keratoacanthoma[26] Actinic keratoses
Malignant lesions	Basal cell carcinomas Bowen's disease Kaposi's sarcoma Lentigo maligna[27,28] Squamous cell carcinomas Palliative treatment

cryosurgery. Wetting the remaining lesion with a piece of cotton or gauze soaked in water will increase cold conductivity.

A second consideration is the use of local anesthesia. If verrucae are small, consider treating them without anesthesia because the injection can be more painful than the cryosurgical treatment. If the lesion is over 3–4 mm, freezing will be prolonged and anesthesia should be given to avoid pain.

Freezing should be carried out with the open technique, with a B or C spraying tip, localizing the spray flow with the use of a plastic disk with four openings of diverse diameters—cones (which are commercially available) or otoscope probes—all of which come in different sizes. Let the freezing front advance just a few millimeters outside the cone area. This reduces the chance of ending up with a ring of verruca at the periphery of the treated lesion once healing has occurred. One freezing cycle is enough.

The treated area should be covered for 2 days, after which the resultant bulla should be removed to hasten healing. The treated area should be cleaned daily with soap and water and local applications of an antibiotic ointment or cream will be sufficient to ensure proper healing.

For multiple condylomata, topical anesthesia can be used (see Chapter 3). If the lesions are few and dispersed, avoid the pain of an injection by pre-treating each lesion with topical anesthesia. Cryosurgery is well tolerated in the genital and perianal areas. One spray cycle is sufficient.

Molluscum contagiosum

Cryosurgery is highly recommended for molluscum contagiosum in people with HIV infection.[31] It avoids curettage and subsequent bleeding. It can be carried out by both the open and closed techniques. In the open technique, use a B or C tip, and spray over the lesion, avoiding pendular or brush painting movements. Point the spray to the center of the lesion. The freezing front has to spread just to the outside margin of the lesion.

For the probe technique, if the lesion is small, use a fine-point probe, such as the eyelid probe, that has been previously frozen to avoid sticking to the surface. This method is faster and allows the treatment of multiple lesions in just one session. No anesthesia is required because it tends to be well tolerated. When treating patients with infectious diseases, such as HIV infection or hepatitis, protect the probe with a latex cover. For larger lesions, we suggest the spraying technique and local anesthesia whenever necessary.

Cryosurgery is not recommended as first-line therapy for children with molluscum contagiosum because other methods are as effective and less time consuming in the postoperative period.

Cutaneous larva migrans

Although cryosurgery is definitely not the first-choice treatment, we have found that cryosurgery can work well for resistant cases or those patients who have difficulty finding or tolerating the oral or local treatments.[32]

Apply a cryotip 3 mm in diameter that has been previously frozen over both ends of the trail and freeze for 5–7 seconds.

Seborrheic keratosis

In seborrheic keratosis, apply the cryospray in an intermittent manner with a B or C tip until the freeze halo covers the whole lesion surface and extends to a maximum of 1 or 2 mm. Let it thaw for a few seconds, until part of the white freeze halo has disappeared and then curettage the frozen lesion; usually one or two curette strokes are sufficient. Remember that freezing is followed by an immediate vasodilator effect. Be ready to apply a hemostatic substance with a cotton swab dipped in aluminum chloride. Curettage of the frozen lesion will speed up recovery, but is not mandatory.

For a very large seborrheic keratosis apply local anesthesia. For small lesions, this procedure is extremely well tolerated. With practice, a large number of seborrheic keratoses can be removed in a single session with extremely satisfying results.

Solar lentigo

Pigmented lesions—lentigines, lentigo simplex, ephelides—are very susceptible to cold. Most of them are superficial and a single freezing cycle carried out with the spray technique is sufficient to cause a small bulla and subsequent sloughing of the macule.

Solar lentigo, ephelides, and lentigo simplex can be treated individually,[33] with the B or C tip, pointed perpendicularly over the pigmented lesion, with intermittent spraying for no more than 3–5 seconds on each one, at a distance of approximately 2 cm. Allow the freeze halo to advance barely outside the outer limit of the macule. If the freezing is not carried out properly, leaving an untreated outer rim, the result may be disappointing, with a residual pigmented ring around the treated area.

For Fitzpatrick skin type III, it is best to treat one or two lesions in less noticeable areas and check for the final appearance. Sometimes, darker skin can hyperpigment with cryosurgery. Likewise, do not treat melasma with cryosurgery because there is a tendency for residual hyperpigmentation.

Acne

Cryosurgery can be helpful for acne and rosacea. Cold has an initial inflammatory effect, but after 24–48 hours, pustules and cysts tend to disappear faster than without any treatment. It is a good alternative during pregnancy, when systemic acne treatments are usually avoided. Spraying should never be carried out over fissured lesions to avoid insufflation of nitrogen and local crepitation similar to that seen in gangrenous areas. Spray for approximately 5–7 seconds, attempting to thinly cover the whole area. There is no need to freeze beyond the outer limit of the lesion. The treated area may drain pus and will need to be covered with antibiotic ointment.

In rosacea associated with rhinophyma, good cosmetic results can be obtained by removing the excess rhinophyma tissue with electrodesiccation. Then a C tip intermittent cryospray is given to the base. Avoid overtreatment. It is better to undertreat and repeat a cryosurgical session than to risk destroying underlying tissue by excess treatment.

Keloids

Cryosurgery for keloids[34] is no better than any other surgical alternative. For earlobe lesions the results can be outstanding.

For earlobe keloids, there are basically two treatment alternatives. The first is to shave the globular lesion and—after hemostasis—to apply a probe over the remaining base of the keloid. A previously frozen tweezers-like probe can be used to grasp the lobe and allow the freezing front to advance 5–7 mm.

The second alternative, for smaller earlobe keloids, is to simply freeze without previously reducing the keloid mass. Spraying can be done with larger tips, A or B, centering the spray at a strategically chosen point and allowing the freezing front to advance slowly until the whole mass is covered. Depending on the size of the tumor, this procedure might take more than 1 minute.

In both cases, the postoperative care should be limited to washing the area with water and soap, and topical hydrogen peroxide and antibiotic ointment applications. Never remove crusts because this could stimulate further keloid growth.

With keloids, there will be a tendency to undertreat rather than overtreat. Keloid tumoral mass is very cold resistant and the thickness variability can cause unpredictable results.

Hemangiomas

Vascular tissue is extremely susceptible to cold. Children with superficial hemangiomas are ideally treated when small. The younger the patient, the better the results.[35] Once a hemangioma appears, usually during the first week of life, it begins to grow, gradually and fast over approximately 1 year, and usually spontaneously involutes over the next 6 or 7 years.

Superficial hemangiomas should always be treated with probes by covering the whole hemangioma area during one single cold application. Cold and pressure are applied together. The pressure will empty the lesion and reduce vascularization (a cause of temperature increase). The probe has to be previously frozen to avoid sticking to the surface, to reduce the risk of breaking this highly vascularized tissue as a result of a sudden involuntary movement of the surgeon or patient. Allow the freeze halo to advance just 1 or 2 mm from the outer limit of the lesion. One freezing cycle is sufficient. It is better to undertreat than to overtreat.

For hemangiomas with both superficial and deep components, it is especially important to apply pressure with the probe as deeply as possible to empty its contents. (An example of a good outcome is shown in Figure 13.4.) We have achieved better results by combining techniques: we inject intralesional steroids into the deep part of the hemangioma and freeze the superficial part. Steroids accelerate regression of the lesion by a mechanism which is not completely clear, but which probably includes the alteration of endothelial cell function and increase of mast cell density.[36]

The corticosteroid is injected first, mixed with local anesthesia, which will reduce the pain of the steroid and will anesthetize the hemangioma that will later be frozen.

Vascular malformations

There are certain vascular malformations for which cryosurgery can be a great help.

Hypertrophic capillary (port-wine stain)

As a port-wine stain hypertrophies, which is a natural process that occurs with time, there is a tendency for the skin to thicken and for vascular nodules to appear over the area. Cryosurgery should not be used for early and flat port-wine stains. After multiple pulsed dye laser treatments have been performed and are becoming less effective, cryosurgery is extremely effective, improving the general appearance of patients with hypertrophic lesions.

Bulky nodules should be treated like hemangiomas (i.e. with probes that fit them as precisely as possible). Previously frozen probes should be applied, exerting pressure to empty blood content, and letting the freeze halo advance barely 1 mm over the outer shape of the lesion.

The hypertrophic area responds well to freezing with the door knob probe (developed by Torre and Garamy at Frigitronics; available through Brymill Cryogenic Systems, www.brymill.com). This curious probe is a teflonized door knob. Previously frozen, it should be applied with pressure, moving along the area and 'ironing' the surface. It is a well-tolerated procedure and can be carried out either without local anesthesia or by previously applying topical anesthesia.

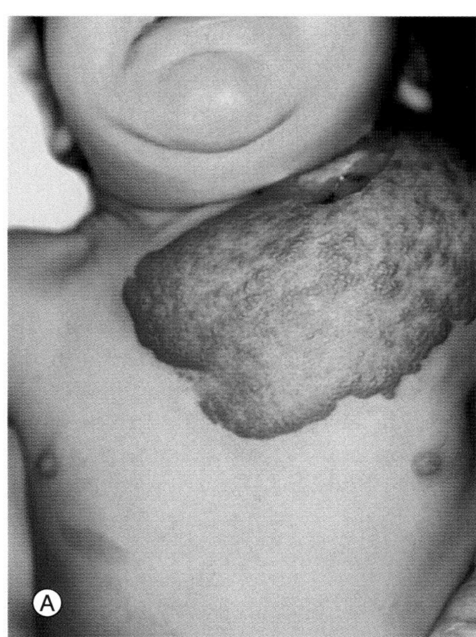

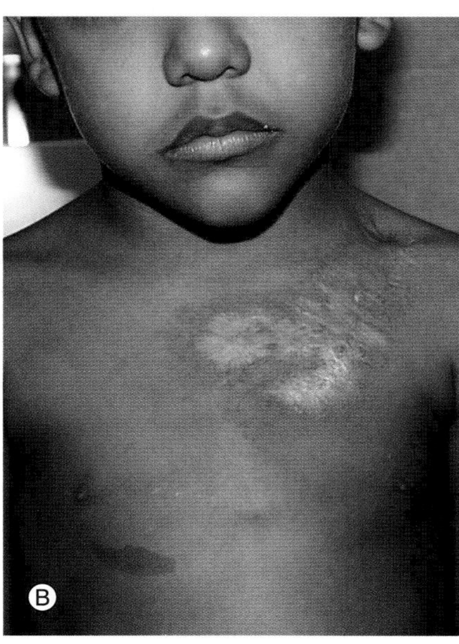

Figure 13.4 (A) A large hemangioma in a 5-month old patient; (B) Postoperative result 5 years later.

The end-result is a clearer and thinner area with extremely satisfying results.

Lymphangiomas

Lymphangiomas tend to be the clinical expression of larger underlying tumors. Probes applied to each individual lesion allow selective destruction with good cosmetic results. Pressure should be applied to each individual lesion to empty the contents. For multiple small lesions, no local anesthesia is necessary. Treat with previously frozen small diameter probes for 5–7 seconds or until the freezing front has reached 1–2 mm outside the outer margin of the lesion.

Mixed malformations (venous–capillary–arterial)

For patients with possible mixed malformations, complete imaging studies—nuclear magnetic angiogram with contrast enhancement, selective arteriography, echosonography, and computed tomography—are performed before treatment to determine the extent of the lesion and vessel diameter.

A multidisciplinary team of head and neck, cardiovascular, plastic, and dermatologic cryosurgeons together with interventional radiologists is needed to provide the expertise to treat such lesions. Many hospitals are forming these teams to help in the treatment of lesions that were until recently considered untreatable. For large vascular tumors fed by big arteries or veins, embolization or ligation will reduce or even eliminate blood flow to the lesion. In the same surgical procedure or in a second attempt, cryosurgery of the residual vascular mass will further destroy the tumor. In general, it is extremely difficult to indicate freeze time for vascular tumors because many factors are involved, such as lesion volume, probe size, and collateral vascularization. In general, there is a tendency to undertreat than to overtreat. Many treatments are usually necessary to eliminate or reduce these tumors.

Actinic keratosis

Cryosurgery is a widely used method for actinic keratosis. It can work very well for isolated or multiple lesions. Some advocate pretreatment of the affected area locally with 5-FU and/or retinoids to expose the lesions and reduce keratin to allow better cold penetrance, but this is not commonly performed. Chiarello[37,38] has shown excellent results with partial and full face cryopeeling. Use an intermittent spray for 5–10 seconds on each actinic keratosis, allowing the freezing front to spread a few millimeters beyond the lesion margin. If the lesion is hyperkeratotic, a longer freezing time will be needed or subsequent freeze/thaw cycles might be necessary.

Basal cell carcinoma

Basal cell carcinoma can be treated with the open or closed technique. A careful dermatopathological evaluation will allow the surgeon to confirm the type of basal cell carcinoma. Once identified as superficial, solid, sclerosing or morpheaform, decide between the open, chamber, or contact technique. We reserve the use of spray for superficial basal cell carcinoma and probes or chambers for the rest.

For all basal cell carcinomas, clean locally and, when necessary, curette the excess tissue that produces bulkiness. Hemostatic solutions applied to the base will stop any local bleeding which tends to increase the local temperature. Apply local anesthesia and prepare to freeze.[39]

For superficial basal cell carcinomas, spray intermittently, pointing at the center of the lesion, and allowing the freeze halo to advance 5 mm outside the margin of the lesion. This can take less than 60 seconds.

For contact freezing, choose a tip that best fits the diameter of the lesion. Apply the probe; begin to freeze in an intermittent manner, until the tip has adhered to the surface. Then, apply a delicate pulling force as if to remove the probe. This will cause a tent-like effect over the tissue. Let the freeze halo advance for the required 5 mm margin for basal cell carcinomas. This is the superficial cycle of treatment (Fig. 13.5). Remove the probe and allow complete thawing. It is very important for tissue to completely thaw from one cycle to the next to ensure total destruction of the area as a result of intracellular ice formation. Then, apply the previously frozen probe, exerting a perpendicular pressure over the area. Care should

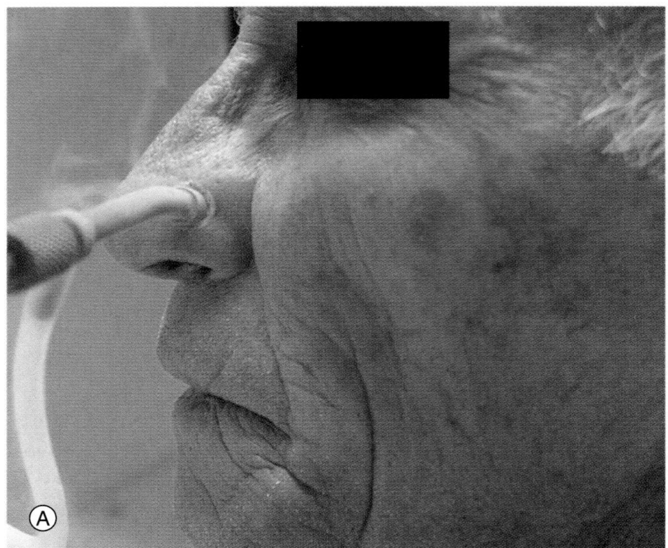

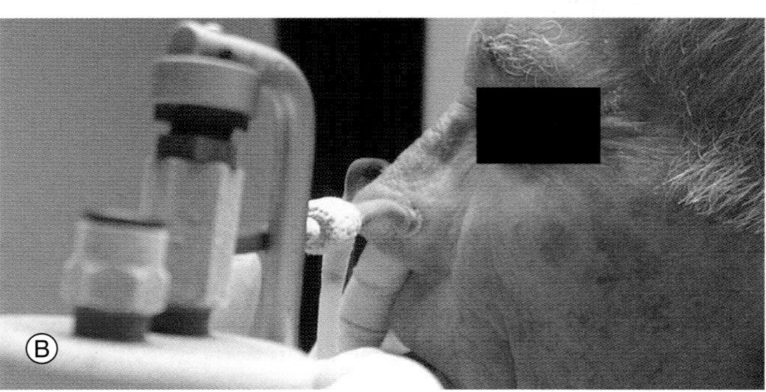

Figure 13.5 Cryosurgery by probe showing treatment of a basal cell carcinoma of the left ala of nose. (A) The superficial component. (B) The deep component treatment—pressure is applied to the underlying tissue.

be taken that the pressure is applied in a perpendicular manner and not bending the probe from one side or another. Start freezing in an intermittent manner until the same freezing halo is obtained. This is the deep component of freezing.

For solid basal cell carcinomas, two cycles,[40] preferably one superficial and one deep cycle should be applied. For squamous or morpheaform tumors, carry out three freeze/thaw cycles, preferably one superficial and two deep.[41]

Kaposi's sarcoma

Kaposi's sarcoma can be a bothersome aesthetic problem when on the face, and because vascular lesions are extremely sensitive to cold, cryosurgery is an excellent treatment alternative.[42]

When Kaposi's sarcoma is persistent and visible in spite of previous treatment with antineoplastic or antiretroviral medication, cryosurgery provides a viable alternative, with results varying from complete disappearance of the original lesion to a faded, less violet and more acceptable spot.

The closed technique is the correct cryosurgery technique for Kaposi's sarcoma, applying a probe that fits the lesion as closely as possible. To protect the probe from contamination, it is convenient to cover it with a rubber slip that will not modify the final temperature or the surface flatness. The easiest way to do so is to obtain a rubber sleeve by cutting out the finger of a latex glove.

One single application, allowing the freezing front to advance just a few millimeters outside the vascular lesion will be sufficient.

Squamous cell carcinoma

For squamous cell carcinoma,[43] teamwork is essential. After the decision has been made that the squamous cell carcinoma is well localized and well differentiated and no local lymph nodes have been invaded, cryosurgery is an option and should preferably be carried out by the closed technique. Probes should be chosen to fit the lesion diameter as closely possible. Triple solid freeze/thaw cycles are indicated.

Palliative treatment

Palliation with cryosurgery is an exciting and growing field. It has opened a new option of treatment for numerous patients with reduced surgical and medical alternatives,[44–47] and is considered when:

- The skin tumor does not respond to conventional treatment (chemotherapy, radiotherapy, or surgical treatment).
- The secondary effects of the above treatments are no longer tolerated by the patient.
- Underlying medical conditions (such as anemia, coagulopathies, heart conditions, diabetes mellitus, and old age) increase the risks of conventional treatments.
- The proposed surgical procedure to reduce or remove the tumor is so disfiguring that the patient rejects it.

Palliative cryosurgery is used to relieve symptoms caused by primary skin tumors or skin metastasis. Some of these tumors can be so destructive and deforming that they cause easy bleeding, local infection, and subsequent foul smell and pain. Cryosurgery can reduce all of these symptoms and thus improve quality of life.

For palliative cryosurgery, the most frequently used technique is the open cryospray because the tumors to be treated tend to be big, solid, and protuberant, and bleed easily. Attempting to shave them (by curettage or electrodesiccation) to reduce their original size, although possible and ideal, is not always advisable because these tumors tend to have an enormous network of neovascularization and patients tend to be weak and anemic (Fig. 13.6).

For certain individual tumors, commercially available cryochambers that fit precisely over the tumor will be an excellent choice. Chamber turbulence allows extremely cold temperatures, which are ideal for highly resistant tumors. They also keep cold within a well defined area. It is very important to apply pressure when using chambers to avoid leakage of liquid nitrogen to the sides of the lesion.

The cryosurgery group from Caracas, Venezuela, has used the most diverse but simple applicators or chambers, including tin cans opened on both sides to build a giant chamber into which liquid nitrogen is directly poured in.

For enormous tumors, cryospray works well. It is important to apply it with the spray fixed at one point and

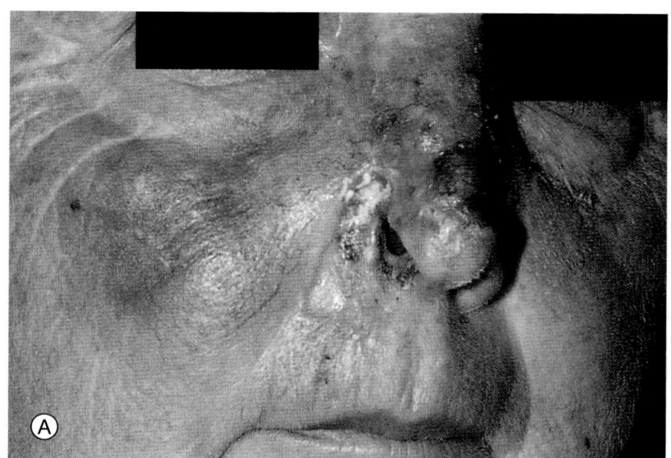

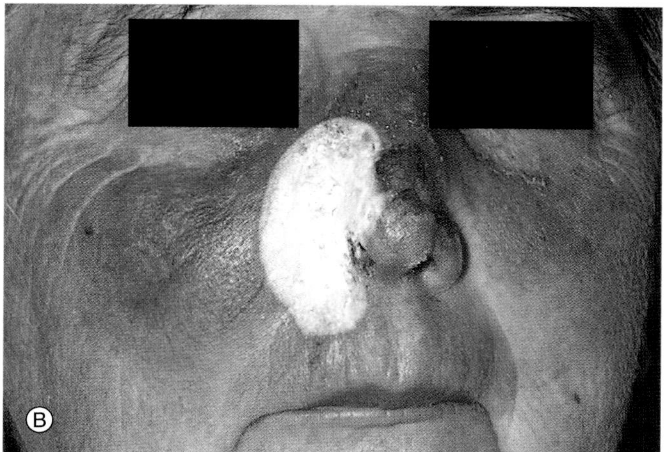

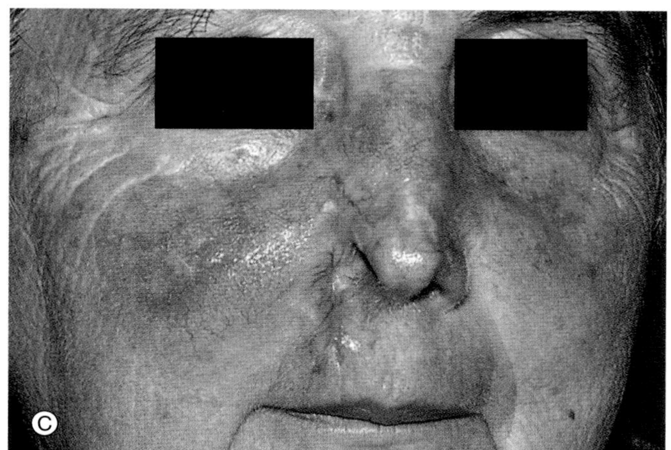

Figure 13.6 (A) A large area with large local destruction in an older woman who has severe underlying medical conditions. (B) The tissue is frozen using a cryospray technique. (C) 2-month postoperative result.

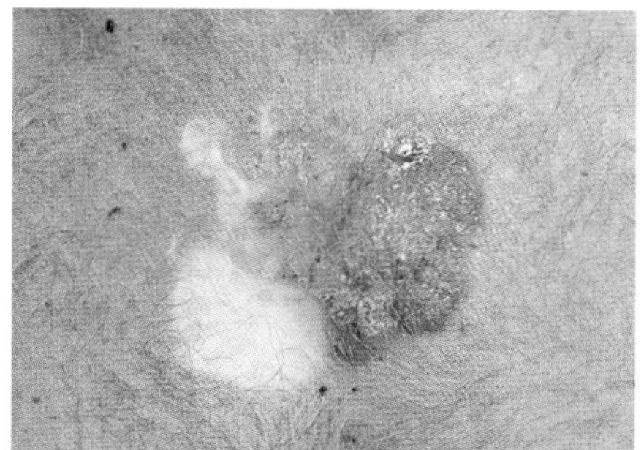

Figure 13.7 Fractional cryosurgery. The white area is the scar left after cryosurgery carried out to only part of this basal cell carcinoma of over 12 cm of diameter on the chest.

allow cold to spread to the periphery. Avoid brushing the spray from one side to the other because this gives the false impression of having obtained the desired low temperatures.

To reassure the surgeon, it is almost impossible to overtreat these lesions. There is a tendency to undertreat them and sessions have to be repeated every 2 weeks until the desired stage at which the main mass has been destroyed and bleeding and pain have been substantially reduced.

Fractional cryosurgery[48] is an excellent alternative—the tumor is gradually reduced in size by treating a small central area at a time and allowing scarring to reduce the tumor (Fig. 13.7). After several treatments, the original tumor will be reduced to a more manageable size. This treatment is extremely useful for large tumoral masses. Weekly follow-ups for debridement are essential. Once a granulating area has been obtained, hydrophilic dressings can be applied.

■ POSTOPERATIVE CARE

Postoperative care in cryosurgery is of extreme importance. It is of much longer duration than for other surgical techniques and patients should be regularly seen at the surgeon's office. In addition, the patient should be aware, before cryosurgery, of all possible secondary effects, and time should be taken to explain the postoperative care to the patient, with the help of carefully written instructions.

The patient keeps the treated area covered at all times to avoid secondary bacterial infection and bothersome exudation into the surrounding tissues or clothing. For simple lesions, care is limited to washing with soap and water with applications of hydrogen peroxide solution (3%).

For more complex lesions, where closed or chamber cryosurgery has been carried out, keep the site clean with water and soap, and use abundant dry gauze dressings and antibiotic ointment. Reserve the use of systemic antibiotics for excessive erythema or pus. These are rare and late events.

The first important postoperative event is local edema. It can be severe in double or triple cycle procedures and the patient should be advised about this to avoid unnecessary anguish and alarmed phone calls. Anti-inflammatory drugs will not reduce it. In areas close to apertures (e.g. nostrils, mouth, and eyelids), the edema can be incapacitating. It lasts a few days, but tends to last longer in skin types I and II.

Remove bullae or vesicles in every case except hemangiomas and keloids. Weeping is expected and will be proportional to the depth of freeze. The deeper the freeze the more prolonged the postoperative weeping.

Once the vesicle has been removed, the denuded area should be cleaned daily with water and soap, and hydrogen peroxide solution (3%) should be applied locally. Keep covered with gauze and tell the patient to clean daily and change dressings as many times as necessary, depending on the amount of weeping.

After an additional 3–10-day period, the lesion starts to dry, tending to form eschar. At this point, the patient should keep the area clean and add an antibiotic ointment. The

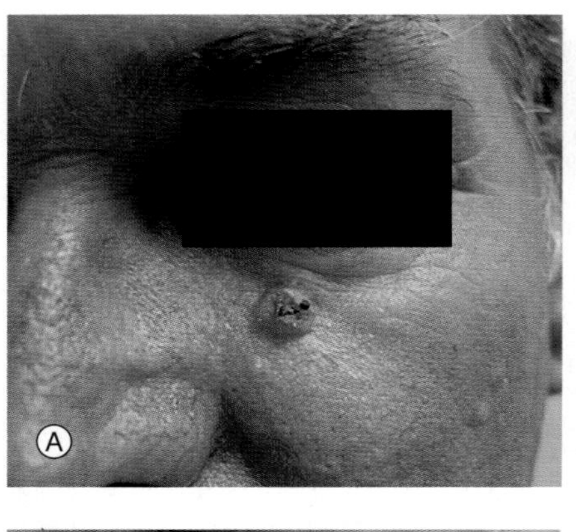

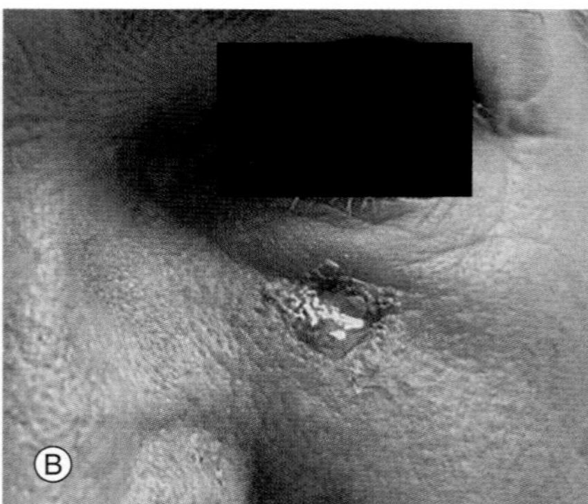

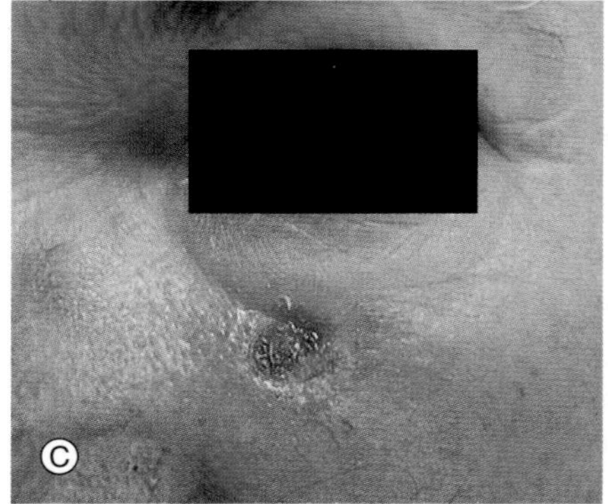

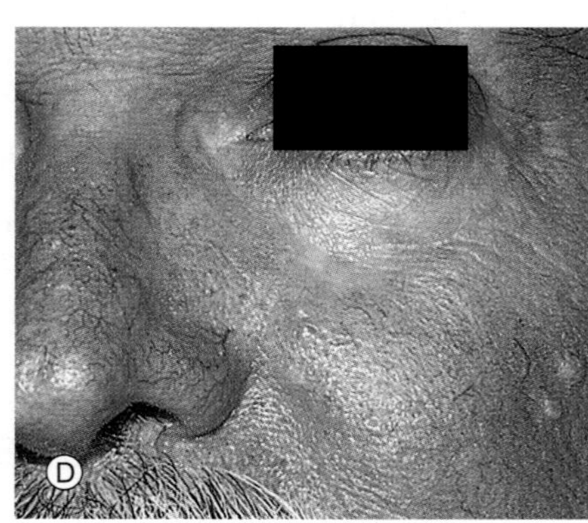

Figure 13.8 (A) Basal cell carcinoma in left cheek, before treatment. (B) 48-hour postoperative edema and redness. (C) 9-day postoperative cryosurgery crust formation. (D) 2-month postoperative cryosurgery result.

cryosurgeon will carry out weekly wound debridement. The postoperative care is crucial because it is the time when there is an increased risk of secondary bacterial infection. Once the ulcer has been freed of any eschar and has appropriate granulation tissue, the use of hydrophilic pads will accelerate healing.

For a superficially sprayed lesion on the face, one could expect 1 week of postoperative time before complete healing. For probe cryosurgery, the deeper the freezing time or the number of cycles, the longer the time it will take to heal. Healing of a probe-treated area on the face can take 3–4 weeks. For a lesion of the same size and treated with the same technique, on the legs, healing can be as long as 2–3 months.

Immediately after healing, the treated area can look erythematous for a variable amount of time. This redness can last weeks and the patient should be strongly advised to use sun protection to avoid hyperpigmentation. Once the redness has disappeared, a hypopigmented area may remain (Fig. 13.8A–D). If the freezing was superficial, as in the case of benign lesions, this hypopigmentation will last just a few weeks and then improve, even resulting in a normally pigmented skin. In deep freezing, such as for skin cancer or hemangiomas, this hypopigmentation tends to last years. In some patients it can take years to repigment while others can be left with a permanent hypopigmented area.

Pseudoepitheliomatous hyperplasia is also a secondary effect of deeply frozen lesions. It does not require treatment and disappears spontaneously after a few months.

Pain can happen minutes after cryosurgery and can last around 45–60 minutes. Then, it will disappear, and regardless of edema, should not be bothersome. The reappearance of local pain several days or weeks after cryosurgery may suggest secondary bacterial infection.

PITFALLS AND THEIR MANAGEMENT

Pitfalls and their management

- Expected occurrences
  - edema and swelling
  - vesicle or bulla formation
  - exudation
  - tissue sloughing
  - eschar formation
  - hypopigmentation
- Occasional temporary cryosurgical events
  - secondary infection
  - inadvertent burn
  - milia
- Occasional permanent cryosurgical events
  - permanent hypopigmentation or achromia
  - retraction
  - notching of ear or ala of nose
  - alopecia
  - nail dystrophy
  - atrophic or depressed scar

As with every method, pitfalls can occur. In cryosurgery, postoperative events may be expected occurrences, occasional temporary events, or occasional permanent cryosurgical events.

Most pitfalls will be reduced if cryosurgery is carried out by appropriately trained surgeons. Most dermatological offices have a cryosurgical unit, and most dermatological training programs include training in this field. Simplicity in any method results from expertise and experience. Even a complicated technique will be simple when carried out by a trained and experienced person. Cryosurgery is no exception.

Expected occurrences

Edema and swelling will be present and proportional to the freeze time. The longer the time, the more cycles applied, the more extensive the local edema. When the procedure has been carried out close to an aperture, the patient may have difficulties in, for example, opening an eye, breathing, or swallowing. The magnitude of edema also depends on the freezing technique and skin type. For fair-skinned and elderly patients, the edema can be very discomforting and longlasting, even though it is not painful. The best treatment in these cases is to reassure the patient. It is better to over-emphasize the expected edema so that the patient is prepared for the worst!

Exudation is also an expected occurrence. For large treated malignancies it can be so extensive that gauze changes are necessary several times a day.

Crust will always tend to form when exudation stops. It is recommended that any newly formed eschar is removed, with the exception of those formed in neovascularized tumors (where removal of the crust could result in bleeding) and keloids (where removal of crust can stimulate further fibroblast activity and growth of the keloid). Weekly debridement by curettage will reduce the risk of secondary bacterial infection.

Hypopigmentation can be expected. It may be temporary and persist for a few weeks or even months. It is proportional to the number and depth of freeze cycles. When the patient has not been strongly advised about it, it can result in a frustrating aesthetic problem.

Occasional temporary cryosurgical events

Secondary infection occurs when postoperative cleaning and debridement have not been properly carried out. It occurs 7–8 days after treatment, once the tissue is not weeping liquid and crust formation allows bacterial colonization. Oral antibiotics should be given for 6–7 days, with cleaning 2–3 times a day, along with the use of local antibiotic ointments or creams.

Care should be taken when freezing using contact probes because cold vapor is emitted from the release hose. If it is not pointed away from the patient, there is always the risk of inadvertently burning the patient.

Milia can easily be eliminated using the point of a needle or a lancet.

■ SUMMARY

Cryosurgery is an extremely versatile method that is indispensable in a dermatologist's office. It is a valid alternative for the treatment of many lesions, such as seborrheic keratosis, actinic keratosis, molluscum contagiosum, and many others. It is as effective as other methods, but with evident cost and time advantages. For other diseases and in certain circumstances (such as advanced age and underlying disease), cryosurgery is the first choice. It allows the treatment of skin conditions under the most adverse conditions, for instance when patients are wheelchair or bedbound, reducing discomfort and unnecessary mobilization.

For palliation, cryosurgery has opened up a whole new field as a simple low-risk procedure to improve symptoms of pain, bleeding, and infection.

■ REFERENCES

1. Hoffmann NE, Bischof JC. The cryobiology of cryosurgical injury. Urology 2002; 20(suppl 1): 40–49.
2. Hoffmann NE, Bischof JC. Cryosurgery of normal and tumor tissue in the dorsal skin flap chamber: Part II—injury response. J Biomech Eng 2001; 123:310–316.
3. Bischof JC. Quantitative measurement and prediction of biophysical response during freezing in tissues. Annu Rev Biomed Eng 2000; 2:257–288.
4. Hoffmann NE, Bischof JC. Cryosurgery of normal and tumor tissue in the dorsal skin flap chamber: Part I—thermal response. J Biomech Eng 2001; 123:301–309.
5. Rubinsky B. Cryosurgery. Annu Rev Biomed Eng 2000; 2:157–187.
6. Kuflik EG, Gage AA, Lubritz RR, et al. History of dermatologic cryosurgery. Dermatol Surg 2000; 26:715–722.
7. Wolf R, Landau M, Berger SA, et al. Transfer of bacteria associated with cryotherapy. Cutis 1993; 51:276–278.
8. Graham GF. Cryosurgery: a useful tool in the treatment of selected infectious diseases. Int J Dermatol 1994; 33:107–108.
9. American Academy of Dermatology Committee on Guidelines of Care. Guidelines of care for cryosurgery. J Am Acad Dermatol 1994; 31: 648–653.
10. Al-Gindan Y, Kubba R, Omer AH, et al. Cryosurgery in old world cutaneous leishmaniasis. Br J Dermatol 1988; 118:851–854.
11. Kenawy MZ, Abadía KF. The clinical picture of six Egyptian cases of cutaneous leishmaniasis. J Egypt Soc Parasitol 1992; 22:453–459.
12. Faber WR. Cryosurgery for cutaneous leishmaniasis. J Dermatol Surg Oncol 1983; 9:354–356.
13. Castro LG, Pimentel ER, Lacaz CS. Treatment of chromomycosis by cryosurgery with liquid nitrogen: 15 years' experience. Int J Dermatol 2003; 42:408–412.
14. August PJ, Milward TM. Cryosurgery in the treatment of lichen sclerosus et atrophicus of the vulva. Br J Dermatol 1980; 103:667–670.
15. Waldinger TP, Wong RC, Taylor WB, et al. Cryotherapy improves prurigo nodularis. Arch Dermatol 1984; 120:1598–1600.
16. Hill AC, Dougherty JW, Torre D. Cryosurgical treatment of dermatofibromas. Cutis 1975; 16:517–518.
17. Bohler-Sommeregger K, Kutschera-Hienert G. Cryosurgical management of myxoid cyst. J Dermatol Surg Oncol 1988; 14:1405–1408.
18. Suhonen R, Kuflik EG.Venous lakes treated by liquid nitrogen cryosurgery. Br J Dermatol 1997; 137:1018–1019.
19. Mullins EA. Cryosurgical therapy of alopecia areata. In: Dyall-Smith D, Marks R, eds. Dermatology at the millennium. New York: Parthenon Publishing Group; 1999; 550–551.
20. Suhonen RE, Kuflik EG. Cryosurgical methods for eyelid lesions. J Dermatol Treatment 2001; 12:135–139.
21. Blume-Peytavi U, Zouboulis CC, Jacobi H, Scholtz A, Bisson S, Orfanos CE. Successful outcome of cryosurgery in patients with granuloma annulare. Br J Dermatol 1994; 130:494–497.
22. Kuflik AS, Schwartz RA. Lymphocytoma cutis: a series of five patients successfully treated with cryosurgery. J Am Acad Dermatol 1992; 26;449–452.
23. Pradel W, Hlawitschka M, Eckelt U, et al. Cryosurgical treatment of genuine trigeminal neuralgia. Br J Oral Maxillofac Surg 2002; 40:244–247.
24. Ocampo-Candiani J, Cueva-Rodriguez JA. Cryosurgical treatment of pearly penile papules. J Am Acad Dermatol 1996; 35:486–487.
25. Dufresne RG, Curlin MU. Actinic cheilitis. A treatment review. Dermatol Surg 1997; 23:490–491.
26. Kuflik EG. Cryosurgery updated. J Am Acad Dermatol 1994; 31:925–944.
27. Kuflik EG, Gage AA. Cryosurgery for lentigo maligna. J Am Acad Dermatol 1994; 31;75–78.
28. Zacarian SA. Cryosurgical treatment of lentigo maligna. Arch Dermatol 1982; 118:89–92.
29. French L, Nashelsky J, White D. What is the most effective treatment for external genital warts? J Fam Pract 2002; 51:313.
30. Connolly M, Bazmi K, O'Connell M, Lyons JF, Bourke JF. Cryotherapy of viral warts: a sustained 10's freeze is more effective than the traditional method. Br J Dermatol 2001; 145:554–557.
31. Vozmediano JM, Manrique A, Petraglia S, et al. Giant molluscum contagiosum in AIDS. Int J Dermatol 1996; 35:45–47.
32. Kaminska-Budzinska G, Krauze E, Pierzchala E, et al .Cutaneous larva migrans—an unusual case. Pol Merkuriusz Lek 2002; 12;232–234.

33. Stern RS, Dover JS, Levin JA, Arndt KA. Laser therapy versus cryotherapy of lentigines: a comparative trial. J Am Acad Dermatol 1994; 30:985–987.
34. Rusciani L, Rossi G, Bono R. Use of cryotherapy in the treatment of keloids. J Dermatol Surg Oncol 1993; 19:529–534.
35. Castro-Ron G, Pasquali P. In: Management of hemangiomas. Special symposium. Pediatr Dermatol 1997; 14:70–71.
36. Hasan Q, Tan S, Gush J, et al. Steroid therapy of a proliferating hemangioma: histochemical and molecular changes. Pediatrics 2000; 105:117–120.
37. Chiarello SE. Cryopeeling (extensive cryosurgery) for treatment of actinic keratoses: an update and comparison. Dermatol Surg 2000; 26:728–732.
38. Chiarello SE. Full-face cryo-(liquid nitrogen) peel. J Dermatol Surg Oncol 1992; 18:329–332.
39. Goncalves JC, Martins C. Debulking of skin cancers with radio frequency before cryosurgery. Dermatol Surg 1997; 23:253–256; discussion 256–257.
40. Mallon E, Dawber R. Cryosurgery in the treatment of basal cell carcinoma. Assessment of one and two freeze-thaw cycle schedules. Dermatol Surg 1996; 22:854–858.
41. Jaramillo-Ayerbe F. Cryosurgery in difficult to treat basal cell carcinomas. Int J Dermatol 2000; 39:223–229.
42. Tappero JW, Berger TG, Kaplan LD, et al. Cryotherapy for cutaneous Kaposi's sarcoma (KS) associated with acquired immune deficiency syndrome (AIDS): a phase II trial. J Acquir Defic Syndr 1991; 4:839–846.
43. Kuflik EG. Cryosurgery for cutaneous malignancies. An update. Dermatol Surg 1997; 23:1081–1087.
44. Biro DE, Biro LB. Cryosurgery in the nursing home. J Geriatr Dermatol 1997; 5:16–19.
45. Pasquali P. Cryosurgical palliation for advanced malignancies. In: Dyall-Smith D, Marks R, eds. Dermatology at the millennium. New York: Parthenon Publishing Group; 1999:564–565.
46. Kuflik EG. Cryosurgery for palliation. J Dermatol Surg Oncol 1985; 11;867–869.
47. Kollender Y, Meller I, Bickels J, et al. Role of adjuvant cryosurgery in intralesional treatment of sacral tumors. Cancer 2003; 97:2830–2838.
48. Goncalves JC. Fractional cryosurgery. A new technique for basal cell carcinomas of the eyelids and periorbital area. Dermatol Surg 1997; 23:475–481.

14 Skin Biopsy Techniques

Carlos Garcia MD

Summary box

- There are several biopsy techniques: shave, saucerization, scissor and punch biopsy, incisional and excisional biopsy.
- The skin biopsy is essential to dermatologic surgery, in diagnosis and in the planning of therapy.
- Preoperative evaluation should emphasize identification of risk factors for complications, particularly bleeding and infection.
- The biopsy site is selected carefully, taking into consideration the size and location of lesions, involvement of the epidermis, dermis and or subcutaneous fat, the cosmetic consequences, and the planned therapy.
- Choice of technique depends upon the type of lesion under investigation.
- Complications are infrequent and can be minimized by careful technique and patient selection.

INTRODUCTION

The skin biopsy is a relatively simple, but essential procedure in the management of skin disorders. Properly performed, it may confirm a diagnosis, remove cosmetically concerning lesions, and provide definitive treatment for a number of dermatoses. The choice of technique depends on the location, depth, and size of the lesion, and its potential for malignancy.

Skin biopsies are indicated to monitor the effectiveness of dermatologic treatment, to remove a neoplasm and check its margins, or to establish a diagnosis. Performance of these procedures places the operator at risk of blood-borne infections. Accordingly, vaccination for hepatitis B is indicated, and universal precautions should be observed by wearing gloves and eye-guards.[1] Used sharp objects (needle, punches, blades) should be disposed in approved Occupational Safety and Health Administration (OSHA) containers. The biopsy site should not be chosen indiscriminately.[2] It is important to consider the purpose (diagnostic versus therapeutic), the suspected clinical diagnosis, the level or depth of pathology, the location of the lesion, and cosmetic implications. For disseminated dermatoses, the arms, upper legs or trunk are the best sites.[3] In general, try to avoid sampling the lower leg, because of poor healing and vascular stasis changes that may complicate the histologic interpretation, and the palms or soles, because the thickness of skin impedes appropriate examination. Hypertrophic scarring tends to occur over the chest and deltoid areas, and secondary infection is common in the axilla and groin. Therefore, biopsies of these areas should be performed only if other sites are unavailable.

Diagnostic biopsies should be taken from the most representative lesion and one with minimal secondary changes. Therapeutic biopsies are indicated in cases where a tumor of appropriate size is suspected or in benign lesions that are of cosmetic concern.

Lesions with epidermal pathology can be shave-biopsied, while dermal lesions are best approached with saucerization, punch, incisional, or excisional techniques.[4] Superficial and pedunculated lesions are suitable for scissor excision, but deeply seated lesions, such as those with involvement of the subcutaneous fat, require incisional or excisional procedures.

Cutaneous tumors are preferably excised *in toto* because examination of the whole specimen is far superior and more rewarding than the analysis of only segments. Yet, incisional biopsies are adequate when the diagnosis is in doubt, the lesion is too large, or if the cosmetic consequences of complete excision are significant. In these cases, the area with the maximum depth of tumor and at least one margin of normal skin should be obtained.

Ulcerative lesions pose special problems and their biopsy may be particularly unrewarding. In general, it is best to sample an area that is several millimeters away from the advancing edge and that includes normal skin. The decision to biopsy an ulcer must be made carefully as there is a propensity for these lesions to show slow healing, or to progress.

For inflammatory conditions, one should avoid traumatized or secondarily infected lesions, and a mature lesion should be selected. Mature lesions should also be selected in cases of infectious and non-infectious granulomatous processes. Punch, incisional, or excisional techniques are preferred in order to obtain epidermis, dermis, and subcutaneous tissue. The central portion of a mature lesion is ideal but the edge is adequate in cases of large plaques or in annular lesions. Traumatized, infected, older, and involuting lesions alter the primary pathology and yield non-specific histologic findings. Vesiculobullous diseases are better diagnosed in early lesions and one must try to avoid sampling well-formed bullae. If only old lesions are available, then the edge of the lesion must be selected. Perilesional skin is appropriate for immúnofluorescence studies.

Bleeding after skin biopsies is usually minimal and can often be controlled with pressure alone. Chemical hemostasia can be achieved with 20% aluminum chloride in absolute alcohol, Monsel's solution (ferric subsulfate), trichloroacetic acid, or silver nitrate. Monsel's solution is the most effective agent but it causes more tissue destruction and may result in unwanted pigmentation of the area.

All biopsy specimens must be carefully labeled, including the names of the patient and physician, the date, location of the lesion, short clinical history, and diagnostic possibilities. In case a tumor was removed, request that margins be checked. For routine light microscopic examination, the specimen is placed in 10% buffered formalin solution. For electron microscopy, glutaraldehyde is used. Frozen tissue is preferred for immunohistochemistry, monoclonal antibodies, and immunofluorescence studies. Biopsies sent for culture are placed in normal saline solution and transported to the laboratory immediately. A special sealed vial is required for anaerobic culture.

The most common light microscopic stains are listed in Table 14.1.

PREOPERATIVE PREPARATION

Preoperative evaluation

As with any other surgical technique, prebiopsy evaluation should be thorough. It is essential to ask about underlying medical problems such as diabetes, peripheral vascular disease, or collagen tissue disorders, as these can interfere with, and significantly delay, the normal wound healing process. Allergies to medications, bleeding disorders, and current medications should be investigated (Table 14.2; see also Chapter 5). Traditionally, patients have been instructed to stop taking coumadin or aspirin in anticipation of their surgery, to avoid bleeding complications. Nevertheless, there is now ample scientific evidence suggesting that these agents do not increase the risk of bleeding after cutaneous surgery, and stopping therapy may place the patient at risk from a thromboembolic event.[5] For instance, a prospective evaluation in 12 patients undergoing Mohs surgery showed that although there was increased intraoperative bleeding, this was easily controlled, and only 1 patient (8%) needed to come back for active intervention.[6] Another prospective study of 16 patients undergoing cutaneous surgery showed that there were no significant bleeding events in patients who continued to take warfarin compared with 77 controls.[7]

Several studies have addressed the use of aspirin by patients undergoing skin surgery. Overall, they show a slightly greater risk of serious bleeding complications but the risk is low, and there is no need to stop the medication. In a prospective study of 40 patients, only three taking aspirin and three controls had excessive bleeding.[8] Another study showed no difference in bleeding between 52 patients on aspirin compared to 119 controls.[9] Finally, a study of 81 patients undergoing Mohs surgery showed that 9 (11.1%) had increased bleeding while taking aspirin, with only 2 (3%) returning for redressing, and 1 (1.5%) requiring another operation, compared to control group values of 2% and 0.5%, respectively.[6]

Informed consent

A succinct but comprehensive informed consent should be obtained before performing skin biopsies. Patients must be told of the rationale and objectives of the procedure, the basic technique to be used, and the potential complications arising from such interventions.[10] At a minimum, we like to include the following points:

- The nature of the biopsy procedure (diagnostic versus therapeutic)
- Pain and/or discomfort may occur during the injection of the anesthetic

Table 14.1 Common stains for light microscopy

Target	Stain
Routine	Hematoxylin and eosin
Glycogen, neutral mucopolysaccharides	Periodic acid–Schiff
Neutral mucopolysaccharides	Periodic acid–Schiff with diastase
Acid mucopolysaccharides	Alcian blue
Mast cells	Giemsa, toluidine blue
Connective tissue	Masson trichrome
Melanin	Silver nitrate, Fontana Masson
Calcium	von Kossa
Amyloid	Congo red, thioflavine T
Lipid	Oil-red-O
Elastic fibers	Verhoeff
Fungi	Periodic acid–Schiff, methenamine silver

Table 14.2 Drug interactions in dermatologic surgery

Phenothiazines	Hypotension and cardiac arrest with use of vasodilating local anesthetics
Monoamine oxidase inhibitors	Hypertensive crisis with use of epinephrine (adrenaline)
Beta blockers	Hypertensive crisis with use of epinephrine (adrenaline)
Tricyclic antidepressants	Hypertensive crisis with use of epinephrine (adrenaline)
Diuretics	Resultant hypokalemia may cause cardiac arrhythmia with use of epinephrine
Immunosuppressive drugs	Delayed wound healing, postoperative infection

- A definitive diagnosis may not be rendered even after adequate biopsy
- A permanent scar will result from the procedure
- Complications are possible but usually minor, including bleeding, infection and dehiscence
- Recurrence of skin lesions is always possible
- Further treatment (surgical and/or medical) may be necessary
- Preoperative photographs will be taken as part of the medical record

A signed informed consent form, with appropriate documentation in the chart, should be available for all types of biopsies. It is important to remember that patients forget information given to them before surgical procedures and some may become litigious if complications arise. We have demonstrated that patients' recall is only 25% at 20 minutes and 1 week after delivery of written and oral information before Mohs surgery.[11]

Preparation of the biopsy site

Small shave, punch, and scissor biopsies are adequately performed using clean or modified-sterile technique. Gowns, face masks, and sterile fields are not strictly necessary, but clean gloves help protect the physician from acquiring blood-borne infections including hepatitis and human immunodeficiency virus (HIV). The infection rate for minor cutaneous surgical procedures is less than 1% and usually related to poor surgical technique. Resident flora in skin includes *Staphylococcus epidermidis*, *Corynebacterium*, *Brevibacterium*, *Propionibacterium* and *Pityrosporum*. Transient flora may include streptococci types A and B and Gram-negative rods, particularly *Pseudomonas*. Colonization with *Staphylococcus aureus* is more common in patients with psoriasis or atopic dermatitis, with intravenous drug users, diabetes, or during isotretinoin therapy.

Topical antimicrobial strategies include preoperative hand washing and surgical scrubbing of the site. Alcohol, chlorhexidine, or iodophors are usually employed. Alcohols are the gold standard. They act rapidly by denaturing proteins but have no residual activity. They are effective against Gram-positive and Gram-negative bacteria, against viruses such as HIV and cytomegalovirus (CMV), and against fungi, but they are not sporicidal. A 10-second alcohol wipe was shown to be as effective as a 1-minute scrub with 1% povidone-iodine or 0.5% chlorhexidine.[12] For larger biopsies, biopsies in 'clean contaminated' fields, such as perineum or axilla, and biopsies in immunosuppressed individuals, chlorhexidine or povidone iodine offers better coverage for Gram-negative bacteria. (For further information, see Chapter 2.)

Chlorhexidine disrupts microbial cell membranes and has an intermediate onset of action. It binds to the skin and therefore has residual activity. This agent also resists an alcohol wipe and is available as a 0.5% hand rinse or 4% detergent. It should be used with caution around ears and eyes because it can produce ototoxicity and keratitis.

Iodophors produce oxidative reactions by releasing free iodine. They require a 2-minute contact time and are stopped by drying or blood. These agents have irritant and allergic potential, may be toxic for human wounds, and have minimal residual activity.

A good surgical hand scrub is required only for sterile technique. It removes debris, transient and resident flora. A 3-minute alcohol wash is equivalent to a 2-minute chlorhexidine scrub. Preoperative showers help reduce the bacterial counts in the skin but shaving of the surgical area is not necessary and may be detrimental.

In spite of the above-mentioned facts, it is worth remembering that skin cannot be truly sterilized. Approximately 90% of the flora resides in periungual areas and 20% in adnexal structures. Even when using sterile gloves our technique may be clean and not sterile. Sterile gloves have a 1.5–3% failure rate, and this increases to 66% after 15 minutes of use. Bacterial counts increase with moisture and there is a 30% incidence of unnoticed punctures during procedures.

Antibiotic prophylaxis

Prophylactic antibiotics are not routine for cutaneous surgery but may be used during skin biopsies if there is a defective immunologic function such as in debilitating underlying disease or very elderly and fragile individuals, if a prolonged procedure is anticipated, or if there is excessive fulguration of tissue during hemostasis. We indicate prophylactic antibiotics for patients with uncontrolled diabetes, alcoholism, malnutrition, and morbid obesity. In order to be effective and truly prophylactic, antibiotics should be administered within 3 hours of the procedure and for no more than 24 hours. Usually, a single preoperative dose is preferred and cephalosporins are the agents of choice.

The American Heart Association's indications for prophylactic antibiotics have been published elsewhere.[13] Currently, prophylaxis is not recommended for people with previous coronary artery bypass surgery, mitral valve prolapse without regurgitation, a history of rheumatic fever without valvular dysfunction, pacemakers or defibrillators, physiologic, functional or innocent heart murmurs, or with a history of Kawasaki's disease without valvular dysfunction.

Anesthesia

Local anesthetics block the sodium channels in axon membranes thereby preventing depolarization. All agents have a lipophilic aromatic component and a hydrophobic amine group connected by an intermediate chain. Two main classes, amides and esters, differ in the structure of the intermediate chain. The former have an amide linkage that is metabolized by microsomal enzymes in the liver and excreted by the kidneys. The latter have an ester linkage that is metabolized by pseudocholinesterase in plasma and excreted by the kidneys.

Sometimes, biopsy procedures can be performed under topical anesthesia. EMLA (eutectic mixture of local anesthetics) is 2.5% lidocaine in eutectic mixture with prilocaine 2.5%.[14] It also contains emulsifiers that increase penetration and/or absorption. It requires a minimum occlusion time of 1 hour for superficial procedures but dermal anesthesia requires 2–3 hours. EMLA may be used without occlusion in genital skin but is ineffective in thick stratum corneum, such as in the palms and soles. There is minimal absorption, with lidocaine being metabolized by the liver, and prilocaine by liver and kidney. Side effects include methemoglobinemia, hypersensitivity reactions, and systemic toxicity. Methemoglobinemia is more common in children younger than 3 months of age due to an immature NADH-reductase system, if there is previous history of methemoglobinemia, or with drugs such as sulfonamides, acetaminophen, chloroquine, dapsone, nitroglycerin, phenobarbital, phenytoin, and quinine.

LMX 4 (Ferndale Laboratories Inc, Ferndale, MI) is lidocaine 4% at pH 7.4. Occlusion times are shorter than with EMLA, with variable effectiveness.[15] Lidocaine in acid mantle is lidocaine powder in a water-miscible vehicle such as mantle (Novartis and Velvachol Health-Point). Both contain parabens, and toxicity has not been studied. Compared to EMLA, it is less effective.

Injection or infiltrative anesthesia includes intradermal, subcutaneous, field blocks, nerve blocks, and tumescent anesthesia.[16] Most frequently, lidocaine alone or in combination with bupivacaine is employed. Epinephrine (adrenaline) 1 in 100 000 is added to improve hemostasis, to decrease absorption, and to prolong duration of anesthetics. Epinephrine (adrenaline) is contraindicated to acral sites such as the tips of the digits, the penis, and the tip of the nose, where a marked vasoconstriction or vasospasm could produce tissue necrosis. Yet, even in these locations, limited amounts are usually used without incident.

Pain on injection of the anesthetic can be minimized by buffering the solution with sodium bicarbonate 8.4% solution (1 in 10 volume), using 30-gauge needles, injecting at a 45° angle from the skin surface, injecting slowly, and pinching the skin before injection.[17] A compassionate demeanor in the physician or nurse is always helpful. Intradermal injection produces immediate and prolonged anesthesia but is very painful. Subcutaneous injection is much less painful but has delayed onset and shorter duration. Nerve blocks are seldom used for biopsy procedures except in digit or nail biopsies. They allow for a higher concentration but decreased volume of anesthetic, cause less distortion of tissues, can anesthetize larger areas, but are without hemostatic effect.

Contraindications for local anesthesia may include a history of allergic reactions to anesthetic agents, pseudocholinesterase deficiency (in case of ester anesthetics), significant liver disease, pregnancy, or breast-feeding.

Adverse reactions may occur with needles, epinephrine (adrenaline), or anesthetic agents. Many patients who report adverse events may have had a vasovagal response with lightheadedness, pallor, sweating, nausea, vomiting, hypotension, and bradycardia.

Needles may provoke pain, fainting, ecchymosis, edema, infection, or hematoma. Epinephrine (adrenaline) has been associated with tissue necrosis, tremors, tachycardia, diaphoresis, palpitations, hypertension, and chest pain. Also, severe hypertensive crises have been reported in patients taking propranolol, or in those with hyperthyroidism.

Adverse reactions to lidocaine may be allergic, anaphylactic, or idiosyncratic. Severe symptoms occur only with high blood levels. These include paresthesias, lightheadedness, drowsiness (>6 μg/ml), muscle twitching, irritability, nystagmus (10 μg/ml), seizures and respiratory arrest (10–20 μg/ml).

Both immediate (type I) and delayed (type IV) hypersensitivity reactions can occur. Type I reactions are more common with ester anesthetics, which are derivatives of the highly allergenic para-aminobenzoic acid (PABA). True allergic reactions to lidocaine are extremely rare and diphenhydramine or sterile saline can be substituted in selected cases. More frequently, the reactions are secondary to preservatives in the anesthetic mixture. Preservative-free lidocaine is available in the single-use vials of regular crash-carts in clinics or hospitals, or can be ordered from specialized pharmacies.

Delayed hypersensitivity reactions are more commonly seen as contact dermatitis to topically applied anesthetics such as benzocaine or PABA.

■ TECHNIQUES

Shave, saucerization and scissor biopsy

The shave technique is adequate for sampling and/or removal of lesions limited to the epidermis and papillary dermis, such as actinic and seborrheic keratoses, warts, sebaceous hyperplasia, superficial and nodular basal cell carcinoma, pyogenic granuloma, and non-pigmented melanocytic nevi (Table 14.3). It is quick, requires little training, and does not require sutures for closure. After preparation of the site, the fingers in the non-dominant hand are used to apply three-point pressure on the skin in order to stretch it taut. Intradermal injection of the anesthetic helps raising a wheal to elevate the lesion from surrounding skin. A #15 surgical blade is held parallel to the skin surface at the base of the lesion and a cutting or sawing motion is used to cut horizontally through the lesion at the level of the mid-dermis.[18] The depth of the biopsy is controlled by the angle of the blade. The edges can then be curetted to remove remaining lesion or improve cosmetic result. An alternative instrument, and the one we favor because it is sharper, is the double-edge razor blade. The blade is gently bent between the thumb and index finger allowing the operator to control the size and depth of the excision by increasing or decreasing the concavity of the blade (Fig. 14.1). Bleeding can be controlled with pressure alone, or by applying aluminum chloride or Monsel's solution. The wound heals by second intention and typically re-epithelializes in approximately 1 week. A small depressed scar the size of the initial lesion is likely to remain.

A saucerization biopsy requires similar technique but the excision includes the skin lesion plus a portion of the surrounding skin down to subcutaneous fat. It is suited for lesions located on epidermis and dermis, such as nevi, basal cell carcinoma, squamous cell carcinoma, or melanoma.

The scissor biopsy is particularly useful for excision of pedunculated skin lesions such as polypoid melanocytic nevi, filiform warts, and skin tags. Reasons for removal include cosmesis, itching, irritation, or a tendency to catch on clothing. After preparation and anesthesia, an iris or Gradle scissor is used to snip the base of the lesion followed

Table 14.3 Indications for shave biopsy

Exophytic benign lesions (warts, skin tags, seborrheic keratoses)
Precancerous actinic keratoses
Superficial neoplasms (basal cell carcinoma, squamous cell carcinoma)
Superficial noduloulcerative processes

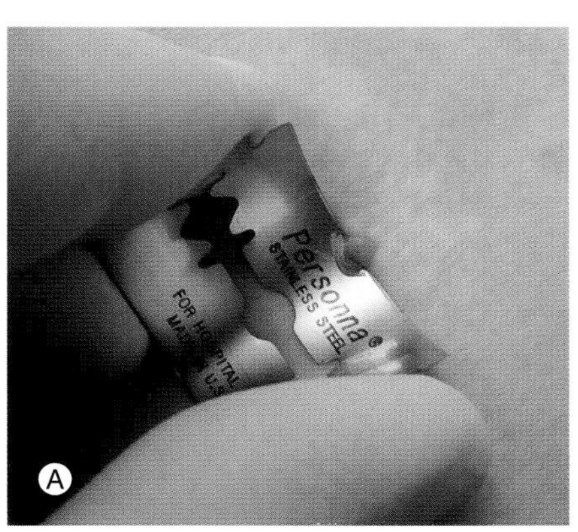

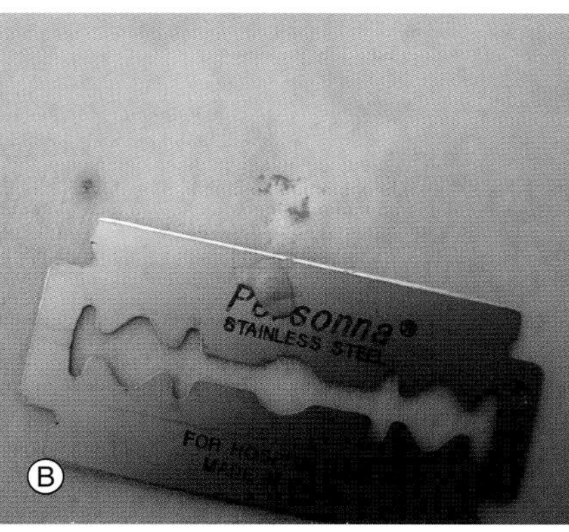

Figure 14.1 Shave biopsy. (A) Local anesthesia is used to elevate the lesion from surrounding skin in order to facilitate the procedure. A double-edged razor blade is gently bent between thumb and index fingers and a sawing motion is employed to obtain the specimen. The operator controls the depth of the excision by increasing or decreasing the concavity of the blade. (B) A shallow wound is produced that heals rapidly by second intention. Hemostasis is achieved with pressure or topical application of aluminum chloride or Monsel's solution.

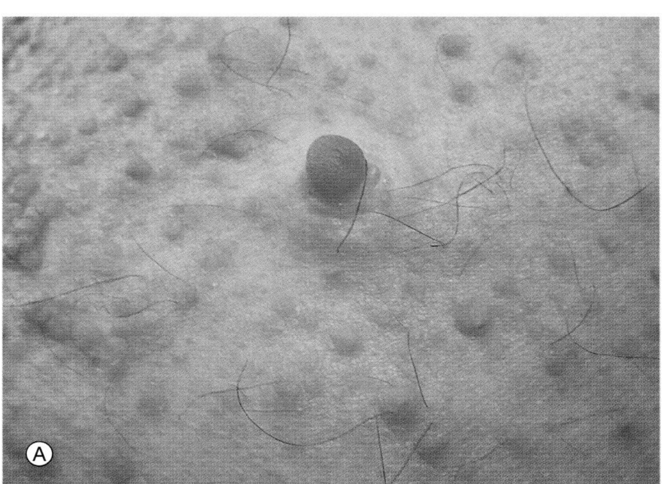

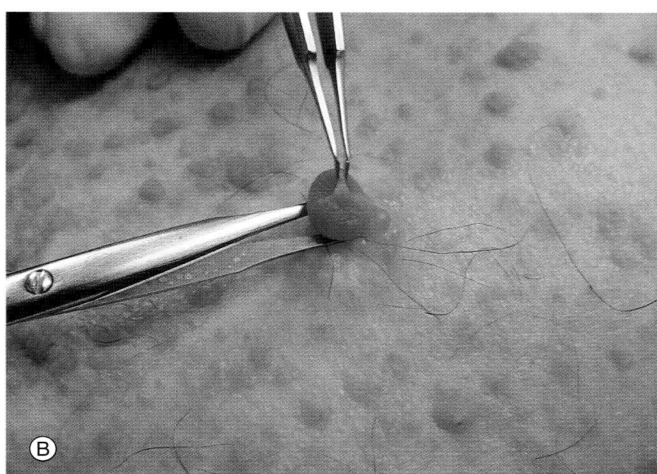

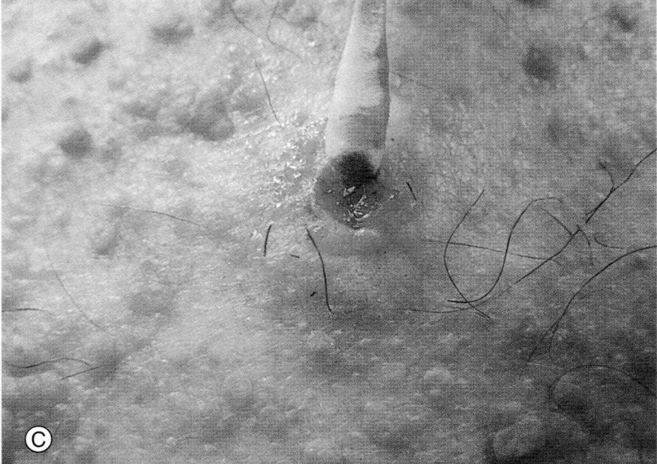

Figure 14.2 Scissor biopsy. (A) The area has been anesthetized and the lesion elevated to facilitate excision. (B) The skin lesion is gently grasped with tissue forceps and its base is sniped with Iris or Gradle scissors. (C) The resulting defect is shallow and hemostasis can be achieved with pressure alone or with the aid of chemicals such as aluminum chloride or Monsel's solution.

by pressure or chemical hemostasis (Fig. 14.2). Very small lesions may be removed without anesthesia.

Punch biopsy

The punch biopsy is the technique most commonly used for obtaining tissue for dermatologic diagnosis but it also has therapeutic applications. It is done with sharp cylindric instruments called punches or trephines. These are available as disposable or reusable instruments, and range in size from 2 mm to 8 mm. Most cutaneous surgeons prefer the disposable punches because they are readily available and are always sharp.

Punch biopsies are easily mastered by physicians, are quick, and have low incidence of significant scarring, non-healing, bleeding, and infection. The distinct advantage of a punch biopsy over the shave biopsy is its ability to sample the full thickness of skin, allowing for evaluation of dermal pathology (Table 14.4). It is widely acknowledged that a punch may not obtain an adequate amount of subcutaneous tissue in cases of panniculitis, in which cases an incisional or excisional specimen is preferred. This concept, however, was recently challenged in a study of 84 cases with various dermatoses.[19] In 79 of them the same histopathologic diagnosis was reached with the 2 mm punch versus the standard ellipse, including two cases of panniculitis. The

Table 14.4 Indications for punch biopsy

Processes involving deep dermis, adnexal structures or superficial subcutis
Inflammatory dermatoses
Direct immunofluorescence
Bullous disorders
Deep noduloulcerative processes
Diffuse eruptions
Small-vessel vasculitis
Infections (tissue culture)

authors concluded that the punch biopsy produces specimens which allow an accurate histological diagnosis to be made in a wide range of dermatological conditions. The 2 mm punch was not appropriate for evaluation of vascular lesions; however, because the authors could not diagnose either of two hemangiomas. It seems that insufficient tissue was present to allow for adequate support of the ectatic blood vessels, with the result that the architecture was not preserved.

Diagnostic techniques available after a punch biopsy include hematoxylin and eosin histopathology, direct immunofluorescence, polariscopic examination, immunohistochemical stains, culture, and electron microscopy. Therapeutic applications are mainly related to reconstructive surgery, hair transplantation, and removal of small skin lesions.

The punch technique produces small wounds with regular and smooth borders. Punch biopsy sites that are 3 mm or less in diameter can be left to heal by second intention, mainly if located in cosmetically irrelevant areas. For wounds that are 4 mm and larger, or those located on the face, suturing with non-absorbable suture produces better aesthetic results.[20]

A punch biopsy tray should include alcohol pads, local anesthetic, gloves, punch instrument (2–6 mm in diameter), forceps, scissors, and gauze. If the lesion is poorly demarcated, its extent can be outlined with a pen before the procedure. After preparation of the site, the fingers in the non-dominant hand are used to apply three-point pressure on the skin in order to stretch it taut. Pulling the skin perpendicular to the direction of the relaxed skin tension lines can produce an oval defect that is easier to close. The punch is held perpendicular to the skin surface and the specimen bored out by pressing down firmly while twirling the punch down to subcutaneous tissue. The punch is withdrawn, and the specimen retrieved by piercing it with the needle from the syringe used for anesthesia or by careful handling with the forceps. If needed, scissors can be used to transect the subcutaneous tissue at its deepest portion (Fig. 14.3). Hemostasis can be achieved with pressure, Gelfoam pledgets, Monsel's solution (ferric subsulfate), or aluminum chloride 25% in isopropyl alcohol 50%.

On the scalp, the punch should be directed at a 20° angle of inclination in order to follow the direction of the hair, and the biopsy should include subcutaneous tissue to ensure sampling of the hair papillae.[21] On the nail apparatus, a 4 mm punch can be used to excise a portion of the nail plate and a 3 mm punch is then used to biopsy the nail bed (Fig. 14.4). For nail matrix biopsies, 2–3 mm punches are taken from the distal matrix in order to minimize complications.[22] The lip and oral mucosa can readily be punch-biopsied with the aid of a chalazion clamp to ensure stability, to help in hemostasis, and provide a flat surface. The tongue can also be sampled while holding its tip with cotton gauze. Obviously, mucosal sites bleed easily and abundantly, and therefore, we recommend placing the suture deeply to encompass the base of the lesion before performing the punch. That way, a series of square knots can be rapidly tied after the biopsy to secure hemostasis in spite of immediate profuse bleeding. Silk remains supple with moisture and is the preferred suture for mucosal sites.

Excisional and incisional biopsy

Excisional biopsies are indicated for removal of cutaneous tumors, lesions larger than 6 mm, for suspected melanomas,

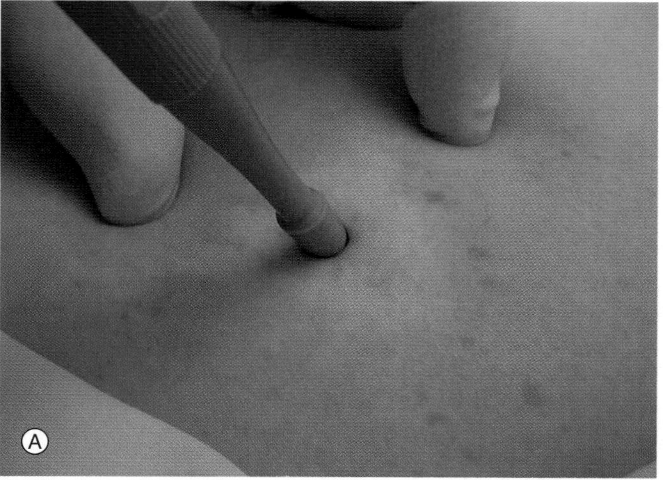

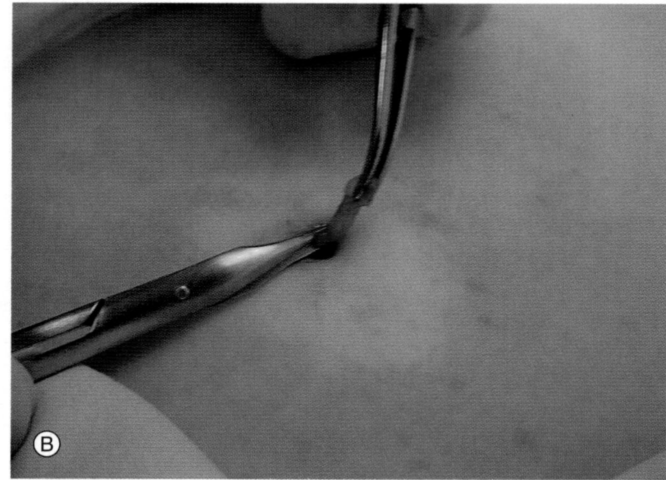

Figure 14.3 Punch biopsy. (A) The skin is held taut with the non-dominant hand and the punch is pushed gently against the skin using a twirling motion. Pulling the skin perpendicular to the skin tension lines produces an oval defect that is easier to close. A sensation of give indicates that the punch has cut through the dermis into subcutaneous tissue. (B) Cut the base of the specimen using Iris scissors and ensuring that a good amount of fat is included.

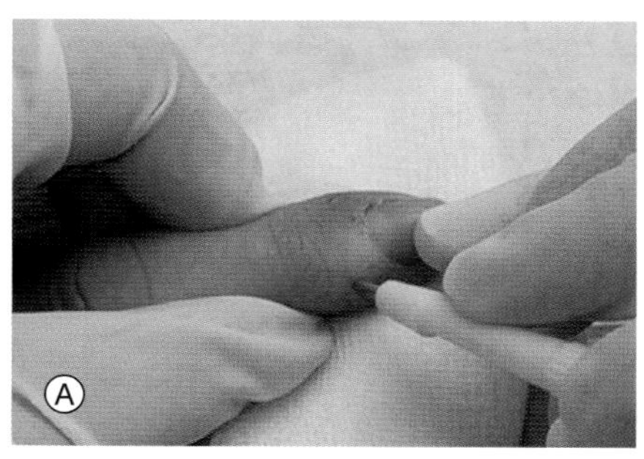

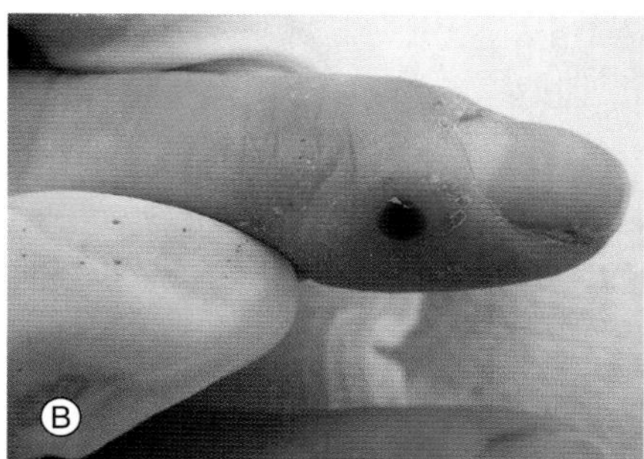

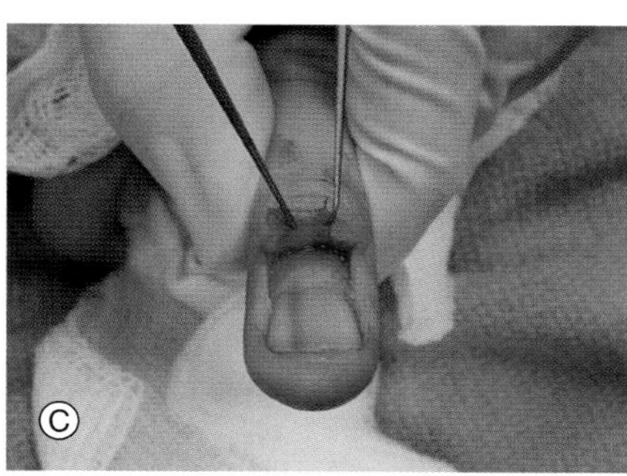

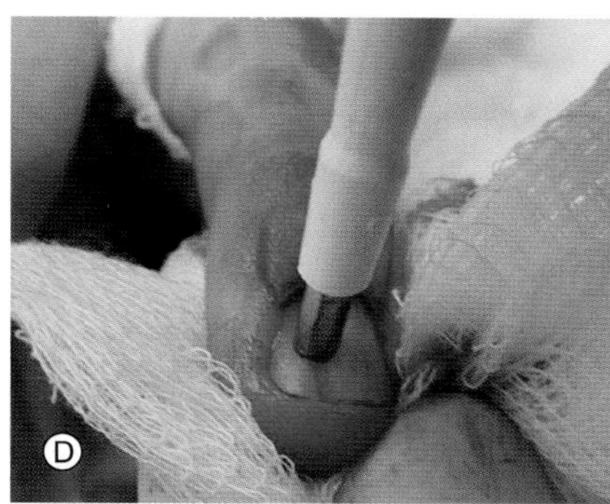

Figure 14.4 Nail biopsy. (A) Nail biopsies are performed after digital nerve and/or paronychial blocks. Use of lidocaine 1–2% without epinephrine (adrenaline) is suggested. A proximal nail fold biopsy is easily performed with 3–4 mm punches. (B) Hemostasis can be achieved with digital pressure on the sides of the fingers or with the aid of a tourniquet if an assistant is not available. (C) Retraction of the proximal nail fold allows direct visualization of the nail matrix. As a general rule, sampling the distal matrix avoids complications and permanent nail deformities. (D) For biopsies of the nail plate and nail bed, we prefer to use the 'double-punch technique' using a 4 mm punch for the plate followed by a smaller (3 mm) punch for the bed.

Table 14.5 Indications for incisional/excisional biopsy

Large vessel vasculitis
Most pigmented lesions
Deep or subcutaneous nodules
Malignant neoplasms
Suspected metastases

or when the presumed pathology involves deep dermis or subcutis (Table 14.5). They require more skill, time, and advanced preparation of instruments. These biopsies pose more risk and discomfort for patients and must be closed with sutures. Their main advantage is the amount of tissue that can be removed, allowing for multiple studies (electron microscopy, immunofluorescence, culture, histopathology) from one biopsy site.

A surgical tray should include alcohol pads, sterile drape and gauze, local anesthetic, surgical pen or Gentian violet, scalpel and surgical blade, forceps, skin hooks, iris scissors, needle holder, suture, and suture scissors. The usual approach involves preparation of the skin and sterile technique as mentioned before. After informed consent and skin preparation, a surgical ellipse is designed with a surgical pen, or with Gentian violet on the wooden end of a cotton-tipped applicator. The ellipse should be oriented parallel to the direction of relaxed skin tension lines to improve cosmesis. Skin tension lines, also referred to as Langer's lines, are formed by pull of muscles at insertion points on the overlying skin. The skin creases in a regular pattern perpendicular to the long axis of the underlying muscle. Studies have shown that skin tension perpendicular to these lines is three times greater than tension parallel. As a result, wounds oriented parallel to Langer's lines close under less tension and result in thinner scars. Also, excisions should be placed and kept on single cosmetic units, to preserve the normal anatomic appearance of the face, and to place scars within normal contour lines.

The ellipse should be three or four times larger than wide, and with 30° angles at the poles, to facilitate closure and reduce the formation of standing cutaneous deformities or 'dog ears'.[23] Drawing the long axis of the ellipse parallel to the long axis of the lesion results in the shortest scar (Fig. 14.5). For most benign lesions, a margin of 1–2 mm is sufficient. For malignant lesions, however, larger margins are indicated. Nodular basal cell carcinomas usually require margins of 4–5 mm, whereas squamous cell carcinomas are better excised with margins of 5–6 mm, and the margins for melanoma vary depending on the depth of the lesion. Curettage can be performed before the excision of basal or squamous cell carcinomas in order to better delineate subclinical involvement. In these instances, a 2 mm margin is recommended (Fig. 14.6).

The surgical technique for excisional biopsy is depicted in the video. Generally speaking, a #15 blade is used for facial and neck lesions, while a #10 blade is more convenient for thick skin on the trunk, scalp, and extremities. The scalpel is held like a pencil in the dominant hand while the other hand applies gentle tension to immobilize the skin around the ellipse. Counter traction by an assistant is also helpful. To begin the incision, the scalpel blade is inserted vertically at the distal apex. It is then lowered to an angle of 45–60° so that the sharpest part of the blade, the 'belly,' cuts along the sides of the ellipse. When approaching the proximal apex, the blade is once again raised to a vertical position. Care should be taken to handle tissue delicately to prevent damage to the epidermis, to cut with enough pressure to reach subcutaneous tissue in one or two strokes to avoid 'staircasing' of the dermis, and to avoid cross-hatching of the tips of the ellipse. For excisions larger than 1 cm, the blade can be angled away from the lesion, slightly undermining the wound edge. This facilitates an easier eversion of the edge during closure. Once incised, the specimen is gently lifted with forceps and

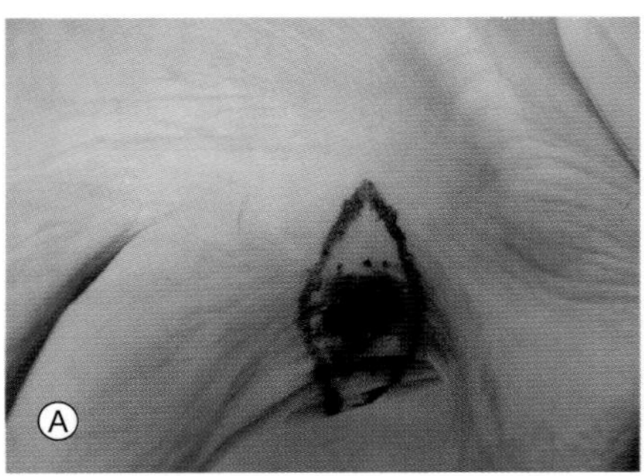

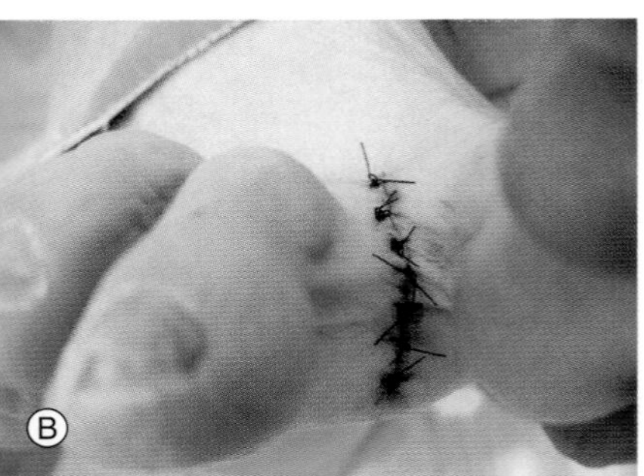

Figure 14.5 Excisional biopsy. (A) An ellipse is designed around the lesion before the infiltration of anesthetic creates distortion of the tissue. In general, margins of 2 mm are used for benign lesions and of 4–6 mm for malignant lesions. The ellipse is three or four times longer than wide and its apical ends have 30° angles to facilitate closure. (B) A simple closure with non-absorbable nylon or Prolene sutures is performed in most cases. An intermediate closure adding subcutaneous absorbable Vicryl is preferred for larger wounds, or if a significant amount of fat has been removed.

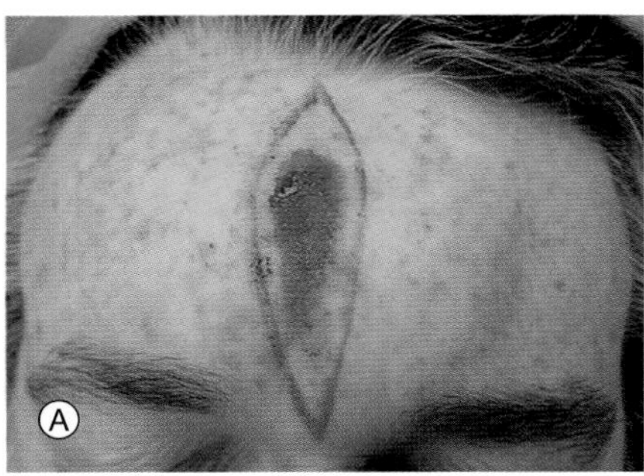

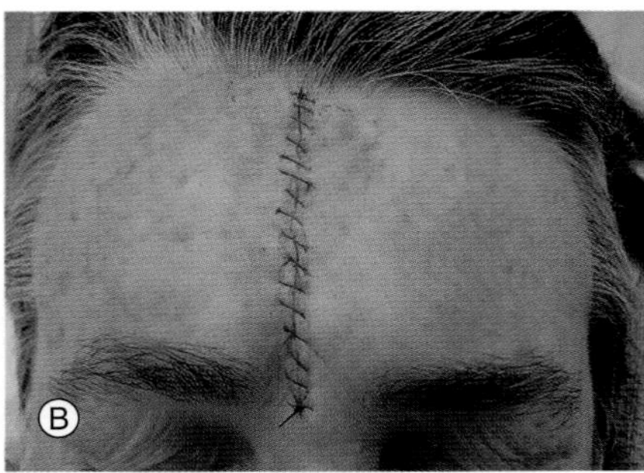

Figure 14.6 Curettage followed by excision. (A) Curettage can be employed prior to the excision in order to better delineate the subclinical extension of malignant skin tumors. A conservative margin of 2 mm is recommended. (B) Layered closure of the resulting defect. Vertical wounds heal with excellent cosmesis in the midline of the forehead.

the subcutaneous fat is cut horizontally, trying to excise the same amount of tissue along the whole base of the wound including the poles.[24] Leaving a larger amount of tissue at the tips creates an unsightly elevation or 'boating' effect at closure. Pressure and Hyfricator hemostasis is then routinely used. In general, lesions of less than 1 cm in diameter can be closed with simple 4-0 or 5-0 non-absorbable cutaneous sutures. Layered closures using subcutaneous Vicryl and cutaneous nylon (or Prolene) are performed only for very deep or large lesions, if marked tension exists in the biopsy site, or to close dead space if significant amount of fat was removed.

Several modifications of the surgical ellipse exist but the two most common are the 'pregnant belly' and the 'S'-plasty. Both are useful in producing curved scars that may follow the skin tension lines more closely. The 'pregnant belly' variation is an excision with one side longer than the other. Closing the wound with the 'rule of halves' will produce the curving of the suture line towards the longer side. The S-plasty involves extending the incisions in slightly curved manner on both ends of the ellipse but on opposite directions. This variation is useful when operating on convex surfaces because it lengthens the scar and reduces the chance of indentation occurring during scar contraction.

Incisional biopsies have similar indications and require identical technique. In this case, however, only a portion of a large lesion is removed. The specimen should include the thickest and most representative area of the lesion, and extend through the edge of a plaque or tumor, into adjacent normal skin. When applied to pigmented lesions, the darkest and most nodular-appearing area of the lesion should be sampled. The incision must be deep enough to sample an adequate amount of fatty tissue but may be only a few millimeters wide. The pathology requisition should include a special request for embedding the specimen for sectioning in the long axis of the specimen. For further information, see Chapter 18.

Undermining

Undermining involves blunt and/or sharp dissection at the subdermal level in order to release tension and promote eversion of wound edges. This technique enhances procedural efficiency, establishment of hemostasis, and cosmesis.[25] The main benefit, though, is the reduction of wound tension. Wounds that heal under excessive tension are at increased risk of necrosis, suture 'tract marks,' dehiscence, infection, and anatomic distortion. In one study, wound tension was reduced between 18.6% and 47.4% after judicious undermining. Other benefits involve orientation of elliptical excisions, mobilization of flaps, and management of standing cutaneous deformities. Undermining in all directions, including the poles of an ellipse, produces a plate-like horizontal fibrotic repair that is less likely to 'pull down' and invert the wound edges, therefore, enhancing the cosmetic outcome of the surgery. For most cutaneous surgical procedures, the plane of undermining is at the level of the subcutaneous fat (Table 14.6). Complications during or after undermining are rare, but careful technique is essential in order to avoid nerve damage (sensory and motor), hematoma formation, impaired cosmesis, and diminished skin edge vascularity. Critical anatomic structures such as spinal accessory, temporal and marginal mandibular nerves are deep to subcutaneous fat and undermining is safe if performed in the high subcutaneous tissue. For further information, see Chapter 18.

Closure of biopsy sites

Shave, saucerization, and scissor biopsies need not be closed. They heal by second intention with acceptable to

Table 14.6 Recommended level for undermining according to anatomic location

Location	Depth
Trunk and extremities	Above muscular fascia
Hands and feet	Immediately subdermal
Neck	Superficial fat
Face	Superficial fat
Scalp	Subgaleal

excellent cosmesis if location and technique were selected appropriately. Punch biopsies smaller than 3 mm located on areas of little cosmetic concern (neck, trunk, extremities) can also be left to heal secondarily. Punches greater than 3 mm and excisional or incisional biopsies require suturing.

Absorbable sutures are placed deep in larger wounds to reduce tension and to provide tensile strength for several weeks. Common options include polyglactic acid (Vicryl; Ethicon Inc, Johnson & Johnson Co, Somerville, NJ), polydioxanone (PDS; Ethicon Inc, Ethicon Inc) and polyglycolic acid (Dexon; Davis and Geck Inc, Tyco Healthcare Group LP, Mansfield, MA). We prefer 6-0 and 5-0 sizes for facial wounds and 4-0 for neck, trunk and extremities.

Non-absorbable sutures are used for skin closure. Generally, 4-0 sutures are used for scalp, trunk and extremities; and 5-0 or 6-0 for the face. Polypropylene (Prolene; Ethicon Inc) and unbraided nylon (Ethilon; Ethicon Inc) are monofilaments and are less likely to harbor infection. Silk and braided nylon are more likely to produce infection but they are stronger and easier to tie. Silk produces a strong inflammatory reaction but is considered the suture of choice for mucosal sites because it remains soft with moisture.

Cutting needles pass easily through tissue and are ideal for skin surgery. For Skin (FS) and Cutting needles (CE) are used for thick skin; whereas Plastic (P) and Plastic Skin (PS) are best for delicate skin. Various sizes are available and we feel comfortable with small P-3 needles for facial sites and larger PS-2 needles (see Chapter 4) for trunk and extremities. C-17 needles were developed specifically to close punch biopsies and are less expensive than P, PS, FS, or CE needles.

In the simple interrupted percutaneous suture, the needle is inserted perpendicular to the skin surface a few millimeters from the wound edge. It is guided through the skin with a turn of the wrist and exits on the other side of the wound a few millimeters away from edge. The suture is tied with a series of square knots. A two-layer closure using buried absorbable sutures is indicated for deep wounds, if a significant amount of fat was removed or if tension exists in the wound.[26]

In the buried interrupted dermal suture, the needle is inserted at the level of subcutaneous tissue and angled superiorly to pass through a small amount of subcutaneous and dermal tissue. The needle is brought out inside the wound parallel to and just beneath the epidermis. The process is repeated in reverse in the other side of the wound beginning just beneath epidermis and ending in subcutaneous tissue.[27] The suture is tied with a series of square knots.

■ OPTIMIZING OUTCOMES

Optimizing outcomes

- Consider the relative contraindications for biopsy in relation to the necessity for it.
- Choose a cleaning agent appropriate to the size, type and location of the lesion.
- Suture punch biopsy sites that are more than 3 mm.
- Undermining can be used to reduce wound tension and improve cosmetic outcome.

Relative contraindications for skin biopsy include severe coagulopathy, known or possible underlying vital structure, severe immunosuppression, distal/acral extremity in patients with diabetes and severe peripheral vascular disease.[28]

■ POSTOPERATIVE CARE

Wound dressing

Occlusive dressings facilitate wound healing and epithelialization. We prefer to apply a thin layer of Vaseline (Unilever, Greenwich, CT) or antibiotic ointment followed by a small piece of non-adherent pad such as Telfa (Kendall, Mansfield, MA), cotton gauze, and paper tape. This dressing is kept undisturbed for 24–48 hours but should be changed daily thereafter. Daily wound care involves gently cleaning with soap and water, application of ointment, and Band-Aids (Johnson & Johnson Co, Somerville, NJ). In hairy areas or oily skin, where tape is difficult to apply, the patient may keep the sutured wound uncovered, but moist, by applying the ointment several times during the day.

Suture removal

It is important to avoid suture marks and dehiscence. The former are a direct consequence of leaving the sutures for too long, and the latter of removing them prematurely. Empirically, we prefer to remove sutures on facial wounds at 5–7 days; from the neck at 7–10 days; from the scalp, trunk, and extremities 10–14 days; and from the palms and soles at 21 days.

■ PITFALLS AND THEIR MANAGEMENT

Avoidance of pitfalls

- Evaluate the patient's current medications to check that none has potential for serious interactions with local anesthetics and epinephrine (adrenaline).
- Use of preservative-free lidocaine will avoid allergic reaction.
- Careful hemostatic technique and compression bandages minimize bleeding and hematoma formation.
- If allergy to ointments or tapes develop, withdraw the ointment or tape and apply topical steroids.

Complications after skin biopsy are extremely infrequent. They include allergic reactions, drug interactions, bleeding, infection, and scars.[29] Allergic reactions to lidocaine are rare and are usually related to preservatives in the mixture. A preservative-free lidocaine is available. An allergy to procaine (Novocain, Sanofi Winthrop Pharmaceuticals, New York, NY) is not a contraindication to the use of lidocaine, since they are chemically different, and cross-reaction is rare.

Bleeding and hematoma formation can be minimized by careful hemostatic technique and the use of compression bandages. Drainage of hematoma is indicated if symptomatic or if there is vascular compromise of the skin. Infection is uncommon and usually associated with *Staphylococcus*, *Streptococcus* or *Candida*. Cephalosporins are our agents of first choice when starting empiric therapy, but the selection must be modified according to culture and sensitivity results. The most significant complication is permanent scarring of the biopsied site. This is less evident after small punches and superficial shaves. Occasionally, patients develop reactions to ointments or tape. The wound turns red, swollen, itchy, and may have vesicles. Treatment involves stopping the ointment and/or tape and applying topical steroids.

■ SUMMARY

The skin biopsy is an essential procedure that allows the dermatologist and cutaneous surgeon to reach a diagnosis and provide therapy for various dermatologic conditions. The preoperative evaluation for patients undergoing such procedures should be thorough and with emphasis on identifying risk factors for complications including bleeding, infection, dehiscence, and unsightly scars. A succinct but comprehensive informed consent must be carried out in every case to help patients make the best decision, and to protect the physician from punitive legal action in case of complications.

Most biopsies can be performed under clean technique, but universal precautions should be followed in all cases to avoid the risk of blood-borne infections. The biopsy site should be selected carefully, taking into consideration the size and location of lesions; if they involve epidermis, dermis, and/or subcutaneous fat; the cosmetic consequences of a permanent scar; and the planned therapy upon confirmation of diagnosis. If possible, avoid biopsies on shoulders (hypertrophic or keloid scars), legs (chronic vascular and stromal changes), or axillae (increased risk of infection).

Inflammatory conditions are best sampled with punch, incisional, or excisional techniques. Epidermal lesions such as seborrheic keratoses or skin tags are adequately removed with shave or scissor biopsies. Pigmented lesions should be excised completely whenever possible, but can be partially punched or incised if they are extremely large, or if the cosmetic consequences of complete excision are significant.

Complications after skin biopsy procedures are infrequent and generally minor, but can be minimized by proper selection of patients and performance of careful technique.

■ REFERENCES

1. Aguire PC, Mathes BM. Skin biopsy techniques for the internist. J Gen Intern Med 1998; 13:46–54.
2. Peters MS, Winkelmann RK. The biopsy. Dermatol Clin 1984; 2:209–217.
3. Robinson JK, LeBoit PE. Biopsy techniques. In: Robinson JK, et al: Atlas of cutaneous surgery. Philadelphia: WB Saunders; 1996.
4. Scott PM. Which technique to biopsy or remove a skin lesion? JAAPA 2001; 14:59–66.
5. Stables G, Lawrence CM. Management of patients taking anti-coagulant, aspirin, non-steroidal anti-inflammatory and other anti-platelet drugs undergoing dermatologic surgery. Clin Exper Dermatol 2002; 27:432–435.
6. Billingsley E, Maloney ME. Intraoperative and postoperative bleeding problems in patients taking warfarin, aspirin and nonsteroidal anti-inflammatory agents. Dermatol Surg 1997; 23:381–385.
7. Alcalay J. Cutaneous surgery in patients receiving warfarin therapy. Dermatol Surg 2001; 27:756–758.
8. Lawrence L, Sakuntabhai A, Tiling-Grosse S. Effect of aspirin and non-steroidal anti-inflammatory drug therapy on bleeding complications in dermatologic surgical patients. J Am Acad Dermatol 1994; 31:988–992.
9. Bartlett GR. Does aspirin affect the outcome of minor cutaneous surgery? Br J Plastic Surg 1999; 52:214–216.
10. Suraj Achar. Principles of skin biopsies for the family physician. Am Fam Physic 1996; 54:2411–2418.
11. Fleischman M, Garcia C. Informed consent in dermatologic/Mohs surgery. Poster presentation. ASDS-ACMMSCO Combined Annual Meeting, Chicago, IL, October 31– November 3, 2002.
12. Dzubow LM, Halpern AC, Leyden JJ, et al. Comparison of preoperative skin preparations for the face. J Am Acad Dermatol 1988; 19:737–741.
13. Osmon DR. Antimicrobial prophylaxis in adults. Mayo Clin Proc 2000; 75:98–109.
14. Lycka BAS. EMLA: A new and effective topical anesthetic. J Dermatol Surg Oncol 1992; 18:859–862.
15. Koppel RA, Coleman KM, Coleman WP. The efficacy of EMLA versus ELA-Max for pain relief in medium-depth chemical peeling: a clinical and histopathologic evaluation. Dermatol Surg 2000; 26:61–64.
16. Auletta MJ, Grekin RC. Local anesthesia in dermatologic surgery. New York: Churchill Livingstone; 1991.
17. Arndt KA, Burton C, Noe JM. Minimizing the pain of local anesthesia. Plast Reconstr Surg 1983; 72:676.
18. Orengo I, Katta R, Rosen T. Techniques in the removal of skin lesions. Otolaryngol Clin N Am 2002; 35:153–170.
19. Todd P, Garioch JJ, Humphreys S, et al. Evaluation of the 2-mm punch biopsy in dermatologic diagnosis. Clin Exper Dermatol 1996; 21:11–13.
20. Zuber T. Punch biopsy of the skin. Am Fam Physic 2002; 65:1155–1158.
21. Madani S, Shapiro J. The scalp biopsy: Making it more efficient. Dermatol Surg 1999; 25:537–538.
22. Clark RE, Madani S, Bettencourt MS. Nail surgery. Dermatol Clin 1998; 16:145–164.
23. Dunlavey E, Leshin B. The simple excision. Dermatol Clin 1998; 16:49–64.
24. Robinson JK. Elliptical incisions and closures. In: Robinson JK et al: Atlas of cutaneous surgery. Philadelphia: WB Saunders; 1996.
25. Boyer JD, Zitelli JA, Brodland DG. Undermining in cutaneous surgery. Dermatol Surg 2001; 27:75–78.
26. Fewkes JL, Cheney ML, Pollack SV. Illustrated atlas of cutaneous surgery. Philadelphia: JB Lippincott; 1992.
27. Roenigk RK, Roenigk HH. Dermatologic surgery: Principles and practice. New York: Marcel Dekker; 1989.
28. Arpey CJ. Biopsy of the skin. Postgrad Med 1998; 103:179–183.
29. Swanson NA. Atlas of cutaneous surgery. Boston: Little, Brown & Co; 1987.

15 Incision, Draining, and Exteriorization Techniques

Jeffrey A Squires MD and Frederick S Fish III MD FACP

Summary box

- Preoperative considerations: incision, draining, exteriorization
- Techniques for removal of lipomas (see also Chapter 47)
- Techniques for removal of various types of cysts (see also Chapter 47)
- Techniques for incision and draining of abscesses and inflamed cysts
- Postoperative care for incisional surgery
- Prevention of adverse sequelae and untoward results

INTRODUCTION

Subcutaneous lesions are a common concern of patients and are often found during the examination of the patient. Through the proper use of incision, draining, and exteriorization techniques, physicians can effectively treat their patients and add an important surgical tool to their armamentarium.

This chapter will cover techniques for incision, draining, and exteriorization of several types of subcutaneous lesions. We will also discuss both the preoperative and postoperative management as well as addressing potential pitfalls and complications to help ensure a successful outcome.

Lipomas, epidermal cysts, and abscesses are the most common lesions treated by these methods. However, once the basic techniques are understood they can be modified and used to treat a number of dermatologic conditions.

HISTORY

Over the years there have been many advancements and refinements in the practice of surgery. However, the practice of incisional surgery has remained essentially unchanged. The origins of incisional surgery date back to 1800 BC, where they can be found in the Egyptian practice of medicine and surgery.[1] In this chapter incisional surgery and draining and exteriorization techniques will be discussed in detail.

Incisional surgery and draining and exteriorization techniques are useful tools in the surgical armamentarium, being widely employed for the removal of various benign subcutaneous neoplasms. Epidermal and pilar cysts, as well as lipomas, are frequently removed by this method. Other less common cystic growths can also be removed utilizing this technique. Incision, drainage and exteriorization of abscesses and infected inflamed cysts can also be accomplished by this method.

PREOPERATIVE PREPARATION

Preoperative evaluation should include a general health and medication history with an emphasis on any medications or health problems which could put the patient at increased risk for bleeding or infection. Preoperative vital signs, including blood pressure and pulse, are always important to obtain.

Most incisional surgeries are performed under local anesthesia. It is important to consider potential complications in order to avoid them. When removing larger lesions avoid anesthetics which are highly concentrated and consider diluting your anesthetic. It is also important to not give excess quantities of anesthetics containing epinephrine (adrenaline) as they can increase blood pressure, pulse, and anxiety level. One must also be aware of the surrounding structures, taking into consideration the underlying nerves, blood vessels, and other important anatomic structures.

Removing subcutaneous masses in certain anatomic sites and conditions can be challenging if one is not familiar with the local anatomy. For example, lipomas on the forehead are frequently found beneath the frontalis muscle and can be much more difficult to mobilize and remove. Lipomas of the upper extremities can infiltrate along the fascial planes and into deeper muscular structures. Cysts, particularly, and other subcutaneous lesions that have been previously treated will often be surrounded by considerable fibrosis and scar tissue complicating their removal. In order to be prepared for the more difficult cases, careful palpation—

using the thumb and forefinger, as well as both forefingers—prior to planning the surgery can help access the mobility and character of the tissue surrounding a lesion to be excised. Areas of scar tissue can be identified as well as larger blood vessels and other underling structures.

Before the anesthetic injection, it is useful to mark both the lateral margins of the lesion to be removed and the anticipated incision line parallel to the relaxed skin tension lines. After the anesthetic is injected, the relaxed skin tension lines may be difficult to see and smaller or deeper subcutaneous lesions may be difficult to palpate or locate.

■ TECHNIQUES

Lipomas

Lipomas are common benign neoplasms. They are a proliferation of histologically normal-appearing adipose tissue that is encapsulated most of the time. They can occur at any age with about 55% occurring in the fourth and fifth decade. Clinically, lipomas are slow growing, mobile masses with lobulations which can range in size from a few millimeters to over 20 cm. Most lesions are asymptomatic, although they can cause discomfort by pressing on nerves and may grow rapidly. They may be solitary or multiple. The most common sites are the subcutaneous tissue of the neck, shoulders and back, followed by the forearms and buttock.[2,3] Lipomas also occur on the forehead, and scalp and these present a special problem for removal.[4] Infiltrating lipomas of the upper extremities may be deep and involve the muscles, as well as neural and vascular structures.[5] Lipomas rarely become inflamed. They are most commonly removed because they become symptomatic or cosmetically objectionable.

After carefully performing the preoperative evaluation, palpate and clinically define the lateral margins of the lipoma by pinching it with the thumb and forefinger (Fig. 15.1) or bimanually with the two index fingers (Fig. 15.2). Carefully mark the lateral margins with a surgical marking pen. The wood shaft of a cotton-tipped applicator broken to a point and dipped into Gentian violet works well also. At the same time also, carefully mark the planned incision line preferably over the center of the lesion within the relaxed skin tension lines.

To achieve local anesthesia, a local anesthetic containing epinephrine (adrenaline) preferably buffered with sodium bicarbonate works well. The buffering helps reduce the pain experienced during injection. Inject the anesthetic slowly to minimize discomfort. The anesthetic should be injected over and around and under the lesion. By injecting all around the lesion and using a good volume of anesthetic, the lesion can to some extent be dissected from the surrounding tissue.

Make the skin incision along the previously inked line, and plan on a length of one-half to one-third of the lesional diameter of the underlying lipoma. Most lipomas will compress or mold with lateral pressure and can be removed through a smaller incision allowing for a smaller more cosmetic scar. If one encounters a considerably larger lesion, fibrosis, or other difficulties, the incision can then be lengthened intraoperatively to facilitate removal.

After an incision has been made, blunt dissection from the surrounding tissue can usually be accomplished with a curved hemostat, Ragnell or Metzenbaum scissors. Lesional tissue will usually be lighter in color and firmer than the surrounding adipose tissue. The lesion may be round or oval but also may have a lobulated shape. Once the lipoma has been dissected free, grasp it with a hemostat (Fig. 15.3) and apply lateral compression to squeeze it through the skin incision. One can extend the incision at this time if the lipoma is too large for removal through the existing incision. Be careful to examine the base of the lipoma as it is removed, to avoid damaging any underlying structures that may still be attached to the base.

After the lipoma is removed, use skin hooks to expose the wound. Examine it for any bleeding and cauterize as necessary (Fig. 15.4). Smaller dead spaces will usually not require any further attention but larger defects may require

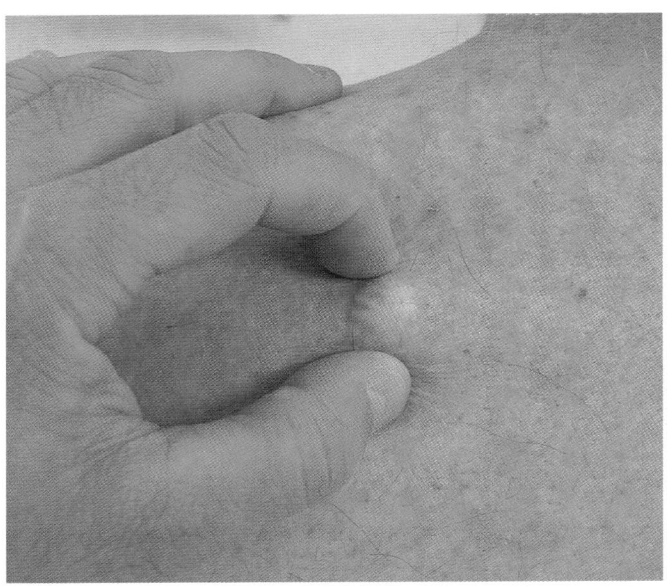

Figure 15.1 Palpation of subcutaneous growth with thumb and forefinger to help delineate margins prior to surgery.

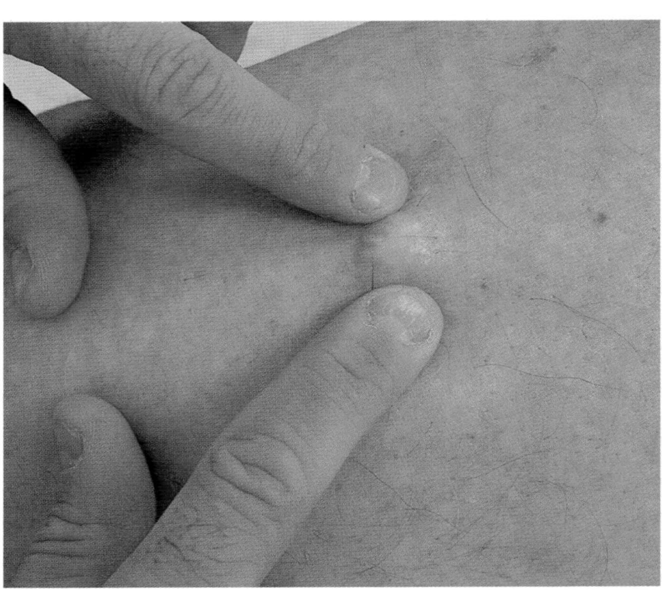

Figure 15.2 Palpation of subcutaneous mass with two forefingers may help further to detect surrounding fibrosis and mobility of the subcutaneous growth.

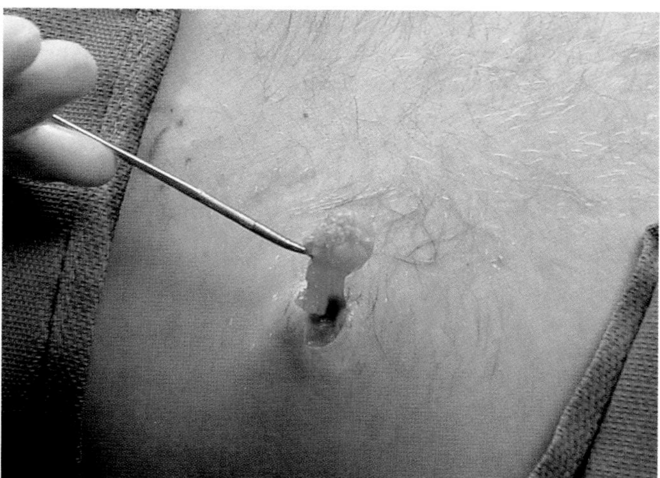

Figure 15.3 Lipoma being grasped with a hemostat to assist with delivery through skin incision.

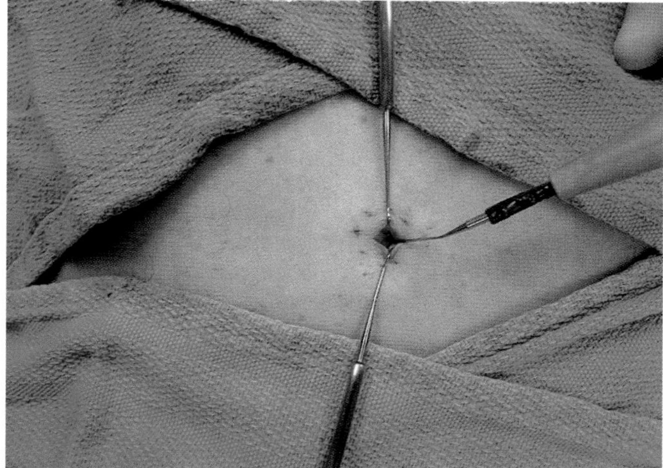

Figure 15.4 Cauterization of bleeding vessels after removal of a lipoma on the neck.

approximation of the subcutaneous tissue to decrease the risk of hematoma and prevent dimpling of the overlying skin.

Wound closure is usually accomplished by approximating the subcutaneous tissue and dermis with an absorbable suture such as Vicryl (Ethicon Inc, Johnson & Johnson Co, Somerville, NJ). The epidermal edges are then apposed with a non-absorbable suture such as Prolene (Ethicon) or Ethilon (Ethicon). Since the overlying skin is not excised, there is little tension on the skin edge. On the face, a running subcuticular closure in combination with Steri-Strips (3M) and an adhesive such as Mastisol (Ferndale

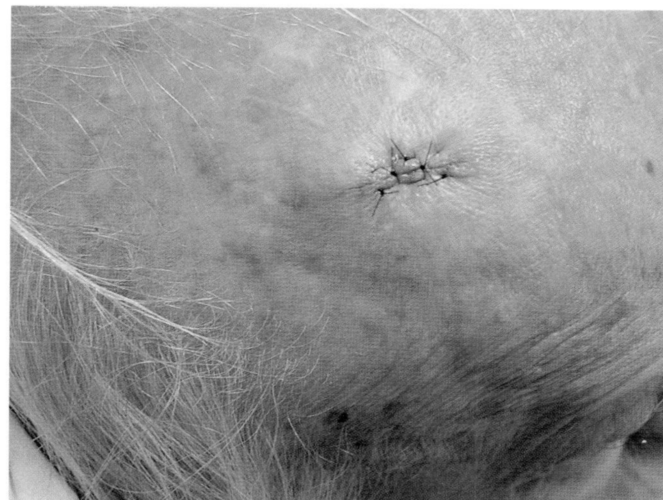

Figure 15.5 Incision closed with a running horizontal mattress suture and simple interrupted sutures. Excellent wound edge eversion is obtained with this closure.

Laboratories Inc., Ferndale, MI) works well. A running horizontal mattress suture also provides good wound edge eversion and gives excellent results (Fig. 15.5).

Lipomas on the forehead present special problems for removal. A clinical entity termed frontalis-associated lipoma of the forehead has been previously described.[5] Forehead lipomas can be found both within the frontalis muscle and between the muscle and submuscular fascia (Fig. 15.6). In removing these lipomas, care must be taken not to cause undue damage to the frontalis muscle (refer to Chapter 1, Surgical Anatomy). Other important structures to consider are the supraorbital and supratrochlear neurovascular bundles. Because these lipomas often lie deep to the frontalis muscle, the supraorbital and supratrochlear neurovascular bundles can be injured if care is not taken during removal. The boundaries of the lipoma need to be carefully marked prior to administering local anesthetic. The local anesthetic will frequently make it very difficult to discern the borders of the lipoma. An incision is made after taking care to optimally place it on the forehead[6] and the frontalis muscle is located and then carefully dissected or partially resected to allow access to the lipoma. Once the capsule of the lipoma becomes evident, careful dissection is carried out to free the lipoma along all of its borders. Blunt scissors or a small hemostat work well. After the superficial surface of the lipoma has been adequately undermined, the deep surface of the lipoma is also thoroughly undermined as well. Frontalis-associated lipomas can be quite adherent to the underlying tissue. Small lesions may be removed intact and larger lesions are sometimes removed in pieces to avoid

Lipomas

- Careful palpation to access depth and size
- Mark planned incision line prior to anesthetic injection
- Attempt to remove through smallest incision possible
- Palpate thoroughly prior to closure to assure complete removal
- Close dead space for larger lesions

Forehead lipomas

- Careful palpation to access depth and size
- Mark planned incision within skin tension lines
- Attempt to dissect frontalis muscle bundles in vertical orientation if possible
- Dissection to free lipoma much more difficult
- Repair muscle and fascial planes if necessary

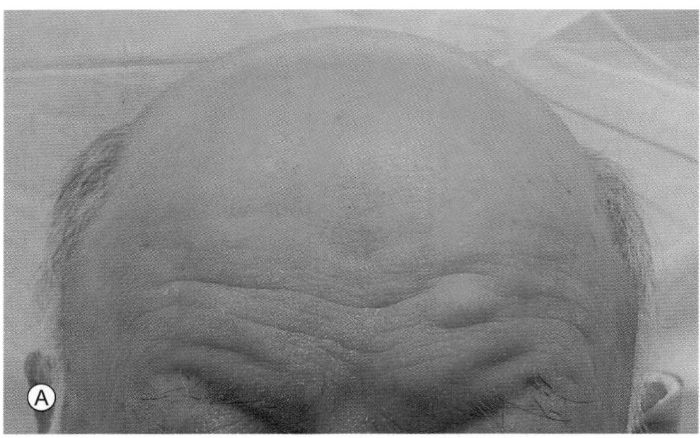

Lipoma: important anatomic structures

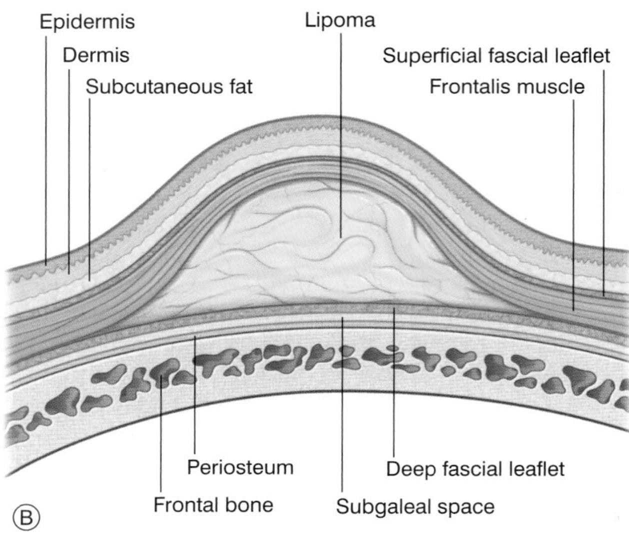

Figure 15.6 (A) Forehead lipoma with (B) diagram highlighting important anatomic structures.

a larger incision. It is important to restore good structural integrity to the forehead after the lipoma has been removed. The submuscular fascia is reapproximated using deep absorbable suture and then the frontalis muscle is also reapproximated prior to closing the subcutaneous tissue. A pressure dressing left on for 24 hours is helpful to avoid accumulation of fluid in the dead space.

Infiltrating lipomas of the upper extremities can be both intermuscular and intramuscular. The intermuscular variant is more common. It arises in the intermuscular fascial septae and may infiltrate into adjacent muscle. Intramuscular lipomas arise within the muscle and are poorly demarcated. These lipomas are frequently firmer than ordinary lipomas.[7,8]

Most infiltrating lipomas of the upper extremities are asymptomatic. However, they may cause pain by compressing adjacent structures. In addition, weakness has been described resulting from compression of nerves. Radiologic studies including CT scans and MRI are very useful in assisting to make the diagnosis and in planning surgical treatment.[7]

It is very important to map out the extent of the lipoma prior to excision, to ensure that it is completely removed. Precise mapping combined with a thorough knowledge of the local anatomy will also help to prevent damage to important structures in and around the lipoma.

These lesions frequently require an incision which is larger than for ordinary lipomas. Great care needs to be taken dissecting these lipomas free from surrounding muscle and neuromuscular structures. A multilayered closure which includes the fascia and subcutaneous tissue allows for optimal results. In larger cases a drain may be appropriate. This is usually removed 24–48 hours postoperatively.

Infiltrating lipomas of the upper extremities

- Difficult to access with palpation
- CT scans and MRI very useful in preoperative planning
- Lesions tend to be large and may be both intermuscular and intramuscular
- Dissect carefully from surrounding muscle and neurovascular structures

Epidermal cysts

Epidermal cysts are commonly encountered benign subcutaneous masses known by many synonyms such as epithelial cysts, keratinous cysts, and sebaceous cysts. These lesions are frequently encountered by the dermatologist and dermatologic surgeon. Epidermal cysts are circumscribed lesions lined by stratified squamous epithelium containing central keratinous material. They arise from the presence of epidermal cells in the dermis. These cells can be implanted by trauma, or existing cells (such as those of the follicular infundibulum) can proliferate and create a cystic mass due to a process such as pilosebaceous occlusion.[9,10]

Clinically, an epidermal cyst usually presents itself as a dome-shaped elevated mass protruding above the skin surface. One may appreciate more of a yellowish white color as the cyst enlarges and stretches the overlying skin. On palpation the cyst is usually freely mobile but may be restricted in movement by surrounding fibrosis and scar tissue. Chronic inflammation and irritation can frequently result in perilesional fibrosis. Acute inflammation can lead to frank purulence and require the cyst to be incised and drained. On the overlying skin surface, a punctum or dilated pore is usually present. It may be located centrally but can be seen at any point on the overlying surface.

Epidermal cysts occur quite commonly in adults, affecting the sexes equally. They are less commonly seen in childhood. Sites of predilection include the face, neck, and trunk. The preauricular area is a commonly affected region as well as the ear lobes. Solitary lesions predominate but multiple lesions can be seen. Multiple lesions may be associated with Gardner syndrome and basal cell nevus syndrome. Individual lesions can vary in size from a few millimeters to many centimeters in diameter.[9,10]

In the removal of an epidermal cyst, the same meticulous preoperative evaluation should be done. Lateral margins should be palpated and marked as previously mentioned. If possible, try to identify the dilated pore in the skin overlying the lesion. Once the pore is identified, it can be marked with surgical ink. The planned incision line is then marked in the relaxed skin tension lines transecting the epidermal pore, if possible.

Injection of a local anesthetic agent will help to dissect the cyst from the surrounding tissue. If considerable fibrosis or scar tissue exists little separation of the cyst from the surrounding tissue will occur. However, care should be taken not to inject directly into the cyst cavity, as this will cause pain, cyst distention, and possible rupture. Local anesthetics containing epinephrine (adrenaline) which have been buffered with sodium bicarbonate help to reduce the pain of injection and provide hemostasis.

Using a #15 blade, make a shallow incision through the pore along the marked line. Some cysts are quite superficial, so be careful not to make the incision too deep. If the cyst has not been previously treated, one should visualize a white-gray sac-like structure that should appear more superficial near the epidermal pore and deeper toward the lateral edges. Once the skin incision is made, beveling the scalpel blade at an angle will decrease the chance of rupturing the cyst wall. If the pore is larger it can be removed. Once the cyst wall has been identified, grasp the epidermal edge with a skin hook (Fig. 15.7) and dissect the cyst wall free from the surrounding skin and subcutaneous tissue with iris or small Gibbs–Gradle scissors. Grasp the cyst with a hemostat and deliver it through the incision if possible. Gentle lateral compression will mold the cyst somewhat allowing the cyst to be delivered through a smaller incision. If the cyst is too large for the incision, it can be decompressed by making a small incision in the wall and with gentle lateral pressure expressing some of the keratinous contents through the incision (Fig. 15.8). The partially collapsed cyst sac can then be more easily delivered through the incision (Fig. 15.9).

During the removal, some cystic contents can contaminate the wound. After removal, one should carefully irrigate the wound with saline and/or an antibiotic solution. Probe the wound gently with a curette to remove any residual keratinous fragments (Fig. 15.10). If any are found, irrigate the wound until none remains.[11] Skin hooks work well to retract the wound edges and thoroughly inspect the margins of the wound for any residual cyst wall because retained portions may lead to recurrence.

In closing the wound one must consider dead space as previously mentioned. Absorbable sutures such as Vicryl (Ethicon) work well to close the subcutaneous tissue. Ethilon (Ethicon) or Prolene (Ethicon) suture can be used to achieve skin closure. Cysts that have been present for a long duration, or which are large in size, can stretch the overlying skin leading to excess or redundant skin. This excess skin may need to be trimmed and removed at the time of wound closure.

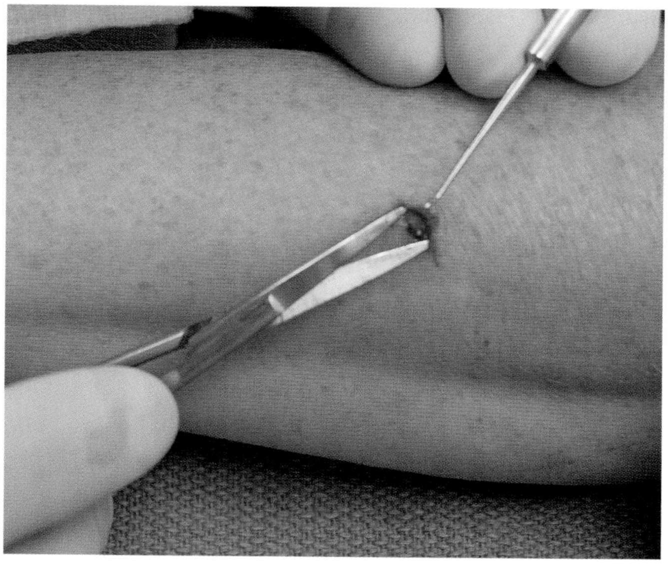

Figure 15.7 Skin hook being used to provide retraction while the cyst wall is dissected free from the subcutaneous tissue with a small curved iris scissor.

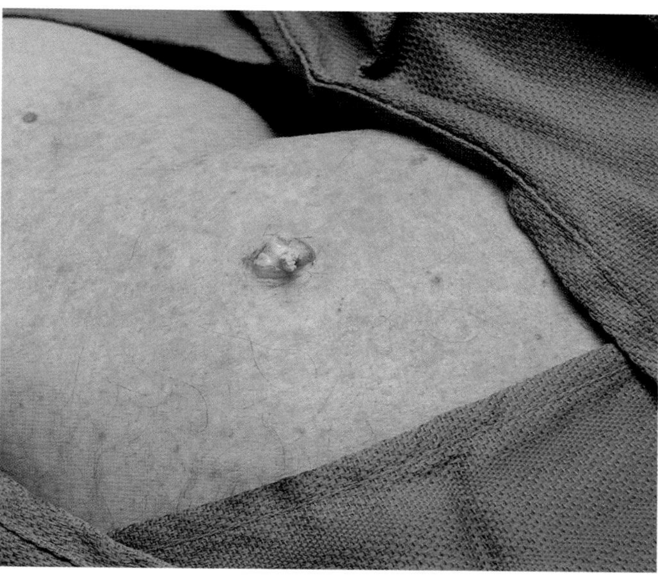

Figure 15.8 After dissecting the cyst free, lateral compression can be used to extrude the cyst. If the incision is too small to allow for easy removal, a small incision can be made in the cyst and a portion of the cyst contents can be removed. This will allow for the collapsed cyst sac to be more easily delivered through the incision.

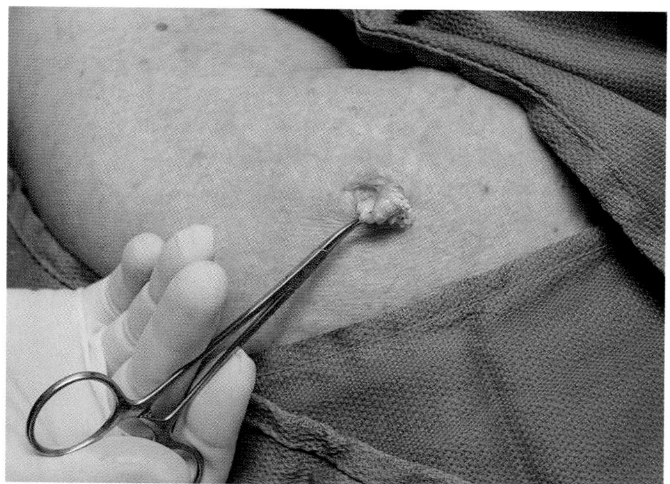

Figure 15.9 Collapsed cyst sac being removed with a hemostat after decompression and removal of the keratinous cyst contents.

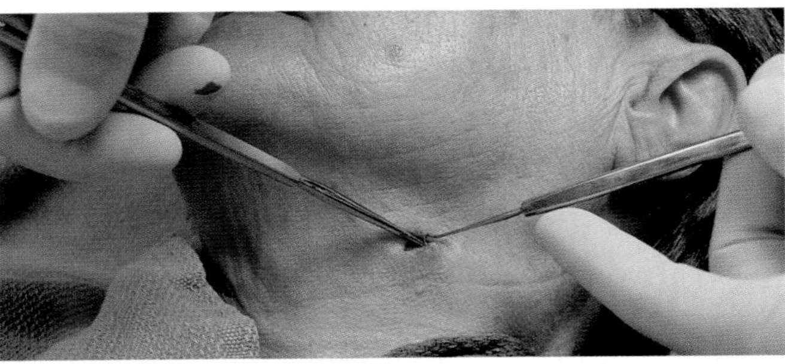

Figure 15.10 After removal of the cyst, the wound should be probed with a curette to make sure that no residual fragments of keratin remain. Irrigating the wound with normal saline solution will help remove any residual keratin fragments.

The use of oral antibiotics is somewhat controversial. It is often reasonable to place the patient on a short course of an oral antibiotic that covers for *Staphylococcus* and *Streptococcus* spp. when excising cysts that are mildly inflamed or have any drainage.

Variations in the technique listed above may need to be employed if the cyst is recurrent or has been previously inflamed and/or drained. These lesions usually have some fibrosis at the periphery making the lateral margins less well defined. They are often adherent to the overlying skin. On careful palpation, a lack of mobility and more ill-defined margins can usually be appreciated. In the absence of clinically palpable fibrosis, one should still anticipate its presence in a recurrent or previously inflamed lesion.

Similar techniques and incision as previously discussed can be used. However, one needs to consider other options if considerable fibrosis is encountered. The best option in some cases is to perform a fusiform excision including the fibrotic area and underlying cyst. This will usually result in a longer scar than desired and more wound tension due to the removal of the fusiform area of tissue. An alternative is to sharply dissect through the fibrotic area, but care must be taken not to rupture the cyst cavity. This can be accomplished with either a scalpel blade or sharp-pointed scissors. Potential problems that may be encountered using this technique include increased difficulty in closing the dead space due to the surrounding fibrosis. There is also a slightly higher risk of contour abnormalities in the overlying skin, and possibly less than ideal healing due to lack of vascularity in the surrounding fibrotic tissue. Careful consideration of these two options depends on lesion size, anatomic location, as well as other factors.

Epidermal cysts

- Palpate to access depth, size, and fibrosis
- Mark punctum and incision line
- Use local anesthetic to aid in dissection from surrounding tissue
- Avoid direct injection into cyst cavity to prevent distention and possible rupture
- Remove intact if possible or decompress if necessary
- Inspect wound margins for retained cyst wall or keratin fragments

Milia

Milia are small, yellowish to white, superficial epidermal cysts usually measuring a few millimeters or less in diameter. They frequently occur on the face of adolescents and adults, but can be seen after trauma associated with burn injuries, dermabrasion, surgical procedures, various subepidermal injuries, and disease processes such as porphyria cutanea tarda and bullous pemphigoid.[12,13] They can usually be easily removed by nicking the overlying skin with a #11 blade and removing the lesion with lateral pressure using a comedone extractor. Alternatively, these lesions can also be removed by making a small incision using the tip of a sterile disposable needle and using the needle to enucleate the cyst.[14] Larger lesions, particularly those around the eyes, may require a slightly longer incision with removal of the sac with a fine forceps. They usually heal well by second intention and topical antibiotic ointment can help to speed healing. New lesions can occur, but treated lesions usually do not recur.

Trichilemmal or pilar cysts

Trichilemmal or pilar cysts represent approximately 15% of excised lesions and occur mainly on the scalp. They are seen more frequently in women.[15] Unlike epidermal cysts, a punctum is usually not found. They can be solitary or multiple and likely are inherited as an autosomal dominant trait when multiple lesions are present.[16] Trichilemmal cysts have many features in common with epidermal cysts but there are some distinct differences which should be considered in their and evaluation and management. One of the most striking differences is the thicker wall of the pilar cyst which, after careful circumferential dissection, frequently allows the cyst to 'pop' out of the incision with lateral compression. This is particularly true with smaller lesions. A thicker wall also frequently prevents rupture. After the cyst has been removed one may encounter a fibrous capsule at the lateral margins surrounding the lesion. This can usually be removed easily with a hemostat, if so desired. Enlargement of pilar cysts on the scalp will manifest as a protruding nodule because of the underlying skull. Over time, stretched redundant skin develops over the cyst. This redundant tissue will often need to be removed at the time of closure (Fig. 15.11). A pilar cyst in the scalp with a size exceeding several centimeters will often have decreased hair or even permanent hair loss over the central portion of the cyst. The hairless skin is usually trimmed and removed at the time of closure.

Pilar cysts

- Palpate to access depth, size, and fibrosis
- Mark margins and planned incision line
- Use local anesthetic to aid in dissection from surrounding tissue
- Thick wall allows for easier delivery through incision
- Decompress prior to removal for larger lesions
- More commonly require removal of redundant overlying skin

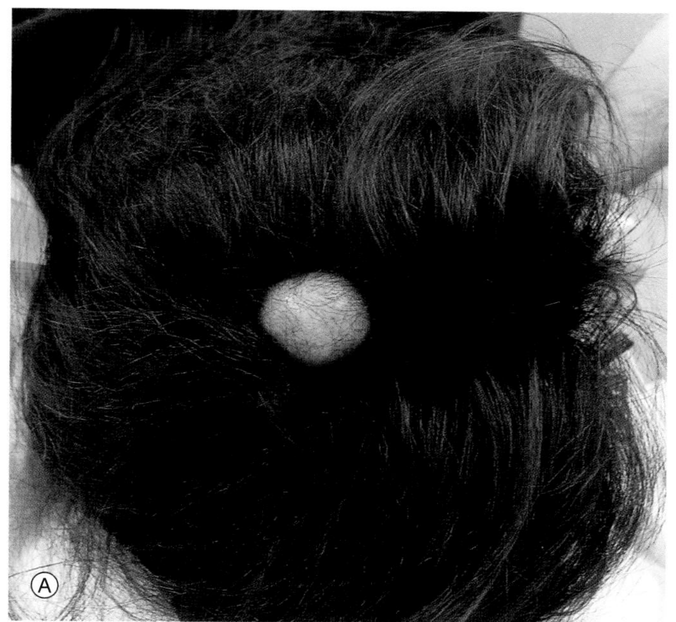
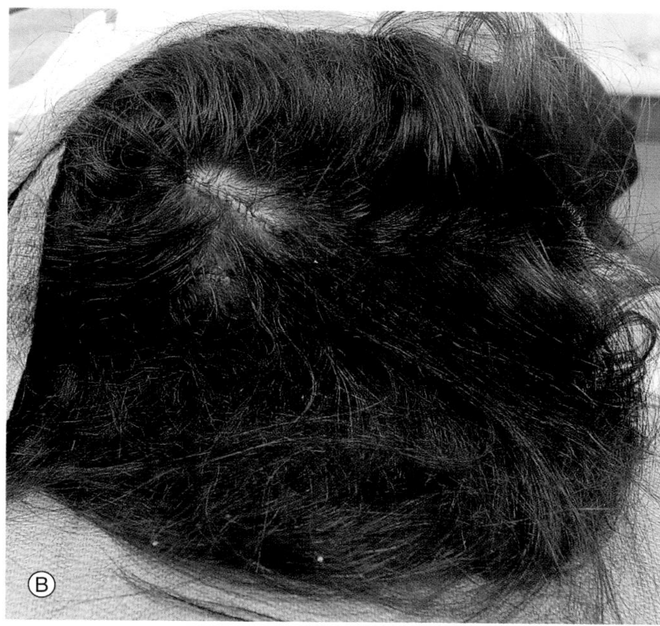

Figure 15.11 (A) Large pilar cyst shown preoperatively with overlying redundant skin. (B) Excess skin was trimmed during the procedure after the cyst was removed to give a fine-line closure.

Steatocystoma

Steatocystoma is the only true 'sebaceous' cyst. It contains sebaceous lobules within the thin wall of the cyst, or it may have sebaceous ducts draining into the cyst cavity. The wall of the cyst is generally quite thin with the contents having an oily consistency and being made up of esters of sebum. Individual lesions are often yellowish-white in color, usually a few millimeters in diameter. Principally they occur on the trunk and proximal extremities with the sternal area being the most common site. Steatocystoma can be a solitary lesion[17] but is seen more frequently as multiple lesions, particularly on the chest. They are commonly inherited as an autosomal dominant condition[18] and occur most frequently in adolescence or early adult life. In contrast to epidermal cysts, the lesions of steatocystoma usually have no overlying epidermal pore, but may be associated with multiple surrounding open comedones.

Individual lesions can be treated by making a small linear incision overlying the cyst and grasping and gently extracting the underlying cyst with fine forceps[19,20] or a skin hook. Care must be taken not to rupture the thin wall of the cyst. Gentle dissection with a small iris or Gradle scissors is occasionally necessary. The skin hook technique utilizes a smaller incision, which is important because when multiple sites are treated there is an increased risk of hypertrophic scars, especially on the chest. One should note that frequently the multiplicity of lesions makes routine incision and removal of all lesions impractical. Sato and associates have reported good success with aspiration drainage of the cysts.[21] The carbon dioxide laser has also been used to exteriorize and destroy these cysts with some success.[22]

Steatocystoma

- Only true 'sebaceous' cyst
- Thin-walled superficial lesions
- Conservative removal is preferred to decrease the risk of scarring

Apocrine hidrocystoma

Apocrine hidrocystomas are most commonly seen in adults. They usually present as bluish-colored papules[23,24] in the periocular region and on the face (Fig. 15.12). The cause of the bluish discoloration has been attributed to the Tyndall phenomenon,[23] extravasated red blood cells,[24] and lipofuscin.[25] The presence of melanin pigment[26] has been reported in one case.

These lesions are frequently asymptomatic but may increase in size and require removal. Usually they are a few millimeters in diameter and rarely exceed 10 mm in size. Although these lesions can be confused with cystic basal cell carcinoma, the surface is usually smoother, contains no telangiectasias, and is somewhat softer in quality. Histologically this lesion consists of a thin lining of apocrine secretory cells. Small lesions of 1–2 mm in size can be incised and drained. Larger lesions can be exteriorized by removing the overlying skin and then taking a sharp delicate scissor and dissecting out the cyst lining. Note that the cyst lining is very fragile and thin and can be easily ruptured, releasing somewhat mucoid material. After the cyst is dissected out, the base is lightly cauterized and topical antibiotic ointment is applied. If the lesion is near the eye an ophthalmic topical antibiotic should be used.

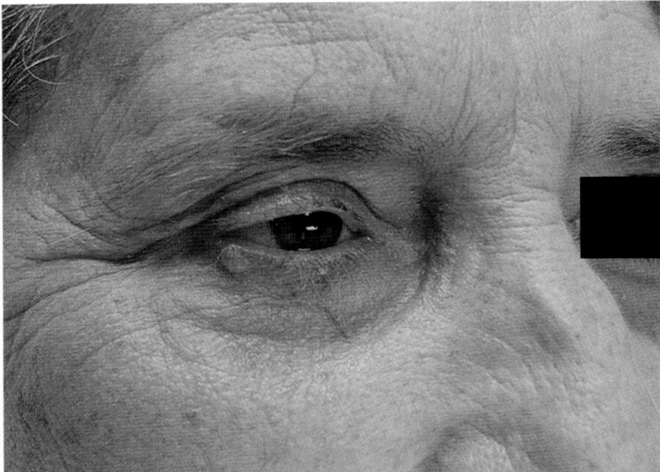

Figure 15.12 Apocrine hidrocystoma on the right lateral lower eyelid. The clinical appearance can mimic a basal cell carcinoma.

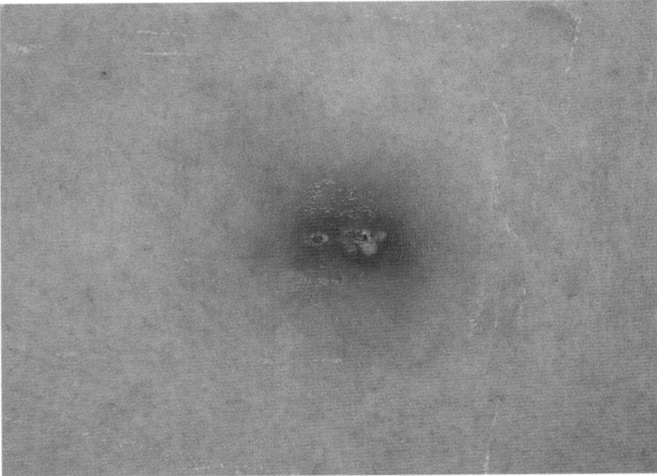

Figure 15.13 Abscess with erythema and induration. The area of maximum fluctuance is identified by gentle palpation.

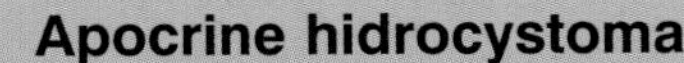

Apocrine hidrocystoma

- May be confused with cystic basal cell carcinoma
- Send tissue fragments for microscopic confirmation
- Care should be taken to avoid injury to the eye when removing periocular lesions
- Ophthalmic antibiotic should be used for periocular lesions

Inflamed and infected cysts and abscesses

Inflamed and infected cysts and abscesses are a common problem. Incision and drainage is frequently used for their treatment. First carefully inspect the area and pay close attention to erythema, induration, and fluctuance (Fig. 15.13). Gently palpate the area as it may be quite tender. If fluctuance is appreciated, then incision and drainage may be necessary. Sterilely prep the area because a culture of the contents may be required for appropriate adjunct oral antibiotic therapy. Prior to the injection of local anesthesia, a topical skin refrigerant may be used to help lessen the discomfort of injection. Inject the anesthetic very slowly as more rapid injection causes abrupt tissue distention, more rapid change in pH, and hence more resultant pain. Local anesthesia is often less effective in infected tissues because of the low pH of infected tissues.[27]

Once the area is adequately anesthetized, make a small stab incision over the point of greatest fluctuance (Fig. 15.14). Make sure you are wearing protective eyewear, masks and clothing as frequently the inflamed lesions are under considerable pressure and decompression can result in the spraying of the contents quite widely. Shielding the area where the stab incision is to be made with sterile gauze helps to minimize spraying of the contents. Immediately after making the stab incision, material should be collected for wound culture if clinically appropriate.

Lateral compression will usually express the contents of the cavity and retained keratinous fragments can be removed by gently probing with a curet. The cavity is then irrigated with saline or antibiotic solution and inspected to remove as much of the contents as possible. A decision is then made whether packing the wound or insertion of a drain is necessary. Packing can be performed with Iodoform or plain gauze (usually one-quarter to one-half inch wide). Packing material is removed from the bottle sterilely with a forceps or hemostat. The wound is then packed using either a forceps or hemostat to advance the material until the inflamed space is appropriately filled to allow for adequate drainage (Fig. 15.15). The packing material is withdrawn a small amount each day when the dressing is changed until it

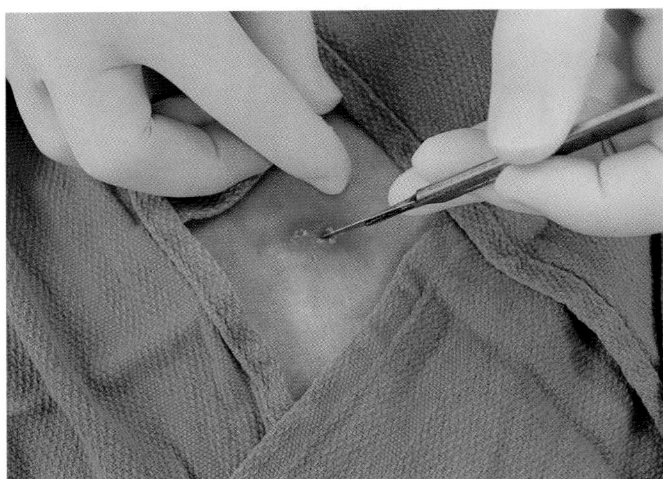

Figure 15.14 After identifying the area of greatest fluctuance, a small stab incision is made to allow for drainage.

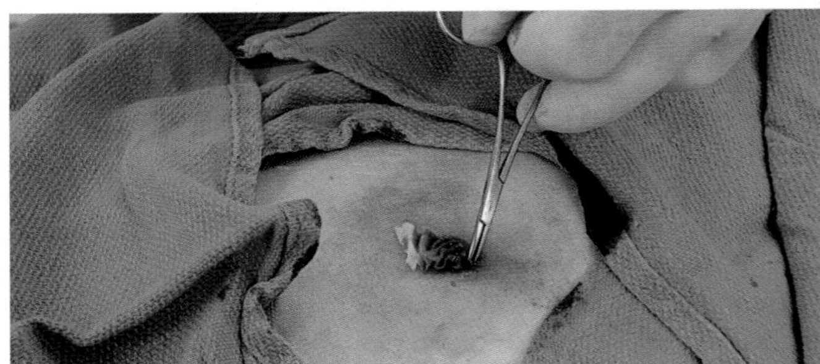

Figure 15.15 Wick of packing material extruding from the wound after packing has been completed.

is completely removed. The wound drains and heals gradually by second intention. If there is concern regarding possible infection, one can prescribe an oral antibiotic. Broad spectrum antibiotics such as cephalosporins or erythromycins are good choices as frequently the lesions can be polymicrobial containing *Staphylococcus* and *Streptococcus* spp.[28] Follow-up in a few days is appropriate to assess healing, check dressing compliance, and correlate culture results with the antibiotic prescribed.

Inflamed and infected cysts and abscesses

- Assess for fluctuance
- Apply topical skin refrigerant to lessen pain of injection
- Local anesthesia may be less effective due to low pH of infected tissue
- Wear protective eye wear, mask, and clothing as contents may be under pressure
- Shield stab incision with sterile gauze to minimize spraying of contents
- Culture contents if appropriate
- Drain cavity and pack if necessary
- Broad spectrum oral antibiotics to cover *Staphylococcus* and *Streptococcus* spp.

Hidradenitis suppurativa

Hidradenitis suppurativa (Fig. 15.16) is a chronic suppurative inflammatory condition that involves skin with apocrine glands and frequently results in scarring, cysts, and sinus tract formation. It frequently involves the axillary, anogenital, and inframammary areas. In the early stages of the disease, patients present with recurrent inflamed cysts and furuncles. Eventually, these progress to chronic low-grade infection with abscess formation and scarring. Fistulas may develop, especially in the anogenital region.[29,30] The histopathology of hidradenitis suppurativa reveals inflammation resulting from rupture of follicular infundibulum distended by keratin. Inflammation of apocrine, eccrine, and sebaceous glands[31,32] appears to be a secondary phenomenon.

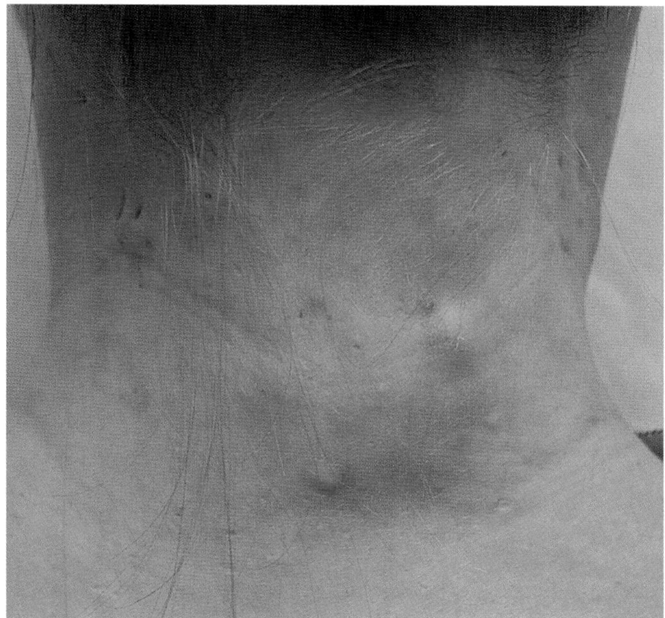

Figure 15.16 Hidradenitis suppurativa on the posterior neck demonstrating inflammatory papules, cysts, and sinus tracts.

Medical treatment of hidradenitis suppurativa includes topical and oral antibiotics. Antibiotics are often rotated to prevent problems with resistant organisms. Systemic and intralesional steroids can also be used as well as isotretinoin.

Surgical intervention is frequently used in the management of this difficult condition. Incision and drainage of newer inflammatory lesions is frequently employed. However, over time this can result in sinus tract formation and marked fibrosis.[33] Exteriorization of cysts and sinus tracks is considered the preferred method of treatment.[34] An incision is made which exposes the area of inflammation. Inflammatory tissue and granulation tissue is curetted and removed. Any overlying tissue is also removed to allow for adequate unroofing. The site is then allowed to heal by second intention. Surgical excision of large scarred sinuses and cysts is sometimes necessary and may be done in conjunction with skin grafting. Large defects are best allowed to granulate.[35]

Hidradenitis suppurativa

- Treat with rotating oral and topical antibiotics to prevent infection with resistant organisms
- Weight reduction is often helpful
- Use incision and drainage sparingly to avoid sinus tract formation and fibrosis
- Exteriorization of cysts and sinus tracts is the preferred method of treatment
- Allow unroofed areas to heal by second intention if possible

OPTIMIZING OUTCOMES

Many factors must be considered to help optimize the outcome when performing incisional surgery and draining techniques. The patient should be made aware of any medications to avoid including blood thinners both preoperatively and postoperatively. Activity restrictions should be thoroughly discussed. Patients with specific medical problems or known scarring problems should be followed closely so that any problems can be detected early and dealt with.

In removing lipomas it is particularly important to spend time in the preoperative planning stage to exactly localize these growths prior to removal. Remember that infiltrating lipomas and forehead lipomas are much deeper than they appear and are often under or between muscle.

In removing cysts with incisional surgery, preoperative marking and planning is again important. Cysts which have been drained previously or which have been traumatized will often have significant scar tissue associated with them. It is important to access this preoperatively so that it can be removed if necessary. Infiltrating local anesthetic in and around a cyst helps to dissect it free from the surrounding tissue. It is important not to inject anesthetic directly into a cyst as this may cause rupture prior to removal. If a cyst is ruptured prior to removal, then every effort should be made to remove all of the wall and the keratinous debris, which may be present.

Cysts which have been present over a long period of time will often have redundant skin overlying them. Sometimes, in the scalp area the redundant skin will lack hair. It is important to trim the redundant skin at the time of closure to ensure an optimum result. Larger cysts will often require multilayered closure.

Incisional surgery for milia, apocrine hidrocystomas, and steatocystoma multiplex cysts is relatively simple. When incising and draining milia, the cyst wall will often be extruded with the keratinous contents with simple pressure from a curette or comedone extractor after a small incision is made. Steatocystomas are somewhat more difficult to remove, but care must be taken not to excessively traumatize the tissue as this may result in excess scar-tissue formation, especially on the chest where many of these lesions occur. Apocrine hidrocystomas respond well to incision and drainage and light electrodesiccation of the base will help to prevent recurrences.

When incising and draining infected or inflamed abscesses occurring as an isolated event or in combination with hidradenitis suppurativa, care must be taken to assure a successful outcome. With solitary inflamed cysts and abscesses, it is important to isolate the area of maximum fluctuance carefully before incising and draining. This will be the area which is most easily incised and allows access to the underlying inflammatory debris and purulent material. When incising an inflamed cyst, care must be taken to remove all of the keratinous fragments and every attempt should be made to remove all fragments of cyst wall. The likelihood of needing to reexcise the lesion later is decreased substantially if all of the cyst wall can be removed.

The incision and drainage performed for hidradenitis is ideally done with the idea of unroofing the area of abscesses formation maximally. This allows it to heal from the inside out by second intention, rather than forming a fistula or scar track, which will become a chronic focus for further inflammation in the future.

■ POSTOPERATIVE CARE

Postoperative care for incisional surgery involves many of the general care guidelines used with any surgery as well as some special instructions for certain situations. It is important to give the patient both written and verbal instructions; if a friend or spouse is present have them listen to the instructions as well. Activity restrictions should be clearly outlined, as well as avoidance of blood thinners or any other medications which may adversely affect healing.

For patients who have had lipomas or larger cysts removed it is important that they avoid any exercise or activity that might cause a seroma or hematoma to form. Ice is very effective for reducing swelling and postoperative bleeding. Instruct the patient to ice the area in cycles of 30 minutes on and 30 minutes off for several cycles immediately postoperatively. Pressure dressings help to prevent postoperative hematoma formation. When removing uncomplicated lipomas and cysts with incisional surgery, postoperative antibiotics are rarely needed. They are, however, helpful in some cases. If there is a concern over contamination or possible inflammation or infection in and around the surgical area, postoperative antibiotics should be considered.

In removing milia, apocrine hidrocystomas, and steatocystomas there is rarely a need for sutures or substantial postoperative care. Frequently topical antibiotic ointment speeds healing. Occasionally, a light dressing is useful for any drainage within the first 24–48 hours.

When incising and draining acute abscesses or inflamed or infected cysts, either isolated or seen in association with hidradenitis suppurativa, postoperative care and dressing maintenance is very important. For larger abscesses and cysts use of a packing material helps to keep the area open and allows for adequate drainage, while allowing healing to occur from the inside out. Either Iodoform (NU Gauze; Johnson and Johnson Medical, A division of Ethicon, Arlington) or plain gauze ribbon can be used to pack larger lesions. A wick of material is left extruding out through the incised and drained area. This is advanced approximately 1 cm daily with each dressing change until it is removed. It is important to use a large amount of absorbent dressing material when bandaging incised and drained abscesses, or infected or inflamed cysts. Drainage can often be heavy for the first few days following the procedure. A dressing consisting of five 8-cm gauze pads stacked over the wound and held in place with a flexible dressing material such as CoverRoll (BSN Medical, Hamburg, Germany) works well. The dressing will often need to be changed daily or sometimes twice daily in the initial stages of healing if drainage is heavy. Antibiotics such as erythromycin or cephalexin are good choices to cover for *Staphylococcus* and *Streptococcus* spp. which can frequently be found in abscesses and infected cysts. Postoperatively, long-term abnormal scarring can occur after incisional surgery. Traditional methods for scar treatment including intralesional steroids and silicone gel sheeting are often helpful. Pulsed dye laser therapy can be useful in some cases.

■ PITFALLS AND THEIR MANAGEMENT

Avoidance of pitfalls

- Lipomas should be completely removed and this can be achieved by clear marking prior to surgery and by thoroughly palpating the area after removal.
- For scarred cysts, the scar tissue and cyst wall should be dissected out.
- Minimal surgery should be carried out when removing milia, steatocystomas, and apocrine hidrocystomas; this should avoid possible excess scar formation.
- For infected cysts and abscesses, occurring either in association with hidradenitis suppurativa or as an isolated event, the inflamed area should be completely drained.
- A frequent complication of hidradenitis suppurativa is chronic sinus tract formation; this can be avoided by unroofing the cavity completely and curetting the base.
- Any material which is going to be taken for culture should be removed immediately upon entering the abscess cavity.

Incisional surgery can have a number of pitfalls which are avoidable if one plans well and uses proper technique. When removing lipomas one of the most common pitfalls is incomplete removal. This frequently results from inadequate marking prior to surgery, or non-thorough palpation of the area after removal to assess for any firm areas which may represent residual lipoma. In removing forehead lipomas, it is especially important to isolate and mark the lipoma well prior to removal. Small lipomas are very easy to miss if not precisely located and marked preoperatively. For infiltrating lipomas of the upper extremities, it is particularly important to identify the precise location of the lipoma prior to removal. MRI scanning for larger lesions helps to avoid injuring neurovascular structures or other structures that may be adjacent to the lipoma.

Scarred cysts are often difficult to remove. Dissecting out the scar tissue as well as the cyst wall frequently gives the best result. If substantial scar tissue is left behind it may be difficult to tell whether there is residual cyst or simply scar tissue after the area heals.

In removing milia, steatocystomas, and apocrine hidrocystomas, minimal surgery should be done to avoid possible excess scar formation. Cautery should also be used minimally as it can cause hypopigmented scarring. Histologic material should be submitted for confirmation of the presumed clinical diagnosis. This is especially true for apocrine hidrocystomas, which frequently can mimic basal cell carcinoma.

In draining inflamed or infected cysts and abscesses occurring either in association with hidradenitis suppurativa or as an isolated event, it is important to completely drain the inflamed area if possible. A hemostat is often useful in spreading the subcutaneous tissue to allow for optimal drainage. In cases associated with hidradenitis suppurativa, unroofing the cavity completely and curetting the base is helpful for avoiding chronic sinus tract formation—a frequent complication of the disease. Incision and drainage for hidradenitis should be used sparingly. Multiple antibiotics are frequently used in treating hidradenitis and a wound culture at the time of the incision and drainage is often quite helpful. If material is going to be taken for culture, it should be removed immediately upon entering the abscess cavity. Initiating empiric antibiotic therapy is frequently appropriate and the antibiotic can be changed if needed when results of the culture and sensitivity testing become available.

■ SUMMARY

Despite the many advancements in medicine and surgery, incision, draining, and exteriorization techniques continue to be an important treatment method for a number of conditions. These techniques can be used to remove a variety of benign subcutaneous neoplasms including lipomas and a variety of cysts. They are also quite useful for incising and draining abscesses and inflamed or infected cysts. Hidradenitis suppurativa, which is a common condition, often ideally requires incision, drainage, and exteriorization of chronically inflamed and infected areas.

For these techniques to be successful, the clinician must adhere to thorough preoperative evaluation and planning. Attention must be given to anatomic location and underlying structures to avoid potential pitfalls.

To ensure optimal results, it is important to utilize sound surgical technique. Spending extra time to thoroughly review postoperative care instructions and answer any of the patients questions helps avoid potential problems and ensure a successful outcome.

■ REFERENCES

1. Breasted JH. The Edwin Smith surgical papyrus. Chicago:University of Chicago Press; 1930.
2. Enzinger FM, Weiss SW. Soft tissue tumors. St Louis, CV Mosby; 1983:199–241.
3. Rhydholm A, Berg NO. Size, site, and clinical insights of lipoma. Act Orthop Scand 1983; 54:929.
4. Truhan AP, Garden JM, Caro WA, et al. Facial and scalp lipomas: case reports and study of prevalence. J Dermatol Surg Oncol 1985; 11:91.
5. Salasche SJ, McCollough ML, et al. Frontalis-associated lipoma of the forehead. J Am Acad Dermatol 1989; 20:462.
6. Andrews K, Ghauami A, Mowlavia, Goldfarb JN. The youthful forehead: Placement of skin incisions in hidden furrows. Dermatol Surg 2002; 5:489–490.
7. Harrington AC, Admot J, Chesser RS. Infiltrating lipomas of the upper extremities. J Dermatol Surg Oncol 1990; 16: 834–836.
8. Kindblom LG, Angervall L, Stener B. Intermuscular and intramuscular lipomas and hibernomas: A clinical, roentgenologic, histologic, and prognostic study of 46 cases. Cancer 1974; 33:754–762.
9. Fitzpatrick TB, Eisen AZ, Wolff K, Freedberg IM, Austen KF. Benign epithelial tumors. In: Dermatology in general medicine, volume I. 4th edn. New York: McGraw-Hill; 1993:866–870.
10. McGavran MH, Binnington B. Keratinous cysts of the skin. Arch Dermatol 1966; 94:499.
11. Krull EA. The 'Little' curet (surgical gems). J Dermatol Surg Oncol 1978; 4:656.
12. Epstein W, Kligman AM. The pathogenesis of milia and benign tumors of the skin. J Invest Dermatol 1956; 26:1–11.
13. Brody MJ. Complications of chemical resurfacing. Dermatol Clin 2001; 19:427–38.
14. Thami GP, Kaur S, Kanwar AD. Surgical pearl: Enucleation of milia with a disposable hypodermic needle. J Am Acad Dermatol 2002; 47:6023.
15. McGavran MN, Binnington B. Keratinous cysts of the skin: Identification and differentiation of pilar cysts from epidermal cysts. Arch Dermatol 1966; 94:499–508.
16. Leppard BJ, Sanderson KV, Wells RS. Herditary trichilemmal cysts: Heredity pilar cysts. Clin Exp Dermatol 1977; 2:23–32.
17. Brownstein MH. Steatocystoma simplex: A solitary steatocystoma. Arch Dermatol 1982; 118:409–411.
18. Noojin RO, Reynolds JP. Familial steatocystoma multiplex: Twelve cases in three generations. Arch Dermatol Syph 1948; 57:1013–1018.
19. Adams BB, Mutashim OF, Nordlund JJ. Steatocystoma multiplex: A quick removal technique. CUTIS 1999; 64:127–130.
20. Kaya TI, Ikozoglu G, Kokturk A, Tursen V. A simple surgical technique for the treatment of steatocystoma multiplex. Int J Dermatol 2001; 40:785–788.
21. Sato K, Shibuya K, Taguchi H, et al. Aspiration therapy in steatocystoma multiplex. Arch Dermatol 1993; 129:35–37.
22. Krahenbuhl A, Eichmann A, Pfaltz M. CO2 laser therapy for steatocystoma multiplex. Dermatologica 1991; 183:294–296.
23. Smith JD, Chernosky ME. Aprocrine hidrocystoma (cystadenoma). Arch Dermatol 1974; 109:700–702.
24. Hashimoto K, Lever WF. Appendage tumors of the skin. Eccrine hidrocystoma. Springfield, IL: Charles C Thomas; 1968:19–25.
25. Cramer HJ. Das schwarze Hidrocystoma (Monfort). Dermatol Monatsschr 1980; 166:114–118.
26. Malhotra R, Bhawan J. The nature of pigment in pigmented apocrine hidrocystoma. J Cutan Pathol 1985; 12:106–109.
27. Bieter RN. Applied pharmacology of local anesthetics. Am J Surg 1936; 34:500–508.
28. Brook I. Microbiology of infected epidermal cysts. Arch Dermatol 1989; 125:1658–1661.
29. Lane JE. Hidrosadenitis axillaries of Verneuil. Arch Dermatol Syph 1933; 28:609–614.
30. Brunsting HA. Hidradenitis suppurativa. Arch Dermatol Syph 1939; 39:108–120.
31. Shelley WB, Cahn MM. Pathogenesis of hidradenitis suppurativa in man: Experimental and histologic observations. Arch Dermatol 1955; 72:562–565.
32. Carmen C-W Yu, Cook MG. Hidradenitis suppurativa: A disease of follicular epithelium, rather than apocrine glands. Br J Dermatol 1990; 122:763–769.

33. Banerjee AK. Surgical treatment of hidradenitis suppurativa. Br J Surg 1992; 79:863–866.
34. Mullins JF. Treatment of chronic hidradenitis suppurativa: Surgical modifications. Postgrad Med 1959; 26:805–808.
35. Morgan WP, Harding KG, Richardson G, Hughes LE. The use of Silastic foam dressing in the treatment of advanced hidradenitis suppurativa. Br J Surg 1980; 67:277–280.

16 Suturing Technique and Other Closure Materials

Sarah Weitzul MD and R Stan Taylor MD

Summary box

- Choice and placement of wound closure materials play critical roles in the outcome of incisional surgery.
- Suture materials have multiple properties which combine to give each suture unique characteristics.
- Sutures must be placed at the same vertical level across the wound to prevent step-off deformity of incision.
- Proper placement of sutures will approximate and evert wound edges.
- Buried sutures are used to close dead space, redistribute tension, decrease dehiscence, and increase wound eversion.
- Time to suture removal varies by location; whenever possible sutures should be removed at the earliest point.

INTRODUCTION

The cutaneous surgeon must become familiar with the various physical properties of sutures and other closure materials in order to make educated choices. In addition, learning the various suture techniques and the appropriate situations in which to use them is essential. This chapter aims to help the cutaneous surgeon accomplish these goals.

PREOPERATIVE EVALUATION

There are many considerations in selecting closure materials and techniques. One of the most important factors is lesion location. In general, finer caliber sutures are used on the face, while larger sutures are used on the scalp, trunk, and extremities. Staples are often used to close wounds of the scalp and trunk. Other important wound characteristics to consider include size, type of planned repair, and anticipated wound tension. Larger caliber sutures are required for wounds under more tension. Another important consideration is patient profile. For example, the surgeon may elect to use absorbable sutures in patients who are unable or unwilling to return for suture removal. Similarly, needle-free tissue adhesives are commonly used instead of sutures to repair simple lacerations in the pediatric population.

Another important preoperative step is selecting instruments of the appropriate type and size. The size of the needle driver should be proportional to the size of the needle and to the size of the wound. Forceps with teeth are preferred when placing suture because the teeth hold the tissue without crushing it. In contrast, forceps without teeth are favored for grasping suture at the time of suture removal. When undermining wound edges, skin hooks are the least traumatic means of stabilizing and mobilizing the wound edges. Suture should be cut with designated suture scissors and not with delicate tissue scissors. Alternatively, special needle holders are available that incorporate a suture cutting function in their design, thereby eliminating the need for the use of a separate pair of suture scissors and shortening the time to perform the closure. Finally, quality needle holders, skin hooks, scissors, and forceps should be used and maintained for ideal surgical results. Educating the surgical staff about these principals is important to optimize efficiency and performance and to preserve the surgical instruments.

CHOOSING A CLOSURE MATERIAL

Suture

Physical properties of suture

Each type of suture has inherent characteristics which affect its handling, tying, and stability in tissue. Characteristics to be considered include configuration, capillarity, tensile strength, size, knot strength, elasticity, plasticity, memory, and flexibility. (See also Chapter 4.)

Configuration

The configuration of suture denotes its composition: monofilament suture is made up of a single strand, and multifilament suture is made up of several strands. Strands of multifilament sutures are often twisted or braided for cohesiveness. Advantages of braiding include increased tensile strength, improved handling and knot tying properties, and decreased fraying of cut ends. However, braided sutures have an increased propensity to retain microorganisms and they encounter more resistance when pulled through tissue.

Coating

Sutures may be coated with various materials to improve the coefficient of friction and thus facilitate passage through tissue. Coating braided sutures with silicone, Teflon (DuPont, Wilmington, DE), and wax decreases friction, allowing the suture to slide more easily through the skin. Newer innovations include suture coatings with either antibacterial or antitumor qualities. For example, Polyglactin 910 has been coated with the antimicrobial agent triclosan and has been shown to prevent in vitro colonization of *Staphylococcus aureus* and *Staphylococcus epidermidis*.[1,2] In addition, monoclonal antibody-coated suture which may enhance a patient's antitumor immune response is under investigation.[3]

Capillarity

Capillarity denotes a suture's ability to wick fluid from an immersed end to its dry end. Sutures with increased capillarity, such as braided sutures, are more likely to harbor bacteria.

Tensile strength

Tensile strength is defined as the weight necessary to break a suture divided by the cross-sectional area. Tensile strength is proportional to the square of the suture diameter, so larger sutures have increased tensile strength. Various factors can affect tensile strength, including twisting or braiding, which, due to shearing forces between the strands, decreases tensile strength. Tensile strength can also be decreased by physical factors including wetness or increased age of sutures. Synthetic sutures tend to have increased tensile strength compared to sutures of natural materials. The exception is stainless steel, which has the greatest tensile strength.[4]

Size

To allow surgeons to compare sutures made of different materials, the United States Pharmacopoeia (USP) assigns a number to all commercially available sutures. This number or 'size' ranks sutures according to tensile strength, represented by a number of zeros. The greater the tensile strength the fewer the zeros. Therefore a 2-0 suture has more strength than a 6-0 suture. As the strength quality inherent in the materials used to make sutures varies, the caliber of a 5-0 nylon will be smaller than that of a 5-0 gut because nylon is a stronger material.

Knot strength

Knot strength refers to the security of a tied knot and is defined by the degree of slippage that occurs in a knot. Sutures with a decreased coefficient of friction slide more easily and have lower knot strength. Sutures vary widely in their knot strength. For example, catgut suture has low knot strength while polyglycolic acid has one of the highest knot strengths.[5]

Memory

Memory is the ability of a suture to regain its former shape after bending. Knots in sutures with increased memory, such as polypropylene and nylon, have a greater tendency to untie themselves, and the surgeon therefore should throw extra ties with these sutures. In general, sutures with increased memory are more difficult to handle.

Elasticity

Elasticity denotes a suture's capacity for returning to its original size and shape after being stretched. This quality may be desirable in selecting a top stitch because tissue usually swells after a trauma such as surgery. Sutures with elasticity can stretch with the tissue, and will also recoil when the swelling subsides. Polybutester is a synthetic non-absorbable suture which exhibits elasticity.

Plasticity

In contrast to elasticity, sutures such as polypropylene exhibit plasticity, and thus have the ability to retain their deformed shape rather than return to their original shape when stretched. As tissues swell, sutures that exhibit plasticity are able to stretch to accommodate the edema. However, as swelling resolves, sutures with plasticity remain stretched, and this can decrease close approximation of tissues. Plasticity may be advantageous in knot tying because deformation of the suture may lead to a more secure knot.

Tissue reaction

All sutures exhibit at least some inflammatory response when placed in tissue, but the degree varies widely. This suture property is very important because exuberant inflammatory reactions have been shown to delay wound healing, to jeopardize wound apposition, and predispose to infection.[6] Many factors contribute to tissue reactivity (Table 16.1). The caliber of suture is directly proportional to its reactivity; thus the greater the suture diameter, the greater the chance of tissue reaction. Configuration also affects a suture's ability to cause tissue reaction: monofilament sutures cause less reactivity than multifilament sutures.[4] Synthetic sutures such as nylon or polypropylene also cause less of an inflammatory response than sutures made of natural materials such as silk and surgical gut.[7] All absorbable sutures—synthetic and natural—induce an immune response which is responsible for their dissolution. Sutures made of natural materials (gut and silk) are degraded by proteolysis, in contrast to synthetic sutures which are degraded by hydrolysis. Proteolysis causes a more brisk immune reaction than hydrolysis. Non-absorbable sutures cause less tissue reaction because they induce a fibrous shell which coats the suture and decreases the host response.[4]

Table 16.1 Suture properties that affect immunogenicity

	More Immunogenic	Less Immunogenic
Material	Natural	Synthetic
Configuration	Multifilament	Monofilament
Absorption	Absorbable	Non-absorbable
Diameter	Large	Small

On rare occasions, true suture allergy may occur, particularly with sutures made of gut. Allergy to gut suture may be due to the foreign collagen or to chromic salts in chromate-sensitive patients.[8] Immediate-type IgE-mediated hypersensitivity reactions have been reported with bovine collagen materials, which may be found in gut suture. In the cases reported, presence of allergen-specific IgE was confirmed by skin-prick testing.[9] Silk can rarely cause an extensive, destructive suppurative and granulomatous response which may be a type of delayed-type hypersensitivity reaction. Such sensitivity to silk can be confirmed or predicted with an intradermal skin test.[10]

Absorption

By definition, absorbable sutures as a group are defined as sutures that lose the majority of their tensile strength within 60 days after placement in living tissue. Nonabsorbable sutures therefore maintain their tensile strength for periods greater than 60 days. All suture materials, excluding stainless steel wire, lose integrity or are absorbed to some degree if left in the skin for long enough. Depending upon the material used, integrity may range from 6 days to 6 months, or longer. The rate of absorption depends on the suture type, the presence of infection, and site of placement. Presence of infection increases suture absorption, as does placement in locations where there is high secretion of proteolytic enzymes, such as mucosa.[11]

Commonly used sutures in dermatologic surgery

Absorbable sutures (Table 16.2)

Surgical gut

Surgical gut is the only absorbable suture made of natural materials. Derived from the intestines of sheep or cows, gut suture is a twisted multifilament suture comprised mostly of collagen. Gut sutures commonly come in three varieties: plain, fast absorbing, and chromic. Plain surgical gut loses much of its tensile strength in 7–10 days and is completely absorbed by 70 days.[12] Fast-absorbing gut is heat-treated for more rapid degradation. This suture is used in facial wound closures or the placement of skin grafts when rapid absorption of suture is desirable. Nearly all of its tensile strength is lost within 7 days, and complete absorption takes 21–42 days. Chromic gut has been treated with chromate salts, which decrease the rate of absorption in tissue. Chromic gut maintains its tensile strength for 10–21 days and is completely absorbed after approximately 90 days. This suture may be used to ligate vessels in open wounds or to suture mucosal wounds. A history of chromate sensitivity should preclude the use of this suture. Disadvantages to gut sutures include unpredictable absorption rates, low tensile strength, and increased tissue sensitivity when compared with other absorbable sutures.

Polyglycolic acid (Dexon S, Dexon II: USSDG, Norwalk, CT)

Polyglycolic acid was the first synthetic absorbable suture, first available in 1970. It is a braided multifilament suture, which creates significant drag when pulled through tissue. To alleviate this problem it is available with a polycaprolate coating; this is marketed as Dexon II. Nonetheless, some surgeons prefer the uncoated Dexon S because it has better knot security. Both coated and non-coated suture retains 65% of its tensile strength 2 weeks after placement and 35% 3 weeks after implantation. It is completely resorbed between 60 and 90 days after placement. Advantages to its use include good handling and knot security and low tissue reactivity.[13] One study showed a decreased incidence of wound infections with polyglycolic acid-sutured incisions when compared with incisions sutured with chromic gut and nylon.[14]

Polyglactin 910 (Vicryl: Ethicon Inc, Somerville, NJ)

Polyglactin was the second synthetic absorbable suture to become available. It is a coated, braided, multifilament suture like polyglycolic acid. Polyglactin 910 consists of a copolymer made from 90% glycolide and 10% L-lactide. This suture has similar handling properties to polyglycolic acid but has more tensile strength.[15] After tissue placement, polyglactin retains 75% of its tensile strength at 2 weeks and 50% at 3 weeks. It is essentially completely resorbed after 56–70 days. Polyglactin 910 is widely used in cutaneous surgery. It has been compared directly with both polydioxanone for use in rhytidectomy reconstruction and polytrimethylene carbonate in Mohs reconstruction without any statistical difference in scar quality.[16,17] Other studies have shown an increased incidence of hypertrophic scars with Polyglactin 910-sutured incision compared to those sutured with either polydioxanone or poliglecaprone 25.[18,19]

Polyglactin 910 also comes in a more rapidly dissolving form called Vicryl-rapide (Ethicon) which was developed to mirror the performance of surgical gut suture. Vicryl-rapide is composed of a polymer material with a lower molecular weight than the regular Polyglactin 910, which increases its absorption rate in tissue. It loses 50% of its tensile strength at 5 days and essentially all tensile strength within 10–14 days. Vicryl-rapide has been shown to have similar performance to nylon in the closure of punch-biopsy sites, without the need for suture removal.[20]

Lactomer (Polysorb; USSDG)

Like Polyglactin 910, lactomer is a coated, braided multifilament suture made of copolymers of lactic and glycolic acids. Lactomer retains 80% of its tensile strength at 2 weeks and over 30% at 3 weeks. It is completely absorbed 56–70 days after implantation. Compared with Polyglactin 910, lactomer has been reported to have superior handling and knot characteristics.[21,22] In one study, lactomer had greater initial tensile strength than Polyglactin 910 and polyglycolic acid, but it lost strength more rapidly than the others after tissue implantation.[22]

Polydioxanone (PDS: Ethicon)

Polydioxanone was introduced in 1982 as the first monofilament synthetic absorbable suture. Its monofilament configuration allows for easier passage through tissue, decreased tissue reactivity, and decreased risk of wound infection. This configuration also confers decreased handling and knot strength due to the decreased coefficient of friction. Polydioxanone has decreased initial tensile strength when compared to Polyglactin 910 or polyglycolic acid. However, polydioxanone is more slowly resorbed and retains its tensile strength for longer. It retains 70% of its

Table 16.2 Properties of absorbable sutures

Suture (Brand Name)	Configuration	Handling	Knot Strength	Tissue Reactivity	Initial Tensile Strength	Longevity of Tensile Strength	Time to Complete Absorption	Comments
Surgical gut, plain	Multifilament Twisted	Interm	Poor	High	Low	Lost in 7–10 days	70 days	Unpredictable absorption rates
Fast-absorbing gut	Multifilament Twisted	Interm	Poor	High	Low	Lost in 3–7 days	21–42 days	High reactivity True allergy possible
Chromic surgical gut	Multifilament Twisted	Interm	Fair	Moderate to high	Low	Lost in 10–21 days	90 days	Unpredictable absorption rates High reactivity True allergy possible to collagen or chromate
Polyglycolic acid (Dexon S)‡	Multifilament Braided	Good	Good	Low to interm	Interm	35% strength at 3 weeks	60–90 days	Uncoated
Polyglycolic acid (Dexon II)‡			Interm					Coated
Polyglactin 910 (Vicryl)†	Multifilament Braided	Good	Good	Low to interm	Quite high	50% strength at 3 weeks	56–70 days	Coated Higher tensile strength than Dexon
Polyglactin 910 (Vicryl Rapide)†		Good	Good	Low to interm		50% strength at 5 days	42 days	
Lactomer (Polysorb)‡	Multifilament Braided	Good	Good	Low to interm	Quite high	>30% strength at 3 weeks	56–70 days	Coated
Polydioxanone (PDS II)†	Monofilament	Poor	Poor	Low	High	50% at 4 weeks 25% at 6 weeks	90–180 days	High memory Very slow absorption
Polytrimethylene carbonate (Maxon)‡	Monofilament	Very good	Very good	Very low	Very high	59% strength at 4 weeks 30% at 6 weeks	60–180 days	Has higher initial tensile strength than PDS but absorbed more quickly
Poliglecaprone 25 (Monocryl)†	Monofilament	Very good	Very good	Very low	Highest	30% at 2 weeks All lost at 3–4 weeks	90–120 days	Highest initial tensile strength Highest knot security of synthetic absorbable sutures
Glycomer 631 (Biosyn)‡	Monofilament	N/D	N/D	N/D	N/D	49% retained at 3 weeks	90–110 days	Decreased coefficient of friction than Monocryl Seldom used in dermatologic surgery

† Trademark of Ethicon
‡ Trademark of USSDG Sutures, US Surgical Corporation
N/D, no data available.
Very low—low—poor—fair—good—moderate—intermediate—relatively high—very high—very good—highest

original tensile strength at 2 weeks, 50% at 4 weeks, and 25% at 6 weeks. Absorption is negligible until the 90th postoperative day, and complete resorption takes approximately 6 months. Therefore, this suture may be useful in wounds under higher tension or wounds that require prolonged dermal support. Indeed, prolonged dermal support for at least 6 months has been associated with decreased scar spreading.[23] The original polydioxanone suture was replaced with an updated product, PDS II, which has improved handling characteristics.

Polytrimethylene carbonate (Maxon: USSDG)

Polytrimethylene carbonate is another monofilament synthetic absorbable suture. It has greater initial tensile strength than polydioxanone. It retains 81% of initial tensile strength at 2 weeks, 59% at 4 weeks, and 30% at 6 weeks.[24] However, polytrimethylene carbonate is absorbed more quickly than polydioxanone; its absorption begins 60 days after implantation compared to 90 days with polydioxanone. Polytrimethylene carbonate has greater knot strength and handling properties compared to polydioxanone, polyglycolic acid, and Polyglactin 910.[12,17]

Poliglecaprone 25 (Monocryl: Ethicon)

This monofilament absorbable synthetic suture became available in 1993 and offers superior handling and tying properties due to its increased pliability. Its knot strength is superior to all of the aforementioned synthetic absorbable sutures.[25] In addition, it has higher initial tensile strength than PDS II or Maxon; however, this strength diminishes more quickly than with the other monofilament synthetic sutures. It retains 60% of its initial tensile strength at 7 days, 30% at 2 weeks, and loses all tensile strength by 3–4 weeks.[26] Like many other absorbable sutures, Monocryl is available in both clear and dyed (violet) sutures; the dyed Maxon sutures retain their tensile strength and remain in tissue slightly longer than the clear sutures. Absorption of both varieties is essentially complete by 3–4 months. When compared to Vicryl-rapide in the closure of breast reduction incisions, Monocryl is associated with smaller, less reactive scars, and with a lower predisposition to form hypertrophic scars.[27]

Glycomer 631 (Biosyn: USSDG)

Glycomer 631 is the newest monofilament synthetic absorbable suture. It dissolves more slowly than poliglecaprone 25. It retains 75% of its original tensile strength at 2 weeks and 49% at 3 weeks. It is completely absorbed between 90 and 110 days. When compared with poliglecaprone 25, glycomer 631 has a decreased coefficient of friction, making its passage through tissue easier, and its knots are slightly less secure.[28] At present, this suture is seldom used in dermatologic surgery.

Non-absorbable sutures (Table 16.3)

Silk (Perma-Hand: Ethicon; Sofsilk: USSDG)

Surgical silk is a multifilament suture composed of braided fibers of protein harvested from the cocoon of the silkworm larva. To improve passage through tissue, the suture is usually coated with wax or silicone. Although surgical silk is classified as a non-absorbable suture, it is slowly absorbed when implanted in tissue, losing almost all its tensile strength 1 year after implantation, and being completely

Table 16.3 Properties of non-absorbable sutures

Suture (Brand Name)	Configuration	Handling	Tensile Strength	Knot Strength	Memory	Tissue Reactivity	Comments
Silk (Sofsilk)‡ (Perma-Hand)†	Multifilament Braided	Excellent	Low	Excellent	Low	High	Use limited by high incidence of tissue reaction Very slowly absorbed in tissue
Nylon (Monosof)‡ (Dermalon)‡ (Ethilon)†	Monofilament	Poor	High	Poor	High	Low	Monofilament nylon may tear through delicate tissue Very slowly absorbed in tissue
Nylon (Nurulon)† (Surgilon)‡	Multifilament	Good	High	Fair	Moderate	Moderate	
Polypropylene (Prolene)† (Surgipro)‡	Monofilament	Poor	Moderate	Poor	High	Low	Does not degrade in tissue
Polyester, uncoated (Dacron)‡ (Mersiline)†	Multifilament Braided	Very good	Very high	Very good	Moderate	Moderate	Expensive and rarely used in dermatologic surgery Very high tensile strength
Polyester, coated (Ticron)‡	Multifilament Braided Silicone-coated	Very good	Very high	Good	Moderate	Moderate to high	If silicone dislodges from suture, significant tissue reaction can occur
Polyester, coated (Ethibond Excel)†	Multifilament Braided Polybutylate-coated	Very good	Very high	Good	Moderate	Moderate	Polybutylate coating very adherent to suture and very seldom breaks off into tissue
Polybutester (Novafil)‡	Monofilament	Good	High	Good	Low	Low	Exhibits elasticity
Polyhexafluoro-propylene-VDF (Pronova)†	Monofilament	N/D	N/D	N/D	N/D	N/D	Low friction coefficient Very seldom used

† Trademark of Ethicon Inc, Johnson & Johnson (Somerville, NJ)
‡ Trademark of USSDG Sutures, US Surgical Corporation (Norwalk, CT)
N/D, no data available.

absorbed within 2 years. Silk suture is very soft, which makes it a good suture to close biopsy sites or small incisions in sensitive locations such as mucosa or intertriginous areas. Although silk suture has superior handling and knot-tying characteristics, its tendency to cause tissue reaction limits its use.

Nylon

Nylon is the most commonly used non-absorbable suture in dermatologic surgery. Nylon suture is available both in monofilamentous (Monosof, Dermalon: USSDG; Ethilon: Ethicon) and coated multifilamentous (Nurulon: Ethicon; Surgilon: USSDG) varieties, with the latter being more common. Both have high tensile strength and are absorbed at a rate of 15–20% per year if left in tissue. Monofilamentous nylon passes easily through the skin and causes minimal tissue reactions but has a high degree of memory, decreasing its pliability, handling, and knot security. It may also tear through delicate tissue. Multifilamentous nylon has improved handling and tying properties, but is associated with higher tissue reactivity and expense. Nylon is made more pliable by moisture, and Ethicon makes a premoistened monofilament nylon suture for cosmetic surgery that has significantly improved handling and tying properties when compared to regular monofilament nylon.

Polypropylene (Prolene: Ethicon; Surgipro: USSDG)

Polypropylene is a monofilament synthetic suture with somewhat lower tensile strength than other synthetic non-absorbable sutures. It is fairly stiff and has high memory, decreasing its handling and tying properties. Polypropylene has low tissue reactivity and an extremely low friction coefficient, making it ideal for running intradermal stitches. This slippery characteristic decreases knot security, and surgeons must take care to throw extra loops in the knots of polypropylene to increase their security.[12] Unlike nylon and silk, polypropylene is not degraded in tissue and may be used when long-term support is useful. For example, clear polypropylene may be used to reapproximate ear cartilage. Polypropylene also exhibits significant plasticity and expands to accommodate swelling tissue. However, when swelling subsides, the suture will not regain its former shape, which may affect wound apposition.

Polyester

Polyester is a braided, multifilamentous, synthetic suture with uses similar to those of multifilamentous nylon. It is soft and pliable and has a high tensile strength; in fact, its tensile strength is only exceeded by metal sutures.[29] Due to its braided nature, uncoated polyester suture (Dacron: USSDG; Mersiline: Ethicon) has significant tissue drag and is therefore available in coated forms. It may be coated with Teflon, silicone (Ticron: USSDG), or polybutylate (Ethibond Excel: Ethicon). Polybutilate adheres well to the suture in contrast to Teflon and silicone, which may break off in tissue, causing an intense immune response.[30] Polyester suture's soft, pliable nature makes it useful for mucosal tissue or in intertriginous areas. However, polyester is costly and is little used in dermatologic surgery.

Polybutester (Novafil: USSDG)

Polybutester is a newer type of polyester which is available in a monofilament suture. It is a copolymer composed of polyglycol terephthate and polybutylene terephthate. Polybutester has a lower coefficient of friction and lower tissue reactivity than the older polyester sutures. It also offers better handling than polypropylene, including lower memory, increased flexibility, and better knot security.[4] Polybutester exhibits elasticity and can regain its former shape when stretched, unlike polypropylene.[31] One study comparing polybutester Novafil with polypropylene showed improved handling, easier removal, and cosmetically superior scars in patients receiving polybutester sutures.[32] Little is written about polybutester in the dermatologic literature, reflecting its rare usage.

Polyhexafluoropropylene-VDF (Pronova: Ethicon)

Polyhexafluoropropylene-VDF is the newest monofilamentous non-absorbable suture, composed of a polymer blend of polyvinylidene fluoride and polyvinylidene fluoride-cohexafluoropropylene. It has a low coefficient of friction, making it easy to pass through and remove from tissue. Very little clinical data is available regarding the use of this suture.

Suture needles

Proper needle selection and needle handling prevents needle damage, minimizes tissue damage, and facilitates suture placement. There is a great variety of needle designs, but a relative few are routinely used by the cutaneous surgeon. Most needles are made of stainless steel and differ in size, degree of tip sharpness, and body design. Needle cost depends on the sharpness and quality of the stainless steel used in its composition. When choosing a needle for cutaneous surgery, one must consider various factors including wound location, tissue type, suture size, and cost.

An ideal needle is malleable, strong, and sharp. Ductility or malleability refers to a needle's resistance to breaking under a given degree of bending. Needle breakage during surgery can be a very difficult situation and every precaution should be taken to avoid this occurrence. Needle strength is determined by how well it resists deformation when being placed repeatedly through tissue. Such needle deformation can cause increased tissue trauma, unnecessary delay, and inadvertent needle-stick injury. In addition, reshaping a bent needle may affect needle's strength or lead to breakage. Tip sharpness is also very important; sharp needles result in less tissue trauma and better cosmetic results. Most needles are machine sharpened, but for very fine work cosmetic surgeons use the more expensive, sharper hand-honed needles. Needle coating can also affect performance. Modern needles are often coated with silicone or other lubricants to improve the ease of needle penetration.

A needle is comprised of three different parts: the shank, the body, and the point (Fig. 16.1). The shank is the portion of the needle that attaches to the suture and it is the weakest part of the needle. Up until the mid-1900s, needles had eyes which were threaded like conventional sewing needles. However, nowadays needles are almost exclusively swaged, meaning they are attached directly to the suture without an eye. This is done by placing one end of the suture in the hollowed end of the needle; then the end, or shank, is crimped down around the needle to secure the suture. Its hollow nature allows seamless connection of the needle to the suture but also imparts weak-

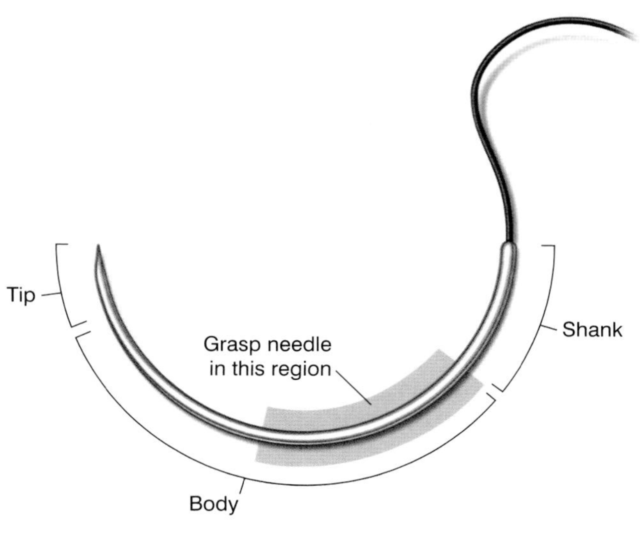

Figure 16.1 The surgical needle is comprised of the tip, body, and shank. The body is the strongest portion of the needle, and should therefore be the portion grasped by the needle holder. The needle should be held one-half way to two-thirds from the tip. (Adapted from Taylor RS. Needles, sutures, and suturing. Atlas Office Proced 1999; 2:53–74.)

ness to this subunit. The shank is the largest part of the needle–suture unit, and hence it determines the size of the suture tract.

The point of the needle extends from the tip of the needle to the largest cross-section of the body. To avoid dulling and injury, the tip should not be handled with the hands or with instruments.

The body is the middle portion of the needle between the shank and point. It is the strongest portion of the needle and this part should therefore be grasped with the needle holder. This prevents damage to the needle tip and crushing of the weaker swaged end of the needle, which leads to bending or breakage. Proper handling of needles is very important to maintain optimum performance. The needle should always be handled by instruments instead of fingers to prevent injury.

Needles may be straight or curved. Curved needles are used almost exclusively in dermatologic surgery. Dermatologic surgeons use the $^{3}/_{8}$ circle needles most frequently, but $^{1}/_{2}$ circle needles may be used to suture small flaps.

Needles come in a wide variety of types that are based on the cross-sectional shape of the body and tip. Most commonly, curved needles with triangular shapes are used. These triangular needles come in two types: conventional cutting and reverse cutting (Fig. 16.2). A conventional cutting needle has its primary cutting edge on the inside of the curve, and when passed through tissue, its tapered puncture is left the closest to the incision. Because the tension vectors go in the direction of the incision, sutures placed with cutting needles may tear through the wound edge. In contrast, reverse cutting needles have their primary cutting edge on the outside of the needle, leaving the tapered point directed away from the wound edge, resulting in less tissue tearing by the suture after tying. Reverse cutting needles are used much more often than conventional cutting needles. Needles can also have a tapered, round shape. These rounded needles cause less tissue tearing than conventional or reverse cutting needles and may be useful for delicate areas or in fascia.

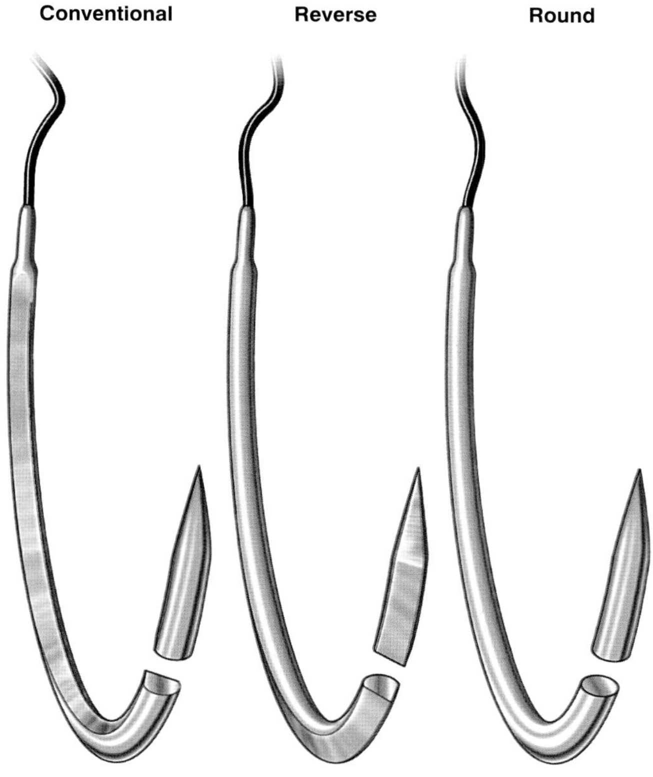

Figure 16.2 Conventional cutting needles have their cutting edge on the inside of the needle arc, and leave their pointed puncture facing the wound incision. Reverse cutting needles have their cutting edge on the outside of the arc, leaving the pointed puncture facing away from the incision which decreases the chance of suture tearing through tissue.

The nomenclature of needles is very confusing and varies by company. The Ethicon Corporation currently manufactures over 80% of the surgical needles used in North America, and a brief description of their needle designations is listed in Table 16.4. Because the company US Surgical bought Davis and Geck Corporation, their suture product line has been merged under the USSDG division. USSDG needle terminology is very difficult to discern, and many needles with the same specifications have different designations. Table 16.5 lists the most common types of sutures used in dermatologic surgery and includes needle designations of the three most prominent suture manufacturers.

Staples

Surgical stainless steel staples offer an efficient means of wound closure and have been used for decades. Staple placement is 80% faster than suture placement, making it

Table 16.4 Ethicon needle abbreviations

Manufacturer	Abbreviation	Meaning	Comments
Ethicon	P	Plastic	Reverse cutting
	PC	Precision cosmetic	Conventional cutting
	PS	Plastic surgery	Reverse cutting
	FS	For skin	Significantly lower-quality honing and steel than P, PC, PS

Table 16.5 Needles commonly used in dermatologic surgery*

Needle Type	Curvature [units?]	Needle Length	Manufacturer		
			Ethicon	USSDG	Look
Premium conventional cutting	$^3/_8$	13 mm	PC-1	PC-10	CP-1
		16 mm	PC-3 CPS-3	PC-11	CP-31
		8 mm	P-6	P-16 (7 mm)	—
Premium reverse cutting	$^3/_8$	11 mm	P-1	P-10 SBE-1	C-1
		13 mm	P-3	P-13 SBE-2 PRE-302	C-3 (12 mm)
		16 mm	PS-3	P-11 PRE-3 SBE-3	PC-34
		19 mm	PS-2	P-12 SBE-4 PRE-304	PC-31
		24 mm	PS-1	P-14 SBE-6	PC-33
	$^1/_2$	8 mm	P-2	P-21 (9 mm)	—
Reverse cutting	$^3/_8$	19 mm	FS-2	C-13	C-6
		24 mm	FS-1	C-14	C-7

**Comparisons are based on latest available manufacturer specifications and do not imply equivalent performance in vivo.*

more cost effective when staff time is factored in.[33] Staples are very strong and have decreased risk of tissue strangulation, reactivity, and infection than sutures.[34] In addition, staples offer excellent wound eversion. Several studies have compared staples to nylon sutures in epidermal closure, and most show equivalent results.[35–37] However, flaps that were stapled had a 62.5% incidence of partial necrosis compared to 20.6% of sutured flaps.[38] In addition, if not removed carefully staples can cause more patient discomfort than sutures.[39] Staples are used most commonly on the trunk and scalp and may be used to secure large full-thickness or split-thickness skin grafts. Usage on the back, over bony prominences, or in intertriginous areas can lead to patient discomfort.

To place staples, the ejecting surface of the stapler is held perpendicular to and flush with the wound surface. Care should be taken to place the staple directly over the center of the incision. The depth of penetration depends on the amount of pressure placed on the stapler against the skin. Releasing the handle of the device disengages the staple. Staple placement requires some practice and technique varies depending on the device used. Disposable staplers are used in dermatologic surgery and come loaded with 5 to 35 staples available in two widths: regular (4–6 mm) or wide (6.5–7.5 mm). The width and height of the staples vary with the manufacturer. Staple extractors are available to facilitate removal.

Skin closure tapes

Modern skin closure tapes are made of a microporous material with an acrylate adhesive and are available in a variety of colors and widths. These tapes are used most commonly to support sutured wounds but can be used alone in very superficial lacerations or for epidermal closure in small tension-free incisions that have been closed with a layer of subcutaneous sutures. Advantages include speed of use, cost savings, and no requirement for in-office removal. However, these strips may cause wound inversion if used without other means of epidermal closure and should not be used alone in cosmetically sensitive areas or wounds closed under tension.

Prior to tape application, the surrounding skin should be degreased with alcohol. For optimal adhesion and durability, a tactifier such as tincture of benzoin or Mastisol (Ferndale Laboratories) is applied around the wound edges where the strips will adhere, avoiding the wound itself. After the tactifier has dried the strips are applied, taking care not to invert or misalign the wound edges. If applied in this way, such skin closure tapes should last 1–2 weeks.

Tissue adhesives

Tissue adhesives are composed of cyanoacrylate compounds. These chemicals rapidly polymerize and bond to various surfaces when applied and pressed into a thin layer. Advantages of tissue adhesive use include rapidity and ease of use, no need for suture removal, and no puncture wounds that could precipitate wound infection or 'track' marks. Liquid adhesives are commonly used to repair superficial lacerations, particularly in the pediatric population. They can also be used for closure of small, superficial, wounds or of low-tension incisions that have been closed with a layer of subcutaneous sutures.

The primary differences between the various cyanoacrylates lies in the length of their alkoxycarbonyl (-COOR) chain.[40] Because of tissue toxicity, short-chain cyanoacrylates have been replaced by longer chain cyanoacrylates.[41] The two cyanoacrylates used in dermatologic surgery are described below.

N-Butyl-2-cyanoacrylate (Indermil: USSDG; Glu-Stitch, Liquid Bandage: Glu-Stitch Inc; Histoacryl: B Braun, Melsugen, AG)

N-butyl-2-cyanoacrylate has a 4-carbon alkyl chain connected to the carboxyl group. It has been studied extensively outside the US since the 1970s and has more rapid polymerization, stronger bond formation, and decreased tissue toxicity compared with the short-chain cyanoacrylates.[40,41] Indermil was FDA approved in 2002 for use as a wound closure material, and is currently the only *n*-butyl-2-cyanoacrylate product in this class with such approval.

Histoacryl and Glu-Stitch are similar products used outside the US. Liquid Bandage is an *n*-butyl-2-cyanoacrylate product marketed in the US for use on unbroken skin. Its approved function is as a skin protectant.

Several studies have shown *n*-butyl-2-cyanoacrylate to be equally efficacious and cosmetically equal to sutures in the repair of lacerations, skin grafts, and wound closures.[42–44]

Octyl cyanoacrylate, N-2-cyanoacrylate (Dermabond: Ethicon)

Dermabond is a long chain cyanoacrylate with an 8-carbon alkyl chain. It was approved by the FDA in 1998 for the closure of superficial lacerations or incisions and was the first tissue adhesive approved for this indication. This adhesive polymerizes in 2.5 minutes, giving the wound strength equivalent to that provided by 5-0 nylon sutures or subcuticular absorbable suture.[45,46]

Octyl cyanoacrylate comes in 0.5 ml single-use ampules which are used to paint on the adhesive in an elliptical manner, starting around the wound edges and working outward. The adhesive should be applied up to the edges of the wound, taking care not to get it in the wound itself, which may slow healing. The adhesive must be applied in three layers, allowing each to dry before application of the next. The first layer polymerizes in 2.5 minutes, and subsequent layers take longer. The polymerization causes generation of heat, which may be slightly uncomfortable for the patient.[41]

Octyl cyanoacrylate has improved flexibility, less tissue toxicity, and at least three times the bonding strength of *n*-butyl-2-cyanoacrylate.[47] However, a randomized clinical trial comparing the two tissue adhesives in repair of pediatric lacerations failed to show any difference between them regarding time of application, patient-perceived pain, physician-perceived difficulty, or cosmetic outcome.[42]

Octyl cyanoacrylate is efficacious for the closure of superficial lacerations, skin grafts, and low-tension incisions.[48–50] Several studies have compared cosmetic outcomes in wounds closed with *n*-2-cyanoacrylate and those closed with sutured; these studies have shown the former to be superior, equivalent, and inferior.[49–51] Although most agree that this and all tissue adhesives give good cosmetic results in laceration repair, they should be used with some caution in excisional surgery in cosmetically sensitive areas because sutures can evert wound edges and hence may give better cosmesis. In addition, tissue adhesives are expensive, and may not be substantially time-saving in cutaneous excisional surgery. In fact, Shamiyeh et al. reported octyl cyanoacrylate was 14 times more expensive than suture and took twice as long to apply when used for skin closure after phlebectomy.[52]

■ SUTURING TECHNIQUES

Knot tying

Suture placement technique greatly affects the cosmetic outcome of wound closure. When planning the closure of a skin defect, the most important aspect to consider is the tension that is created across the wound when closure is attempted. This more than any other factor determines the ultimate functional and cosmetic outcome. Whenever possible, tension should be taken off the wound edges, allowing them to heal together without strain, because significant wound tension in a sutured incision increases the chances of dehiscence and of creating a more obvious, widened scar. Careful placement of removable top stitches, buried stitches, or a combination of both can successfully minimize wound-edge tension and provide a good cosmetic result.

Instrument-tied knots are used almost exclusively in dermatologic surgery, and should be perfected by those wishing to perform cutaneous surgery. The most commonly used knot is the square knot shown in Figure 16.3. The needle driver is held by the non-dominant hand while the suture is looped around the closed tips of the needle driver (Fig. 16.4). The suture is then pulled off the needle driver in a direction that makes the looped suture lie flat against the wound surface. The initial double throw helps secure the suture, preventing slippage while the second loop is being thrown. Second, third, and sometimes fourth single-throw loops are subsequently made to ensure a secure knot, which is especially important when using monofilament sutures with decreased friction coefficients. Each throw should be pulled taught in a direction directly opposite to the last, in order to square and secure the knot. Failing to do so will create a less secure knot. The needle should be carefully held in the non-dominant hand while tying the knot to prevent needle-stick injuries to the surgeon or assistants. The knot should be tied tightly enough to create a slight eversion of the wound edges without causing strangulation. The surgeon must remember that the tissue will swell, which will cause the suture to be even tighter.

Proper positioning and handling of instruments is critical to correct suture placement. After locking the needle into the tip of the holder, the holder is grasped in a palm grip, as one would hold a screwdriver. This allows rotation of the wrist when advancing the needle through the skin. The index finger can be placed down the shaft of the needle

Square knot

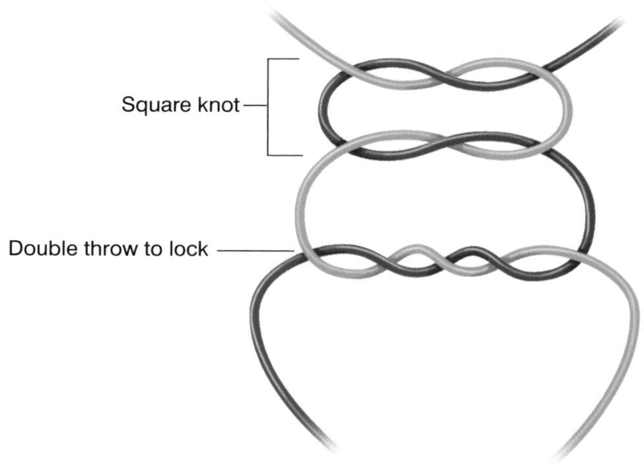

Figure 16.3 Illustration of the square knot. The initial double throw keeps the suture from slipping during tying. (Adapted from Taylor RS. Needles, sutures, and suturing. Atlas Office Proced 1999; 2:53–74.)

The instrument tie

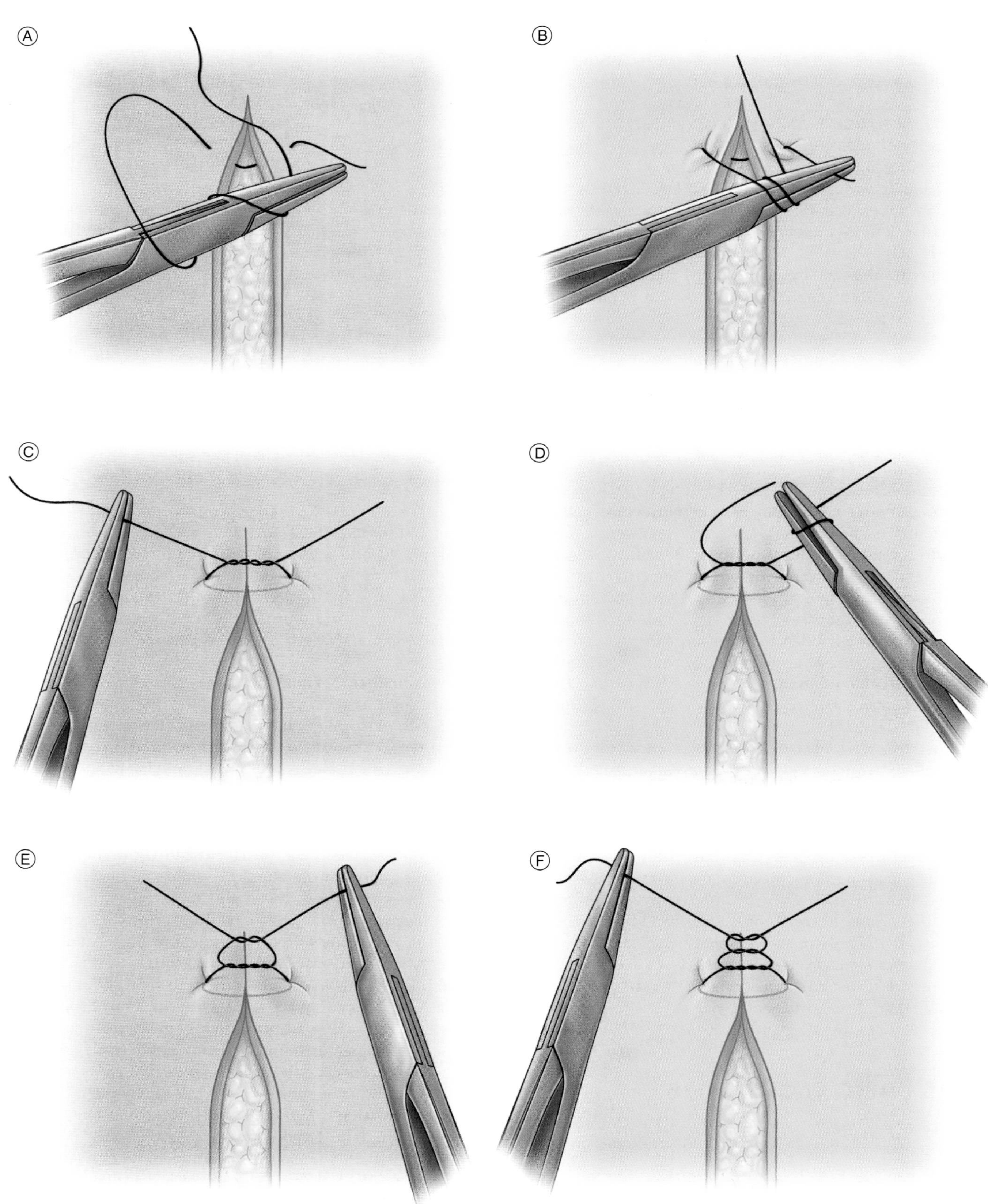

Figure 16.4 How to perform the instrument tie. (A) The long portion of the suture is held in the non-dominant hand and wrapped twice around the end of the needle driver. (B) The needle driver grasps the short end of the suture. The two ends of the suture are pulled taught in opposite directions (C), causing the tied suture to lie flat against the closing incision. (D) The long end is wrapped once around the jaws of the needle holder. (E) The suture is again pulled taught in opposite directions. (F) A third throw is placed in the same fashion. (Adapted from Taylor RS. Needles, sutures, and suturing. Atlas Office Proced 1999; 2:53–74.)

holder to guide placement of the sutures. Surgeons must limit finger contact with the needle to minimize the risk of injury. Forceps with teeth facilitate advancement of the needle through the tissue by grasping, stabilizing, and elevating the wound edges. To minimize tissue trauma, the forceps should grasp the skin with only light pressure. If used correctly, visible forceps indentions should not be present on the skin after suturing; alternatively, skin hooks may be used which offer the least risk of tissue trauma.

Simple interrupted stitches

Simple interrupted stitches are the most basic and widely used stitches in cutaneous surgery and are used to close punch biopsy sites, simple lacerations, and small, low-tension incisional wounds. They may also be used as the epidermal stitch, or top stitch in layered closures, flaps, and grafts. In addition, this stitch can be used to fine-tune wounds that are sutured with other techniques. For example, depth placement can be used to correct a step-off deformity caused by uneven suture placement.

To place a simple interrupted stitch, the needle is placed 3–5 mm from the wound edge, perpendicular to the skin surface. The needle is then directed downward into the skin with a single motion (Fig. 16.5). When the needle is in the middle-to-deep dermis, it is rotated through the tissue to the opposite wound edge, following the inherent arc in the needle with a rolling wrist motion. In larger wounds, larger amounts or 'bites' of tissue are taken, and it may be necessary to reload the needle in the center of the wound before placing it across the wound. Whether the suture is placed in one bite or two, great care should be taken to place needle and suture at the exact same vertical level on both sides of the wound edge to prevent uneven wound edge approximation—so-called 'step-off.' As the needle exits the wound, it is grasped with forceps (taking care not to grab the tip). Once secured with forceps, the needle holder releases the needle, which is then pulled through with the trailing suture. The surgeon may use the needle holder to regrasp the needle near—but not on—the tip to pull the needle through the tissue. The needle is then loaded back on the needle driver with the forceps for the next stitch.

Simple interrupted stitches should be placed to create a pear-shaped loop when the knot is tied (Fig. 16.6). This is accomplished by directing the needle away from the wound opening once introduced through the epidermis and looping a large piece of dermis before exiting to the opposite epidermal edge. The needle should exit the epidermal surface at the same distance from the epidermal wound edge as the epidermal entry point. Incorrect suture

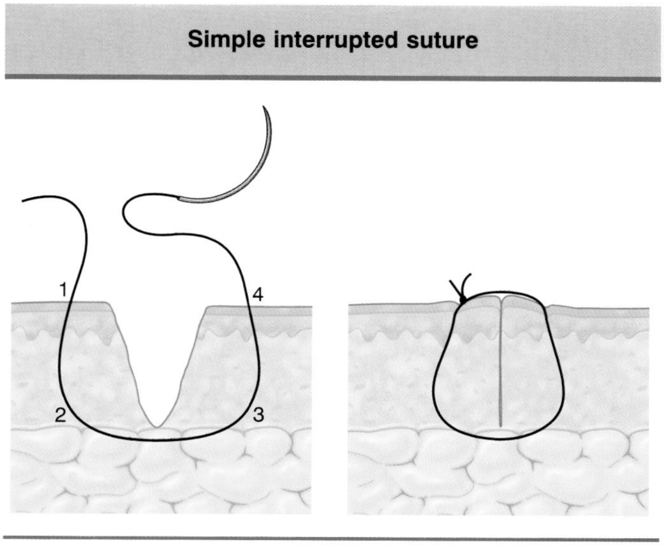

Simple interrupted suture

Figure 16.5 Placement of the simple interrupted suture. The needle penetrates the epidermis (1) and is rotated slightly outward through the dermis and subcutaneous tissue in certain wounds (2). The needle then crosses the wound, looping a substantial portion of dermis and possibly subcutaneous tissue before being redirected upwards (3). The needle then exits the epidermis where the suture is then tied (4).

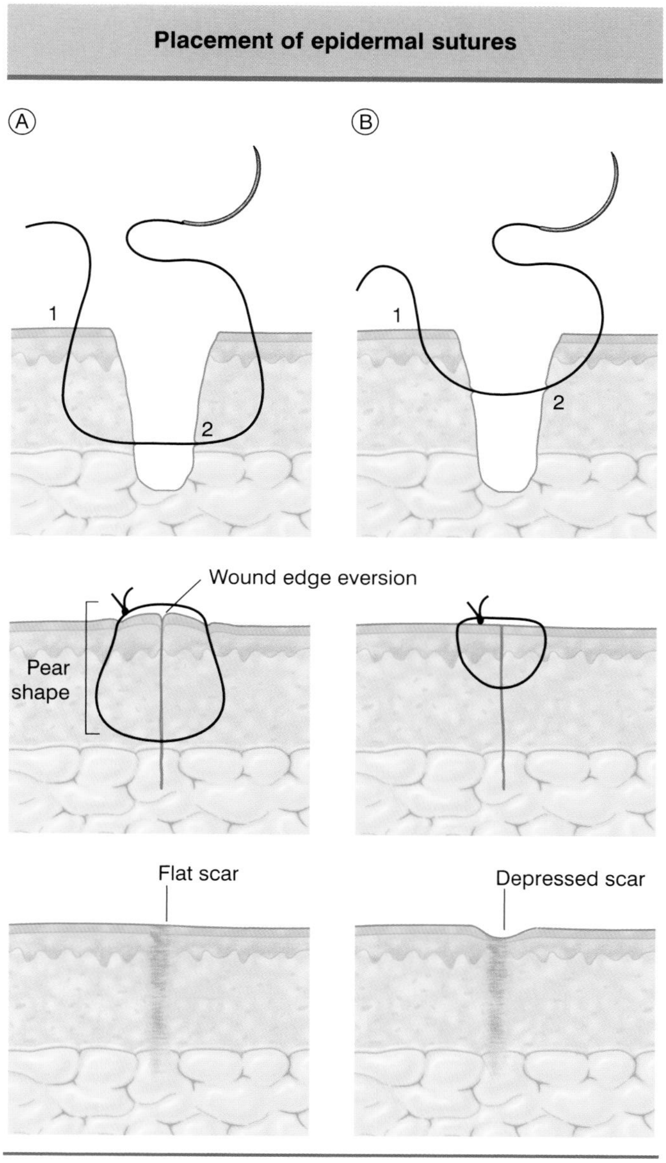

Placement of epidermal sutures

Figure 16.6 Proper placement of epidermal sutures involves looping a larger portion of the dermis and/or subcutis than the epidermis. This creates a pear-shaped suture which everts wound edges (A). Failure of wound edge eversion often leads to a more depressed, noticeable scar (B). Numbers indicate entry points of the needle. (Adapted from Taylor RS. Needles, sutures, and suturing. Atlas Office Proced 1999; 2:53–74.)

placement, characterized by a larger bite of epidermis than dermis, produces a loop that resembles a balloon or upside-down pear. This may result in a wound with well-approximated edges but, once healed, vertical contraction of the scar will cause a slight inversion of the edges, resulting in a depressed, more noticeable scar. The same wound contraction occurs with proper suture placement, but the everted wound edges settle to a flattened position, which is much less visible than a sunken scar.

Vertical mattress stitches

Vertical mattress stitches effectively decrease wound tension, and provide significant closure support while everting wound edges. This stitch is also very useful for closing dead space. The vertical mattress stitch begins with penetration of the epidermis 5–10 mm away from the wound edge (the far entry point) (Fig. 16.7). The larger and tighter the wound, the farther the needle is placed from the wound edge. Then the needle is directed downward, taking a generous bite of dermis before exiting the vertical edge of the wound near the base of the defect. Crossing the defect, the needle is introduced into the base of the contralateral wound edge and is directed upwards toward the epidermis (the far exit point). The far entry and exit points should be equidistant from the wound edge. The direction of the needle is then reversed in the needle driver and introduced through the skin 1–3 mm from the epidermal edge (the near entry point) on the same side of the wound as the far exit point. A small bite of epidermis and dermis is taken before exiting into the wound opening. Crossing the wound, the needle is introduced into the opposite wound edge at the same level as its last exit. Another small bite of dermis and epidermis is made before exiting the epidermis 2–3 mm from the wound edge. The suture is then gently tied to approximate the wound edges. The sequence of far–far–near–near is repeated for subsequent vertical mattress sutures. For optimal results, all needle entry and exit points should be placed to lie along one vertical line perpendicular to the wound edge. Care must be taken when tying this suture to prevent strangulation and subsequent necrosis of the epidermal wound edge. In wounds under significant tension, bolsters made of cardboard, cotton, or rubber can be placed between the exposed loop of suture and the skin to prevent trauma to the underlying epidermis, which can occur when postoperative edema ensues. Although they are useful in many situations, vertical mattress stitches are more time consuming than simple interrupted stitches.

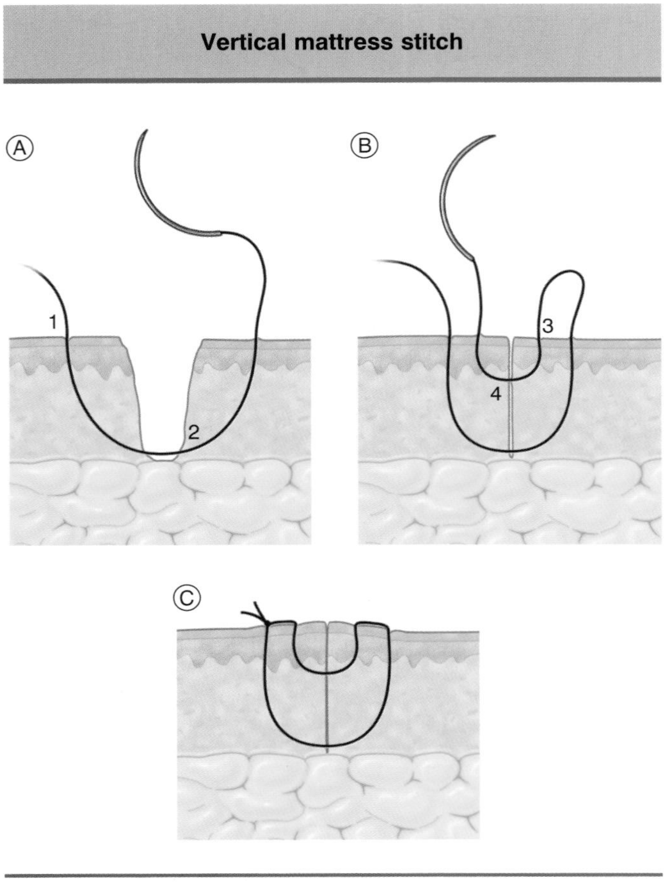

Vertical mattress stitch

Figure 16.7 Placement of the vertical mattress stitch. (A) The needle is placed 5–10 mm from the wound edge, and a deeply-seated simple interrupted suture is placed (1) (2). Numbers indicate entry points of the needle. (B) The needle is redirected back across the wound more superficially, penetrating the skin edge 2–4 mm from the wound on both sides (3). (C) Final appearance of this suture after tying. (Adapted with permission from Robinson JK. Technique of suture placement. In: Robinson JK, Arndt KA, LeBoit PE, Wintroub BU, eds. Atlas of cutaneous surgery. Philadelphia: WB Saunders 1996; 79–90.)

Horizontal mattress stitches

The horizontal mattress stitch is very useful to decrease and redistribute wound tension, to close dead space, and evert wound edges. Its tension-relieving properties make it a good retention suture to close larger wounds or flaps so that subsequent sutures can be placed with less tension. To place a horizontal mattress suture, place the needle 4–10 mm from the wound edge, passing it through the dermis or subcutaneous tissue to the contralateral side (Fig. 16.8). Exit through the opposite epidermis at a distance from the wound edge which is equal to that taken in the initial side. Re-enter the epidermis 3–5 mm lateral to the last point of exit. Direct the needle back across the wound edge, coming out of the epidermis on the same side as the initial puncture site. Then gently tie off the suture, taking care not to strangulate tissue. When completed, the exposed suture runs parallel to the incision. There is a greater theoretical risk of strangulation of a larger portion of the dermal plexus with this stitch compared with simple interrupted or even vertical mattress stitches. Thus, it is usually not used in poorly vascularized wounds or in suturing flaps. When used in situations of significant tension, bolster material such as gauze or cotton is placed between the exposed suture loops and the skin surface to prevent the suture from cutting into the epidermis.

Half-buried horizontal mattress (tip) stitch

Horizontal mattress stitches can also be placed with half of the suture buried in the dermis. This stitch can be beneficial for decreasing the risk of suture marks and epidermal strangulation while still closing dead space and everting wound edges. The first bite is like a simple interrupted

Horizontal mattress stitch

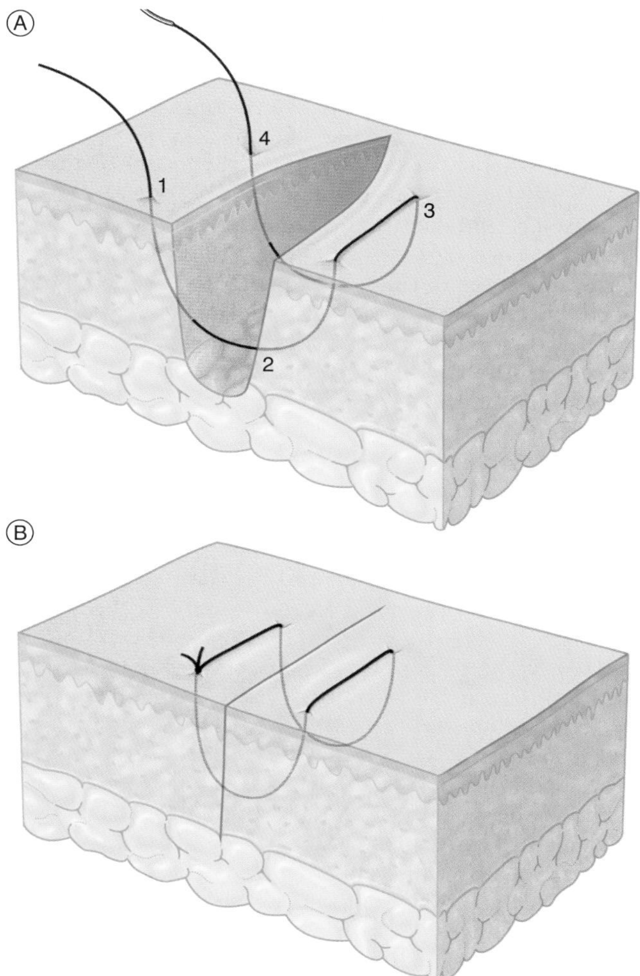

Figure 16.8 Horizontal mattress suture. (A) To place this suture, begin with a widely-spaced simple interrupted suture (1) (2). Numbers indicate entry points of the needle. Move laterally down the wound 3–5 mm, and place another interrupted suture in the opposite direction as the first (3) (4). (B) The appearance of this suture when tied. (Adapted with permission from Robinson JK. Technique of suture placement. In: Robinson JK, Arndt KA, LeBoit PE, Wintroub BU, eds. Atlas of cutaneous surgery. Philadelphia: WB Saunders 1996; 79–90.)

Half-buried horizontal mattress tip stitch

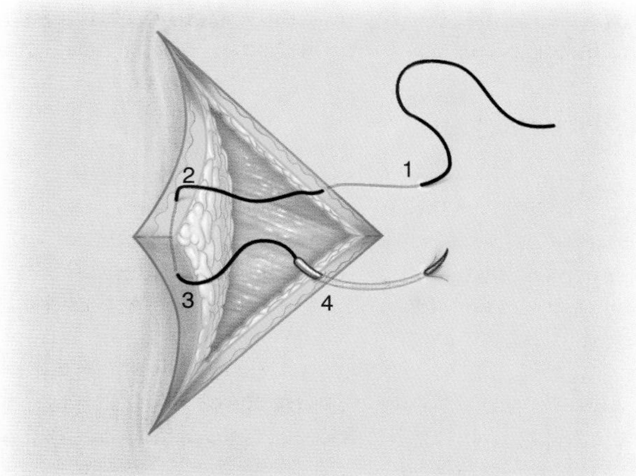

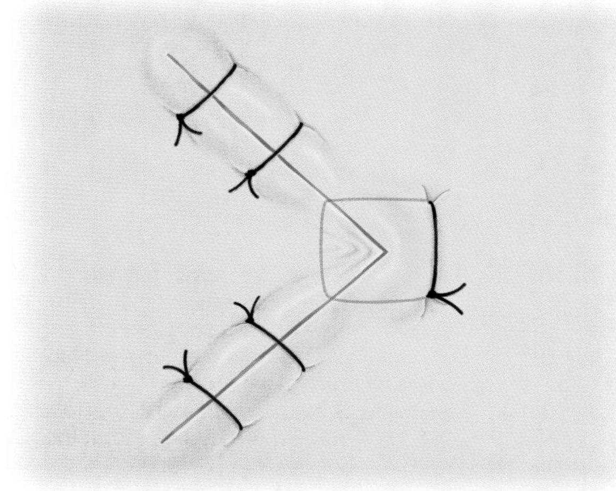

Figure 16.9 Half-buried horizontal mattress tip stitch. (A) This suture is started as an interrupted suture (1) on the 'V' portion of the wound crossing over to the tip of the flap (2). A horizontal bite is made through the dermis of the tip (3). The needle is then directed back across the wound and tied (4). (B) Final appearance of this suture after placement. Numbers indicate entry points of the needle. (Adapted with permission from Robinson JK. Technique of suture placement. In: Robinson JK, Arndt KA, LeBoit PE, Wintroub BU, eds. Atlas of cutaneous surgery. Philadelphia: WB Saunders 1996; 79–90.)

horizontal mattress stitch but the second bite is taken of the opposing wound edge, directing the needle parallel to the epidermal surface, entering and exiting at the dermal wound edge. The third bite is taken of the opposite wound edge, and the needle is then directed back up through the epidermis, lateral to the initial epidermal entry site.

This half-buried horizontal mattress stitch is often used as a 'tip stitch' to secure the triangular tips of flaps or M-plasty incisions. The buried portion of the tip stitch is thus placed through the dermis of the pointed flap tip, and the transepidermal sutures are placed on the V-shaped contralateral wound edge (Fig. 16.9). When performed correctly, the tip stitch perfectly sets the pointed tip of a wound into its recipient angular wound bed, without placing puncture holes through a small and fragile tip. In addition, this half-buried tip stitch provides increased blood flow to flap tips compared to simple interrupted sutures.[53]

Step-off correction

A step-off deformity occurs when a wound is closed by suture that is placed at different levels in the edges of the wound. Although severe step-off correction requires removal and replacement of the offending sutures, mild or moderate disparity can be corrected with a corrective top stitch. To place such a stitch, a simple interrupted suture is placed that goes deeper into the dermis on the lower side and remains more superficial on the higher side (Fig. 16.10). Once tied, this will bring the lower wound edge up to meet the higher wound edge. Sometimes more than one correcting suture is necessary.

Running stitches

In a running or continuous stitch, individual stitches are placed in succession without interruption by knots. Placement of running stitches is much faster than for interrupted stitches. However, a running epidermal stitch is not quite as strong as an interrupted stitch and should be used with caution when it is the sole means of wound closure. Running stitches should not be used alone in wounds under moderate or significant tension because the running loops of suture would be pulled tightly and strangulate the superficial and possibly deep dermal vascular plexus that could damage tissue. However, when used in the appropriate circumstance, running stitches are very efficient and offer excellent cosmetic results. Most epidermal stitches, including simple and mattress stitches, can be placed in a continuous fashion.

The running simple stitch is the easiest of the continuous stitches to perform (Fig. 16.11). To begin, a simple interrupted stitch is placed and tied at the end of the wound, but the suture is not cut free from the needle. The needle is then introduced into the epidermis next to the interrupted stitch and directed diagonally across and down the length of the wound. A healthy bite of dermis and fat is taken from both sides of the wound and the needle exits approximately 3–5 mm from the epidermal edge of the opposite side of the wound. The needle is then introduced through the epidermis at the same distance from the epidermal edge on the opposite side of the wound. The needle is passed through the dermis from one side of the wound to the next as the needle is directed diagonally down the length of the wound. These steps are repeated by placing pairs of opposing exit and entry points 3–7 mm apart until the entire wound is closed. The surgeon must hold enough tension on the suture during the stitching process so that the wound remains closed, but not enough to cause strangulation of the wound edges. Upon reaching the end of the wound, the suture is tied off on itself.

When stitching wounds with a high risk of postoperative bleeding, such as the scalp or posterior ear, the running simple stitch can be modified to place consistent pressure to the wound edges. In this technique, the needle is passed through the remaining suture loop with each stitch. This locks segments of the suture connecting the loop segments above the skin surface, instead of allowing them to be looped in the dermis (Fig. 16.12).

Step-off correction

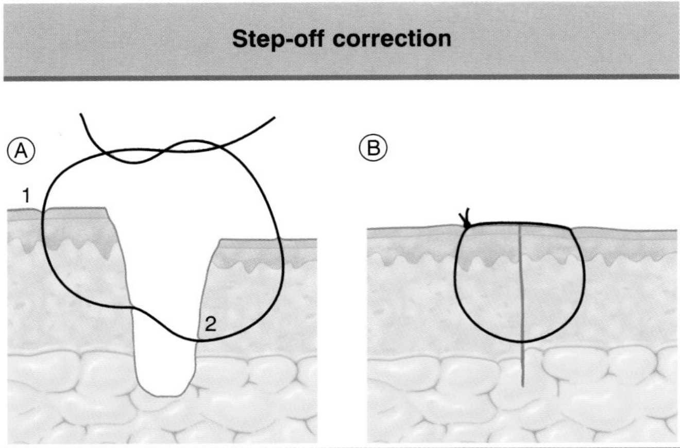

Figure 16.10 Step-off correction. (A) To correct a step-off deformity, place a simple interrupted suture superficially on the higher wound edge (1) and deeply on the lower wound edge (2). (B) Tying this suture results in even wound edges. Numbers indicate entry points of the needle. (Adapted with permission from Robinson JK. Technique of suture placement. In: Robinson JK, Arndt KA, LeBoit PE, Wintroub BU, eds. Atlas of cutaneous surgery. Philadelphia: WB Saunders 1996; 79–90.)

Running simple suture

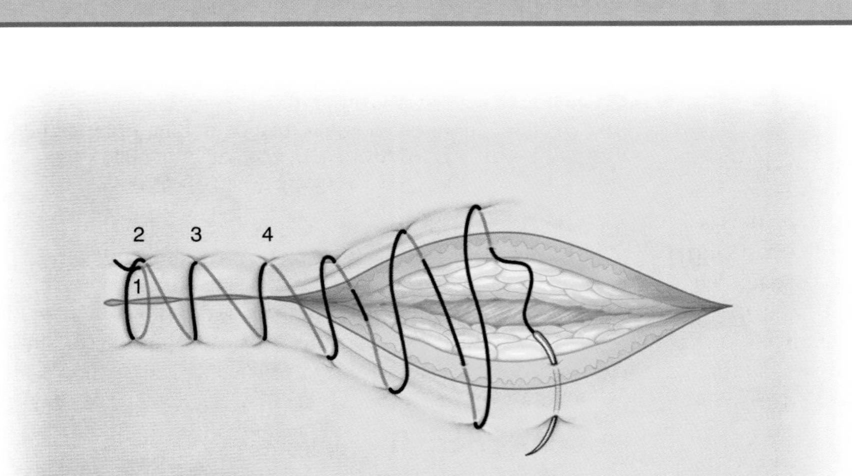

Figure 16.11 Running simple suture. Multiple simple sutures are placed in succession, allowing for rapid closure of wounds. Numbers indicate entry points of the needle. (Adapted from Taylor RS. Needles, sutures, and suturing. Atlas Office Proced 1999; 2:53–74.)

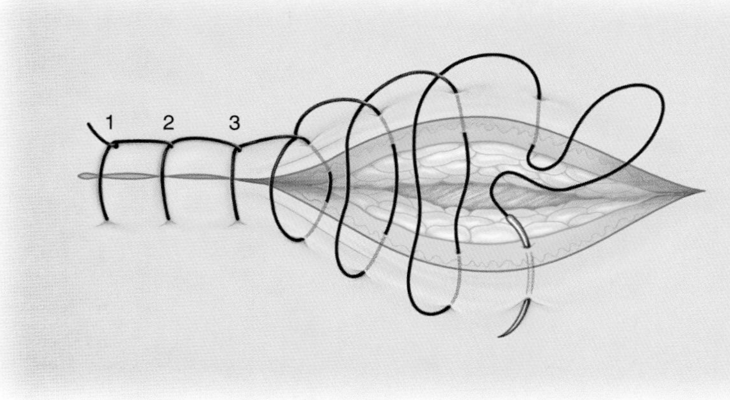

Figure 16.12 Running locked suture. A running simple suture is placed, passing the needle through the loop created by the last suture. This locking suture facilitates hemostasis. Numbers indicate entry points of the needle. (Adapted from Taylor RS. Needles, sutures, and suturing. Atlas Office Proced 1999; 2:53–74.)

Running variations of the horizontal and vertical mattress stitches can also be performed. Because running mattress stitches can be difficult to visualize in a healed incision, it is advisable to place a simple running stitch between every two or three mattress sutures for easier removal.

Running subcuticular stitch

Using a suture with a low friction coefficient, such as polypropylene, the running subcuticular stitch can achieve excellent cosmetic results. The benefit of this stitch is that epidermal puncture points are minimized, allowing suture to be left in place longer; this improves wound healing and decreases the possibility of suture-track scars. To place this stitch, begin by placing the needle approximately 1 cm distal to one end of the wound, passing the needle into the apex of the wound opening, at the level of the dermis (Fig. 16.13). The suture tail is then secured with tape strips or held by an assistant to be tied once the entire stitch is run. The needle is then introduced into the vertical wound edge at the level of the dermis and threaded, taking a horizontal bite, through the dermis into the wound edge at the same dermal plane, exiting 1–1.5 cm distally down the wound. Next, introduce the needle into the opposite side of the wound at the same dermal plane but 2–3 mm behind the previous dermal exit point. By backtracking this way, the suture assumes a zigzag configuration in the skin, ensuring apposition of the dermal edges and complete closure. These steps are repeated down the length of the wound until the end of the wound is reached. Once reaching the distal wound apex, exit the epidermis approximately 1 cm from the wound opening. Tighten the suture so the wound edges are well approximated, but do not tighten so much that the skin bunches. Finally, secure the tail either by tape or by tying it back on itself. Alternatively, an absorbable suture can be placed to avoid the need for removal. In this scenario, the ends are tied off to themselves underneath the skin surface.

Traditional buried stitches

Subcutaneous stitches are invaluable for closing dead space, for redistributing wound tension, and for apposing wound edges. Their placement gives prolonged dermal support that dramatically decreases the chance of wound dehiscence and improves scar cosmesis. Proper placement is critical for optimal results. If placed too high in the dermis, buried sutures may extrude or 'spit' from the surface, delaying wound healing. If placed unevenly, vertical disparity of wound edges, or step-off, will occur. Although not absolutely necessary, undermining wound edges greatly facilitates the placement of buried sutures.

The buried suture is placed by entering the deep aspect of the wound in the subcutaneous tissue. In undermined wounds, it is ideal to enter the under-surface of the flap in the subcutaneous tissue. The needle is then directed up through the reticular dermis, following the arc of the needle to exit through the mid-dermis of the wound edge (Fig. 16.14A). A mirror image of the preceding step is then performed. The needle enters the mid-dermis of the opposite wound edge at the same level in the dermis it just exited. Continuing in an arc through the dermis, the needle exits through the subcutaneous tissue at the base of the wound. Keeping the suture at the same vertical level on both wound edges prevents a step-off deformity (Fig. 16.15). The suture is then pulled and tied, redistributing the tension to the surrounding tissues, away from the wound edge. Placing the suture in the order described above will ensure the knot is buried deeply in the tissue, decreasing the chance the knot will travel to the surface during healing and 'spit' out of the skin. Excess suture is cut on the knot, because leaving the tail as short as possible will decrease wound reaction. Buried sutures alone are almost always used in combination with some form of epidermal closure, such as sutures, wound adhesives, or staples.

In small wounds where tying off one subcutaneous suture makes it difficult to place others, several buried sutures may

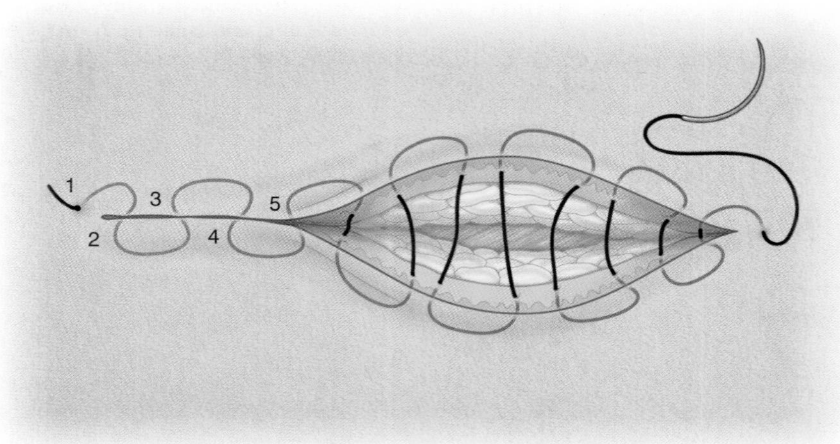

Figure 16.13 Running subcuticular suture. Multiple horizontally placed dermal sutures are placed in succession on alternating wound edges. This results in epidermal and dermal closure without visible suture marks. Numbers indicate entry points of the needle. (Adapted from Taylor RS. Needles, sutures, and suturing. Atlas Office Proced 1999; 2:53–74.)

be placed in succession without tying them. The suture is cut long and held by hemostats or by an assistant for future tying. When all sutures are placed, they are tied starting at one wound end, moving down to the other.

Buried vertical mattress suture

The buried vertical mattress suture offers the advantage of prolonged wound eversion in addition to the other benefits of buried suture. This stitch is placed by placing the curved needle in the subcutaneous tissue and making an arc upwards toward the superficial dermis, continuing the arc and exiting through the mid-dermis (Fig. 16.14B). A mirror image of this step is repeated on the opposite side: enter through the mid-portion of the dermis, make an upward arc toward the upper reticular dermis, and continue the curve downward to exit the subcutaneous surface. Looping of the dermis in this way causes wound edge eversion when the suture is tied.[54]

Buried butterfly suture

The buried butterfly suture results in even greater wound eversion than the buried vertical mattress suture.[55] Wound edges must be undermined prior to its placement. This stitch is placed by entering the under-surface of the flap in the subcutaneous tissue, directing the needle up through the reticular dermis, and following the arc of the needle and exiting on the under-surface of the flap in the subcutaneous tissue (Fig. 16.14C). Next, this process is repeated on the opposite wound edge: the under-surface of the flap is entered, directing the needle up through the dermis, and exiting at a point farther from the wound edge than the entry point. The suture is then pulled and tied, the closure tension is distributed to the surrounding skin, away from the wound edge. This redistribution may create dimpling in the surrounding skin and will cause elevation or ridging

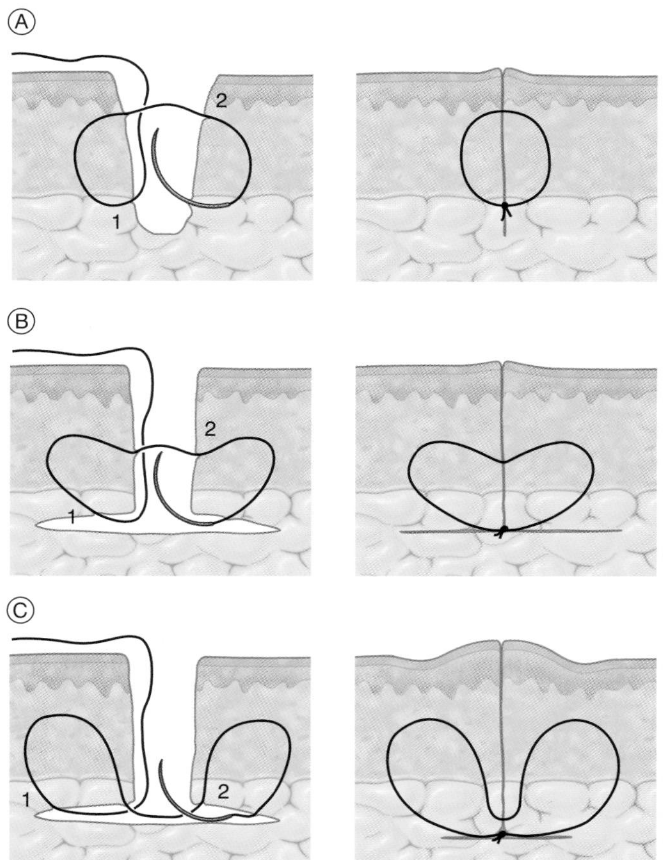

Figure 16.14 Buried dermal sutures. (A) Conventional buried suture placement results in mild wound eversion. (B) Buried vertical mattress suture placement results in moderate to significant wound eversion. (C) Buried butterfly suture placement results in the greatest degree of wound eversion. Numbers indicate entry points of the needle.

Step-off deformity

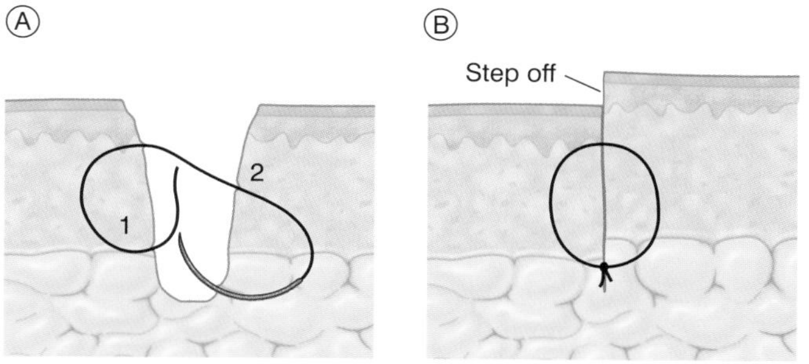

(A) (B) Step off

Figure 16.15 Step-off deformity. (A) Uneven placement of sutures across the wound (B) results in a step-off deformity. Numbers indicate entry points of the needle. (Adapted from Taylor RS. Needles, sutures, and suturing. Atlas Office Proced 1999; 2:53–74.)

along the closure line as the epidermal edges are intentionally everted. These distortions disappear as the skin stretches and the buried stitches lose integrity. Such wound eversion facilitates the creation of a fine-line scar by removing all tension from the wound edge.

Purse string suture

A variation of the buried dermal suture called the purse string suture is very good for closing dead space and decreasing the diameter of a wound. Instead of vertical bites described in the traditional buried subcutaneous suture, the purse string suture involves multiple horizontally-oriented bites spaced 5–10 mm apart, placed continuously along the circumference of the wound edge. The stitch is placed at the level of the mid-dermis or deep dermis, taking care to maintain the same vertical level with each bite. When the last bite has been taken, the suture is pulled taught, which clinches the tissue together. An assistant holds the tissue together while the knot is tied. This stitch may partially or completely close a wound. Wounds that are partially closed in this manner may be left to granulate or may be completely closed with an overlying skin graft.[56]

Running subdermal stitch

The buried running subdermal stitch is a rapid means of closure that can be used in wounds under mild tension or moderate tension. Begin by placing a buried interrupted vertical stitch, cutting only the free suture tail. Then introduce the needle into the side of the wound at the base of the defect, 5–10 mm down the length of the defect. Advance the needle up in a vertical fashion, exiting directly above the entry point after looping through subcutaneous fat and dermis. Moving to the opposite vertical wound edge, loop the needle downward through dermis and fat. This sequence is repeated down the wound edge, keeping enough tension to close the wound without clinching it too tightly. This suture should not be used in wounds under moderate to severe tension because it offers less strength than interrupted sutures, and if one strand breaks the entire wound may dehisce.

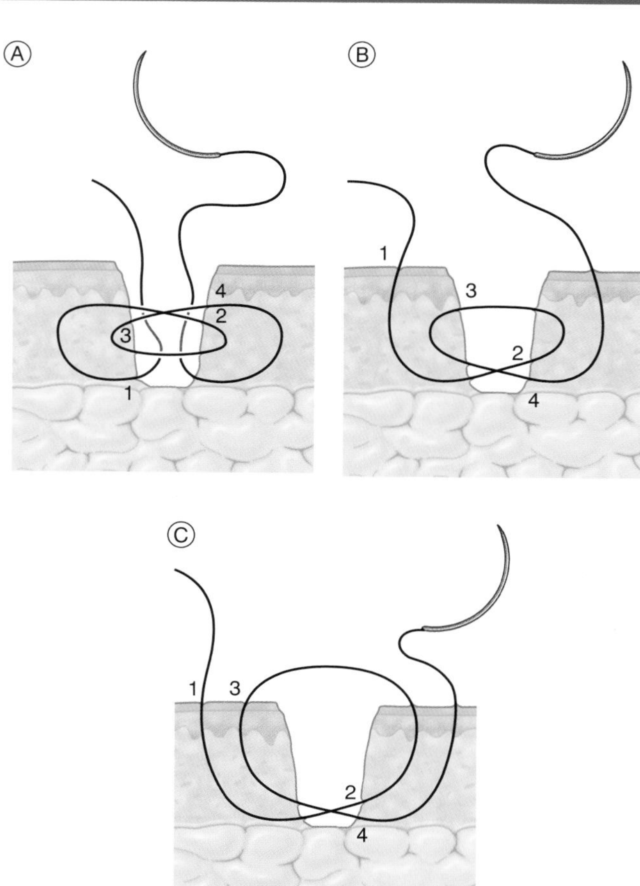

Figure 16.16 Pulley stitches (A) Buried pulley stitch. (B) Partially buried pulley stitch. (C) Epidermal pulley stitch. Numbers indicate entry points of the needle.

Pulley stitch

The pulley stitch allows closure of wounds under tension. It is commonly used to close wounds on the scalp or large wounds of the trunk. Several ways of placing the stitch have been described, similar to the vertical mattress stitch.[57] Key to the design of this stitch are the multiple passes through the tissue. This creates enough resistance so that when the suture is placed and pulled to close the wound, and then released to tie, the suture does not slip. Figure 16.16 shows the suture paths that can be used.

■ OPTIMIZING OUTCOMES OF SUTURED WOUNDS

The appropriate wound closure material and method should be chosen based on the wound characteristics, such as size, location, wound tension, and type of repair. In addition, high-quality instruments of the proper size must be used and maintained.

Skin surgeons often close wounds under tension. Large wounds, or wounds in areas of the body were the skin does not readily move, can force a closure under varying degrees of tension. Proper placement of buried stitches in a wound with undermined edges can distribute tension away from wound edges, but placement of the initial stitch can be problematic. Assistants can be taught to push and hold wound edges together while the first knot is being thrown. Three wraps around the needle driver—instead of two—can also be used for the first throw to prevent the knot from slipping while the second and subsequent throws are being performed. The pulley stitch was designed to be used in these situations. Finally, a towel clamp can be used to hold the wound edges together while placing suture, but this approach will leave puncture scars on either side of the wound.

When closing the epidermis the surgeon should select suture of the finest caliber to close the wound adequately, in order to minimize puncture marks and suture tracks. If the closure is under any tension the surgeon should consider using a buried absorbable suture that is at least one suture size larger than the epidermal suture. While the epidermal suture should be placed to provide precise epidermal wound edge approximation, the stitch chosen for placement of the buried suture should redirect tension away from the wound edge and provide good wound edge eversion.

Placement of suture requires practice, skill, and attention to detail. Buried suture should be placed at even levels across the wound to prevent step-off deformity. Prior to placing the epidermal or top stitch, all tension should be off the wound edges so they can be easily approximated. When placing the top stitch, care must be taken to tie the suture tight enough to approximate wound edges without tissue strangulation. In addition, the wound edges should be handled very carefully, either using toothed forceps or skin hooks to avoid crushing.

Surgeons must also train their assistants in the optimal ways to cut suture. Buried sutures should be cut on the knot to minimize the amount of suture material being left in the wound. The tails of surface stitches should be cut to a length that provides ease of grasping at the time of removal. When placed in the periorbital areas, tails should be secured by taping to the skin, cutting shorter tails, or securing under other sutures to prevent damage to the eye.

■ POSTOPERATIVE CARE

Sutures should be removed at a time that is long enough for the development of initial wound healing and strength. However, sutures left in too long will promote wound infection, delay wound healing, and promote suture-track formation.[58] These track marks, which can look like 'railroad' scars and only occur when the epidermis is punctured, are formed when keratinocytes form a complete tract around the suture material. Formative epithelialization of suture occurs even in the first days after suture placement, but complete suture-tract formation, which takes 8–12 days, is responsible for the track marks.[59] Therefore, sutures should be removed earlier rather than later whenever possible. To remove interrupted sutures, grasp the tail of the suture knot with forceps. Lifting the suture away from the wound, cut the suture underneath the knot (Fig. 16.17). After cutting, continue lifting the tail of the suture to complete its removal. It is important to only cut one end of the suture under the knot; cutting both ends

Suture removal

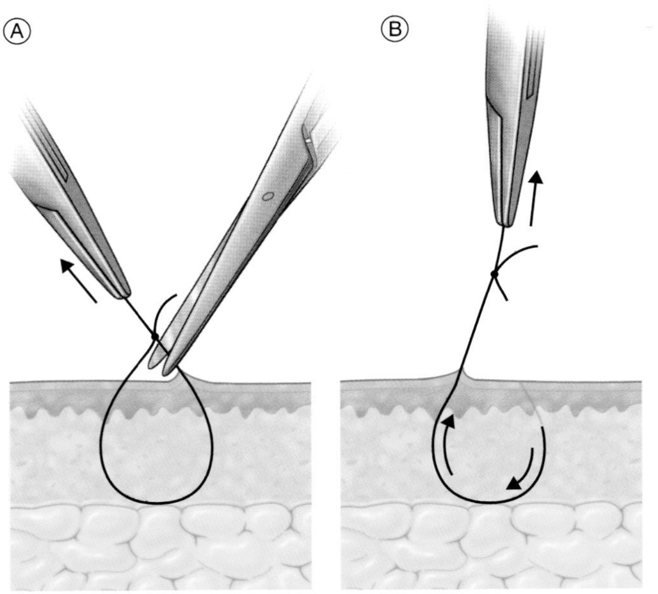

Figure 16.17 Suture removal. (A) Pull the tail of the suture away from the wound and with one side of the suture underneath the knot. (B) The cut suture is lifted straight up from the incision for complete removal.

Table 16.6 Recommended suture removal times

Area Sutured	Removal Times
Eyelid	2–4 days
Face	4–6 days
Neck	5–7 days
Scalp	5–7 days
Trunk	7–12 days
Extremities	10–14 days

of the suture underneath the knot will prevent the buried portion of the suture from being removed. Running sutures can be removed in the same fashion if the incision is relatively small. To prevent patient discomfort from pulling long continuous sutures out, the suture can be cut at shorter intervals along the incision and removed in a similar manner.

If necessary, wound adhesive strips may be used after suture removal to reinforce the wound. Incisions that have been closed with subcutaneous sutures allow for earlier removal. However, wounds under significant tension or in high-movement areas such as the extremities may require staged suture removal. For example, every other suture may be removed first, with complete removal following several days later. Recommended suture removal time varies by location (Table 16.6).

■ PITFALLS AND THEIR MANAGEMENT

Most pitfalls in surgical repair can be avoided by proper preparation, knowledge, and technique (Table 16.7). Corrections of any detectable imperfections should be

Table 16.7 Pitfalls: Causes and management		
Pitfall	**Possible Causes**	**Prevention/Management**
Suture breaking during tying	Choice of suture material with too low tensile strength or too fine caliber High tension wound	Use suture with more tensile strength or larger caliber If possible undermine wound edges farther
Knot slippage	Use of suture with high friction coefficient High tension wound	Increase number of initial throws of knot Have assistant hold together wound during knot tying Undermine more widely
Incision step-off	Uneven placement of sutures	If severe, remove and replace offending sutures If mild, place corrective interrupted suture(s)
Needle bending	Using too small a needle Not using arc motion to place suture	Use larger size needle Rotate needle through arc while placing suture
Wound edge inversion	Incorrect placement of buried and/or top sutures	Ensure eversion by looping portion of dermis with buried suture Ensure eversion by arcing needle slightly away from wound edge when placing topstitch Use corrective everting topstitches such as interrupted vertical mattress
Suture tracks	Sutures left in place too long Needle and suture caliber too large Sutures tied too tightly	Remove sutures at earliest possible time Use epidermal suture with smallest caliber possible Tie knot only tight enough to approximate wound edges, do not strangulate

made at the earliest possible time, preferably during surgery. It is much easier to remove and replace improperly placed sutures than to revise a scar at a later date.

■ SUMMARY

Acquiring a working knowledge of wound closure materials and their appropriate use are important components of the surgeon's education. Attention to detail and meticulous execution of suturing techniques can vastly improve the cosmetic and functional surgical results. Similarly, proper training and use of the surgical staff is an important step to ensure that optimum outcomes are achieved.

■ REFERENCES

1. Rothenburger S, Spangler D, Bhende S, et al. In vitro antimicrobial evaluation of coated VICRYL plus antibacterial suture (coated Polyglactin 910 with triclosan) using zone of inhibition assays. Surg Infect (Larchmt) 2003; 3(Suppl 1):79–87.
2. Storch M, Perry LC, Davidson JM, et al. A 28-day study of the effect of coated VICRYL plus antibacterial suture (coated Polyglactin 910 suture with triclosan) on wound healing in guinea pig linear incisional skin wounds. Surg Infect (Larchmt) 2003; 3(Suppl 1):89–98.
3. Shibuya TY, Wei WZ, Zormeier M, et al. AntiCD3/AntiCD28 monoclonal antibody-coated suture enhances the immune response of patients with head and neck squamous cell carcinoma. Arch Otolaryngol Head Neck Surg 1999; 125:1229–1234.
4. Bennett R. Materials for wound closure. In: Bennett RG, ed. Fundamentals of cutaneous surgery. St Louis, MO: Mosby 1988; 274–309.
5. Tera H, Aberg C. Strength of suture knots after one week in vivo. Acta Chir Scand 1976; 142:1–7.
6. Brunius U, Zederfeldt B. Suture materials in general surgery a comment. Prog Surg 1970; 8:38–44.
7. Hurty CA, Brazik DC, Law JM, et al. Evaluation of the tissue reactions in the skin and body wall of koi (*Cyprinus carpio*) to five suture materials. Vet Rec 2002; 14:324–328.
8. Engler RJ, Weber CB, Turnicky R. Hypersensitivity to chromated catgut sutures: a case report and review of the literature. Ann Allergy 1986; 56:317–320.
9. Mullins RJ, Richards C, Walker T. Allergic reactions to oral surgical and topical bovine collagen. Anaphylactic risk for surgeons. Aust N Z J Ophthalmol 1996; 24:257–260.
10. Hocwald E, Sichel JY, Dano I, et al. Adverse reaction to surgical sutures in thyroid suture. Head Neck 2003; 25:77–81.
11. Van Winkle W, Hastings JC, Barker E, et al. Effect of suture materials on healing skin wounds. Surg Gynecol Obstet 1975; 140:7–12.
12. Terhune M. Materials for wound closure. http://www.emedicine.com/derm/topic825.htm 13. Accessed March 2002.
13. Auerback R, Pearlstei MM. A comparison of polyglycolic acid (Dexon), nylon and silk sutures in skin surgery. J Dermatol Surg 1975; 1:38–40.
14. Wetter LA, Dinneen MD, Levitt MD, et al. Controlled trial of polyglycolic acid versus catgut and nylon for appendectomy wound closure. Br J Surg 1991; 78:985–987.
15. Rodeheaver GT, Thacker JG, Edlich RF. Mechanical performance of polyglycolic acid and Polyglactin 910 synthetic absorbable sutures. Surg Gynecol Obstet 1981; 153:835–841.
16. Guyuron B, Vaughan C. Comparison of polydioxanone and Polyglactin 910 in intradermal repair. Plast Reconstr Surg 1996; 98:817–820.
17. Moy RL, Kaufman AJ. Clinical comparison of polyglactic acid (Vicryl) and polytrimethylene carbonate (Maxon) suture material. J Dermatol Surg Oncol 1991; 17:667–669.
18. Hohenleutner U, Egner N, Hohenleutner S, Landthaler M. Intradermal buried vertical mattress suture as sole skin closure: evaluation of 149 cases. Acta Derm Venereol 2000; 80:344–347.
19. Niessen FB, Spauwen PH, Kon M. The role of suture material in hypertrophic scar formation: Monocryl vs Vicryl-rapide. Ann Plast Surg 1997 39:254–260.
20. Gabel EA, Jimenez GP, Eaglstein WH, et al. Performance comparison of nylon and an absorbable suture material (Polyglactin 910) in the closure of punch biopsy sites. Dermatol Surg 2000; 26:750–752.
21. Faulkner BC, Gear AJ, Hellewell TB, et al. Biomechanical performance of a braided absorbable suture. J Long Term Effect Med Implants 1996; 6:167–179.

22. Debus ES, Geiger D, Sailer M, et al. Physical, biological and handling characteristics of surgical suture material: a comparision of four different multifilament absorbable sutures. Eur Surg Res 1997; 29:52–61.

23. Elliot D, Mahaffey PJ. The stretched scar: the benefit of prolonged dermal support. Br J Plast Surg 1989 42:74–78.

24. Katz AR, Mukherjee DP, Kaganov AL, et al. A new synthetic monofilament absorbable suture made from polytrimethylene carbonate. Surg Gynecol Obstet 1985; 161:213–222.

25. Trimbos JB, Niggebrugge A, Trimbos R, et al. Knotting abilities of a new absorbable monofilament suture: poliglecaprone 25 (Monocryl). Eur J Surg 1995 161:319–322.

26. Bezwada RS, Jamiolkowski DD, Lee IY, et al. Monocryl suture, a new ultra-pliable absorbable monofilament suture. Biomaterials 1995; 16:1141–1148.

27. Niessen FB, Spauwen PH, Kon M. The role of suture material in hypertrophic scar formation: Monocryl vs Vicryl-rapide. Ann Plast Surg 1997; 39:254–260.

28. Molea G, Schonauer F, Bifulco G, et al. Comparative study on biocompatibility and absorption times of three absorbable monofilament suture materials (Polydioxanone, Poliglecaprone 25, Glycomer 631). Br J Plast Surg 2000 53:137–141.

29. Herrmann JB. Tensile strength and knot security of surgical suture materials. Am Surg 1971; 37:209–217.

30. Conn J, Beal JM. A study of polybutilate lubricated polyester sutures. Surg Gynecol Obstet 1977; 144:707–709.

31. Rodeheaver GT, Shimer AL, Boyd LM, et al. An innovative absorbable coating for the polybutester suture. J Long Term Effect Med Implants 2001; 1–2:41–51.

32. Bang RL, Mustafa MD. Comparative study of skin wound closure with polybutester (Novafil) and polypropylene. J R Coll Surg Edin 1989 34:205–207.

33. Orlinsky M, Goldberg RM, Chan L, et al. Cost analysis of stapling versus suturing for skin closure. Am J Emerg Med 1995; 13:77–81.

34. Bennett RG. Selection of wound closure materials. J Amer Acad Dermatol 1988; 18:619–637.

35. Medina dos Santos LR, Freitas CA, Hojaij FC, et al. Prospective Study using skin staplers in head and neck surgery. Am J Surg 1995; 170:451–452.

36. Khan A, Dayan PS, Miller S, et al. Cosmetic outcome of scalp wound closure with staples in the pediatric emergency department: A prospective, randomized trial. Pediatr Emerg Care 2002; 18:171–173.

37. Meiring L, Ciliers K, Barry R, et al. A comparison of a disposable skin stapler and nylon sutures for wound closure. S Afr Med J 1982; 62:371–372.

38. Coupland RM. Sutures versus staples in skin flap operations. Ann R Coll Surg Engl 1986; 68:2–4.

39. Stockley I, Elson RA. Skin closure using staples and nylon sutures: a comparison of results. Ann R Coll Surg Engl 1987; 69:76–78.

40. Leonard F, Hodge JW, Houston S, et al. Alpha-cyanoacrylate adhesive bond strengths with proteinaceous and nonproteinaceous substrates. J Biomed Mater Res 1965; 3:281–289.

41. Ammirati CT. Advances in wound closure materials. Adv Dermatol 2002; 18:313–338.

42. Craven NM, Telfer NR. An open study of tissue adhesive in full-thickness skin grafting. J Amer Acad Dermatol 1999; 40:601–611.

43. Naik SS, Wright V, Timmons J, et al. A single blind, prospective, randomized trial comparing n-butyl-2-cyanoacrylate tissue adhesive (Indermil) and sutures for skin closure in hand surgery. J Hand Surg 2001; 26B:264–265.

44. Goktas N, Karcioglu O, Coskun F, Karaduman S, et al. Comparison of tissue adhesive and suturing in the repair of lacerations in the emergency department. Eur J Emerg Med 2002; 9:155–158.

45. Penoff J. Skin closures using cyanoacrylate tissue adhesives. Plastic Surgery Educational Foundation DATA Committee. Device and Technique Assessment. Plast Reconstr Surg 1999; 103:730–731.

46. Shapiro AJ, Dinsmore RC, North JH. Tensile strength of wound closure with cyanoacrylate glue. Am Surg 2001; 67:1113–1115.

47. Quinn J, Wells G, Sutcliffe T, et al. A randomized trial comparing octyl-cyanoacrylate tissue adhesive and sutures in the management of lacerations. JAMA 1997; 277:1527–1530.

48. Osmond MH, Quinn JV, Sutcliffe T, et al. A randomized, clinical trial comparing butylcyanoacrylate with octylcyanoacrylate in the management of selected pediatric facial lacerations. Acad Emerg Med 1999; 6:171–177.

49. Tamez OA, McGuff HS, Prihoda TJ, et al. Securing meshed split-thickness skin grafts with 2-octylcyanoacrylate. Otolaryngol Head Neck Surg 1999; 121:562–566.

50. Toriumi DM, O'Grady K, Desai D, et al. Use of octyl-2-cyanoacrylate for skin closure in facial plastic surgery. Plast Reconstr Surg 1998; 102:2209–2219.

51. Bernard L, Doyle J, Friedlander SF, et al. A prospective comparison of octyl cyanoacrylate tissue adhesive (Dermabond) and suture for the closure of excisional wounds in children and adolescents. Arch Dermatol 2001; 137:1177–1180.

52. Shamiyeh A, Schrenk P, Stelzer T, et al. Prospective randomized blind controlled trial comparing sutures, tape, and octylcyanoacrylate tissue adhesive for skin closure after phlebectomy. Dermatol Surg 2001; 27:877–880.

53. Kandel EK, Bennett RG. The effect of stitch type on flap tip blood flow. J Amer Acad Dermatol 2001; 44:265–272.

54. Zitelli JA, Moy RL. Buried vertical mattress suture. J Dermatol Surg Oncol 1989; 15:17–19.

55. Breuninger H, Keilbach J, Haaf U. Intracutaneous butterfly suture with absorbable synthetic suture material. Technique, tissue reactions, and results. J Dermatol Surg Oncol 1993; 19:607–610.

56. Harrington AC, Montemarano A, Welch M, et al. Variations of the pursestring suture in skin cancer reconstruction. Dermatol Surg 1999; 25:277–281.

57. Snow SN, Dortzbach R, Moyer D. Managing common suturing problems. J Dermatol Surg Oncol 1991; 17:502–508.

58. Bennett R. Basic excisional surgery. In: Bennett RG, ed. Fundamentals of cutaneous surgery. St Louis, MO: Mosby 1988; 381–411.

59. Panek PH, Prusak MP, Bolt D, et al. Potentiation of wound infection by adhesive adjuncts. Am Surg 1972; 38:343–345.

17 Hemostasis

Tri H Nguyen MD

Summary box

- Physiologic hemostasis occurs in three interrelated phases: initiation (thrombin formation), amplification (platelet aggregation and activation), and propagation (fibrin formation and clot stabilization).
- A focused preoperative history is the most valuable screen for patients at higher risk of bleeding.
- In general, prescribed anticoagulation for secondary thrombotic prophylaxis should not be discontinued with dermatologic surgery.
- Optimizing hemostatic anesthesia, alleviating anxiety and situational hypertension will significantly reduce the risk of perioperative bleeding.
- Some physiologic hemostatic agents have benefits beyond hemostasis and may promote wound healing and skin graft survival.
- Electrosurgery and suture ligation for hemostasis should be precise to minimize excessive collateral tissue injury.

INTRODUCTION

With all incisional surgeries, exsanguination will occur as blood vessels are disrupted. Hemostasis is defined as the arrest of bleeding through physiologic or surgical intervention. Inadequate hemostasis will compromise even the most meticulous of techniques, leading to intra- and post-operative bleeding and the terrible tetrad of hematoma, dehiscence, necrosis, and infection. Historically, dermatologists have had few difficulties with surgical bleeding because procedures were often small and limited to biopsies, excisions, and closures of simple defects. As dermatologic surgery evolves, however, cutaneous surgeons increasingly perform complex procedures and encounter intricate medical issues and medications in their patients. Achieving adequate hemostasis requires careful evaluation and management of these issues throughout the perioperative period.

PREOPERATIVE PREPARATION

Hemostatic process

A basic knowledge of physiologic hemostasis is helpful in understanding newer anticoagulants and in using hemostatic agents. The coagulation process is a highly evolved system that involves the interactions of endothelial cells, coagulation factors (Factors I–XIII), and platelets. Precipitating this process is endothelial injury (i.e. incision), which exposes collagen and tissue factor (TF) in subendothelial fibroblasts. Traditionally, the coagulation cascade was described as two separate reactions—the intrinsic and extrinsic pathways—which converged into a common pathway. This model evolved from in-vitro studies of clotting, but is not consistent with in-vivo observations. A deficiency of Factor XII (intrinsic pathway), for example, markedly prolongs activated partial thromboplastin time (aPTT), but there is no clinical bleeding.

A newer perspective on coagulation depicts three phases of hemostasis; initiation, amplification, and propagation.[1]

Initiation (thrombin formation)

This phase begins with endothelial injury and TF exposure. Exposed TF binds to circulating Factor VII and activates it (VIIa). This TF–VIIa complex then activates Factor X and Factor IX, generating small amounts of thrombin (Factor II).

Amplification (platelet aggregation and activation)

Platelets serve four functions: they adhere to sites of endothelial injury; store essential clotting cofactors (Factors V, VIII); aggregate with other platelets to form a primary clot; and provide a surface for coagulation reactions.

Platelet aggregation begins when circulating von Willebrand factor (vWF) detects and binds to exposed endothelial collagen. vWF then serves as a glue to attract platelets to the endothelial wound. This early platelet plug is unstable, is not sufficient for hemostasis, and must be stabilized by fibrin in the third stage.

Thrombin, produced during the initiation phase, activates aggregated platelets. Once activated, the platelet enzymes cyclooxygenase and thromboxane synthase generate thromboxane A2, which stimulates the release of clotting cofactors (adenosine diphosphate [ADP], Factor V, Factor VIII) from its granules. Factors V and VIII serve as cofactors for further production of Factor X and thrombin.

Propagation (fibrin formation and stabilization of the platelet clot)

In this final phase, thrombin (now present in increasing quantities) converts soluble fibrinogen into an insoluble fibrin meshwork, which is polymerized and stabilized by Factor XIII and calcium. It is this firm fibrin network that stabilizes the early platelet clot and secures the arrest of bleeding. Calcium is essential throughout these reactions by helping proteins bind to surfaces. Overall, the final hemostatic plug derives 55% of its strength from platelets and 45% from the fibrin network.[2]

Evaluation

A focused history is the most useful screen for patients with bleeding tendencies. Routine laboratory studies for all patients undergoing surgery are not indicated, and often yield false-positive or false-negative results.

The preoperative evaluation should concentrate on identifying underlying disorders and medications that may increase surgical bleeding. Inquiries must be specific to be informative because one-third of patients with von Willebrand disease (VWD) deny a bleeding diathesis.[3] Bleeding in coagulation disorders is excessive for the injury, prolonged, and recurrent. Physicians may consider these three strategic questions as they interview their patients: Is the bleeding real? Is the bleeding consistent with platelet or coagulation factor abnormalities? Is it an acquired or inherited condition?

Physicians may enhance the specificity of positive responses by clarifying the severity and frequency of symptoms. Table 17.1 lists useful questions for eliciting a bleeding history. Patients with coagulation factor disorders (hemophilia) have prolonged surgical bleeding and hemorrhage deeply into muscles and joints. These patients usually have an established personal and family history of bleeding and are easily identified. Patients with VWD and platelet abnormalities, on the other hand, bleed from mucocutaneous surfaces. A variety of disorders may impair hemostasis and are listed in Table 17.2.

VWD is the most common inherited bleeding disorder, affecting up to 1% of the population. Affected individuals are most challenging to diagnose because symptoms are quite variable and vWF levels vary with exercise, stress, and even blood type. Symptoms may be mild and never manifest if patients have never had surgery. vWF not only facilitates platelet aggregation, but also acts as a carrier for Factor VIII, protecting it from premature destruction. Consequently, people with VWD have platelet-type bleeding (mucocutaneous) and may also have abnormalities in Factor VIII.[4] Patients with known or suspected VWD are best

Table 17.1 Interview questions for bleeding history

General questions	Have you ever had prolonged bleeding after surgery? Have you required transfusions after surgery?
Women	Do your periods last longer than 7 days? Is your menstrual flow heavy for 3 days or more? Have you ever had anemia or required iron supplements as a result of menstrual bleeding? Have you ever needed transfusions after childbirth because of excessive bleeding?
Coagulation factor abnormalities (delayed bleeding and deep hemorrhage into joints and muscles)	Have you ever had delayed bleeding after surgery (>3 days postoperatively)? Do you have a family history of bleeding problems? Have you ever bled into joints or muscles? (coagulation factor deficiency)
Platelet type bleeding (mucocutaneous bleeding)	Have you had bleeding after dental surgery? Did the bleeding require stitching or packing? Did the bleeding occur immediately or the next day? Have you ever had a nosebleed? If so, how frequent are they and do they ever require emergency or hospital care? Do you have excessive bruising (>5 cm, truncal locations, absence of injury)?

Table 17.2 Common disorders affecting hemostasis[4,37]

Disorders affecting platelets	Comment (bleeding time is not predictive of bleeding risk for any condition; some disorders may affect both platelets and coagulation factors)
Severe renal disease	Uremia may impair platelet function Heparin considerations with dialysis
Immune thrombocytopenia	Antibody-mediated platelet destruction
Splenomegaly	Platelet sequestration
Bone marrow failure	Platelet production problem
VWD	*Type 1* (70–80%) Low levels of vWF and Factor VIII *Type 2a* Abnormal vWF protein, levels normal *Type 2b* vWF 'hyperactivity', causing platelet aggregation without endothelial injury Mild thrombocytopenia *Type 3* Homozygous deletion Zero levels vWF and Factor VIII Deep joint bleeding similar to hemophilia
Disorders affecting clotting factors	**Comment**
Severe hepatic insufficiency	Impaired synthesis of vitamin K-dependent clotting factors
Alcoholism (liver, vasodilatation)	Hepatic insufficiency Direct vasodilator
Vitamin K deficiency	Clotting Factors II, VII, IX, X
Hemophilia A	Factor VIII deficiency
Hemophilia B	Factor IX deficiency

referred to hematologists for management in the perioperative period.

Thrombocytopenia is rarely an issue for cutaneous surgeons. Platelets serve as the primary hemostatic plug as well as the focus of many hemostatic reactions. Abnormalities may be in the quality and/or quantity of platelets. Platelet function may be affected by medications, which usually impair the amplification phase of hemostasis (Table 17.3). Moderate thrombocytopenia (50 000–100 000) should not affect hemostasis in cutaneous surgery. Even counts of 20 000–50 000 may be acceptable if patients do not have clinical signs and symptoms of bleeding (i.e. large bruising, petechiae, gingival bleeding), and if complex reconstruction (interpolation flaps or bone or cartilage grafting) is not anticipated. Levels below 20 000, or clinically excessive bleeding regardless of levels, should warrant caution and consultation with a hematologist.

Medications and agents impairing hemostasis

Increasingly, patients present with complex anticoagulation regimens. Even nonprescription medications and herbal and vitamin supplements may impair hemostasis. These agents and their potential effects are reviewed in Table 17.3. A continuing controversy among dermatologic surgeons is whether anticoagulation should be discontinued before surgery. The sequelae of bleeding complications can be serious and may be divided into three types:

- Type 1—life-threatening bleeds that result in intracranial, cardiac, or airway compromise (e.g. expanding cervical hematoma after neck liposuction).
- Type 2—major (not life-threatening but serious) bleed resulting in a reduction of hematocrit, a need for transfusion or surgical intervention, and functional compromise.

Table 17.3 Oral medications and supplements affecting hemostasis

Medication	Mechanism of action	Comment
		Platelet inhibition
Aspirin	Irreversible inhibition of cyclooxygenase, affecting platelet release of clotting cofactors	Discontinue 10–14 days preoperatively
Non-steroidal anti-inflammatory drugs	Reversible inhibition of cyclooxygenase	Variable, depending on specific drug (usually 2–3 days preoperatively)
Clopidogrel (Plavix)	Oral inhibitor of platelet aggregation	Discontinue 5 days preoperatively
Ticlopidine (Ticlid)	Oral inhibitor of platelet aggregation and adhesion. Also inhibits fibrinogen binding to platelets	Discontinue 10–14 days preoperatively
Dipyridamole (Persantin)	Phosphodiesterase inhibitor with mild vasodilatory and anti-platelet activity	Dipyridamole alone has no clinical effects on hemostasis Aggrenox is dipyridamole with 25 mg aspirin and does impair hemostasis as a result of the aspirin component
		Coagulation factor inhibition
Warfarin	Oral vitamin K antagonist (inhibits clotting factors Factor II, Factor VII, Factor IX, and Factor X)	Discontinue 3–4 days preoperatively (lowers the International Normalized Ratio [INR] ratio to near normal)
Herbs and supplements—all enhance anticoagulation effects of warfarin; garlic and vitamin E have additional effects		
Feverfew		For migraine headaches, arthritis, rheumatic disease
Garlic	Inhibits platelet aggregation and thromboxane B2 in vitro. Enhances fibrinolysis in vivo	For lowering cholesterol, triglycerides, and blood pressure
Ginger		For reducing nausea, vomiting, vertigo
Ginkgo		For increasing blood circulation and oxygenation, memory
Ginseng		For increasing physical stamina and mental concentration, immune function
Dong Quai root		For antispasmodic, anticlotting, laxative, analgesic effects
Bilberry		For diuretic, astringent effects
Chondroitin		For arthritis
Vitamin E	Decreases platelet adhesion Impairs platelet aggregation only in patients with abnormal platelets	Mild anticoagulant effect may be significantly increased when taken with aspirin, garlic

- Type 3—minor bleed where the outcome is not affected but requires additional physician visits or nonsurgical intervention (e.g. compression).

In dermatologic surgery, type 1 and 2 events are extremely rare. The consequences of thrombotic events (stroke, myocardial infarction, pulmonary embolus) with discontinuation of anticoagulants, however, are devastating.

For most cutaneous procedures, medically necessary anticoagulation (for secondary prevention of previous thrombotic events) should not be discontinued perioperatively. Supporting this position are data from recent studies that emphasize four key points: the risk of any complications with dermatologic surgery is already low;[5] the risk for major bleeding or complications with dermatologic surgery is not increased in patients who are taking aspirin or warfarin;[6–8] the risk of thrombotic events is substantially elevated in patients who discontinue their anticoagulation;[9,10] and finally the severity of real thrombotic events surpasses any perceived bleeding risk from cutaneous surgery.[11] Inferring from these studies that aspirin and warfarin do not affect hemostasis is incorrect. These agents do impair the coagulation process. However, any increased bleeding during cutaneous surgery is negligible and easily controlled with direct measures (i.e. electrocoagulation and ligation). Although warfarin may be continued, the INR should not exceed 3.0 if possible. Despite a general recommendation to continue anticoagulation, each patient requires an individualized approach. For patients who do not have a history of thrombotic events, but are taking aspirin and supplements for primary rather than secondary prevention, discontinuation is permissible.

■ TECHNIQUES

General approach to intraoperative bleeding

Despite all precautions, some degree of intraoperative bleeding will occur with any surgery. Beginning surgeons are often overwhelmed with surgical bleeding. Where do I start? What do I do first? Do I electrocoagulate or ligate? What do I do if I cannot see the bleeding vessel? These and other questions arise simultaneously and cause great anxiety.

Vessels initially spasm and constrict with injury. This is rapidly followed by vasodilatation unless epinephrine (adrenaline) has been used. With profuse bleeding, compression by an assistant proximal to the bleeding vessels will slow hemorrhage and allows time to retrieve supplies or rethink strategies. Pressure may then be slowly released to identify the offending vessel(s).

At times, bleeding may occur at so many sites as to be overwhelming. To maintain focus, the bleeding area should be mentally divided into several quadrants. While compressing the other quadrants, the surgeon may achieve hemostasis, one section at a time. In general, hemostatic efforts should be directed from arteries to veins, from larger to smaller vessels, and from superior to inferior sections of the wound. Efforts at hemostasis actually begin before the first incision, with proper patient positioning and effective anesthesia. The degree of bleeding and wound depth will influence the specifics of intervention.

Preparing the surgical field

Visibility and accessibility are critical to the effective management of intraoperative bleeding. Proper patient positioning will enhance surgical hemostasis as well as execution of technique. Lighting should be bright and sufficient. Gauze, Q-tips, and the electrosurgery unit should all be prepared and ready. Patients should be relatively flat with the surgical plane at a slight incline (15°). The mild incline will cause any bleeding to drain inferiorly towards a gauze, reducing blood pooling at the superior end. This permits the surgeon to concentrate on hemostasis at the more visible (superior) portion of the field. If the incline is too steep (>15°) however, then surgical technique may be compromised because the wrist or neck is bent into a nonergonomic position. Anticipating which sites are more prone to bleeding (i.e. scalp, nose, ears, lips, and digits) will assist in equipment preparation.

Hemostatic anesthesia

Epinephrine (adrenaline) added to injectable local anesthetics provides vital vasoconstriction in dilutions of 1 : 100 000 or 1 : 200 000. A more dilute concentration of epinephrine (1 : 1 000 000) in tumescent anesthesia is also effective and will provide pronounced and prolonged vasoconstriction. The tumescent effect (tissue swelling) itself aids hemostasis by temporarily compressing small vessels. Tumescent anesthesia is ideal for large reconstruction, liposuction, hair transplantation, and full face laser resurfacing.

To maximize the vasoconstrictive effects of epinephrine, at least 15 minutes should pass before the first incision. Clinically, a diffuse blanched appearance to the skin usually reflects effective hemostasis. More concentrated epinephrine formulations (1 : 2000 dilution) are available and are useful with mucosal procedures. Topical lidocaine with epinephrine (TLE—lidocaine 5% plus epinephrine 1 : 2000), for example, soaked on a dental roll is effective for intranasal hemostasis. Epinephrine may also be used alone. Packaged as Adrenelin, epinephrine may be diluted and injected to improve hemostasis. Caution is warranted in patients with severe coronary artery disease because cardiac ischemia may develop with significant systemic absorption.

Epinephrine has traditionally been avoided at acral sites, especially the fingers and toes, for fear of ischemic necrosis or injury. Several studies now refute this dogma and epinephrine appears to be safe, at least as a digital block, for fingers and toes.[12,13] To enhance the safety of epinephrine use in the digits, the following guidelines are offered: epinephrine dilutions should be ≥1 : 200 000; inject small volumes (1.5 mL or less per side); avoid circumferential ring blocks; inject as far as possible from the surgical site; and avoid in patients with peripheral vascular disease, diabetes mellitus, or vasospastic/thrombotic conditions.

Intravenous regional anesthesia (IVRA) or the Bier's block provides complete anesthesia and profound hemostasis. IVRA may anesthetize complete regions on extremities, such as from the elbow to fingers or from the knee to toes. The treated extremity is raised for 5–10 minutes to exsanguinate venous channels. A specialized tourniquet (not a standard blood pressure cuff) is placed proximal to the treated region (arm above elbow or thigh above knee) and inflated to 250 mmHg. Dilute 0.5–1%

plain lidocaine is then injected slowly and intravenously on the dorsal hand or dorsal foot of the treated limb (the intravenous line having been secured preoperatively).[14] A total lidocaine dose of 3 mg/kg should not be exceeded. Onset of anesthesia is within 5 minutes and complete in 15–20 minutes. The entire region, from the proximal tourniquet to the distal digits, is completely anesthetized. The elevated tourniquet tamponades both arteries and veins and no pulses are felt. A variety of procedures (excisions and incisions, carbon dioxide laser destruction, and botulinum toxin injections) may now be carried out in a bloodless field.[15] The limit to IVRA is time because tourniquet inflation is limited to 90 minutes. Serious lidocaine toxicity may develop if lidocaine leakage occurs either during injection or during cessation of therapy.[16] The minimal requirement for the injected lidocaine to be tissue distributed and protein bound is 30 minutes.[17] Tourniquet deflation before 30 minutes is therefore contraindicated (even if the surgery has finished) because a systemic lidocaine bolus may result. Bruising and local pain at the tourniquet site may occur, especially if compression duration exceeds 60 minutes. IVRA may be especially useful for surgery on extremity lesions that have a strong vascular component.

Compression

The simplest, but most often overlooked measure for hemostasis is manual compression. Firm pressure over a bleeding wound for 15–20 minutes will achieve hemostasis for most vessels, unless large vessels are involved. Pressure directly compresses vessels and permits time for either physiologic clotting or time for other interventions. Pressure is necessary when topical hemostatic agents are applied, or to facilitate electrosurgery. Compression is often applied downward, but may also project upwards to tamponade vessels near hollow openings. Brisk bleeding is often encountered with incisions on the nasal ala, for instance. By applying upward pressure from within the nasal vestibule, the alar surface is stabilized for incisions and blood vessels are compressed (Fig. 17.1). Upward pressure may be achieved with moistened Q-tips, a dental roll, or an inflated Foley catheter.[18] A chalazion clamp may similarly provide both stabilization and hemostasis for surgery on the mucosal lip (Fig. 17.2).

An extension of manual pressure is tourniquet compression. The judicious use of tourniquets can greatly reduce intraoperative bleeding and improve the control of bleeding vessels, especially on fingers and toes. Tourniquets may be fashioned from the cut finger of a surgical glove or a Penrose drain (Figs 17.3–17.5).[19–21] Although proximal tourniquets at the forearm or distal thigh are generally safe for up to 2 hours,[22] the pain with prolonged compression is usually intolerable without sedation. Tourniquet use without sedation should therefore be limited to 60 minutes or less. Elevating the extremity or digit for 10 minutes before tourniquet placement will achieve venous exsanguination, which may improve on hemostasis.

Topical hemostatics

Topical caustics, such as zinc chloride paste, silver nitrate, ferric sulfate (Monsel's solution), or aluminum chloride are useful as adjuncts to hemostasis.[23] These agents have in common a protein coagulation effect that causes varying degrees of tissue necrosis and leads to eschar formation and hemostasis. These styptic agents are rubbed onto the wound base for a hemostatic effect with either gauze or a Q-tip applicator. Wounds should be dried of blood immediately before application. Aluminum chloride is the least likely to leave pigment particles, which may stain the skin, unlike silver nitrate or ferric sulfate.

A number of topical noncaustic hemostatic agents are also available (Table 17.4). The ingredients of each agent vary widely as do their origin (plant, bovine, human) and mechanism of action. Although all are relatively absorbable, the physiologic hemostatics are resorbed most completely.

Physical hemostats (gelatin sponge, oxidized cellulose, microfibrillar collagen hemostat) act as a physical mesh onto which coagulation can occur and are the most practical, as well as cost-effective for dermatologic surgery. A physical hemostat that is readily available to consumers is Urgent QR Powder. QR contains hydrophilic polymers and potassium salts that form an artificial scab when applied to bleeding wounds. Because of the variable granulomatous reaction that may occur with the physical hemostatics, these products should be avoided near the conjunctiva and should be removed with layered closure.

Physiologic hemostatics use natural components of the coagulation cascade to augment either the amplification or

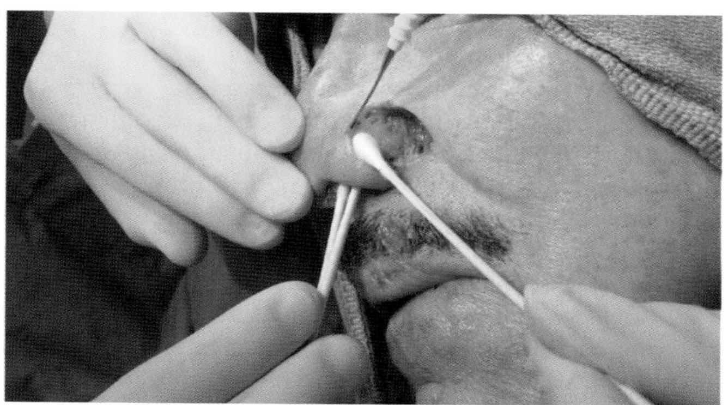

Figure 17.1 Nasal stabilization and hemostasis with Q-tips.

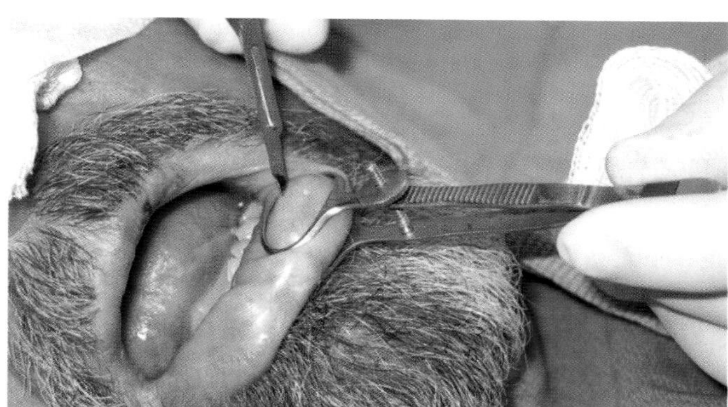

Figure 17.2 Lip stabilization and hemostasis with a chalazion clamp

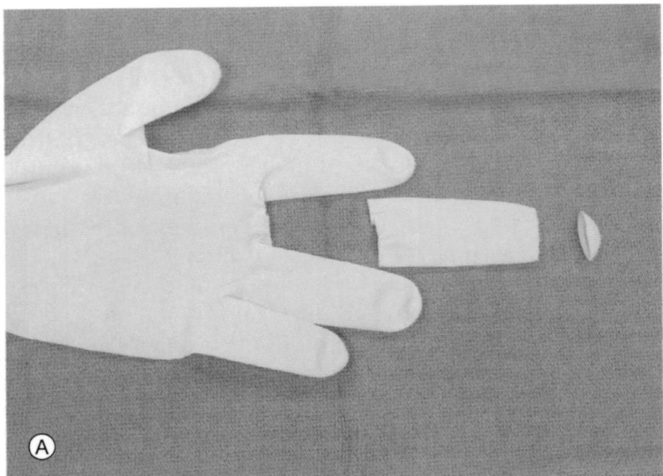

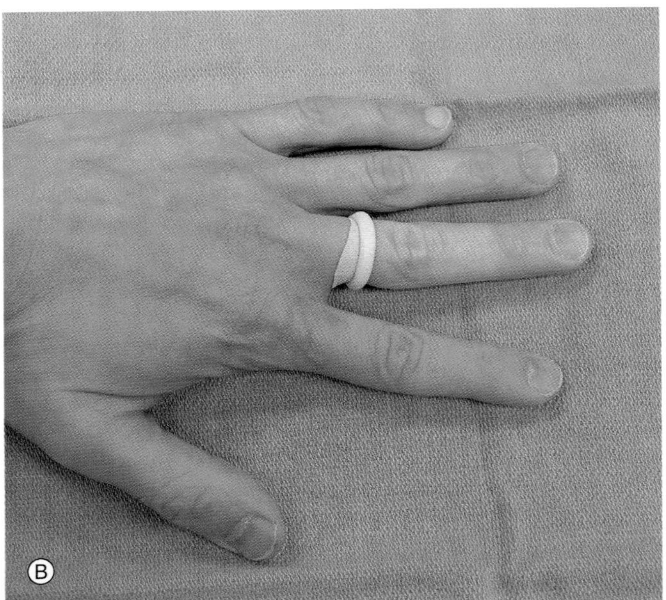

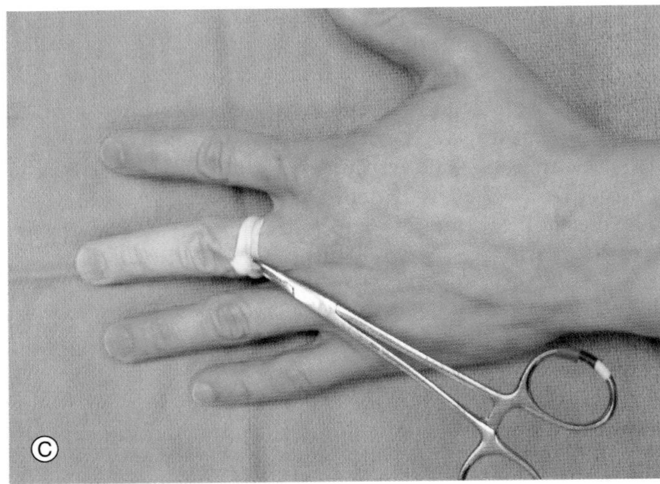

Figure 17.3 Surgical glove tourniquet. (A) The middle finger from a surgical glove is severed at both its base and its tip; (B) The finger glove is placed over the treated digit and rolled back proximally, forming the tourniquet. (C) A curved hemostat grasps the ring tourniquet with the loops facing away from the surgical field (optional step—provides additional compression and ensures tourniquet is not forgotten and left in place).

propagation phase of hemostasis. Some products such as fibrin sealant (Tisseel, Baxter Healthcare) have benefits beyond hemostasis. Fibrin sealant significantly improves split-thickness skin graft survival in difficult locations[24] and may promote wound healing. Fibrin sealants have been used for suture support (reduce operating time, increase suture integrity), tissue sealing (minimize dead space and fluid leakage), and for delivery of tissue-engineered skin.[25] Physiologic and antifibrinolytic hemostases are prohibitively expensive (several hundred to several thousand dollars per application) for routine use in cutaneous surgery.

Laser surgery

The continuous wave carbon dioxide laser is a valuable tool for hemostasis. At a wavelength of 10 600 nm, the carbon dioxide laser targets water and nonspecifically destroys tissue. It may be used in a focused (tissue incision) or defocused (tissue vaporization) mode while also sealing blood vessels of 0.5 mm in diameter.[26] There is reduced bleeding when compared to scalpel surgery. This incisional hemostasis is advantageous in procedures such as blepharoplasty, where meticulous hemostasis is mandatory. Optimal power output for most purposes is 5–10 watts. The dilemma with carbon dioxide laser hemostasis is that any blood or moisture in the field will absorb the laser energy and prevent effective coagulation. Therefore, laser hemostasis is best applied to slow capillary bleeding because with more brisk hemorrhage it is difficult to achieve a dry field. Mastering the carbon dioxide laser for surgery and hemostasis requires a high learning curve as well as significant investment in equipment and safety. As a result, it is not routinely used as the primary method of hemostasis.

Another laser for hemostasis is the continuous wave neodymium: yttrium aluminum garnet (Nd:YAG) laser (1064 nm wavelength). In the continuous wave mode, this laser generates diffuse thermal damage to several chromophores such as melanin, hemoglobin, and water. It may be used with a sapphire tip, which permits cutting with direct tissue contact, simulating a scalpel.[27] The Nd:YAG energy penetrates to a depth of 4–6 mm and diffuses widely, causing significant thermal coagulation peripherally.

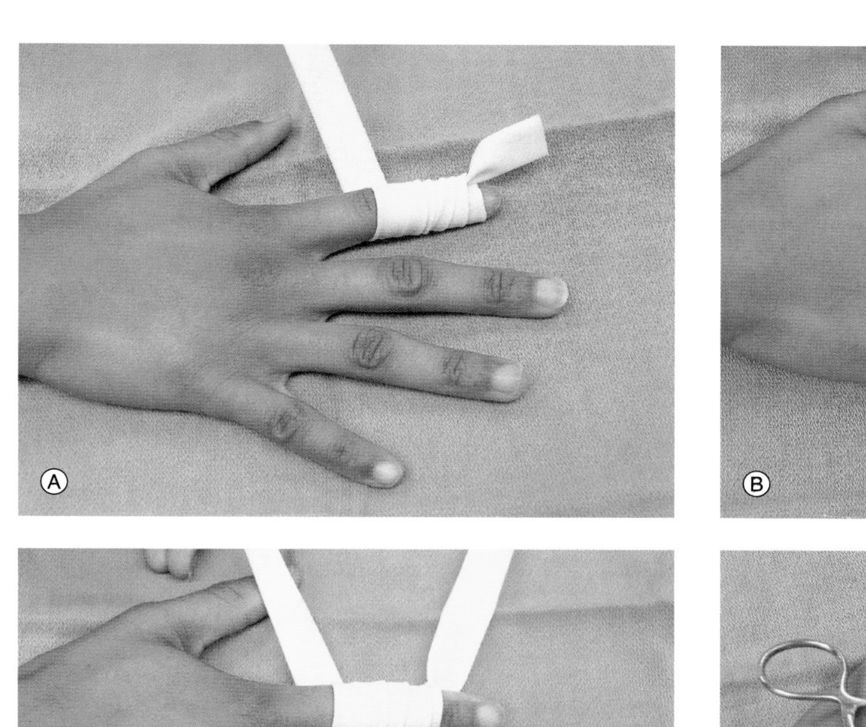

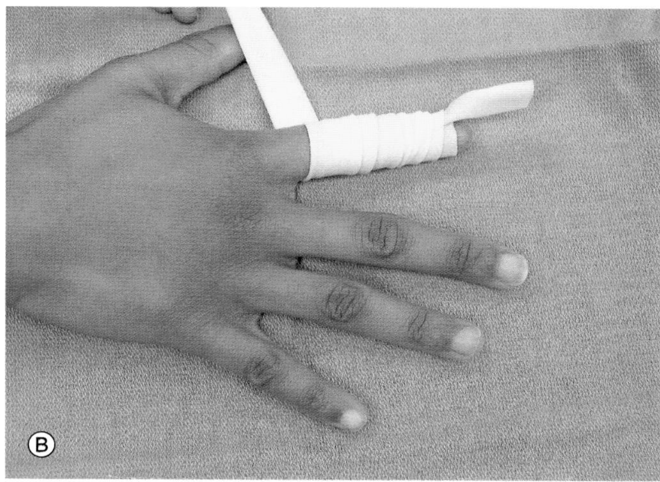

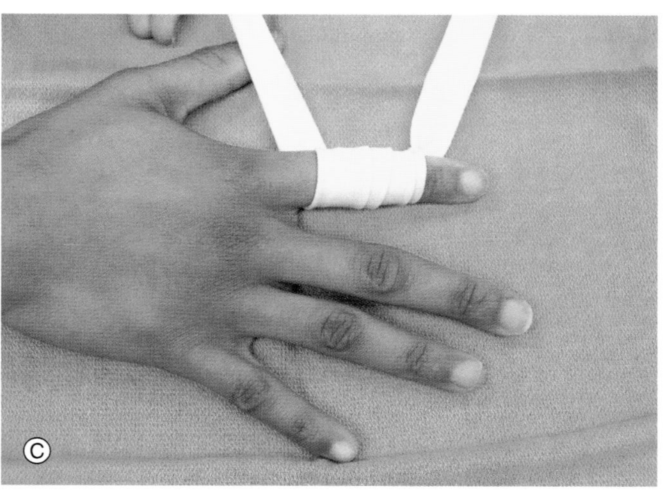

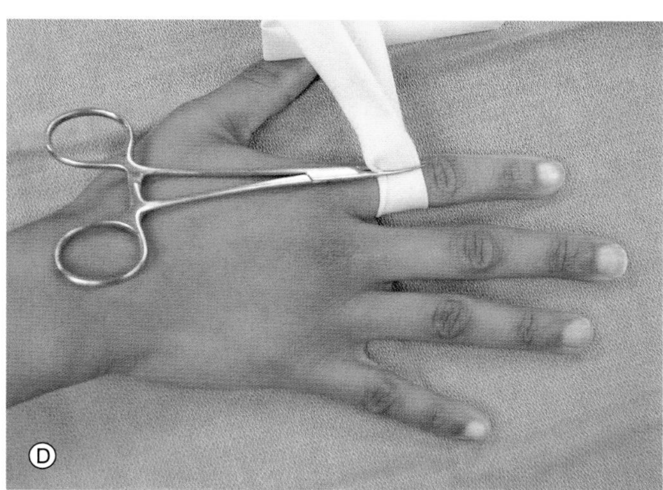

Figure 17.4 Exsanguinating tourniquet. (A) A Penrose drain is wrapped around the distal fingertip with a length exposed; (B) The drain is wrapped proximally under tension with overlapping layers. The wrap should extend beyond the surgical site, leaving an exposed end proximally as well as distally; (C) The distal end is now unwound slowly and until it reaches the proximal exposed end; (D) A hemostat secures both ends to form the tourniquet.

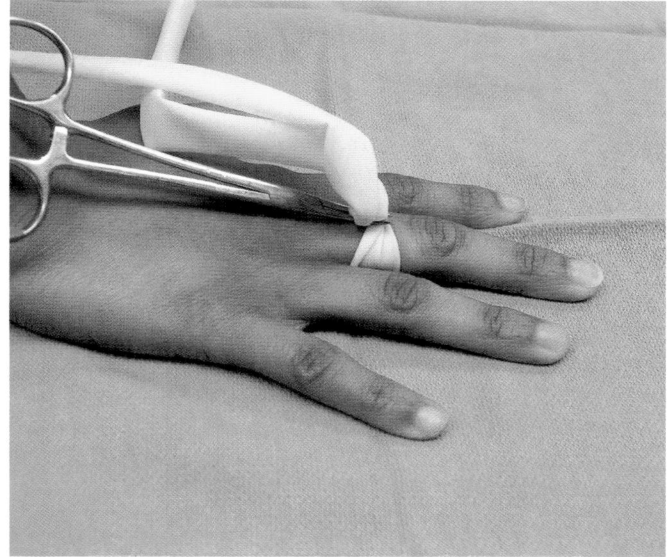

Figure 17.5 Penrose drain tourniquet. A Penrose drain is wrapped around the digit proximal to the treated site, stretched and secured at its base with a curved hemostat.

Given its diffuse and deep destruction, the Nd:YAG should be avoided as the sole instrument for hemostasis.

Electrosurgery

Electrosurgery is an effective method for surgical hemostasis. Monoterminal electrosurgery includes electrofulguration or electrodesiccation and provides adequate hemostasis for superficial procedures. It uses high voltage through a single electrode to desiccate tissue and thrombose small blood vessels (<2 mm diameter).[28]

Biterminal electrosurgery is known as electrocoagulation. Electrocoagulation generates a low voltage current and has two electrodes that may be applied in a unipolar or bipolar fashion. With all electrosurgery, the treatment electrode and current are applied directly to the bleeding vessel. Alternatively, the current may flow indirectly through a metal forceps or clamp that grasps the vessel. Bipolar electrocoagulation is the safest for patients with implantable defibrillators because the current is isolated between the two tips of the bipolar forceps and there is no distal dispersion of electricity. Further, it achieves hemostasis with the least tissue destruction, causing three times less

Table 17.4 Topical hemostatic agents[2,23,38–42]

Hemostatic agents—generic (trade name)	Formulation (manufacturer)	Comment
Caustic hemostatics—cause protein coagulation and precipitation, enhancing thrombus formation and occlusion of small vessels		
Zinc chloride paste	Paste	Not readily available, painful tissue necrosis
Silver nitrate	10–50% topical solution (Gordon Laboratories) Topical swabs/sticks (Arzol, Raway Pharmacal)	May stain skin, causes thick eschar.
20% ferric sulfate (Monsel's solution)	Solution	Iron particle stains, tattoo effect
Aluminum chloride hexahydrate, 20–70% (Drysol, Hypercare)	Solution (Hypercare, Stratus Pharmaceuticals; Drysol, Person & Covey)	Least likely to leave residual pigment.
Physical hemostatics—provide structural mesh that facilitates platelet aggregation and coagulation; relatively absorbable, but granulomatous foreign body reaction may occur		
Gelatin (Gelfoam)	Available as foam sponge or powder. Foam strips most practical and easy to handle for cutaneous surgery (Pharmacia & Upjohn)	Sponge may be used alone or soaked in thrombin. Absorbs several times its weight. Partially resorbable but granulomatous foreign body reaction if left in wound
Oxidized cellulose (Surgicel, Spongostan)	Mesh, gauze, fibrillar tufts, sponge (Johnson & Johnson)	Plant cellulose. Acts as physical mesh that facilitates clotting. Antibacterial. Absorbable in 1–6 weeks depending on formulation
Microfibrillar collagen hemostatic (Avitene)	Flour (shredded fibrils), sheets, sponge (Ultrafoam, Bard CR Inc)	Purified bovine collagen. Wound sponged dry and product directly applied with overlying pressure. For control of bleeding only. Should not be used as surface dressing or for packing wounds
Urgent QR powder	Powder dispenser (Biolife)	Forms artificial scab (Hematrix™). Powder sprinkled onto wound and pressure applied
Physiologic hemostatics—use components of coagulation cascade (fibrin, thrombin, calcium, etc) to augment physiologic hemostasis; products are completely resorbed without foreign body reaction		
Fibrin sealant (Tisseel, Fibrin Sealant FS)	Injectable dual syringe kit, spray (Baxter Hyland Immuno)	Enhances propagation phase of hemostasis. Tisseel contains calcium chloride, human fibrinogen, human thrombin, and bovine aprotinin. Fibrin Sealant FS has no bovine ingredient (aprotinin deleted)
Thrombin (Thrombin-JMI)	Powder reconstituted into solution. Minimum effective concentration for hemostasis is 100 U/mL (range 100–600 U/mL) (Gen Trac Inc)	Enhances propagation phase of hemostasis. Either the powder form or solution may be used. Powder is applied onto wound, followed by compression. Site must be relatively dry. Solution may be directly sprayed, applied with gauze, or soaked in Gelfoam and applied
Platelet gels	Prepared individually for each patient (SmartPReP)	Augments amplification phase of hemostasis. Autologous concentrate of platelet-rich plasma from differential centrifugation. Rich source of platelets and growth factors that may enhance hemostasis and wound healing

(continues on next page)

tissue necrosis than an equivalent current through a unipolar electrode.[29] In electrocautery, there is no electrode and sealing of blood vessels occurs through a hot wire device. It is effective only for the most minimal of bleeding.

With all electrosurgical methods, charring and collateral tissue damage may occur and is greater with electrodesiccation and electrofulguration than with electrocoagulation (see also Chapter 12). Precise application of current is essential to minimize excessive tissue charring, which then leads to poor wound healing and possible infection. Precision is mandatory in periorbital areas and with exposed perichondrium. The periorbital skin is thin and deeper structures may be damaged with excessive voltages. The perichondrium is also vulnerable and easily injured, necrosed, and inflamed. Haphazard and generalized coagulation is inappropriate. The lowest effective current setting should be used.

A 'wet' field (presence of blood) disperses electric current and causes excess charring. Drying the field is critical and may be achieved with proper use of a Q-tip or dental roll. The 'roll back' rather than the 'dabbing' method is best for precise electrocoagulation. In the first technique,

Table 17.4 (*Continued*) Topical hemostatic agents[2,23,38–42]

Hemostatic agents—generic (trade name)	Formulation (manufacturer)	Comment
Antifibrinolytic hemostats—counteract clot dissolution by preventing or delaying lysis of fibrin; these products are traditionally used systemically (intravenous or oral), but topical application has been reported		
Aminocaproic acid (AMICAR)	Syrup 1.25 g/5mL, tablet 500 mg, injectable (IMMUNEX USA)	Prevents conversion of plasminogen to plasmin. Most useful in bleeding as a result of hyperfibrinolysis. Prophylactic use in hemophiliacs undergoing dental surgery (maybe used orally or soaked in oxidized cellulose)
Aprotinin (Trasylol)	1.4 mg/mL (100, 200 mL) (Bayer Corp)	Serine protease inhibitor (inhibits plasmin, plasma kallikrein). Bovine origin. Has been used topically
Tranexamic acid (Amstat)	100 mg/mL (10 mL) (Glaxo)	Competitive inhibitor of plasmin (displaces plasmin from fibrin surface). Oral swish as bleeding prophylaxis in oral surgery
Miscellaneous hemostats		
Cocaine hydrochloride	Powder (packet 1 mg); solution, topical 4% (10 mL), 10% (10 mL); epinephrine—cocaine solution (epinephrine 1 : 2000 plus cocaine 11.8%, Roxane Laboratories) Extemporized preparations—epinephrine—cocaine gel (1.5 mL of epinephrine—cocaine solution mixed with 0.15 mg methylcellulose powder); TAC (tetracaine 0.5%, epinephrine 1 : 2000, cocaine 11.8% gel)	Potent vasoconstriction, anesthesia, and decongestion. Onset of action within 1 minute. Duration of 20–60 minutes. Decongestive and vasoconstrictive effects. 1 mg/kg maximum dose for most procedures. A 4% solution should not be exceeded topically as a result of systemic absorption and CNS stimulation. Intranasal use is most common. Caution with cardiac ischemia

a Q-tip compresses the bleeding area and slowly rolls back towards the surgeon. As the Q-tip rolls back, bleeding vessels should be immediately coagulated and sealed. This 'roll back' approach is more effective than 'dabbing', where the Q-tip dabs on and off at the bleeding site and permits a 'wet' field in between dabs.

Inadvertent wound edge necrosis is common with electrosurgery. Electrical current will conduct indiscriminately through any uninsulated metal and cause damage. If the device is held slanted (like a pen), for example, the proximal metal electrode may brush against the epidermal edge and cause necrosis. Adequate skin edge retraction and holding the device vertically will minimize this risk. Commercially made insulating needles (only the distal electrode tip is exposed) or extemporized insulating devices are also helpful.[30]

When grasping a bleeding vessel (either with a forceps or mosquito clamp), there is a tendency to clamp a large cuff of perivascular tissue. This results in excessive tissue damage when electrosurgery is subsequently applied. Ideally, only the vessel should be secured or at least the minimum tissue necessary. This may be accomplished by using two forceps, where the first clamps the general area to arrest bleeding, and the second localizes the bleeding vessel to be electrocoagulated.

Suture ligation

Hemorrhage from vessels of all sizes may be arrested with appropriate suture techniques. Vessels greater than 2 mm in diameter should generally be ligated because other methods of hemostasis are not as secure. If a vessel is transected, then each end may be clamped and ligated individually. Curved mosquito clamps (Halsted clamps) are preferred for securing larger vessels. As in electrosurgery, only the minimum of tissue should be clamped and ligated. Sutures that will be buried should be absorbable (i.e. polyglactin 910 [Vicryl, Ethicon Inc, Johnson & Johnson Co, Somerville, NJ]).

Different suture techniques are available for hemostasis (Figs 17.6–17.10). One of the most difficult situations in hemostasis is a bleeding vessel that is not visible. This may occur when a blood vessel spasms with injury and retracts behind the wound edge. It may also occur when punch biopsies are performed in highly vascular areas (scalp) and bleeding develops deep to the wound. For either situation, more undermining may reveal the retracted vessel for ligation or electrocoagulation. If further undermining is not possible, then ligation is necessary without identifying the offending bleeder. A figure-of-eight suture or a square stitch around the bleeding site is effective. Compressing the skin proximal to the area of hemorrhage will temporarily reduce bleeding sufficiently for suture intervention.

Excisions of vascular lesions (e.g. hemangiomas, port-wine stains) are inherently difficult. There may be diffuse bleeding, which limits visibility. A useful technique to control such bleeding is a double imbricating suture.[31] This method, which consists of two modified vertical purse-string sutures, is applied peripheral to the area of excision. The tension is adjusted by pulling on either ends of the suture, which constricts the central area of surgery and permits controlled hemostasis (see Fig. 17.7).

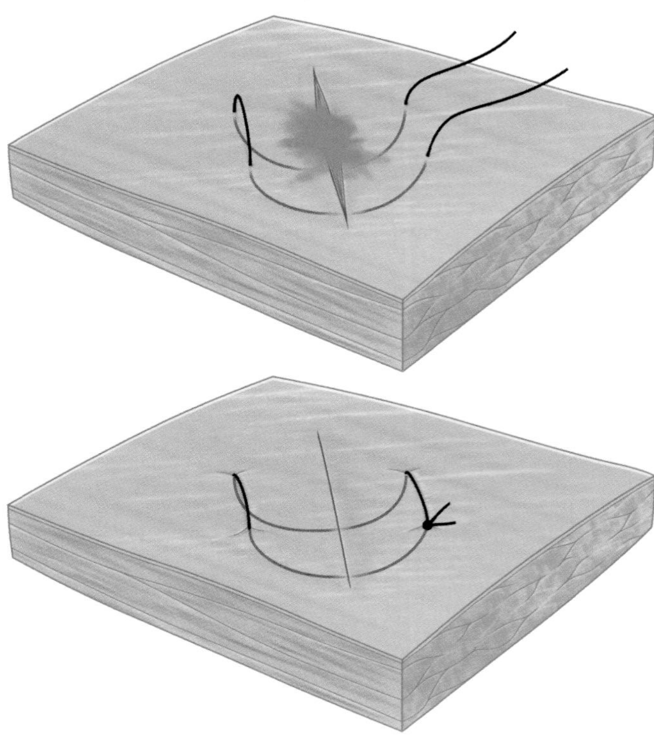

Figure 17.6 Horizontal mattress suture. As an epidermal suture, the horizontal mattress is useful for nonspecific epidermal oozing along the wound edge.

■ OPTIMIZING OUTCOMES

Hypertension and anxiety

Optimizing medical issues and anxiolysis before surgery are helpful strategies to decrease the risk of bleeding. Uncontrolled hypertension elevates intravascular pressure, which aggravates surgical bleeding. Patients with untreated hypertension should be stabilized before surgery, especially if systolic pressures exceed 180 mmHg. Sustained systolic hypertension above 180 mmHg is dangerous and may lead to myocardial infarction or stroke as well as bleeding. For many patients already on treatment, hypertension on the day of surgery is often situational and anxiety related. Calming music, soft and reassuring voices, and distraction are all useful methods to calm and relax patients. Medications, however, have a role if more rapid and effective anxiolysis is required. In patients with anxiety accompanied by situational hypertension, clonidine 0.1 mg orally is especially effective. Clonidine provides antihypertensive, sedative, and anxiolytic effects.[32] Its antihypertensive effect is prolonged (12 hours), which is an advantage in the immediate postoperative period when the risk of bleeding is greatest with hypertension. Further, clonidine reduces analgesic needs after surgery and lowers tachycardia through its alpha-2 agonist effects.[33] Clonidine should be given 60 minutes before surgery. It should be avoided in patients with a preoperative systolic pressure less than 100 mmHg or pulse rate less than 60/minute. If hypertension is absent, however, but anxiolysis is still significant, then oral midazolam (Versed) 5–10 mg will provide rapid anxiolysis within 20 minutes and has no hemodynamic benefits.[34] More important than its rapid onset, however, is its short half-life of 2 hours, which is an advantage in elderly patients. Initial doses of both clonidine (0.1 mg) and midazolam (5 mg) should be low in the elderly to avoid excess sedation.

Anatomic location and hemostasis

Experienced surgeons will anticipate sites that are prone to greater bleeding and prepare appropriately. Hemorrhage during cutaneous surgery usually involves random vessels, although named arteries may be transected in the head and neck and fingers or toes. Hemostasis in periorbital procedures must be meticulous and complete. The consequences of orbital hemorrhage are disastrous. The dorsal nasal artery, inferior and superior labial arteries, angular artery (and nasal branches), and superficial temporal artery are most vulnerable to injury in cutaneous reconstruction. Familiarity with these arteries and their paths will assist the surgeon in hemostasis. Arterial circulation is usually not compromised on the head and neck because there is extensive arborization of vessels and collateral supply. On the digits, however, extreme vigilance is necessary to preserve the two sole arteries (palmar or plantar digital arteries) to each finger or toe. The scalp is extensively vascularized above the galea. Numerous arterial perforators from the posterior auricular artery supply the anterior auricular surface. On both the scalp and ear, even minor punch biopsies may result in significant bleeding and should be anticipated. Finally, incisions involving muscles may result in profuse bleeding.

Appropriate undermining can greatly reduce surgical bleeding. Undermining below the galea on the scalp (above periosteum) and below the nasalis muscles on the nose (above perichondrium) is almost bloodless because the vascular planes are not violated.

Procedural hemostasis

With most planned procedures, appropriate precautions will reduce the bleeding risk. For example, out of town patients undergoing a complex procedure may be asked to stay locally overnight to permit rapid intervention if needed. For all layered closures, the closure of dead spaces is essential for hemostasis to prevent hematoma formation. Certain procedures in dermatologic surgery are especially prone to bleeding. Interpolation flaps for reconstruction tend to bleed at the proximal pedicle. Bleeding may be delayed for several hours if epinephrine has been used with local anesthesia. The surgeon may either avoid using epinephrine or monitor the patients for several hours after flap closure. The author prefers monitoring because meticulous technique is difficult without the vasoconstrictive benefits of epinephrine. Hair transplantation is also an inherently vascular procedure. The occipital arteries and its branches are invariably severed during donor harvesting. Tumescent anesthesia, directed compression, and the 'Ex' suture described in Figure 17.8 will optimize hemostasis in hair transplantation. Finally, plantar wart destruction is particularly prone to bleeding. Intravenous regional

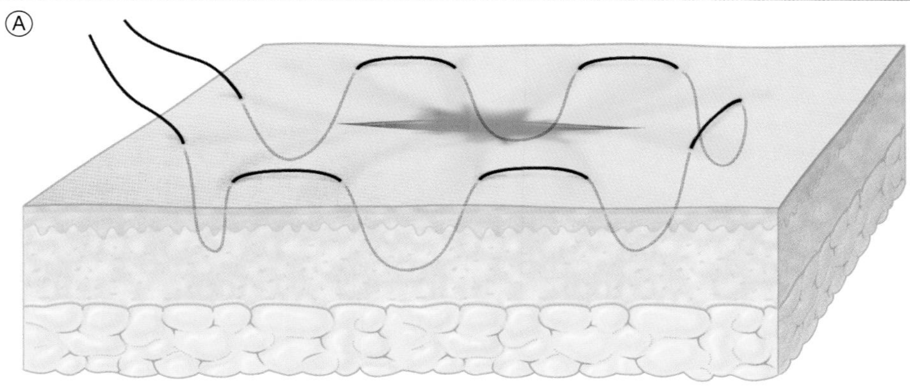

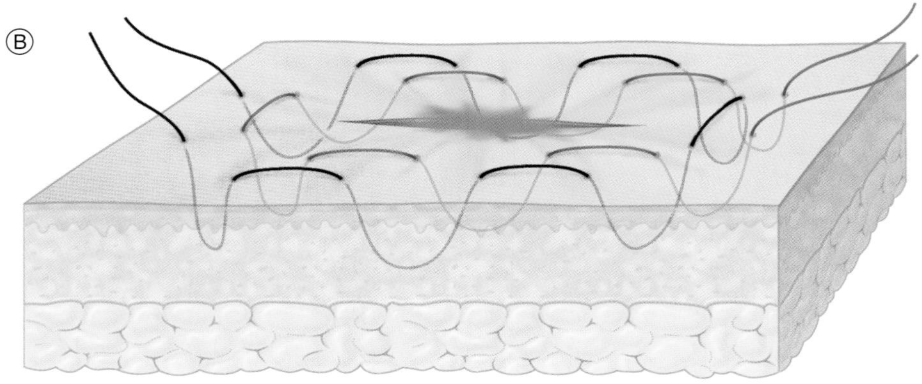

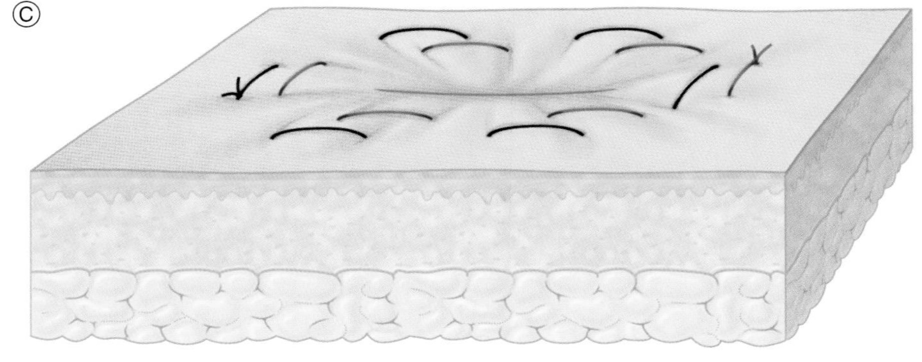

Figure 17.7 Double purse-string or imbrication suture. A 3-0 Prolene (Ethicon Inc, Johnson & Johnson Co, Somerville, NJ) suture with PS-2 needle is most useful for this technique. (A) First purse string is placed around the central lesion, with both ends of suture terminating on one side of the lesion; (B) Second purse string is begun on opposite end of the first suture and placed around the central lesion. (C) Hemostasis is achieved as both purse-string ends are cinched tight, tamponading the vessels peripheral to the centrally excised lesion.

anesthesia with its tourniquet compression is ideal for this procedure, creating a relatively bloodless field.

■ POSTOPERATIVE CARE

Patients must have detailed instructions on activity restrictions and wound care in the postoperative period (Table 17.5). Hemostasis may be compromised if patients are excessively active after surgery. The risk of postoperative bleeding is greatest in the first 48 hours, and especially within the first several hours. Acute bleeding occurs either with trauma or with rebound vasodilatation when the effect of epinephrine dissipates. Cold packs, elevation, and rest are important in this initial period. Cold packs will stimulate vasoconstriction and reduce swelling. Elevation and rest will reduce dependent blood flow and risk of bleeding. The purpose of wound care is to minimize bleeding, promote wound healing, and prevent infection. There are as many variations of wound dressings as there are dressing materials. To minimize bleeding, however, all dressings should provide effective compression. A compressive dressing not only provides pressure to close vessels but also immobilizes the wound and prevents external trauma. Dressings on the digits (fingers and toes) must be modified. Pressure ischemia or necrosis is a complication with excessive and circumferential compression. By using an elastic mesh such as Surgitube (Western Medical Ltd, Tenafly, NJ), SurgiGrip (Western Medical Ltd), or Surgilast (Western Medical Ltd), dressings may be kept in place without excess constriction. A splint, sling, or brace for the extremities and digits may also be useful. These devices remind patients of activity restrictions and provide wound

Ex suture

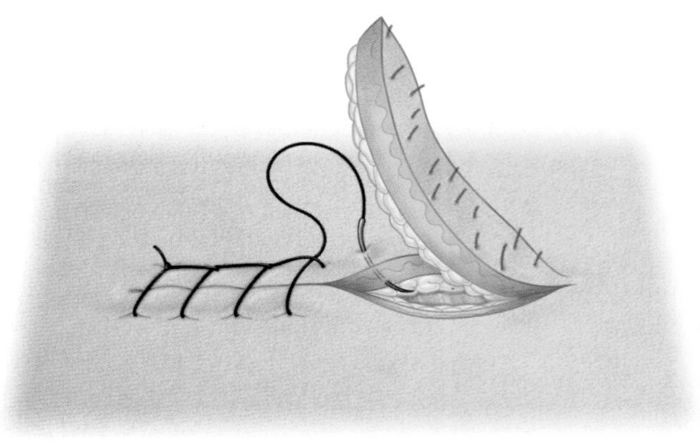

Figure 17.8 Ex suture—as the hair graft ellipse is excised, an assistant places a running locked suture behind the removed graft, securing hemostasis.

Square or U stitch

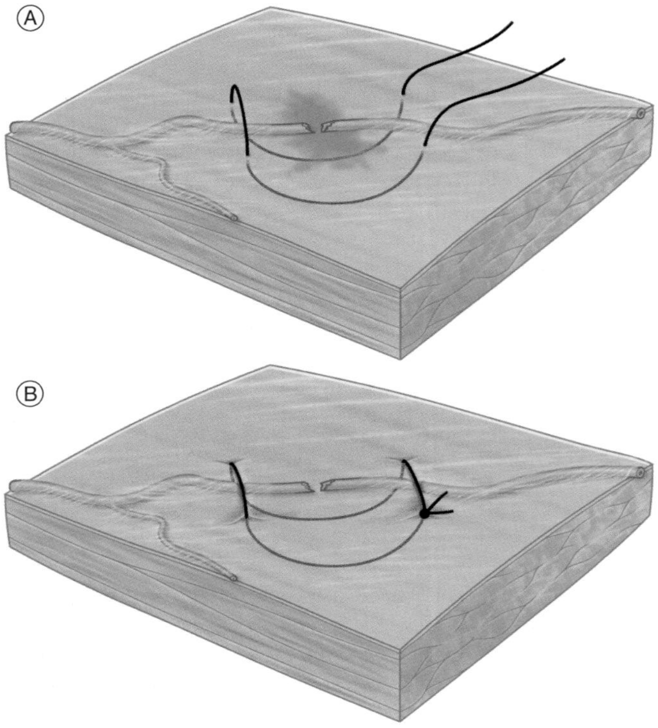

Ⓐ

Ⓑ

Figure 17.9 Square or U suture—this is similar to the horizontal mattress suture, but can be placed deep with an absorbable suture.

protection. For procedures on the extremities, a compression stocking (20–30 mm Hg) provides added support to the primary wound dressing. Stockings are especially helpful for patients with venous insufficiency to decrease wound swelling.

Figure of eight suture

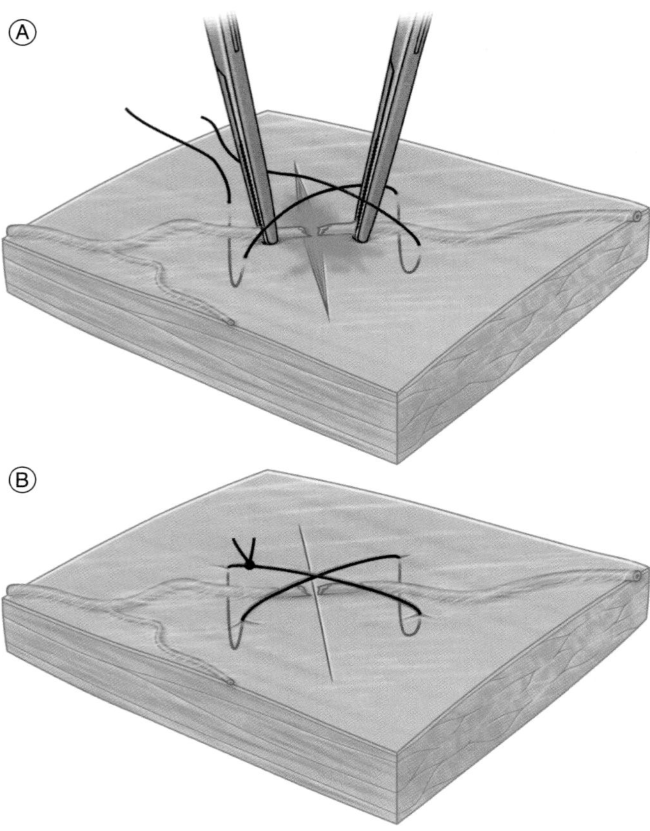

Figure 17.10 Figure-of-eight suture—this technique may secure hemostasis either as a top (nonabsorbable) or as a deep (absorbable) suture. The figure of eight crisscross configuration tamponades the underlying bleeding vessel.

■ PITFALLS AND THEIR MANAGEMENT

Pitfalls and their management

- The risk of bleeding is highest in the first 48 hours after surgery, especially within the immediate postoperative period.
- A new onset of painful swelling within a previously stable and asymptomatic wound is an expanding hematoma until proven otherwise.
- Expanding hematomas require intervention and are medical emergencies in periorbital and cervical locations.
- Evacuation of a hematoma is not always necessary, especially if it is small, stable, and not compromising tissue viability.
- Intervention may require wound exploration, irrigation, aspiration, and or drain placement.
- Bromelain may be given orally to expedite hematoma resolution.

Table 17.5 Postoperative patient instructions for hemostasis

Bleeding Bleeding after surgery rarely occurs, but if it does, it usually occurs during the first 48 hours after surgery. Following the activity restrictions below will help minimize your risk of bleeding. If you have any bleeding, please follow these instructions: 1. Lie down, elevate the area if possible, and apply firm pressure to the site for at least 15 minutes. If a bulky dressing has been placed over the wound, it should be removed 2. **Direct, firm pressure should be applied for 15 minutes to the gauze or towel next to the wound**. Do not stop applying pressure until 15 minutes have passed 3. If bleeding continues after 15 minutes, remove the pad, change it to a clean one, and hold pressure for an additional 15 minutes 4. If the bleeding has not stopped after three applications of pressure, please call the contact number on your wound care instruction sheet
Activities after surgery Decrease your overall physical activity, especially physical activity that pulls or stretches your wound and physical activity that will increase your heart rate. Avoid any activity that may traumatize your surgical site Do not use alcohol for 2 days after surgery. Alcohol dilates your blood vessels and may increase your risk of bleeding Lifting—avoid lifting anything greater than 10 lb (4.5 kg) and do not bend down to lift Facial surgery—avoid bending down below your waist. Elevate your head with one to two extra pillows when sleeping or lying down Hand, feet, arm, or leg surgery— elevate the area as much as possible above your waist when you are resting Lip surgery—eat soft foods. Keep your lip well lubricated with petrolatum ointment (Vaseline petrolatum, Aquaphor, or Bacitracin)
When to call your physician Contact your physician if you notice any of the following: • Bleeding not controlled by direct pressure • Pain that increases each day or is not relieved by over-the-counter medications • Rapid or increasing swelling within the wound • Reopening of the wound at any time • Increased redness, warmth, or pain around the wound

Despite all precautions, bleeding complications will occur if enough surgeries are performed. Bleeding emergencies are rare in cutaneous surgery. Dermatologic surgeons rarely penetrate the deep fascia to injure larger arteries. However, protective layers in the neck of elderly patients may be thin or atrophied and more caution is warranted during incision and undermining. With a large arterial bleed, the same principles of intervention apply. Immediate compression, identification of the vessel, and clamping will prevent further exsanguination. The patient should be transferred as soon as stable to a more appropriate setting where surgical exploration may be performed if needed.

A more likely scenario for dermatologic surgeons is an expanding hematoma. This is often because of continued bleeding within a closed wound, especially when there is a dead space. For small bleeders, the hematoma expansion may eventually tamponade the open vessel(s), which prevents further bleeding. However, if there is continued bleeding, the hematoma will progressively enlarge and cause compression injury to adjacent tissues. Wound necrosis, dehiscence, and infection are all potential sequelae of hematomas. Nowhere is this more dangerous than in the periorbital and cervical regions. An expanding hematoma in the orbit, for instance, will quickly result in blindness without treatment. Intervention requires performing a lateral canthotomy (the lateral canthal tendon is divided into a superior and inferior tendon) and cantholysis (the inferior canthal tendon is severed from its periosteal attachment) of the affected eye, which immediately relieves orbital pressure. In the neck, an expanding hematoma may compromise the airway if the wound is not explored and ligated. Intubation for airway protection may be necessary as hemostatic efforts are initiated. Anticoagulated patients undergoing procedures such as cervicofacial liposuction or rhytidectomy and platysmal plication are at risk. Patients must know emergency phone numbers and be aware of dangerous signs and symptoms. A new onset of painful swelling within a previously stable and asymptomatic wound is an expanding hematoma until proven otherwise.

The management of a stable hematoma depends on its stage, size, and associated symptoms.

Hematoma evolution

Hematomas evolve through four stages as outlined below.

First stage—early development

This occurs within hours with active hemorrhage and early blood accumulation. Clinically, the wound is swollen, warm, and fluctuant. Regardless of size, intervention is recommended to prevent progression. Suture removal and opening of part or the entire wound may be necessary to identify the bleeding areas. Most often, several bleeding foci are encountered rather than one offending vessel. Suction is useful to increase visibility. Following hemostasis with electrosurgery or ligation, the wound should be examined, irrigated with normal saline, and re-examined for more bleeding. If the wound is not contaminated, then all layers should be resutured. A drain may be considered if the risk of rebleeding is high or if complete hemostasis was not possible. Drains should be removed within 24 hours to minimize the risk of infection. For diffuse oozing, not responsive to electrosurgery or ligation, fibrin sealants or thrombin hemostats should be strongly considered.

Second stage—gelatinous phase

Hematomas quickly become gelatinous with physiologic clotting. The wound becomes more spongy than fluctuant and there may be a purplish hue. If a gelatinous hematoma is small, asymptomatic, and not threatening tissue viability, then observation is appropriate. Otherwise, evacuation is necessary and is similar to intervention in the first stage.

Third stage—organization

Within several days, the hematoma becomes organized into a rubbery, adhesive clot and the wound feels solidly firm. The adhesive clot is more difficult to remove completely at this stage and deferring intervention until the fourth stage may be best.

Fourth stage—liquefaction

After 7–10 days, the organized hematoma begins to liquefy

with fibrinolysis and is eventually resorbed. The wound again feels fluctuant. Resorption of the hematoma may require months depending on the hematoma's size. Intervention at this stage is simpler and does not require wound opening. The liquefied clot may be aspirated with a 16 or 18-gauge needle.[35] After the first stage, the decision whether or not to resuture the wound is subjective. If active infection is present or if the risk is high, then second intention healing with antibiotics is recommended with possible scar revision in the future. Bromelain (Ananase, Delta Labs, Traumanase, Aventis) is an oral concentrate of proteolytic enzymes derived from the pineapple plant, *Ananas sativus*. It inhibits plasma exudation and has anti-inflammatory and fibrinolytic effects. Bromelain may be given to expedite hematoma resolution at a dose of 500 mg three to four times daily until resolution.[36] Bromelain should be given cautiously to patients who have coagulation disorders or severe liver and renal disease.

■ SUMMARY

Successful hemostasis requires careful forethought throughout the perioperative period. Patients must be properly evaluated preoperatively, prepared appropriately intraoperatively, and followed carefully postoperatively. Advances in the understanding of physiologic hemostasis have resulted in better interventions for surgical bleeding. Most patients may continue their anticoagulation with dermatologic surgery. A wide array of hemostatic agents and techniques is available to locally manage perioperative bleeding. Pre-emptive strategies of reducing hypertension and anxiety and optimizing hemostatic anesthesia are helpful adjuncts. Bleeding complications, however, must be quickly recognized and managed to avoid patient morbidity and poor surgical outcome.

■ REFERENCES

1. Veldman A, Hoffman M, Ehrenforth S. New insights into the coagulation system and implications for new therapeutic options with recombinant Factor VIIa. Current Medicinal Chemistry 2003; 10:797–811.
2. Bhanot S, Alex JC. Current applications of platelet gels in facial plastic surgery. Facial Plast Surg 2002; 18:27–33.
3. Miller CH, Graham JB, Golden LR, et al. Genetic analysis of classic von Willebrand's disease I. Phenotypic variation within families. Blood 1979; 56:117–136.
4. DeLoughery T. Hemostasis and thrombosis. Georgetown TX: Landes Bioscience 1999.
5. Cook JL, Perone JB. A prospective evaluation of the incidence of complications associated with Mohs micrographic surgery. Arch Dermatol. 2003; 139:143–52.
6. Billingsley EM, Maloney ME. Intraoperative and postoperative bleeding problems in patients taking warfarin, aspirin, and nonsteroidal anti-inflammatory agents: a prospective study. Dermatol Surg 1997; 23:381–383.
7. Shalom A, Wong L. Outcome of aspirin use during excision of cutaneous lesions. Ann Plast Surg 2003; 50:296–298.
8. Stables G, Lawrence CM. Management of patients taking anticoagulant, aspirin, non-steroidal anti-inflammatory, and other anti-platelet drugs undergoing dermatologic surgery. Clin Exp Dermatol 2002; 27:432–435.
9. Kovich O, Otley CC. Thrombotic complications related to discontinuation of warfarin and aspirin therapy perioperatively for cutaneous operation. J Am Acad Dermatol 2003; 48:233–237.
10. Kearon C, Hirsh J. Current concepts: Management of anticoagulation before and after elective surgery. New Eng J Med 1997; 336:1506–1511.
11. Otley CC. Continuation of medically necessary aspirin and warfarin during cutaneous surgery. Mayo Clin Proc 2003; 78:1392–1396.
12. Denkler K. A comprehensive review of epinephrine in the finger; to do or not to do. Plast Reconstr Surg 2001; 108:114–124.
13. Willhelmi BJ, Blackwell SJ, Miller JH, et al. Do not use epinephrine in digital blocks: Myth or truth? Plast Reconstr Surg 2001:107:393–397.
14. Reuben SS, Steiberg RB, Lurie SD, et al. Intravenous regional anesthesia using lidocaine and clonidine. Anesthesiology 1999; 91:654–658.
15. Blaheta HJ, Vollert B, Xuder D, et al. Intravenous regional anesthesia (Bier's block) for botulinum toxin therapy of palmar hyperhidrosis is safe and effective. Dermatol Surg 2002; 28:666–672.
16. Grice SC, Morell RC, Balestrieri FJ, et al. Intravenous regional anesthesia: Evaluation and prevention of leakage under the tourniquet. Anesthesiology 1986; 65:316–320.
17. Tucker GT, Boas RA. Pharmacokinetic aspects of intravenous regional anesthesia. Anesthesiology 1971; 34:538–549.
18. Alcalay J, Goldberg LH. Intraoperative nasal ala stabilization using the foley catheter. J Dermatol Surg Oncol 1991; 17:957–958.
19. Smith IM. Austin OM, Knight SL. A simple and fail safe method for digital tourniquet. J Hand Surg [Br] 2002; 27:363–364.
20. Tucker S, Harris PC. The unforgettable finger tourniquet. Injury 2002; 33:76–77.
21. Salasche SJ. Surgery. In: Scher R, Daniel CR, eds. Nails: therapy, diagnosis, surgery, 2nd edn. Philadelphia: WB Saunders 1997; 326–349.
22. Wakai A, Winter DC. Street JT, et al. Pneumatic tourniquets in extremity surgery. J Am Acad Orthop Surg 2001; 9:345–351.
23. Larson P. Topical hemostatic agents for dermatologic surgery. J Dermatol Surg Oncol 1988; 14:623–632.
24. Vibe P, Pless J. A new method of skin graft adhesion. Scand J Plast Reconstr Surg 1983; 17:263.
25. Currie LJ, Sharpe JR, Martin R. The use of fibrin glue in skin grafts and tissue-engineered skin replacements: A review. Plast Reconstr Surg 2001; 108:1713–1726.
26. Dover JS, Arndt KA, Geronemus RG, Alora MB. Continuous and pulsed carbon dioxide laser surgery. In: Dover JS, Arndt KA, Geronemus RG, Alora MB, eds. Illustrated cutaneous and aesthetic laser surgery, 2nd edn. Stamford: Appleton & Lange 2000; 23–80.
27. Apfelberg DB, Maser MR, Lash H, et al. Sapphire tip technology for YAG laser excisions in plastic surgery. Plast Reconstr Surg 1989; 84:273–279.
28. Khouri S, Lodha R, Nouri K. Electrosurgery. In: Khouri S, Nouri K. eds Techniques in dermatologic surgery. Philadelphia: Mosby Elsevier 2003; 81–83.
29. Edlich RF, Reddy VR. 5th Annual David R Boyd, MD lecture: Revolutionary advances in wound repair in emergency medicine during the last three decades. A view toward the new millennium. J Emerg Med 2001; 20:167–193.
30. Nichter LS, Goldstein LJ, Bush AM, et al. A simple method for preventing misplaced electrocauterization. Plast Reconstr Surg 1987; 80:307.
31. Harahap M, Siregar AS. Method of minimizing hemorrhage in excising hemangiomas. J Dermatol Surg Oncol 1989; 15:1077–1080.
32. Klein J. *Ancillary pharmacology* In Klein J, ed. Tumescent liposuction. St Louis: Mosby 2000; 196–209.
33. Beer GM, Spicher I, Seifert B, et al. Oral premedication for operations on the face under local anesthesia: A placebo-controlled double blind trial. Plast Reconstr Surg 2001; 108:637–643.
34. Otley CC, Nguyen TH, Phillips PK. Anxiolysis with oral midazolam in pediatric patients undergoing dermatologic surgical procedures. J Am Acad Dermatol 2001; 45:105–108.
35. Salasche SJ. Acute surgical complications: Cause, prevention, and treatment. J Am Acad Dermatol 1986; 15:1163–1185.
36. Petry JJ. Surgically significant nutritional supplements. Plast Reconstr Surg 1996; 97:233–240.
37. Peterson SR, Joseph AK. Inherited bleeding disorders in dermatologic surgery. Dermatol Surg 2001; 27:885–889.
38. Micromedex Healthcare series. www.micromedex.com
39. Sweetman SC. Martindale: The Complete Drug Reference. London: Pharmaceutical Press; 2002.
40. Casdorph DL. Topical aminocaproic acid in hemophiliac patients undergoing dental extraction. DICP 1990; 24:160–161.
41. Product Information. Urgent QR™.www.biolife.com.
42. Bonadio WA, Wagner VR. Adrenaline-cocaine gel topical anesthetic for dermal laceration repair in children. Ann Emerg Med 1994; 23:1435–1438.

18 Ellipse, Ellipse Variations, and Dog-ear Repairs

Samuel E Book MD, Sumaira Z Aasi MD, and David J Leffell MD

Summary box

- The best results in ellipse excision are achieved by:
  - designing the simplest repair that will achieve optimal cosmesis
  - avoiding unnecessary flaps or grafts
  - undermining only as needed.
- The repair type is selected according to patient need and clinical circumstance, including:
  - consideration of the patient's age, health, and level of activity
  - consideration of second intention healing if cosmetic outcome is likely to be superior to reconstructive repair.
- An understanding of cosmetic units and skin characteristics of the anatomic location are important in elliptical excision.
- There are a number of variations on the ellipse and when to apply them depends on the circumstances.
- Even the best-planned ellipse may result in standing cones (dog-ears); there are several techniques to repair these.

INTRODUCTION

The increasing practice of skin surgery by dermatologists has introduced to the world of dermatologic surgery a philosophy of reconstruction that reflects an understanding of the biology of the skin. From less invasive skin biopsy to complex local reconstruction, office-based surgery—advanced by dermatologists under local anesthesia—has led to refinements and improvements in a range of common procedures. Chief among the surgical procedures performed on skin is the ellipse, or fusiform, excision. It is used for the therapeutic removal of benign and malignant lesions and is critical to the proper diagnosis of pigmented lesions and inflammatory diseases of the skin. The elliptical excision comprises all the fundamental elements of more advanced procedures such as local flaps, skin grafts, and cosmetic procedures. Those elements which must be learned thoroughly, understood instinctively, and practiced continually, include a knowledge of local anatomy, skin type, cosmetic units, incision technique, tissue handling, suture selection and placement, and wound management. All of these essentials are the bedrock of more advanced procedures. Learn the ellipse and perform it flawlessly and all else will follow. The goal of the elliptical excision, as with all other repairs, is a cosmetically excellent result; the scar should be hairline in thickness and well concealed within natural contours.

PREOPERATIVE PREPARATION

History

In skin surgery, as in most endeavors which are not by their very nature spontaneous, thorough preparation is paramount. Every skin lesion is associated with a patient, and that patient needs a complete, and directed medical history as a prerequisite to excellent care and an optimal result. The history must include (but is not limited to) significant medical conditions, current medications, drug allergies (including allergy to local anesthetic and latex), and history about past healing. Any medications that cause immunosuppression or alterations in bleeding (warfarin, clopidogrel bisulfate, aspirin, non-steroidal anti-inflammatory medication) must be documented, and the surgery modified accordingly. It is not unusual to encounter excess bleeding and oozing in patients taking 'natural' supplements such as vitamin E, ginkgo biloba, and garlic. It must be clarified whether or not these were prescribed by a physician for medical reasons. In view of recent studies and our own experience over 15 years, we generally do not discontinue any prescribed anticoagulants and/or platelet inhibitors prior to surgery.[1] However, if a patient takes aspirin without a medical indication, it should be discontinued 10–14 days prior to surgery. Meticulous hemostasis usually suffices in patients in whom antiplatelet drugs or warfarin could not be discontinued. In general, the risk of stroke or myocardial infarction outweighs the disadvantages of a cutaneous hematoma, which can be evacuated easily if necessary.

Patients with electronic cardiac devices present another problem during skin surgery. Confirmation should be sought to ascertain whether the patient has a pacemaker or an implantable cardioverter–defibrillator (ICD). Most newer pacemakers have filters that block extraneous electrical current, permitting the routine use of short bursts of electrocautery, but ICDs can be adversely affected by any electrical impulses. The options for these patients include disabling the ICD temporarily, using heat cautery, or using bipolar forceps to confine the current to a very small local area.[2]

Most of the medical history can be obtained on the day of surgery. One exception is information about an artificial heart valve or another condition that may require antibiotic prophylaxis.[3] While the issue of antibiotic prophylaxis remains controversial, the American Heart Association currently recommends prophylaxis only for contaminated skin wounds or those that have been open for more than 2 hours. The risk of bacteremia leading to endocarditis from a clean skin biopsy or similar minor procedure is extremely low and prophylaxis is not currently recommended.

Evaluation

Once the history has been satisfactorily obtained and clearly documented, evaluation of the individual who presents for facial excision should be done under proper lighting, with the patient in a sitting position.

First, any landmarks, cosmetic units, and relaxed skin tension lines that can be used to help camouflage the scar are identified. Examination and planning are not passive activities: inspection, palpation and gentle manipulation are necessary to confirm relaxed skin tension lines and to determine the impact of a particular repair on adjacent structures. The patient can be asked to 'show' their teeth, in preference to being asked to 'smile' as most patients are anxious, and not naturally disposed to cheerfulness when a surgeon looms over them, poised to incise. Observe the patient making specific facial expressions to accentuate the natural facial lines. Pursing the lips and raising the brow are two important maneuvers for studying the lip area and forehead and brow region.

The importance of understanding cosmetic units cannot be emphasized strongly enough. A longer scar limited to one cosmetic unit will be less noticeable than a shorter one that crosses the border between two units. It is important to recognize potential functional problems, such as the risk of ectropion, elevation or depression of the lip, or collapse of the nasal ala. Often the extent of potential ectropion can be estimated by asking the patient to look upward. This exaggerates the pull on the lower lid as the globe rotates upward. If the proposed repair lacks sufficient laxity under these circumstances, it is likely that an ectropion will result, even if it initially seems the wound is small enough to repair otherwise.

Although relaxed skin tension lines are useful guidelines, variations in skin laxity, previous surgery, and skin texture may often suggest alternative preferred scar alignment parameters. If the optimal direction for the ellipse is unclear, it may be helpful to excise the lesion as a simple circle, undermine as needed, and then observe which direction, independent of relaxed skin tension lines or cosmetic units, will provide for the most cosmetically elegant repair. Often, excision of the redundant cones of excess skin will be performed in a way that achieves a well-concealed scar.

Informed consent

Once the surgeon decides on the nature of the excision to be performed, and understands its impact, the risks and benefits of the procedure must be discussed in detail with the patient. First, give a clear description of the diagnosis and the need for the procedure. For cosmetic procedures it should be emphasized that the procedure is not medically indicated; in this circumstance, the risks are especially germane because they are affected by the benefit that accrues to the patient. The greater the medical need, the more risk the reasonable person would assume. The inverse is true for cosmetic procedures. Next, simple terms should be used to explain exactly what will happen during surgery and what can be expected during the postoperative period. The use of medical jargon should be avoided. Remember that while the surgeon gives informed consent many times a day and the process may feel routine, for the patient it is all new information. Therefore care must be taken to avoid words that are likely to frighten or confuse, and all discussions should be direct but compassionate. An instinctive assessment of the patient's level of comprehension should be made. Do not quote an endless stream of statistics—they generally are only meaningful to options traders, actuaries, and gamblers. If the risk of infection is 1%, explain that in your experience 'only one out of a hundred' patients is likely to get an infection, but add that this can usually be treated easily with antibiotics. Spend a few minutes discussing the issue of 'scarring'. This issue is of great concern to patients, often because of an unrealistic expectation of the final aesthetic result and familiarity with others who have had suboptimal skin surgery.

In our experience, scarring is the outcome of greatest concern to most patients. It is important to be explicit about the fact that there will be a scar and that it is the natural consequence of healing. We explain that scarring is actually the end result of the amazing ability of the body to heal. And we explain that the issue is not whether there will be a scar—there will most definitely be one. The issue is whether it will be noticeable. Explained in these terms, we are comfortable that the patient is best prepared for the healing process that will ensue.

As part of the informed consent procedure, we provide a hand-held mirror so that the patient can see the extent of the lesion and probable length of the scar that we outline. It is important to explain the concept of dog-ears and that in order to correct such 'darts' (a term well-understood by people who sew) the scar may be lengthened. No one likes surprises in this situation which is why it is valuable to give an explicit description of what the surgeon will be doing and why it is good medicine. The informed consent discussion and written consent should include references to the risk of bleeding, infection, recurrence of the lesion, damage to pertinent nerves, and an unsatisfactory cosmetic result. Other treatment options should also be described, at least verbally. Finally, offer to answer any remaining questions and have the patient sign the informed consent.

In the case of an adverse outcome, the patient might claim that they did not understand what they were signing, but a proper and detailed discussion can prove such a claim to be false.

Anesthesia

Introducing the local anesthesia is often a source of great anxiety for the patient. There are many techniques to minimize the fear induced by the 'needle' and 'injection.' Before proceeding with this step, which often requires patience and much skill, the lesion must be carefully marked and the excision outlined with respect to the evaluation already performed. Mark important landmarks, such as the vermillion border, which might be distorted by the introduction of the local anesthetic. The most popular markers are Gentian violet and indelible felt-tipped markers. The latter offer the advantages that they are slow to dry out and do not spill. Gentian violet markers have a limited and unpredictable lifespan. Dry markers are ineffective. In addition, Gentian violet may 'tattoo' if not cleaned off before closing the wound.

The method used to inject the anesthesia will be remembered by the patient more than anything else the surgeon or surgical assistants do. The patient will recall whether the procedure was gentle or not, whether it was very painful or minimally so, and whether it was done with compassion. All patients fear needles, and fear accounts for a great proportion of perceived pain. With an enhanced anesthetizing procedure, the patient will do well throughout the rest of the operation. Follow these simple guidelines:

- If lidocaine with epinephrine (adrenaline) is used as the anesthetic, buffer it with 8.4% sodium bicarbonate to reduce the acidity and minimize the burning and stinging sensation caused by the injection; mixing one part of 8.4% sodium bicarbonate with ten parts of lidocaine with epinephrine (adrenaline) will raise the pH to above the neutral range[4]
- Use a 2.5-cm 30-gauge needle to permit wide distribution of the anesthetic
- Gently pinch the area to be injected, taking advantage of the gate theory of pain, and inject slowly because some pain is associated with tissue expansion caused by the solution[5]
- Do not perform multiple needle-sticks through the epidermis—introduce the needle only once, using a fan-like method to distribute the anesthetic throughout the surgical field, injecting slowly while the needle is advanced around the lesion.
- If the lesion is large and multiple sticks are unavoidable be sure that the second injection is in an area that is already numb (a ring block is especially helpful for very large excisions because it limits the amount of anesthetic used and decreases the risk of toxicity)
- Remember basic skin anatomy and target the dermal neural plexus for maximally efficient anesthesia
- In anatomic areas of concern, such as the temple, the surgeon may want to add anesthetic solution to swell or tumesce the area to protect underlying structures

Prepping and draping

After the patient is anesthetized, the surgical area should be prepped with antiseptic and draped. This is a critical step, but it should be noted that the risk of serious infection in skin surgery is quite low and that the level of antisepsis used for general surgical cases is not achieved in the office setting nor, apparently, is it required. However, every effort should be made to prepare the surgical site in an appropriate fashion. Popular prepping agents include povidone-iodine, chlorhexidine, and pHisoDerm (Chattem Inc, Chattanooga, TN). Povidone-iodine can cause contact allergies[6] and chlorhexidine can cause keratitis with prolonged contact.[7] Ototoxicity has been reported from chlorhexidine gaining access to the middle ear.[8]

The surgical site should be cleansed in an outward-spreading spiral, which begins from the center of the planned surgery. The cleansing agent should remain on the skin for the requisite period of time necessary for full effectiveness.

■ TECHNIQUES

Elliptical excision

The classic simple excision is most commonly known as the ellipse or fusiform excision. The procedure is based on a design that bears a length to width ratio of 3 to 1 or 4 to 1 with the apical angles ranging from 30° to 75° (Fig. 18.1).[9] This design is intended to eliminate any redundancies or dog-ear formation at the apices as the circular defect is transformed into a linear closure. The final result of such an excision should be a long thin scar which conforms to anatomic contours. As mentioned earlier, the excision should be designed to take advantage of anatomic 'hiding places'. Rhytides, relaxed skin tension lines, and borders of cosmetic units can all be used to advantage. In most instances, excision along the relaxed skin tension lines is

An ellipse or fusiform excision line

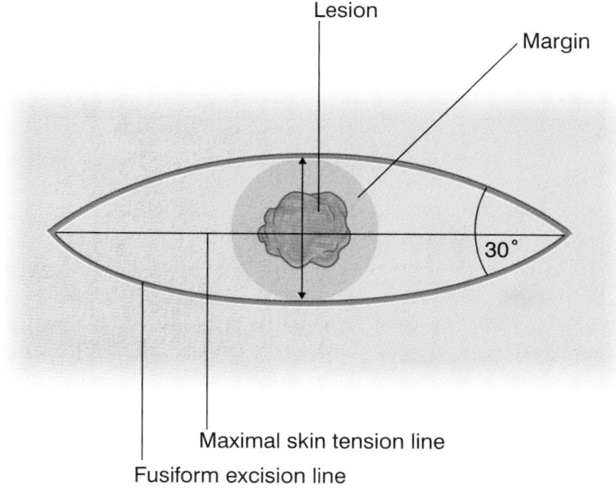

Figure 18.1 An ellipse or fusiform with a length to width ratio of 3 to 1 or 4 to 1 and 30° to 75° angles at the apices. Modified with permission from Leffell DJ, Brown M. Manual of skin surgery. New York: Wiley-Liss; 1997: 154. Copyright © John Wiley & Sons.

advantageous (a notable exception is the forehead where a mid-forehead excision perpendicular to the relaxed skin tension lines—a vertical excision—may offer a superior result).

When designing the ellipse, the size of the lesion, including the margins of normal skin necessary for appropriate removal, must be considered. Basal cell and squamous cell carcinomas that are well demarcated should be excised with a minimum margin of 4 mm if the Mohs micrographic surgery technique is not used.[10] It is generally considered that severely atypical nevi and melanoma in situ require a 5-mm margin.[11] Margins for invasive melanoma are based on the Breslow level of invasion. For optimal closure all excisions must be extended into the subcutis or else approximation of wound edges will be impeded.

After the surgical site has been marked, anesthetized, and prepped and draped, the surgeon's technique becomes paramount. The incision must be directed, smooth, and confident. In our experience, novice skin surgeons tend to make short, ragged incisions along the length of the ellipse when in fact a smooth incision at approximately 10° to the outside of the wound is required (Fig. 18.2). The point of the blade makes the initial cut at the apex, then quickly the sharper belly is used to move along the arc. Traction of the surrounding area is critical and if no assistants are available the surgeon must learn how to use the non-dominant hand, or must rest the fifth finger of the dominant hand on adjacent skin to apply mild tension on the surgical site. The incision should be carried down to subcutis on the first pass. On the back, where the dermis is very thick, this is not always possible although use of a #10 blade can facilitate a smooth percutaneous incision. The specimen can be marked with a suture for orientation either while the specimen is still in situ (to avoid errors), or after it has been completely removed. Using a toothed forceps, grasp the specimen at one of the apices and gently elevate it. Then dissect in an even plane, using scalpel for sharp dissection, or scissors for blunt dissection. If properly executed, there should be a fusiform defect with smooth, even walls and base.

Bleeding is normal, especially in more vascular areas such as the scalp and face. Meticulous hemostasis should be achieved. Do not underestimate the effectiveness of direct pressure. Holding firm pressure over the area with gauze even for a few minutes will significantly decrease the amount of oozing. When pressure alone is insufficient, the use of electric or heat cautery should be employed. While heat cautery will work in a wet field, electrocautery is only

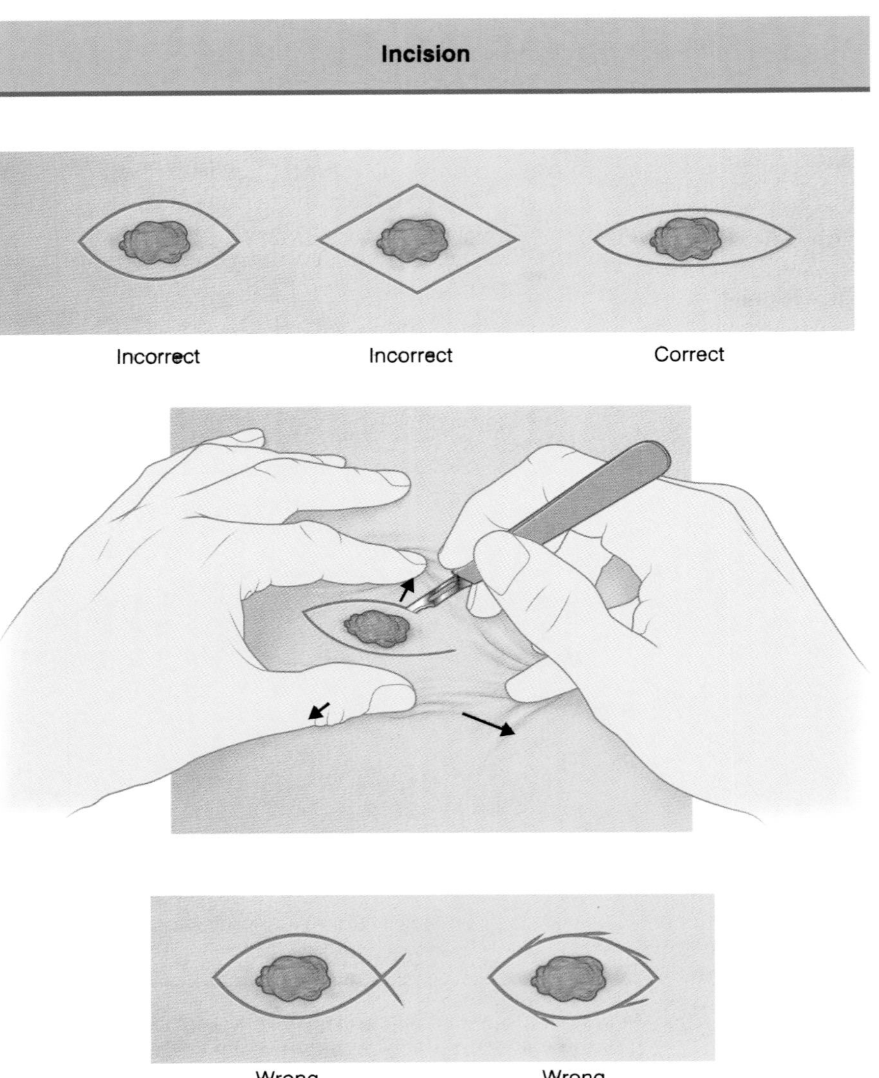

Figure 18.2 Incision. In order to avoid a jagged edge, use firm confident strokes. Using the non-dominant hand to provide tension is also helpful. Modified with permission from Leffell DJ, Brown M. Manual of skin surgery. New York: Wiley-Liss; 1997:156. Copyright © John Wiley & Sons.

effective in a dry field. Quickly dabbing the area with gauze or rolling a cotton-tipped applicator over the area prior to cautery enhances its effectiveness. Vacuum suction is often required to obtain a clear field if there is moderate to severe bleeding. To help decrease unnecessary tissue damage and char, pinpoint cautery is preferred. Remember the phrase 'visualize—then cauterize.' The surgeon cannot treat what the surgeon cannot see. Random cautery is ineffective and may be harmful because it causes unnecessary thermal tissue damage. For larger vessels, cautery may not suffice and the vessel should be ligated with 4-0 or 3-0 absorbable suture. A hemostat can be used to identify and isolate the bleeding end of the arteriole or artery prior to ligating.

Once hemostasis is achieved, repair of the defect can begin. It is not unusual to have persistent wound-edge bleeding from the dermal plexus, especially in individuals with ruddy skin. It is not necessary to cauterize this tissue as the bleeding will stop promptly once the wound is sutured closed. While cautery enhances outcomes and minimizes bleeding complications, it should always be used judiciously.

It is a widely held belief that undermining the surrounding skin is required to close any wound. In fact, undermining is only needed to the extent that it is necessary to minimize tension on the wound. If the skin surrounding the surgical site is intrinsically lax from photodamage or chronologic aging, and the wound can be approximated without undermining, it is quite appropriate to do so. Moreover, in patients on anticoagulants or platelet inhibitors, excess undermining increases the risk of bleeding and hematoma. In some larger, deep defects, absorbable sutures can be placed in the subcutis to decrease the tension and eliminate the need for undermining.[12]

When undermining is required, it must be done carefully and meticulously. Regardless of whether sharp or blunt techniques are used, the surgeon must have in mind a clear understanding of the local anatomy: severing motor nerves or large vessels because of poor technique is an adverse outcome. Use of a skin hook is very helpful when undermining as it allows lifting of the wound edge with minimal tissue damage. The hook should be held perpendicular to the surface of the wound to permit maximal exposure of the wound bed. Some prefer to use a forceps, but care must be taken to avoid crushing the wound edge. If needed, undermine around the whole ellipse, including the apices. Often undermining alone at the apices will obviate the need for excising small dog ears. To evaluate the adequacy of the undermining, use two skin hooks and bring the sides together. If they do not come together easily, further undermining might be helpful. After the undermining is complete inspect the base of the wound and the undersurface of the undermined tissue for bleeding. Remember that when epinephrine (adrenaline) is used as an anesthetic ingredient, vessels can go into spasm, only to relax and bleed 2–3 hours after surgery. For this reason the surgeon must identify and cauterize any vessels that might be at risk.

With the wound properly prepared, and hemostasis complete, the layered closure can be initiated. This consists of the use of absorbable deep sutures and a non-absorbable superficial suture. There are variations with respect to how the epidermis can be closed and some defer epidermal closure completely if approximation of wound edges is otherwise excellent.

If there is little tension on the wound, closure by halves is the rule. The first suture is placed in the center of the wound. Next, each half of the remaining defect is repaired in a similar fashion. If there is tension on the wound it might be beneficial to simulate the 'zipper' effect: start suturing at the apex and close the wound incrementally by placing a deep dermal suture every 3 mm. This helps reduce the tension as the repair advances down the defect. The buried vertical mattress suture is suggested by some to provide optimal wound eversion (Fig. 18.3).[13] The buried suture, regardless of the technique used, is the foundation of the repair and will have the greatest impact on the final result. Precise placement is critical. Remove improperly placed sutures and reposition as needed.

Once the buried sutures have been placed, proceed with the superficial epidermal layer. The goal of this component is epidermal approximation. In areas with no tension and good subcutaneous approximation, these additional sutures may not be needed. In such cases adhesive tapes such as Steri-strips (3M Surgical Products, St Paul, MN) applied with an adhesive such as Mastisol (Ferndale Labs, Ferndale, MI) can be used. Alternatively, octylcyanoacrylate tissue adhesive (Dermabond (Ethicon, Summerville, NJ) is expensive but popular. Glustich (Glustitch Inc, Delta, BC, Canada) is a similar medical adhesive and is much less expensive.

The typical epidermal sutures can range from 4-0 to 6-0 monofilament. On the lip, silk may be used. Where additional hemostasis is not a concern, a running suture effectively achieves rapid, excellent approximation (Fig. 18.4). Because tension is less predictable with this method, simple interrupted sutures should be used if better approximation or hemostasis is required (Fig. 18.5). Similarly, if it becomes necessary to open the wound to find the source of postoperative bleeding or to place a drain, it will be possible to open a few sutures and not have to remove an entire running suture. All sutures should be snug, but not so tight that they strangulate the tissue.

Running locking sutures, which provide additional hemostasis may be used on the ear or genitals where blood supply is plentiful and unlikely to be compromised by the locking suture (Fig. 18.6). Finally, in areas where the skin naturally inverts (e.g. forehead creases) vertical mattress

Buried vertical mattress suture

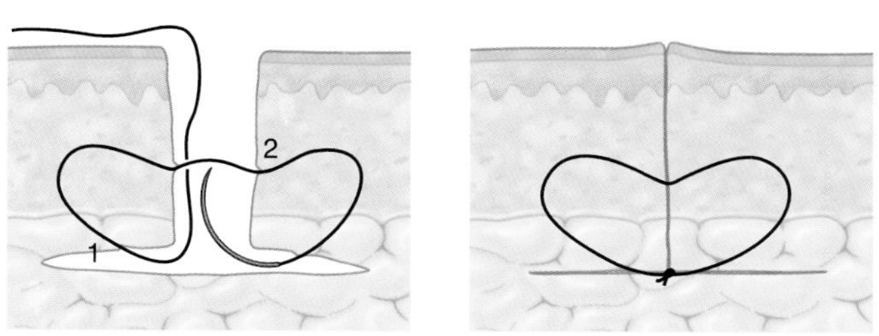

Figure 18.3 Buried vertical mattress suture. Placement of buried suture using the vertical mattress technique may enhance wound eversion resulting in an improved final result. Numbers indicate entry points of the needle. (See also Fig. 16.14.) Modified with permission from Zitelli JA, Moy RL. Buried vertical mattress suture. J Dermatol Surg Oncol 1989; 15:17–18.

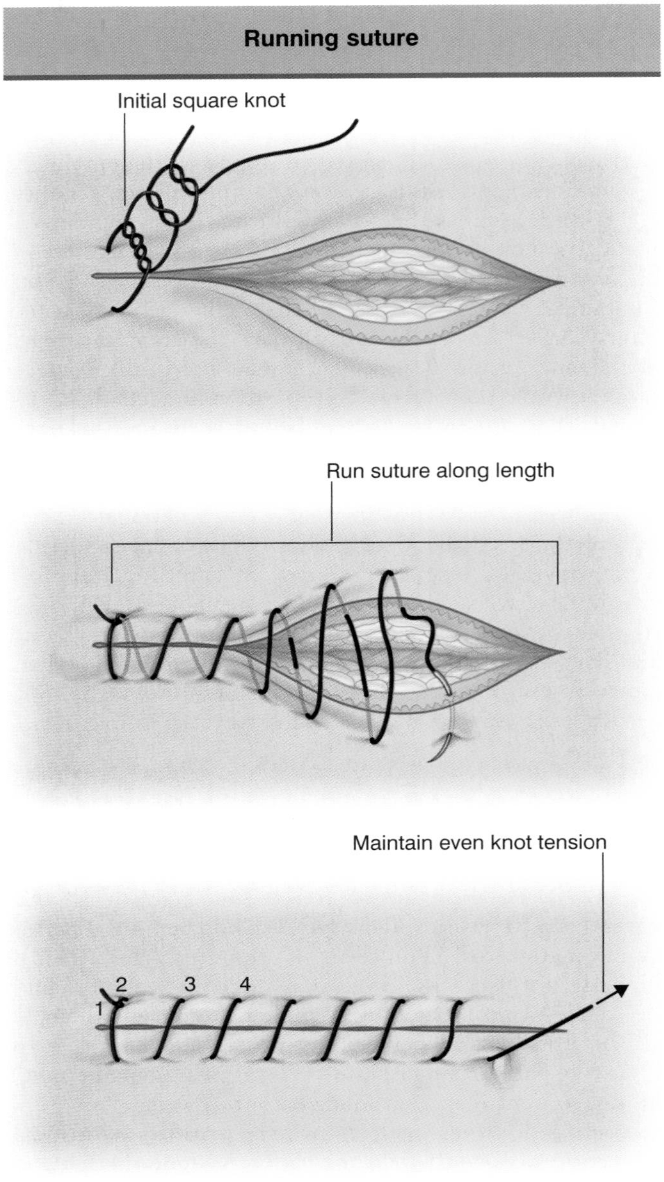

Running suture

Initial square knot

Run suture along length

Maintain even knot tension

2 3 4
1

Figure 18.4 Running suture. The running suture should be placed approximately 1 mm from the wound edge and advanced down the linear repair every 2–3 mm. If the repair is long (>3 cm) it is advisable to tie off the suture at intervals and continue running the suture. The tie provides more knot security and enhances suture tension. Numbers indicate entry points of the needle. (See also Fig. 16.11.) Modified with permission from Leffell DJ, Brown M. Manual of skin surgery. New York: Wiley-Liss; 1997:169. Copyright © John Wiley & Sons.

Placement of epidermal sutures

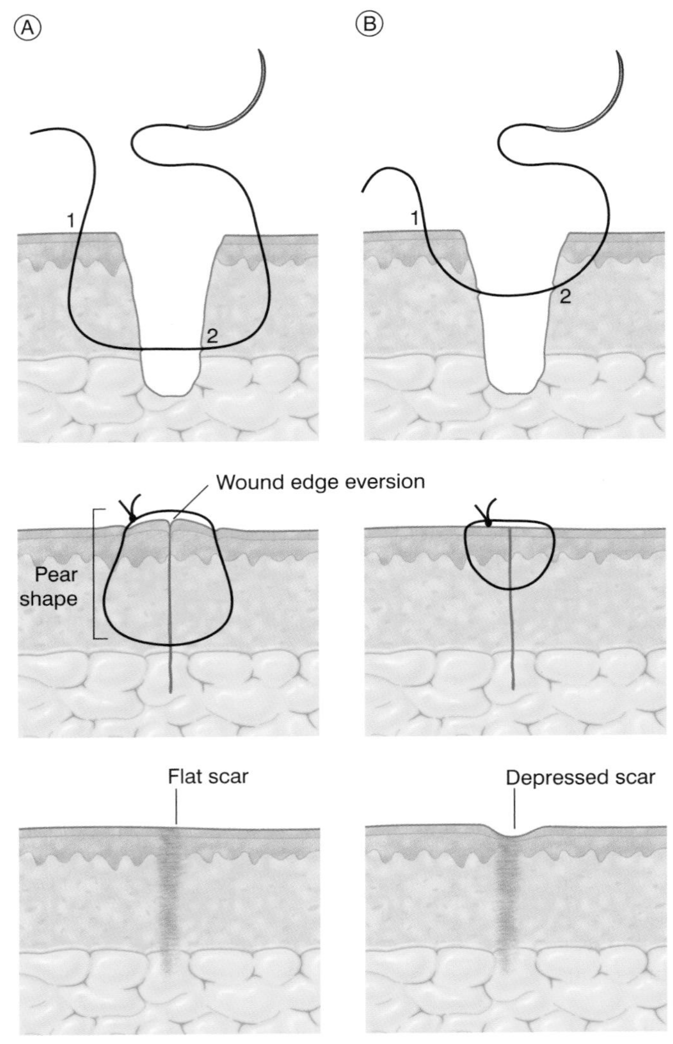

Figure 18.5 The simple suture is the workhorse of all cutaneous surgery. A square knot is used to secure the wound edges and the knot should be placed off to the side rather than overlie the incision where the suture material can interfere with healing. Numbers indicate entry points of the needle. (See also Fig. 16.16.) Modified with permission from Leffell DJ, Brown M. Manual of skin surgery. New York: Wiley-Liss; 1997:168. Copyright © John Wiley & Sons.

Optimizing outcomes

- Remember that a shorter scar is not necessarily a less noticeable scar; the choice of technique should be based on location, the patient's needs, and their level of activity.
- If there is uncertainty about the proper orientation of the final repair, first excise the lesion as a circle and observe the actual relaxed skin tension lines.
- Consider second intention healing if the cosmetic result is likely to be superior to reconstructive repair.
- Crescent excision takes advantage of sides of unequal length and is helpful on the cheek or chin.
- M-plasty is a useful method when the scar would otherwise encroach on neighboring functional or cosmetic structures.
- S-plasty achieves a superior cosmetic result on convex surfaces such as the jaw and extremities.

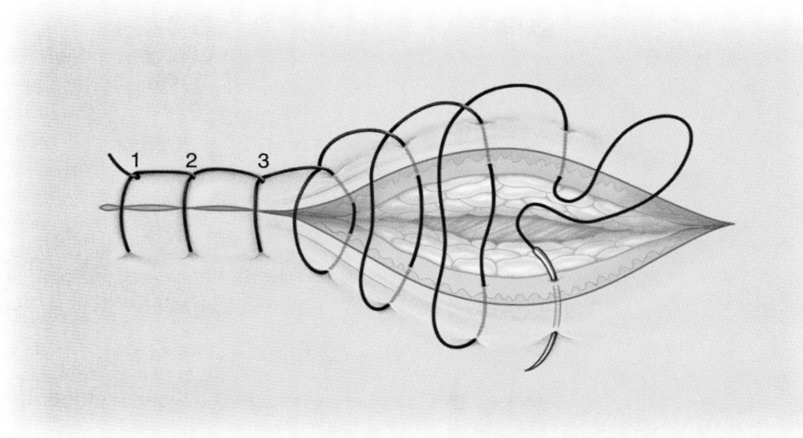

Figure 18.6 Running locked stitch. The running locking suture provides added hemostasis in areas of substantial blood supply and at risk of oozing, it is also helpful in certain situations for patients on anticoagulants and/or platelet inhibitors. Numbers indicate entry points of the needle. (See also Fig. 16.12.) Modified with permission from Leffell DJ, Brown M. Manual of skin surgery. New York: Wiley-Liss; 1997:169. Copyright © John Wiley & Sons.

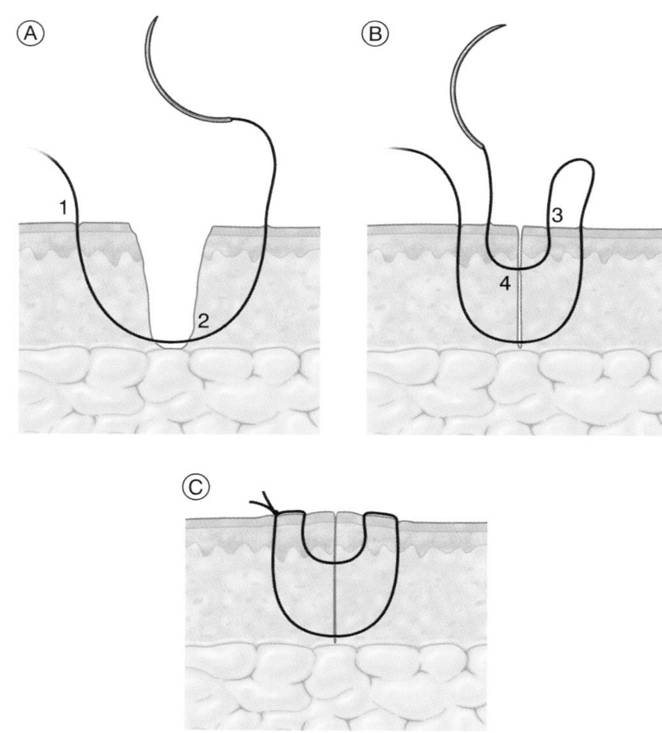

Figure 18.7 The vertical mattress suture. The vertical mattress suture is effective at enhancing wound eversion. This facilitates a finer final scar where natural wound edge inversion is a tendency. Numbers indicate entry points of the needle. (See also Fig. 16.7.) Modified with permission from Leffell DJ, Brown M. Manual of skin surgery. New York: Wiley-Liss; 1997:170. Copyright © John Wiley & Sons.

sutures are very helpful. An occasional vertical mattress stitch may help in proper eversion (Fig. 18.7).

After the suturing is complete ensure that there is no active bleeding. This is best accomplished by firmly rolling a cotton-tipped applicator along the suture line. There should be only minimal oozing which disappears with subsequent rolls. If there is continued bleeding, apply firm pressure with gauze for 5 minutes by the clock. Finally, if bleeding through the wound persists, it must be opened and the wound bed examined for any active sources of bleeding.

Crescent excision

There are variations to the standard ellipse that may provide superior results, depending on location or specific situations. The crescent excision which takes advantage of sides of unequal length, can result in a shorter curvilinear scar which can be cosmetically superior to a longer straight scar. The crescent repair is a versatile one that is often helpful on the cheek and around the chin. When evaluating the patient in the sitting position, note the natural rhytides. The arc of the crescent will determine the final result so orient the arc in the direction of the natural lines (Fig. 18.8). These must be closed by the rule of halves in order to avoid any redundancies. Even with this approach small redundancies at either end of the wound may have to be removed. If so, direct the final scars so they are well hidden.

M-Plasty

The M-plasty is a simple and effective method for reducing the length of the scar when it otherwise would encroach on neighboring functional or cosmetic structures. Instead of extending the fusiform excision beyond its apex, as one would normally do to excise the redundant cone of skin or dog ear, an M-plasty can be designed to remove the excess skin while allowing the limbs of the repair to be well-concealed (Fig. 18.9). The M-plasty can be designed prior

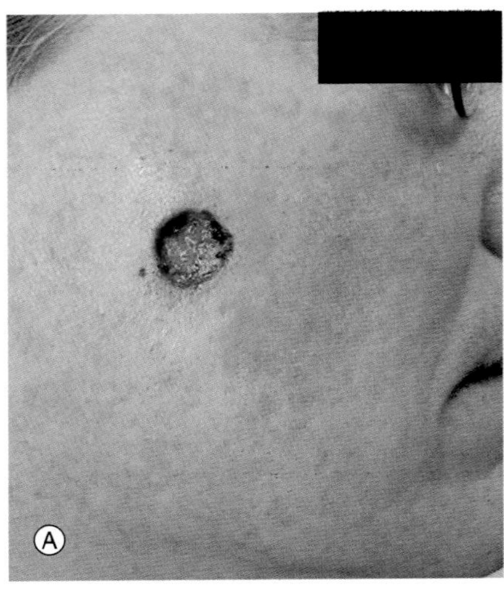

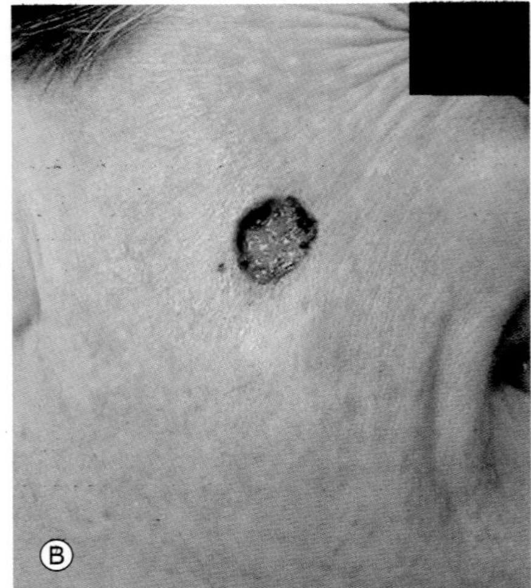

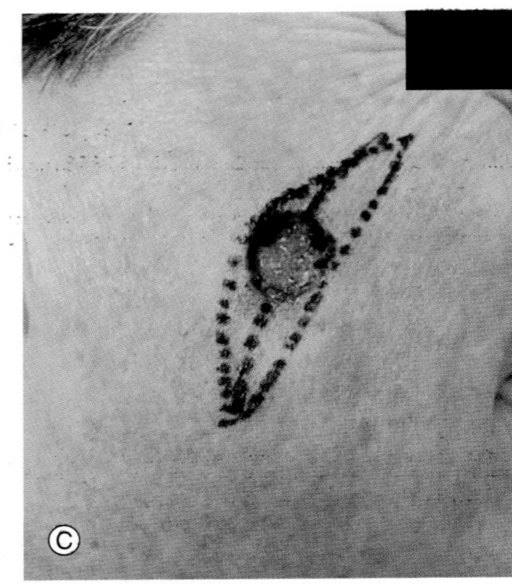

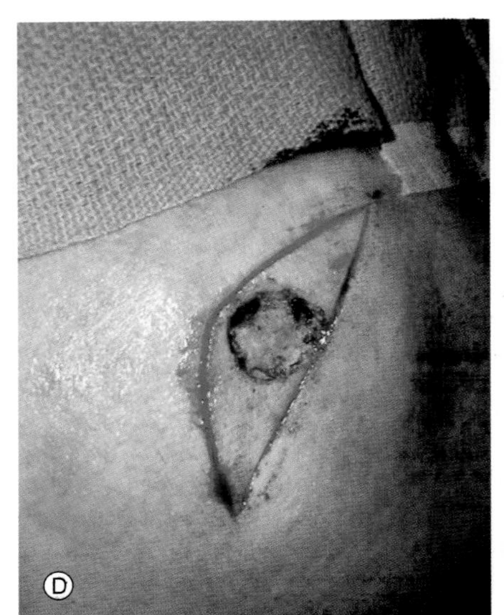

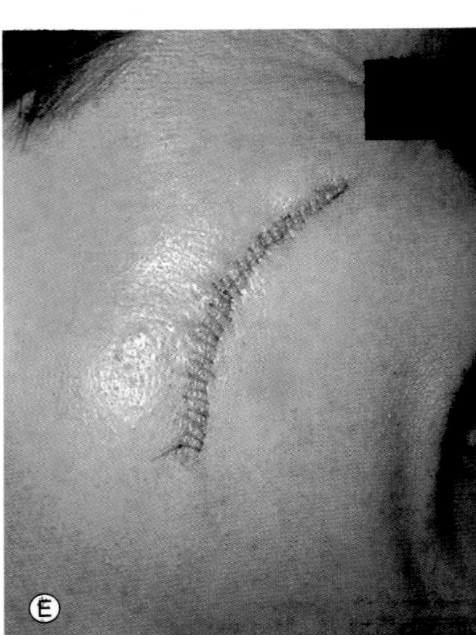

Figure 18.8 (A) Circular defect on the cheek following removal of a basal cell carcinoma utilizing the Mohs method. (B) The patient is asked to show his teeth to accentuate the natural lines of expression. (C–D) Crescent designed to result in a curvilinear line that follows the natural relaxed skin tension lines. (E) The crescent repair permits a final scar that is well-hidden within the natural lines of facial expression. Note that the original circular wound is modified so that the sides of the repair have unequal lengths. Reprinted with permission from Leffell DJ, Brown M. Manual of skin surgery. New York: Wiley-Liss; 1997. Copyright © John Wiley & Sons.

to the excision, or if indicated, during the completion of the repair. When planning the excision, envision a typical ellipse but draw an 'M' shape instead of the apical tip at approximately one quarter of the length of the ellipse. When used to remove a dog ear, the 'M' shape is formed by lifting the excess tissue with a skin hook and making incisions with 45° angles on both sides of the standing cone. Proceed by draping the tissue over the incision lines and remove the redundant triangles on each side. A tip stitch is helpful when performing an M-plasty.

S-Plasty

Another variation of the ellipse is the S-plasty or Lazy S repair. This repair is used to achieve a superior cosmetic result when working on convex surfaces such as the jaw and extremities (Fig. 18.10). Although a standard fusiform will heal well initially, as the scar contracts over time the repair may become depressed or buckled. By elongating the scar through the use of an S-plasty, where both sides of the ellipse are designed in the shape of the letter 'S,' the contraction will occur over a greater length, which will minimize buckling of the scar. This is important to understand since all scars can contract up to 30% in length over time.

Partial closure

When excising benign lesions one should be careful to calculate that a complete closure is possible so that the final cosmetic result is superior to the appearance of the lesion itself. With malignant tumors, the defect is determined by the extent of the cancer. At times the health of the patient, or the patient's wishes, suggest consideration of second intention healing. Although most wounds will heal well by second intention, this process can often be facilitated by performing a partial closure. One option is to begin the closure at the apex where there is the least amount of tension and to proceed to close like a zipper. When the wound edges can no longer be approximated, the closure can be commenced at the opposite apex, working towards the center of the wound. Often, as the repair progresses, tissue creep will allow complete closure at the center. A pulley stitch (3-0 monofilament) left in place for approximately 20 minutes prior to closure may also enhance complete approximation. Finally, even if it is not possible to join the wound edges completely at the center, satisfactory healing will usually occur at this site by second intention healing (Fig. 18.11). The final scar will usually take on the linear conformation of the sutured ends of the wound.

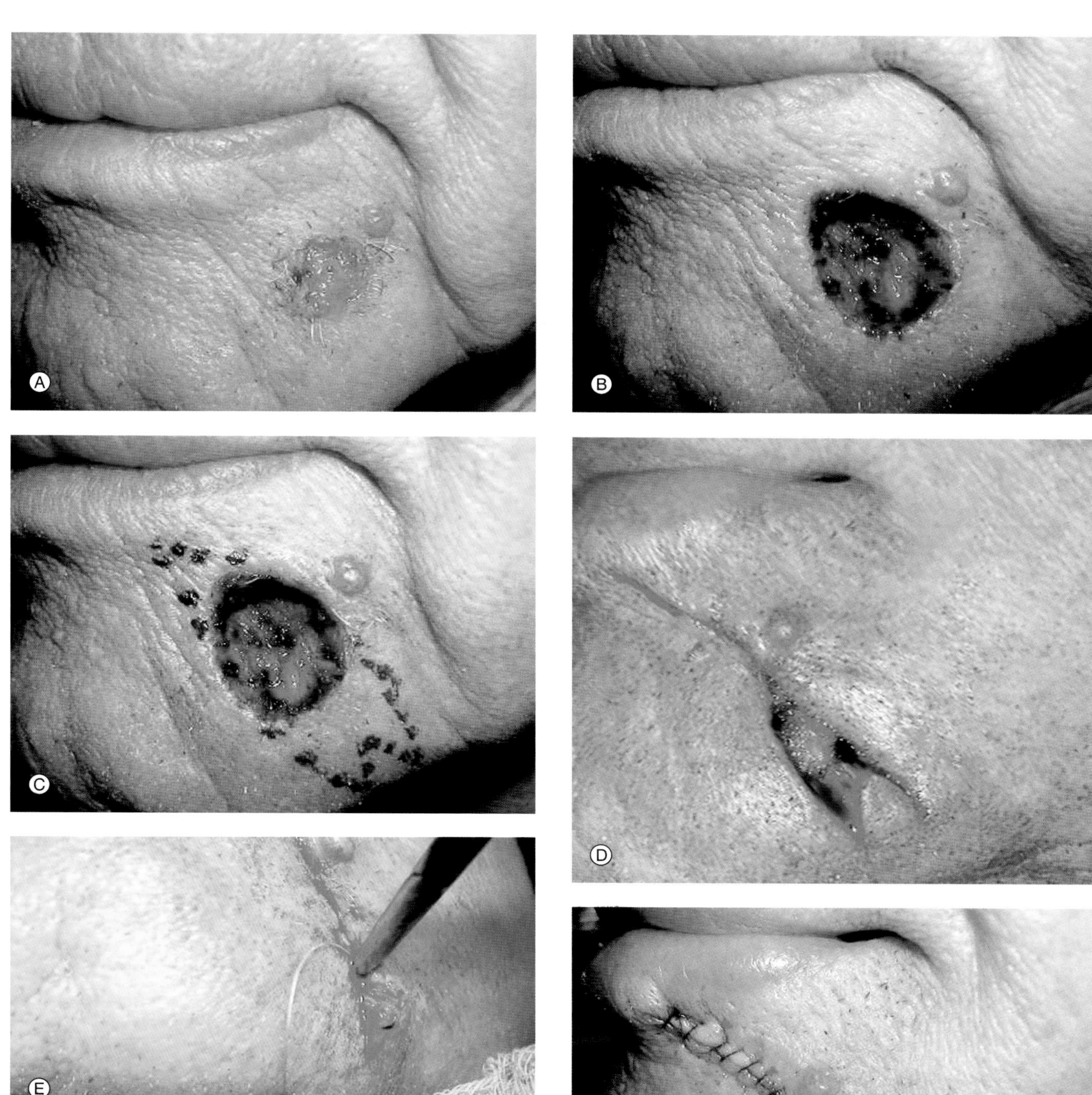

Figure 18.9 (A) Basal cell carcinoma on the chin. (B) Circular defect status after Mohs micrographic surgery. (C) M-plasty designed to avoid crossing over into a new cosmetic unit. (D)–(E) A tip stitch may be used to complete the M. (F) Final result shorter scar remains within one cosmetic unit. Reprinted with permission from Leffell DJ, Brown M. Manual of skin surgery. New York: Wiley-Liss; 1997. Copyright © John Wiley & Sons.

Dog-ear repairs

Even the best-planned and designed ellipse may result in redundancies at one or both ends. The dog-ear repair will correct these imperfections, which can be quite noticeable and distracting even when small. Skillful management of standing cones of redundant skin, created by the transformation of a circular defect into a linear repair, will contribute substantially toward a superior cosmetic result. The novice surgeon is frequently fearful of excising excess 'normal' skin. However one must remember that it is not the length of the scar that is important but how noticeable it is when finally healed. A long fine line with no protrusions is far superior to a shorter scar with puckers. The removal of even a few millimeters of excess will greatly improve the

Lazy-S repair

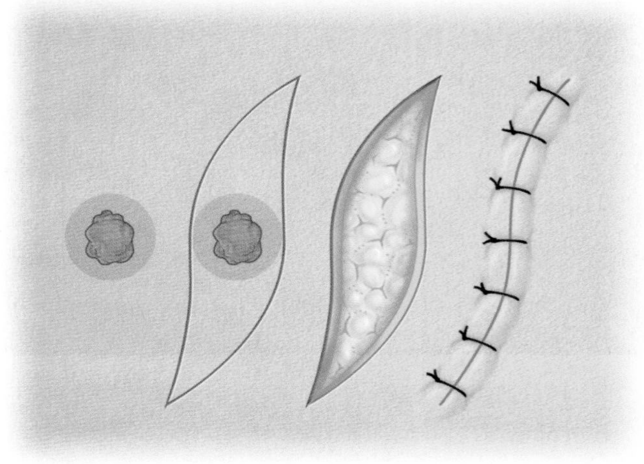

Figure 18.10 The Lazy-S repair is designed by juxtaposing two S-shaped incisions around the defect. By approximating the center of each slightly offset S to the other, the final repair becomes a smooth serpentine line which contracts over convex surfaces with minimal buckling. Reprinted with permission from Leffell DJ, Brown M. Manual of skin surgery. New York: Wiley-Liss; 1997. Copyright © John Wiley & Sons.

outcome. It is helpful to explain this concept to the patient so there is less surprise at what is inevitably a longer 'scar' than they might have expected. Remind them that over time the scar will become less noticeable. Repair of dog ears can be accomplished in several ways

Most often the standing cone of excess tissue can be removed in a linear fashion by extending the incision. To do this, lift the apex of the cone with a skin hook or just gently squeeze the excess between the thumb and index fingers of the non-dominant hand. Using the scalpel, make a straight incision from the apex through the center of the cone. There should now be two individual triangles which, when incised at their bases, will extend the original incision line linearly (Fig. 18.12). An alternative to this method is excision of another small ellipse at the point of redundancy.

In many instances, a curved line will be less conspicuous than a linear one. This is especially true when dealing with excisions on the face where there are natural rhytides, smile lines, and relaxed skin tension lines. The hockey-stick or curved method of dog-ear repair allows the surgeon to take advantage of these natural creases and create an optimal outcome (Fig. 18.13). Once again start by elevating the apex of the excess tissue with a skin hook or forceps. Gently pull the cone in the direction of the desired final incision. Start from the end of the original excision and make a curved incision in the desired location. The

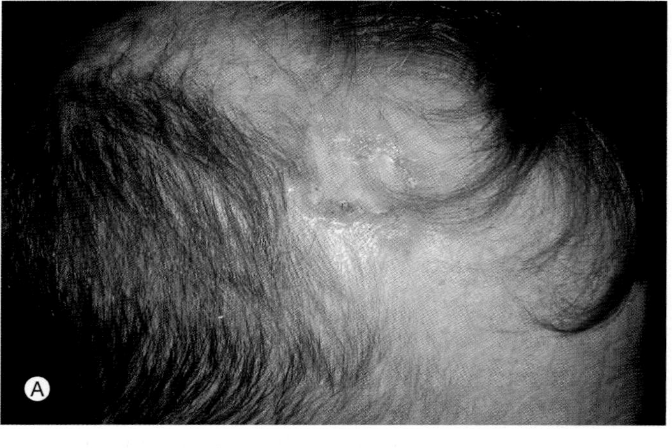

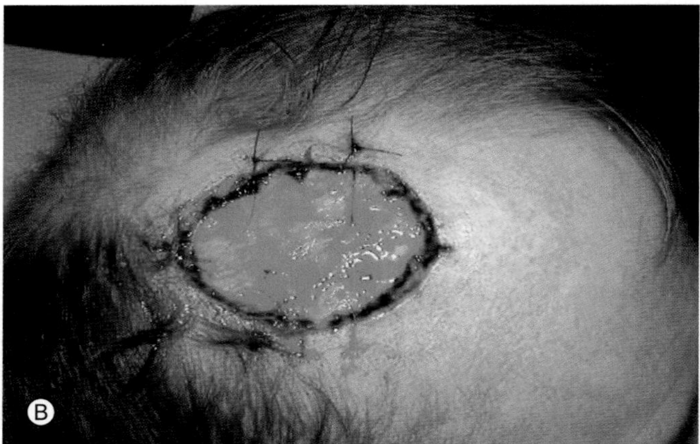

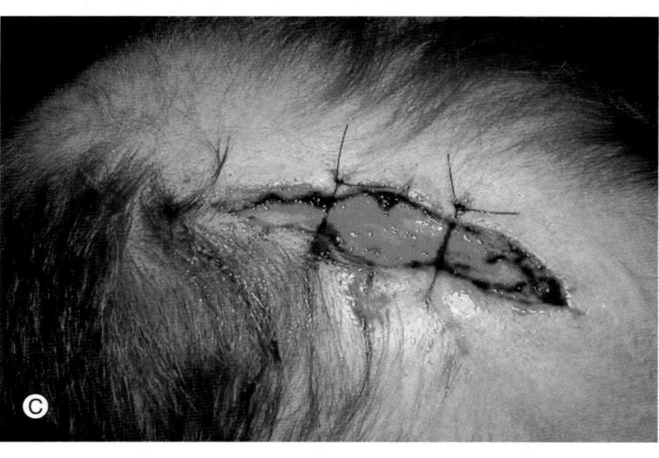

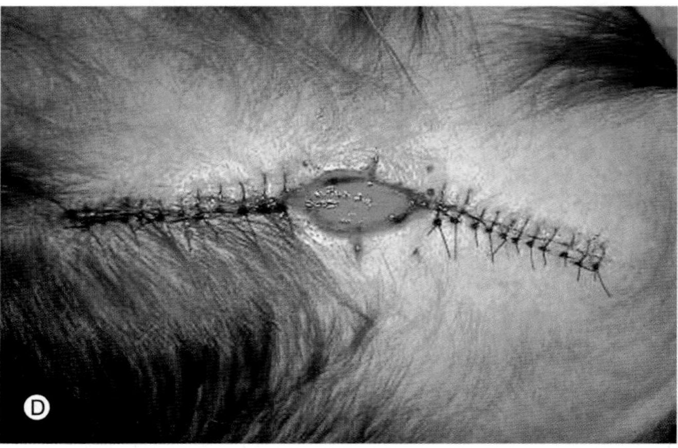

Figure 18.11 (A) Large basal cell carcinoma on the parietal scalp. (B) Defect after Mohs micrographic surgery. (C) Pulley stitches act as an intraoperative tissue expander. (D) Closing the wound from the apices and "zippering" towards the center leaves only a small wound to heal by second intention, thus reducing healing time. Reprinted with permission from Leffell DJ, Brown M. Manual of skin surgery. New York: Wiley-Liss; 1997. Copyright © John Wiley & Sons.

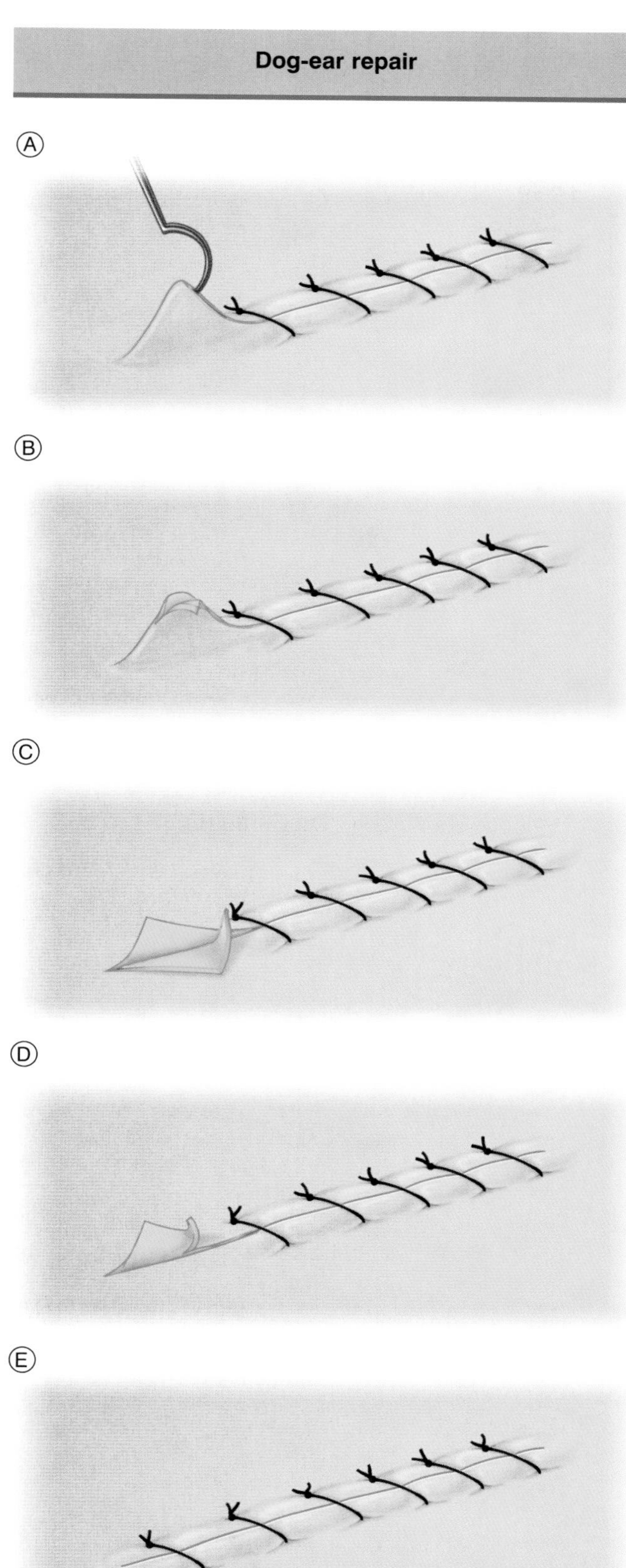

Figure 18.12 In this dog-ear repair, the excess cone of skin is incised so that the final scar is an extension of the linear closure.

remaining triangle of skin can then be draped down over this curved incision line and excised along the curved line. Remember that the first incision will determine the direction of the line. It may be helpful to lightly score the tissue with the scalpel prior to making a full-thickness cut. Some prefer to score with a scalpel and then excise the dog ear with a sharp scissors.

An L-shaped repair is similar to the curved repair but after lifting the cone at the apex, an incision is made at a 90° angle to the original suture line, forming an 'L' shape. The triangle is draped over the incision and removed at its base. The T-shaped correction is the same, but is bilateral so as to form a 'T.' In most instances a curved repair gives a superior result.

■ POSTOPERATIVE CARE

When the closure is complete, a pressure dressing is placed on the wound and postoperative instructions are given to the patient. There are many bandage variations but they all generally consist of triple antibiotic ointment layer, followed by a non-adhesive layer (e.g. Telfa (Kendall, Mansfield, MA)), a pressure layer (gauze), and a semi-elastic surgical tape. Alternatively, skin glue or paper adhesive strips may be used in place of epidermal sutures or in conjunction with absorbable epidermal sutures such as fast-absorbing gut sutures. In these cases daily wound care is not required. Regardless of the dressing used, application of pressure to the wound site in the first 24 hours is, in our experience, beneficial. After removing the dressing the wound should be cleansed with tap water to gently remove any crust. We avoid hydrogen peroxide despite its continued popularity as it has been shown to be cytotoxic to cells *in vitro* and adds no benefit to the healing process. Patients should be instructed to pat dry and reapply a thin layer of ointment, a non-stick gauze, and paper tape. Should there be a thick adherent crust, a wet gauze should be placed on the wound for 5–10 minutes. This will help loosen the crust and allow it to be removed with minimal discomfort or damage. The patient may shower after the first 24 hours but should be careful not to allow the forceful stream of water to hit the wound directly. Advise the patient that there may be swelling and bruising as well as some oozing from the wound. This is especially true for excisions in the periocular region.

These basic wound care instructions should be given both orally and in writing. If a family member or friend will be handling the care, be sure to review it with them. Potential adverse events such as bleeding and infection, and steps to take if they occur, should be thoroughly reviewed. Be sure to provide a contact number so that the patient can bring up any questions or concerns.

Sutures on the face and neck are generally removed in 5–7 days and those on the trunk and extremities can be removed at 7 days if adequate buried sutures have been placed. Leaving sutures in too long will result in permanent suture marks which are unsightly. When removing the sutures it is best to have the patient in a comfortable supine or prone position. After carefully removing the sutures, apply a liquid adhesive (e.g. Mastisol) and wound closure tapes (e.g. Steri-strips). The strips help keep the epidermal edges approximated and occluded allowing for additional epidermal proliferation. The strips can be removed in

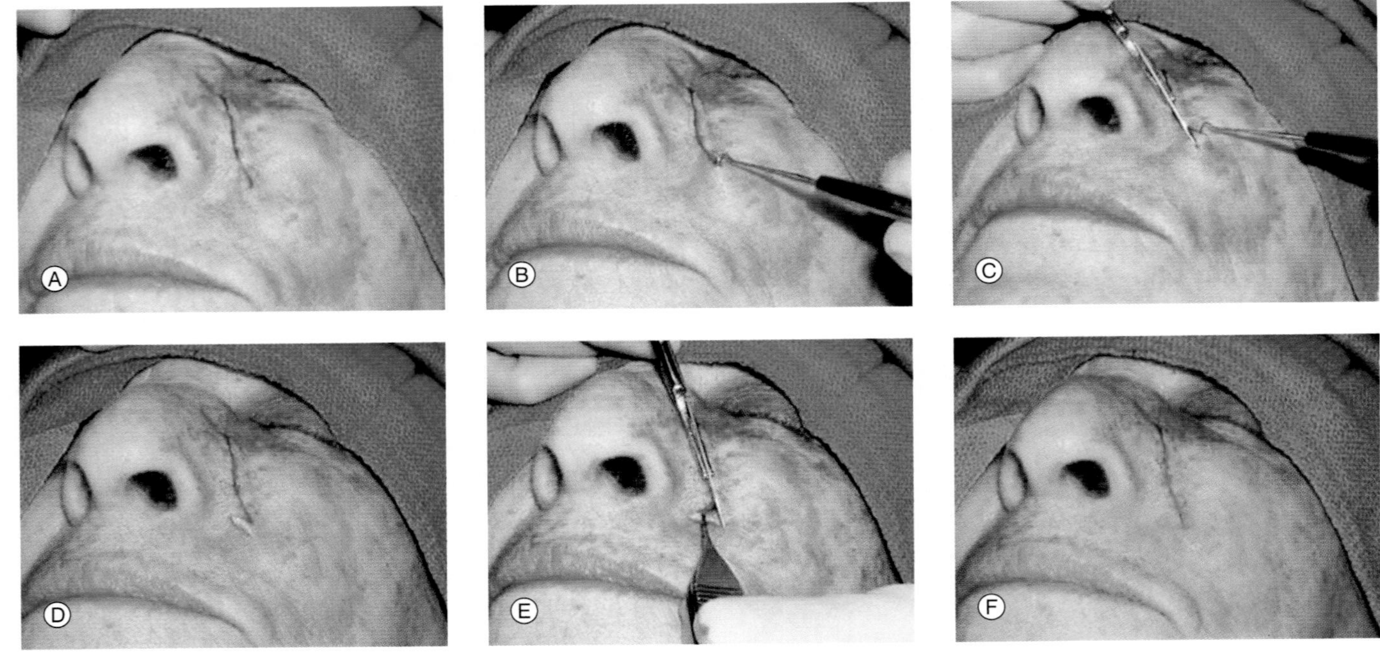

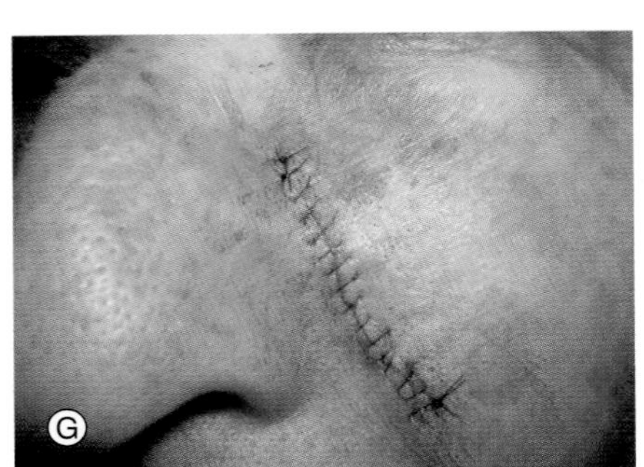

Figure 18.13 (A) Excess tissue after a linear closure of a wound on the medial cheek. (B) Using a skin hook or forceps the apex is pulled to one side and (C) a curved incision is made. (D) The tissue is then draped over the incision line, and (E) the redundancy is removed along the curved cut edge of the incision. (F)–(G) Suturing is then completed. Reprinted with permission from Leffell DJ, Brown M. Manual of skin surgery. New York: Wiley-Liss; 1997. Copyright © John Wiley & Sons.

3–5 days and the patient may apply make-up at that point if desired. Remind the patient that the final outcome of the scar cannot be determined until a full year has elapsed. Patients will very often ask about the use of vitamin E or other products to enhance wound healing. There is no evidence that vitamin E enhances the appearance of the final scar or the 'speed' of healing but it is so ingrained in the popular imagination that we do not strongly discourage it. Massage and the application of polyurethane foam or silicone patches may be beneficial in some patients in the early stages of healing.

PITFALLS AND THEIR MANAGEMENT

When surgeons operate frequently enough they eventually experience complications; that is the nature of the imperfect discipline of medicine. With the elliptical excision and its variants there are four major categories of complications: bleeding, infection, dehiscence, and scarring. The importance of clear and explicit communication with the patient both preoperatively and postoperatively cannot be overstressed. If the patient is clearly informed about the possibility of complications, and how they can be managed, the impact of any complication will be minimized. The surgeon should always remain accessible to patients, so that problems or potential problems can be heard at an early point when they might be easier to resolve.

Intraoperative bleeding was discussed earlier, but if there was extensive bleeding during the surgery one must anticipate the possibility of postoperative bleeding as well. The placement of a drain at the surgical site may help prevent the collection of fluid and hematoma formation.

Avoidance of pitfalls

- Extensive intraoperative bleeding increases the possibility of postoperative bleeding; placement of a drain may help prevent fluid collection and hematoma formation.
- Scrupulous use of sterile technique, careful tissue handling, and closure without tension reduce the likelihood of infection.
- In the areas more prone to infection (intertriginous areas, the extremities, and exposed cartilage) use acetic acid soaks and/or antibiotic prophylaxis.
- If infection does occur treat it empirically with antibiotics for Staphylococcus aureus, the most likely cause of infection, but if there is drainage send specimen for culture and modify antibiotic choice accordingly.
- Advise patients preoperatively that at least some scarring will occur, particularly where there is significant tension as on the shoulders and upper back.
- Warn patients that incompletely dissolved sutures are not uncommon and that they should return for prompt treatment if this happens.

The surgeon can use either a Penrose drain or a gauze wick for this purpose. If a drain was not placed and the wound continues to bleed despite firm pressure for 15 minutes, or if there is an expanding collection of blood beneath the suture line, surgical intervention is necessary. The patient should be positioned comfortably, prepped and draped. Local anesthetic may be needed, but avoid using one containing epinephrine (adrenaline) as it can cause vasoconstriction and mask the source of the bleed. Remove the sutures and open the wound. Clean out any collection of blood and irrigate with saline. Carefully search for any obvious arterial pumper that may be the cause. Most of the time the source is less obvious and there is generalized oozing. Be thorough in the search for the source of the bleeding as it may be coming from beneath an undermined edge. Use cautery and suture ligation to stop the bleeding. During the first 24 hours one can safely resuture the wound but it may be preferable to leave it open to heal by second intention. After it has healed completely a scar revision can be performed. In either case the patient should be placed on antibiotics to avoid infection.

When the bleeding is slower a hematoma may develop over a few days and only become apparent to the patient several days later as an enlarging tender (or non-tender) mass. If the hematoma is small and stable and there is no concern about infection, observation is acceptable. Alternatively, draining the hematoma will facilitate healing and avoid the development of excess scar tissue. If any compromise of wound healing is suspected, the surgeon must remove it. Although an 18-gauge needle is usually sufficient to aspirate the hematoma, opening the wound may be necessary. If the wound is open at this point, it should be left to heal by second intention.

Infection rates in office-based skin surgery range from 1–3%.[14,15] While mild wound infections with erythema and swelling are most common, abscess formation and even systemic infection can occur. Immunocompromised patients are obviously at greater risk but the operative technique and anatomic location also play a role. Using sterile technique, prepping the patient properly, careful handling of the tissue, and closure without tension will all decrease the chance of infection. Intertriginous areas such as the perineum and axillae, as well as the lower extremities, are more susceptible to infection.

Exposed cartilage, especially on the ear, is likewise at an increased risk of infection, particularly *Pseudomonas* infection in diabetic patients.[13] Thus, in such instances acetic acid soaks and/or prophylactic anti-pseudomonal antibiotics are recommended. Although it may be difficult to distinguish routine postoperative erythema and swelling from true infection, if the postoperative pain is increasing rather than decreasing, and other classic signs of infection are present, one must suspect infection and treat appropriately.

Most superficial skin wound infections are caused by *Staphylococcus aureus* so empiric treatment with the appropriate antibiotic is reasonable. If there is drainage a specimen should be sent for culture, and sensitivity and antibiotic coverage modified if necessary once the culture results are obtained. Any collection of fluid or abscess formation should be drained and sutures should be removed. The wound should be packed with iodoform gauze and changed daily until there is no more drainage. Once again, the wound should be left to heal by second intention and repaired in the future if necessary.

There is no such thing as scarless surgery but there is such a thing as an optimal scar. Never promise the patient that there will be no scar. In fact it is best to be explicit about the fact that there will be a scar but that every effort will be taken to make it minimally noticeable. The patient must understand that a scar is unavoidable and that in many instances the final outcome is not in the hands of the surgeon, but is subject to the impact of genetics and anatomic location.

Hypertrophic scars and keloids are thickened, raised scars (see also Chapter 44). Keloids are in fact tumors of scar tissue that extend beyond the wound margins. Hypertrophic scars tend to resolve with time. Both tend to occur in areas of high tension, such as the chest, upper back, and shoulders. Those with a personal or family history are at greater risk. In either case, scar revision may lead to worsening of the condition and therefore treatment generally consists of intralesional steroids, and topical pressure devices or garments.

If a thickened scar is anticipated, preventive intralesional steroid injections as well as pressure dressings may help reduce its severity.

In areas of significant tension, the scar may spread or widen rather than thicken. This occurs most often on the shoulders and upper back. Patients should be advised of the likelihood of this outcome.

Erythema and telangiectasias may also develop as the scar matures and these can quite easily be treated with a pulsed dye laser. Alternatively, electrocautery at the lowest possible setting using an insulated epilating needle can be used to eradicate these small vessels. Patients should understand that in most cases the redness will resolve with time.

Incompletely dissolved or 'spitting' sutures are not uncommon and patients should be educated about this possibility. Spitting buried sutures usually occur at 3–6 weeks postoperatively and appear as small pimples, pustules, crusting, or blood blisters along the suture line. When not warned about this in advance, patients are quite concerned that this is an infection or a recurrence of the lesion. Treatment consists of removal of the suture fragment. It is important to do this early so that it does not fester and cause an unsightly, persistent foreign body reaction.

■ SUMMARY

The ellipse or fusiform excision is the workhorse of cutaneous surgery. It is the foundation and basis for all other advanced surgical techniques. A thorough understanding of the ellipse and its variations is essential for anyone involved in surgery of the skin. The surgical result will be optimized by careful planning, and this should include attention to detail as highlighted by the maxim 'measure twice—cut once.'

■ REFERENCES

1. Kovich O, Otley C. Thrombotic complications related to discontinuation of warfarin and aspirin therapy perioperatively for cutaneous operation. J Am Acad Dermatol 2003; 48:233–237.
2. LeVasseur JG, Kennard CD, Finley EM, Muse RK. Dermatologic electrosurgery in patients with implantable cardioverter–defibrillators and pacemakers. Dermatol Surg 1998; 24:233–240.

3. Dajani AS, Taubert KA, Wilson W, et al. Prevention of bacterial endocarditis: recommendations by The American Heart Association. Clin Infect Dis 1997; 25:1448–1458.
4. Stewart JH, Cole GW, Klein JA. Neutralized lidocaine with epinephrine for local anesthesia. J Dermatol Surg Oncol 1989; 15:1081–1083.
5. Arndt KA, Burton C, Noe JM. Minimizing the pain of local anesthesia. Plast Reconstr Surg 1983; 72:676–679.
6. Marks JG. Allergic contact dermatitis to povidone-iodine. J Am Acad Dermatol 1982; 6: 473–475.
7. Hamed LM, Ellis FD, Boudreault G, et al. Hibiclens keratitis. Am J Ophthalmol 1987; 104:50–56.
8. Bicknell PG. Sensorineural deafness following myringoplasty operations. J Laryngol Otol 1971; 85:957–961.
9. Mody BR, McCarthy JE, Sengelmann RD. The apical angle: a mathematical analysis of the ellipse. Dermatol Surg 2001; 27:61–63.
10. Thomas DJ, King AR, Peat BG. Excision margins for non-melanotic skin cancer. Plast Reconstr Surg 2003; 112:57–63.
11. Consensus Development Panel on early melanoma. Diagnosis and treatment of early melanoma. JAMA 1992; 268:1314–1319.
12. Dzubow LM. The use of fascial placation to facilitate wound closure following microscopically controlled surgery. J Dermatol Surg Oncol 1989; 15:1063–1066.
13. Zitelli JA, Moy RL. Buried vertical mattress suture. J Dermatol Surg Oncol 1989; 15:17–19.
14. Futoryan T, Grande D. Postoperative wound infection rates in dermatologic surgery. Dermatol Surg 1995; 21:509–514.
15. Cook JL, Perone JB. A prospective evaluation of the incidence of complications associated with Mohs micrographic surgery. Arch Dermatol 2003; 139:143–152.

19 Layered Closures, Complex Closures with Suspension Sutures and Plication of SMAS

Edgar F Fincher MD PhD, Hayes B Gladstone MD, and Ronald L Moy MD

Summary box

- Facial skin is divided into discrete cosmetic subunits whose aesthetic characteristics are derived from regional variations in the composition of the underlying tissue layers. Careful attention to restoring these subunits during reconstruction is critical.
- The human face is composed of an interrelated functional unit of muscle, connective tissue, and overlying skin that should be treated as a single unit to obtain optimal results.
- Layered closure is crucial in optimizing the ultimate outcome of cutaneous reconstruction. Careful re-approximation of the individual tissue layers to restore the disrupted integrity of skin must be obtained.
- Human skin has both viscoelastic and anisotropic characteristics. Understanding these tissue properties and their effects during flap manipulation and skin closure are fundamental principles of cutaneous surgery.
- Suspension sutures are effective in stabilizing the skin against the opposing vector forces of the elastic dermis and the forces of gravity, and are used in both reconstructive and cosmetic surgery.
- Performing complex closures often requires the use of a combination of techniques (flaps, grafts and primary closure) to obtain optimal results.

INTRODUCTION

Successful surgical reconstruction and enhancement of the face requires a comprehensive knowledge of the anatomy of the skin and its underlying support structures as well as an understanding of tissue biomechanics and the tension vector forces at play. Surgeons must combine this knowledge with skilled wound closure techniques to maximize the outcome.

The responsibility of the surgeon, whether it be for reconstruction of a defect following tumor extirpation or for cosmetic enhancement of the aging face, is to recreate or enhance the normal anatomy to ensure proper form and function. Many times, this simply requires the re-approximation of existing landmark structures without disruption of any underlying deep tissue. However, the surgeon is often faced with reconstructing a large full-thickness defect after tumor excision or alternatively, is asked to recreate what time and nature has altered. To achieve optimal functional and cosmetic results, tissue layers must be moved, repositioned, and reconstructed in a manner that will overcome tissue deficits or redundancies and forces opposing wound closure.

This chapter will examine the functional anatomy and biomechanics of the skin and will review fundamental principles that are applicable to complex wound closures. An approach to treating the skin as an integrated multi-layered structure will be presented along with relevant surgical techniques that have been developed for the reconstruction and enhancement of this integrated unit. Special consideration will be given to surgical reconstruction and enhancement of the head and neck.

HISTORICAL VIGNETTE

In 1976, Mitz and Peyronie published their landmark paper[1] identifying the presence of a subcutaneous musculoaponeurotic system (SMAS) in the head and neck. In this report, they proposed the benefits of using suspension sutures from the SMAS flap to the pretragal area to provide superior results in both rhytidectomy and repair of facial nerve palsy. This concept revolutionized approaches to facial rejuvenation and reconstructive surgery of the head and neck.

PREOPERATIVE PREPARATION

Fundamental objectives of wound closure

Successful design of wound closure begins with an understanding of cosmetic subunits, tissue biomechanics, and anatomical layers of the skin and subcutaneous tissues. Structurally, the integument is best thought of as a multi-layered unit of epidermis, fibrous connective tissue, subcutaneous adipose tissue, and muscle that provides structure and texture to the skin. Regional variations in the relative composition of these layers provide the characteristic textural qualities of various anatomical sites. These regional variations in skin quality and texture and their resultant qualitative effect upon the aesthetic appearance of the skin are most notable in the head and neck region. Careful attention to these regional variations is paramount for planning a reconstruction that best recreates the natural appearance. When primary closure is not an option, careful selection of local skin flaps and skin grafts that match both tissue color and texture of the recipient site will provide the best cosmetic outcome.

A second fundamental principle that should be obeyed when planning closures on the head and neck is to respect the natural lines of demarcation. Aesthetically, the face is composed of multiple cosmetic subunits (Fig. 19.1). Natural skin folds, variations in tissue thickness and composition, and the underlying bony structure collectively create the natural lines of demarcation along these subunits. In most cases, these subunits have a corresponding symmetrical unit on the contralateral face. These natural undulations and demarcations of the face define the individuality of the patient and the primary challenge to the reconstructive surgeon is to restore this symmetry and individuality to the patient. Planning a reconstruction so that incision lines fall within the boundaries between these cosmetic subunits will provide the least conspicuous scar.[2] A scar that passes within a single subunit or that crosses lines of demarcation between two subunits can disrupt the natural contour and symmetry of the face and will be most apparent. Adhering to this fundamental principle often means using larger than necessary tissue flaps or resecting extra tissue so that suture lines can be placed within the boundary to avoid disrupting the subunit. Although this technique can be more laborious and may create a larger than necessary defect, ultimately it will yield a superior cosmetic result.

Defects that cross boundaries between cosmetic subunits, are often best repaired using a combination of flaps (complex repairs) or special suturing techniques (i.e. tacking or suspension sutures) to redefine the disrupted lines of demarcation. Complex repairs and suspension sutures in reconstructive surgery are the primary focus of this chapter and a more thorough discussion of the principles and applications of these techniques will be presented in later sections.

Functional facial anatomy

A comprehensive knowledge of anatomy is a prerequisite for successful reconstructive or cosmetic surgery. Tissue layers consist of epidermis, dermis, subcutaneous adipose, fascia, and muscle. Each of these layers has its own inherent specific characteristics, but it is the collective contribution of these different layers that contributes to the overall integrity and texture of the skin. In the head and neck, these layers are interconnected through a series of interdigitating adhesions that enable the human face to function as an integrated unit. The activity of specific combinations of facial muscle groups is transferred to the overlying skin through this connective tissue scaffolding and provides the functional capacity to perform complex maneuvers such as eating, drinking, kissing, and speech. These coordinated movements also provide humans with their characteristic ability for emotional expression through complex animated facial movements.

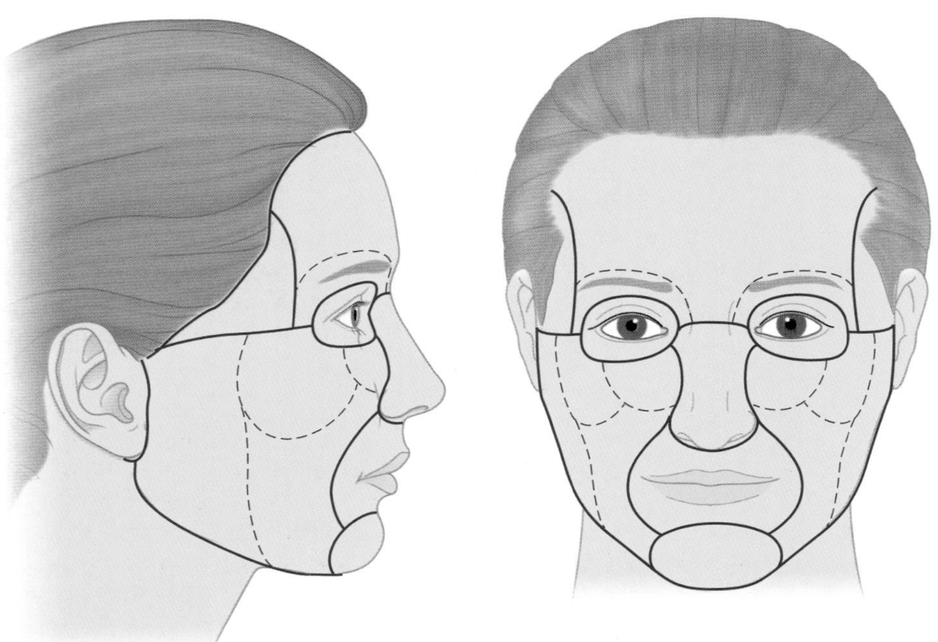

Figure 19.1 The major cosmetic units of the face, which are the cheek, nose, temple, forehead, periorbital area, perioral area, and the chin, may be subdivided. (For additional information, see Fig. 1.4.)

Before embarking upon a discussion of techniques for complex closures, it is pertinent to briefly review the major structural anatomy of the face. The underlying framework of the human face begins with the concrete origins of the bony skeleton. The topography of the cranium consists of prominences and valleys that not only create the aesthetics and individuality of the human face, but also serve as key anchoring points for facial muscles. For example, the forehead anchors the frontalis muscle against gravity and enables raising of the brow, the orbital rim provides structural support for the delicate sphincter muscles that protect the orbit, and the malar prominence and zygomatic arch are the anchor points that permit elevation of the upper lip. These and many other key anchoring points provide support for the facial structures, offset the forces of gravitational pull on the face, and permit normal functioning of the facial muscles.

Overlying the cranium and facial muscles is a continuous fascial layer. In 1976, Mitz and Peyronie[1] performed an elegant anatomical, histologic, and radiographic description of a fibromuscular fascial layer of the head and neck that they termed the superficial musculoaponeurotic system or SMAS.[1] This layer has attachments to the cranium and invests the facial musculature, forming an interconnected sling that both provides support to the facial structures and acts to integrate the functional activity of facial movements. The SMAS begins in the forehead as a continuation of the galea aponeurotica. It progresses inferiorly, being continuous with the temporalis fascia and zygoma laterally, and with the superficial parotid fascia and malar prominence in the preauricular zone and mid-face, respectively. The SMAS then crosses over the mandible to become continuous with the platysma and inserts into the clavicle, the pectoralis fascia and sternocleidomastoid fascia of the neck (Fig. 19.2). The SMAS is the unifying structural component of the face linking muscles of facial expression as an integrated network that enables the countless numbers of facial maneuvers. Facial muscles are linked to the SMAS through direct interdigitations as well as via several well-defined mid-facial ligaments.[3–5] These connections permit mimetic actions to be transferred to the SMAS and subsequently to the overlying skin.

The functional importance of the SMAS along with an understanding of the major bony attachments of the cranium cannot be overemphasized to the surgeon attempting complex closures of the face. Manipulation of these structures is crucial to overcoming opposing vector forces that resist closure of cutaneous defects to achieve optimal cosmetic results.

Functional skin biomechanics

The heterogeneous cutaneous anatomy contributes to the unique biomechanical properties of skin. Although most of these properties are derived from the dermal collagen and elastin, the subcutaneous fat, blood vessels, and nerves also play a role. Interestingly, the epidermis plays only a small role in skin deformation. Understanding these biomechanical characteristics not only enables the surgeon to choose the best option for a particular defect, but also to perform more precise closures.

Unlike other static materials such as steel, skin's stress–strain relationship varies with time. Skin is both viscoelastic and anisotropic meaning that its 'stretchability' is nonlinear. Movement of skin is also characterized by it's ability to stretch over time ('creep'), and at a certain point in the stress–strain curve to almost completely relax ('stress relaxation').[6] This quality is most likely because of the breakage of collagen fibers. Although studies have investigated these properties in porcine models, cadavers and intact human skin rather than incised living skin, the application of these principles to living skin biomechanics during cutaneous surgery has a number of important clinical implications. More recently, the use of computer-generated finite element modeling has increased our understanding of human skin biomechanical properties.[7–9]

The primary axiom of closing a wound without tension derives from these tissue mechanics. Increased tissue stretch affects the skin's microcirculation, most likely through a combination of narrowing of blood vessel lumina and by causing shear fractures.[7,8] This tension may also result in venous congestion that can compromise closures. While highly vascularized regions may withstand some degree of tension, poorly perfused areas are susceptible to necrosis. Knowledge of the regional anatomy is critical for understanding the appropriate tissue plane to undermine to reduce tension. Additionally, recognizing that after a certain point, undermining will not reduce closure tension, but will in fact increase the risk of adverse effects such as hematomas or nerve damage, is equally important.

Once the inherent properties and limitations of skin biomechanics are understood, it becomes evident that the properties of time-dependent creep and stress relaxation can be manipulated to aid in the closure of difficult defects. For example, the surgeon can take advantage of these properties when closing a linear defect whose width to length ratio is less than the optimal 1 : 3 proportions (i.e. excessive width). Multiple techniques are often applied to take advantage of the elastic properties of skin. Intraoperative tissue expansion can be performed by a number of methods. The rule of halves may be applied in suturing with each subsequent stitch leading to a progressive reduction of the tension across the wound. Or initially an interrupted suture or 'pulley-stitch' may be placed at the center of the wound to reduce tension while the remainder of the wound is closed. With the tension across the wound decreased, buried sutures can be placed more easily and more accurately. Once the deep layer has been sutured, the pulley stitch is no longer needed and can be replaced by a new layer of epidermal sutures. Alternatively, in many instances, one can begin suturing from one end of the wound toward the opposite pole. By approaching the closure in this manner, the surgeon is taking advantage of sequential wound creep.

Layered closures

The objectives for wound closure should be restoration of functional anatomy, recreation of anatomic form, and minimization of the visible scar. To achieve these ends, surgeons have employed a variety of suturing techniques and layered wound closure. Layered closure allows the surgeon to recreate the tissue planes that have been disrupted and provides strength to the wound as it heals.

Wound strength and elasticity are predominantly factors of the cross-linked dermal collagen and elastin fibers. The

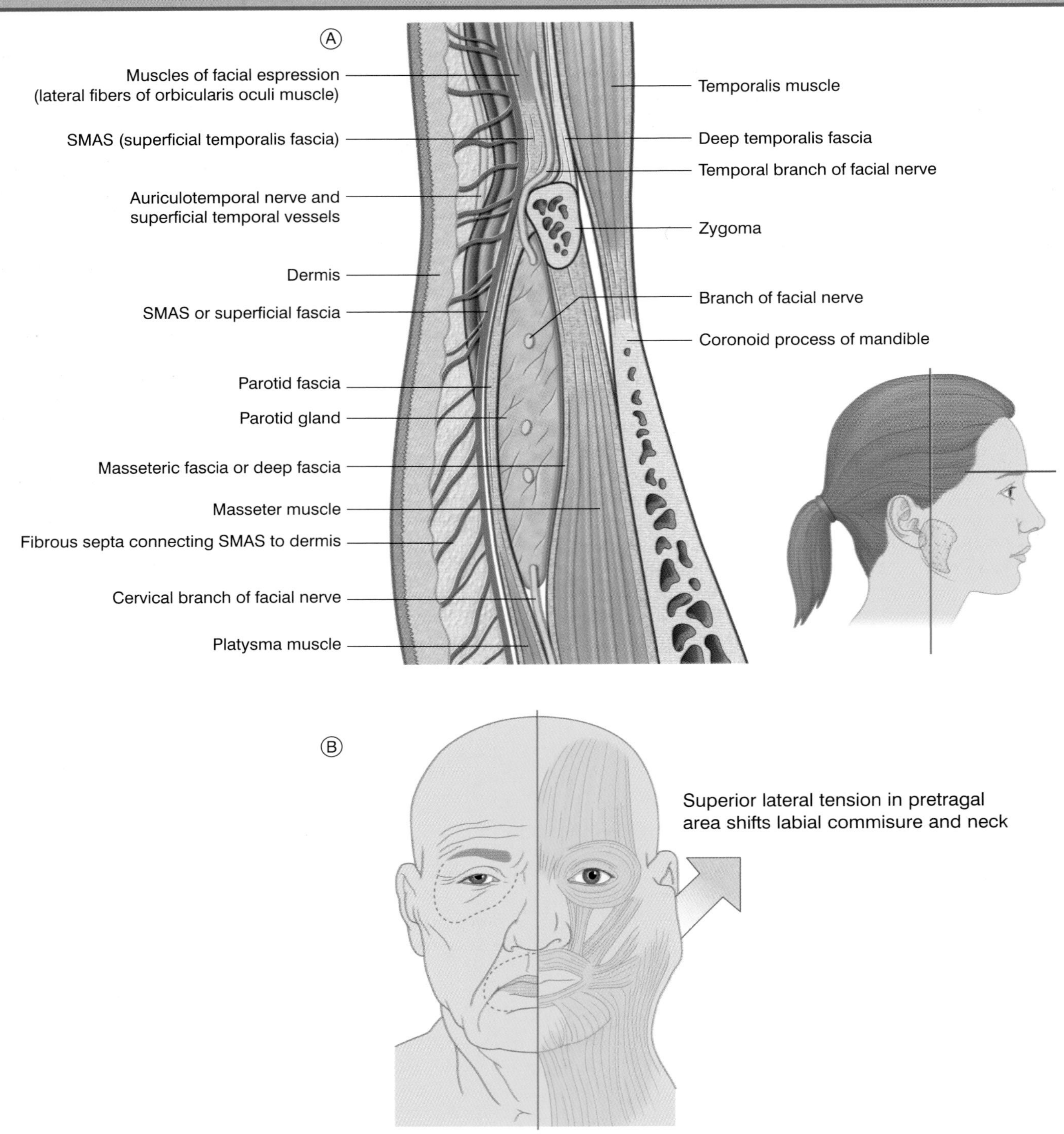

Figure 19.2 (A) Although the subcutaneous musculoaponeurotic system (SMAS) is a single connective tissue layer intricately connected to the muscles of facial expression, the scalp and forehead seem to be discontinuous with the lower face. The red pretragal line shows the location of the anatomical cross section. The blue line at the level of the brow indicates this demarcation of the scalp and forehead from the lower face. (B) The labial commissure and anterolateral neck skin are mobilized and shifted by tension on the SMAS in the pretragal area below the zygomatic arch (the area indicated by the red line in Fig. 19.2a).

inherent elasticity of the dermis becomes obvious upon disruption of these connective tissue layers. A full-thickness wound that severs the dermis leads to retraction of the wound edges with a net tension vector perpendicular to the direction of the wound or incision. As a result of this dermal retraction, the overlying epidermal wound edge becomes inverted into the wound. If left to heal naturally, the tendency will be for a wound to heal with a wide depressed scar. Successful wound closure must counteract these intrinsic forces to achieve acceptable cosmesis. Failure to do so can lead to poor tensile strength, scar retraction, and spreading.

Proper suturing technique of both dermal and epidermal layers is the key to successful wound closure. The dermal wound edges must be realigned in both horizontal and vertical orientations and the epidermis must be re-approximated accurately to create a wound without any visible step-off or undulations. Layered closure allows the surgeon to achieve these fundamental goals. First, a deep layer of sutures is used to close dead space and reestablish the elastic tensile strength/holding strength of the dermis. A superficial layer of sutures is then used to finish the wound. This superficial layer re-approximates epidermal wound edges to minimize scarring and provide maximal cosmesis. Because the deep layer holds tension and provides strength to the wound, the superficial layer can be placed under minimal tension and can be removed after 5–7 days after epithelialization has occurred and before any suture marks are left on the skin.

■ TECHNIQUES

Basic techniques of wound closure

The most unobtrusive scars are those that are narrow and smooth. These scars are best obtained through wound eversion and careful re-approximation of the edges (Fig. 19.3). Failure to evert a wound leads to a depressed scar following normal wound contraction. Poor alignment of the wound edges creates a high–low phenomenon that, upon healing,

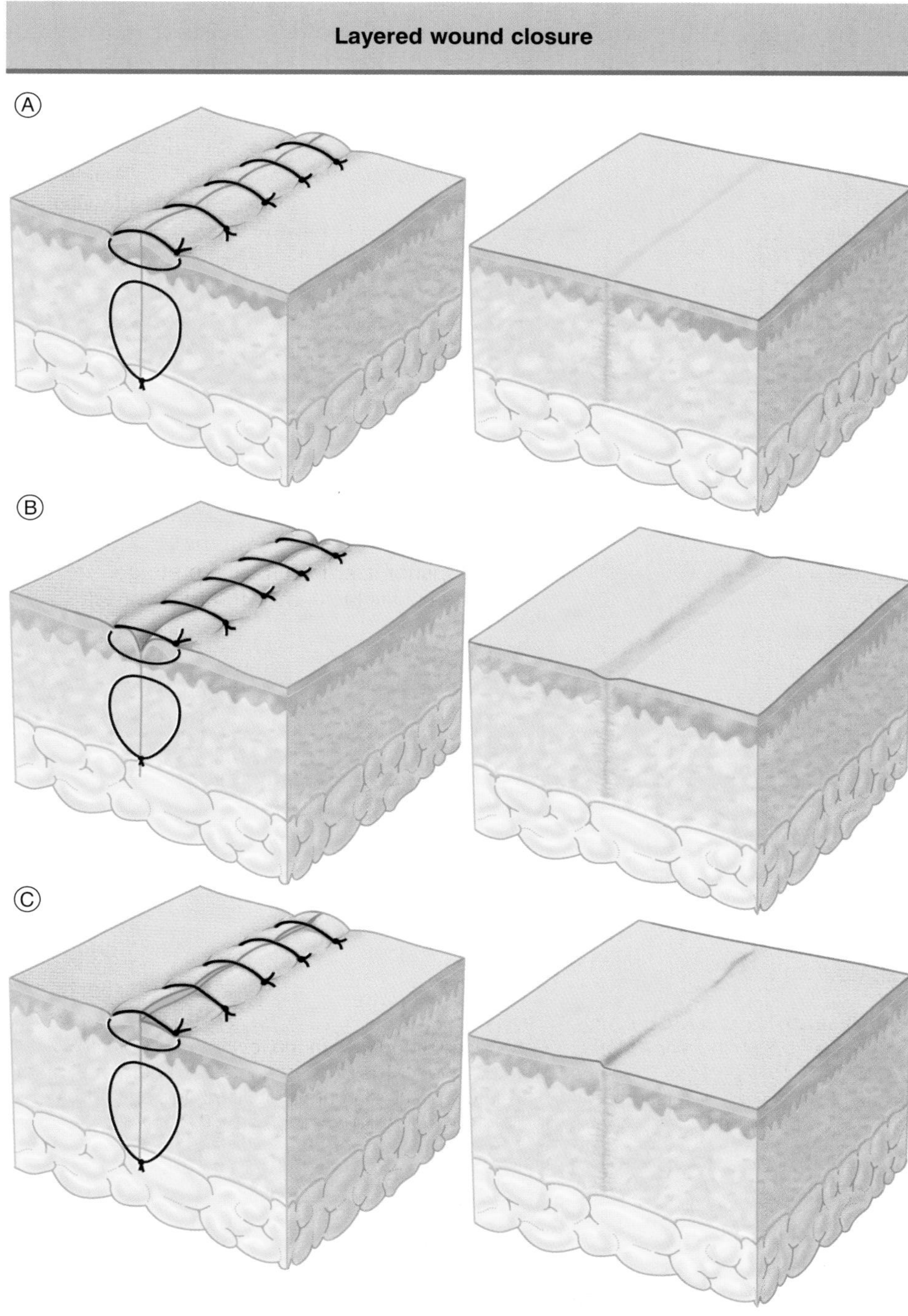

Figure 19.3 Layered wound closure. (A) Careful alignment of the deep layer of sutures and the wound edges results in wound eversion and a smooth scar. (B) Failure to evert the wound edges by proper placement of deep sutures results in inverted wound edges and a depressed scar. (C) Uneven closure of the depth of the wound results in misaligned wound edges and variation in the elevation of the scar with some areas appearing high and others low. The uneven scar casts noticeable shadows.

leads to a step-off across the scar. These irregularities along the scar cause ambient light scattering and perceptible shadows that emphasize the presence of the scar. Wound eversion is the key to achieving a smooth scar and is primarily accomplished through proper execution of deep layer (dermal) sutures. It is emphasized, however, that eversion must also be achieved along the epidermal layer to maximize cosmesis.

Deep layer sutures

Deep layer or dermal sutures function to close dead space, re-approximate the tissue layers, provide tensile strength to the healing wound, and if performed properly, evert the overlying epidermis. Deep layer suturing is best achieved through the use of a buried absorbable suture such as Vicryl (Ethicon Inc, Johnson and Johnson Co, Somerville, NJ), Dexon (Davis and Geck, Danbury, CT) or Maxon (Davis and Geck, Danbury, CT) placed within the dermis. The half-life of these suture materials provides tensile strength for 4–6 weeks of healing—sufficient time for early collagenesis to begin rebuilding the dermis. The stitch most commonly utilized for this purpose is the buried vertical mattress suture.[10]

The buried vertical mattress is placed in an inverted fashion so that the knot is tied deep in the wound placing the bulk of the suture material farther away from the surface to avoid extrusion of the suture material. The suture path is structured so that the superficial curvature of the loop is wider than its deeper portion creating an inverted flask-shape through the tissue (Fig. 19.4). Upon tightening of the suture, the incorporated deep tissue forces eversion of the overlying wound edges. Deep sutures are spaced evenly along the wound edge so that tension is distributed equally along the wound and tension across any single suture is minimized. It may be argued that a wound need only be closed with a single layer of appropriately placed buried sutures. When properly performed, the wound edges will be approximated and everted with minimal tension so that the epidermal sutures function only as a finishing layer to correct small inequalities.

Epidermal sutures

A variety of suturing techniques can be utilized for closure of the epidermis. These include interrupted or running sutures, simple sutures, or vertical and horizontal mattress sutures.[11] Tensile strength, wound eversion, the degree of tissue ischemia imparted upon the wound edge, the risk of permanent suture marks (railroad tracking), and the ease of application and efficiency of the suture are all factors that must be taken into account when selecting the most appropriate suture technique to employ.

Proper epidermal suture technique begins with the first throw of the needle entering the skin at a perpendicular or acute angle relative to the wound (Fig. 19.5). The needle is then rotated through its arc creating a flask-shaped path that will provide eversion to the wound edge. Using the forceps to lift up on the near edge of the wound, forcing the angle of entry to become more acute, and pressing down on the far side of the wound distal to the exit point of the needle again forcing an acute exit angle aids in achieving eversion.

Simple interrupted suture

The simple interrupted suture is the most fundamental and perhaps the most common of all suture techniques. It is a single throw that begins and ends equidistant from opposite sides of the wound. A surgeon's knot is tied to complete the stitch and the knot is positioned to rest to one side of the wound to avoid irritation of the scar (see Fig. 19.5). This stitch provides the surgeon with a great deal of flexibility in closure. Varying amounts of eversion or high–low correction can be achieved with each suture placed allowing the surgeon to tailor the entire closure. Other advantages are that individual sutures may be removed without compromising the entire wound. For example, in the case of a hematoma, or infection, a few sutures may be removed to explore the wound, evacuate the hematoma, or to permit drainage while leaving the remainder of the wound undisturbed, thus minimizing the overall scarring. The major disadvantage of this stitch is that for each pass of the suture a knot has to be tied and this greatly increases the overall closure time. Furthermore, the increased number of knots also increases the net suture bulk across the wound and thus the tendency for more prominent suture marks (railroad tracks) and skin irritation.

Running sutures

An alternatives to interrupted sutures is the continuous running suture. These begin and end with a single knot

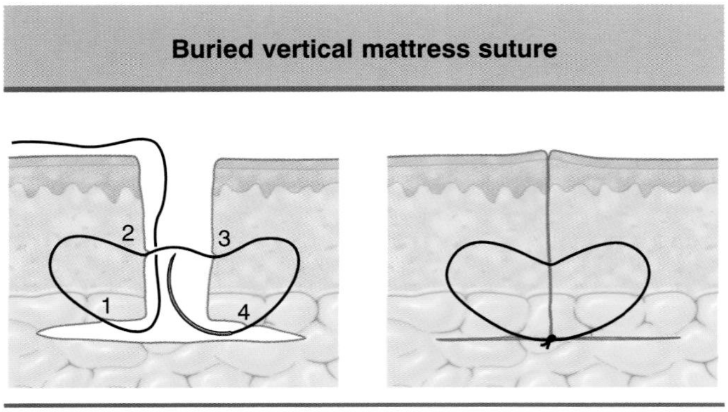

Buried vertical mattress suture

2 3 1 4

Figure 19.4 Buried vertical mattress suture. Numbers indicate sequence of insertion and passage of the needle. (Adapted from J Dermatol Surg Oncol 1992; 18(9): 785–795.)

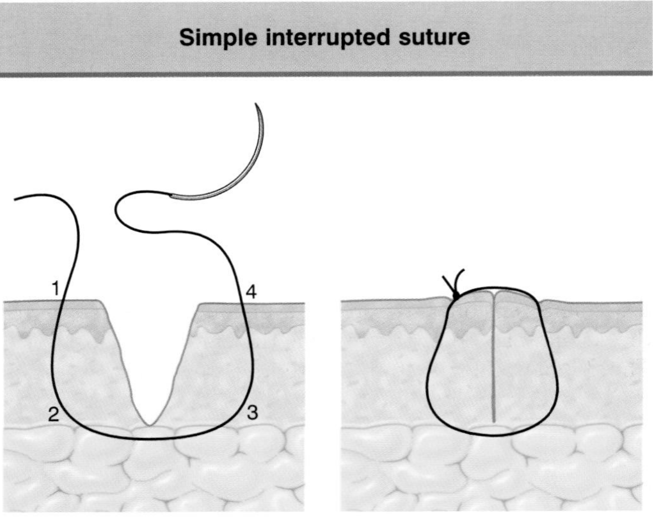

Figure 19.5 Simple interrupted suture. Numbers indicate sequence of insertion and passage of the needle. (Adapted from J Dermatol Surg Oncol 1992; 18(9): 785–795.)

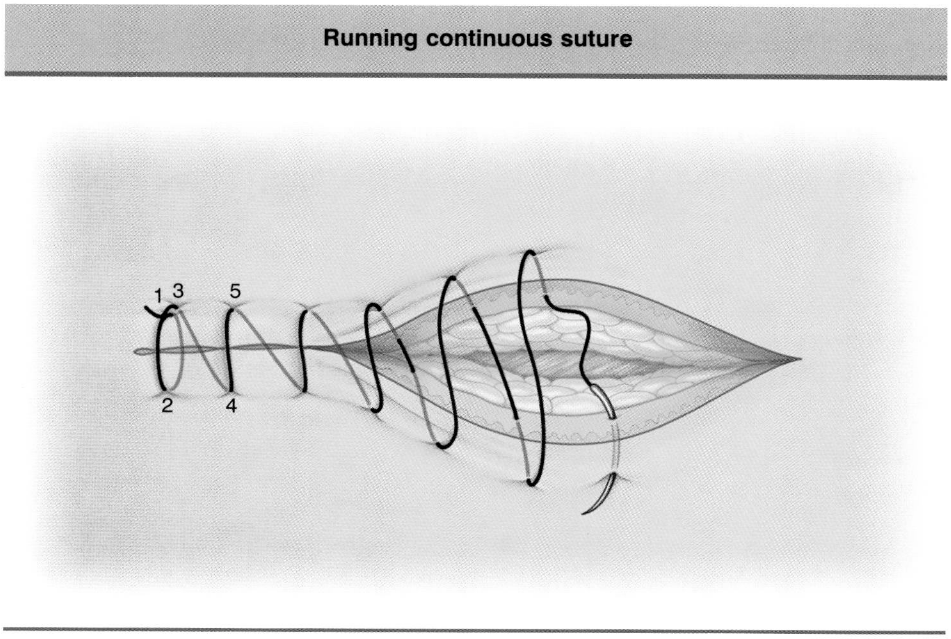

Running continuous suture

Figure 19.6 Running continuous suture. Numbers indicate sequence of insertion and passage of the needle. (Adapted from J Dermatol Surg Oncol 1992; 18(9): 785–795.)

placed at each end of the wound. The wound edge is re-approximated by a series of continuous throws of the needle along the incision line (Fig. 19.6). Again, the basic principles of closure are obeyed with the needle path following a flask-shaped path through the tissue to achieve eversion and the needle exits and enters the wound edge at equivalent depths to avoid any high–low mismatch. The continuous suture is an excellent choice for wounds with minimal residual tension where deep sutures have successfully re-approximated wound edges. The disadvantages of this suture are that its integrity depends solely upon the knots at either end. If a break in the suture occurs, then the entire wound is compromised and may dehisce. The running suture is also not indicated in areas of high tension or mobility because this suture permits some degree of shifting to occur under these circumstances and may result in a less desirable scar. It should be mentioned, however, that this can be avoided or minimized by the addition of surgical tapes across the wound.

Vertical mattress suture

The vertical mattress suture (far-far-near-near stitch) is a specialized stitch that is useful for providing extra wound closing tension and eversion when needed. The first throw of the needle begins at a distance from the wound and finishes equidistant on the opposite end. The needle is then reversed and a second, more superficial pass back across the wound is performed. The suture path thus forms two loops through the tissue with the first, deeper and longer pass dispersing tension and forcing eversion of the tissue and the second pass re-approximating the epidermis (Fig. 19.7). The double-pulley system created by the vertical mattress provides unmatched wound eversion and distributes the closing tension across a longer path. These factors make the vertical mattress an excellent choice for closing wounds under high tension or for areas of high mobility such as the extremities where limb motion and increased tension may disrupt the wound. The main disadvantage to this stitch is its tendency to leave permanent suture marks on the skin. Because it forms two loops through the epidermis, there is

Verticle mattress suture

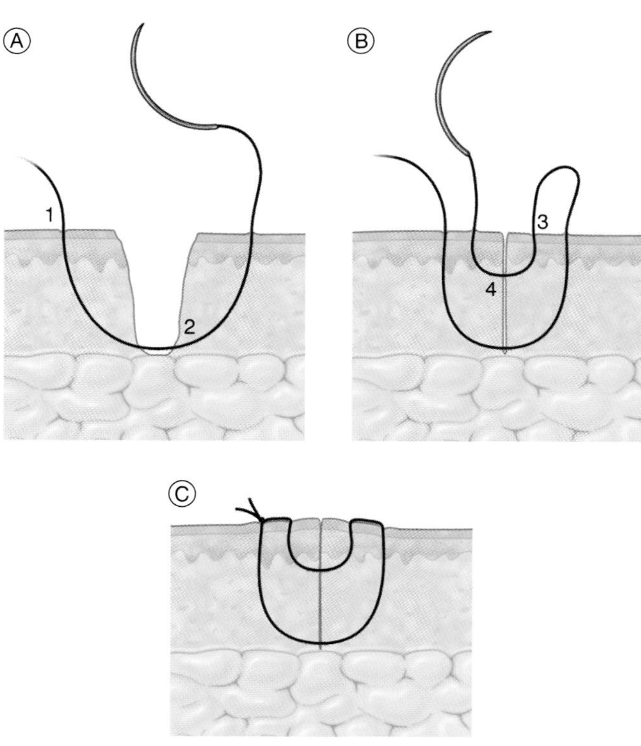

Figure 19.7 Vertical mattress suture. Numbers indicate sequence of insertion and passage of the needle. (Adapted from J Dermatol Surg Oncol 1992; 18(9): 785–795.)

an increased amount of suture contacting the surface and thus a higher likelihood of leaving permanent marks.

Horizontal mattress suture

The horizontal mattress is another specialized suture that is also useful for providing increased holding tension and wound eversion. It can be executed in either a running or interrupted mode. Each segment of the horizontal mattress must begin and end equidistant from the wound edge to maintain equal tension and a smooth finish to the closure. This stitch is actually two linked simple interrupted sutures passing across the wound in opposite directions. The first throw passes through the deep tissue and exits equidistant from the edges. The suture is then advanced parallel to the wound before initiating the second pass. The second throw passes through the deep tissue and exits at an equal distance from the wound as the point of origin. This stitch can then be tied to achieve a single stitch or can be continued in a running fashion along the wound with progressive and equal advances down the length of the wound. The horizontal mattress provides excellent wound eversion and holding tension and is useful in tight situations where a vertical mattress may not be possible. The major argument against using this suture has been that it causes significant tissue ischemia and railroad tracking, especially following tissue edema.

A variation of this suture is the 'tip stitch' or half-buried vertical mattress.[12] This suture is useful for closing corners of tissue flaps where careful tissue re-approximation is needed to counteract wound contracture that commonly leads to visible spreading of the surgical scar. The 'tip stitch' begins on the recipient side of the wound with a half throw through the deep tissue. The needle is then reloaded before initiating the second pass. The second pass is placed horizontally through the dermis of the flap corner a few millimeters from the tip edge. The needle is again reloaded before performing the final throw back through the deep aspect of the recipient edge on the opposite side (Fig. 19.8). The knot is then tied to lie across the recipient tissue side to minimize excess ischemia to the tip of the flap. The key to successful completion of this stitch is ensuring that the entry and exit points through the dermis of the flap and recipient sides are all in the same plane, otherwise a step-off mismatch of the wound edge will be apparent.

Running subcuticular suture

Another option for epidermal closure is the running subcuticular suture. This is an excellent choice for closing wounds that have minimal tension and mobility. This suture is performed entirely within the subepidermal plane and has the advantage of avoiding any suture marks along the skin. If necessary, the suture may be left in place for an extended period of time because there is no risk for railroad tracking on the epidermis. Absorbable or permanent sutures may be used for this stitch.

Many options exist for executing this suture including the use of absorbable sutures with the knots buried subcutaneously, nonabsorbable suture material with knots loosely fixed to the epidermis, or free ends of the suture fixed to the epidermis via tape. The absorbable suture with buried knots has the advantage of permitting prolonged holding tension across the epidermis, but this must be weighed against the risk of tissue reactivity, suture granuloma formation and the possibility of the suture spitting through the epidermis. The best results are usually obtained using a minimally reactive nonabsorbable suture such as coated polypropylene and taping the knotted ends to the skin to minimize epidermal reactivity. The suture passes along a superficial dermal plane alternating from one side to the next (Fig. 19.9). The length of the throw as well as the distance from the wound edge must be exact, otherwise tissue bunching will occur. The drawbacks to using this suture are that it is more technically demanding and usually requires more time to execute. Additionally, it is not recommended for use in areas of high tissue mobility where the suture and skin edges are likely to shift and buckle resulting in a poor cosmetic result.

Half-buried horizontal mattress tip stitch

Ⓐ

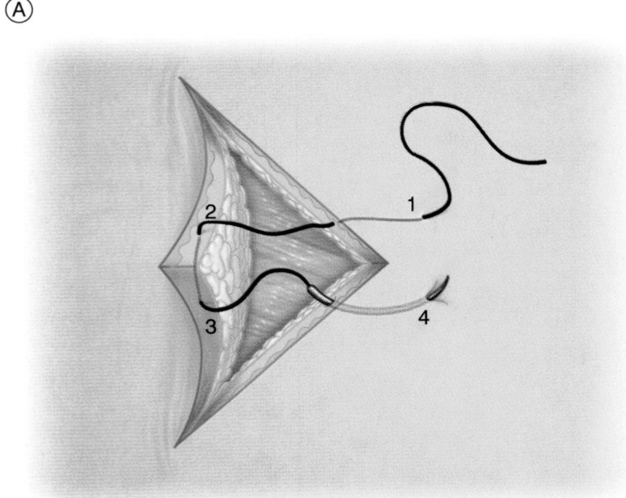

Ⓑ

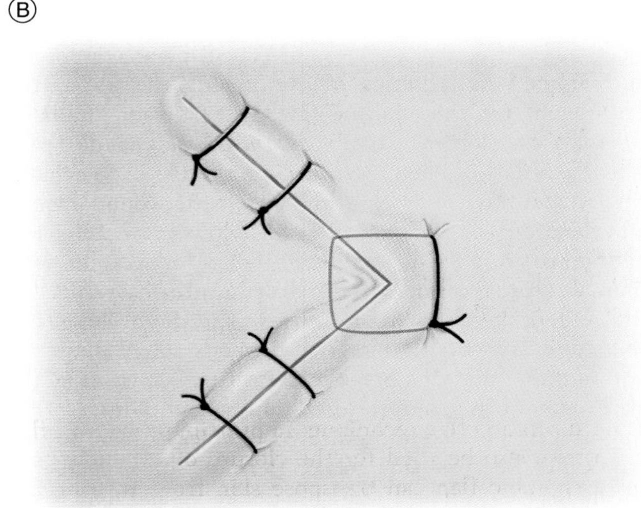

Figure 19.8 Half-buried horizontal suture used to align the tip of a flap (the tip stitch). Numbers indicate sequence of insertion and passage of the needle. (Adapted from J Dermatol Surg Oncol 1992; 18(9): 785–795.)

Complex closures

Although most surgical defects can be closed with standard multilayered linear closures, flaps, or skin grafts, including the use of suspension sutures as an adjunct, some wounds defy the conventional wisdom because of their large size involving multiple cosmetic units, or a critical structure such as the eyelid. The most important aspect of designing a closure for these types of defects is to simultaneously

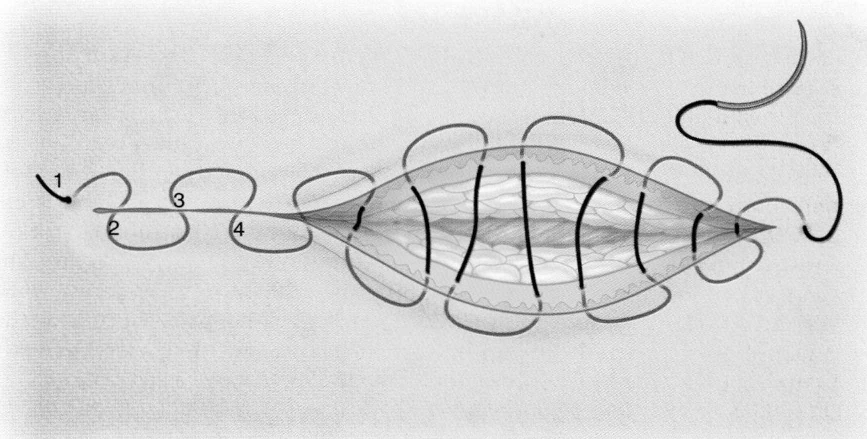

Figure 19.9 Running subcuticular suture. (Adapted from J Dermatol Surg Oncol 1992; 18(9): 785–795.)

follow the principles of cutaneous biomechanics and geometry while not being constrained by the dogma of the standard closures. In short, it is necessary to understand where there is the most tissue laxity and the biomechanics of that region, to use one's experience, investigate how others have closed analogous wounds, and to ultimately 'think out of the box'. The head and neck has an excellent vascular supply that permits the use of very large surface areas for tissue transfer. One such example, the cervico-facial rotation flap, appears technically demanding with elevation of the entire cheek as well as the lateral neck skin (Fig. 19.10). However, when reduced to its fundamental technical components it is merely an extension of the standard rotation flap technique. In principle, any basic flap design may also be used for the closure of larger defects, thus a rhombic flap can transpose skin from the neck to repair a large cheek defect. Another option is utilizing a bilobed flap, most commonly performed for small-to-medium distal nasal defects to repair large cheek defects with the neck acting as the donor reservoir.

When available, tissue reservoirs are limiting or anatomical constraints impose physical limitations, it may be necessary to use multiple flaps or combinations of closures to repair a single defect. As an example, one can consider the options for repair of a large scalp defect. On the scalp, the amount of adjacent skin available for transfer is severely limited by the inherent inelasticity of the regional skin. The pinwheel closure (O–Z flap) consisting of multiple rotation flaps is an option because it distributes the amount of donor tissue over two separate regions. Another alternative in this area would be to borrow from the hair restoration experience, and perform multiple transposition flaps,[13–16] again utilizing two separate regions to donate suitable tissue that would otherwise be insufficient from a single adjacent region.

Other alternatives for complex closure include a combination of a flap and a full-thickness skin graft. This combination is frequently used on the cheek with excellent results. As an example, a combined cheek and temple defect that crosses two cosmetic subunits with distinctly different skin textures and thicknesses requires a large

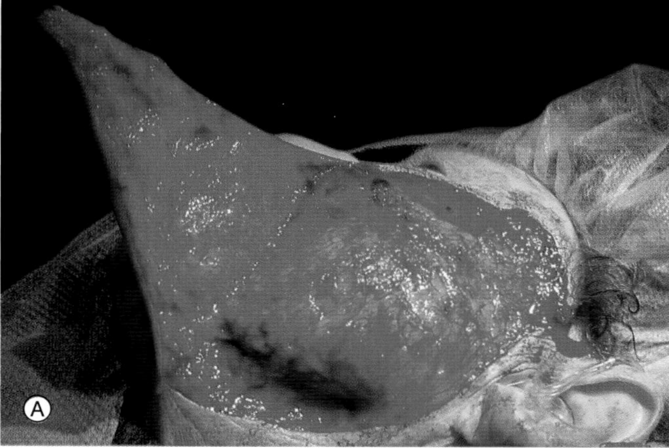

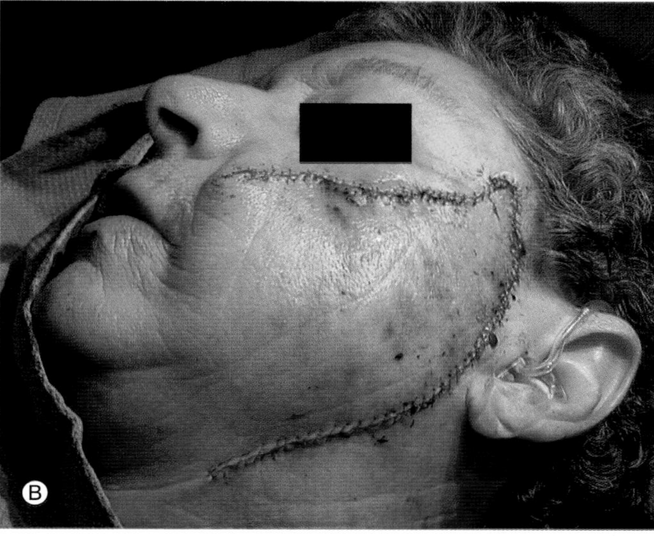

Figure 19.10 Cervicofacial flap. (A) Flap elevated before closure. (B) Flap sutured into place. A suspension suture anchors the flap to the zygoma.

surface area of tissue for repair. A combination of a cervicofacial rotation flap utilizing a suspension suture anchoring the flap to the zygoma to cover the cheek component and a skin graft to close the adjacent temple defect is an excellent solution. The forehead is another region that often requires complex closures to repair moderate-to-large defects due to the inelastic nature of the local skin and the limited amount of adjacent skin reservoirs. In this situation combination flaps or flaps combined with skin grafts offer excellent options.

While small, complex closures of defects involving the anterior lamella of the upper eyelid extending onto the periorbital skin still require an intricate understanding of tissue biomechanics and wound contraction to predict how it will affect the natural eyelid anatomy. Second intention healing can lead to contraction and distortion of the eyelid. A full-thickness skin graft has a high risk for failure given the continual rapid movement of the eyelid. A flap from the lateral inferior aspect of the area near to the wound will likely distort the lateral canthus. One viable solution would be a supraorbital transposition flap. This method utilizes adjacent skin offering good color and thickness match as well as an excellent vascular pedicle. Tissue transposition results in a low tension closure with minimal risk of distorting the eyelid (Fig. 19.11). Because the supraorbital flap is a thin flap, the secondary defect can be left to heal by second intention with a good functional and cosmetic result.

Although these complex skin maneuvers are extremely useful and yield excellent results when used in the appropriate setting, often the most simplistic approach is the best choice. Healing by second intention is an excellent choice for wound closure, either when used alone or in combination with flaps. The utility of second intention healing is well documented in the history of Mohs surgery.[17]

One final technique that can be considered for wound closure is the use of artificial skin equivalents. Advances in tissue engineering have led to a variety of skin equivalents that are commercially available for surgical applications. These devices are available in a variety of compositions including human-, bovine- or porcine-derived tissues. They are either living tissues composed of fetal foreskin fibroblast and keratinocyte bilayers (Apligraf, Organogenesis Inc, Canton, MA), or are tissue-derived collagen matrices—Integra (Johnson and Johnson, New Brunswick, NJ) and Dermagraft (Smith and Nephew plc, London, UK). Successful use of these tissue equivalents for both burn wound closure and surgical wound reconstruction is widely reported.[18–20] Although these skin equivalents are only temporary tissue grafts, they do aid in accelerating wound closure and decreasing postoperative pain. Currently, their use is limited by their high cost, but their effectiveness in repairing complex wounds should not be overlooked. (See also Chapter 8.)

Suspension sutures

Dermatologic surgeons are often faced with the challenge of re-approximating large tissue defects, either as the result of tumor extirpation or to enhance the natural facial contour. These situations often require closure of wounds where large opposing vector forces are present. This high tension across the wound, if not properly dealt with, can lead to scar spreading or wound dehiscence and an unsightly outcome. A second challenge for the surgeon is to maintain or recreate natural demarcations along cosmetic subunits. Maintaining these natural boundaries is paramount for re-establishing the symmetry of the face and for creating a natural appearance. The use of deep anchoring sutures,

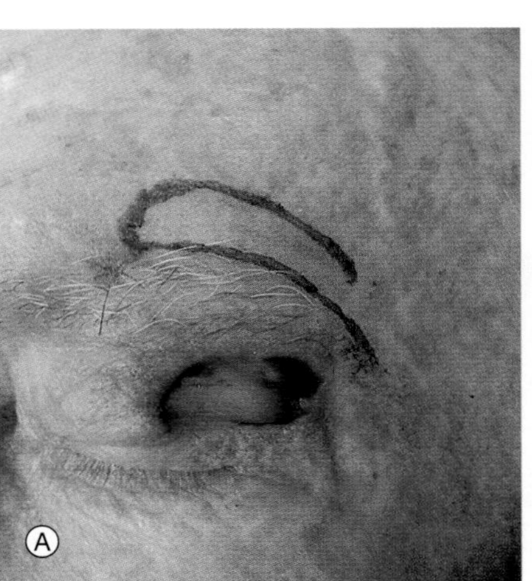

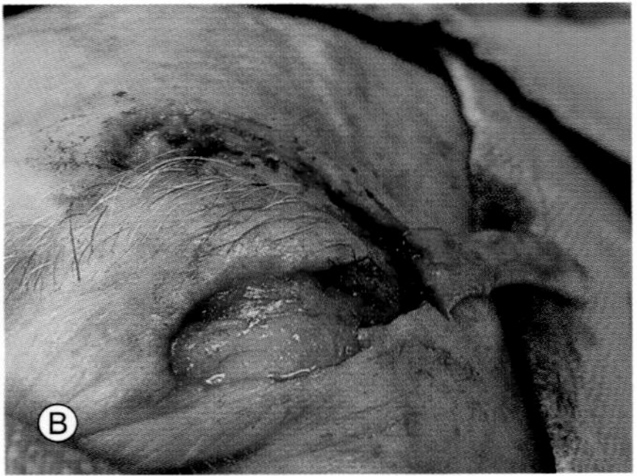

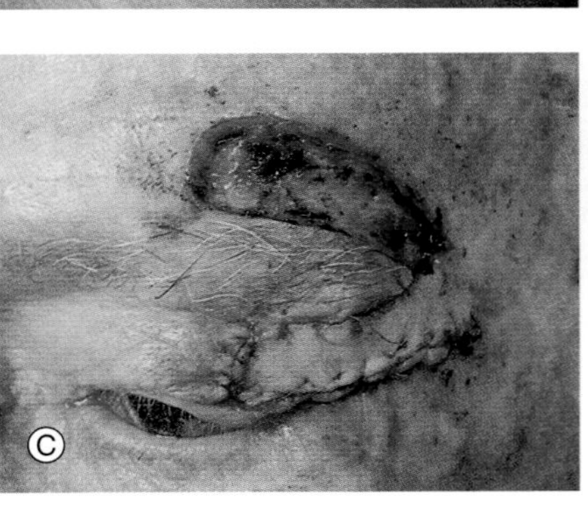

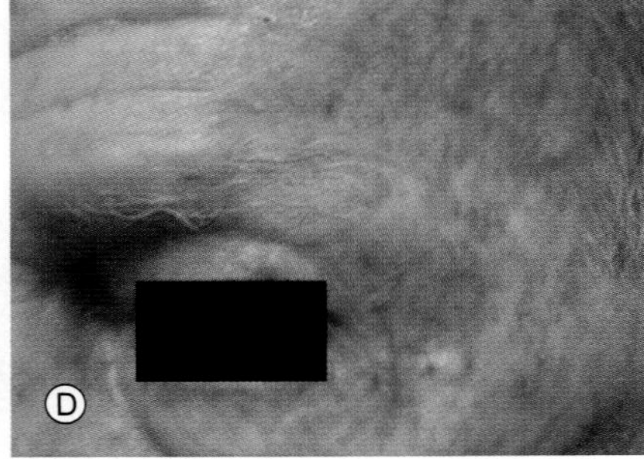

Figure 19.11 The supraorbital transposition flap for closure of complex upper eyelid defects. (A) Postoperative defect with planned suprabrow transposition flap outlined. (B) Transposition flap elevated before placement and suturing. (C) Transposition flap sutured in place. Complex wound is closed without tension on eyelid and minimal risk of disrupting the normal anatomy. (D) Secondary defect healed by second intention.

Bone anchoring points for suspension sutures

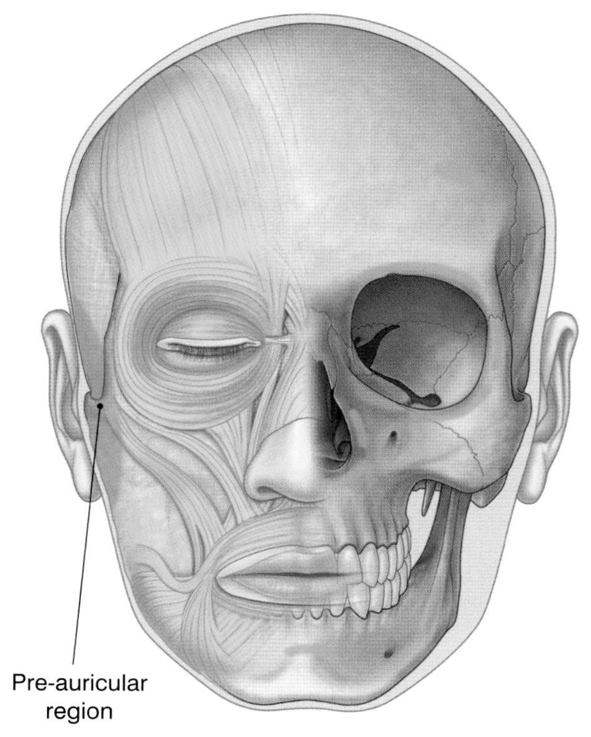

Figure 19.12 Bone anchoring points for suspension sutures. Bone anchoring points are shown in blue.

Suspension suture placement technique

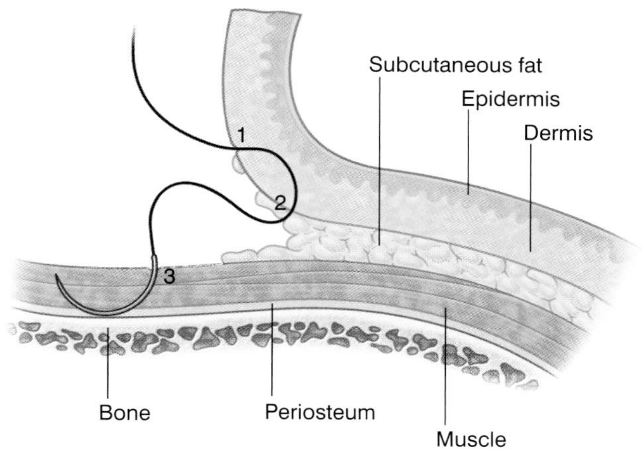

Figure 19.13 Suspension suture placement. (Adapted from J Dermatol Surg Oncol 1987; 13(9): 973–978.)

tacking, or suspension sutures is an effective means of offsetting these opposing vector forces and achieving the desired outcome. Suspension sutures are placed between the deep fascia or periosteum and the overlying dermis and provide fixation to a static structural support, thus preventing migration or slippage of the closure. The anatomical location of these anchoring points and their use in facial reconstructive surgery are well documented in the dermatology literature[21–25] (Fig. 19.12). This section will review the basic technique for utilizing suspension sutures and will provide specific examples to highlight their usefulness in cutaneous surgery.

Basic technique

The basic technique utilizes a buried suture passing between the leading edge of the wound and an underlying fixation point. The first throw of the needle is an inverted pass placed approximately 5–7 mm from the wound edge that is under the greatest tension. This pass should be placed through the reticular dermis such that a stable bite is obtained and so that no slippage occurs. Too superficial a pass will cause dimpling of the overlying skin and an undesirable outcome. The second throw of the needle passes through the deep subcutaneous tissue at the position of the desired point of wound closure. The needle is advanced until its point contacts bone, at which time it is then reversed and redirected in a slightly more superficial plane to catch a substantial bite of periosteum and deep tissues. The surgeon then rotates the needle through its remaining radius exiting the deep tissue. The suture is then tightened such that the wound edge is advanced into the appropriate position for closure (Fig. 19.13). Because this second pass proceeds blindly through deeper tissue structures, it is emphasized that the surgeon has a solid understanding of the local anatomy to avoid injury to neurovascular structures that may lie in these deep tissue planes. The simple act of anchoring the advancing edge of a skin flap to the underlying periosteum will advance tissue to fill the surgical defect and remove tension from the wound edge. Furthermore, with proper closing tension applied, a deep tacking suture can even be used to create a downward force that inverts tissue to recreate a natural skin fold.

Regional applications of suspension sutures

Forehead

The forehead and eyebrow region of the human face is primarily under the control of the frontalis and orbicularis oculi muscles and the overlying SMAS. These structures create a sling that suspends the overlying skin during periods of rest and mobilizes the upper face and eyebrows during facial expression. As such, the position of the eyebrows and upper eyelids are a direct result of the joint action of these structures.[26] A compromised frontalis muscle resulting from temporal branch disruption, facial nerve palsy, or a relaxed SMAS secondary to the natural course of aging, results in a ptotic brow and a drooping eyebrow and upper eyelid. Temporal nerve disruption occurring after tumor excision creates an asymmetry compared to the normal contralateral face and, in severe cases, may obstruct normal vision. An aged ptotic brow creates bilateral sagging and gives the patient a sleepy, tired appearance. Each of these scenarios results from downward gravitational forces acting on the brow and are common presentations to the cutaneous surgeon. Surgical intervention with a brow lift is required for correction of the abnormality.

Many different techniques have been devised to lift the brow and range from a simple elliptical skin excision, to endoscopic procedures or a coronal incision brow lift.[27–29] Although these procedures differ significantly in their degree of difficulty, they all employ the use of single or multiple suspension sutures as a unifying concept to elevate and resuspend the ptotic brow. Rafaty et al.[27] described a direct browlift in 1975 performed through a simple elliptical excision of skin placed just above the eyebrow. Although designed as a simple procedure, these authors do recognize the need to offset gravitational forces to prevent scar stretching and wound dehiscence. They describe the use of multiple nonabsorbable suspension sutures anchoring eyebrow skin superiorly to the frontalis fascia and periosteum of the forehead. The net effect of these suspension sutures is to create an upward pull on the eyebrow and to reset the position of the eyebrow and upper eyelid. Erol et al.[30] described a minimally invasive technique for applying suspension sutures to correct brow ptosis. This technique introduces multiple suspension sutures through small stab incisions placed at the temporal hairline and at the orbital rim to provide excellent lifting of the ptotic brow with limited scarring.

Lower eyelid

The thin skin of the lower eyelid makes it exquisitely sensitive to deformities resulting from aberrant tension forces. Several situations exist that may alter the normal vector forces upon the eyelid. Abnormal forces can result from increased directional tension secondary to wound contracture following tumor excision on the cheek or eyelid or may occur following lower lid blepharoplasty or laser rhytidectomy. Furthermore, gravitational pull resulting from natural changes in the aging face will also lead to increased downward or inferolateral forces on the lower lid. Each of these situations may lead to lid eversion and downward migration with a resultant ectropion and sequela of a dry eye. Of these, scar contraction is probably the most common concern for the cutaneous oncologic surgeon. The potential for cicatricial ectropion must always be considered when operating on the upper cheek and eyelid. Incisions and subsequent repairs in this area must be planned carefully to avoid these complications. In the same manner, the cosmetic surgeon is frequently consulted for correction of a lower lid ptosis or sagging lateral canthal angle and specific surgical techniques must be employed to offset these altered forces and to achieve the desired outcome.

The orbicularis oculi muscle forms a sphincter overlying the orbit. Its fibers attach to the superior orbital rim and interdigitate with the frontalis muscle. Laterally and medially the fibers of the orbicularis oculi condense to form thickened fibrous attachments to the orbital rim. These lateral and medial canthal tendons provide the primary structural support for the sphincter function and their relative positioning is responsible for establishing the canthal angle. The normal youthful position of the lateral canthal angle places the lower eyelid in line with the inferior edge of the pupil. Normal aging or scarring can lead to dehiscence of the lateral canthal attachments and a downward displacement of the lower lid. This downward displacement leads to increased scleral show, a ptotic or tired appearance of the eye and, if excessive, may cause dysfunction of eyelid closure.

Suspension of the lower eyelid to counteract downward forces and prevent or correct ectropion can be accomplished by the placement of a suspension suture at the lateral canthus. The various techniques and indications for lateral canthopexy have been reviewed recently by McCord et al.[31] Lateral canthopexy is accomplished by attaching single or multiple suspension sutures from the conjoined tendon of the lower lid traveling superiorly and laterally to anchor in to the periosteum of the inner aspect of the orbital rim (Fig. 19.14). Suture tension is then set to align the lower lid with the inferior edge of the pupil. The net effect of this suspension is to create an upward and lateral pull on the lower eyelid that re-establishes the normal youthful position of the lower lid. This suture also provides anchoring of the lid to the orbital rim so that functional eyelid closure is re-established.

Mid-face and preauricular zone

The anatomy of this area has received a great deal of attention mostly because of the focus on enhancing and maintaining the youthful appearance of the face. The mid-face is bounded by the zygomatic arch superiorly, the preauricular area laterally, the mandible inferiorly, and the melolabial junction and nose medially. The malar eminence along with the zygomatic arch forms the major structural component of the mid-face and forms the basis for the cosmetic subunit of the cheek. The structure of the cheek is further defined by a prominent malar fat pad which overlies the zygoma and whose position is maintained by the collective contributions of the overlying SMAS and several musculocutaneous ligaments.[4,5] Through the natural process of aging, the skin loses elasticity and succumbs to the forces of gravity and repetitive motion of the facial muscles. Additionally, the malar fat pad begins a downward migration that further accentuates the nasolabial fold and jowling. This downward migration creates a hollowed atrophic appearance in the superior aspect of the cheek and a prominent nasojugal fold. The net result of these processes is the formation of jowls, the accentuation of skin lines, and an overall aged appearance to the face.

These dramatic changes and the associated stigmata of an aged appearance cause many patients to seek surgical correction in an effort to regain their lost youthful

Lateral canthopexy/canthoplasty

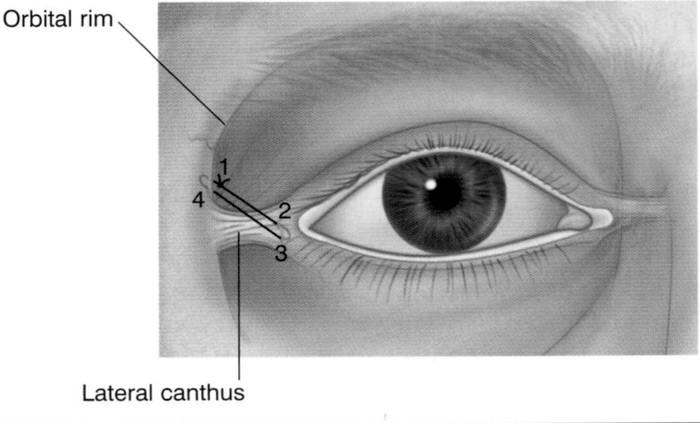

Figure 19.14 Lateral canthopexy. Horizontal mattress sutures are placed between the lateral canthal tendon and the periosteum of the orbital rim. The tension created by the suture creates an upward and lateral repositioning of the lower eyelid.

appearance. In the practice of cutaneous oncology, surgeons are often faced with the challenge of reconstructing the normal contour of the cheek following the excision of large tumors. To meet these challenges, surgeons have developed techniques that involve raising cutaneous flaps and repositioning the tissue to restore the pre-existing state. These procedures employ various suspension techniques to tighten the preauricular skin, recreate the malar prominence and nasolabial crease to restore definition to the cheek.

The face lift or rhytidectomy is the hallmark procedure for repositioning the mid-face and has undergone many modifications over the years in an effort to perfect this aim. The facelift and the S-lift are two similar procedures that are commonly performed to tighten the mid-face and jawline in an effort to restore the youthful anatomy of the face.[32–35] (See also Chapter 41.) Although there are significant technical distinctions between these two procedures, for the purpose of this chapter they will be considered as one method with attention focused upon the preauricular and cheek area. A preauricular incision is made and continued inferiorly around the earlobe into the postauricular area. Next, working in a subcutaneous plane, a skin flap is developed that has the SMAS as its floor and the subcutaneous fat and skin as the roof (Fig. 19.15). This flap can be safely developed without concern for damage to the facial nerve since its course in the preauricular area lies within the body of the parotid gland. Once the skin flap is raised and the SMAS exposed, one of two techniques, plication, or imbrication of the SMAS, is performed to mobilize and tighten the mid-facial structures.[36] Imbrication involves excising the redundant SMAS followed by suturing the two free ends together. This technique carries with it a risk of injury to the underlying facial nerve and thus the alternative method of plicating the SMAS has become more common. Plication of the SMAS is accomplished by placing a series of interrupted suspension sutures from the SMAS overlying the cheek passing superiorly and posteriorly in a 45° direction to the deep temporal or preauricular fascia (Fig. 19.16). The sutures are tightened causing an upward mobilization and suspension of the SMAS and facial structures. By elevating the SMAS and securing it to the fixed structural support of the preauricular fascia, all of the tension is transferred to the static bony structures of the face alleviating tension on the overlying cutaneous flap. This prevents tension across the incision line and avoids scar stretching and the possibility of dehiscence. Moreover, it accomplishes the goal of tightening the facial skin to correct jowling and better define the contour along the jaw.

Plication of the subcutaneous musculoaponeurotic system

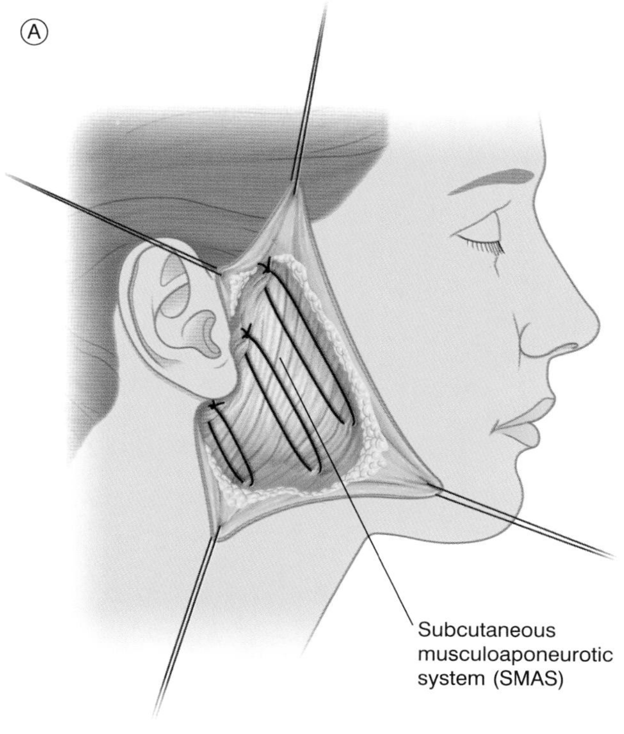

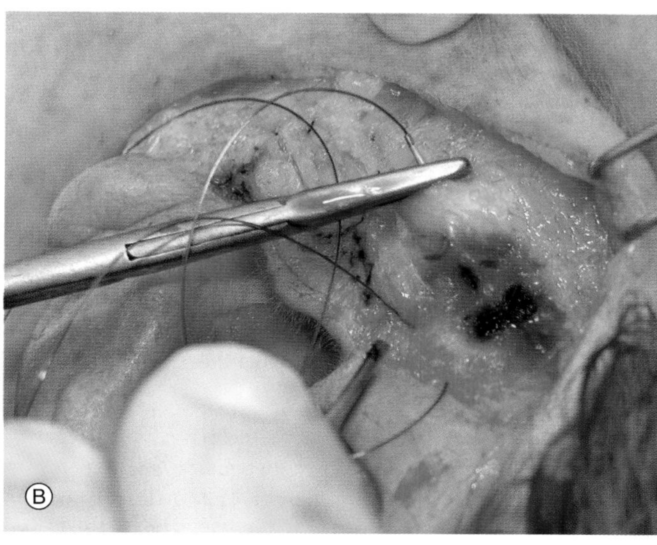

Figure 19.16 Plication of the SMAS. (A) A series of suspension sutures plicate the SMAS and create lift during rhytidectomy. Sutures are placed at a 45° angle. (B) The technique of placing suspension sutures in the SMAS and anchoring this to the preauricular fascia.

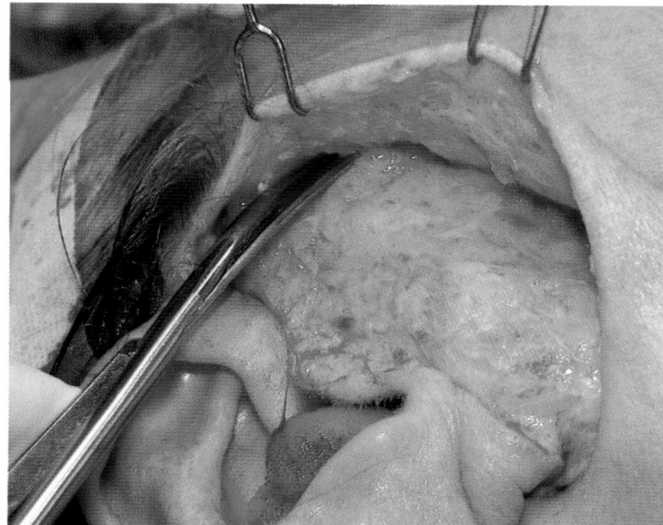

Figure 19.15 SMAS flap during facial rhytidectomy. The skin flap is dissected from the underlying SMAS. The SMAS is the floor of the wound and the subcutaneous fat and skin are the roof over the cavity.

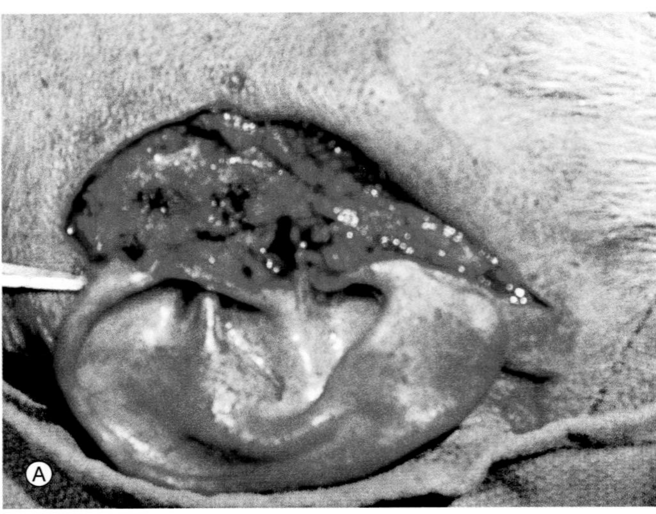

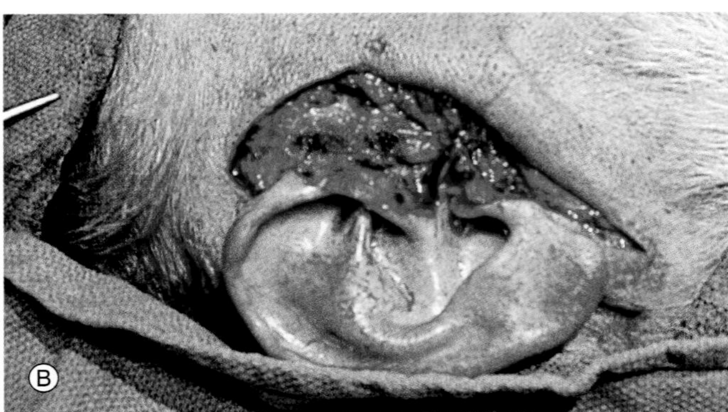

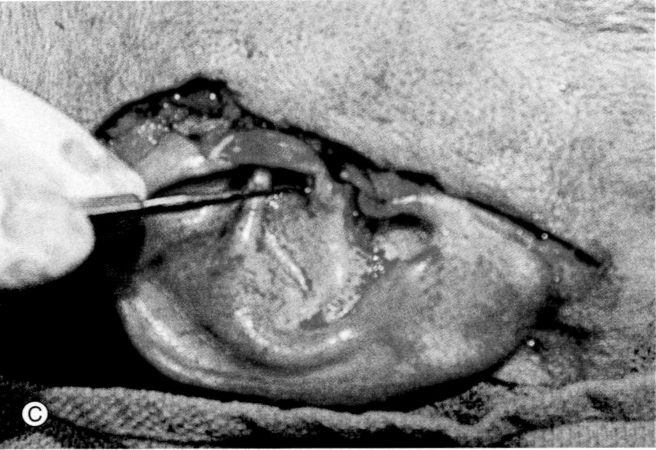

Figure 19.17 Preauricular suspension sutures in wound closure. (A) Direct closure of this wound would create sufficient tension as to risk wound dehiscence and flap necrosis. (B) SMAS plication by suspension sutures anchoring the SMAS to the preauricular fascia. Tightening the suture advances the skin flap into the defect. (C) After placing a series of SMAS plication sutures, the flap is advanced into the wound and tension is reduced.

Mid-face suspension lift

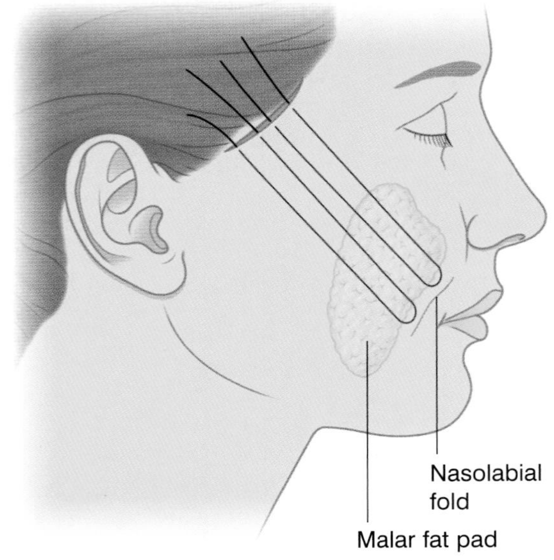

Figure 19.18 Mid-face suspension lifting sutures. This minimally invasive procedure elevates the malar fat pad and rejuvenates the mid-face with percutaneous placement of a series of suspension sutures. (Adapted from Arch Facial Plast Surg 2002; 4(1) 20–25.)

The same principles of SMAS suspension are extremely useful for closure of preauricular or cheek defects under high tension. Reconstruction of large defects in the mid-face requires the mobilization of tissue flaps to cover the defect. These are most often accomplished using cervicofacial rotation or transposition flaps with the lower face and neck as the tissue reservoir.[37] Despite wide undermining, these flaps still retain a high degree of oppositional tension that must be offset to achieve a successful closure. This tension can be attenuated by stable anchorage to the preauricular fascia much in the same manner as described with a face-lift procedure. Placement of suspension sutures from the flap to the preauricular fascia or periosteum of the orbital rim will advance the flap into the primary defect, will alleviate tension from the wound edge and, if properly placed, can aid in recreating the normal contour of the cheek. Additionally, in the case of a large cervicofacial rotation flap, this suspension technique has the added benefit of redirecting tension forces in the superolateral direction such that a downward pull on the lower eyelid and the potential for ectropion is avoided. The use of SMAS plication is applicable even for small elliptical incisions along the preauricular zone. With the removal of small amounts of tissue, this area may be subject to closure against high tension. Placement of one or two plicating sutures in the preauricular SMAS will help to approximate the wound edges and reduce tension across the defect (Fig. 19.17).

Recently, several minimally invasive cosmetic procedures that utilize suspension sutures for repositioning the malar fat pad and redefining the mid-facial contour have been described.[38–42] Terms such as the mid-face lift, the puppet face lift, or SOOF (suborbicularis oculi fat) lift have been coined for these procedures. The basic technique employed with these procedures is the percutaneous introduction of multiple suspension sutures at the nasolabial fold, which then tunnel superiorly in a subcutaneous plane toward the zygomatic arch or orbital rim. The positioning of these sutures encompass the malar fat pad and the soft tissues of the cheek incorporating them into a sling that can then be suspended from a more cephalad fixation point such as the deep temporal fascia, the zygomatic arch, or the orbital rim (Fig. 19.18). Tension placed upon these sutures results in elevation and repositioning of the malar fat pad in a superior direction to its normal youthful location to restore the natural contour of the mid-face. In the case of the special APTOS (KMI, Corona, CA) threads developed by Sulamanidze et al,[43] unidirectional barbs incorporated into the sutures prevent migration of the suture and thus may enhance their function.

Nasolabial junction

The natural concavity that exists at the nasolabial junction is a defining landmark between two cosmetic facial subunits. Preservation of this landmark is essential for maintaining facial symmetry and normal contour. Reconstruction of a medial cheek or low nasal sidewall defect often requires advancement of tissue from the cheek to perform the repair. The cheek advancement flap is an excellent option for this repair because it provides a large reservoir of tissue for wound closure and the incision lines of the flap are easily disguised within the natural skin folds. However, in the process of elevating a cheek flap and mobilizing it medially the loss of deep tissue connections combined with the retrograde tension forces on the flap will cause tenting of the tissue (Fig. 19.19). If not properly addressed, healing in this manner will cause blunting of the melolabial fold and a resultant asymmetry. This situation is a classic example of where a tacking or suspension suture can be used to recreate a natural skin fold. A single absorbable (Vicryl or Dexon) suture is placed through the reticular dermis of the advancing skin flap at a position that coincides with the point of maximum concavity of the repositioned tissue, the nasolabial fold. The second pass of the suture is then anchored to the underlying periosteum at the medial aspect of the maxilla. The knot is next tightened to the appropriate tension such that the newly created nasolabial fold is symmetric with the contralateral face. The suspension suture transfers tension to the periosteum so that tension across the scar line and the risk of dehiscence or scar spreading is minimized.

Other sites where this basic technique of utilizing suspension or tacking sutures to recreate natural skin folds and lines of demarcation include the alar crease and the mental crease. These are critical lines of demarcation that separate major cosmetic subunits and as such, are landmarks that must be preserved to restore the natural appearance. Facial reconstruction of tumor defects by mobilization of skin flaps into these regions will be greatly enhanced by first placing a tacking suture to the underlying periosteum. This tacking suture or suspension suture will redefine the cosmetic subunit, appropriately position the tissue flap, and eliminate tension across the flap that can lead to tenting of the flap and distortion of the subunit.

Optimizing outcomes

- Plan a reconstruction to fall within the boundaries between cosmetic units.
- Excise extra tissue so the line can be placed at the boundary.
- Suture precisely to evert wound edges with minimal tension.
- Use vertical mattress sutures in wounds under tension for the areas of high mobility.
- For wounds with minimal tension and lower mobility that may have the suture in place for an extended period, use a running subcuticular suture to avoid suture marks.
- Use suspension sutures to minimize tenting of flaps across natural concavities.

POSTOPERATIVE CARE

Surgical tapes across the wound minimize mobility and tension in the postoperative period.

■ SUMMARY

Human skin is an elastic and malleable structural unit that allows the reconstructive surgeon the ability to manipulate these properties to fashion flaps and grafts for the closure of surgical defects. The skin on the human face has distinct regional variations that reflect the specific composition of the underlying tissue and bony layers. Careful attention should be paid to these distinct subunits not only for preservation of aesthetic appearances, but also for planning appropriate closures. Each region has its own specific physical properties (i.e. variable thickness, stretch, and texture) that must be matched or maintained to achieve optimal results. Successful planning of wound closure begins with a firm understanding of these physical properties and their subtle regional variations across different anatomical subunits.

When assessing options for wound closure, a variety of techniques should always be considered. Tissue flaps, skin grafts, primary closure, and healing by second intention can all be excellent options in specific settings. When planning the closure of complex wounds one should always consider the use of combinations of flaps, grafts, and second intention healing. The use of suspension sutures to stabilize tissue against opposing vector forces is a valuable technique for both reconstructing surgical defects as well as for use in various cosmetic enhancement procedures. When selecting the most appropriate closure for a particular defect, the surgeon should consider multiple options and utilize either single or combined techniques tailored to meet the specific challenges and requirements to achieve optimal results.

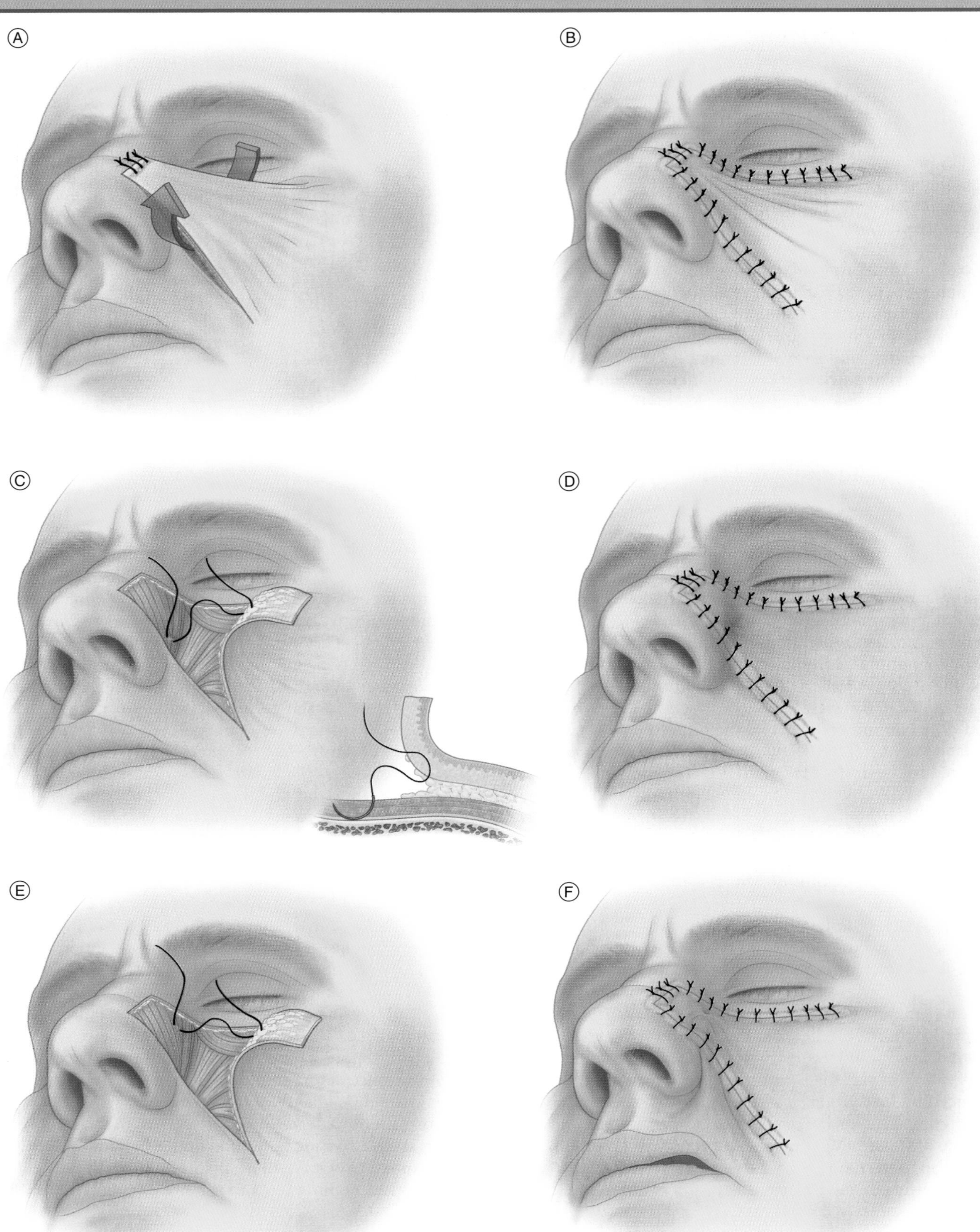

Figure 19.19 Cheek advancement flap. (A–B) Cheek advancement flap without the use of suspension sutures. (A) Arrow shows the area of tenting created by pulling the cheek skin directly across the concave junction of the nose and the cheek. (B) Closure without tacking the flap. The depth of the nasofacial sulcus leaves the flap elevated with blunting of the sulcus and a potential dead space for a seroma to develop. (C–D) Cheek advancement flap with suspension suture used to place the flap into the concave junction of the nasofacial sulcus. (E–F) The placement of tension on the suspension suture can be varied. When placed too far superior and with too much tension, the suspension suture elevates the flap, raises the lip, and distorts the oral commissure. (Adapted from J Dermatol Surg Oncol 1987; 13(9): 973–978.)

Pitfalls and their management

- Incisions crossing lines of demarcation between geometric units disrupt the natural contour and facial symmetry.
- Functional skin biomechanics – closure of wounds under high tension can result in poor wound re-approximation, scar spreading, or wound dehiscence unless appropriate techniques are utilized. Skin is elastic and 'stretchable' and thus allows for intraoperative or delayed tissue expansion to assist in wound closure.
- Basic techniques of wound closure – the deep layer sutures are critical for re-approximating wound margins. Failure to achieve adequate wound eversion with deep layer sutures can lead to a widened and depressed scar with poor cosmesis.
- Epidermal sutures – securing the knots of epidermal sutures with the appropriate tension is crucial for achieving quality cosmetic results: a knot that is too loose can lead to poor wound re-approximation; one that is anchored too tight will constrict tissue and lead to permanent 'railroad tracking' on the skin surface. The surgeon must allow for local tissue edema during healing that may further contribute to tissue constriction when calculating the appropriate tension of the knots.
- Complex closures – many postoperative wounds are challenging to repair because available tissue reservoirs are limited and attempts to close these wounds using a single flap or graft can lead to an undesirable cosmetic outcome or can cause deformities in adjacent anatomic structures. These complex wounds are best repaired using a combination of techniques to restore the natural appearance of the tissue subunits.
- Mid-face and preauricular zone – suspension of the cheek tissue during a face-lift procedure or a cervicofacial rotation flap for reconstruction is integral for restoring the natural appearance, and achieving the appropriate suture tension is critical for achieving the desired results. A suture placed too loose will result in a failed procedure; alternatively, too much tension can lead to dimpling of the skin flap, focal tissue necrosis and a poor cosmetic outcome.
- Nasolabial junction – mobilizing tissue across a surface concavity can lead to blunting of the normal anatomy unless specific techniques are used to redefine the natural appearance. Suspension or tacking sutures are ideal for achieving this goal. Anchoring the tissue flap to the underlying periosteum will recreate the natural concavity and will help advance the tissue flap into position.

REFERENCES

1. Mitz V, Peyronie M. The superficial musculo-aponeurotic system (SMAS) in the parotid and cheek area. Plast Reconstr Surg 1976; 58:80–88.
2. Dzubow LM, Zack L. The principle of cosmetic junctions as applied to reconstruction of defects following Mohs surgery. J Dermatol Surg Oncol 1990; 16:353–355.
3. Barton FE, Gyimesi IM. Anatomy of the nasolabial fold. Plast Reconstr Surg 1997; 100:1276–1279.
4. Ozdemir R, Kilinc H, Unlu RE, Uysal AC, Sensoz O, Baran CN. Anatomicohistologic study of the retaining ligaments of the face and use in face lift: retaining ligament correction and SMAS plication. Plast Reconstr Surg 2002; 110:1134–1147.
5. Mendelson BC, Muzaffar AR, Adams WP. Surgical anatomy of the midcheek and malar mounds. Plast Reconstr Surg 2002; 110:885–895.
6. Wilhelmi BJ, Blackwell SJ, Mancoll JS, Phillips LG. Creep vs. stretch: a review of the viscoelastic properties of skin. Ann Plast Surg 1998; 41:215–219.
7. Larrabee WF. A finite element model of skin deformation. I. Biomechanics of skin and soft tissue: a review. Laryngoscope 1986; 96:399–405.
8. Larrabee WF, D Sutton. A finite element model of skin deformation. II. Experimental model of skin deformation. Laryngoscope 1986; 96:406–412.
9. Larrabee WF, JA Galt. A finite element model of skin deformation. III. The finite element model. Laryngoscope 1986; 96:413–419.
10. Zitelli JA, Moy RL. Buried vertical mattress suture. J Dermatol Surg Oncol 1989; 15:17–19.
11. Moy RL, Waldman B, Hein DW. A review of suturing techniques. J Dermatol Surg Oncol 1992; 18:785–795.
12. Starr J. Surgical pearl: the vertical mattress tip stitch. J Am Acad Dermatol 2001; 44:523–524.
13. Juri J. Use of parieto-occipital flaps in the surgical treatment of baldness. Plast Reconstr Surg 1975; 55:456–460.
14. Juri J, Juri C, Arufe HG. Use of rotation scalp flaps for treatment of occipital baldness. Plast Reconstr Surg 1978; 61:23–26.
15. Orticochea M. Four flap scalp reconstruction technique. Br J Plast Surg 1967; 20:159–171.
16. Orticochea M. New three-flap scalp reconstruction technique. Br J Plast Surg 1971; 24:184–188.
17. Zitelli JA. Wound healing by secondary intention. J Am Acad Dermatol 1983; 9:407–415.
18. Eaglestein WH, Iriondo M, Laszlo K. A composite skin substitute (Graftskin) for surgical wounds. Dermatol Surg 1995; 21:839–843.
19. Moiemen NS, Staiano JJ, Ojeh NO, Thway Y, Frame JD. Reconstructive surgery with a dermal regeneration template: clinical and histologic study. Plast Reconstr Surg 2001; 108:93–103.
20. Prystowsky JH, Siegel DM, Ascherman JA. Artifical skin for closure of wounds created by skin cancer excisions. Dermatol Surg 2001; 27:648–654.
21. Salasche SJ, Jarchow R, Feldman BD, Devine-Rust MJ, Adnot J. The suspension suture. J Dermatol Surg Oncol 1987; 13:973–978.
22. Dzubow, LM. The use of fascial plication to facilitate wound closure following microscopically controlled surgery. J Dermatol Surg Oncol 1989; 15:1063–1066.
23. Zitelli JA. Tips for wound closure: pearls for minimizing dog-ears and applications of periosteal sutures. Dermatol Clinics 1989; 7:123–128.
24. Robinson JK. Suspension sutures aid facial reconstruction. Derm Surg1999; 25:189–194.
25. Robinson JK. Suspension sutures in facial reconstruction. Derm Surg 2003; 29:386–393.
26. Knize DM. An anatomically based study of the mechanism of eyebrow ptosis. Plast Reconstr Surg 1996; 97:1321–1333.
27. Rafaty RF, Goode RL, Fee WE. The brow-lift operation. Arch Otolaryngol 1975; 101:467–468.
28. Costantino PD, Hiltzik DH, Moche J, Preminger A. Minimally invasive brow suspension for facial paralysis. Arch Facial Plast Surg 2003; 5:171–174.
29. Knize DM. Limited incision foreheadplasty. Plast Reconstr Surg 1999; 103:271–284.
30. Erol OO, Sozer SO, Velidedeoglu HV. Brow suspension, a minimally invasive technique in facial rejuvenation. Plast Reconstr Surg 2002; 109:2521–2532.
31. McCord CD, Boswell CB, Hester TR. Lateral canthal anchoring. Plast Reconstr Surg 2003; 112:222–236.
32. Fulton JE, Saylan Z, Helton P, Rahimi AD, Golshani M. The S-lift facelift featuring the U-suture and O-suture combined with skin resurfacing. Derm Surg 2001; 27:18–22.
33. Saylan Z. The S-lift for facial rejuvenation. Int J Cosmet Surg 1999; 7:18–23.
34. Tonnard P, Verpaele A, Monstrey S, et al. Minimal access cranial suspension lift: a modified S-lift. Plast Reconstr Surg 2002; 109:2074–2086.
35. Duminy F, Hudson DA. The mini rhytidectomy. Aesth Plast Surg 1997; 21:280–284.
36. Webster RC, Smith RC, Papsidero MJ, Karlow WW, Smith KF.

Comparison of SMAS plication with SMAS imbrication in face lifting. Laryngoscope 1982; 92:901–912.
37. Herbst, AM, Benedetto AV. The use of spanning suspension suture in facial reconstruction. Dermatol Surg 2002; 28:337–339.
38. Gunter JP, Hackney FL. A simplified transblepharoplasty subperiosteal cheek lift. Plast Reconstr Surg 1999; 103:2029–2035.
39. Olver JM. Raising the suborbicularis oculi fat (SOOF): its role in chronic facial palsy. Br J Ophthalmol 2000; 84:1401–1406.
40. Keller GS, Namazie A, Blackwell K, Rawnsley J, Khan S. Elevation of the malar fat pad with a percutaneous technique. Arch Facial Plast Surg 2002; 4:20–25.
41. Sasaki GH, Cohen AT. Meloplication of the malar fat pads by percutaneous cable-suture technique for midface rejuvenation: outcome study (392 cases, 6 years' experience). Plast Reconstr Surg 2002; 110:635–654.
42. Yousif NJ, Matloub H, Summers AN. The midface sling: a new technique to rejuvenate the midface. Plast Reconstr Surg 2002; 110:1541–1553.
43. Sulamanidze MA, Fournier PF, Paikidze TG, Sulamanidze GM. Removal of soft tissue ptosis with special threads. Dermatol Surg 2002; 28:367–371.

20 Repair of the Split Earlobe, Ear Piercing, and Earlobe Reduction

Sirunya Silapunt MD and Leonard H Goldberg MD

Summary box

- Because the earlobe is composed only of skin and fibrous and fatty tissue, it is easily split as a result of trauma, and it is prone to keloid and hypertrophic scar formation.
- A wide variety of techniques are available for split earlobe repair, with or without preservation of the canal for an earring, where the choice of technique depends upon the nature of the split (whether full or partial) and whether the canal is to be preserved.
- Ears can be pierced using a one-needle or a two-needle technique; commercial kits have no advantages over these methods.
- Drooping earlobes can be congenital or caused by aging, gravity, and certain diseases, and they can be reduced by several reduction techniques.

The ear plays a significant role in appearance, particularly the earlobe, which has traditionally been adorned with earrings. The auricle consists of skin and cartilage whereas the earlobe consists of skin, fibrous and fatty tissue and is devoid of cartilage. The ears and especially the earlobes are prone to the formation of hypertrophic scars and keloids.

SPLIT EAR LOBES

■ INTRODUCTION

Split earlobes and enlarged pierced earlobe canals are common problems that may have a congenital or traumatic cause.[1–3] Traumatic causes of split earlobes include sudden pulling of an earring, wearing heavy earrings, pressure necrosis caused by clip-on earrings, the weight of a telephone receiver on an earring, an infection, an allergic reaction, multiple piercings, and a piercing site too low in the earlobe.[4–7] The partially split earlobe usually occurs following ear piercing and the wearing of heavy earrings. The completely split earlobe usually results from the gradual downward progression of the partially split earlobe, or a sudden trauma. Several repair options have been described to restore these defects.[8]

■ PREOPERATIVE PREPARATION

Patient evaluation should include taking a history of hypertrophic scars or keloids. Enquiries should be made about the patient's expectations of the cosmetic outcome, and whether there will be a continuing desire to wear earrings. Antiseptic cleansing is required on both sides of the split earlobe before the procedure is begun.

A general dermatologic surgery tray with a #15 surgical blade, a chalazion clamp (which stabilizes the split earlobe and provides hemostasis), and local anesthesia is then applied to the split earlobe until it becomes firm and pale; this is achieved by lidocaine injection with a 30-gauge needle. Non-absorbable 5-0 or 6-0 suture is used for cutaneous closure. Absorbable 5-0 or 6-0 suture may be required for subcutaneous closure.

■ TECHNIQUES

Repair of partially split earlobes

Side-to-side closure

This technique is illustrated in Figures 20.1 and 20.2. The split earlobe can be stabilized with a chalazion clamp during the cutting. Both sides of the epithelialized skin of the split are excised with narrow margins anteriorly and posteriorly with a #15 surgical blade. Care is taken to avoid cross-hatching of the excision at the ends of the split, and excising unequal length of the split edges, which will result in a dog-ear deformity. The resulting defect is closed with simple side-to-side interrupted sutures on both the anterior and posterior surface of the earlobe. Absorbable 5-0 or 6-0 subcutaneous suture may also be used but is not necessary.

Punch technique (Tan's technique)[9]

The punch technique (Fig. 20.3) is used only for enlarged round pierced canals of less than 4 mm. The epithelium-

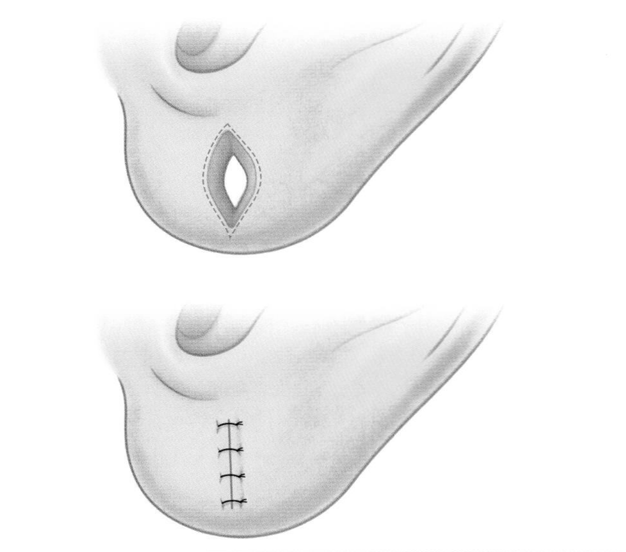

Figure 20.1 Repair of the partial split with side-to-side closure after de-epithelializing the split area.

lined edges of these pierced canals are excised by a punch. The earlobe is stabilized with a chalazion clamp. An appropriately sized punch is applied perpendicular to the enlarged pierced canals. The incision is carried from the anterior-through-posterior surface of the earlobe resulting in a round defect. Interrupted sutures are placed on both the anterior and posterior surface to close the defect. This technique is not recommended for a split larger than 4 mm in diameter because dog-ear deformities arise upon suturing. The suture line may be vertical or horizontal depending on the shape of the ear, but the horizontal line may be more supportive of the earring load in the future.

Parallel opposed flaps (Reiter and Alford's technique)[10]

Two opposing flaps are created on the anterior and posterior surface of the earlobe. Each flap is based alternately on the medial edge or the lateral edge of the split. The flaps are pulled through the split and attached to the freshened surface on the opposite side, which resulted from the creation of the other flap (Fig. 20.4).

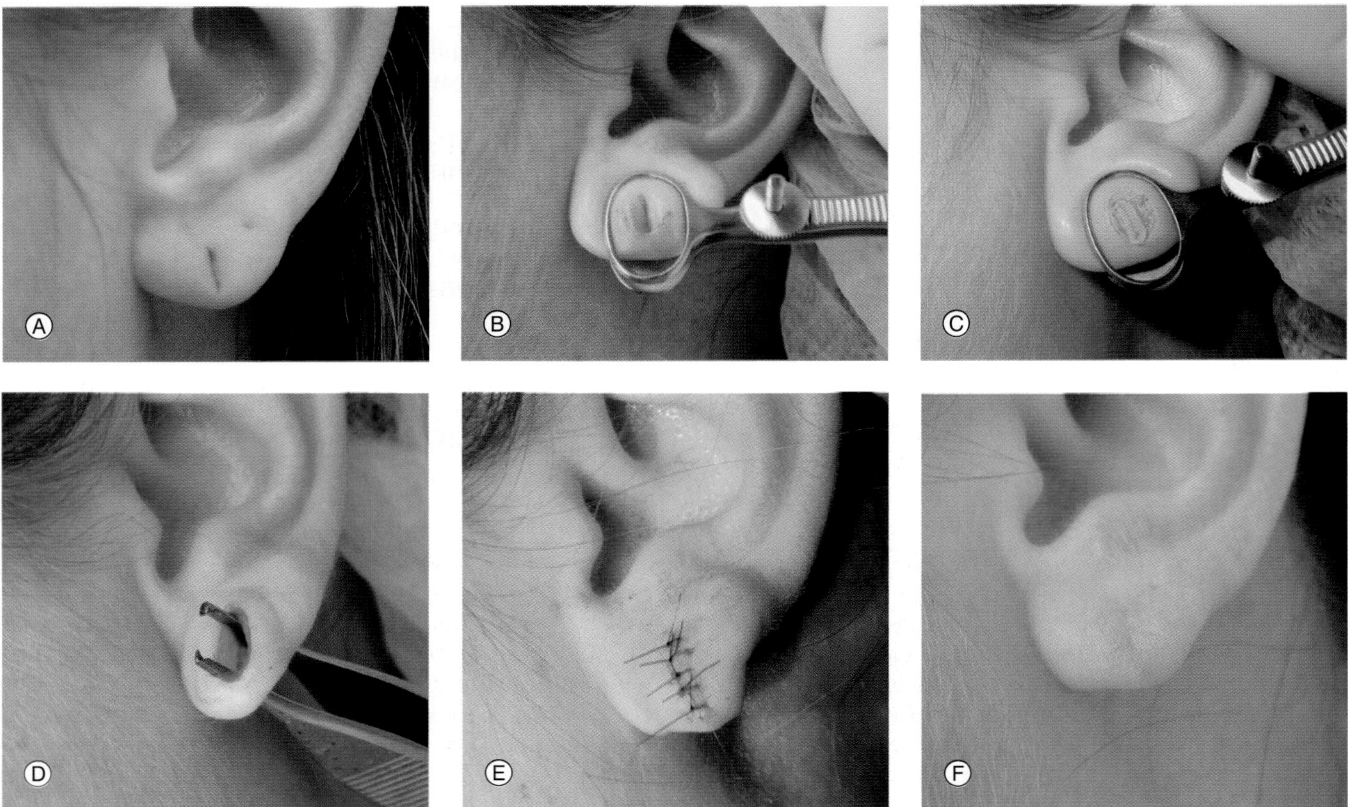

Figure 20.2 (A) Partial split earlobe in a 24-year-old woman. (B) A chalazion clamp is applied to stabilize the earlobe. (C) The epithelialized edges of the split are dissected and excised. Bleeding is well controlled with the chalazion clamp. (D) The resulting defect of anterior-through-posterior excision of the split edges. (E) Simple interrupted sutures placed on the anterior and posterior aspects of the earlobe. (F) At 2-months follow-up.

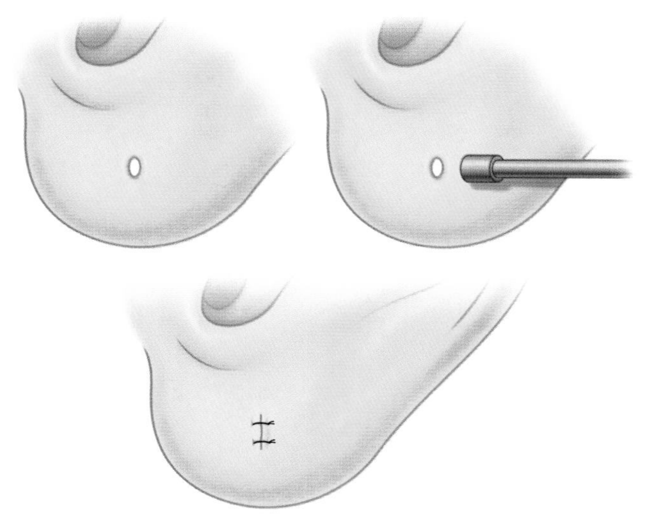

Figure 20.3 Punch technique to de-epithelialize the split area (Tan's technique).

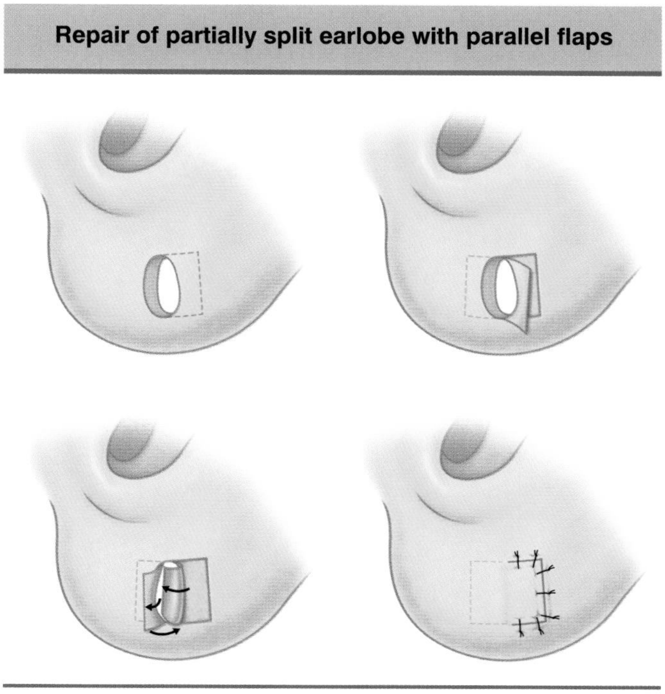

Repair of partially split earlobe with parallel flaps

Figure 20.4 Parallel flaps are created on the anterior and posterior surfaces of the earlobe (Reiter and Alford's technique).

Repair of completely split earlobes

Completely split earlobes are more difficult to repair, as there is a loss of the inferior margin of the earlobe. Notching at the inferior rim of the earlobe may occur after repair. The indentation occurs from scar contraction and it can be prevented by several techniques such as Z-plasty, L-plasty, V-flap, and Lap-joint. The canals for earrings may be left in place by not excising the skin edges of the superior portion of the split, or may be constructed simultaneously with the repair of the split using a superiorly based skin flap. Some prefer to make the repair without preservation of the pierced canals; if desired, ear piercing may be performed 6 weeks later.

Repair of the completely split earlobe without preservation of the pierced canal

Side-to-side closure with vertical or horizontal mattress at the inferior end of the suture line

The epidermal surface of the split is excised with narrow margins, being careful to attain equal length of the split edges. Vertical or horizontal mattress sutures are placed on the inferior rim of the earlobe to create wound eversion and reduce the risk of notching. Simple interrupted or mattress sutures may be used for the rest of the surgical line (Fig. 20.5).

Undermining wound edges and side-to-side closure (Apesos' technique)[11]

The wound edges may be undermined prior to approximation to maximize wound eversion (Fig. 20.6). The skin edges of the split are excised. The anterior and posterior skin edges are undermined 1 mm. The skin edges are everted and stitched with interrupted simple sutures.

Side-to-side closure with Z-plasty at the inferior margin of the earlobe (Casson's technique)[12]

The skin at the edges of the split earlobe is excised (Fig. 20.7). The freshened edges of the defect are approximated and simple interrupted sutures are placed on the anterior and posterior surfaces. The Z-plasty is applied on the inferior margin of the closure. The vector of the wound contraction is redirected to decrease the risk of the earlobe notching. Tip stitches are not required because the tips of the flaps are very small. The scar line of the Z-plasty is concealed within the inferior rim of the earlobe.

Z-plasty of the earlobe (Tromovitch's[13] *and Reiter and Alford's techniques)*[10]

The epithelialized surface of the split is excised. A through-and-through Z-plasty is designed to create a side-to-side repair of the defect.[13] The scar is lengthened and the direction of wound tension is rearranged. Scar formation and contraction are diminished, which further reduces the risk of notching (Fig. 20.8).

Z-plasty may be used on the anterior skin of the earlobe and a vertical linear closure on the posterior surface (Fig. 20.9).[10]

L-plasty (Fatah's technique)[14]

This technique can be used with or without reconstruction of the pierced canal. The split area is excised through the

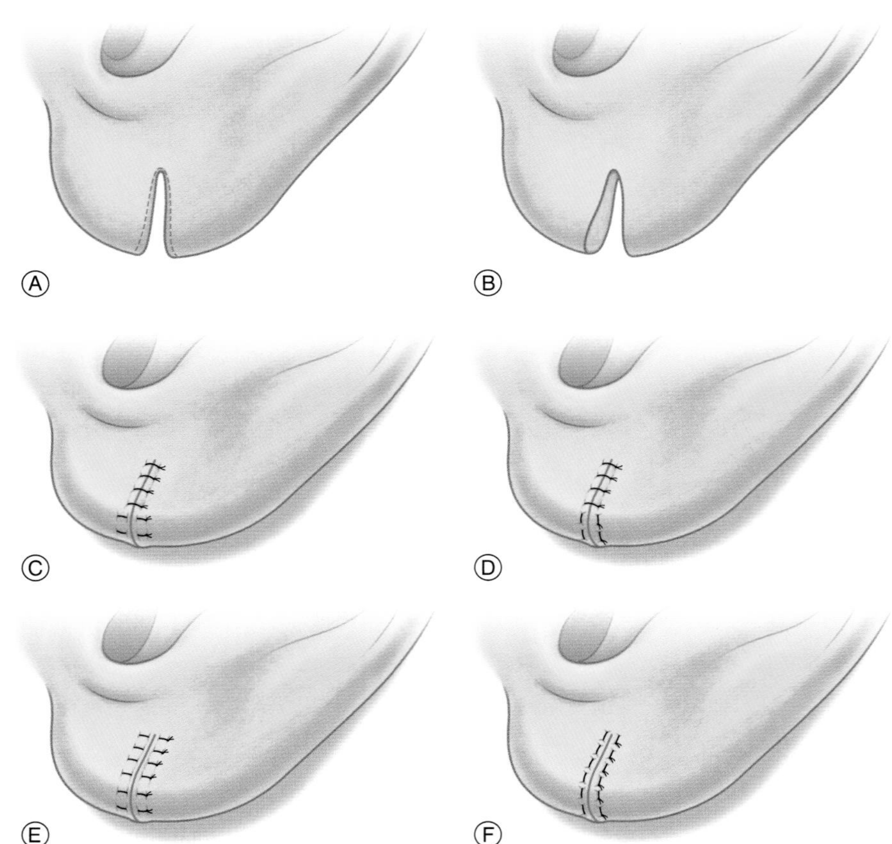

Figure 20.5 Use of vertical or horizontal mattress sutures to close the area. (A–B) Split earlobe. (C) Repair of rim with vertical mattress sutures and remainder of split with simple interrupted sutures. (D) Repair of rim with horizontal mattress sutures and remainder of defect with simple interrupted sutures. (E) Repair of entire split with vertical mattress sutures. (F) Repair of entire split with horizontal mattress sutures.

full thickness of the earlobe to create an L-shaped flap on one side and a complementing L-shaped defect on the other side (Fig. 20.10). The flaps are advanced, complementarily joined to each other, and stitched with simple interrupted sutures. If a canal is desired, a small flap at the superior end of the split is preserved and turned over and stitched on the anterior and posterior aspects. The L-plasty repair prevents notching at the inferior border of the earlobe because the line of scar contracture is broken up.

V-flap (Kalimuthu's technique)[15]

The edges of the split are excised. A 3-mm V-shaped socket is cut from the fat on one side of the split earlobe. On the other side of the split earlobe, an inverted V-shaped joint is cut into the fat to receive the opposite side. The flaps are stitched with simple interrupted sutures (Fig. 20.11).

Overlapping posterior–anterior flaps (Harahap's technique)[16]

The epithelium-lined edges of the split are excised (Fig. 20.12). A triangular flap is created on the anterior surface of one edge. The posterior surface of the other edge is cut in the same way with a similar amount of tissue excised. The resulting triangular flaps overlap. Sutures are placed on the anterior and posterior sides with the consequent Z-suture line at the inferior rim of the earlobe. This technique staggers the scar on the free border of the earlobe to avoid notching.

Partially incised Y-plasty (Arora's technique)[17]

With this technique the split is repaired and the earlobe's thickness is augmented. Two triangular areas are defined along the edges of the split. The base of the triangle is placed on the inferior rim of the earlobe and its apex pointed to the superior part of the split. The first triangular area is placed on the anterior surface of one side of the split, and the second triangular area is defined on the posterior aspect of the other. These two triangular areas are de-epithelialized and the raw areas are moved to overlap each other, resulting in an increased thickness of the earlobe. The suture lines are placed on the anterior and posterior surface and they run obliquely rather than overlap each other (Fig. 20.13).

Rotational flap (Effendi's technique)[18]

The edges of the split are excised. The lower border and the lateral edge of the lateral part of the split are excised to a distance that will fit a rotational flap from the medial part of the split (Fig. 20.14).

Various Repairs of the Completely Split Earlobe

Undermining wound edges

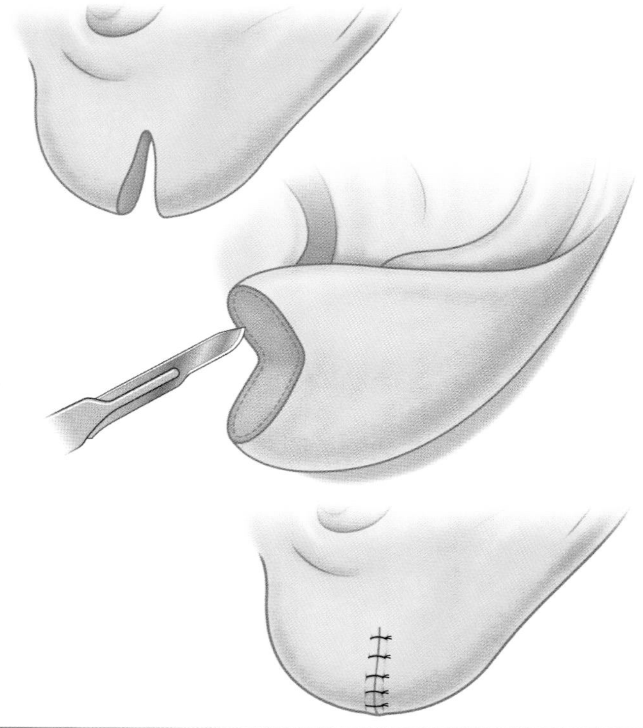

Figure 20.6 Undermining of the wound edge (Apesos's technique).

Z-plasty on full-thickness of earlobe

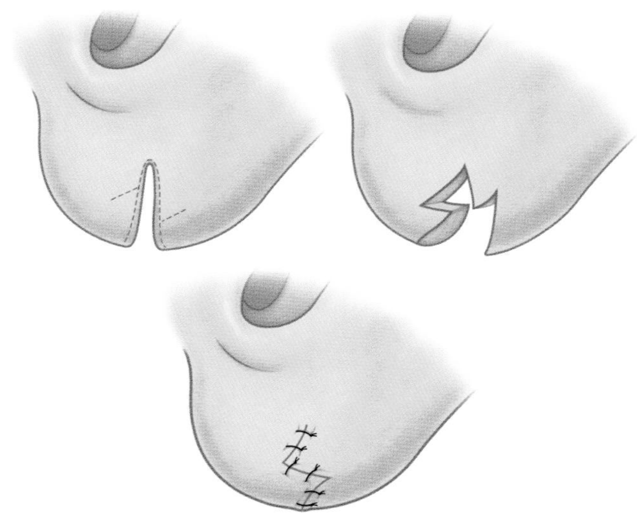

Figure 20.8 Z-plasty of the full thickness of the earlobe.

Z-plasty at the inferior margin

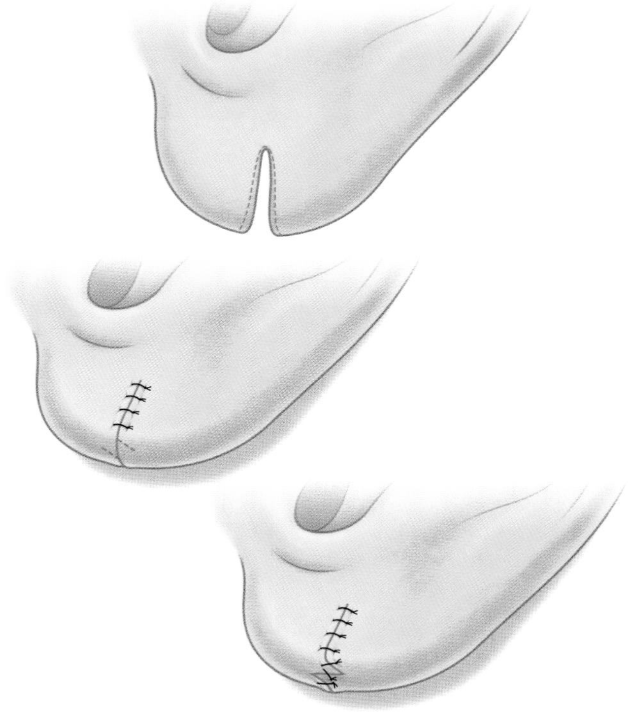

Figure 20.7 Side-to-side closure with Z-plasty at the rim of the lobe (Casson's technique).

Z-plasty on partial-thickness of earlobe

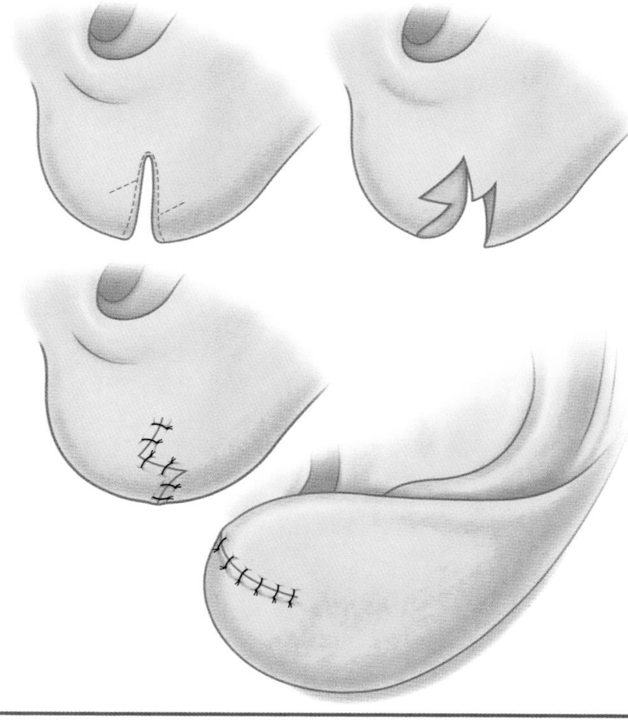

Figure 20.9 Z-plasty on the partial thickness of the anterior earlobe (Reiter and Alford's technique).

Various Repairs of the Completely Split Earlobe

L-plasty: medial and lateral

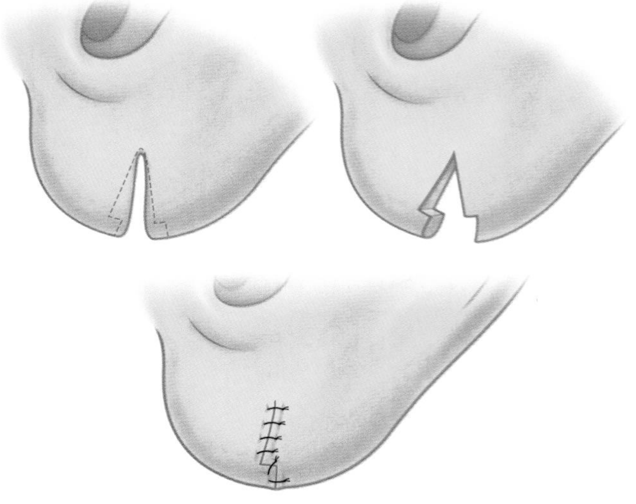

Figure 20.10 Interlocking L-incisions of the medial and lateral positions of the split earlobe (Fatah's technique).

L-plasty: anterior and posterior

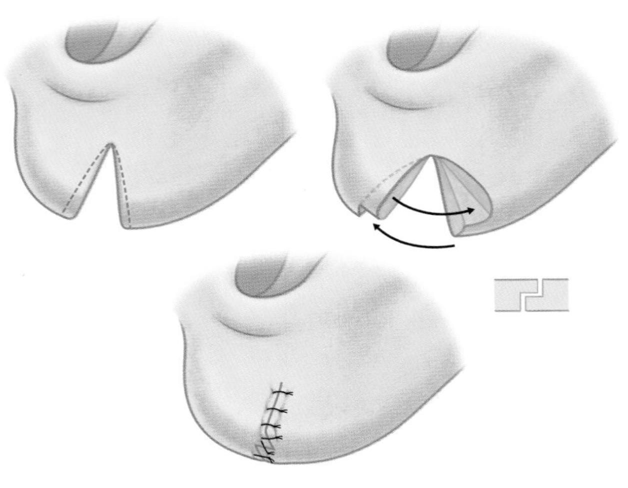

Figure 20.12 Interlocking L-plasty flaps formed by partial incision anteriorly and posteriorly (Harahap's technique).

Interlocking V-incisions

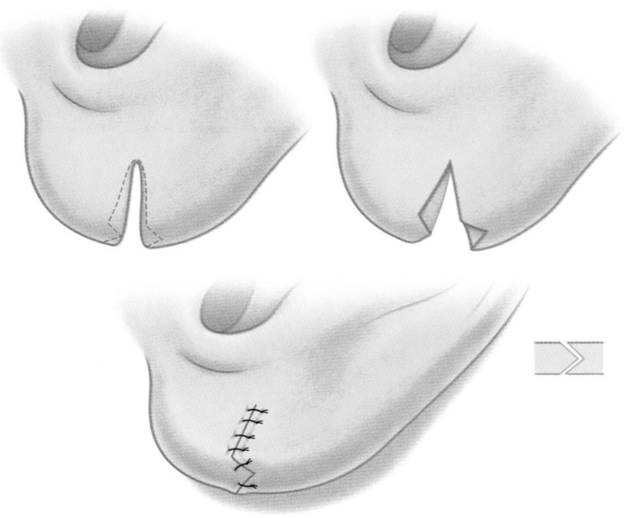

Figure 20.11 Interlocking V-incisions of the medial and lateral portions of the split earlobe (Kalimuthu's technique).

Partially incised V-plasty: anterior and posterior

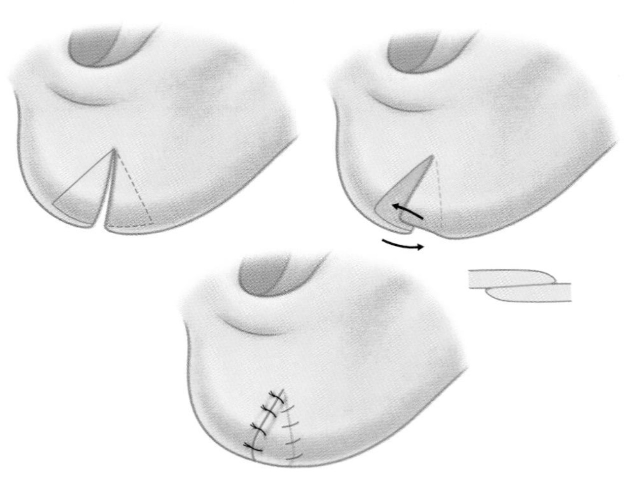

Figure 20.13 Partially incised V-plasty of the anterior and posterior flaps (Arora's technique).

Rotational flap

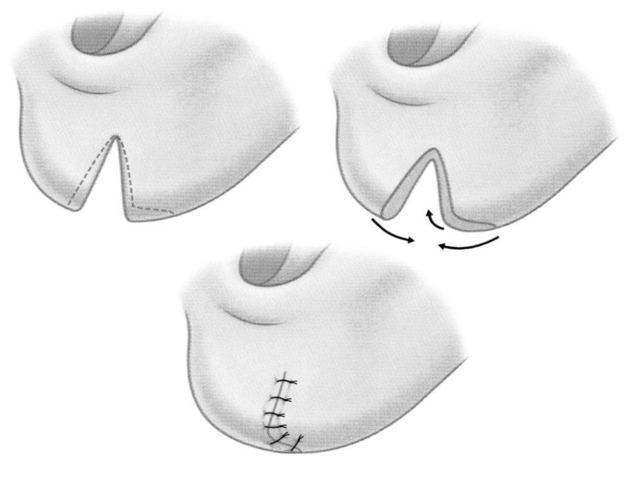

Figure 20.14 De-epithelialization of the wound edges (Effendi's technique).

Preservation of apical skin of the split lobe

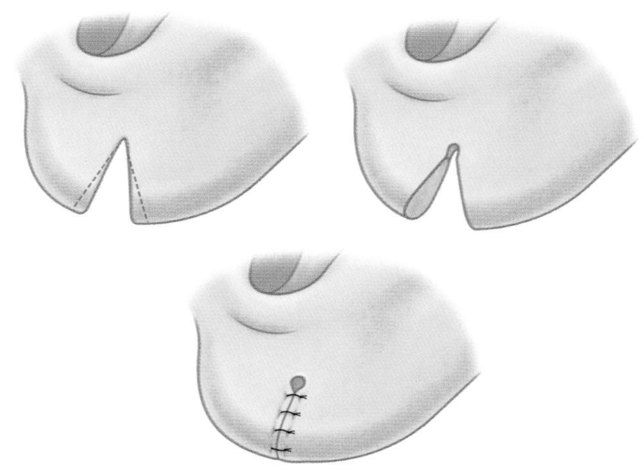

Figure 20.15 Only the inferior portion of the split earlobe is de-epithelialized leaving a tract for the earring (Boo-Chai's technique).

Repair of the completely split earlobe with preservation of the pierced canal

There are several techniques to repair the split earlobe with preservation of the pierced canal—for example, the skin edges can be joined below the pierced canal, or a flap can be used to create an epithelialized canal. These techniques may be used in the repair of partially split earlobes if desired. Earrings, or a non-absorbable material such as nylon 1-0 or 2-0, are used to maintain the newly formed canal.

Preservation of skin at apex of the split earlobe (Boo-Chai's technique)[1]

The skin at the apex of the split is preserved. The freshened edges below the apex of the split are joined side-to-side with the sutures placed on the anterior and posterior aspects of the earlobe (Fig. 20.15). This technique leaves a canal lined with freshened skin, as with ear piercing

Creation of flap from lateral portion of split lobe (Pardue's technique)[6]

The edges of the split are excised and the skin at the upper end of one side of the split is preserved to form a flap (Fig. 20.16). This superior based skin flap is trimmed to the appropriate length, turned, and sutured to the opposite side of the split to form a pierced canal. A stitch is not placed at the floor of the newly formed canal so that the risk of recurrence of the split may be minimized. The rest of the excised edges are stitched on the anterior and posterior surfaces.

Creation of a flap from the lateral portion of the split lobe and a Z-plasty (Walike and Larrabee[19] and Hamilton and La Rossa[3] techniques)

The skin is removed from the margin of the split, preserving skin superiorly on one side of the split. A new aperture for the earring is formed with the created skin flap. Z-plasty is used at the inferior border of the earlobe to prevent notching (Fig. 20.17).

Creation of flap from lateral portion of the split lobe

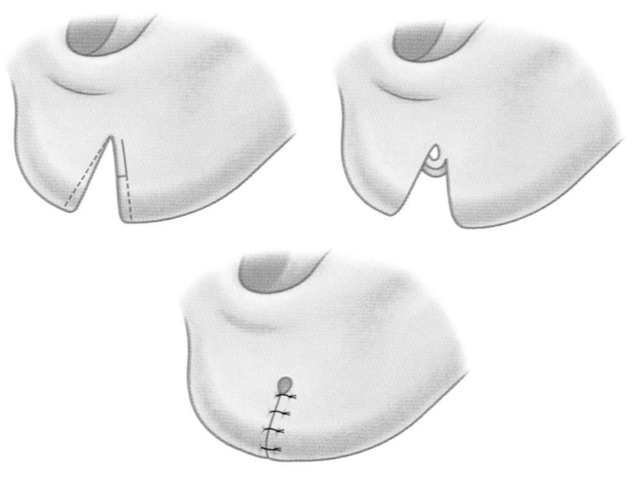

Figure 20.16 Creation of a flap from the lateral portion of the split lobe forms a tract for the earring (Pardue's technique).

Bilateral flap from posterior and lateral portion of the lobe (Buchan's technique)[20]

The epithelium-lined skin of the split is excised but a small superiorly based flap on the posterior aspect of one side of the split is preserved. This flap is drawn through the split to form the floor of the formed canal. The remaining edges of

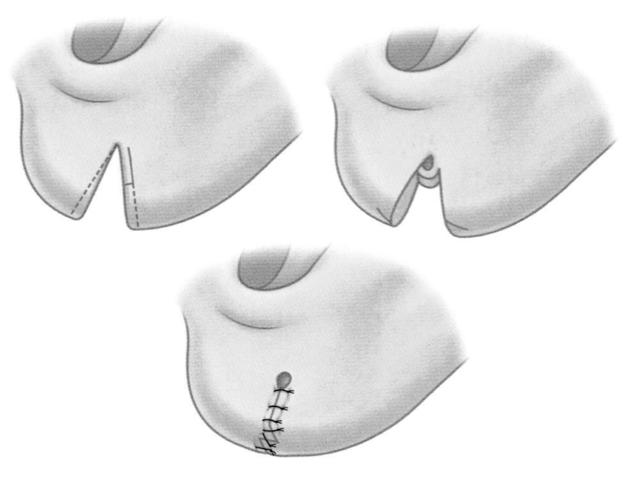

Figure 20.17 Creation of a flap from the lateral part of the split lobe and a Z-plasty on the rim of the lobe (Hamilton and La Rossa's, and Walike and Larrabee's techniques).

the split are stitched together. A Z-plasty or a lap-joint technique is used at the inferior margin of the closure (Fig. 20.18).

Lap-joint technique (Argamaso's technique)[21]

The epithelialized sides of the split are excised leaving a strip of skin at the apex. Triangular flaps are created on the anterior half of one side of the split (Fig. 20.19). The depth of excision is a half of the earlobe thickness. The excision is performed in the same way on the posterior half of the other edge. The two triangular flaps are overlapped and stitched. This technique prevents the formation of a notch and creates holes for earrings.

Rectangular flaps on anterior and posterior sides of the split lobe (Zolite's technique)[22]

The skin edges of the split are excised with preservation of the skin at the apex of the split to form a lining for the pierced canal. Broadly based rectangular flaps are created on the anterior half of one side of the split and the posterior half of the other side (Fig. 20.20). The length to width ratio of the flap is 1–1 or 1–2. The flaps are overlapped and sutured. The technique of using broadly based flaps avoids an earring situated on a potentially less stable scar.

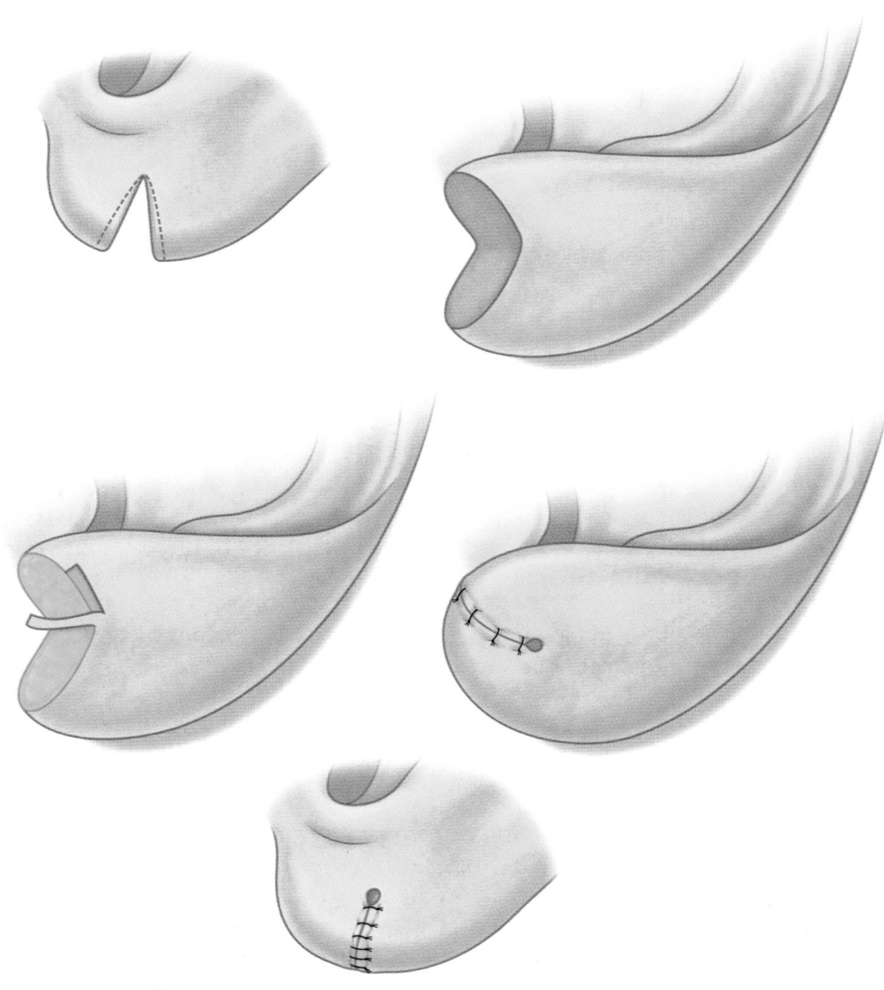

Figure 20.18 Creation of a flap from the posterior and lateral part of the lobe (Buchan's technique).

Repair of the Completely Split Earlobe with Preservation of the Pierced Canal

Lap-joint flaps

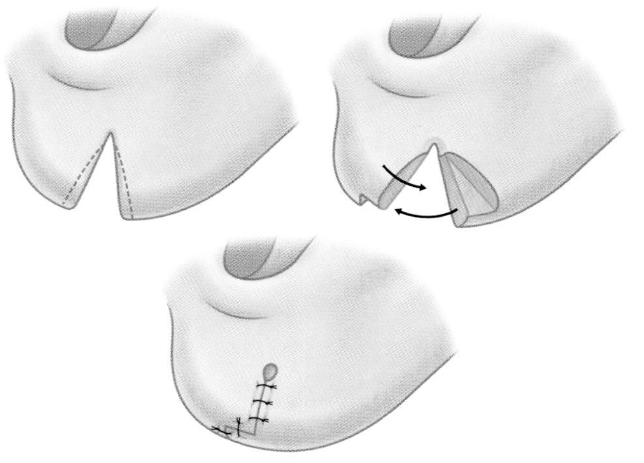

Figure 20.19 Overlapping joining flaps from the anterior and posterior flaps preserve an epithelialized portion for the earring (Argamaso's technique).

L-shaped flaps

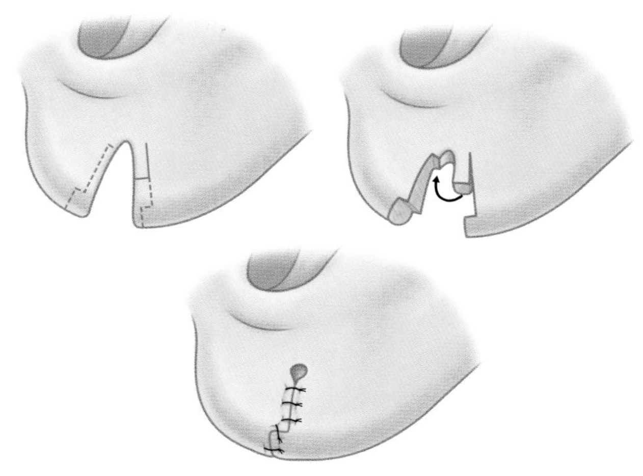

Figure 20.21 Creation of the tract for the earring by a posterior flap with an L incision to repair the split lobe (Fatah's technique).

Rectangular flaps on the anterior and posterior sides of the split lobe

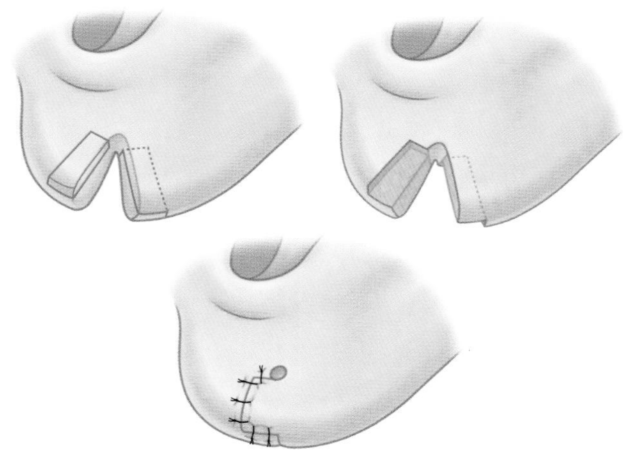

Figure 20.20 Parallel opposed flaps from the anterior and posterior flaps preserve an epithelialized portion (Zolite's technique).

Superiorly based skin flaps

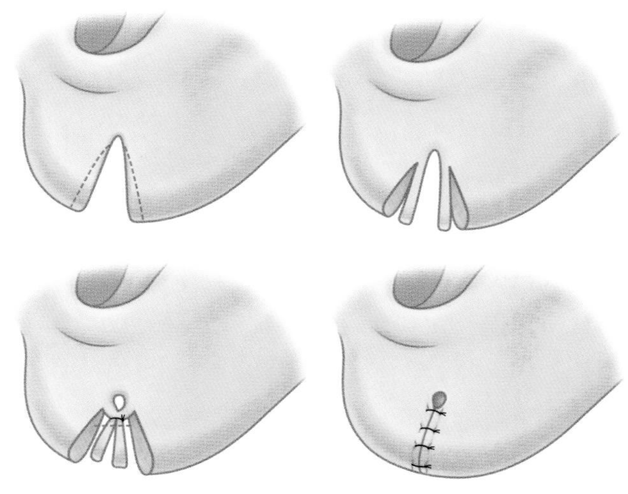

Figure 20.22 Creation of the tract for the earring (Elsahy's technique).

L-shaped flaps (Fatah's technique)[14]

L-shaped flaps are created on both sides of the split while preserving a small skin flap at the superior end of one edge. The skin flap is then rotated and stitched with the other side of the split (Fig. 20.21).

Superiorly based skin flaps (Elsahy's technique)[23]

The margins of the split are excised with preservation of the skin at the superior portion of both edges. The two superiorly based skin flaps are stitched together and the remaining parts of the flap are excised (Fig. 20.22). The freshened edges of the split are approximated with simple interrupted sutures.

Superior strip repair of tract and two Z-plasties to repair split lobe (Fayman's technique)[24]

The split margins are excised with a strip of skin at superior portion of one edge is preserved to reconstruct an earring canal. Two Z-plasties are performed to mid-thickness of the earlobe, anteriorly and posteriorly (Fig. 20.23). The first Z-plasty is placed on the anterior aspect of the earlobe, and the second is performed on the posterior aspect in the opposite direction to the first.

Modifications

- Excision of the split edges:
  - avoid cross-hatching of the inverted 'V' excision at the superior end of the complete split, and at both ends of the partial split
  - if the length of the split edges is different, a triangular excision may be placed at the apex of the split to compensate for the difference in length and to prevent dog-ear formation.
- When a partial split is nearly complete and the excision of epithelialized tract at the inferior border is difficult, the tissue at the inferior margin of the split may be discarded and the repair carried out as for a completely split earlobe.
- If the split occurs on one earlobe only, it may be closed completely and the earlobe can be re-pierced to match the other earlobe after 6 weeks. If the hole is left in place, it should be at the superior edge of the split.
- Some prefer re-piercing at 6 weeks after the repair of the split earlobe. Techniques that preserve the pierced canal by allowing the weight of the earrings to be carried directly on the scar may result in a recurrence of the split.
- The re-pierced site should be placed adjacent to, but not directly over, the repair scar line.

■ POSTOPERATIVE CARE

Regular daily wound care is advised. Suture removal is performed 7–14 days after the procedure. Re-piercing within the first 6 weeks after the repair is not

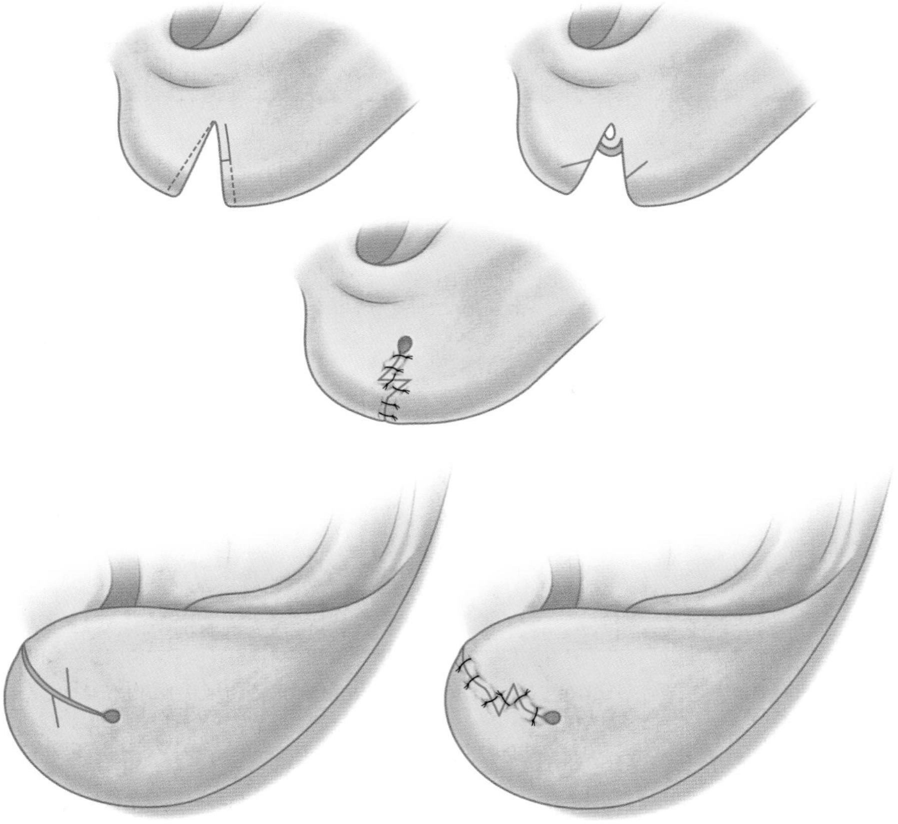

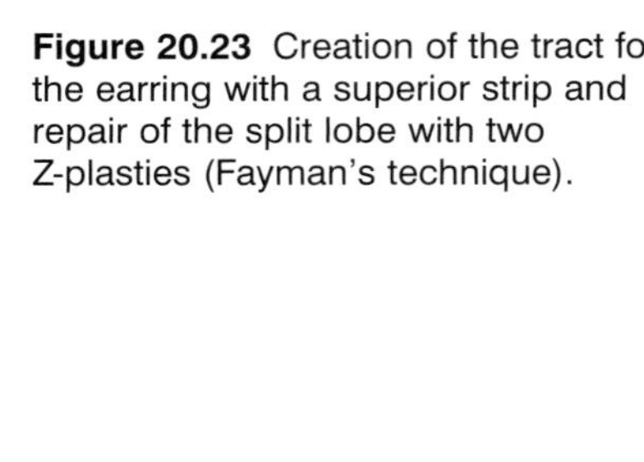

Figure 20.23 Creation of the tract for the earring with a superior strip and repair of the split lobe with two Z-plasties (Fayman's technique).

recommended. In the long term, wearing heavy earrings should be avoided. The shape and size of the earlobe are generally well preserved, and no notching occurs.

PITFALLS AND THEIR MANAGEMENT

The potential complications of split earlobe repair include bleeding, infection, notching of earlobes, hypertrophic scars, and keloids. Methods to manage these complications are summarized below.

Management of pitfalls

- Bleeding is managed by external compression.
- Infection requires antibiotics and wound care.
- Notching of earlobes can occur and will require scar revision.
- Hypertrophic scars can be treated with intralesional corticosteroids, silicone gel sheeting, cryotherapy, or laser therapy.[25,26]
- Keloids (see Chapter 44) require combination therapy, including some or all of the following: surgical excision, intralesional corticosteroids, intralesional interferon, silicon gel sheeting, cryotherapy, and laser therapy.[26–36]

SUMMARY

Symmetrical and rounded earlobes give the ears a good aesthetic appearance. An individually tailored approach to the repair of a split earlobe, as well as an understanding of surgical techniques and wound healing, improves the chance of a cosmetically acceptable outcome.

EAR PIERCING

INTRODUCTION

Several techniques of ear piercing are available, such as the intravenous cannula stent, the needle, and the spring-loaded piercing gun.[37–44] Ear piercing in the cartilaginous portion of the ear may be complicated by chondritis, cartilage necrosis, and auricular deformity.

PREOPERATIVE PREPARATION

The evaluation should include taking a history of hypertrophic scar or keloid formation, finding out about allergic reactions to metallic components of earrings, and asking about the desired site of piercing. Patients with earlobe less than 4 mm in thickness should be informed about the increased risk of developing split earlobes and the need to be careful about the weight of earrings.[10] Nickel-free stainless steel earrings are preferred; these should be cold-sterilized in alcohol for 30 minutes. With respect to the instruments, a 16-gauge or 18-gauge needle will be required.

Both sides of the earlobes are cleansed with antiseptic and the desired piercing site is marked. Local anesthesia to the earlobe is provided by lidocaine injection with a 30-gauge needle. An ice-cube or cooling spray on the earlobe may be used to numb the area prior to any piercing procedure.

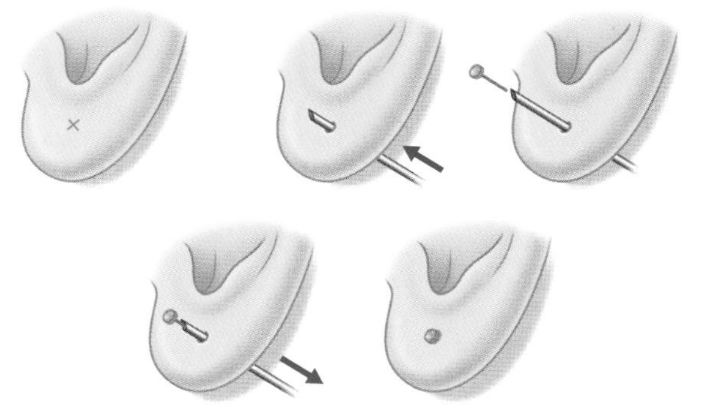

Figure 20.24 One-needle technique for ear piercing.

NEEDLE TECHNIQUES

One-needle technique

The points on the anterior and posterior surface of the earlobe where the earring is to be placed are marked with Gentian violet or a marking pen. The marking should be made in the middle of the earlobe and the patient should be allowed to see and approve this mark using a handheld mirror. The earlobe is anesthetized with 1% lidocaine. A 16-gauge or 18-gauge needle is inserted at the posterior surface of the earlobe in a plane perpendicular to it (Fig. 20.24). The needle is directed and advanced anteriorly to exit at the marked point on the anterior surface of the earlobe. The post attached to the earring stud is then inserted into the barrel of the needle, and this is then drawn back through the earlobe. The needle is removed from the earring post, which protrudes from the posterior surface of the earlobe. The earring clasp is attached to the earring post.[42]

Two-needle technique

The desired piercing sites are marked anteriorly and posteriorly on the earlobe, and anesthetized. A 30-gauge needle is inserted through the earlobe in the anterior-to-posterior direction. Local anesthesia may be injected with the insertion of the 30-gauge needle (Fig. 20.25).[44] A 16-gauge or 18-gauge is slipped over the 30-gauge needle at the posterior aspect of the earlobe. Both needles are drawn toward the anterior surface of the earlobe, and the 30-gauge needle is then removed from other needle. The earring post is inserted into the lumen of this remaining needle, and drawn posteriorly through the earlobe. The needle is removed and the earring clasp is fastened onto the earring post.

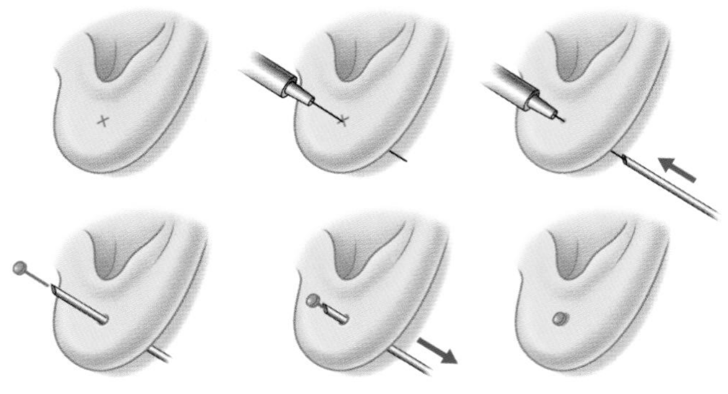

Figure 20.25 Two-needle technique for ear piercing.

■ EAR-PIERCING KITS

Commercial ear-piercing kits are more convenient but offer no advantages over these methods. Two available ear-piercing kits are the Steri-Quick ear-piercing kit (Roman Research, Norwell, MA) and the Debut Prestige ear-piercing kit (H&A Enterprises Inc, Whitestone, NY). Embedded earrings may be associated with the use of ear-piercing guns. Care must be taken to ensure that the earring clasp is not too tightly fixed against the earlobe.

Modifications

- Some patients have asymmetric earlobes, with one earlobe more pendulous than the other.[45] The piercing sites of both earlobes should be adjusted to prevent one earring from appearing higher than the other
- To avoid drooping of the earrings, the needle is advanced slightly superiorly toward the anterior surface of the earlobe in the one-needle technique or directed slight inferiorly toward the posterior surface of the earlobe in the two-needle technique

■ OPTIMIZING OUTCOMES

The aim of ear piercing is to ensure accurate placement of the earrings and to ensure that the patient is satisfied with the piercing site. Therefore it is important to ensure that both earrings are on the same horizontal level. The pierced canal should become fully re-epithelialized so that earrings can be worn without difficulty. There should be no evidence of allergic reaction, of infection, of hypertrophic scars or of keloids.

■ POSTOPERATIVE CARE

The earrings should be kept in place until the tract has epithelialized, which usually occurs in 2–3 weeks. The person should be advised to clean both sides of the ears underneath the earrings with sterile saline or hydrogen peroxide twice a day for 2 weeks or until the tract has epithelialized, and to rotate the earrings twice a day to prevent the formation of adhesions. The piercing earrings may be removed and another pair inserted after 4–6 weeks. People should be warned that long-term wearing of heavy earrings is best avoided due to the likelihood of developing split earlobes—especially if they have thin earlobes.

■ PITFALLS AND THEIR MANAGEMENT

The complications of ear piercing are listed in Table 20.1.[46–79] Methods to manage these complications are summarized in the box.

> **Management of pitfalls**
>
> - Use scrupulous aseptic technique and select appropriate earrings to reduce complications such as infection and embedding of earrings in the earlobe.
> - Advise patients on daily wound care and prescribe local and systemic antibiotics if infection occurs.
> - Recommend that patients use nickel-free posts to avoid development of allergic contact dermatitis.
> - Screen out patients who have thin earlobes, because they are most at risk for split earlobes and elongation of the piercing tract.

Embedded earrings

Earrings may become embedded in the earlobe, especially when the earlobes are thick. This complication occurs more frequently with the use of spring-loaded ear-piercing instruments.[60,61] Patients present with a tender cyst or keloid-like nodule within the earlobe.[62,63] Embedded earrings can be avoided by using aseptic technique, confining ear piercing to the earlobe, using earrings with larger clasps and longer posts, not securing the clasp too tightly against the earlobe, and removing the earrings if infection develops.

Management includes the removal of the embedded earrings under local anesthesia. An incision may be required to assist the extraction. Thereafter, the area should be cleansed daily and topical antibiotics applied. Earrings can be reinserted after the swelling and tenderness have disappeared. In some cases, the ear may need to be re-pierced at a later date.

Infections

Local bacterial infection is the most common complication of ear piercing. Purulent drainage, swelling, persistent redness, and delayed healing are evident. Staphylococcal sepsis, toxic shock syndrome, acute poststreptococcal glomerulonephritis, osteomyelitis, viral hepatitis, and tuberculosis have been reported after ear piercing.[46,47,51–53,80–82] Potentially, human immunodeficiency virus (HIV) can be transmitted by ear piercing.[83]

Management includes daily wound care and the removal of earrings so that drainage can occur. Topical and systemic antibiotics should be given. The tract may be occluded after the infection subsides. Re-piercing should only be performed after the wound completely heals.

Table 20.1 Complications of ear piercing

Complications		References
Bleeding and hematoma formation		
Infection	Staphylococcal and streptococcal infection	46,47
	Pseudomonas chondritis	48
	Tetanus	49
	Viral hepatitis	50–52
	Primary tuberculosis of the earlobe	53
	Botryomycosis	54
Hypersensitivity and allergic contact dermatitis to metal		55–59
Embedded earrings		60–63
Hypertrophic scars and keloids		25,64,65
Elongation of ear-piercing tract and split earlobe		66–70
Lymphoplasia		71–73
Cyst formation		74
Granulomatous reaction		75
Localized argyria		76
Frostbite		77
Lipoma		78
Postauricular pressure sores		79

Piercing of the auricular cartilage may lead to perichondrial infection, auricular chondritis, cartilage necrosis, and resultant auricular deformity.[84–86] The responsible organisms most commonly found in these patients are *Pseudomonas aeruginosa* and *Staphylococcus aureus*.[48,85,87] Management of these infections includes an appropriate systemic antibiotic. In addition, incision and drainage, wound debridement, and subsequent auriculoplasty may be required.[87,88]

Hypersensitivity and allergic contact dermatitis

Ear piercing is an important risk factor for nickel sensitization.[89–92] Therefore it is recommended that patients start with earring posts that are nickel-free and made of either stainless steel or 24-carat gold. The use of an intravenous catheter as an earring-post sheath allows nickel-sensitive individuals to wear earrings in pierced ears on a limited basis.[93]

Hypertrophic scars or keloid formation

Hypertrophic scars may be treated with intralesional corticosteroids, silicone gel sheeting, cryotherapy, pulsed-dye laser, or a combination of these methods.[25–26] In addition, for keloids these treatments may be combined with surgical excision, intralesional interferon, and external compression.[26–36] (See also Chapter 44.)

Elongation of ear-piercing tract and split earlobes

These complications are likely to occur in patients who have earlobes of less than 4 mm in thickness and who wear heavy earrings.[10]

■ SUMMARY

Patients who undergo ear piercing should be screened carefully. The thickness of the earlobe should be evaluated. The lack of aseptic technique and improper postoperative care contribute significantly to the complications associated with ear piercing.

EARLOBE REDUCTION

■ INTRODUCTION

Earlobes droop and broaden as a result of gravity and of aging, or as a consequence of some diseases such as contact dermatitis and leprosy. Unusually large earlobes may occur congenitally. Several techniques for reducing the size of the earlobes have been described.

■ PREOPERATIVE PREPARATION

Patient evaluation should include taking a history of hypertrophic scars or keloids, and inquiring about the patient's wishes about the size of the newly formed earlobe, and expectations of the cosmetic outcome. The equipment to be prepared in advance includes a general dermatologic surgery tray with a #15 surgical blade, a chalazion clamp, non-absorbable 5-0 or 6-0 suture for cutaneous closure, and absorbable 5-0 or 6-0 suture for subcutaneous closure. Antiseptic cleansing of both sides of the earlobes is required. Local anesthesia is then injected into the earlobe.

■ TECHNIQUES

A chalazion clamp can be used to stabilize the earlobe and control bleeding. Simple interrupted sutures may be used to close the resulting defect. At the earlobe margin, a

Z-plasty may be used to reduce scar contraction and subsequent notching of the earlobe.

Wedge excision

The wedge excision may be performed on the medial, lateral, or inferior portion of the enlarged earlobe. The preferred location is the inferior portion of the enlarged earlobe because of the superior vascular supply (Fig. 20.26).

Elliptical excision

The ellipse may be performed at the inferior, medial, or lateral border of the earlobe. The technique of McCoy, Stark and Tipton allows the scar line to be hidden on the posterior surface of the earlobe.[94–96] The incision is made at an oblique angle to the anterior surface so the scar is placed on the posterior surface and a rounded appearance of the new margin of the earlobe is achieved (Fig. 20.27).

Techniques used at the lateral portion of the earlobe

The redundant earlobe is repaired by the desired technique (Joseph, Denecke, Tanzer, Enna and Delgado, and Lewis techniques) (Fig. 20.28).[97–100] Local anesthesia is given and the full thickness of the marked tissue is excised. The resulting defect is stitched with simple interrupted sutures. A notch may develop with any of these techniques as the end of the suture line remains on the lateral free margin of the earlobe.

Wedge excision

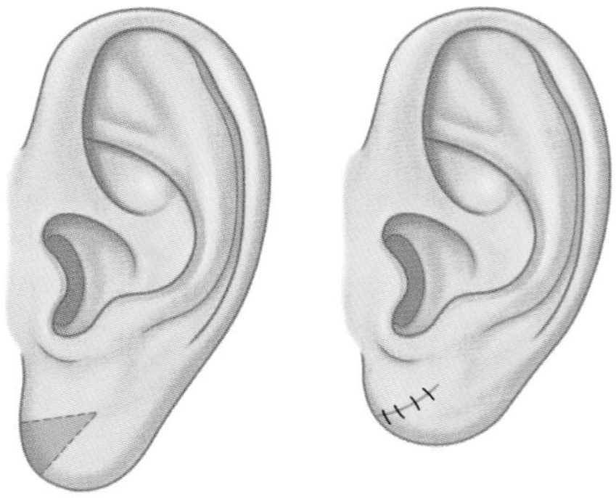

Figure 20.26 Wedge excision to remove redundancy.

Crescentic excision of redundant earlobe

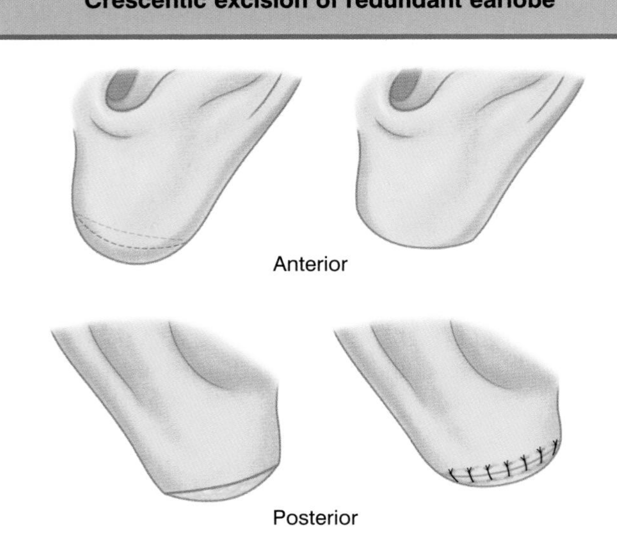

Figure 20.27 Crescentic excision to remove redundancy (McCoy, Stark and Tipton's technique).

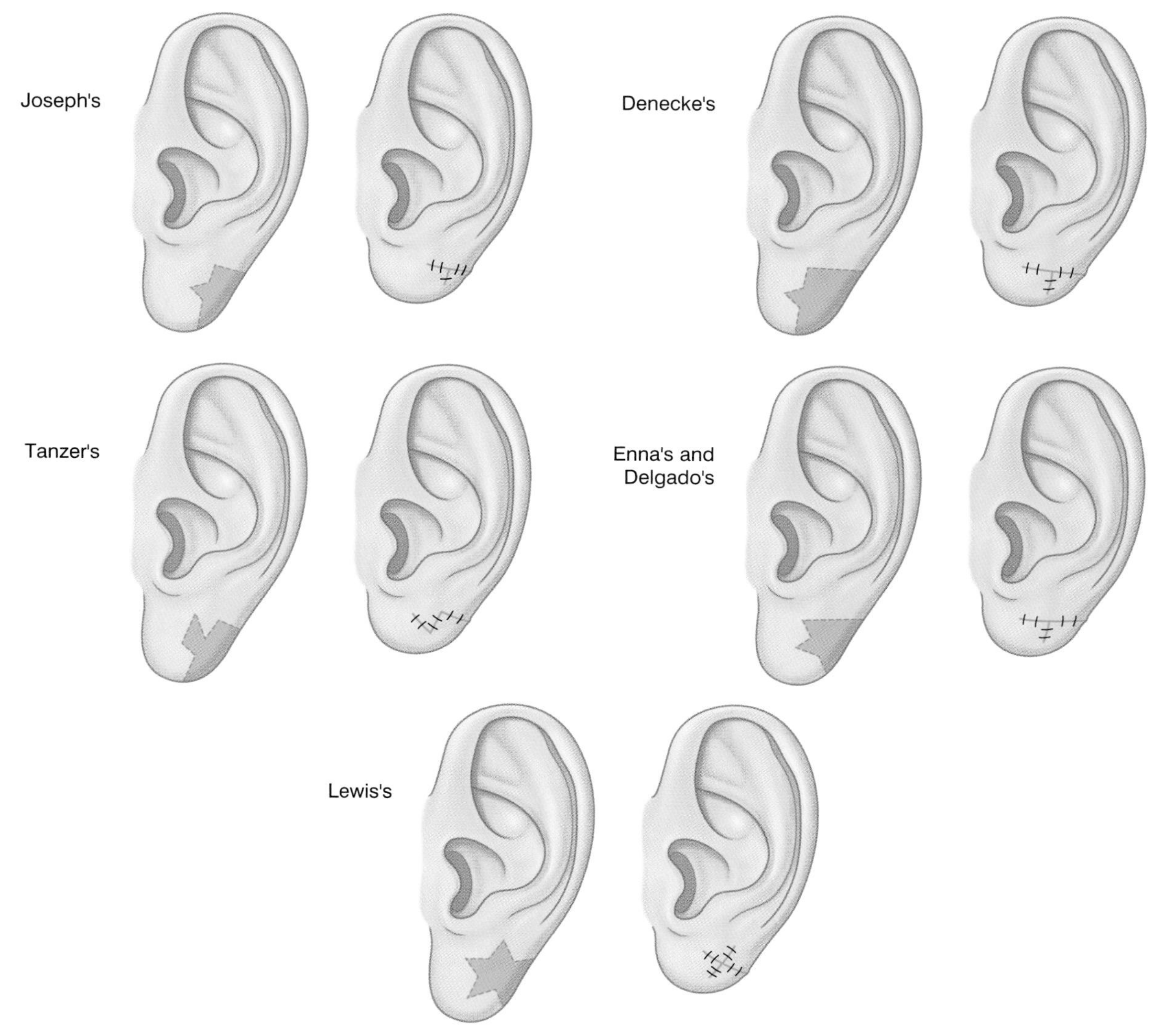

Figure 20.28 Techniques from the lateral portion of the earlobe. (A) Joseph's technique; (B) Denecke's technique; (V) Tanzer's technique; (D) Enna and Delgado's technique; (E) Lewis's technique.

Techniques used at the medial portion of the earlobe

These techniques prevent notching because the end of the suture line is on the anterior margin of the earlobe. The excess earlobe is marked and excised. Techniques used are those of Eitner, Miller, Rubin, Loeb, Guerrero-Santos, Constant, Lassus or McCollough (Fig. 20.29).[101–107] Care must be taken to avoid pulling the earlobe outward, as this results in an increased angle between the earlobe and the jawline. The scar line may be seen with these techniques, as well as with the techniques applied to the posterior portion of the earlobe.

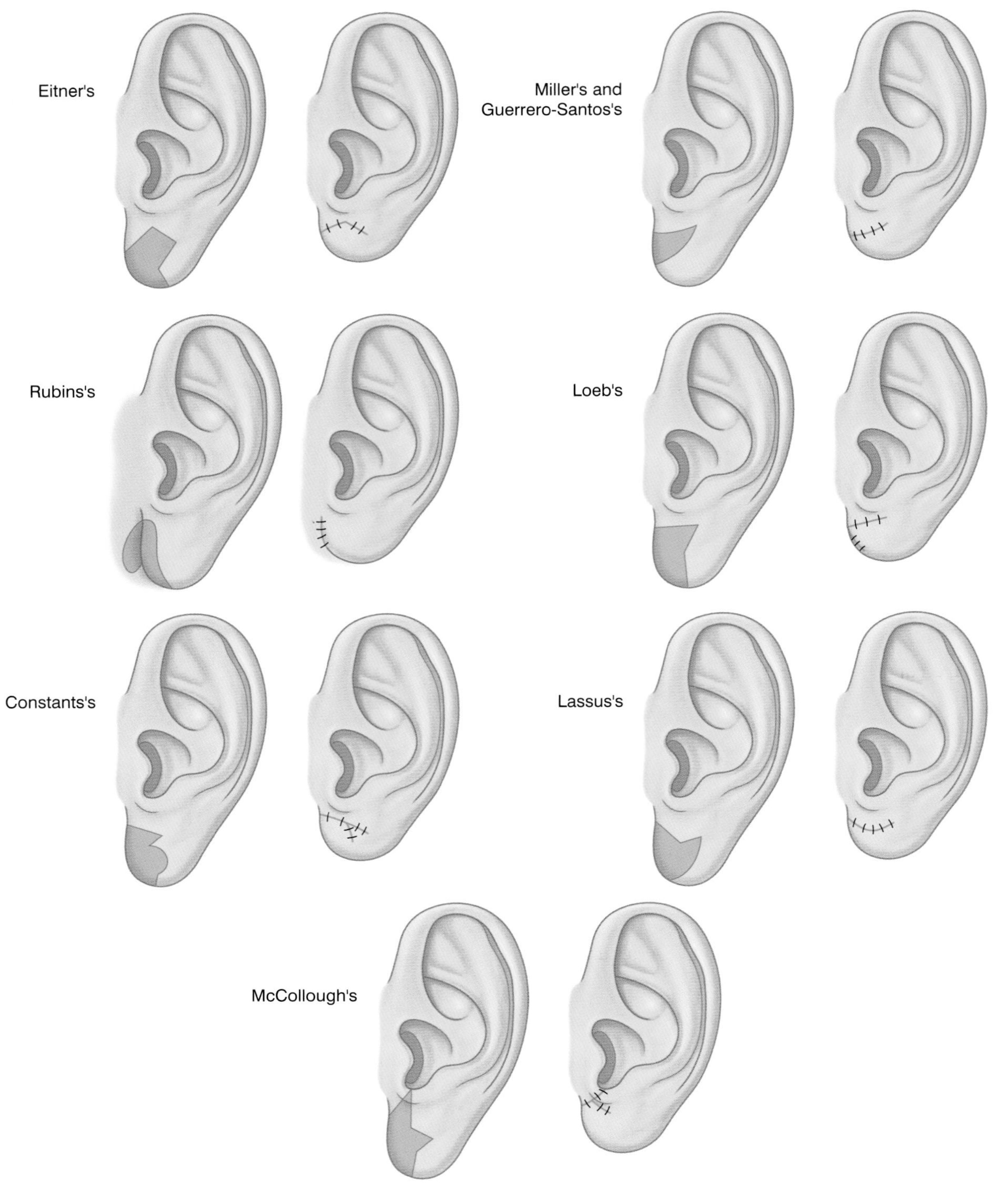

Figure 20.29 Techniques from the medial portion of the earlobe. (A) Eitner's technique; (B) Miller and Guerrero-Santos's technique; (C) Rubin's technique; (D) Loeb's technique; (E) Constant's technique; (F) Lassus' technique; (G) McCollough's technique.

Earlobe reduction at the inferior portion of the earlobe

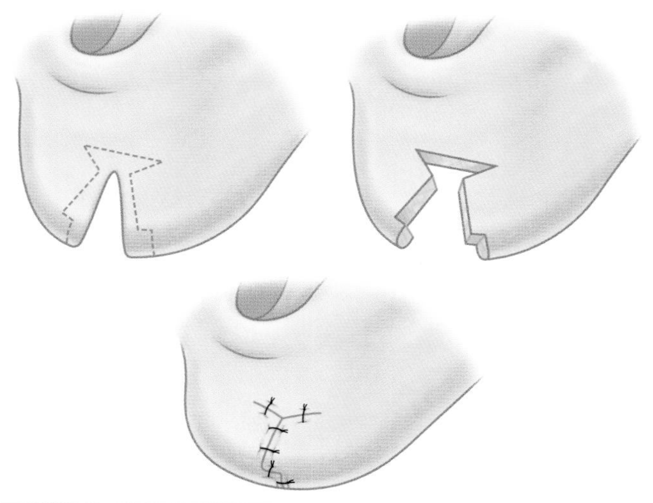

Figure 20.30 Inferiorly based earlobe reduction with an L-plasty with superiorly based wedge (Fearson's technique).

L-plasty with a superiorly based wedge (Fearson's technique[108])

The addition of a superiorly based wedge excision to the L-plasty permits an earlobe reduction (Fig. 20.30). This technique is suitable for the simultaneous repair of split earlobe and reduction of the earlobe size.

■ OPTIMIZING OUTCOMES

The enlarged earlobe is reduced according to the patient's desired size and shape. The scar line is concealed within the crease of the earlobe. No notching occurs.

■ POSTOPERATIVE CARE

The wound must be cleaned daily. Sutures can be removed after 7–14 days.

■ PITFALLS AND THEIR MANAGEMENT

These are the same as for repair of the split earlobe.

■ SUMMARY

Reduction of the earlobe is a simple surgical procedure giving pleasing results with the techniques described above.

■ REFERENCES

1. Boo-Chai K. The cleft ear lobe. Plast Reconstr Surg 1961; 28:681–688.
2. Kitayama Y, Yamamoto M, Tsukada S. Classification of congenital cleft ear lobe. Keisei Geka 1980; 23:663–670.
3. Hamilton R, LaRossa D. Method for repair of cleft earlobes. Plast Reconstr Surg 1975; 55:99–101.
4. McLaren LR. Cleft ear lobes: a hazard of wearing ear-rings. Br J Plast Surg 1954; 7:162–165.
5. Wallace AF, Garrets M. A case of necrosis of the earlobes. Br J Plast Surg 1960; 12:64–66.
6. Pardue AM. Repair of torn earlobe with preservation of the perforation for an earring. Plast Reconstr Surg 1973; 51:472–473.
7. Altchek E. Tearing of an earlobe by weight of a telephone earpiece on an earring. Plast Reconstr Surg 1977; 59:564.
8. Blanco-Davila F, Vasconez HC. The cleft earlobe: a review of methods of treatment. Ann Plast Surg 1994; 33:677–680.
9. Tan EC. Punch technique: an alternative approach to the repair of pierced earlobe deformities. J Dermatol Surg Oncol 1989; 15:270–272.
10. Reiter D, Alford EL. Torn earlobe: a new approach to management with a review of 68 cases. Ann Otol Rhino Laryngol 1994; 103:879–884.
11. Apesos J, Kane M. Treatment of traumatic earlobe clefts. Aesthetic Plast Surg 1993; 17:253–255.
12. Casson P. How do you repair a split earlobe? J Dermatol Surg 1976; 2:21.
13. Tromovitch TA, Stegman SJ, Glogau RG. Flaps and grafts in dermatologic surgery. St Louis: Mosby; 1989.
14. Fatah MF. L-plasty technique in the repair of split ear lobe. Br J Plast Surg 1985; 38:410–414.
15. Kalimuthu R, Larson BJ, Lewis N. Earlobe repair: a new technique. Plast Reconstr Surg 1984; 74:299–300.
16. Harahap M. Repair of split earlobes. A review and a new technique. J Dermatol Surg Oncol 1982; 8:187–191.
17. Arora PK. Reconstruction of the middle-aged torn earlobe: a new method. Br J Plast Surg 1989; 42:118.
18. Effendi SH. Reconstruction of the middle-aged torn earlobe: a new method. Br J Plast Surg 1988;41:174–176.
19. Walike J, Larrabee WF Jr. Repair of the cleft ear lobe. Laryngoscope 1985; 95:876–877.
20. Buchan NG. The cleft ear lobe: a method of repair with preservation of the earring canal. Br J Plast Surg 1975; 28:296–298.
21. Argamaso RV. The lap-joint principle in the repair of the cleft earlobe. Br J Plast Surg 1978; 31:337–338.
22. Zoltie N. Split earlobes: a method of repair preserving the hole. Plast Reconstr Surg 1987; 80:619–621.
23. Elsahy NI. Reconstruction of the cleft earlobe with preservation of the perforation for an earring. Plast Reconstr Surg 1986; 77:322–324.
24. Fayman MS. Split earlobe repair. Br J Plast Surg 1994; 47:293.
25. Ketchum LD, Cohen IK, Masters FW. Hypertrophic scars and keloids. A collective review. Plast Reconstr Surg 1974: 53:140–154.
26. Babin RW, Ceilley RI. The freeze-injection method of hypertrophic scar and keloid reduction. Otolaryngol Head Neck Surg 1979; 87:911–914.
27. Griffith BH, Monroe CW, McKinney P. A follow-up study on the treatment of keloids with triamcinolone acetonide. Plast Reconstr Surg 1970; 46:145–150.
28. Ashbell TS. Prevention and treatment of earlobe keloids. Ann Plast Surg 1982; 9:264–265.
29. Griffith BH. The treatment of keloids with triamcinolone acetonide. Plast Reconstr Surg 1966; 38:202–208.
30. Hirshowitz B, Lerner D, Moscona AR. Treatment of keloid scars by combined cryosurgery and intralesional corticosteroids. Aesthetic Plast Surg 1982; 6:153–158.
31. Shons AR, Press BH. The treatment of earlobe keloids by surgical excision and postoperative triamcinolone injection. Ann Plast Surg 1983; 10:480–482.
32. Brent B. The role of pressure therapy in management of earlobe keloids: preliminary report of a controlled study. Ann Plast Surg 1978; 1:579–581.
33. Salasche SJ, Grabski WJ. Keloids of the earlobes: a surgical technique. J Dermatol Surg Oncol 1983; 9:552–556.
34. Pollack SV, Goslen JB. The surgical treatment of keloids. J Dermatol Surg Oncol 1982; 8:1045–1049.
35. Kantor GR, Wheeland RG, Bailin PL, Wlaker NP, Ratz JL. Treatment of earlobe keloids with carbon dioxide laser excision: a report of 16 cases. J Dermatol Surg Oncol 1985; 11:1063–1067.
36. Shepherd JP, Dawber RP. The response of keloid scars to cryosurgery. Plast Reconstr Surg 1982; 70;677–682.

37. Inoue T, Kurihara T, Harashina T. Ear-piercing technique by using an eyelet-type Teflon piercer (eyelet-Piercer). Ann Plast Surg 1993; 3:159–161.
38. Zackowski DA. An i.v. cannula stent for ear piercing. Plast Reconstr Surg 1987; 80;751.
39. Matarasso SL, Glogau RG. Surgical pearl: ear piercing facilitated by magnetic earrings. J Am Acad Dermatol 1994; 31:485–486.
40. Duffy MM. A simple instrument for ear piercing. Plast Reconstr Surg 1967; 40:92–93.
41. Goff WF. Ear piercing—by whom? Eye Ear Nose Throat Mon 1975; 54:319.
42. Bennett RG. Fundamentals of cutaneous surgery. St Louis: Mosby; 1998.
43. Goldman L, Kitzmiller KW. Earlobe piercing with needles and wire. Arch Dermatol 1965; 92:305–306.
44. Landeck A, Newman N, Breadon J, Zahner S. A simple technique for ear piercing J Am Acad Dermatol 1998; 39:795–796.
45. Nakamura M, Ikeda T, Shioya N. Side-to-side earlobe variation with respect to surface area and shape: a quantitative study. Aesthet Plast Surg 1995; 19: pp. 561–565.
46. George J, White M. Infection as a consequence of ear piercing. Practitioner 1989; 233:404–406.
47. Ahmed-Jushuf IH, Selby PL, Brownjohn AM. Acute post-streptococcal glomerulonephritis following ear piercing. Postgrad Med J 1984; 60:73–74.
48. Turkeltaub SH, Habal MB. Acute *Pseudomonas* chondritis as a sequel to ear piercing. Ann Plast Surg 1990; 24:279–282.
49. Mamtani R, Malhotra P, Guptal PS, Jain BK. A comparative study of urban and rural tetanus in adults. Int J Epidemiol 1978; 7:185–188.
50. Van Sciver AE. Hepatitis from ear piercing. J Am Med Assoc 1969; 207:2285.
51. Johnson CJ, Anderson H, Spearman J, Madson J. Ear piercing and hepatitis. Non-sterile instruments for ear piercing and the subsequent onset of viral hepatitis. J Am Med Assoc 1974; 227:1165.
52. Hayes MO, Harkness GA. Body piercing as a risk factor for viral hepatitis: an integrative research review. Am J Infect Control 2001; 29:271–274.
53. Morgan LG. Primary tuberculosis inoculation of an earlobe. J Pediatr 1952; 40:482–485.
54. Olmstead PM, Finn M. Botryomycosis in pierced ears. Arch Dermatol 1982; 118:925–927.
55. Cortese TA, Dickey RA. Complications of ear piercing. Am Fam Physician 1971; 4:66–72.
56. Fisher AA. Ear piercing and sensitivity to nickel and gold. J Am Acad Dermatol 1987; 17:853.
57. Christensen OB. Nickel dermatitis. An update. Dermatol Clin 1990; 8:37–40.
58. Fisher AA. Ear piercing and nickel allergy. Cont Dermatit 1986; 14:328.
59. Boss A, Menne T. Nickel sensitization from ear piercing. Cont Dermatit 1982; 8:211–213.
60. Muntz HR, Pa-C DJ, Asher BF. Embedded earrings: a complication of the ear-piercing gun. Int J Pediatr Otorhinolaryngol 1990; 19: pp. 73–76.
61. Cockin J, Finan P, Powell M. A problem with ear piercing. BMJ 1977; 2:1631.
62. Saleeby ER, Rubin MG, Youshock E, Kleinshmith DM. Embedded foreign bodies presenting as earlobe keloids. J Dermatol Surg Oncol 1984; 10:902–904.
63. Smith RB. Earring clasp as a foreign body in the earlobe. Plast Reconstr Surg 1978; 62:772.
64. Cheng LH. Keloid of the ear lobe. Laryngoscope 1972; 82:673–681.
65. Cosman B, Wolff M. Bilateral earlobe keloids. Plast Reconstr Surg 1974; 53:540–543.
66. McLaren LR. Surgery of the external ear. J Laryngol Otol 1974; 88:23–38.
67. Jay AL. Ear-piercing problems. BMJ 1977; 2:574–575.
68. Pardue AM. Repair of torn earlobe with preservation of the perforation for an earring. Plast Reconstr Surg 1973; 51:472–473.
69. Harahap M. Repair of split earlobes. A review and a new technique. J Dermatol Surg Oncol 1982; 8:187–191.
70. Buchan NG. The cleft ear lobe: a method of repair with preservation of the earring canal. Br J Plast Surg 1975; 28:296–298.
71. Iwatsuki K, Tagami H, Moriguchi T, Yamada M. Lymphadenoid structure induced by gold hypersensitivity. Arch Dermatol 1982; 118:608–611.
72. Iwatsuki K, Yamada M, Takigawa M, Inoue K, Matsumoto K. Benign lymphoplasia of the earlobes induced by gold earrings: immunohistologic study on the cellular infiltrates. J Am Acad Dermatol 1987; 16:83–88.
73. Aoshima T, Oguchi M. Intracytoplasmic crystalline inclusions in dermal infiltrating cells of granulomatous contact dermatitis due to gold earrings. Acta Derm Venereol 1988; 68:261–264.
74. Ellis DA. Complication and correction of the pierced ear. J Otolaryngol 1976; 5:247–250.
75. Mann RJ, Peachey RD. Sarcoidal tissue reaction—another complication of ear piercing. Clin Exp Dermatol 1983; 8:199–200.
76. Van den Nieuwenhuijsen IJ, Calame JJ, Bruynzeel DP. Localized argyria caused by silver earrings. Dermatologica 1988; 177:189–191.
77. Noble DA. Another hazard of pierced ears. BMJ 1979; 1:125.
78. Castellani A. Minor tropical diseases. J Trop med 1932; 35:24–26.
79. Phelan WJ. Complications of earrings in an infant. JAMA 1980; 243:2288.
80. George J, White M. Infection as a consequence of ear piercing. Practitioner 1989; 233:404–406.
81. Lovejoy FH Jr, Smith DH. Life-threatening staphylococcal disease following ear piercing. Pediatrics 1970; 46:301–303.
82. Shulman BH. Ear piercing and sepsis. Clin Pediatr (Phila) 1973; 12:27A.
83. CDCP (1998) Centers for Disease Control and Prevention. Can I get HIV from getting a tattoo or through body piercing? http://www.cdc.gov (17 Dec 2003).
84. Margulis A, Bauer BS, Alizadeh K. Ear reconstruction after auricular chondritis secondary to ear piercing. Plast Reconstr Surg 2003; 111:891–897, 898.
85. Yahalom S, Eliasher R. Perichondritis: a complication of piercing auricular cartilage. Postgrad Med J 2003; 79:29.
86. Widick MH, Coleman J. Perichondrial abscess resulting from a high ear-piercing-case report. Otolaryngol Head Neck Surg 1992; 107:803–804.
87. Cicchetti S, Skillman J, Gault DT. Piercing the upper ear: a simple infection, a difficult reconstruction. Br J Plast Surg 2002; 55:194–197.
88. Iida N, Hosaka Y, Ogawa T. Correction of auricular deformity caused by high ear-piercing: case report. Ann Plast Surg 2003; 50:82–84.
89. Nakada T, Iijima M, Nakayama H, Maibach HI. Role of ear piercing in metal allergic contact dermatitis. Cont Dermatit 1997; 36:233–236.
90. McDonagh AJ, Wright AL, Cork MJ, Gawkrodger DJ. Nickel sensitivity: the influence of ear piercing and atopy. Br J Dermatol 1992: 126:16–18.
91. Nielsen NH, Menne T. Nickel sensitization and ear piercing in an unselected Danish population. Glostrup Allergy Study. Contact Dermatitis 1993; 29:16–21.
92. Dotterud LK, Falk ES. Metal allergy in north Norwegian schoolchildren and its relationship with ear piercing and atopy. Cont Dermatit 1994; 31:308–313.
93. Cornetta AJ, Reiter D. Ear piercing for individuals with metal hypersensitivity. Otolaryngol Head Neck Surg 2001; 125:93–95.
94. Tipton JB. A simple technique for reduction of the earlobe. Plast Reconstr Surg 1980; 66:630–632.
95. McCoy FJ. Macrotia. In: Masters FW, Lewis JR Jr , eds. Symposium on aesthetic surgery of the nose, ears and chin, St Louis: Mosby; 1973: pp. 160–164.
96. Stark RB. Plastic surgery. New York: Harper and Row; 1962.
97. Barsky A. Principles and practice of plastic surgery. Baltimore: Williams & Wilkins; 1950.
98. Tanzer RC. Congenital deformities of the auricle. In: Converse JM, ed. Reconstructive plastic surgery. Philadelphia: Saunders; 1964: p. 1084.
99. Enna CD, Delgado DD. Surgical correction of common facial deformities due to leprosy. Plast Reconstr Surg 1968; 42:422–432.
100. Lewis JR Jr. Atlas of aesthetic plastic surgery. Boston: Brown; 1973.
101. Miller CC. Cosmetic surgery: the correction of featural imperfections. Philadelphia: Davis; 1925.
102. Rubin LR, Bromberg BE, Walden RH, Adams A. An anatomic approach to the obtrusive ear. Plast Reconstr Surg 1962; 29:360–370.

103. Loeb R. Correction of hypertrophy of the lobule of the auricle. Rev Latinoam Cir Plast 1965; 9:186–192.

104. Guerrero-Santos J. Correction of hypertrophied earlobes in leprosy. Plast Reconstr Surg 1970; 46:381–383.

105. Constant E. Reduction of the hypertrophic earlobe. Plast Reconstr Surg 1979; 64:264–267.

106. Lassus C. Another technique for the reduction of the earlobe. Aesth Plast Surg 1982; 6:43–45.

107. McCollough EG, Hom DB. Correction of the enlarged earlobe: auricular lobuloplasty—an adjunctive face-lift procedure. Laryngoscope 1989; 99:1193–1194.

108. Fearon J, Cuadros CL. Cleft earlobe repair. Ann Plast Surg 1990; 24:252–257.

21 Random Pattern Cutaneous Flaps

Jonathan L Cook MD and Glenn D Goldman MD

Summary box

- Random pattern flaps are ideal closures for surgical wounds that will neither predictably heal by second intention nor be easily repaired by direct linear closure.
- For each operative wound, several flaps may be suitable, but one will likely be optimal. To improve outcomes, a reconstructive surgeon must be able to match an appropriate repair to a given surgical defect.
- Flap execution requires attention to minute details in design and small changes in the sizes or angles of flaps may result in substantial improvements in outcomes. This is particularly true for transposition and rotation flaps.
- The plane of flap elevation is crucial. Some flaps should be elevated within the subcutis, some just above the superficial fascia, and others at the deep fascia, perichondrium, or periosteum.
- Most surgical complications associated with random pattern flap reconstructions are preventable with proper flap design and meticulous operative technique.
- There is a great deal of literature on surgical reconstruction, and the art of flap repair requires lifelong learning.

INTRODUCTION

Most operative defects in dermatologic surgery can be closed linearly or allowed to heal by second intention. Certain shallow wounds can be aesthetically repaired with full-thickness skin grafts. Deeper and more critically located wounds present greater challenges to the reconstructive surgeon, and often require the skillful execution of a local tissue rearrangement (a flap). A flap is a moving construct of skin and subcutaneous tissue created from tissue near an existing surgical defect (Table 21.1). In distinction to skin grafts, flaps retain vascularized connections to underlying tissues at their bases. Flaps provide the surgeon with opportunities not only to restore function by filling and closing operative wounds, but to more elegantly restore natural appearances.

Historically, there have been many classification schemes for surgical flaps. Flaps have been categorized by their vascular supply (random or arterial/axial), their primary motion (advancement, rotation or transposition), their configurations (rhomboid or bilobed, for example), their eponymous designations (e.g. Rieger, Mustarde), and their locations (local, regional or distant).

In this chapter, flaps are classified by their primary motion. Such a classification scheme is traditionally attractive and conceptually simplistic, but most flaps combine several different types of tissue motion. For example, many rotation flaps incorporate tissue advancement, and the classic nasolabial transposition flap involves substantial unidirectional cheek advancement.

Random pattern flaps are geometrically designed surgical repairs based on either deep or lateral vascular pedicles that do not necessarily involve the use of larger caliber named arteries or the formation and subsequent division of delayed pedicles. The base of a random pattern flap is supplied by deeper unnamed musculocutaneous arteries, and the elevated portion of the flap is perfused by the highly anastomotic subdermal and dermal vascular network. To survive, random pattern flaps capitalize on the fact that the vascular supply to skin is amazingly redundant. Because the normal perfusion of skin is approximately ten times the blood flow needed to provide basic nutritional support,[1] appropriately designed flaps can predictably survive. Although the term 'random' might seem to add a sense of casualness to these flap repairs, the design and execution of successful flap reconstructions is anything other than random. Only appropriate flap design and proper surgical technique can ensure reliable operative results.

Considerable skill is needed to perform a flap reconstruction. The effective reconstructive surgeon must have a thorough knowledge of the reconstructive literature, a detailed understanding of anatomy and the biomechanical properties of skin, an eye for geometry and aesthetics, appropriate manual dexterity, surgical confidence, the

Table 21.1 Defect definitions

Primary defect	The surgical wound to be repaired (often the site of a skin cancer excision)
Secondary defect	The 'new' surgical wound created by harvesting and moving the primary lobe of the flap
Dog-ear redundancy	Tenting of tissue at the periphery of a flap created when the flap is moved
Primary lobe	That portion of the flap that is designed to cover the primary defect
Secondary lobe	An additional lobe of the flap that is used to cover the secondary defect
Tension vector	The direction of force that is required to move the flap into the primary defect
Pivot point	The point at the flap's base around which the flap rotates or transposes
Primary motion	The main direction of flap motion
Secondary motion	Movement that is other than that imagined as the primary motion of the flap

ability to prevent and manage common surgical complications, and, perhaps most importantly, the mentorship of a dedicated instructor. This chapter mainly considers facial wound reconstruction, but the flap principles and techniques can and should be extrapolated to other anatomical sites of the body.

■ HISTORY

Dermatologists' interests in reconstructive surgical techniques have dramatically accelerated during the past several decades, but the rudiments of facial reconstruction date to the antiquities. As early as 700 BC, Indian surgeons used local flaps in nasal reconstruction. Celsus and Galen, in ancient Rome, described the use of multiple facial repairs, including advancement and island pedicle flaps. In Renaissance Italy in the 1500s, both Gaspare Tagliacozzi and the Braca family used local and pedicle flap reconstructions for the repair of auricular and nasal wounds. In the late 1700s the Indian forehead flap technique was first published in an English language journal. Carupe, an English surgeon, published his experience with the forehead flap in 1816, and his manuscript was widely circulated throughout Europe.[2] This publication was an extraordinary admission by a European physician that the historic practice of surgery by apprenticed workers in India could result in the impressive reconstruction of a diseased or traumatized nose. It is remarkable to realize that these early efforts at facial reconstruction were carried out without aseptic technique, antibiotic prophylaxis, advanced instrumentation, or the use of effective local or general anesthesia. Nonetheless, many of the surgical results were outstanding, particularly when the results are viewed in their historic context. These early surgeons demonstrated a thorough knowledge of anatomy and an impressive attention to the aesthetic subtleties of the face.[3]

Modern facial reconstruction began in the military theater in World War I. As advances in general medical and surgical care promoted the survival of soldiers who had been seriously injured, increasing attention was placed on the complete rehabilitation of the war's wounded. Surgeons became much more interested in surgical techniques to reconstruct the damaged face, and many of the currently used techniques in facial reconstructive surgery can trace their origins to this important period in the early 20th century.

Historically, the greatest inputs to the field of reconstructive surgery have come from plastic surgeons and otorhinolaryngologists. In the past several decades, however, there has been an explosion of interest and innovation from the nascent field of dermatologic surgery. Dermatologic surgeons have contributed greatly to the field of facial reconstructive surgery, and many currently used facial flaps owe their developments and refinements to dermatologists who have acquired high levels of expertise in the repair of facial surgical wounds.

PREOPERATIVE PREPARATION

When a surgical flap is used to repair a wound resulting from the removal of a cutaneous malignancy, confirmation of the adequacy of tumor removal should first be obtained. It is undesirable to complete a surgical reconstructive procedure only to learn that tumor persists at a lateral or deep surgical margin. Additionally, because flap reconstructions cover operative defects with inherently thick pieces of tissue, the clinical manifestations of persistent or recurrent disease may be concealed from the patient and physician for several years. Clinically apparent tumor recurrence following flap reconstruction is therefore often advanced and may be difficult to treat.

The Mohs micrographic surgical technique (see Chapter 48) offers the highest cure rates for the extirpation of most cutaneous tumors.[4–6] It also conserves appreciable amounts of normal tissue.[7,8] The use of Mohs surgery therefore provides a reliably complete, yet conservative, excision. For these reasons, most surgical flaps carried out in the authors' practices follow Mohs surgical excisions of various types of skin cancers.

Cutaneous flaps offer several important advantages in the repair of facial wounds. Flaps can prevent the functionally and aesthetically significant distortion that can occur when wounds are allowed to heal by second intention, and can also restore a three-dimensional facial form that would be impossible to achieve with the application of a skin graft when there is significant tissue loss. Flaps move adjacent tissue of similar color, texture, and thickness into operative defects, and the aesthetic results from flap reconstructions often exceed the aesthetic results that would have resulted from simpler reconstructive alternatives. Because properly designed flaps have reliable perfusion, flaps can also be used to successfully cover relatively avascular tissues such as cartilage or bone. With proper planning and surgical technique, the healing from flap repairs is often much more rapid than the healing of granulation or skin grafting. The morbidity and complications associated with skillfully performed surgical flap reconstructions should be similar to those of skin grafting procedures.

However, like all surgical interventions, flap reconstructions have several potential disadvantages. Because most flaps are used to repair conspicuous facial wounds, the surgeon should provide proper preoperative counseling and obtain detailed informed consent. The artful design and proper execution of facial flaps are acquired skills honed over many years of surgical practice. Even a minor miscalculation in flap design can result in flap failure, postoperative morbidity, and functional or aesthetic compromise. For proper mobilization, flaps generally require relatively long incision lines and generous undermining. Poorly designed or improperly implemented flaps may therefore lead to scarring and distortion far beyond the area of the original surgical defect. Surgical morbidities such as postoperative hemorrhage or damage to underlying facial motor nerves may result from poor surgical technique, a lack of knowledge of the underlying anatomy, or patient-related factors. Failure of a surgical flap as a result of ischemia can lead to a large and complex wound with a protracted healing course and a poor aesthetic outcome. Finally, the costs associated with large flap repairs can be greater than the costs associated with less complicated reconstructive alternatives.

Proper patient selection is critical to flap success. An appropriate screening of a patient's suitability for a flap repair should precede any operative intervention. Following tumor removal, random pattern flap reconstructions can typically be safely performed in all but the most debilitated and medically fragile patients. Because most procedures by dermatologic surgeons are carried out in an ambulatory setting with the use of only local anesthesia, systemic complications associated with flap repairs are rare.

A large randomized trial has demonstrated that for cataract surgery, a formal preoperative screening evaluation with laboratory tests, electrocardiogram and chest radiography confers no benefit to the patient or to the physician, and such medically unnecessary testing certainly adds great expense.[9] Dermatologic reconstructive procedures could be conceptualized as analogous to these ophthalmologic procedures, and the need for extensive preoperative evaluation in most patients undergoing outpatient reconstructive surgery for small and moderately sized wounds remains unproven. Unless a patient has a history of serious, unstable cardiac disease, a significant bleeding disorder, or concurrent severe medical disease such as profound immunosuppression or malnutrition, the patient's preoperative evaluation for tumor extirpation and flap reconstruction can typically consist of a well-documented medical history and a competent physical examination.

In addition to verifying general health, the cutaneous surgeon should also properly assess the patient's anatomy for suitability of a flap reconstruction. This is particularly true when assessing facial defects because minor degrees of asymmetry, particularly in the central face, are quite common. These asymmetries should be demonstrated to the patient before initiation of the flap procedure. Failure to do this can lead the patient to believe that the reconstructive procedure caused the distortion.

When possible, flaps should be designed so that incision lines do not cross convexities with underlying bone such as the ramus of mandible, the zygomatic arch, or the clavicle because hypertrophic scarring is more common in these situations.

The physician should determine the quality and laxity of the patient's skin adjacent to the surgical defect. The mobility of the skin varies tremendously from location to location and from patient to patient. A proper evaluation of the skin's laxity can be easily accomplished by the surgeon's probing hands. The quality of the skin should also be carefully assessed. Many elderly patients have surprisingly atrophic skin and subcutaneous tissue, and flaps that require relatively high wound closure tensions should be avoided in these patients because the tensile strength of the thinned dermis will be unable to support the required wound closure tensions. Conversely, areas of thick, sebaceous skin should also be noted. Highly sebaceous skin has a low compliance, does not easily stretch or bend, and can be brittle to work with. In addition, it is generally advantageous to avoid placing incision lines within thick, sebaceous skin because the resultant suture lines frequently track and invert. Finally, when possible, flaps should not rely on pedicles based on previously scarred or irradiated skin because in addition to the inelastic nature of this tissue, the perfusion of this skin is often suboptimal and usually unpredictable.

Most surgical complications that follow reconstructive facial surgery involve difficulties in hemostasis,[10] and there are therefore many historic suggestions that medications that promote bleeding should be routinely discontinued in the perioperative period. The issue of whether or not to continue the use of anticoagulants during the perioperative period in patients undergoing facial reconstructive surgery is an active area of discussion among dermatologic surgeons, especially because there have been reports of thrombotic complications (including strokes and myocardial infarctions) when anticoagulants have been withheld for cutaneous surgical procedures.[11] The risk of major bleeding following flap reconstruction in patients who are anticoagulated with warfarin may be slightly higher than the risk of bleeding without anticoagulation, but the likelihood of catastrophic hemorrhage remains low. If the surgeon does elect to continue the use of anticoagulants during the perioperative period, it is reasonable to check a recent International Normalized Ratio (INR). If the patient has a markedly elevated INR, warfarin may be withheld for several days to bring the INR back into the normal therapeutic range. The authors of this chapter discontinue warfarin for 3–5 days in selected patients in whom large flap reconstructions are needed. It is advisable that the surgeon works with the patient's primary physician when medication adjustments are desirable.

Medications that adversely affect platelet function may also complicate reconstructive surgery. Because aspirin irreversibly inhibits cyclooxygenase,[12] an enzyme crucial to proper platelet function, the drug's effects on hemostasis last for up to 2 weeks, and any aspirin use may therefore predispose to intraoperative and postoperative bleeding. Many older individuals take daily aspirin as prophylaxis against myocardial infarction and stroke. For patients who have never had a vascular event this is primary prevention. Patients with a history of a medically significant vascular event are taking aspirin for secondary prevention. Both authors discontinue aspirin 1 week before surgery for patients on aspirin for primary prevention, but not for individuals on aspirin for secondary prevention of further stroke or heart attack. If a large surgery is planned, it is advised that the surgeon consults with the primary care doctor before recommending discontinuation of aspirin for patients in this latter group.

Smoking is not a contraindication to flap reconstruction, but smokers do have higher incidences of flap failure and distal flap necrosis,[13] wound dehiscence[14] and wound infection.[15] The adverse relationship between smoking and facial surgery was initially described in rhytidectomy patients. Among these patients, smokers had significantly increased chances of flap necrosis.[16] In studies from the dermatologic literature, smokers have also been shown to have higher risks of focal flap loss than their age-matched, nonsmoking controls[17] (see Chapter 5). As a result of potential ischemia of the distal or peripheral margins of a flap, the scars that accompany reconstructive surgery in smokers tend to be more visible than the scars in nonsmokers. When feasible, it is therefore advisable for patients to discontinue smoking several weeks before and for at least 1 week after flap repairs. Of course, many patients fail to comply with a physician's suggestions to abstain from the use of all tobacco products. These individuals should be advised that their continued smoking during the perioperative period puts them at higher risk of operative complications. In addition, large, aggressive flaps should generally be avoided or undertaken only with extreme caution. Nonetheless, with conservative appropriate flap design and gentle, meticulous operative technique, the dermatologic surgeon can perform most reconstructive procedures in smokers with safety and reasonable aesthetic success.

Preoperative patient counseling is critically important in reconstructive surgery, especially facial surgery. The patient's aesthetic expectations should be carefully evaluated. Patients should prospectively understand that facial flaps can be relatively complex reconstructions and that occasionally long and complicated incision lines are required for proper tissue mobilization. The undermining required for flap mobilization frequently causes bruising and some postoperative discomfort. It is important to stress that flap reconstructions may take months to mature and that, although uncommon, surgical revisions may be necessary. In areas prone to sensory disturbance such as the forehead or upper lip, it is also essential to inform patients about likely postoperative numbness, paresthesias and the potential for developing neuropathic-type pain. Fortunately, most sensory disturbances associated with flap repairs are temporary. Because of recent mass media efforts to glamorize many plastic surgery procedures as painless, bloodless and risk free, many patients require substantial education before the flap's incisions are made. The physician's explanations that are provided preoperatively constitute informed consent; those that are provided postoperatively are often viewed by patients as self-protecting excuses.

■ TECHNIQUES

Advancement flaps

Tissue may be advanced to close an operative wound either as a linear repair or as a flap. Many, if not most, surgical defects are best handled by simple, direct side-to-side closure, particularly in anatomic areas that have abundant loose skin adjacent to the primary defect. Such linear repairs typically distribute tension perpendicular to the line of closure. In many locations, the resultant fine linear scar is aesthetically ideal and generally well tolerated, particularly if the scar runs within or parallel to one of the facial relaxed skin tension lines. When an operative defect lies near a free margin such as the vermilion border or close to a defined facial boundary such as the nasolabial fold, any proposed linear repair may violate the free margin or the facial boundary and may therefore be technically infeasible or aesthetically undesirable. In such cases, an advancement flap frequently allows for optimal closure.

The advancement flap is conceptually the simplest of all flap repairs. In most cases, the tissue movement associated with these flaps is a unidirectional, uncomplicated advancement of the flap's leading edge. In addition to moving adjacent tissue into the operative defect, advancement flaps displace the tissue redundancies (dog-ears) created by tissue movement to locations from which they can be excised with less cosmetic burden. The ideally designed advancement flaps allow for a limb of the repair to run along a free margin or within a defined facial boundary. Importantly, advancement flaps do not generally recruit much additional tissue laxity, and the tension vector of the flap repair remains parallel to the primary motion of the flap. Therefore, in distinction to rotation and transposition flaps, advancement flaps do not have the advantage of being able to redirect wound closure tensions to a more favorable axis.

Because a pure advancement flap does not recruit much more tissue laxity than would be available with a simple linear closure of the wound, some degree of secondary motion near the flap's insertion point is often required. If the primary defect is near a facial structure that cannot be displaced without undesirable distortion, this potential reliance upon secondary motion should be anticipated.

H-plasty

The classic advancement flap involves the creation of a rectangular pedicle or bilateral rectangular pedicles (H-plasty). As the flap is advanced, tissue redundancies develop at the pedicle base (Figs 21.1, 21.2). If the ideal skin contour is to be preserved, these dog-ear redundancies must be excised, which adds further complexity to the simple U-shaped scar of the traditional advancement flap. Historically, simple advancement flaps were frequently used to repair nasal bridge defects from a superior glabellar base and forehead defects from a lateral base on the adjacent forehead or temple. Because nasal skin is largely inflexible and noncompliant, simple advancement flaps to repair distal nasal defects must often rely upon secondary motion at the nasal tip to close the wound. This motion produces an unaesthetic elevation of the nasal tip, and more appropriate flap repairs can nearly always be designed.

The leading edge of an advancement flap always requires undermining to free deep restraints. Wide undermining of the pedicle base does not necessarily increase mobility[18] because this does little to liberate the lateral, superior and inferior restraints on flap motion. A pure rectangular advancement flap with a longer length-to-width ratio is more easily mobilized than a wider flap,[19] and early advancement flap designs were long unilateral advancements with 3 : 1 length : width ratios advocated. These length : width ratios were often touted as appropriate designs to minimize the risks of distal flap necrosis. In reality, it is uncommon to need an advancement flap with such length, and in clinical practice, narrow flaps that are excessively long or sutured under unacceptably high wound closure tensions are no more subject to ischemia than wider flaps created under equally undesirable conditions.[20]

When sufficient tissue laxity does not exist to allow for a simple unilateral advancement flap, a bilateral advancement

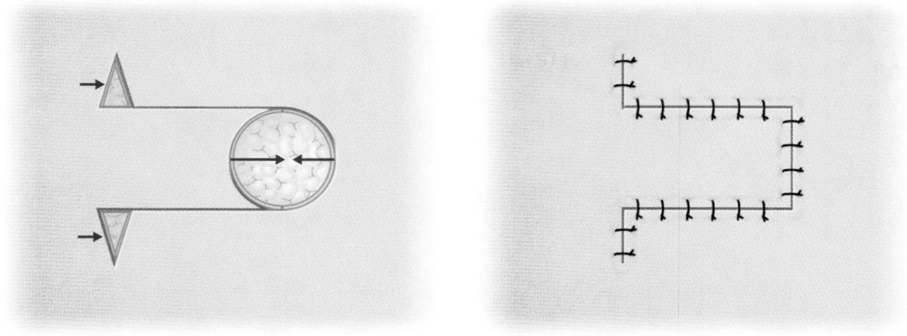

Figure 21.1 A unilateral advancement flap displaces dog-ears and creates a U-shaped scar.

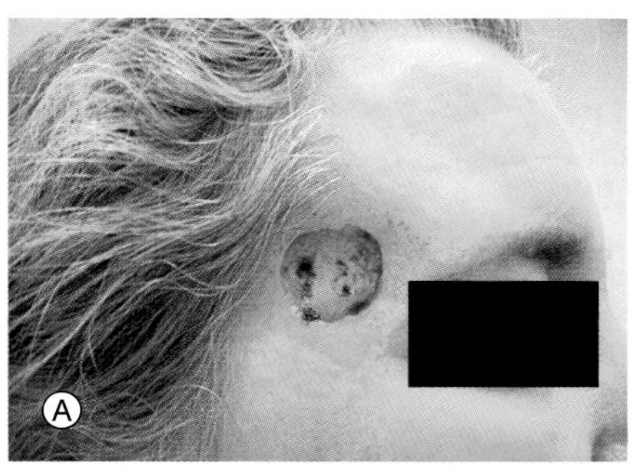

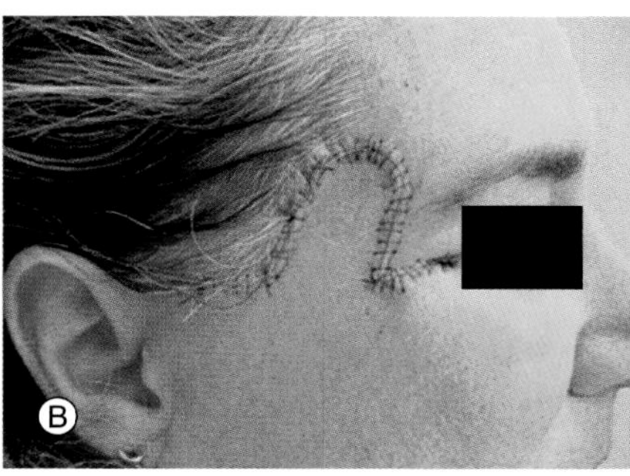

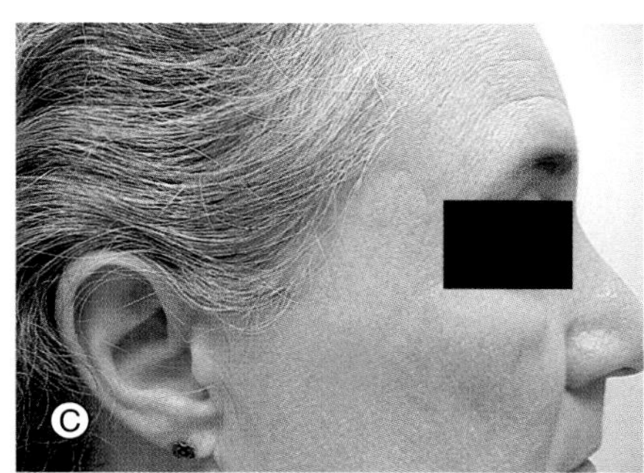

Figure 21.2 (A) A traditional advancement flap has placed one incision line along a normal anatomic boundary (the hairline) and (B) placed a dog-ear within the normal lines of the lateral canthus. (C) One year after surgery.

Bilateral advancement flap

Figure 21.3 Bilateral advancement flap (H-plasty) is most suitable for repair of defects within the eyebrow where scars can be readily hidden. Elsewhere the H-plasty produces a complex scar and other repairs are generally favored.

flap may be designed such that each flap advances half as far to meet in the center of an operative wound (Fig. 21.3). The standard bilateral rectangular advancement flap (known as the H-plasty) is most useful for eyebrow defects, where the horizontal and vertical scars can be hidden adjacent to and within the brow, respectively. Often a unilateral advancement flap with short broad limbs will suffice to close an eyebrow wound that historically would have been closed with lengthy bilateral advancements.[21] As such, once an H-plasty is designed, it makes sense to elevate one flap side at first to determine whether unilateral tissue movement will be adequate to close the defect before incisions are made bilaterally.

The H-plasty repair has limited applications in other facial locations because of the complexity of the required incision lines. Although the bilateral advancement flap has been historically suggested as an appropriate repair of forehead wounds, the horizontally oriented 'H' scar resulting from bilateral tissue advancement is often quite visible. Excision of the dog-ear redundancies that result from tissue advancement further complicates the rather unaesthetic arrangement of the scar. Also, if there is any ischemia of the

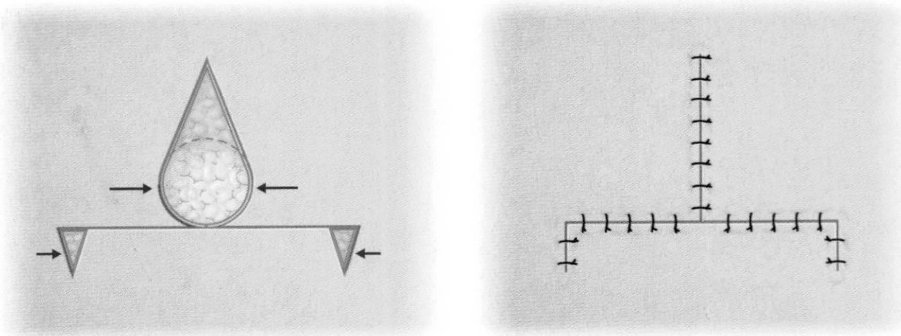

Figure 21.4 A classic A–T bilateral advancement flap allows for the base of the flap (the horizontal portion of the T) to be placed within an existing rhytid or facial boundary.

flap's advancing edge(s), this vertical closure is likely to leave behind a slightly depressed scar. Simpler closures, even a vertically oriented linear repair, are frequently more suitable. If there is sufficient laxity to allow the direct advancement of two adjacent flaps, there is nearly always sufficient laxity to allow a primary linear closure. For selecting the more appropriate simple linear repair, the surgeon is rewarded with simplicity of design and operative ease, and the patient is rewarded with a lower risk procedure, less (if any) sensory loss above the closure, and a more visually pleasing scar.

Bilateral T-plasty (A–T flap)

The standard bilateral T-plasty repair or A–T (A to T) flap can be a great improvement over the unilateral and bilateral rectangular advancement flaps in most facial locations. In the A–T repair, a linear repair of the operative wound is designed perpendicular to a free margin or to a pre-existing cosmetic junction (Fig. 21.4). Instead of extending a primary linear repair across a cosmetic boundary or free margin, incisions are designed along the margin of the operative defect, a free margin or a cosmetic boundary, perpendicular to the linear repair axis. In this manner, one line of the repair is hidden in a cosmetic junction or dynamic rhytid.[22]

Closely related to the A–T advancement flap is the O–T rotation flap. Conceptually similar, the flaps both create a T-shaped incision. Where the A–T flap relies upon linear tissue advancement, the O–T flap relies upon flap rotation. The A–T flap is useful for peri-alar defects where the top of the T can be hidden in the alar crease and the vertical limb of the T can be hidden in the nasolabial fold. Above the brow or on the forehead, the base of an inverted T can be hidden either just above or just below the brow or within a horizontal forehead rhytid. The vertical scar that results from this repair may be somewhat visible, but it generally fades nicely over time if the flap is not closed under tension. Although the classic A–T flap is rather simplistic from a design perspective, great care must be taken to align the advancing tissue edges. If the leading edges of the advancement(s) traverse a great distance to close a large defect, distracting dog-ear redundancies can be produced. Sometimes these tissue redundancies need to be excised in the areas that the surgeon was initially reluctant to manipulate, so undermining flap utility. Often, a single limb advancement flap will suffice to displace a dog-ear far away from a free margin into a natural crease. Whenever possible a single limb advancement flap is favored because its inherent simplicity in design minimizes suture lines.

As with all facial flaps, advancement flaps are most useful when the incisions of the flap can be hidden within cosmetic unit boundaries or along natural facial expression lines. Commonly used sites for advancement flaps are the nasal sidewall superior to the alar crease, the upper lateral lip superior to the vermillion border and the supraorbital forehead lateral to the mid-pupillary line. For defects in these areas a vertical limb extends superiorly from the operative defect and a horizontal or nearly horizontal limb extends laterally along a free margin (the alar crease, vermilion border, brow or forehead furrow) (Figs 21.5, 21.6). A dog-ear is then removed laterally either within the alar groove or nasal fold, the oral commissure or the lateral canthus or crow's feet.

This Burow's-type advancement flap can be viewed simplistically as a flap that displaces the inferior dog-ear redundancy that would have resulted from a linear closure to an anatomic site from which it may be much more appropriately excised.[23,24] A similar advancement modification, first described by Webster,[25] is often used along the nasofacial sulcus for operative defects of the lateral nasal sidewall and cheek or for defects adjacent to the nasal ala. In this case, a superior dog-ear is removed nearly vertically along the nasofacial sulcus while the inferior limb of the flap curves around the ala as a crescent. A crescent of redundant tissue is removed inferiorly to allow proper tissue advancement (Fig. 21.7). The concept of the crescentic advancement flap may be extended to other common defects. This technique obviates the need for dog-ear resection because this is accounted for in flap design with a crescent of excess skin to be excised. Removing this crescent of tissue prevents unsightly tissue protrusion in the area of flap harvesting.

Island pedicle flap

The island pedicle flap is a specialized advancement flap. The island pedicle flap differs from other traditional advancement flaps in that most of its vascular supply derives from a subcutaneous pedicle. Additionally, all dermal margins of the flap are severed as the flap is advanced (hence the appropriate 'island' nomenclature). The first island pedicle flap was described by Celsus, but the first

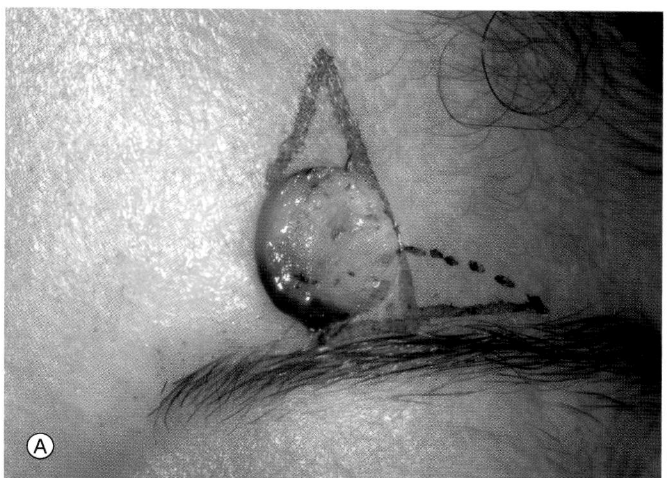

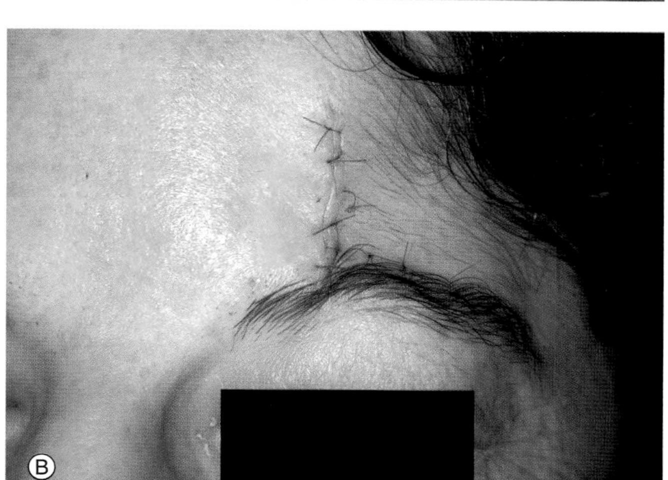

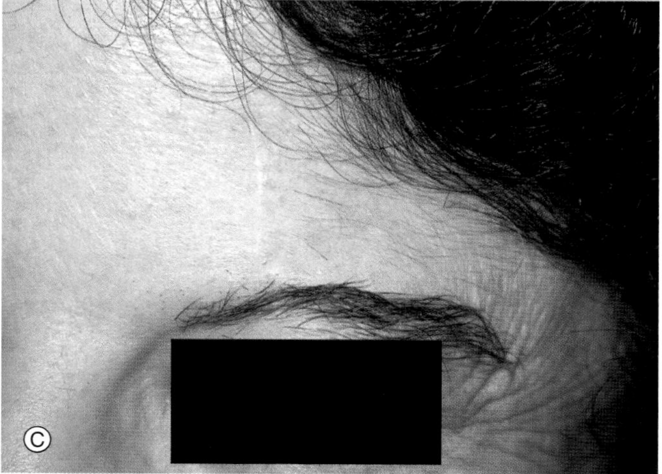

Figure 21.5 (A) A unilateral advancement flap hides the scar line along the superior brow. (B) In this case, a dog-ear redundancy was avoided by removing a crescent of tissue above the brow. (C) One year after surgery the mature incision line is hypopigmented.

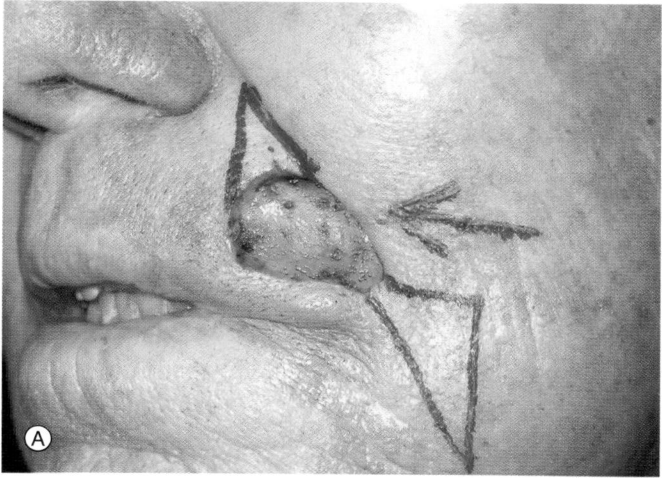

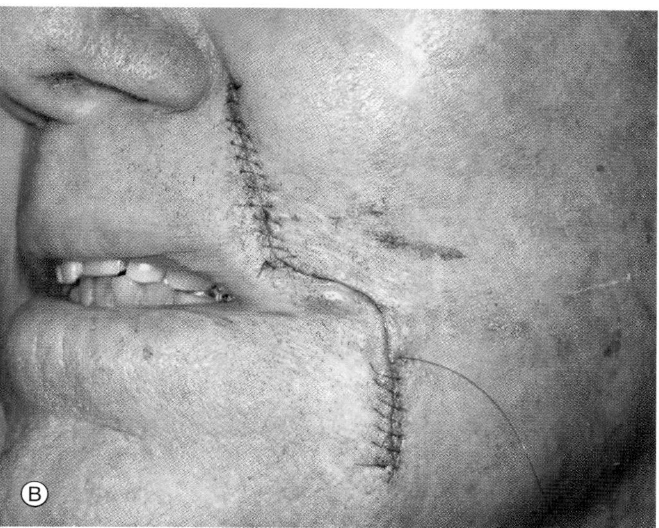

Figure 21.6 (A) A Burow's advancement flap allows for dog-ear removal lateral to the oral commissure and for approximate recreation of the nasolabial fold. (B) This flap is useful in displacing the dog-ear to an area from which it may be more appropriately excised.

modern use of the island pedicle flap was by Esser in 1917.[26] Since the 1940s, many types of island pedicle flaps have been described, the most common of which is a triangular flap that derives its blood supply from a deep and mobile subcutaneous or muscular pedicle, which remains attached to the central portion of the flap.[27,28] In the plastic surgery literature, this traditional island pedicle flap is frequently referred to as a V to Y advancement flap.[29]

The island pedicle flap is remarkable because the flap can be advanced as far as the motion of the deep pedicle allows. This mobility is frequently much greater than a similarly designed flap would advance if dermal margins that restrain flap motion were retained at the peripheral margins of the flap (Fig. 21.8). In addition, the island pedicle has a rich blood supply from underlying vessels and musculature and is not forced to rely solely upon the anastomotic vascular network of the dermis for perfusion. As such, the island pedicle flap is remarkably impervious to ischemia, even when the flap is inserted under considerable wound closure tensions.

Because the traditional island pedicle flap has a conspicuous kite-shaped outline, its greatest use is in locations where one or two of the margins of the flap can be hidden within a contour line or aesthetic unit boundary. Surgical defects on the upper lip near the nose–lip–cheek junction and on the lateral nasal sidewall are particularly well-suited for repair with an island pedicle flap (Figs 21.9, 21.10). Additionally, the island pedicle flap is useful in the

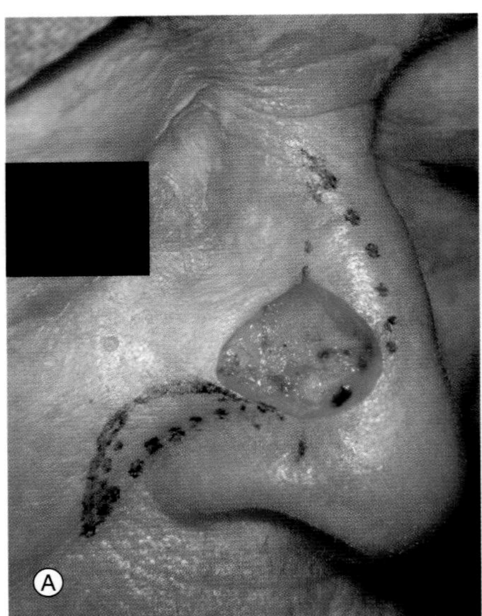

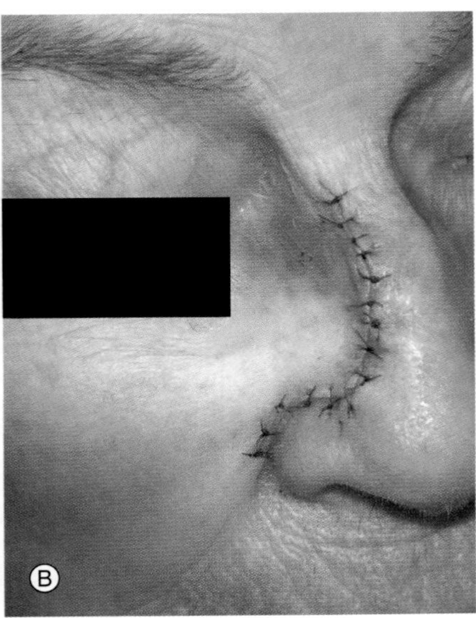

Figure 21.7 (A) A crescentic advancement flap for nasal sidewall defects offers the ability to hide one curvilinear aspect of the repair within the alar crease and preserves this prominent cosmetic junction. (B) The curvilinear crescent of tissue that is excised prevents dog-ear formation.

Island pedicle flap

(A)

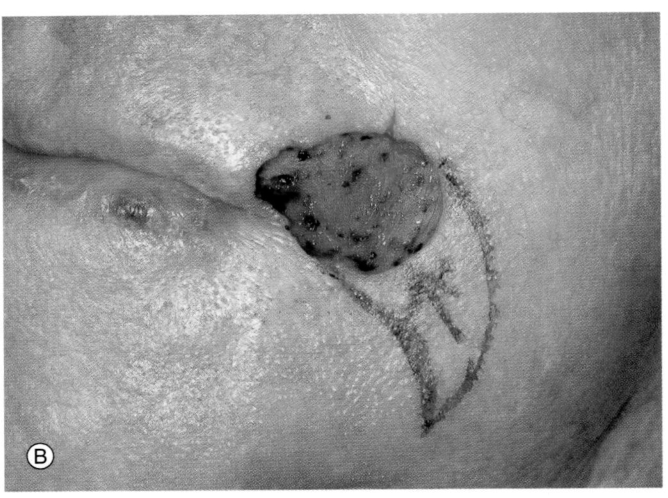

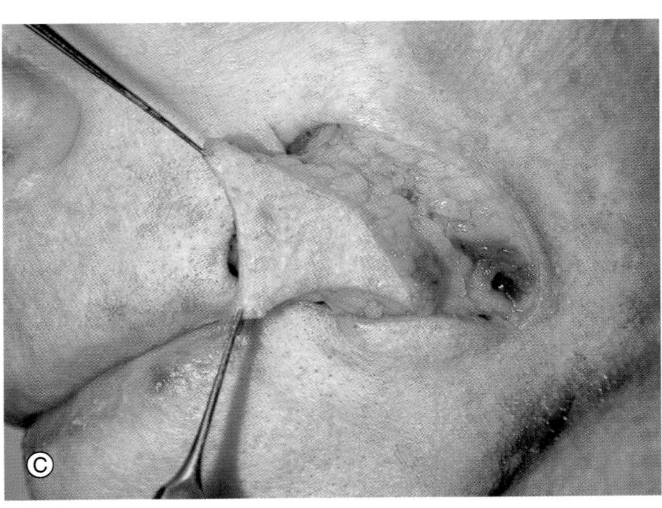

Figure 21.8 (A) Schematic of flap. (B) Island pedicle flap in progress. (C) All lateral ties have been severed leaving all deep connections intact. The flap has great mobility on an underlying muscular and fatty pedicle.

reconstruction of the eyebrow, where the flap can advance the remaining brow medially to recreate brow continuity and central facial symmetry. Certain defects of the temple and forehead are likewise amenable to closure with either a single or bipedicle island flap repair; however, in many of these cases, alternative flaps that produce less conspicuous scars than the triangular-shaped scars of the island pedicle flap are available.

In designing and executing the island pedicle flap, it is essential to predict the amount of mobility that will be

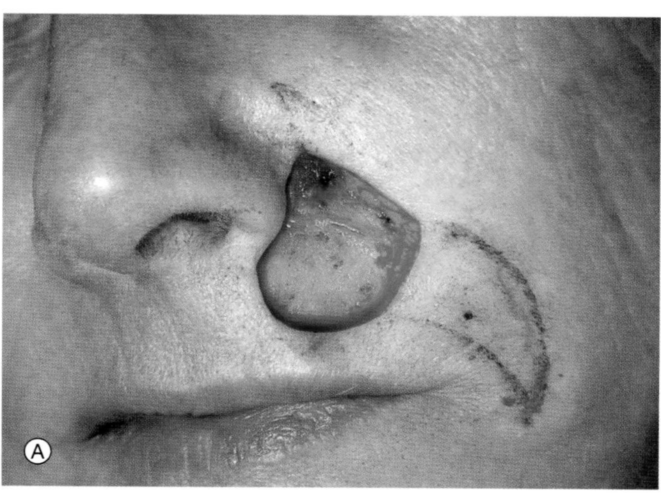

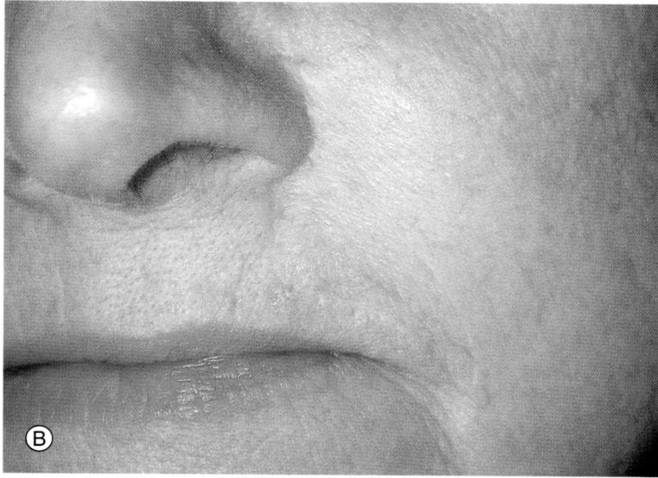

Figure 21.9 (A) Island pedicle repair of perinasal upper lip defect. Note that the flap is slightly undersized. Large wounds of the upper lip can be predictably repaired with an island pedicle flap based on the rich vascular supply of the underlying orbicularis oris. (B) One year after surgery there is no retraction of the lip.

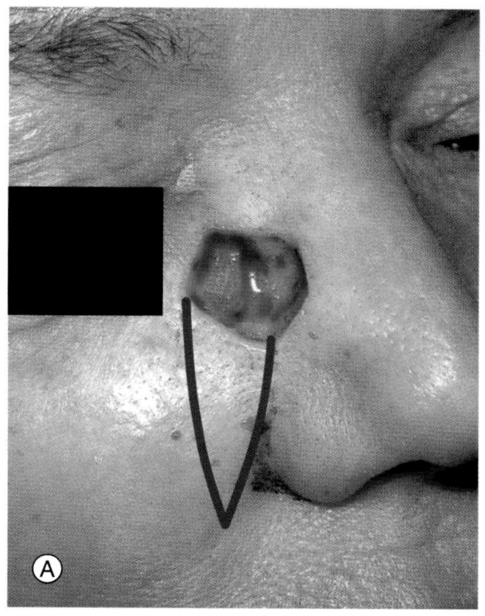

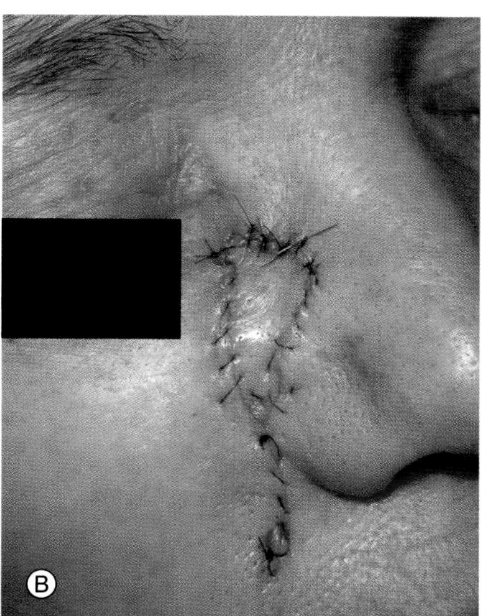

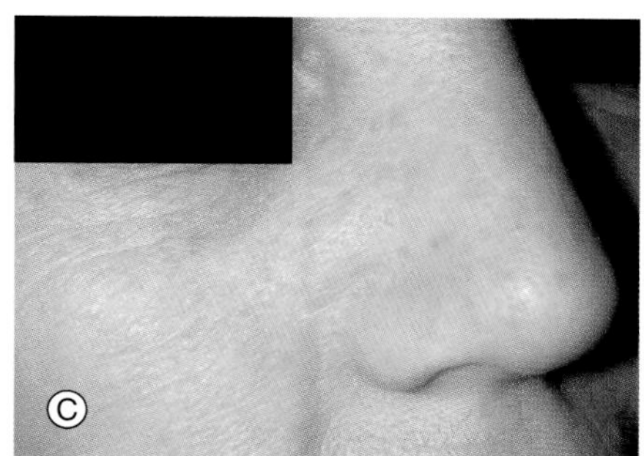

Figure 21.10 (A) Island pedicle repair of perinasal cheek defect. The flap can be advanced a great distance on a nasalis muscular swinging pedicle, which provides reliable blood supply. (B) Note that although the flap was undersized, the surrounding tissues were undermined, and the flap was inset at the time of repair. (C) There is slight flap elevation, a trapdoor deformity, at 6 months.

achieved when all peripheral margins of the flap have been severed. Two centimeter in diameter or even larger wounds of the perinasal area of the upper lip can be repaired with an island pedicle flap, but in general, defects on the nose amenable to island pedicle flap repairs tend to be smaller (given the poor compliance of stiff nasal skin and the inability to rely on secondary motion at the flap's insertion point without producing distracting nasal asymmetry). The island pedicle flap is particularly well suited to deeper operative wounds because it carries all tissue layers with it including skin, subcutaneous tissue and some skeletal muscle. Additionally, the flap's rich vascular supply makes it appropriate for repairs in areas of compromised skin vascularity (such as areas of chronic radiation damage).

Proper design and execution of an island pedicle flap are necessary for an aesthetic repair. Because the flap has a thick base, it is particularly subject to developing a protuberant appearance (the pin-cushioned or trapdoor deformity) during the early postoperative period. The development of the trapdoor deformity with this flap is common when the flap is used to repair wounds on the medial cheek and lip, and this globular appearance may be permanent. One solution may be to design a flap that has a smaller breadth than the diameter of the primary surgical defect and will still generally allow for closure of the operative wound by relying upon secondary motion of the skin edge of the wound. This slight flap undersizing places modest wound tension on the lateral aspects of the island pedicle flap, which theoretically diminishes postoperative contraction of the flap and the risk of developing a subsequent trapdoor deformation.[30] The flap is incised with either strictly vertical incisions or with slightly outwardly beveled incisions that include the adjacent deep subcutaneous fat or underlying muscle. The peripheral margins of the flap's incisions are widely undermined, as is the primary defect. The tapering tail (approximately the distal third) of the flap must be freed completely from any lateral or deep restraint, either by blunt or sharp undermining. This tethering of the tail of the flap is usually the primary area of restraint that inhibits the flap's mobility.

Because the flap must be deeply undermined vertically but not across its base to allow proper flap mobility, a thorough knowledge of the underlying anatomy is required. This undermining is generally carried out just over the superficial fascia. In addition to freeing the flap's tail, the surgeon may need to undermine the leading edge of the island pedicle flap to some extent (rarely more than 1 cm) to allow the flap to advance with minimal wound closure tension and to prevent inversion as a result of tethering of the leading edge. Failure to minimize the flap tension can result in unanticipated and undesirable secondary motion near the flap's insertion point. In critical areas, such as along the free margin of the eyelid, this secondary motion can produce aesthetically significant distortion (an ectropion, for example).

The flap itself should be inset slightly into the operative defect and secured with several deep sutures, and a flap that is initially slightly concave will eventually heal as a flap that is appropriately flush with the surrounding skin. This flap recession can be routinely achieved, as mentioned above, by slightly undersizing the flap and by suturing the flap under slightly increased wound tension.

In addition to the traditional design, many variants of the island pedicle flap have been discussed in the reconstructive literature. Curved island pedicle flaps can be particularly useful on the nose, where the incision lines can be placed along the alar groove.[31] De-epithelialized flaps or even flaps that have the entire pedicle buried in a subcutaneous tunnel can occasionally be quite useful in the repair of deep nasal or medial canthal wounds.[32,33] Regardless of the design nuances, all island pedicle flaps have as their chief advantage a healthy and protected vascular supply.

Mucosal advancement flap

For operative wounds restricted to the glabrous portion of the pink lip, repair choices are often limited. Partial-thickness wounds that do not cross the vermilion border can be allowed to heal by second intention with minimal scarring. For broader wounds, an advancement flap from the remaining intraoral mucosa is often an appropriate repair. The mucosal advancement flap is designed so that the incision line traverses the entire horizontal length of the border between the cutaneous and the mucosal portions of the lip. The flap is incised, and the flap is undermined between the plane of the minor salivary glands and the underlying orbicularis oris musculature.[34] This undermining plane protects the perfusion of the flap while preserving the function of the underlying muscle. The flap is sharply undermined from anterior to posterior, following the natural curvature of the lip. Extensive undermining may be necessary into the intraoral mucosa to achieve proper flap mobility; undermining is generally extended to the area where the mucosa reflects onto the mandible. Using the principles of simple tissue advancement, the generously liberated flap can then be advanced to cover even broad wounds on the lower lip. Because the actual length of tissue advancement is relatively small and because the mucosa is quite forgiving, dog-ear redundancies that result from tissue advancement are not typically significant enough to require complete removal. Although the incision scar of the mucosal advancement flap is often quite subtle, the modest tension required to advance the flap typically results in a slightly flattened appearance of the lower lip.

Alternatively, an island pedicle flap can be designed by advancing mucosal skin anteriorly to fill full-thickness defects of the pink lip that do not cross the vermilion border. Advancement must proceed with minimal tension in the direction of primary movement or lip distortion ensues. One adverse effect of moving mucosal lip onto the exposed pink portion of the lip is long-term peeling of this new lip skin as a result of metaplasia.

Bipedicle advancement flap

The bipedicle flap is a variant of a linear closure technique that also relies upon local tissue advancement. The flap has its greatest use on the upper forehead[35] and temple, where a simple linear repair of a large defect may be associated with unacceptably high wound closure tensions or with the production of lateral canthal distortion. The flap is constructed as a rectangular advancement of tissue that basically shares the diameter of the original surgical defect equally between primary and secondary defects.

To design the flap, the surgical defect is envisioned as an elliptical side-to-side closure. To minimize the tension that would be required to close the wound, a parallel incision of equal length is placed several centimeters lateral or superior to the primary defect. When both incisions have been made, a bipedicled, easily mobile flap is created (Fig. 21.11). The pedicled portion of skin between the defect and parallel incision is not undermined such that it maintains a rich blood supply. The other aspects of the defect and incision, however, are undermined to allow tissue advancement and closure with minimal tension. Therefore, the diameter of the primary defect is effectively shared with the secondary defect, and secondary motion around the original wound is minimized. The scars that result from the construction of the flap consist of two fine parallel lines.

Rotation flaps

Many surgical wounds that cannot be closed side-to-side or with local tissue advancement may be repaired by recruiting adjacent tissue laxity while directing wound closure tension vectors away from the primary surgical defect. This redirection of wound closure tension is the primary purpose of a rotation flap.

The design of a traditional rotation flap uses a curvilinear incision along an arc adjacent to the primary surgical defect. As a rotation flap is created, the direction of wound closure tension is effectively changed (Fig. 21.12). This allows a rotation flap to use abundant donor tissue located a considerable distance from the primary defect to close wounds in areas in which tissue availability is minimal. In addition to reorienting tension vectors, rotation flaps also frequently allow for displacement of dog-ears to more favorable locations. If well-designed, rotation flaps create scar lines that are hidden along facial boundaries or within relaxed skin tension lines or are camouflaged within hair-bearing skin (Figs 21.13, 21.14).

As the rotation flap is raised and undermined, the laxity of the adjacent tissue allows the flap to be rotated into the primary defect. Like all flaps, rotation flaps are hindered in their movements by the inherent stiffness of the tissue especially at the flap's pivot point. Because of this pivotal restraint, the tip of the rotation flap will not extend

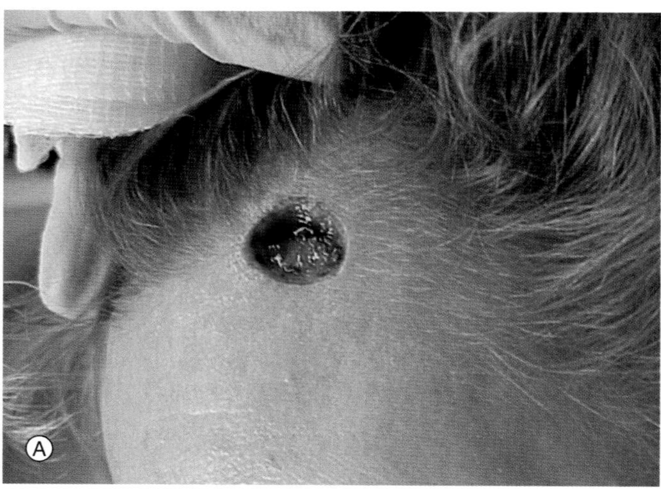

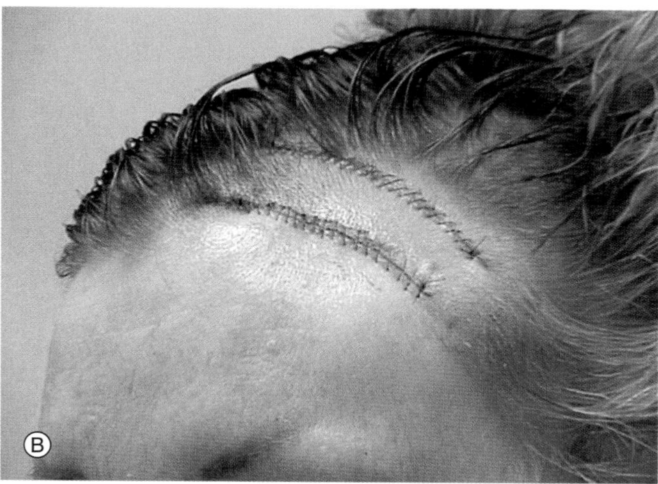

Figure 21.11 (A) Defect on the forehead at the hairline. (B) A bipedicled flap is used to repair a forehead wound. The tightness of the forehead precluded a simple linear repair, and the wound closure tensions have now been shared between the primary and secondary defects.

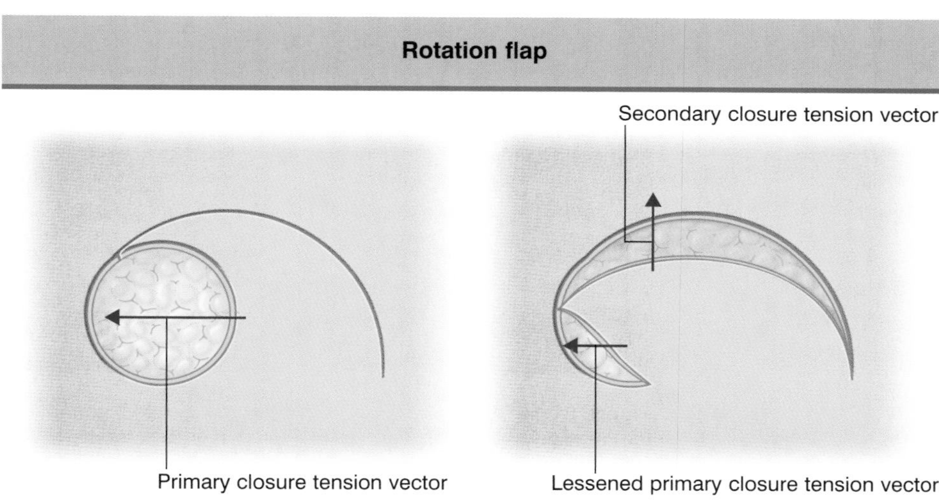

Figure 21.12 A rotation flap recruits laxity and creates motion in several directions, so diminishing closure tension at the primary defect.

to the distal margin of the operative defect unless the tip of the flap is also advanced under some tension and/or the recipient edge is mobilized toward the flap tip (secondary motion). To compensate for pivotal restraint, minimize tension on the flap, and eliminate the need for secondary motion around the operative defect, the arc of the rotation can be oversized and offset so that it extends vertically beyond the distal extent of the operative defect[36] (Fig. 21.15). When the flap's rotation is subsequently executed, the extended tip of the flap then rests without tension where it meets the distant point of the primary defect. A rotation flap can often be closed without undermining beneath the point of pivotal restraint; however, for optimal flap motion, this area of restraint should be undermined (Fig. 21.16). This is particularly important with the dorsal nasal flap, where maximal rotation is required to close a defect in the inelastic skin of the distal nose.

Occasionally, a backcut into the rotation flap's body can improve flap mobility (Fig. 21.17), particularly on relatively immobile skin such as the scalp. This must be done conservatively because cutting too far into the pedicle base may interfere with blood supply to the flap. In addition to reorienting tension vectors, rotation flaps also serve to exchange primary defects for displaced secondary defects.

Random pattern flaps do not 'create' new tissue, and the entire purpose of any flap, including the rotation flap, is to trade the existing primary surgical defect for an adjacent secondary defect that can be more easily closed. The management of the secondary defect created upon flap movement is often the most challenging part of a rotation flap repair. If a rotation flap with a short arc is designed, the width of the secondary defect created upon flap rotation will be proportionally larger, and the potential for unacceptable secondary motion and inappropriately high wound closure tension is magnified.

A longer arc of flap rotation allows easier closure of the narrowed secondary defect, and the likelihood for flap survival is increased to a point as a result of the minimization of wound closure tensions. Of course, if the pedicle is very long compared to its base width, flap survival may be impaired.

Typically the incision lines for a rotation flap need to be longer than one would initially expect if the flap is to be placed under minimal tension and to avoid unwanted displacement of structures surrounding the primary defect.

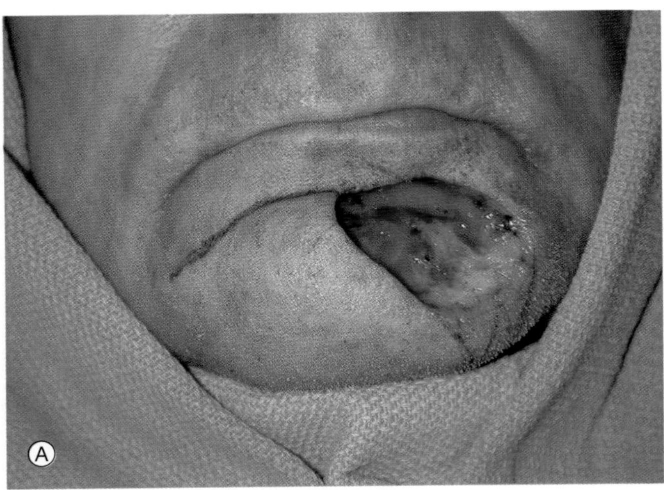

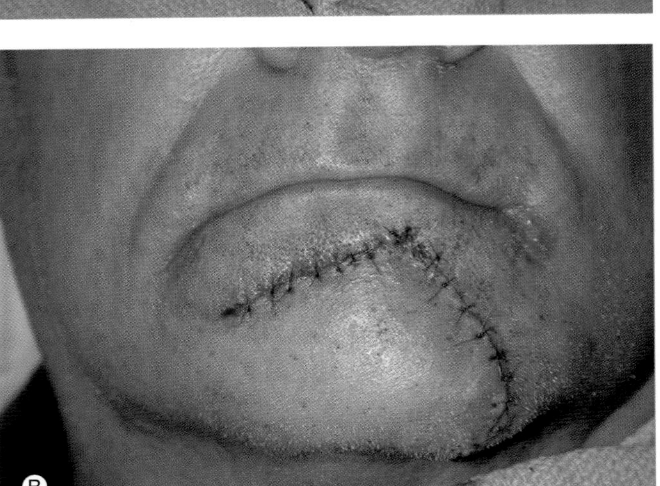

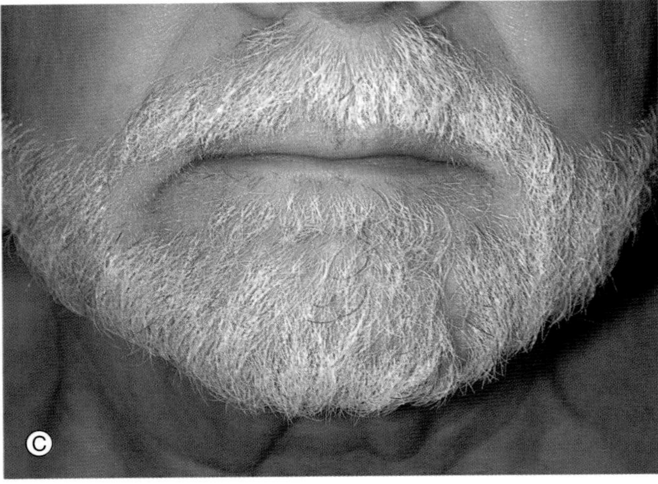

Figure 21.13 (A) Rotation flap on the chin allows for repair of a large defect. (B) Most of the scar is hidden in the mental crease. (C) Minimal hair loss is noted along closure line.

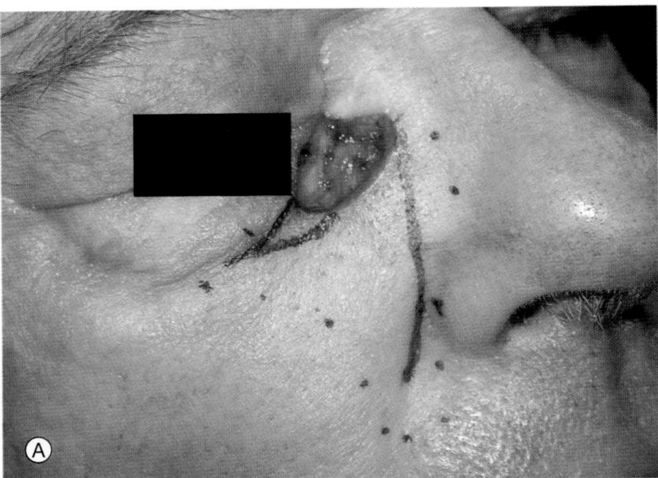

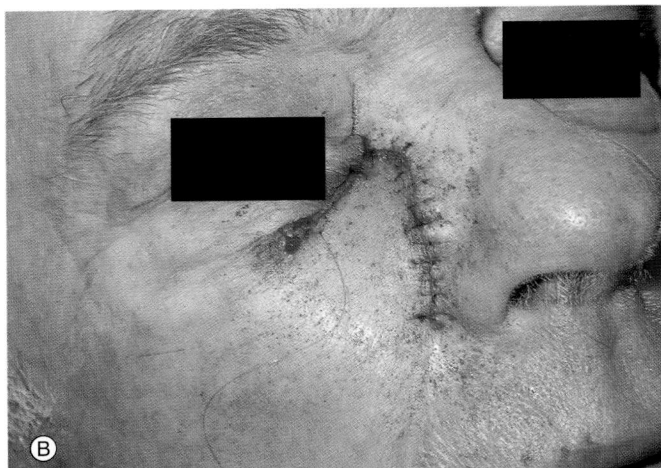

Figure 21.14 (A) A rotation flap for repairing a defect spanning the medial lower eyelid and cheek. Tension is directed by a suspension suture placed from the dermis of the tip of flap to the nasal periosteum. (B) Curvilinear scars along the nasofacial sulcus and infraorbital crease will be minimally visible.

However, ischemic failure of a well-designed rotation flap, handled gently and closed under minimal tension, is quite rare.

Because rotation flaps require long incision lines to achieve appropriate flap motion, in many facial locations, other flap options that are often more palatable. Rotation flaps have their greatest use in the closure of scalp, temple and cheek defects and other nonfacial areas. In selected cases, rotation flaps can be useful on the nose. On the scalp, a lack of adjacent skin mobility requires rotation flaps to be especially long to close even small-to-moderate sized operative wounds. On the cheek, rotation flaps are particularly useful to repair medially located wounds, because the rotation flap can effectively mobilize the large reservoir of loose skin in the entire area of the lateral cheek.[37] Infraorbital wounds on the eyelid and cheeks can be closed with rotation flaps that recruit substantial laxity from the temple.

Special rotation flaps

Dorsal nasal rotation flap

In 1967 Rieger introduced the dorsal nasal rotation flap as an alternative to island or nasolabial flaps for the reconstruction of distal nasal wounds.[38] The dorsal nasal flap is most useful for medium-sized defects that are too large to be repaired with bilobed transposition flaps or too small to warrant the use of two-staged pedicled flaps. The flap described by Rieger is a full-thickness rotation of the entire nasal dorsum with a glabellar back-cut to improve flap mobility. The flap is designed with a long sweeping arc that

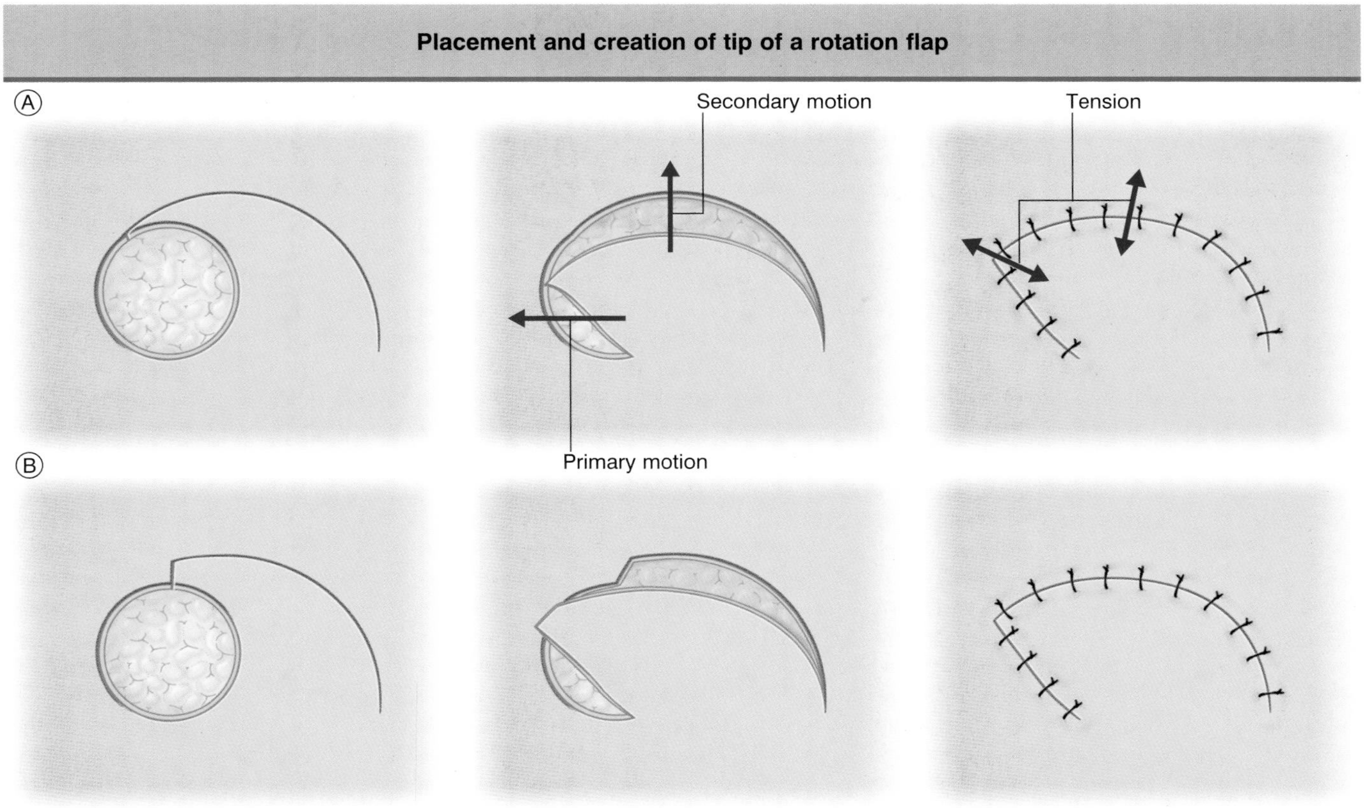

Placement and creation of tip of a rotation flap

(A) Secondary motion Tension

Primary motion

(B)

Figure 21.15 (A) If the rotation flap is designed as a simple arc taken off a round operative defect, the tip rotates and falls short of its destination – it will only meet the far edge of an operative wound if the flap tip is advanced in a secondary motion. (B) Oversizing the tip and leading edge of the rotation flap beyond the extent of the operative defect compensates for pivotal restraint and allows for closure of the primary defect without tension on the tip of the flap and without much secondary motion.

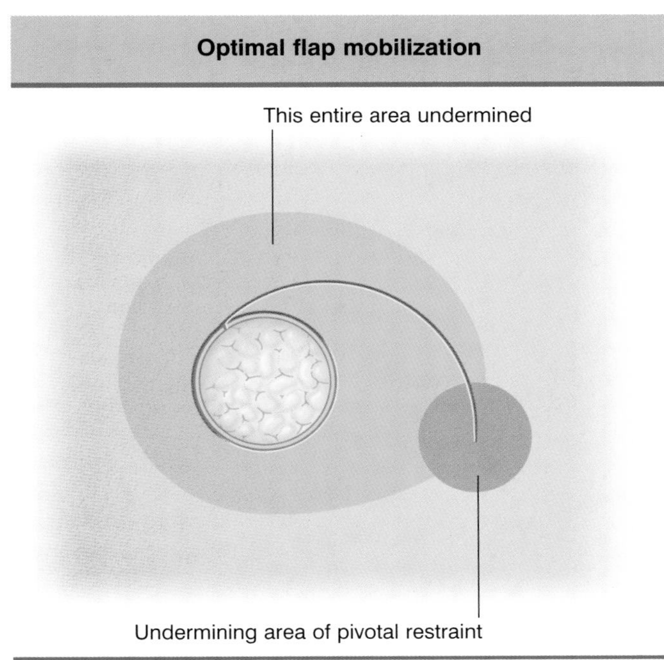

Figure 21.16 For optimal flap mobilization, the base of a rotation flap is undermined to minimize pivotal restraint.

extends from the distal aspect of the defect contralaterally to the nasofacial sulcus, past the contralateral medial canthus and to a midpoint just superior to the glabella (Fig. 21.18). To include the abundantly perfused underlying nasal musculature, the flap is elevated at the level of the perichondrium and periosteum. The inclusion of facial musculature in the base of the flap makes distal ischemia unlikely. The point of pivotal restraint with the dorsal nasal flap is in the areas of the ipsilateral medial canthal tendon and the attachment of the nasal musculature to the nasofacial sulcus. As with all rotation flaps, undermining in the area of pivotal restraint can improve flap mobility, but this undermining should be cautiously performed given the need to protect the flap's vascular input at its base. Properly performed, the dorsal nasal flap can be used to repair distal nasal defects up to 2 cm in diameter. Of course, the dorsal nasal flap can be suitably modified for smaller defects. With such smaller flaps, it is not always necessary to extend the backcut superiorly onto the glabella or to extend the flap's curvilinear excision far laterally onto the contralateral nasal sidewall except to hide the scar.

Because of the inherent stiffness of sebaceous nasal skin, the rotation of the nasal dorsum required to close wounds with this flap can introduce significant potential for developing alar asymmetry. By understanding the basic principles of

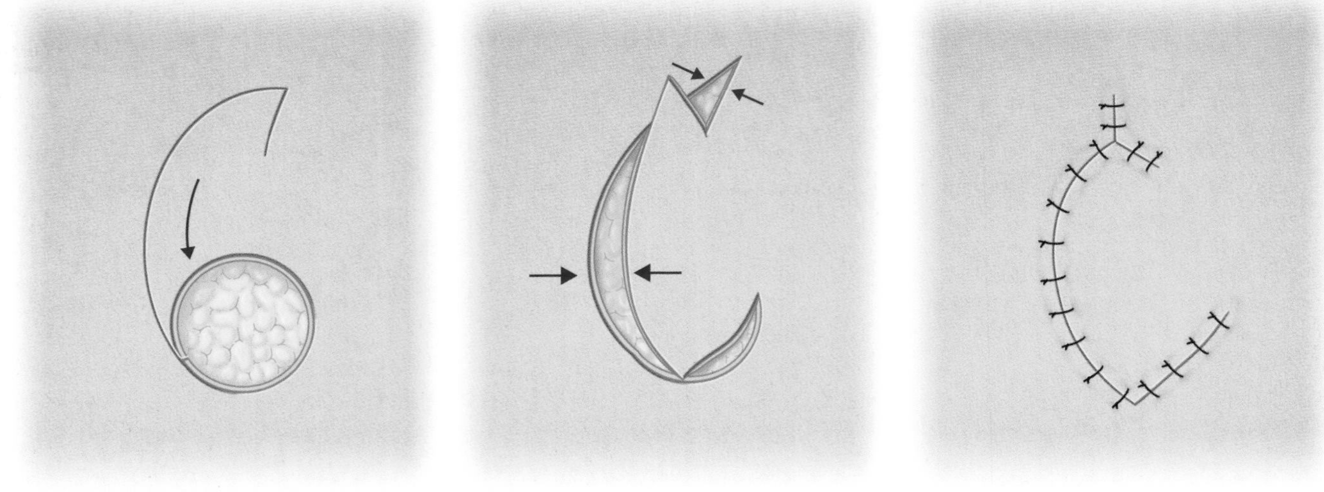

Figure 21.17 A backcut on a rotation flap facilitates closure by introducing an added component of flap advancement (arrows) and diminishing pivotal restraint. If the backcut is too large, decreasing pedicle size may affect flap viability.

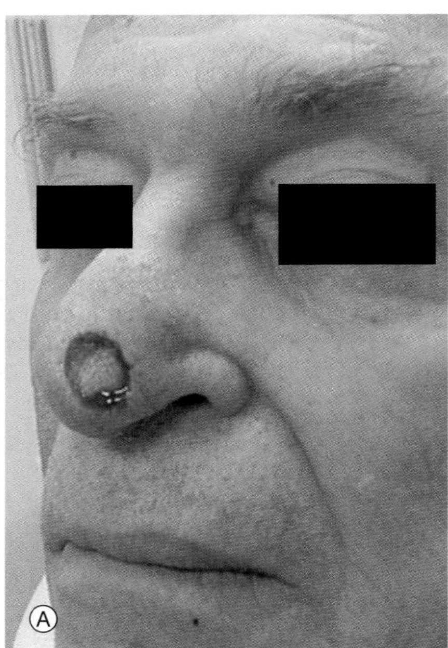

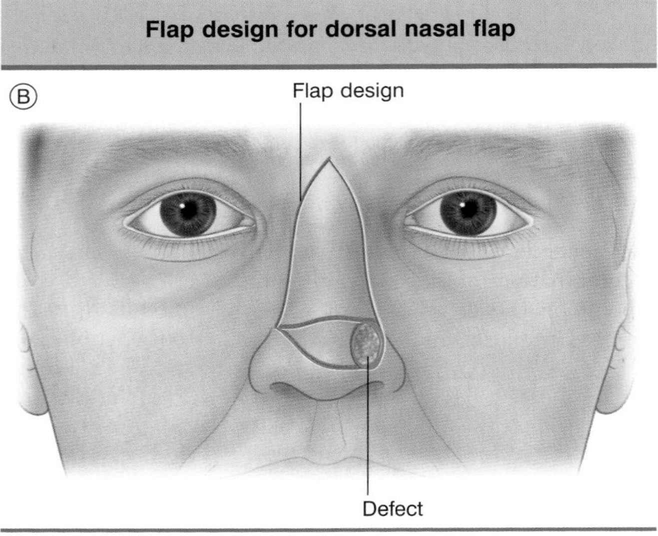

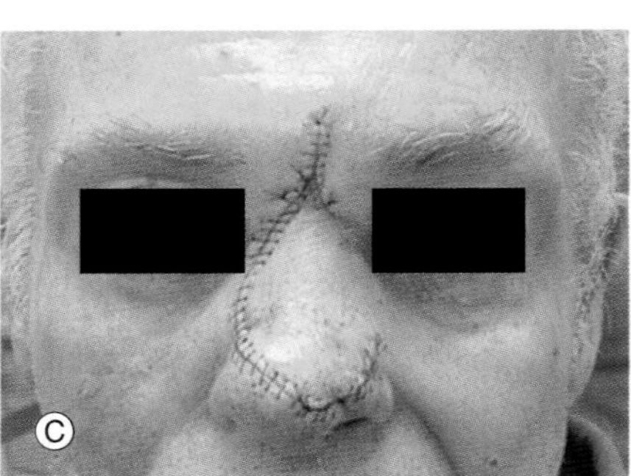

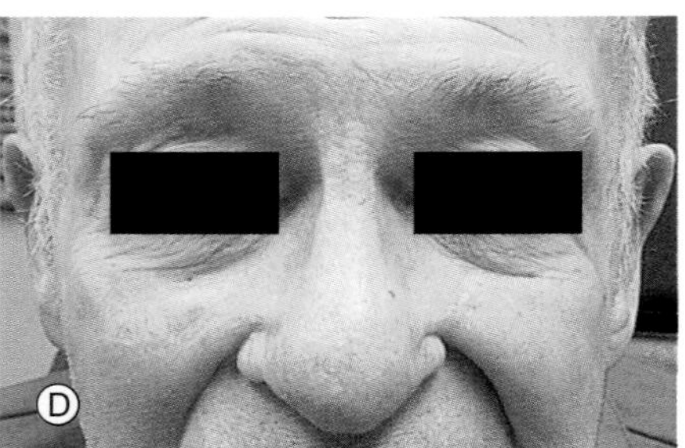

Figure 21.18 (A)–(B) A dorsal nasal flap is used to repair a distal nasal defect. (C) Despite the long incision line required to create the flap, the final aesthetic result is favorable. (D) One year postoperatively.

rotation flap reconstruction, the surgeon can prevent this untoward effect in most cases.[39] To prevent this distortion, the restraint of the flap in the area of the pivot point needs to be addressed. Adequate undermining of the rotation axis alleviates pivotal restraint, which allows the flap to redrape over the distal nasal defect under minimal tension. When undermining the pedicle, it is essential to be at the level of the periosteum to preserve the sizeable arterial branches that perfuse the flap. To reduce the likelihood of nasal distortion, most of the flap's secondary defect is distributed along the flap's arc of rotation along the nasofacial sulcus where there is considerable tissue mobility. Side-to-side closure can be easily achieved in this area by proper undermining of the adjacent cheek tissue. Although longer incision lines may create aesthetic concerns in the early postoperative period (particularly along the more sebaceous, distal areas of the nose), a longer arc of flap rotation will minimize the width of the secondary defect at any particular point, and this minimization will reduce the likelihood of the alar or medial canthal distortion that can result from an improperly designed dorsal nasal flap repair. In essence, longer Reiger flaps often produce superior aesthetic results.

Tenzel and Mustarde rotation flaps

In 1966, Mustarde described a cheek rotation flap for lower eyelid reconstruction.[40] In 1975, Tenzel and Stewart described a similar rotation flap from the temple to repair full-thickness lower eyelid defects.[41] The classic Mustarde flap is a large rotation of cheek and temple skin with extension of the flap incision into the preauricular cheek. The classic Tenzel semicircular flap is a similarly designed rotation of skin and orbicularis oculi muscle from the temple and lateral canthal areas. The classic Tenzel flap also incorporates a cantholysis of one crus of the lateral canthal tendon to promote easier flap rotation. Originally described by the author as an advancement flap, the Tenzel flap actually constitutes a combination of advancement and rotation about a pivot point on the zygoma. A superiorly arcing semicircular incision lateral to the canthus allows recruitment of adjacent tissue to reconstruct the lower lid. Both the Mustarde and Tenzel flaps use the primary rotational motion of the flap to support the eyelid, and both flaps direct all wound closure tensions toward the temple superolaterally and toward the cheek medially. Unwanted vertical tension along the eyelid margin is avoided, and the appropriate position of the lower lid is maintained. Similar to the design of the rotating dorsal nasal flap, the Mustarde and Tenzel flaps' long arcs of rotation allow redistribution of the volume of the primary defect along a narrowed secondary defect. Because the secondary defect with both these flaps is within the compliant and mobile skin of the temple and cheek, distortion of the surrounding structures is minimized.

These useful rotation flap reconstructions have been commonly modified,[42] and they are reliable flaps to repair defects of the lower eyelid. The most commonly used flap variant is a modified Tenzel flap to repair skin defects of the mid to lateral lower eyelid (Figs 21.19, 21.20). From the superior extent of the surgical defect, a curvilinear rotation is extended laterally and superiorly past the lateral canthus and onto the temple. As with the traditional rotation flaps mentioned above, the superior extension of the flap's design allows the flap's rotation to overcome the 'shortening' associated with pivotal restraint. If the arc of rotation is not extended superiorly, the eyelid may be required to undergo secondary motion to meet the leading edge of the flap. If any of this tension is vertically oriented, an iatrogenic ectropion can develop. The flap is elevated just above the orbicularis oculi superomedially, above the medial insertions of the superficial musculoaponeurotic system (SMAS) inferiorly, and over the superficial temporal fascia superolaterally. All tension is directed horizontally along the vector of the primary motion to support the lower eyelid and prevent ectropion formation. It is important to thin the superior aspect of the flap adequately to avoid placing a thick flap adjacent to the remaining thin tissue on the lower eyelid. The modified Tenzel flap often produces temporary edema of the lower lid because of the obstruction of the laterally draining lymphatic channels, but this edema rarely persists beyond several weeks. A similarly modified Mustarde flap can be used for extensive cheek defects.

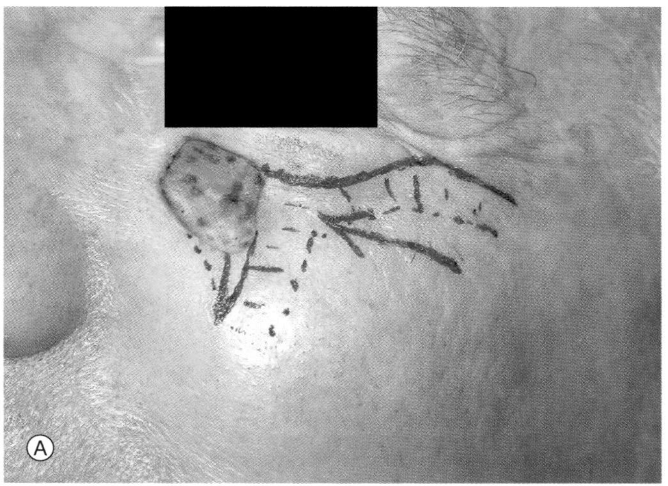

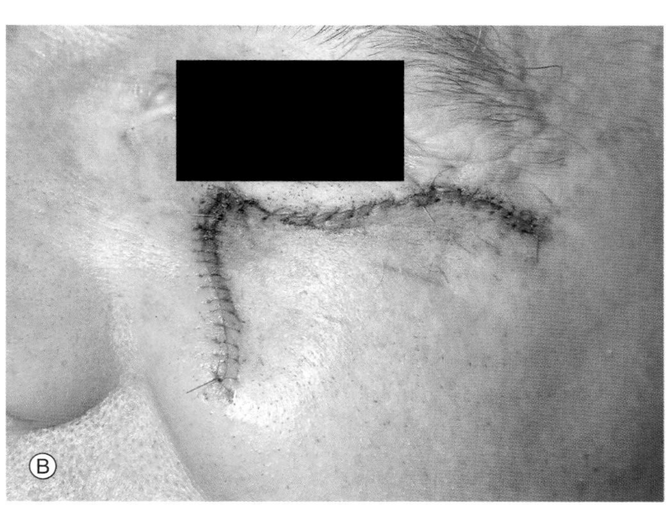

Figure 21.19 (A) A modified Tenzel flap combines features of rotation and advancement. The direction of flap motion is indicated by an arrow, and the likely extent of flap undermining is also detailed. (B) A rotation flap is placed without tension on the lower lid.

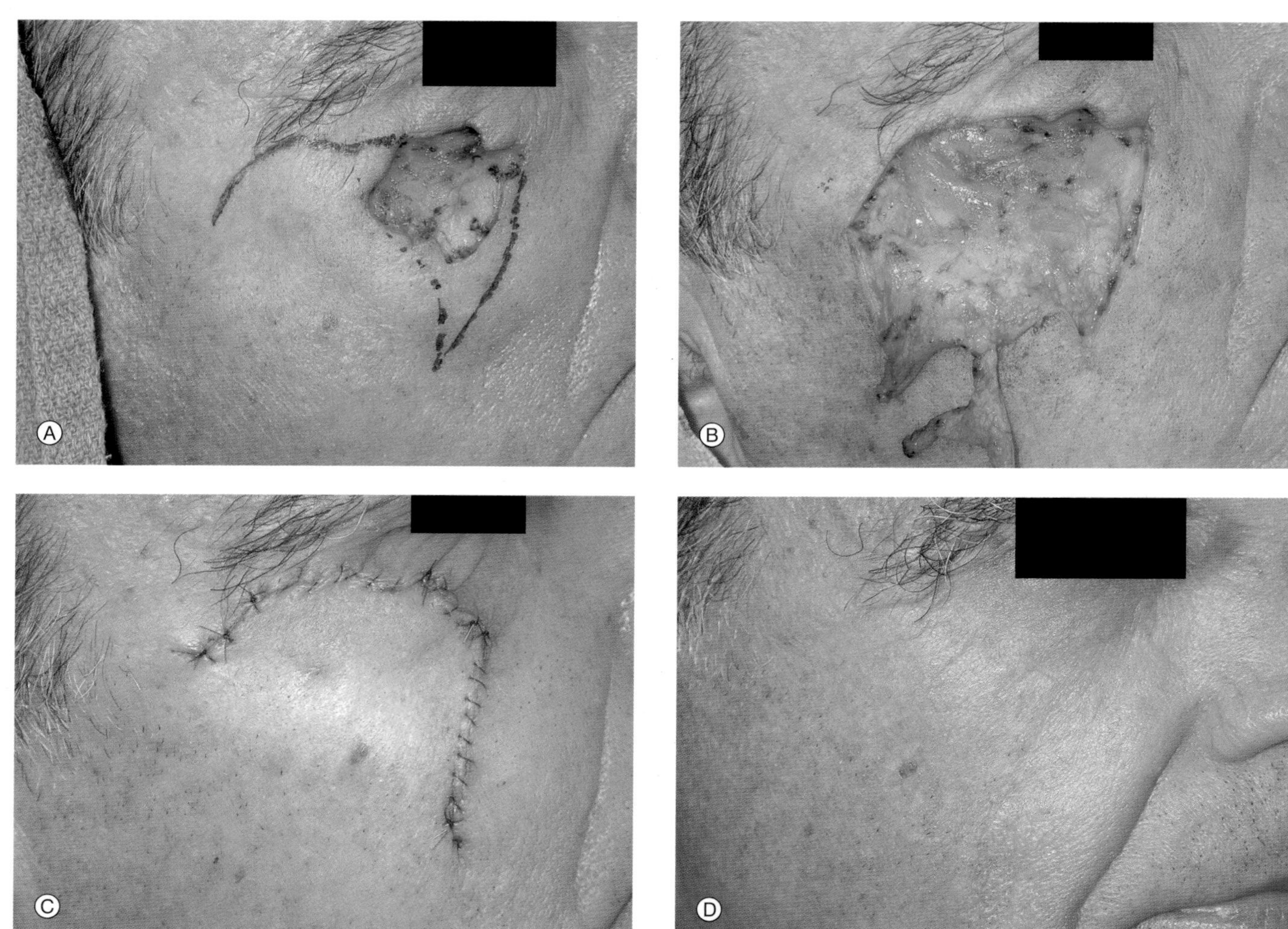

Figure 21.20 (A) With infraorbital rotation flaps, extending the incision superiorly near the lateral canthus oversizes the flap and supports the eyelid, preventing the tendency to produce an ectropion. (B) The flap is undermined just above orbicularis musculature superiorly and above the SMAS inferiorly. The flap is folded back to expose the level of undermining. (C) The site immediately postoperatively. (D) 90 days postoperatively.

O–Z (O to Z) rotation flap

When there is insufficient laxity to close a surgical defect with a single rotation flap, bilateral rotation flaps can be created. Because bilateral rotation flaps convert a circular operative defect into a Z-shaped incision line, this com-bination of rotation flaps is often called an O–Z flap. The construction of an O–Z flap is similar to the construction of a traditional rotation flap; therefore, attention should be directed toward compensating for the pivotal restraint of the flaps. The flap lengths should also be sufficiently long to minimize the width of the secondary defects because this will facilitate flap closure and minimize wound tensions. In the design of the O–Z flap, however, there is great flexibility. The paired flaps can be designed to rely upon pure rotational movement, or there can be varying amounts of flap advancement introduced into the operative design. The surgeon should appropriately select how much tissue advancement or rotation can be accomplished without producing anatomic distortion of the surrounding structures and in such a way as to hide scars. As with traditional rotation flaps, the movement of O–Z flaps produces paired dog-ear redundancies near the flaps' pivot points, and these redundancies should be excised to produce proper flap contour. This adds another dimension to the O–Z flap's potentially distracting incision lines. The O–Z repair has its greatest application on the scalp,[43] where the prominent incision lines are hidden beneath a blanket of hair (Fig. 21.21).

Transposition flaps

In design, transposition flaps are the most complex of the random pattern flaps. Transposition is an inherently more complicated tissue movement than simple advancement or rotation, and the less experienced surgeon typically has a more difficult time envisioning the proper design and predicting the tension vectors of these flaps. Tissue transposition is used when the characteristics of a surgical wound preclude closure by a simpler method of flap repair. Transposition flaps allow for complete redirection of wound closure tension by moving tissue from an area of surplus to an area of need by transposition of skin across intervening islands of unaffected tissue. Because the transposition flap effectively redirects wound closure tension, the flap can be used to close difficult wounds near free margins such as the ala, lip, proximal helix, or eyelid. For example, in a nasolabial transposition flap, loose tissue in the area of the medial

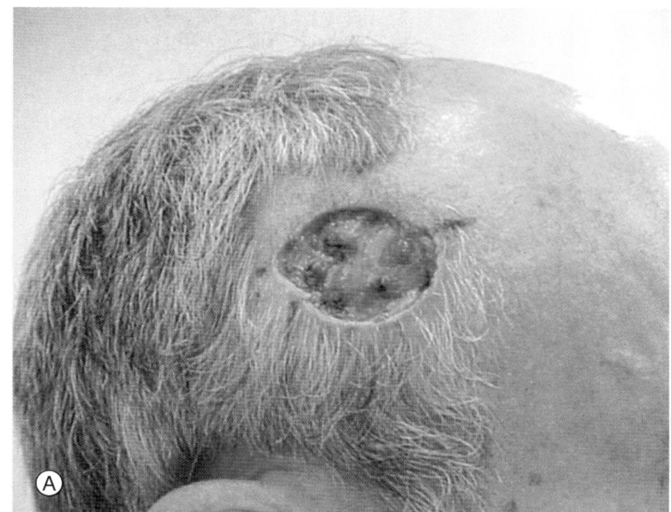

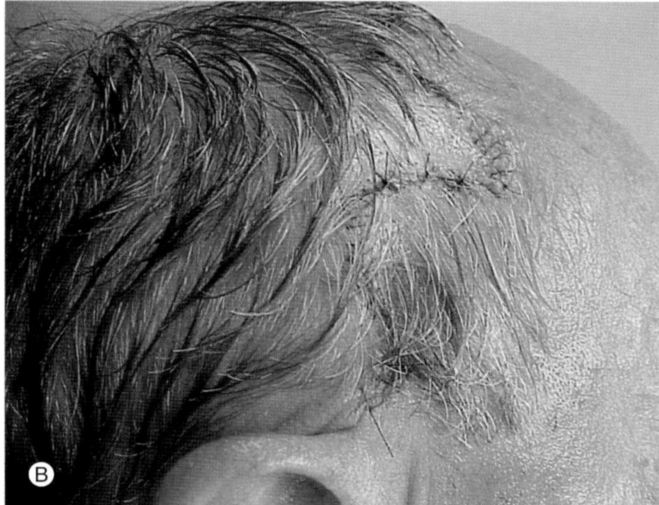

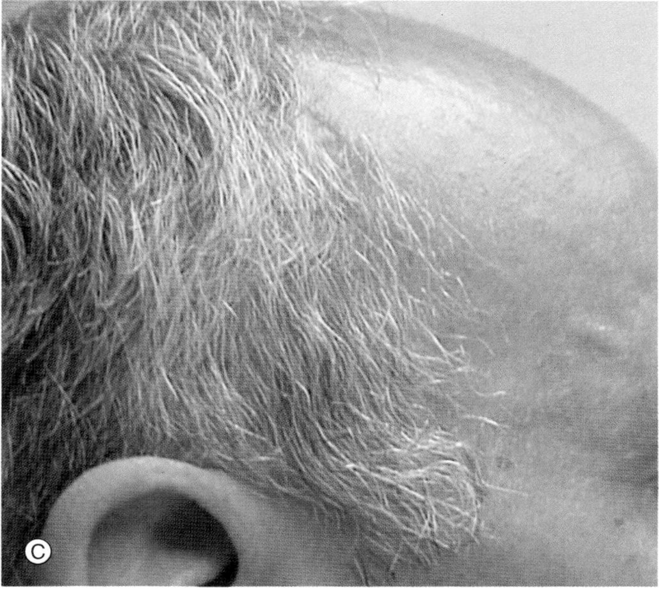

Figure 21.21 (A) An O–Z rotation flap used to repair a scalp defect. (B) The incision lines of the flap are well hidden within the adjacent hair. (C) The final result 6 months after surgery shows no disruption of hair beneath the skin.

cheek can be transposed over an unaffected lateral ala to cover a more medially located nasal ala or nasal tip wound. Because the cheek transposition flap is not directly advancing or rotating into the surgical defect on the medial ala, the important nose–cheek–lip junction is maintained instead of blunted.

Transposition flaps are affected by pivotal restraint in a manner analogous to rotation flaps. This pivotal restraint causes the transposed flap to 'fall short' of its intended target (the primary defect) unless the restraint is accounted for in proper flap design and undermining. Transposition flaps are defined by greater degrees of flap movement, which produces greater degrees of effective flap 'shortening'. As such, the surgeon who is just beginning to perform these more difficult transposition flap repairs should make the primary lobe of the flap slightly longer than initially considered appropriate until a more complete understanding of the nuances of flap transposition and pivotal restraint can be achieved.

The most commonly used transposition flaps are the rhomboid (rhombic) transposition flap, the bilobed transposition flap, the banner transposition flap and the nasolabial transposition flap. Many challenging surgical wounds can be reconstructed with these repairs, and their skillful execution is an essential technique for the advanced reconstructive surgeon.

Rhombic transposition flap

Probably the most well known of the random pattern flaps is the rhomboid or rhombic transposition flap. Limberg described the rhomboid transposition flap (Fig. 21.22) in 1946, and his work was translated into English in 1966.[44] Modifications of the Limberg flap were introduced in 1962 by Dufourmentel.[45] A rhombus is an equilateral parallelogram. The classic rhomboid flap is only suited to rhomboidal-shaped defects with equally sized sides and angles of 60° and 120°. The flap is designed by bisecting one of the 120° angles and extending a line equal to the length of one side of the rhombus from the tip of this angle away from the rhombus. From the distal extent of this line, a line of equal length is extended in either direction parallel to one side of the rhombus. By following this strategy for rhombic flap design, four separate flaps may be drawn for a single rhomboidal-shaped defect. The selection of the one flap most appropriately suited to repair the surgical defect is dictated by the laxity of adjacent skin and the presence of various anatomic structures in the vicinity of the wound.[46]

The great advance of the rhomboid flap was the ability to direct all tension away from one axis of a given defect. As the rhomboid transposition flap is elevated and transposed, all tension on the flap is directed toward closing the secondary defect. By suturing closed the secondary defect first, the flap is essentially 'pushed' into place in the primary defect without the need for secondary movement around the primary defect. This is particularly beneficial for defects that extend near a free margin that might be distorted by simpler reconstructive alternatives. A rhomboid flap is satisfactorily executed only when substantial tissue laxity exists or can be created adjacent to the defect at the base of the flap, therefore allowing easy closure of the secondary defect. There should also be sufficient tissue laxity so that the flap can transpose into the primary defect without undue tension. This usually requires that a line that bisects

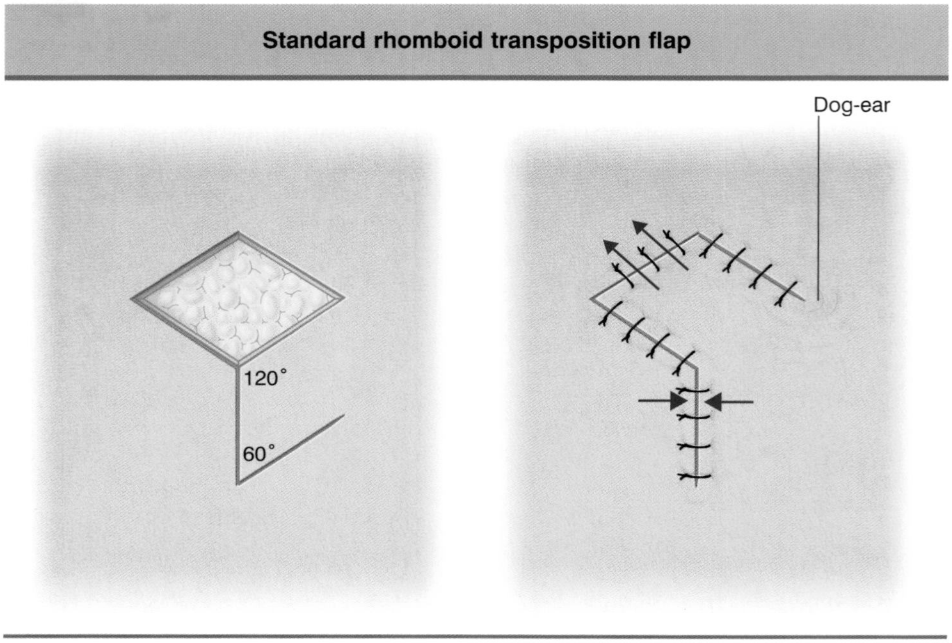

Standard rhomboid transposition flap

Figure 21.22 The standard rhomboid transposition flap as designed by Limberg. The major advantage of the rhomboid flap is to redirect tension away from the operative wound to a secondary area of laxity straddling a relaxed skin tension line.

the apex of the flap runs along or parallel to a relaxed skin tension line.[47] The basic rhomboid flap is useful for defects of the medial canthus, upper nose, lower eyelid, temple and peripheral cheek.[48–50] If classically designed with 60° angles at the apices of the rhomboidal defect, the transposition flap will produce dog-ear redundancies. This flap is also prone to developing trapdoor phenomena. It is therefore essential to undermine circumferentially beneath the base of the flap and around the margin of the primary defect.

Although the classic rhomboid flap is often avoided because of the limitations that the flap's design imposes, a modified rhomboid flap can be particularly useful in the closure of some facial defects (Figs 21.23 and 21.24). Instead of the geometrically complicated traditional flap design, a modified transposition flap is taken at a tangent off the circular primary defect. Attention is placed upon keeping the apex angle of the flap to a minimum, ideally less than 30°, so that a dog-ear redundancy near this point is accounted for. The modified flap is easily transposed into the primary defect, and the flap effectively redirects wound closure tensions. This modified transposition flap is commonly used in the reconstruction of lateral nasal sidewall and lateral brow defects.

Throughout the 1970s the rhomboid transposition flap enjoyed great popularity in the surgical literature. Tumor removal and closure were planned so that a rhomboidal defect could be initially created. The surgical literature from that era is replete with examples of rhomboid transposition flaps that were used to close many defects that could have been repaired in a simpler manner had the tumor been excised and the margins checked before planning a reconstructive procedure. Numerous reports that detailed the use of multiple small rhomboid flaps to close rather uncomplicated facial wounds on the nose or cheek also followed.[51] Although the creation of the flaps certainly testified to the surgeon's command of geometric principles, the flaps often created unnecessarily complicated incision lines, and simpler more aesthetically pleasing reconstructive alternatives could usually have been selected.

In its most suitable applications, the rhomboid transposition flap is an elegant repair, with the scar from the primary defect hidden within a cosmetic line and with wound closure tensions appropriately redirected away from the primary defect. At its worst, the flap is an unnecessarily complicated repair that leaves as its sequela a large, unaesthetic question mark-shaped scar surrounding a protruding, pin-cushioned flap.

Bilobed transposition flap

The bilobed flap, initially described by Esser in 1918[52] and refined by Zitelli in 1989,[53] is particularly useful for repairing difficult wounds on the distal nose (Fig. 21.25). Conceptually, the flap is more complicated than simple transposition flaps. After all, the bilobed flap is an intricate arrangement of two connected transposition flaps, and the potentials for misjudging pivotal restraint and the management of the secondary and tertiary defects are therefore magnified. Although the bilobed flap is categorized as a transposition flap, like the rhombic flap, there are significant degrees of flap rotation incorporated into the flap's design. When properly used, the bilobed flap offers an unparalleled opportunity to restore sebaceous skin to the convexity of the distal nose, and the flap is useful for repairing nasal wounds up to approximately 1.5 cm in diameter. Despite the bilobed flap's potentials for aesthetic success, the flap can produce dramatic distortion of the alar margins and apparent incision lines when poorly designed or executed.

As with all flaps, the bilobed flap's true value lies in its ability to recruit tissue from an area in which it is abundant (i.e. the proximal nasal dorsum) and transfer it to an area in which it is limited (i.e. the nasal tip). The usefulness of the bilobed flap is significantly increased by the flap's great flexibility in design. Depending on the stiffness and availability of nasal skin, the surgeon can alter the primary and secondary lobes' sizes, origination points, locations and angles of motion.[54] Although this seemingly adds great complexity to the bilobed flap's design, this flexibility

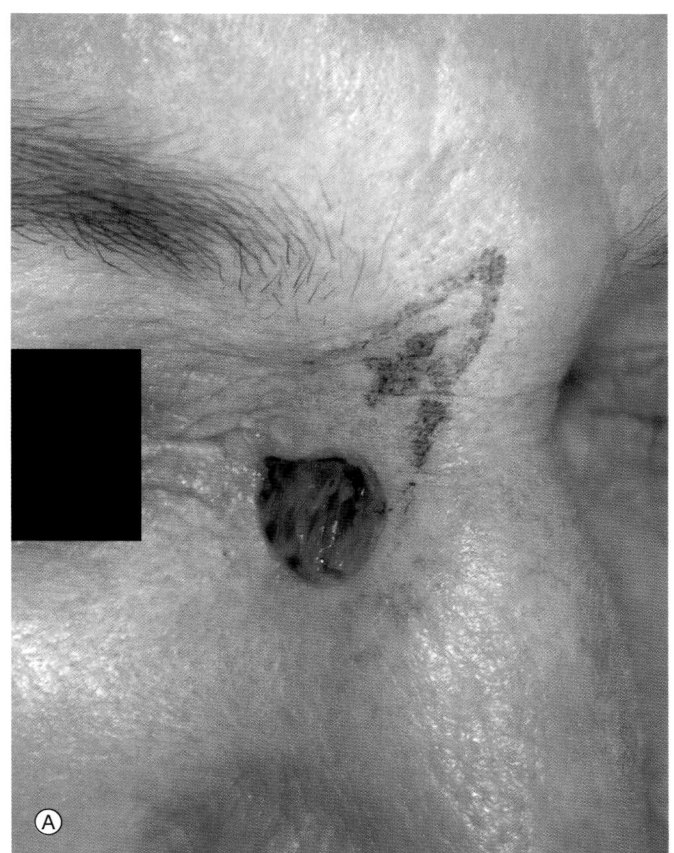

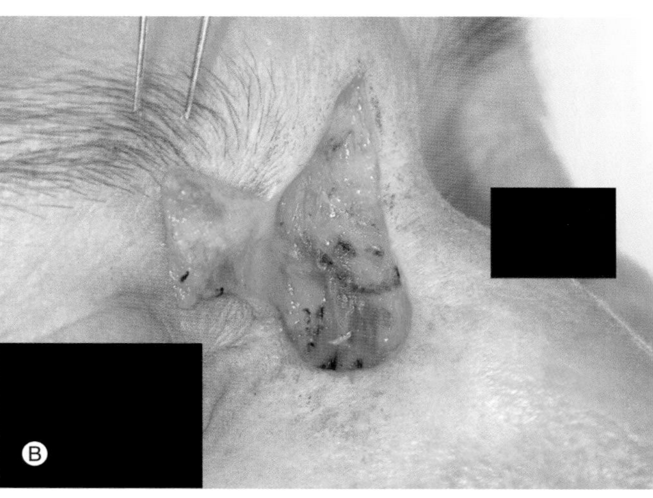

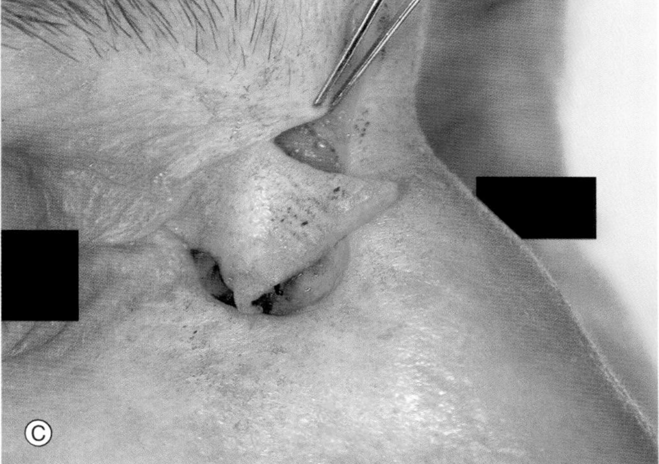

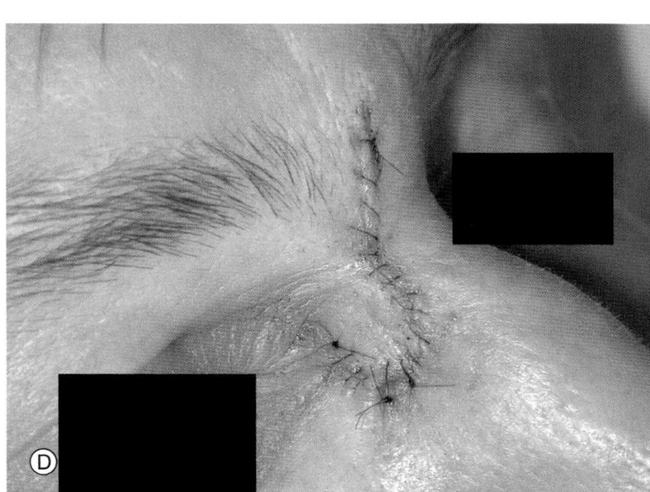

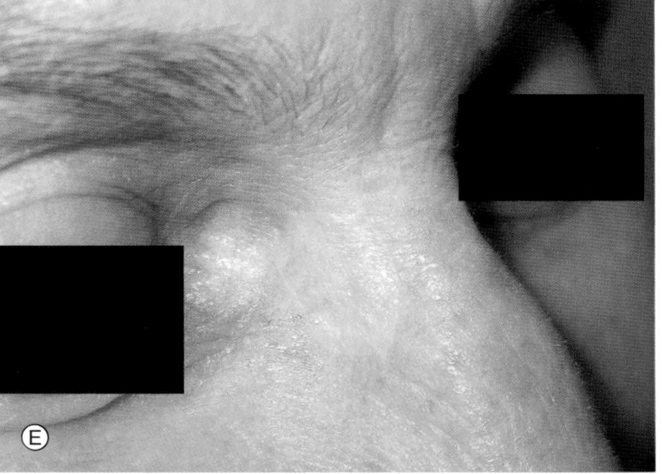

Figure 21.23 (A) Modified rhomboid flap for repair of a medial canthal wound. The flap is taken at a tangent to the operative wound and the angle of the flap is more acute than the traditional 60°. This design facilitates closure of the secondary defect within a glabellar fold. Closure of the secondary defect 'pushes' the flap into the primary defect and prevents the epicanthal web formation caused by tension at the medial canthus. (B) Flap undermined. (C) Closure of the secondary defect first "pushes" the flap into the primary defect. (D) Flap placed. (E) 90 days postoperatively.

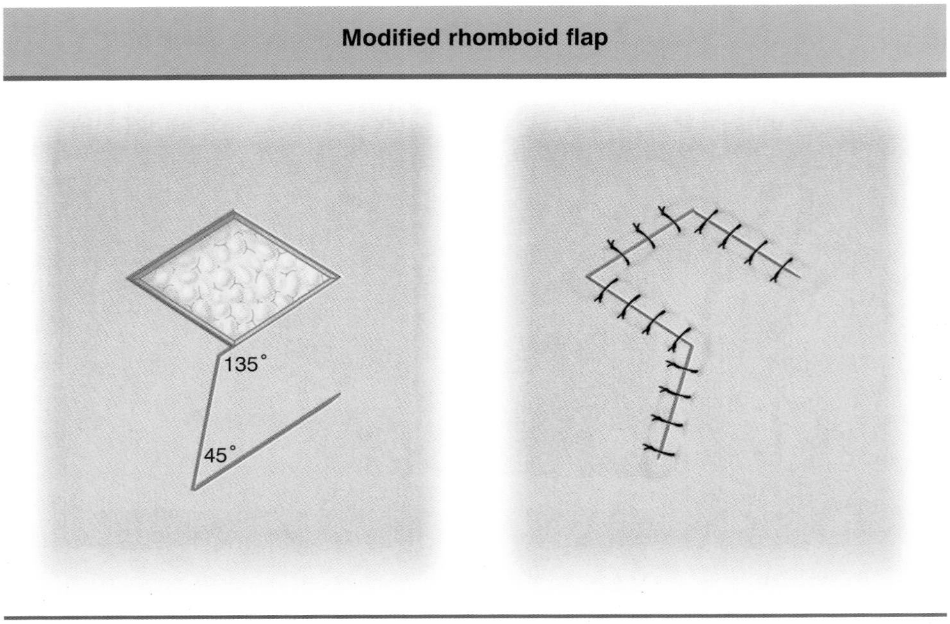

Modified rhomboid flap

135°

45°

Figure 21.24 Pivotal restraint requires a component of advancement for the tip of a standard Limberg flap to reach its destination. Lengthening all sides of the flap and decreasing the angle at the apex of the secondary defect can reduce pivotal restraint and allow for more facile closure.

allows the surgeon to expertly use the flap to reconstruct difficult nasal wounds.

After the appropriate bilobed flap design has been selected, the flap is sharply incised. Critical to the predictability of the flap's perfusion is the inclusion of nasalis musculature in the base of the flap. Wide undermining promotes flap mobility, minimizes wound closure tensions, and helps prevent inferior displacement of the ipsilateral alar margin as the stiff, sebaceous flap moves distally (Figs 21.26, 21.27). If the lobes of the flaps have been ideally sized (in general the first lobe measures approximately 75% of the area of the defect, the second lobe approximately 40% of the area of the primary lobe to allow for a modest degree of secondary movement) and if the entire nasal dorsum is widely undermined, the bilobed flap easily extends even to the infratip lobule of the nose to fill a defect. Because the incision lines of the bilobed flap are geometric and do not fall into already existing facial lines, great attention must be paid toward securing the flap with expert surgical technique if the flap is to be well hidden.

Although the bilobed flap is most commonly used to reconstruct distal nasal wounds, the flap, because of its abilities to transfer skin from distant areas into a surgical defect, also has a use in the reconstruction of difficult wounds on the chin, the lateral cheek, the hand and the posterior ear. In these extranasal sites, the surgeon can take advantage of the ability to use secondary motion to assist in the closure of the flap donor wounds, and great variances can therefore be made in the sizing of both the primary and the secondary lobes of the flap to accommodate the surgeon's needs for tissue transfer.

Banner transposition flap

Banner flaps are long, narrow, transposition flaps with a high length-to-width ratio, usually measuring 3 : 1 to 5 : 1. These flaps are designed and elevated along existing facial junctions or relaxed skin tension lines and are transposed 90° (or even more) to cover adjacent operative wounds. Because of their large length-to-width ratio, banner flaps must be elevated in areas with a predictable vascular supply, and they must have substantial mobility and laxity at their bases. The banner flap is particularly suited to oval or oblong defects that are oriented essentially perpendicular to the line of harvest of the flap. Defects of the upper helical rim are amenable to reconstruction with banner flaps elevated either from the postauricular or preauricular sulcus[55] (Fig. 21.28). Nasal bridge and medial canthal defects are also frequently closed in elegant fashion by glabellar banner flaps, the originations of which are hidden within glabellar creases[56] (Fig. 21.29). Medial lower eyelid defects are suitable for repair with a banner flap transposed from the nasofacial sulcus. Finally, lateral lower eyelid defects may be repaired with banner flaps harvested from the ipsilateral upper eyelid.[57] These flaps are also useful to close extremity wounds. The nasolabial flap is essentially a banner flap with approximately 60° of transposition, and is discussed in detail below.

The base of a banner transposition flap must be sufficiently undermined to allow for ideal transposition and to promote circumferential wound contraction during healing. Although banner flaps are ideal repairs for certain wounds, they are highly prone to developing the trapdoor deformity. When repairing a wound with a banner flap (and most flaps for that matter), it is useful to slightly undersize the flap and to undermine the recipient defect. It may also be useful to firmly tack the flap to the underlying wound in one or several locations to prevent the development of a potential dead space along the lengthy flap.

Nasolabial transposition flap

Used to reconstruct lateral and central alar wounds, the nasolabial transposition flap is often touted as a 'workhorse' flap for the reconstructive surgeon. Despite its simple design, the nasolabial flap is often a difficult flap with which to achieve reproducibly excellent results, and takes considerable experience to use properly. The flap is harvested from the relatively sebaceous skin in the medial cheek just adjacent to the ipsilateral melolabial fold. The flap is thinned as it is raised, and once undermined (to the superior base as well as circumferentially around the primary and secondary

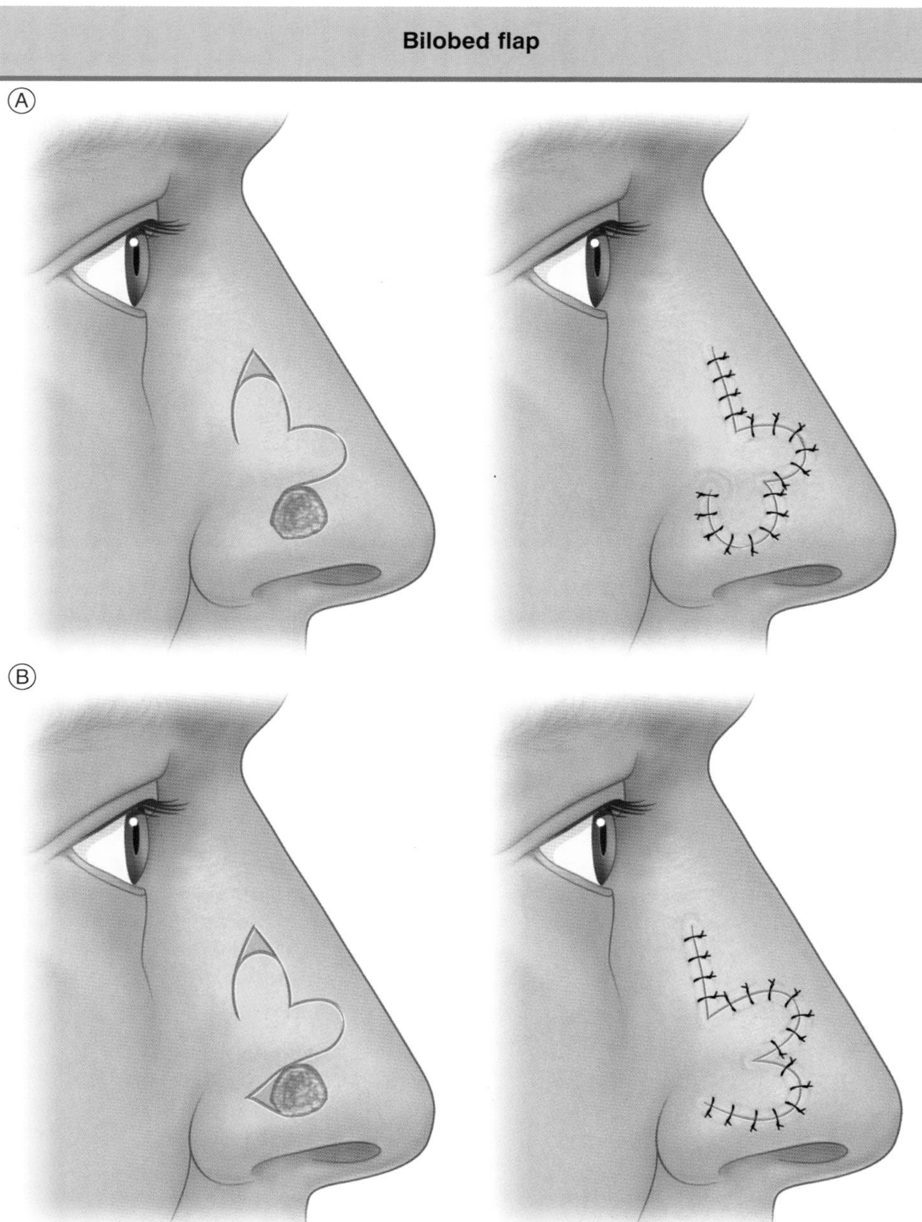

Figure 21.25 The bilobed flap was initially described by Esser (A), and Zitelli significantly improved the flap's design (B) by introducing the prospective removal of the Burow's triangle and reducing the angles of flap transposition required to close the primary and secondary defects.

defects) it is transposed into the alar wound. The anticipated dog-ear redundancy superior to the primary defect can be prospectively removed to facilitate flap motion and restore contour (Fig. 21.30).

Historically, the nasolabial flap has been a two-step surgical reconstruction of the nose. After the initial flap transfer, a revision procedure was required to thin the inevitably protuberant flap. However, with proper attention to flap design and technique, the nasolabial flap can be an appropriate single-stage repair.[58] To achieve predictable results, the superior dog-ear above the primary defect should be designed to be tall and narrow with no more than a 30° apical angle. The flap's origin within the melolabial fold should extend far enough inferiorly to compensate for the 'shortening' that occurs as the flap is transposed onto the nose. Importantly, the flap's donor site on the cheek should be widely undermined so that medial advancement of the cheek occurs readily and deep tacking sutures can be used to anchor the pivot point of the flap (which is superolaterally-based) to the piriform aperture near the junction of the lateral ala to the isthmus of the upper lip. Once the flap has been suitably anchored, the flap should basically fall into place with minimal tension to fill the alar defect. The distal portion of the flap that will be inset into the defect should be thinned (almost to the dermis) to prevent the unsightly pin-cushioning of the flap that is rather common. Additionally, the flap should be carefully trimmed to fit the defect and prevent retraction of the alar margin.

Similar to the design flexibility seen with the bilobed transposition flap, the nasolabial flap has numerous modifications that can enhance the usefulness of the flap. Bilateral nasolabial flaps can be used to repair larger nasal wounds, although the paramedian forehead flap is typically a more aesthetically appropriate reconstructive alternative for these difficult defects. For full-thickness alar defects, the nasolabial flap can also be designed with a long enough

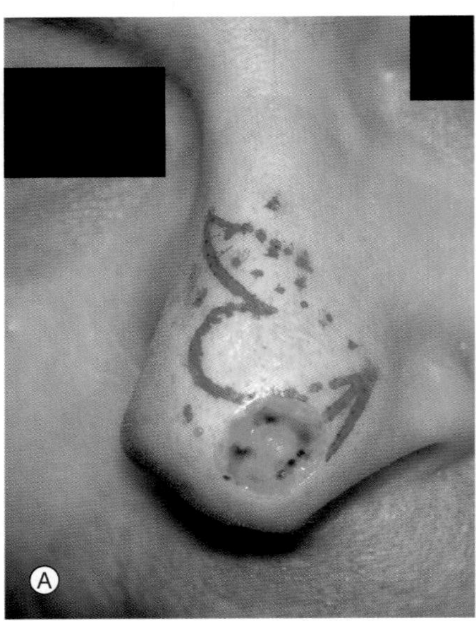

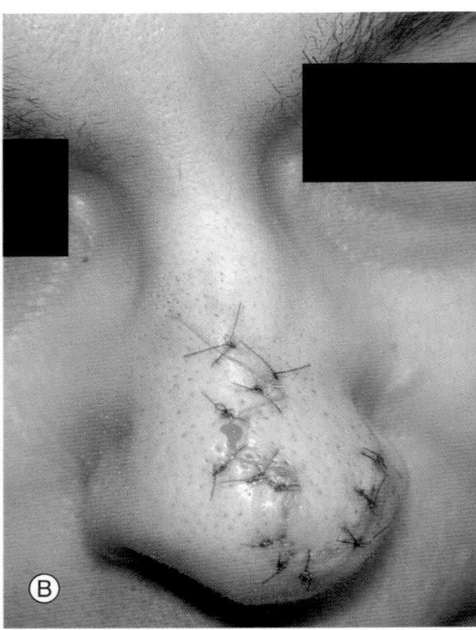

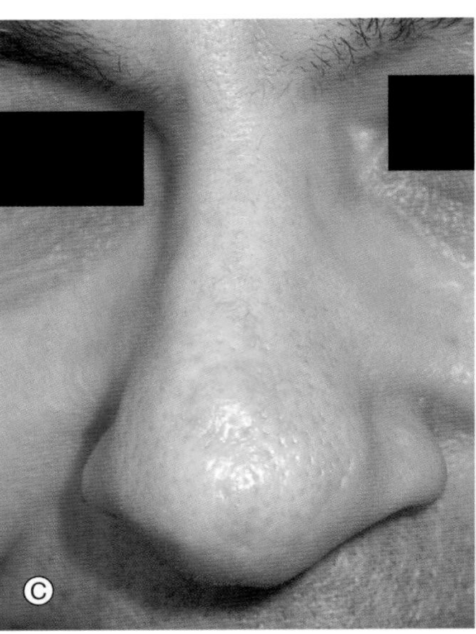

Figure 21.26 A bilobed flap for a distal nasal defect is designed with a 90° axis for facile transposition. The arc of transposition and rotation of the flap is carefully delineated to appropriately size the primary and secondary lobes. Superolateral orientation of the dog-ear removal at the inferior aspect of flap prevents alar distortion. (A) Flap design. (B) Execution. (C) Final result 90 days postoperatively, no revision. Dermabrasion or laserbrasion may be used to improve the contour of the incision line.

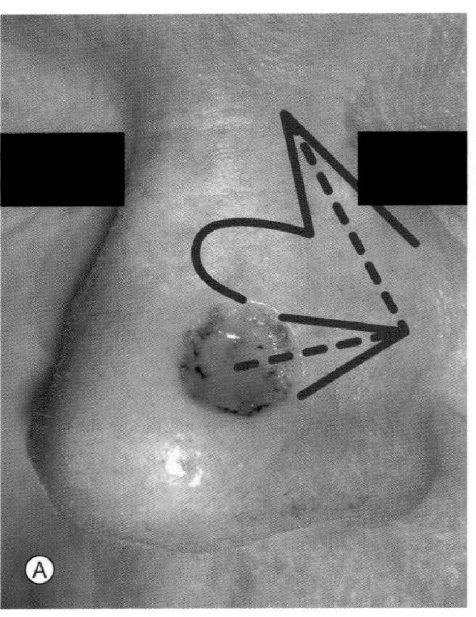

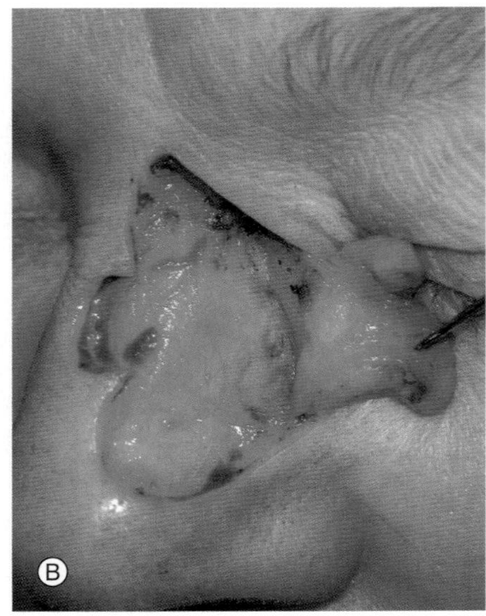

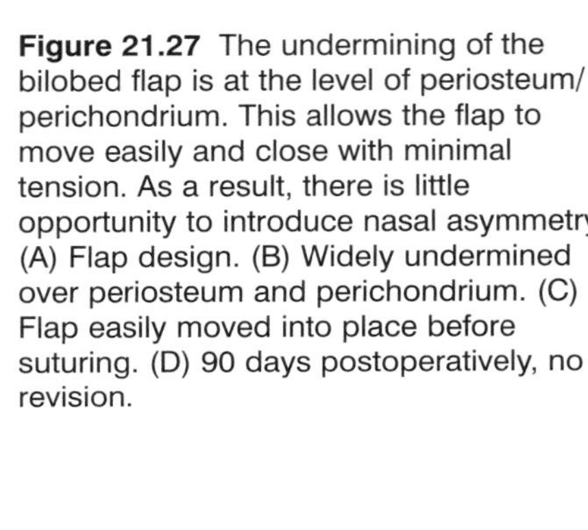

Figure 21.27 The undermining of the bilobed flap is at the level of periosteum/perichondrium. This allows the flap to move easily and close with minimal tension. As a result, there is little opportunity to introduce nasal asymmetry. (A) Flap design. (B) Widely undermined over periosteum and perichondrium. (C) Flap easily moved into place before suturing. (D) 90 days postoperatively, no revision.

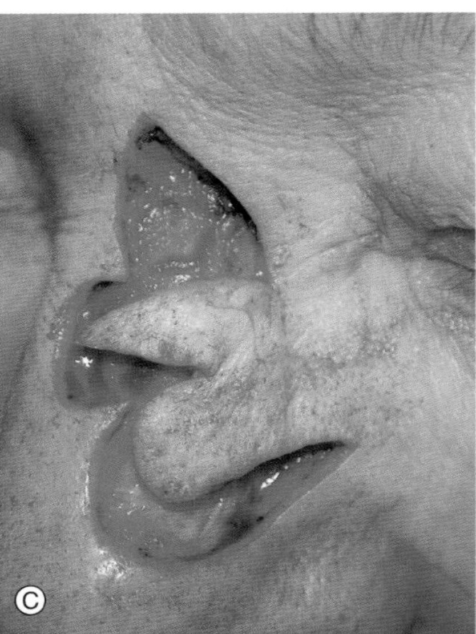

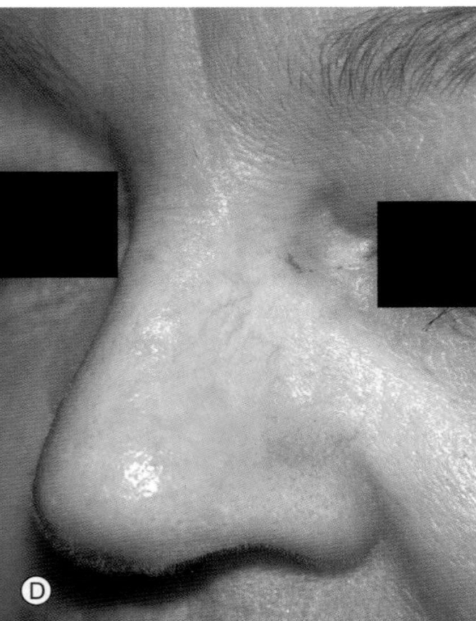

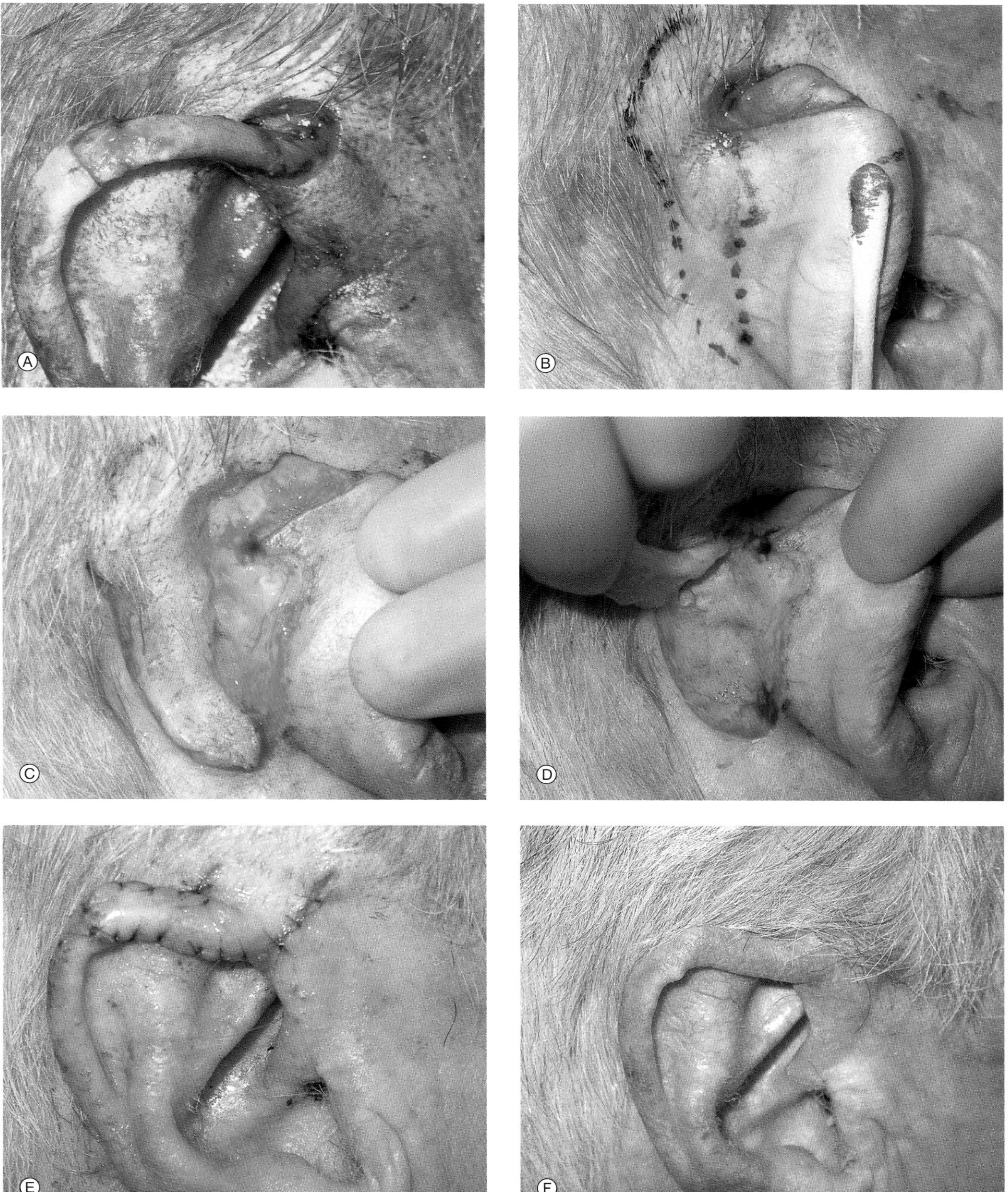

Figure 21.28 Proximal helical rim defects can be repaired with a long, thin banner flap from the preauricular or postauricular sulcus. These flaps are based on a rich vascular supply from branches of the temporal artery. The base of the flap is undermined at the superficial fascia, but the distal portion of the flap may be thinned to dermis to recreate a suitable thickness for the helical rim. No tension should be placed on the distal flap, and the flap should simply drape over the exposed cartilage. (A) Defect. (B) Banner flap designed into postauricular sulcus. (C) Flap developed by undermining at the level of the fascia in the sulcus. (D) Flap elevated to show the level of undermining, which is proximally at level of superficial fascia and distally just below dermis. (E) Flap inset into defect and closed under minimum tension. (F) Final result after one year.

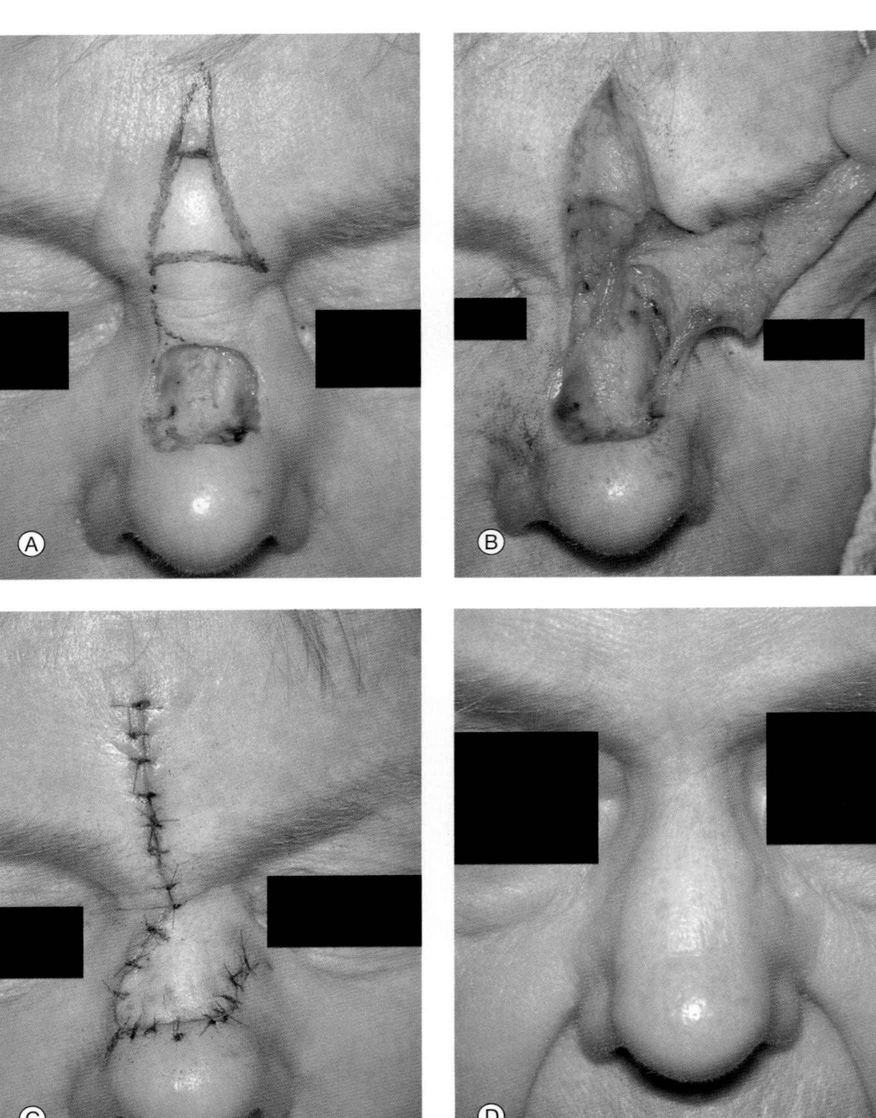

Figure 21.29 (A) Nasal banner flap hides donor scar within a glabellar crease. (B) This flap is elevated above the level of the procerus and corrugator muscles to expose the area undermined over muscle and bone. (C) Flap executed. (D) 90 days postoperatively, no revision.

pedicle so as to 'fold' upon itself at the alar margin. With this folding nasolabial flap, the donor tissue along the medial cheek can serve as both the internal nasal lining and the external nasal coverage.[59] The predictability of the nasolabial flap's perfusion is well demonstrated by the manipulations that these folded flaps can undergo without suffering ischemia.[60]

The pedicled transposition flap is yet another modification that can be used for defects of the lateral nose that are more medial and are not immediately adjacent to the nasofacial sulcus. In these scenarios, when a nasolabial flap is deemed desirable, it must transpose over the lateral alar segment that is intact to be inset. As such, a pedicle of skin bridges this gap and the flap must later be divided. Division of a pedicled flap occurs only once flap viability has been ascertained, which generally occurs at around 3 weeks.

The disadvantages of the nasolabial flap are readily apparent. Long, complex incisions are required to raise the flap, and because it originates at the melolabial fold it has a potential to place terminal beard hair onto the nose in male patients. The flap predictably flattens the alar groove, and a secondary procedure to reintroduce the shadowed concavity of this area is required to maximize the final aesthetic outcome. Finally, the flap is highly prone to developing the trapdoor deformity (Fig. 21.31) and appropriate attention should be placed on meticulous operative technique with undermining at the recipient site, insetting the flap with deep sutures and not oversizing the flap. For these reasons, pedicled flaps from the cheek occasionally offer more predictable results in nasal reconstruction. However, the single-staged nasolabial flap remains an important, if somewhat more difficult to master, reconstructive alternative for challenging alar wounds.

■ OPTIMIZING OUTCOMES

The purpose of performing any flap repair is to return the skin and soft tissues to a configuration that is as near normal as the dynamics of the surrounding tissue will allow. With experience, flap reconstructions can be conceptualized and executed with safety and reproducibly good functional and aesthetic results. Designing and executing flap repairs requires meticulous attention to detail at all steps, from planning the reconstruction to placing the final suture.

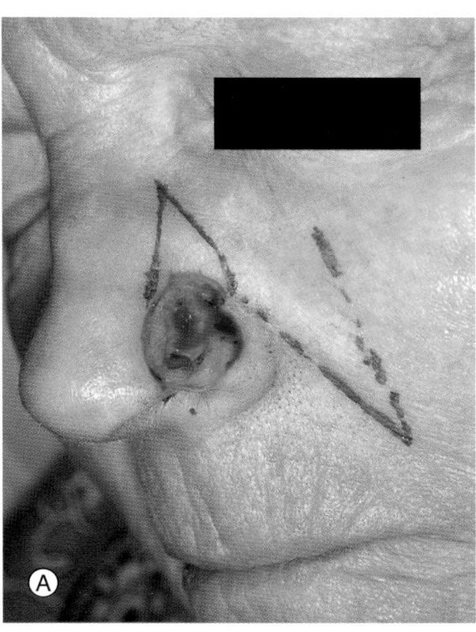

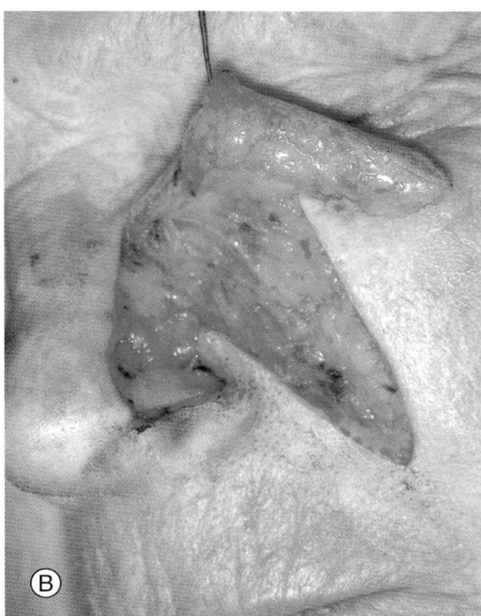

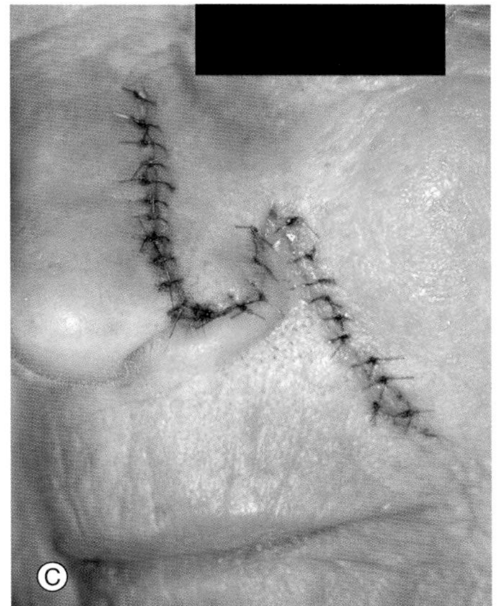

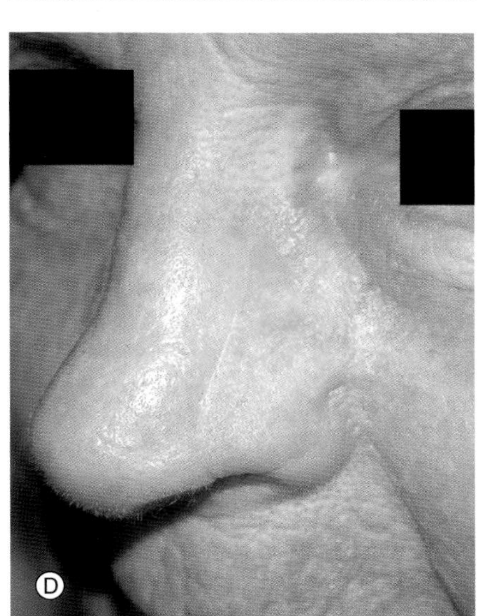

Figure 21.30 The nasolabial flap is elevated lateral to the nasolabial fold. It is elevated at the depth of the subcutis within the larger looser fat lobules overlying the facial musculature. The portion of the flap to be inserted into the operative defect is thinned to the superficial subcutis. The alar crease may be recreated with a tacking suture. A typical result is shown in which the border of the flap is slightly visible. In this case, a cartilage graft was also used to stabilize the ala. (A) Nasolabial flap design. (B) Flap undermined in deep subcutaneous tissue. (C) Flap inset and closure done. (D) 90 days postoperatively, no revision.

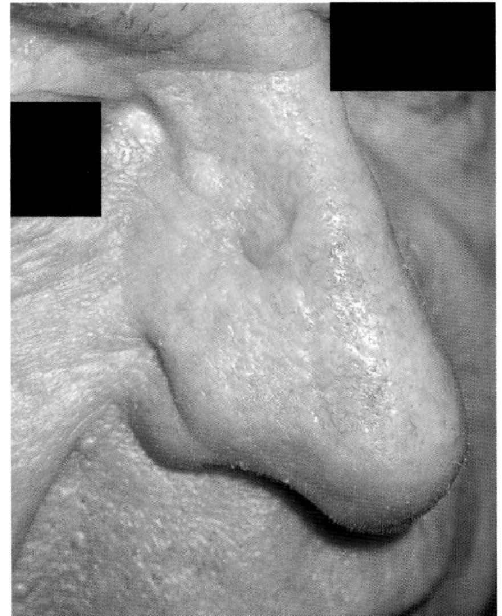

Figure 21.31 Trapdoor (or pincushion) deformity of a nasolabial flap forms 4 months after surgery despite meticulous design and operative technique. This may respond to intralesional corticosteroid injections, otherwise surgical revision procedure may be required.

Surgical planning

A properly performed flap reconstruction will close a wound without undue tension or distortion of a free margin. A critical aspect of surgical planning and informed consent is to inform the patient why the flap is needed and what the flap repair entails. Some patients will have low aesthetic expectations and will accept any reasonable surgical outcome. Other patients will expect essentially bloodless, painless, scarless and complication-free surgery and postoperative course. Although many surgeons rationalize that elderly patients have lower aesthetic demands than younger patients, recent dramatic increases in the numbers of older patients undergoing elective cosmetic surgery[61] suggest that they also have high aesthetic expectations. Therefore, reconstructive surgeons should strive for a good cosmetic outcome in all patients willing to consider a flap repair.

The concepts of skin grafting and direct wound closures are often easily understood by the lay public, flap repairs involve complicated geometric tissue rearrangements; many patients will not readily understand why so many incisions are required to close what they perceive to be a relatively small wound. As part of the informed consent process, the surgeon should discuss the proposed reconstructive procedure with the patient with the aid of a mirror. Not surprisingly, some patients will refuse to view an operative wound, and the informed consent can therefore be achieved with only a thorough discussion of the anticipated flap procedure. In addition to an explanation of the flap's design and execution, the reconstructive surgeon should also inform the patient of predictable surgical sequelae including transient hemorrhage, bruising, swelling, discomfort and suture line visibility as well as less likely sequelae including nerve injury, infection, tumor recurrence and contour deformity.

The planning of a surgical flap as a reconstructive alternative first involves the exclusion of simpler wound management strategies such as second intention healing, primary linear closure or skin grafting. If the surgical wound is large, deep or complicated, a flap reconstruction is likely to offer aesthetic and functional results superior to the results of other reconstructive alternatives. The most simple flap option should always be selected. Despite their advantages, flaps do require long incision lines that can be quite noticeable, and all attempts to limit the visibility of these incision scars should be undertaken. Because the entire premise of a flap reconstruction involves relocation of the primary surgical defect to an area in which there is more tissue availability and less cosmetic penalty, the surgeon should initially carefully assess the laxity and quality of the tissue immediately surrounding the primary defect. Wound closure tensions should be appropriately directed away from critical anatomic structures such as the eyelid or eyebrow margin, the vermilion border, or the alar rim. The tension required to close the donor site of the flap should also be carefully assessed before initiation of the surgical procedure to verify that these structures will not be distorted. Finally, the most appropriate flap should be demarcated using marking ink with the patient upright and demonstrating relaxed skin tension lines and facial expression lines where incision lines can be hidden. This should be done before distorting the area with the infiltration of local anesthesia.

In addition to planning for the surgical repair and preparing the patient, the surgeon should also properly prepare himself or herself to optimize operative outcomes. The experienced dermatologic surgeon with a competent assistant can complete many moderately complex random pattern flap reconstructions in less than 90 minutes, but appropriate scheduling of operative procedures should be allowed so that the surgeon is not unnecessarily rushed. The accurate performance of flap reconstructive procedures depends upon the surgeon's ability to perform consistently. Distractions during this process need to be minimized. The surgical tray should be arranged in a predictable manner, and the comfort of the surgeon should be assured before the operation. The operating room must be designed for ergonomic comfort because there are suggestions in the literature that the motions associated with the frequent performance of medical procedures can result in repetitive use injuries in physicians (see Chapter 5).[62,63]

Anesthesia

Most random pattern facial reconstructions can be carried out using only local anesthesia. A combination of facial nerve blocks and local infiltration anesthesia will allow for the repair of all but the largest and most complicated surgical defects. The most common anesthetic used by the dermatologic reconstructive surgeon is 1% lidocaine with 1 : 100 000 parts epinephrine (adrenaline). A longer-acting local anesthetic such as bupivicaine may be added if the anticipated surgical procedure will be lengthy. For large surgical defects, there is occasionally a need for tumescent anesthesia using larger volumes of diluted lidocaine (known as tumescent anesthesia).[64] Tumescent anesthesia offers the benefit of excellent local anesthesia, enhanced hemostasis and lower peak serum levels of anesthetic, but the larger volumes of injected anesthetic can cause tissue distortion and tension intraoperatively as well as prolonged postoperative facial edema.

Epinephrine (adrenaline) is routinely added to the anesthetic solution to provide suitable hemostasis, and the use of epinephrine greatly facilitates the speed and safety of facial reconstructive procedures. Additionally, the duration of anesthesia is prolonged and the peak serum levels of anesthetic are minimized with the addition of epinephrine to a certain point. Historically, there have been concerns that the profound pharmacologic vasoconstriction associated with the use of epinephrine can result in flap death or even necrosis of adjacent tissue in watershed areas such as the nasal tip, ear lobe, penis, or digit, but reconstructive procedures carried out with the use of epinephrine in these anatomic areas have not been associated with higher levels of tissue ischemia or surgical complications in those without peripheral vascular disease (see Chapter 5). In fact, even digital block anesthesia with the use of epinephrine has been shown to be undeniably safe.[65] Additionally, the early concerns that the concomitant administration of β-blockers and epinephrine would result in unopposed α-adrenergic stimulation and serious hypertension were proven to be unfounded.[66] The use of epinephrine may blanch a flap and the surrounding tissues during an operative reconstruction, but this relative intraoperative pallor does not indicate prolonged ischemia and does not predict flap failure.

Local anesthesia is safe and appropriate for the overwhelming majority of skin cancer reconstructive procedures including complicated pedicled flaps. By avoiding the use of general anesthesia or conscious sedation, patient postoperative recovery can be hastened, overall morbidity diminished, and operative expenditures minimized. Especially in those with a history of anxiety or panic disorder, and occasionally for nervous patients, oral anxiolytics or analgesics can be used, but most patients can tolerate extensive reconstructive facial flap surgery with the use of only injected local anesthetics. This must be assessed on a case-by-case basis.

Incision

After sufficient anesthesia is obtained, the operative site is prepped and draped in a standard surgical manner. Because flap reconstructive procedures involve the introduction of foreign materials (suture) into the operative site, these procedures should be carried out only under strictly sterile conditions to minimize the risk of postoperative wound infection. To improve the accuracy of flap surgery, the physician should surgically prepare the entire face so that any intraoperative complications such as the development of facial asymmetry can be recognized and corrected. Thereafter, the flap is incised with a scalpel. Lateral traction on the skin during the incision facilitates the creation of an even wound edge. Definitive incisions to the subcutaneous fat should be performed initially to prevent fraying of the flap's incised margins. During the incision and liberation of the flap, all efforts should be made to minimally handle the tissue. Tissue forceps with teeth and skin hooks are much less traumatic than forceps with flat blades, and should be used exclusively to manipulate tissue. Any unnecessary manipulation of the wound's edges can cause subtle degrees of tissue ischemia that can impact on the aesthetic quality of the final scar.

Plane of flap elevation and surgical undermining

A flap needs to be freed from its attachments to the deeper subcutaneous tissues before it can be effectively transferred to a recipient site. Flap elevation loosens the flap from its restricting connections and undermining minimizes the wound closure tensions on the flap. Because elevated wound closure tensions accurately predict the risk of ischemic flap loss,[67] adequate undermining should always be performed. Undermining is effective, and animal studies have demonstrated that the force required for a one-dimensional closure of a linear repair of an in-vivo porcine operative wound is reduced between 18.6% and 47.4% with simple undermining of the wound's edges.[68] Undermining of the flap, the tissue surrounding the flap and the primary defect may also minimize the risk of developing pin-cushioning in the later postoperative period because the wound contractile forces are distributed in more directions and over much greater distances.[69] Undermining comes at a cost, however. Undermining, particularly at a flap's base, can transect vital arterial input to the flap, and overly aggressive undermining can therefore introduce an ischemic risk. Paradoxically, undermining that is too extensive can also impede tissue movement.[70] The successful dermatologic surgeon therefore approaches flap undermining as carefully as flap design. For rotation and transposition flaps, undermining is even more vital, because the flap must move a greater distance and must do so in two or even three dimensions.

Undermining may be carried out either bluntly or sharply. Sharp undermining with a scalpel or iris or Shea undermining scissors under direct visualization is preferred by many surgeons because the flap can be elevated within a uniform and predictable plane.[71] Sharp undermining produces less blunt force trauma and shear force on surrounding structures and can limit postoperative swelling. Blunt undermining on the other hand can be useful when undermining near vital neurovascular structures that need to be spared. When a fascial plane such as the SMAS or muscular plane is encountered, undermining can often be accomplished with great precision using electrosection.

Flaps are elevated and undermined in defined planes based on anatomic location (Table 21.2, Fig. 21.32). For

Table 21.2 Undermining planes in flap reconstructions

Location	Preferred undermining plane	Structures to be aware of
Nose	Submuscular fascia/perichondrium/ periosteum	Nasociliary nerve, angular artery
Lip	Just above orbicularis oris	Multiple branches of labial artery
Ear	Just above perichondrium	
Eyelid	Just above orbicularis oculi	
Scalp	Just above or just beneath galea	Scalp arteries
Cheek	Mid to deep subcutaneous fat	Parotid duct, buccal branches of the facial nerve
Forehead	Just above frontalis	Supraorbital and supratrochlear arteries and nerves
Temple	Just above superficial fascia	Temporal branch of facial nerve, superficial temporal artery

ideal flap repairs, the thickness of the elevated flap should closely match the depth of the primary surgical defect except when the defect is deeper than the plane desired. Cheek flaps are usually elevated within the subcutaneous fat. Flaps that are elevated within the subcutis should generally be undermined in the larger, looser fat lobules near the mid to deep subcutis. The fat lobules of the superficial subcutis are smaller, laced with fibrous tissue, and richly vascularized, making flap elevation more challenging. Thicker subcutaneous flaps have a more predictable pattern of perfusion, and elevation just above a superficial fascial plane will often produce greater flap mobility than elevation in the superficial subcutaneous plane. This plane of dissection is also used for all closures on the neck, trunk, and extremities as well.

The cutaneous surgeon should have a well-honed knowledge of the underlying anatomic structures because deeper undermining introduces significant risks of transecting vital structures. Flaps on the forehead are typically elevated just above the frontalis musculature. Although this plane of elevation requires careful separation of the subcutis from the underlying skeletal muscle, it prevents the numbness and arterial transection that can occur with deeper flap elevation. Scalp flaps are most appropriately elevated beneath the galea in the bloodless tissue plane immediately above the periosteum. Because the flap elevated under galea has limited tissue mobility/stretch, incision in the galea or excisions of a portion of the galea may be useful to provide an added component of tissue advancement.

Many lip flaps are elevated just above the orbicularis oris. Some small nasal flaps are elevated above the nasal musculature, while more complicated flaps, such as the bilobed transposition flap and the dorsal nasal flap are most appropriately elevated just above the perichondrium. This deeper plane of undermining on the nose is associated with far less hemorrhage than undermining within the nasalis musculature, and the inclusion of richly perfused skeletal muscle with the bases of these flaps makes the flaps nearly immune

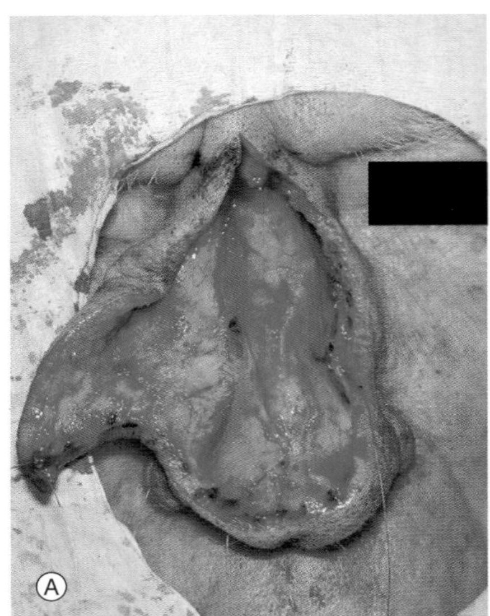

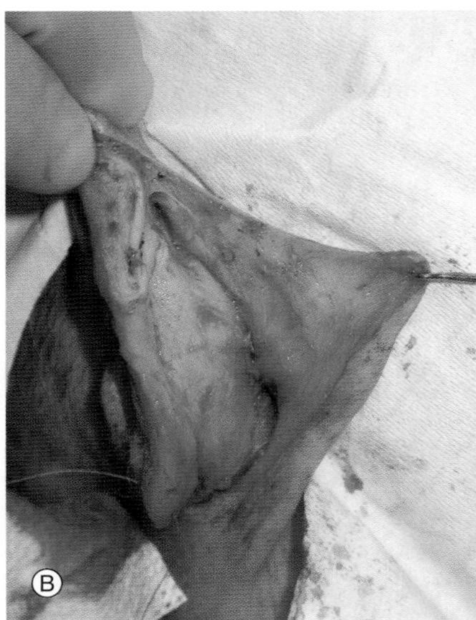

Figure 21.32 Preferred flap elevation planes. (A) Nose: perichondrium and periosteum. (B) Ear: perichondrium. (C) Forehead: just above the frontalis muscle. (D) Lower eyelid: just above the orbicularis oculi muscle.

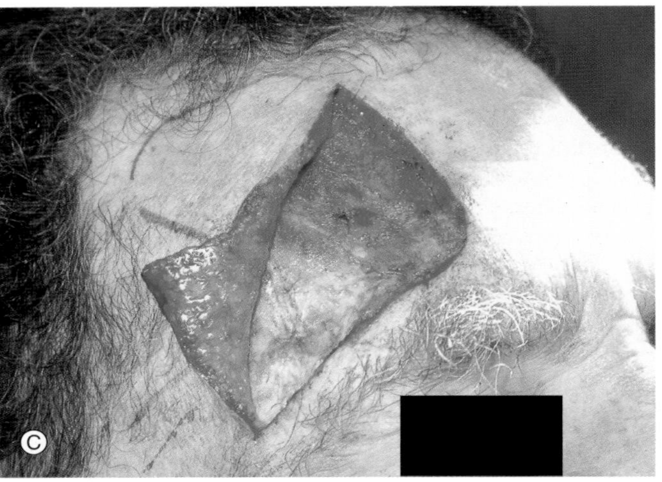

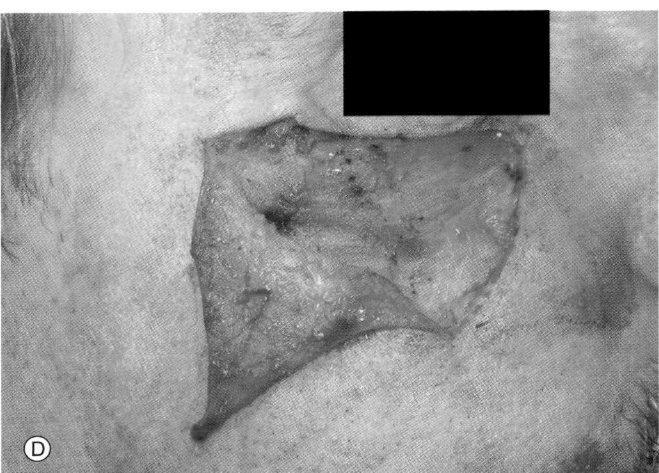

to ischemia. Rhinoplasty surgeons also choose this plane of undermining because they consider that this plane allows the most proper tissue movement while minimizing the scar formation that inevitably accompanies any surgical intervention.[72] Flaps on the ear should be undermined over perichondrium while those involving periorbital skin should be undermined just above orbicularis oculi musculature.

Hemostasis

Because flaps often require wide undermining for creation, they typically have higher rates of associated bleeding complications than side-to-side or skin graft repairs. Animal studies and clinical observations have demonstrated that hemorrhagic complications associated with flap reconstructive procedures dramatically increase the likelihood of ischemic flap failure.[73] Postoperative hemorrhage is also traumatic to the patient, and frequently painful. With meticulous intraoperative hemostasis, the risk of postoperative hemorrhagic complications can be minimized. Before closure, all visibly bleeding vessels should be effectively addressed. Small-caliber bleeding vessels can be sealed with electrocoagulation or bipolar cautery interventions, but vessels with a visible lumen are routinely ligated with a 4-0 or 5-0 absorbable suture to prevent a delayed hemorrhage if the small seal provided by the use of a cautery apparatus should dislodge. Although surgical drains are often used in other disciplines to minimize the risk of hematoma formation, the type of flap reconstructions used to repair even larger facial defects do not typically require the use of drains if strict hemostasis has been achieved. Pressure bandages are not a substitute for appropriate surgical hemostasis because studies have demonstrated that the amount of pressure that such bandages can apply is minimal. Furthermore, the pressure associated with the application of bandage materials rapidly falls in the immediate postoperative period.[74]

Suturing

After thorough hemostasis has been achieved, all flaps are sutured into place with at least two distinct layers of tissue closure. Buried sutures are important for securing the flap into place and for minimizing wound closure tensions on epidermal edges. If the deeper subcutaneous tissues and dermis are not adequately apposed, the epidermal sutures will be placed under unacceptable tension, which may strangulate wound edges and lead to unaesthetic scars.

Eversion of the wound's edges (important to prevent the development of an inverted, trough-like scar) is largely a reflection of the accurate placement of the subcutaneous sutures. Approximation and eversion of the wound's edges can be obtained by using buried vertical mattress sutures[75] although there are many variations in this technique. In general, the authors prefer Vicryl (Ethicon Inc, Johnson & Johnson, Somerville, NJ) or Monocryl (Ethicon Inc, Johnson & Johnson, Somerville, NJ) sutures for subcutaneous or fascial closure. The suture knots should be placed deeply enough to minimize the likelihood of later extrusion. Although wound edges should be well-approximated and dead space minimized, buried sutures should be placed sparingly because they are foreign bodies capable of producing inflammatory reactions in the dermis.

Suspension or tacking sutures are sutures that anchor a portion of a flap to underlying immobile structures such as the periosteum. This technique is used to shift tension away from the edges of a flap, to reorient the tension vector of a flap, or to tack a flap down at a point of facial concavity where the flap would otherwise tent and create a potential dead space.[76] Tacking for facial closures is usually carried out with a 4–0 absorbable or clear non-absorbable suture. The frontal bone, lateral orbital wall, zygomatic arch, nasal bones and medial maxilla are the most frequently used anchoring sites for tacking sutures. A classic example of how a tacking suture may be used to redirect tension is a medial cheek rotation flap used to close an infraorbital wound. The dermis of the advancing edge of the flap is tacked to the nasal sidewall at the superior and medial extent of the rotation. This single suture effectively closes the primary defect and takes all tension off the leading edge of the flap, therefore preventing a vertical tension vector at the medial lower lid and ectropion formation (see Fig. 21.14). Similarly, it is often useful to tack large cheek and temple rotation flaps to either the zygoma or to the lateral orbital rim or temple (Fig. 21.33). One flap that frequently benefits from a tacking suture is the nasolabial flap. Tacking from the center of the flap to the underlying maxilla at the alar crease can help avoid tenting of the flap and may assist in maintaining an otherwise ablated alar crease. In placement of this suture through the flap pedicle, care must be taken to keep the bite rather small and vertically aligned with flap blood supply to prevent excessive ischemic strain on the flap. For larger flaps, this is rarely a compromising factor.

Nylon, polypropylene, or fast-absorbing gut sutures are typically used for epidermal closure. Interrupted sutures are occasionally used for key sutures and for adjusting small discrepancies in the wound edges, but most of the flap's incision lines can be closed with a running suture. Running sutures are time efficient and offer an ability to distribute wound closure tensions evenly. In our experience, epidermal everting sutures, such as the horizontal or vertical mattress sutures, can produce subtle wound edge ischemia when used on the face and are therefore avoided.

■ POSTOPERATIVE CARE

After the flap procedure has been completed, an appropriate sterile dressing should be applied. An initial layer of lubricating ointment is applied to the sutures, followed by an overlying nonstick dressing that conforms to the flap's outline and is secured with a bolster of dry gauze and hypoallergenic paper tape. Patient acceptance of the bandage is significantly improved if flesh-colored paper tape is used. Prophylactic antibiotics are used if the risk of wound infection is unacceptably high. Studies that have examined the benefit of systemic antibiotics in these clean or clean-contaminated types of flap repairs are conflicting,[77,78] and more carefully designed studies are required to determine whether or not systemic antibiotics improve the inherently low risk of infection associated with these procedures.

Surgeons use many different postoperative wound care regimens following flap repairs, and much has been written about proper postoperative care. Two techniques are most commonly used. In the first, the patient cleans the suture line several times each day with either hydrogen peroxide or saline and applies a bland petrolatum-based ointment and a bandage. This technique of frequent wound care has the benefit of removing any crusted blood that accumulates on the incision line during the early postoperative period. Hydrogen peroxide is particularly effective for removing encrusted blood, and should not impede wound healing as long as the wound has been closed primarily. Some believe that manual debridement of the suture line may promote more rapid epithelialization of the wound's edges. Patients can feel involved in their own medical care, and it may be helpful to have them marvel at how quickly they heal. After removing the hemorrhagic crust that invariably accompanies any sutured wound, liberal lubrication of the incision line with an ointment promotes healing and makes suture removal easier. Antibiotic ointments are commonly used, and data from an emergency room study suggested that traumatic wounds treated with antibiotic ointment had lower wound infection rates than similar wounds treated with only bland petrolatum.[79] A placebo (petrolatum)-controlled study in the dermatologic literature demonstrated, however, that the infection rates of clean wounds treated with the petrolatum were no higher than the infection rates of sutured wounds treated with an antibiotic-containing preparation.[80] For that reason, simple petrolatum ointment is usually sufficient for proper wound care, particularly for patients with a history of allergic contact dermatitis to topical antibiotics.

As an alternative to this open-wound care regimen, the original dressing can be left in place for the entire 5–7 days before suture removal or wound check. With this closed-wound care regimen,[81] the epidermal layer of sutures is often a fast-absorbing plain gut. Adhesive tape strips are carefully applied over the sutured wound. This is then covered with a pressure dressing secured with a mesh or cloth tape. In contrast to the daily wound care required with the open technique, this closed technique requires the bandage to stay dry and intact for the entire 5–7 days that the sutures are in place. This minimal care technique is useful for patients for whom compliance is an issue. Most surgeons agree that the two wound management strategies produce roughly equivalent aesthetic results.

Suture removal must occur punctually, particularly for flaps on the face. If the epidermal nonabsorbable sutures are allowed to remain in place for an extended period, a distracting cross-hatched scar is often the final result. For that reason, the sutures of facial flaps are routinely removed 4–7 days postoperatively. With proper wound care, suture removal should occur readily. Care is taken not to exert unnecessary tension on the flap's edges because the healing

Eyelid repair at the lateral canthus

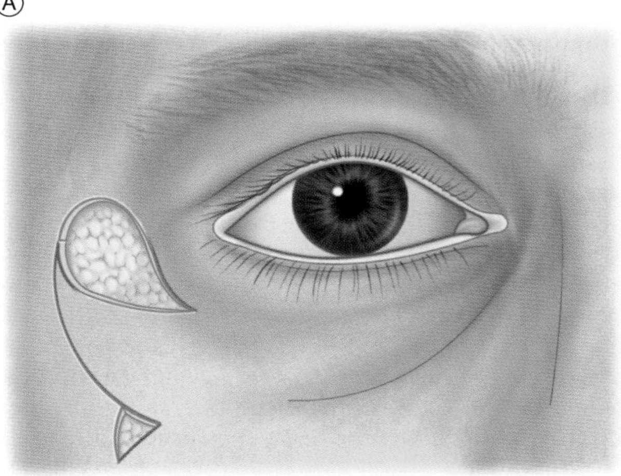

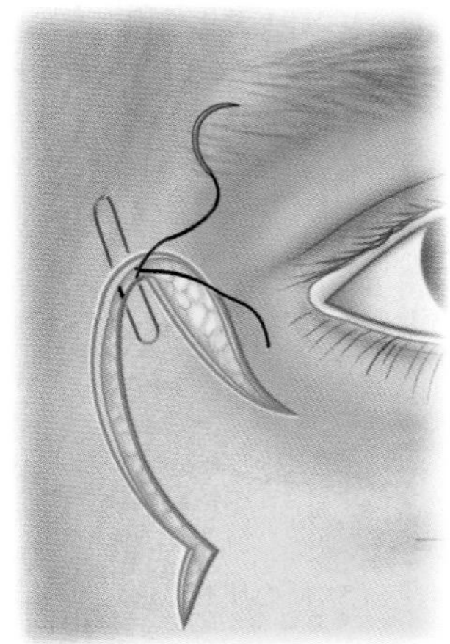

Eyelid

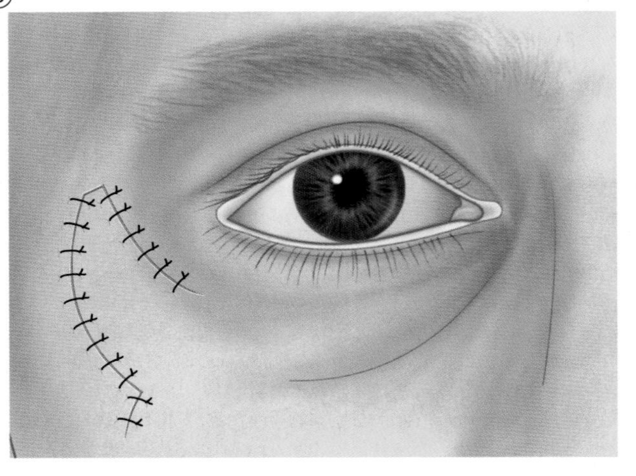

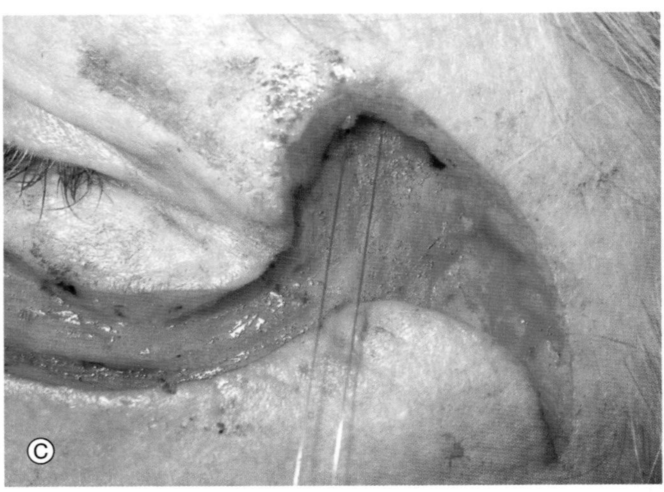

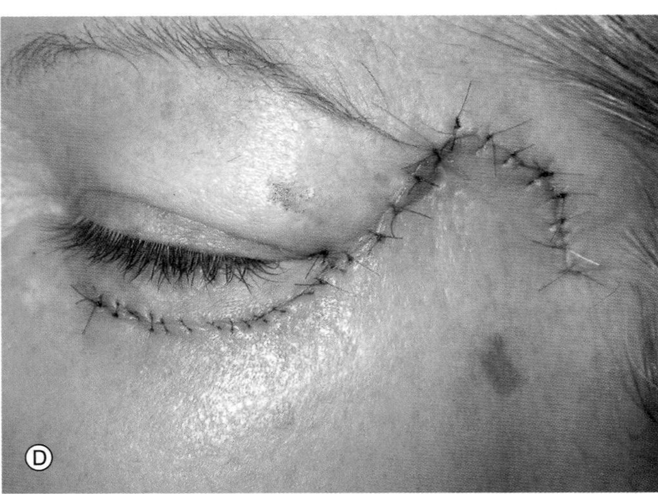

Figure 21.33 (A)–(D) By tacking the leading tip of a rotation to periosteum with a suspension suture, all tension is removed from the closure of primary and secondary defects. A suspension suture from the flap dermis to the periosteum of the temple supports the weight of the flap lateral to the eyelid to prevent ectropion formation. The flap combines elements of rotation and advancement. Slight lateral displacement of the lateral canthus will resolve when the local anesthesia dissipates.

Optimizing outcomes

- A minor miscalculation in flap design can result in flap failure, postoperative morbidity and functional or aesthetic compromise. The surgeon should provide proper preoperative counseling and obtain detailed informed consent.
- Most flap failures on the face can be traced to crucial errors in flap design or poor surgical practices. The successful creation of facial flaps involves finding the correct balance between flap liberation and vascular preservation. For proper mobilization, flaps generally require relatively long incision lines and generous undermining.
- Surgical morbidities such as postoperative hemorrhage or damage to underlying facial motor nerves may result from poor surgical technique, a lack of knowledge of the underlying anatomy or patient-related factors. Proper patient selection and surgical expertise and knowledge are critical for flap success.
- Most surgical complications that follow facial flap repairs result from difficulties in hemostasis. Careful attention should be placed on proper patient selection, the occasional use of preoperative screening laboratory tests, and thorough intraoperative hemostasis.
- Pin-cushioning is easier to prevent than to manage. The most important technique to reduce the risk of this complication is to properly size the flap.

wound has a low tensile strength during this early post-operative period.

After the sutures have been removed, the edges of the flap are supported with adhesive tape strips. The patient is given detailed information about the anticipated changes in the flap that will occur over the following months. Facial flaps occasionally require months to 'settle', and the patient should be informed that erythema, edema and incision line visibility all improve with time. Scar massage can be initiated after the first postoperative month to soften the flap and hasten the resolution of any textural irregularities that result from the placement of the buried sutures.

PITFALLS AND THEIR MANAGEMENT

There are many potential complications associated with random pattern flap reconstruction. With appropriate training and experience, the overall risk of encountering major surgical complications should be quite low. Most of these complications are the same as those seen with any surgical procedure (bleeding, wound infection, tissue necrosis and dehiscence), but some are particularly apparent with the use of facial flaps (poor aesthetic outcome, functional deficit with or without cutaneous motor nerve injury, and flap pin-cushioning). Most complications are much easier to avoid than to rectify, and emphasis should be placed on the need for careful flap design and meticulous operative technique.

Most surgical complications that follow facial flap repairs result from difficulties in hemostasis.[10] As mentioned above, careful attention should be placed upon proper patient selection, the occasional use of preoperative screening laboratory tests, and thorough intraoperative hemostasis. With proper care, only a small number of patients will experience significant postoperative hemorrhage, usually as the vasoconstrictive effects of epinephrine (adrenaline) subside in the early hours after completion of the flap repair. Most minor bleeding can be controlled with simple compression, and the patient should be told that the bruising that accompanies cutaneous surgery is strictly temporary. Sudden, often painful, violaceous swelling in the operative field heralds the formation of a hematoma. Because hematomas are associated with an increased risk of flap ischemia and tissue death, hematoma that compromises wound integrity should be evacuated. Interestingly, the cause of flap death associated with the formation of a hematoma is not because of hydrostatic compression of the flap's vascular input. Rather, the accumulated blood is an abundant source of iron, which catalyzes the formation of tissue-injuring free radicals.[82] When a dynamic hematoma is detected, the sutures are immediately removed, the bleeding is addressed, the wound is copiously irrigated, and the flap is resutured. Prophylactic antibiotics are appropriate in cases where a static hematoma is detected as well as when the wound needs to be re-opened to control surgical hemorrhage.

Wound infections that accompany flap reconstructions on the face are particularly uncommon.[10,83] With sterile preparation of the skin and aseptic operative technique, the risk of infection is even further reduced. The use of prophylactic antibiotics with flap repairs is a debated topic, and the clinician is encouraged to use antibiotics when the risk of wound infection is deemed to be higher than acceptable. Clinical experience and laboratory evidence[84] have shown that ischemic flaps are more prone to surgical wound infections, so the importance of proper flap design and gentle surgical technique cannot be overstated. When wound infections occur, most are caused by *Staphylococcus aureus*, and empiric antibiotic therapy should be commenced until culture results become available. If abundant purulent debris is present, the surgeon should consider removing buried sutures (a nidus for infection) and allowing the wound to granulate. Because surgical complications are so closely interwoven, it is not uncommon for the infected skin flap to then undergo wound dehiscence. The resulting poor aesthetic result can be revised after the wound has entirely healed by second intention.

Dehiscence of a wound is defined as the separation of previously apposed wound edges. One of the leading causes for wound dehiscence is the presence of a surgical wound infection. Dehiscence can also occur as a result of poor wound apposition. One example would be a simple closure without deep sutures in a dependent area such as the ear lobule. If infection is avoided and the flap has been properly closed with buried sutures, the risk of dehiscence is minimal.

Distal flap tissue necrosis is occasionally seen with flap reconstructions. Of paramount importance in avoiding flap necrosis is the minimization of wound closure tensions. Tension on the leading edge of a flap causes circulatory collapse at its vulnerable distal portion. In the authors' opinions, most flap failures on the face can be traced to crucial errors in flap design or to poor surgical practices. The successful creation of facial flaps involves finding the correct balance between flap liberation and vascular preservation. With experience, the incidence of flap necrosis should be low (<5–10%).[10] When cutaneous flaps fail, tissue loss is usually heralded by a dusky purple–blue and white discoloration at the time of closure. It may be difficult to judge flap perfusion in the immediate postoperative period as a result of vasoconstriction associated with the use of epinephrine-containing anesthetic solutions, and some dusky flaps will survive without necrosis. When a portion of a flap does fail as a result of ischemia, the tissue either sloughs or forms a dense black eschar at the affected distal tip of the flap. Although there are sophisticated ways (such as color Doppler evaluations[85]) to evaluate tissue perfusion after flap creation, these techniques are rarely carried out in daily practice.

If a flap is thought to be failing in the immediate postoperative period, many pharmacological interventions are available to attempt to rescue the ischemic flap. Unfortunately, most of these interventions have proven to be of little or no benefit when they have been appropriately examined with carefully constructed clinical trials.[86] Superficial epidermolysis of the distal flap will not typically affect the eventual appearance of the healed wound, but full-thickness necrosis of the flap will produce a deep wound that is most appropriately allowed to heal by second intention. Because an accurate assessment of the depth of tissue necrosis in the failing flap cannot be obtained with a simple visual inspection, the surgeon should resist all temptation to manually debride the wound, even if a densely adherent dry eschar is present. Continued wound care is required until the entire flap has healed. Surgical revision procedures can be contemplated later for aesthetic refinement.

Flaps are desirable reconstructive options, because they offer opportunities to aesthetically reconstruct the face. In a quest for providing aesthetic balance, the reconstructive surgeon should remember that many areas of the face have important physiologic functions. Poorly designed or maneuvered facial flaps can cause complications such as an ectropion or eclabium, and these problems can produce functional as well as cosmetic concerns. Specialized techniques can be helpful in preventing functional deficits. For example, the alar rim often needs to be supported by a cartilage graft to ensure patency of the airway before covering the complicated distal nasal wound with a flap. Similarly, the eyelids and the mouth serve obvious functions, and reconstructive alternatives should therefore be carefully selected. Functional compromise associated with flap reconstruction can be difficult to revise later and should be avoided whenever possible.

Once proper function has been maintained or restored, patients will then concentrate on the aesthetic success of their flap repair. One complication that produces an unaesthetic result of any flap repair is the development of the trapdoor (or pin-cushioned) deformity (see Fig. 21.31). This globular, protuberant appearance of a flap commonly appears at 3–6 weeks and is particularly common and apparent on the nose. Many postsurgical phenomena (e.g. lymphatic obstruction) have been postulated as the cause of the trapdoor deformity, but the most reasonable explanation for the development of this tissue protrusion involves the circumferential contraction of the scar surrounding the flap's recipient site.[87] As the scar contracts, the flap decompresses anteriorly, the only direction in which the flap is not tightly anchored. Transposition flaps (particularly the nasolabial flap) are especially prone to developing the trapdoor deformity, and the risk of the deformity is elevated when the procedures are carried out on thick, sebaceous skin. Like most surgical complications, pin-cushioning is easier to prevent than to manage. The most important technique involved in reducing the risk of this complication is to properly size the flap. If too much flap is 'stuffed' into the primary defect, the flap has little hope of escaping the trapdoor deformity as scar maturation occurs. Accordingly, the flap should be trimmed to just the right size to minimize tissue redundancy. The ideal flap should be even with the adjacent skin's surface (or even slightly recessed) at the completion of the reconstructive procedure. Additional interventions that have been suggested to minimize the development of protuberant flaps include widely undermining the flap's recipient site[70] and 'squaring off' the flap's edges,[88] both of which could conceivably disperse or reorient tension vectors. If the flap undergoes pin-cushioning despite these techniques, intralesional corticosteroids, after allowing the flap to 'settle', may help to improve the flap's contour. When corticosteroids are used in an attempt to introduce subcutaneous atrophy and contour refinement, especially in thick-skinned areas, relatively high concentrations must be used. Several monthly injections may be required before significant improvement can be detected. Additionally, aggressive massage along the scar line can help to improve the appearance of the flap. Rarely, a surgical revision procedure is required to lift the flap and subsequently sculpt the underlying tissues to restore a more appropriate contour.

Even if the surgeon has meticulously planned and expertly performed a flap in a healthy patient who practices diligent wound care, some flaps fail to meet patient and physician expectations. In such cases, flap revision procedures can be contemplated if the patient has appropriate aesthetic expectations and if the surgeon can offer reasonable hope for improvement. On occasion, the incision lines of flaps can be improved with laser resurfacing or dermabrasion. Manual dermasanding[89] with sterilized, industrial-grade sandpaper typically works as well as the mechanical dermabrasion with diamond fraises, and the ideal time to abrade a wound for aesthetic refinement is between the fourth and eighth postoperative weeks.[90] Resurfacing procedures may be complicated by the production of textural alterations and distracting hypopigmentation of the skin (even in the absence of the use of refrigerants designed to produce skin firmness and vasoconstriction before the dermabrasion procedure).

If improper flap design or unanticipated flap contracture produces bothersome distortion, a Z-plasty procedure can effectively reorient wound tensions and relocate adjacent structures. The Z-plasty technique offers seemingly endless flexibility, and accurate degrees of tissue motion can be accomplished if the Z-plasty's arms and angles are thoughtfully constructed. On occasion, flap redundancies can be addressed with secondary procedures designed to thin the flap and restore a more appropriate contour. When these interventions are planned, all operative incisions should be placed through pre-existing scars or along natural anatomic boundaries so that additional cosmetic burdens are not introduced. Some flaps, because they necessarily blunt anatomic structures such as the alar groove, need planned revision procedures to reintroduce normal facial structures.

■ SUMMARY

Excellence in random pattern flap design and creation requires education, dedication and perseverance. These skills are most appropriately learned with the aid of a suitably trained mentor. Flaps offer unequaled opportunities to restore the appearance of the face after the excision of cutaneous malignancies. Flap techniques can be safely and predictably performed only if the surgeon has an in-depth understanding of skin flap designs and biomechanics, a thorough knowledge of basic and advanced surgical techniques and anatomy, and suitable operative experience. When appropriately designed, flaps are extremely safe and predictable options for facial reconstruction. The aesthetic results of flap procedures commonly exceed the results obtained from second intention healing or skin grafting procedures, and flap repairs are therefore firmly entrenched in the practices of all physicians who attempt to balance the needs to surgically manage skin malignancies with the desires to restore appearance and function.

■ REFERENCES

1. Guyton A. Textbook of medical physiology, 5th edn. Philadelphia: WB Saunders; 1976.
2. Carupe JC. Account of two successful operations for restoring a lost nose from the integuments of the forehead, London, Longman, 1816. Reprinted in Plast Reconstr Surg 1966; 37:167–183.
3. Zelac DE, Swanson N, Simpson M, et al. The history of dermatologic surgical reconstruction. Dermatol Surg 2000; 26:983–990.
4. Rowe DE, Carroll RJ, Day CL. Long term recurrence rates in previously untreated (primary) basal cell carcinoma: Implications for patient follow-up care. J Dermatol Surg Oncol 1989; 15:315–328.
5. Rowe DE, Carroll RJ, Day CL. Mohs' surgery is the treatment of choice for recurrent (previously treated) basal cell carcinoma. J Dermatol Surg Oncol 1989; 15:424–431.
6. Rowe DE, Carroll RJ, Day CL. Prognostic factors for local recurrence, metastasis, and survival rates in squamous cell carcinoma of the skin, ear, and lip: implications for treatment modality selection. J Am Acad Dermatol 1992; 26:976–990.
7. Bumstead RM, Ceilly RI. Auricular malignant neoplasms. Arch Otolaryngol 1982; 108:225–231.
8. Downes RN, Walker NP, Collin JR. Micrographic (Mohs') surgery in the management of periocular basal cell epitheliomas. Eye 1990; 4:160–168.
9. Schein OD, Katz J, Bass EB, et al. The value of routine preoperative medical testing before cataract surgery. Study of medical testing for cataract surgery. N Engl J Med 2000; 342:168–175.
10. Cook JL, Perone JB. A prospective study of complications associated with Mohs micrographic surgery. Arch Dermatol 2003; 139:143–152.
11. Kovich O, Otley CC. Thrombotic complications related to discontinuation of warfarin and aspirin therapy perioperatively for cutaneous operation. J Am Acad Dermatol 2003; 48:233–237.
12. Vane JR, Botting RM. The mechanism of action of aspirin. Thromb Res 2003; 110:255–258.
13. Nolan J, Jenkins RA, Kuhihara K, et al. The acute effects of cigarette smoke exposure on experimental skin flaps. Plast Reconstr Surg 1985; 75:544–551.
14. Manassa EH, Hertl CH, Olbrisch RR. Wound healing problems in smokers and nonsmokers after 132 abdominoplasties. Plast Reconstr Surg 2003; 111:2082–2087.
15. Sorensen LT, Karlsmark T, Gottrup F. Abstinence from smoking reduces incisional wound infections: a randomized controlled trial. Ann Surg 2003; 238:1–5.
16. Rees TD, Liverett DM, Guy CL. The effect of cigarette smoking on skin-flap survival in the face lift patient. Plast Reconstruct Surg 1984; 73:911–915.
17. Goldminz D, Bennett RG. Cigarette smoking and flap and full-thickness graft necrosis. Arch Dermatol. 1991; 127:1012–1015.
18. Kox KW, Larrabee WF. A study of skin flap advancement as a function of undermining. Arch Otolaryngol 1982; 108:151–155.
19. Larrabee WF, Sutton D. The biomechanics of advancement and rotation flaps. Laryngoscope 1981; 91:726–734.
20. Milton S. Pedicled skin flaps: the fallacy of the length-width ratio. Br J Plast Surg 1970; 57:502–508.
21. Dzubow LM. Chemosurgical report: indications for a geometric approach to wound closure following Mohs surgery. J Dermatol Surg Oncol 1987; 13:480–486.
22. Hirshowitz B, Mahler D. T-plasty technique for excisions in the face. Plast Reconstr Surg 1966; 37:453–458.
23. Gormley DE. A brief analysis of the Burow's wedge/triangle principle. J Dermatol Surg Oncol 1985; 11:121–123.
24. Gormley DE. Use of Burow's wedge principle for repair of wounds in or near the eyebrow. J Am Acad Dermatol 1985; 12:344–349.
25. Webster JP. Crescentic peri-alar cheek excision for upper lip flap advancement with a short history of upper lip repair. Plast Reconstr Surg 1955; 15:434–464.
26. Barron JN, Emmett AJJ. Subcutaneous pedicle flaps. Br J Plast Surg 1965; 18:51–78
27. Dzubow LM Subcutaneous island pedicle flaps. J Dermatol Surg Oncol 1986; 12:591–596.
28. Tomich JM, Wentzell JM, Grande DJ. Subcutaneous island pedicle flaps. Arch Dermatol 1987; 123:514–518.
29. Zook EG, Van Beek AL, Russell RC, et al. V–Y advancement flap for facial defects. Plast Reconstr Surg 1980; 65:786–797.
30. Cook J. Commentary on V–Y nasolabial advancement flaps in the repair of central facial defects. Dermatol Surg 2001; 27:659–660.
31. Rybka FJ. Reconstruction of the nasal tip using nasalis myocutaneous sliding flaps. Plast Reconstr Surg 1983; 71:40–44.
32. Yildrim S, Akoz T, Akan MD, et al. Nasolabial V–Y advancement for the closure of midface defects. Dermatol Surg 2001; 27:656–658.
33. Hairston BR, Nguyen TH. Innovations in the island pedicle flap for facial reconstruction. Dermatol Surg 2003; 29:378–385.
34. Cook JL. Reconstruction of the lower lip. Dermatol Surg 2001; 27:775–778.
35. Stoner JG, Swanson NA. Use of the bipedicled scalp flap for forehead reconstruction. J Dermatol Surg Oncol 1984; 10:213–215.
36. Dzubow LM. The dynamics of flap movement: effect of pivotal restraint on flap rotation and transposition. J Dermatol Surg Oncol 1987; 13:1348–1353.
37. McGregor IA. Local skin flaps in facial reconstruction. Otolaryngol Clin NA 1982; 15:77–98.
38. Rieger RA. A local flap for repair of the nasal tip. Plast Reconstr Surg 1967; 40:147–149.
39. Dzubow LM. Dorsal nasal flaps. In: Baker SR, Swanson NA, eds. Local flaps in facial reconstruction. St Louis: Mosby 1995; 225–246.
40. Mustarde JC. The use of flaps in the orbital region. Plast Reconstr Surg 1970; 45:146–150.
41. Tenzel RR, Stewart WB. Eyelid reconstruction by the semicircle flap technique. Ophthalmology 1978; 85:1164–1169.
42. McGregor IA. Eyelid reconstruction following subtotal resection of upper or lower lid. Br J Plast Surg 1973; 26:346–354.
43. Albom MJ. Repair of large scalp defects by bilateral rotation flaps. J Dermatol Surg Oncol 1978; 4:906–907.
44. Limberg AA. Design of local flaps. In: Gibson T, ed. Modern trends in plastic surgery. London: Butterworth & Co 1966; 38–61.
45. Dufourmentel C. Le fermeture des pertes de substance cutanée limitées : Le lambeau de rotation en L pour losange' det 'LLL'. Ann Chirurgie Plast 1962; 7:61–66.
46. Borges AF. Choosing the correct Limberg flap. Plast Reconstr Surg 1978; 62:542–545.
47. Borges AF. The rhombic flap. Plast Reconstr Surg 1981; 67:458–466.
48. Shotton FT. Optimal closure of medial canthal surgical defects with rhomboid flaps: 'rules of thumb' for flap and rhomboid defect orientation. Ophthal Surg 1983; 14:46–52.
49. Bullock JD, Flagg SV. Rhomboid flap in ophthalmic plastic surgery. Arch Ophthalmol 1973; 90:203–205.
50. Gunter JP, Carder HM, Fee WE. Rhomboid flap. Arch Otolaryngol 1977; 103:206–211.
51. Jervis W, Salyer KE, Vargas Busquets MA, et al. Further applications of the Limberg and Duforurmentel flaps. Plast Reconstr Surg 1974; 54:335–339.

52. Esser JSF. Gestielte locale Nasenplastik mit zweiplifgem Lappen, Deckung des sekundaren Defektes vom ersten Zipfel durch den zweiten. Dtsch Z Chir 1918; 143:385–390.
53. Zitelli JA. The bilobed flap for nasal reconstruction. Arch Dermatol 1989; 125:957–959.
54. Cook JL. A review of the bilobed flap's design with particular emphasis on the minimization of alar displacement. Dermatol Surg 2000; 26:354–362.
55. Lawson VG. Reconstruction of the pinna using preauricular flaps. J Otolaryngol 1984; 13:191–193.
56. Field LM. The glabellar transposition 'banner' flap. J Dermatol Surg Oncol 1988; 14:376–379.
57. Field LM. Surgical flaps: The upper-to-lower eyelid transposition flap. J Dermatol Surg Oncol 1983; 9:809–811.
58. Zitelli JA. The nasolabial flap as a single-stage procedure. Arch Dermatol 1990; 126:1445–1448.
59. Spear SL, Kroll SS, Romm S. A new twist to the nasolabial flap for reconstruction of lateral alar defects. Plast Reconstr Surg 1987; 79:915–920.
60. Cook JL. Reconstruction of a full-thickness alar wound with a single operative procedure. Dermatol Surg 2003; 29:956–962.
61. http://abcnews.go.com/sections/GMA/GoodMorningAmerica/GMA20131Downagingfeature.html, July 27, 2003.
62. Wright ME. Long term sickness absence in an NHS teaching hospital. Occup Med 1997; 47:401–406.
63. Magnavita N, Bevilacqua L, Paoletta M, et al. Work-related musculoskeletal complaints in sonologists. J Occup Environ Med 1999; 4:981–988.
64. Field LM. Alternative and additional techniques for facial tumescent anesthesia. Dermatol Surg. 2002; 28:442.
65. Wilhelmi BJ, Blackwell SJ, Miller JH, et al. Do not use epinephrine in digital blocks: myth or truth? Plast Reconstr Surg 2001; 107:393–397.
66. Dzubow LM. The interaction between propranolol and epinephrine as observed in patients undergoing Mohs' surgery. J Am Acad Dermatol 1986; 15:71–75.
67. Larrabee WF Jr, Holloway GA Jr, Sutton D. Wound tension and blood flow in skin flaps. Ann Otol Rhinol Laryngol 1984; 93:112–115.
68. McGuire MF. Studies of the excisional wound: I. Biomechanical effects of undermining and wound orientation on closing tension and work. Plast Reconstr Surg 1980; 66:419–427.
69. Koranda FC, Webster RC. Trapdoor effect in nasolabial flaps. Causes and corrections. Arch Otolaryngol 1985; 111:421–424.
70. Larrabee WF Jr, Sutton D. Variation of skin stress–strain curves with undermining. Surg Forum 1981; 32:553–558.
71. Boyer JD, Zitelli JA, Brodland DG. Undermining in cutaneous surgery. Dermatol Surg 2001; 27:75–78.
72. Tardy ME. Topographic anatomy and landmarks. In: Tardy ME, ed. Surgical anatomy of the nose. New York: Raven Press 1990; 1–23.
73. Chang N, Mathes SJ. Comparison of the effect of bacterial inoculation in musculocutaneous and random-pattern flaps. Plast Reconstr Surg 1982; 70:1–10.
74. Swada Y. Alterations in pressure under elastic bandages experimental and clinical evaluation. J Dermatol 1993; 20:767–772.
75. Zitelli JA, Moy RL. Buried vertical mattress suture. J Dermatol Surg Oncol 1989; 15:17–19.
76. Salache SJ, Jarchow R, Feldman BD, et al. The suspension suture. J Dermatol Surg Oncol 1987; 13:973–978.
77. Bencini PL, Galimberti M, Signorini M, et al. Antibiotic prophylaxis of wound infections in skin surgery. Arch Dermatol 1991; 127: 1357–1360.
78. Baran CN, Sensoz O, Ulusoy MG. Prophylactic antibiotics in plastic and reconstructive surgery. Plas Reconstr Surg 1999; 103:1561–1566.
79. Dire DJ, Coppola M, Dyer DJ, et al. Prospective evaluation of topical antibiotics for preventing infections in uncomplicated soft-tissue wounds repaired in the ED. Acad Emerg Med 1995; 2:4–10.
80. Smack DP, Harrington AC, Dunn C, et al. Infection and allergy incidence in ambulatory surgery patients using white petrolatum vs. bacitracin ointment: a randomized controlled trial. JAMA 1996; 276:972–977.
81. Cook JL. Low-maintenance wound care. Skin Aging 1999; 2:77–78.
82. Angel MF, Narayanan K, Swartz WM, et al. The etiologic role of free radicals in hematoma-induced flap necrosis. Plas Reconstr Surg 1986; 77:795–803.
83. Whitaker DC, Grande DJ, Johnson SS. Wound infection rates in dermatologic surgery. J Dermatol Surg Oncol 1988; 14:525–528.
84. Phillips LG, Mann R, Heggers JP, et al. In vivo ovine model to evaluate surgical wound infection and tissue necrosis. J Surg Res 1994; 56:1–4.
85. Choi CM, Bennett RG. Laser Dopplers to determine cutaneous blood flow. Dermatol Surg 2003; 29:272–280.
86. Goding GS, Hom DB. Skin flap physiology. In: Baker SR, Swanson NA, eds. Local flaps in facial reconstruction. St Louis: Mosby 1995; 15–30.
87. Hosokawa K, Susuki T, Kikui T, et al. Sheet of scar causes trapdoor deformity: a hypothesis. Ann Plast Surg 1990; 25:134–135.
88. Field LM. Peripheral tissue undermining is not the final answer to prevent trapdooring in transposition flaps. J Dermatol Surg Oncol 1993; 19:1131–1132.
89. Poulos E, Taylor C, Solish N. Effectiveness of dermasanding (manual dermabrasion) on the appearance of surgical scars: a prospective, randomized, blinded study. J Am Acad Dermatol 2003; 48:897–900.
90. Yarborough JM Jr. Ablation of facial scars by programmed dermabrasion. J Dermatol Surg Oncol 1988; 14:292–294.

22 Axial Pattern Flaps

Joel Cook MD and John A Zitelli MD

Summary box

- The increasing incidence of facial melanoma and non-melanoma skin cancers means more surgical treatment that requires the reconstructive dermatologic surgeon to fully understand all reconstructive options.
- Although most facial surgical defects may be repaired with primary closure, skin graft, or random pattern cutaneous flaps, larger or more complex facial defects may need more advanced reconstructive techniques.
- Axial pattern flaps are cutaneous flaps based on a named nutrient vessel. The predictable arterial supply increases the reliability of the flaps and allows for aesthetic and functional repairs of even the most challenging surgical wounds.
- Axial pattern flap repairs are usually staged surgical procedures with significantly more operative complexity and morbidity than alternative reconstructive techniques.
- Axial pattern flaps are durable and aesthetically pleasing repairs with minimal risks for surgical complications if properly designed and executed.
- Axial pattern flaps are unsurpassed options for repairing complex lower nasal defects, especially if multiple other procedures (cartilage grafts, lining flaps, other flaps) are needed.

INTRODUCTION

The incidence of non-melanoma skin cancer is increasing 8–10% per year in the US.[1] There are many treatment options for non-melanoma and melanoma skin cancers, including destruction by various techniques, surgical excision, Mohs micrographic surgery (MMS), topical and systemic chemotherapies, radiation therapy, and photodynamic therapy. The obvious goal of skin cancer treatment is to provide effective tumor removal in a manner that is not only of low morbidity but is also cost-effective. The predominance of skin cancers on the face demands that functional and aesthetic outcomes be optimized.

The gold standard of skin cancer treatment is surgical excision with or without intraoperative margin control. Previously published studies have documented the unsurpassed success of Mohs surgery for most non-melanoma and melanoma skin cancers.[2–5] Mohs surgery affords significantly higher cure rates for skin cancer treated with this technique when compared to conventional surgical resection—especially with tumors located in challenging anatomic areas, tumors with aggressive histologic subtypes, and large or recurrent tumors. Moreover, the Mohs technique has proven to be cost-effective and tissue sparing (see also Chapter 48).[6–8]

Whether utilizing conventional techniques or Mohs surgery, the cutaneous surgeon will invariably produce a wound that must be addressed. The appropriate management of these surgical defects requires skill, knowledge, and experience to achieve superior results. A firm understanding of operative techniques is requisite for the treating physician. The potential undesirable cosmetic impact of any surgical defect must be recognized and efforts should be extended to restore a normal appearance. Following confirmation of successful tumor extirpation, the resulting surgical wound's characteristics must be carefully analyzed. The missing anatomic structures are identified and plans are formulated to provide suitable replacement. The potential for functional impairment must be critically weighed. Significant anatomic distortion, functional loss, or poor cosmetic outcomes may challenge the dermatologic surgeon. If all operative variables are assessed and accounted for, cutaneous reconstructive surgeries can be safe and reliable procedures with tremendous potential to impact a patient's wellbeing and appearance. Any surgical defect will have numerous repair options. The repair that preserves function and restores appearance will prove superior.

Paramount to achieving successful repair of a surgical wound is complete tumor extirpation. Reconstructive procedures should not proceed without first obtaining accurate and clear surgical margins. The clinical appearance of a tumor recurrence of a previously resected neoplasm buried underneath a cutaneous flap reconstruction may be delayed for some time. This delay in definitive treatment, secondary to the failed initial treatment, may prove to increase the extent of subsequent repairs or increase the incidence of locoregional aggressive disease. The failure to completely remove a skin cancer before reconstruction may result in significantly increased operative morbidity or poor end-results with a requirement for additional surgical procedures.

After confirming tumor removal, the surgeon must meet the dual goals of preserving or restoring function and optimizing cosmesis. A careful assessment of function is made prior to considering any reconstructive option. Repairs may vary significantly in complexity, operative morbidity, and end-results. The physician must clearly predict a patient's expectations. Concomitant health problems that increase operative complications must be recognized and manipulated, if possible.

Although most surgical wounds on the face are repaired, in certain circumstances second intention healing may provide an acceptable or even ideal result. Zitelli has previously shown that the aesthetic success of such healing is largely dependent upon anatomic location.[9] Concave areas typically heal better with second intention than convex areas. A wound of the alar crease, conchal bowl, or medial canthus, for example, may heal with excellent results with second intention healing. However, wounds of the helical rim, nasal tip, or mid-cheek would need to be repaired to achieve the optimal results (Fig. 22.1). Although at times providing good results, second intention healing may fail to restore contour and may result in significant anatomic distortion when predictable postoperative wound contraction occurs. This anatomic distortion, if near a mobile eyelid, lip, or ala may provide unacceptable final cosmesis.

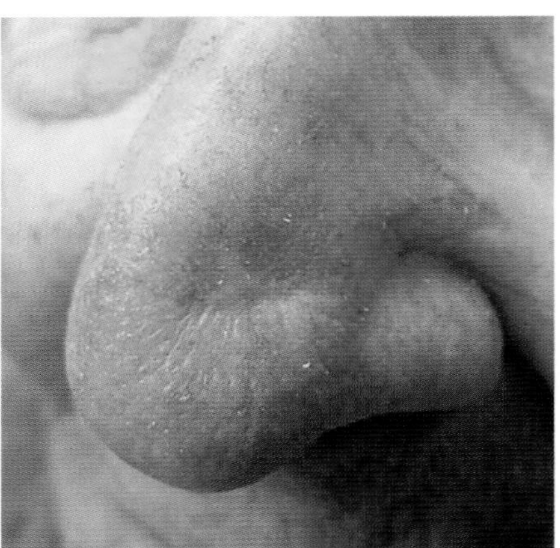

Figure 22.1 A depressed cicatrix following second intention healing of a distal nasal defect showing suboptimal cosmesis. Surgical repair would likely have produced an improved aesthetic result in this anatomic location.

Small surgical defects with sufficient regional tissue laxity and low risk of anatomic distortion may be repaired with primary closure. Although primary or linear closure may achieve elegant functional and cosmetic restoration with some defects, it is typically not an option with larger or more complex facial surgical wounds. Split- or full-thickness skin grafts are uncomplicated surgical procedures that, at times, may offer excellent outcomes. However, skin grafts may not effectively repair more complex surgical defects without a risk of complications secondary to lost function or poor cosmesis (Fig. 22.2). Skin grafts are repairs with low operative morbidity that may be used in situations in which flaps or other closures may have an excessive risk of failure. However, skin grafts are not typically favored over skin flaps when the reconstructive surgeon strives to achieve ideal facial reconstructive results. Although, the final cosmetic result for skin grafts at times may prove elegant, grafts rarely match the aesthetic results seen with flap reconstructive procedures (Fig. 22.3).

Cutaneous flaps

Because of the limitations of second intention healing, primary closures, and skin graft repairs, surgeons have increasingly turned to the use of cutaneous flaps in many

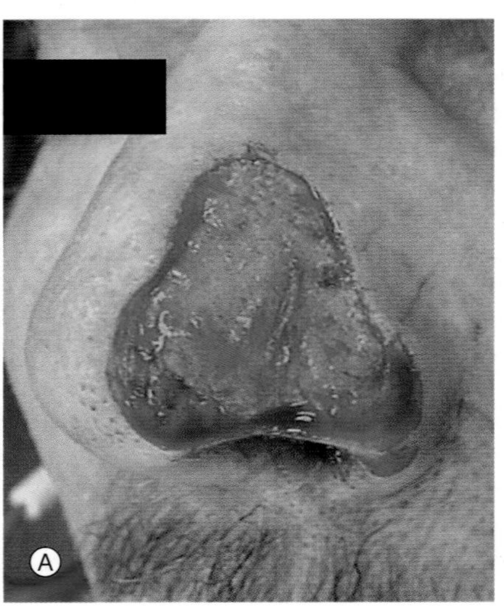

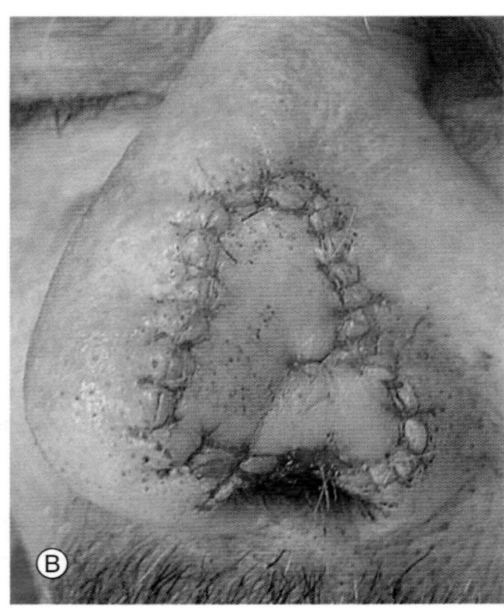

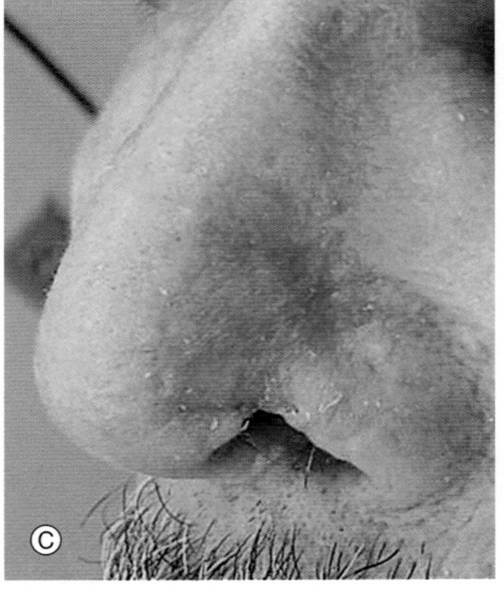

Figure 22.2 (A) A moderate, but shallow, wound of the ala following Mohs micrographic surgery. The close approximation of the surgical wound to the alar rim mandates careful attention to surgical repair. Second intention healing would fail to achieve correct nasal contour with postoperative wound contraction. (B) The patient shown refused two-staged flap restoration and elected to have the wound repaired with a supraclavicular full-thickness skin graft. (C) The graft has contracted in the postoperative period and allowed cephalic alar retraction with a subsequent poor cosmetic result.

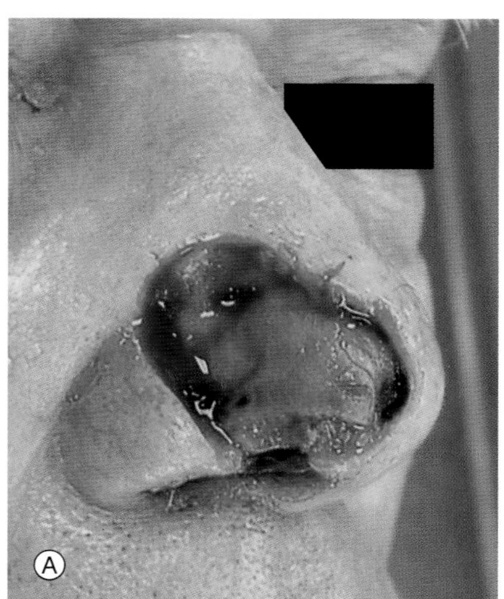

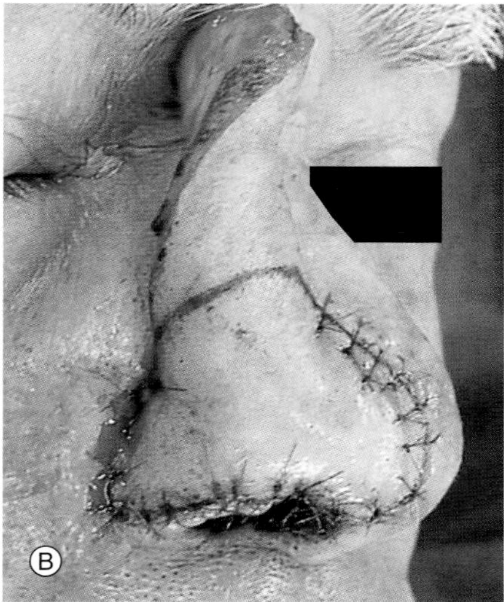

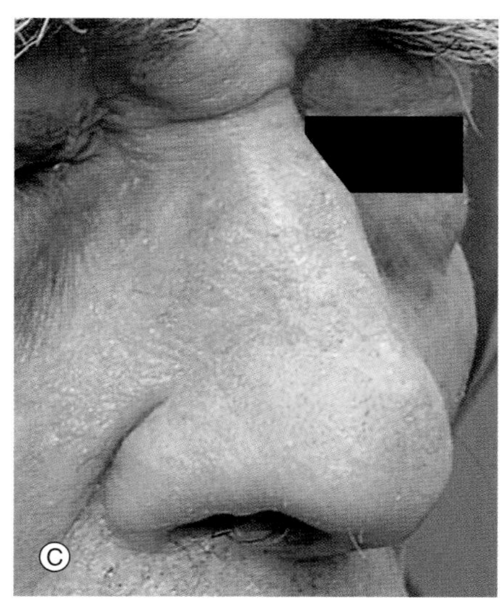

Figure 22.3 (A) A similar surgical wound of the ala as presented in Figure 22.2. A moderate-sized nasal defect extends from the alar rim to portions of the lower nasal sidewall. The lining of the nasal cavity has not been surgically resected. To resist the cephalic alar displacement seen with a contracting surgical wound, a cartilage batten graft is harvested from the ear and inserted into the base of the surgical defect. The margins of the surgical wound are expanded as the rest of the alar cosmetic unit is removed before flap placement. The surgical defect is enlarged to the borders of the nasal aesthetic subunits to improve scar camouflage. (B) A paramedian axial forehead flap is harvested and inset into the defect of the ala. (C) The forehead flap has afforded excellent cosmetic and functional repair of the ala.

reconstructive situations. Cutaneous flaps are unparalleled in their ability to repair simple-to-complex defects. With proper design, skin flaps can overcome the shortcomings of alternative reconstructive techniques. Cutaneous flaps are robust and versatile reconstructive methods that allow excellent long-term surgical results.

The survival of any flap is ultimately dependent upon cutaneous blood flow. Adequate blood flow into a flap supplies the necessary nutritional support of the transferred skin and soft tissue. The minimal nutritional requirements of skin afford the creation of cutaneous flaps of varied design with excellent chances of complete tissue survival.[10,11] The richly anastomotic vascular supply of the face predicts flap survival when surgical procedures are performed in this area. The goal of the cutaneous surgeon when performing flap reconstructive surgery should therefore be to ensure adequate blood flow to the nascent flap. Sufficient perfusion is requisite for the survival of the flap, especially the distal portions. It is well recognized that blood flow is reduced when traversing a flap from proximal to distal.[12] This reduction of blood flow and the resulting relative tissue hypoxia challenge flap survival. The amount of blood supply to a flap ultimately depends upon the arteriolar pressure of the vessels supplying the flap and the distal flow. Flap execution must be based on geometric principles of design to protect the blood supply and thus to ensure flap survival. If the critical capillary closing pressure of the tissue is not surpassed by the flap's blood inflow, necrosis will result. The initial incision and elevation of flap tissue will always cause significant blood flow reductions and physiologic stress. Upon insertion of the flap into its recipient site, this blood flow gradually increases. Skin can withstand prolonged periods of ischemia, but the prompt restoration of blood flow improves the survival of transferred tissues. Neovascularization begins at 5–7 days in the postoperative period.[13] Most of these new vessels result from growth of cutaneous vasculature into the flap. The rich anastomotic subdermal plexus will provide, with proper design, the vascular support required to achieve flap survival until adequate new tissue perfusion has been achieved.

The strain of relative hypoxia that flap elevation creates can usually be overcome. Other significant variables may also influence flap survival. Maximal effort must be extended to ensure that adequate nutrient vessels are included in the flap's base. Flaps that have excessive length : width ratios may undergo distal necrosis. Flaps inset under heightened tension show predictably reduced perfusion.[14] Efforts must be made to minimize wound closure tensions by proper flap design, undermining, and suture technique. Additionally, other variables may limit operative success. Exposure to tobacco has deleterious effects on flap survival. Rhytidectomy patients who smoke have significantly higher rates of flap failure and operative complications than nonsmoking controls.[15] Experimental animal flap studies have also demonstrated reduced flap viability in the setting of smoke exposure.[16,17]

When contemplating surgery, the physician must assess all flap repair variables. Patient risk factors increasing the risk of surgical failure must be weighed. Cutaneous flaps should be created under sterile conditions because postoperative infections increase the risk of flap failure. Moreover, flaps with sufficient blood flow have reduced rates of infection and thus improved survival. This even further underscores the importance of proper flap design. Hemostasis is important to minimize postoperative complications. Gentle tissue handling further reduces the risk of surgical complications. Flaps are generally inset and sutured into place using layered closures. Excellent results may be predictably reproducible with proper operative technique for flap design and creation. Many patient variables contribute to the success of cutaneous flap reconstructive surgery. Poor nutrition, previous radiation therapy, concomitant medical conditions, and many other factors may increase operative risk.

Random pattern versus axial pattern flaps

In cutaneous surgery, flaps are typically characterized based upon one of two classification systems. One classification system is based on movement (e.g. transposition, rotation). An alternative method of classifying cutaneous flaps is based on vascular supply (e.g. random pattern, axial pattern). Most flaps utilized in dermatologic surgery are random pattern cutaneous flaps. The richly anastomotic unnamed musculocutaneous plexus of small vessels supplies these random pattern flaps, which are widely used in facial and nonfacial reconstruction, and constitute most flaps commonly utilized. Many published works have detailed modifications in the design of random pattern flaps that improve operative outcomes.

Although versatile and robust, random pattern cutaneous flaps have significant limitations that at times may prove insurmountable. The precipitous decrease of blood flow with advancing length of any flap makes random pattern cutaneous flaps poor choices for selected facial wounds. Large or full-thickness wounds of the nose may require reconstructive tissue in volumes that a random pattern cutaneous flap may not be able to successfully provide. In distinction to random pattern flaps, axial pattern flaps (arterial cutaneous flaps) include a named septocutaneous artery within the flap's longitudinal axis. This larger vessel included in the flap's base yields significantly enhanced blood flow. Thus, flap length may be increased beyond that of a random pattern cutaneous flap without such risk of necrosis.

Axial pattern flaps are the workhorse reconstructive options for larger complex nasal wounds. Unfortunately, however, the limited availability of direct cutaneous named arteries reduces axial flap options in reconstructive dermatologic surgery. Axial pattern flaps that are commonly used in facial reconstruction include the median and paramedian forehead flaps, the dorsal nasal flap (DNF) based upon the inner canthus, and the Abbe flap. All these flaps share a luxurious vascularity as a result of septocutaneous vessels being included in the flaps' bases. The longitudinal vessels included in the bases of the flaps supply most of the vascular inflow. However, the most distal portions of the flaps may, to some degree, depend on random pattern cutaneous vascularity. The inclusion of a larger named vessel provides the cutaneous surgeon with a flap that is not only larger, but also more predictably perfused. For this reason, these flaps are important to any dermatologic surgeon hoping to offer the most appropriate surgical procedures.

Flaps for nasal reconstruction

Cancer of the skin is the most common human malignancy.[1] Many of these cancers are on the nose. In dermatologic surgery, axial pattern flaps are largely used to reconstruct nasal defects following tumor extirpation. The goals of nasal reconstruction after tumor removal are to restore contour, to replace missing skin and soft tissue with that of similar character, and to preserve or restore nasal function, ensuring patent unrestricted air flow. The complex topography, functional importance, and aesthetic prominence of the nose demand careful attention to operative plans and detail. Burget and Menick detailed the complicated geometry of the nasal surface in 1985.[18] The nose is subdivided into aesthetic units based upon the underlying bone and cartilaginous framework. Reconstructive experience has demonstrated that improved cosmetic results may be obtained by understanding the visual significance of these nasal subunits. When most of a nasal subunit has been removed with tumor extirpation, the optimal reconstructive result may be achieved by replacing the entire subunit (Fig. 22.4, see Fig. 22.28).

The removal of an entire subunit or units may produce a complex nasal wound incapable of being repaired with a local random pattern nasal flap. For nasal defects greater than 2 cm, alar or distal nasal defects, or full-thickness wounds, local nasal flaps may prove unable to provide effective repair. The random pattern cutaneous flap, although robust, may not provide sufficient vascular support in these situations. Moreover, if large portions of exposed cartilage devoid of perichondrium, or bone devoid of periosteum are present, skin grafting may fail to adequately reconstruct the surgical defect because of the lack of a sufficiently perfused wound bed.

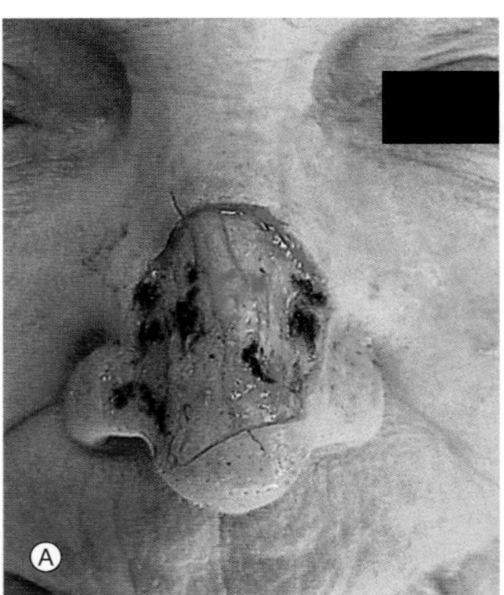

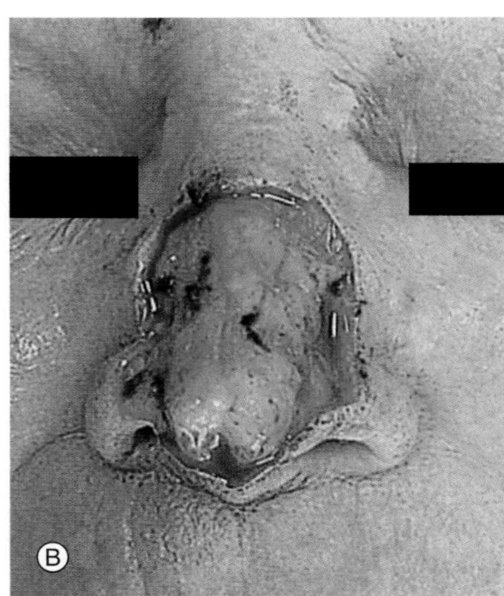

Figure 22.4 (A) A large wound of the lower nose involving several entire cosmetic units and portions of others. (B) Before surgical repair, the defect is enlarged to extend to the borders of the defined nasal cosmetic unit.

Early reconstructive experience demonstrated that full-thickness defects of the nose must be approached by laminar reconstructive techniques. Surgeons found that repairing nasal defects without internal flap lining produced exaggerated postoperative flap contraction with resultant nasal distortion.[19] Larger or more complex defects—especially full-thickness defects—may mandate replacement with a lining layer of skin or mucosa, a supporting cartilage or bone framework, and aesthetically proper external skin and soft tissue coverage. The placement of this trilaminar reconstruction usually requires the predictable vascular support of an axial, not random pattern, cutaneous flap (Fig. 22.5).

Cutaneous reconstructive surgeons have struggled with lower nasal defects. Skin of similar character must be used to achieve optimum results. For smaller (<2 cm) wounds, a random pattern flap may prove ideal because such amounts of loose skin may be effectively harvested from the laxity of the nasal dorsum with success (bilobed flap and others). However, the amount and mobility of nasal dorsum skin has limited the role of random pattern flaps when repairing larger defects in this area.

The aesthetic repair of nasal wounds must not only restore contour and function but also replace missing skin with skin of similar color, texture, and thickness. If contour is restored, appropriately placed surgical incisions will be better camouflaged. To resist the forces of wound contraction, contour restoration may require the addition of cartilage batten grafts. Surgeons have long recognized local tissue reservoirs of skin on the face that may be harvested with

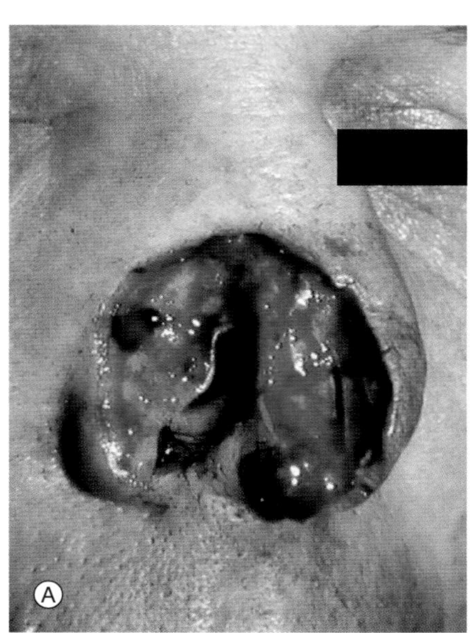

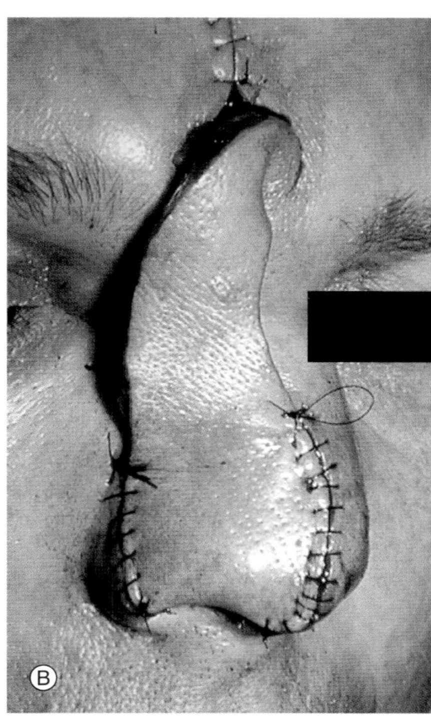

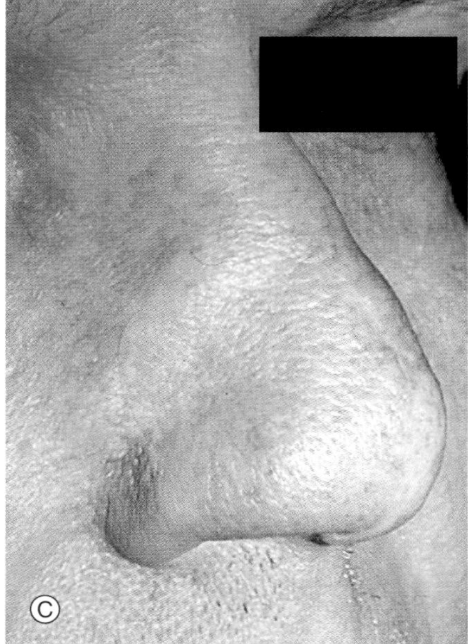

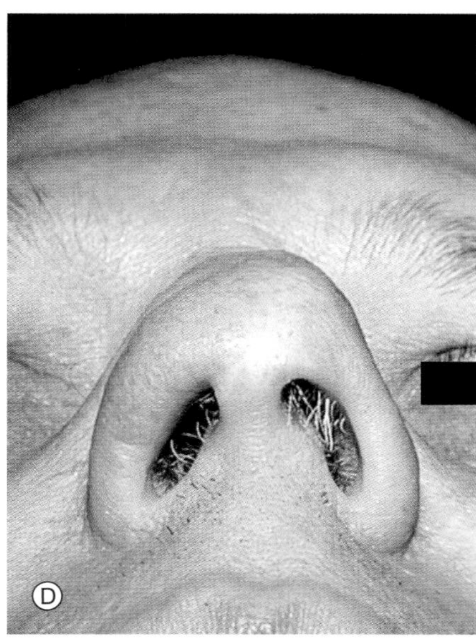

Figure 22.5 (A) Defect following Mohs surgery for skin cancer. (B) The defect has been lined with a mucosal flap harvested from the distal nasal septum. A conchal cartilage graft is then placed over the lining flap. A paramedian forehead flap is used to provide soft tissue coverage. (C) One year after surgery the right oblique view and (D) the basilar view.

minimal morbidity and transferred to the nose to repair soft tissue deficiencies. Such reservoirs exist on the mid-cheek and mid-forehead. Both may supply ample quantities of skin with a quality similar to that of surrounding nasal skin to rebuild the nose. The forehead is generally preferred for nasal reconstruction when insufficient dorsal nasal skin is found.

Forehead skin may be recruited for nasal reconstruction with minimal morbidity, minimal donor scarring, and significant operative versatility. The lower cheek may be used, in a similar fashion, to repair defects of the ala (Fig. 22.6). Both the paramedian forehead flap and the cheek melolabial interpolation flap are staged procedures. They are both interpolation flaps—the base of the flap's pedicle resides some distance away from the surgical wound (noncontiguous). Each may prove to be an excellent reconstructive option for distal nasal defects. Both reconstructive interpolation flaps may yield durable and predictable results if properly executed. The principal differences are that unlike the cheek (melolabial) interpolation flap, the forehead flap is a true axial pattern flap with a named dedicated vascular supply—the supratrochlear artery. This improved vascularity allows larger flaps to be harvested with better chances for survival than the random pattern vascular supply of the cheek interpolation flap. The cheek interpolation flap is largely used to repair defects of the ala or lower nose (not the tip). The forehead flap's design versatility allows for better reconstruction of the tip, supratip, and dorsum. The choice of repair option is dependent upon wound character, patient factors, and surgeon preference. A significant majority of the axial pattern flaps commonly used in facial reconstruction are paramedian forehead flaps. The DNF (Rieger flap) and axial lip flaps will also be discussed.

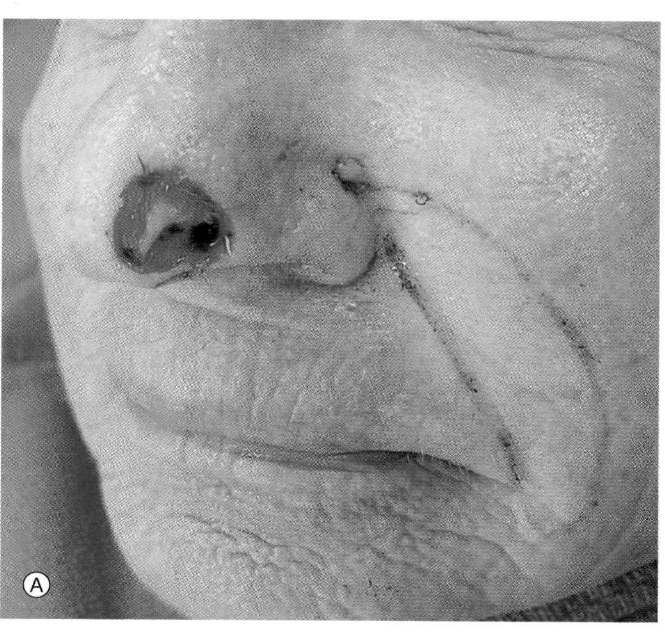

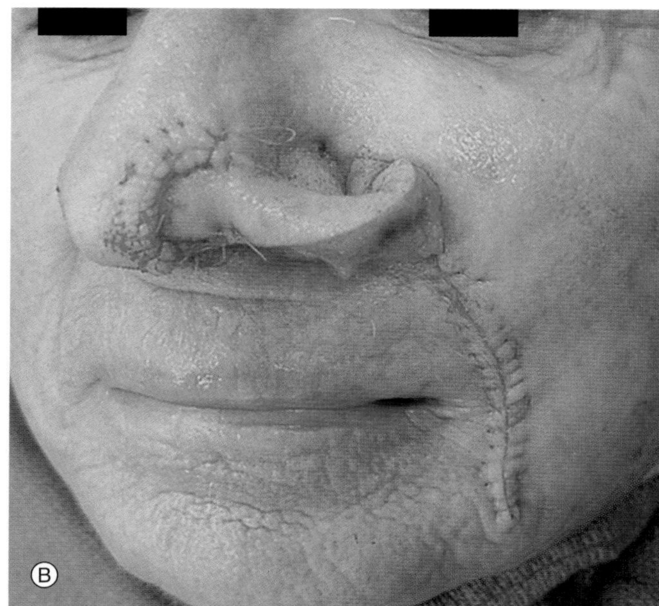

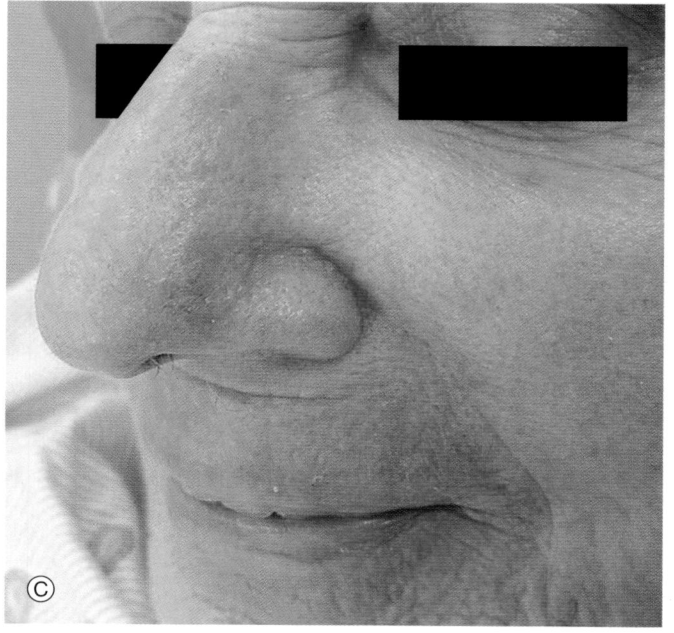

Figure 22.6 (A) A partial-thickness defect of the anterior left nasal tip. (B) The defect has been repaired with a two-stage cheek interpolation flap. Like the forehead flap, the cheek interpolation is a staged pedicled flap. However, it is best viewed as a random pattern cutaneous flap and lacks the predictable axial vascular supply of its paramedian forehead flap counterpart. The propensity of the cheek interpolation flap to contract in the postoperative period limits its use principally to the reconstruction of smaller defects of the ala. The cheek interpolation flap cannot be used to successfully repair defects of the nasal dorsum, tip, or columella. (C) Postoperative result 1 year after surgery.

■ HISTORICAL VIGNETTE

Forehead flaps in nasal reconstruction were first detailed in an Indian work entitled Sushruta Samita over 2000 years ago. A group of Indian potters transferred forehead skin to the nose to repair missing distal noses amputated as punishment for a variety of crimes. Confined largely to the Indian subcontinent for centuries, the forehead flap was subsequently adopted in Europe by the Italian Antonio Beanca in the 15th century.[20] Later, the flap experienced a resurgence of interest in Europe following an operative description published in *Gentleman's Magazine* in 1894.[21] Carpue then published his forehead flap repair results on patients after perfection of the technique on cadaveric specimens.[22] In the 1800s, numerous authors detailed the use of the forehead flap in distal nasal reconstruction almost simultaneously. Like most plastic surgical procedures, the carnage of warfare in the 20th century accelerated the flap's surgical refinement.

The vascular supply of the forehead is supplied by four paired arteries—the dorsal nasal (angular) arteries, the supratrochlear arteries, the supraorbital arteries, and the superficial temporal arteries. Multiple interconnecting anastomoses between these vessels provide this region with tremendous vascularity. Kazanijan was the first to confirm the axial basis of the forehead flap in the 1930s. His mid-forehead flap design, exactly placed in the forehead center, utilized the paired vascular supply from both the supraorbital and supratrochlear vessels.[23] Subsequently, cadaveric studies with the injection of facial vessels have confirmed the vascular distributions of these vessels.[24] Mangold demonstrated that in a median and paramedian location, the forehead flap was supplied by the supratrochlear artery with secondary filling from the dorsal nasal and supraorbital arteries.[25]

Early reconstructive surgeons placed the forehead flap in the midline to increase the flap's vascular supply. After all, a midline location would conceivably harvest both the right and left supratrochlear arteries. Also, it was felt that, in this location, mimetic defects were minimized because the frontalis muscle shows a natural discontinuity in this area. Although this midline design generated large flaps, the broad pedicle resulted in less effective flap rotation. This restriction of movement increased closure tension and produced secondary tissue movement and subsequent nasal distortion. Additionally, an unnecessarily large donor forehead scar resulted in significant reductions in the final aesthetic result. Labat is credited as the first to shift the flap's pedicle from a median to a paramedian location.[26,27] The relocation of the flap to a paramedian location at approximately the medial end of the brow was postulated to be successful based on the predictable location of the vertically oriented supratrochlear artery. This modification in the base of the flap's origin produces distinct advantages. In the 1970s and 1980s, Menick and Burget further advanced the refinements of the paramedian forehead flap.[27–31] The axial basis and paramedian location allowed the flap's pedicle to be narrowed to 10–20 mm. The reduction of pedicle width allows greater flap movement and lowers closure tensions with improved results on the distal nose. Moreover, less of a standing cutaneous deformity in the glabella and lower closure tensions of the donor site on the forehead have improved the aesthetic success of the paramedian flap when compared to its median predecessor.

Because the paramedian forehead flap can be extended across the orbital rim, a longer flap is produced. The increased length produced by shifting the flap to a paramedian location eliminated the curved orientation of many early median forehead flaps or the extension of the flap onto hair-bearing scalp in efforts to recruit additional flap length—both improving the chance for aesthetically successful nasal reconstruction. Although widely regarded as an axial flap, the true dependency of the paramedian forehead flap on a patent supratrochlear artery has been debated. McCarthy's anatomic studies showed that the interconnecting forehead arteries are so redundant that even complete occlusion of the supratrochlear artery resulted in adequate demonstrable collateral flow through principally the dorsal nasal artery.[24] This may prove important when considering such a repair in a patient who has had previous surgery of the forehead or glabella.

The anatomic basis of the paramedian flap is the key to its success. The supratrochlear artery, the flap's perfusion source, exits the superior medial orbit 1.7–2.2 cm lateral to the midline. At its origination near the superior orbit, the artery is sandwiched between the corrugator supercilii and frontalis muscles. At approximately the level of the eyebrow, the vessel assumes a more superficial, vertically oriented location in the subcutaneous tissues. Doppler studies have confirmed the consistent location and course of the vessel.[32] Undermining in a subfascial plane just superior to the periosteum near the flap's origination ensures inclusion of the nutrient vessel within the body of the elevated flap. McCarthy's anatomic studies[24] and the experience of Menick and Burget have shown that the richly anastomotic vasculature of the medial canthus allows extension of the flap inferior to the orbital rim if necessary to further increase its effective length. This flap design places the superior aspect of the flap (the future nasal tip) within the non-hair-bearing forehead skin obviating the need for secondary depilatory procedures of a hair-bearing flap transposed to the nose. Because the terminal branches of the supratrochlear artery travel superficial to frontalis 1 cm above the brow, the distal flap can be aggressively thinned of frontalis muscle and subcutaneous tissue—even in smokers (albeit more conservatively). The reliability, ease of transfer and contouring, and axial vascular supply have positioned the paramedian forehead flap as a stable of reconstructive choices. The excellent color and textural match of forehead skin to the nose allows for unsurpassed aesthetic and functional repairs.

■ PREOPERATIVE PREPARATION

The forehead flap is considered with larger (over 2 cm) or complex nasal defects not amenable to second intention, local flap, or skin graft repair. The axial pattern paramedian forehead flap is not a simple repair to execute, and the proper utilization of the flap requires significant operative knowledge and experience (Fig. 22.7). A surgeon's preoperative planning is the most critical element for success. For proper informed consent, the patient must be counseled about the multiple steps required, the scars that will inevitably result, the risks of the surgery, the alternative reconstructive options, and the need to have realistic expectations. All patients view the defect prior to initiation of the repair, and are also shown photographs of representative flap cases to better understand the procedure. Digital photographs are taken to document the operative procedure.

It is of utmost importance to obtain clear surgical margins before the initiation of reconstructive procedures. All the defects presented in this chapter resulted from the excision of melanoma and non-melanoma skin cancers using the Mohs micrographic surgical technique. The authors perform almost all of these repairs in an office setting environment without the use of general anesthesia or conscious sedation. The safety and cost-effectiveness of such surgery in the office has been previously documented.[33,34] Oral benzodiazepines may be used for anxiolysis as required. Preoperative antibiotics are typically administered—especially if the flap is used to cover a cartilage graft. Preoperative assessment of nasal symmetry, concomitant patient risk factors for a poor outcome (e.g. anticoagulation, smoking), nasal valve function, and other pertinent information is obtained. West et al.[35] have shown that discontinuation of anticoagulants before surgical repair is probably not necessary. Based on intraoperative findings, physicians were unable to predict which patients were anticoagulated. Moreover, complications in anticoagulated patients undergoing cutaneous surgical procedures were no more frequent than complications in control patients.[36] The discontinuation of anticoagulation may be associated with thromboembolic perioperative events of significant consequence.[36] For this reason, medically necessary anticoagulant medicines are uncommonly withheld before reconstructive efforts. In our experience, no significant perioperative complications have been experienced in anticoagulated patients undergoing such repairs.

The patient's face is carefully studied. Neurologic function is tested and documented. An assessment of effective respiratory airflow is made. The forehead is carefully studied. Vertical height from the brow to the hairline is assessed to ensure that a flap of sufficient length may be generated. If necessary, extension of the flap below the brow or orbital rim to gain length may be required. The incision should not go below the brow unless necessary because this may increase the risk of distal flap necrosis. Surgical scars of the forehead may predict increased operative risk. It is the authors' opinion that previous forehead surgery does not eliminate the potential for paramedian forehead flap repair, but such scarring does increase the operative risk of flap necrosis. This may be especially relevant in patients who smoke.

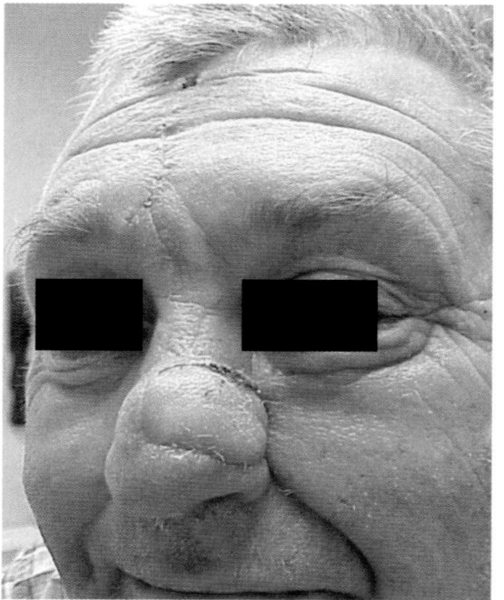

Figure 22.7 An excessively bulky and large forehead flap has been used to repair a nasal defect. Cosmetic success, in this case, may require significant additional procedures. The flap has been harvested from the hair-bearing frontal scalp, transposing the hair onto the nose. Also, the flap has been used to fill the missing portion of the cheek cosmetic unit obscuring normal anatomic boundaries.

■ TECHNIQUES

Paramedian forehead flap repair

First stage

The patient is placed in a supine position. The face is prepped and draped with standard operative technique. Local anesthesia is instilled with a buffered solution of 1% lidocaine with 1 : 100 000 epinephrine (adrenaline). Supraorbital nerve blocks are used to provide longer lasting anesthesia and diminish the discomfort of procedures required to close the donor area. The authors, in distinction to Burget, infiltrate the donor site with epinephrine (adrenaline) and lidocaine and think that it does not significantly impact flap survival and yields a defect of the forehead that may be more easily repaired.[37]

The flap is designed based on the known location of the supratrochlear vessels at approximately the medial end of the eyebrow (Fig. 22.8). The flap's base or pedicle is designed to be ideally 1.2–1.7 cm in width (Fig. 22.9). Too narrow a pedicle may fail to incorporate the nutrient vessel. Paradoxically, too wide a pedicle may result in kinking and reduced rotation with a subsequent reduction of vascularity and a poor result. The flap's pedicle is designed in a true vertical axis to ensure that the maximum length of the named vessel is included. If adequate length cannot be gained with vertical placement of the flap's long axis, the surgeon may consider a curved flap axis, extension of the flap donor tissue into the hair-bearing scalp, or flap extension below the level of the eyebrow. Some surgeons utilize Doppler examination to ensure the patency and location of the supratrochlear artery. We do not typically use Doppler localization of the artery and feel that in all but exceptional cases ultrasound confirmation of the vessel is unnecessary.

The flap's recipient site on the nose is then prepared. If the repair follows Mohs micrographic surgical resection, the edges of the wound may need to be freshened or excessive dermis trimmed to provide a 90° skin angle. Burget, Menick, and others have championed the principles of subunit reconstruction.[29] The nasal subunits are identified and

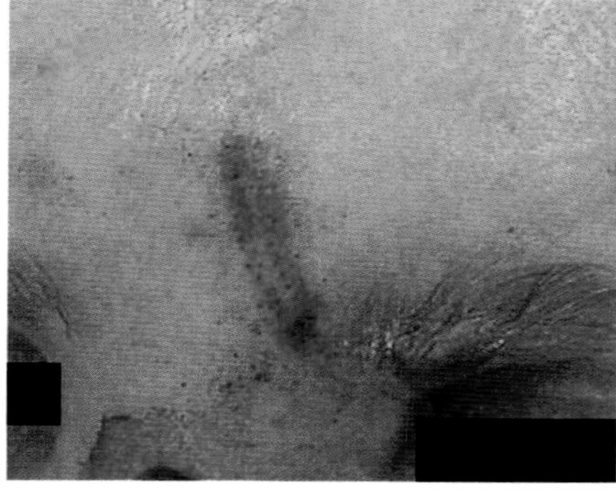

Figure 22.8 The approximate location of the left supratrochlear artery.

demarcated with surgical ink. Typically, the flaps are designed to reach the borders of such subunits—even if excess skin must be resected. Improved results are usually seen when the margin of the flap is placed along the border of a cosmetic subunit. However, this is not requisite for operative success. If only a small portion of a subunit has been removed the forehead flap may still provide excellent results without the further removal of nasal tissue. The surgeon must weigh the potential benefit of enlarging the nasal defect to reach cosmetic borders with the potential for creating a larger forehead donor scar. Any curvilinear incisions on the nose are preferentially changed to more acute angles to minimize the potential for postoperative trapdoor deformity.

A template of the nasal defect is made from the foil of a suture pack or other suitable material. The template must exactly match the size and three-dimensional quality of the nasal defect. An oversized flap will pincushion and not provide suitable contour reconstruction. Conversely, a flap that is too small will result in significant anatomic distortion when secondary tissue movement of the alar margin or nasal tip is required to close the wound.

Full-thickness defects or defects near the free alar margin may require the placement of cartilage graft(s) to maintain nasal patency and to resist the forces of postoperative wound contraction. Although there are many potential sites for donor cartilage (ear, nasal septum, costal cartilage, and others), the authors use, almost exclusively, auricular cartilage given its ease of harvest and its minimal donor site morbidity (Fig. 22.10). The primary sources of auricular cartilage are the conchal bowl and antihelix. Both may yield significant amounts of cartilage to reconstruct the lower nose (Fig. 22.11).

If lining flaps and/or cartilage grafts are utilized, the template should be constructed after their placement so a more accurate conceptualization of the true form of the nose can be appreciated. The template is then transferred to the upper forehead (Fig. 22.12). The pattern is reversed to compensate for the rotational axis change with inter-

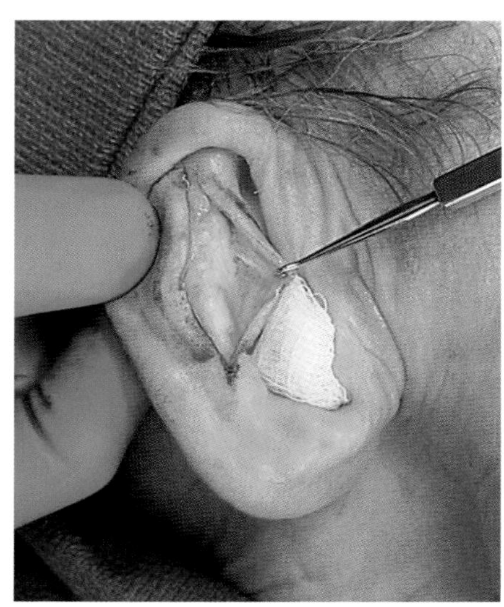

Figure 22.10 An appropriately sized cartilage graft may be harvested from the antihelix with surprisingly little cosmetic deformity.

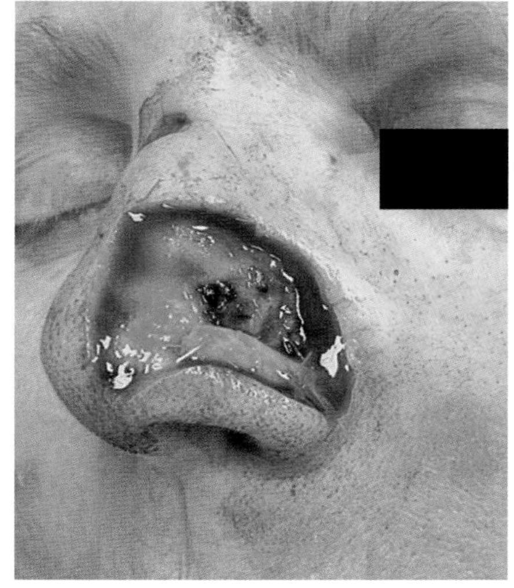

Figure 22.11 A large auricular cartilage graft has been placed into a pocket created in the fibrous tissue of the lateral ala. The anterior aspect of the cartilage graft is sutured to the remnant of the left lower lateral cartilage at the genu. This cartilage graft proves important to maintain the neutral position of the ala as postoperative wound contraction occurs.

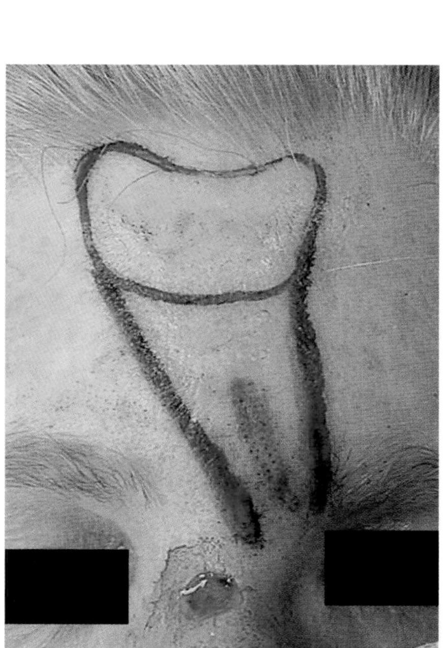

Figure 22.9 The paramedian forehead flap is designed in a near true vertical axis.

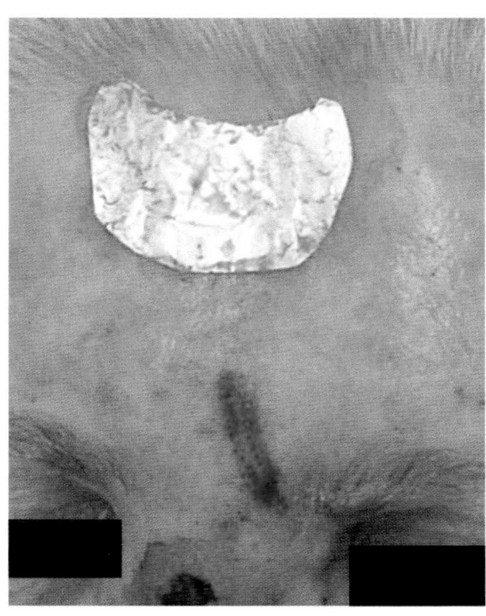

Figure 22.12 Because the vertical dimension of the forehead is short, the template may need to be placed in the hair-bearing frontal scalp. It is preferred, however, to extend the flap below the brow to gain additional length because the placement of hair-bearing tissue on the distal nose may jeopardize the cosmetic outcome.

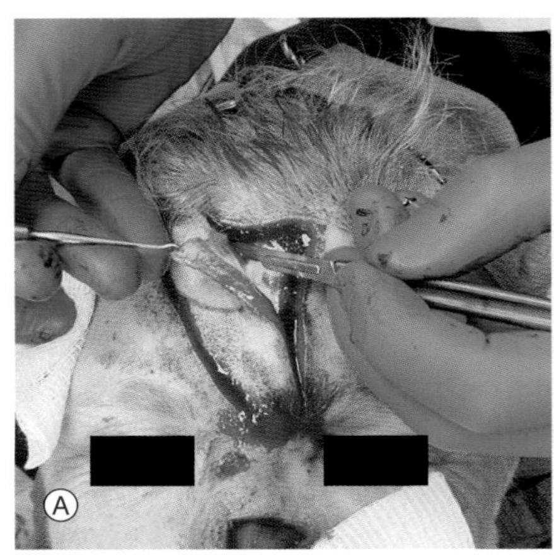

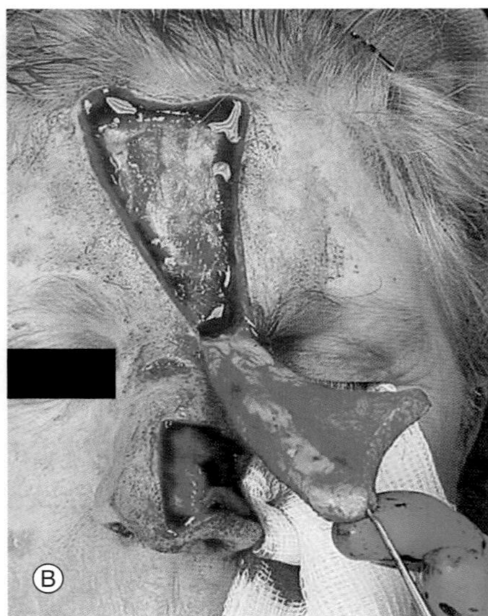

Figure 22.13 (A)–(B) Elevation of the paramedian axial flap.

polation. The transferred template and designed pedicle are then placed to ensure that adequate length may be gained to insert the flap under minimal wound closure tension. A cotton gauze is held at the flap's base and pivoted onto the nose to test for adequate pedicle length before any incisions are made. Using particular attention to maintain a 90° angle of the scalpel blade, the template and pedicle are then incised. The incision is extended through skin, subcutaneous tissue, muscle, and fascia. The flap is then elevated from a cephalic to caudad direction just above the frontal bone's periosteum (Fig. 22.13). The surgeon should avoid removal of calvarial periosteum because this significantly slows second intention healing at the flap's donor site.

At the origination point of the pedicle flap, the corrugator supercilii muscle is encountered and elevated off the periosteum of the frontal bone. The nutrient vessels exit the medial orbit sandwiched between the corrugator supercilii and frontalis muscles. Thus, when the proximal portion of the flap is elevated just above the periosteum of the calvarium, the nutrient vessels are preserved to ensure the axial vascular support of the nascent flap. If the flap is extended past the orbital rim in efforts to gain additional rotational length, skin and subcutaneous tissue only are excised in this area. Particular attention must be given when undermining the most proximal aspect of the flap to prevent unwanted anatomic injury. Typically significant resection of the corrugator supercilii muscle is necessary to gain the flap mobility required. This has surprisingly little postoperative mimetic effect.

Once elevated, the flap is covered and attention directed to the donor site of the forehead. Donor site closure is assisted by wide undermining of the forehead in a subfascial plane from the most lateral aspect of the forehead. If necessary, galeatomies may improve the mobility of the forehead skin. Hemostasis is achieved as needed with electrocautery. The frontalis muscle and galea of the forehead are then repositioned. The donor site is closed as a vertical linear layered closure (Fig. 22.14). For larger nasal reconstructions, primary closure of the cephalic portion of the defect may not be possible. It is the authors' opinion that this defect is best managed by second intention healing. Additional flaps or grafts are unlikely to improve the aesthetic outcome when repairing the donor site at the cephalic margin of the wound on the forehead. Such additional procedures also introduce increased operative morbidity and cost.

The forehead is covered after repair and attention is then directed to the nasal defect. The axial vascular support allows the surgeon to significantly alter the distal flap. Even in smokers, the distal aspect of the axial flap may be aggressively thinned of all muscle and nearly all subcutaneous tissue to the underlying dermis (Fig. 22.15). This allows the flap to drape over the native or replaced cartilaginous framework to restore nasal contour.

Once significant subcutaneous tissue has been removed and hemostasis achieved, the flap is transposed. The surgical defect of the nose is then conservatively undermined just above the periosteum and perichondrium before insertion of the flap. This undermining may prevent postoperative trapdoor deformity. The flap is then inset into the nasal defect and sutured into place. It is retained with only a few subcutaneous Vicryl (Ethicon Corp, Johnson and Johnson Co, Somerville, NJ) sutures and a running cuticular suture (Fig. 22.16). Any small bleeding vessels of the pedicle are then electrocoagulated with care not to disrupt the underlying vascular supply.

Some surgeons have advised covering the flap's pedicle with a skin graft to minimize this risk of bleeding. We think, however, that this is not indicated and may add to the morbidity and/or expense of the reconstruction. The wounds are then dressed. The exposed pedicle is wrapped in petrolatum gauze. The donor and recipient sites are then covered with petrolatum, nonstick bandages, and occlusive paper tape dressings. Antibiotics and narcotic analgesics are prescribed. Patients are usually discharged to home and only infrequently admitted to the hospital. Hospital admission may be necessary for a patient living alone or residing a significant distance from medical care. Appropriate restrictions on bending, lifting, or exertion are dispensed.

Wound care is either with a closed technique (all dressings remain in place until the time of suture removal) or an open technique (clean with soap and water and application of petrolatum once or twice daily). We have found that many patients prefer the closed technique with all

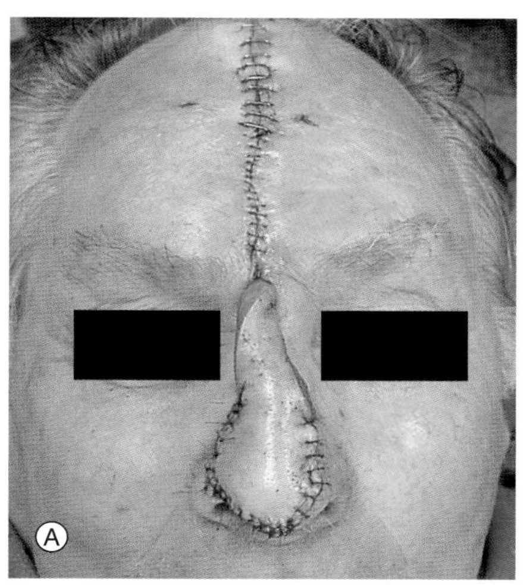

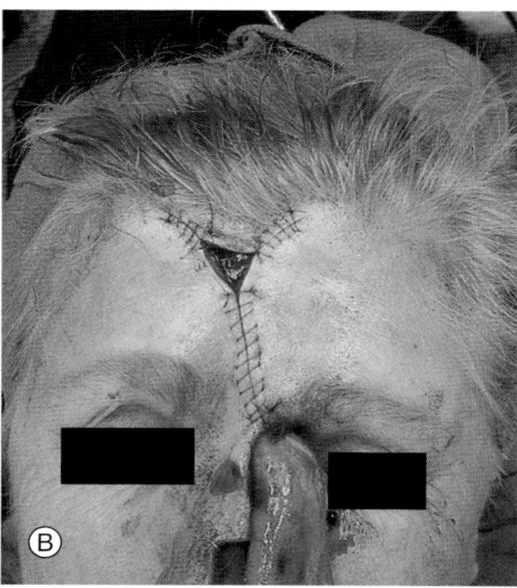

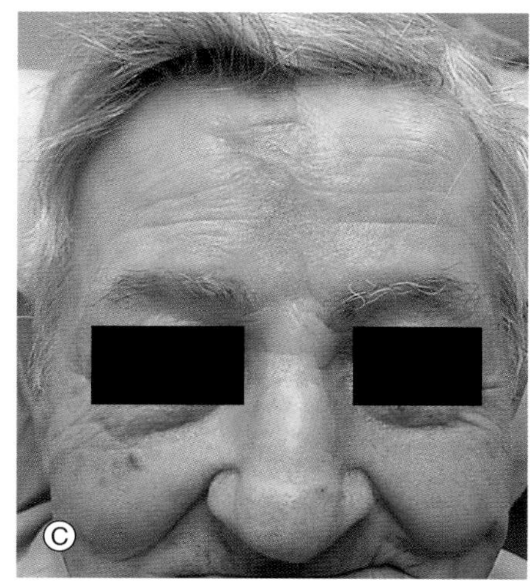

Figure 22.14 The laxity of the forehead is variable in individual patients. (A) The inferior half may nearly always be closed after extensive subfrontalis undermining. The cephalic margin, depending upon the size of the template required to reconstruct the nose may prove too large for primary closure. (B) The portion of the donor defect not closed is best allowed to heal by second intention. Additional flaps or grafts are unlikely to improve cosmetic result. (C) The cosmetic end-result from skin graft closure of the surgical wound shows no better, and perhaps an inferior, result than that with second intention healing.

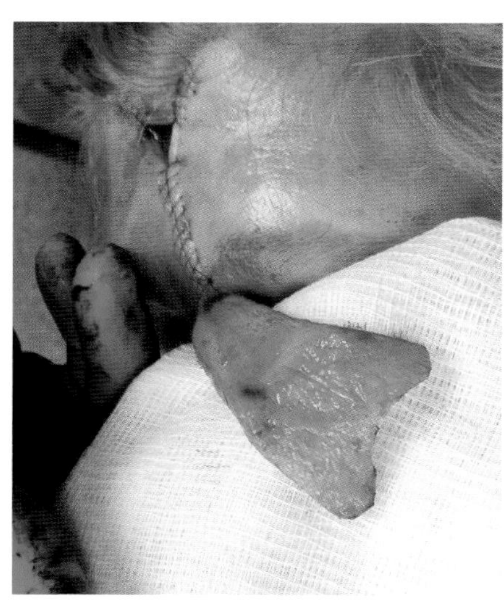

Figure 22.15 The distal flap may be thinned of all frontalis muscle and nearly all subcutaneous tissue.

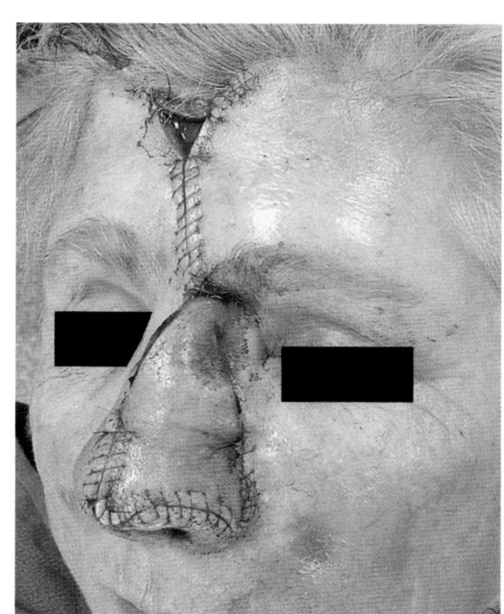

Figure 22.16 The thinned forehead flap is then inset into the nasal defect and sutured into place.

dressing changes done in the office. A significant amount of reassurance may need to be provided to the patient at this stage and reviewing photographs of completed repairs may prove helpful. The sutures are removed from the reconstruction at a postoperative interval of 5–7 days. If the forehead site is allowed to heal by second intention, it is bandaged and the dressing changed daily until this healing has been completed (typically 4–6 weeks).

Second stage

The ideal interval for flap division and insertion has been questioned. The delay of flap pedicle division allows for adequate collateral circulation to be established. Ideally, the pedicle is severed as soon as this collateral circulation has been achieved because the bulky pedicle and bandage associated with the flap may significantly disrupt the patient's ability to work or wear glasses. Animal studies have supported the fact that physiologically the pedicle may be safely divided at approximately postoperative day 11.[38,39] However, we customarily divide the pedicle as a second stage procedure at approximately postoperative day 21. It is thought that this interval of time allows adequate collateral vascularization to be established, which enhances the survivability of the transected pedicle flap.

The patient returns at week 3 of the postoperative period for the second stage of the repair (Fig. 22.17). The preoperative assessment and preparation are identical to those of the first stage of the repair. At the time of division and insertion, a surgical defect surrounding the flap's origin is created in the glabella in the shape of an inverted V (Fig. 22.18). The cephalic portion of the transected pedicle is thinned and inset into this defect to mimic glabellar rhytids once healing has been completed. The remaining portion of the dorsal nasal or other aesthetic subunit of the nose is then resected to the underlying periosteum or perichondrium and the caudad margin of the pedicle is trimmed and inset into the nasal defect using a layered closure (Fig. 22.19).

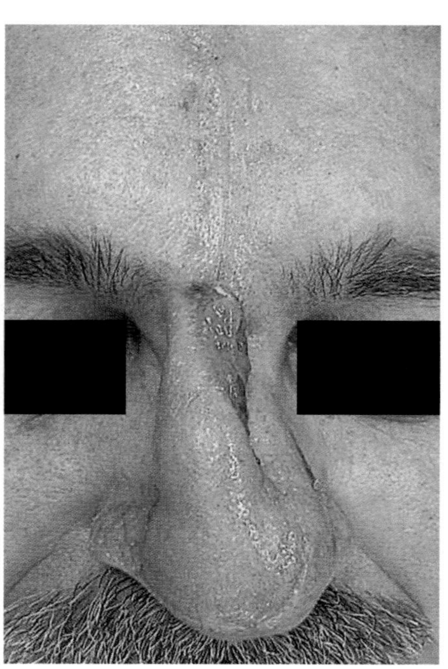

Figure 22.17 Three weeks after surgery the flap is well vascularized and ready to divide the pedicle.

Additional interim stage

Menick has described an additional stage in the forehead flap reconstruction of the nose.[40] In this interim step, the flap is nearly totally elevated except for a portion of the most distal flap near the nasal tip. The flap and underlying nasal tissue are then aggressively thinned and sculpted. The interpolation flap is returned to position and resutured into place without division. A third step entailing division and insertion of the pedicle as detailed above is then performed at an appropriate postoperative interval (Fig. 22.20).

Whether as a second or third stage after division and insertion of the pedicle flap, the wounds are bandaged and care prescribed as noted above. Sutures are again removed at an interval of 5–7 days following the procedure.

Dorsal nasal flap

In distinction to the paramedian forehead flap, the DNF is a single staged repair that can be utilized to repair defects of the nasal tip, supratip, or dorsum/sidewall that are less than 2.5 cm in diameter. Rieger is attributed with the

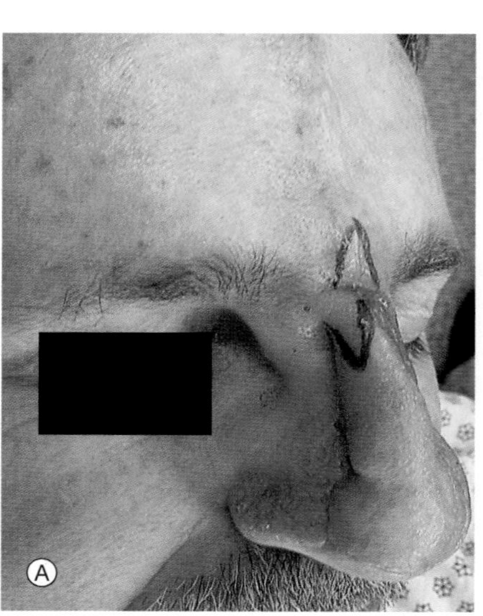

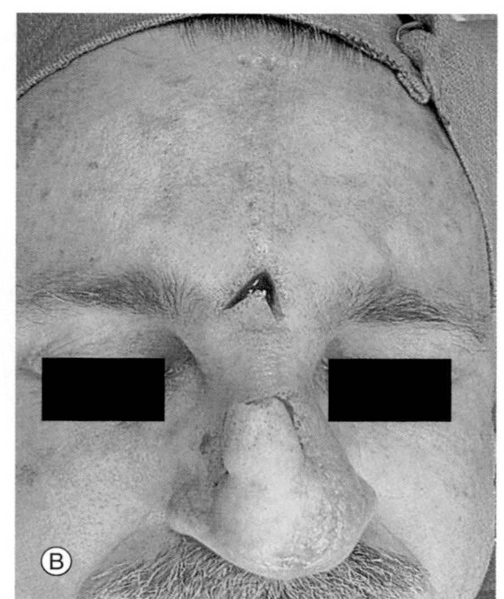

Figure 22.18 The pedicle is transected in the midportion. (A)–(B) A surgical defect in the shape of an inverted V is created in the glabella. The proximal portion of the flap is trimmed to meet this defect and sutured into place. The proximal pedicle is typically not simply excised for this may cause the medial aspects of the brows to be too close together. Particular attention is given at this stage to ensure that the medial ends of the eyebrows are positioned well to preserve facial symmetry.

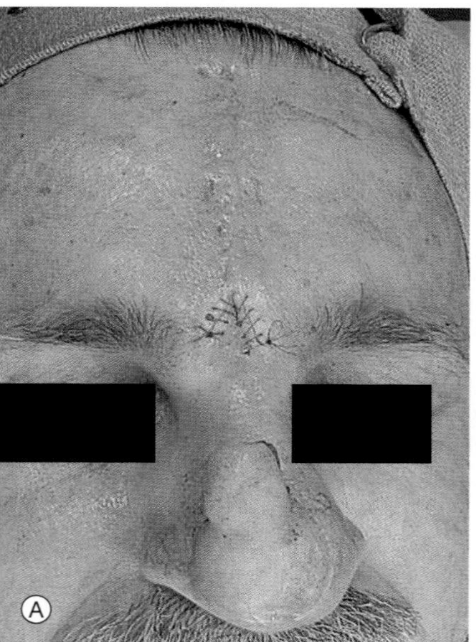

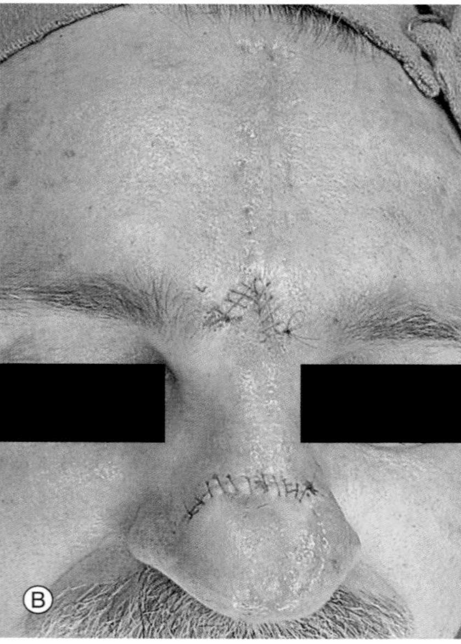

Figure 22.19 (A)–(B) The nasal portion of the pedicle is thinned and inset into the nasal defect.

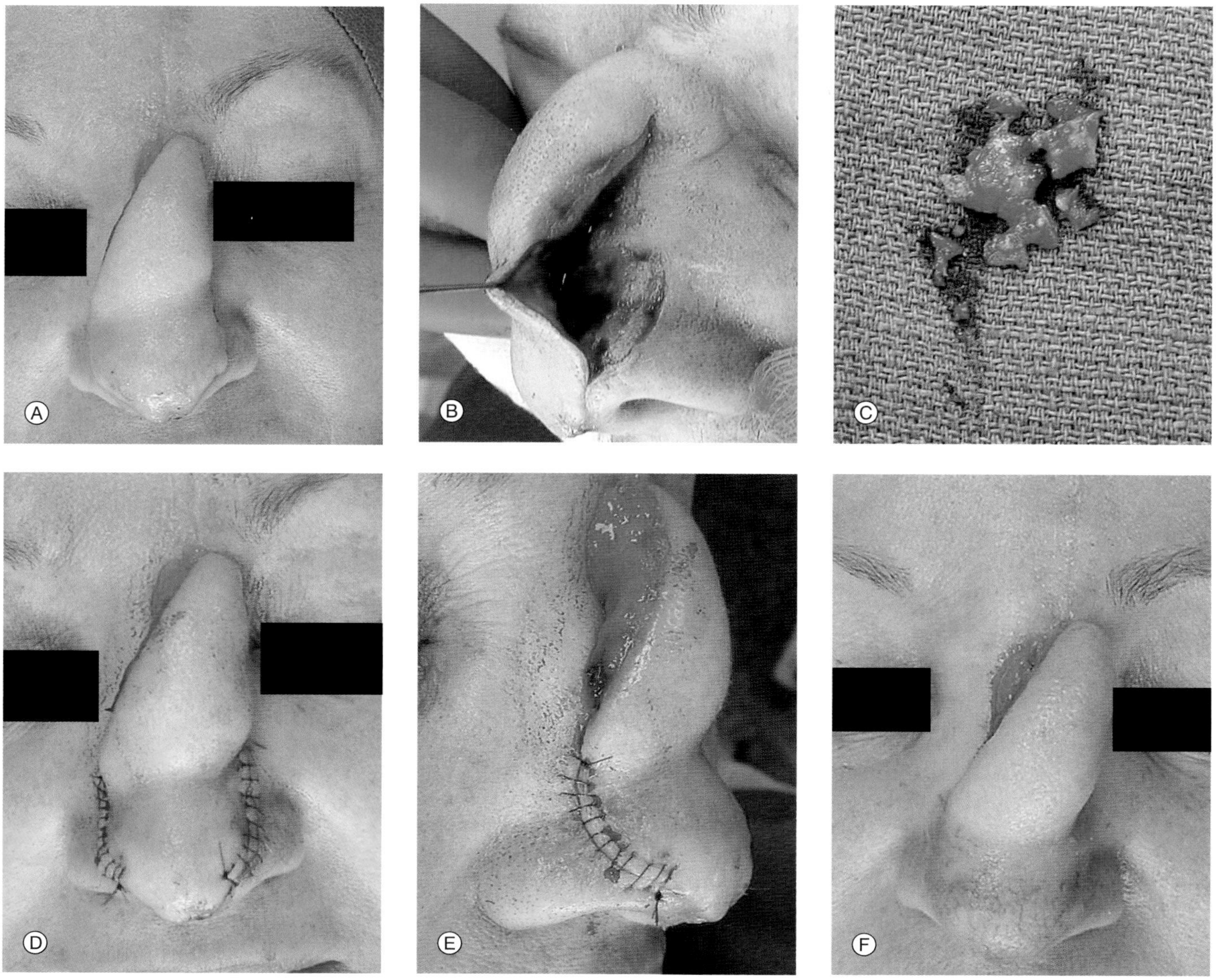

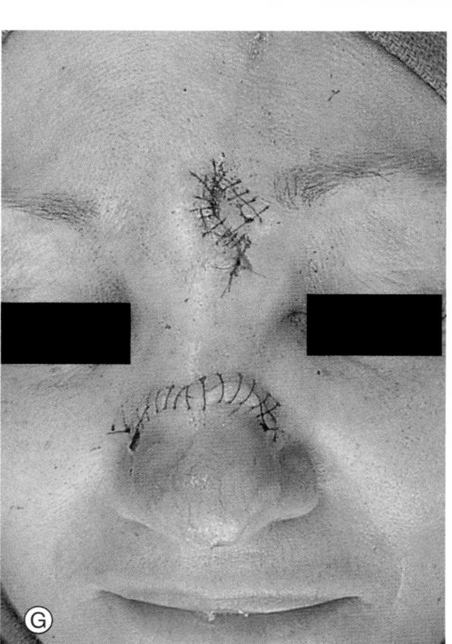

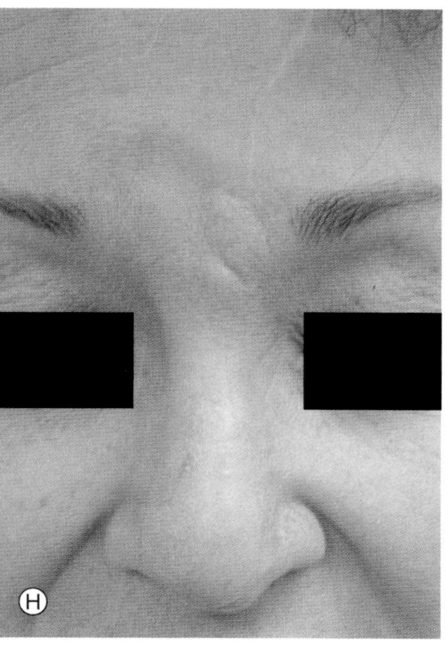

Figure 22.20 (A) At 3 weeks postoperatively the flap appears excessively bulky with loss of the normal nasal contour. (B) The forehead flap is incised along its margin except an attachment at the columella. The pedicle is not divided at this interim stage. The flap and 2–3 mm of underlying tissue are elevated. (C) Scar tissue, residual frontalis muscle, and subcutaneous tissue are then resected from the base of the wound on the nose. (D)–(E) The flap is resutured into place. (F) An additional period of 3 weeks is allowed for re-establishment of the vascular support. (G) At 6 weeks after the initial reconstructive procedure the pedicle is divided and inserted. (H) The reconstructive result at 3 months following initial repair efforts.

design modification of the DNF currently widely used.[41] When utilized on the lower sidewall and not centered about a base in the medial canthus, the DNF is a random pattern cutaneous flap as discussed in Chapter 21. Marchac and Toth modified the DNF to pivot about a pedicle based on the inner canthus, thus establishing an axial basis for the flap.[42] The inclusion of the angular artery in the flap's base provides the same preservation of perfusion seen with the paramedian forehead flap, and this design represents a significant advancement in the evolution of the flap. By including a named vessel in the base, the vascular support is improved, allowing a more generous back-cut, which improves the flap's mobility. This improved mobility allows the flap to be inset under less tension, lowering the risk of flap necrosis or associated nasal tissue distortion. By including a named nutrient vessel, many of the pitfalls of the random pattern DNF may be surmounted.

The DNF is best used for defects on or near the midline of the lower nose less than 2.5 cm in diameter. Broader wounds cannot typically be covered with a DNF without introducing unaesthetic alar or tip distortion. In these instances, a forehead flap is preferred. The flap's success is dependent entirely on the laxity of dorsal nasal skin, which allows the flap to be rotated to cover the primary defect under minimal tension. If the surgeon misjudges nasal laxity or misdesigns the flap's lines of incision, nasal distortion results. As the DNF is rotated, its effective length shortens, increasing closure tensions. This increased closure tension may contribute to more conspicuous scarring or anatomic distortion, both of which are poorly tolerated in the aesthetically demanding patient.

The nose is prepped and draped in routine fashion. Local anesthesia is achieved with lidocaine with 1 : 100 000 epinephrine (adrenaline). The flap is designed with the standing cutaneous deformity carefully positioned to avoid alar lifting with closure. As previously discussed by Dzubow, the critical element for success is designing the leading edge of the flap.[43] It is important for the leading edge to extend past the defect to compensate for flap shortening with rotational movement. The arc is then designed in the alar crease and up along the nasofacial junction. The arc of flap design is then continued through the medial canthus onto the superior glabella. The more the flap extends into the glabella, the easier the flap and secondary defect are to close without introducing anatomic distortion. A generous backcut to improve flap mobility is allowed when incorporating the angular artery. To preserve this vascular supply of the flap, the incision of the backcut should not extend inferior to the medial canthal tendon.

Upon incision, the flap is then elevated just above the periosteum and perichondrium of the nasal framework (Fig. 22.21). This plane of undermining incorporates the nasalis muscle and its associated vascular supply into the flap. Particular care is given when undermining the origination of the flap in the medical canthus to ensure protection of the nutrient vessel. Hemostasis is achieved with care to avoid electrocoagulation of the skin edges, which may result in epidermal necrosis. Wide undermining laterally to the nasal facial junction facilitates wound closure of the flap's donor area with minimal tension. The donor site of the glabella is then closed. The remaining portion of the flap is then sutured into place using a layered closure with particular emphasis on avoiding anatomic distortion. The standing cutaneous deformity of the glabella that has been rotated into the medial canthus is then amputated and the thinned flap is inset into the medial canthus and sutured into place (Fig. 22.22). The thick forehead skin of the glabella must be significantly thinned before insertion into the medial canthus. The wound is then bandaged and care instructions dispensed as previously discussed. Antibiotics may be prescribed as needed—especially for patients with a higher risk for postoperative wound infection.

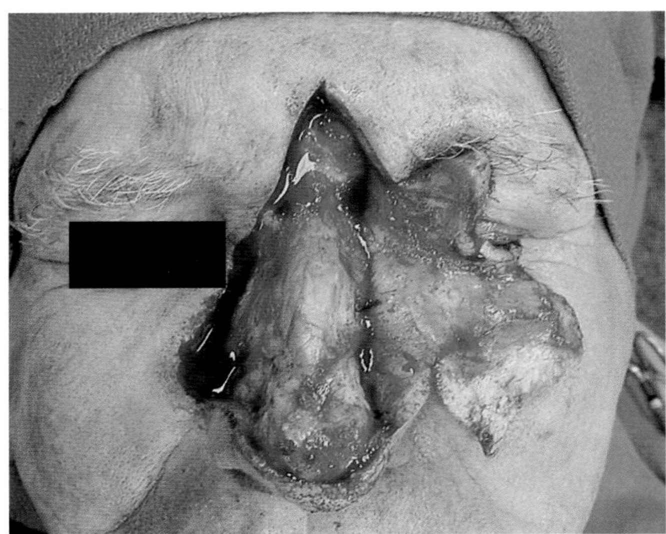

Figure 22.21 Submuscularis undermining of the dorsal nasal flap.

If properly designed and inset, secondary procedures are rarely needed. Dermabrasion may improve noticeable scars, particularly on thick sebaceous skin. Perhaps the greatest limitation of the DNF is the transposition of the thick glabellar skin into the medial canthus. This may be improved with secondary revision. The flap offers one-staged reconstruction of small-to-medium sized lower nasal defects, avoiding the complexities of staged reconstructive procedures. Although this axial pattern flap is robust and reproducible, the large arc of rotation for even smaller defects generally limits its use to defects less than 2.5 cm in diameter. The flap cannot be used for subtotal nasal reconstruction or with extensive cartilage grafts or lining flaps with success. In these cases, superior results are achieved with the staged interpolation flaps.

The limited availability of named nutrient facial vessels limits the use of axial pattern flaps. Most axial flaps used in dermatologic surgery are based on variants of the forehead flap and DNF. Axial pattern flaps in nasal reconstructions offer unsurpassed viability, particularly in patients with concomitant risk factors or requiring multiple reconstructive procedures. The versatility of axial flaps can offer the dermatologic surgeon durable and predictable repairs.

Lip flaps

The lips share significant aesthetic and functional importance with the nose. The relatively high prevalence of non-melanoma skin cancer on the lips demands that reconstructive surgeons have techniques for successful reconstruction. The functional importance of the lips is of

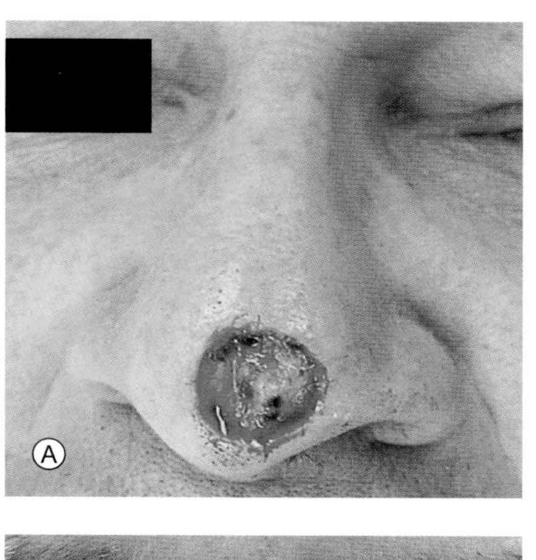

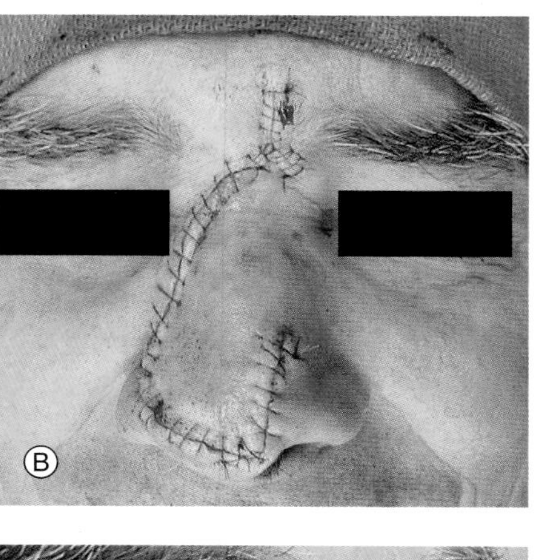

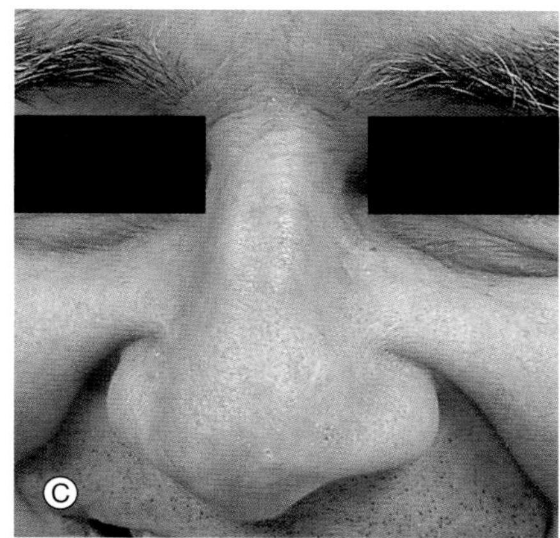

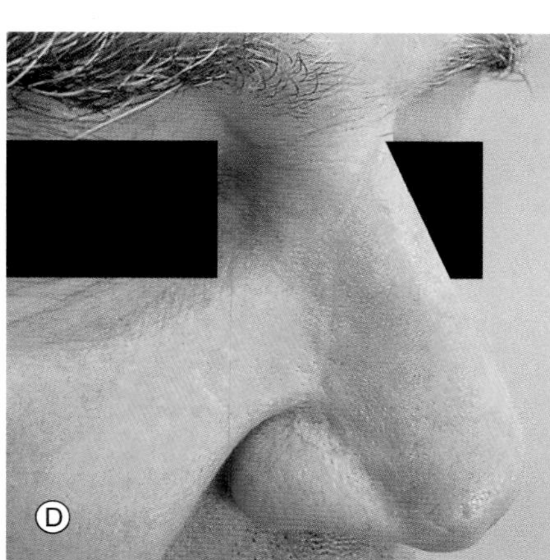

Figure 22.22 (A)–(D) The Rieger flap repair of a lower nasal defect. No additional procedures undertaken.

paramount concern. Oral competence must be preserved or restored to achieve operative success. Oral competency allows for proper phonation, eating, expression, and respiration. Smaller wounds of the lip may be repaired with primary closure or local flaps as discussed elsewhere in this text. Larger wounds resulting in removal of significant volumes of lip tissue may not be closed by direct apposition without an inordinate risk of microstomia and its associated complications. The potential loss of motor function and the resulting complications limits the usefulness of repairing lip defects with tissue harvested from the laxity of the cheek or chin.

Abbe cross-lip flap

With larger lip wounds, the underlying orbicularis oris musculature should be repaired to allow coordinated motor activity and preservation of function. The restoration of coordinated muscular function is critical for the lower lip to maintain oral competence. Larger lip defects may present the risk of functional compromise secondary to resected orbicularis muscle. For this reason, effective functional and aesthetic repair must utilize flaps that supply orbicularis muscle in addition to skin and soft tissue to achieve optimum results. Cross-lip flaps may provide an effective reconstructive option. Abbe, in 1899, described the full-thickness transposition of lower lip tissue to repair a defect of larger diameter on the upper lip.[44] Similarly, a flap may be harvested from the upper lip to repair a defect of larger size on the lower lip. The Abbe cross-lip flap is a pedicled axial pattern flap supplied by the labial artery. The labial artery is between orbicularis oris muscle and mucosa posterior to the vermilion. Its course may become more tortuous and superficial with advancing age. The labial artery is identified and preserved in this flap to provide axial vascular support. The flap is incised and rotated to fill the defect of the opposing lip with a preserved vascular pedicle. The pedicle is then divided in a second staged procedure at an appropriate postoperative interval.

The patient undergoes the usual preoperative counsel after successful tumor extirpation. Routine prepping and draping and local anesthesia are then undertaken. A pedicled flap is then designed. The flap is undersized to fill the defect. The flap harvested should be approximately 75% of the surgical defect's diameter. The flap's full-thickness is then incised with emphasis to preserve the pedicle at either the medial or lateral aspect of the flap, and hemostasis is achieved with electrocautery. The flap is then rotated 180° to fill the defect of the opposing lip and sutured into place. The donor site is closed with identical technique (Fig. 22.23). Careful re-approximation of all layers is important to achieve success.

For motor function of the lip to be restored the orbicularis oris muscle should be visualized and re-approximated with slowly absorbing or nonabsorbable sutures. The mucosa, subcutaneous tissue, and skin are then carefully approximated and closed in layers with care to ensure the neutral position of the vermilion.

Circumoral axial advancement flaps

As an alternative to cross-lip or Abbe flaps, various modified advancement flaps have been championed for lip repair. Most of these flaps are axial in nature and specifically

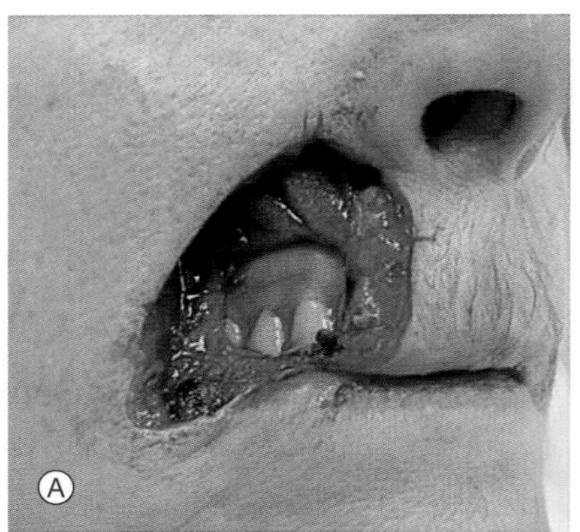
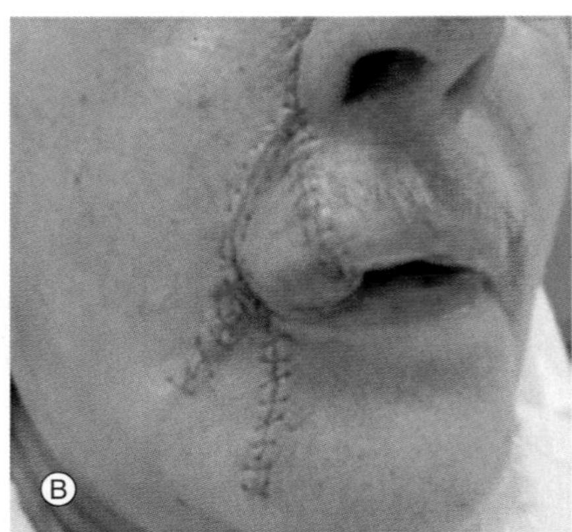

Figure 22.23 (A)–(B) Abbe flap reconstruction of a large full-thickness upper lip defect.

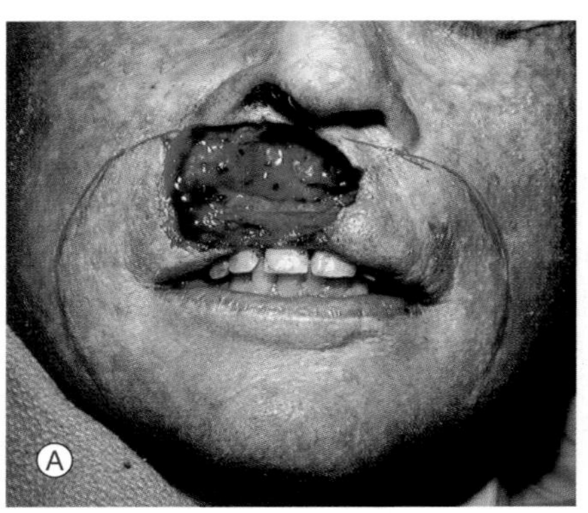
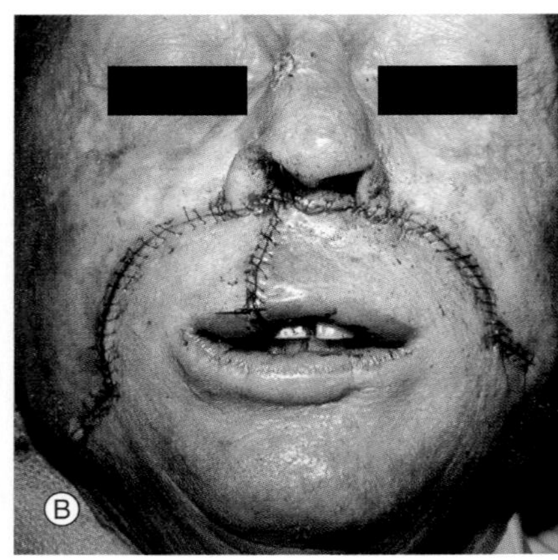
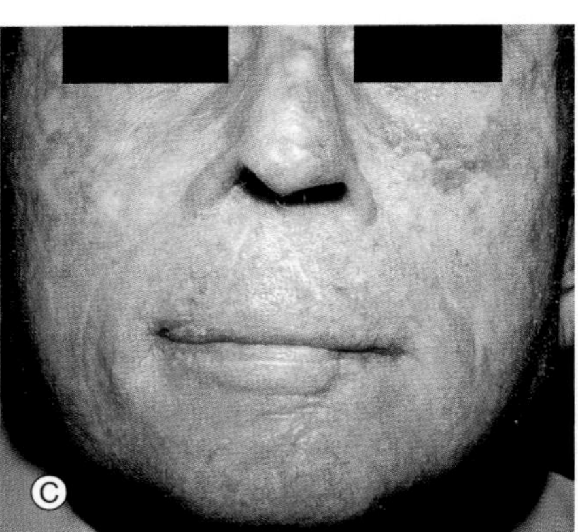

Figure 22.24 (A)–(B) A large central upper lip defect. Circumoral advancement flaps are designed and incised. The vascular supply is identified and preserved. (C) Postoperative result shows restoration of the soft tissue defect and preservation of lip function.

preserve the integrity of the labial vessels to improve the flap's vascular supply. Von Bruns first described circumoral advancement flaps in 1857 (Fig. 22.24).[45] Karapandzic in 1974 detailed extensive efforts in circumoral advancement flap repairs to preserve, through direct visual dissection, the neurovascular support to ensure the flap's vascular support.[46] His modifications have improved operative outcomes in challenging lip repairs. The circumoral axial advancement flaps are robust flaps typically used for larger lip reconstructions. The dermatologic surgeon undertaking such advanced reconstructive procedures must be well versed in managing all potential complications including microstomia, oral incompetence, and others.

■ POSTOPERATIVE CARE

Paramedian forehead flap repair

As with any facial reconstructive procedure, significant changes occur in the postoperative period of a paramedian forehead flap repair. The end-result of this reconstructive technique may not be seen for a period of several months and early surgical revisions are best delayed until scar maturation has been completed. Lymphedema and postoperative trapdooring are best managed with massage, intralesional corticosteroids, and simple observation (Fig. 22.25). Nearly all of the early flap elevation or pincushioning can be successfully managed with such minimally disturbing techniques. The repair is then allowed to mature for 6–12 weeks. At that time, dermabrasion may be done to assist in scar camouflage. Secondary procedures to address flap contour issues are infrequently needed. However, at times surgical revisionary efforts may be required to correct more noticeable deficiencies including nasal malalignment, persistent trapdooring, or others (Fig. 22.26). Other more involved tertiary procedures to recreate an alar groove or change tip or ala position may be undertaken to correct topographic problems (Fig. 22.27). Epilatory procedures may be required if the distal portion of the flap was harvested from hair-bearing scalp. Laser-assisted hair removal may prove significantly less risky than surgical microepilation as described by others. However, with extension of the flap's origin below the orbital rim such procedures are uncommonly needed because the flap's tissue may be harvested from the forehead and not the anterior scalp.

The axial paramedian forehead flap is a robust flap. Total ischemic flap failure is uncommon. However, in the event of such flap loss, the surgeon may be faced with a rather significant reconstructive challenge. The flap is versatile and may cover small, complex, or large nasal defects. Perhaps the only common postoperative event is continued oozing

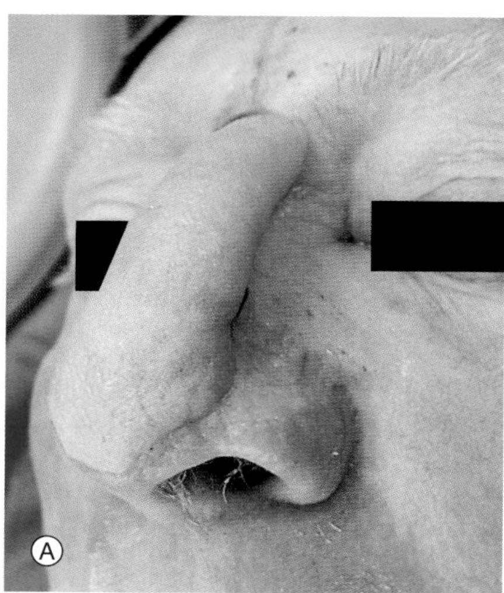

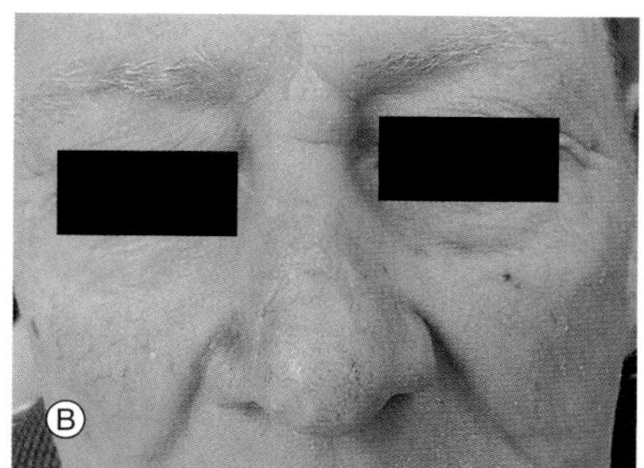

Figure 22.25 (A) The flap frequently appears bulky at the time of division and insertion. (B) The contour irregularity typically resolves without surgical intervention.

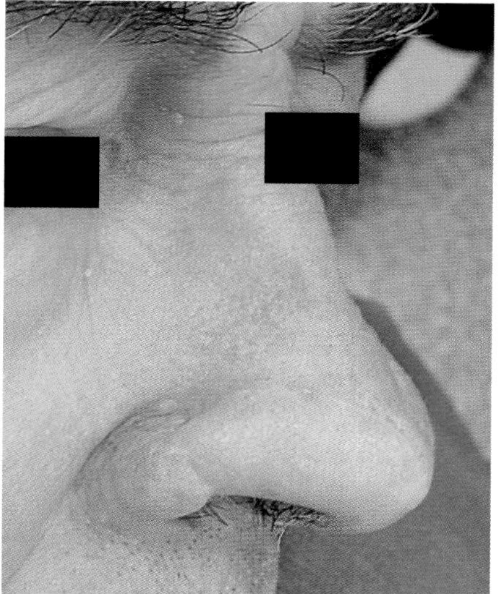

Figure 22.26 The forehead flap's contractile force has overcome the undersized cartilage graft placed at the time of the repair and elevated the alar rim producing a notch. Secondary revision may be desired to correct the topographical shortcoming. Surgical intervention may be required in the presence of reduced inspiratory airflow.

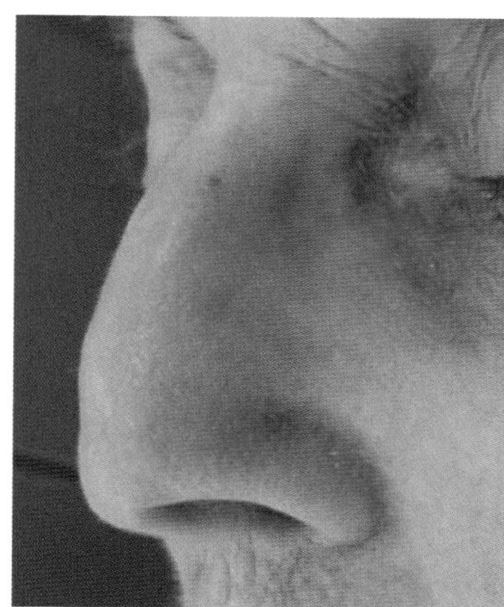

Figure 22.27 Failure to adequately repair the missing lower lateral cartilages has limited the success of this forehead flap repair.

from the transected pedicle near the glabella. Patients must be counseled to expect some degree of minor postoperative hemorrhage from this area. It typically responds to compression with minimal blood loss. The surgeon should thoroughly understand the operative technique to ensure aesthetic and functional repair.

The paramedian forehead flap has few equals in total or subtotal nasal reconstruction. The complexity of operative technique is rewarded with unsurpassed end results (Fig. 22.28). However, the morbidity and expense of this operation should be considered. Smaller or less complex nasal defects are better repaired with more simple operative techniques (random pattern flaps or skin grafts) discussed in Chapter 21.

Abbe cross-lip flap

The Abbe cross-lip flap is somewhat prone to trapdooring but cannot be effectively thinned at operative time without a significant risk of necrosis. After the flap has been inset and the donor site repaired, the wounds are bandaged and cared for as previously discussed. The patient must be counseled to avoid excessive strain on the flap. Soft foods are recommended and gentle oral hygiene is reviewed. The sutures are removed 5–7 days following the procedure. Much like with other interpolation flap procedures, division of the pedicle is delayed to allow neovascularization to proceed. After an appropriate interval has passed, the patient returns for division and insertion of the flap.

Flap revisions may be necessary in the postoperative period to correct malpositioning of the lip or persistent trapdooring. Both may prove difficult to correct completely without compromising the functional competence of the lip. The principal disadvantage with cross-lip flaps is the obvious problem if the flap fails. However, complete ischemic loss is unusual because of the axial blood supply. The horizontal dimension of both lips has been reduced and symptomatic problems related to postoperative microstomia may prove challenging to manage. Nevertheless, for large full-thickness lip defects, the Abbe flap provides functional repair in a procedure of low relative morbidity when compared to alternative reconstructive techniques.

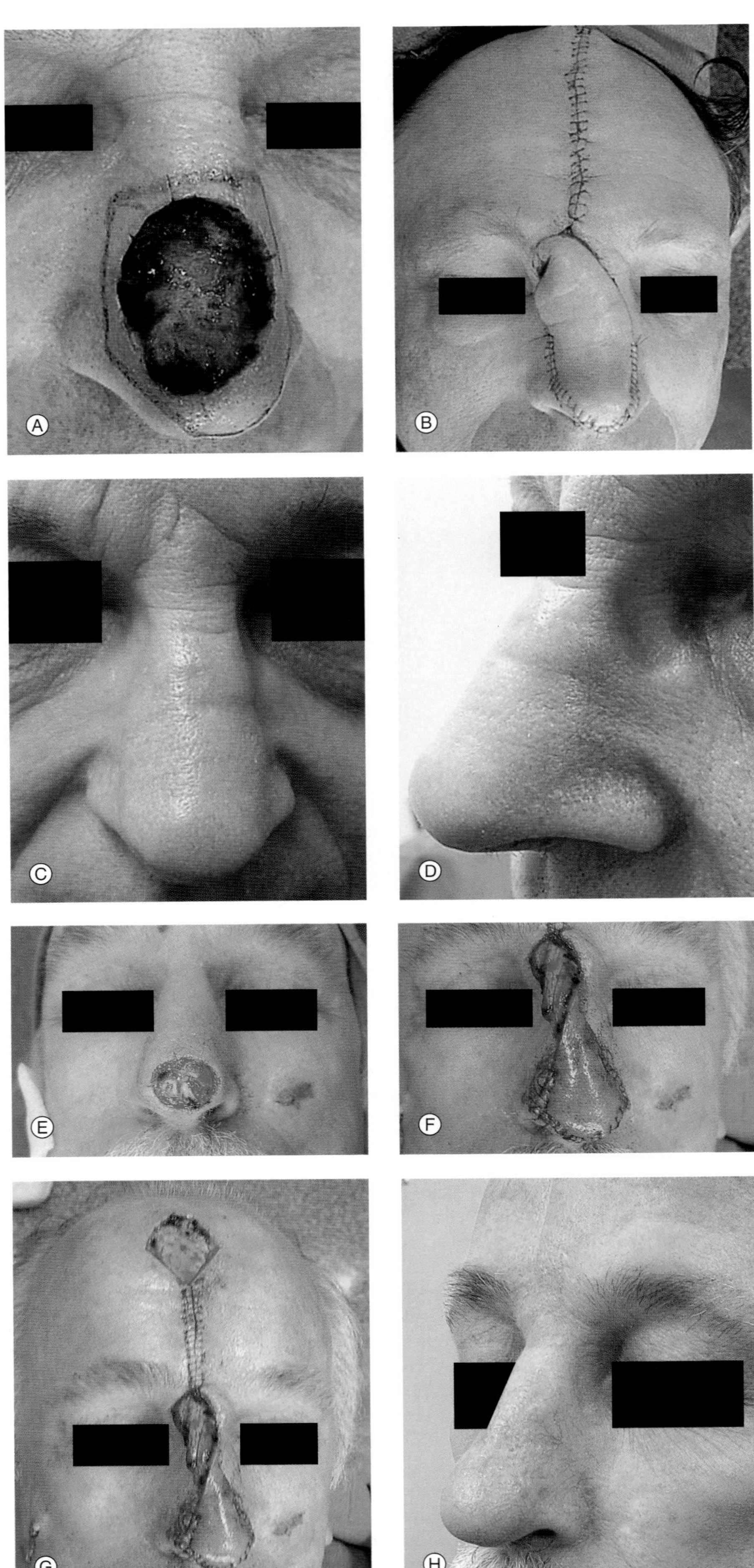

Figure 22.28 Case 1. (A) Preoperative defect; (B)–(D) Forehead flap repair. Case 2 (E) Preoperative defect; (F)–(H) Forehead flap repair.

Optimizing outcomes

- Preoperative planning is the most critical element for success—the patient must be counseled about the multiple steps required, the scars that will inevitably result, the risks of the surgery, the alternative reconstructive options, and the need to have realistic expectations.
- Paramedian forehead flap
  - the base or pedicle is designed ideally to be 1.2–1.7 cm in width—if too narrow it may fail to incorporate the nutrient vessel, and if too wide kinking and reduced rotation may reduce vascularity and lead to a poor result
  - the pedicle is designed in a true vertical axis to ensure that the maximum length of the named vessel is included
  - any curvilinear incisions on the nose are preferentially changed to more acute angles to minimize the potential for postoperative trapdoor deformity
  - conservatively undermining the surgical defect of the nose just above the periosteum and perichondrium before insertion of the flap may prevent postoperative trapdoor deformity
  - dividing the pedicle as a second staged procedure at approximately postoperative day 21 is thought to allow adequate collateral vascularization to be established, which enhances the survivability of the transected pedicle flap.
- Dorsal nasal flap
  - the inclusion of the angular artery in the base improves the vascular support, allowing a more generous back-cut, which improves the flap's mobility and so the flap can be inset under less tension, lowering the risk of flap necrosis or associated nasal tissue distortion
  - wide undermining laterally to the nasal facial junction facilitates wound closure of the flap's donor area with minimal tension.
- Lip procedures
  - with larger lip wounds, the underlying orbicularis oris musculature should be repaired to allow coordinated motor activity and preservation of function.

Pitfalls and their management

- Paramedian forehead flap
  - the axial pattern paramedian forehead flap is not a simple repair, and its proper use requires appreciable operative knowledge and experience
  - discontinuation of anticoagulation may be associated with thromboembolic perioperative events, so medically necessary anticoagulant medicines are rarely withheld before reconstruction
  - scarring from previous forehead surgery increases the operative risk of flap necrosis, and this may be especially relevant in the patient who smokes
  - an oversized flap will pincushion and not provide suitable contour reconstruction
  - a flap that is too small will result in significant anatomic distortion when secondary tissue movement of the alar margin or nasal tip is required to close the wound
  - when elevating the flap, avoid removal of calvarial periosteum because this significantly slows second intention healing at the flap's donor site
  - total ischemic flap failure is uncommon, but if it occurs the surgeon may be faced with a major reconstructive challenge
  - the only common postoperative event is continued oozing from the transected pedicle near the glabella—patients must be counseled to expect some degree of minor postoperative hemorrhage from this area. it typically responds to compression with minimal blood loss.
- Dorsal nasal flap
  - the DNF's success is dependent entirely on the laxity of dorsal nasal skin, which allows the flap to be rotated to cover the primary defect under minimal tension—if the surgeon misjudges nasal laxity or misdesigns the flap's lines of incision, nasal distortion results
  - as the DNF is rotated, its effective length shortens, increasing closure tensions, which may contribute to more conspicuous scarring or anatomic distortion
  - the critical element for success is designing the leading edge of the flap—it is important for the leading edge to extend past the defect to compensate for flap shortening with rotational movement
  - hemostasis is achieved with care to avoid electrocoagulation of the skin edges, which may result in epidermal necrosis.

■ SUMMARY

Cutaneous neoplasia is commonly treated with surgical excision resulting in defects that must be repaired. The dermatologic surgeon is faced with many reconstructive options for any given soft tissue defect. Cutaneous flaps are unparalleled in their ability to restore form and function. Most wounds requiring flap closure may be repaired with random pattern cutaneous flaps. Large or more complex reconstructions require advanced reconstructive techniques. Axial pattern flaps are cutaneous flaps based on a named nutrient vessel. These robust flaps are versatile in repairing larger or more challenging wounds. Although axial pattern flaps involve significantly more surgical risk and complexity than random pattern flaps, they are unsurpassed in their ability to provide functional and aesthetic reconstruction of significant facial defects.

■ REFERENCES

1. Jemal A, Murray T, Samuels A, et al. Cancer Statistics 2003. CA Cancer J Clin 2003; 53:5–26.
2. Rowe DE, Carroll RJ, Day CL. Long term recurrence rates in previously undetected (primary) basal cell carcinoma: implications for patient follow up care. J Dermatol Surg Oncol 1989; 15:315–328.
3. Rowe DE, Carroll RJ, Day CL. Mohs' surgery is the treatment of choice for recurrent (previously treated) basal cell carcinoma. J Dermatol Surg Oncol 1989; 15:424–431.
4. Rowe DL, Carroll RJ, Day CL. Prognostic factors for local recurrence, metastasis, and survival rates in squamous cell carcinoma of the skin, ear, and lip: implications for treatment modality selection. J Am Acad Dermatol 1992; 26:976–990.
5. Zitelli JA, Borwn C, Hanusa B. Mohs micrographic surgery for the treatment of primary cutaneous melanoma. J Am Acad Dermatol 1997; 37:236–245.
6. Bumstead RM, Ceilly RI. Auricular malignant neoplasms. Arch Otolaryngol 1982; 108:229–231.
7. Downes RN, Walker NP, Collin JR. Micrographic (Mohs') surgery in the management of periocular basal cell epitheliomas. Eye 1990; 4:160–168.
8. Cook J, Zitelli JA. Mohs micrographic surgery: a cost analysis. J Am Acad Dermatol 1998;34:698–703.
9. Zitelli, JA. Wound Healing by second intention, a cosmetic appraisal. J Am Acad Dermatol 1983; 9:407–415.
10. Cuttino CA. Critical closing and perfusion pressures in flap survival. Ann Plast Surg 1982; 9:524.
11. Ferrigan CL, Daniel RK. Critical ischemia time and the failing skin flap. Plast Reconstr Surg 1982; 69:986–989.
12. Milton SH. Pedicled skin flaps: the fallacy of the length : width ratio. Br J Surg 1970; 57:502–508.
13. Tsur H, Daniller A, Strauch B. Neovascularization of skin flaps: route and timing. Plast Reconstr Surg 1980; 66:85–90.
14. Larrabee WF Jr, Holloway GA Jr, Sutton D. Wound tension and blood flow in skin flaps. Ann Otol Rhinol Laryngol 1984; 93:112–115.
15. Rees TD, Liverett DM, Guy CL. The effect of cigarette smoking on skin-flap survival in the face lift patient. Plast Reconstr Surg 1984; 73:911–915.
16. Mosely LH, Finseth F, Goody M. Nicotine and its effect on wound healing. Plast Reconstr Surg 1978; 61:570–575.
17. Nolan J, Jenkins RA, Kurihara K, et al. The acute effects of cigarette smoke exposure on experimental skin flaps. Plast Reconstr Surg 1985; 75:544–551.
18. Burget GC, Menick FJ. The subunit principle in nasal reconstruction. Plast Reconstr Surg 1985; 76:239–247.
19. Gillies HD. Plastic surgery of the face based on selected cases of war injuries of the face including burns with original illustrations. London: Oxford Medical Publication 1920; 8.
20. Mazzola RF, Marcus S. History of total nasal reconstruction with particular emphasis on the folded forehead flap technique. Plast Reconstr Surg 1983; 72:408–413.
21. Letter to the Editor. Gentleman's Magazine, London, October 1794; 891. Reprinted in Plast Reconstr Surg 1969; 44:67–69.
22. Carpue JC. An account of two successful operations for restoring a lost nose from the integuments of the forehead. London: Longman; 1816. Reprinted in Plast Reconstr Surg 1969; 44:175–185.
23. Kazanjian VH. Repair of nasal defects with the medial forehead flaps. Surg Gynecol Obstet 1946: 83:37–43.
24. McCarthy JG, Lornec ZP, Lotting C, et al. The median forehead flap revisited: the blood supply. Plast Reconstr Surg 1985; 76:866–689.
25. Mangold V, Lierse N, Pfeifer G. The arteries of the forehead as the basis of nasal reconstruction with forehead flaps. Acta Anat (Basel) 1980; 107:18–25.
26. Labat M. De la rhinoplastic, art de restaurer ou de refaire completenent la NBF (dissertation). Paris: 1834.
27. Menick FJ. Aesthetic refinements in the use of the forehead for nasal reconstruction: the paramedian forehead flap. Clin Plast Surg 1990; 17:607–622.
28. Burget GC. Aesthetic restoration of the nose. Clin Plast Surg 1985; 12:463–480.
29. Burget GC, Menick FJ. The subunit principle in nasal reconstruction. Plast Reconstr Surg 1985; 76:239–247.
30. Burget GC, Menick FJ. Nasal reconstruction: seeking a fourth dimension. Plast Reconstr Surg 1986; 78:145–157.
31. Burget GC, Menick FJ. Nasal support and lining: the marriage of beauty and blood supply. Plast Reconstr Surg 1989; 84:189–203.
32. Shumrick KA, Smith TL. The anatomic basis for the design of forehead flaps in nasal reconstruction. Arch Otolaryngol Head Neck Surg 1992; 118:373–379.
33. Cook JL, Perone JB. A prospective study of complications associated with Mohs micrographic surgery. Arch Dermatol 2003; 139:143–152.
34. Carditello A, Mule V, Milone A, et al. One day surgery: results of 3000 surgical procedures. G Chir 2001; 22:269–272.
35. West SW, Otley CG, Nguyen TH, et al. Cutaneous surgeons cannot predict blood thinner status by intraoperative visual inspection. Plast Reconstr Surg 2002; 110:98–103.
36. Kovich O, Otley CG. Thrombotic complications related to discontinuation of warfarin and aspirin therapy preoperatively for cutaneous operations. J Am Acad Dermatol 2003; 48:233–237.
37. Burget GC, Menick FJ. The paramedian forehead flap. In: Aesthetic reconstruction of the nose. St Louis: Mosby 1994; 57–91.
38. Klingenstrom P, Nylen B. Timing of transfer of tubed pedicles and cross-flaps. Plast Reconstr Surg 1966; 37:1–12.
39. Gatti JE, LaRossa D, Brousseau PA, et al. Assessment of neovascularization and timing of flap division. Plast Reconstr Surg 1984; 73:396–402.
40. Menick FJ. A ten-year experience in nasal reconstruction with the three-stage forehead flap. Plast Reconstr Surg 2002; 109:1839–1855.
41. Rieger RA. A local flap for the repair of the nasal tip. Plast Reconstr Surg 1967; 40:679–684.
42. Marchac D, Toth B. The axial frontonasal flap revisited. Plast Reconstr Surg 1985; 765:686–694.
43. Dzubow LM. Dorsal nasal flaps. In: Baker SR, Swanson NA, eds. Local flaps in facial reconstruction. St Louis: Mosby 1995; 225–246.
44. Abbe RA. A new plastic operation for the relief and deformity due to double harelip. Medical Record 1899; 53:477.
45. Renner G. Reconstruction of the lip. In: Baker SR, Swanson NA. Local flaps in facial reconstruction. St Louis: Mosby 1995; 364–367.
46. Karapandzic M. Reconstruction of lip defects by local arterial flaps. Br J Plast Surg 1974; 27:13–97.

23 Skin Grafting

Dane R Christensen MD, Christopher J Arpey MD, and Duane C Whitaker MD

Summary box

- A skin graft is a portion of skin that has been separated from its vascular supply.
- Full-thickness grafts (epidermis and dermis plus adnexal structures) generally give better results than split-thickness grafts (epidermis and partial-thickness dermis only) because they give better retention of skin function, but split-thickness grafts are more appropriate where a large area is to be grafted.
- The choice of donor site involves a balance between that which gives the best match with the recipient skin, and that which ensures both concealment and adequate healing of the donor site scar.
- Re-establishment of vascular supply at the recipient site is vital for graft survival, and impeccable technique is, therefore, essential for outcome.
- The potential role of skin substitutes in general is under investigation, however porcine grafts already have a role in second intention healing and in delayed repairs.

INTRODUCTION

Skin grafting has been performed for several centuries, with the first reports of skin grafting dating back 3000 years to India when gluteal grafts were used to reconstruct noses that had been amputated as punishment for crimes such as adultery or theft.[1,2] The early reports of skin grafting did not appear in western literature until several thousand years later in the mid-to-late 19th century.[3–5] Skin grafts have evolved over the last century from being a reconstructive option used as the last resort, to a routinely performed closure technique in dermatologic surgery.

With the increasing popularity and description of new flaps in the medical literature, the use of skin grafts by dermatologic surgeons as a surgical repair technique appears to be declining. Although perceived by some surgeons as consistently inferior to flaps or primary closure, grafts continue to offer several surgical advantages. They are technically simpler to execute than most flaps, and nearly any wound with a vascularized bed will function well as a recipient site. Grafts offer great variability in their size and shape to allow for closure of a wide variety of defects. Multiple donor sites are available, enabling selection of the closest tissue match. Disadvantages include the creation of a second surgical site and suboptimal tissue color and texture match if an improper donor site is selected. Additionally, complete denervation of the graft occurs such that patients rarely experience full sensation at the recipient site, even after prolonged periods. Despite some shortcomings, skin grafting continues to be a viable, useful, and versatile closure option, and in some instances it is the repair method of choice.

Definitions

By definition, a skin graft is a portion of skin that has been completely separated from its vascular supply. Several types of skin grafts exist. Full-thickness skin grafts contain the entire epidermis and dermis and preserve adnexal structures. Split-thickness skin grafts are composed of the epidermis and partial-thickness dermis with few or no adnexal structures. Composite grafts consist of skin and a second type of tissue; in dermatologic surgery, composite grafts most often contain cartilage, although occasionally they include adipose tissue. An autograft is a graft taken from a donor site on an individual and placed at a recipient site on the same individual, while a homograft is taken from one individual and transplanted to another of the same species. The final type of graft is a xenograft (heterograft) which is a graft that is transplanted between species (e.g. from pig to human).

Skin graft physiology

Since skin grafts are completely removed from their underlying vasculature, re-establishing a blood supply at the recipient site is essential for graft survival. The study of skin grafts has identified three stages of graft survival.[6]

Imbibition is the first stage and is an ischemic period that lasts for the first 24–48 hours.[7] The graft becomes

edematous and increases in weight by up to 40%. During this time fibrin serves to attach the graft to its new bed and the graft is sustained by the plasma exudate from the wound bed. Nutrients are obtained by passive diffusion. Ultimately the fibrin 'glue' is replaced by granulation tissue that more permanently fixes the graft to the recipient bed.

The second stage is inosculation. This is a process of revascularization that results in the linkage of dermal vessels in the graft to those present in the recipient bed.[8–11] This process begins as early as 48–72 hours and lasts for 7–10 days. This phase requires a healthy microvasculature at the recipient base and also explains why exposed bone and cartilage serve as poor substrates for grafts. Delayed grafting at sites initially devoid of periosteum or perichondrium, however, allows for the development of overlying granulation tissue and an improved chance of subsequent graft survival through successful inosculation.

The final stage of graft survival is neovascularization, which occurs through capillary ingrowth to the graft from the recipient base and sidewalls.[6,10] This phase often occurs temporally in conjunction with inosculation. The rate at which a skin graft revascularizes is a function of both the graft thickness and the vascularity of the recipient bed. Under optimal healing conditions, full circulation can be restored to the graft between the fourth and seventh day.[6]

The re-establishment of lymphatic flow occurs concurrently with the restoration of the blood supply and is usually completed by the end of the first week of graft healing.[12,13] Upon return of lymphatic drainage, the graft begins to lose the weight that was acquired during imbibition and likewise begins to lose the bulkiness noted clinically by patients and surgeons early in the healing process. Reinnervation is a much slower process that begins within 2 months but may not be complete for many months or years, and full sensation may never completely return.[14,15]

■ PREOPERATIVE PREPARATION

Preoperative consultation between the patient and surgeon is essential for a successful surgical outcome. This interaction allows the physician to assess the patient as a surgical candidate from both physical and psychological standpoints. When counseling a patient preoperatively it is important to keep in mind that from their point of view an 'explanation' offered initially is often interpreted as a 'reason' and the same explanation offered after the fact is considered to be an 'excuse.' In addition to the information outlined in Chapter 5, the medical issues particularly relevant to skin grafting include coagulation abnormalities (both primary abnormalities and those secondary to medications), alcohol consumption, smoking, vascular disease, metabolic derangements, and poor nutrition.[16–18] These issues need to be specifically addressed preoperatively because hematoma formation, or insufficient oxygenation or nutrient supply to the graft may result in graft failure.

The consultation visit also allows the surgeon to assess the individual patient's cosmetic expectations and the likelihood of postoperative compliance. While patients regularly state that they are not concerned about the surgical scar, we find this is rarely the case in reality. Postoperative compliance with wound care instructions is also essential to graft survival because certain physical activities or graft site manipulation in the immediate postoperative period may result in shearing forces between the graft and the recipient bed with subsequent graft failure. An open discussion regarding the postoperative healing time, surgical scars, and potential complications establishes a relationship between the surgeon and the patient, and also educates the patient regarding realistic postoperative expectations. We have found that patients who are well informed regarding the variety of surgical outcomes are more compliant with postoperative wound care and more satisfied over the long term.

■ TECHNIQUES

Full-thickness skin grafts

Full-thickness skin grafts (FTSG) are indicated as a repair consideration for surgical defects that cannot be apposed primarily or with a flap, and where healing by second intention is likely to result in poor cosmesis or functional deficits. Full-thickness skin grafts have a better overall cosmesis when compared to split-thickness skin grafts (STSG), resulting in less wound contracture.[19,20] However, the increased thickness of FTSG results in an increased metabolic demand and a higher rate of graft failure. This fact also limits the overall size of a FTSG that can be utilized (typically 4–5 cm) while STSG can be used to repair very large defects. Sites where FTSG are commonly utilized in dermatologic surgery include convexities and concavities of the nasal tip and alar, helix, the medial canthus, digits, and extremities, although a graft can cover nearly any site where a proper recipient bed exists.[13]

The equipment needed for performance of full-thickness skin grafting includes:

- a sterile marking pen or Gentian violet with sterile toothpick
- a #15 or #15C blade with handle
- iris scissors
- suture scissors
- Adson or Paufique toothed forceps
- a needle driver
- curved hemostats
- Telfa (Kendall, Mansfield, MA) or foil wrapping from the suture package to develop the graft template
- 5-0 fast-absorbing gut suture or mild chromic gut suture for securing the graft, and closing the donor site
- 4-0 silk suture for securing bolster (optional in some instances) and closing the donor site
- a sterile Petri dish containing saline
- bolster material (cotton balls, dental rolls, or foam)
- antibiotic ointment
- non-adherent dressing such as Adaptic (Johnson and Johnson Medical, Arlington, TX) or Xeroform (Johnson and Johnson Medical, Arlington, TX)
- mineral oil to moisten cotton balls of the bolster dressing.

Performance of full-thickness skin grafts

In the setting of oncologic surgery, before an FTSG repair is performed it is essential to ascertain the tumor-free

margins. Tumor-free margins prior to skin grafting are most commonly obtained by either Mohs micrographic surgery or through surgical pathology frozen sections. Once this type of graft is selected as the repair of choice, a donor site must be selected. When selecting a donor site, the primary goal is to best match the donor skin with the skin surrounding the recipient site. Concealment of the donor site scar and the ability to primarily close the donor site wound are highly desirable objectives. Several factors contribute to the selection process, including skin color, tissue texture, the amount of photodamage, and the presence or lack of hair. The most common donor sites include preauricular skin, postauricular skin, skin from the clavicular and inner upper arm regions, and from the upper eyelids. These areas serve as ideal tissue reservoirs for several reasons. They provide areas of tissue redundancy that have a range of tissue textures, of photodamage, and thickness. In addition, donor wounds at these sites are typically apposed easily with relatively concealed postsurgical closure lines. Finally, it is important to select a donor site that will not result in the transplantation of terminal hairs to a non-hair-bearing recipient area. This mistake most commonly occurs when too large a graft is harvested from the preauricular region that includes sideburn hair.

Once a donor site has been selected, it is anesthetized, scrubbed, and draped in a sterile fashion. A template of the defect is then made (Fig. 23.1A). A Telfa pad, or the foil packaging of suture material, serve as excellent materials for making an imprint of the defect (Fig. 23.1B). The template is laid over the donor site and outlined with a surgical marking pen or Gentian violet. We recommend oversizing the graft by 10–20% to prevent obtaining too small a graft.[21] This slight oversizing accounts for graft contracture after harvesting, and also any defect irregularities or measuring inaccuracies, without affecting donor site closure. An ellipse is subsequently drawn to include the outlined template (Fig. 23.1C). Excision of the donor site, including subcutaneous adipose, is performed, paying particular attention to handling the tissue gently and at the ellipse tips so as to cause minimal trauma to the graft tissue. The graft is quickly transferred into a basin, such as a Petri dish, containing sterile saline. Once the graft is excised it is important to work quickly and efficiently to prepare the graft for placement on its recipient bed so that nutrient diffusion can begin. To facilitate this we recommend performing only essential hemostasis at the donor site and then covering the defect with saline-soaked gauze, with final repair of the donor site occurring after the graft is fully secured in place.

Defatting of the graft is effectively performed with curved iris scissors. It is important to perform this process as soon as possible after harvesting to allow the stage of imbibition to begin. The least amount of time in the Petri dish—if any time at all—is highly desirable. The graft is held with the non-dominant hand with the subcutaneous fat exposed. The fat globules are removed by tangential cuts with the scissors (Fig. 23.1D). Some patience is required to ensure that the fat is thoroughly removed until the glistening white dermis is broadly exposed. A poor technical job during this stage results in a graft with a higher likelihood of necrosis because any remaining adipose serves as a further barrier to nutrient diffusion between the recipient bed and the graft dermis. It is very difficult to damage or remove dermis with this approach. Remoistening the graft periodically with sterile saline or local anesthetic during the defatting procedure is recommended to prevent desiccation.

In preparation for the graft application, the wound edges of the recipient site should be undermined several millimeters. This serves to minimize potential postoperative pin cushioning while allowing for uniform wound contracture, and also permits precise epidermal approximation of the donor and graft epidermis that is essential with full-thickness skin grafting. Meticulous hemostasis of the donor site is crucial because even a small amount of persistent oozing can elevate the graft from its nutrient-providing bed. Excessive electrocoagulation of the wound bed must be avoided, however, so abundant devitalized tissue is not present. We find the use of bipolar electrocautery allows for more precise pinpoint hemostasis while producing less tissue damage than monopolar units.

The graft is now ready for transfer to the recipient site. The oversized graft is draped onto the defect with the dermis side down (Fig. 23.1E). No buried sutures are required in anchoring the graft as they would introduce unnecessary foreign material into the graft base where intimate apposition is critical. They also increase the risk of hematoma formation through injury of underlying vessels during their placement. One edge of the graft is finely approximated with the apposing skin edge and sutured in place. (Fig. 23.1F). Absorbable suture such as 5-0 fast-absorbing gut or mild chromic gut are recommended. These dissolve quickly over several days and eliminate the risk of graft disruption by not requiring suture removal. The optimal suturing technique is with the needle entering the graft first, 2–3 mm from the edge, and then exiting in the adjacent recipient site skin and subsequently tied with three or four throws of a square knot. We favor the needle penetrating the graft first, because the motion is downward and results in less 'lifting' tendency of the graft from its new base. The distance between sutures is usually 3–4 mm. Simple interrupted sutures are recommended as we feel these allow for more precise apposition of the epidermal edges, although a running stitch can be used. The sutured margin serves as an anchoring point to provide for accurate trimming of the graft for an optimal fit for the defect. Gentle and precise trimming of the graft is now performed. Alternate trimming and suturing not to exceed 20% of the margin at any one time is recommended, which helps ensure an exact fit by preventing overtrimming (Fig. 23.1F–G).[22]

Basting sutures may be placed to anchor the central portion of the graft with 5-0 or 6-0 gut suture if so desired.[23,24] They are placed directly through the central portion of the graft into the recipient bed and should be positioned at least 1 cm apart. They can be useful for securing the central portion of the graft, protecting it from shearing forces and helping to maintain close contact with the recipient bed. We do not routinely find basting sutures necessary with the exceptions of large grafts or grafts placed over concave surfaces. If basting sutures are placed, we recommend this occur before peripheral sutures are placed. This approach allows inspection of the central region for inadvertent puncturing of a vessel, and coagulation if necessary, without having to remove peripheral sutures to investigate.

A tie-over bolster is now considered. While almost universally performed in the past, recent studies have

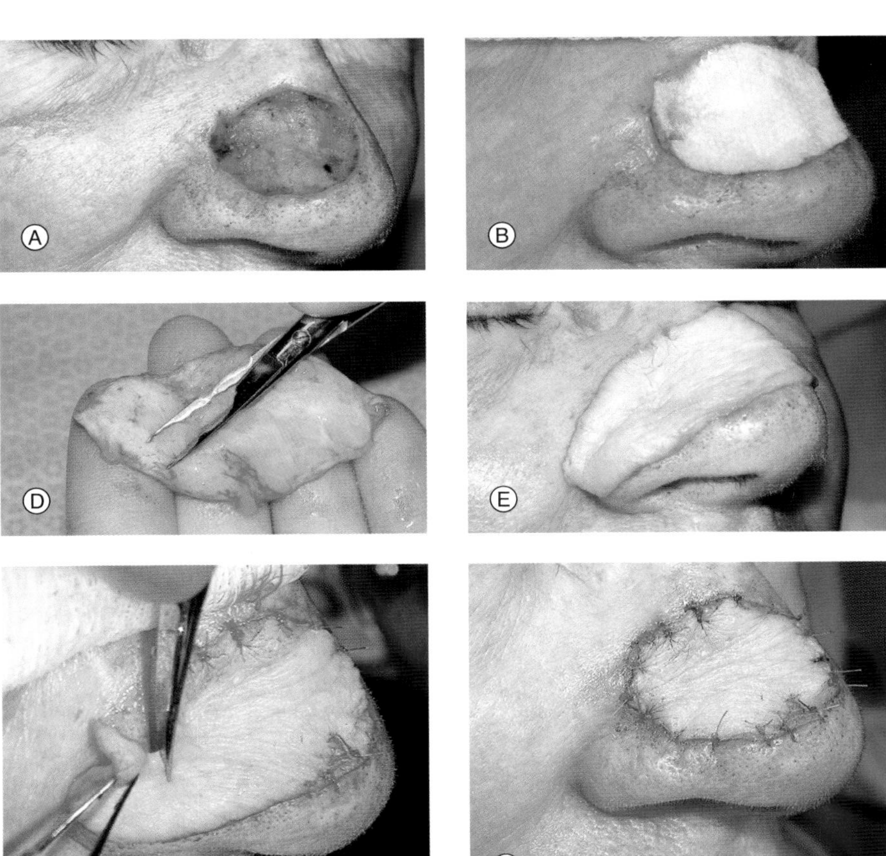

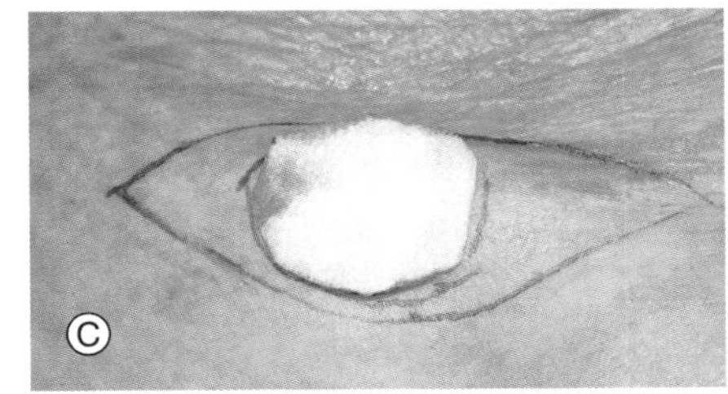

Figure 23.1 (A) Surgical defect resulting from Mohs micrographic surgery of an infiltrative basal cell carcinoma. (B) A template of the defect made from Telfa is cut to fit the defect. (C) The right clavicular skin is chosen as the donor site because of the large defect size. A slightly oversized ellipse is drawn around the template. (D) The adipose is gently trimmed away with a scissors to expose the glistening white dermis. (E) The graft is draped over the recipient site after complete defatting of the dermal side. (F) Alternating suturing and trimming is performed to obtain a perfect fit for this full-thickness skin graft. (G) The graft is now fully secured with 5-0 fast-absorbing gut sutures.

shown that bolsters are not essential for a good surgical outcome.[25,26] Advantages include further promotion of graft adherence to its recipient bed through the application of constant, direct pressure, and bolsters also help to minimize patient manipulation and inadvertent trauma of the graft. The disadvantages of a bolster are the much bulkier dressing for the patient to have to endure for a full week, and the additional time and cost required to place it. In most instances, compliant patients with small grafts in anatomically stable locations do not require bolsters, however we continue to use bolsters regularly for grafts on the extremities, or for patients who may be less reliable at avoiding trauma to their graft sites.

In preparation for the bolster dressing, tie-over sutures may be placed, although occasionally a small bolster can be securely fastened with a reliable adhesive tape such as Hypafix (Smith & Nephew Inc, Largo, FL). Silk suture performs ideally for this task with its excellent knot security and handling properties. Pairs of 4-0 caliber suture are placed opposite each other with one of the suture tails left 6–8 cm long which will be used to tie across the dressing to its paired suture on the opposite side. Larger bolsters over broader areas may require 3-0 or 2-0 caliber suture. Smaller caliber bolster sutures are much more likely to snap with the tension required to affix them. The number of sutures required varies with the size of the graft, with the optimal number being sufficient to prevent tangential movement of the bolster materials. Small full-thickness skin grafts may require only two pairs (four sutures) while larger grafts may require up to four pairs (eight sutures). Tie-over sutures can be anchored in one of two locations. They can be placed entirely within the surrounding recipient skin (Fig. 23.2A) or between the simple interrupted sutures anchoring the graft (Fig. 23.2B). Both provide for equal bolster security, but the former is favored because it does not carry the risk of further disruption of the graft either during suture placement or removal.

A bolster also consists of a thick layer of antibiotic ointment or petrolatum applied over the graft followed by a non-adherent contact layer with a product such as Xeroform (Johnson and Johnson Medical, Arlington, TX), Adaptic (Johnson and Johnson Medical, Arlington, TX), or another petrolatum-impregnated gauze.[27] A bulky material such as dental roll, layered gauze, foam, or cotton balls make up the final layer. Sutures at opposite poles are then hand tied across the bolster dressing. To ensure adequate pressure it is helpful to have an assistant apply pressure with a hemostat across the knot after the first throw of the square knot, so it does not loosen while the second throw is being performed. The hemostat is then removed as the second throw is about to be cinched down. Each suture pair is then tied in a similar fashion (Fig. 23.3). An additional protective dressing may then be applied, if so desired, over the bolster with fluffed gauze and an elastic tape such as

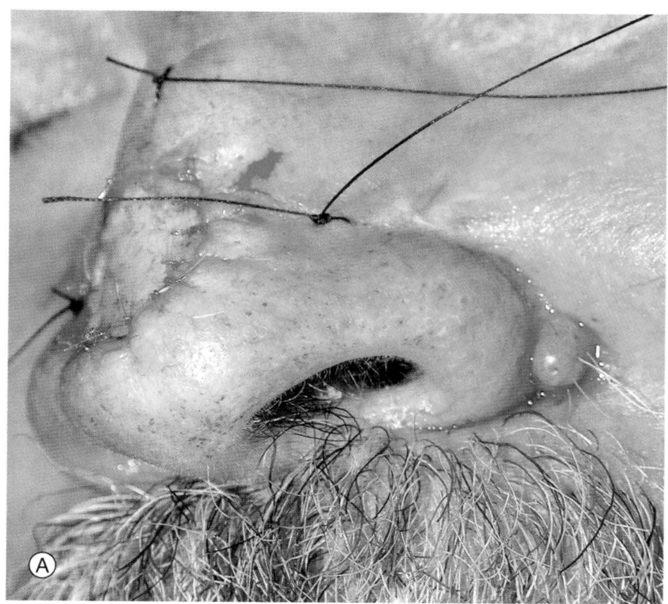

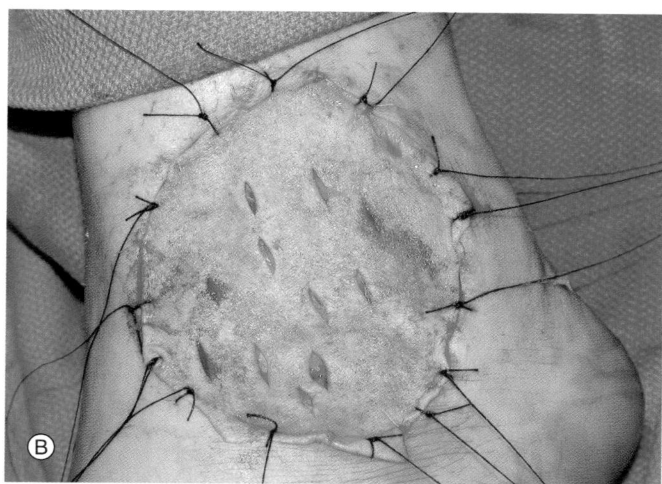

Figure 23.2 (A) Silk tie-over sutures are placed in the skin adjacent to the full-thickness skin graft. The advantage of placement of these sutures in this location is decreased risk of disrupting the graft during tie-over suture placement and removal. (B) Tie-over sutures bridging graft and recipient skin are placed between the absorbable sutures anchoring the graft.

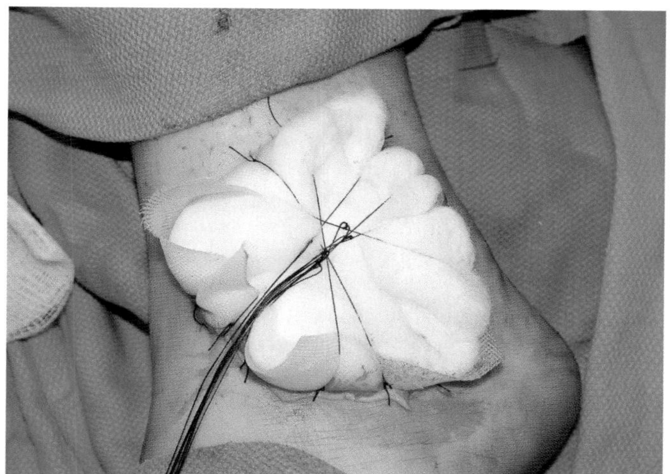

Figure 23.3 Bolster consisting of antibiotic ointment (Adaptic) and cotton balls moistened with mineral oil anchored with 3-0 silk tie-over suture.

Hypafix (Smith & Nephew Inc, Largo, FL), or Coban wrap (3M, St Paul, MN), which is particularly useful on the extremities.

After the graft is securely placed, attention is turned to the donor site for closure. This is most often closed in a layered fashion, as for any standard fusiform wound (Chapter 18). This repair should be performed carefully, attempting to conceal the scar in natural skin lines, so as to maximize the cosmetic outcome of this second scar.

In defects with a depth that cannot be adequately replaced by a full-thickness skin graft alone, several options exist. A delayed graft can be performed and this is described in detail later in this chapter. Two other options that have been described are the use of a subcutaneous hinge flap or a myocutaneous hinge flap which will more fully occupy the base of the recipient site with well-vascularized tissue.[28,29] These flaps borrow adjacent subcutaneous adipose and/or muscle tissue that is freed up and hinged like the page of a book over into the primary defect, thereby reducing the overall depth of the defect (Figs 23.4A–B). A full-thickness graft can then be placed directly over the hinge flap given that an adequate vascular bed for reliable graft survival is present (Fig. 23.4C).

Burow's graft

A Burow's graft—or island graft—is a full-thickness skin graft in which the grafted tissue does not originate from a distant donor site, but instead is obtained from skin adjacent to the defect.[30–32] They are most commonly utilized when the primary repair does not provide enough movement to fully close the defect, or if full closure would result in distortion of a free anatomic margin. In these situations, tissue removed from the dog-ear repair of the partial primary closure that would normally be discarded is instead used to repair the residual defect. The technical approach to the graft is identical to that of a conventional full-thickness skin graft. Because the standing tissue cone from adjacent skin is utilized for the Burow's graft, an excellent tissue color and texture match can be expected. Another advantage is that there is only one surgical site and thus no secondary donor defect and resultant scar.

Hair-bearing grafts

While flaps for defects in hair-bearing regions usually present the ideal closure option, hair-bearing grafts can be performed if necessary. Several important points are worth remembering when using these grafts. The donor site should possess hair that is of the same density and caliber as that of surrounding skin. For example, beard skin should be used for beard defects and scalp skin for scalp defects. The occipital and temporal regions are most commonly used as donor sites on the scalp as these areas are least likely to undergo androgenetic alopecia. In contrast to FTSG of non-hair-bearing skin, these grafts should be defatted minimally,

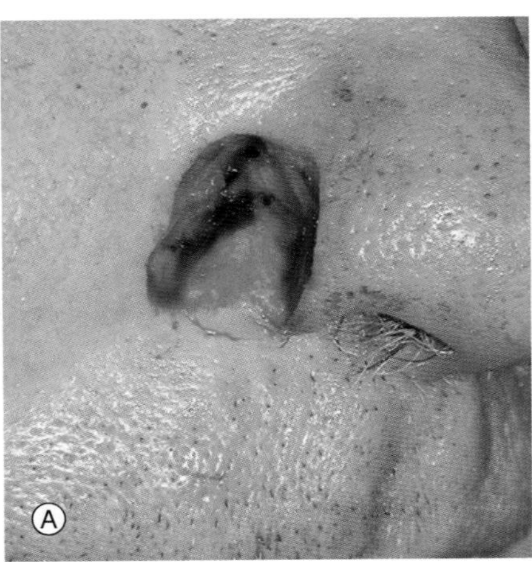

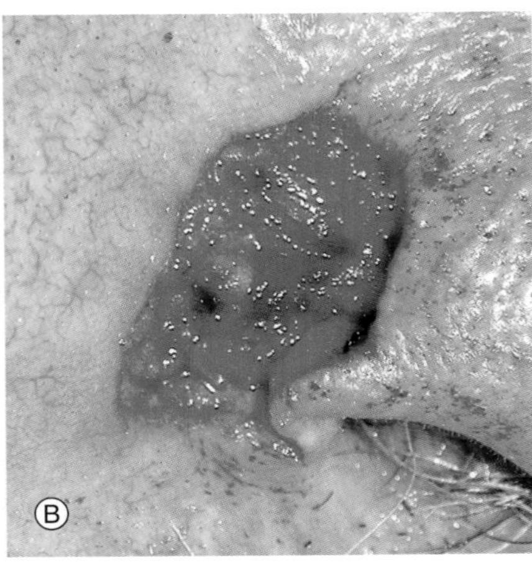

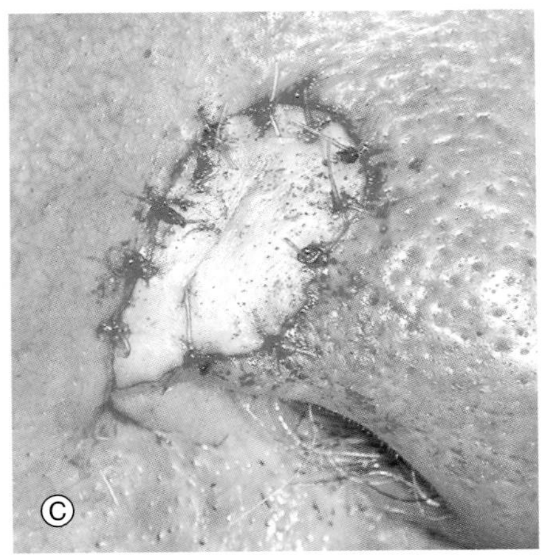

Figure 23.4 (A) Deep surgical defect after Mohs micrographic surgery of an infiltrative basal cell carcinoma involving the right nasal ala and medial cheek. (B) A significantly more shallow defect is created after a hinge flap was performed with adjacent subcutaneous tissue from the medial cheek. In this case, the hinge flap permits immediate repair of the wound with a graft, rather than a delay that would be necessary to allow granulation tissue to form. (C) Full-thickness skin graft from preauricular skin is sutured in place directly over the hinge flap with an even surface contour.

or not at all. The follicles that are to be preserved are located in the subcutis and diffuse defatting results in alopecia of the graft. Therefore, if defatting is to be performed, fat should be removed only between the hair bulbs.[22] This requires increased patience and good technique and significantly increases graft preparation time. Visualization of the follicular bulbs can be increased with the aid of surgical loupes. Even in instances where inter-follicular defatting is minimal, survivability of hair-bearing grafts is surprisingly common. Finally, it is important to orient the graft in the defect such that the hair will exit the skin in the direction of those shafts residing in the surrounding skin. An improperly oriented hair-bearing graft can result in a patched appearance. The remainder of this grafting technique is identical to that described for FTSG.

Split-thickness skin grafts

Split-thickness skin grafts (STSG) contain full-thickness epidermis and a variable amount of dermis. They generally lack adnexal structures and therefore do not produce sweat or sebum and do not grow hair. They are subclassified by their overall thickness in millimeters or thousandths of an inch, and are dependent on the amount of dermis included in the graft. Subdivisions include thin (0.125–0.275 mm), medium (0.275–0.4 mm) and thick (0.40–0.75 mm).[13] The majority of the grafts harvested for use in the head and neck region are typically 0.3–0.4 mm (0.012–0.016 inches) thick, while slightly thicker grafts of 0.5–0.6 mm (0.020–0.024 inches) are more commonly utilized for defects on the trunk and extremities.

As with all surgical repairs, split-thickness skin grafts have benefits and limitations. Major advantages include the ability to cover very large defects (>5 cm) and the higher likelihood of graft survival under suboptimal circumstances as nearly any wound bed can provide adequate nutritional support for such thin tissue. Occasionally, exposed bone or cartilage will support an split-thickness graft, but some vascularization of the bed is still highly desirable, and delayed STSG are as much an option as delayed FTSG in order to allow for an improved chance of survival. In addition, because these grafts are thin they allow for earlier detection of tumor recurrence in the setting of cutaneous oncology. Therefore, they are particularly useful at surgical sites where there are concerns about clear surgical margins or in situations where, because of an aggressive-behaving tumor or other extenuating circumstances, the risk of recurrent malignancy is believed to be higher. STSG also may be fenestrated; this allows for expansion of the surface area of the graft, a smaller portion of donor skin to be harvested, and for egress of serum or blood in patients with coagulopathy or lymphatic drainage impairment.

Disadvantages of split-thickness grafts include a less cosmetically desirable color or texture match with surrounding skin and the need for specialized equipment. The degree of contracture is more significant than with FTSG and this fact is particularly important to consider if STSG are being used to repair defects around a free anatomic margin. Finally, this repair creates a significant second granulating surgical site, which requires further postoperative care.

Equipment necessary for the performance of split-thickness grafts includes:

- a general dermatologic surgery tray
- graft-harvesting instrumentation
- a #10 or #15 scalpel blade, or a Weck blade (Pilling Weck Surgical Inc, Port Washington, PA), or an air-driven or electric dermatome
- a graft mesher or #11 blade to hand-mesh (optional)
- 5-0 fast-absorbing gut or mild chromic gut suture
- bolster materials
- mineral oil.

Harvesting of split-thickness grafts

Split-thickness grafts can be harvested by one of three techniques. For small defects the necessary tissue can be obtained with the free-hand use of a #10 or #15 blade. One advantage is that this can be performed quickly without the use of additional equipment.[33] A significant disadvantage is that it is much more difficult to obtain a graft with a uniform dermal thickness with this technique. For this reason we prefer harvesting the majority of our grafts with the use of a Weck blade or a powered dermatome.

The Weck blade (Fig. 23.5) is a specialized free-hand knife that has accompanying templates which allow selection of various graft thicknesses. The graft is obtained by holding the donor skin taught and then a sawing motion is performed while placing moderate downward and forward pressure across the blade. The blade is virtually parallel to the skin surface during harvesting. This is a relatively simple technique that is easily learned and the equipment is very inexpensive and easy to maintain. Harvesting skin with a Weck blade is analogous to performing a large shave biopsy with a single-edged razor blade on a handle.

Air-driven or electric dermatomes are used when split-thickness grafts are necessary to cover larger defects that are several centimeters in size or greater. Brown developed the first of these devices in the 1940s.[34] These pieces of equipment have continued to evolve and the newest models, such as the Zimmer electric dermatome (Zimmer Inc, Warsaw, IN) (Fig. 23.6) allow for varying thicknesses and widths. Graft thickness is adjusted by a control lever on the side of the dermatome that allows for grafts up to 0.75 mm in thickness (Fig. 23.7). Four width plates are available that deliver grafts that are 25 mm, 50 mm, 75 mm or 100 mm wide and these plates are easily attached to the underside of the dermatome with the crossed-head screwdriver provided. The graft obtained (Fig. 23.8) can be further enlarged with the use of a meshing device. Meshing can increase the ability to cover a defect by 25–35% and it also increases the flexibility of the graft so it can be used over mobile surfaces such as joints.

The typical mesher contains a flat bed with a roller that compresses the harvested skin on a plastic carrier with a predetermined 'grid' pattern etched into the plastic with available expansion ratios of 1.5 : 1, 2 : 1, 3 : 1, and 4 : 1 (Fig. 23.9). Once the plastic carrier is compressed between

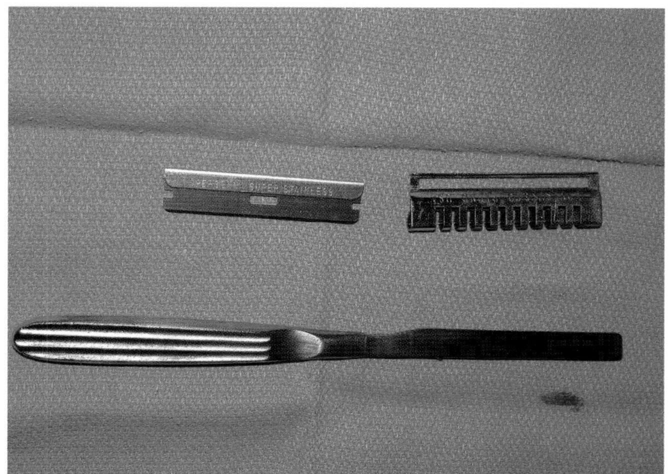

Figure 23.5 Weck blade components including the knife handle, blade, and a template that controls the split thickness skin graft.

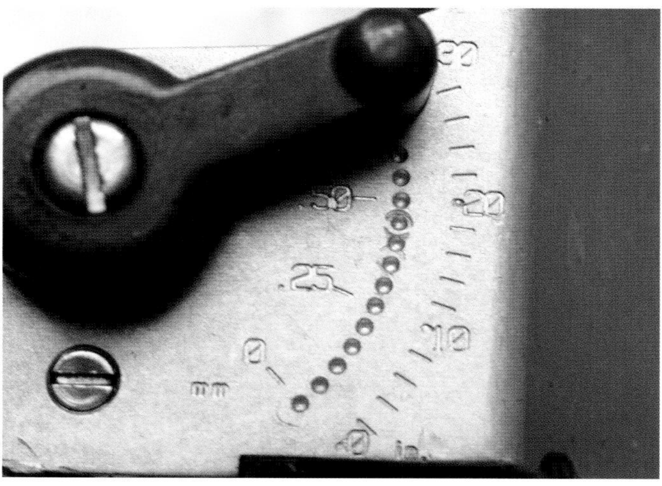

Figure 23.7 The control lever on the side of the dermatome allows for easy and precise selection of graft thickness. It is scaled in both millimeters and thousandths of an inch.

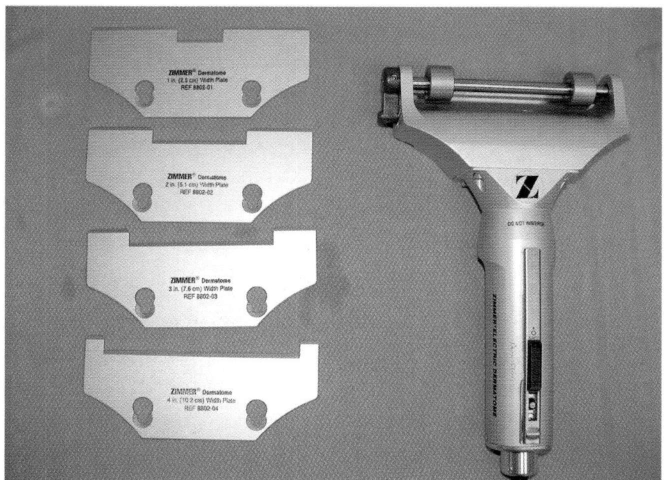

Figure 23.6 The Zimmer electric dermatome and its four width plates.

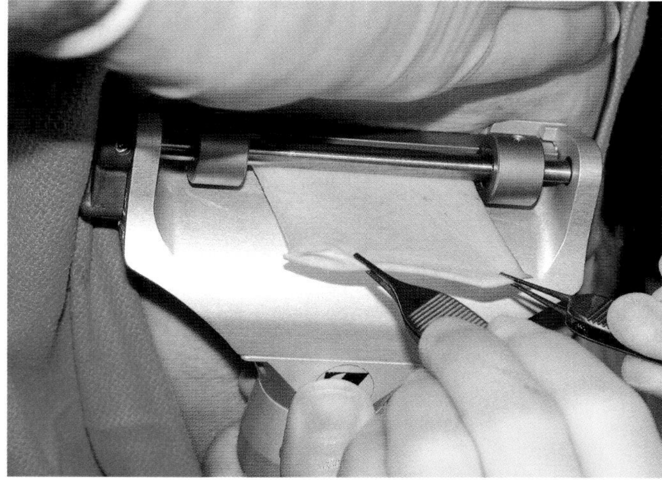

Figure 23.8 Harvesting of a graft with the Zimmer electric dermatome from the anterolateral thigh. The surgeon applies pressure with the non-dominant hand distal to the advancing dermatome while an assistant delivers the graft with toothed forceps.

the steel roller and its bed, the graft emerges on the opposite side with uniform fine fenestrations. Other meshers function similarly, but make use of rollers with variably placed serrations that create the fenestrations. Once a roller of desired expansion is selected it is inserted directly into the meshing device and with this technique the graft is delivered through the machine on a skin graft carrier. The whole process takes minutes, and the major caveat is that the graft should be maintained flat as it is compressed such that it does not become stuck in the roller mechanism. The likelihood of this can be lessened by the application of several drops of sterile saline or mineral oil to the harvested tissue, and this also prevents desiccation. Smaller and fewer fenestrations can be easily accomplished with a #11 blade.

Performance of split-thickness skin grafts

When split-thickness skin grafting is indicated for repair, the initial step is selection of a donor site.[35] Various donor sites are available and typically include the upper thigh (medial, anterior, and lateral portions), lateral hips, inner aspect of the upper arms, low back, and abdomen. For large defects requiring the use of a powered dermatome we prefer the proximal anterior thigh. This donor site provides a broad tissue reservoir that can be easily flattened manually during tissue harvesting. Additionally, this site is easily accessible to the patient for performing the necessary postoperative wound care and is hidden under clothing for cosmetic camouflage. For small defects such as those involving the ear, the skin over the mastoid process or superior medial arm provide ample tissue reservoirs that are well concealed postoperatively.

The donor site should be prepared and draped in the normal sterile fashion and local anesthesia obtained. A template should be utilized to assure the harvested graft is of adequate size. Recall that when attempting to cover very large defects a meshing device can be utilized so that the donor site can be undersized by 25–35%.

A thin layer of mineral oil, antibiotic ointment, or other skin lubricant should be applied to moisten the donor site if a mechanical dermatome is to be used because this decreases friction and eases graft harvesting. Utilization of an assistant makes graft harvesting much more efficient and is essential for graft extraction using a powered dermatome. The donor skin must be pulled taught and flat and this is best accomplished with the surgeon's non-dominant hand, while the dominant hand operates the dermatome. The mechanical dermatome is then engaged with the skin at a 30–45° angle and persistent downward and forward pressure is applied to the dermatome until the end of the template is reached. Failure to correctly perform this step can result in an uneven graft or even premature graft transection. As the graft begins to appear through the dermatome delivery port, the assistant uses two toothed forceps on the corners of the emerging skin to gently lift the graft off of the dermatome with light tension, thus preventing it from folding on itself, until harvesting is complete (Fig. 23.8). The graft is then promptly transferred into a sterile saline-containing Petri dish or directly onto the recipient site. The donor site should be temporarily covered with gauze soaked in 1% lidocaine with epinephrine (adrenaline) while attention is quickly turned back to the graft. The epinephrine (adrenaline) in the solution promotes hemostasis in this acute, abrasion-like donor site.

If meshing is desired it should be performed at this time. We recommend mechanical meshing of grafts that are being used to cover defects >8 cm in diameter or when extensive serosanguineous drainage is anticipated. One limitation of mechanical meshing is a less desirable cosmetic outcome as often this procedure results in a honeycombed graft appearance that is usually not seen with hand-meshed smaller grafts. Smaller grafts can be easily hand meshed while the graft is soaking in the Petri dish or after suturing with the use of a #11 blade.

The graft is then quickly transferred to the recipient site (Figs 23.10A–C). The graft is trimmed as necessary to fit the defect, however this does not need to be performed as precisely as with FTSG because any graft tissue that overhangs the adjacent epidermis will quickly slough off. Peripheral placement of 5-0 fast-absorbing gut or mild chromic gut suture affixes the graft (Figs 23.10D–E). We most often make use of simple sutures placed at 5–6 mm intervals although a running suture can be utilized after a few anchoring sutures have been placed. Staples offer another method of securing the graft to the recipient bed, although subsequent removal is then required, as opposed to the absorbable sutures suggested above.[36,37] A bolster or pressure dressing as described under FTSG should then be applied.

Attention is subsequently turned to the donor site that is best treated as a superficial abrasion (Fig. 23.10F). Further hemostasis is usually not necessary. A moist occlusive dressing is applied making use of antibiotic ointment or petrolatum and a polymer film such as Tegaderm (3M, St Paul, MN) or Opsite (Smith & Nephew Inc, Largo, FL).[38] A pressure dressing or wrap can be applied to reduce trauma and diminish serum exudate, if so desired. Such moist occlusion significantly decreases postoperative pain at the site and promotes re-epithelialization. Often there is significant drainage at the donor site over the initial 48 hours, and patients are instructed to either focally lance the film dressing at the site of fluid collection to allow for drainage or to simply perform more frequent dressing changes. This surgical site re-epithelializes over 2–3 weeks

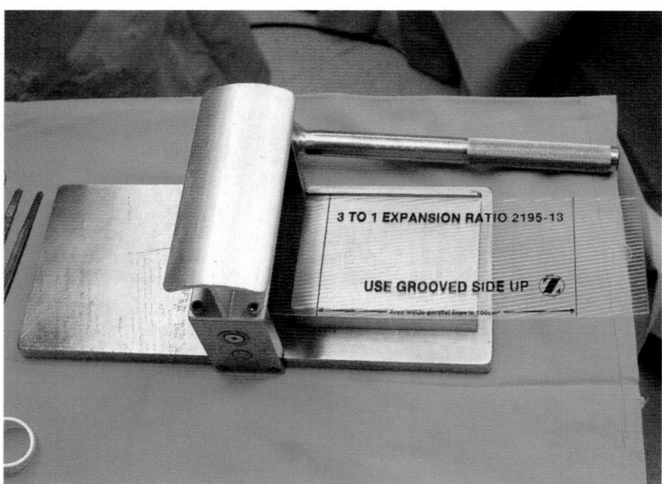

Figure 23.9 A Zimmer meshing device (Zimmer Inc, Warsaw, IN). The single use plastic carrier contains a grid that determines the expansion ratio. The harvested graft is spread onto the carrier and advanced through the mesher by the attached ratchet.

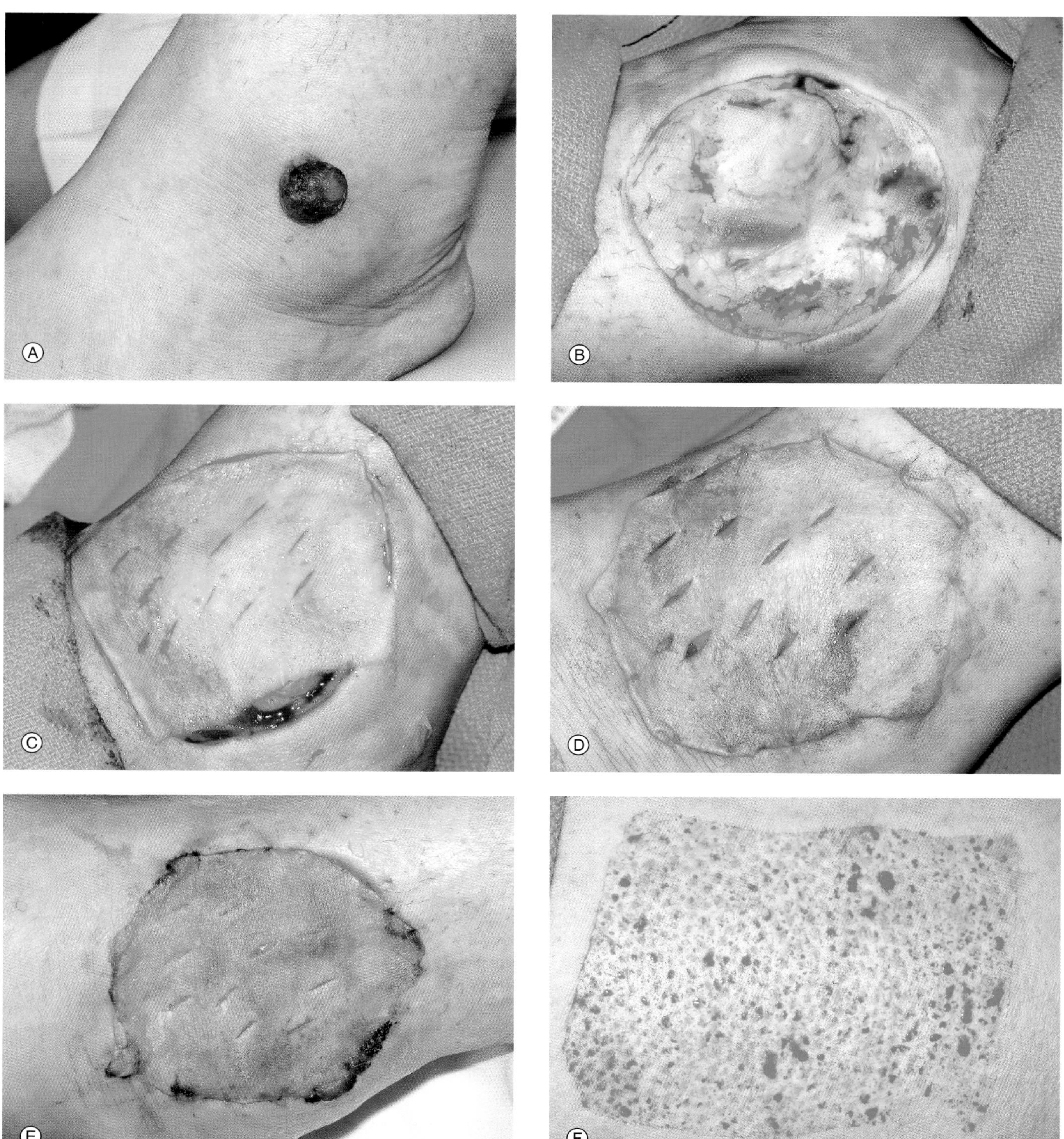

Figure 23.10 (A) Preoperative photograph of large nodular melanoma over the left lateral malleolus. (B) Postoperative defect after wide local excision with 3-cm margins. (C) A 0.45-mm thickness split-thickness skin graft was harvested with an electric dermatome from the left thigh, hand meshed, and placed over the recipient site. (D) The graft is trimmed and sutured to fit the defect. (E) Appearance of the graft at the time of bolster removal and dressing change 1 week after surgery. (F) Pinpoint bleeding is present at the donor site; however, further hemostasis beyond the direct pressure from the dressing is not required.

and typically remains pink for several months and later becomes hypopigmented.

Composite grafts

In the head and neck region, cartilage contributes significantly to maintaining the anatomic structure and function of the nose and ears. Occasionally, cartilage in these areas must be sacrificed during cancer surgery, resulting in both structural and functional deficits requiring repair. In most situations where the loss of cartilage results in a functional deficit the cartilage should be replaced in order to provide patency of the nostrils or ear canals. One method of restoring the lost structure is with a composite graft.

A composite graft is simply a modified FTSG that contains more than one tissue component. In the realm of dermatologic reconstructive surgery, the additional tissue is most often cartilage. However, the survival of composite grafts is more tenuous than FTSG. Revascularization of FTSG occurs from vessels throughout both the base and edges of the graft, while composite grafts only obtain their new vascular supply from the subdermal plexus of the wound and graft edges.[39] Given the limited pattern of revascularization of composite grafts, their size is limited. Authors addressing this subject suggest maximum graft diameters ranging from 1–2 cm to minimize the risk of necrosis.[40–42] As suggested by Burget and Menick[42] one should strive for maximum graft diameters of approximately 1.5 cm, such that no point of the graft is more than 0.75 cm from a vascular source. Fortunately, in the two locations where these grafts are most often utilized, the nose and ear, a rich vascular network exists.

The use of composite grafts is most often utilized in dermatologic surgery to repair defects of the nasal ala. The loss of alar cartilage can result in incompetence of the nasal valve and decreased stability of the ala, such that during inspiration nasal tissue is pulled inward toward the nasal septum resulting in decreased airflow and functional compromise. Cartilage is utilized as part of the graft to restore structure and to maintain proper function by preventing alar collapse during inspiration. The ear usually serves as the donor site, with the crus of the helix being most commonly employed, although the helical rim and concha can also be utilized.[43] These grafts have the best tissue match with that of the nasal ala, namely thin and flexible cartilage with relatively thin overlying skin and subcutis.[42] If the tissue surrounding the alar defect is sebaceous and bulky, the tissue match will undoubtedly be poor and another reconstructive option should be considered, including placement of cartilaginous struts alone followed by a local flap or delayed skin grafting after granulation over the cartilage occurs.

In an attempt to increase composite graft survival, some surgeons have suggested increasing the surface area for revascularization by developing the tongue-in-groove technique.[44] This technique involves converting the defect into a wedge that fits geometrically with the groove created on the composite graft. Others have suggested modifying this concept, utilizing a reverse tongue-in-groove technique, and this is the design we currently favor for the repair of full-thickness nasal ala defects.[45]

This reverse tongue-in-groove approach requires 5–10% oversizing of the graft when compared to the defect site. The skin and cartilage of the helical crus are harvested en bloc as a skin–cartilage–skin 'sandwich' graft. The graft should be handled very diligently and the graft should be kept moist at all times. A small amount of skin is removed from each end of the graft so the remaining skin will perfectly fill the surface defect. This leaves exposed cartilage 'pegs' at each end of the graft. A pocket is then made with a hemostat or scalpel medially and laterally in the soft tissue of the recipient site that will be filled with the cartilage pegs of the graft. This process results in interlocking of the recipient and graft tissues. The nasal mucosal side of the graft is sutured with 6-0 mild chromic gut or fast-absorbing gut suture. The skin surface is then sutured with 6-0 non-absorbable sutures. If the mucosal lining is still intact after tumor clearance, it provides a viable base for graft placement. In this situation, the only modification to the above description is that the harvested composite graft needs only to contain one layer of skin. If small, the donor site can be left unrepaired with acceptable cosmetic results. This site can also be repaired with an upward advancement or rotation flap or transposition flap avoiding the use of hair-bearing skin whenever possible.[46] A 1-week dressing making use of non-stick products such as Adaptic or Xeroform is applied and should be positioned to apply support in the nasal vestibule. The gentle use of ice packs is encouraged to minimize tissue swelling. Regular use of postoperative antibiotics in these patients is recommended because of heavy bacterial colonization of the nares. Suture removal is performed at 1 week.

Delayed grafts

Periodically it is necessary for the dermatologic surgeon to make use of a delayed graft.[47,48] The characteristics of the recipient bed and understanding the nutritional requirements of skin grafts determine when this technique should be utilized. Defects that most commonly necessitate a delayed graft are those that have a significant amount of exposed bone or cartilage, where greater than 25% of the periosteum or perichondrium is lacking. These recipient bases often provide inadequate nutrition, and grafts placed directly over them are at increased risk of necrosis. A second scenario where this repair option is useful is in a deep primary defect with a depth that cannot be adequately filled by an FTSG at the time of initial surgery. A relatively simple solution to this dilemma is the utilization of a delayed graft.

The wound is allowed to granulate for 1–3 weeks, depending on the patient's rate of wound healing, at which time delayed grafting is performed. As these defect sites often contain exposed cartilage or bone, we encourage the use of dilute acetic acid for wound cleansing, as it is less desiccating. To reduce cost, patients can mix and refrigerate their own acetic acid using a ratio of 15 ml of white table vinegar to 1 liter of clean tap water.[49] They then soak or clean the wound twice daily with a cotton-tipped applicator to gently remove any debris. The granulation tissue that develops provides a well-vascularized bed that is much more likely to promote graft survival. Preparation for delayed grafting involves beginning oral antibiotics, such as dicloxacillin or cephalexin (500 mg twice daily), or clindamycin (150 mg three times daily in penicillin-allergic patients), 1 day prior to the procedure and continuing for 4 days postoperatively.

On the day of surgery for the delayed graft, the recipient site is scrubbed vigorously with a sterilizing agent such as povidone-iodine or chlorhexidine as these wounds are likely to be colonized with some bacteria, despite antibiotics. Care should be taken during cleaning, however, not unwittingly to debride excess granulation tissue, perichondrium, or periosteum. The recipient base should be 'freshened' and any eschar present should be removed with an iris scissors or scalpel blade, particularly at the peripheral margins where apposition of graft dermis and epidermis will occur. The remainder of the grafting technique is identical to those described for routine FTSG and STSG.

Skin substitutes

The potential for use of skin substitutes in dermatology has been increasing recently. The initial products were used in the late 1970s, and the initial application of these products was in treating non-healing ulcers or burn wounds.[50,51] A more recent application in dermatology has been treating the wounds of patients with dystrophic epidermolysis bullosa as well as postsurgical wounds.[52–54] In 1998, Apligraf (Organogenesis Inc, Canton, MA) became the first biomedical device containing living human cells approved for use by the Food and Drug Administration (FDA). Epidermal, dermal, and composite or bilayer (epidermal and dermal) skin substitutes exist and this classification is based on their components. These products can be further subdivided into temporary or permanent; synthetic/biosynthetic or biological; and allogeneic/xenogeneic or autogeneic.[55]

While there are no definitive indications for use of these products in dermatologic surgery currently, work to evaluate their potential roles in treating postsurgical wounds is ongoing. Shelf-life and cost are two potential limitations when considering clinical utility of these products in the realm of dermatologic surgery. The cost of a single bioengineered graft can range from several hundred to more than a thousand dollars. Shelf-life also will play a role because in dermatologic surgery it is not always possible to predict preoperatively when a skin substitute might be utilized. For this reason, products with a short shelf-life are not practical for most dermatologic surgeons to stock in their clinics or surgical facilities. However, products such as Oasis (porcine small intestine submucosa; Cook Inc, Bloomington, IN) and Mediskin 1 (porcine STSG; Brennan Medical Inc, St Paul, MN) are products that provide surgeons flexibility in clinical practice because of their long shelf-life and relative affordability. We have found porcine xenografts to have the most versatility among this group of products. These biological dressings are described in greater detail in the following section.

Porcine xenografts

Porcine xenografts, while temporary, can play an important functional role in dermatologic surgery. The two situations where these grafts are most commonly utilized in dermatologic surgery are in second intention healing and in delayed repairs. These grafts are occlusive biological dressings that promote granulation and may remain in place for 7–10 days. Essentially they require no wound care from the patient.[56–58] These grafts can be particularly useful in the elderly or incapacitated patients where home wound care would be especially difficult. Other advantages include covering vital structures such as bone, cartilage, tendons, and nerves, and the use of these grafts decreases postoperative pain at the granulating surgical site. These grafts also function to predict potential autograft survival. Healthy appearing porcine heterografts at 1 week suggest the presence of a good environment for autograft viability, while a necrotic-appearing heterograft often predicts subsequent failure for an autograft. Additionally, these grafts are inexpensive (approximately US$20 per graft, for 5 × 5 and 7.5 × 10 cm sizes) and are easily applied. Disadvantages include the need to be replaced approximately 1 week after initial application, with subsequent reapplication of a new heterograft if additional granulation of the base is desired. These grafts may become malodorous after several days and should not be used in patients with pork-meat allergy or hypersensitivity.

Porcine xenografts are prepared from domestic swine and harvested as split-thickness skin grafts with a thickness of 0.25 mm with a dermatome. They are sterilized, packaged, and frozen, and can be stored in a medicinal freezer for up to 2 years. Such grafts are also available in room temperature forms at a comparable cost, although their shelf-life is limited to 18 months.

In anticipation of application, the graft is removed from the freezer and thawed which is easily performed in less than 5 minutes by warming the package between the hands. The graft is then removed from its packaging. Attention should be paid to the folded side of the graft as the fold is toward the dermal side of the xenograft. While maintaining sterile technique, the dermal side of the graft is placed down onto the wound base. The graft does not need to be extensively trimmed as any excess graft will simply desiccate and slough, in a similar way to autologous STSG. The graft is then sutured in place with a few 5-0 fast-absorbing or mild chromic gut and a light pressure dressing is applied (Figs 23.11a–b).

The graft should be inspected at 5–7 days. A healthy appearing graft that has received adequate nutrition is dried and shriveled at the edges with a white to pink center that is adherent to the wound base. An unhealthy graft is dark colored or necrotic and malodorous (Fig. 23.11c). The latter appearance is an indication that the wound base is not likely to support an autograft. One should not mistake a small underlying hematoma, or a focal 'bruised' appearance of portions of the graft, for necrosis. The graft should be removed after 7 days and the wound inspected and cleansed. Depending on the clinical situation, a secondary repair can be performed or another xenograft can be placed if so desired, and this can be repeated weekly as necessary, based on the patient's progress. Additional granulation can also be accomplished at this stage by moist occlusive wound care in the absence of a new heterograft depending on host factors and clinical judgment.

■ POSTOPERATIVE CARE

The postsurgical care for all grafts is essentially the same. It is most important to avoid shearing forces on the graft and its new bed so that neovascularization can occur without interruption. The biggest risk to graft survival comes from the patients themselves. There is a natural curiosity about

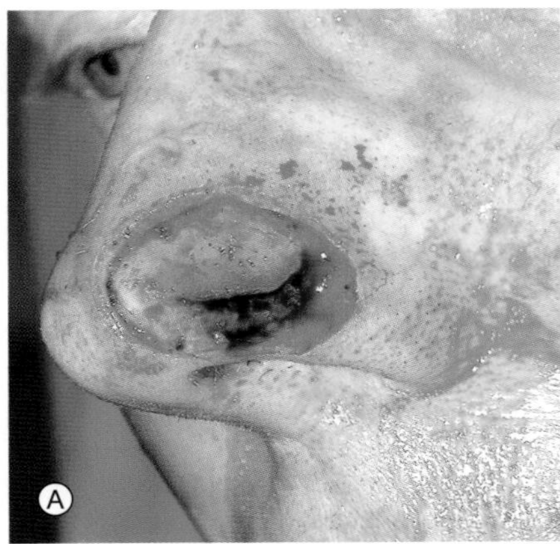

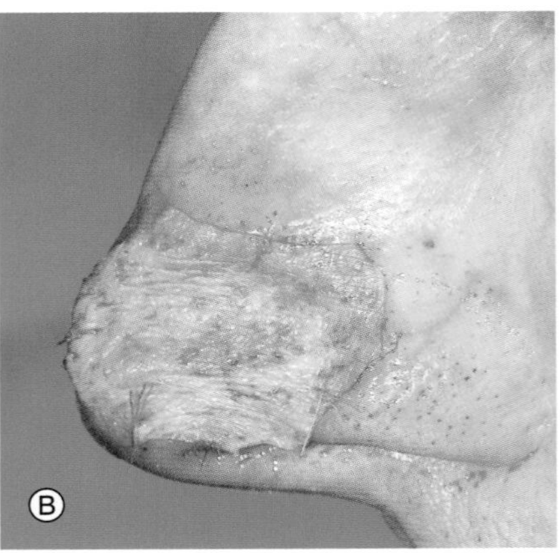

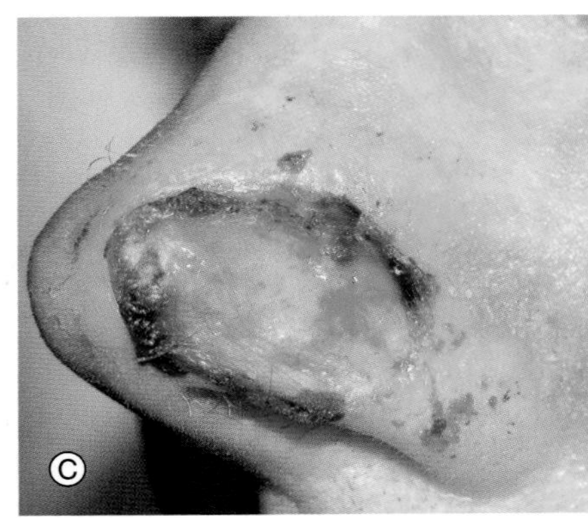

Figure 23.11 (A) Surgical defect of the left ala resulting from Mohs micrographic surgery for an invasive squamous cell carcinoma. A large portion of the lateral crus of the greater alar cartilage is exposed. (B) A delayed full-thickness skin graft repair is planned and therefore a porcine xenograft is trimmed and anchored with several fast-absorbing gut sutures. (C) Healthy appearing xenograft at 1 week with a white center that is adherent to the wound bed.

the surgical site and the graft, so the patient must be definitively counseled about the importance of not manipulating the dressing or graft as this can compromise its survival. This may also be a challenge because the site may be pruritic or uncomfortable. Strenuous activities must be avoided so that physical stress is not placed on the graft and marked elevation of blood pressure is avoided. The goal is to reduce the risk of bleeding and hematoma formation. Decreased ambulation though the use of crutches and leg elevation are essential in lower extremity grafts. Splints or slings can be used on the hand and upper extremity sites to protect grafts at sites of movement, and these also function as a constant reminder to the patient to avoid trauma to these areas.

The graft site should be kept dry for 1 week at which time patients return for bolster or dressing removal and inspection of the donor and recipient sites. Any tie-over sutures are removed, and the dressing is gently assessed for adherence to the graft. Quick removal of an adherent dressing by an unsuspecting surgeon or assistant may lift the graft off its base. Simply moistening the contents of the dry bolster with saline will loosen the dressing from the graft. One edge of the dressing can then be elevated slowly and removed across the breadth of the graft.

At 1 week FTSG are typically violaceous in appearance (Fig. 23.12). This can be alarming to the patient and reassurance should be provided that this is the expected and natural progression of graft healing. In the uncommon situation where the graft is more black and potentially necrotic appearing, the temptation for quick debridement must be resisted.[18] In this clinical situation, there may still only be partial graft loss, and watchful waiting for an additional 5–7 days may lead to an improvement in appearance. Even in the worst-case scenario, where the entire graft does become necrotic, it functions as a biologic dressing that will function to promote healing over the near term. Often when a graft appears particularly dusky, the epidermis sloughs over a viable dermis and re-epithelialization occurs from the appendageal structures. One of the clues that the surface of a FTSG is truly necrotic is a 'gummy' or 'spongy' feel upon gentle pinching of the surface with toothed forceps. In instances where a graft fails to survive, it is imperative that the surgeon and patient consider the potential cause or causes of failure. Of particular interest are host factors such as recipient bed bleeding, vascular compromise, or lack of nutrients in the base, or infection, trauma, or tobacco use. Surgeons should also consider their own graft techniques—harvesting, trimming, and suturing. All of these factors will influence whether a second graft is also likely to fail, and whether an alternative repair method should be considered.

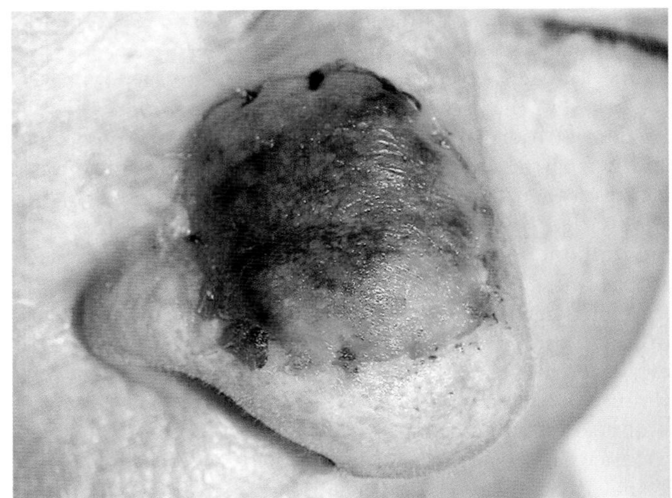

Figure 23.12 The typical violaceous appearance of a healthy full-thickness skin graft on the right nasal tip on postoperative day 7.

After bolster removal, the site is cleansed with half-strength hydrogen peroxide or saline compresses. A dressing composed of antibiotic ointment, non-stick gauze, and adhesive tape is then applied. This dressing is kept dry and in place for another 2–3 days. Daily wound care is begun with twice daily cleansing with hydrogen peroxide to remove any debris, and the site should remain covered with antibiotic ointment or petrolatum and a bandage. If the patient is not going to be doing the wound care, it is important to have the primary caregiver present for instructions regarding ongoing management of donor and recipient sites. Patients having difficulty caring for their grafts often benefit from home health nurses for early dressing changes.

At 2 weeks, most grafts undergo a transition from the early violaceous color to pink, and subsequently toward a more normal appearance. Continued use of a thick emollient, such as plain petrolatum, may help to keep the graft moist, particularly in those patients who tend to form more crust around wound margins. After 2–3 weeks, however, topical therapy is optional for most individuals. A bandage is no longer required unless the patient desires one or the patient is in a dirty environment. Patients are reminded of the importance of continuing to avoid trauma to the surgical site. At 1 month, wound care may be stopped and the patient can begin to treat the site as normal skin, including the use of cosmetics.

STSG differ only in that they are pink to skin colored as early as the 1-week dressing change, and this may influence patient counseling (Fig. 23.13A). If the graft had been oversized, the excess peripheral tissue is dry and sloughing at this point and can be painlessly trimmed off if desired. Re-epithelialization of fenestrations of extensively meshed grafts can require up to 6–8 weeks, and patients should be advised accordingly. STSG have a tendency to become dry, scaly, and hyperkeratotic over time and therefore the liberal use of emollients such as plain petrolatum is recommended (Fig. 23.13B).

PITFALLS AND THEIR MANAGEMENT

Avoidance of pitfalls

- Routine antibiotics are not necessary in the perioperative period provided that proper sterile technique is used at donor and recipient sites; however, treat any early signs of postoperative infection promptly to avoid graft failure.
- To avoid elevation of the graft due to fluid collection at its base, use meticulous hemostasis and, if possible, discontinue anticoagulants before and during surgery.
- Educate the patient to refrain from physical activities that may provoke bleeding, e.g. exercise and heavy lifting.
- Advise the patient that cool compresses over the dressing and, for craniofacial grafts, sleeping with an extra pillow will reduce swelling.
- Maturation of grafts takes many months therefore postoperative follow-up and reassurance are important.

Postoperative complications can be divided into those relating to short-term graft failure and functional or aesthetic long-term problems.[59]

The most common complication leading to loss of any graft is fluid collection at the graft base that elevates it from the recipient bed. This most commonly occurs with hematoma formation but a seroma can produce the same unwanted result. Meticulous hemostasis is essential for this reason and when medically possible, the discontinuation of anticoagulants should be considered. Aspirin should be discontinued for 2 weeks, and non-steroidal anti-inflammatory drugs avoided for 5–7 days prior to surgery. If cessation of warfarin is possible, we stop it 2–4 days prior to surgery and restart it the day following surgery. Some recent studies have shown no increased risk of complications in patients where anticoagulants were not discontinued preoperatively. We do perform skin grafts on patients in this setting; however, if consultation with the prescribing physician reveals no contraindications, we temporarily discontinue anticoagulants when possible.[60,61]

It is imperative that the patient does not engage in physical activities such as exercising or heavy lifting, which may increase blood pressure and promote bleeding. The patient may use cool compresses over the dressing to decrease swelling. In addition, sleeping with the head elevated on an extra pillow for a few nights also may reduce swelling in patients with craniofacial grafts. A few small incisions can be placed in the graft with a #11 or #15 blade to allow fluid that may accumulate to drain, instead of collecting below the graft and elevating it. A tie-over bolster or compression dressing also helps prevent this complication.

Proper surgical and sterile techniques at both the donor and recipient sites result in a very low rate of infection. For this reason we do not routinely prescribe antibiotics in the perioperative period with the exception of delayed grafts, or in cases where the surgical wound had been open for a prolonged period secondary to lengthy cancer surgery. Early signs of infection postoperatively, however, should be treated quickly with appropriate oral antibiotics, because untreated infection will likely result in graft failure.

Long-term complications include poor cosmesis and functional deficits. The maturation of skin grafts, particularly FTSG, to their final appearance takes many months, and long-term remodeling extends for years. Therefore, education of the patient prior to surgery and postoperative follow-up and reassurance are of particular importance. STSG are nearly always aesthetically inferior

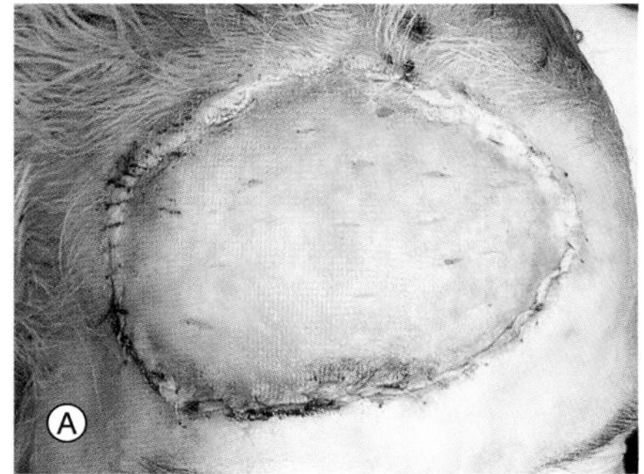

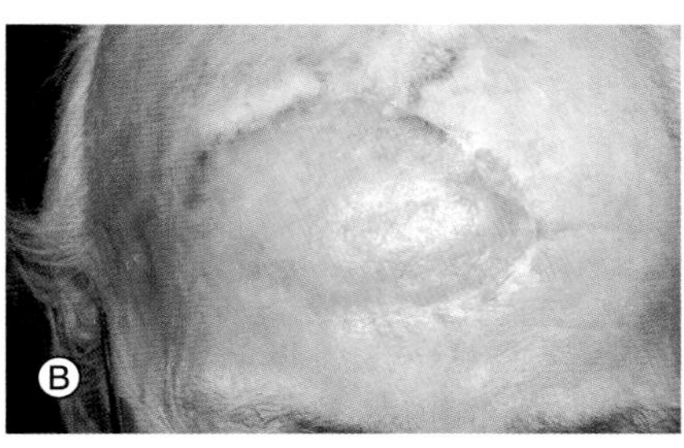

Figure 23.13 (A) Hand-meshed split-thickness skin graft (STSG) 1 week after repair of a large forehead defect resulting from a staged angiosarcoma excision. Donor site was the right thigh. Note the skin colored appearance at 1 week that distinctly contrasts with the violaceous appearance of a full-thickness skin graft at 1 week as in Figure 23.12. (B) At 5 months, the STSG from Figure 23.13a has an acceptable color match. Note the persistence of xerosis and hyperkeratosis requiring the use of emollients. As anticipated with deep defects repaired with STSG, the site continues to be depressed.

to FTSG. The color and texture mismatch of STSG are expected outcomes. Contour, texture, and color abnormalities of FTSG can be significantly improved postoperatively with the use of spot dermabrasion.[62] This can be performed as early as 6 weeks, but we tend to wait to intervene with this modality until the graft has significantly matured for 3–4 months. By this time, much of the transient edema and textural changes have abated, requiring either less intervention or no intervention. While a hand engine can be used for localized dermabrasion (or resurfacing lasers) we have had excellent results using a sterilized medium-grade drywall-sanding screen wrapped around a 3 ml syringe. We use this to manually spot dermabrade the graft site and its adjacent cosmetic unit.[62–64]

Contraction occurs with both FTSG and STSG but is much more significant in the latter as graft contracture increases as the thickness of the graft decreases. This fact is important to remember when considering grafts near free anatomic margins or over joints. In reconstructive dermatologic surgery, the anatomic sites most likely to be susceptible to the effects of graft contracture are the eyelid, the vermilion border of the lip, and the nasal ala.

■ SUMMARY

Considered by some as a repair option of the last resort, skin grafts continue to be an effective and versatile closure technique in dermatologic surgery. Selection of the proper patient and clinical situation are imperative in achieving success with skin grafts. Graft survival is generally more tenuous when compared to skin flaps because the vascular supply is minimal in the early stages of healing. However, with meticulous hemostasis, a compliant patient, and strict attention to detail, graft loss is a rare occurrence and the cosmetic and functional outcome can be excellent. Ongoing skin substitute and wound healing research will undoubtedly lead to additional advances in skin grafting over the next several decades.

■ REFERENCE

1. Davis J. The story of plastic surgery. Ann Surg 1941; 113:641–656.
2. Hauben DJ, Baruchin A, Mahler A. On the history of the free skin graft. Ann Plast Surg 1982; 9:242–245.
3. Wolfe JR. A new method of performing plastic operations. BMJ 1875; 2:360–361.
4. Krause F. Ueber die transplantation grosser ungestielter hautlappen. Verhandle Deutsch Ges Chir 1893; 22:46.
5. Hill TG. The evolution of skin graft reconstruction. J Dermatol Surg Oncol 1987; 13:834–835.
6. Smahel J. The healing of skin grafts. Clin Plast Surg 1977; 4:409–424.
7. Converse JM, Uhlschmid GK, Ballantyne DL Jr. 'Plasmatic circulation' in skin grafts. The phase of serum imbibition. Plast Reconstr Surg 1969; 43:495–499.
8. Converse JM, Smahel J, Ballantyne DL Jr, Harper AD. Inosculation of vessels of skin graft and host bed: a fortuitous encounter. Br J Plast Surg 1975; 28:274–282.
9. Birch J, Branemark PI, Nilsson K. The vascularization of a free full thickness skin graft. 3: An infrared thermographic study. Scand J Plast Reconstr Surg 1969; 3:18–22.
10. Zarem HA, Zweifach BW, McGehee JM. Development of microcirculation in full thickness autogenous skin grafts in mice. Am J Physiol 1967; 212:1081–1085.
11. Clemmesen T, Ronhovde DA. Restoration of the blood supply to human skin autografts. Scand J Plast Reconstr Surg 1960; 2:44–46.
12. McGregor IA, Conway H. Development of lymph flow from autografts and homografts of skin. Transplant Bull 1956; 3:46.
13. Johnson TM, Ratner D, Nelson BR. Soft tissue reconstruction with skin grafting. J Am Acad Dermatol 1992; 27:151–165.
14. Waris T, Rechardt L, Kyosola K. Reinnervation of human skin grafts: a histochemical study. Plast Reconstr Surg 1983; 72:439–447.
15. Skouge JW. Skin grafting. New York: Churchill Livingstone; 1991: pp. 2–3.
16. Goldminz D, Bennett RG. Cigarette smoking and flap and full-thickness graft necrosis. Arch Dermatol 1991; 127:1012–1015.
17. Pollack SV. Wound healing: a review. IV. Systemic medications affecting wound healing. J Dermatol Surg Oncol 1982; 8:667–672.
18. Hill TG. Enhancing the survival of full-thickness grafts. J Dermatol Surg Oncol 1984; 10:639–642.
19. Brown JB, McDowell F. Skin grafting. Philadelphia: JB Lippincott; 1958: pp. 346–347.
20. Mir Y, Mir L. Biology of the skin graft. Plast Reconstr Surg 1951; 8:378–389.
21. Hill TG. Contouring of donor skin in full-thickness skin grafting. J Dermatol Surg Oncol 1987; 13:883–888.
22. Arpey CJ, Whitaker DC, O'Donnell MJ. Skin grafting. New York: McGraw-Hill; 1997: pp. 155–194.
23. Adnot J, Salasche SJ. Visualized basting sutures in the application of full-thickness skin grafts. J Dermatol Surg Oncol 1987; 13:1236–1239.
24. Kent DE. Full-thickness skin grafts. New York: McGraw-Hill; 1996: pp. 297–308.
25. Davenport M, Daly J, Harvey I, Griffiths RW. The bolus tie-over 'pressure' dressing in the management of Full-thickness skin grafts. Is it necessary? Br J Plast Surg 1988; 41:28–32.
26. Langtry JA, Kirkham P, Martin IC, Fordyce A. Tie-over bolster dressings may not be necessary to secure small Full-thickness skin grafts. Dermatol Surg 1998; 24:1350–1353.
27. Salasche SJ, Winton GB. Clinical evaluation of a non-adhering wound dressing. J Dermatol Surg Oncol 1986; 12:1220–1222.
28. Fader DJ, Wang TS, Johnson TM. Nasal reconstruction utilizing a muscle hinge flap with overlying full-thickness skin graft. J Am Acad Dermatol 2000; 43:837–840.
29. Johnson TM, Baker S, Brown MD, Nelson BR. Utility of the subcutaneous hinge flap in nasal reconstruction. J Am Acad Dermatol 1994; 30:459–466.
30. Zitelli JA. Burow's grafts. J Am Acad Dermatol 1987; 17:271–279.
31. Chester EC Jr. Surgical gem. The use of dog-ears as grafts. J Dermatol Surg Oncol 1981; 7:956–959.
32. Chester EC Jr. Closure of a surgical defect in a nose using island grafts from the nose. J Dermatol Surg Oncol 1982; 8:790–791.
33. Snow SN, Stiff M, Lambert D, Tsoi C, Mohs FE. Freehand technique to harvest partial-thickness skin to repair superficial facial defects. Dermatol Surg 1995; 21:153–157.
34. Bennett JE, Miller SR. Evolution of the electro-dermatome. Plast Reconstr Surg 1970; 45:131–134.
35. Rigg BM. Importance of donor site selection in skin grafting. Can Med Assoc J 1977; 117:1028–1029.
36. Larson DL. Rapid application of skin grafts over large areas. Ann Plast Surg 1980; 5:244–245.
37. Kaplan HY. A quick stapler tie-over fixation for skin grafts. Ann Plast Surg 1989; 22:173–174.
38. James JH, Watson AC. The use of Opsite, a vapour permeable dressing, on skin graft donor sites. Br J Plast Surg 1975; 28:107–110.
39. McLaughlin CR. Composite ear grafts and their blood supply. Br J Plast Surg 1954; 7:274–278.
40. Maves MD, Yessenow RS. The use of composite auricular grafts in nasal reconstruction. J Dermatol Surg Oncol 1988; 14:994–999.
41. Ruch MK. Utilization of composite free grafts. J Int Coll Surg 1958; 30:274–275.
42. Burget GC, Menick FJ. The use of composite auricular grafts. Aesthetic reconstruction of the nose. St Louis: Mosby; 1994: pp. 212–225.
43. Field LM. Nasal alar rim reconstruction utilizing the crus of the helix, with several alternatives for donor site closure. J Dermatol Surg Oncol 1986; 12:253–258.
44. Davenport G, Bernard FD. Improving the take of composite grafts. Plast Reconstr Surg 1959; 24:175–182.
45. Ratner D, Katz A, Grande DJ. An interlocking auricular composite graft. Dermatol Surg 1995; 21:789–792.
46. Field LM. Nasal alar rim reconstruction utilizing the crus of the helix with several alternatives for donor site closure. J Dermatol Surg Oncol 1986; 12:253–258.

47. Bumsted RM, Panje WR, Ceilley RI. Delayed skin grafting in facial reconstruction. When to use and how to do. Arch Otolaryngol 1983; 109:178–184.
48. Ceilley RI, Bumsted RM, Panje WR. Delayed skin grafting. J Dermatol Surg Oncol 1983; 9:288–293.
49. Arpey CJ, Whitaker DC. Postsurgical wound management. Dermatol Clin 2001; 19:787–797.
50. Burke JF, Yannas IV, Quinby WC Jr, Bondoc CC, Jung WK. Successful use of a physiologically acceptable artificial skin in the treatment of extensive burn injury. Ann Surg 1981; 194:413–428.
51. Rue LW IIIrd, Cioffi WG, McManus WF, Pruitt BA Jr. Wound closure and outcome in extensively burned patients treated with cultured autologous keratinocytes. J Trauma 1993; 34:662–667.
52. Falabella AF, Valencia IC, Eaglstein WH, Schachner LA. Tissue-engineered skin (Apligraf) in the healing of patients with epidermolysis bullosa wounds. Arch Dermatol 2000; 136:1225–1230.
53. Eaglstein WH, Iriondo M, Laszlo K. A composite skin substitute (graftskin) for surgical wounds. A clinical experience. Dermatol Surg 1995; 21:839–843.
54. Eaglstein WH, Alvarez OM, Auletta M, et al. Acute excisional wounds treated with a tissue-engineered skin (Apligraf). Dermatol Surg 1999; 25:195–201.
55. Bello YM, Falabella AF. Use of skin substitutes in dermatology. Dermatol Clin 2001; 19:555–561.
56. Davis DA, Arpey CJ. Porcine heterografts in dermatologic surgery and reconstruction. Dermatol Surg 2000; 26:76–80.
57. Elliott RA Jr, Hoehn JG. Use of commercial porcine skin for wound dressings. Plast Reconstr Surg 1973; 52:401–405.
58. Papp GM. The use of porcine skin in partial and full-thickness skin loss. J Am Osteopath Assoc 1976; 75:951–957.
59. Skouge JW. Skin grafting. New York: Churchill Livingstone; 1991: pp. 60–63.
60. Kovich O, Otley CC. Thrombotic complications related to discontinuation of warfarin and aspirin therapy perioperatively for cutaneous operation. J Am Acad Dermatol 2003; 48:233–237.
61. Alcalay J. Cutaneous surgery in patients receiving warfarin therapy. Dermatol Surg 2001; 27:756–758.
62. Yarborough JM Jr. Ablation of facial scars by programmed dermabrasion. J Dermatol Surg Oncol 1988; 14:292–294.
63. Zisser M, Kaplan B, Moy RL. Surgical pearl: manual dermabrasion. J Am Acad Dermatol 1995; 33:105–106.
64. Gillard M, Wang TS, Boyd CM, Dunn RL, Fader DJ, Johnson TM. Conventional diamond fraise vs manual spot dermabrasion with drywall sanding screen for scars from skin cancer surgery. Arch Dermatol 2002; 138:1035–1039.

24 Regional Reconstruction: Trunk, Extremities, Hands, Feet, Face (Perioral, Periorbital, Cheek, Nose, Forehead, Ear, Neck, Scalp)

Camille L Mason MD, Christopher J Arpey MD, and Duane C Whitaker MD

Summary box

- There are four major wound closure options: second intention healing, primary closure and its variations, skin grafts, and local or distal flaps.
- Choice of which option to use depends on the nature of the defect, the site of the repair and the patient's age, concomitant medications and diseases, irradiation history and tendency for multiple tumors; factors related to the patient's self image and expectations about wound appearance should also be taken into account.
- The detailed approach to excision and repair in each of the different body regions varies as a result of the differing skin characteristics at each site; for example, near the eye the highly mobile nature of the lower eyelid has to be taken into account.
- Patient education about the likely outcome is important to assuage patients' fears and to avoid disappointment with the result.

INTRODUCTION

In broadly approaching the repair of cutaneous defects, it is important to realize that all generalizations must be uniquely applied to the individual patient. A similar sized wound in an identical location on two different patients may not be managed the same way due to unique patient factors outlined in Table 24.1.[1]

From the initial meeting between the patient and the skin surgeon, it is important to emphasize the priorities of treatment, which are oncologic cure, maintenance of important structures and their function, and finally the best cosmetic result given the prior two factors. A patient may be more likely to accept a suboptimal cosmetic outcome if a careful explanation of these priorities is given prior to the procedure.

For cutaneous defects, there are four major wound closure options considering both the surgical defect and patient factors: second intention healing, primary closure and its variations, skin grafts, and local or distant flaps. These options will be briefly discussed in increasing order of complexity.

Healing

Secondary intention healing

Second intention healing can be an ideal closure option in select patients or select locations (see also Chapter 7). The critical stages and factors necessary for wound healing will be briefly described to provide a framework for managing and advising patients whose wounds heal by granulation. The wound-healing process has been divided into three primary stages.[2] The first stage is described as the inflammatory phase. It begins at the time of incision and lasts approximately until day 5. A number of cellular and humoral factors are involved in early healing, including platelets, polymorphonuclear leukocytes, macrophages, fibrin, fibronectin and other clotting factors, and growth factors. Capillary growth in the direction of the wound space also begins in the initial phase. At approximately day 4, fibroblasts appear. The tensile strength of the wound is approximately only 6% of normal skin at this stage.[3]

Table 24.1 Factors influencing choice of wound closure option

Subjective	Objective
Patient self image	Age
Patient's occupational image	Drugs: anticoagulants, antiplatelets immunosuppressants
Patient's social situation	Illnesses: bleeding diathesis, diabetes, peripheral vascular disease
Patient's fears	Tobacco and alcohol use
Patient's expectations	Obesity
Patient's tolerance for the appearance of the wound	Previous or concurrent irradiation
Tendency for multiple tumors	

The granulation phase occurs from day 6 to day 14. There is a proliferation of fibroblasts, which take on the phenotype of contractile myofibroblasts with subsequent wound contracture. As more fibroblasts reach the wound site, more collagen is deposited forming a structural framework. Neovascularization continues and is necessary for ongoing fibroplasia. An understanding of the process allows us to reassure our patients that granulation tissue and significant wound contracture are unlikely to occur until week 2. The tensile strength at this stage is 6–14% of normal skin primarily due to the deposition of collagen.

Finally, the maturation phase begins at approximately day 15. At this time, there is a reduction in the number of macrophages and fibroblasts and an increase in remodeling of newly formed collagen. The wound breaking strength of skin reaches 45% of normal at day 70 and 50% of normal at day 120.[2] Over time the wound will mature, with continued remodeling of collagen, attenuation of angioneogenesis, scar relaxation, color change, and contour alteration. These changes frequently take up to 1 year or longer and this should be addressed early in the patient's care to allay any fears over the immediate appearance of the wound.

Re-epithelialization of granulating wounds depends on the size, depth, anatomic location, and host factors such as smoking status, but in general can occur as early as 5 days or as late as 60 days or longer.

Primary closure

The most important factor for choosing granulation as a repair method is location of the defect. Healed wounds are often imperceptible on concave surfaces of the nose, eyes, ears, and temple. On convex surfaces of the nose, lips, cheeks, chin, and helix of the ear, superficial wounds heal with an acceptable appearance, but deep wounds can heal with depressed or hypertrophic scars. On the forehead, antihelix, eyelids, and remainder of the nose, lips and cheeks, the scar can be variable in appearance but is often flat and hypopigmented.[4] Wounds on the trunk and extremities yield variable results but often the scars are thicker and remain erythematous for a longer period of time (Table 24.2).

Many skin defects can be closed primarily with a fusiform excision or with a fusiform variation such as a curvilinear closure, M/W-plasty or V-to-Y closure. The resultant scar is linear with a generally smooth contour and pleasing cosmetic outcome. In an apposed wound, re-epithelialization begins as early as 24 hours and is complete in 48–72 hours. Care should be taken to carefully evaluate for any distortion of free margins, such as eyelids, nasal alae, and lips, when performing an excision. Also, the side-to-side closure should be executed to minimize the wound tension and conceal the scar in a fold, crease, or the border between anatomic subunits. As delineated in previous chapters, knowledge of regional relaxed skin tension lines and facial cosmetic units as well as palpation of tissue is imperative in reconstruction efforts.

Skin grafting

The third closure option is skin grafting (see also Chapter 23). In skin grafts, full-thickness or split-thickness grafts are removed from the donor site and underlying vascular supply and used to repair a recipient wound site. The blood supply must be restored at the recipient site to achieve graft viability. Virtually any wound with a vascularized bed will accept a graft, providing a great deal of flexibility to the skin surgeon. Full-thickness skin grafts are often cosmetically superior to split-thickness grafts because they more effectively prevent wound contracture; however, the bulkiness of the graft may conceal tumor recurrences. Care must be taken to provide the best color and textural match and the patient must be informed that the graft can occasionally look like a 'patch.' Occasionally, grafts may be depressed or alternatively pin-cushioned, and there may be long lasting dyschromia.

Flaps

Flaps provide a unique method for wound closure (see also Chapters 21 and 22). A flap allows for the movement of skin and subcutaneous tissue with its own underlying vascular supply to cover a surgical defect. Flaps are often classified based on the primary movement of the tissue as advancement, rotation, or transposition flaps. Another general classification is axial-patterned flaps, which are based on a major named artery or random-patterned flaps, which are based on the subdermal arterial plexus.

■ TECHNICAL ASPECTS

These alternative repair options will now be explored by region, starting in the cephalad location and moving in a centrifugal and caudad direction, although the upper and lower extremities are examined together, as are the hands and feet. In general, the order of repair options in each section parallels the preferred order of repair in that particular region.

Scalp

The scalp proper is a broad area extending from the supraorbital rims anteriorly to the superior nuchal line posteriorly. The scalp consists of five layers. Underlying the skin layer is the connective tissue, which contains the blood vessels and nerves. The next layer is the galea aponeurotica, a fibrous sheet that covers the vault of the skull and unites the occipitalis and frontalis muscles. These first three layers act functionally as one unit because they are fused via fibrous septae. Deep to the galea and superficial to the periosteum is the loose connective tissue forming the subaponeurotic space or subgaleal plane, a relatively avascular plane where undermining is frequently performed.

Defects of the scalp up to approximately 3 cm in greatest diameter may be closed primarily, although redundant tissue repairs in larger scalp wounds are often much more extensive than those of comparable wounds elsewhere on the body. Larger wounds or wounds under tension can often be closed primarily due to the rich vascular supply of the scalp and the fibrous support of the galea, especially if some of the buried sutures encompass a small amount of galea. The relaxed skin tension lines of the scalp are variable and palpation prior to planning the orientation of the surgical excision is crucial to take advantage of any areas of extra mobility. The long axis of the fusiform excision should parallel the lines of least tension.

Table 24.2 Ideal selection factors for second intention healing

1. Location amenable to second intention healing
2. Shallow wounds
3. Fair-skinned patients
4. Need for long-term monitoring for cure (recurrent or large tumors)
5. Older patients
6. Ability to perform or have assistance in wound care
7. Wounds in previously irradiated skin
8. Patients who drink alcohol to excess, or smoke
9. Patients who are on anticoagulants
10. Patients who are immunosuppressed

Prior to excision, the hair should be trimmed to several millimeters or less, and adjacent hair should be pinned or slicked back with petrolatum to improve visibility and minimize the possibility of hair entrapment and foreign body response in the wound. Lidocaine with epinephrine (adrenaline) should be locally infiltrated 10–15 minutes prior to repair to minimize bleeding. The important cleavage plane to identify when working on the scalp is the subgaleal space located between the galea and the pericranium, which allows for relatively bloodless dissection. Care should be taken not to interrupt the periosteum and inadvertently expose bone of the skull, which has poor osteogenic properties in adults. Bleeding should be impeccably controlled with electrocoagulation to avoid hematoma formation. Typically 3-0 or 4-0 caliber suture is used as buried suture, although large lesions under more significant wound closure tension may require larger caliber suture. Epidermal edges are typically approximated with 4-0 or 5-0 monofilament non-absorbable suture. Wound care typically consists of hydrogen peroxide applied twice daily to the surgical site, followed by liberal application of antibiotic ointment. Dressings are typically not utilized secondary to poor adherence to hair-bearing skin.

The second-favored method of scalp closure is granulation (Fig. 24.1). If the periosteum is intact, the scalp heals well, with good contraction of the wound circumference. Again, due to the poor ability of the bony skull to spontaneously regenerate with injury, defects with exposed bone heal slowly. If bone is exposed, cleansing with dilute (0.25%) acetic acid compresses rather than hydrogen peroxide is recommended, followed by generous amounts of topical antibiotics to maintain a moist, clean environment. Care should be taken to monitor for signs of

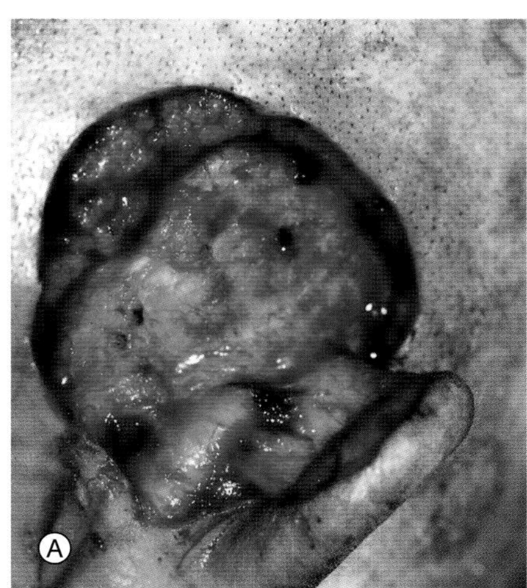

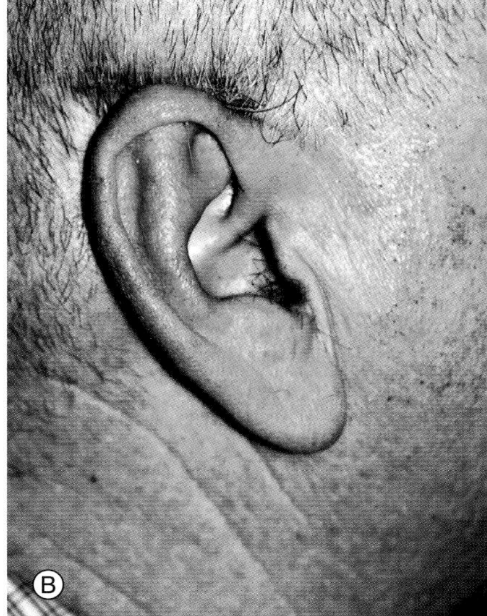

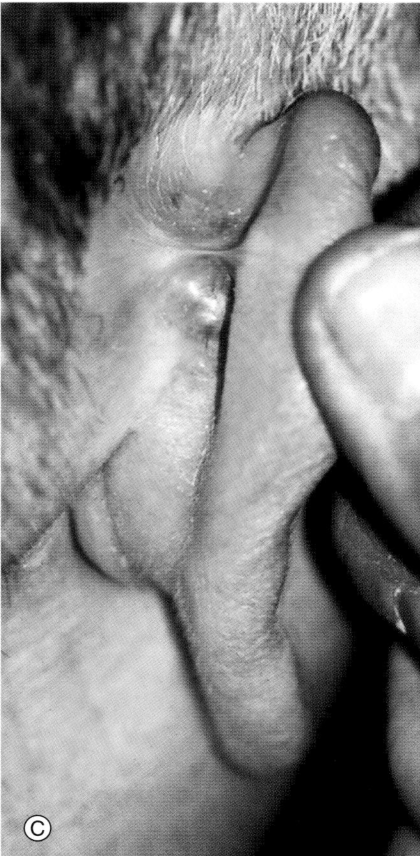

Figure 24.1 (A) A large surgical defect of the posterior ear, postauricular sulcus, and postauricular scalp with intact periostium and perichondrium. (B) Long-term follow-up of lateral view without distortion and acceptable cosmesis. (C) Long-term follow-up of posterolateral view showing slight webbing but no functional deformity.

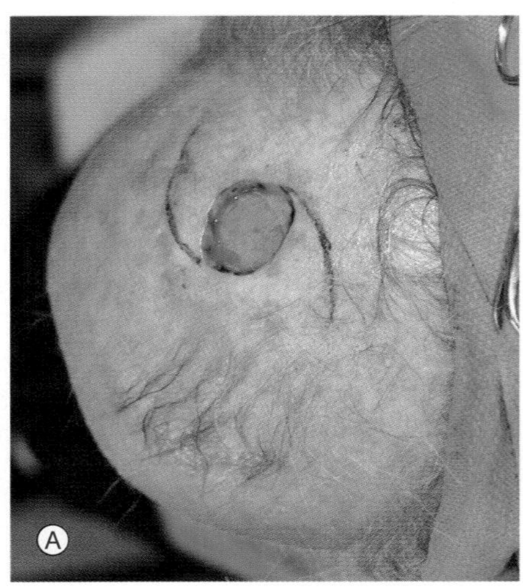

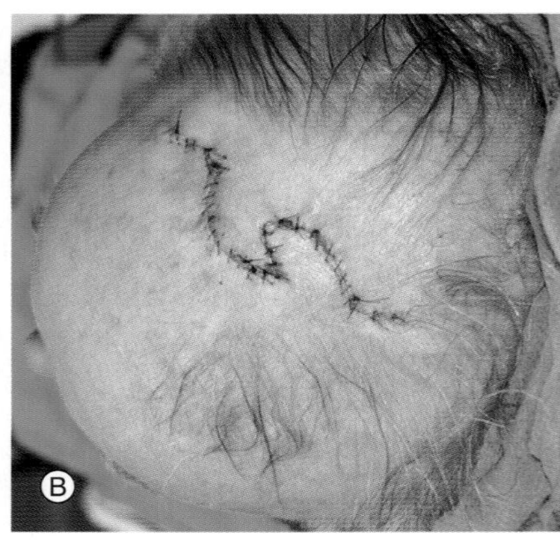

Figure 24.2 (A) An O-to-Z flap (bilateral rotation flap) is designed for a circular defect of the frontal scalp. (B) The sutured defect is shown. The O-to-Z repair recruits more scalp tissue for repair and overcomes the relative inelasticity of the tissue.

osteomyelitis including pain, increased drainage, or slowed healing. Osteonecrosis can also occur, the signs of which are often yellow-gray discoloration, and a 'mushy' texture to the outer table of the cranium when probed with forceps or curette. The patient should be counseled regarding the protracted healing time, often 8–12 weeks or longer with several centimeters of exposed bone.

If skin grafting is used, as previously discussed in Chapter 23, there are several unique considerations for hair-bearing areas. The preferred donor site for the scalp is scalp skin usually derived from the occipital or temporal areas, because the donor site can be more readily approximated primarily, and hair from these locations is unlikely to be affected by androgenetic alopecia. The graft should have minimal defatting or no defatting in order to preserve the hair follicles localized to the subcutaneous tissue. The graft should be placed so that the hairs exit the skin in the same direction as the hairs in the surrounding recipient bed.

Several additional considerations exist for skin grafting. The graft can be directly placed on pericranium. The drawback to this approach is that the normal laxity of the scalp is lost in the grafted area because the graft becomes fixed to the underlying tissue. Any force applied to the graft, even minor force, can lead to skin graft ulceration or loss. Another option is to perform delayed skin grafting of the area. The recipient site can be allowed to granulate for several weeks until a nice vascular base is achieved and then a delayed graft can be successfully placed.

Local random flaps used for scalp reconstruction include advancement, rotation and transposition. The unique anatomy of the scalp demands special considerations in comparison to similar flaps used on other areas. The density of the galea limits the distensibility of the scalp, particularly in areas where there is no investment of muscle, such as over the vertex of the scalp. In addition, the thickness of the skin in the scalp area limits the ability to stretch or drape the skin over a given defect. Direction of hair growth or absence of hair growth must also be taken into consideration so that a blended appearance is achieved. An important underlying concept is that the scalp has its more mobile segments primarily located along the periphery in a 'hatband' distribution, where the galea invests musculature and is much more distensible; the vertex of the cranium is less distensible, where there is no underlying muscle and the galea forms a thick band.

As a result of scalp immobility, rotation flaps (Fig. 24.2) are useful because of their high flap to defect ratio, which provides a well-vascularized pedicle and less secondary tissue movement. The flap is most successful when the length of the arcing incision is at least four times the width of the defect at its greatest diameter. Backcuts are often necessary due to the inelasticity of the scalp, and in some cases multiple backcuts oriented perpendicular to the arcing incision are required to lengthen the flap and conform it to the spherical configuration of the scalp. Aggressive reduction of standing tissue deformities is not recommended at the time of flap transfer. Over time the deformities tend to flatten, and persistent deformities can be addressed once the flap is viable and well vascularized, typically after 6 weeks.

Transposition flaps have been used successfully in reconstruction of scalp defects and scalp reduction in the setting of alopecia. Generally, the length to width ratio of the flap should not exceed 4 : 1 (length to base) unless the pedicle has a known arterial and venous vascular supply. If possible, the base of the flap should be within a looser area of the scalp. Extending the arc of the pivot beyond 90° limits the effectiveness of the flap because a larger standing deformity is created and the effective length of the flap is decreased.[5]

There is little benefit in using an advancement flap on the scalp due to the resistance of the galea to tissue distention or stretching.

Forehead and temple

Anatomically, the upper forehead resembles the scalp, often complete with an anterior extension of the galea aponeurotica. The primary muscle of the forehead is the frontal belly of the occipitofrontalis muscle. The muscle fibers run vertically and thus result in the transverse orientation of relaxed skin tension lines of the forehead. The glabellar lines, however, may be vertical or oblique. The nerve most at risk during surgery of the forehead is the temporal branch of the VIIth cranial nerve (facial nerve),

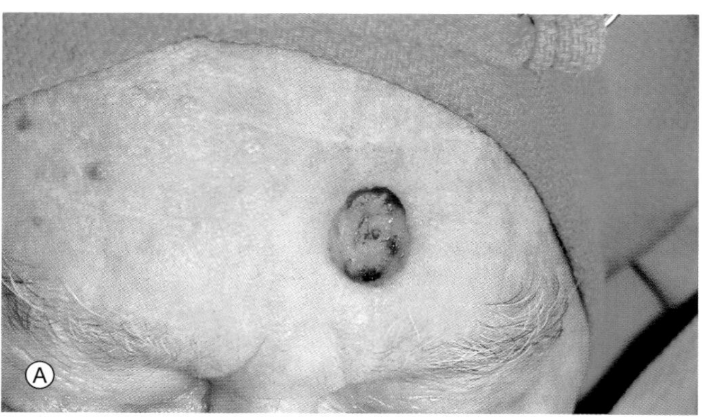

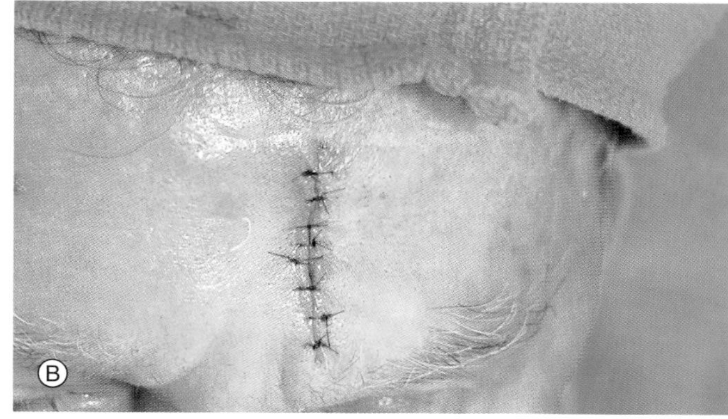

Figure 24.3 (A) Forehead defects are often easily closed primarily. Care must be taken to prevent elevation of the eyebrow greater than 1 cm. (B) A vertical closure of the forehead defect is chosen to prevent eyebrow elevation. Lower forehead and glabellar defects are often closed vertically rather than horizontally.

particularly as its course becomes superficial over the zygomatic arch. Upon actually reaching the forehead, the nerve enters the frontalis muscle from the deep side, reducing the risk of inadvertent transection. If this nerve branch is severed, the patient will be unable to raise the ipsilateral eyebrow or to wrinkle the ipsilateral forehead. The major sensory nerves of the forehead are the supraorbital and supratrochlear nerves exiting over the mid-pupillary line and the medial eyebrow respectively. The nerves then pierce the overlying muscle and extend cephalad in the subcutaneous tissue. Undermining in this region should be performed in the mid-subcutaneous tissue plane to avoid inadvertent injury resulting in anesthesia distal to the point of transection. It is important to warn the patient that anesthesia in the general region of these nerves can lead to temporary paralysis or numbness so that they do not become unduly alarmed.

Primary repairs of forehead defects are often possible especially in patients with tissue laxity secondary to age or sun damage. The scar should be camouflaged in relaxed skin tension lines, the brow, or along the hairline for the best cosmetic effect. Mid-line defects of the forehead are often closed in a vertical fashion (Fig. 24.3). It is also crucial to maintain motor and sensory nerve function unless transection of the nerve is required to obtain complete oncologic cure.

Forehead excisions often result in brow elevation, especially with procedures performed in close proximity to the eyebrows. With time the affected brow frequently resumes its normal position due to gravity. This is especially true if the elevation is less than 1 cm. However, elevations greater than 1 cm can lead to permanent asymmetry and distortion. Elevations less than 1 cm in younger people can also lead to asymmetry and distortion due to the increased elasticity of the tissue. Care should be taken to assess the effect of primary and secondary tissue movement on the brow. If elevation occurs, one should not pursue immediate intervention but promote watchful waiting until the final resting point of the brow can be determined. Another note of caution when treating near the brow is that eyebrow hair should not be shaved due to slow regrowth. Incisions through the eyebrow should be obliquely parallel to the angle created by the hair shaft as it exits the skin to minimize transection of the hair with subsequent alopecia. When closing fusiform excisions of the forehead, most buried sutures are of 4-0 or 5-0 caliber and the non-absorbable epidermal sutures are of 5-0 or 6-0 caliber. Sutures are typically removed in 7 days.

The results of granulation of forehead wounds vary by location. If the forehead is divided into thirds, starting at the extreme lateral forehead and ending at the mid-line, a pattern of second intention healing can be appreciated that goes from excellent results to less predictable results. In general, wounds (including deep and large wounds) of the extreme lateral forehead and temples heal with an excellent cosmetic result. Moving medially to the middle third of the forehead, the results become intermediate. Finally, the central forehead heals with the least predictable results providing in many cases a suboptimal scar.

Flaps are an excellent repair option when primary closure or granulation (depending on the location) is not a suitable option. It is probably best when considering flap reconstruction options to divide the forehead conceptually into medial and lateral segments. Advancement flaps, including unilateral, bilateral, and island pedicle flaps, are the most commonly utilized flaps for the central forehead. The advancement flap is ideally suited for this location because an adequate reservoir of tissue can usually be recruited, and the scars can be easily camouflaged in the horizontal forehead creases. The amount of tissue extension with the advancement flap can be easily visualized. The outcome can generally be predicted by visually and manually testing the tissue movement prior to actual closure. Very infrequently, advancement flaps provide more movement than is perceived during preplanning.[6,7] Incisions for the flap are made horizontally with an approximate 3 : 1 or 4 : 1 ratio of length to width. Flaps are dissected in the mid-subcutaneous plane. Burow's triangles can be removed anywhere along the length of the flap. For defects of the central forehead, particularly upper mid-forehead defects, inferolaterally based double rotation flaps can be designed to rotate large quantities of tissue into a defect, while camouflaging the scar in hair-bearing areas of the temporal and frontal hairline. In other locations of the central forehead, rotation flaps may be less ideal because of lengthy incision lines. Transposition flaps are also less than ideal because of the resultant multidirectional scars in a region where most visible skin lines are unidirectional (horizontal).

The lateral forehead begins at the mid-brow and extends to the extreme lateral forehead and temples. A-T closure is often effective for lateral suprabrow defects. In this procedure, single-arm bilateral advancement flaps are extended horizontally from the base of the defect in relaxed skin tension lines, or along the upper border of the brow. The vertical aspect will then be the only portion not camouflaged. Other options include a unilateral rotation flap of the lateral forehead based laterally and inferiorly to hide the scar along the temporal hairline, and a double rotation flap. As with the medial forehead, transposition flaps are not used as frequently on the lateral forehead, although small rhombic flaps or their variants are sometimes useful on the temple.

Skin grafts provide a ready source of tissue replacement but are considered to be the least optimum repair option on the forehead due to difficulties in obtaining an ideal color and textural match. However, for large defects where prolonged granulation may not be tolerable, split-thickness grafts are occasionally necessary.

Periorbital region

Fusiform excisions can be performed near the eye with forethought given to the highly mobile nature of the lower eyelid. A cicatricial ectropion caused by a poorly oriented repair is not only unsightly but may also lead to epiphora and eventual corneal damage. To avoid postoperative ectropion, fusiform excisions near the eyes should be oriented so that the long axis is perpendicular or slightly oblique to the lid margin. This leads to vectors of tension predominantly directed lateral to medial, and avoids inferiorly directed tension on the lower lid. To minimize the amount of normal tissue removed in a normal fusiform excision, a double-S ellipse can be designed to reduce the amount of tissue sacrificed by half.[8]

Granulation of select eye defects is a viable repair option. A number of investigators have found that for smaller Mohs defects of the lower eyelids second intention healing in this location is beneficial. In looking at color, contour, and scar cosmesis, surgeons in one such study felt that partial-thickness or small full-thickness lower-eyelid wounds healed with excellent cosmetic and functional results. The patients also rated the areas as healing with excellent results.[9] In another study, skin defects following excision of lid and periocular tumors in 24 [white] patients were allowed to heal by granulation. The locations included lower eyelid (n = 10), upper lid (n = 6), medial canthus (n = 5), nasojugal fold (n = 2), lateral canthus (n = 1) and brow (n = 1). Four patients had involvement of the lid margin. The size of the initial defect, time taken to heal, discomfort during healing, the functional and cosmetic results both from the surgeon's and the patient's perspectives, complications, secondary intervention if any, and patient satisfaction were studied. Good functional and cosmetic results were obtained in 23 of the 25 lesions (92%). Healing by second intention of large defects following excision of periocular tumors is an effective alternative to primary or staged reconstruction in selected cases.[10] Defects of both the medial and lateral canthus heal very well by granulation. This is especially true if approximately 50% of the wound is located above and 50% below the canthus proper because wound contraction will occur in a symmetric fashion, minimizing the risk of ectropion. In the medial canthus, defects up to 1 cm often heal well, but as the defect approaches the nasal root, increased webbing between the canthus and nasal root may occur.[11]

For uncomplicated defects, the standard rotation (Fig. 24.4), advancement, and transposition flaps can be utilized. For circular defects, especially of the lower lid, O-Z double rotation flaps allow repair with minimal tension, and allow tension to be directed parallel to the lid margin. Unilateral advancement flaps consisting of skin and (orbicularis) muscle can be used to repair defects of the upper and lower eyelids and eyebrows. Small transposition flaps, particularly rhombic-shaped and their variants, are useful for repairing medial canthal defects[12] and lateral periorbital defects. As for any eyelid repair, care must be taken when designing the flap to prevent distortion of the eyelid margins or brow. The wound-closure tension vector should always be directed parallel to the lower lid margin. When working in the canthal regions, the wound-closure tension vector can be perpendicular to the lid margin as long as no distortion is transmitted to the lids.

Grafts are occasionally a repair option for smaller defects of the eyelids proper, or for wounds that can be apposed only partially. In such instances, the best donor skin is typically the contralateral eyelid if there is sufficient laxity. Harvesting such skin requires the same decision-making process involved in blepharoplasty candidates, including adequacy of tarsal plate strength and absence of excessive lid lag on 'snap testing.' If sufficient contralateral eyelid skin is present, the color match and thickness are usually very good. Skin grafts still carry a risk of contraction and circular or oval scar lines at the periphery, making them less desirable than flaps in most instances.

Nose

When approaching repair options for the nose, it is best to consider a division into the superior two-thirds (dorsal nose and paired lateral sidewalls) and the lower one-third (nasal tip, soft triangles, columella, and alar lobules). In general, the concavities of the nose are more amenable to granulation. The perinasal folds, alar grooves, and alar creases often heal with excellent cosmetic results, even with deep defects. However, the function of the nasal valve must always be considered, as well as possible distortion of the nasal passageways, alar rims, and columella. If a hypertrophic scar develops in the alar crease, the lateral nasal cartilage or lateral wing of the alar cartilage may be pushed into the nasal passageway, causing deformity and obstruction to airflow. The nasal alae also heal well if the defects are shallow. From a practical standpoint, defects closer than 3–4 mm from the alar rim may cause unsightly retraction of the free margin after healing by granulation is complete; defects with depths greater than 2–3 mm have a greater risk of hypertrophic scarring and nasal valve compromise. Granulation of the upper nose, including the midline bridge of the nose, and the convex portion of the tip may result in depressed, or occasionally hypertrophic, scars.

Fusiform excisions of the lower nose, especially of the nasal tip, are possible if the excision is narrow and the tissue overlying the perichondrium sufficiently mobile. The

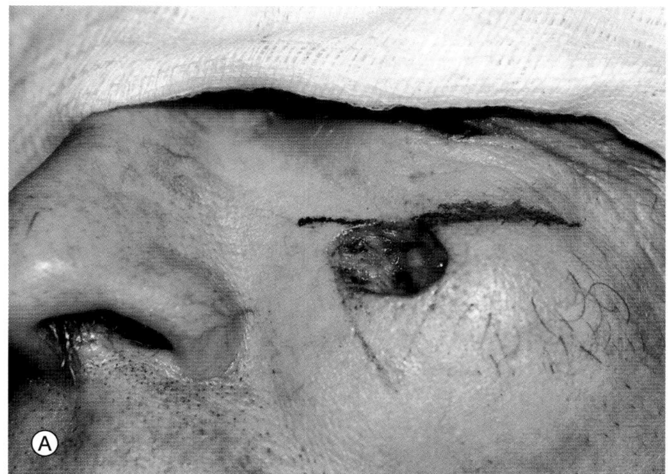

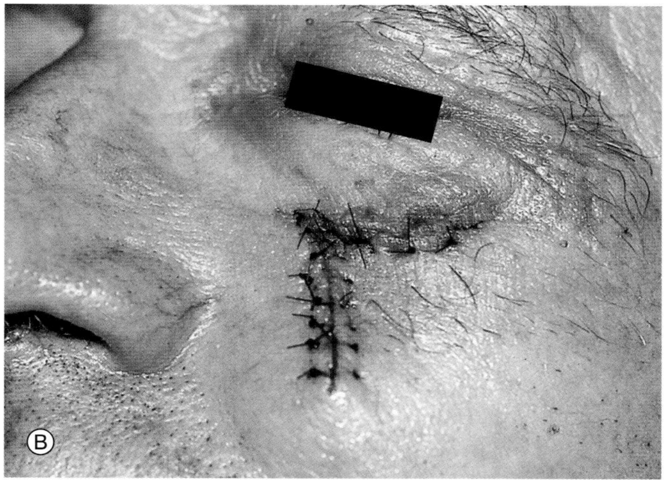

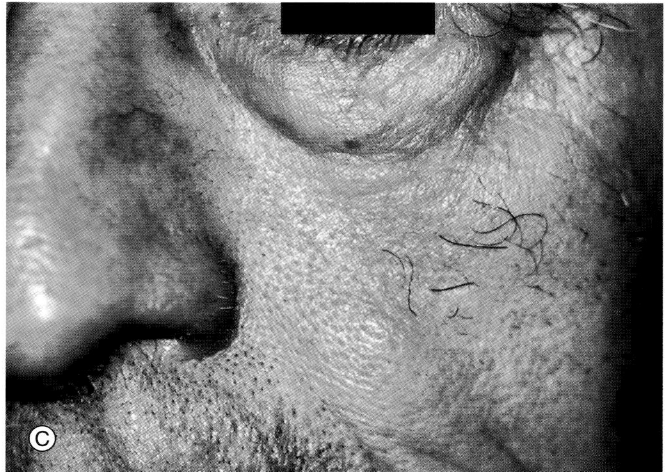

Figure 24.4 (A) a An O–T bilateral advancement flap is designed for a circular defect of the lower eyelid at the junction with the cheek. (B) The defect is closed by advancing two flaps in opposite directions with the horizontal lines placed at the junction of the aesthetic units. (C) Follow-up at 6 months without ectropion of the lower lid because the tension vector of the vertical limb of the flap is directed horizontally with respect to the eyelid margin.

typical orientation is oblique or vertical. The upper nose is more amenable to fusiform excisions with primary closures oriented either vertically or horizontally, depending on the patient's tissue laxity. Closures on the nasal root should most often be oriented transversely. Sebaceous skin of the nose presents a cosmetic challenge because the skin is thicker and heals with an increased risk of scar widening and dehiscence. It is important to advise patients of this risk prior to any repair or procedure. Often the buried sutures used on nasal skin are oriented horizontally or obliquely within the dermis rather than vertically. Non-absorbable sutures are typically removed after 7 days.

Bilobed flaps are ideal for small defects, up to approximately 1.5 cm in size, of the lateral nasal tip, lower sidewall, or medial alae (Fig. 24.5). The transferred lax tissue from the superior sidewall and dorsum is often an ideal color and textural match. The base of the flap is typically directed laterally. However, the base can be directed medially for laterally based defects. Modifications of the classic flap design (transposing skin 180°) include rotation of each lobe of the flap only 45° (total 90°–100°), the use of a Burow's triangle at the point of rotation, and wide undermining to minimize initial problems with pin-cushioning and tissue protrusions.[13] The nasal flap is undermined deep to the nasalis muscle and above perichondrium, in a relatively avascular plane. The tertiary defect is repaired first, followed by the secondary defect, and finally the primary flap and original defect.

The superiorly based nasolabial flap is another useful transposition flap for small to large defects of the lower sidewall and ala (Fig. 24.6). In this flap, the medial incision lies in the melolabial sulcus. The lateral incision is designed on the cheek with the incision being no higher than the most inferior part of the nasal defect. Modifications to reduce some of the undesirable outcomes of the flap technique include removal of a large Burow's triangle above the initial wound, wide undermining, significant thinning of the donor flap, and the use of a deep tacking suture to recreate the nasofacial sulcus.[14] The greatest disadvantage to this flap, even with modifications, is blunting of the sulcus along with occasionally lateral compression of the nasal valve.

In general, advancement and rotation flaps are not frequently used on the lower nose. For the upper two-thirds of the nose, the transposition flap is often used because it allows redirection of tension vectors and is often smaller than advancement or rotation flaps. Nasal tissue can be recruited to provide the ideal color and textural match. Small rotation flaps of nasal skin can be performed but are less than ideal for repair of large defects because of the relative length of the flap in relation to the width of the defect.

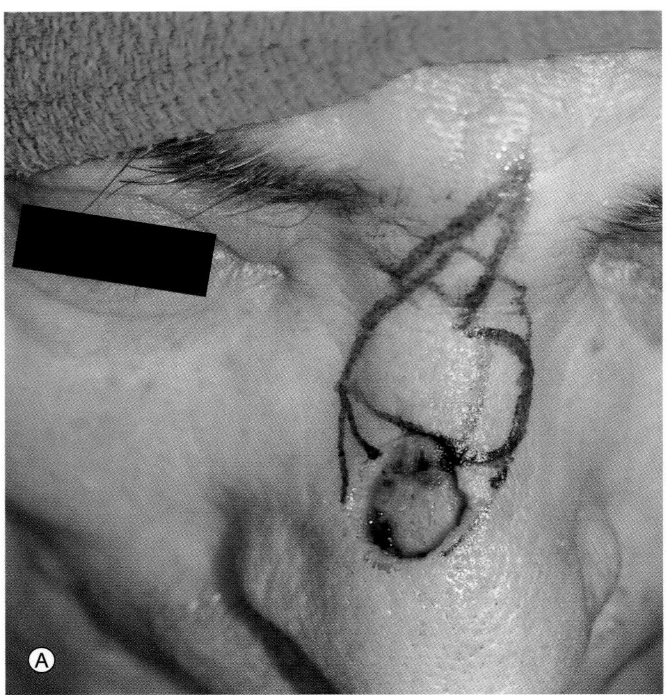

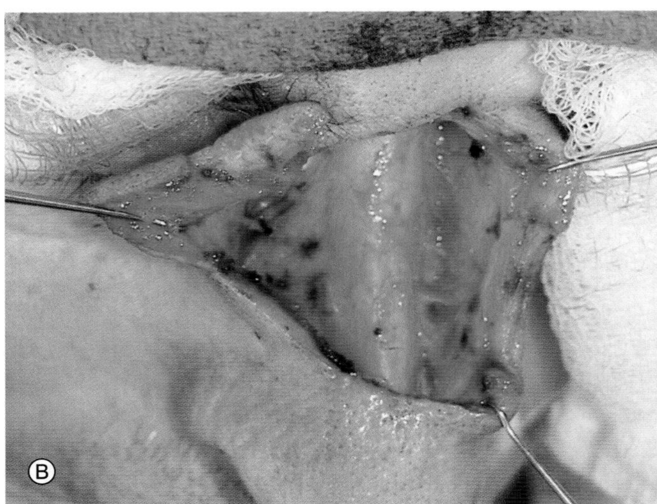

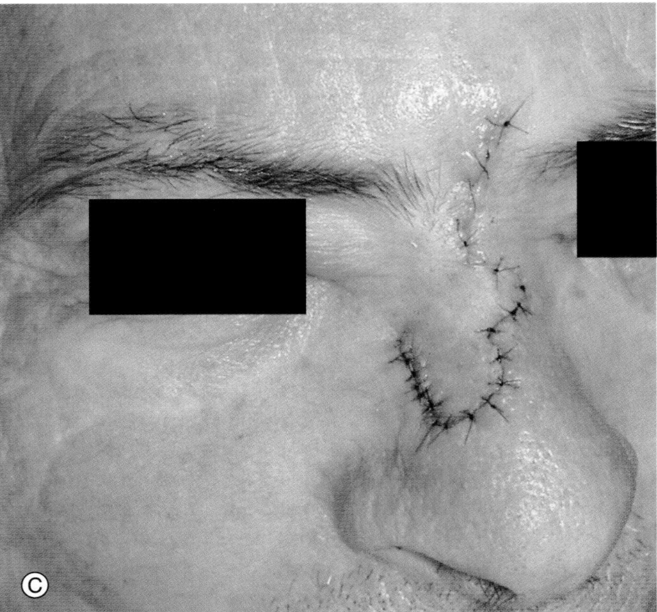

Figure 24.5 (A) A circular nasal defect less than 1.5 cm in size and localized to the side wall of the nose is shown. A bilobed flap is outlined. (B) The defect should be widely undermined deep to nasalis and superficial to perichondrium to reduce wound tension and the chance of trapdoor deformity. (C) The sutured defect is shown. This flap provides tissue of a similar texture and color. Loose glabellar tissue is utilized and the repair is localized in a cosmetic unit.

If nasal tissue cannot be utilized, the glabella is often a good source of donor tissue for constructing a flap. Two major advantages of tissue from this region are that the relaxed skin tension lines tend to run vertically, and there is excellent blood supply from the supratrochlear and supraorbital vessels. A glabellar transposition flap can be designed as a single transposition flap or a double transposition flap, as in bilobed repairs, to repair defects primarily of the lateral nasal root. For defects of the root, the dorsum, and for medially located sidewall defects, glabellar rotation flaps, often with a backcut, are utilized. Glabellar tissue can be thicker and more sebaceous than the tissue on the bridge of the nose. This can be addressed by thinning the flap. Also, there can be a flattening of the natural concavity of the dorsal root with recruitment of tissue from the glabella. This is usually not a cosmetic limitation if the flap is oversized and good technique is used in fixation of the flap with suspending sutures to underlying deep tissue.

Grafts can provide satisfactory results in the upper two-thirds of the nose. The texture and slightly shiny appearance of this skin is easier to match (although there may be slight variations in color due to hypo- or hyper-pigmentation) than the more highly sebaceous tissue of the lower nose. A full-thickness graft from preauricular skin is often selected for repair. Skin grafts of the lower nose are more likely to have a 'patched' appearance because of the textural and color differences between the recipient and

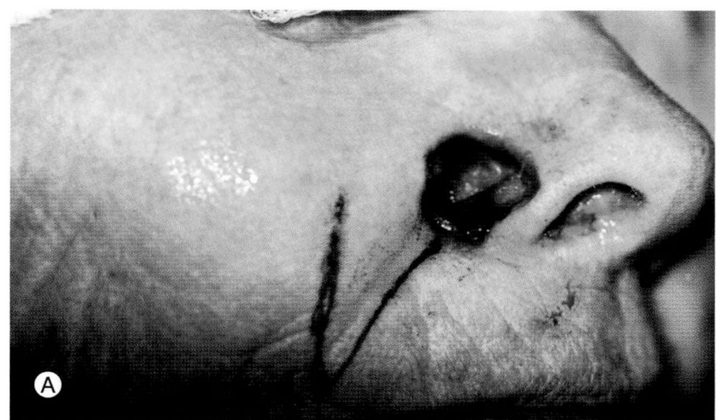

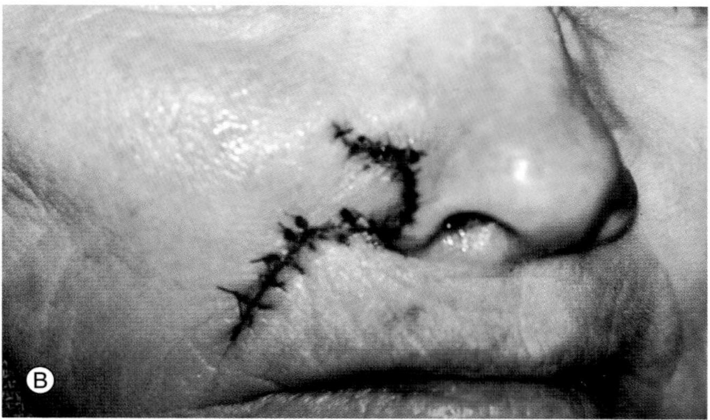

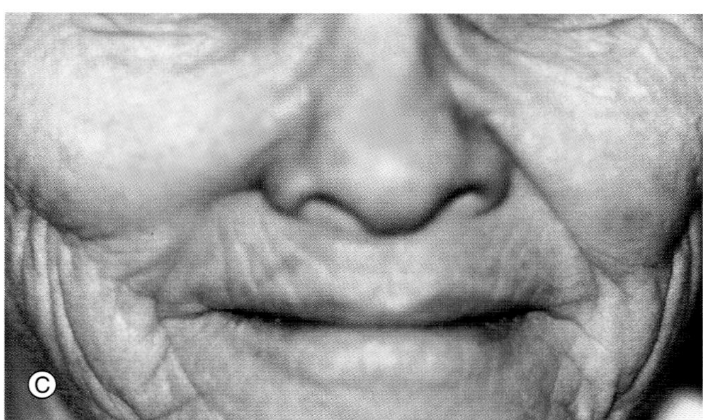

Figure 24.6 (A) A defect of the right nasal ala following Mohs surgery is shown with a superiorly based melolabial flap outlined. The medial aspect of the designed flap lays in the melolabial fold. The width of the flap extending from the medial to lateral aspect should be equivalent to the height of the defect. (B) The flap is sutured after wide undermining of the cheek skin and excision of standing cutaneous cone deformities. (C) Postoperative result at 6 months showing symmetry of the ala and minimal blunting of the sulcus.

donor skin. Delayed skin grafting of the nasal tip and ala with denuded cartilage may improve graft survival and may also improve the ultimate contour for initially deeper defects, because partial granulation of the base fills some of the void. Typical duration of the delay is 10–14 days.[15]

Cheeks

The cheek typically has a reservoir of excess tissue, laterally and inferiorly, making primary closure the treatment of choice for most small cheek defects. The skin lines of the cheek run obliquely in most areas, although anterior to the ear the skin lines are more vertical and they are more circumferential around the eyes. Care must be taken to avoid tension on the highly mobile lower eyelid, oral commissure, or the distensible nasal ala. Because the cheek is highly visible and composed of multiple anatomic units, long scars that cross anatomic units are easily noticed and less cosmetically acceptable. Most mid-cheek lesions are oriented obliquely. Undermining can be done at the level of the upper to mid-subcutaneous fat. In men, undermining should be performed below the level of the hair follicles. Typically 4-0 or 5-0 buried absorbable suture is utilized with 5-0 or 6-0 non-absorbable epidermal sutures. Sutures may be removed in 7 days.

Although the cheek is one of the regions less susceptible to procedural morbidity, there are some danger zones. Deep excisions performed laterally may expose the parotid gland. If the parotid gland is exposed focally, often its overlying fascia can simply be reapposed with smaller caliber absorbable suture. For larger areas of exposed parotid it is often helpful to allow its surface to granulate in place of its original fascia. This reduces the likelihood of fistula formation to the skin surface, containing saliva, from denuded parotid surface. The parotid (Stenson's) duct exits the parotid gland in the mid-cheek and courses above and perpendicular to the masseter muscle, then pierces the buccinator muscle, finally opening into the oral cavity opposite the second upper molar. A draining sinus will develop if the duct is injured and left unrepaired. Coursing over the mandibular ramus below the inferior margin of the parotid and adjacent to the facial artery and vein is the marginal mandibular branch of the facial nerve. In this location, the nerve is covered only by skin and platysma muscle, both of which may be thin. Transection of the nerve will result in an inability to evert the vermilion or retract the lip inferolaterally on the same side as the injury. To the observer, the resultant facial deformity is apparent drooping of the contralateral lower lip. The temporal branch of the facial nerve is also at risk as it crosses the zygomatic arch and has been previously discussed.

When primary closure is not an option, a local flap should be used in most instances to repair cheek defects. Because of the mobility of cheek skin, all three flap movements (advancement, rotation, and transposition) can be utilized. Transposition flaps are very useful for small to moderately sized defects of cheek and eyelid areas (Fig. 24.7). If the flap is positioned properly, the tension vectors are directed parallel to the eyelid margin avoiding a possible ectropion. Double transposition flaps (bilobed flaps) may also be used anywhere on the cheek. However, given the number of incisions, the scars may not fall into cosmetic units and may be cosmetically disappointing. Melolabial flaps, as previously discussed for nasal repair, can also be used for

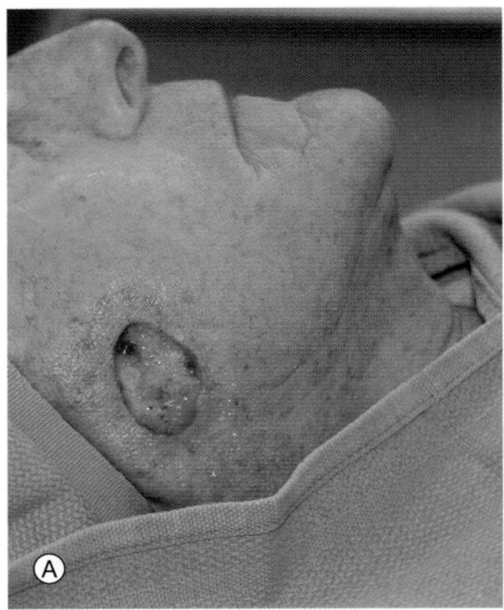

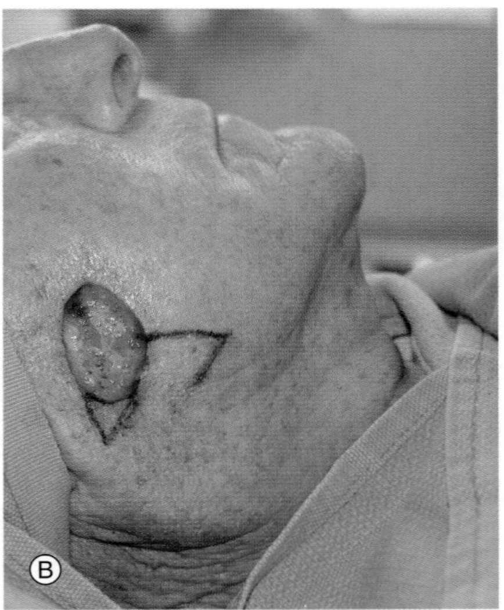

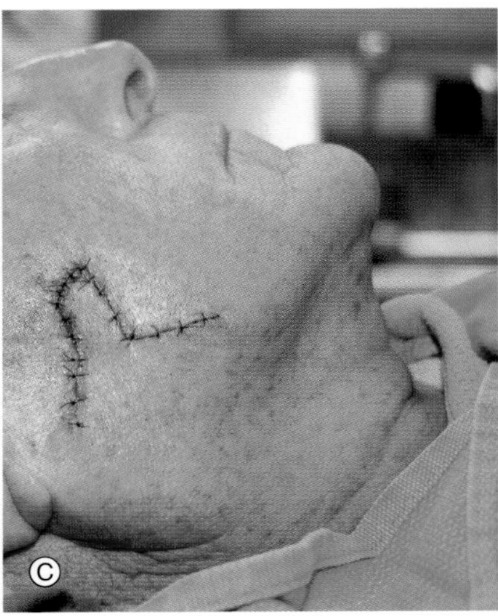

Figure 24.7 (A) A circular defect of the lateral cheek from micrographic surgery. (B) A Limberg transposition flap is designed to utilize inferolateral tissue laxity. (C) The sutured defect after excision of the standing tissue cone deformity.

small to moderately sized defects of the upper, middle, or lower medial aspects of the cheek and can be inferiorly or superiorly based. Advancement flaps (typically designed as single arm), unilateral flaps, or island pedicle flaps are useful for defects of the preauricular cheeks, medial cheeks, and upper medial cheeks. Rotation flaps are very useful for larger defects of the preauricular area and upper medial and mid-cheek. The tissue is typically recruited from the lower cheek/upper neck and lateral cheek/upper cheek, respectively. When designing a flap for an upper mid-cheek defect, a key point taken from the concept of the Mustarde flap used in lower eyelid reconstruction[16,17] is that the superior edge of the flap must include some skin of the temple. This will maintain the elevation and position of the lower eyelid skin, minimizing the possibility of ectropion.

Skin grafts are rarely used as a long-term repair option given the poor cosmetic outcome. However, if surveillance for tumor recurrence is of importance, a simple skin graft could be initially utilized and reconstructed later. Typical donor sites are the postauricular skin, preauricular skin, or supraclavicular areas to obtain the best color match. Split-thickness grafts should not be used near the eyelid because as the graft contracts it will pull down on the eyelid, possibly causing an ectropion. If grafting is performed on bearded areas of the chin or cheeks of a man, the donor site should be bearded skin to obtain the quantity and caliber of hairs identical to the surrounding skin. Little or no defatting of such grafts helps preserve the terminal hair bulbs originating in the subcutis. Skin grafts are occasionally necessary for very large cheek defects where other options are exhausted, or to repair smaller residual defects after much of the repair has been accomplished by a more favorable primary or flap repair.

Allowing a small, superficial cheek wound to heal by second intention is an acceptable repair option. Care must be taken that deformity of the eyelids or lips will not occur, making selection of appropriate wounds the critical step. The cosmetic result is typically satisfactory on concave areas of the cheeks and more variable laterally.

Perioral region

The upper and lower lips are important cosmetic units of the lower face and have several important motor, as well as sensory, functions. Distortion or asymmetry may be aesthetically displeasing, as well as functionally compromising. The anatomical margins of the lips include the base of the nose superiorly, the melolabial sulcus on each side, and the mental crease inferiorly. Relaxed skin tension lines run vertically or slightly obliquely, extending radially from the lips and the commissures; they are oblique or horizontal. Lip tissue is best viewed as a six-layered 'sandwich' lying sideways, with the skin and mucosal surfaces as the 'bread.' The layers are—in order—skin, subcutis, muscularis, minor salivary glands, submucosa, and mucosa. The best tissue for lip repair is lip tissue. In general, lip tissue can be recruited for repair as long as the defect is approximately one half or slightly more of either the upper or lower lip. When the defect is larger, tissue is usually recruited from the cheek or chin.

When reconstructing the lip, it is crucial that the vermilion borders are perfectly aligned. The vermilion border should be marked with ink or Gentian violet before anesthesia is injected. It is also important to preserve, if possible, the cosmetically important central philtrum—Cupid's bow—of the upper lip created by the union of the bilateral philtral crests. On a practical note, patients who wear dentures should remove them prior to surgery.

For defects encompassing approximately one half of either the lower lip or lateral upper lip, the defect should be closed primarily. For simple lesions, particularly partial-thickness lesions, a fusiform excision oriented so that the long axis parallels relaxed skin tension lines with primary closure is ideal. Every attempt should be made to confine the scar to the anatomic subunit as described above. M-plasty designs may be utilized if the size of the fusiform excision would extend beyond the anatomic subunit. The ellipse is incised deep to the base of the fat for skin or deep to the minor salivary glands for mucosal lesions. Hemostasis is best achieved by electrocoagulation. Special attention

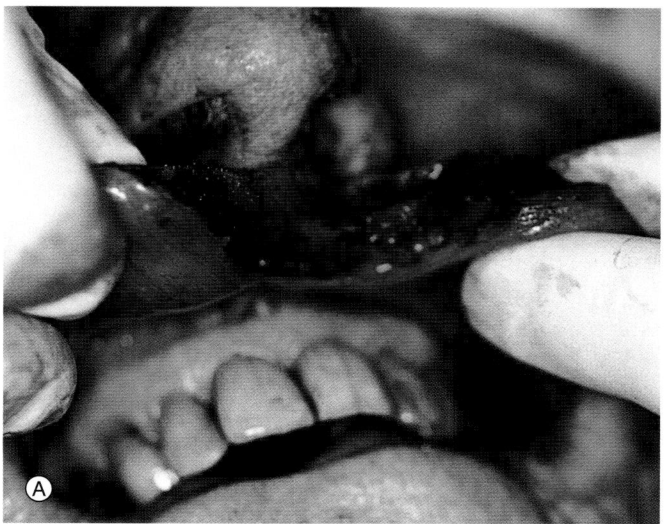

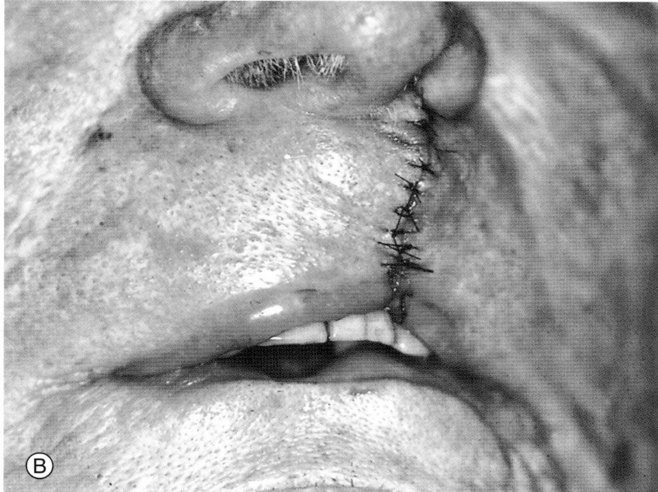

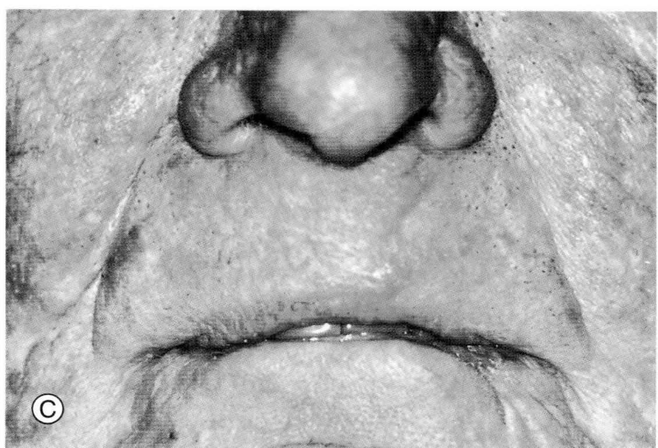

Figure 24.8 (A) A full-thickness wedge defect of the upper lip is shown. (B) The mucosal followed by muscular layers are apposed in full-thickness lip excisions prior to vermilion and cutaneous closures. Care is taken to perfectly align the vermilion as demonstrated in the sutured defect. (C) At 2-month follow-up the vermilion is aligned and there is no distortion of the lips or free margins.

should be directed to the labial artery, which runs horizontally in the loose areolar tissue and minor salivary glands. If transected, the vascular supply of the lip should not be compromised. The artery should be electrocoagulated or ligated while an assistant compresses the cut ends of the artery. For closures of cutaneous lip, monofilament nylon or polypropylene suture is typically utilized. For closures of the vermilion or mucosal surfaces, soft, braided, 5-0 coated polyester is ideal. Silk is typically not utilized because of its inflammatory properties. When the vermilion has been incised, it is important that the first sutures perfectly align the previously inked vermilion margins. This is best achieved by using 5-0 braided, coated polyester suture to perform a vertical mattress suture. Subsequently the cutaneous lip should be repaired in layered fashion, followed by repair of the vermilion proper and mucosa. Any redundancies should be removed on, or in very close proximity to, the vermilion/mucosal margin to provide the best possible cosmetic result. Typically the redundancies are removed parallel to the lip margin. Postoperative care consists of cleansing cutaneous wounds with hydrogen peroxide followed by generous application of antibiotic ointment after the petrolatum-gauze dressing is removed at 48–72 hours. For wounds on the vermilion or mucosa, the patient should swish and expectorate half-strength hydrogen peroxide three or four times daily. In order to prevent postoperative dehiscence, patients should be advised to avoid excessive speech, wide opening of the mouth, and foods that are difficult to chew for 3–4 weeks. They should adhere to a soft diet for the first 7–10 days. Non-absorbable suture is removed at 7–10 days. Increasing tenderness, edema, pain, or fever should prompt immediate evaluation for infection, particularly if the mucosa was incised.

For full-thickness defects of the lips, many of the principles described above apply. In planning a full-thickness upper-lip excision, the excision is drawn as a triangle with the base at the vermilion/mucosal margin, and the apex directed toward the cutaneous lip (Fig. 24.8). The length of the triangle should be approximately one-and-a-half times the width of the base and the tip should have a 30° angle. This type of repair is not appropriate for defects where the base of the triangle would be more than about one-quarter of the length of the upper lip because subsequent oral patency and overall appearance become compromised. For the lower lip, the configuration is a pentagon rather than a triangle to account for the concavity between the vermilion and the chin. Again the base of the pentagon is at the vermilion/mucosal margin and the apex directed toward the mental crease. The angle at the peak

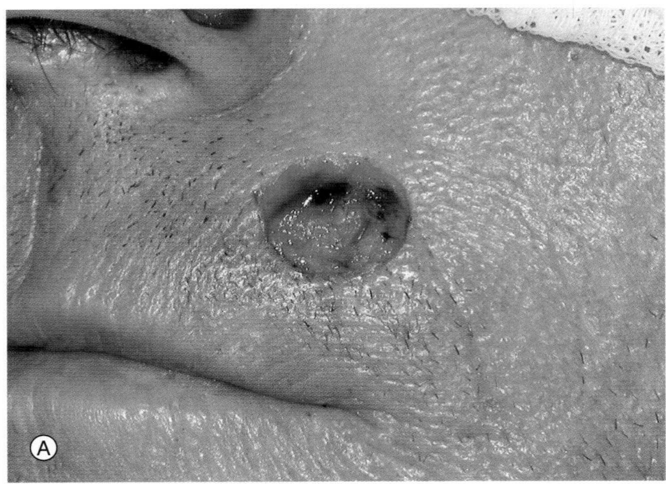

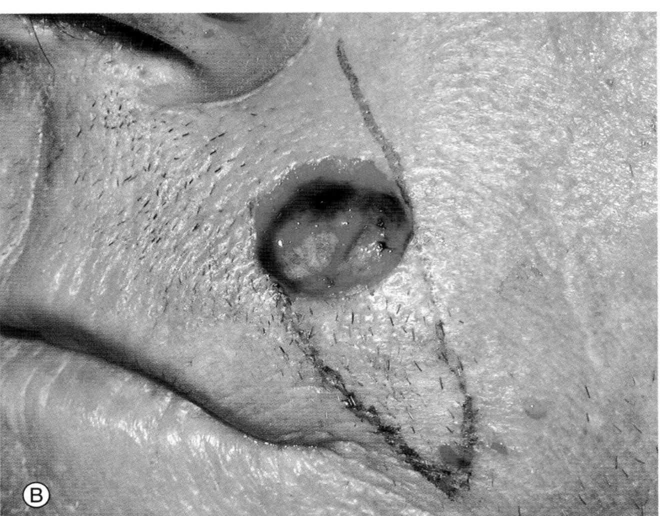

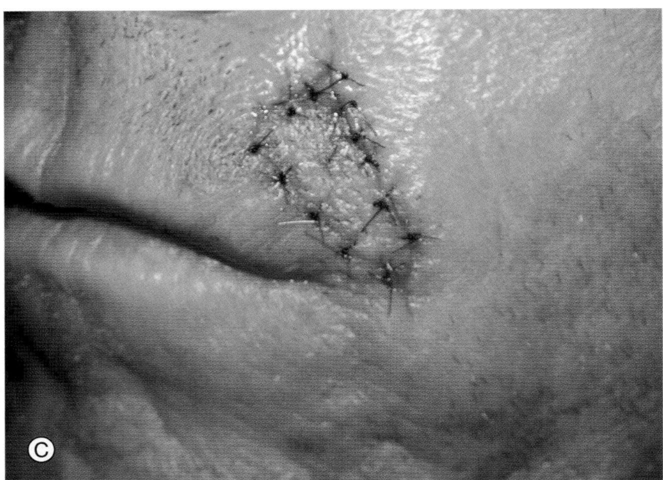

Figure 24.9 (A) A defect of the upper cutaneous lip is created following micrographic surgery. (B) An island pedicle advancement flap is designed. An island of skin with a vascularized pedicle attached to muscle is advanced toward the recipient site. Undermining is performed around but not underneath the flap. (C) The sutured defect shows excellent matching of tissue color and texture. There is no distortion of surrounding cosmetic boundaries.

varies from 60°–100° depending on the width of the base. For mid-line lower-lip lesions the sides of the pentagon are equal, whereas for more lateral lesions the pentagon becomes asymmetric. This type of repair is not appropriate for defects where the base of the pentagon would be greater than one-third the length of the lower lip, or for defects nearly abutting the oral commissure, for both functional and cosmetic reasons. Closure of the defect should begin with the apex of the triangle or pentagon, followed by the mid-portion, and finally the vermilion. When suturing on the mucosal surface, it is important that the absorbable suture knots are well buried and directed away from the mucosal surface (toward the center of the 'sandwich').

When performing a flap in the perioral region, particular attention should be given to the primary and secondary movements and the effects on the free margins of the lips and nose. An ideal place to hide transverse incision when working at the vermilion–cutaneous border is the white roll, a smooth, reflective, linear band just above the vermilion of the upper lip. Advancement and transposition flaps are useful in repair of perioral wounds because of their ability to precisely align vectors or primary and secondary movements. For small to large defects of both the upper and lower lips, advancement flaps can be designed to advance lateral lip tissue or medial cheek tissue. On the upper lip, the incisions can often be hidden in the white roll or at the junction of the nose and cutaneous lip. On the lower lip, the incisions can be hidden at the vermilion border and along the mental crease. Smaller defects of either the upper or lower lip can be repaired with A-to-T type advancement flaps. The horizontal component of the flap can be hidden in junction lines as previously discussed, while the vertical component can be hidden in the relaxed skin tension lines. An island pedicle flap can be designed to repair defects of the superior and lateral upper cutaneous lip (Fig. 24.9). Transposition flaps are often used to repair larger defects of the upper and lower lip with medial cheek tissue. Small defects of the mid- to lateral upper lip may be repaired with rotation flaps directing the arc along the melolabial fold. Tissue redundancies are excised along skin tension lines. If a minor eclabium is produced, it will usually correct within 1–2 months. Larger defects of the upper and lower lips can require more extensive repair. For example, defects from one-half to two-thirds of the lip can be closed with a 'lip-switch' flap (a full-thickness pedicled flap) or with the Karapandzic flap, a large cheek–lip advancement flap.[18] Defects away from the commissure can be closed with an Abbe flap, a full-thickness flap from the opposite lip pedicled on the vermilion border and containing the labial artery.[19] The Estlander flap was designed for defects near the commissure of the mouth.[20] Especially in men, the use of cheek skin for flaps of the upper lip results in a bald spot within the moustache, and should be used as a last resort. Protection of philtrum symmetry is particularly important. Finally, intact commissures and a contiguous orbicularis oris muscle are paramount because these structures are critical for speech, eating, and sphincter function.

Repair by grafts or with second intention healing are not the preferred options on the lips. Second intention healing can be used for shallow defects of the vermilion, philtrum, or melolabial folds. Skin grafts can sometimes be employed in the replacement of an entire cosmetic subunit of the lip, such as philtrum, or the triangular area between philtrum, nose, and melolabial fold. Grafts in this area often contract with resultant eclabium, and do not blend well with hair-bearing skin, confining their use almost exclusively to women. Donor sites for graft skin in this area are most often periauricular, supraclavicular, or the melolabial-fold region.

Chin

Fusiform excisions with primary closure are an excellent choice for repair on the chin. Relaxed skin tension lines extend radially from the vermilion border, so excisions on the chin can be planned whereby the final orientation of the scar is vertical or oblique to the vermilion border. This also directs tension vectors toward a horizontal plane, preventing possible depression of the lip. An exception to vertical scar placement is in the mental crease and adjacent areas, where horizontal placement allows for better scar concealment. The risk of horizontal scar placement is the resultant vertical tension vectors, which could potentially depress the lower lip. Ellipses in this region should spare the vermilion borders, when possible, to preserve the important contours of the lips. Also, one should strive for maximal eversion of the wound edge when suturing on the chin because the thick sebaceous skin often heals with a depressed appearance.

There are no major anatomic danger zones in this region, although deep incision of the lateral chin may result in trauma to the facial artery or mental nerve. Anesthesia of the chin and lower lip can be achieved by regional block of the mental nerve, located in the middle portion of the mandible at the mid-pupillary line. Buried absorbable suture in this region is typically 4-0 or 5-0 caliber and superficial non-absorbable suture 5-0 or 6-0. Sutures may be removed in 7–10 days.

Because of the geometric and curved lines of the chin, advancement and rotation flaps are most useful. For larger central defects of the chin, bilateral subcutaneous island pedicle flaps can be used with excellent results. Adjacent tissue, but not the flap itself, is undermined just deep to the hair follicles. The double rotation flap, or O-to-Z flap, is also used to close central chin defects. The double rotation allows more tissue movement, which is especially useful on the chin where the tissue is less mobile. Local flaps that redirect tension vectors to a horizontal plane, preventing possible lip depression, are optimal.

Grafts of the chin have the disadvantage of poor color and texture match. Wrinkling of the graft can occur due to the constant movement from speech and chewing. Hypertrophic scarring or pin-cushioning can also occur.

Variable cosmetic results occur with second intention healing of defects on the convex surfaces of the chin, making other repair options as listed above more desirable.

Ear

Malignant tumors less than 1 cm in diameter located on the helix, antihelix, or scapha can be treated with ear wedge excisions. Prior to excision, anesthesia is obtained by a field block of the auricle using 1% lidocaine with 1 in 100 000 epinephrine (adrenaline). To improve hemostasis and prolong anesthesia, anesthetic is then infiltrated locally at the excision site. After appropriate margins have been established, the wedge is planned with an angle of approximately 30°. Larger angles create circumferential tension, which increases the risk of infection, dehiscence, or cup deformity. Numerous modifications can be made to the wedge excision if large lesions are being treated, thus avoiding creation of an angle greater than 30°. The wedge can be excised with tissue scissors or a scalpel. Meticulous electrocoagulation is then performed to obtain hemostasis while avoiding damage to the underlying cartilaginous structures. Buried absorbable suture in this region is typically 4-0 caliber and is directed in a horizontal, rather than vertical, fashion. Epidermal edges are closed with interrupted 5-0 or 6-0 suture with the goal of margin eversion. Even with proper eversion of the wound edges, notching may occur. To reduce the risk of notching, vertical mattress sutures may be used over the helical rim. Alternatively, Z-plasty of the helical rim can be performed to redistribute the vectors of scar contraction at the incision line. Postoperative analgesia is often required for the several days following the procedure. Increasing pain and/or edema requires prompt evaluation for infection or chondritis.

Certain subsites of the ear are very amenable to healing by second intention. The concavities of the ear, including the scapha, triangular fossa, and conchal bowl, heal well by granulation, as does the posterior helix and postauricular sulcus. If the perichondrium is absent, the granulation process can be markedly prolonged. In these cases, fenestration of ear cartilage using a 2–3 mm punch biopsy to access intact perichondrium on the other surface of the ear is beneficial in forming islands of granulation tissue. Fenestrations should be spaced to leave at least 5 mm of intact cartilage between fenestration sites and should not be closer than 5 mm to the wound edge. Fenestrated cartilage requires meticulous wound care consisting of cleansing with moist compresses of dilute acetic acid (0.25%), application of generous amounts of topical antibiotics, and occlusion where possible. Granulation of the internal auditory meatus should be avoided as a stricture of the ear canal may develop.

The lateral surface of the ear is irregularly concave and presents numerous eminences and depressions. Defects of this surface with intact cartilage are often best treated by skin grafts. The donor site is often the contralateral postauricular skin or preauricular skin. A petrolatum-impregnated bolster should be used for graft immobilization. If perichondrium is absent, fenestrations should be performed as outlined above. Once healthy islands of granulation tissue have formed, a delayed split-thickness or full-thickness skin graft may be applied.

For defects of the conchal bowl lacking skin and cartilage, a retroauricular island transposition flap is an alternative to

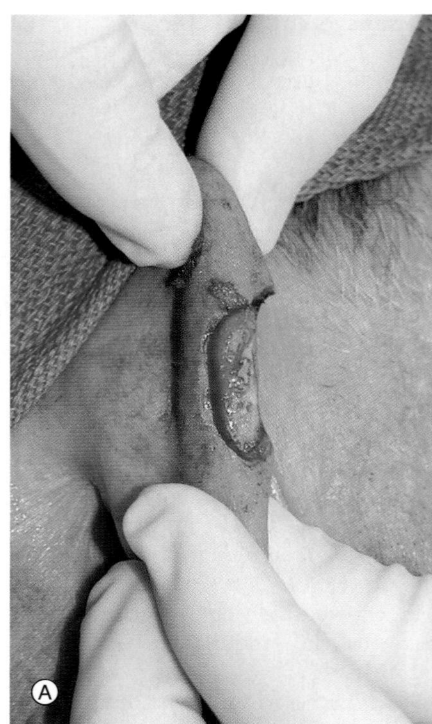

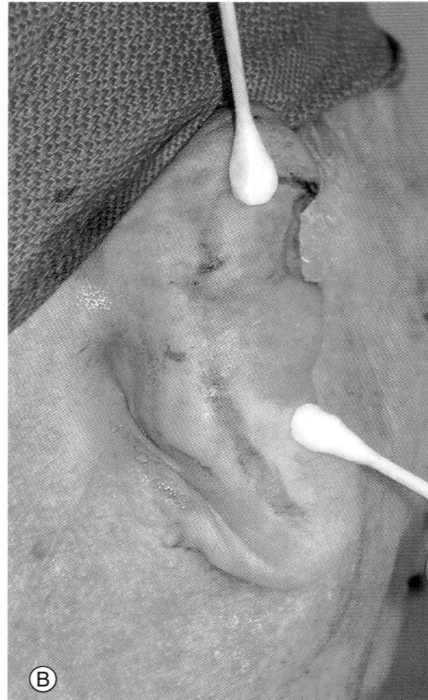

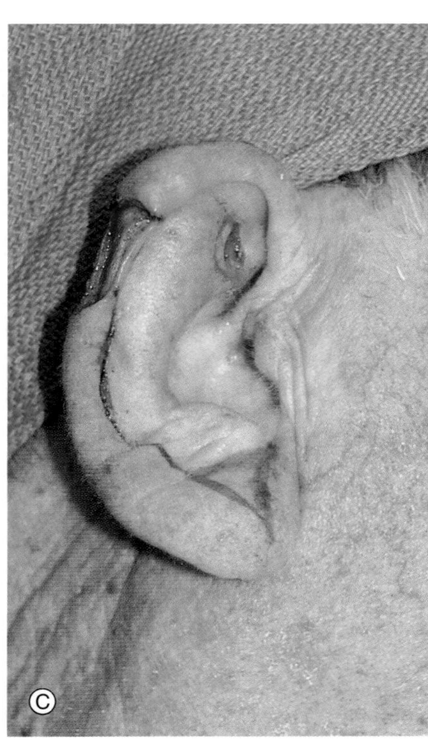

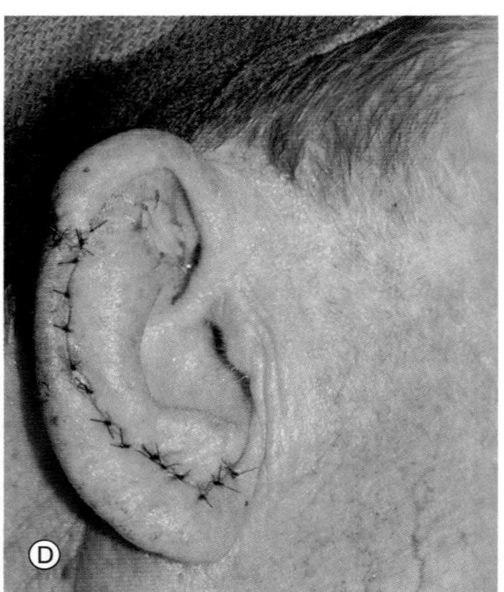

Figure 24.10 (A) Micrographic surgery defect of the right mid-helix. (B) The posterior aspect of the outlined through-and-through incision of the classic helical rim advancement flap. (C) The first incision will extend from the inferior aspect of the defect into the lobule. The most important suture is placed first and approximates the margins of the helical defect. (D) Flap replaces the tissue with minimal alteration of the ear profile and no cupping.

full-thickness skin grafting. Skin of the postauricular ear is transposed anteriorly as an island flap into the defect, followed by primary closure of the postauricular donor site. Defects of the upper and middle one-third of the ear greater than approximately 0.15 cm but less than 2.5 cm can be closed with the helical chondrocutaneous advancement flap as described by Antia,[21] with the posterior skin left intact to increase vascularity of the pedicle (Fig. 24.10). Larger defects are often closed with a retroauricular or preauricular tubed flap in a multistaged procedure. The first stage requires formation of a skin tube with superior and inferior attachments. The second stage involves attachment of the tube to the auricle. The third stage involves flap inset. Small lateral skin defects of the upper and middle ear can be closed with rotation/advancement flaps. Defects of the lower third of the ear are often amenable to advancement flaps. Extensive defects require cartilage grafting techniques. Flap repairs of the posterior (medial) ear can be based on the availability of excess tissue in the postauricular area. Traditional rotation flaps or transposition flaps are the most useful.

Flap repair serves an important role in auricular reconstruction. Again, preservation of form and function is critical. The skin of the lateral ear is tightly adherent to the perichondrium and lacks subcutaneous tissue. The skin of the medial (posterior aspect of the ear) ear is loose and subcutaneous tissue is present. Undermining should be performed superficial to the perichondrium. Both advancement and transposition flaps are useful in repairing defects of the ear.

Neck

The favored methods of closure on the neck include primary closure and flaps. The relaxed skin tension lines of the neck are oriented obliquely on the lateral sides of the neck and become more horizontal anteriorly and posteriorly. Anatomically, the posterior triangle of the neck is a danger zone that the cutaneous surgeon must respect. The posterior triangle of the neck is bounded by the posterior border of the sternocleidomastoid muscle, the anterior border of the trapezius muscle, and the superior border of the clavicle. Its roof is formed by the platysma and the investing layer of the deep cervical fascia. The spinal accessory nerve (XIth cranial nerve) enters the triangle from the posterior border of the sternocleidomastoid coursing diagonally and posteriorly along the levator scapulae muscle, before exiting deep to the trapezius muscle. Within the posterior triangle, the nerve courses superficially, covered only by skin and adipose. Transection or damage of this nerve results in a loss of function of the trapezius muscle. The patient will clinically have a dropped shoulder, inability to abduct the shoulder greater than 80°, paresthesia, and chronic pain. The entrance point of the nerve known as Erb's point is localized by 'dropping' a vertical line approximately 6 cm from the mid-point of a line drawn from the mastoid process to the angle of the mandible.

The skin of the anterior and lateral sides of the neck is relatively mobile, so primary closures are usually performed. Undermining occurs at the level of the superficial subcutaneous adipose tissue. Buried absorbable suture is usually of 3-0 or 4-0 caliber and superficial non-absorbable suture is usually of 4-0 or 5-0 caliber. Standard wound care and dressings are used. Sutures can typically be removed in 10–14 days.

For larger defects of the neck or defects of the thicker posterior neck, flaps may be utilized. All three flap movements can be designed. Again, care should be taken to avoid injury to deeper structures of the neck. Careful hemostasis must be employed after flap surgery because the frequent movement of the neck increases the risk of postoperative hematoma formation. Postoperative bleeding in the neck area can lead to compression of vital underlying structures.

Trunk

The trunk is an area of the body commonly treated with fusiform excisions or fusiform variations, and subsequently closed primarily. The relaxed skin tension lines vary by location on the trunk and should be determined prior to planning the excision to determine the directions of skin laxity and tension. The long axis of the fusiform excision should parallel the relaxed skin tension lines. There are few danger zones on the trunk making it a relatively forgiving site. However, patients should be forewarned of the possibility of hypertrophic or keloidal scarring particularly on the chest and presternal area, as well as less frequently on the shoulders and upper back. People with a history of keloids or hypertrophic scarring, or Asians, African–Americans, and those with a family history of adverse scarring should be carefully counseled regarding the possibility of exuberant scar tissue formation, especially prior to elective procedures.

Closure of a surgical wound is achieved either with one or two layers of absorbable suture. Usually the subcutis and deep dermis are closed with absorbable 2-0 or 3-0 caliber suture while the more superficial dermis is closed with absorbable 3-0 or 4-0 suture. Larger caliber suture may be required for wounds under more tension. For final skin closure, typically 4-0 caliber monofilament non-absorbable suture is used, although surgical staples are also a reasonable option. Standard wound care measures and dressings are utilized. Sutures are typically removed in 14 days. Physical limitations may have to be placed on the patient depending on the degree of wound tension to prevent dehiscence.

Since there is a large reservoir of tissue on the trunk, all three flap movements can be designed. Again, physical limitations may have to be placed. Either full-thickness or split-thickness grafts can be used for repair of defects on the torso that cannot be repaired primarily or with a flap. Full-thickness grafts are cosmetically and functionally superior to split-thickness grafts and are used more frequently for smaller defects on the torso that cannot be completely apposed primarily or do not granulate fully. Split-thickness grafts are used for wounds too large for full-thickness skin grafts, and also allow for close inspection and palpation of the site if there is a risk of tumor recurrence. Granulation on the trunk often results in a scar that is thicker and more persistently erythematous. When cosmetic concerns are of minimal importance, granulation is a reasonable option.

Extremities

The extremities have a curved shape, which often results in tissue redundancies after excisional surgery. The relaxed skin tension lines of the extremities are often oblique although they become more horizontal near the antecubital and popliteal fossae. Again, it is important to palpate the tissue prior to designing the excision or flap to fully determine the directions of greatest skin laxity. Although there are few anatomic danger zones on the extremities, there are anatomic considerations that must be discussed with the patient prior to surgery. Any surgical wound near a joint is at an increased risk for dehiscence. Activity should be minimized for 3–4 weeks postoperatively. Occasionally, splints, crutches, or slings are required to minimize movement.

Curvilinear closures such as a 'lazy S' excision are useful over the convexities of the extremities. The excision is designed as an ellipse with 30° angles at the tips, but the tips are twisted in opposite directions. When oriented longitudinally along the extremities, this excision more evenly distributes tension and reduces the tissue redundancies at the tips of the excision.

For lower extremity lesions not amenable to primary closure, skin grafts rather than flaps are typically utilized because the dependent nature of the legs often leads to varying degrees of edema. Edematous tissue is known to heal slowly and poorly, and the additional incision lines of flaps may be adversely affected. However, for occasional small defects where tension redistribution or redirection is desirable, rhombic transposition flaps, and A–T flaps are useful, particularly on the dorsal hands and dorsal feet. Caution is required for repairs on extremities as a result of possible inadequacies of circulation, especially of the lower legs and feet. Split-thickness skin grafts are used more frequently than full-thickness grafts because of the higher risks of graft failure on the lower leg. Patients should be aware that split-thickness grafts will not produce sweat or hair and are usually hypopigmented in comparison to the surrounding skin.

On the arm, flaps of all types are used more frequently

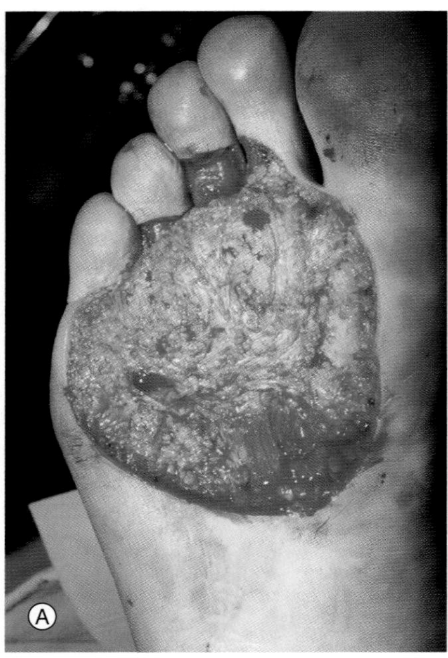

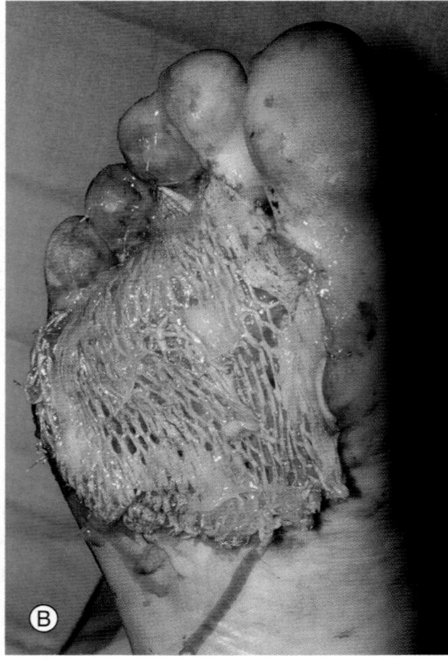

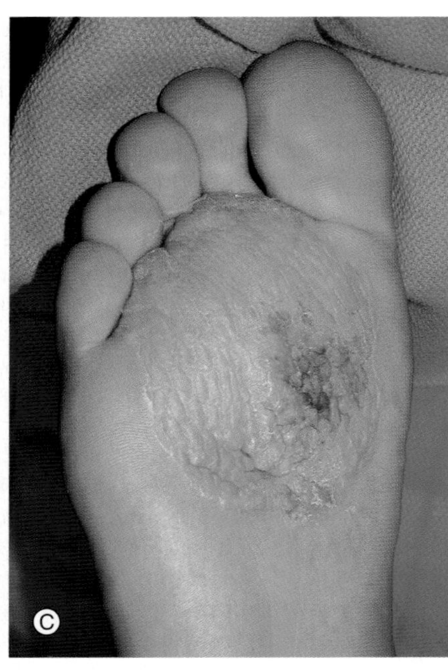

Figure 24.11 (A) A large defect of the plantar foot with an intact fat pad. (B) A split-thickness skin graft is utilized in this location because the fat pad is preserved and provides cushioning and protection of the underlying tendons. (C) 7-month follow-up showing good epithelialization with minor crusting at the medial aspect corresponding to localized daily pressure.

than grafts. All three tissue movements are possible. Immobilization of the arm may be required in the postoperative period.

Granulation is typically not a primary repair option on the extremities because the scars tend to be bulkier and more erythematous. However, granulation of a wound can be used as an adjunctive measure prior to delayed skin grafting.

Hands, feet, and digits

The hands and feet are unique in comparison to other sites because of the frequent, often repetitive and intricate movements that occur in these locations. The hands and feet are particularly challenging because of the small circumferences of the digits and the repetitive stresses that are unavoidable with daily activities and ambulation, which make wounds prone to dehiscence. In addition, the subcutaneous tissue is relatively thin, especially in the elderly, and vital structures such as vessels, bone, and tendon can easily be compromised. Relaxed skin tension lines can vary but are usually oriented horizontally or obliquely. Careful observation along with palpation is required to determine laxity and appropriate direction of closure. It can be helpful to ask the patient to gently flex and extend the wrist and fingers or ankle and toes intraoperatively to determine likely tension on the wound; this may aid in suture placement or decisions as to the necessity of soft casting or splinting if intraoperative measures fail to relieve excess tension. Smaller excisions are frequently conducted with standard fusiform design with primary apposition. Larger excisions, excisions over the lateral surfaces of the hands and feet, and excisions closer to web spaces are more often repaired with a 'lazy S' design as previously discussed. Regardless of the design, redundancies at the excisional tips are more common on the dorsal hands and feet than elsewhere. Because these areas remodel well, redundancies are typically not 'chased' across the dorsal surfaces, and patients should be counseled to expect these standing cones to resolve more readily over time than would be expected elsewhere on the body.

All incisions should be superficial with attention to the deep structures. Undermining should be immediately deep to the dermis. Buried absorbable sutures of a 4-0 or 5-0 caliber are typically used. Often the buried suture is directed in an oblique or horizontal fashion rather than a vertical fashion so that more surface area of the supportive dermis is in contact with the suture. For the epidermis, 4-0 or 5-0 non-absorbable suture is used. For especially thin skin, Ethibond suture (Ethicon Inc, Johnson & Johnson Co, Somerville, NJ) may result in less tearing of the fragile skin. While suturing, one should focus on keeping the suture pathways superficial, to avoid inadvertent trapping of a tendon in the suture material which can result in significant physical impairment requiring physical therapy. Patients should be cautioned to avoid heavy lifting and to minimize hand movements. Casting or splinting may be utilized when necessary. Standard wound care and pressure dressings are used. Sutures are typically removed in 10–14 days.

For defects that cannot be closed primarily, rhombic transposition flaps and A-T flaps are useful, particularly for small defects where tension redistribution or redirection is desired. Skin grafting is utilized on the dorsal hands if a defect is not amenable to primary closure or repair with a flap. On the dorsal foot, grafts, especially split-thickness grafts, are more often employed because of the high risk of graft/flap failure in this location.

For the palmar and plantar surfaces, defects should be repaired primarily whenever possible using the same considerations as outlined above. When primary repair is not possible, split-thickness skin grafts harvested from elsewhere on the palm or sole or upper-inner arm or thigh are utilized (Fig. 24.11). Avoiding trauma and weightbearing are paramount for reducing complications such as dehiscence, hematoma, tissue necrosis, and future hypertrophic scarring. Most patients should protect distal extremities in this fashion for 3–4 weeks, and several weeks longer for larger repairs.

For defects of the digits, split-thickness skin grafts are the repair option of choice. For the small grafts used in these locations, non-mechanical harvesting of donor skin is typically performed using a Weck blade or #10 scalpel blade with a smooth, slicing motion tangential to the donor site surface. Graft survival of a split-thickness skin graft is higher in this location than a full-thickness skin graft.

SUMMARY

It can be seen that there are a large number of considerations to make when choosing the best reconstruction technique to use in any one body region. The authors' preferences, region by region, are given in Table 24.3. Wherever feasible, primary closure and its variants are the preferred option.

The treatment priorities for each patient have to be considered, along with other health factors. The patients' attitudes are also important, and they need to be given a full understanding of the rationale behind the choice of technique, especially when disease considerations necessitate a technique that has a suboptimal cosmetic outcome.

Avoidance of pitfalls

- Scalp: careful hemostasis is required because the subgaleal space is a potential reservoir for postoperative hematoma formation.
- Central forehead excisions: warn the patient that these can result in superior retraction of the eyebrows, and advise that in most instances gravity returns them to their normal position in 6–12 months.
- Lateral forehead or temple: to prevent undue alarm, warn the patient that anesthesia can result in temporary paralysis of the local musculature.
- Periorbital region and cheeks: educate the patient about the expected edema and non-indurated ecchymosis that occurs when working around the eyes.
- Perioral region: to prevent wound dehiscence, advise the patient against excess postoperative movement of the mouth; discuss dietary and speaking limitations prior to the surgery.
- Chin: to prevent wound dehiscence advise the patient to avoid excessive speech, wide opening of the mouth, and foods that are difficult to chew for 3–4 weeks.
- Ear: closely monitor the ear for postoperative infection and/or perichondritis, and inform the patient that the ears will no longer look symmetrical because the circumference and vertical height of the treated ear will be reduced.
- Neck: unavoidable neck movement increases the possibility of postoperative hematoma formation, therefore undermining should be limited on the neck with careful attention to hemostasis.
- Trunk: discuss the possibility of hypertrophic or keloidal scarring.
- Extremities: advise the patient that activity should be minimized for 3–4 weeks postoperatively; occasionally splints, crutches or slings will be required to minimize movement.
- Hands and feet: avoid wound dehiscence and other complications due to physical activity by intraoperative assessment of wound tension; patients may require the support of physical therapists or occupational therapists after surgery to the hands or feet (this possibility should be discussed prior to the surgery).

Table 24.3 Preferred closure options by region

Location	Closure options ranked in order of preference	Pitfalls
Scalp	1. Primary closure and variants 2. Granulation 3. Grafts 4. Flaps	The subgaleal space is a potential reservoir for postoperative bleeding. Careful hemostasis is advised to prevent postoperative hematoma formation.
Forehead, central	1. Primary closure and variants 2. Partial closure 3. Flaps/granulation 4. Grafts	Forehead excisions can result in superior retraction of the eyebrows. In most instances, time and gravity return the eyebrows to their normal position in 6–12 months.
Forehead, lateral	1. Primary closure and variants 2. Granulation/flaps 3. Grafts	Anesthesia of the lateral forehead or temple can result in temporary paralysis of the local musculature. The patient should be cautioned of this beforehand to prevent undue alarm.
Periorbital region	1. Primary closure and variants 2. Flaps 3. Granulation (in select lesions) 4. Grafts	Patients should be educated regarding the expected edema and non-indurated ecchymosis that occurs when working around the eyes.
Nose, upper	1. Primary closure and variants 2. Flaps 3. Grafts 4. Granulation (concavities)	
Nose, lower	1. Granulation if shallow (assess nasal valve function) 2. Flaps/grafts	
Cheeks	1. Primary closure and variants 2. Flaps	Patients should be educated regarding the expected edema and non-indurated ecchymosis that occurs when working around the eyes.
Perioral region	1. Primary closure and variants 2. Flaps 3. Grafts (for replacement of an entire subunit) 4. Granulation (for shallow vermilion lesions)	Patients with dentures should remove them prior to surgery. Ink the vermilion margins prior to infiltration of anesthesia so the borders can be perfectly aligned during reconstruction. Patients need to avoid excess movement of the mouth postoperatively to prevent dehiscence. Dietary and speaking limitations should be discussed prior to the surgery.
Chin	1. Primary closure and variants 2. Flap 3. Graft (infrequently)	In order to prevent postoperative dehiscence, patients should be advised to avoid excessive speech, wide opening of the mouth, and foods that are difficult to chew for 3–4 weeks.
Ear	1. Wedge and variants 2. Granulation (for posterior, concave lesions) 3. Grafts/flaps (depending on location and size)	Perform a field block of the auricle and then infiltrate anesthesia locally at the excision site to improve hemostasis and prolong anesthesia. The wedge excision should not exceed one-quarter of the auricular circumference to reduce distortion and excessive cupping. Closely monitor in the postoperative period for infection and/or perichondritis. Inform patients that the ears will no longer look symmetrical. The circumference and vertical height of the treated ear will be reduced.
Neck	1. Primary closure and variants 2. Flaps	The unavoidable movement of the neck increases the possibility of postoperative hematoma formation. Undermining should be limited on the neck with careful attention to hemostasis.
Trunk	1. Primary closure and variants 2. Grafts/flaps 3. Granulation (when appearance is not an issue	Discuss the possibility of hypertrophic or keloidal scarring.
Extremities	1. Primary closure and variants 2. Grafts: lower extremities, split-thickness > full-thickness skin graft/flaps (upper extremities) 3. Granulation as adjunctive measure	Activity should be minimized for 3–4 weeks postoperatively. Occasionally, splints, crutches or slings are required to minimize movement.
Hands, dorsum	1. Primary repair, especially curvilinear design 2. Flap 3. Graft	Surgical wounds on the hands and feet are more prone to dehiscence and other complications because of physical activity. During any operative procedure, it is helpful to have the patient gently flex and extend the wrist and fingers or ankle and toes to determine the tension on the wound. This may aid in suture placement or if necessary determine the necessity of soft casting or splinting if intraoperative measures fail to relieve excess tension. Patients may require the support of physical therapists or occupational therapists after surgery to the hands or feet. This possibility should be discussed prior to the surgery.

(Continued on next page)

Table 24.3 Preferred closure options by region—continued

Location	Closure options ranked in order of preference	Pitfalls
Hands, palmar	1. Primary repair 2. Split-thickness skin grafting (donor site from palm or upper, inner arm)	
Feet, dorsum	1. Primary repair 2. Graft 3. Flap 4. Granulation (rare)	
Feet, plantar	1. Primary repair 2. Split-thickness skin grafting	
Digits	1. Split-thickness skin grafting	

REFERENCES

1. Bucknall TE, Ellis H. Wound healing for surgeons, East Sussex: Baillière Tindall; 1984.
2. Falcone PA, Caldwell MD. Wound metabolism. Clin Plast Surg 1990; 17:443.
3. Moy RL, Waldman B, Hein DL. A review of sutures and suturing techniques. J Dermatol Surg Oncol 1992; 18:785.
4. Zitelli JA. Wound healing by secondary intention. A cosmetic appraisal. J Am Acad Dermatol 1983; 9:407.
5. Panje WR, Minor LB. Reconstruction of the scalp. In: Baker SR, Swanson NA, eds. Local flaps in facial reconstruction. St Louis: Mosby 1995; 481–514.
6. Leshin B, Whitaker DC, Swanson NA. Preoperative evaluation in dermatologic surgery. J Am Acad Dermatol 1988; 19:1081–1088.
7. Dzubow LM. Chemosurgical report: indications for a geometric approach to wound closure following Mohs surgery. J Am Acad Dermatol 1987; 13:480–486.
8. Patel BC, Flaharty PM, Anderson RL. Reconstruction of the eyelids. In: Baker SR, Swanson NA, eds. Local flaps in facial reconstruction. St Louis: Mosby 1995; 275–303.
9. Deutsch BD, Becker FF. Secondary healing of Mohs defects of the forehead, temple, and lower eyelid. Arch Otolaryngol Head Neck Surg 1997; 123:529–534.
10. Shankar J, Nair RG, Sullivan SC. Management of peri-ocular skin tumours by laissez-faire technique: analysis of functional and cosmetic results. Eye 2002; 16:50–53.
11. Arpey CJ. Wound management. In: Arpey CJ, Whitaker DC, O'Donnell MJ, eds. Cutaneous surgery: illustrated and practical approach. New York: McGraw Hill 1997; 73–96.
12. Shotton F. Rhombic flap for medial canthal reconstruction. Ophthalmic Surg 1983; 14:46.
13. Zitelli JA. The bilobed flap for nasal reconstruction. Arch Dermatol 1989;125:957–959.
14. Zitelli JA. The nasolabial flap as a single stage procedure. Arch Dermatol 1990; 126:1445–1448.
15. Robinson JK, Dillig G. The advantages of delayed nasal full-thickness skin grafting after Mohs micrographic surgery. Dermatol Surg. 2002; 28:845–851.
16. Callahan MA, Callahan A. Mustarde flap lower lid reconstruction after malignancy. Ophthalmology 1980; 87:279–286.
17. Mustarde JC. Repair and reconstruction in the orbital region. Edinburgh: Churchill Livingstone 1991; 125–190.
18. Karapandzic M. Reconstruction of lip defects by local arterial flaps. Br J Plast Surg 1974; 27:93–97.
19. Baker SR. Malignancy of the lip. In: Gluckman, J, ed. Otolaryngology. Philadelphia: WB Saunders; 1988.
20. Estlander JA. Eine methods aus der einen lippe substanzverluste der anderen zu ersetzen. Arch Klin Chir 1872; 14:622.
21. Antia NH, Buch VI. Chondrocutaneous advancement flap for the marginal defect of the ear. Plast Reconstr Surg 1967; 39:472.

25 Scar Revision

Ken K Lee MD, Annalisa K Gorman MD, and Neil A Swanson MD

Summary box

- There are four major wound closure options: second intention healing, primary closure and its variations, skin grafts, and local or distal flaps.
- Choice of which option to use depends on the nature of the defect, the site of the repair and the patient's age, concomitant medications and diseases, irradiation history and tendency for multiple tumors; factors related to the patient's self image and expectations about wound appearance should also be taken into account.
- Scar revision methodology includes intralesional steroids, non-ablative lasers, surgical excision, and dermabrasion and ablative lasers and is sometimes as simple as allowing more time for the original scar to heal.
- Fusiform elliptical excision is the simplest surgical technique but the resultant scar is always longer than the original scar.
- W-plasty, geometric broken-line closure, and Z-plasty each use irregular lines, to give a less visible scar.
- Z-plasty, V-to-Y repair, and Y-to-V repair are useful to lengthen contracted scars.
- Dermabrasion superficially abrades the scar and can improve uneven scar edges and raised grafts and flaps; pulsed ablative laser produces similar results.
- Ectropion repair requires special considerations as it has implications beyond cosmetic appearance.

INTRODUCTION

Scar formation is an inherent aspect of surgery. Frequently, the aesthetic appearance of a scar is the single most important determinant used by patients and physicians alike, to judge surgical outcome. The ideal scar is a nearly imperceptible fine line that is level with the skin and blends with the natural creases and folds. The scar's appearance, however, can vary greatly due to surgical technique including final orientation and shape of the scar, as well as the location on the body. Scars with poor cosmetic results include those that are wide, raised, depressed, red, pigmented, or those that transect natural relaxed skin tension lines. Depending on the type of abnormality, different techniques are used to improve the overall cosmetic appearance.

PREOPERATIVE PREPARATION

In the majority of cases proper surgical technique at the time of the initial surgery obviates the need for scar revision. Below we discuss the various components involved in order to maximize cosmetic outcome of surgical scars.

Suturing technique

Wound eversion, critical to create a superior scar, results from meticulous suture technique. Everted wound edges eventuate in thinner and flatter scars. The majority of wound eversion results from proper placement of buried dermal sutures. In specific regions that have a tendency to form depressed scars, such as the forehead creases, additional measures are employed to further evert the upper dermis. Such measures include vertical mattress sutures placed in the cuticular suture layer (see Chapter 16). At the time of suture removal Steri-strips (3M Surgical, St Paul, MN) are applied to augment the wound as it is only at a fraction of the final strength.

Relaxed skin tension lines

Relaxed skin tension lines (RSTL) constitute a series of curvilinear lines that form naturally and predictably on the skin. Scars that run parallel to the RSTL reduce the tension across the wound, resulting in a thinner scar. Whenever possible, incisions should be placed along the RTSL. Even in complex flaps with geometric shapes, the design should place tension vectors along the RSTL to minimize scar spread.[1]

Flap refinements

Despite the confusing nomenclature in current use, local flaps may be simply divided into two categories: sliding and lifting. Sliding flaps include advancement and rotation flaps, as local tissue slides into the defect to be closed. Lifting flaps include transposition, interpolation, and bilobed flaps, as the designed flaps are lifted over adjacent tissue into the defect. The primary motion of a flap is the movement of the flap into the defect. The secondary motion is the movement of the surrounding skin that results from the flap being placed into the defect. These motions need to be understood in order to avoid complications that arise from errant flap design near free margins, including the eye, nasal ala, and oral commissure.[2]

A commonly seen flap complication is bulkiness or thickening of the flap above the level of the surrounding skin. This results from a flap that was cut too thick or from trapdooring. Trapdooring or pin-cushioning is a dramatic 'quilt-like' deformity, which results from contraction of the flap wound bed during healing causing the flap to buckle (Fig. 25.1).[3,4] Flaps should generally lay flat or slightly inset with the surrounding skin at the time of surgery. To inset the flap, its subcutaneous tissue may be thinned with care, guarding against aggressive defatting which may compromise vascularity. Additionally, the defect can be deepened to receive and accommodate an inset flap. Trapdooring is accentuated in rounded or U-shaped flaps. It can be minimized by widely undermining the defect so that the flap and the surrounding skin contract together during the wound healing process. Lastly, flaps may be designed with squared edges to reduce the trapdoor effect.

Cosmetic units

Cosmetic units are an important aspect of facial dermatologic surgery. These units divide the face into distinct regions and are divided by landmarks, contours, lines, and skin texture differences. Occasionally defects are enlarged so that a graft or flap may be designed to encompass an entire cosmetic unit, thus leading to a less apparent scar. Placing incision lines at the cosmetic unit junctions can optimize scar appearance.

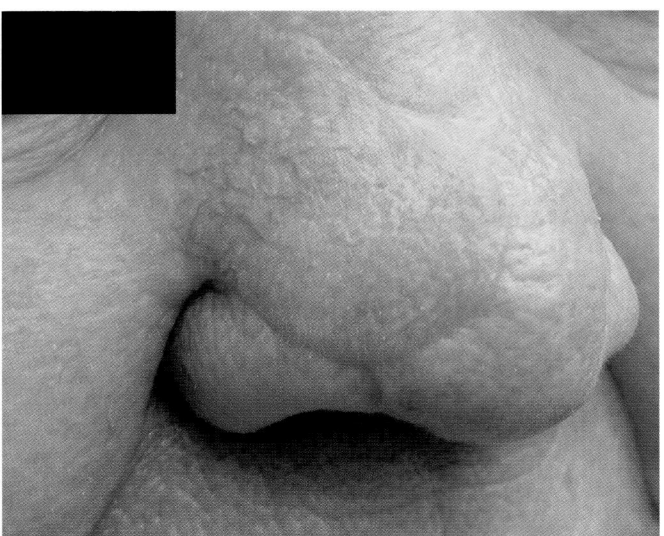

Figure 25.1 Trapdoor effect.

Timing of scar revisions

Scars can take 1 year to mature as collagen continues to remodel during this period. While the vast majority of healing is complete by 1 year, the final appearance of a scar can improve even beyond this period. It is therefore imperative to give adequate time for the natural healing and remodeling process and not to institute invasive revision procedures prematurely. However, occasional situations may arise where early scar revision is necessary to avoid a functional impairment.[5] Patients can actively participate in the healing process of their scars by gently massaging the scar, beginning approximately 1 month postoperatively. This can hasten resolution of the induration associated with newly healing wounds.

■ TECHNIQUES

Intralesional steroids

Hypertrophic linear scars, as well as bulky grafts and flaps, are ideal for intralesional corticosteroids. Injections can be instituted at approximately 1 month postoperatively when fatty tissues become fibrofatty. A small amount (as little as 0.1 ml) of low-dose Kenalog (triamcinolone acetonide) (Bristol-Myers Squibb, Princeton, NJ) at 5–10 mg/ml is injected into the scar and can be repeated monthly until the scar has flattened. However, this will not affect the width of the scar. The injection is placed into the bulkiest region of the scar, at the level of the deep dermis or subcutaneous fat. One must be cautious not to be overly aggressive with quantity, frequency, or strength of Kenalog injections, as significant atrophy may occur.[6]

Non-ablative lasers

Ablative techniques such as dermabrasion and carbon dioxide laser ablation have been widely used for scar improvement (see below). Non-ablative lasers are now becoming popular in the treatment of scars. They have the obvious advantage of improving scars without incision or wounding, thereby minimizing downtime. Multiple lasers have been used to refine scars. The flashlamp-pumped pulsed dye laser has been used most extensively. The pulsed dye laser works through absorption by oxyhemoglobin, causing direct destruction of the blood vessels and an indirect effect on the surrounding collagen. This vascular laser improves the appearance of the scar by reducing the overall redness caused by the scar's vascularity, as well as by promoting collagen remodeling and scar softening. The collagen remodeling has been shown to be most effective at lower subpurpuric fluences.[7–9] It is probably best suited for red hypertrophic scars or for telangiectasias surrounding scars, but the treatment has even been initiated as soon as suture removal to improve immediate scar appearance.[10] Newer non-ablative lasers with wavelengths of 532 nm,

1064 nm, 1390 nm, and 1450 nm are also being used to promote collagen remodeling. Further advancements in technology should continue to enhance the ability to treat scars in a minimally invasive fashion.

Fusiform elliptical excision

One of the simplest methods of surgical scar revision is the re-excision of the scar in a linear or slightly curvilinear fashion. This technique is best suited for spread, or depressed scars that usually result from excess tension and/or poor wound eversion at the time of the initial surgery. The scar should ideally be designed to run parallel to RSTL. Re-excision is best performed on a mature scar, not a newly placed scar under tension. This allows for reapproximation, with less resultant scar spreading, and better wound eversion. A fusiform ellipse is outlined around the scar with the ideal 30° at the tips to promote blending. The scar is excised and the surrounding skin appropriately undermined to relieve surrounding tension. In sebaceous skin, scarring can be minimized by beveling one edge and counterbeveling the other, creating a 'tongue and groove' effect when sutured. Proper placement of deep and superficial sutures will again allow for wound eversion. In areas such as the trunk where suture track marks are more likely to appear, running subcuticular sutures should be used.

A re-excised scar will always be longer than the original scar. This is an important point to discuss with patients prior to the re-excision (Fig. 25.2).

In larger scars, fusiform elliptical excisions are frequently performed serially in stages to minimize tension on the wound. For example, split thickness skin grafts are sometimes used as a temporary closure because of large defect size or for tumor surveillance. If the scar is cosmetically unacceptable to the patient after it has fully matured, it may be serially excised. By waiting for the wound tension to subside and elasticity to return, the final scar length can be made shorter than that of a single-staged excision. The fusiform ellipse is oriented within the width of a broad scar, resulting in an increasingly narrowed scar width with each stage (Fig. 25.3).[11]

W-plasty

Both the W-plasty and geometric broken-line closure (see below) techniques rely on the similar principle that an irregular line is less visible than a straight line. This is especially advantageous when the scar is not along the RSTL, and might therefore be more visible and spread.

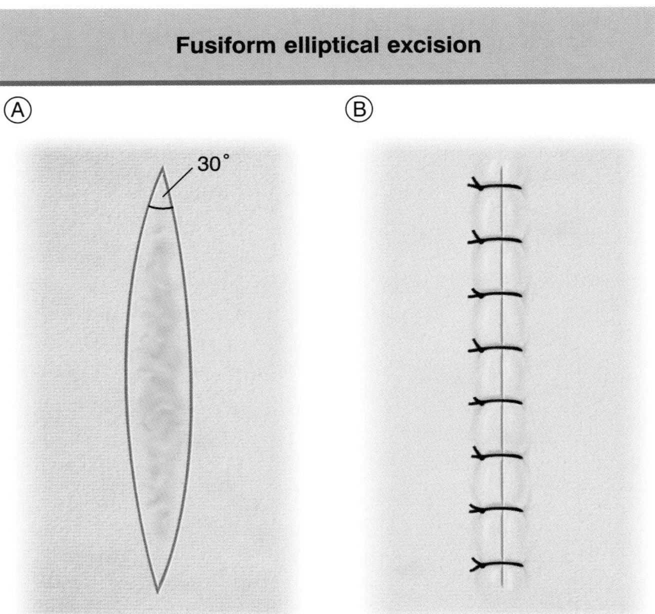

Figure 25.2 Fusiform elliptical excision. A spread linear scar is excised using a fusiform ellipse. The tips of the excision should be 30° to minimize standing cutaneous cones. The wound is closed using a two-layered closure. The resultant scar is longer than the initial scar.

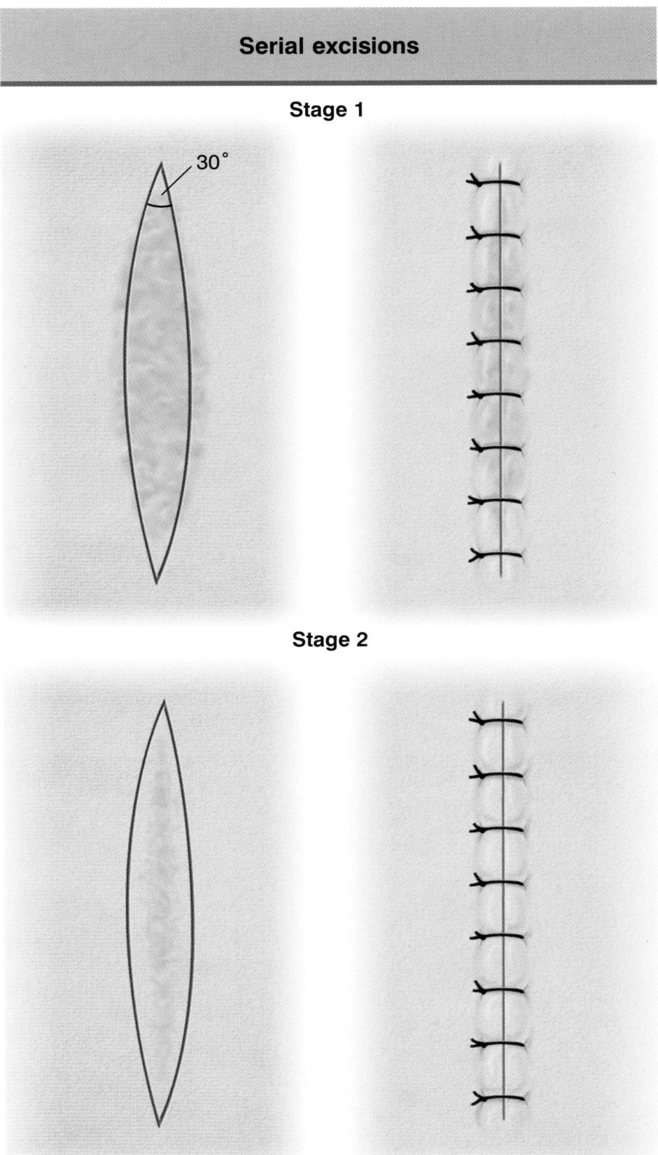

Figure 25. 3 Serial excisions. The scar is serially excised in stages. The length of the final scar is shorter than a single stage excision.

W-plasty is performed by outlining a zigzagging line on one side of the scar, then a mirror image line on the opposite side (Fig. 25.4). The tips of the 'W' should run parallel to the RSTL as the scar is running perpendicular it. The scar is excised along these lines then reapproximated so that the mirror images coincide and form a single zigzagging line. The width of each triangular cut out should be approximately 5 mm to achieve a visibly irregular line. The incision is carefully reapproximated using a combination of dermal three-point tip sutures and cuticular sutures. The advantage of the W-plasty is reduced with longer scars because the regularity of the zigzags makes it more noticeable. In these cases, the geometric broken-line closure is preferable.[12,13]

W-plasty

Ⓐ Ⓑ

Relaxed skin tension lines

Figure 25.4 W-plasty.

Geometric broken-line closure

Geometric broken-line closure (GBLC) is a more elaborate version of the W-plasty.[14] It is preferable for longer scars to provide a less predictable irregularity to the incision line. An outline is made along one side of the scar using various geometric designs (such as semicircles, triangles, and squares) and the mirror image is made on the opposite side. The pattern should appear random (Fig. 25.5). The scar is excised along the drawn outline and adequately undermined. It is then carefully reapproximated using dermal and cuticular sutures so that the mirror images coincide.

Z-plasty

Z-plasty is a useful technique for revising scars. As with W-plasty and geometric broken lines, Z-plasty creates irregular lines that make the scar less visible. Additionally, it has other unique benefits: it alters the direction of a prominent scar placed perpendicular to the RSTL parallel to the RSTL. Furthermore, it has the advantage of lengthening a contracted scar. The latter is particularly important with visible deformation of free margins, including the eye, nasal ala, or lip. It is therefore an essential technique for scar revision. Moreover, understanding the Z-plasty helps the surgeon with many aspects of cutaneous flap surgery.

The geometry of the Z-plasty is often considered to be quite complex. In essence, Z-plasty is two zigzagging triangular flaps that are transposed into the shape of a Z. (For those more familiar with flap surgery, a rhombic transposition flap is an asymmetric Z-plasty.)

Two points in the construction of the Z-plasty are critical to its understanding and performance: the angle size and

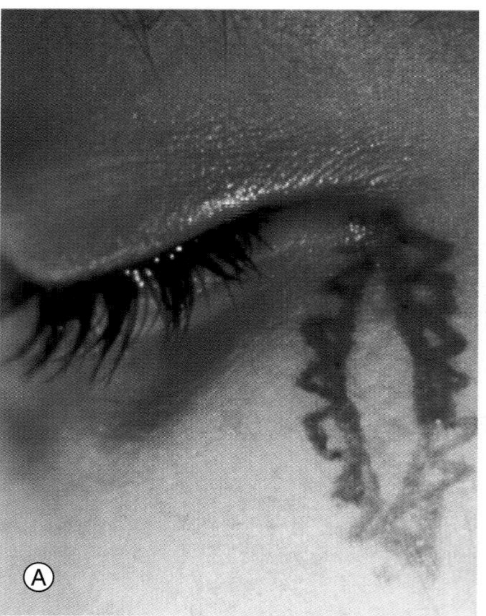

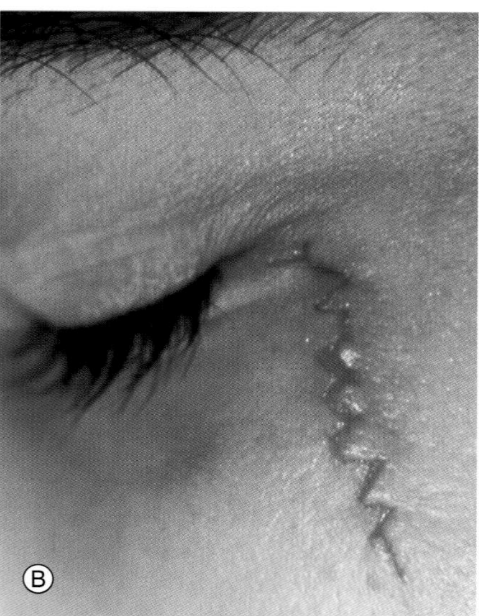

Figure 25.5 Geometric broken-line closure. (A) The spread scar is outlined using various geometric shapes. (B) The wound is carefully reapproximated to match the mirror images.

60° Z-plasty

Figure 25.6 60° single Z-plasty. (A) The central scar is the common diagonal. (B) Incisions result in two triangular flaps which are lifted and transposed. (C) 60° Z-plasty results in a 75% gain in tissue length.

length of the common diagonal (also referred to as the common limb or the common member) (Fig. 25.6).[15–17] In scar revision, the central diagonal is the scar. Two arms that are of the same length as the common diagonal are extended from the ends in opposite directions. The 'angle' is determined by the arm and common limb. The angle of the designed triangle determines the degree of tissue lengthening, whereby larger angles result in greater gains. The length of the central diagonal also determines tissue gain but this is less variable as it is usually predetermined by the length of the scar. The classic 60° Z-plasty angle results in a 90° change in scar direction and a 75% gain in tissue length. The Z-plasty is performed by making an incision along or around the scar and the outlined arms. The skin is widely undermined and the scar loosened. The tips of the triangular flaps are then transposed to change the direction of the common diagonal into the transverse diagonal. A trick is to mark one tip with a marking pen and make sure it changes position during the transposition. Thus, a single Z-plasty effectively changes the direction of the scar and lengthens the scar simultaneously. As the length of the common diagonal and arms become longer, the tension placed across the transverse diagonal critically increases, especially in inelastic skin. Furthermore, the resultant scar can be quite noticeable because of the larger 'Z' configuration. In these cases, multiple Z-plasty has the advantage of better hiding the 'Z' shape by using multiple smaller 'Z' shapes along the scar line, as well distributing the tension across multiple smaller transverse diagonals (Fig. 25.7).

Z-plasties are frequently used to correct contracted or asymmetric anatomic landmarks such as an elevated or depressed oral commissure (Fig. 25.8).

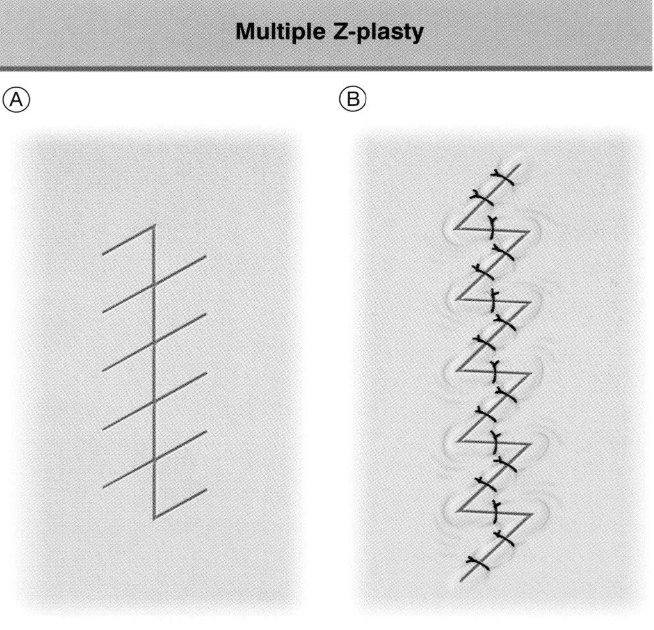

Figure 25.7 Multiple Z-plasty. (A) Multiple smaller 'Z' incisions are made along the scar. (B) The flaps are lifted and transposed in a staircase fashion.

V-to-Y repair and Y-to-V repair

When confronted with a contracted scar, V-to-Y repair is another technique used to lengthen the scar. It is particularly useful near free margins such as around the eyes and mouth when a scar has caused an ectropion or an eclabion, respectively.

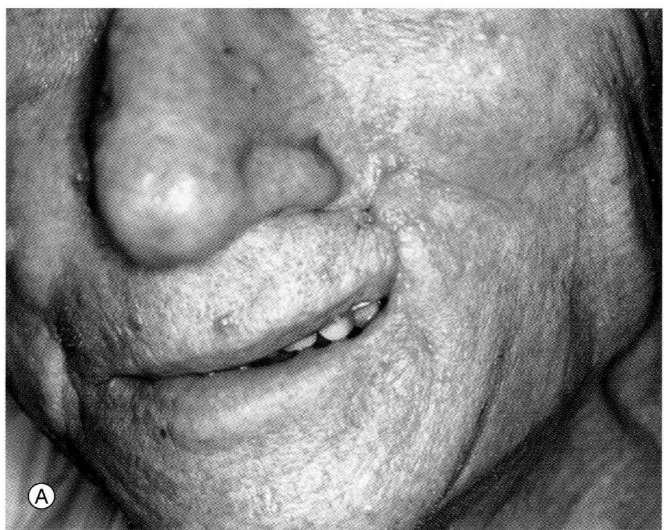

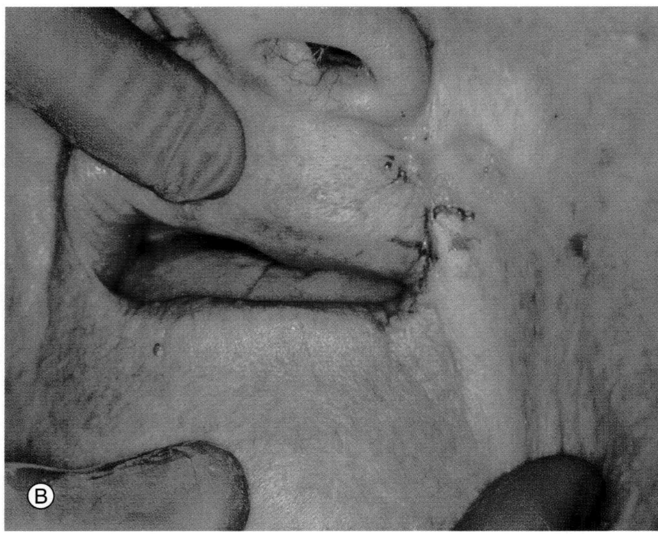

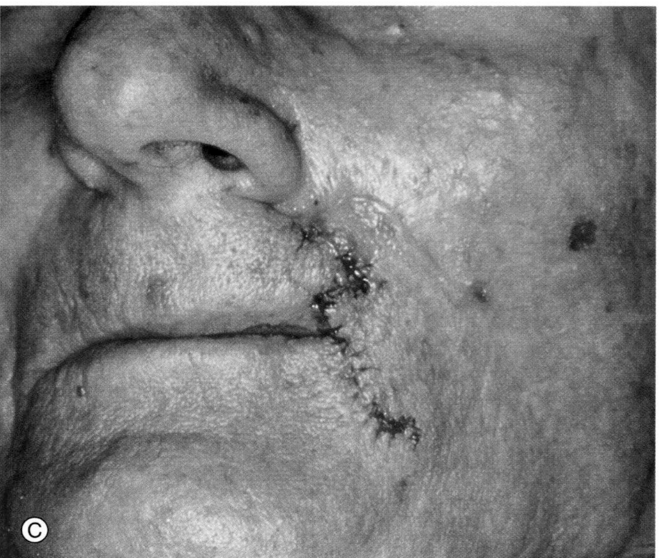

Figure 25.8 Z-plasty to correct oral commissure. (A) Upturned oral commissure. (B) Outline of single Z-plasty. (C) Z-plasty converts the commissure into neutral position.

The technique is performed by making a V-shaped incision along the length of the contracted scar. The wound is then widely undermined to loosen the scar. The V-shaped flap is then pushed away from the incision to relieve the tension and simultaneously lengthen the scar. The newly created defect is then closed such that the two sides the defect are brought together to form a straight line along the initial scar line (Fig. 25.9). V-to-Y repair is helpful for relatively smaller contractions. Just as the V-to-Y repair can raise an anatomic point, a Y-to-V repair can be used to lower it. The initial incision is made in a Y-shaped and similarly converted to form a 'V'.

Trapdoor deformity repair

Mild trapdoor deformities can usually be managed with intralesional steroids beginning at approximately 1 month postoperatively. If the wound edges blend well with the surrounding skin then the flattening that results from intralesional steroids is all that would be required. If the deformity is pronounced, however, surgical revision may be additionally required. An incision is made along the curvature of the flap. Because the entire flap does not need to be lifted, the portion of the scar that is the most uneven or spread is selected for placement of the incision. The incised flap is then reflected back. The undersurface is thinned, as well as the base deepened (Fig. 25.10). A technical trick is to use a #69 Beaver blade (Becton-Dickinson, Franklin Lakes, NJ), rounded at the tip, to remove the disc of fibrofatty tissue. The flap can be thinned to a greater extent than it was at the time of the initial reconstruction because there is reduced tension, better vascularity, and less disruption of the flap base and pedicle. Any excessive flap tissue is trimmed and the wound edges are undermined to widen the scar base. The wound edges are widely undermined. The flap is then gently draped back and placed slightly inset to the surrounding skin.[18,19]

Ectropion repair

Ectropion is a complication that deserves special mention. Unlike most other scars, it has implications beyond the cosmetic appearance. Patients with ectropion complain of irritation, tearing, and conjunctival injection, which demands immediate consideration of scar revision. How-

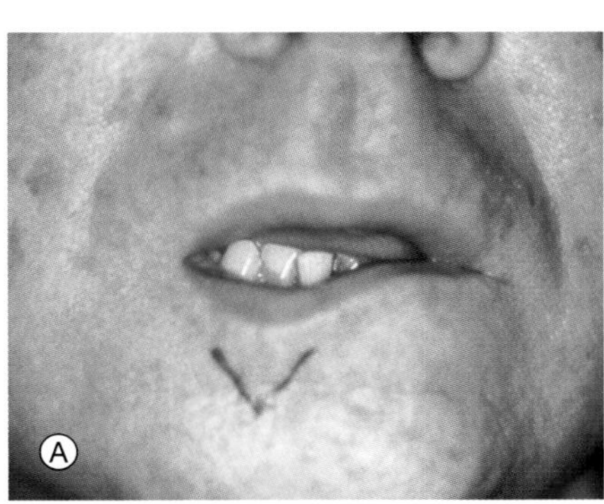

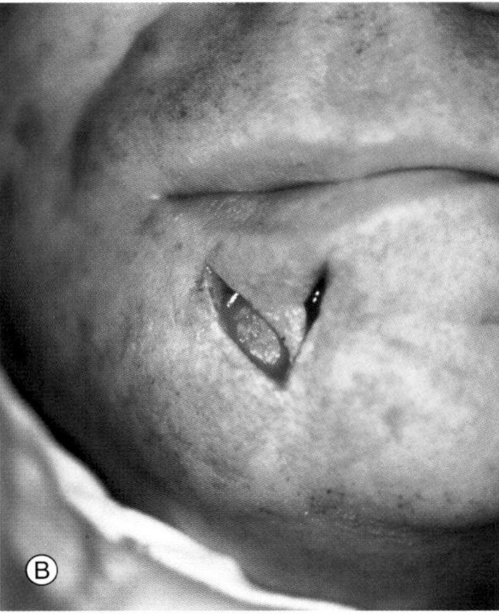

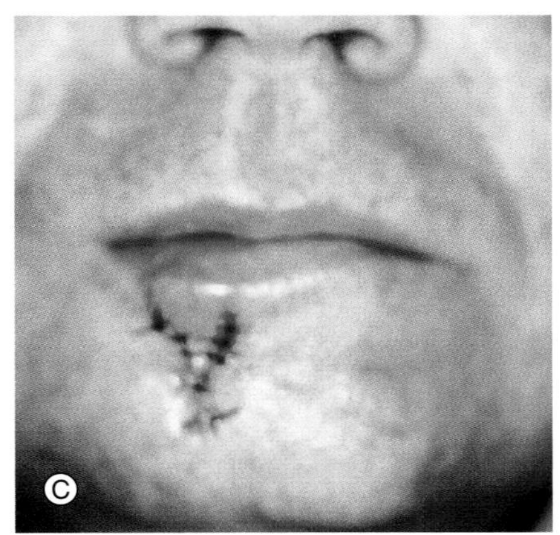

Figure 25.9 V-to-Y repair. (A) Retracted lower lip. (B) 'V' incision made inferiorly and scar undermined. (C) The lip is pushed up and the 'V' is converted into a 'Y'.

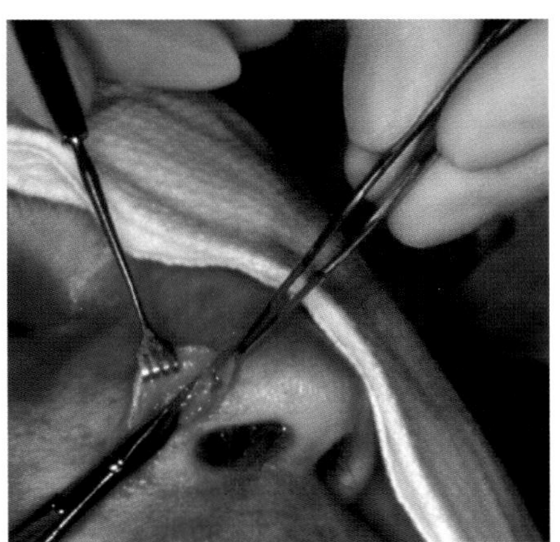

Figure 25.10 Flap debulking. An incision is made along a bulky flap. The scar is carefully trimmed to reduce the bulkiness.

ever, keep in mind that a mild ectropion frequently resolves spontaneously over several weeks postoperatively.

Ectropion can be difficult to repair therefore its prevention through careful planning and surgical technique is paramount at the time of the initial surgery. Scars should be oriented perpendicular to the lower lid margin. Grafts should be oversized up to double the defect size to compensate for the massive contraction that occurs with thinner grafts in this region. Flaps should be sized generously in order to push the inferior lid up, such as in an inferiorly based rhombic transposition flap. The flap's tension vector can also be designed to pull up on the lower lid as is seen in a laterally based advancement flap that is incised above the level of the lateral canthus in order to pull up on the lower eyelid. Additionally, periosteal tacking sutures can be placed to suspend flaps to the bony orbit to prevent pull on the lower lid. If excessive lid laxity is present then the lower lid should be tightened preventatively by removing a full-thickness triangular wedge of the lower lid.[20] Additionally, canthoplasty can be performed by making a horizontal incision several millimeters lateral to the lateral canthus, exposing the lateral canthal ligament, then tacking down this ligament to the superior orbital rim, thereby resulting in a tightening of the lower lid skin.

Once an ectropion has developed, however, other techniques need to be performed to release the contracture causing the ectropion. V–Y repair is helpful for a mild ectropion.[21] For more prominent ectropia, a full-thickness skin graft is the good option to restore the lower eyelid. The ideal donor site is the upper lid skin. The graft should be oversized to up to double the defect size.[22] If the original scar is present near the lower lid margin than an incision is made through the scar and undermined to lift the lower lid into proper position thus releasing the ectropion. The graft is then inserted into the defect created by the release. If the original scar is distant from the lid margin, then the incision is made horizontally at the subciliary line. In severe cases, the lower lid is tacked to the eyebrow in order to suspend the lower lid in an elevated position for approximately 3 weeks. This maneuver can be performed alone without a skin graft for mild to moderate ectropia (Fig. 25.11).

Dermabrasion and ablative lasers

Spot dermabrasion is an ideal technique to improve subtle textural abnormalities associated with scars. This can be performed on a scar as the sole scar revision technique or used in combination with a re-excision. The ideal timing for dermabrasion is 6–12 weeks postoperatively.

Dermabrasion superficially abrades the scar and the surrounding skin to the level of the papillary dermis in a precise and controlled manner. This results in a smoother texture and evens out any irregularities along the scar surface. Dermabrasion can improve the appearance of uneven scar edges as well as raised grafts and flaps by leveling the irregular contours.[23,24] Even in aesthetically acceptable scars, dermabrasion can help to blend the scar into the surrounding skin. Dermabrasion is performed in multiple different ways. Larger areas usually need a power dermabrader with local anesthesia and freezing. Smaller scars, however, can be lightly dermabraded to the point of

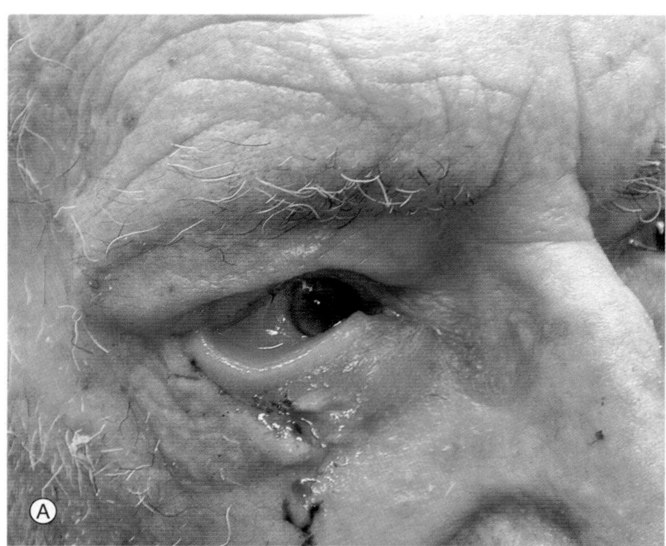

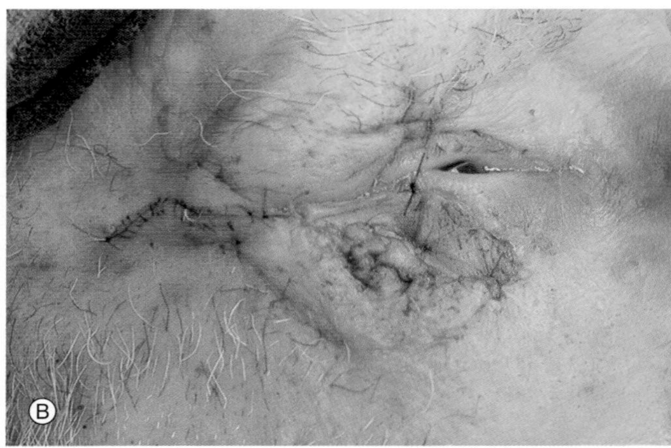

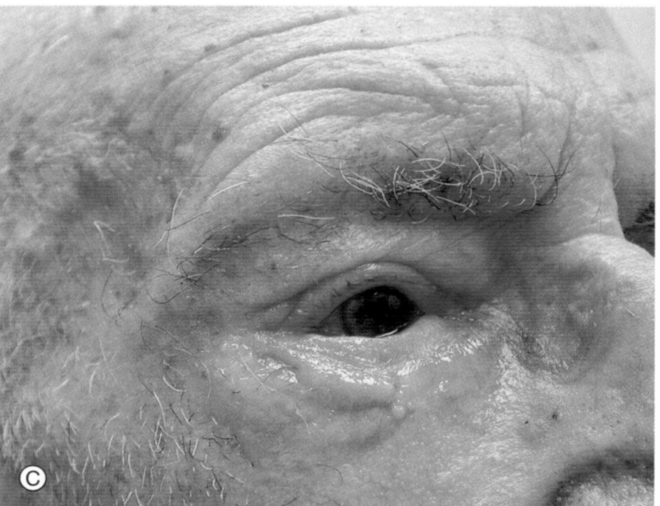

Figure 25.11 Ectropion repair. (A) Severe ectropion. (B) Scar is loosened, the lower lid is tacked to the eyebrow, and an oversize full-thickness skin graft from contralateral upper eyelid placed into the defect. (C) Results 2 months postoperatively.

pinpoint bleeding using sterile 300–400 grit sandpaper wrapped on a dental roll. One must be cautious not to go too deeply into the dermis, thus causing a depression that is difficult to repair. The margins along the scar undergoing dermabrasion should be extended and feathered into normal surrounding skin, including an entire cosmetic unit or subunit, because pigmentary alteration occasionally resulting from dermabrasion may lead to a more conspicuous treated area (Fig. 25.12).

Pulsed ablative lasers (carbon dioxide and erbium:YAG) can provide similar results as dermabrasion by superficially ablating the scar.[25] Each laser has its distinct advantages. Erbium:YAG has a higher affinity for water, so it is more precise in ablating raised scar edges. The carbon dioxide laser causes more thermal necrosis and thus promotes more wound contraction and collagen remodeling. Surgical scar revision and laser resurfacing can be combined into a single-step procedure where the cosmetic unit surrounding the scar is lasered first, immediately followed by scar re-excision.

All ablative procedures including both dermabrasion or laser ablation carry a slight risk of worsening a scar from overly aggressive treatment or from pigmentary alteration. Patients need to be fully informed and consented for this potential risk.

■ POSTOPERATIVE CARE

After scar revision, care is the same as that for other skin incisions. For further detail on wound healing, see Chapter 7, and on dressings and postoperative care, see Chapter 8.

■ SUMMARY

Meticulous planning and technique will lead to superior scars. Even the best surgeons must confront scars that are aesthetically unacceptable. Often, just waiting may be the best treatment as wound healing is not a static process. Sometimes, surgical intervention is needed to optimize the appearance of the scar. With careful assessment of the scar, various scar revision techniques can be applied to create an aesthetically pleasing scar.

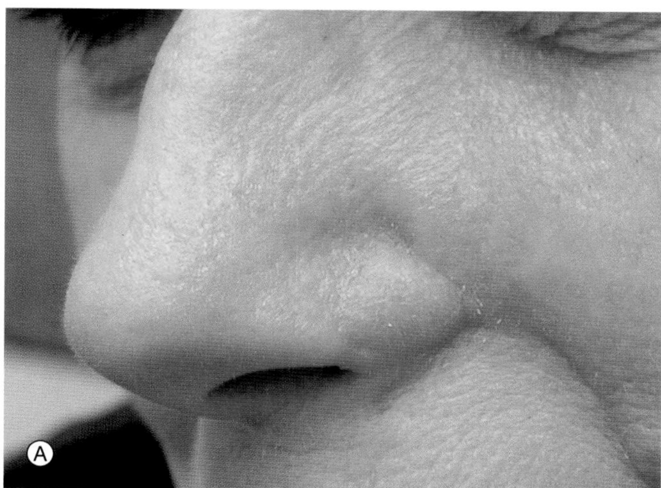

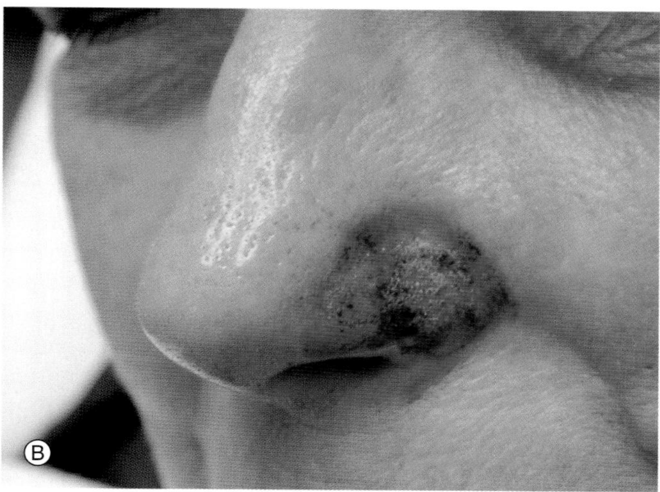

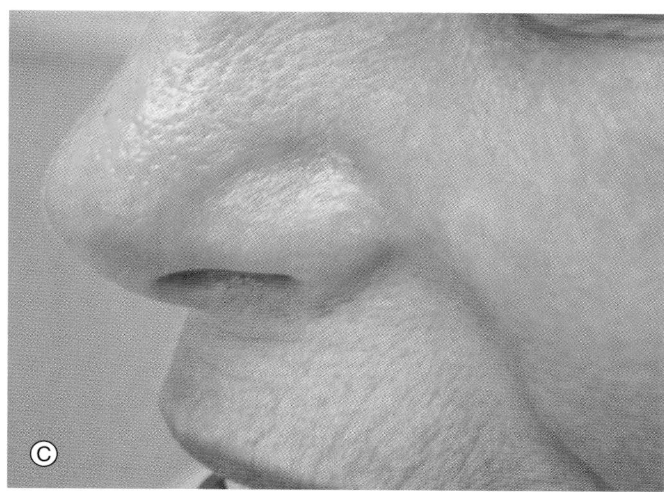

Figure 25.12 Dermabrasion. (A) Bulky flap on lateral nasal ala. (B) The entire alar subunit is dermabraded. (C) Good cosmetic blend 2 months postoperatively.

REFERENCES

1. Borges AF. Relaxed skin tension lines (RSTL) versus other skin lines. Plast Reconstr Surg 1984; 73:144.
2. Baker SB, Swanson NA. Local Flaps in Facial Reconstruction. St Louis: Mosby; 1995.
3. Koranda FC, Webster RC. Trapdoor effect in nasolabial flaps. Arch Otolaryngol 1985; 111:421.
4. Webster RC, Benjamin RJ, Smith RC. Treatment of 'trapdoor deformity.' Laryngoscope 1978; 88:707.
5. Borges AF. Principles of scar camouflage. Facial Plast Surg 1984; 1:181–190.
6. Goslen JB. The role of steroids in preventing scar formation. In: Thomas JR, Holt GR, eds. Facial scars: incision, revision, and camouflage. St Louis: Mosby; 1989: 88–89.
7. Alster TS. Improvement of erythematous and hypertrophic scars by the 585 nm flashlamp pumped pulsed dye laser. Ann Plastic Surg 1994; 32:186–190.
8. Alster TS, Williams CM. Treatment of keloid sternotomy scars with 585 nm flashlamp pumped pulsed dye laser. Lancet 1995; 345:1198–1200.
9. Manuskiatti W, Fitzpatrick R, Goldman M. Energy density and numbers of treatment affect response of keloidal and hypertrophic sternotomy scars to the 585 nm PDL. J Am Acad Dermatol 2001; 45:557–565.
10. Nouri K, Jimenez GP, Harrison-Balestra C, Elgart GW. 585 nm pulsed dye laser in treatment of surgical scars starting on the suture removal day. Dermatol Surg 2003; 29:65–73.
11. Thomas JR. Scar analysis. In: Thomas JR, Holt GR, eds. Facial scars: incision, revision, and camouflage. St Louis: Mosby; 1989:88–89.
12. Borges AF. Improvement of antitension lines scars by the 'W' plastic operation. Br J Plast Surg 1959; 12:29–43.
13. Thomas JR, Frost TW. Scar revision and camouflage. In: Baker SB, Swanson NA, eds. Local flaps in facial reconstruction. St Louis: Mosby; 1995:587–595.
14. Webster RD, Davidson TM, Smith RC. Broken line scar revision. Clin Plast Surg 1977; 4:263–274.
15. Swanson NA. Atlas of cutaneous surgery. Boston: Little Brown & Co; 1987: 118–123.
16. Borges AF. Z-plasty. In: Borges AF, ed. Elective incisions and scar revision. Boston: Little Brown & Co; 1973.
17. Frodel JL, Wang TD. Z-plasty. In: Baker SB, Swanson NA, eds. Local flaps in facial reconstruction. St Louis: Mosby; 1995: 131–148.
18. Hosokwawa K, Susuki T, Kikui T, et al. Sheet of scar deformity: a hypothesis. Ann Plast Surg 1990; 25:134.
19. Salache SJ. Complications of local flaps. In: Baker SB, Swanson NA, eds. Local flaps in facial reconstruction. St Louis: Mosby; 1995: 581.
20. Young VL, Bartell TH. Burns of the face. In: Thomas JR, Holt GR, eds. Facial scars: incision, revision, and camouflage. St Louis: Mosby; 1989: 238–239.
21. Tromovich TA, Stegman SJ, Glogau RG. Flaps and grafts in dermatologic surgery. Chicago: Mosby-Year Book 1989:217.
22. Skouge JW. Skin grafting. New York: Churchill-Livingstone; 1991.
23. Hill TG. Enhancing the survival of full-thickness grafts. J Dermatol Surg Oncol 1984; 10:639.
24. Robinson J. Improvement of the appearance of full-thickness skin grafts with dermabrasion. Arch Dermatol 1987; 123:1340.
25. Wheeland RG: Revision of full-thickness skin grafts using the carbon dioxide laser. J Dermatol Surg Oncol 1988; 14:130.

PART 3

Aesthetic Surgical Procedures

26 Psychosocial Issues and the Cosmetic Surgery Patient

Dee Anna Glaser MD and Jason Layman BS

Summary box

- Psychosocial factors are important in cosmetic surgery patient selection.
- An appropriate preoperative psychiatric exam is essential.
- By recognizing the key features of common personality and mental disorders, cosmetic surgeons can plan effective treatment for each individual patient.
- Body dysmorphic disorder is one of the more common psychological disorders seen in people seeking cosmetic surgery.
- Surgical success rates are poor for patients who have body dysmorphic disorder and cosmetic surgery is generally contraindicated for such patients.

■ INTRODUCTION

Over the years there has been a growing interest in determining the actual rates of psychiatric conditions present in a typical cosmetic surgery practice. One such study by Ishigooka et al. indicates that just under half (47.7%) of a sample of 415 patients seeking cosmetic surgery suffer from at least one serious mental disorder.[1] Among the major diagnoses were schizophrenia, persistent delusional disorders, major depressive episodes, neurotic disorders, hypochondriacal disorder, paranoid personality disorder, and histrionic personality disorder. In addition, over half of the patients surveyed suffered from poor social adjustment (56%), indicating that many patients are turning to surgery as a way of obtaining social acceptance. Furthermore, the researchers also found that the men in this sample tended to suffer from a greater number of mental conditions, including dysmorphophobia, a disease that will be discussed in great length later in this chapter.

Of course, many people whom we would consider to be typical cosmetic surgery patients suffer from at least one diagnosable psychological disorder including—but not limited to—social inhibition, moderate self-consciousness, anxiety, and depression.[2] In fact, aesthetic surgery would be contraindicated for any patient whose psychological health could not be improved in one way or another through the desired operation. In most cases, upon completion of an appropriately indicated treatment, and possibly some minor psychological counseling, the patient should have a positive outlook on the procedure and should be able to function as a normal member of society. In some cases, however, patients may be much more psychologically disturbed, suffering from severe depression, personality disorders, neurosis, and other psychoses. In any of these cases, it is important that the surgeon is able to immediately recognize the presence of these more severe conditions so that appropriate treatment can be obtained.

■ TECHNICAL ASPECTS

The psychiatric exam

The importance of obtaining the mental status of a patient is unique in its ubiquity. It is a mainstay of every examination regardless of where the patient encounter takes place—the exam table in the emergency room, or on the psychiatrist's couch. Even though the psychiatrist and the emergency room physician will undoubtedly have very different goals for their evaluations, the general structure of the exam and the information obtained are generally the same. Here we will describe the basic steps to the psychological evaluation of a patient and the information that is necessary for the cosmetic surgeon to obtain before proceeding with any cosmetic procedure.

The psychological exam is also unique as it begins the moment the patient walks into the office. With bizarre patients, nurses and office staff often alert the physician that the patient may be acting strangely or unusually. In any case, the physician should begin to evaluate the mental status of the patient from the moment they meet, throughout the visit, until the moment the patient walks out the door. For most physicians, and in particular cosmetic surgeons, this is a simple task, as a highly developed power of observation is warranted by their chosen occupation.

The first thing any physician will notice is the appearance of the patient. Taken alone, appearance means next to nothing in our society as fashion and grooming style are no longer accurate indicators of occupation, intelligence, or mental status. However, the appearance of a patient may give the physician clues as to the line of questions that will be most appropriate in obtaining information about this particular patient. More often than not the most informative indicator of appearance is their clothing, which might be dirty or disheveled, tight or flashy, grotesque or gothic, or seductive. For instance, a female patient who is very neat and well dressed, with a blouse that precisely matches her earrings, nail polish, and shoes might be considered for screening for obsessive–compulsive disorder. It is, of course, important to remember that these are not concrete associations that can be stereotyped, but such observations may lead a physician to specific lines of questioning.

The next attribute the physician will typically notice is the patient's orientation to time and place. Normally orientation is not an issue that needs direct questioning unless patients appear to be noticeably confused or vague about their surroundings. Even in cases where this does appear to be a problem, a few simple questions can often confirm whether or not this lack of orientation will significantly impact the outcome of the procedure to be performed. In situations where questioning is warranted, it is probably not best to proceed by asking patients directly if they know the year, or who the current president of the United States is. Nevertheless, most physicians will inadvertently ask questions where proper orientation is inherently required to respond succinctly. If lack of orientation is found, it may not be much of an issue for minor procedures, but caution should be used before undertaking extremely arduous and invasive surgeries on such patients.[3]

Having noted appearance and orientation, the next and possibly most important factor to consider is the patient's mood and affect. Occasionally, the patient may actually tell you about their current mood if attention is paid to such phrases as 'I've been a little down' or 'I'm happier than I have been.' When not told directly the physician must rely on observation. In some cases, such as mania or severe depression, the behavioral signs are straightforward. With depression there may be signs of sadness, indifference to the questioning with reluctance to answer questions at length, or use of a monotonous voice. At the other extreme, those with mania often express inappropriate happiness and extreme eagerness to answer questions, sometimes preventing the doctor from getting a word in edgewise. At this point, it may be appropriate to question patients about their use of psychiatric services or other mental health services. This may seem like a very direct and personal question, but those who are not being treated will simply say no, while those who are being treated are usually no more embarrassed than someone undergoing treatment for a disease such as diabetes or hepatitis. In any case, the information gained by asking this question is far more valuable than any temporary embarrassment or discomfort one would cause to the patient. It may be useful to have questions on a medical intake form that assesses current and past psychiatric conditions. Naturally, this would not replace the techniques described above but would provide some indication that something may be awry.

As mentioned above, depression and mania are usually readily recognized by physicians. Other conditions, such as schizophrenia, require a heightened level of psychiatric observational skill. To identify schizophrenics, the doctor should look for what are called colorless affects. These affects include monotonous speech and other non-reactive, non-responsive behaviors. In these cases, it is very important to distinguish between patients truly suffering from schizophrenia and those who may be too scared or too nervous to ask many questions or to respond appropriately. For this reason it is important that physicians do not guide the patients' answers too much, and close attention should be paid not just to the content of the speech, but also to how the patient speaks.

The next part of the psychiatric exam deals with establishing the patients' thought processing ability and judgment and insight. Again, certain psychological diagnoses can be gleaned from observed patterns of behavior. For example, those affected by mania will often be very flighty and skip from one idea to another, unable to stay focused on one topic. On the other hand, severely depressed people typically find it harder to answer questions and will have slower response times. Other abnormalities may be noticed if the patient is excessively concerned with details or is not interested in anything past an overly generalized description of the procedure. Understanding the patient's background may also be helpful in investigating these attributes. The purpose of evaluating the patients' thought processes, judgment, and insight is to determine if they are able to arrive at a rational decision independently. In all these areas it is important for the physician to focus on asking specific but open-ended questions, so that more of the patient's personality and character will come through in the answers.

With some procedures it may be worthwhile to evaluate the patient's intelligence and level of comprehension. If a patient is to undergo an extensive procedure that may lead to dramatic alterations of appearance, or that carries a risk of significant untoward effects, the physician must be confident that the patient possesses the intellect to process and understand the details of the procedure. Most of the time the screening described above will allow a reasonable assessment of cognitive ability. If there is doubt, however, several mental status exams have been developed that can be used by non-psychiatrists to screen patients with limited cognitive function. One of the more widely used is that developed by Folstein called the Mini-mental Status Exam.[4] Tools such as these provide a simple and efficient way for physicians to ensure that only mentally fit patients are selected for procedures.

Using these techniques and by asking questions pertinent to the requested procedure, the doctor should be able, by the end of the first appointment, to ascertain the following:

- How long they have been dissatisfied with the relevant body part.
- Why surgery is requested at this particular time.
- What their motivations are for requesting the surgery.
- What their expectations are: what the surgery will do for them and how will it influence their life.
- What surgeries or procedures they have undergone in the past, and what these experiences were like; whether

there were real or perceived problems with the procedures or physician.

- Whether they are having some form of life crisis.
- Whether they suffer from any known psychiatric condition that would preclude them from undergoing the procedure.
- If the physician or office staff are suspicious of an unreported or unrecognized psychiatric condition that would reduce surgical candidacy.
- Whether family and friends support the surgery and how they will react.

By taking the time to go through these aspects of the initial interview and receiving relevant answers, the surgical team will be able to reduce significantly the amount of complications due to psychiatric factors on behalf of the patient. The very best time to screen patients for the presence of these conditions is during preoperative consultation.

■ OPTIMIZING OUTCOMES

Personality identification

Some may question the need to perform a thorough psychiatric screening in a cosmetic surgery setting. Under most conditions the personality type of the patient will have little or no effect on the major outcome of the indicated procedure. However, by identifying certain personality characteristics in patients, the physician will be able to estimate what level of care the patient will require throughout the course of treatment, how to best handle any questions or problems that may arise, and how to ensure that both doctor and patient view the procedure as a success. Below we will describe some common personality characteristics and some generalizations about the type of care each type of personality prefers or elicits.

Passive–aggressive patients

- These patients have an increased need for postoperative nurturing.
- Whining and childish behavior may frustrate the nursing and supporting staff.
- Physicians may need to direct staff to withdraw somewhat from the patient to avoid indulging the behavior.

Hostile and angry patients

- Paranoid patients will project feelings onto the doctor and staff.
- In reality the vast majority of these patients are simply frightened.
- Strong and confident reassurance is needed in the postoperative period.
- Honest and thorough answers should be given to all the patient's questions.
- Do not simply tell patients 'Everything will be alright.' Patients will do much better if all information is given in a forthright manner.

Sociopathic patients

- The doctor must maintain an authoritative presence.
- The doctor is in charge with regard to the surgical treatment and postoperative management.

Obsessive–compulsive disorder patients

- The patients will need a concrete plan.
- The details are extremely important (How long? How severe? How much?).

■ PITFALLS AND THEIR MANAGEMENT

Avoidance of Pitfalls

- Cosmetic surgery is a team effort.
- Be wary of the patient who cannot point out or verbalize the defect or problem that they would like improved.
- Be wary of the patient who requires a magnifying mirror to pick out the problematic defect.
- It is crucial that a thorough history includes all past consultations and treatments.
- Make sure you understand exactly what the patient expects of the procedure.
- Be wary of the patient who demands one particular treatment and is unwilling to contemplate other options suggested by the physician.
- Be wary of the cosmetic surgery patients who are 'price-shoppers' and try to push you into performing a less effective treatment because it costs less.
- Perhaps, most importantly, know yourself.

Most patients presenting to a dermatology practice have a normal mental health history and have realistic expectations. There are several helpful hints that we have found to be useful from our experiences in the clinical setting.

Cosmetic surgery is a team effort. The physician should listen to the concerns raised by those of the office and nursing staff who have encountered the patient. The patient who appears pleasant in the presence of the physician, but is degrading or unreasonable with the staff, can easily turn this same frustration and anger toward the physician or surgical procedure. In cases such as these, it is important to take a more detailed look at the patient before proceeding with surgery.

Be wary of the patient who cannot point out or verbalize the defect or problem that they would like improved. These patients may make broad hand gestures around the face or accusingly ask the physician questions such as 'Can't you see the problem?'. A common scenario is the patient who enters the office and says 'I want to look better' or 'I want to look younger.' Despite well-performed procedures, these patients frequently are unhappy with the results and feel that they do not look any better or younger.

Be wary of people who require a magnifying mirror to pick out the problematic defect. This is often encountered with scars or wrinkles that are so obscure that neither the patient nor the doctor can find them without great effort. These patients may even make excuses as to why the deformity is not visible during the consultation. For example, they may claim that this particular defect can only be seen at a certain time of day, perhaps under certain lighting. In our practice, we have found that these patients tend to have higher dissatisfaction rates with treatments.

It is crucial that a thorough history includes all past consultations and treatments. It is important to find out if and why so many different physicians have treated the patient and, more importantly, if it was for the same problem. Be wary of patients who speak poorly of or blame previous physicians. Ask about past treatments and their outcomes. We also ask 'Were there any problems or complications?' In situations where the outcome was satisfactory but the patient perceived complications or a prolonged postoperative course, you may anticipate similar perceptions during the care that you provide.

Make sure you understand exactly what the patient expects of the procedure. Despite a detailed consultation on the fine points of a procedure, such as the risks and possible outcomes, some patients have ongoing unrealistic expectations. These patients may repeatedly ask their doctor questions such as 'But *I* will get results, won't I?' or 'But *I* won't have any complications, right?'. These patients may be able to develop a better communication pattern with another physician and it should be suggested that the patient obtain a second opinion.

Be wary of the patient who demands one particular treatment and who is unwilling to contemplate other options suggested by the physician. This can often lead to a situation where either the patient or physician will be disappointed with the outcome, or other unforeseen complications arise. For example, a patient insisting on laser treatment for leg telangiectasia should not be treated with that modality if the doctor feels a different option is superior or less risky.

Be wary of cosmetic surgery patients who are 'price-shoppers' and try to push you into performing a much less effective treatment because it costs less. This can lead to dissatisfaction and it is important to counsel the patient on the expected outcome and likely degree of improvement. A 60-year-old woman with significant jowling is not going to be satisfied with a TCA (trichloroacetic acid) peel if she expects to eliminate the laxity, even though it costs significantly less than a face-lift and is more suited to her budget. In these cases the best course of action is to not perform the requested procedure, even if some benefit may be gained, because it will not achieve what the patient desires. In the example given here, the woman may have lentigos or other lesions amenable to the peel, but if she continues to express concerns about the jowling and skin laxity these must be addressed in the treatment plan. Physician should refer such patients to a colleague if they cannot provide a treatment that will affect the deformity that the patient wants to improve. Most patients will respect the physician's integrity and honesty when referred elsewhere for a superior treatment. We have found that such patients will not only return to our office but will refer their friends and family as well. Other examples might include a referral for a surgical procedure that you do not provide such as a face lift or blepharoplasty, or a referral for laser treatment that may be superior for treating a particular problem for which you lack the proper equipment or expertise.

Perhaps most importantly: know yourself. Recognize your own personality, strengths, and style. Some patients are excellent candidates for cosmetic surgery but may simply have a 'better fit' with a different physician. We frequently suggest that patients have a second consultation with a colleague for another opinion. This colleague could be another dermatologist or a plastic surgeon. Again we have found that in the end this enhances the patients' experiences—and your practice—because patients who may not fare as well in your environment can be avoided. In addition, patients will usually respect your honesty and the fact that you truly consider their welfare as paramount—they may become your best referrer in the future.

■ PRACTICAL APPLICATIONS

Body dysmorphic disorder

Clinical Vignette

B.D. is a 48-year-old white man who complained of ingrown hairs on his neck and face, especially his middle and lower cheeks. During his first visit to the office 4 years previously, he was diagnosed with pseudofolliculitis barbae and underwent treatment with the long-pulsed Nd:YAG laser to reduce hair growth in the affected area. Historically, he had also been treated with 13-cis retinoic acid and was currently using topical cleocin and oral doxycycline, prescribed by other physicians with minimal improvement. B.D. stated that the laser helped with the darker hairs, but made the 'bumps' worse. He described needing to 'work' everyday for 1–2 hours with a needle in order to get out the ingrown hairs. Upon examination, extensive scarring and self-inflicted wounds were observed, the most notable being a 1 cm laceration on his right mandible, which had been closed with three white nylon sutures (Fig. 26.1). Upon questioning, we learned that the sutures, rather large for facial repairs, were actually done with fishing line and had been placed by the patient himself. It was not uncommon for the patient to require suturing due to the extent of the wounds he induced.

One of the more common if not *the* most common psychological disorders that presents in a dermatology office is body dysmorphic disorder. This disorder, also known as dysmorphophobia, was formally recognized as a distinct disorder in 1987,[5] even though the clinical features of body dysmorphic disorder were first described over a century ago.[6] Since that time, articles related to this disease have been published under various categories including dysmorphic syndrome, dermatologic hypochondriasis, dermatologic non-disease, monosymptomatic hypochondriasis non-disease, and monosymptomatic hypochondriasis. According to the DSM-IV (Diagnostic and Statistical Manual of Mental Disorders), the current diagnostic manual of the American Psychiatric Association, a diagnosis of body dysmorphic disorder is based upon three major criteria.[7] First, the patient must show a preoccupation and excessive concern with an imagined defect, or a defect that is slight and unnoticeable at normal conversational distance. Second, this preoccupation must cause some hindrance to the patient in terms of normal social or occupational functioning; examples of this include poor performance at school or work and difficulty in dating or maintaining other relationships. Finally, this preoccupation must not be explainable by another comorbid

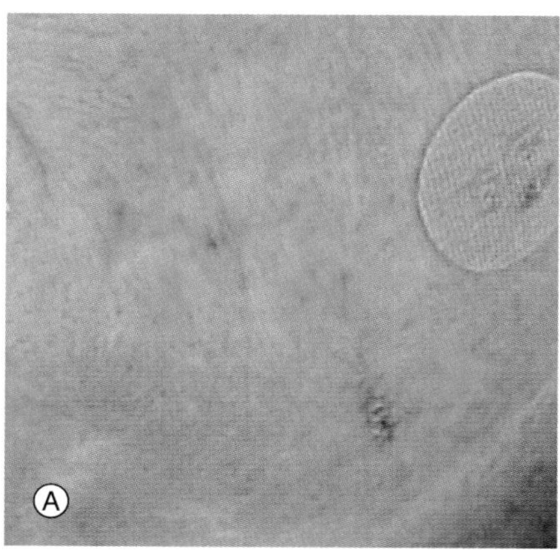

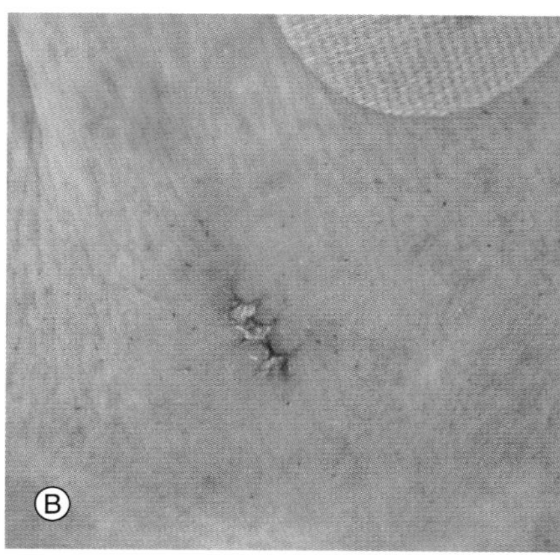

Figure 26.1 (A) Man with body dysmorphic disorder has significant scarring but no evidence of 'ingrown hairs' or acne that drives him to spend many hours 'working' on the hairs under the skin. (B) Close-up view of patient with fishing-line sutures that the patient placed himself.

Table 26.1 Criteria for diagnosis of body dysmorphic disorder

1. Preoccupation with an imagined or overemphasized defect
2. Imagined defect is a source of severe social or occupational dysfunction
3. Patient engages in repeated behaviors such as picking in order to improve the defect

condition such as anorexia nervosa or transsexualism. These criteria can be found summarized in Table 26.1.

Although the DSM-IV criteria maintain that the patient may be preoccupied with any part of the body, the most common complaints tend to involve the skin, face, and nose.[8] Body dysmorphic disorder has been described in many different cases and apparently has several variations. For example, one such variation is known as muscle dysmorphia. In this type of dysmorphic disorder, usually seen in men, the patient feels as though his body is weak and scrawny, when in fact he is typically very large and muscular.[9] Body dysmorphic disorder is listed under the rubric of hypochondriasis, with the difference that there is no other underlying mental disorder in this disease. Unfortunately, even though this disorder is one of the most commonly seen, it can be one of the most difficult to treat.

Epidemiology

Although several studies have been conducted to establish the prevalence of body dysmorphic disorder, there is a tremendous amount of disagreement. Because we have all been concerned with a particular part of our bodies at one time or another, determining what exactly qualifies one as suffering from body dysmorphic disorder can be very difficult. The best estimate for the presence of this disorder in the general population is around 1% in the United States, although rates ranging from 0.7% to 2.3% have been reported.[10] As would be expected, the overall rates of body dysmorphic disorder appear to be much higher in dermatological and cosmetic surgery settings. In cosmetic surgery, rates have been reported ranging from 7% to 15%,[11] while in dermatology, one of the largest studies which involved screening 268 patients for body dysmorphic disorder revealed a rate of 11.9% (95% confidence interval, 8.0% to 15.8%).[12] In addition, it is believed that body dysmorphic disorder effects men at an equal or slightly higher rate than women, although the presentation of the disease varies slightly in men and women. Affecting around 1 in every 10 patients, it is apparent that dermatologists see a great number of patients suffering from this disorder, many of whom continue to be undiagnosed.

In terms of their overall appearance, it is interesting that cosmetic surgery patients are no more dissatisfied, critical, or preoccupied than the general population.[8] But when questioned about their perception of the specific body part for which they seek cosmetic surgery a much greater level of dissatisfaction is found compared with non-cosmetic surgery seeking counterparts. This finding has led some to believe that it is not dissatisfaction with overall appearance that leads a body dysmorphic patient to seek out cosmetic surgery, but dissatisfaction with one particular cosmetic feature. This hypothesis would also explain why patients with body dysmorphic disorder often present to dermatologists with one chief complaint, such as hair loss or severe acne.

Etiology and pathophysiology

As with most other psychological disorders, the exact physiologic cause of body dysmorphic disorder has yet to be determined. For the most part, body dysmorphic disorder, like other obsessive–compulsive disorders, is thought to result from a neurochemical imbalance, mainly involving serotonin.[13] This explains the improvement that some patients experience when treated with selective serotonin reuptake inhibitors. However, recent studies have attempted to elucidate the pathogenesis of this disease. One such case describes a 24-year-old man who began showing symptoms of body dysmorphic disorder after suffering an inflammatory brain process 3 years previously.[14] During clinical evaluation and treatment, neuroimaging determined that the patient had suffered significant atrophy in the frontotemporal region of his brain. Although this isolated case does not give absolute proof, the correlation of this focal atrophy along with the onset of body dysmorphic disorder has given credence to the idea that a specific area of the brain is responsible.

In another recent study, magnetic resonance imaging was used to compare the brains of eight women suffering from body dysmorphic disorder with eight unaffected women.[15] The preliminary results of this study show a predominant leftward shift in caudate asymmetry and a greater amount of total white matter in the group with body dysmorphic disorder compared to the control group. These findings are consistent with brain scans of those who suffer from similar obsessive–compulsive disorders. Although both these studies have limited applications at this time, it is hoped that similar studies will one day allow for the development of more specific diagnostic tests and treatments for this disease. The current treatments for body dysmorphic disorder will be discussed later in this chapter.

Clinical features

The clinical presentation of body dysmorphic disorder can be divided into two general areas: the preoccupation with the imagined defect and the performance of repetitive compulsive behaviors. As mentioned earlier, the preoccupation has been shown in several studies to be primarily with the skin, followed by the hair and nose. Based on this preoccupation with the skin and hair, most doctor-shopping by these patients occurs within the field of dermatology. Interestingly, there have been reports that sex differences exist in terms of the nature of the complaints about the most often 'obsessed over' body parts. For example, regarding hair 'defects' most women might complain about their hair being the wrong color, being asymmetrical, too curly, or too straight, while men are mostly concerned about hair thinning or balding.[9] In addition, women are more frequently concerned over the presence of excess body hair than men are.[9] In terms of overall body appearance, women tend to be more preoccupied with their weight and the size of their hips, while men tend to suffer more from muscle dysmorphia (see above). Furthermore, men appear to have greater preoccupation with the size of their genitals, mainly believing that their penis is too small.[9] Interestingly, women do not share the same preoccupation with their genitals.[9]

Body dysmorphic disorder and its variants have been described by physicians in all disciplines of medicine and in all parts of the world. Two such interesting international variants include a delusional belief that the penis is shrinking (Koro) by people in the Chinese community, and an obsession with eyelids seen in Japanese people.[16] Regardless of the specifics of the apparent 'deformity' the underlying theme in all cases is that the concern is trivial or nonexistent, and causes much more distress in the patient than it would if it were present in the rest of the population.

The second manifestation of the disease, repetitive compulsive behavior, can be directly attributed to the presence of the imagined or exaggerated defect. For example, because in most cases the preoccupation is with some blemish present on the skin, a common behavior will be obsessive skin checking in the mirror (Fig. 26.2). Some patients may present to dermatologists with excoriations, due to constant picking and rubbing at their imagined blemishes. In these cases, lesions on the patient's skin will actually be present due to the patient's own destruction. Cases such as these often complicate the physician's physical assessment of the patient's condition and make the diagnosis of body dysmorphic disorder even more difficult. Other obsessive behaviors seen in cases of body dysmorphic disorder include excessive grooming, camouflaging the defect with make-up, hair, clothes, or posture, measuring the disliked body part, persistent questioning of others about the defect, and, of course, constantly seeking out surgical, dermatologic, or other medical treatment, even though other people and physicians have explained to them that there is nothing to treat.

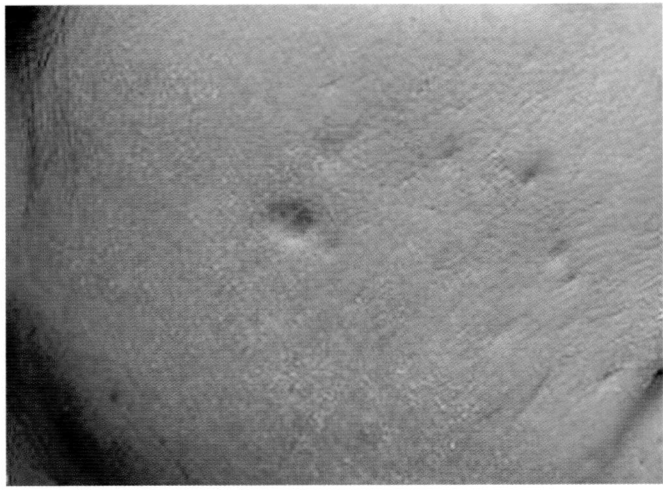

Figure 26.2 A deep crater-like scar is noted in addition to a few ice-pick type scars on the face of a woman. The crater-like scar was induced by the patient's persistent 'attention to' and picking of the pimple and scar.

Evaluation

The first step in diagnosing the disease lies in listening to the patient. As most physicians already have discovered, however, listening to the patient can often be both the best and the worst thing to do. One of the most frequently heard initial warning signs is that the patient has been to countless doctors for this same problem. If after listening to the patient's chief complaint you can find no sign of the defect to which they are referring, the best plan of action is to probe the patient by further questioning about what aspects of the defect bothers them. Another option is to have the patient complete a standard body dysmorphic disorder questionnaire (BDDQ). Many forms of questionnaires have been published, but most of the standards are aimed at establishing the presence of the criteria set forth by the DSM-IV. An example of a typical BDDQ is shown in Figure 26.3.

The results of this questionnaire in no way serve to definitively diagnose body dysmorphic disorder. The survey simply attempts to ascertain whether a severe physical preoccupation exists, what the extent of the severity is, and if the severity can be attributed to another condition such as anorexia nervosa. Upon completion, the physician should have a fairly good understanding as to whether or not the patient meets the DSM-IV criteria for body dysmorphic disorder, and if treatment should be pursued. When there is a psychological disease such as body dysmorphic disorder, the patient is most likely not going to be very amenable to any discussion that makes them seem mentally ill. Therefore, great care must be taken to ensure that enough evidence is present to confront any patient with the possibility of this diagnosis (see Table 26.2).

Complications and psychiatric comorbidity

Although body dysmorphic disorder may sound fairly trivial, the comorbid conditions associated with it are not only damaging to the patient's quality of life, but also carry the risk of physical harm to the patient and others. O'Sullivan et al. report of a woman with body dysmorphic disorder who self-inflicted an almost mortal wound by skin picking.[17] Self-inflicted skin wounds, also called neurotic excoriations, are a fairly common finding with body dysmorphic disorder, but can also be present with various other conditions such as trichotillomania and obsessive–compulsive disorder.[17] At the time of the incident, this 48-year-old woman had a 4-year history of skin picking and had been seen by several dermatologists and family practitioners for the treatment of severe skin wounds and infections. The patient claimed to be trying to eradicate pimples and bumps from her face, arms, and legs, which she would obsess about for up to 4 hours daily. On several occasions, it was necessary to hospitalize the patient for treatment of wounds that would not resolve on their own. Even though the patient received psychiatric therapy for her condition, the symptoms of body dysmorphic disorder did not seem to improve, and the picking continued. After the removal of a small occlusion cyst of the neck (unrelated to body dysmorphic disorder) the patient continued to pick at the surgical defect because she thought it 'just didn't feel right.' Described by her as a pimple, she proceeded to pick at the wound with her fingernails, and eventually a pair of tweezers. She continued to dissect through her dermis, subcutaneous tissue, and musculature until she had exposed her carotid artery. When the patient's husband discovered her, he noted what he described as a 'bullet hole' in her neck and immediately rushed her to the hospital where the wound was properly treated. In this dangerous incident, the patient suffered from no psychiatric condition other than body dysmorphic disorder.

Despite the danger body dysmorphic disorder patients pose to themselves through skin picking and other compulsive acts, there is also a significant level of psychiatric comorbidity that can put the patient in mortal danger when the angst and despair may lead to suicide. The treating physician may also be at risk of being harmed by the disturbed patient because of feelings of frustration and retribution. Among these comorbidities, severe depression usually tops the list, often leading to rates of suicidal tendencies that far exceed the general population. In one study, 22% of patients who had presented to a dermatology clinic with body dysmorphic disorder had attempted suicide.[12] Furthermore, when these patients are assessed for mental health status, they frequently score lower than patients suffering from a variety of severe chronic illnesses such as diabetes, depression, and myocardial infarction.[18] Along with suicide and depression, body dysmorphic disorder has also been shown to be positively correlated with other psychiatric and medical illnesses such as anxiety disorder, heart disease, diabetes, panic disorder, obsessive–compulsive disorder, substance use, and manic–depressive illness.[18] In most cases, the social phobias develop prior to body dysmorphic disorder, while depression and substance use begin after the onset of the disease.[19] Some studies have also reported gender differences regarding specific comorbid conditions. More specifically, women with body dysmorphic disorder are often reported to suffer from panic attacks, bulimia, and generalized anxiety disorder, while men are more likely to suffer from bipolar disorders.[20]

Table 26.2 Resources for information on body dysmorphic disorder

Internet Resources	Books
The Body Image Program http://www.bodyimage program.com Last accessed: 1 June 2004	The broken mirror: Understanding and treating body dysmorphic disorder. Phillips KA. New York: Oxford University Press; 1996[26]
National Alliance for the Mentally Ill http://web.nami.org/youth/ dysmorphic.html Last accessed: 1 June 2004	The Adonis complex: The secret crisis of male body obsession. Pope HG, Phillips KA, Olivardia R. New York: The Free Press; 2000[27]
Body Dysmorphic Disorder Central http://www.bddcentral.com Last accessed: 1 June 2004	

Along with risk to the patient there may be significant danger to the patient's family and treating physician. As might be expected, the continuous doctor-shopping and seeking out of treatments can often lead to a heightened level of frustration for the patient. As treatments continue to fail, patients can lash out at their loved ones, especially their spouse or significant other, for being unable to help them find the treatment they feel they need. In addition, surgeons who have performed cosmetic surgery on these patients, especially male patients, have reported cases of extreme violence after being disappointed with the outcome of the surgery. In some of these more tragic cases the aggression toward the surgeon has even resulted in murder.[11]

Treatment options

In most patients with body dysmorphic disorder, the rate of surgical success is exceedingly poor. In addition, after the surgery has taken place and the area has healed, the patient will claim that the surgery failed to improve the defect. If, by chance, the surgeon is able to convince the patient that the surgery has ameliorated any imperfection the patient may have had, the patient will not be convinced for long, and will soon turn attention to another part of the body. This pattern greatly contributes to the excessive doctor-shopping as seen in many body dysmorphic disorder patients who continually request surgeries and extensive workups that the physician knows will do no good in fixing the patient's apparent defect.

Because of the risks involved and this recurrent pattern of dissatisfaction, the performing of any cosmetic surgery on these patients is generally contraindicated. Even in cases where a deformity has been present, such as a large nose or an area of excessive body hair, the completion of surgery rarely improves the patient's outlook on the situation and most will be unhappy with the results. There have been some reports that these patients can be considered good surgical candidates, but an extreme caveat must be taken to ensure that the best interest of the patient and the physician is being taken into consideration before any cosmetic procedure is undertaken. In most cases, the performing of simple restorative cosmetic procedures such as botulinum toxin injections show little risk of severe psychological complications when compared to permanent structural change procedures such as rhinoplasties, where the entire general appearance of the patient is altered.[21]

Body dysmorphic disorder questionnaire (BDDQ)

1

This questionnaire asks about concerns with physical appearance. Please read each question carefully and circle the answer that is true for you. Also, write in answers where indicated.

NAME:.. **TODAY'S DATE:**..

1. Are you very worried about how you look? Yes No

If yes: Do you think about your appearance problems a lot and wish you could think about them less? Yes No

If yes: Please list the body areas you do not like: ....

....

....

Examples of your disliked body area include: your skin (for example: acne, scars, wrinkles, paleness, redness); hair; the shape or size of your nose, mouth, jaw, lips, stomach, hips, etc.; or defects of your hands, genitals, breasts, or any other body part.

If the answer to either of the above questions was **No**, you are finished with this questionnaire. Otherwise, please continue.

2. Is your *main* concern with how you look that you are not thin enough or that you might get too fat? Yes No

3. How has this problem with how you look affected your life?

Has it often upset you *a lot*? Yes No

Has it gotten in the way of doing things with friends or dating? Yes No

If yes, please describe how: ....

....

....

Has it ever caused problems with school? Yes No

If yes, what are they? ....

....

....

Are there things you avoid because of how you look? Yes No

If yes, what are they? ....

....

Continued on next page

Figure 26.3 Body dysmorphic disorder questionnaire.

BDDQ questionnaire (continued)

2

4. How much time a day do you usually spend thinking about how you look? Please circle one.

a) Less than 1 hour a day

b) 1–3 hours a day

c) More than 3 hours a day

You're likely to have BDD if you give the following answers on the BDDQ:

Question 1: Yes to both parts

Question 3: Yes to any of the questions

Question 4: Answer b or c

Figure 26.3, *continued*.

On the other hand, there are physicians who believe that many surgeons are 'passing up' patients who may actually be helped by a combined surgical and medical approach. Nonetheless, current research indicates, on the whole, that most patients suffering from body dysmorphic disorder do *not* benefit from cosmetic surgery and frequently suffer from a worsening of symptoms as treatment proceeds.[22]

Interestingly, there is little research evaluating the percentage of cases of body dysmorphic disorder that start out as common cosmetic repairs or enhancement. For instance, in rhinoplasty surgery a significant percentage of the population would probably consider the patient's nose structure to be cosmetically unappealing. In these instances, cosmetic surgery is almost always indicated, with the patient usually approving the final outcome. However, there are some cases where the first surgery is just the start. Once the repair has been made, the patient will insist that more work needs to be done until it seems they become addicted to the changes and potential enhancement of cosmetic surgery. Some physicians have speculated that some celebrities who appear to be addicted to cosmetic surgery probably suffer from body dysmorphic disorder; there are some very poignant examples of what can happen when a serious mental condition is combined with millions of dollars.

In cases such as these, it is difficult to say whether the patient suffered from body dysmorphic disorder before undergoing the initial procedure or because of disapproval of the initial surgical results. Clearly, more research will have to be done to investigate the pathogenesis of body dysmorphic disorder in these people.

In most cases, dermatologists and cosmetic surgeons lack the experience and training necessary to treat a patient for this type of psychological condition. Once the presence of body dysmorphic disorder is confirmed through questionnaires or other means, the most appropriate step is a referral to a psychiatrist. What follows are some general guidelines adapted from Katharine Phillips' guide[23] for dermatologists and plastic surgeons as to how one should proceed with a patient suspected of having body dysmorphic disorder:

Provide education

- Inform the patient of your suspicion of body dysmorphic disorder, explaining in simple terms what that means.
- Recommend reading material (e.g. fliers, the internet) where the patient may obtain more information (a list of appropriate web sites is given in Table 26.2).
- Do not downplay any of the patient's concerns about their appearance as this may have a significant negative impact on their recovery.
- If appropriate, educate any family members who may be involved or are able to help.

Behavior modification

- Do not try to talk patients out of picking their skin or being worried about their appearance.
- Attempts to end the patient's compulsive behaviors often leads to further depression, frustration, and lack of recovery.

- Do not encourage the patient to use make-up or any other concealing methods to hide their deformity as this has also been shown to interfere with recovery.

Appropriate referral

- Explain to the patient that the disorder cannot be effectively treated by dermatologists or with cosmetic procedures.
- Attempt to refer the patient to a psychiatrist, emphasizing the amount of time they spend worrying about their appearance and how it affects their life.
- If the patient is worried about taking antipsychotic medications, explain that therapies that do not include the use of medications may be available.
- If the patient is suicidal or severely depressed, attempt no other referral than to a psychiatrist, as treatment with antipsychotic medications is the best approach.

Once referred to a psychiatrist or other mental health specialist, the patient can expect to encounter two forms of treatment: pharmacotherapy and cognitive-behavioral therapy (CBT), a form of psychotherapy. For over 10 years the mainstay of treatment for body dysmorphic disorder has been pharmacological with selective serotonin reuptake inhibitors (SSRIs).[24] In most situations, dermatologists and plastic surgeons are not qualified to monitor the patient's progress under the influence of these medications. If the physician feels that treatment for body dysmorphic disorder is warranted, a referral to a qualified psychiatrist is most likely the best course of action.

Although most research indicates that surgery should be contraindicated in patients with severe psychological conditions, there are some physicians who feel that surgeons are bypassing these patients unnecessarily, and that they might actually be benefited by combining surgical and psychological therapies for treatment. In some studies patients were selected who screened positive for the presence of body dysmorphic disorder or other psychological disturbances, and then cosmetic surgery was performed. After being followed for several years, only a small percentage of patients experienced negative outcomes from the surgery, with no reports of lawsuits, suicide, or further induced psychological complications.[25] Thus, although most surgeons prefer not to perform cosmetic procedures on psychologically disturbed patients, in the end it is up to the individual surgeon to decide whether or not the patient is a good candidate for the desired cosmetic surgical procedure.

SUMMARY

Evaluating the psychosocial status of a patient is a crucial component of every medical specialty. However, dermatologists and cosmetic surgeons undoubtedly encounter patients with certain psychological disorders at a much higher frequency than many of their colleagues. At its most superficial level, the underlying goal of any cosmetic surgery procedure is to provide some sort of psychological benefit to the patient.[25] More specifically, the surgeon should be able to lead the patient to greater emotional health.[25] Because of the inextricably intertwined relationship of cosmetic surgery and psychology, the psychosocial health of every cosmetic surgery patient must be thoroughly evaluated in order to ensure that no serious underlying psychological disorders exist that would preclude that patient from an aesthetic procedure. As such, any doctor performing cosmetic procedures should have a working knowledge of the presentation, etiology, and treatment options for many of the common diseases that may be encountered. Consequently, the team will be able to develop the most appropriate plan of action for treatment, ultimately helping the patient to attain a more physically and emotionally appealing state. Furthermore, the dermatologist will also be able to help identify patients in need of counseling or psychiatric treatment, and avoid performing surgeries that would otherwise be contraindicated due to the presence of various mental conditions.

REFERENCES

1. Ishigooka J, Iwao M, Suzuki M, Fukuyama Y, Murasaki M, Miura S. Demographic features of patients seeking cosmetic surgery. Psychiatry Clin Neurosci 1998; 52:283–287.
2. Brawman-Mintzer O, Lydiard RB, Phillips KA, et al. Body dysmorphic disorder in patients with anxiety disorders and major depression: a comorbidity study. Am J Psychiatr 1995; 152:1665–1667.
3. Goin J, Goin M. Changing the body: psychological effects of plastic surgery. Baltimore: Williams & Wilkins Co; 1981.
4. Folstein MF, Folstein SE, McHugh PR. 'Mini-mental state.' A practical method for grading the cognitive state of patients for the clinician. J Psychiatr Res 1975; 12:189–198.
5. Hollander E, Allen A, Kwon J, et al. Clomipramine vs desipramine crossover trial in body dysmorphic disorder: selective efficacy of a serotonin reuptake inhibitor in imagined ugliness. Arch Gen Psychiatr 1999; 56:1033–1039.
6. Phillips KA, Albertini RS, Rasmussen SA. A randomized placebo-controlled trial of fluoxetine in body dysmorphic disorder. Arch Gen Psychiatr 2002; 59:381–388.
7. AMA. Diagnostic and statistical manual of mental disorders, 4th edn. Washington, DC: American Psychiatric Association; 1994.
8. Sarwer DB, Wadden TA, Pertschuk MJ, Whitaker LA. Body image dissatisfaction and body dysmorphic disorder in 100 cosmetic surgery patients. Plast Reconstr Surg 1998; 101:1644–1649.
9. Phillips KA, Diaz SF. Gender differences in body dysmorphic disorder. J Nerv Ment Dis 1997; 185:570–577.
10. Phillips KA, Dufresne RG Jr. Body dysmorphic disorder: a guide for primary care physicians. Prim Care 2002; 29:99–111; vii.
11. Phillips KA, Grant J, Siniscalchi J, Albertini RS. Surgical and nonpsychiatric medical treatment of patients with body dysmorphic disorder. Psychosomatics 2001; 42:504–510.
12. Phillips KA, Dufresne RG Jr, Wilkel CS, Vittorio CC. Rate of body dysmorphic disorder in dermatology patients. J Am Acad Dermatol 2000; 42:436–441.
13. Slaughter JR, Sun AM. In pursuit of perfection: a primary care physician's guide to body dysmorphic disorder. Am Fam Physician 1999; 60:1738–1742.
14. Gabbay V, Asnis GM, Bello JA, Alonso CM, Serras SJ, O'Dowd MA. New onset of body dysmorphic disorder following frontotemporal lesion. Neurology 2003; 61:123–125.
15. Rauch SL, Phillips KA, Segal E, et al. A preliminary morphometric magnetic resonance imaging study of regional brain volumes in body dysmorphic disorder. Psychiatr Res 2003; 122:13–19.
16. Cotterill JA. Body dysmorphic disorder. Dermatol Clin 1996; 14:457–463.
17. O'Sullivan RL, Phillips KA, Keuthen NJ, Wilhelm S. Near-fatal skin picking from delusional body dysmorphic disorder responsive to fluvoxamine. Psychosomatics 1999; 40:79–81.
18. Phillips KA. Quality of life for patients with body dysmorphic disorder. J Nerv Ment Dis 2000; 188:170–175.
19. Gunstad J, Phillips KA. Axis I comorbidity in body dysmorphic disorder. Compr Psychiatr 2003; 44:270–276.
20. Perugi G, Akiskal HS, Giannotti D, Frare F, Di Vaio S, Cassano GB. Gender-related differences in body dysmorphic disorder (dysmorphophobia). J Nerv Ment Dis 1997; 185:578–582.
21. Castle DJ, Honigman RJ, Phillips KA. Does cosmetic surgery improve psychosocial wellbeing? Med J Aust 2002; 176:601–604.

22. Sarwer DB, Crerand CE, Didie ER. Body dysmorphic disorder in cosmetic surgery patients. Facial Plast Surg 2003; 19:7–18.
23. Phillips KA, Dufresne RG. Body dysmorphic disorder. A guide for dermatologists and cosmetic surgeons. Am J Clin Dermatol 2000; 1:235–243.
24. Phillips KA, Najjar F. An open-label study of citalopram in body dysmorphic disorder. J Clin Psychiatr 2003; 64:715–720.
25. Edgerton MT, Langman MW, Pruzinsky T. Plastic surgery and psychotherapy in the treatment of 100 psychologically disturbed patients. Plast Reconstr Surg 1991; 88:594–608.
26. Phillips K. The broken mirror: Understanding and treating body dysmorphic disorder. New York: Oxford University Press; 1996.
27. Pope HG, Phillips KA, Olivardia R. The Adonis complex: The secret crisis of male body obsession. New York: The Free Press; 2000.

27 Evaluation and Management of the Aging Face

Lisa M Donofrio MD

Summary box

- Evaluation of the aging face must take into account changes that occur in all levels of tissue.
- Young faces are characterized by arcs and fullness, not merely by the absence of wrinkles.
- The morphologic changes that occur in the aging face are due mostly to the redistribution of fat and changes in muscle tone (both increased and decreased) but bony remodeling also plays a role.
- Gravitational aging is in all likelihood a myth – it is elucidative, not causative.
- Structural fat augmentation and other methods of soft tissue augmentation can reapproximate the contours of the youthful face; chemodenervation is a useful adjunctive treatment in achieving this goal.

INTRODUCTION

Evaluation of the senescent face requires that one look deeper than the rhytides and dyschromia of photoaged skin, into the structural alterations that occur below the skin surface. Throughout life the face, like the body, changes shape. Certainly some of these changes are due to bony growth and remodeling and changes in muscle mass and tone, but fat seems to be the most substantial contributor to soft tissue changes. When examining a face for rejuvenation procedures, the physician must think of the face in 'layers' and approach the aging changes in each layer separately. Aging occurs both as an extrinsic and intrinsic phenomenon. External aging occurs through ultraviolet (UV) and oxidative damage and most characteristically takes the form of dyschromia, telangectasias, and textural changes. Internal aging is likely hormonally and genetically regulated and is responsible for bone and soft tissue remodeling, including dermal changes. In essence, 'wrinkles' occur secondary to intrinsic and extrinsic aging.

TECHNICAL ASPECTS

Epidermal and dermal aging

Cumulative UV exposure decreases skin collagen content, aggregates elastic fibers, disrupts cutaneous immune surveillance, stimulates melanogenesis and angiogenesis, and disorganizes epidermal cell maturation.[1–6] Clinically this translates into coarsened pores, sebaceous hyperplasia, telangectasias, keratosis, and skin cancers. A clinical correlation can be made between ultrastructural changes in the collagen and elastin and textural changes such as a crepe paper-like appearance and fine rhytides. Coarse rhytides or folds are more reasonably explained by soft tissue atrophy or muscular movement.

Mimetic muscle aging

Sarcopenia, or skeletal muscle wastage with age, is a selective event affecting some but not all muscle of the body. For instance, the quadriceps muscles lose up to 21% of their mass with advancing age, but the muscles of the arm remain unchanged.[7,8] This loss is also somewhat attenuated by exercise. While a widely recognized theory to explain aging, to date there is no evidence to substantiate that the facial mimetic muscles atrophy with age. In fact, evidence exists to the contrary. For example, MRI studies reveal that there is no significant change in length or projection of the levator labii superioris or the zygomaticus muscles between young and old subjects.[9]

The skin/muscle interaction

In youth, the mimetic muscles are separated from the overlying cutis by a diffuse layer of subcutaneous fat. This serves to attenuate the muscular 'pull' on the skin and acts as a glide plane between the skin and muscle. Animation of a young face is followed by a relaxation of the muscular impression on the skin. In an old face, the undersurface of the dermis lies in close juxtaposition to the mimetic musculature and investing superficial musculoaponecrotic system (SMAS). Trabeculae of the reticular dermis attach

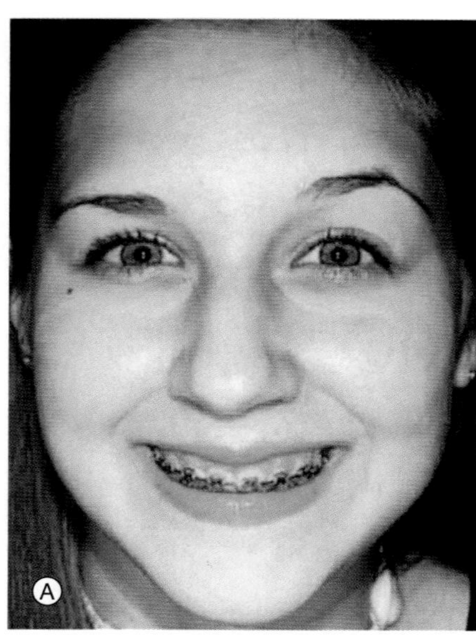
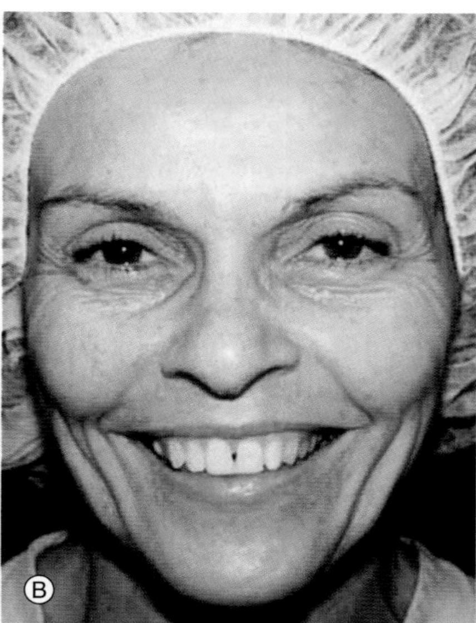

Figure 27.1 (A) Due to the thickness of subcutaneous fat, animation in the young face produces few wrinkles in the overlying skin. (B) Lack of subcutaneous fat in the aging face allows the mimetic muscles to pull the skin along. Courtesy of Lisa M Donofrio.

to the underlying muscles.[10] The skin is tugged along with each facial expression. Repeated facial animation over time in conjunction with chronic sun exposure serve to permanently fibrose the skin to the muscle and set in the dermal component of the rhytides.[4] A helpful analogy is to think of the face as a Roman shade or blind. When young, the Roman shade is made of foam, so any tugging on the cord only minimally raises and wrinkles the shade. With age, the shade becomes like tissue paper so even a minor pull on the cord produces a number of creases (Fig. 27.1). Botulinum toxin halts the tugging on the cord, but only volume replacement can replenish the thickness of the shade.

Craniofacial skeletal aging

Significant aging changes take place in the facial bones. These include changes in contour of the maxilla, increase in vertical maxillary dimension with retrusion of the lower maxillary skeleton, a slight overall widening of the face, and a decrease in the overall facial height. This causes a 'concertina effect' with compression of the soft tissue and relative redundancy of skin. Skeletal remodeling in adulthood changes the facial dimensions to that of an infant with an increase in the ratio of the maxillary height to the orbital height (Fig. 27.2).[11,12] These changes are even more dramatic in edentulous people.[13] Aging also causes the orbital rim and anterior cheek to move posterior relative to the cornea, changing the relationship of the orbit to the mid-face and causing the eye to appear proptotic.[14] In young adulthood, however, there is a balance between the bony facial skeletal support and the soft tissue envelope and so aesthetic harmony ensues.[15]

Structural fat remodeling with age

An infant has a characteristic distribution of fat, displaying jowls, tear trough deformity, and submental fullness. Interestingly, these patterns are seen again in the adult face, but all too often gravity is erroneously named as the culprit. It is more likely that fat redistribution is responsible for the hallmark shape of the aging face, so that aging, like infancy, can be considered a state of facial fat dysmorphism.

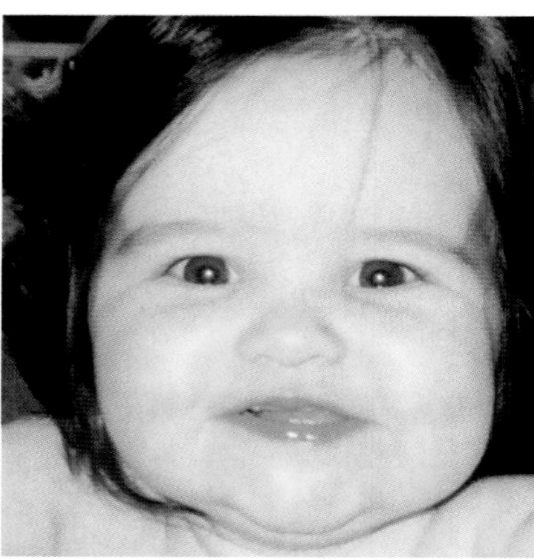

Figure 27.2 The facial fat distribution of an infant is similar to the dysmorphism seen in aging adults. Photo property of Lisa M Donofrio.

The face of the middle to late 20s is the standard in desirability of aesthetics. The rounded fullness of the teenage years is lost and the face becomes mildly sculpted in the subzygoma area. Overall, there is a homogeneity to the fat distribution. Topographically, the facial contour is like a gently rolling plain and the facial fat appears balanced. There is a seamless connection between the cosmetic units of the face and a near absence of shadows. The upper third of the face is broad with a convexity in the temples and a projection of the forehead and brow away from the underlying frontal bone. The lower lid is supported with ample fat and this fat is contiguous with the anteriorly projecting malar eminence. There may be fullness or slight flatness of the buccal fat area; however, hollowing is not seen in most healthy young adults. In profile, the cheek, like the forehead, arcs forward giving the face a strong anterior projection (Fig. 27.3). The lower third of the face is arced on with a sweep of the jawline from ear to ear (Fig. 27.4). The jaw itself is full with an anterior projection that then wraps inferiorly forming an obtuse angle with the neck. The prementum is full and projects forward and superiorly thus shortening the distance between the lip and the nose. Overall the shape of the young face is triangular with the apex of the triangle occurring at the mentum and the base at the temples (Fig. 27.5).

The aforementioned contours occur because of ampleness in the deep fat compartments. On a more subtle level,

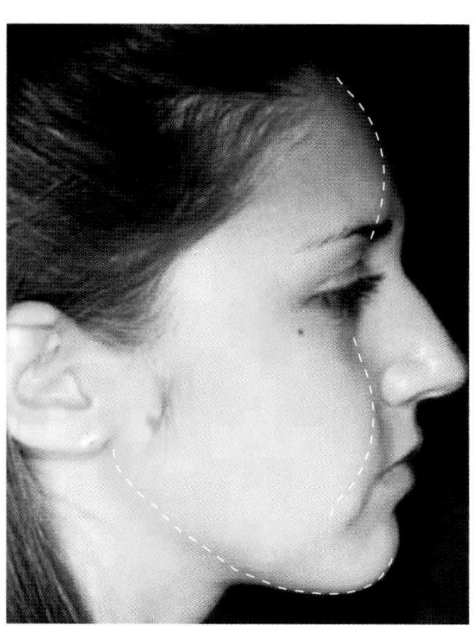

Figure 27.3 The profile arcs of the young face. Photo property of Lisa M Donofrio.

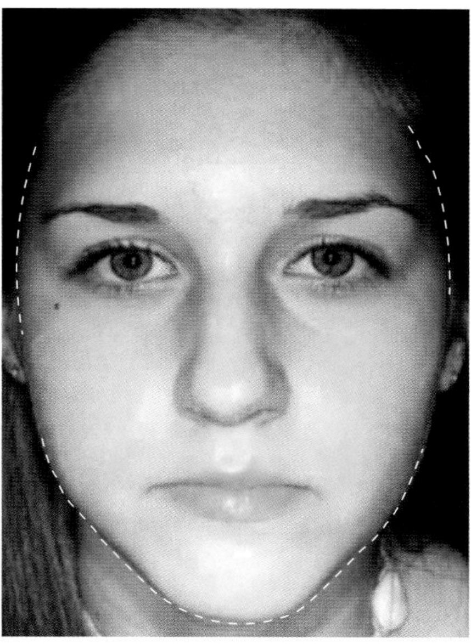

Figure 27.4 The frontal arcs of the young face. Photo property of Lisa M Donofrio.

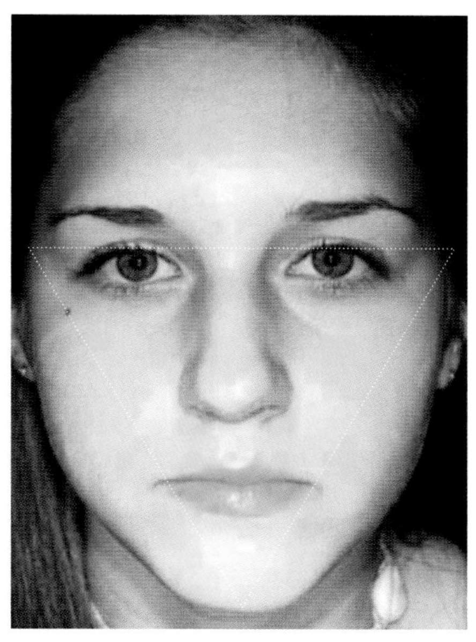

Figure 27.5 Due to a generous distribution of fat in the upper third of the face, a young face is like a triangle with the apex lying at the level of the mentum. Photo property of Lisa M Donofrio.

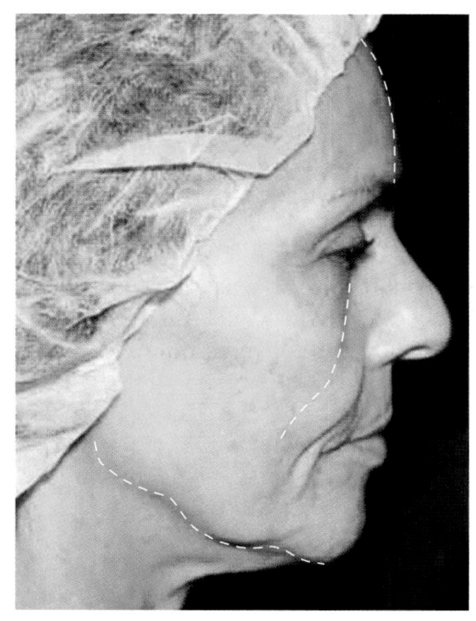

Figure 27.6 Loss of profile arcs in the aging face. Photo property of Lisa M Donofrio.

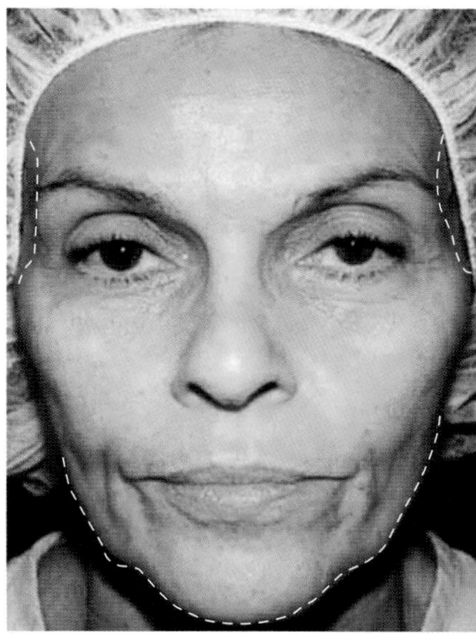

Figure 27.7 Loss of frontal arcs in the aging face. Photo property of Lisa M Donofrio.

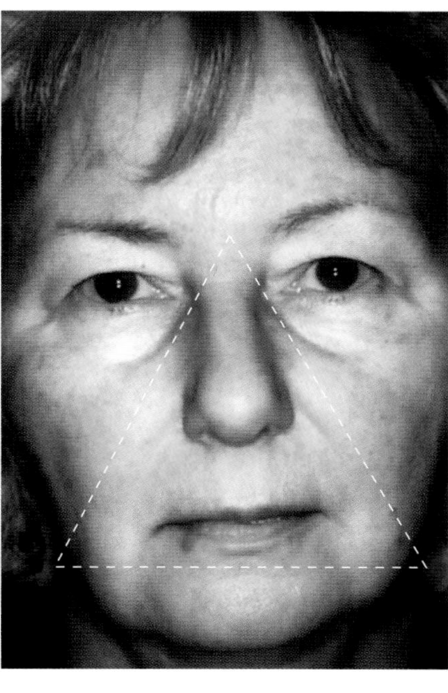

Figure 27.8 Due to a preponderance of fat in the lower third of the face and loss of fat in the upper third of the face, the aging face is like a triangle with the apex lying at the level of the glabella. Photo property of Lisa M Donofrio.

the presence of a diffuse layer of subcutaneous fat lends suppleness and opacity to a young face and hides the insertion and pull of the mimetic musculature. In contrast, the aging face is a contradiction in terms. There is unbalancing of the fat with areas corresponding to fat hypertrophy and/or fat atrophy. This leads to a hill and valley topography and an abundance of shadows. The anterior projection of the forehead and cheek is lost causing these areas to flatten and result in a downward displacement of tissues (Fig. 27.6). The temples become concave, as does the lateral third of the face. The sweep of the anterior jawline arc is replaced by an undulating curve due to submental fat accumulations, with loss of definition with respect to the neck (Fig. 27.7). The cosmetic units no longer flow but show separation with demarcation at underlying bony landmarks. The overall shape is 'bottom heavy' and the triangular shape flip-flops, with the apex lying at the level of the glabella and the base at the jawline (Fig. 27.8).

Life as art

Painters and sculptors are cognizant of the structural changes in the face that occur throughout life and use them as ways to denote the age of their subject. A sculptor will groove in shadowed areas and a painter will brush in a darker color to represent the valleys of hill and valley contours. Seeing as artists, we can surmise the age of a subject without seeing surface changes such as wrinkling, lentigines, or telangectasias because what tells us how old someone is the contours of their face. An illustrator will have to make a two-dimensional representation of age by painting a flattened cheek and more angularity as a subject ages. Conversely, a young nubile face is represented by fullness, arcs, and many points of highlight (Fig. 27.9).

Human beings have evolved to 'look their age.' There must have been a distinct advantage to looking different with every decade for this trait to have survived Darwinian evolution. It makes sense that if age could be assessed from a distance, then the threat of the on-comer could effectively be evaluated. Those who 'looked older' represented less of a threat and therefore were left alive to pass on their genes. Phenotypically aging is a gross event, evident from 3 meters away, not a microscopic one. That is why artist renditions are so successful at denoting age.

PITFALLS AND THEIR MANAGEMENT

Avoidance of pitfalls

- The aging face must not be addressed superficially, by treating only the epidermal and dermal components; treat all layers of the face as separate entities, and titrate treatment to the individual—and do not forget to treat the structural components of aging (bone and fat remodeling).
- It is important to take into account the patient's current weight and how that affects the aging face; look at photos taken in their youth and ask how their body weight compares, perhaps weighing the patient, obtaining body fat measurements, or suggesting a weight-loss regimen to optimize rejuvenation.
- It is wrong to assume that gravity is to blame for facial aging, and to address skin as an 'excess' phenomenon; take into account the alterations in three-dimensional projection and the shape of the face, and how filling the face with autologous fat can restore youthful projection.
- Fat does best as a pan-facial filler; recommendations to achieve longevity and predictability include blunt infiltration, multilayer low-pressure injection, global, dynamic filling, and under-correction with 'touch-up' procedures.

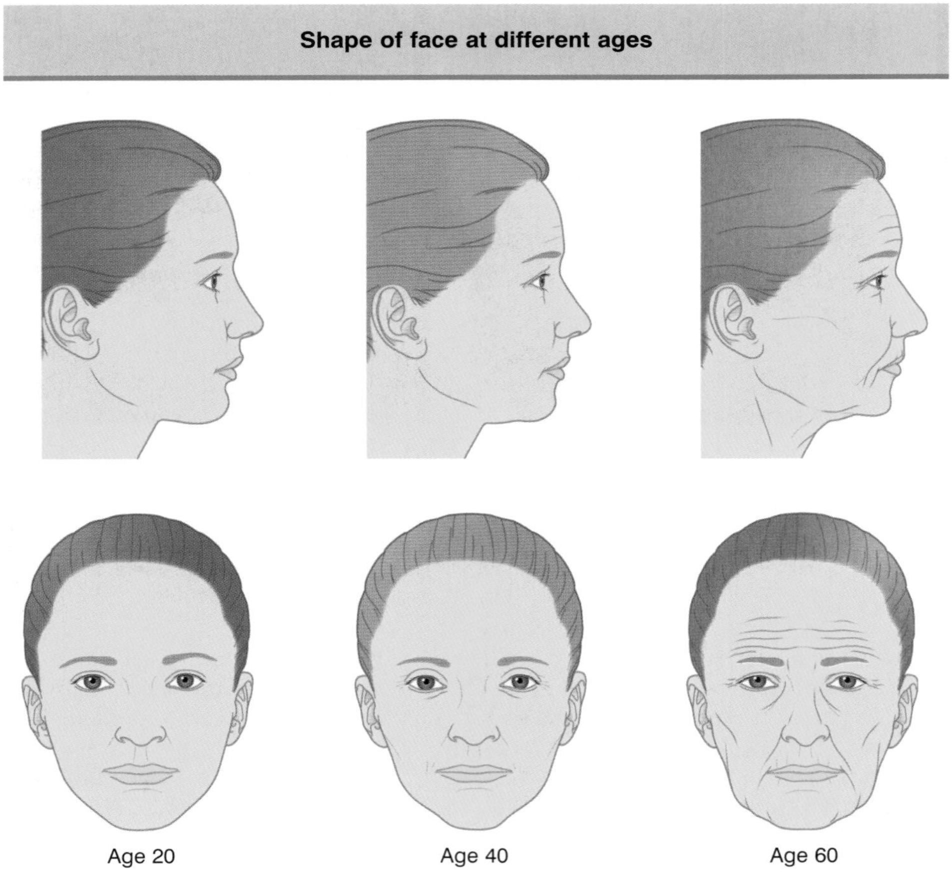

Figure 27.9 Merely by changing the angularity of the face and the appropriation of light and shadow, an artist can render the age of their subject.

The myth of gravitational aging

To date, gravitational aging is the premise for all traditional cosmetic surgery, but accepting gravity as a significant influence of sagging is probably erroneous. Since at least one third of our life is spent in a recumbent position, the downward 'force' should be somewhat mitigated by a perpendicular one. There exist no animal models for gravitational descent of tissues. Sagging occurs in the animal kingdom as a phenotypic expression, not an age-related one. For instance, parrots in their sixth decade show no signs of gravitational descent of tissues, and baby elephants display convoluted sagging of skin. In humans, aging leads to fibrosis of connective tissues and a stiffening against the forces of gravity.[16] With the exception of ptosis of the reproductive organs in multigravida women, advancing age does not bring about descent of internal organs. The pericardium and diaphragm do not sag. Gravity has also been blamed for the descent of the malar fat pad, as if somehow standing upright allowed fat to separate itself from surrounding tissues and 'slide' inferiorly.[17]

If this was true then dependent areas of the body, such as the dorsum of the hand, would 'collect' fat with age. Of course the opposite is true with the posterior aspect of the hands becoming devoid of fat with age. Therefore, if gravity were the cause of sagging it would have to be selective. Perhaps the strongest argument against gravitational aging is the fact that we all age differently. If gravity was the cause of sagging, then every 60-year-old should sag the same, but in fact we all age very differently, with prominent cross cultural variation in sagging. Gravity is not causative in facial aging but merely elucidative. The cause of morphologic aging occurs within the soft tissues and especially subcutaneous tissues which atrophy and hypertrophy relative to other structures.

Facial fat mirrors body fat

A common mistake when evaluating a patient for rejuvenation is to ignore their total body fat status. A 55-year-old with 46% body fat will have a very differently shaped face compared to a 55-year-old with 20% body fat (Fig. 27.10). Similarly, two 30-year-old faces will look very different with overall body fat of 20% versus 46%. The main difference between heavy faces of different ages is where the fat goes. Patterns of facial fat atrophy and fat hypertrophy are changes that are relative to each other. A hypertrophic area only appears such because it abuts a neighboring area of atrophy (Fig. 27.11).[18] An overweight 30-year-old has the ability to gain fat diffusely in all areas of the face. The facial fat is 'balanced' and so the face becomes rounded and homogeneously full. In contrast a 55 year old with a high body fat percentage can only gain weight in patterns that correspond to the hypertrophic areas of the face. Cadaver and MRI studies have noted an increase in fat lateral to the nasolabial and labiomental creases in aging adults, consistent with a hypertrophic fat storage pattern.[9] The areas that correspond to the atrophic areas stay as such. The heavier the face, the more discrepancy between these two areas. In contrast, a lean woman in her early 30s, while having ample subcutaneous fat, will have a more ascetic look. If she stays the same weight while she ages, her face will experience little if any of the hypertrophic fat storage patterns and instead show only atrophy. In this case, increased shadowing is from bony demarcation and angularity. When a 60-year-old patient brings in a photo of herself when she was 45 with a desire to 'turn back the clock' it is important to evaluate the difference in weight that has occurred in the previous 15 years. Since most North Americans gain weight throughout life, this has a profound effect on the shape of the face and what the patient can reasonably expect.

Paradoxically, both lean and heavy aging faces exhibit sagging as a direct result of fat distribution. Fat accumulations will hang in the direction of gravity. In the aging face of a heavy person, this fat collects in the lower third of the face leading to jowls and prominent submental fat. In contrast, a lean aging face being devoid of fat will hang empty and collapsed in the direction of the gravitational force (Figs 27.12, 27.13). What is true of fat distribution on the face is also seen on the body. With the abdomen, the skin is closely apposed to underlying rectus fascia at birth, and only becomes pendulous with excessive fat accumula-

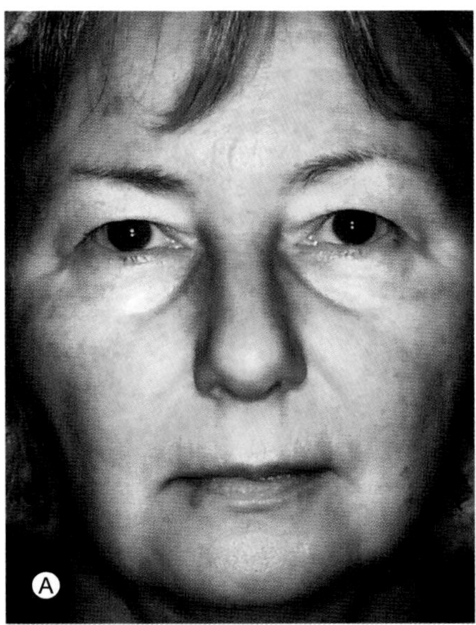

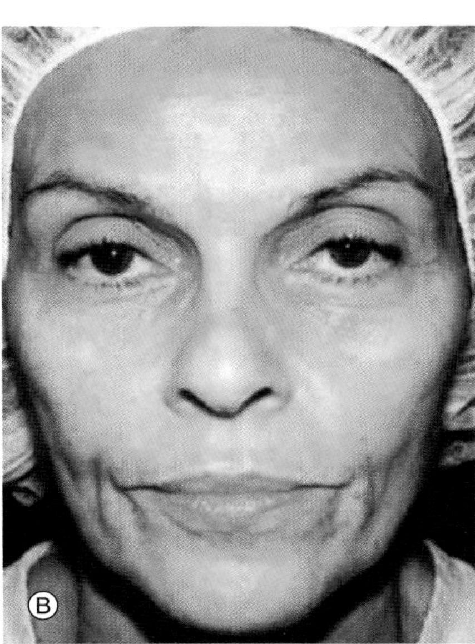

Figure 27.10 (A) The heavy aging face. (B) The lean aging face. Courtesy of Lisa M Donofrio.

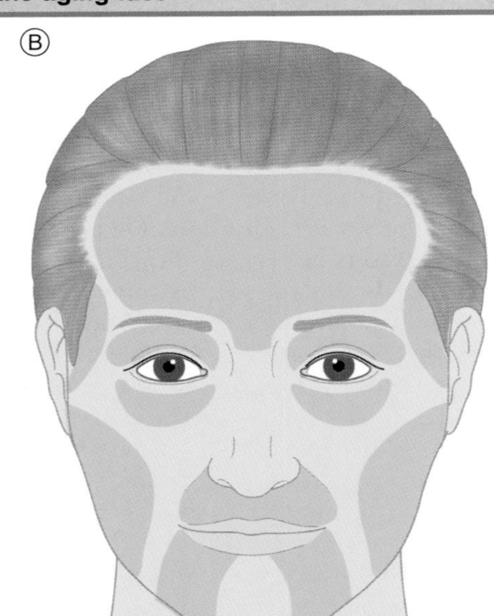

Figure 27.11 (A) Areas prone to relative hypertrophy in the aging face. (B) Areas prone to atrophy in the aging face.

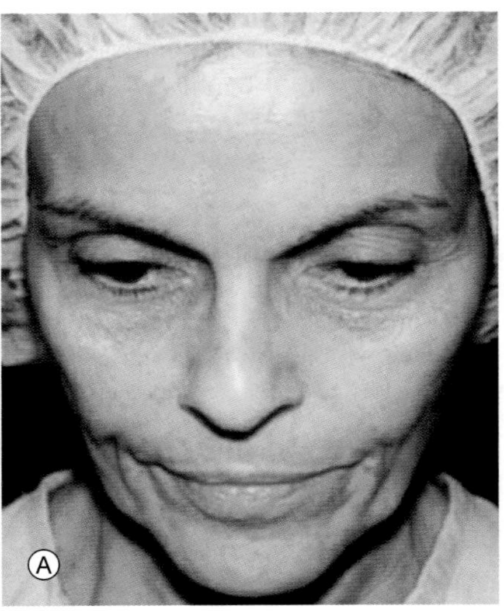

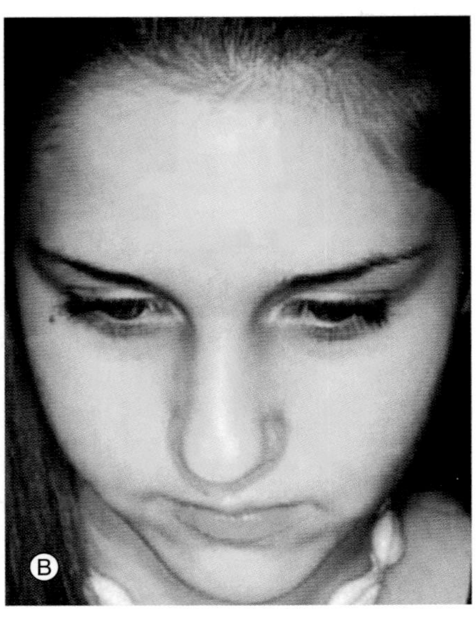

Figure 27.12 (A) Due to the loss of support from deep fat atrophy, a lean aging face with collapse in the direction of gravity. Photo property of Lisa M Donofrio. (B) A young face with ample subcutaneous and deep fat will hold its shape regardless of the direction of gravitational pull. Photo property of Lisa M Donofrio.

tion. A pendulous abdomen will be displaced downward due to the sheer weight of the panniculus. Liposuction of this area removes the fat so the skin can retract.[19] Similarly, suction of submental and jowl fat in the presence of good skin tone can markedly correct sagging by removing the offending pocket of fat. With the breast, the skin envelope develops a relative redundancy because glandular breast tissue, which grows during puberty, atrophies with aging. The common complaint of breast sagging is often remedied by 'filling up' the breast skin pocket with an implant. This serves to increase the anterior projection of the breast and take up the redundant tissue. In the same way, re-establishing the anterior projection of the cheek can serve to 'lift' the face forward and correct sagging (Fig. 27.13).

Baseline elasticity

There is an 'optimal' elasticity of skin, a point at which it is neither stretched nor deflated, which is seen in youth when the face is appropriately full of fat at an ideal body weight. This is the point where the skin has the ability to 'snap' back to its original position when stretched—referred to as elastic recoil. Elastic recoil has been studied in pleural tissue and molecularly corresponds to intact elastic fibers and organized bundles of collagen.[20] At this point, the underlying 'tension' on the skin relies on filling by soft tissues, especially subcutaneous fat, so that the overlying tissues appear taught. If a young person loses this subcutaneous layer, the overlying skin responds to the changes underneath

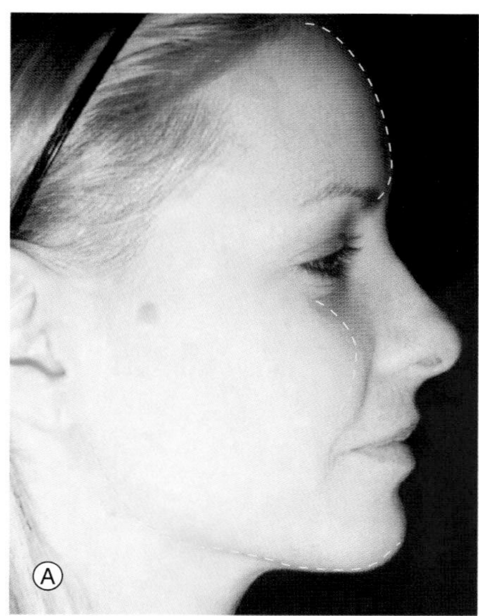

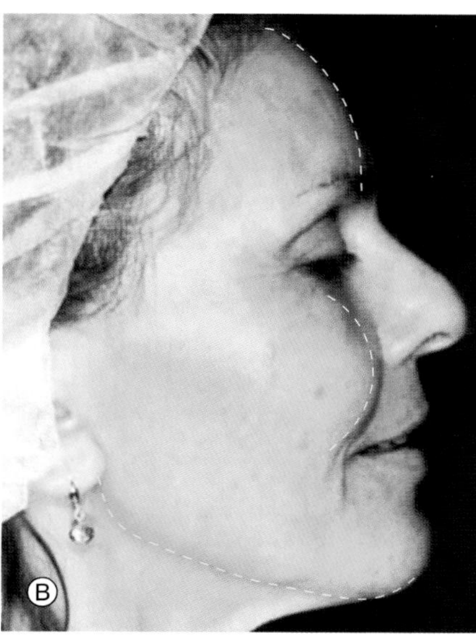

Figure 27.13 (A) The profile arcs of the young face. (B) The same patient as seen in Figure 27.6 after structural fat replacement. Note reapproximation of arcs of face and restoration of forward projection. Courtesy of Lisa M Donofrio.

by exhibiting 'supercontraction' and in essence shrinks to accommodate the changes without slackening. This can be demonstrated in a young face that has facial hemiatrophy, where the skin has an ability to contract past its baseline elasticity clinging to the skeletal framework below. However, an old face has lost this capability. The contractile properties of the skin become impaired such that it hangs in folds in response to underlying atrophic changes in the fat. Atrophy in the adult face can be seen as a normal part of the aging process or can also occur iatrogenically, secondary to overaggressive liposuction or removal of buccal fat pad. Photoaging is at least partially responsible for the inelasticity of aged skin, with its inability to respond to atrophic insults in an aesthetic manner.

■ OPTIMIZING OUTCOMES

Figure 27.14 summarizes how an aging face can be made to look younger.

■ PRACTICAL APPLICATIONS

Cosmetic management of the aging face

Cosmetic improvement of the changes that occur with aging must be specific to the structure or level of skin in which the aging occurred (Fig. 27.14). Dyschromia and poikilodermatous changes are epidermal and dermal events that must be treated with resurfacing tools (lasers, peels or topical therapies). Wrinkles must be subcategorized into fine or coarse, superficial or deep, and then further into those present at rest or only with movement. Dynamic wrinkles that disappear at rest are best treated with botulinum toxin. In those with an 'at rest' component to the wrinkle, superficial augmentation (e.g. with collagen) or resurfacing are needed for optimal results.[21] Very fine wrinkles at rest that are superficial in nature respond to intervention with tretinoin, glycolic acid, or superficial resurfacing like that achieved with TCA (trichloroacetic acid) peels or erbium:YAG laser.[22,23] Most problems in the delegation of appropriate cosmetic procedures come when treating coarse or deep rhytides. Coarse rhytides resulting from severe elastotic solar damage are often ashen or yellow in color and should be treated with deep resurfacing such as wire brush dermabrasion, carbon dioxide laser resurfacing, or deep peeling agents, such as with higher strength trichloroacetic acid or phenol. A clue to the etiology of this subset of wrinkles is the presence of exaggerated pores and comedones in the periocular region and a history of carcinomatous changes of the skin. Most aging patients have some degree of solar elastosis, but what separates those best treated with resurfacing is that the wrinkles appear superficially, as creases in the skin, rather than causing skin involutions. Involutional changes like the folds occurring in the nasolabial area or mid-cheeks are due to relative excess of skin secondary to shrinkage of the framework of the face, and pulling from underlying muscle with failure of the skin envelope to adapt. These wrinkles are ameliorated by either traditional rhytidectomy procedures that lift the skin, or structural augmentation procedures. Sagging, like folding of the skin, is an atrophic event, occurring in the direction of gravity. Face and neck lifts and skin-contracting lasers and radiofrequency devices are efficient at shrinking the skin to again fit the face, but they can unmask the bony framework of the face and accentuate the angularity that is so uncharacteristic of youth (Fig. 27.15). Care must be taken to reapproximate, not only the texture and color of youthful skin, but the shape and arcs of the young face as well.

Structural facial rejuvenation

Structural facial rejuvenation is that which replaces the scaffolding of the face—the bone and soft tissue—so that the skin can assume draping without redundancy.

True rejuvenation can only be accomplished by restoration of the young arcs of the face and rebalancing the fat and bony compartments. Options include mid-face lifting procedures that re-establish forward cheek projection (Chapter 41), synthetic and injectable implants to approximate mid-face volume and jawline definition (Chapters 28 and 30), and autologous fat transfer (Chapter 33). Implants available for augmenting the zygoma, maxilla, mandible, and chin, and injectable substances such as calcium hydroxylapatite can reapproximate the shape of the young bony facial skeleton. The former may ultimately become demarcated and visible through the skin with age. Since much of the loss of the young architecture of the face

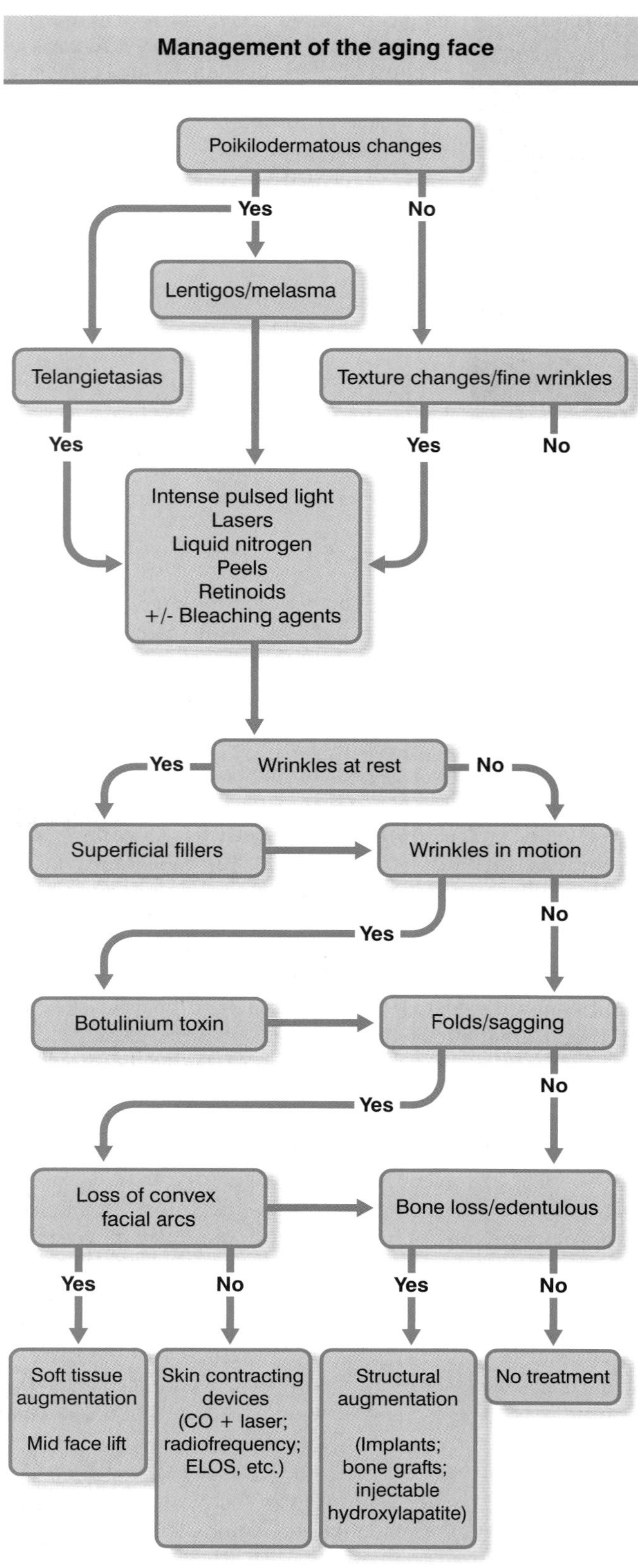

Figure 27.14 Algorithm for management of the aging face.

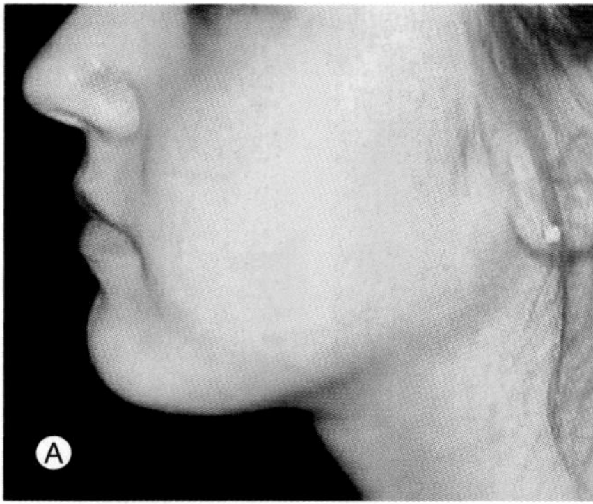

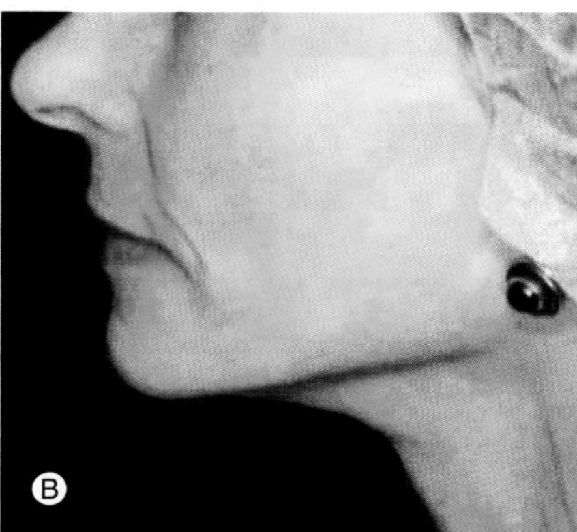

Figure 27.15 (A) The youthful jawline is full and rounded. (B) After lower facelift the jawline is ascetic with an acute angularity. Courtesy of Lisa M Donofrio.

is due to the redistribution of fat, autologous fat transfer is a useful option and a versatile choice.[24] Fat removed from extra deposits on the body can be used to reconstruct youthful facial contours (Figs 27.16, 27.17, 27.18). In addition, areas of fat hypertrophy on the face can be suctioned out to level off unevenly projected areas (Figs 27.19, 27.20). This requires the surgeon to think like a sculptor. Examination of photographs of the patient when younger is an invaluable tool that can help to plan a 'blueprint' of the surgery (Fig. 27.21). In this way, the fat compartments of the face can be 'rebalanced' to the fat distribution of youth. Careful staged fat transplantations can bring about a gradual improvement and may enhance 'take' of the fat graft[25] (Chapter 33). Any suction performed on the face should be done with microcannulae and hand-generated negative pressure. Undercorrection via a staged removal of fat is advised to minimize the risk of poor skin contraction secondary to an atrophic insult in photodamaged skin.

■ SUMMARY

Successful rejuvenation occurs when the physician takes into account all of the changes that have occurred in the aging face, and their etiologies. The clinician must remember that aging is an intrinsic event with shrinkage of the underlying framework and an extrinsic event with alterations in the dermis and epidermis. Creams that reduce the appearance of fine lines are not appropriate when the concern of the patient is the nasolabial fold or wrinkles that occur with movement.

Judicious tailoring of the procedure to treat the etiology ensures the best outcome and a satisfied patient.

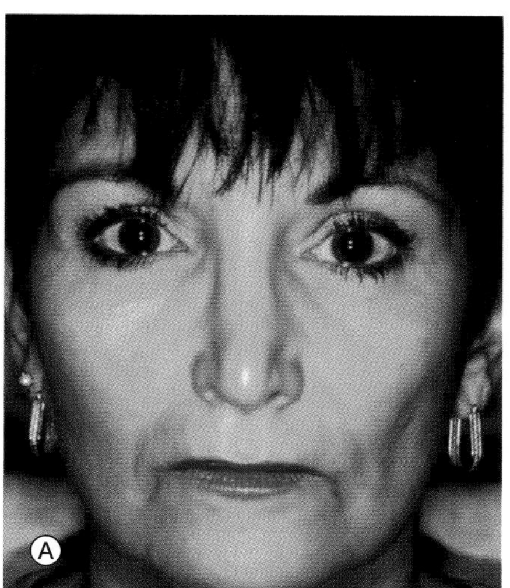
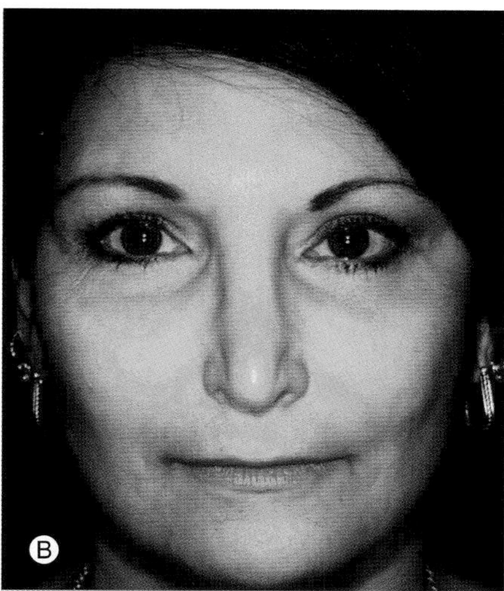

Figure 27.16 A 55-year-old lean-faced woman (A) before and (B) after structural fat augmentation. Courtesy of Lisa M Donofrio.

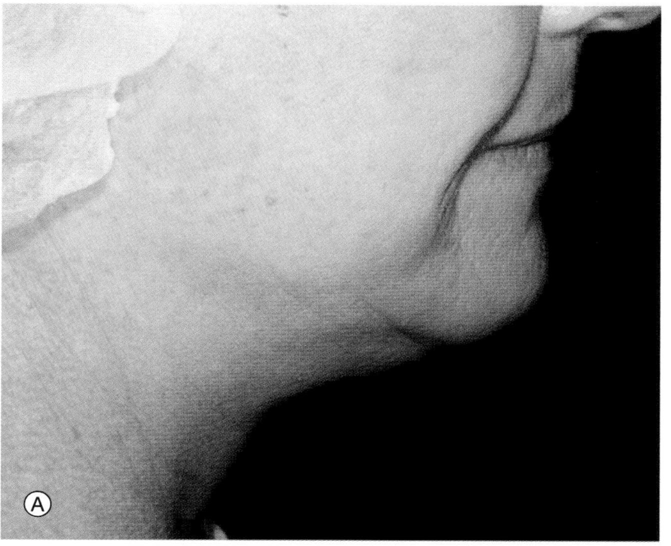
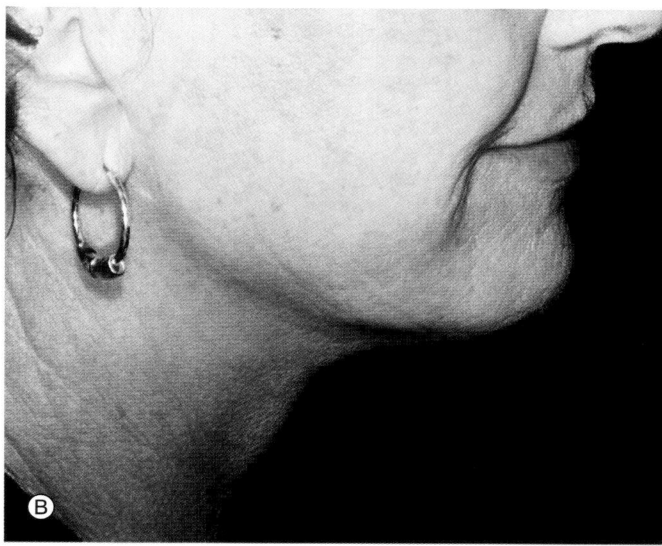

Figure 27.17 (A) Before and (B) after structural fat augmentation of face and jawline without suction. Note how jawline is full and rounded and more closely approximates the shape of the young jawline seen in Figure 27.15a. Courtesy of Lisa M Donofrio.

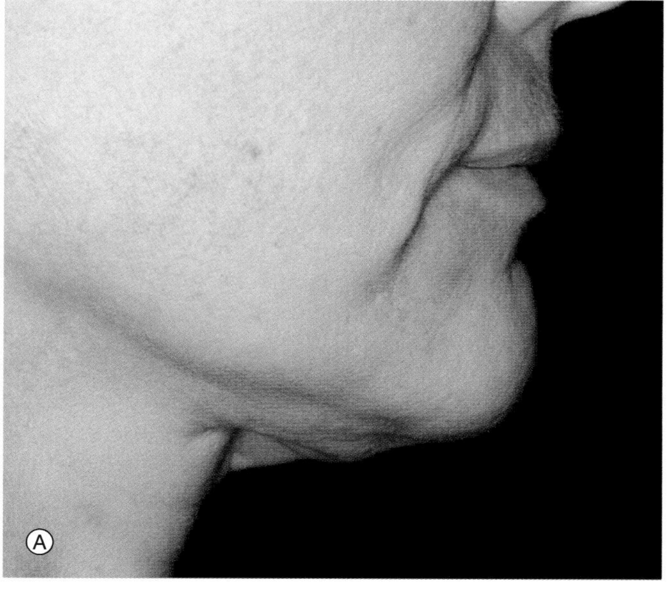
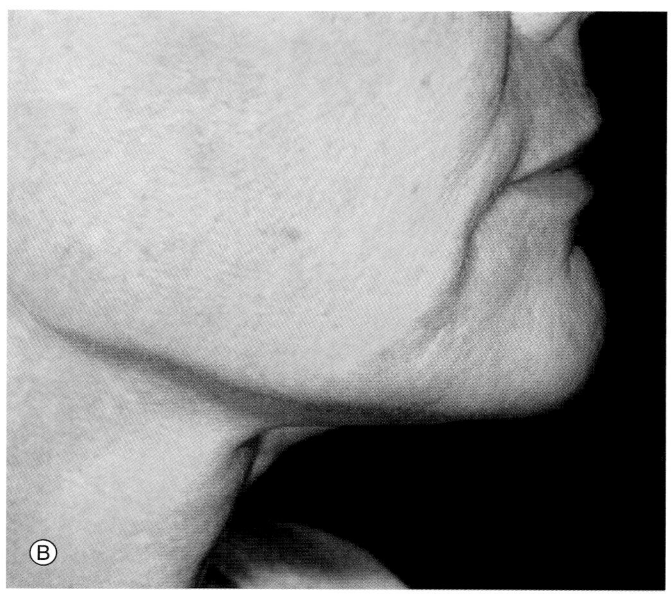

Figure 27.18 (A) Before and (B) after structural augmentation of the jawline and face. Note how 'excess skin' has been redraped over new framework. Courtesy of Lisa M Donofrio.

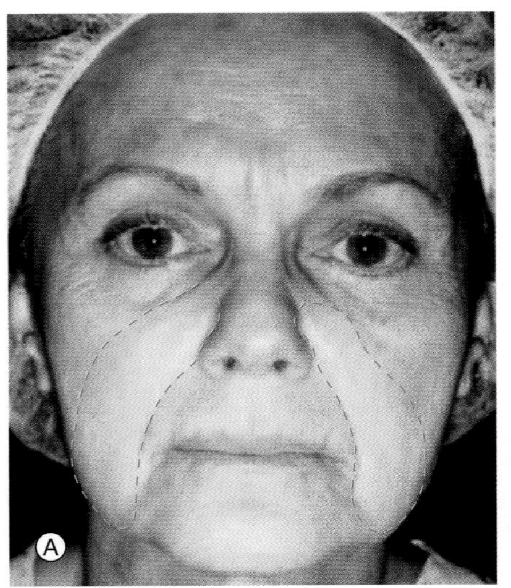

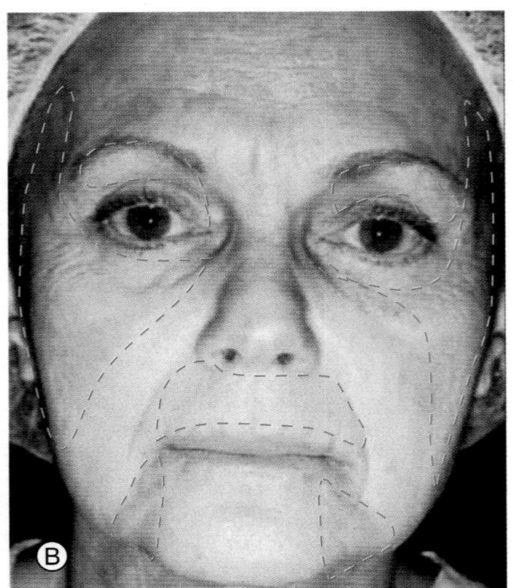

Figure 27.19 Outlined areas of hypertrophy (A) and atrophy (B) in aging woman's face. Courtesy of Lisa M Donofrio.

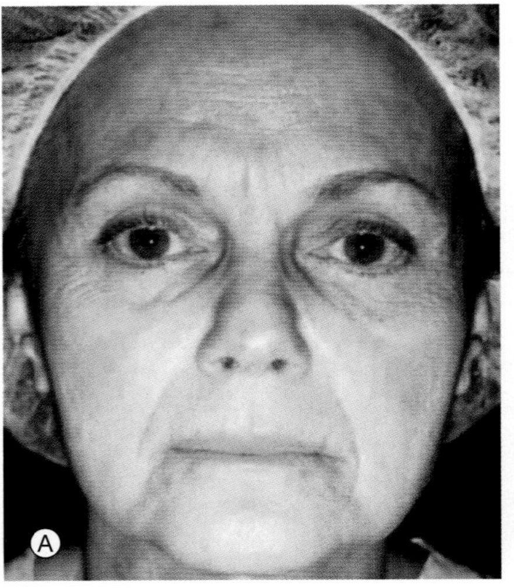

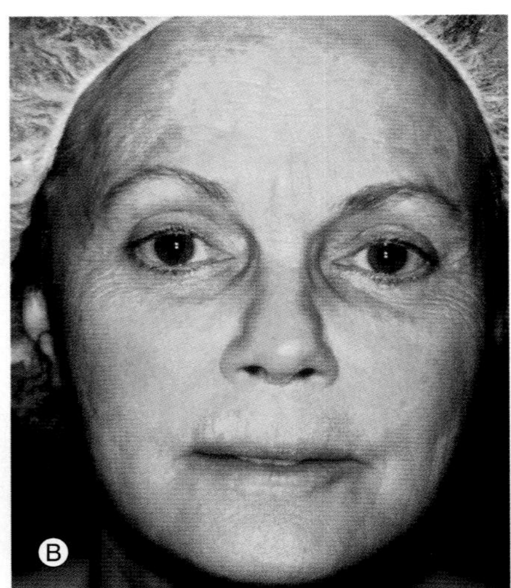

Figure 27.20 Before (A) and after (B) facial fat rebalancing via a combination of microsuction of the hypertrophic areas and structural augmentation of the atrophic areas seen in Figure 29.19. Courtesy of Lisa M Donofrio.

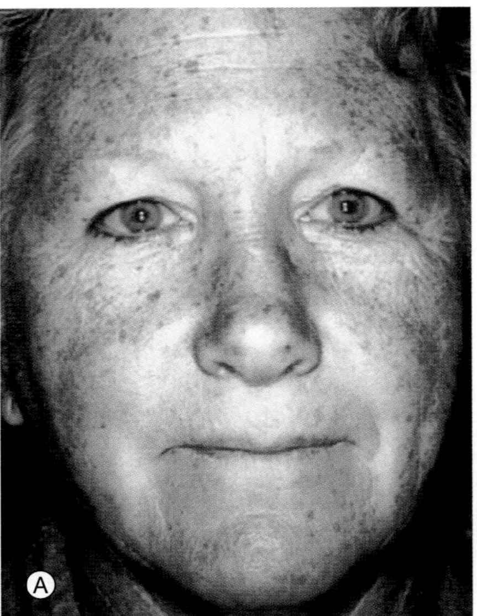

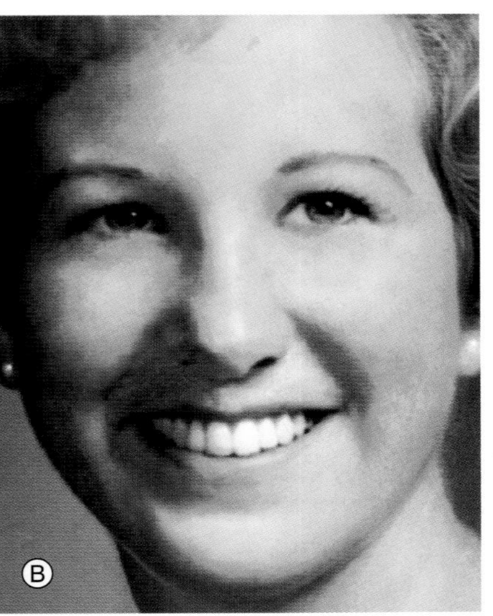

Figure 27.21 (A) Surface changes such as wrinkles and lentigos best treated by resurfacing are easy to see in this 52-year-old woman's face. It is not until examining a photograph of (B) of the same woman in her 20s that the striking change in facial contours is appreciated. Courtesy of Lisa M Donofrio.

■ REFERENCES

1. Bertazzo A, Favretto D, Costa CV, Allegri G, Tralsi P. Effects of ultraviolet irradiation of melanogenesis from tyrosine, dopa and dopamine: a matrix-assisted laser desorption/ionization mass spectrometric study. Rapid Commun Mass Spectrom 2000; 14:1862–1868.
2. Whitmore SE, Morison WL. The effect of suntan parlor exposure on delayed and contact hypersensitivity. Photochem Photobiol 200 Jun; 71:700–705.
3. Warren R, Garstein V, Kligman AM, Montagna W, Allendorf RA, Ridder GM. Age, sunlight and facial skin: a histologic and quantitative study. J Am Acad Dermatol 1991; 25:751–760.
4. Contet-Audonneau JL, Jeanmaire C, Pauly G. A histological study of human wrinkle structures: comparison between sun-exposed areas if the face, with or without wrinkles, and sun protected areas. Br J Dermatol 1999; 140:1038–1047.
5. Kambayashi H, Yamashita M, OdakeY, Takada K, Funasaka Y, Ichihashi M. Epidermal changes caused by chronic low-dose UV irradiation induce wrinkle formation in hairless mouse. J Dermatol Sci 2001; 27(Suppl 1):S19–S25.
6. Toyoda M, Nakamura M, Luo Y, Morohashi M. Ultrastructural characterization of microvasculature in photoaging. J Dermatol Sci 2001; 27(Suppl 1):S32–S41.
7. Reimers CD, Harder T, Saxe H. Age-related muscle atrophy does not affect all muscles and can partly be compensated by physical activity: an ultrasound study. J Neurol Sci 1998; 159:60–66.
8. Morley JE, Baumgartner RN, Roubenoff R, Mayer J, Nair KS. Sarcopenia. J Lab Clin Med 2001; 137:231–243.
9. Gosain AK, Amarante MT, Hydede JS, Yousif NJ. A dynamic analysis of changes in the nasolabila fold using magnetic resonance imaging: implications for facial rejuvenation and facial animation surgery. Plast Reconstr Surg 1996; 98:622–636.
10. Pierard GE, Lapiere CM. The microanatomical basis of facial frown lines. Arch Dermatol. 1989; 125:1090–1092.
11. Pessa JE, Zadoo VP, Mutimer KL, et al. Relative maxillary retrusion as a natural consequence of aging combining skeletal and soft-tissue changes into an integrated model of midfacial aging. Plast Reconstr Surg 1998; 102:205–212.
12. Bartlett SP, Grossman R, Whitaker LA. Age-related changes of the craniofacial skeleton: an anthropometric and histologic analysis. Plast Reconstr Surg 1992; 90:592–600.
13. Kingsmill VJ. Postextraction remodeling of the adult mandible. Crit Rev Oral Biol Med 1999; 10:384–404.
14. Pessa JE, Desvigne LD, Lambros VS, Nimerick J, Sugunan B, Zadoo V. Changes in ocular globe-to-orbital rim position with age: implications for aesthetic blepharoplasty of the eyelids. Aesthetic Plast Surg 1999; 23:337–342.
15. Pessa JE, Zadoo VP, Yuan C, et al. Concertina effect and facial aging: nonlinear aspects of youthfulness and skeletal remodeling, and why, perhaps, infants have jowls. Plast Reconstr Surg 1999; 103:635–644.
16. Lindner J, Grasedyck K. Age-dependant changes in connective tissue. Arzneimittelforschung 1982; 32:1384–1396.
17. De Cordier BC, de la Torre JI, Al-Hakeem MS, et al. Rejuvenation of the midface by elevating the malar fat pad: review of technique, cases, and complications. Plast Reconstr Surg 2002; 110:1526–1536.
18. Pessa JE, Garza PA, Love VM, Zadoo VP, Garza JR. The anatomy of the labiomandibular fold. Plast Reconstr Surg 1998; 101:482–486.
19. Pollack SV. Liposuction of the abdomen. The basics. Dermatol Clin 1999; 17:823–834; vii.
20. Lemos M, Pozo RM, Montes GS, Saldiva PH. Organization of collagen and elastic fibers studied in stretch preparations of whole mounts of human visceral pleura. Anat Anz 1997; 179:447–452.
21. Carruthers J, Carruthers A, Maberley D. Deep resting glabellar rhytides respond to BTX-A and Hylan B. Dermatol Surg 2003; 29:539–544.
22. Nyirady J, Bergfeld W, Ellis C, et al. Tretinoin cream 0.02% for the treatment of photodamaged facial skin: a review of two double-blind clinical studies. Cutis 2001; 68:135–142.
23. Khatri KA, Machado A, Magro C, Davenport S. Laser peel: facial rejuvenation with a superficial erbium:YAG laser treatment. J Cutan Laser Ther 2000; 2:119–123.
24. Donofrio LM. Fat distribution: a morphologic study of the aging face. Dermatol Surg 2000; 26:1107–1112.
25. Donofrio LM. Structural autologous lipoaugmentation: a pan-facial technique. Dermatol Surg 2000; 26:1129–1134.

28 Soft-tissue Augmentation

Roberta D Sengelmann MD, Stacey Tull MD MPH, and
Sheldon V Pollack MD

Summary box

- The ideal augmentation material would be characterized by the following properties: safety, efficacy, reproducibility, ease of administration, low abuse potential, non-carcinogenicity, non-teratogenicity, non-migratory, cost-effective, physiologic, permanent, and government-sanctioned.
- A large variety of materials are currently available worldwide for dermal filling.
- These have varying levels of implantation, biodegradability, allergenicity, and durability.
- Indications include atrophic scarring, contour defects due to soft tissue loss, lip atrophy and static rhytids.
- Appropriate patient expectations are improvement of atrophic scar and contour deformities, lip fullness, and wrinkle reduction.
- Understand limitations of the technique and potential side-effects in order to maximize outcomes.

■ INTRODUCTION

As people live longer and healthier lives, more seek physicians to help them to achieve a more youthful appearance. The skin's natural aging process is manifested as contour changes and rhytids secondary to ptosis and atrophy of soft tissues, including muscle and subcutaneous fat and loss of skin resistance as dermal collagen, hyaluronic acid, and elastin are depleted (see Chapter 27).

Traditionally, rejuvenation has been achieved with surgical resection of the skin. Today, a multitude of minimally invasive procedures, of which soft-tissue augmentation is one, rejuvenate without the risks, recovery time, and expense of major surgery. The development and popularity of Botox Cosmetic (Allergan Inc, Irvine, CA) (see Chapter 31) has opened the door for equally non-invasive, adjunctive treatments for rhytids and other signs of facial aging.

Soft-tissue augmentation has become a popular means of addressing volume loss and contour defects that result from aging, photodamage, trauma and/or scarification, and disease. Dozens of filling agents now exist in our armamentarium with varying degrees of durability and viscosity. The physician makes a choice to select the one best suited to address each patient and their particular problem. Currently, injectable fillers tend to offer a more temporary improvement as compared to implants which allow for semi-permanent and permanent augmentation.

Significant strides have been made toward the development of an ideal filler/implant which would be characterized by the following properties: safety, efficacy, reproducibility, high use potential, low abuse potential, non-carcinogenicity, non-teratogenicity, non-migratory, cost-effective, physiologic, permanent, and approved for human use by government agencies. This chapter provides an overview of currently available dermal filling agents that are used for augmentation of superficial contour irregularities and subdermal fillers and soft-tissue implants that correct contour defects where volume is needed.

■ HISTORICAL ASPECTS

The search for an ideal dermal filler for the correction of facial lines and wrinkles has spanned a century. The first organic injectable material used for this purpose, at the turn of the 20th century, was injectable paraffin. This material proved unacceptable and was abandoned due to the appearance of paraffinomas.[1] A refined form of liquid silicone (medical grade 360) introduced in the 1960s by the Dow Corning Corporation (USA) was adopted by a number of American clinicians for use in correction of facial deformities, lines, and wrinkles.[2] During the following three decades, various forms of injectable silicone were used in the management of tens of thousands of patients. When injected through a fine-bore needle using a 'microdroplet' technique, there were relatively few reported complications. Unfortunately, numerous severe complications arose from the use of adulterated or impure silicones and, on occasion, following the use of purified liquid silicones as well.[3] These problems, coupled with the lack of approval for use in this form by the Food and Drug Administration

(FDA) in the United States and the Health Protection Branch (HPB) in Canada, significantly limited injectable silicone use in North America. Since the recent (2002) FDA approval of 1000 centistoke liquid silicone for intraocular injections, the off-label use of this injectable silicone oil as a permanent soft-tissue filler for facial rejuvenation has increased in the United States.[4] This may establish efficacy and safety data that will support approved use of injectable silicone for cosmetic purposes in the near future.

After extensive premarketing trials, injectable bovine collagen was introduced in 1981 by the Collagen Corporation (Palo Alto, CA). This material (Zyderm, Zyplast), currently marketed by Inamed Aesthetics (Santa Barbara, CA), is easily administered, safe and effective in short-term soft-tissue augmentation.[5–8] Injectable bovine collagen products are also available in Japan (Kokenatelocollagen implant, Koken Co, KTD, Tokyo) and Europe (Resoplast, Rofil Medical International BV, Bredia, Netherlands) and have similar indications to Zyderm and Zyplast collagen. However, the possibility of allergy to bovine collagen products and their limited tissue longevity have fueled the ongoing search for a more ideal dermal filler.[9–11] For many physicians, the development of Cosmoderm and Cosmoplast, which are analogous to the Zyderms and Zyplast, but are human collagens, have replaced treatment with bovine collagen as they negate concerns for allergenicity.

A readily available augmentation material is the patient's own dermis and fat. While autologous fat transfer was first employed over a century ago by Neuber,[12] the use of autologous tissue for subcutaneous augmentation was attempted with varying results throughout the 20th century.[13–18] Dermis and fat were most commonly used but variable degrees of resorption following implantation render outcomes unpredictable.[19] The modern use of fat as a filling substance dates to its reintroduction by Fournier as 'microlipoinjection' in the late 1970s.[20] The longevity of contour correction following autologous fat injection appears to be somewhat variable. It may be dependent on several factors including whether fat is fresh or frozen, which affects the viability of fat cells, the technique used, amount of fat injected, location of recipient site, and type of defect being treated. Recent independent innovations in technique by Coleman and Amar appear to have improved the longevity of correction.[21] Although early results are promising and there is an inherent intuitive benefit to using an autologous agent for soft-tissue augmentation, it is not clear that autologous fat will be the long-sought ideal soft-tissue agent [22] and it is not indicated for correction of dermal defects. A complete discussion of fat transfer is presented in Chapter 33 of this book.

In 1957, Spangler first published his studies on the use of 'fibrin foam' to treat depressed scars.[23] Based on this work and modifications by Gottlieb[24] a new product, Fibrel, was developed by Serono Laboratories and introduced in 1985. It was later marketed by Mentor Corporation. Fibrel is a mixture of gelatin powder, epsilon-aminocaproic acid, and plasma from the patient. The gelatin forms scaffolding upon which collagen synthesis occurs. The enzyme inhibitor epsilon-aminocaproic acid blocks fibrinolysin, which turns off collagen synthesis degradation, thus increasing collagen production to fill the clot matrix. Blood plasma provides a supplemental source of fibrinogen and other clotting factors that enhance the collagen matrix. Although venipuncture and centrifugation of the patient's blood made Fibrel preparation tedious, reported results were generally favorable.[9,25–27] Nonetheless, a corporate decision was made by the Mentor Corporation to discontinue marketing of this product, which at the current time remains unavailable.

The search for an ideal, injectable, soft-tissue filler continues. We have numerous wonderful options on the market today to help us accomplish our patients' goals.[28–30] Dozens of new products have appeared worldwide during the past two decades and new additions appear each year. Many of the injectable fillers incorporate biologically compatible ingredients such as hyaluronic acid gels (Restylane, Hylaform), human fibroblasts (Isolagen), fibroblast-derived human collagen (Cosmoderm, Cosmoplast), fascia lata (Fascian), acellular human collagen (Alloderm, Cymetra), elastin, and other human dermal products. Others have introduced substances such as Dextran (Reviderm Intra), polyethylene beads (Profill), silicone polymers (Dermagen), polymethylmethacrylate (Artecoll), polyacrylamide gel (Formacryl, Outline), or polylactic acid (New-Fill/Sculptra) to increase tissue residence time. Of these newer materials, the most widely used worldwide have been a variety of hyaluronic acid gels and Artecoll, a product in which polymethylmethacrylate (PMMA) is suspended in bovine collagen.[31]

Balazs and Denlinger established that insoluble, injectable, cross-linked hylan gels derived from hyaluronic acid exhibited a prolonged residence time in soft tissues and were as biocompatible as natural hyaluronan.[32] Hylan B, first developed in the mid-1980s, is produced by introducing sulfonyl-bis-ethyl cross-links between hydroxyl groups of the polysaccharide chain of hyaluronan. Intra-articular injections of this material were found to be helpful for knee pain associated with osteoarthritis.[33] Subsequently, it was evaluated and used for soft-tissue augmentation.[34] Hylan B gel has a number of attributes that are favorable for an intradermal injectable implant material. It is water insoluble, resists degradation and is unlikely to migrate. The high water content mimics the natural hydrating function of native hyaluronan in the skin. The elastic properties of the gel render it soft and natural feeling and provide elastic protection (shock absorption) to the cutaneous soft tissue.[34] The physical properties of hyaluronic acid gels are controlled by the molecular weight and the concentration of the material and by the degree of cross-linking.[35] The most commonly used sources of hyaluronic acid are rooster combs (Hylaform), bacterial cultures (Restylane), as well as human umbilical cord, vitreous humor, tendons, and skin.[36]

PMMA was first synthesized in 1902 by the German chemist Rohm and was patented as Plexiglass in 1928. It has had medical applications since 1945, commonly used in bone cement, intraocular lenses, dental prostheses, and repair material for craniofacial surgery. In addition to being immunologically inert and biocompatible, PMMA has never demonstrated degradation or carcinogenicity. Professor Gottfried Lemperle (St Markus Hospital, Frankfurt, Germany) developed the concept of using PMMA microspheres for tissue augmentation.[37,38] The initial product tested, Arteplast, was heterogeneous, containing various PMMA monomers, spheres of various sizes, and even some impurities. This led to several instances of granuloma formation, consisting of swelling and inflammation. Artecoll (formerly Artefill), which has been available in Europe for a decade, contains only smooth microspheres of 30–40 microns in size and 99% of the remaining monomers have been removed during processing. These changes in the product appear to have significantly reduced the incidence of granuloma formation.[39]

In 1971, Robert and William Gore developed expanded polytetrafluoroethylene (e-PTFE) as an expanded, fibrillated form of Teflon (PTFE). This was originally used as a vascular prosthesis in bypass surgery[40–42] but rapidly found uses in a variety of other surgical procedures, such as the treatment of facial lines and wrinkles, and lip augmentation.[43–49] It was approved for use in facial and reconstructive surgery in 1993. Softform and its softer, more pliable second generation counterpart, Ultrasoft (Tissue Technologies Inc, San Francisco, CA) are sheets, strips, and tubes of e-PTFE used as facial implants to treat depressed scars, lip atrophy, and deep furrows such as nasolabial folds and marionette lines.[50] Advanta[51,52] (Atrium Medical Corporation, Hudson, NH) is the newest of these products. It is a dual-porosity e-PTFE which is marketed as a softer, smoother implant which comes in a wider variety of shapes and sizes. It has been available since 2001, with preliminary studies showing encouraging results in the treatment of marionette lines (the vertical grooves extending downwards from oral commissures to the mental area) nasolabial folds, and lip augmentation.[53]

Alloderm (LifeCell Corporation, Palo Alto, CA) is acellular human cadaveric dermis that has been freeze-dried. Alloderm is processed as sheets and was widely used in the treatment of full-thickness burns, blistering conditions such as epidermolysis bullosa, and in reconstructive surgery for patients with urinary incontinence. It is also used as an implant in soft-tissue augmentation procedures such as rhinoplasty, lip augmentation, glabellar contouring, and scar revision.[54–56] Cymetra (LifeCell Corporation, Palo Alto, CA) is the injectable form of Alloderm.[57] Alloderm and Cymetra have been available since the mid-1990s.

Most recently, Radiesse (previously Radiance, but renamed when referring to its cosmetic usage) (Bioform, Franksville, WI) is composed of calcium hydroxylapatite microspheres suspended in polysaccharide gel. It has been used off label as a semipermanent injectable filler for several years. Currently, it is FDA approved in the treatment of urinary incontinence (bladder neck bulking)[58] and in vocal cord augmentation. It is approved in Europe for craniofacial restoration by subdermal injection. A recent study in Italy (unpublished at the time of press) showed excellent cosmetic results in 40 patients treated for augmentation of the zygomatic region, lips, nasolabial folds, and the under-eye region.

A comprehensive listing of injectable dermal fillers available at the time of this writing appears in Table 28.1. Of these products, those deemed by the authors to be of most immediate importance to the reader are discussed below and presented in Table 28.2.

■ PREOPERATIVE PREPARATION

In general, minimal preoperative preparation is required for the patient undergoing soft-tissue augmentation. With a

Table 28.1 Table of commercially available products

Products	Trade/Brand name	Products	Trade/Brand name
Animal-derived	Bovine Endoplast-50 Resoplast Zyderm I Zyderm II Zyplast Porcine Permacol Surgisis	Polymethyl methacrylate	Artecoll Meta-Crill
		Silicone-based	AdatoSil 5000 Bioplastique Dermagen Silikon 1000
		Biocatayst	Dermacellagen New-Fill/Sculptra Reviderm Intra
Hyaluronic acid	AcHyal Acrylic Hydrogel Hyal-System Hylaform Fine Line Hylaform Hylaform Plus Hylan Rofilan Gel Juvederm (18,24,30) MacDermol Macrolane Restylane Fine Line Restylane Perlane Rofilan	Other injectable synthetic	Kopolymer (sterile plastic fatty acid gel) Profill (polyethylene beads) Radiance/Radiesse (calcium hydroxylapatite)
		Autologous	Autologen Autologous grafts (fat, dermis, dermis-fat, tendon, scar, fascia) Isolagen Plasmagel
		Human-derived	Alloderm Biocell Ultravital Cosmoderm I (Cosmoderm II) Cosmoplast Cymetra Dermaplant Fascian Human placental collagen Recombinant human collagen
Polyacrylamide gel	Amazing Gel Aquamid Argiform Bio-Alcamid Bioformacryl Dermalive DermaDeep Evolution Formacryl Outline (fine, regular, ultra)	Synthetic implants (e-PTFE)	Advanta Gore-Tex (strings, strands) Softform/Ultrasoft

Table 28.2 Most commonly used products (by injection/implant level)

Product	Trade/Brand Name
Dermal fillers	
Superficial/mid-dermis	Cosmoderm I Zyderm I
Mid-dermis	Autologen (Cosmoderm II) Hylaform Restylane Zyderm II
Deep dermis	Artecoll Cosmoplast Dermalive Hylaform Plus Perlane Reviderm Intra Zyplast
Versatile dermal levels	Fascian Hylan Rofilan Gel Isolagen Juvederm 18,24,30
Subdermal fillers	Cymetra Radiesse (calcium hydroxylapatite) Dermadeep New-Fill/Sculptra
Subdermal implants	Advanta Alloderm Gore-Tex Softform/Ultrasoft Autologous grafts (fat, dermis, dermis-fat, tendon, scar, fascia)

variety of products available, it behooves the physician to advise patients of the strengths and potential pitfalls of the various products and come to a mutual agreement regarding which product would best suit the patient's needs and risk tolerance. The patient should have realistic expectations of side effects, longevity of correction, and adverse reactions (Table 28.3) prior to undergoing treatment. It is advisable that informed consent be obtained from patients undergoing cosmetic procedures of any kind.

When medically appropriate, patients should discontinue the use of blood thinners including non-steroidal anti-inflammatory drugs (NSAIDs), acetylsalicylic acid (i.e. aspirin)-containing products, warfarin (coumadin), high doses of vitamin E and most herbal medicines at least 1 week prior to treatment to minimize the risk of ecchymosis, especially when treating thin skin around the eyes and lips.

Injectable fillers

Some products, such as Zyderm, Zyplast, Cosmoderm, and Cosmoplast, contain a local anesthetic, mitigating the need for preoperative local anesthesia. However, the patient should know that the needle stick will still be uncomfortable for them. The pain of the needle stick can be diminished by pretreating the area with a topical anesthetic such as Betacaine (Betacaine, Tampa, FL) or LMX (Ferndale Laboratories Inc, Ferndale, MI).[59] Perioperative cold packs may help minimize discomfort and bruise formation. In patients with particularly low pain thresholds, a regional nerve block with an injectable local anesthetic, such as 1% lidocaine will be helpful. Infraorbital and mental nerve

Table 28.3 Pitfalls of soft-tissue augmentation

Discomfort
Bruising
Vasovagal reactions
Incomplete correction
Bluish discoloration (Tyndall effect)
Beading
Granuloma formation
Swelling
Hematoma
Asymmetry
Hypersensitivity
Palpability in skin
Scarring
Infection
Extrusion
Neuropraxia
Skin necrosis (intra-arterial injection)
Blindness

blocks, which decrease sensation around the midface and upper and lower lips, are particularly helpful (see Chapter 3). Robust local infiltration of anesthesia is not recommended as it causes tissue swelling, which makes it difficult to assess the endpoint of treatment. The swelling of local anesthesia also causes the patient undue anxiety about the immediate outcome.

All make-up should be removed prior to treating the sites. Areas to be injected should be prepared with an antiseptic such as isopropyl alcohol, Betadine (Purdue, Wilson, NC) or benzalkonium chloride (Hibiclens, Regent Medical, Norcross, GA) solution. For injectable fillers, patients are seated comfortably with head support; either upright or leaning back at no more than an angle of 45°. This position allows the physician to appreciate the effects of gravity on soft tissues. Overhead lighting will accentuate the shadowing where treatment is needed.

Soft implants

For patients having soft-tissue implants, anesthesia is infiltrated, with the patient supine and the treatment site prepped and draped in a sterile fashion. Possibly the most important preoperative factor to consider with soft-tissue implants is whether the patient has an understanding of the expected appearance with their chosen filler or implant. For this reason, it may be helpful if they have initial augmentation with a temporary filler that will yield similar results. Patients may consider Radiesse or Alloderm if long-lasting, but not permanent, results are desired. Patients should also realize that their lips will be quite swollen postoperatively and that the swelling may persist for a couple of weeks. Setting reasonable expectations pre-operatively will optimize patient satisfaction.

Other preoperative aspects to consider with soft-tissue implants include antibiotic and/or antiviral prophylaxis. History of recurrent orolabial herpesvirus infection should prompt use of antiviral prophylaxis, especially for procedures performed around the mouth. Perioperative systemic antibiotics should be considered any time that a foreign body, such as a solid implantable device, is used in a patient.

Choice of anesthesia is important depending on the level of implantation and anatomical location. Regional nerve blocks are encouraged whenever possible with minimal local anesthesia for vasoconstrictive field effect. Excessive amounts of locally infiltrated anesthesia may obscure tissue planes and impair precision of implantation. Additionally, mild sedation is recommended as vigorous manipulation of soft tissues, which can cause patient anxiety, are often involved with implantation.

■ TECHNICAL ASPECTS AND OVERVIEW OF COMMONLY USED PRODUCTS

Dermal fillers

Bovine collagen

A large variety of injectable dermal fillers is now available worldwide. Regulation of use of devices in some countries, notably the United States, limits their use by clinicians (Table 28.4). These products may be delivered into the very superficial (papillary) dermis for fine line improvement, into the (mid)reticular dermis for moderate-depth wrinkles, and into the deep dermis for treatment of deep grooves or folds (Fig. 28.1). The bovine collagen products, Zyderm I, Zyderm II, and Zyplast (Inamed Aesthetics, Santa Barbara, CA), demonstrate a family of products, each with increasing viscosity, that are designed to be implanted at these three respective levels, and will serve as an example for the discussion that follows.

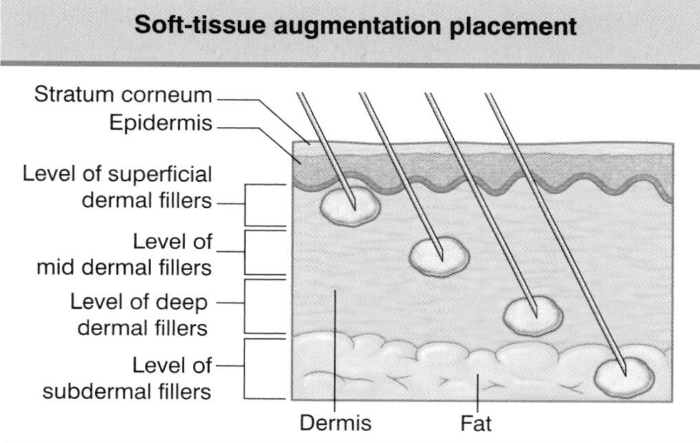

Figure 28.1 Soft-tissue augmentation placement.

Bovine collagen was the first device approved for soft-tissue augmentation in the United States, and it remains the gold standard against which all other dermal implants are measured.[60] Since its introduction in 1981, over 1 million patients have been treated. Results have been reported to last up to 18 months, but in the authors' experience, repeat treatment is usually required in 3–5 months (Fig. 28.2). The material is derived from the hides of an isolated domestic herd of cattle, thereby minimizing the possibility of contamination with the bovine spongiform encephalopathy virus or prion that causes 'mad cow disease.'[61]

Zyderm I is 3.5% bovine dermal collagen by weight, suspended in physiologic phosphate-buffered sodium chloride solution with the addition of 0.3% lidocaine. It contains 95–98% type I collagen and the remainder is type III collagen. It is injected into the papillary dermis for treatment of superficial rhytids anywhere on the face, including those around the eyes, lips, glabellar region, and cheeks. It is also used in depressed acne scars and can be overlaid on a more viscous substance, such as Zyplast or Cosmoplast, for lip augmentation. Overcorrection by approximately 100% is required to offset absorption of the saline.

Zyderm II is identical to Zyderm I except that it is 6.5% bovine dermal collagen by weight, and slightly more viscous. It is injected into the upper reticular dermis for treatment of more coarse rhytids as well as for acne scars and lip augmentation. Less overcorrection (approximately 50%) is required than for Zyderm I because of a higher concentration of collagen and less saline absorption.

Zyplast, like Zyderm I, is 3.5% bovine dermal collagen, but it is cross-linked with glutaraldehyde to form a lattice-work and a more viscous compound. It is less immunogenic

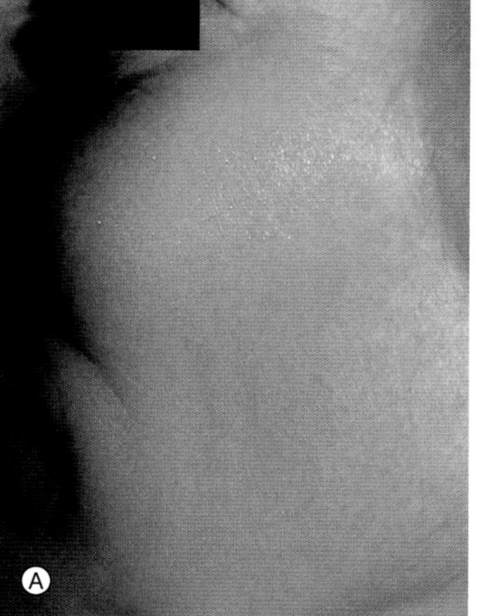

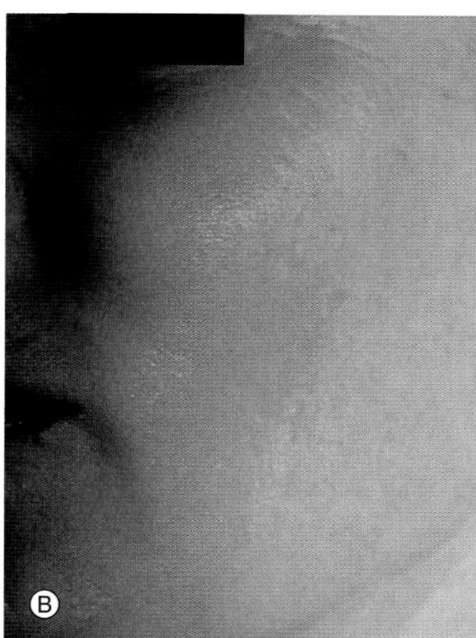

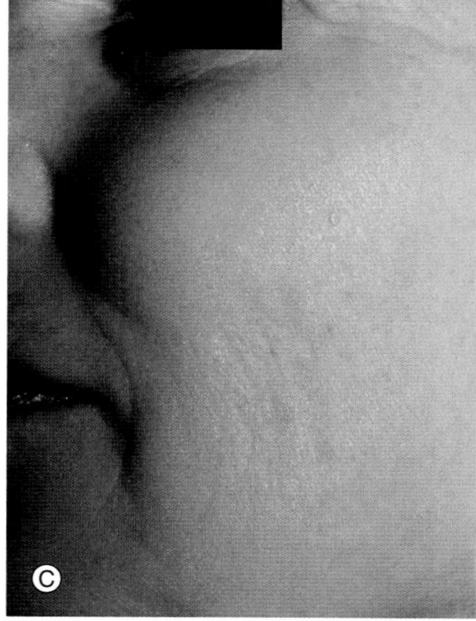

Figure 28.2 Preoperative photograph of a middle-aged woman shows secondary and tertiary nasolabial lines at the cheek prior to Zyplast bovine collagen implant. (B) After three treatments of 0.5 ml of Zyplast each. (C) After 7 months; the lines are beginning to reappear as the bovine collagen is eliminated.

Table 28.4 Injectable dermal fillers available worldwide

Category and Manufacturer	Units, Shelf life, Storage, and Cost (US $)	Availability and FDA Approval	Composition and Mechanism	Duration of Effect	Indications and Contraindications (CI)	Pretesting	Related Studies
Superficial dermal fillers							
Zyderm I *Inamed Corp* *Santa Barbara, CA* *Tel +1 800 766 0171* *http://www.inamed.com*	0.5, 1.0, 1.5-ml syringe Shelf life 3 years Refrigerate $145 for 1 ml	Worldwide	3.5% bovine dermal collagen and lidocaine	3–4 months	For superficial rhytids, scars, layering CI: Hypersensitivity to bovine collagen, lidocaine	Two skin tests 2–4 weeks apart Wait 4 weeks from time of second skin test to treatment	Klein[95]
Cosmoderm I *Inamed Corp* *Santa Barbara, CA* *Tel +1 800 766 0171* *http://www.inamed.com*	1-ml syringe Shelf life 3 years Refrigerate $175–205	USA Canada Europe South America Asia	Human collagen and plain lidocaine	3–4 months	For superficial rhytids, scars, layering CI: Lidocaine hypersensitivity	None	N/A
Hylaform Fineline *Inamed Corp* *Santa Barbara, CA* *+1 800 766 0171* *http://www.inamed.com*	0.4-ml syringe Shelf life 2 years Refrigerate at room temperature $250–750	Europe Canada USA (pending)*	Hyaluronic acid derived from rooster comb	3–6 months	For superficial rhytids, scars, layering CI: None	None	N/A
Restylane Fine Line US: *Medicis* *Scottsdale, AZ* *+1 602 808 8800* *http://www.medicis.com* Europe: *Q-Med Laboratories* *Uppsala, Sweden* *+46 18 474 9000* *http://www.q-med.com*	0.4-ml syringe Shelf life 18 months Refrigerate at room temperature $250–500	Europe UK Canada Australia South America USA (pending)*	Hyaluronic acid (20 mg/ml) in small gel particle size derived from bacterial fermentation	3–6 months	For superficial rhytids, scars, layering CI: None	None	Friedman et al.[94]
Mid dermal fillers							
Zyderm II *Inamed Corp* *Santa Barbara, CA* *Tel +1 800 766 0171* *http://www.inamed.com*	0.5, 1-ml syringe Shelf life 3 years Refrigerate $150 for 1 ml	Worldwide	6.5% bovine dermal collagen and plain lidocaine	3–4 months	For mid-dermal rhytids, layering CI: Hypersensitivity to bovine collagen and lidocaine	Two skin tests 2–4 weeks apart Wait 4 weeks from time of second skin test to treatment	Klein[95]
Hylaform *Inamed Corp* *Santa Barbara, CA* *Tel +1 800 766 0171* *http://www.inamed.com*	0.7-ml syringe Shelf life 2 years Refrigerate or room temperature. $145–199	Europe Canada USA	Hyaluronic acid (small particle) derived from rooster comb (5.5 mg/mL)	3–6 months	For moderate rhytids, layering, early folding, lip augmentation CI: None	None	Pollack[31] US Food and Drug Administration[82]

Table 28.4 Injectable dermal fillers available worldwide—*cont.*

Category and Manufacturer	Units, Shelf life, Storage, and Cost (US $)	Availability and FDA Approval	Composition and Mechanism	Duration of Effect	Indications and Contraindications (CI)	Pretesting	Related Studies
Mid dermal fillers (continued)							
Restylane US: *Medicis* *Scottsdale, AZ* *+1 602 808 8800* *http://www.medicis.com* Europe: *Q-Med Laboratories* *Uppsala, Sweden* *+46 18 474 9000* *http://www.q-med.com*	0.4 ml, 1-ml syringe Shelf life 18 months Refrigerate or room temperature $230–250	Europe UK Canada Australia South America USA	Hyaluronic acid (20 mg/ml) in medium gel particle size derived from bacterial fermentation	4–6 months	For moderate rhytids, folds and lips CI: None	None	Pollack[31] Olenius[84] Narins[85]
Autologen *Collagenesis Inc* *Beverly, MA* *Tel +1 978 23 9333*	3-ml syringe Shelf life ≤ 5 years with manufacturer $1200–4000 for 3 ml Stored frozen with manufacturer until needed Storage costs: free, $500 for first ice, $100 additional ices	USA Canada Europe	Autologous human collagen derived from patient's skin Harvested during cosmetic or reconstructive procedure Processed at the manufacturer	4–9 months	For rhytids, lip and fold augmentation, sensitivity to bovine collagen CI: None	None	Sclafani and McCormick[96]
Deep dermal fillers							
Zyplast *Inamed Corp* *Santa Barbara, CA* *Tel +1 800 766 0171* *http://www.inamed.com*	1.0, 1.5, 2.0, 2.5-ml syringes Shelf life 3 years Refrigerate $165 for 1 ml	Worldwide	3.5% bovine collagen cross-linked with glutaraldehyde and plain lidocaine	3–5 months	For deep rhytids and folds, lip augmentation, layering CI: Hypersensitivity to bovine collagen and lidocaine	None	Klein[95]
Cosmoplast *Inamed Corp* *Santa Barbara, CA* *Tel +1 800 766 0171* *http://www.inamed.com*	1.0, 1.5-ml syringe Shelf life 3 years Refrigerate $199–235 for 1 ml; $270 for 1.5 ml	Worldwide	Human collagen cross-linked with glutaraldehyde and plain lidocaine	3–4 months	For deep rhytids and folds, off label lip augmentation CI: Lidocaine hypersensitivity	None	N/A
Hylaform Plus *Inamed Corp* *Santa Barbara, CA* *Tel +1 800 766 0171* *http://www.inamed.com*	0.7-ml syringe Shelf life 2 years Refrigerate or room temperature $165–219	Europe Canada USA	Hyaluronic acid (medium particle) derived from rooster combs	3–6 months	For deep rhytids and folds, lip augmentation CI: None	None	US Food and Drug Administration[103]
Perlane US: *Medicis* *Scottsdale, AZ* *+1 602 808 8800* *http://www.medicis.com* Europe: *Q-Med Laboratories* *Uppsala, Sweden* *+46 18 474 9000* *http://www.q-med.com*	0.7-ml syringe Shelf life 18 months Refrigerate or room temperature $250–500	Europe UK Canada Australia South America USA (pending)*	Hyaluronic acid (20 mg/ml) in large gel particle size derived from bacterial fermentation	3–9 months	For deep facial lines, folds and lips CI: None	None	Friedman et al.[94]

Table 28.4 Injectable dermal fillers available worldwide—*cont.*

Category and Manufacturer	Units, Shelf life, Storage, and Cost (US $)	Availability and FDA Approval	Composition and Mechanism	Duration of Effect	Indications and Contraindications (CI)	Pretesting	Related Studies
Deep dermal fillers (continued)							
New-Fill/Sculptra US: *Dermik Laboratories* *Berwyn, PA* *Tel +1 800 340 7502* *http://www.dermik.com* Europe: *Biotech Industry SA* *Luxembourg* *Tel +352 26 259 462* *http://www.new-fill.com)*	150 µg powder for reconstitution with 3–5 ml sterile water and 1 ml lidocaine Room temperature $480	Europe (New-Fill) USA (Sculptra)	Poly-L-lactic acid in gel carrier	Permanent	For rhytids of variable depth, lip augmentation, lipoatrophy (New-Fill) For HIV associated lipoatrophy (Sculptra)	None	Berry[99]
Artecoll *Artes Medical Inc* *San Diego, CA* *Tel +1 858 550 9999* *http://www.artecoll-usa.com*	0.5-ml syringe Shelf life 2 years Refrigerate $400–900 per 1 ml (4-pack of 1-ml syringes filled with 0.5 ml product)	Europe Canada Mexico South America USA (pending)*	Homogeneous polymethylmethacrylate beads in 3.5% bovine collagen suspension Mixed with plain lidocaine	Permanent	For deep rhytids and folds, acne scars, lip augmentation CI: Hypersensitivity to bovine collagen and lidocaine	One skin test 30 days before treatment	Pollack[31]
Dermalive *Derma Tech* *Paris, France* *Tel 00 33 1 49 24 06 86* *http://www.dermatech.fr*	0.8-ml syringe Shelf life 3–5 years Room temperature $400–600	Europe South America Africa Middle East	40% acrylic hydrogel suspended in 60% hyaluronic acid	Permanent	For deep rhytids CI: Autoimmune diseases, healing disorders, areas with another filling material present	None	Bergeret-Galley and Illonz[97]
Reviderm Intra *Rofil Medical International* *Broda, The Netherlands* *Tel +31 76 531 5670* *http://www.fenix.cz*	1-ml syringe $300–750	Europe Canada	Flexible dextran microbeads suspended in super-coiled, stabilized hyaluronic acid (non-animal origin)	12–18 months	For deep rhytids CI: Keloids, autoimmune diseases	None	Lemperle et al[104]
Variable dermal fillers							
Juvederm (18, 24, 30) *LEA Derm* *Paris, France* *Tel +33 149 240 686* *http://www.juvederm.com*	Two 0.6-ml syringes $250–500	Europe USA (pending)*	Viscoelastic hyaluronic acid gel (18 mg/g, 24 mg/g or 30 mg/g)	3–6 months	For superficial (18), mid-level (24), and deep (30) rhytids, lip augmentation, layering CI: Autoimmune diseases	None	Bergeret-Galley and Illonz[97]
Fascian *Fascia Biosystems LLC* *Beverly Hills, CA* *Tel +1 888 3FASCIA* *http://fascian.com*	0.25, 0.5, 1.0, 2.0 µm particulate size in 80-mg 3-ml syringes Hydrated to 3 ml with saline or lidocaine Shelf life 2 years Room temperature $500–2000	Worldwide	Injectable irradiated human cadaveric preserved particulate fascia lata (varying particle size)	3–6 months	For rhytids of variable depth (by particulate size), acne scars, lip augmentation CI: Hypersensitivity to polymyxin B sulfate, bacitracin, gentamicin	None	Burres[74]

Table 28.4 Injectable dermal fillers available worldwide—*cont.*

Category and Manufacturer	Units, Shelf life, Storage, and Cost (US $)	Availability and FDA Approval	Composition and Mechanism	Duration of Effect	Indications and Contraindications (CI)	Pretesting	Related Studies
Variable dermal fillers (continued)							
Hylan Rofilan Gel *Rofil Medical International* *Broda, The Netherlands* *Tel 00 31 76 531 5670* *http://www.fenix.cz*	1-ml syringe Shelf life 2 years Refrigerate or room temperature $250–500	Europe Canada USA (pending)*	Viscoelastic stabilized non-animal hyaluronan gel	3–6 months	For rhytids of variable depths, lip augmentation CI: None	None	N/A
Isolagen *Isolagen* *Houston, TX* *Tel +1 713 780 4754* *http://www.isolagen.com*	3-mm punch biopsy sent to lab for fibroblasts culture Frozen and stored for future culturing Live cultured fibroblasts injected ≤ 48 h of leaving lab $1000–1500	Europe USA Australia¶	Cultured autologous human fibroblasts	Unclear (months or years)	For rhytids, acne scars, lip augmentation CI: None	One test dose 2 or more weeks before treatment	Watson and Lask[98]
Subdermal fillers							
Cymetra *Life Cell Corp* *Branchburg, NJ* *Tel +1 908 947 1100* *http://www.lifecell.com*	330 mg dried acellular particulate dermal matrix in 5-ml syringe Reconstituted to 1 ml Shelf life 2 years Room temperature $600–900 per 1 ml	Worldwide	Micronized acellular human cadaveric dermis	3–6 months	For deep rhytids, acne scars, lip augmentation CI: Hypersensitivity to gentamicin, collagen vascular disease, avascular or infected recipient site	None	N/A
Radiesse *Bioform* *Franksville, WI* *Tel +1 262 835 9800* *http://www.bioforminc.com*	1-ml syringe Shelf life 2 years Room temperature $500	Europe USA¶¶	Calcium hydroxylapatite microspheres suspended in aqueous polysaccharide gel	9 months–5 years	For deep rhytids and folds, lip augmentation, acne scars, lipoatrophy CI: None	None	Drobeck et al[101]
Subdermal implants							
Alloderm *Life Cell Corp* *Branchburg, NJ* *Tel +1 908 947 1100* *http://www.lifecell.com*	Freeze-dried sheets of variable size/thickness 1 × 2 cm to 4 × 12 cm Shelf life 2 years Room temperature $135–1500 per sheet	Worldwide	Acellular human cadaveric dermis	12–24 months	For deep rhytids, acne scars, lip augmentation, skin grafting, rhinoplasty CI: Hypersensitivity to gentamicin, collagen vascular disease, avascular or infected recipient site	None	Sclafani et al.[100]
Advanta *Atrium Medical Corp* *Hudson, NH* *http://www.atriummed.com/whatsnewframe.ht*	Implants of variable shape and size with or without preattached trocars Shelf life 5 years Room temperature $310–420 per implant	Europe Canada USA	Dual porosity e-PTFE	Permanent (Easy to remove if placed within 90 days)	For nasolabial folds, marionette lines, lips CI: Infection at recipient site	None	Truswell[51]

Table 28.4 Injectable dermal fillers available worldwide—*cont.*

Category and Manufacturer	Units, Shelf life, Storage, and Cost (US $)	Availability and FDA Approval	Composition and Mechanism	Duration of Effect	Indications and Contraindications (CI)	Pretesting	Related Studies
Subdermal implants (continued)							
Gore-Tex (strings, strands) *Gore Advanced Technologies Worldwide, Newark, DE* *Tel +1 410 506 7787 or 888 914 4673 (US)* *http://www.gore.com*	Tubes and strings of variable size Shelf life 5 years Room temperature $300–350 per implant	Worldwide	e-PTFE	Permanent (easy to remove)	For deep rhytids, lip augmentation CI: Infection at recipient site	None	Maas and Denton[102]
Softform/Ultrasoft *Tissue Technologies San Francisco, CA* *Tel +1 415 771 7960* *http://www.tissuetechnologies.com*	Tubes of variable length and thickness Shelf life 5 years Room temperature $300–500 per implant	Worldwide	Tubular e-PTFE	Permanent (easy to remove)	For deep rhytids, lip augmentation CI: Infection at recipient site	None	Miller et al.[50]
Autologous grafts (fat, dermis, dermis-fat, tendon, scar, fascia)	$2000–5000 per treatment	N/A	Fat with or without dermis, tendon, scar or fascia Harvested from the patient	Fat 6–24 months; tendon potentially permanent; dermis unknown; fascia unknown	For lipoatrophy, lip augmentation, folds CI: None	N/A	Krauss[30]

CI, contraindications; e-PTFE, polytetrafluoroethylene.
**Pending FDA approval in the USA.*
†See Gottlieb.[24]
‡See Krauss.[30]
§Italian study: 3-year follow-up of 21 000 soft tissue augmentation procedures.
¶Australia currently not accepting biopsy specimens from new patients until FDA approved.
¶¶Available off-label in the USA.

than either Zyderm I or Zyderm II, and is more resistant to degradation. Zyplast is injected into the mid to deep reticular dermis for treatment of deeper rhytids and contour defects, including nasolabial folds, marionette lines, and significant lip augmentation (Fig. 28.3). No overcorrection is required. It is often overlayered with Zyderm I or Zyderm II for full-thickness dermal augmentation and longer-lasting results. Zyplast is not recommended for implantation into the glabellar region due to the possibility of intra-arterial injection causing local tissue necrosis (Fig. 28.4)[62] as well as a rare risk of partial blindness.[63]

As compared to many of the newer products in which host antibody production is rare and skin testing is unnecessary, use of bovine collagen carries a 1–3% risk of hypersensitivity (Fig. 28.5A). Internal postmarketing surveillance by Inamed showed a 3% prevalence of circulating antibodies to bovine collagen. According to the company, only one of six patients in the 3% showed clinical symptoms. For this reason, skin testing is required before treatment. Two skin tests performed 2–4 weeks apart is now standard.[64,65] A positive skin test result is defined as erythema, induration, tenderness, or swelling that persists for more than 6 hours after implantation and more typically arises 2–3 days after implantation as a delayed hypersensitivity reaction (Fig. 28.6). According to the manufacturer, fewer than 3% of patients who have had negative test results will develop an allergic reaction. If hypersensitivity occurs, it usually does so within 2 weeks following treatment. Such reactions manifest as erythema and induration, with or without pruritus in the area treated. The treatment of hypersensitivity is usually not required, because the inflammatory reaction will eventually eliminate the offending material and the reaction will cease. In our experience, most patients are very upset by this and will press for an intervention. If treatment of hypersensitivity reaction is necessary, this may take the form of intralesional steroids, topical tacrolimus 0.1% ointment (or similar compound) twice daily,[66] systemic cyclosporin,[67] or systemic steroids. Treatment should be

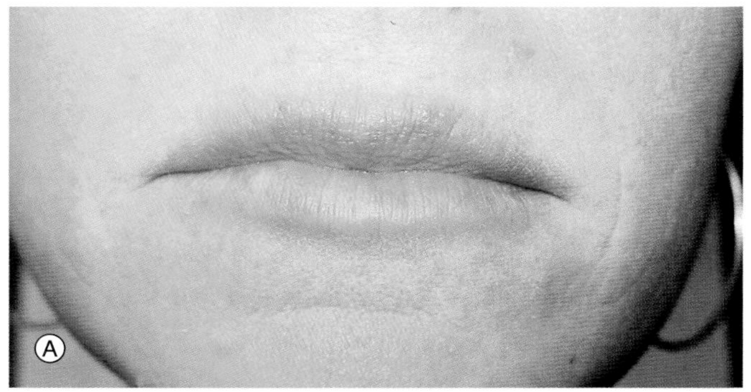

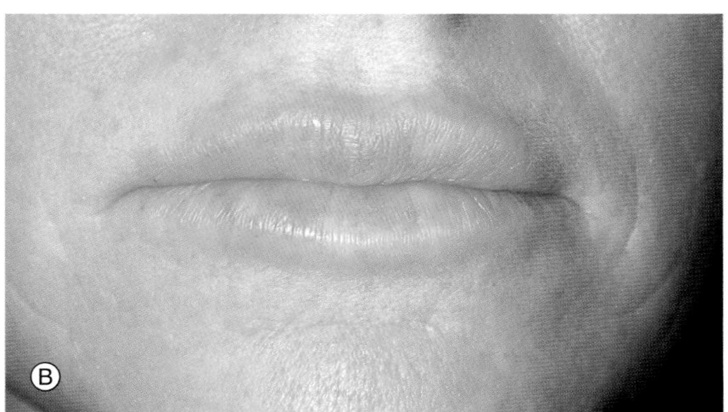

Figure 28.3 Lips. (A) Before Zyplast injection. Note pulling down at oral commissures and thinning of lips with accentuation of vertical lip lines. (B) Lip enhancement remains 3 months following Zyplast 1 ml. Improved fullness, eversion, and elevation at angles of mouth.

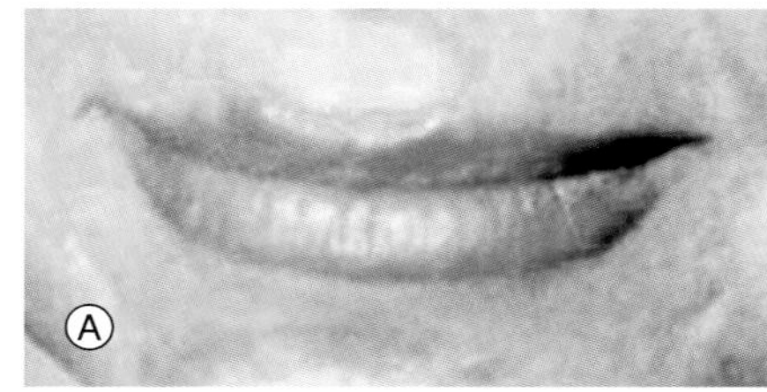

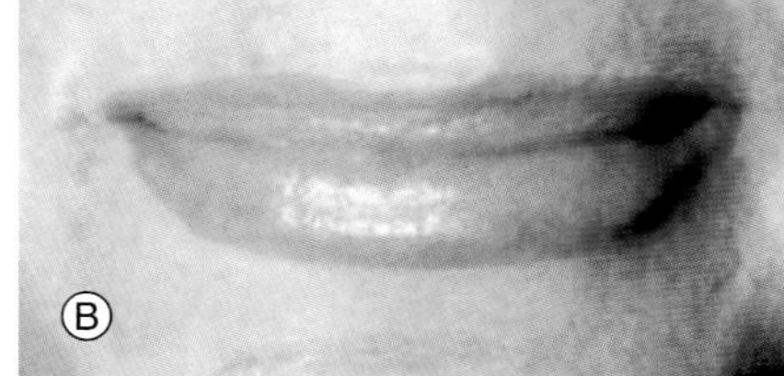

Figure 28.5 Bovine collagen hypersensitivity. (A) Reaction 1 week following treatment. Two pretreatment skin tests were negative. (B) 2 weeks later: bovine collagen hypersensitivity reaction resolved. Patient used topical 0.1% tacrolimus twice daily.

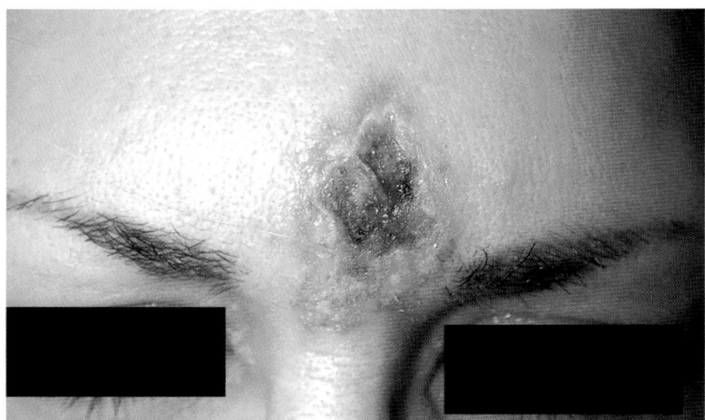

Figure 28.4 Cutaneous necrosis after bovine collagen (Zyplast) injection into the glabella. This patient was injected by a non-physician 10 days prior to this.

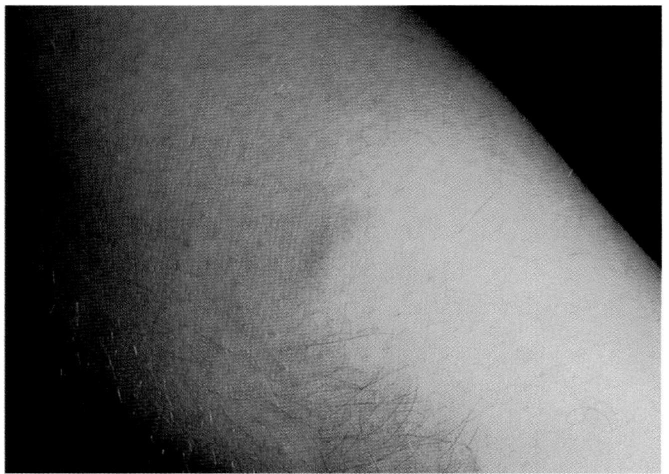

Figure 28.6 A positive reaction to a bovine collagen skin test.

stopped once the local reaction is tolerable to the patient. Occasional flares occur while the remaining product is absorbed. In rare, severe reactions, sterile abscesses and scarring have been known to occur but no other long-term sequelae have been recognized (Fig. 28.5B).

Contraindications to using injectable bovine collagen include a history of an anaphylactic event of any cause, prior hypersensitivity to bovine collagen, lidocaine sensitivity, pregnancy, lactation, and active infection at the treatment site. Although no formal testing has been completed, the manufacturer states that patients undergoing hormonal fluctuation, such as that in pregnancy or during menopause, may have an increased risk of hypersensitivity.

With any injection technique, the skin should be held taut with the free hand and the patient's head supported by a backrest (Fig. 28.7). Although many of the products discussed herein will work best when injected in a particular customized fashion, the bovine collagen products mentioned above are appropriate examples to use in discussing basic injection techniques. In general, these products are injected with a 27-gauge to 32-gauge needle (depending on the viscosity of the product) with the needle angled nearly parallel to the skin for superficial lines and wrinkles (Fig. 28.8), and at a gradually greater angle for lines and grooves of greater depth (Fig. 28.9). Serial punctures are generally made along or adjacent to the fold or wrinkle being treated, with small aliquots of material injected through each puncture site, advancing in the direction of filling to minimize loss of the product through the previous entry site (Fig. 28.10B). Once

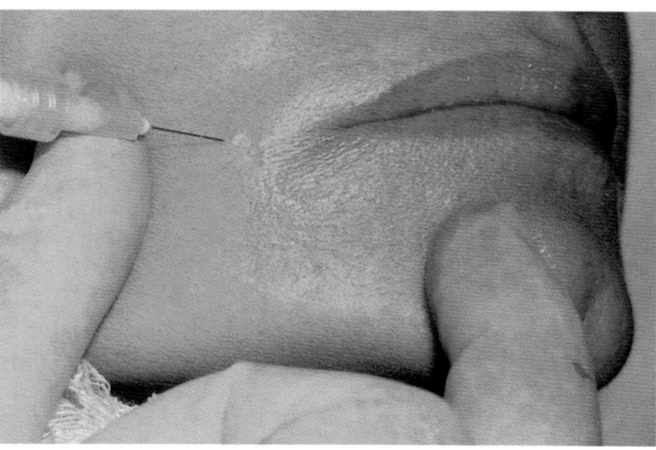

Figure 28.7 During injection of any dermal filler it is crucial that the patient's head be supported and the area under treatment be held taut and stabilized as shown here. Note also, that the needle is supported on one of the fingers of the stabilizing hand. This will prevent the needle from penetrating too deeply in the event of a sudden movement by the patient.

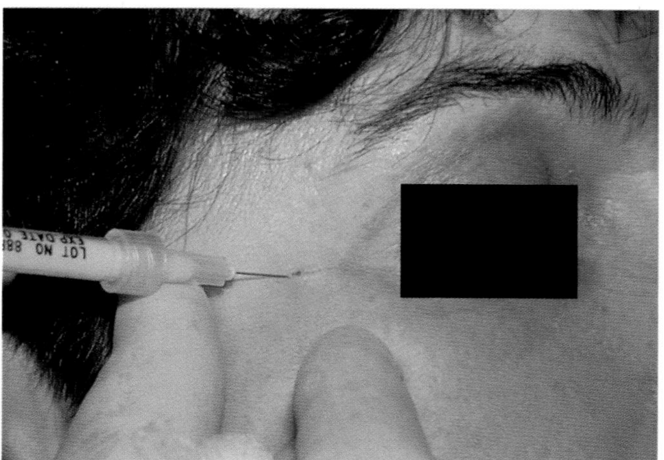

Figure 28.8 Injection of superficial lines (crow's feet) using Zyderm I bovine collagen. Note the very acute angle of the needle, which is almost parallel to the skin surface.

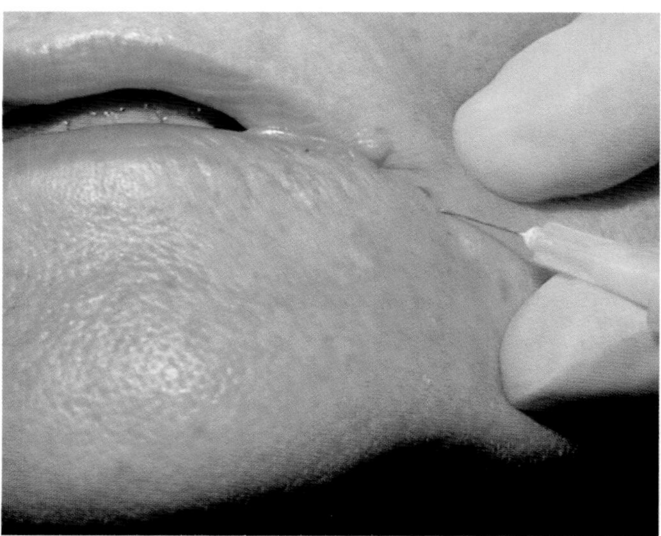

Figure 28.9 Injection of deeper skin lines using Zyplast bovine collagen implant. Note that the needle is held at a less-acute angle when treating deeper lines.

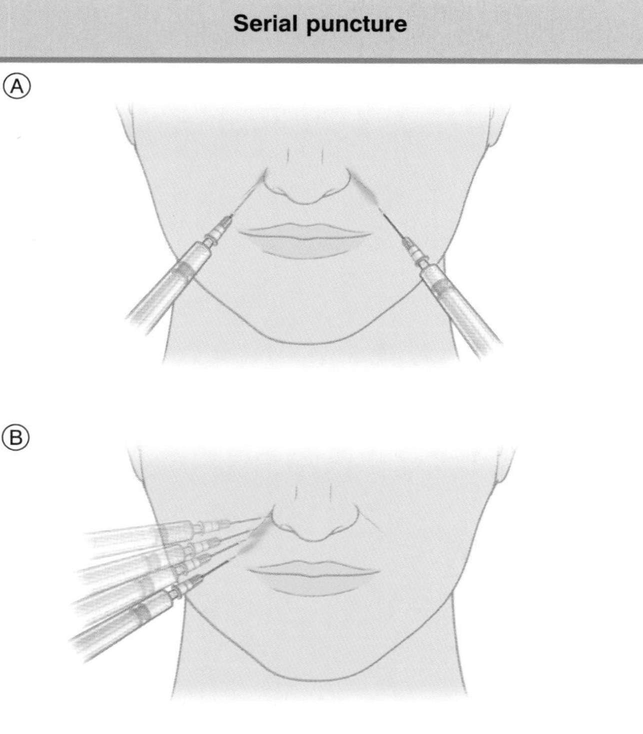

Figure 28.10 Injection technique. (A) Threading. (B) Multiple puncture technique.

injected, gentle massage can mold the collagen at the treatment site to be sure that the final result is even and smooth. If required, additional injections can be given. For deeper rhytids, the needle may be placed more perpendicular to the skin surface. Care is taken to insure placement at the base of the furrow, rather than at the shoulder of overhanging redundant skin. Another option is the 'threading' technique where a longer needle may be used and advanced for some distance under the rhytid with injection as the needle is withdrawn (Fig. 28.9). A threading approach is used routinely with injections of Hylan B gels as well as the more viscous collagens – Zyplast and Cosmoplast.

Following treatment with injectable bovine collagen, some bleeding may occur through punctures and is easily controlled after a few minutes of gentle pressure. If a patient is particularly prone to bruising, an icepack may be applied for 5 minutes postoperatively. Another caveat is the need to inject at the medial side of the nasolabial fold and marionette lines in order to avoid further 'heaviness' laterally. The 'crow's feet' should be approached with care to avoid overfilling and potential lumpiness (Fig. 28.11). The orbital area is very prone to bruising. Just barely place the needle tip below the skin before injecting and perform thorough massage in the orbital area.

Autologous collagen

Fournier, a leader in microlipoinjection, reasoned that the extracted adipose tissue contained intracellular fat contents, adipocyte cell walls, and intercellular fibrous septae.[68] He processed harvested autologous fat by mixing it with sterile distilled water and then froze it, leading to the rupture of adipocytes. This resulted in an oily fraction of intracellular triglycerides, which was disposed of, and a solid fraction representing lipocyte cell walls and connective tissue amenable to soft-tissue injection. Injection of this 'autologous collagen' was reportedly comparable to bovine collagen injections in terms of longevity.[68,69] It has been suggested that centrifugation of the tissue prior to separating the oily and solid fractions yields better results and this step is added by many clinicians using this 'autologous collagen' method.[65]

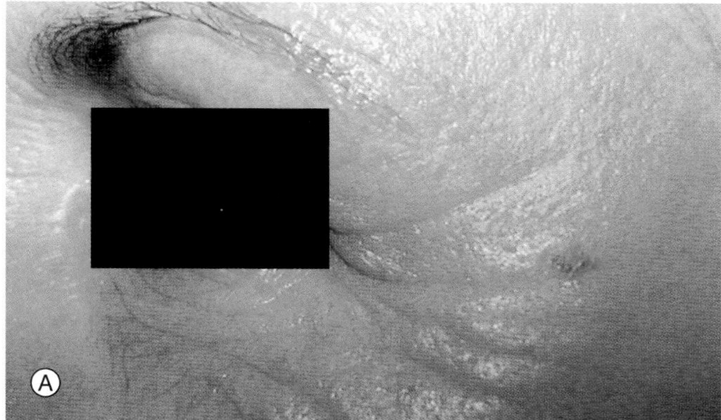

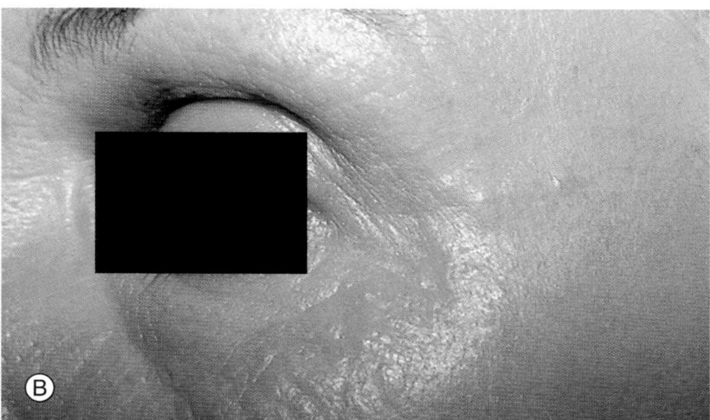

Figure 28.11 (A) Preoperative photograph of deep 'crow's feet' in a middle-aged woman prior to injection with Zyplast bovine collagen implant. (B) Following treatment, the lines are much improved, but 'beading' has occurred at a number of injection sites. This would have been avoided if Zyderm I or Zyderm II was used instead of Zyplast.

The major disadvantage of this technique is that the injected material is quite viscous, requiring injection through a needle of at least 25-gauge, if not larger. As a result, local anesthesia is necessary and needle marks can persist for several days. It is difficult with autologous collagen to precisely place the material at the required dermal level, and much more bruising is seen as compared with bovine collagen injected through a finer needle. Nonetheless, the autologous nature of this material is a distinct advantage in that antigenicity is not a concern and an abundant supply of donor material exists for each patient. Autologous collagen can be used to overlay furrows augmented by microlipo-injection. Fat can be harvested and some used unmodified to fill subcutaneous defects, while the rest is converted into autologous collagen for dermal augmentation. In fact, 'autologous collagen' is primarily made up of ruptured lipocyte cell walls and contains very little collagen.[70] Injection of this material is believed to cause considerable dermal inflammation that, in turn, results in the deposition of new collagen in the recipient area.[70]

Isolagen (Isolagen Technologies Inc, Houston, TX) is an injectable in vitro culture of autologous fibroblasts in an extracellular matrix that replenishes the dermis and subcutaneous tissues that have lost collagen and fibroblasts as a result of photodamage, aging, or scarring.[71] A 3-mm punch biopsy is obtained from the patient and then sent to the manufacturer to be grown in culture. Processing usually takes 6 weeks at which time a test dose is sent back to the physician to be administered to the patient. If no reaction occurs 2 weeks following this test injection, Isolagen can be administered. Expansion of the implant may be seen for many months after augmentation, presumably by new collagen production from the fibroblasts.

Isolagen needs to be injected into multiple levels of the dermis for best results in the treatment of rhytids and scars and for use in lip augmentation. The product should be administered within 24 hours of receipt, a situation that can pose a significant logistic challenge to patients and clinicians alike. Two to three treatments have been shown to yield persistent therapeutic results for as long as 22 months.

Since growth factors are used to culture the cells, it has now been determined that Isolagen must be regulated by the Food and Drug Administration (FDA) in the USA. Therefore, at the time of writing, the manufacturer has temporarily halted production and is not accepting biopsy specimens from new patients. Clinical trials are underway that may eventually lead to FDA approval.

In recent years, several new injectable filling materials have been introduced into the marketplace in the USA, with varying success. Included in this group are autologous injectable human collagen (Autologen; Collagenesis Inc, Beverly, MA) which is processed from skin surgically excised from the patient.[72,73] This makes the most sense for patients undergoing concomitant rhytidectomy surgery. The major problem in using this agent is the recurrent requirement for a substantial volume of donor tissues. Following one to four injection sessions, correction of scars has persisted for 1–2 years.

Newer dermal filler products

Fascian (Fascia Biosystems LLC, Beverly Hills, CA) is particulate freeze-dried, irradiated cadaveric fascia lata prepared in a variety of injectable particle sizes (0.25 mm, 0.5 mm, 1.0 mm and 2.0 mm).[74] The product is provided preloaded in a 3-ml syringe containing 80 mg of fascia lata and must be rehydrated prior to injection. Local anesthesia is recommended before injection, to minimize discomfort. The company reports results lasting 6–8 months.

In the enthusiastic rush to find the ultimate filler product, dozens of new contenders have appeared in Europe. Most of these have not yet become available in North America. Among the most notable of these is New-Fill (Biotech Industry SA, Luxembourg), which has recently been approved in the US as Sculptra (Dermik Laboratories, Berwyn, PA). New-Fill/Sculptra is a non-animal-derived polylactic acid touted to be biocompatible, biodegradable, and immunologically inert. It is distributed freeze-dried, can be stored at room temperature, and is reconstituted with sterile water. New-Fill/Sculptra is injected into the deep dermis or dermal–subcutaneous junction to treat lipoatrophy of the face and hands, liposuction contour deformities, and atrophic lips. While New-Fill/Sculptra is not intended for direct filling of rhytids (it is too bulky to be injected superficially), when injected to recontour the face, it causes a three dimensional augmentation which serves to lift the face and stretch rhytids and tissue redundancies. In July 2004, Sculptra received FDA approval for use in treating HIV associated lipoatrophy. Use as a general cosmetic soft tissue filler is pending further investigation and approval by the FDA but has had success (marketed as New-Fill) internationally since 1999.

Recently, two forms of high-viscosity liquid silicone, AdatoSil-5000 (Chiron Vision Corporation, Irvine, CA) and Silikon-1000 (Alcon US, Fort Worth, TX) have been approved as ophthalmologic devices. Some physicians in the US have used these forms of injectable silicone for off-label purposes for facial dermal filling.[4]

The newest human-tissue-derived product to come to market in the US is injectable human collagen derived from longstanding fibroblast culture lines. Cosmoderm and Cosmoplast (Inamed Aesthetics, Santa Barbara, CA) are not yet available in Europe, but were approved for marketing by both the Canada Health Protection Branch and the US FDA in early 2003. They were felt to be substantially similar to prior approved bovine collagen fillers in terms of injection technique and anticipated longevity. However, the demonstrated lack of antigenicity of this material makes pretreatment skin testing unnecessary. Like Zyderm and Zyplast, these products contain lidocaine, which minimizes the discomfort associated with injection.

In the manufacture of these products, expanded human fibroblast cultures are seeded onto nylon mesh and placed inside special bottles, called bioreactors, which simulate *in vivo* conditions. The cells grow until the nylon mesh is covered and tissue develops. The tissue is then removed from the bottles and tested for a variety of pathogens and contaminants. Subsequently, the collagen is isolated from the tissue, subjected to additional viral inactivation, and purified for injection (see soft tissue fillers video clip).

A number of novel injectable filler materials have been approved for marketing in Canada after first being introduced in Europe. These include injectable hyaluronic acid derivatives Hylaform, Hylaform Plus, Hylaform Fine Line (Inamed Aesthetics, Santa Barbara, CA), Restylane Perlane, Restylane Fine Lines (Q-Med, Uppsala, Sweden), Rofilan (Rofil Medical International, Breda, The Netherlands) and Artecoll (which will be marketed as Artefill in the US), a suspension of polymethylmethacrylate microspheres in bovine collagen (Rofil Medical International, Breda, The Netherlands). Hylaform, Restylane, and Hylaform Plus were approved by the US FDA recently (2004), while the remaining products are currently under FDA evaluation. They have undergone extensive clinical evaluation in Canada by one of the authors (S.V.P.) and their introduction into the United States, in the near future, is anticipated. They are discussed in detail below.

Hyaluronic acid gels

Hyaluronic acid (hyaluronan) is a naturally occurring glycosaminoglycan biopolymer which is a component of all connective tissues. It exhibits no species or tissue specificity because the chemical structure of this polysaccharide is uniform throughout nature. Therefore, there is no potential for immunologic reactions to hyaluronan in humans. In nature, the primary biologic function of hyaluronan is to provide stabilization to the intercellular structures and to form the elastoviscous fluid matrix in which collagen and elastic fibers become embedded. In addition, the hyaluronan matrix regulates the transport of solutions in the extracellular space,[75] regulates cell movement and functions,[76] and plays a role in developing and remodeling tissues.[77] Hyaluronan has a very large average molecular weight (4–5 million Daltons in all human tissues) and consists of repeating diasaccharides of D-glucoronic acid and *N*-acetyl-D-glucosamine arranged in long, unbranched polyanionic chains. These molecular chains form highly hydrated random coils that entangle and interpenetrate each other, producing highly elastoviscous solutions.

The amount of hyaluronic acid in the skin progressively decreases with age,[78] and loss results in reduced dermal hydration and increased skin folding.[79] With its unique elastoviscosity, immunologic compatibility, and natural role as a structure-stabilizing, space-occupying, cell-protecting connective tissue matrix filler, hyaluronan would at first sight appear to be an ideal material for soft-tissue augmentation.[80] However, with a tissue half-life of only 1–2 days, hyaluronan turns over too quickly to be of value in this regard. Exogenous hyaluronic acid is rapidly cleared from the dermis and degraded in the liver to carbon dioxide and water.[81] For this reason, investigators sought modifications of hyaluronan that would render it more stable following injection while preserving its biocompatibility.

Hylaform Fine Line, Hylaform and Hylaform Plus (Inamed Aesthetics, Santa Barbara, CA) are a family of viscoelastic Hylan B gel products marketed in Europe and Canada for the treatment and correction of soft-tissue defects of the face. This material is extracted from rooster combs and is supplied in preloaded sterilized syringes which contain either 0.75 ml (Hylaform, Hylaform Plus) or 0.4 ml (Hylaform Fine Line) of transparent gel. Like Zyderm I, Zyderm II, and Zyplast, each product has a different viscosity and indication, dependent on the depth of the tissue defect. Hylaform Fine Line is injected through a 32-gauge needle into the upper dermis for treatment of fine lines and wrinkles such as those on the upper lip and periorbital region. For deeper wrinkles, Hylaform is injected into the mid-dermis, using a 30-gauge needle. Deep dermal placement of Hylaform Plus is useful for deep lines and grooves, including the nasolabial folds and deep oral commissures. The greater viscosity of this latter product requires the use of a 27-gauge needle. Both Hylaform and Hylaform Plus are FDA approved in the US. Hylaform Fine Line is pending FDA approval at the time of press.

Preclinical studies established that this material was non-immunogenic, non-cytotoxic, non-pyrogenic, non-inflammatory, non-mutagenic, non-hemolytic, non-thrombogenic, and non-teratogenic.[80] In studies in which Hylaform and collagen implants were injected intradermally in guinea pigs, histologic persistence of the Hylan B gel was evident at the end of the 52-week observation period whereas most of the collagen implants were resorbed by 26 weeks.[80] Radiotracer studies in animals yielded a calculated half-life of more than 9 months, suggesting that Hylaform is stable in dermal tissue for extended periods of time.

To determine the safety and efficacy of Hylaform as a dermal augmentation device, a multicenter, open-label, 12-month study was conducted in six sites.[80] A total of 216 patients were enrolled in the trial and 177 completed the entire follow-up period of 1 year. One to four facial sites (wrinkles/folds or scars) were treated in each patient with touch-up reinjections at the same site or sites allowed after 2 and/or 4 weeks. Of the 724 treatment sites, 86% were facial folds or wrinkles. Thirty percent of all of the sites received only one injection, 53% received a second injection, and 17% required a third injection. 'Success' was defined as 60% of all sites showing at least a 33% degree of correction. This degree of improvement was noted in both wrinkles/folds and scars at 18 weeks. Linear regression analysis of the degree of correction by facial location and type of defect showed a mean effectiveness of 22 weeks (18–26 weeks) for wrinkles/folds and 23 weeks (13–48 weeks) for all scars. Treatment reactions were as expected and included transient and mild erythema, itching, swelling, and pain. Related reactions, occurring in less than 2% of all treatments, included persistent erythema, acne papule formation, and ecchymotic changes, among others. All resolved without sequelae. No known immunogenic responses were observed and skin testing is, therefore, not required prior to this therapy.

Hylaform received FDA approval for the treatment of nasolabial folds based on a study under an investigational protocol comparing Hylaform to Zyplast.[82] Two hundred and sixty-one patients were randomized to either Hylaform or Zyplast for the treatment of prominent nasolabial folds. Each patient received one treatment followed by a touch-up at 2 weeks if indicated. Of the 133 patients who were randomized to the Hylaform arm, 96 (72%) received a touch-up. Patients were seen in follow-up at 3 days, 2, 4, 8, 12, and 14 weeks following the initial treatment. Blinded investigators used an Independent Panel Review of photographs taken at the 12- and 14-week follow-ups and found efficacy and safety to be comparable between the two study groups.

Restylane Fine Lines, Restylane, and Perlane (Q-Med, Uppsala, Sweden), like the Hylaform products mentioned above, are a family of stabilized hyaluronic acid gels.[83] As with the Inamed products, the molecule sizes of these three products are increasingly larger, resulting in a viscosity gradient. There are, however, some differences between the two products. Whereas Hylaform contains a concentration of 6 mg/ml of Hylan B, Restylane contains 20 mg/ml. The production of the two materials also differs. Hylaform is extracted from rooster combs while Restylane is manufactured using a bacterial fermentation process. Hylaform has a higher molecular weight and its viscoelastic properties have a more elastic tendency compared to the more viscous tendency of Restylane.

In an Italian study of the efficacy of Restylane,[83] 158 patients received intradermal Restylane injection for correction of facial wrinkles/folds or for lip augmentation. Patients reported a 73.4% incidence of moderate or marked improvement after 8 months, independent of the treatment area. Treatment reactions of a localized and transient nature occurred after 12.5% of treatments. The most commonly reported were bruising, tenderness, discomfort, edema, and erythema at the treatment site (Fig. 28.12). Thirteen patients complained, particularly after lip augmentation, of an intermittent swelling of the implanted material.

Evaluation of paired implants of Restylane and Zyplast collagen on the volar forearms in five volunteers,[83] showed a gradual shrinkage of the Zyplast implant between weeks 12 to 24. At week 24, only two of ten Zyplast implant sites were visually recognizable by hyperpigmentation over the resorbed implant sites although histological examination revealed normal skin. At week 52, none of the Zyplast implants was present. By comparison, Restylane implants maintained their spot size in weeks 12 through 24. At week 52 four of ten implants were still clearly visible under the skin. Staining for hyaluronic acid revealed the presence of such material but with a significantly more watery appearance than that seen in earlier biopsies. This is explained by a property of hyaluronic acid gel referred to as

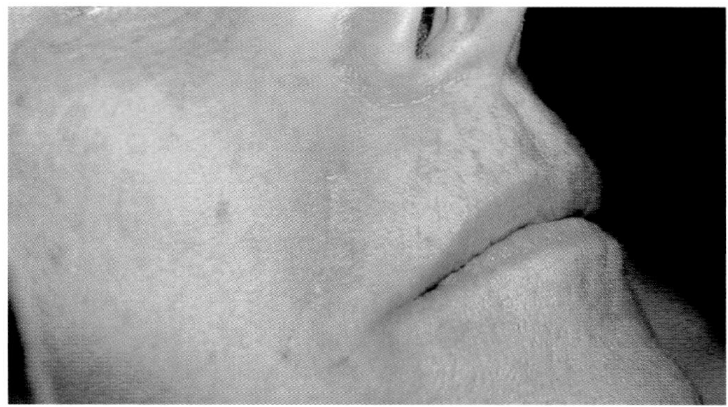

Figure 28.12 Following injection of hyaluronic acid gel, slight erythema and swelling may persist for a few hours. At this point, many patients will apply a small amount of make-up and carry on with normal schedules.

isovolemic degradation,[36] which dictates that such gels bind greater quantities of water as their concentration diminishes. It should be pointed out that this property is also responsible for a rather sudden disappearance of contour correction when the final molecules of hyaluronic acid gel are finally resorbed.

In a Swedish study of Restylane, 113 patients received intradermal implants of Restylane into 285 facial locations.[84] Patients received either one or two treatments, depending on the response to treatment. Sixty-six percent of the treatment sites received a second treatment 2 weeks following the initial therapy. All patients were followed for up to 26 weeks and, at that point in time, evaluation by physicians revealed an overall 69% correction, compared with the patient assessment of 61%. Unfortunately, only 20 patients were randomly selected for a 1-year follow-up and the results, although comparable to those at 26 weeks, cannot be considered reliable due to the small follow-up sample number. In the same study, injection-related adverse events were noted in 8.4% of the treatment sites and resolved within 1 week. These included erythema, swelling, darkening of the treatment site, and slight pain. Red spots, bumps, and hematoma were encountered in approximately 5% of treatment sites and were felt to be associated with the technique used during implantation of the device.

In the pinnacle study that earned its FDA approval for the treatment of nasolabial folds, Restylane was compared to Zyplast. One hundred and thirty-eight patients were randomized to receive either Restylane or Zyplast and received treatments at 2-week intervals to achieve 'optimal' results. The total number of treatments ranged from 1–3 with a mean of 1.4 for both products (difference not significant). Once this outcome was achieved, patients were considered to be at 'baseline'. Blinded investigators evaluated clinical outcome at 2, 4, and 6 months following baseline using the Wrinkle Severity Rating Scale and Global Aesthetic Improvement Scale. Assessments at 6 months after baseline indicated that hyaluronic acid gel was superior in 56.9% and 62.0% of patients, respectively, while Zyplast was rated as superior in 9.5% and 8.0% of patients, respectively. Additionally, the mean total injection volume required to achieve optimal results was 1 mL of Restylane, compared with 1.6 mL of Zyplast.[85]

Hylaform and Restylane products handle in a comparable fashion during injection and have similar 'feels' for the injector. Injections are generally administered using a threading technique: the needle is advanced along the line to be treated and injection is made with constant pressure on the syringe plunger as the needle is withdrawn and possibly also as it is advanced (Fig. 28.13). Pressure is relieved just prior to the needle exiting the skin, to avoid leakage and wastage of gel. The needle should be kept quite superficial in the dermis, with the aim being to inject into the mid dermal plane. If injected too superficially, a bluish discoloration will be seen through the skin (Tyndall effect), which may require lancing to extrude product. Although Duranti et al.[83] and Olenius[84] suggest that the needle bevel be up, this is probably not essential. As it is injected, the material will be noted to 'spread' through the upper dermal tissue plane, providing a natural-appearing plumping of the treatment area. At this point, the injected 'thread' may be kneaded gently, along the line of injection, to be certain that the implant is smooth and uniform. Successive 'threads' of injected material are laid down adjacent to previous injections, until the entire line, fold, or wrinkle has been treated.

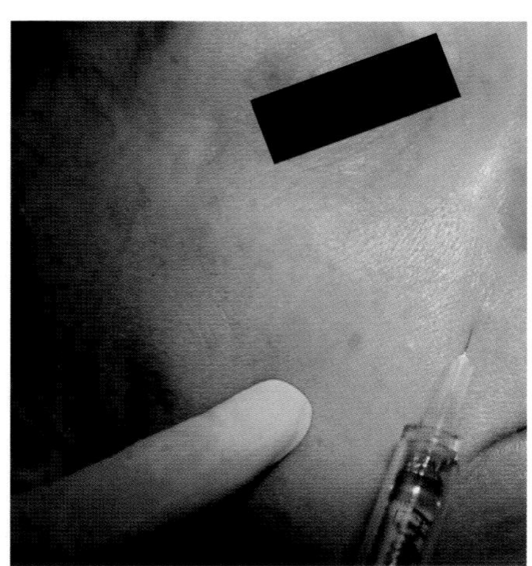

Figure 28.13 Same patient as in Figure 28.12. Treatment of a nasolabial fold with hyaluronic acid (Hylaform) in a middle-aged woman. The hyaluronic acid is injected with uniform pressure during withdrawal of the needle. The injected material will flow easily into the upper dermal plane as shown here.

In the nasolabial fold, for example, where there is a triangular-shaped concavity at the upper aspect (the isthmus of the lip), two or three threads of implantation, arranged in a fan-like array, can be used to uniformly fill this area. The lower portion of the line is treated with threads of injected material placed one below the next (always staying medial to the crease in the case of nasolabial folds) in a continuous row. If the fold is excessively wide, two parallel rows of implantation may be made, with gentle massage after each thread is placed. Oral commissures, marionette lines, and glabellar frown lines may be treated in the same manner. If correctable by tissue stretch, forehead lines can also be treated. Often this is done in combination with *botulinum toxin* injections (see Chapter 31).[86]

Lip enhancement has become one of the most sought-after procedures today. Hyaluronic acid gels are particularly effective in this regard (Fig. 28.14). The usual technique is to define the lip margin by gently injecting along the vermilion border, administering a row of successive, thread-like aliquots of hylan gel in five or six 'threads' for each lip margin. Approximately 0.3–0.4 ml is used for lip-edge definition. The remainder is injected, again using a threading technique, along the 'wet line' of the red lip—the line at which the dry outer mucosa meets the moist inner mucosa. Again, a spreading effect is noted as the material spreads through the plane of injection. Gentle massage should be performed throughout the treatment to insure uniformity and smoothness of the implant. Significant postinjection swelling will often be noted in this area and, frequently, some degree of bruising, particularly on the red of the lip, will occur. Whereas the swelling generally resolves within a day or two, bruising may persist for up to a week.

Many injectors have found topical anesthetics to be useful for minimizing discomfort during injection. Alternatively, small aliquots of local anesthetic may be administered quickly into the nasolabial folds, commissures, or glabella, prior to injection. While some patients tolerate treatment without any anesthetic, perioral injections can be quite uncomfortable and we recommend nerve blocks in this area. Prior to lip enhancement, infraorbital and mental nerve blocks or a ring block are virtually always required (see Chapter 3).

The longevity of correction is approximately 4–6 months following one or two treatments although some patients

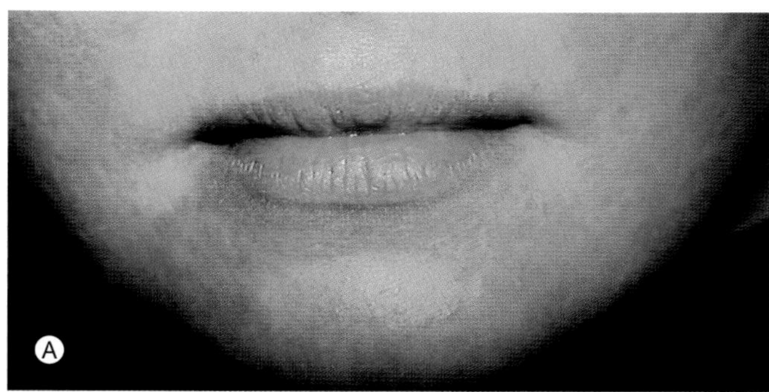

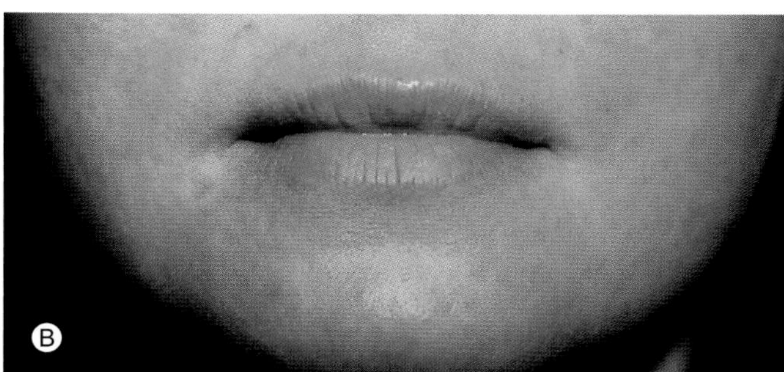

Figure 28.14 (A) Preoperative photograph of the upper lip in a young woman shows a slightly diminutive upper lip with poor definition of the lip margin. (B) Immediate postoperative photograph of the same woman, following injection of 0.7 ml of hyaluronic acid gel (Restylane) into the upper lip. Equal amounts of material were implanted into the lip margin and bulk of the lip.

require retreatment sooner. In our experience, retreatment after one injection session is usually required 4 months after Hylaform injection and 5–6 months after Restylane injection. Occasional patients in whom correction has persisted for longer than expected have also been encountered.

A number of other hyaluronic acid derivatives have been marketed worldwide. These include Rofilan (Rofil Medical International, Breda, The Netherlands) and Juvederm (LEA. Derm, Paris, France).

Artecoll (formerly Artefill)

In September 1998, after almost a decade of use in Europe and other parts of the world, Artecoll (Rofil Medical International, Breda, The Netherlands) became the first permanent dermal filling material to be approved by Canada's Health Protection Branch (HPB). This product utilizes partly denatured 3.5% bovine collagen (Resoplast; Rofil Medical International, Breda, The Netherlands) as a carrier substance in which tiny spheres of polymethylmethacrylate (PMMA) are evenly suspended. The final injection mixture contains a 1 : 3 ratio of microspheres to atelocollagen with an average concentration of 0.3% lidocaine hydrochloride. The bovine collagen is biodegraded in several weeks, leaving behind spheres of PMMA with a smooth surface and measuring approximately 30–40 mm in diameter (Fig. 28.15). These spheres are inert and non-biodegradable. They stimulate tissue fibroblasts to produce a fibrotic capsule, which essentially 'cements' the PMMA in place. In this way, the material is easily incorporated into the treatment site.

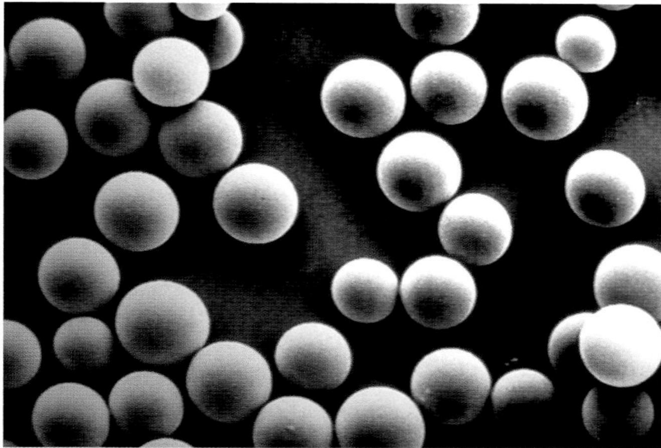

Figure 28.15 PMMA microspheres of 30–40 μm in diameter and surface smoothness as seen by electron microscopy.

Although the manufacturer states that the amount of new host collagen synthesis roughly equals the shrinkage from lost bovine collagen, the authors feel that clinically there is some obvious shrinkage of the implant noted 2 months after treatment. Therefore, prior to treatment patients are told that this treatment should be thought of as 'four steps forward and three back' in terms of the correction achieved with each treatment. Patients are also advised that correction is best achieved over two to four treatments with intervals of at least 6–8 weeks between injection sessions (Fig. 28.16). This allows time for dissolution of the collagen carrier and initial encapsulation of the PMMA spheres. During this time, patients will note some diminution of the initial correction (as the collagen is degraded) followed by renewed correction of the defect (as collagen encapsulation of the PMMA spheres proceeds). This gradual correction of skin defects allows for a more natural, smoother and balanced result. Too rapid a correction is more likely to result in irregularities in contour, which may be permanent.

To minimize the chance of developing any of these problems, physicians should be extremely conservative as they begin to use Artecoll. There is a definite 'learning curve' which occurs during the first few dozen treatments. It is suggested that initially only one or two 0.5-ml syringes of material be used at any given treatment session until experience with the product has been achieved. One 0.5-ml syringe is sufficient to treat one deep nasolabial fold or two less accentuated skin folds. An upper or lower lip may be treated with one syringe. Several acne or surgical scars may be treated with 0.5 ml of Artecoll. Marionette lines and glabellar frown lines, unless very deep, require a total of 0.5 ml for treatment of both areas. Depending on the degree of improvement achieved with the initial treatment, an equal or lesser amount of Artecoll is injected at the second treatment session about 2 months later. A third treatment session should be thought of as an opportunity to 'fine tune' the results and even out any mild imbalances or irregularities. A fourth treatment may be required, especially if several sites are being treated concomitantly. Although it is assumed that implanted PMMA microspheres reside permanently at the treatment sites, facial lines are dynamic in nature and therefore may deepen with time. This is particularly true for gravity-dependent areas such as the

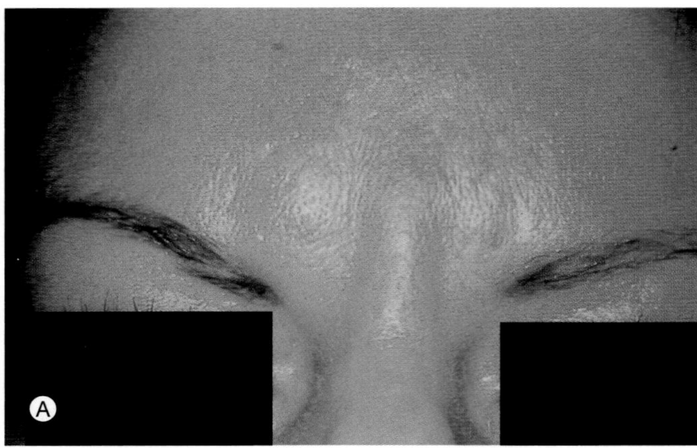

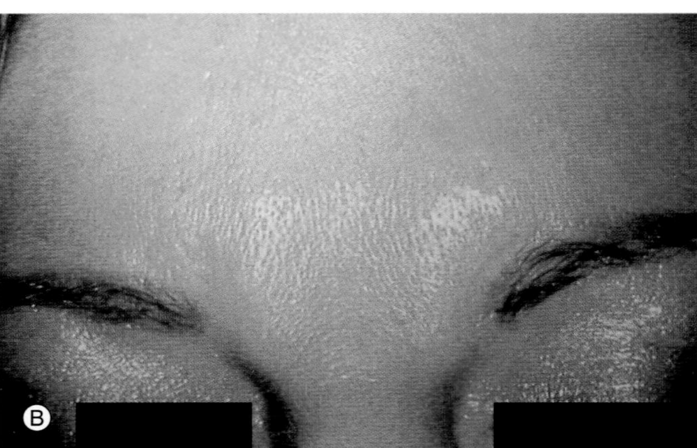

Figure 28.16 (A) Preoperative photograph of glabellar frown lines in a woman following BOTOX injections but prior to Artecoll treatment. Photo courtesy of G Lemperle. (B) 81 months after having received a total of 0.5 ml of Artecoll, the frown lines are still improved. Intradermal augmentation of frown lines is usually supplemented with injections of BOTOX. Photo courtesy of G Lemperle.

nasolabial folds and marionette lines. Patients need to understand that touch-up treatments may be required intermittently in the future to maintain optimal correction of lines and folds.

Due to the high viscosity of Artecoll, a 26-gauge needle is recommended for injection. The needle should be threaded under the skin in a manner similar to that described above for hyaluronic acid gels. However, the plane is deeper for Artecoll, with the goal being to administer the implant into the deepest aspect of the dermis. It is better to err on the side of being too deep than to risk superficial placement of PMMA spheres. Material placed in the subcutaneous fat may not provide contour correction but can act as a platform upon which future implants may be deposited. Nodule formation can occur if Artecoll is injected into muscle.[39] Lemperle describes an injection procedure in which the needle is advanced and withdrawn in a 'to and fro' motion two or three times to form a tunnel-like channel into which the Artecoll is evenly deposited as the needle is finally withdrawn.[38] Treatment of the nasolabial folds, glabellar frown lines, oral commissures, and marionette lines are easily performed using the technique just described. Aliquots of approximately 0.1 ml of Artecoll are deposited uniformly into each channel as the needle is withdrawn. For all gravity-dependent sites, one should take care to inject just along the medial aspect of the expression line to prevent further lateral 'overhang' from occurring immediately following injection. Injecting too laterally can actually result in accentuation of these unwanted lines. For treatment of oral commissures, Lemperle suggests injecting a small amount of material horizontally into the lateral vermilion border, with the injection beginning just lateral to the commissure and directed medially. The track so created tends to cross the commissure at a 90° angle, causing an additional lifting effect at the level of the vermilion. This technique may also be used for other dermal fillers.

Treatment of the lips requires particularly careful technique. There are two aspects to lip enhancement, as presented above in the discussion of hyaluronic acid gels. The first is improvement of lip line definition by injecting along the vermilion border; the second is actual lip enlargement, achieved by direct injection into the bulk of the lip, just above the muscle and along the 'wet line' of the lip mucosa. In both instances, Artecoll should be injected in minute quantities with no more than 0.5 ml being used per lip during a single sitting. For complete lip enlargement and enhancement of lip definition, the author will generally inject about 0.25 ml along the vermilion border, in five threads of about 0.05 ml each. The remaining 0.25 ml is injected into the bulk of the lip, along the 'wet line' of the mucosa, in four or five thread-like injections of 0.05 or 0.06 ml each. Be sure to inject uniformly as the needle is withdrawn from the track to avoid clumping of the injected material. Obviously, injection should cease just prior to needle withdrawal in order to avoid too-superficial placement of Artecoll at the proximal end of the track. As with other anatomic sites, patients should be advised that at least two treatments will be necessary to achieve the best outcome (Fig. 28.17). Swelling and erythema will usually last for a few days. Patients are also reassured that since the implant will shrink over the first few days, they should not be concerned if the immediate result seems too extreme. In our experience, bruising occurs in about 20% of lip-augmentation patients, despite postoperative icepacks for 5 minutes, and resolves in about 1 week. Whereas hyaluronic acid derivatives have finite residence times in the dermis following implantation, the acrylic polymethylmethacrylate used in Artecoll can persist indefinitely. If performed conservatively, slowly and carefully, Artecoll therapy can be quite gratifying for both physicians and patients. Patients need to understand that small, incremental improvements are the rule, and not rapid overnight correction.

A novel 'middle ground' approach taken by Rofil Medical International (Breda, The Netherlands) has been to suspend dextran beads in hyaluronic acid in an attempt to provide a product with an intermediate longevity (1–2 years). This product, Reviderm Intra, is also available in Canada and Europe, but we await clinical results that corroborate the manufacturer's claim of extended longevity.

Subdermal fillers and implants

Radiesse (Bioform, Franksville, WI) is composed of calcium hydroxylapatite microspheres suspended in a polysaccharide carrier which holds the microspheres in place until reabsorbed and fibroblast-driven collagenation takes place. The hydroxylapatite takes on characteristics of the local environment as cellular growth occurs in and

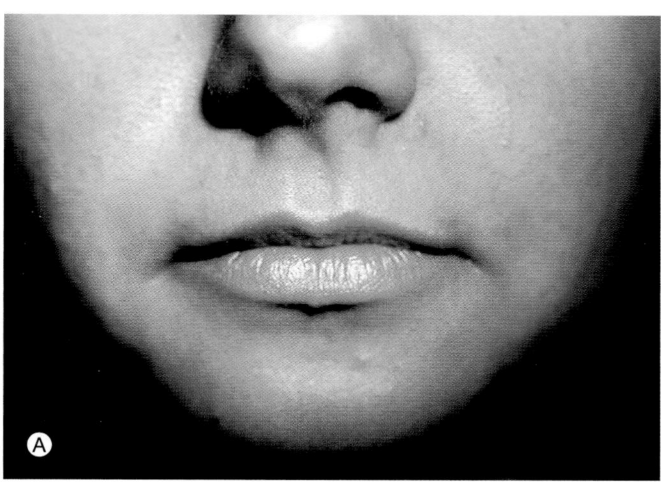
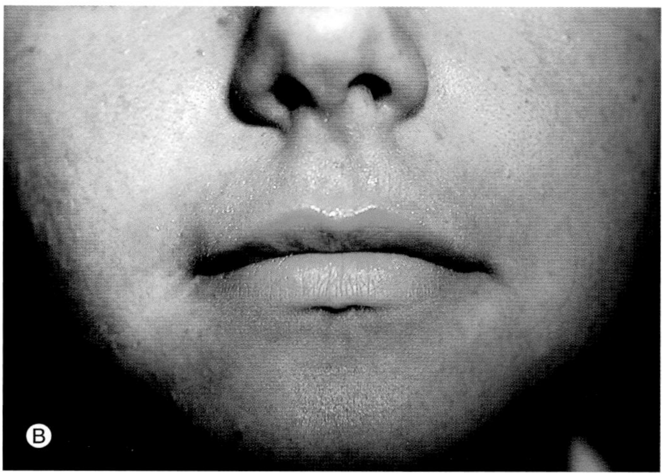

Figure 28.17 (A) Preoperative photograph of a young woman prior to Artecoll enhancement of the upper lip. (B) Immediately following the second of two treatments during which a total of 1.0 ml of Artecoll was injected into the upper lip. Half of the material was injected into the lip bulk and half into the lip margin. Some swelling and redness commonly persist for 1–2 days.

around it. Radiesse has been used off label (FDA approved as Radiance for treatment of urinary incontinence and vocal cord paralysis) in the treatment of HIV-associated lipoatrophy of the temples and cheeks, acne scars, lip augmentation, and in obscuring nasolabial folds and marionette lines. Allergy testing is not needed and results typically last for 9 months to several years. The product has a shelf life of approximately 2 years and does not require refrigeration.

Patients are advised to use a topical anesthetic preoperatively. Those with a history of frequent orolabial herpes simplex virus (HSV) infection should be placed on antiviral drugs. Regional blocks and/or small amounts of local anesthesia will make patients more comfortable. The skin is prepped with isopropyl alcohol, Betadine, or chlorhexidine (Hibiclens) solution. With the patient seated upright but leaning against a headrest, a 23-gauge to 25-gauge needle is directed into the subdermal plane and slow, gentle pressure is applied to the plunger upon withdrawal to distribute a thin, even layer of 0.1–0.2 ml per pass. This is repeated so that several layers or threads are juxtaposed. Overcorrection is not advised. Once injected, mold or smooth the material to achieve the desired effect. Since this product is semipermanent, conservative augmentation with reinjection as necessary is recommended. Approximately 0.5–1 ml is used to treat each nasolabial fold and 0.5 ml is used for an upper or lower lip with no more than 1 ml of product used per treatment site. Patients should be told to expect swelling for several days following treatment (see soft tissue fillers video clip).

Alloderm (Life Cell Corporation, Branchburg, NJ) is an acellular human (cadaveric) allograft collagen implant that may be used in multiple sheets to augment deeper defects of structure, and in single sheets for smaller acne scars and lip augmentation.[54] Stringent controls over cross-infection from cadaveric donors are required. Rejection is minimized by removing all cellular material and longevity and nonresorption are among its best characteristics.[87] After being fully rehydrated in a sterile solution and manipulated to the surgeon's preferred shape, Alloderm is then surgically implanted in a sterile field under local or general anesthesia. The technique for soft-tissue augmentation of lips and nasolabial folds is not unlike that of e-PTFE except that this product comes in the form of sheets, not a tube, and requires manipulation. The sheet can either be pulled through the subdermal plane such that it folds on itself naturally or the surgeon may choose to suture the sheet into a tube-like shape prior to implantation (i.e. for lip and nasolabial fold augmentation).[89] A tendon passer (Fig. 28.18) is inserted through the subdermal plane from exit to entry site. There, the implant is grasped and pulled through the tissue in this plane. Redundant Alloderm is trimmed at either end. When suturing the entry and exit sites closed, one author likes to anchor the implant in place to prevent migration during early wound healing. Significant swelling can occur in the first postoperative week. Results last for anywhere from 6 months to 12 months in most but have been known to persist for several years.

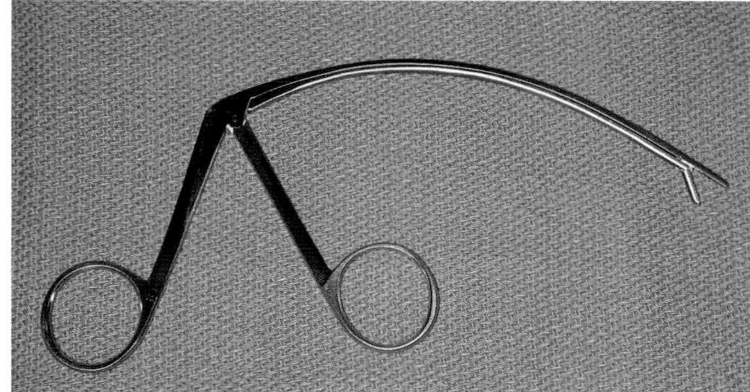

Figure 28.18 Tendon passer.

Cymetra (Life Cell Corporation, Branchburg, NJ) is the micronized, injectable form of Alloderm.[57] It is reconstituted in the physician's office with lidocaine, which can take up to 15 minutes. Like Alloderm, no allergy testing is required according to the manufacturer, and no known hypersensitivity to the product has been reported. It is injected into the deep dermis just over the dermal–subcutaneous junction to treat deeper rhytids, acne scars, and for lip augmentation, and produces a very smooth result. According to the company, results typically last 3–6 months. Because of its high viscosity, it has a tendency to clump in the needle

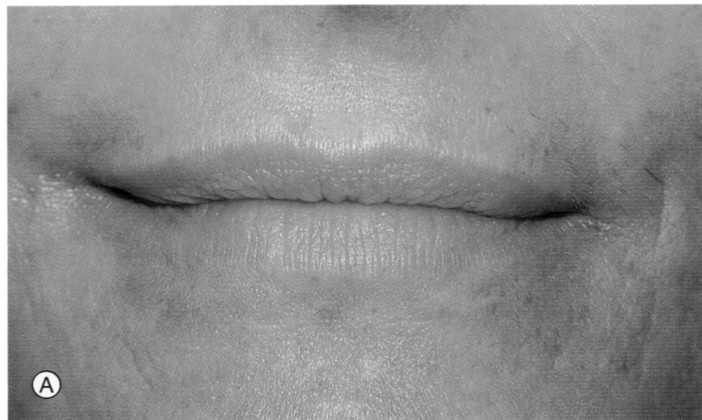

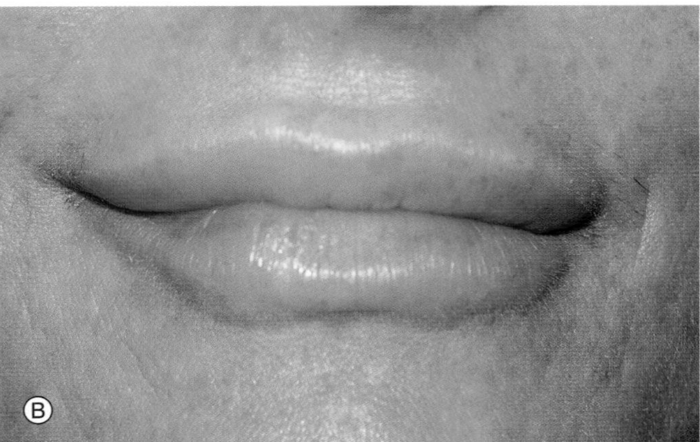

Figure 28.19 (A) Lips before Cymetra injection. (B) Lip augmentation immediately following Cymetra 1 ml. Note lip eversion and fullness.

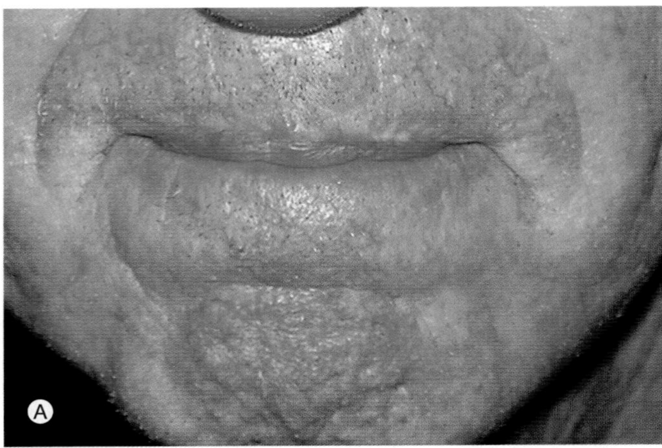

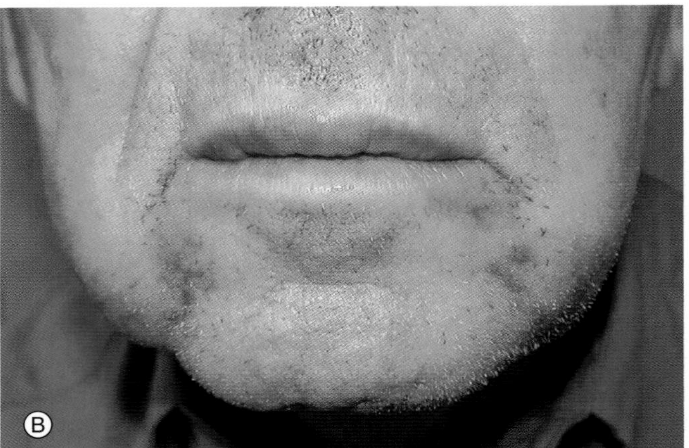

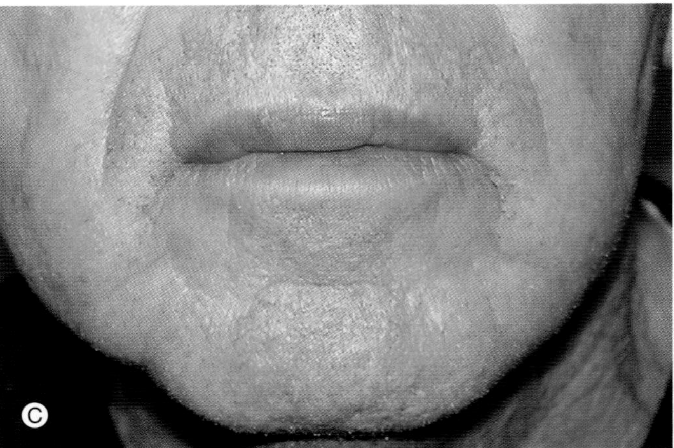

Figure 28.20 (A) Marionette lines and turned down oral commissures before Softform implants. (B) Five days following Softform implants into marionette lines. Minor bruising and swelling is noted. (C) Improvement in marionette lines and elevation of oral commissures at 6 months after operation. Patient did note mild palpation of implants.

during injection. Consequently, administration via a 25-gauge or 27-gauge needle is recommended (Fig. 28.19).

Contraindications to using Alloderm or Cymetra include allergy to gentamicin, collagen vascular disease, and an avascular or infected recipient site. The authors do not recommend use of Cymetra in the glabellar region due to risk of arterial occlusion.

Subdermal implants

Softform and its second generation counterpart Ultrasoft (Tissue Technologies Inc, San Francisco, CA) are tubes of expanded polytetrafluoroethylene (e-PTFE , or Gore-Tex), used as facial implants to treat depressed scars, lip atrophy, and deep furrows such as nasolabial folds and marionette lines. Because the material is porous, it allows ingrowth of fibroblasts thereby preventing migration and providing permanent correction. Because of the permanent nature of the implant, it is advisable that the patient be treated with a temporary filler first to insure that they like the result (Figs 28.20–28.21) (also see the video clip of implants). Gore-Tex Strings or Strands (Gore Advanced Technologies Worldwide, Newark, DE) come as single thread-like cylindrical rubber bands or as a combination of solid ends flanking shredded central strings (facilitating the incorporation of tissue and allowing more flexibility in areas such as the lips). e-PTFE implants are generally used for deeper defects and as such are implanted just below the dermis at its junction with the fat.

Advanta (Atrium Medical Corporation, Hudson, NH) is a newer generation dual porosity e-PTFE. It combines a soft, highly porous center with a smooth, medium-porosity outer surface. The dual-porosity design more closely mimics the natural healing response by readily incorporating endogenous collagen.[52] Because of this extensive tissue integration, adverse effects such as extrusion and migration are less likely. Alternatively, implant removal has been shown to be

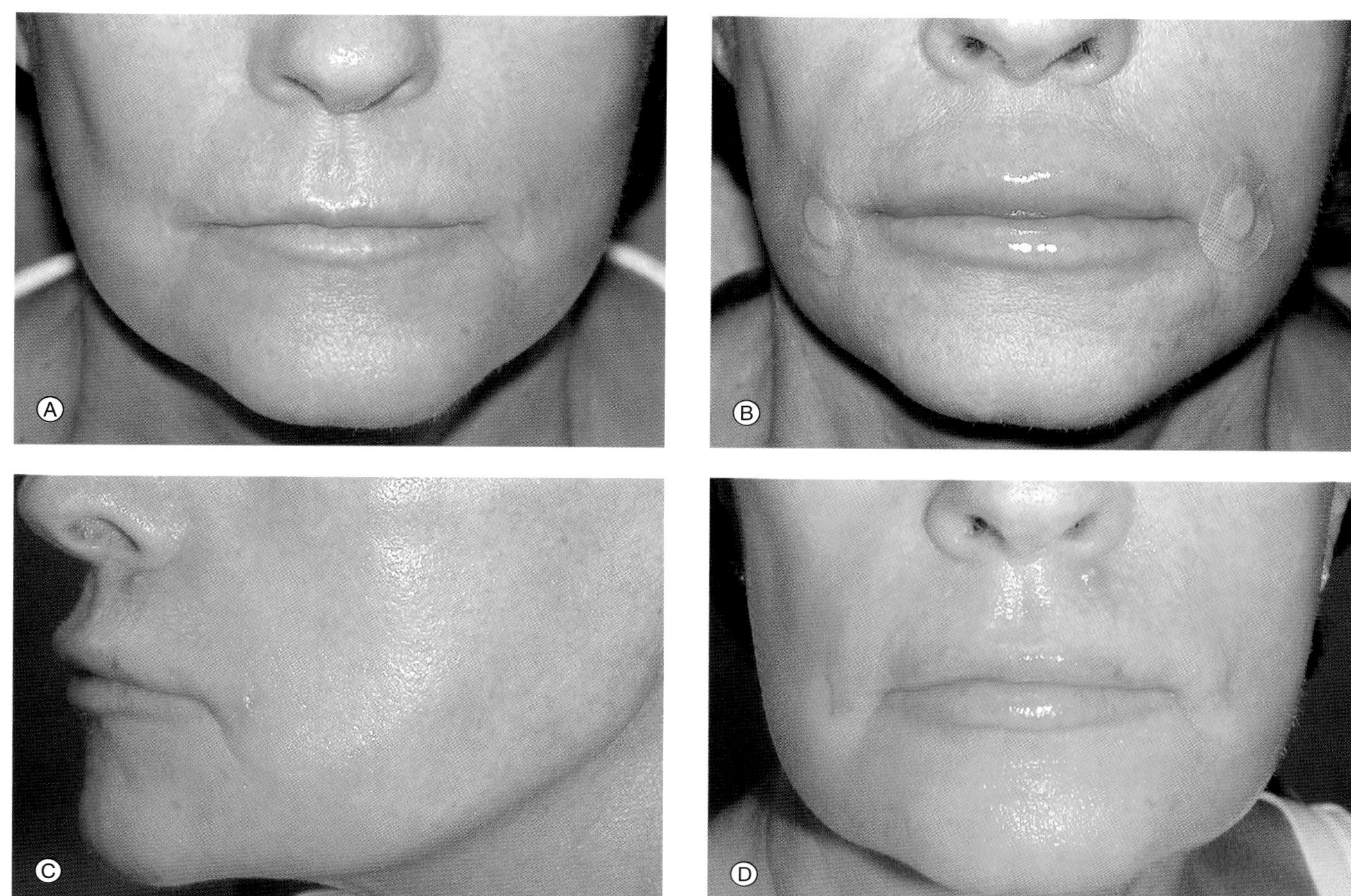

Figure 28.21 Softform sequence. (A) Before Softform implants. (B) Four days after Softform to nasolabial fold and lips. (C) Three weeks after Softform implantation. (D) Lateral view after 3 weeks.

more difficult after 90 days, potentially requiring longitudinal dissection. Additionally, the extremely soft nature of the material, the wide variety of sizes and shapes of implants, and the low-complication and high-satisfaction rates make this a superior product.

Patients undergoing subdermal implant procedures are advised to be accompanied by a family member or friend when possible for moral support. When the patient has a driver, they are offered an anxiolytic preoperatively. All patients should take perioperative antibiotics, to cover skin flora, and antivirals starting on the morning of surgery. Areas to be treated are marked preoperatively and patient expectations and risks are reviewed. Regional blocks are always utilized with local anesthesia for hemostasis to minimize perioperative swelling and ecchymoses.

The patient is prepped and draped in the usual sterile fashion and placed in a supine position. Entry and exit sites for implant placement are created approximately 3–5 mm in length with a #11 scalpel blade. For nasolabial fold implantation, one author recommends entry at the most inferior aspect of the defect in a pre-existing rhytid and exit at the uppermost aspect and possibly inside the nares. For lip augmentation, incisions for entry and exit sites are made perpendicular to the vermillion border just behind the 'wet line' of the lip so as not to be noticeable and approximately 2–4 mm from the oral commissure bilaterally. For most patients, one implant will nicely span the entire upper or lower lip, giving a natural look depending on the size of the implant chosen. However, for those people with an extremely sculpted cupid's bow, it is advisable to enter at the oral commissure and exit at the cupid's bow on either side so as not to flatten it creating a 'sausage lip' look, unless that is the desired goal. Products can be obtained in many sizes and shapes, many of which come with a trochar device for ease of placement. In this technique, the trochar is carefully pushed from entry to exit site through the soft tissues, twisting as it is advanced. Once correctly placed evenly in the subdermal plane, the trochar is released. (This maneuver varies depending on the implant used.) The tissue is then maximally stretched over the implant (and guide wire, if present). If a guide wire is present, it can then be carefully removed while maintaining a strong hold on the implant. The tissue is once again stretched over the implant, the ends are tapered obliquely, such that 3–5-mm tips are implanted into the tissue below. Sutures are used to close the entry and exit sites. As long as the implant tails are positioned deeply in tissue, this suture may be used to anchor the implant in place to stabilize it during the inflammatory phase of wound healing.

Soft-tissue implants are placed just under the dermis at the dermal-fat interface. Whether the implant is made of an e-PTFE tube (Advanta, Ultrasoft), Gore-Tex threads, or acellular human collagen sheets (Alloderm), careful placement at this junction is critical. When implants are placed too high, they become visible and when too deep, they negate the positive effects that patients expect.

■ OPTIMIZING OUTCOMES

It is important that both clinicians and patients recognize the limitations of injectable therapy in the treatment of facial lines and wrinkles. Specific surgical techniques are a more appropriate and effective therapy than are injectables or soft implants in instances where significant solar elastosis and/or cutaneous laxity is present. The yellowish plaques that characterize severe solar elastosis often have furrows running through them, between the papules of elastotic material. Some clinicians may be tempted to inject these lines with the materials discussed in this chapter. The results are usually disappointing. A more appropriate treatment is to remove the elastotic material, which is generally confined to the papillary dermis, by dermabrasion, chemical peeling, or laser resurfacing. Likewise, injectables cannot be expected to counter the effects of gravity and are entirely ineffective in treating 'jowls' or other problems associated with significant skin laxity. In such cases, rhytidectomy procedures, with or without liposuction, should be recommended to patients (see Chapter 41). Additionally, deep dynamic rhytids will not be improved as well with fillers alone as they would with botulinum toxin and fillers combined. It is our experience that filling substances tend to be more durable in areas that have been treated with botulinum toxin. Deeper lines and folds may require implants such as those made of e-PFTE.

Prior to treatment, the physician should give the patient a handheld mirror and ask him or her to point out areas where improvement is desired and to note any facial asymmetries. It is also advisable to allow the patient to help determine the endpoint of therapy. This will decrease the number of 'touch up' procedures and dissatisfied patients.

Layering of soft-tissue augmentation materials of varying viscosity allows for slow, natural, smooth augmentation which minimizes the risk of clumping and asymmetry. Patients without prior experience with soft-tissue augmentation should consider temporary fillers before investing physically, emotionally and financially in permanent fillers. While implants can be removed, no surgery is without risks or downtime. Some of the newer semipermanent (Radiesse, New-Fill/Sculptra) and permanent (Aretecoll/Artefill) products cannot be removed.

A touch-free technique should be used with all implants to maintain sterility. Depending on the implant used, it may need to be soaked preoperatively and kept in antibiotic solution until ready to be placed (i.e. Alloderm).[90] The patient should not be allergic to the antibiotic used. Proper placement of fillers and implants in the soft tissue is important; if placed too superficially, they may extrude or be palpable and implants may cause a tethering of the overlying skin.

■ POSTOPERATIVE CARE

Patients may help to reduce postoperative swelling by applying cold compresses to the affected areas regularly for the first 24–48 hours. Courses of perioperative antibiotics and antivirals should be completed. Care should be taken to minimize aggressive movement in order to avoid dislodging the filler or implant and causing additional inflammation. Patients should also be instructed to avoid manipulation of their fillers or implants. Bruising is to be expected, but patients should be instructed on signs and symptoms of hematoma and infection so that early and aggressive intervention can be made if necessary. Patients are allowed to resume anticoagulants 24 hours after their procedure. Following soft tissue implantation only, they are instructed not to exercise vigorously for 4 days and to follow-up at 5–7 days for evaluation and suture removal if applicable. The next follow-up visit for soft implant patients and first time filler patients should be at 2–6 weeks for evaluation and touch-up if indicated.

■ PITFALLS AND THEIR MANAGEMENT

Avoidance of pitfalls

- Skin test twice before treatment with bovine-based collagen products (e.g. Zyderm and Zyplast) to avoid an allergic response.
- Pretreat patients with a low pain threshold with topical or injectable anesthesia to minimize pain associated with treatment.
- Patients should be asked to fill in a consent form, so they are aware of the fact that they may palpate the implant under the skin, either as a thread-like or beaded area.
- Administer treatment to the patient in a reclined or tilted position to help avoid a vasovagal episode.
- Careful injection of Artecoll into the deep dermis and avoidance of treating very thin skin will minimize the risk of ridging.
- The appearance of lumps and bumps can be prevented by gently kneading the treatment sites as the implants is placed, smoothing any irregularities as they are encountered.
- If the implant should become infected, try initially treating with oral antibiotics; if the infection does not resolve, the implant must be removed.
- Foreign body granulomas may be initially treated with intralesional steroids before considering surgical intervention.

Since approximately 1–3% of the general population may have an allergic reaction to bovine collagen, an effort to develop less antigenic filling materials has been made over the past decade. Many of the newer materials, such as the hyaluronan-based gels, carry a much lower risk of allergic response and skin testing is not required. Nonetheless, since these products do contain minute amounts of foreign protein, which can act as antigenic determinants, reactions can occasionally occur. Treatment with bovine-based Zyderm and Zyplast collagen products is preceded by two skin tests. However, patients should be warned that allergic reactions have been reported, on rare occasion, even after two negative skin tests.

In a series of 290 patients treated with Artecoll (which also contains bovine collagen), Lemperle[39] noted an acute allergic reaction in one woman who had received Zyderm collagen 2 years earlier. However, after repeated testing for sensitivity, there was no reaction noted in a patient with a prior history of a delayed cell-mediated immune response to Zyderm 4 years earlier. Since the collagen used in Artecoll is intended to act as a carrier rather than a filler, it is partially denatured to insure more rapid dissolution. It is also processed in such a way that it has a much lower quantity of potentially sensitizing non-collagen protein. The reported allergy rate with Artecoll collagen is 0.78% compared to approximately 1–3% for Zyderm/Zyplast. Although Health Canada does not require skin testing prior to Artecoll treatment, the distributor of Artecoll in Canada (Canderm Pharma, Saint-Laurent, Quebec) currently recommends a single skin test to the collagen component of Artecoll. If no reaction occurs, Artecoll treatment may be administered 1 month following skin test placement. Two patients out of approximately 250 tested by one of the authors (S.V.P.) have reported temporary (1 week or less) reactions at skin test sites. Although methylmethacrylate monomers, such as those found in adhesives, can be sensitizing, totally polymerized PMMA—such as that found in Artecoll—is not known to cause sensitization.

With most injectables, appropriate patient preparation will eliminate the potential problems associated with predictable short-term side effects. For example, patients with a low pain threshold should be pretreated with topical and injectable anesthetic to avoid undue anxiety and minimize the amount of pain associated with treatment. Gently telling the patient what to expect, in a reassuring and calm voice, goes a long way in relaxing them. Patients should also be made aware of reasonable outcomes, and need to understand that additional treatment sessions may be required to reach an entirely satisfactory outcome. Treatment should be administered with the patient in a reclined or tilted position, preferably on an adjustable chair or table, which can be placed into Trendelenburg position in the event of a vasovagal episode.

Signs of an impending vasovagal episode include the rapid appearance of facial skin pallor, diaphoresis, lightheadedness, and nausea. At the first sign of such an event, the patient should be placed in a fully reclined position, preferably with the legs higher than the upper body, and measures taken to prevent bodily injury. Since these patients usually experience a brief loss of consciousness and, frequently, a mild seizure, they should not be left alone. A moist cloth or cool pack is placed on the brow until recovery occurs. Patients should be gradually placed into an upright position as their lightheadedness settles. Too rapid a return to the upright position can lead to orthostatic hypotension and further significant lightheadedness. Anecdotally, one author has found this to be much more common in patients who have not eaten on the day of treatment.

Some patients are concerned by the fact that they can palpate the implant under the skin, either as a thread-like or beaded area. In general, although these can be felt by the patient, they are not visible. Whereas initially these may feel quite hard, they tend to soften over time as the fibrotic response matures and softens. Patients are best forewarned of this common finding in a pretreatment information sheet or informed consent form. Occasionally, irregularities in the form of small beads of injected material will occur, especially in the soft tissues of the lips.

With most injectable dermal fillers, acute postinjection swelling and/or erythema may persist for 1–2 days, while bruising, if present, can last for 1 week. Inflammation postinjection is more common with the hyaluronans than with collagen products. Asymmetry may occur if injections are not performed in a balanced fashion. This can usually be corrected with supplemental injections to even out the contour defect. Occasional late side-effects with bovine collagen injections have included persistent redness, tissue necrosis at the glabella (presumably due to vascular occlusion), abscess or granuloma formation, and contour irregularity. One case of partial blindness has been reported with Zyderm collagen treatment near the eye,[63] but is a possible sequela with any of the filler products used in the glabellar region if not properly implanted.

Similar mild adverse events have been noted with most of the other temporary intradermal fillers in current use. Artecoll deserves special mention since it is a permanent filler and, as such, can give rise to more longstanding complications similar to those that were seen with silicone in the past. The appearance of a raised, whitish-blue ridge at the treatment site is indicative of too superficial placement of this material, which should ideally be placed in the deep dermis. Careful injection into the deep dermis and avoidance of treating very thin skin will minimize the risk of ridging. Should blanching be observed following a too superficial injection, the implant should be massaged aggressively to disperse and flatten the injected material. If a wrinkle is too superficial to be erased totally with Artecoll, collagen or hyaluronic acid gels can be implanted intradermally above the Artecoll implant in order to improve the result.[39]

There is evidence to suggest that the appearance of lumps and bumps, presumably associated with clumping of material, is more likely to occur in the lips, especially with Radiesse or Artecoll. These are generally quite subtle and are not usually of significant cosmetic concern. In the case of Radiesse, these will eventually go away, although it may take months to years. Intralesional injections of triamcinolone acetonide 2.5–5.0 mg/ml will help soften and shrink such lumps but unless they are of considerable concern to the patient, they are best left alone to soften with time. If they are substantial in size, they can be surgically excised with minimal scarring when approached from the mucosa lip. This complication can be partially prevented by gently kneading the treatment sites as the implant is placed, smoothing any irregularities as they are encountered and by diligent mouth rest on the patient's part post-treatment.

The only significant complication reported with PMMA microsphere implant has been granuloma formation with a reported incidence of up to 1 in 1000.[91,92] In this situation, rather than normal encapsulation of the PMMA beads occurring, a granulomatous response to the implant ensues with areas of chronic redness, inflammation, and swelling. In one animal study, the biocompatibility of Artecoll was questioned, in particular its potential for inciting immune reactions.[92] However, work by Aracil Kessler et al.[93] indicated no detectable change in the immunoglobulins IgE and IgG and triptase following Artecoll implantation in New Zealand rabbits.

Additional complications that are more common to soft implants than fillers include infection, extrusion, migration, shrinkage, hardening, and development of foreign body granulomas. If the implant should become infected, try initially treating with oral antibiotics. If the infection does not resolve, the implant must be removed. Should extrusion of the implant occur, trim the extruding material under sterile conditions and close the exit site loosely, allowing for drainage. Inform the patient that as little movement as possible of the lip is best to allow optimal healing. Antibiotic ointment also aids in healing. Material that has shrunken, hardened, or migrated necessitates replacement. This is less common with the newer implants such as Ultrasoft and Advanta, which allow tissue ingrowth. Foreign body granulomas may be treated with intralesional steroids before considering surgical intervention. In our experience, swelling and temporary postoperative distortion are common sequela, followed by bruising. Only rarely do we see hematoma, infection, and extrusion.

■ SUMMARY

Since the introduction of injectable bovine collagen in 1982, injectable fillers and soft implants have been an integral part of dermatologic surgery. The proven safety and efficacy of these products encouraged a large number of biotechnology companies to seek to develop the 'ideal' filler material. Patient demand and the desire of dermatologists to respond to the demand have helped a large number of new products to gain acceptance in the international medical market-place over the past several years. Some of these have greater potential than others by virtue of their simplicity of use, prolonged tissue longevity, and minimal risks. The 'ideal' filler may not yet be available, but devices will continue to improve over time.

Clinicians should be aware of the variety of soft-tissue augmentation devices available and in which situations each is most useful. Patients must be educated about their treatment options and reasonable expectations, with regard to treatment outcomes, need to be discussed. An awareness of limitations and potential side-effects is useful for both physicians and patients. When significant solar elastosis and cutaneous laxity is present, surgical techniques are more appropriate and effective therapy than are injectables or soft implants alone.

■ REFERENCES

1. Heidingsfeld ML. Histo-pathology of paraffin prosthesis. J Cutan Dis 1906; 24:513–521.
2. Ashley FL, Braley S, Rees TD, et al. The present status of silicone fluid in soft-tissue augmentation. Plast Reconstr Surg 1967; 39:411–420.
3. Duffy D. Injectable liquid silicone: New perspectives. In: Klein AW, ed. Tissue augmentation in clinical practice: Procedures and techniques. New York: Marcel Dekker; 1998:237–267.
4. Benedetto AV, Lewis AT. Injecting 1000 centistoke liquid silicone with ease and precision. Dermatol Surg 2003; 29: 211–214.
5. Klein AW. Implantation techniques for injectable collagen: Two-and-one-half years of personal clinical experience. J Am Acad Dermatol 1983; 9:224–228.
6. Kaplan EN, Falces E, Tolleth H. Clinical utilization of injectable collagen. Ann Plast Surg 1983; 10:437–451.
7. Tromovitch TA, Stegman SJ, Glogau RG. Zyderm collagen: Implant techniques. J Am Acad Dermatol 1984; 10:273–278.
8. Castrow FFII, Krull EA. Injectable collagen implant—update. J Am Acad Dermatol 1983; 9:889–893.
9. Clark DP, Hanke CW, Swanson NA. Dermal implants: Safety of products injected for soft-tissue augmentation. J Am Acad Dermatol 1989; 21:992–998.
10. Siegle RJ, McCoy JP Jr, Schade W, Swanson NA. Intradermal implantation of bovine collagen: Humoral responses associated with clinical reaction. Arch Dermatol 1984; 120:183–187.
11. Keefe J, Wauk L, Chu S, DeLustro F. Clinical use of injectable bovine collagen: a decade of experience. Clin Mater 1992; 9:155–162.
12. Neuber F. Fat grafting. Cuir Kongr Verh Otsum Ges Chir 1893; 20:66.
13. Thompson N: Tissue transplantation. In: Grabb W, Smith J, eds. Plastic surgery. Boston: Little, Brown 1973; 106–130.
14. Sattler G, Sommer B. Liporecycling: a technique for facial rejuvenation and body contouring. Dermatol Surg 2000; 12:1140–1144.
15. Coleman SR. Structural fat grafts: the ideal filler? Clin Plast Surg 2001; 28:111–119.
16. Coleman WP IIIrd, Lawrence N, Sherman RN, et al. Autologous collagen? Lipocytic dermal augmentation. A histopathologic study. J Dermatol Surg Oncol 1993; 19:1032–1040.
17. Sclafani AP, Romo T IIIrd. Collagen, human collagen, and fat: the search for a three-dimensional soft tissue filler. Facial Plast Surg 2001; 17:79–85.
18. Swinehart JM. Dermal grafting. Dermatol Clin 2001; 19:509–522.
19. Gormley DE, Eremia S. Quantitative assessment of augmentation therapy. J Dermatol Surg Oncol 1990; 12:1147–1151.
20. Fournier PF. Microlipoextraction et microlipoinjection. Rev Chir Aesthet Lang Franc 1985; 10:36–40.
21. Coleman SR. Long-term survival of fat transplants: Controlled demonstrations. Aesthetic Plast Surg 1995; 19:421–425.
22. Dzubow L, Goldman G. Introduction to soft-tissue augmentation: A historical perspective. In: Klein AW, ed. Tissue augmentation in clinical practice: Procedures and techniques. New York: Marcel Dekker 1998; 1–22.
23. Spangler AS. New treatment for pitted scars. Arch Dermatol 1957; 76:708–711.
24. Gottlieb S. GAP repair technique. Poster presentation. Annual meeting of the American Academy of Dermatology, Dallas, TX, 1977.
25. Millikan L. Long-term safety and efficacy with Fibrel in the treatment of cutaneous scars—results of a multicenter study. J Dermatol Surg Oncol 1989; 15:837–842.
26. Gold MH. The Fibrel mechanism of action study. A preliminary report. J Dermatol Surg Oncol 1994; 20:586–590.
27. Treatment of depressed cutaneous scars with gelatin matrix implant: a multicenter study. J Am Acad Dermatol 1987; 16:1155–1162.
28. Cheng JT, Perkins SW, Hamilton MM. Collagen and injectable fillers. Otolaryngol Clin North Am 2002; 35:73–85.
29. Ashinoff R. Overview: soft-tissue augmentation. Clin Plast Surg 2000; 27:479–487.
30. Krauss MC. Recent advances in soft-tissue augmentation. Semin Cutan Med Surg 1999; 18:119–128.
31. Pollack S. Some new injectable dermal filler materials: Hylaform, Restylane, and Artecoll. J Cutan Med Surg 1999; 3(Suppl.4):s27–s35.
32. Balazs EA, Denlinger JL. Clinical uses of hyaluronan. In: Evered D, Whelan J, eds. The biology of hyaluronan (Ciba Foundation Symposium #143). Chichester and New York: John Wiley 1989; 265–280.
33. Hamburger MI, Lakhanpal S, Mooar PA, Oster D. Intra-articular hyaluronans: A review of product-specific safety profiles. Sem Arthrit Rheum 2003; 32:296–309.
34. Piacquadio DJ, Larsen NE, Denlinger JL, Balazs EA. Hylan B Gel (Hylaform) as a soft-tissue augmentation material. In: Klein AW, ed. Tissue augmentation in clinical practice: Procedures and techniques. New York: Marcel Dekker 1998; 269–291.
35. Balasz EA, Bland PA, Denlinger JL, et al. Matrix engineering. Blood Coag Fibrin 1991; 2:173–178.
36. Goa KL, Benfield P. Hyaluronic acid. A review of its pharmacology and use as a surgical aid in ophthalmology, and its therapeutic potential in joint disease and wound healing. Drugs 1994; 47:536–566.
37. Lemperle G, Ott H, Charrier U, et al. PMMA microspheres for intradermal implantation: Part I: Animal research. Ann Plast Surg 1991; 26:57–63.
38. Lemperle G. Hazan-Gauthier N, Lemperle N. PMMA-microspheres (Artecoll) for skin and soft-tissue augmentation. Part II: Clinical investigations. Plast Reconstr Surg 1995; 96:627–634.
39. Lemperle G, Gauthier-Hazan N, Lemperle N. PMMA-microspheres (Artecoll) for long-lasting correction of wrinkles: Refinements and statistical results. Aesth Plast Surg 1998; 22:356–365.
40. Soyer T, Lempier MA, Cooper P, et al. A new venous prosthesis. Surgery 1972; 72:864–872.
41. Florian A, Cohn LH, Dammin GJ, Collins JJ Jr. Small vessel replacement with Gore-Tex (expanded polytetrafluoroethylene). Arch Surg 1976; 111:267–270.

42. McAuley CE. Seven year follow-up of expanded polytetrafluoroethylene in femoro-popliteal bypass grafts. Ann Surg 1984; 199:57–60.
43. Bauer JJ, Salky BA, Gelernt IM, Kriel I. Repair of large abdominal wall defects with expanded polytetrafluoroethylene (EPTFE). Ann Surg 1987; 206:765–769.
44. Maas CS, Gnepp DR, Bumpous J. Expanded polytetrafluoroethylene (Gore-Tex) in facial bone augmentation. Arch Otolaryngol Head Neck Surg 1993; 119:1008–1015.
45. Waldman RS. Gore-Tex for augmentation of the nasal dorsum: A preliminary report. Ann Plast Surg 1991; 26:520–525.
46. Lassus C. Expanded PTFE in the treatment of facial wrinkles. Aesth Plast Surg 1991; 15:167–174.
47. Conrad K, Reifen E. Gore-Tex implant as a tissue filler in cheek-lip groove rejuvenation. J Otolaryngol 1992; 21:218–222.
48. Cisneros JL, Singla R. Intradermal augmentation with expanded polytetrafluoroethylene (Gore-Tex) for facial lines and wrinkles. J Dermatol Surg Oncol 1993; 19:539–542.
49. Ellis DA, Trimas SJ. Gore-Tex implants for correction of thin lips. Laryngoscope 1995; 105:207–209.
50. Miller PJ, Levine J, Ahn MS, Maas CS, Constantinides M. Softform for facial rejuvenation: historical review, operative techniques, and recent advances. Facial Plast Surg 2000; 16:23–28.
51. Truswell WH. Dual-porosity expanded polytetrafluoroethylene soft tissue implant: a new implant for facial soft-tissue augmentation. Arch Facial Plast Surg 2002; 4:92–97.
52. Hanke CW. A new e-PTFE soft tissue implant for natural-looking augmentation of lips and wrinkles. Dermatol Surg 2002; 28:901–908.
53. Coleman WP. Soft-tissue augmentation. In: Ratz JL, ed. Textbook of dermatologic surgery. Philadelphia: Lippencott-Raven 1998; 565–577.
54. Terino EO. Alloderm acellular dermal graft: applications in aesthetic and reconstructive soft tissue augmentation. In: Klein AW, ed. Tissue augmentation in clinical practice: Procedures and techniques. New York: Marcel Dekker; 1998:349–377.
55. Rubin PA, Fay AM, Remulla HD, Maus M. Ophthalmic plastic applications of acellular dermal allografts. Ophthalmology 1999; 106:2091–2097.
56. Abenavoli FM, Corelli R, Vittori I. Use of AlloDerm for lip reaugmentation. Ann Plast Surg 2002 ; 48:447–448.
57. Sclafani AP, Romo T 3rd, Jacono AA. Rejuvenation of the aging lip with an injectable acellular dermal graft (Cymetra). Arch Facial Plast Surg 2002; 4:252–257.
58. Mayer RD, Lightfoot M, Jung I. Preliminary evaluation of calcium hydroxylapatite as a transurethral bulking agent for stress urinary incontinence. Urology 2001; 57:434–438.
59. Raveh T, Weinberg A, Sibirsky O, et al. Efficacy of the topical anaesthetic cream, EMLA, in alleviating both needle insertion and injection pain. Ann Plast Surg 1995; 35:576–579.
60. Klein AW. Collagen substitutes: bovine collagen. Clin Plast Surg 2001; 28:53–62.
61. Carruthers J, Carruthers A. Mad cows, prions, and wrinkles. Arch Dermatol. 2002; 138:667–670.
62. Hanke CW, Jolivette D, Stegman SJ, et al. Abscess formation and local necrosis following treatment with Zyderm or Zyplast collagen implant. J Am Acad Dermatol 1991; 25:319–326.
63. Cucin RL, Barek D. Complications of injectable collagen implants. Plast Reconstr Surg 1983; 71:731.
64. Klein AW. In favor of double skin testing. J Dermatol Surg Oncol 1989; 15:263.
65. Hanke CW, Coleman WP III. Dermal filler substances. In: Coleman WP III, Hanke CW, Alt TH, Asken S, eds. Cosmetic surgery of the skin: Principles and techniques, 2nd edn. St Louis: Mosby Year Book 1997; 217–230.
66. Moody BR, Sengelmann RS. Topical Tacrolimus in the treatment of bovine collagen hypersensitivity. Dermatol Surg 2001; 27:789–791.
67. Baumann LS, Kerdel F. The treatment of bovine collagen allergy with cyclosporine. Dermatol Surg 1999; 25:247–249.
68. Fournier P. Facial recontouring with fat grafting. Dermatol Clin 1990; 8:523–537.
69. Zocchi M. Methode de production de collagene autologue par traitment du tissu graisseax. J de Med Aesthet Chirurg Dermatol 1990; 17:105–114.
70. Coleman WP III, Lawrence N, Sherman RN, et al. Autologous collagen: lipocytic dermal augmentation. A histopathologic study. J Dermatol Surg Oncol 1993; 19:1032–1040.
71. Boss WK Jr, Marko O. Isolagen. In: Klein AW, ed. Tissue augmentation in clinical practice: Procedures and techniques. New York: Marcel Dekker 1998; 335–347.
72. Fagien S. Facial soft-tissue augmentation with autologous and homologous injectable collagen (Autologen and Dermalogen). In: Klein AW, ed. Tissue augmentation in clinical practice: Procedures and techniques. New York: Marcel Dekker 1998; 97–124.
73. Fagien S. Facial soft-tissue augmentation with injectable autologous and allogeneic human tissue collagen matrix (Autologen and Dermalogen). Plast Reconstr Surg 2000; 105:362–373.
74. Burres S. Soft-tissue augmentation with Fascian. Clin Plastic Surg 2001; 28:101–110.
75. Comper WD, Laurent TC. Physiological function of connective tissue polysaccharides. Physiol Rev 1978; 58:255–315.
76. Balazs EA, Darzynkiewicz Z. The effect of hyaluronic acid on fibroblasts, mononuclear phagocytes and lymphocytes. In: Kulonen E, Pikkarainen J, eds. Biology of the fibroblast. London: Academic Press 1973; 237–252.
77. Feinberg RN, Beebe DC. Hyaluronate vasculogenesis. Science 1983; 220:1177–1179.
78. Ghersetich I, Lotti T, Campanile G, Grappone C, Dini G. Hyaluronic acid in cutaneous intrinsic aging. Int J Dermatol 1994; 33:119–122.
79. DeVore DP, Hughes E, Scott JB. Effectiveness of injectable filler materials for smoothing wrinkle lines and depressed scars. Med Prog Technol 1994; 20:243–250.
80. Piacquadio DJ, Larsen NE, Denlinger JL, Balazs EA. Hylan B Gel (Hylaform) as a soft-tissue augmentation material. In: Klein AW, ed. Tissue augmentation in clinical practice: Procedures and techniques. New York: Marcel Dekker 1998; 269–291.
81. Reed RK, Laurent UB, Frazer JR, et al. Removal rate of [3H] hyaluronan injected subcutaneously in rabbits. Am J Physiol 1990; 259:H532–535.
82. US Food and Drug Administration (FDA) homepage. New Medical Device Approvals – Hylaform (hylan B gel). http://www.fda.gov/cdrh/mda/docs/p030032.html (last accessed May 2004).
83. Duranti F, Salti G, Bovani B, et al. Injectable hyaluronic acid gel for soft-tissue augmentation. A clinical and histological study. Dermatol Surg 1998; 24:1317–1325.
84. Olenius M. The first clinical study using a new biodegradable implant for the treatment of lips, wrinkles, and folds. Aesth Plast Surg 1998; 22:97–101.
85. Narins RS, Brandt F, Leyden J, Lorenc ZP, Rubin M. Smith S. A randomized, double-blind, multicenter comparison of the efficacy and tolerability of Restylane versus Zyplast for the correction of nasolabial folds. Dermatol Surg 2003; 29:588-595.
86. Carruthers A, Kiene K, Carruthers J. Botulinum A exotoxin use in clinical dermatology. J Am Acad Dermatol 1996; 34:788–797.
87. Livesey S, Herndon D, Hollyoak M, et al. Transplanted acellular allograft dermal matrix: Potential as a template for the reconstruction of viable dermis. Transplantation 1995; 60:19.
88. Eppley, BL. Experimental assessment of the revascularization of acellular human dermis for soft-tissue augmentation. Plast Reconstr Surg 2001; 107:757–762.
89. Mang WL, Sawatzki K. Fremdkörperreaktion nach implantation von PMMA (Polymethylmethacrylat) zur weichteilaugmentation. Zeitschr Hautkrankheiten H+G 1998; 73:42–44.
90. Adams WP Jr, Conner WC., Barton FE Jr, et al. Optimizing breast pocket irrigation: an in vitro study and clinical implications. Plast Reconstr Surg 2000; 105:334–338.
91. Hoffmann C, Schuller-Petrovic S, Soyer P, et al. Adverse reactions after cosmetic lip augmentation with permanent biologically inert implant materials. J Am Acad Dermatol 1999; 40:100–102.
92. McClelland M, Egbert B, Hanko V, et al. Evaluation of Artecoll polymethacrylate implant for soft-tissue augmentation: biocompatibility and chemical characterization. Plast Reconstr Surg 1997; 100:1466–1474.
93. Aracil Kessler JP, Diaz Torres JM, Martin Garcia RF. Artecoll: An experimental study. Cir Plast Ibero-Latinoamer 1997; 23:389.
94. Friedman PM, Mafong EA, Kauvar AN, et al. Safety data of injectable non-animal stabilized hyaluronic acid gel for soft-tissue augmentation. Dermatol Surg 2002; 28:491–494.
95. Klein AW. Collagen substances. Facial Plast Surg Clin North Am 2001; 9:205–218.
96. Sclafani AP, McCormick SA. Autologous collagen dispersion (Autologen) as a dermal filler: clinical observations and histologic findings. Arch Facial Plast Surg 2000; 2:48–52.

97. Bergeret-Galley C, Illonz YZ. The value of a new filler material in corrective and cosmetic surgery: Dermalive and Dermadeep. Aesthet Plast Surg 2001; 25:249–255.

98. Watson D, Lask GP. Autologous fibroblasts for treatment of facial rhytids and dermal depressions. A pilot study. Arch Facial Plast Surg 1999; 1:165–170.

99. Berry J. New-Fill for an old face. Positively Aware: The Monthly Journal of the Test Positive Aware Network 2002; 13:34–35.

100. Sclafani AP, Romo T IIIrd, Jacono AA, et al. Evaluation of acellular dermal graft (Alloderm) sheet for soft-tissue augmentation: a 1-year follow-up of clinical observations and histological findings. Arch Facial Plast Surg 2001; 3:101–103.

101. Drobeck HP, Rothstein SS, Gumaer KI, et al. Histologic observation of soft tissue responses to implanted, multifaceted particles and discs of hydroxylapatite. J Oral Maxillofac Surg 1984; 42:143–149.

102. Maas CS, Denton AB. Synthetic soft tissue substitutes: 2001. Facial Plast Surg Clin North Am 2001; 9:219–227.

103. US Food and Drug Administration (FDA) homepage. New Medical Device Approvals – Hylaform Plus. http://www.fda.gov/cdrh/pdf3/p030032s001.html (last accessed October 2004).

104. Lemperle G, Morhenn V, Charrier U. Human histology and persistence of various injectable filler substances for soft tissue augmentation. Aesthetic Plast Surg 2003; 27:354–366.

29 Chemical Peels

Sue Ellen Cox MD and Kimberly J Butterwick MD

Summary box

- Chemical peeling is the application of one or more exfoliating agents, usually an acid, to produce a controlled partial-thickness injury to the skin.
- After healing, the skin has improved color and texture.
- Indications include photoaged skin, various pigmentation disorders, epidermal growths such as actinic and seborrheic keratoses.
- Peels may be superficial, medium, or deep, depending on the indication.
- Most peels are carried out on the face, but body peeling can also be carried out, usually using a lower concentration of exfoliating agent.
- Complications increase with depth of peel, the most common being irregular pigmentation; hyperpigmentation is usually transient, but hypopigmentation is an expected sequela of deep peels.

INTRODUCTION

Chemical peeling is the application of one or more exfoliating agents to the skin, to produce a controlled partial-thickness injury. The agent, usually an acid solution, destroys varying amounts of epidermis depending on the strength, and affects dermal collagen.[1] Partial-thickness wounds heal by second intention with overlying skin acting as a biologic dressing before it sloughs. Wound repair consists of epidermal regeneration by migration from adnexal structures or epithelium derived from adjacent uninjured skin.[2] Replacement of epidermis and dermal connective tissue results in skin rejuvenation. The results include an improvement in skin color, texture and removal of actinically related growths.

Long-term sun exposure accounts for a significant amount of the damage that we associate with aged skin. Most of this damage is from overexposure to ultraviolet (UV) light. The sun and artificial tanning lights are both sources of light that can be harmful to the skin.[3] The skin is primarily affected by UVA and UVB in the wavelengths of 320–400 nm and 290–320 nm respectively. The UVA radiation penetrates deeper in the skin and damages the elastic tissues deeper in the dermis than UVB. In the UVA range, light is absorbed by proteins and lipid. In the UVB range, absorption affects the DNA.[4] In photoaging, the skin surface is rough and dry because of an accumulation of corneocytes. Chronically, photo-induced changes of the skin include thickening, sallowing and a coarsely wrinkled appearance.

The level of injury and the depth of penetration into the skin quantify superficial, medium, and deep peels (Fig. 29.1, Table 29.1). It is important to match the skin pathology to the chemical agent. For instance, a patient with extensive actinic keratoses would be better served by a medium-depth peel; whereas a patient with acne would do better with more superficial agents such as glycolic acid or salicylic acid peels.

Preparation of the skin before chemical peeling is extremely important. In the author's opinion, the simplest skin care program consists of patient education about sun avoidance, the use of effective sunscreen on a daily basis and pre-treatment with tretinoin or tazarotene and/or alpha hydroxy acids (AHAs) (Table 29.2).

HISTORY

Aesthetic improvement of the skin dates back to ancient Egypt. Papyruses contain descriptions of the use of acids, balms and oils for chemical peeling. Greek, and later Roman, physicians used sour milk, grape juice and lemon extracts for rejuvenation. The active ingredients in these substances were the AHAs—lactic acid, tartaric acid, and citric acid.[5] Light mechanical exfoliation similar to current popular microdermabrasion was performed in India with pumice to exfoliate the stratum corneum.

Dermatologists pioneered the therapeutic use of chemical peeling in the latter half of the 19th century. In 1882, the German dermatologist Unna described using salicylic acid, resorcinol, phenol and trichloroacetic acid (TCA) for chemical peeling.[5] In England, a British

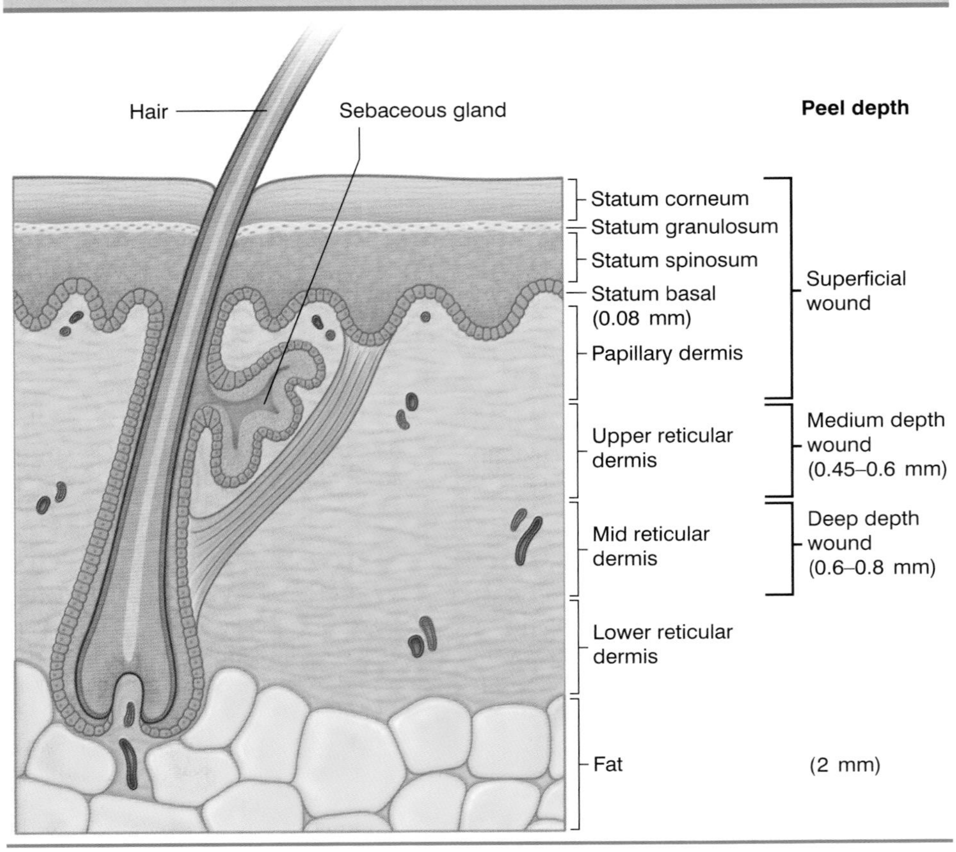

Peel depths

Hair
Sebaceous gland
Peel depth
Statum corneum
Statum granulosum
Statum spinosum
Statum basal (0.08 mm)
Papillary dermis
Upper reticular dermis
Mid reticular dermis
Lower reticular dermis
Fat
Superficial wound
Medium depth wound (0.45–0.6 mm)
Deep depth wound (0.6–0.8 mm)
(2 mm)

Figure 29.1 Peel depths.

Table 29.1 Classification of chemical peels

Type	Depth of penetration
Superficial	Epidermis to papillary dermis
Medium	Papillary dermis to upper reticular dermis
Deep	Mid-reticular dermis

Table 29.2 Preoperative preparations for chemical peeling

Sun avoidance
Tretinoin/tazarotene
Alpha hydroxy acids (AHAs)
Sunscreen
Hydroquinone (as indicated by skin type and depth of peel injury)
Antiviral medication (as indicated by skin type and depth of peel injury)

dermatologist named Mackee used phenol as a peeling agent to treat acne scarring as early as 1903 and published 50 years of experience with these peels in 1952.[6] During World War I, LaGasse used phenol to treat facial gun-powder burns.[3] His daughter Antoinette, a non-physician, brought phenol chemical peeling to the US. During this time chemical peels offered by salons often resulted in extensive skin sloughing and scarring.[5]

In the 1940s, physicians made great strides in advancing the knowledge of chemical peeling. Highlights include Eller and Wolff's description of peeling agents including sulfur, resorcinol, salicylic acid, phenol and carbon dioxide (CO_2) slush.[5] In the 1940s and 1950s a 'secret' formula that contained phenol was brought by 'lay peelers' to the US from Eastern Europe. Litton, Baker and Gordon provided the scientific clinical works demonstrating the dramatic effects following phenol facial peels.[7–10] Monash described his use of TCA for treating scarring.[11] Later, Ayres combined the TCA experiments of Monash with his own clinical experience and histology comparing TCA to phenol.[11]

In the early 1960s, otolaryngologists, dermatologists and plastic surgeons published works on clinical experience with phenol formulas. It is Baker and Gordon's modified phenol peel that is the standard deep chemical peel used today.[12]

In the early 1980s Stegman's comparison of different wounding agents based on histology set the stage for a more academic approach to chemical peeling.[13] Simultaneously, VanScott and Yu published extensively on the effects of AHAs on the stratum corneum.[14] This led to the widespread use of superficial AHA peels by dermatologists in the 1990s.

Brody and Hailey introduced the concept of using two superficial peeling agents to produce a medium-depth peel in 1986. They combined solid CO_2 followed by TCA to produce skin injury to the level of upper reticular dermis.[15] In 1989, Monheit described the use of Jessner's solution followed by the application of 35% TCA. This medium-depth peel is extremely popular and reproducibly safe and effective.[16] Coleman published on the combination of glycolic acid plus TCA to produce medium-depth injury to the skin.[17]

■ PREOPERATIVE PREPARATION

Preparing the skin for chemical peeling

Tretinoin

Numerous benefits may be seen with the use of topical tretinoin on photodamaged skin. Tretinoin improves skin texture and reduces fine wrinkling and mottled hyperpigmentation.[18–21] Histologically, tretinoin increases epidermal layer thickness, decreases melanin content and causes stratum corneum compaction.[16,22] Tretinoin also increases dermal collagen production and stimulates angiogenesis.[23,24] These effects may account for the improved wound healing in patients that are pretreated before resurfacing procedures.

Topical tretinoin pretreatment accelerates wound healing after medium-depth chemical peels. In a double-blind, placebo- controlled, prospective, randomized study, 16 men with actinically damaged skin were treated daily with tretinoin 0.1% versus placebo cream to the left and right halves of the face and the left and right forearms and hands, respectively, for 14 days before a 35% TCA peel.[25] After peel healing was evaluated on days 3, 5, 7, 9, 11 and 14, the appearance of intact, pink skin after the brown desiccated skin had sloughed off was an indication of re-epithelialization. In 94% of the patients, the sloughing occurred earlier and was more uniform, regardless of body location, in skin pretreated with tretinoin than with placebo treated skin. The differences between tretinoin and placebo, respectively, in healed skin were maximal after 5 days for the face (68% vs 52%), after 11 days for the forearms (72% vs 24%) and after 9 days for the hands (61% vs 29%).[25,26]

The American Academy of Dermatology (AAD) Guidelines Outcomes committee developed 'Guidelines of Care for Chemical Peeling' to enhance quality of care for patients having cosmetic procedures. This AAD committee recommended tretinoin pretreatment as preparation for skin that is undergoing chemical peeling. The committee also recommended postoperative tretinoin to enhance wound healing and maintain results.[27]

Tretinoin should be started in advance of the chemical peel. Six weeks or more is preferable. Once re-epithelialization has occurred tretinoin should be re-started initially using a low concentration emollient or cream preparation such as 0.02% Renova (Ortho Pharmaceutical Corporation, Raritan, NJ) or 0.025% tretinoin cream. Newer retinoic acid receptor creams such as tazarotene can be used before and after peels and may be more effective then tretinoin.[28]

Alphahydroxy acids

AHAs have been used both before peels and as a superficial chemical peeling agent. They exert their epidermal effect at the level of the stratum corneum and granulosum junction. A thinner stratum corneum with a normal-appearing basket weave pattern is achieved by reducing corneocyte cohesion. This produces a smoother, more supple skin surface.[29]

The use of AHAs has been shown to reverse histologic signs of photoaging. AHAs used regularly for 6 months resulted in a 25% increase in epidermal thickness and papillary dermal thickness. There was also an increase in mucopolysaccharides, improved quality of elastic fibers and increased collagen density. Additionally there was a reversal in basal cell atypia, dispersing melanin pigmentation and normalization of the rete pattern of the dermoepidermal junction.[30]

AHAs have also been used as an adjunct to tretinoin therapy without increasing adverse sequelae.[31–33]

Sunscreens

Sunscreens work by absorbing, reflecting and scattering UV light. The effectiveness of the sunscreen is indicated by a sun protection factor (SPF), which represents the ratio of the amount of radiation needed to produce erythema with and without sunscreen.[34] A sunscreen should be chosen that blocks both UVA and UVB radiation. The main objective is to diminish the degree of baseline pigmentation and lessen the potential for developing hyperpigmentation. The decrease in UV damage allows the skin to rest before the peel. This should be started at least 3 months before the peel and continued indefinitely after the peel.[35]

Hydroquinone

Many surgeons advocate the use of pretreatment with hydroquinones to reduce the risk of postinflammatory hyperpigmentation following resurfacing procedures. Hydroquinone is cytotoxic to melanocytes; it decreases melanosome formation by inhibiting tyrosinase. Alster and West carried out a randomized study of 100 patients pretreated with topical skin lightening agents versus placebo 2 weeks before laser resurfacing. There was no significant difference in the incidence of hyperpigmentation after resurfacing in the pretreated groups or the placebo group.[36] The use of hydroquinones postoperatively for post-inflammatory hyperpigmentation is effective.[37]

Antiviral prophylaxis

All resurfacing procedures have the potential to reactivate herpes simplex virus (HSV). Active HSV infection is a contraindication to proceeding with a chemical peel. Because many patients are unaware of their exposure to the HSV, it is prudent to use prophylaxis for all patients before a medium-depth peel. Antiviral agents have been shown to be effective in reducing reactivation. A recent study looked at infection rates following laser resurfacing after using prophylactic valacyclovir 500 mg twice a day beginning the day before the procedure and continuing for 10 or 14 days following the procedure; of 120 patients, no patient developed an HSV infection or recurrence.[38]

Photography

All patients should have preoperative photographs taken to document the degree of actinic damage and facial dyschromia. Additionally, patients tend to forget their preoperative appearance and it is helpful for them to appreciate the degree of improvement by looking at their preoperative photographs. To this end, in our office (SEC) we use the Mirror Image Suite version 6.1.0 by Canfield Imaging Systems (see also Chapter 6).

Consent

Patients are educated and given the opportunity to ask questions before signing a consent form for chemical peeling.

The consent specifies the most common risks associated with peels. These include stinging, burning sensation of the skin, visible peeling, scaling, pigmentary changes, infections, and rarely, scarring.

Consultation

At the consultation it is important to identify the patients' motivation for improvement (Table 29.3). It is the physicians' responsibility to direct the patient to the most effective treatment based on the individual's problems and risk tolerance. The physician needs to explain the limitations of each type of peel and make sure that the patient has realistic expectations. It is essential that the physician explains the postoperative course, especially with medium and deep peels. It is helpful for patients to see photographs taken after a peel so that they can visualize the healing process. In our experience, verbal descriptions are rarely adequate. It is also important to stress the post-operative care needed to ensure a good result. It is important to ascertain the patient's lifestyle with regard to recreational activities and sun exposure. It is necessary to stress to patients that it is their responsibility to protect their skin from sun exposure before the peel, during the healing phase and thereafter to ensure that dyschromia and postinflammatory hyperpigmentation do not occur.

A questionnaire filled out by the patient before the consultation is helpful so that the physician is aware of pertinent medical history. Relevant history includes HSV infection immunosuppression, radiation exposure, keloid formation or previous development of postinflammatory hyperpigmentation. Active viral, bacterial or fungal infection preclude chemical peeling until completely resolved. Additionally, the use of oral minocycline during skin injury can cause hyperpigmentation.

Medications and past medical and surgical history should be carefully reviewed. Patients who have been on isotretinoin within the past 6–12 months should not be resurfaced. Isotretinoin produces atrophy of the pilosebaceous unit. Re-epithelialization originates from these adnexal structures so their alteration can impair wound healing and increase the risk of scarring. Similarly, patients who have had exposure to previous facial radiation therapy have fewer adnexal structures and have a higher risk for scarring after dermal injury.

Although immunosuppression can increase the risk of infection after resurfacing and therefore delay healing and scarring, these risks can be mitigated by the use of prophylactic antivirals, antibiotics and antifungals. Immunosuppression is not therefore a strict contraindication.

Previous recent facial surgery in which the blood supply to the skin has been compromised by surgical undermining, such as in facial rhytidectomy or a large flap repair for skin cancer, is a contraindication for mid-level and deep peels that affect the dermis. We recommend delaying resurfacing for at least 6 months in these circumstances.

Smokers have impaired microcirculation to the skin and increased rates of infection. Additionally, smoking damages the elastic fibers and collagen, producing an increase in wrinkling and actinic damage. Smokers can benefit from chemical peeling, but need to be educated about realistic expectations and complications.

SUPERFICIAL CHEMICAL PEELS

Superficial chemical peeling is the application of wounding agents to injure part or all of the epidermis, which may in turn lead to mild stimulation of collagen production in the superficial papillary dermis. Many agents of varying strengths can accomplish this goal (Table 29.4). The indications for superficial peeling include melasma, postinflammatory hyperpigmentation, ephelides, acne vulgaris, solar lentigines, photoaging and fine rhytides. The popularity of superficial peels underscores the many advantages of light peels (Table 29.5). The rapid healing, relatively low cost and minimal risk, even in darker skin types offsets the limitations of the procedure for most patients (Table 29.6). Unfortunately, marketing hyperbole about 'lunchtime peels' has created unrealistic patient expectations. It is important to set appropriate patient expectations at the outset. Superficial peels are helpful in the treatment of acne and may improve melasma. They provide smoothness and luster to photo-damaged skin, but will not usually eliminate fine lines or actinic keratoses.[39] Solar lentigines lighten, but may not resolve. Pore size may or may not diminish.

Table 29.3 Patient evaluation to optimize outcomes

Physician—patient relationship
Patient's realistic expectations
Fitzpatrick skin type
Active infection
Tobacco use
Medications: minocycline, isotretinoin
History of herpes simplex virus (HSV) infection
History of keloid formation
History of previous radiation exposure
History of immunosuppression
History of postinflammatory hyperpigmentation
Recent facial surgery

Table 29.4 Superficial peeling agents

Trichloroacetic acid (TCA) 10–25% (35% [one coat])
Jessner's solution: resorcinol/salicylic acid/lactic acid
Modified Unna's resorcinol paste
Solid carbon dioxide (CO_2) slush
Salicylic acid
AHAs
Tretinoin solution

Table 29.5 Advantages of superficial peels

Excellent safety record
May be used on all Fitzpatrick skin types
Rapid healing, minimal downtime
Repeated peels provide cumulative effects
Amplifies effects of topical rejuvenating agents
Can be combined with laser modalities
May be performed by trained nurses, medical technicians and aestheticians
Affordable
No anesthesia needed

Table 29.6 Limitations of superficial peels

Little clinical effect with one peel
Multiple superficial peels do not equate to one mid-level or deep peel
Media has created unrealistic patient expectations
Minimal effect on medium-to-deep rhytides
Return to before-peel condition within 2 years without topical agents

Patients need to be educated that one peel may have little effect alone. Rather, the combination of a series of three to six peels is likely to produce the best results in conjunction with a topical regimen at home. A common misconception among patients is that multiple superficial peels will produce the same result, as one deeper peel.[13]

Realistic benefits are particularly important to clarify when discussing the outcome of superficial peeling on rhytides and deep acne scarring. If the patient has Glogau group II or III photoaging, multiple superficial peels will not achieve the same results as a medium or deep peel on medium-to-deep rhytides (Table 29.7). Similarly, patients with deep acne scarring will have little benefit from superficial peeling and should be advised accordingly. Patients with both superficial and deep melasma can expect only partial improvement. A Wood's lamp can be used to detect epidermal melasma,[40] but in one study the response to a superficial peel was difficult to predict on the basis of this test.[41]

Ideally, the skin is conditioned before superficial peeling. Patients should be using a sunscreen and avoid active tanning. Tretinoin used topically before peeling accelerates healing, but should be stopped 2–4 days before superficial peeling to ensure an intact epidermis. It is best to start a bleaching agent before peeling in patients with darker skin types or pigmentary disorders. Although the study by Alster and West[36] showed no benefit to using bleaching creams before laser peels, this effect has not been studied for superficial peels. In addition, if an irritant or allergic contact dermatitis develops to hydroquinone or other agents, it is helpful to know this in advance. In general, antiviral agents are prescribed preoperatively in patients with a history of facial herpetic eruptions.

■ TECHNICAL ASPECTS

Superficial peeling varies from producing a very superficial slough of only a few layers of the stratum corneum to producing a slough of the entire epidermis and papillary dermis. The depth of the peel is determined not only by the particular agent and the concentration, but also by the area treated, skin preparation, method of application and the sebaceous quality of the patient's skin (Table 29.8). These variables may change during the course of successive peeling in the same patient and need to be evaluated before each peel.

The technique of application is a significant determinant of the depth of the peel. The type of applicator and the degree of saturation of the applicator determines the amount of peel solution applied. Commonly used applicators include 4 × 4 gauze, 2 × 2 gauze, cotton-tipped applicators and sable brushes. Of these, the sable brush was found to deliver the greatest quantity of solution in one study.[2] The degree of rubbing or pressure and also the number of coats applied further determine the response to the peel. The practitioner should become familiar with one technique and remain consistent when using a particular agent to develop predictability of a given peel.

The condition of the skin and the skin preparation technique similarly influence the depth of peeling. If the patient's epidermal barrier is disrupted for any reason, such as retinoid dermatitis, seborrheic dermatitis or active acne with erosions, the peeling solution may penetrate more deeply and result in a medium-depth peel when a superficial peel was intended.[39] The depth of the peel is also altered by the choice of the skin preparation technique. If the patient has oily skin or advanced photoaging, vigorous degreasing with Septisol (Calgon–Vestal Laboratories, St Louis, MO), alcohol or acetone (one, a combination, or all) may be used for more uniform penetrance of the peel. (The skin may appear lightly frosted after thorough cleansing, manifested by scattered flecks of white frost throughout the pink surface of the skin.) Peikert et al. noted no

Table 29.7 Glogau's classification of photoaging groups

Group	Severity	Age group (years)	Features
I	Mild	Usually 28–35	No keratoses Little wrinkling Little or no make-up
II	Moderate	Usually 35–50	Early actinic keratoses—slight yellow skin discoloration Early wrinkling—parallel smile lines Small amount of make-up
III	Advanced	Usually 50–65	Actinic keratoses–obvious yellow skin discoloration with telangiectasia Wrinkling—present at rest Wears make-up always
IV	Severe	Usually 60–75	Actinic keratoses with skin cancers have occurred Wrinkling—much cutis laxa of actinic, gravitational and dynamic origin Wears make-up that does not cover, but cakes on

Table 29.8 Variables of peeling
Agent selected
Concentration of agent
Technique of application
Skin preparation technique
Previous use of tretinoin
Sebaceous gland density
Integrity of epidermal barrier
Frequency of peeling
Area treated

difference in evenness among four commonly used degreasing agents; acetone, rubbing alcohol, Freon skin degreaser, or Hibiclens.[42] Because of the flammability of acetone, the other agents are preferred. If the patient has thin sensitive skin or a disrupted epidermis, light cleansing with a cotton ball and gentle cleanser is recommended, especially when peeling with AHAs.

The area being treated is also a variable. The central face including the forehead, nose and cheeks has a higher density of sebaceous glands and can usually tolerate more vigorous cleansing and application of the peeling agent than other facial areas, yet heal in the same time interval as areas treated more conservatively. In general, the thicker and more sebaceous the skin, the less susceptible it is to the peeling agent. Nonfacial areas such as the neck, forearms and dorsum of the hands have significantly fewer sebaceous glands and other adnexal structures from which to regenerate new skin. As a result of delayed healing and a tendency to scar, these areas must be peeled conservatively and only with superficial peeling agents repeated over time. With successive peeling, the concentration of the agent applied may be titrated up, depending on the reaction to the peel.

Each practitioner develops a specific pattern for peeling the face, which may differ for superficial, medium or deep peels. In one author's practice (KB), the superficial peeling agent is applied to the forehead first. If the patient is unusually sensitive or has an unusually rapid response to the peeling agent, it is helpful to know this in advance of treating other less sturdy areas. Next, the outer aspects of the face are treated in a clockwise rotation from one temporal region to the other. The nose, cheeks and perioral regions are next treated, and the infraorbital region is treated last. The patient is instructed to keep the eyes closed throughout. Moistened gauze may be placed over the eyes for further protection.

This author's (KB) preferred applicator for superficial peeling is wrung out 4 × 4 gauze for TCA or Jessner's peels. Saturated cotton balls are used for glycolic peeling because they are less abrasive. The infraorbital region is always treated with saturated cotton-tipped applicators regardless of the agent and care is taken to minimize drip or splash exposure to the eyes. The level of discomfort is generally quite tolerable. A handheld fan can be used to minimize discomfort. Occasionally, with 50–70% glycolic acid, the patient experiences more than mild discomfort. With this agent, significant pain is an important sign that the peel is penetrating more deeply and the peel should be neutralized sooner than anticipated with sodium bicarbonate soaked cotton balls.

Superficial peeling agents

Trichloroacetic acid 10–25%

TCA is one of the most commonly used and time-honored agents for superficial peeling. It has no known systemic toxicity. The depth of cutaneous penetration varies with concentration. TCA 10–25% will produce necrosis of superficial layers by precipitation of proteins, clinically causing a mild epidermal slough. Many classify one-coat TCA 35% in the superficial category.[43] However the depth of penetration of this concentration will vary with patient factors and technique, and an intermediate-depth peel can be produced.[27] Aqueous solutions of distilled water mixed with TCA crystals are prepared by the pharmacist and are stable for 6 months at room temperature in amber glass bottles.[44] A solution of TCA 25% consists of 25 g (United States Pharmacopeia, USP, crystals) in 100 ml of distilled water. It is important in mixing that the weight/volume technique of composing is used because tremendous variation in concentration has been noted with other methods.[45,46]

The application method of TCA may be single-to-multiple coats to prepped skin. This author (KB) prefers to use a wrung out 4 × 4 gauze to apply with pressure. With lower concentrations, mild erythema or whitish speckling may be evident. With concentrations of 25% or greater, a distinct white frost is seen. If this does not appear uniform, repeated applications can be made to areas that do not frost. If the frost is unexpectedly rapid or intense, alcohol neutralization may dilute the effect if applied within 30–90 seconds.[47] Patients are told stinging will crescendo for 2 minutes and then subside. Unlike glycolic acid peels, which must be neutralized, TCA peels achieve a depth of penetration based on strength. Cold wet compresses are applied immediately after the peel. Antibiotic ointment is then applied. The white frosting resolves within 2 hours if not sooner.

Light peels can be performed weekly or biweekly at concentrations of 10–15% for acne vulgaris with minimal downtime whereas applications of 25–35% TCA may take 5–7 days to heal with darkening of the face for 2–3 days and fine desquamation on days 3–6. These are predictable peels that can be adjusted to the patient's pathology and available downtime by the concentration used. For pigmentary problems such as postinflammatory hyperpigmentation or melasma one must proceed with caution, especially in darker skin types because results may be variable with TCA and the problem may even worsen. Starting with lower concentrations and/or performing test patches is recommended.[48]

Jessner's solution

Jessner's solution (also known as Combes' formula) consists of 14 g each of resorcinol, salicylic acid and lactic acid in ethanol (Table 29.9). It was formulated by Jessner in the 1940s to reduce the concentrations of salicylic acid and resorcinol and so minimize their respective side-effects—tinnitus with salicylic acid and syncope and thyroid suppression with resorcinol.[49] The result is a good keratolytic that breaks intracellular bridges with minimal side-effects.

Jessner's solution is applied to prepped skin and rubbed in or painted on, depending on the degree of penetration desired. It is not necessary to neutralize this peel. The first

Table 29.9 Jessner's solution formula

Resorcinol 14 g
Salicylic acid 14 g
Lactic acid 14 g
Ethanol 95% qs ad 100 ml[1]

peel usually consists of just one coat, with subsequent peels of two to three coats as dictated by the patient's pathology and available downtime. There is usually no frosting, just erythema and white speckling. A Jessner's peel will usually result in 2–3 days of light white desquamation, which often serves as a pleasing demonstration to the patient that the peel is effective. In one study, Jessner's peels were found to be comparable to 70% glycolic peels in efficacy for the treatment of melasma, and had fewer side-effects.[41]

Jessner's solution has been combined with topical 5-fluorouracil (5FU) weekly for 8 weeks for the treatment of actinic keratoses and photoaging, with 88% clearing in one series.[50] The ability of Jessner's peel to disrupt the epidermal barrier has also been used to enhance penetration of other agents; with TCA 35% for a medium-depth peel[51] or with resorcinol paste 53% for penetration to the deep papillary dermis.[52]

Alpha hydroxy acids

AHAs are naturally occurring organic acids extracted from fruit, sugar cane and other foods.[53] Glycolic acid is the smallest AHA and the most commonly used in superficial peeling. The choice of available formulations ranges from 20% to 70%. AHAs are keratolytic at low concentrations and cause epidermolysis with increasing concentrations and duration of contact time. In some studies, serial glycolic peels have been found to have a long-term effect on both the epidermis and dermis with an increase in dermal and epidermal glycosaminoglycans, an increase in dermal collagen and an increase in epidermal thickening.[49] These beneficial effects on the papillary dermis occur without tissue necrosis at that level.[54] This may account for more clinical improvement than one would predict with the level of injury sustained. They are reported to be of particular benefit in treating postinflammatory hyperpigmentation, solar lentigines and melasma, even in Fitzpatrick IV–VI skin types.[55,56] Indeed, monthly glycolic acid 70% peels are one author's (KB) treatment of choice for melasma of any depth in combination with topical bleaching agents (Fig. 29.2). In one of the few comparison studies, a series of six glycolic acid 20% peels was preferred by patients over six microdermabrasion treatments, although efficacy was similar and quite minimal because both treatments resulted in only mild improvement.[57] In another comparison study, 70% glycolic acid peels were equivalent to Jessner's solution for efficacy in active acne, yet caused less exfoliation and downtime and were preferred by patients.[58] These peels have also proven efficacious in photoaging.[59]

Many other properties of glycolic acid solutions also affect penetration, rendering this agent somewhat unpredictable in any given patient (Table 29.10).[60] Low pH solutions (pH < 2) appear to create more necrosis without improving efficacy.[61] Most physicians use 70% glycolic acid unbuffered and unneutralized.[62] It is important for the practitioner to gain experience with one formula and technique and to be consistent with peeling methods to gain predictability with these peels. In addition, the depth of penetration of glycolic peels appears to be more dependent on the degree to which skin is degreased and the condition of the epidermis at the time of the peel. An irritated or inflamed epidermis or one which has been aggressively degreased will have minimal resistance to penetration. In the former, it is often best to delay treatment until the barrier is intact. An abrasive skin-cleansing regimen is avoided.

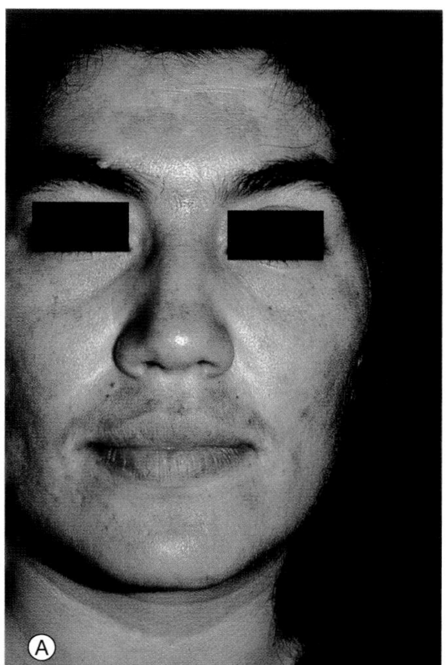

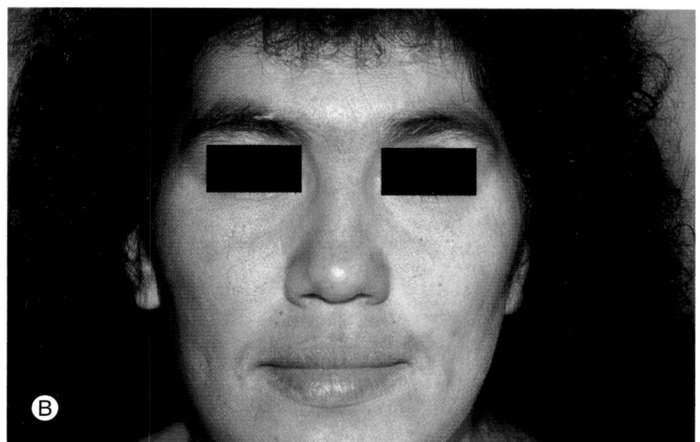

Figure 29.2 Glycolic acid 70% peel. (A) Before; (B) After.

Table 29.10 Factors affecting the penetration of AHAs

Acid concentration (pH)
Bioavailability
Degree of buffering
Volume of agent applied
Duration of time acid remains on skin
Condition of the epidermal barrier
Extent of degreasing

In this author's practice (KB), the patient cleans his or her face with a gentle cleanser without an abrasive cloth using only fingertips. The solution is applied with cotton balls rather than gauze to avoid abrasive effects of rubbing.

Time dependency is a unique aspect of glycolic acid peeling. The agent is left on anywhere from 15 seconds to 3 minutes maximum for the first peel. With subsequent peels, the solutions may be left on 15–30 seconds longer, up to 7 minutes maximum. The nurse assistant monitors the time and announces each 15–30 second time interval. The peel is neutralized with water or a 5–10% solution of sodium bicarbonate with multiple rinses. Pinpoint frosting, edema, or microvesiculation is sometimes seen selectively around acne lesions. Indicators to neutralize the solution include an unusual degree of patient discomfort, mild erythema, or adequate time interval. For patients with pigmentary disorders and type IV or higher skin type, the time interval is more conservative to minimize the risk of postinflammatory hyperpigmentation. Patients are advised that minimal peeling will occur. However, because cellular stimulation occurs even without appreciable desquamation, pigment will improve. To further minimize potential postinflammatory hyperpigmentation in these patients, a topical hydrocortisone ointment is applied immediately after the peel. Topical bleaching agents are applied between peels for optimal lightening.

Salicylic acid

Salicylic acid (ortho-hydroxybenzoic acid) is a beta hydroxyl acid that has been used in low concentrations for decades by dermatologists to treat acne, a variety of skin disorders and aging. It has been used for years as a component of Jessner's solution at 14%. It has been used more recently as a solo agent in 20–30% solutions for superficial peeling. There are few reports in the literature about salicylic acid peels. Kligman developed the 30% salicylic acid peel and noted several advantages over glycolic acid peels.[63] Salicylic acid offers the advantage of uniform application because the peel causes an immediate white precipitation and skip areas are readily visible. The peel is self-limited and there is no need for timing or neutralization. Because of the anesthetic property of salicylic acid, there is very little discomfort immediately following the procedure. Berger noted less subjective irritation with salicylic acid peels compared to AHA peels.[64] However, both Kligman and Ashinoff described more stinging during the salicylic acid peel compared to glycolic acid peeling despite its anesthetic properties.[63,65] Theoretically, this peel may benefit acne more than other peels, because besides being keratolytic, it is comedolytic. The peel has been used successfully in Fitzpatrick V and VI skin types, although it is advised to start with the 20% peel and to resume hydroquinone topically 48 hours after the peel.[66] Swinehart has reported on a 50% salicylic acid ointment under occlusion for photoaging of the dorsa of the hands and forearms.[67] Much maceration and desquamation ensues and the process may take 4 weeks to heal. In this author's (KB) experience, this peel causes needless morbidity and in one patient, a few fine reticulated scars.

Solid carbon dioxide (CO_2)

Although popular for the treatment of acne for many years, the solid CO_2 slush is now rarely used. A 5–10-inch block of dry ice at –78.5 °C can be purchased inexpensively from ice plants and other manufacturers and stored in an office ice chest. A piece is then broken off, wrapped in a towel and dipped in a solution of acetone and alcohol 3 : 1, which melts or slushes the tip. It is then brushed with light or firm pressure against the skin for less than 10 seconds. The tip requires ongoing softening and is frequently dipped in the solution during the peel. More or less pressure can be applied to the skin, which will affect the depth to which the epidermis is injured. Mild erythema or bullae formation can ensue depending on the time and pressure. However unlike potential adverse reactions with liquid nitrogen at –185.6 °C, hypopigmentation and scarring are generally not problematic. Solid CO_2 application has also been described by Brody as an enhancement step preceding application of TCA 35% for a uniform medium-depth peel.[15] This obviously carries a learning curve and depth is operator-dependent.

Tretinoin

Topical tretinoin (all-trans retinoic acid) has been a mainstay of acne therapy and photoaging for many years. It has also been used to prepare the skin before peeling or to prolong results after peeling. The use of tretinoin as a superficial peeling agent has been more recent. Cuce et al. reported improvement in melasma, ephelides and acne after a series of five superficial peels with tretinoin 0.05–1%.[68] Histology revealed an increase in epidermal thickness and a reduction in stratum corneum thickness. Topical tretinoin imparts a yellowish coloration after application, making it easier to see the treatment. In 48–72 hours, the skin undergoes noticeable fine white desquamation. In this author's (KB) experience, tretinoin solution 1.0% can be layered over other superficial peeling agents to enhance desquamation.[69] It is a very safe peel that does not require neutralization or timing.

■ OPTIMIZING OUTCOMES

Optimizing outcomes of superficial peeling

- Target superficial pathology.
- Perform a series of light peels.
- Perform maintenance peels as needed.
- Recommend a topical regimen before and after the peel.
- Choose the most superficial peel for sensitive skin or dark skin types.
- Combine with other modalities.

It is important that the goals of treatment not exceed the capability of the superficial peel series. Multiple superficial peels, rather than one or two, need to be carried out to achieve the best improvement. Some disorders, such as melasma or acne vulgaris, may be recurrent or chronic during a patient's lifetime. It is best to advise these patients that the problem may require periodic maintenance peeling after the initial series for long-term control. Indeed, maintenance peeling should be discussed with all patients in advance because the effects of superficial peels are not permanent. Studies have shown a return to the before-peel state within 60 days to 6 months[70,71] when maintenance therapy is not incorporated.

Topical regimens are essential to successful long-term results. In one study, superficial peels that were not followed up with topical regimens had only temporary results.[72] Skin biopsies showed that the skin returned to its before-peel condition within 2 years. Sunscreens, retinoids, bleaching agents, low concentration AHAs, antioxidants and other appropriate agents should be recommended by the physician.[18] Not only are retinoids helpful after treatment, but pretreatment with topical retinoids has been shown to accelerate healing from the peel and should be prescribed routinely with the deeper superficial peels.[35]

For patients with sensitive skin or dark skin types (Fitzpatrick skin types IV–VI), the peels will be optimized by avoiding a problem at the outset. It is essential to assess the integrity of the epidermis and avoid peeling inflamed skin in these patients to avoid 'hot spots' of deeper penetration. Start with light peeling and build with successive peels. A starting peel may consist of one pass of Jessner's solution lightly rubbed in, TCA 10%, or glycolic acid 50% left on 30 seconds or less, or 20% salicylic acid. Remind patients they do not need to see dramatic peeling to achieve results over time. Although all Fitzpatrick skin types may be peeled successfully with superficial peels, one must proceed cautiously and conservatively in those patients. In the literature, glycolic acid, salicylic acid and Jessner's peels appear to be effective for Fitzpatrick skin types IV–VI with the fewest side-effects, particularly if combined with a topical bleaching agent.[41,55,56,66]

For patients with deeper pathology, combination therapies may yield the best results. These may include layering a therapeutic agent over a superficial peel. For actinic keratoses, the literature describes 5FU solution applied either over Jessner's[50] or glycolic acid peels.[73] Efficacy is similar with both peels: 88% clearing of actinic keratoses with Jessner's solution and 5FU, and 91.9% clearing with glycolic acid 70% and 5FU. Cosmetic improvement in photoaging was noted in both series. Topical tretinoin can also be used as a topical agent for acne vulgaris or melasma; this can enhance effects when layered over various superficial peeling agents.[65]

Another combination technique to optimize outcome and minimize risk is to use different concentrations of the same solution, different preparation techniques or even different peeling solutions concurrently in the same patient, depending on the cutaneous pathology to be treated. One could more vigorously treat acne scars on the cheeks or periorbital lines with an abrasive preparation and TCA 25%, and treat other areas with a conservative preparation and TCA 10%. Matarraso recommends that the peel chosen be individualized for each particular patient.[1]

Combinations of laser therapy and superficial peels may offer the most targeted intervention and the least downtime for patients with more than superficial pathology. Lee et al. have suggested the combination of Q-switched alexandrite laser with concomitant superficial TCA peeling to treat recalcitrant pigmentary disorders.[74] Although the peeling agent was applied after lasering in that study, it seems prudent to apply the peel before the laser procedure to avoid deeper penetration in the laser treated areas. For patients with multiple solar lentigines and diffuse dyschromia, this author (KB) often treats the lentigines first with a Q-switched yttrium-aluminum-garnet (YAG) or alexandrite laser, followed a few weeks later by three successive monthly glycolic acid peels for overall improvement. Weiss described the combination of microdermabrasion and nonablative 1320 nm resurfacing for acne scars.[75] The combination was found to be synergistic with results superior to either modality alone. Rather than microdermabrasion, a superficial peeling agent could be used before noninvasive laser therapies. These and other novel combinations await further investigation.

■ POSTOPERATIVE CARE

Immediate postoperative care is minimal with superficial peeling. A thin coat of petrolatum or antibiotic ointment is applied after most peels. A topical corticosteroid ointment may be used instead if the skin reaction has been brisk and or the patient's skin type is Fitzpatrick IV or greater to reduce the risk of postinflammatory hyperpigmentation. The newly peeled skin appears mildly to moderately erythematous for a few hours to a few days. Superficial desquamation then occurs over the following few days to a variable degree depending on the peel. The patient is instructed to cleanse twice daily with gentle, nondetergent cleansers and to resume regular skin care as soon as the skin seems back to normal. This healing time will vary from 1 to 7 days depending on the depth of the superficial peel. Patients with a history of facial HSV infection are given prophylactic antiviral therapy. Oral antibiotics are not routinely prescribed. Patients are instructed to avoid sun exposure and to wear sun-blocking agents as soon as the skin will tolerate them.

MEDIUM-DEPTH PEELS

Medium-depth peeling is defined as injury to the skin at or through the level of the papillary dermis. The injury is associated with coagulation necrosis of the epidermis and part of the papillary dermis with inflammation to the reticular dermis. Indications for this type of peel include epidermal growths such as actinic keratoses (Fig. 29.3), seborrheic keratoses, lentigines, other pigmentary dyschromia, and skin rhytides.[76]

TCA has long been the gold standard wounding agent to achieve a medium-depth injury to the skin, with medium-depth peeling concentrations ranging from 35 to 50%. However, 45–50% TCA may produce an unpredictable response. In an attempt to reduce the morbidity of higher concentrations of TCA, combinations of chemical peeling agents should be used. These combination peels produce a more even and predictable wounding agent than a higher concentration of TCA (Table 29.11)

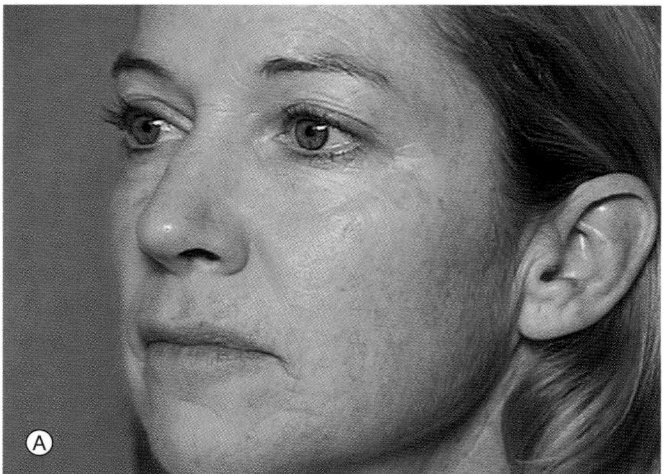

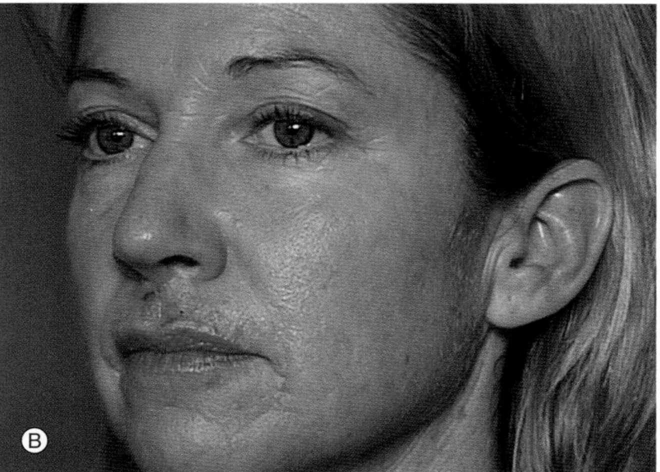

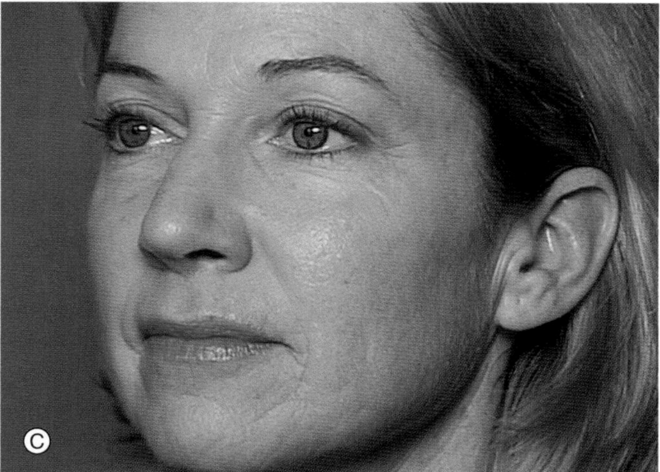

Figure 29.3 TCA peel for actinic keratosis. (A) Before. (B) 13 days after. (C) 26 days after.

The most common combination peels include solid CO_2 ice freezing with 35% TCA, Jessner's solution with 35% TCA, and glycolic acid 70% with 35% TCA. Whichever technique is chosen, it is important to be consistent to be confident of obtaining good results.

Table 29.12 shows indications for proceeding with medium-depth peeling. Benefits are seen in patients with moderate actinic damage and sallow discoloration of the skin without significant wrinkling. Lawrence and Cox showed a 75% reduction in the number of actinic keratoses after a medium-depth peel with Jessner's solution and 35% TCA. This was equal to the results one could achieve with 5FU topical therapy[77] (Fig. 29.4). Other indications include atrophic acne scars,[78] and pigmentary dyschromias such as lentigines and melasma. Blending of facial areas in conjunction with other areas following deeper resurfacing methods can optimize the outcome of a medium-depth peel. Other acids such as bichloroacetic acid can be carefully used as spot treatments for conditions such as trichodiscomas (Fig. 29.5), sebaceous hyperplasia, syringomas and trichoepitheliomas. TCA in higher concentrations (50% or more) can be used to spot treat thick actinic keratoses.

Table 29.11 Medium-depth chemical peeling agents
50% TCA
Solid CO_2 + 35% TCA
Jessner's solution + 35% TCA
70% glycolic acid + 35% TCA
88% phenol
Pyruvic acid

Table 29.12 Indications for medium-depth peel
Actinic damage
Epidermal growths
Pigmentary dyschromias
Superficial scarring
Superficial rhytides
Blending sun-damaged skin with deeply resurfaced skin

TECHNICAL ASPECTS

The technique this author (SEC) finds most predictable is the Jessner plus 35% TCA peel. The technique of medium-depth peeling with Jessner's solution and 35% TCA includes pretreatment conditioning of the skin as described previously in this chapter.

The patient is asked to come in without make-up and cleanses the skin with a gentle cleanser on the day of treatment. With the patient in the upright-seated position, the inferior edge of the mandible is marked so that when the patient is supine the 35% TCA can be feathered below this point. The neck can be treated with Jessner's solution at the same time as a medium-depth facial peel to blend the areas. The author uses 4 × 4 gauze and acetone to degrease the skin with a moderate pressure scrub. This is repeated until no residual oils are apparent on the skin (usually 2–5 passes).

After cleansing is complete, Jessner's solution is applied with large cotton-tip applicators or 2 × 2 gauze. The cotton applicators are not as easily saturated and deliver less acid to the skin. One to two coats of Jessner's solution, with several minutes in between, is applied to achieve a scattered white precipitate. The uniformity of the peel solution can be identified using a Wood's lamp. The salicylic acid in the

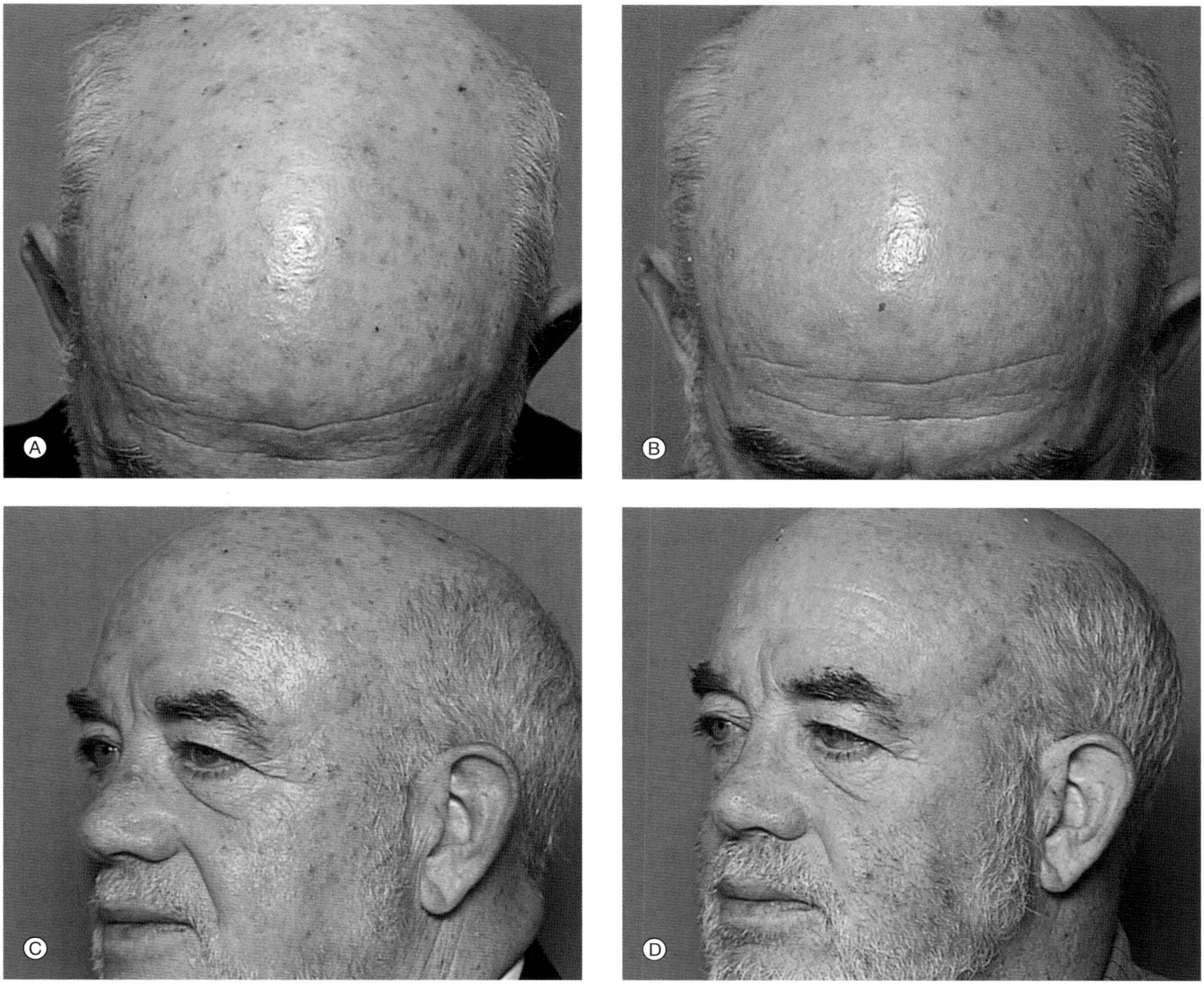

Figure 29.4 TCA medium-depth peel for actinic keratosis. (A) Before; (B) 19 days after; (C) Before; (D) 19 days after.

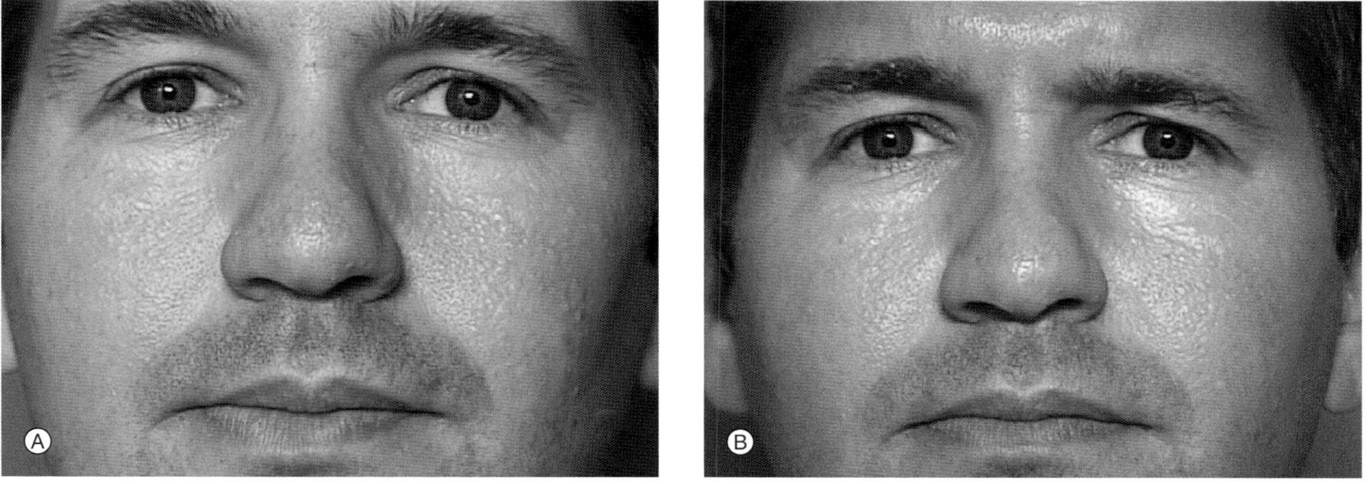

Figure 29.5 Treatment of trichodiscomas on the nose and cheeks. (A) Before; (B) After bichloracetic acid spot treatment.

Jessner's solution fluoresces under the Wood's light, giving the physician another method for ensuring even coverage of the solution.[79] With this, patients usually experience a mild stinging and burning sensation. The skin appears slightly erythematous with speckled areas of whitening.

The use of Jessner's solution disrupts the barrier function of the skin allowing a uniform penetration of TCA. 35% TCA is applied starting from the mid-face, where there is the highest concentration of sebaceous glands. The author uses several large cotton-tipped applicators to gently apply the acid. The applicator is more saturated initially, this is the rationale for starting in the central face where there is less risk of scarring. Care should be taken not to drench the applicator and cause drippage of acid. The entire face should be treated, with feathering into the hairline and below the jawline to ensure no lines of demarcation occur between treated and untreated areas. The reaction of precipitated protein coagulation is manifested as a 'frost' or whitening and it takes 1–2 minutes to be complete. The time it takes for the skin to frost is directly related to how well the skin has been pretreated and degreased. Additional factors include the amount and concentration of the TCA used, the sebaceous quality of the skin being treated, and the degree of actinic damage. Coarser, more sun-damaged skin will react more slowly and requires more heavily applied acid. Areas where frosting is patchy, may be retreated with a minimally saturated cotton-tipped applicator. The more heavily saturated the applicator the deeper the penetration of the acid. For this reason when treating the lower eyelid skin, it is important to use a minimally damp fine cotton-tipped applicator (like a Q-tip). Additionally, an assistant should hold two small dry cotton-tip applicators at the medial and lateral canthus of the eye to catch any tears that may develop and prevent trickling of the acid into the eye. Artificial tear solution, for rapid flushing of the eyes, should be readily available. This author (SEC) likes to hold a dry 4 × 4 gauze so that acid does not drip onto an untreated areas. If the patient has deep vertical upper lip lines and one is not using a deeper peeling agent or laser resurfacing, an assistant should stretch out the lip lines while the peel solution is applied with a small cotton-tip applicator. This allows even coating and prevents pooling of acid into rhytides.

Hyperkeratotic growths, such as thick seborrheic keratoses and actinic keratoses, can be curetted or frozen with liquid nitrogen before or following the peel (the latter is recommended to decrease the risk of deeper penetration of acid in de-epithelialized tissue). Thinner lesions can be treated simply by applying extra peel solution and rubbing it directly into the lesions.[80] Within seconds of applying the TCA, there is a burning sensation on the skin that escalates briefly (30–90 seconds). Whitening appears and the intensity of the burning decreases within minutes. As previously mentioned, there is no neutralization of TCA peels. Once the solution has been applied, there is about a 30-second window in which it can be diluted before keratocoagulation and the frosted appearance. Ice-soaked gauze is applied directly on the skin to relieve the burning sensation and cool packs are placed over this gauze to decrease the hot sensation. Once the patient feels comfortable, Vaseline petrolatum based ointment (Chesebrough-Ponds Inc., Greenwich, CT) or Aquaphor ointment (Beiersdorf Inc) is applied. The patient may be given an injection of corticosteroid or a tapering schedule of prednisone. The indications for this include decreasing post procedure edema.

■ OPTIMIZING OUTCOMES

All of the caveats presented in the 'Optimizing Outcomes' section for superficial chemical peels apply here and become even more important guidelines to follow because the risks associated with this more aggressive peel are greater—albeit so are the benefits in properly selected cases. It is this author's (SEC) experience that the adjunctive use of botulinum toxin injections (Botox, Allergan Inc, Irvine, CA) 7–10 days before the peel enhances peel results. Botox denervates the underlying muscles of facial expression that cause dynamic wrinkling. The onset of action occurs 24–72 hours after injection and lasts 3–6 months.[81] New collagen formation can then be laid down over a stationary area allowing the fabric of the skin to heal without reinforcing the creation of the wrinkles. This effect has been substantiated in patients undergoing periorbital laser resurfacing when pre-treating the area with Botox (see Chapter 31).

Other ancillary procedures such as injectable fillers will enhance the results. Laser resurfacing to the deeper perioral rhytides complements medium-depth peeling. It allows the practitioner to individualize the peel and optimize results.

■ POSTOPERATIVE CARE

Within 20–30 minutes after the peel the skin appears erythematous and there is a sunburn-like sensation. Edema occurs within the first 2 days. The patient is instructed to keep the skin greasy with a mild ointment at all times until desquamation is complete, generally within 5–7 days. Acetic acid 0.25% and cool water soaks are used for 10–20 minutes three to five times daily for the first few days soothe the area and encourage peeling. Alternatively, patients can splash or spray cool water on their face or take cool showers several times a day. By 24 hours after the peel, the skin has a light brown appearance (Fig. 29.6). Areas of pigmentary dyschromia and freckling appear darker than at baseline. Desquamation begins around the mouth and in the central portion of the face. The last areas to peel are usually along the hairline and preauricular area. Peeling, begun within the first 2–3 days, is generally complete within 1 week, leaving behind subtle to moderate erythema. If peeling has occurred too quickly the skin will appear blotchy and redder then expected. It is important to counsel patients not to facilitate the peeling process by scrubbing or picking at the skin. It is also important to warn them against coming in contact with harsh chemicals or cleaners that may be aerosolized and irritate the newly epithelialized skin (Fig. 29.7). Patients can wear make-up within 7–10 days after the peel and the erythema fades over 2–4 weeks (Fig. 29.8). Sun avoidance is necessary throughout and the use of a sunscreen is required once re-epithelialization is complete provided it does not cause skin irritation. We recommend seeing patients in follow-up on day 3 and day 7, to reassure them and review postoperative care. AHAs may be restarted 3 weeks after the peel and tretinoin 4–6 weeks after the peel if the skin is not too sensitive.

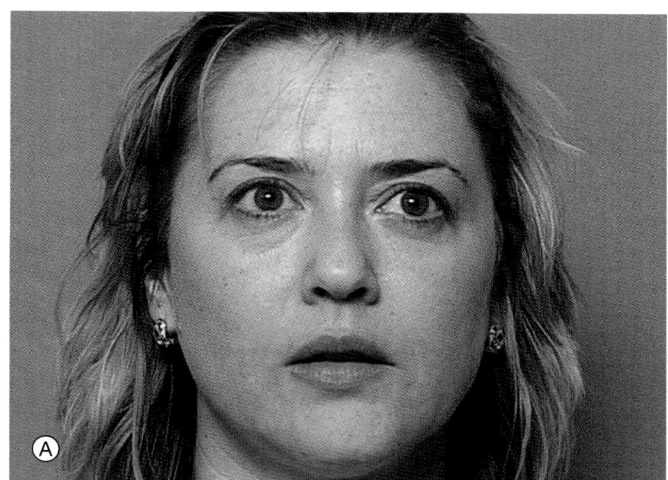

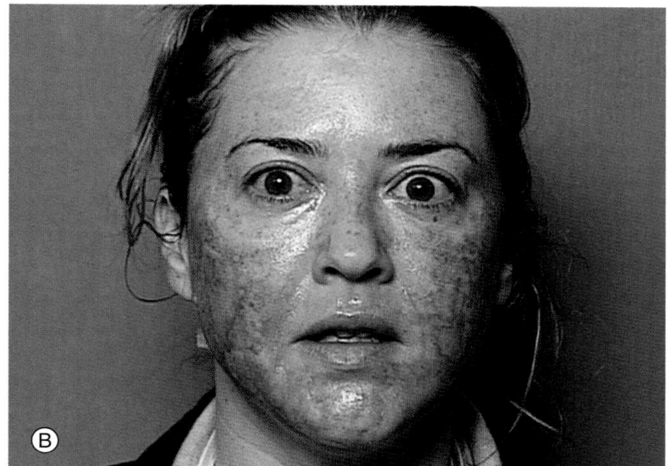

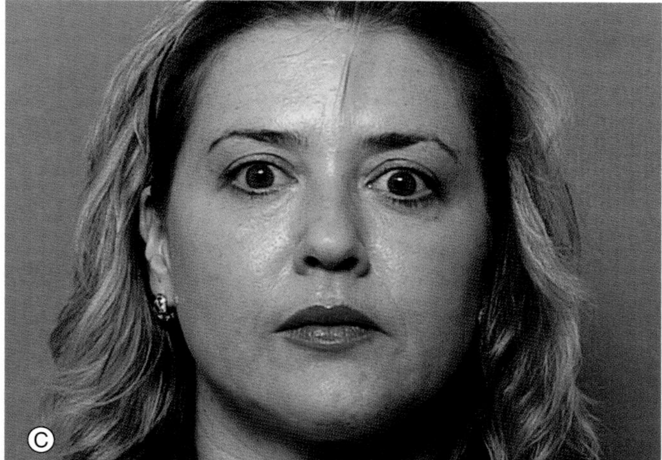

Figure 29.6 TCA medium-depth chemical peel and glabellar botox. (A) Before; (B) 2 days after. (C) 12 days after.

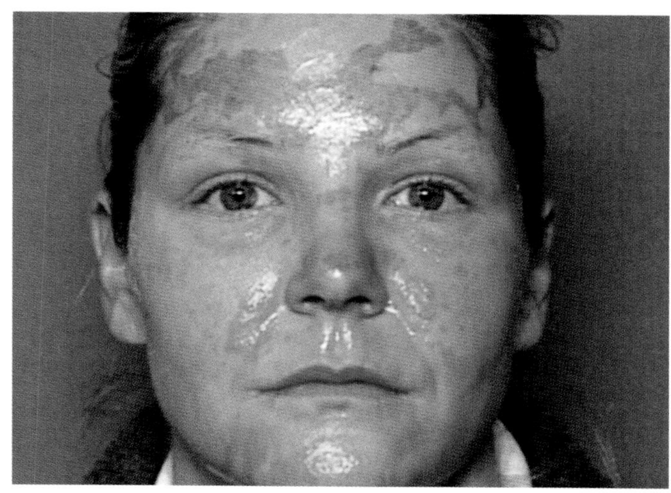

Figure 29.7 7 days after TCA medium-depth chemical peel. Contact dermatitis as a result of Tilex cleaning solution exposure. Note the patchy erythema on chin and area superior to the nasolabial folds.

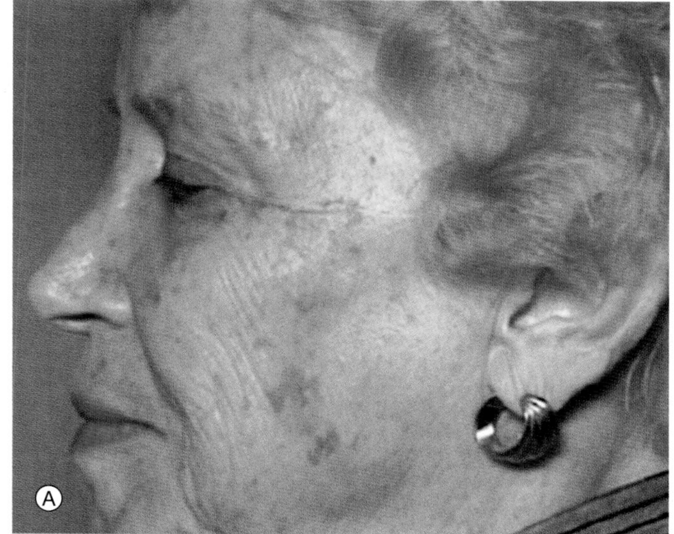

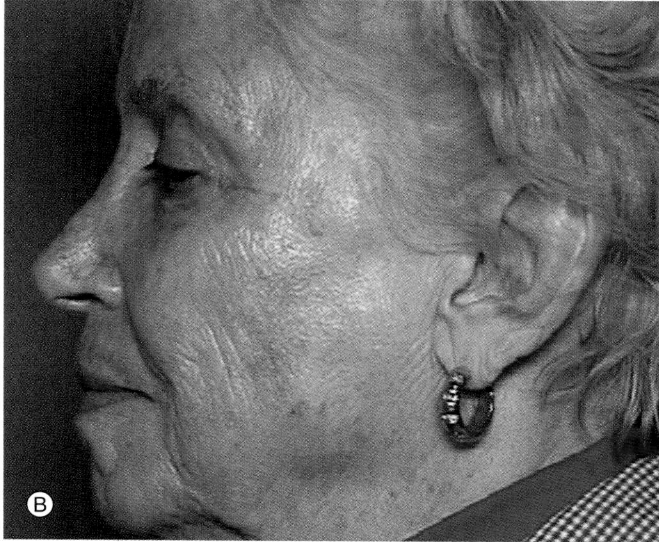

Figure 29.8 TCA medium-depth chemical peel for actinically damaged skin actinic keratoses and lentigines. (A) Before; (B) 28 days after.

DEEP CHEMICAL PEELS (PHENOL PEELS)

Phenol (also known as carbolic acid) is a keratocoagulant originally used as a disinfectant. Phenol represents the only deep chemical peeling agent that has been widely used and understood. The discussion here therefore revolves only around the nuances of chemical peeling with phenol. Because of its ability to penetrate deep into the dermis, patient selection is critical to a good outcome; the risks are considerable, but the results can be quite dramatic.

Clinical and histologic changes in the epidermis and dermis persist for as long as 15–20 years.[79] Histologically, there is improvement in the dermal architecture, and a grenz zone measuring 2–3 mm thick develops between the epidermis and the underlying elastotic tissue.

■ TECHNICAL ASPECTS

Adequate cleansing of the face and removal of deep facial oils is imperative especially if an open technique is used instead of taping the skin postoperatively. For a discussion of the virtues of taped vs open technique, Beeson has written an excellent chapter in *Skin Resurfacing*.[82] The use of Septisol is advocated as the astringent of choice because of its keratolytic properties. Following facial cleansing, acetone is used to further remove facial oils.

Intravenous sedation is standard when full-face phenol chemexfoliation is being carried out. Adequate hydration is necessary to avoid renal toxicity. The recommended hydration consists of 500 ml of Ringer's lactate before applying the solution followed by an additional 1000 ml of fluid during the operative and immediate postoperative period.[82]

Phenol is known to be cardiotoxic. To avoid cardiac arrhythmias, a full-face peel should extend over a 60–90 minute period. No more than 50% of the face should be treated during a 30-minute period to limit systemic absorption.[83] Cardiac monitoring is necessary during and after the procedure.

'Baker's formula' developed by Baker and Gordon, is the most widely used deep peeling agent (Table 29.13). This solution consists of 3 ml phenol USP (88%), 2 ml distilled water, 3 drops croton oil, 8 drops 0.25% Septisol (liquid hexachlorophene soap in alcohol). The solution should be freshly prepared and stirred constantly before and during the application to ensure an even peel.

After proper degreasing with Septisol, cleansing with water and wiping the skin with acetone, the peel may begin. Fresh Baker's solution is mixed to provide a turbid emulsion. It is then applied using cotton-tipped applicators that have been pressed against the rim to remove excess solution. The solution is applied slowly over aesthetic units, allowing 10–15 minutes to elapse between regions to minimize absorption great enough to be toxic to the heart. The skin immediately turns white as a result of frosting as the phenol solution causes keratolysis and keratocoagulation. The initial pain felt subsides within minutes, but then returns later in the day as the initial sedation and the anesthetic effect of the phenol subside. The solution is feathered beyond the margins of the peeled areas to reduce lines of demarcation. Adjacent areas (i.e. neck, chest) must likewise be rejuvenated much of the time so that skin color and texture remain in balance.

Table 29.13 Baker/Gordon phenol formulation

Phenol USP 88% 3 ml
Distilled water 2 ml
Septisol liquid soap (8 drops)
Croton oil (3 drops)

Periorbital areas must be treated cautiously to avoid intraocular injury, which may increase absorption and cause significant injury. When applying the solution in the periocular area there should be no excess solution on the applicator. Upper eyelid peeling should not be carried out below the superior tarsal fold. Lower eyelid peeling should be carried out with the patient gazing upward. Cotton-tipped applicators should be placed in the medial and lateral canthi to blot tears. Perioral peeling should be carried out by stretching out the vertical rhytides so that the peel solution can be applied evenly. A broken wooden applicator can be used to apply more solution to the deepest crevices.

■ OPTIMIZING OUTCOMES

Proper patient selection is the most important aspect of obtaining satisfactory results with phenol peeling. The ideal patient is a thin-skinned woman with fair complexion and fine generalized wrinkling. These individuals are less likely to have lines of demarcation between peeled and unpeeled skin. The conditions that are most successfully treated are fine facial wrinkles (especially in the periocular and periorbital regions), pigmentary dyschromia, actinic keratoses and superficial, shallow acne scars.[82]

■ POSTOPERATIVE CARE

Postoperatively, the patient should be monitored for cardiac arrhythmias for 1 hour.[84] Several authors have switched from using a closed technique of taping to an open technique.[83–85] The advantages of an open technique include less pain, halting further penetration of phenol, lower risk of scarring, quicker re-epithelialization and decreased risk of infection.

Petrolatum should be applied to the peeled areas and be liberally reapplied during the subsequent week. The patient gently washes or soaks the skin as described previously and reapplies the ointment to prevent dehydration and crust formation that could retard healing. This process is repeated six times a day until re-epithelialization is complete, usually within 7 days. The skin appears erythematous for up to 12 weeks. Sun avoidance for 3–6 months is important to prevent hyperpigmentation.

BODY PEELING

Peeling techniques have traditionally been limited to the face because standard techniques in nonfacial areas have inconsistent results. Nonfacial skin has a decreased number of hair follicles, sebaceous glands and dermal vessels, which relative to facial skin, means impaired wound healing. As such, neck, trunk and limb skin has a narrower margin for error than the face. Traditionally peeling of these areas requires lower concentration acids and serial treatments (see superficial chemical peels).

One chemical peel technique for nonfacial skin using 70% glycolic acid gel combined with 35% or 40% TCA has given

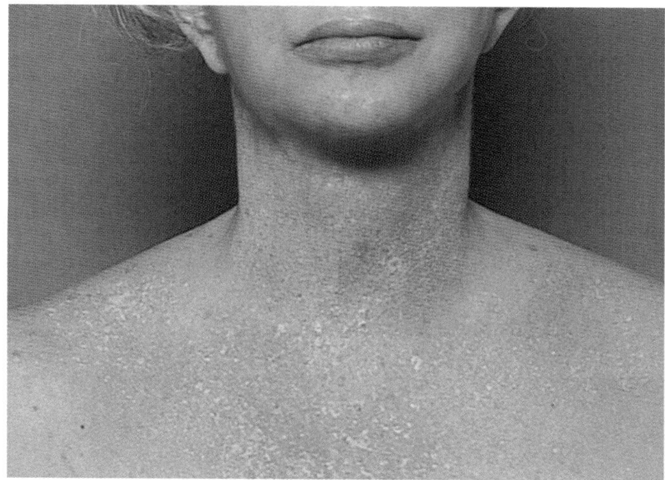

Figure 29.9 Frosting from Cook body peel.

consistently good results on the arms, hands, chest, neck, back and legs. This peel is easy to implement and produces a peel in which the depth can be controlled more precisely, ranging from light to medium. The technique, named after its developers, is the Cook total body peel.[86] The skin is degreased with acetone, 70% glycolic acid gel is applied to the skin using 4 × 4 gauze, followed immediately by 40% TCA applied in the same manner. The skin is carefully monitored so the physician can neutralize the peel at the desired depth with copious amounts of 10% sodium bicarbonate solution as soon as stippled frosting is noted. The typical endpoint desired is characterized by erythema with scattered white speckles (Fig. 29.9). Certain areas may require more time or more TCA to achieve the desired endpoint as controlled by the physician. Blending can be easily achieved with this technique. It is important to use glycolic acid gel rather than liquid, because the gel acts as a partial barrier to the TCA penetration. Liquid glycolic acid could result in increased penetration of the TCA and resultant scarring.

After this body peel, the skin will flake for 2–4 weeks depending on the area (Fig. 29.10). As with all skin peeling procedures, hydrating the skin with liberal use of an emollient after treatment helps during the healing phase. Clinical results produce smoother skin texture, decreased wrinkling and fading of lentigines and macular seborrheic keratosis (Fig. 29.11). This author (SEC) has also used the Cook peel to reduce actinic keratoses and disseminated superficial actinic porokeratoses with some success (Fig. 29.12).

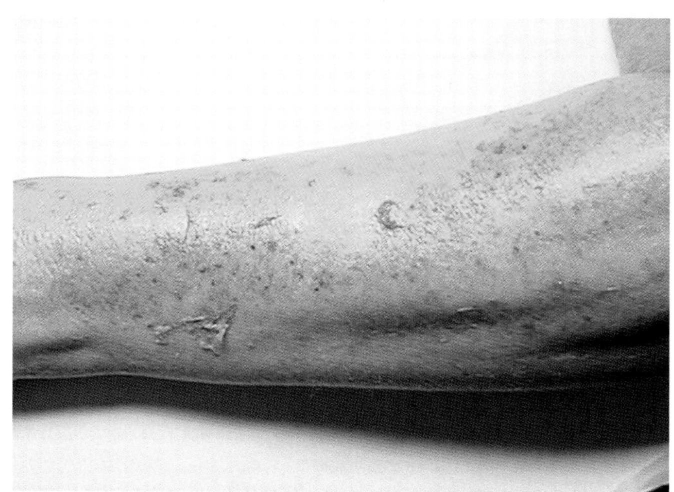

Figure 29.10 Peeling 7 days after Cook body peel.

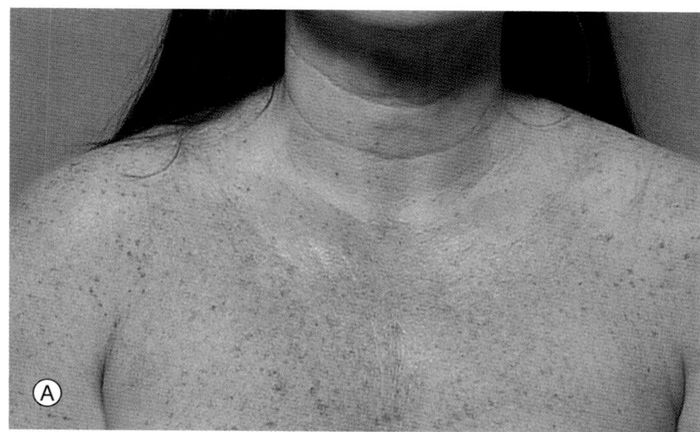

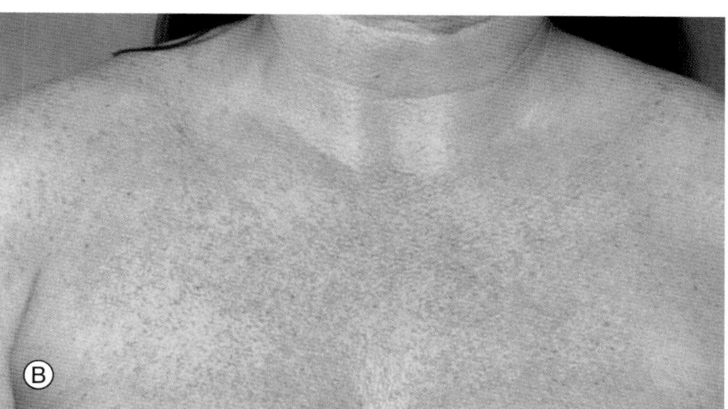

Figure 29.11 Cook body peel. (A) Before; (B) 21 days after.

Other peeling options for nonfacial skin include low concentrations of TCA varying from 20 to 25% and carrying out serial treatments over time. Brody has advocated the use of 35% TCA for acne scarring of the back with the placement of 50% TCA to the elevated peripheral scar edges.[87] Serial Jessner peels and 50% salicylic acid ointment under occlusion described by Swinehart[67] may also be used.

PITFALLS AND THEIR MANAGEMENT

Avoidance of pitfalls

- Careful patient selection is essential, and screening for risk factors, especially those that increase the risk of scarring (such as recent isotretinoin, previous radiation therapy, and recent surgery that has compromised vascular supply to the skin).
- Advise patients about sun protection after the peel to avoid dyschromia and postinflammatory hyperpigmentation.
- For deep peels, advise patients to expect hypopigmentation.
- Institute meticulous wound hygiene to reduce the risk of infection.
- For mid to deep peels, use antiviral prophylaxis in all patients who are immunocompromised or have a history of HSV infection.

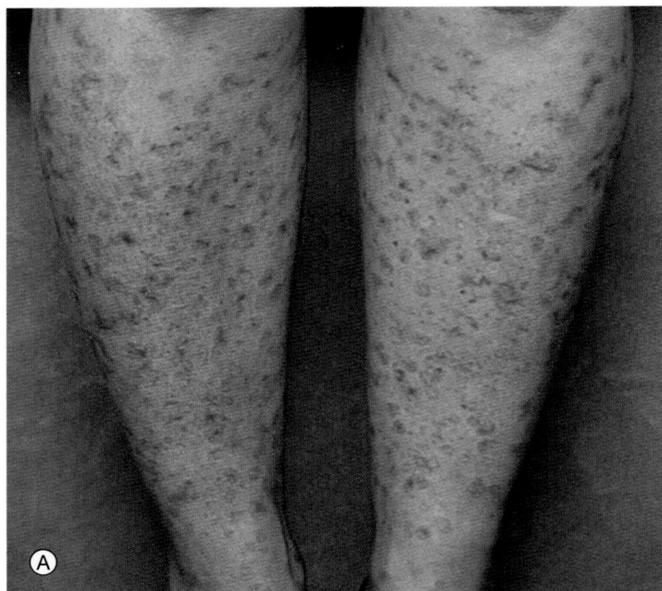

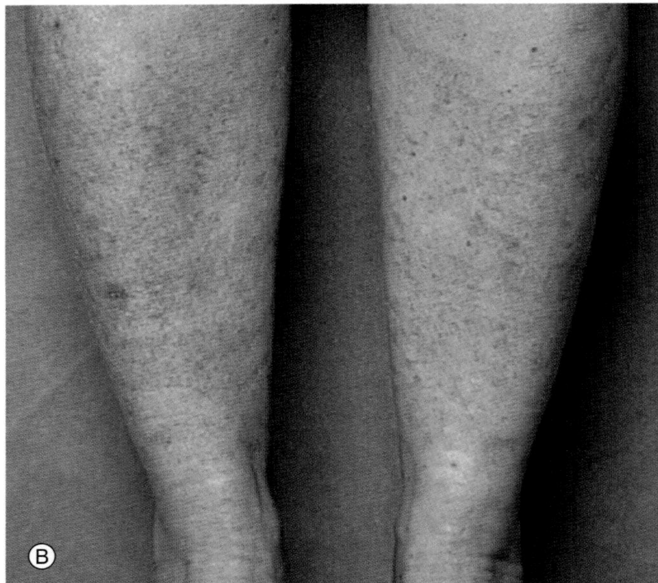

Figure 29.12 Cook body peel for disseminated superficial actinic porokeratosis. (A) Before; (B) After two treatments.

The risk of complications from peels (Table 29.14) increases proportionately with the depth of wounding. Superficial peels carry the lowest risk of adverse reactions and if they occur are usually pigmentary in nature. Medium-depth peels can likewise cause pigmentary changes and occasionally even scarring. Deep phenol peels are associated with these risks, as well as systemic toxicities.

Pigmentation (hypopigmentation/ hyperpigmentation)

The most common complication of chemical peeling is irregular pigmentation. Lighter peels are more likely to be associated with hyperpigmentation and deeper peels with hypopigmentation. Hyperpigmentation is almost always transient and is best treated with hydroquinone bleaching agents, retinoic acid or tazarotene cream, and a physical barrier sunscreen such as titanium dioxide. Some advocate a further superficial peel and aggressive skin care for the best results. Exogenous estrogens, photosensitizing medications and direct sun exposure during the first 6 weeks after a peel increase the risk of hyperpigmentation (Fig. 29.13).

Table 29.14 Complications of chemical peeling

Pigmentary alteration
Scarring
Infection
Milia
Persistent erythema
Atrophy
Textural changes
Cardio, renal and hepatotoxicity; laryngeal shock; toxic shock syndrome (limited to phenol peels)

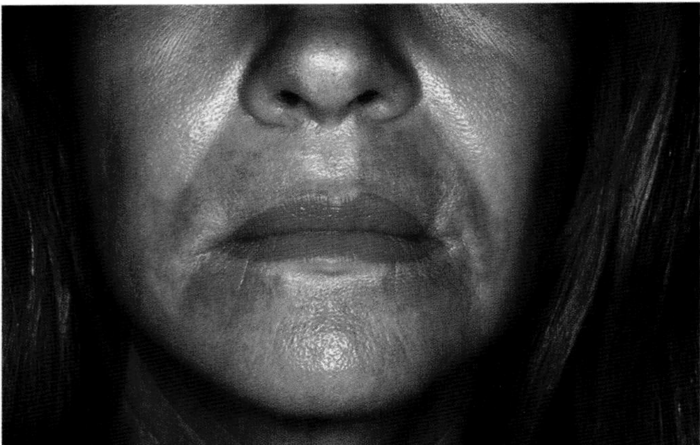

Figure 29.13 Postinflammatory hyperpigmentation.

Hypopigmentation is an expected sequela of phenol peels and deeper resurfacing procedures. It is essential to educate patients pursuing deeper peels that hypopigmentation and/or a line of demarcation between peeled and nonpeeled areas is a trade-off for smoother, more youthful skin. Accentuation of pigmented nevi may also occur after chemical peeling because they appear more prominent against the light-skinned background.

Milia

Milia result from occlusion of the pilosebaceous unit, usually within the first 1–3 months after a peel. They may occur because of the use of petrolatum-based ointments applied to the skin during the early healing process. However, this is not problematic enough to consider not using ointments that are so helpful in wound healing. Milia are easily treated with an 18-gauge needle and comedone extractor once the skin is fully epithelialized and otherwise back to normal.

Prolonged erythema

Persistent erythema is more closely associated with deeper resurfacing procedures, but may be seen after medium-depth peels and rarely after superficial peels. When erythema is localized and persists for more than 2 weeks, one needs to consider both contact dermatitis and early impending scarring (Fig. 29.14).

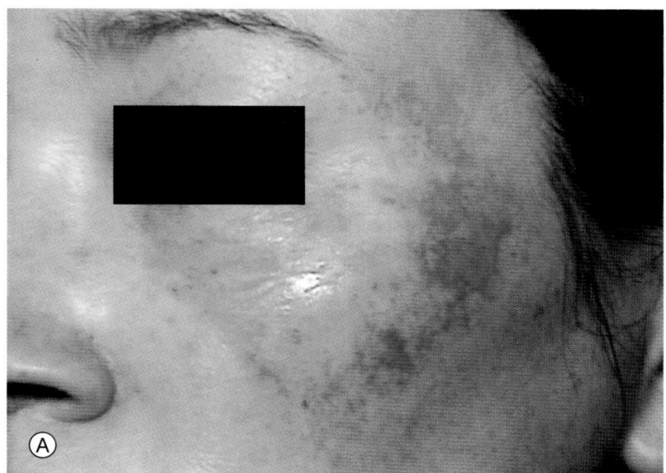

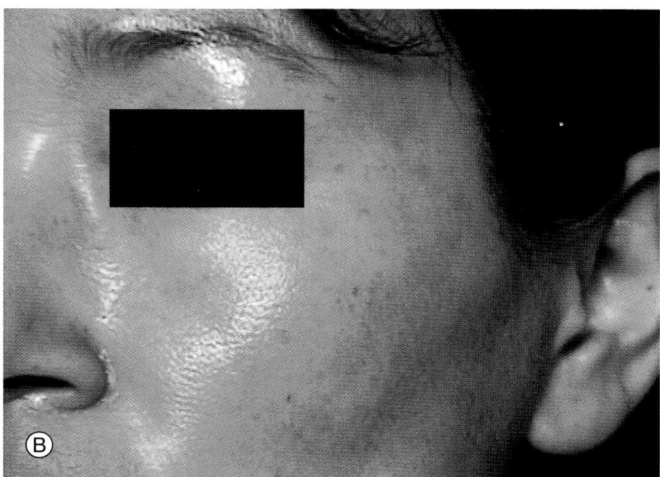

Figure 29.14 (A) Persistent erythema 1 month after 70% glycolic acid peel; (B) After two treatments with pulse dye laser.

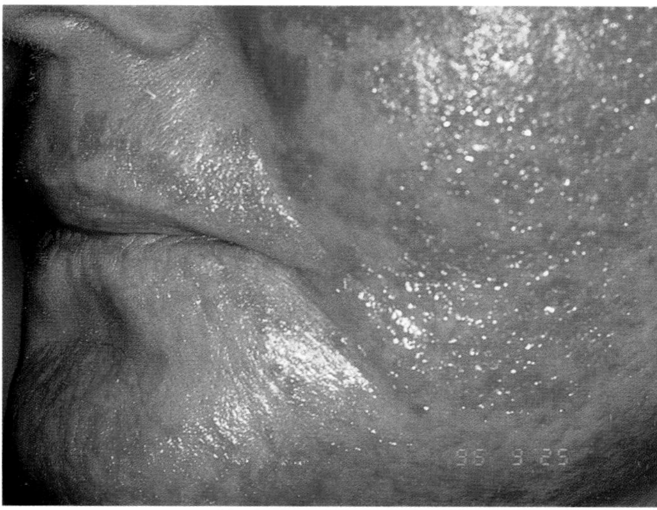

Figure 29.15 Bacterial infection after peel.

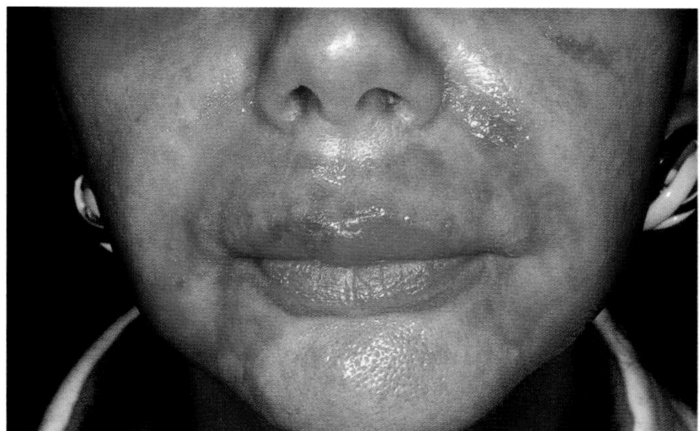

Figure 29.16 Perioral herpes simplex virus (HSV) infection after resurfacing.

Maloney et al. evaluated the etiology of persistent erythema after chemical peeling and devised a successful treatment plan in all 196 cases reviewed.[88] Suggested treatment included avoidance of possible irritants, and the utilization of bland emollients, mild topical corticosteroids, 0.25% acetic acid soaks and if needed, systemic corticosteroids. In the author's (SEC) practice, low-energy long-pulsed dye laser treatment is also initiated if the erythema persists beyond 6 to 8 weeks or if textural changes occur. Intralesional corticosteroids are rarely necessary.

Infection

Infection is rare following chemical peels, and while both TCA and phenol are bactericidal,[89] this is generally not a factor because infection usually sets in several days after the peel. Poor wound care is what most frequently contributes to bacterial infection after a peel. Occlusive ointments may promote folliculitis that may be secondarily infected with staphylococci or streptococci (Fig. 29.15). Pseudomonas is another pathogen that can be identified with poor wound hygiene. When infection is suspected, cultures should be taken and broad-spectrum antibiotics and frequent acetic acid soaks should be instituted immediately. Toxic shock syndrome has been associated with phenol-based peels.[90]

Chemical peeling may activate HSV (Fig. 29.16). The development of postoperative HSV infection cannot be predicted based on a previous history of a 'cold sore.' This supports the policy of prescribing antiviral prophylaxis for all patients undergoing mid-to-deep facial peels and immunosuppressed patients regardless of past HSV history.[91] The onset of HSV infection is often heralded by severe facial or perioral burning pain. Within 24 hours vesicles develop and these give way to well demarcated punched out ulcers. Untreated infection readily spreads to the de-epithelialized areas. Despite oral HSV prophylaxis, patients occasionally develop infection. The prophylaxis that this author (SEC) adheres to is valacyclovir 500 mg twice a day beginning the day before the procedure and until completely re-epithelialized, usually 7 days after treatment. If a herpetic infection does develop the dose is increased to 1000 mg every 8 hours and continued until fully healed.

Cutaneous candida infection may be seen after chemical peeling (Fig. 29.17). Tiny pustules develop, usually periorally, and rapidly spread to adjacent areas. Patients complain of an itching or burning sensation. Topical or systemic antifungal agents can be used to treat this superficial infection. Perleche, concomitant vaginal candidiasis and recent oral antibiotics may be predisposing risk factors. For

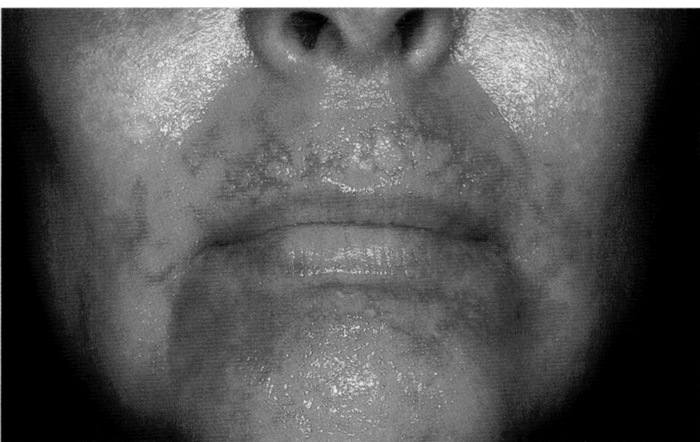

Figure 29.17 Cutaneous candida infection after peel.

this or any suspected infection, cultures should be sent before commencing therapy when possible.

Scarring

Scarring is one of the most dreaded complications of chemical peeling. The risk of scarring increases with the depth of the peel (Fig. 29.18). TCA at concentrations greater than 50% demonstrates an unpredictable pattern of penetration and can lead to scarring. Factors that may increase the risk of scarring include a history of isotretinoin treatment within a 6-month period, poor nutritional status, chronic disease state, and tobacco use. Surgery that involves large areas of undermining may increase the risk of sloughing if carried out at the same time as a peel. Previous medium or deep peels, dermabrasion and laser resurfacing within the preceding 6–12 months can increase the risk for scarring. Hereditary predisposition or connective tissue disease, such as the mild form of Ehlers–Danlos syndrome, can cause delayed wound healing.[88]

Early scarring manifested as indurated, patchy erythema should be treated aggressively, as discussed above, with pulsed dye laser, and topical, intralesional or oral corticosteroids.

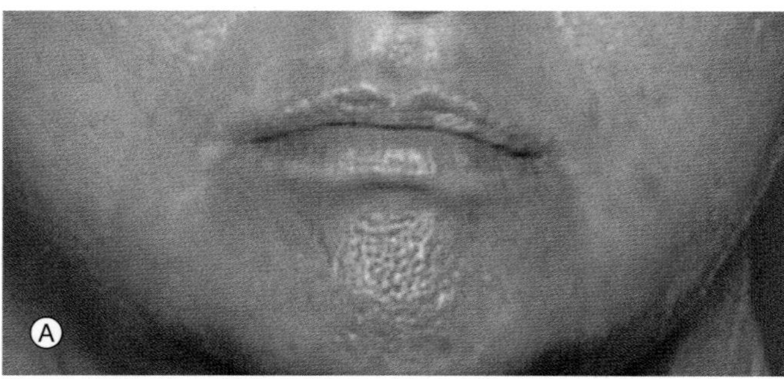

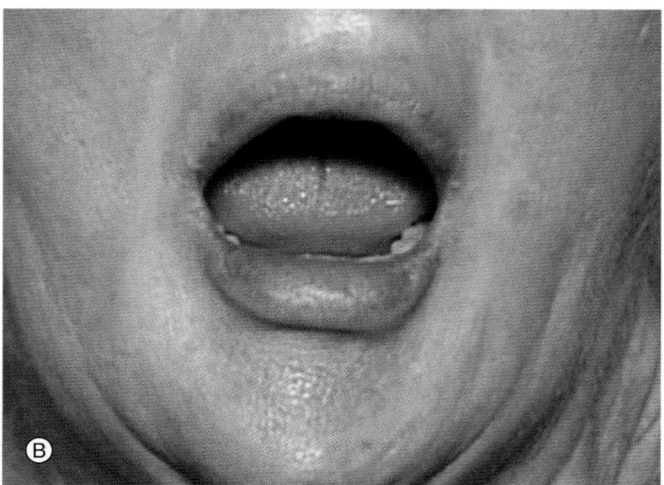

Figure 29.18 (A)–(B) 7 weeks after perioral phenol peel with decreased oral aperture and early scarring.

Systemic complications

Systemic complications may be seen with phenol peeling. Phenol applied quickly can produce cardio-, hepato-, and nephrotoxicity. It is suggested that peeling the skin in segments and intervals allows metabolism of the absorbed phenol and so decreases the chance of arrhythmias as well as kidney and liver toxicities.[83] Cardiac monitoring is therefore extremely important. Intravenous hydration assists in clearing the phenol from the circulation and decreases the likelihood of toxicity.

■ SUMMARY

Chemical peeling is an effective technique to combat the effects of photoaging, a variety of pigmentary disorders and epidermal growths. Given the media hyperbole, it is particularly important that patients are fully aware of the efficacy of single superficial peels. Provided patients are educated to expect realistic outcomes and patient selection is careful, the results for all depths of peel are highly satisfactory.

■ REFERENCES

1. Matarasso SL, Glogau RG. Chemical face peels. Dermatol Clin 1991; 9:131–149.
2. Brody HJ. Skin response to chemical peeling. In: Coleman W, Lawrence N, eds. Skin resurfacing. Philadelphia: Williams and Wilkins 1998; 37–44.
3. De Leo VA. Prevention of skin cancer. J Derm Surg Oncol 1988; 14:902–906.
4. Steinsapir KD. The chemical peel. Int Ophthalmol Clin 1997; 37:31–96.
5. Coleman W, Lawrence N. The history of skin resurfacing. In: Coleman W, Lawrence N, eds. Skin resurfacing. Philadelphia: Williams and Wilkins 1998; 3–6.
6. Mackee GM, Karp FL. The treatment of post acne scars with phenol. Br J Dermatol 1952; 64:456–459.
7. Baker TJ, Gordon HL. Chemical face peeling. Surg Rejuvenation of the Aging Face 1986; 37.
8. Baker TJ, Gordon HL, Mosienko P, et al. Long-term histological study of skin after chemical face peeling. Plast Reconstr Surg 1974; 53:522.
9. Baker TJ, Gordon HL, Seckinger DL. A second look at chemical face peeling. Plast Reconstr Surg 1966; 37:487.
10. Litton C. Chemical face lifting. Plast Reconstr Surg 1962; 29:371.
11. Brody HJ. History of chemical peels. In: Chemical Peeling. Mosby 1992; 1–5. Sponsoring editor: Anne S Patterson, St Louis, MO.
12. Baker TJ. Chemical face peeling and rhytidectomy. Plastic Reconstruct Surg 1962; 29:199.
13. Stegman SJ. A comparative histologic study of the effects of three peeling agents and dermabrasion on normal and sundamaged skin. Aesthetic Plastic Surg 1982; 6:123.
14. Van Scott EJ, Yu RJ. Hyperkeratinization, corneocyte, and alpha hydroxy acids. J Am Acad Dermat 1984; 11:867–879.

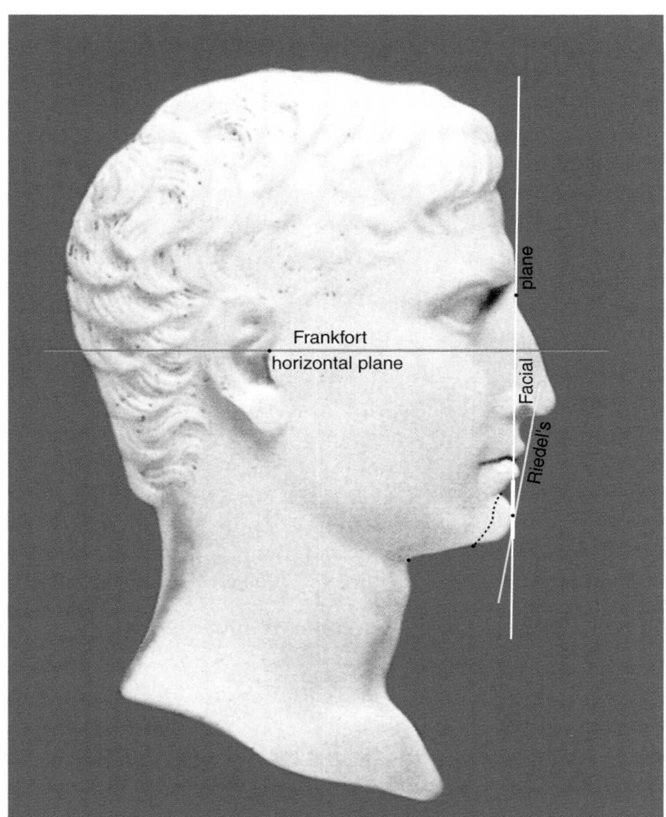

Figure 30.2 Augustus Caesar. Demonstrates ideal facial proportions for chin projection (Gonzalez-Ulloa), upper and lower lip–chin relationship (Riedel), and chin–lower lip relationship (vertical line from vermillion of lower lip) (increased width of vertical white line).

Bone and soft tissue structures of the neck also contribute to aesthetic appreciation of the profile. The hyomandibular angle[16] is formed by the submental line (horizontal line), tangential to the submental area, intersecting with the anterior cervical line, tangential to the vertical portion of the neck. Their intersection is the cervical point.

An ideal 'sculpted' neck has a sharp angulation, approaching a hyomandibular angle of 85°–90°.[16] However, if the hyoid bone is low and anteriorly located, the hyomandibular angle is made obtuse. This blunting of the hyomandibular angle created by a low anterior hyoid bone contributes to the perception of a small chin.

Redundant skin, muscle, and adipose tissue also contribute to making the hyomandibular angle blunted and not attractive. These soft tissues that define the anterior cervical line and submental line can be retracted and elevated, improving the neck angulation, with submental liposuction, face lift, and/or platysmaplasty.

A low anterior hyoid and weak chin can limit this improvement. The hyoid position cannot be changed, but chin position can be with chin augmentation. The most anterior soft tissue part of the chin is the pogonion, and the menton is the most inferior soft tissue point of the chin. By surgically augmenting the chin, shifting both these landmarks anteriorly, the submentum is lengthened and the submental line or horizontal line is made more horizontal, improving the hyomandibular angle. By creating a greater distance between the hyoid bone and pogonion the illusion that the hyoid bone is not as anterior nor as blunting to the hyomandibular angle is achieved,[16] and a more pleasant neck can be achieved. In analyzing results of neck sculpting procedures, it can be seen that in aesthetically pleasing necks, virtually all patients have 'good' chins either from nature or surgery.

Anatomy

Anatomic considerations of importance to augmenting the mandible include bone, bony foramina, muscle, motor and sensory nerves, blood vessels and skin.

The mental protuberance is the thick bone at the medial and inferior aspect of the mandibular body, with mental tubercles raised on each side. The upper border of the mandible is the alveolar part, containing alveoli for the roots of the teeth. The oblique line runs posteriorly from each tubercle along the inferior mandibular border[17] (Fig. 30.3A).

The mental foramen is a bilateral structure through which exits the mental nerve and vessels. The horizontal position of the mental foramen is variably described as inferior and slightly anterior to the second premolar tooth,[17] or just posterior to a line drawn down from the oral commissure,[18] or below the apex of the second premolar tooth in the mid-pupillary line, approximately 2.5 cm from the midline,[19] though it may range from 1.5–4.5 cm from the midline.[20] A study of 100 adult mandibles revealed the foramen to be at the level of the root of the second premolar (bicuspid) in 50%, between the first and second premolar (bicuspid) in 20–25% and posterior to the second premolar (bicuspid) in 24%.[21]

The mental nerve provides sensation to the skin of the chin and lower lip, as well as to the mucosa of the lip and adjacent gum (Fig. 30.3B). It is a branch of the mandibular nerve of the third division of the trigeminal nerve (see Chapter 1), running superiorly as it exists the mental foramen, surrounded by a fibrous sheath. The bony angle of the mental foramen allows the lower labial branch to run upward toward the lip, while the mental branch travels anteriorly and medially to the skin of the chin.[22]

The muscles of the chin are the mentalis, the depressor anguli oris, and depressor labii inferioris (Fig. 30.3C). The paired mentalis muscle originates from the anterior mandible at the level of and below the roots of the incisors, running downward inserting into the skin of the chin. It elevates the lower lip indirectly (its fibers do not enter the lip), draws the lower lip against the gums and teeth, and protrudes the lower lip (as in a pout).[23] The depressor muscles originate from bone at the oblique line and insert into skin and mucosa of the lower lip and orbicularis oris muscle. They pull the lower lip downward and laterally; the depressor labii inferioris also everts the lip.

The marginal mandibular nerve, a branch of the facial nerve, provides motor innervation to the muscles of the chin and lower lip. It enters these muscles deeply on their lateral undersurface, after coursing medially under the superficial musculo-aponeurotic system (SMAS) and platysma until it is crosses superficial to the facial artery and vein at the medial border of the masseter muscle. Approximately 2 cm lateral to the oral commissure it lies in the soft tissue overlying the dissection plane.

If the marginal mandibular nerve is injured during surgery, the patient is unable to perform chin muscle

Skeletal anatomy of the chin

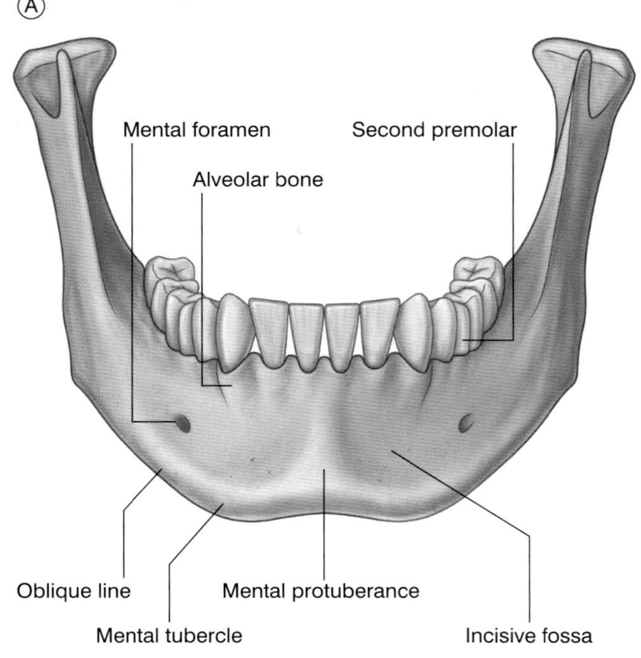

Muscular anatomy of the chin

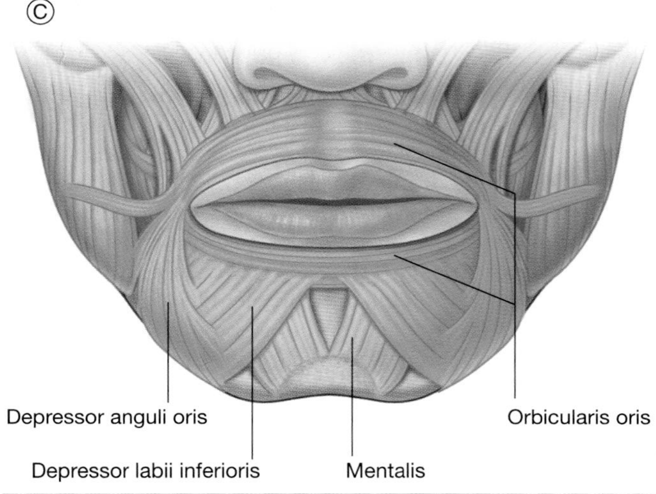

Mental nerve

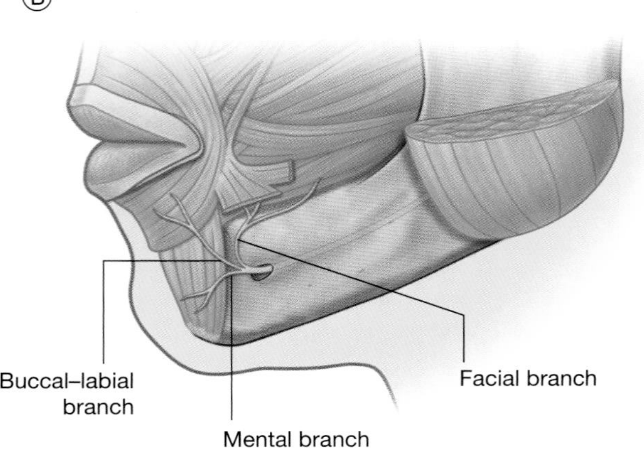

Age related changes of the mandible

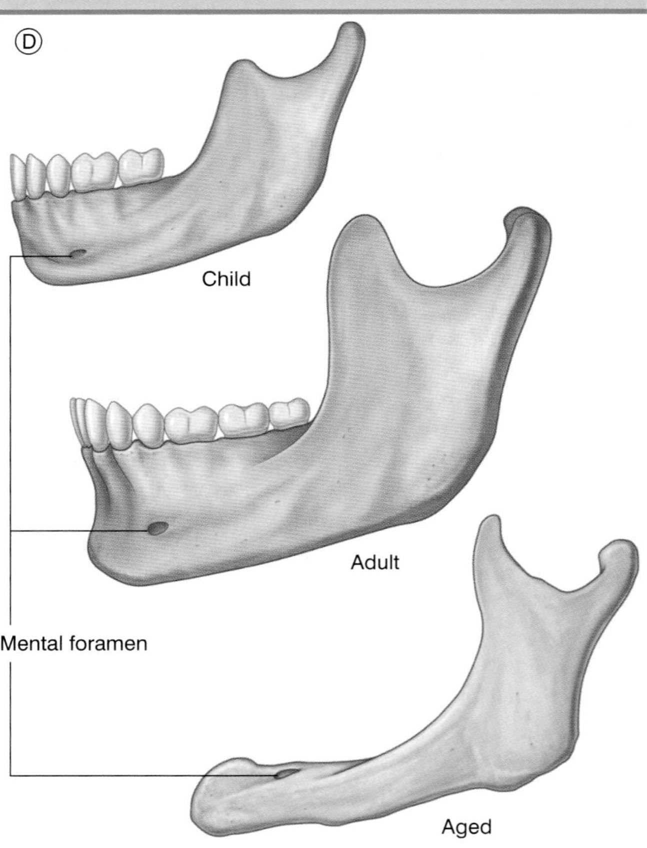

Figure 30.3 (A) Skeletal anatomy of the chin. (B) Mental nerve. (C) Muscular anatomy of the chin. (D) Age-related changes of the mandible.

functions on that side. With smiling, that side of the lower lip remains up, unable to be drawn downward and laterally and the vermillion border cannot be everted on that side.[24] This is not apparent with the mouth at rest.

Age-related changes affect the vertical position of the mental foramen (Fig. 30.3D). In adults, it is mid-way between the upper and lower borders of the mandible. In older, edentulous patients, because of atrophy of the alveolar ridge, its relative position is nearer the superior border.[25] Its distance from the inferior mandibular margin remains constant, at least 8–10 mm.[11] Also with aging, bony resorption of the mandible at its inferior aspect below the mental foramen results in a depression, named the anterior mandibular groove by Mittelman.[26]

Soft tissue changes also occur with age. A soft tissue depression, the pre-jowl sulcus,[26] develops between the jowl and chin. This overlies the anterior mandibular groove, accentuating the pre-jowl sulcus. Atrophy of chin musculature and the alveolar ridge also contribute to less anterior projection of the chin.

■ PREOPERATIVE PREPARATION

Evaluation and exam

The surgeon must be able to recognize a chin deficiency to be able to improve it and to know when chin augmentation is the appropriate procedure. This requires aesthetic judgment and a systematic approach, because few patients present with 'weak chin' as their primary area of concern. They may think that their neck is not well defined and needs liposuction, or that their nose is too large.

Patients are often unaware of the imbalance of their own profile because they typically view themselves from the frontal view, not the profile view. Occasionally, a person will recognize their chin weakness in candid, unposed family photographs, or recognize it in others, especially if it is a hereditary feature. To appreciate a chin deficiency, the physician must consistently examine the profile, using mirrors, instant photography, digital photos, or computer imaging, and present it to the patient in such a way that the chin deficiency and its role in facial balance is understood.

The profile view is only helpful and accurate if the head is positioned consistently for evaluation and photos. The Frankfort horizontal plane described above is that consistent head position. The inclusion of the tragus is thus required in photos or the plane is uncertain. Unfortunately, it is common for the patient with a chin deficiency, excess submental fat, or low, anterior hyoid to hold his or her head in a position which is more flattering, projecting the chin anteriorly by tilting the head slightly upward[27] (Fig. 30.4). Slouching also encourages anterior positioning of the mandible.[28] These things must be recognized, and the patient asked to sit erect without leaning back in a chair during the examination.

If this naturally assumed, subconscious compensatory posture is unrecognized and not addressed by the evaluating surgeon, the opportunity to improve the profile with chin augmentation may be missed.

The position of the hyoid bone and hyomandibular angle should be noted and considered, because a low, anteriorly positioned hyoid, which is not surgically correctable, may limit improvements attainable by face lift, by

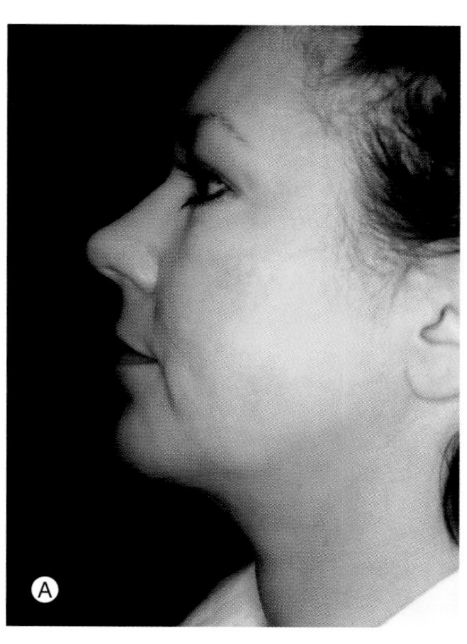

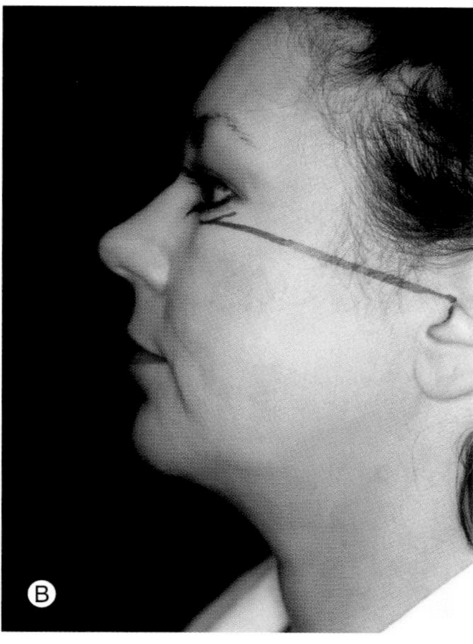

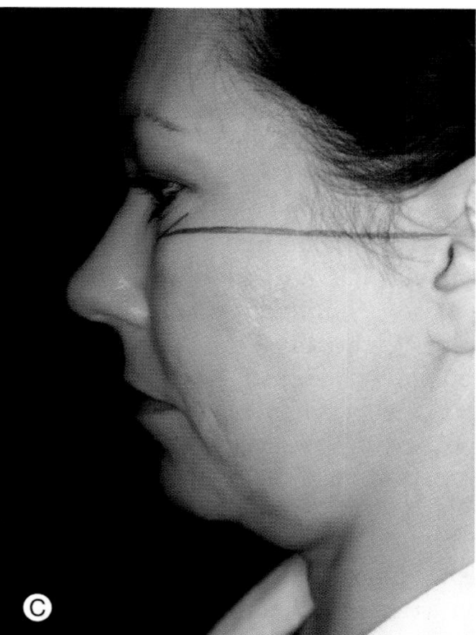

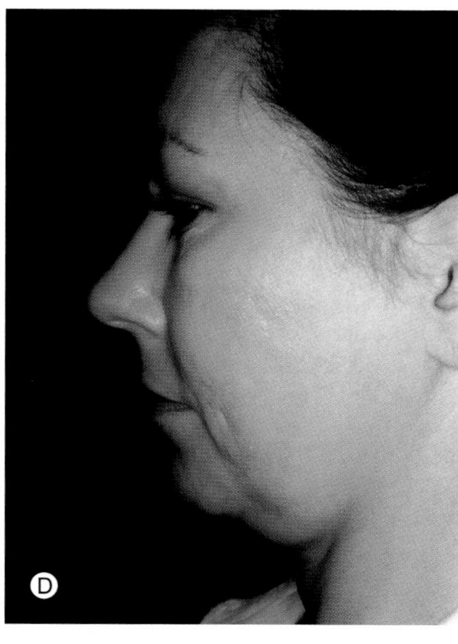

Figure 30.4 (A) Head position naturally assumed by this patient with a full neck, or obtuse hyomandibular angle. Chin is projected anteriorly, falling in a plane drawn vertically from the lower lip. (B) However, the Frankfort plane is not horizontal when the patient holds her head in this compensatory position. (C) The patient's head is then positioned in the Frankfort horizontal plane revealing the chin deficiency; (D) by using the vertical line of Gonzalez-Ulloa, at an angle of 90° to the Frankfort plane, or a line drawn from the lower lip with the head in the Frankfort plane. This patient was not initially offered chin augmentation, previously undergoing only submental liposuction. This suboptimal outcome was a missed opportunity to enhance the facial balance with a chin implant.

platysmaplasty, or submental liposuction. A chin implant improves aesthetically pleasing angles by lengthening and subsequently making more horizontal the submental line from cervical point to menton.[16]

Muscle function should be evaluated and photographically documented with the patient smiling, as asymmetry is not uncommon.

Lip posture is assessed at rest and in animation. In patients with more severe retruded chins, dimpling of the skin of the chin often accompanies labial incompetence as the mentalis muscles 'overwork,' attempting to create lip closure at rest.[29] This is a relative contraindication to chin augmentation with implants because of a higher rate of complications (see Pitfalls and their Management).

Other notable features of the physical exam are the presence of submental scars, skin thickness, a dimple or cleft, vertical height, pre-jowl sulcus, ptosis (witch's chin), and symmetry.

Intraorally, hygiene, occlusion, and the presence or absence of teeth or dentures is documented.

Chin/mandibular implants are appropriate for patients with mild microgenia (small chin) and normal or near-normal dental occlusion, and/or a pre-jowl sulcus. Microgenia is the result of underdevelopment of the mandibular symphysis with an adequate mandible.[17] Micrognathia is hypoplasia of various parts of the jaw with malocclusion. Patients with micrognathia, or microgenia with greater degrees of malocclusion, should be offered orthodontic or surgical correction—not chin augmentation with implants. Patients requiring more than 0.5 cm augmentation (approximately 0.8 cm anterior dimension implant) may develop complications from too large an implant; consideration should be given to horizontal osteotomy with mandibular advancement.[22] Increased or decreased vertical height, and bony asymmetries, are also better addressed by orthognathic procedures.

A surgeon who performs cervical liposuction or other neck and face contouring procedures will enhance satisfaction by educating patients on the role of their chin in facial balance and harmony.

Implant selection

Implant materials used historically include paraffin, gold, silver, ivory, bone, cartilage, dermis, and fat. Unpredictable absorption, reaction, and rejection have been some of the problems that have prompted surgeons to search for predictable and safe implants.

Alloplastic materials used with documented experience include silicone,[28,30,31] polymethacrylate (hard acrylic),[32] porous materials such as Mersiline mesh (Ethicon, Sommerville, NJ),[33] Proplast (polytetrafluorethylene, withdrawn from the market by the FDA in 1992), Medpor[18] (polyethylene; Porex Industries, Fairburn, GA), and more recently Gore-Tex (expanded polytetrafluorethylene; e-PTFE, WL Gore, Flagstaff, AZ).[18,34,35] (For general reading on implant materials see Choe and Stucki-McCormick,[18] Romo et al.,[34] Binder et al.[36])

The ideal implant material (Table 30.2) should be well tolerated with a non-palpable, natural feel, be stable and resist resorption and infection, be non-immunogenic and non-carcinogenic and be easily removed, as well as straightforward to insert and modify, flexible enough to conform to the underlying bony surface, and capable of being folded for placement through a relatively small incision.

Table 30.2 Ideal chin implant

Well tolerated
Non-palpable
Natural feel
Stable, resistant to resorption and infection
Non-immunogenic
Non-carcinogenic
Easily removed
Straightforward to insert and to modify
Flexible enough to conform to the underlying bony surface, and to be folded for placement through a relatively small incision

Silicone

Silastic is solid silicone rubber, which satisfies criteria for an ideal chin implant.[28,30,31,37,38] Silastic is flexible enough to be able to bend, allowing it to be inserted through a 2–3 cm incision. It is soft enough to suture through, to place holes, and to modify with a blade or scissors. At the same time, it is firm enough to approximate a natural feel to the chin, as its consistency is between that of hard bone and soft tissue. It maintains its shape, resisting resorption indefinitely. A thin fibrous capsule forms around the non-porous implant; there is no tissue ingrowth as in porous implants, making silastic easy to remove if necessary and unlikely to harbor bacteria. It is heat stable, allowing removal and resterilization if necessary. Holes are manufactured in some implants, and can be made on the others, to allow fibrous tissue ingrowth for stabilization.

This capsule does not distort the implant as a fibrous capsule may do to a silicone gel breast implant because the implant is solid, not gel, and is spread over bone. The capsule is even thought to help stabilize the implant to the surrounding tissues.[39]

Design of silastic implants has evolved and improved over the past two decades with the development of the extended mandibular implant. Formerly, implants were designed to augment the mandible in its anterior dimensions only, confined to a region between the mental foramina (thus, they are called 'central' implants). This anterior-only augmentation led to the term 'button' chin and, by augmenting only centrally, these implants often further deepened and accentuated the pre-jowl sulcus (Fig. 30.5 (top panel) and Fig. 30.11).

Mittelman[26] recognized that the anatomy of the aging mandible required augmentation in the pre-jowl sulcus, the depression formed by the bony anterior mandibular groove and soft tissue atrophy in the pre-jowl region. Central implants did not extend far enough laterally to augment this area. By designing a thicker extended lateral limb in the region of the pre-jowl sulcus, his Prejowl Chin Implant (Implantech; Ventura, CA) was able to address this anatomic deficiency in addition to anterior augmentation (Fig. 30.5 (bottom)).

For the patient with adequate anterior chin projection but needing pre-jowl augmentation alone to create a smoother, stronger jawline, Mittelman designed the Prejowl

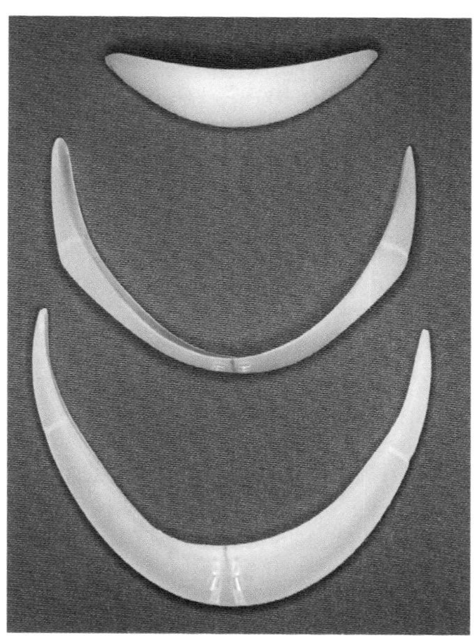

Figure 30.5 Silastic implants. From top to bottom: central implant; Mittelman Prejowl Implant; Mittelman Prejowl Chin Implant.

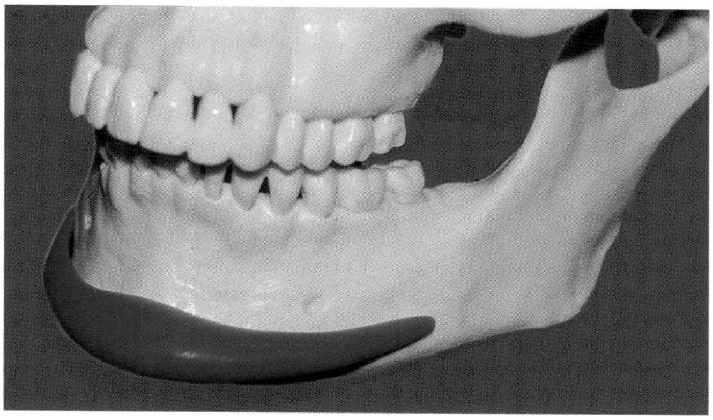

Figure 30.6 Proper position of an extended implant (blue sizer) over thick cortical bone of the mental symphysis, along the inferior mandibular border under the mental foramen, tapering laterally.

Implant with a thin central portion, providing minimal anterior projection, with thickness-confined to the pre-jowl sulcus (Fig. 30.5 (middle)). In his experience, 75% of face lift patients have a treatable pre-jowl sulcus and 40% have microgenia improvable with anterior augmentation as well.[11] Because the pre-jowl sulcus has a bony as well as a soft tissue component, face lift tightening of soft tissues alone is often insufficient to significantly smooth the entire sulcus; the thickening in pre-jowl sulcus of these implants helps to augment this defect.

Flowers[28] hand-sculpted implants from silicone blocks and later designed preformed extended implants with slightly softer consistency, greater flexibility, and different dimensions. He addressed the variety of angles of incline of the anterior face of the mandible, noting that an implant with a straight vertical back (as many central implants have) can cause problems in positioning. His implant, the Flowers Mandibular Glove (Implantech, Ventura, CA), has a caudal lip allowing vertical tilt, helping to create a smooth transition from implant to the non-augmented adjacent mandibular body.

Extended implants address the anatomy which results in chin and pre-jowl deficiencies; at the same time, they introduce additional considerations and features.

Dissection of a pocket to place these laterally extended implants requires care to avoid the mental and marginal mandibular nerves (Fig. 30.6). The limited lateral extent of central implants does not require dissection in these danger zones (Fig. 30.5 (top)). Chin Implant Style 3 (Allied Biomedical Corporation, Goose Creek, SC) has preformed cutouts on its superior aspect below the mental foramina, allowing more space (safety zone) between implant and mental nerve. Other design characteristics include fenestrations medially or laterally. These holes allow tissue ingrowth to help stabilize the implant, and the medial holes may be used as well for suture fixation. Fenestrations for tissue ingrowth and stabilization can be created by using a small (1.5 mm) trephine or punch biopsy instrument.

Because implants are commercially manufactured in a limited number of sizes, some modification may be performed on the implants if necessary. The implants may be trimmed superiorly to allow more clearance for the mental nerve, or to prevent pressure on dentures. Trimming laterally may facilitate insertion and prevents augmenting the jowl itself if a significant portion of the implant extends beyond the pre-jowl sulcus. Care must be taken to smoothly taper the lateral wings when trimming as sharp edges may result in extrusion. Another method of shortening an implant is to remove a central portion and to suture the two remaining halves together. This can give an implant the same length as if trimmed bilaterally, while preserving the thin tapers of the lateral edges. A pre-jowl implant can be sewn to a pre-jowl chin implant to provide additional pre-jowl augmentation without additional anterior projection.

To add augmentation to an already manufactured implant centrally only, a Glasgold Wafer (Implantech, Ventura, CA), a 2 mm disc without lateral extensions, can be positioned underneath the implant and sutured to the implant with non-absorbable sutures.[12] If any uncertainty exists regarding size, the smaller implant is inserted and if necessary, a wafer added. This avoids the time and additional surgical manipulation when using sizers.

■ TECHNIQUES

Surgical technique

Two surgical approaches have been utilized for placing a chin/mandibular implant—the intraoral (transoral) and submental (extraoral). Because a submental incision is used in neck contouring procedures such as liposuction, platysmaplasty and often in face lift, it will be discussed here. The intraoral technique is described elsewhere.[20] Its primary advantage is that there is no external incision; disadvantages include more difficult placement of extended implants laterally under the mental nerve, and more difficult suture fixation to the inferior border of the mandible. A review of over 100 cases of adverse events after chin implant augmentation stated 'almost all chin implant problems that the senior author has seen were caused by implants placed transorally'.[13] Training and experience of the surgeon certainly contribute to choice of approach as well.

Submental approach

The scar from the submental approach usually heals well and is inconspicuous since it is on the underside of the chin and not visible from the front or side.

Anesthesia may be accomplished in a variety of manners. If the surgeon and patient choose intravenous sedation or general anesthesia, 1–2% lidocaine with 1 in 100 000 or 1 in 200 000 epinephrine (adrenaline) is infiltrated by injecting through the skin with a 30-gauge 1 inch needle in a perpendicular manner to bone and periosteum, along the soft tissue adjacent to the periosteum, and skin and subcutaneous tissue at the incision line.

If the patient will be sedated orally, or not sedated at all, a bilateral mental nerve block may be administered prior to local infiltration.

Prior to surgical prep, the midline is marked on the chin and submental area across the proposed incision. The position of the mental foramen may be marked after locating it by intraoral palpation at the base of, or anterior or posterior to the second premolar, approximately halfway down the mandible.[22]

The incision is made in the submental crease, or slightly posterior to it. Because the incision and resulting scar is so well hidden, it is not necessary to minimize the incision. A longer incision will provide better exposure, facilitate implant insertion, and allow the periosteal elevator to remain on bone when it advances laterally as the mandible curves posteriorly. A 2–3 cm incision is carried through skin and subcutaneous tissue to the mandible. The periosteum is exposed, then incised horizontally with the blade, and a subperiosteal plane developed superiorly with a Freer periosteal elevator. The bony surface should be clearly seen (Fig. 30.7). The feel and sound of the elevator on bone should be present during the entire dissection of the pocket. When superior pocket elevation has reached 1.5 cm or the labiomental sulcus, a Joseph periosteal elevator is used to develop the lateral pocket along the inferior border of the mandible (Fig. 30.8A). The non-dominant hand is essential to externally palpate the elevator, guiding it and providing feedback that it is indeed hugging the inferior mandibular border, avoiding the mental nerve and not levering upward into the overlying soft tissues.

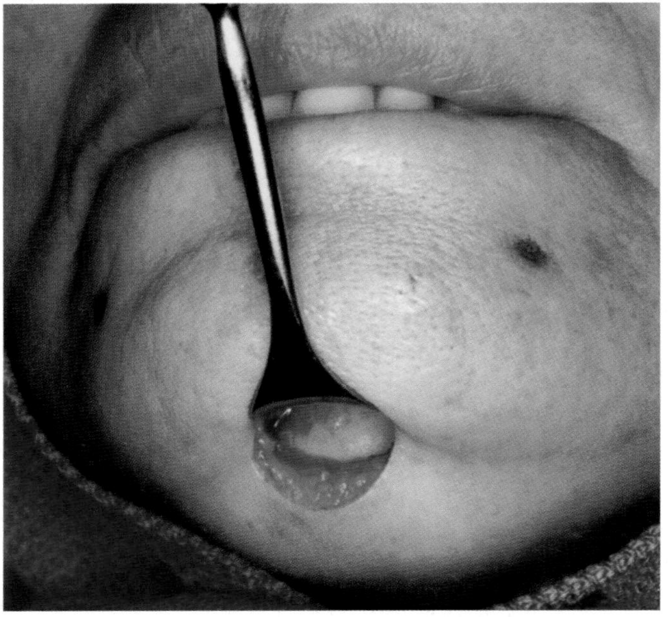

Figure 30.7 Bone exposed after subperiosteal dissection.

The mental foramen and nerve lie 1.5 cm superior to the inferior mandibular border in younger patients.[12,34] In the aging mandible, 8–10 mm of distance remains.[11] Therefore the width of the elevator should be 8 mm in an older patient to avoid injury to the nerve (up to 1 cm in younger patients). The implant should have a height of 6–8 mm in this area.[11] The superior border of the implant may be trimmed with scissors if necessary.

Opinion is divided regarding the necessity to visualize the mental nerve and foramen. Terino[20] recommends an Aufricht fiberoptic light retractor for direct visualization to prevent injury. On the other hand, if the dissection is carefully guided using knowledge of anatomic landmarks, (palpation and marking of the mental foramen), staying on bone, and on the inferior mandibular border (and not below it) at all times, it may not be necessary to visualize the mental nerve and foramen.[22,28] Using these principles, and the non-dominant hand, the lateral dissection may proceed without direct visualization of the developing pocket.

The lateral extent of the pocket is judged by knowing the dimensions of the implant. Most extended lateral implants have a posterior surface of 9–12 cm long, so the lateral dissection must at least be 4.5–6.0 cm on either side of the midline. The pocket should be made slightly larger, around 5 mm, than the dimensions of the implant to accommodate it comfortably.

A sizer implant can be placed on the skin to give a close idea of the size and extent of the pocket (Fig. 30.9A), keeping in mind that the thickness of the skin and anterior dimensions of the implant will require a more laterally extended pocket on bone than is apparent from marking around an implant placed on skin. Before placing an implant, the pocket is examined using an Aufricht retractor for any bleeding or irregularities. A gentamicin solution in which the sizers and implant are placed is then used to generously irrigate the pocket. Sizer implants may be used to assess the adequacy of the pocket, and the appropriate size of implant for the patient. Sizers are manufactured in identical sizes to the permanent implants, and are intended for insertion, inspection, and then removal once the ideal size has been chosen. It must be kept in mind that in the supine position, the mandible retracts. A jaw thrust can advance the mandible for better size assessment. Local anesthesia may also distort the volume of the soft tissue of the chin; minor adjustments must also be made for this.

The procedure for inserting a sizer (Fig. 30.9) is identical to that of inserting the permanent implant (with suture fixation following insertion for the permanent implant).

One limb of the sizer/implant is grasped with an Adson dressing forceps and directed through the incision into the far-side pocket, exposing and opening the pocket with the Aufricht retractor (Figs 30.8B, 30.9B). When it has been advanced as far as it can go, the middle of the implant is grasped with a hemostat or Adson forceps near the midline and stabilized. This maneuver helps keep the first side from slipping out of the incision while the second side is inserted. When both ends are in their respective lateral pockets, the center of the flexible implant may still be buckled outside the incision. The center can be pressed down toward the

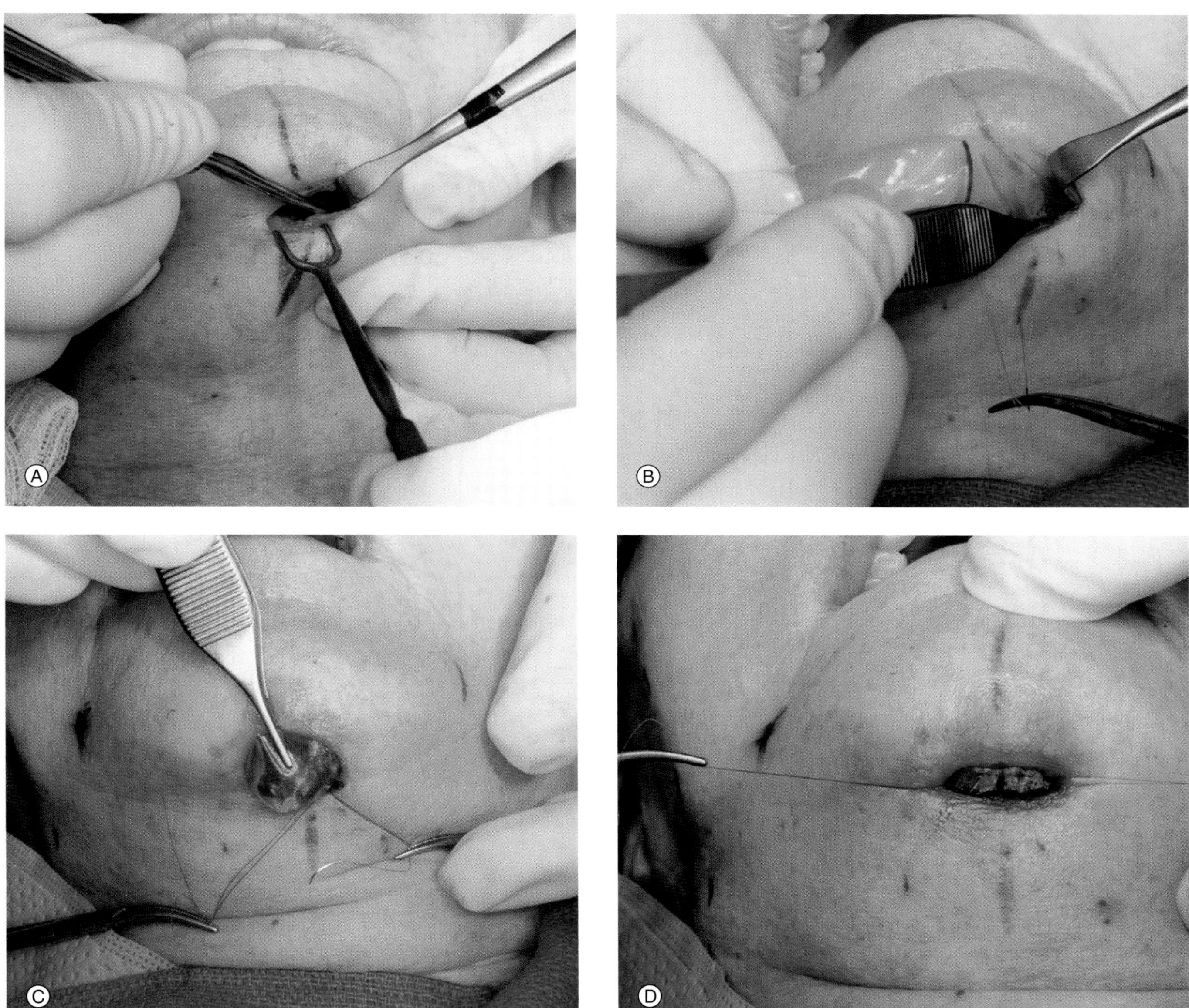

Figure 30.8 (A) Dissection of lateral pocket at inferior mandibular border with Joseph periosteal elevator. (B) Insertion of implant into pocket. (C) Buckled center of implant pressed toward bone. (D) Midline marker of implant aligned with midline skin markings, with sutures on either side prior to placement.

bone, pushing each tip outward toward the full lateral extent of the pocket (Figs 30.8C, 30.9C).

After an implant has been placed, it should lie flat without lifting away from bone, which would indicate too small a pocket, or ends misplaced in soft tissue irregularities, preventing full lateral extension along the bony surface. To assure that the ends are not folded, curled, or in a 'false tunnel',[20] a flat elevator can be advanced laterally above and below the implant to unfold it.

Next, the midline marker of the implant is aligned with the midline previously marked on the skin. If no midline marker is on the implant, the midline must be marked on the implant with a notch prior to insertion. Once its midline position is established, the implant should be stabilized in at least two places. One 5-0 Vicryl (polydioxanone) (Ethicon, Sommerville, NJ) suture is placed on each side of the midline (Fig. 30.8D), either through prefabricated holes, or by placing the curved needle directly through the implant. This is sutured to the inferior cuff of periosteum and soft tissue. For all implants, the inferior aspect of the overlying soft tissues is incorporated in the closure with inferior periosteum to cover the implant. The remainder of the deep tissue and muscle is closed with 6-0 Vicryl in two layers and the skin closed with a suture of choice. Steri-strips (3M, St Paul, Minnesota) are applied over the closure and the chin is covered in a sling or hammock-like dressing with Steri-strips or Elastoplast (Johnson and Johnson, New Brunswick, NJ) tape, left on for 3–5 days.

■ OPTIMIZING OUTCOMES

The subperiosteal dissection plane has been chosen for description here because of its several advantages. Bone is the surgeon's guide to safety. It is a well-defined plane,

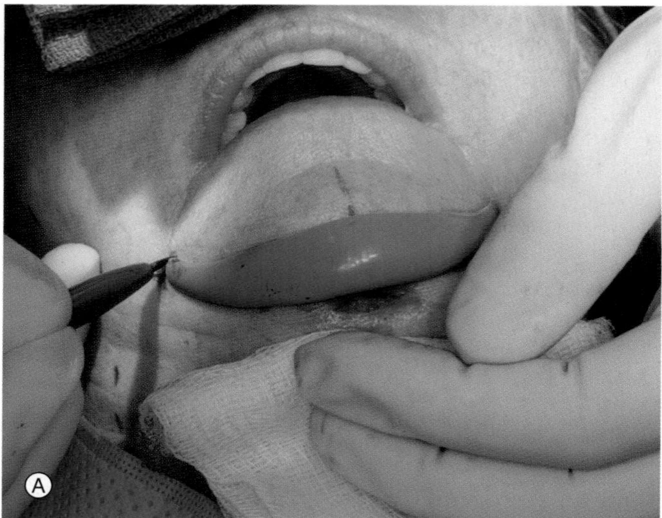

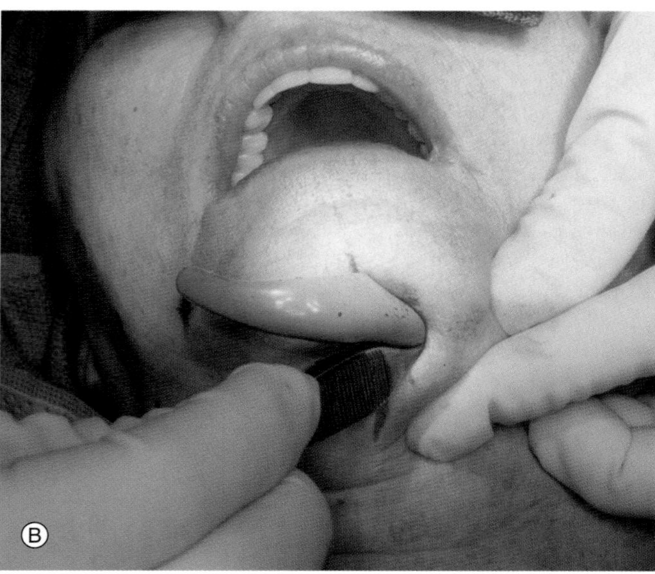

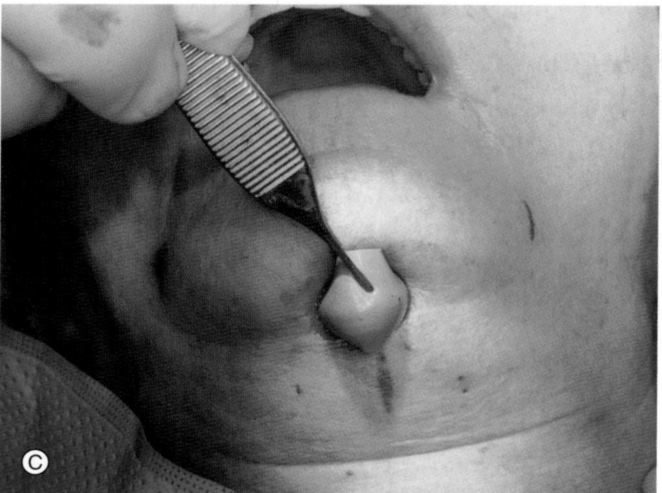

Figure 30.9 Insertion of a blue sizer. (A) Size of pocket estimated by marking with sizer on skin. (B) Adson dressing forceps directing sizer into lateral pocket. (C) The opposite limb of the sizer has been inserted into its pocket. The center of the flexible sizer is grasped in its center, and pushed down toward bone.

easily identifiable with exposed bone at the entire floor of the space. Bone also adds to stability to the implant,[11,18] as does the overlying periosteum.[40] The dissection plane is relatively avascular. Another safety feature is created by confining the dissecting instrument to contact with bone, using audible, palpable, and visual feedback, thereby dissecting deeper and further away from the marginal mandibular nerve, which lies in the overlying soft tissues between periosteum and muscle.

The subperiosteal dissection becomes somewhat technically difficult 1.5–2 cm lateral to the midline because of dense connective tissue,[28] the anterior mandibular ligament.[20]

A theoretical disadvantage to the subperiosteal plane is bone resorption (see Complications under Pitfalls and their Management). Some surgeons, concerned with bone resorption under implants placed directly on bone (subperiosteal), prefer a supraperiosteal pocket (especially for the medial portion of the implant), to prevent bone resorption. The supraperiosteal plane, however, has the disadvantages of being more vascular and closer to the marginal mandibular nerve, and the implant is visible in thin skin. Because a supraperiosteal plane allows increased mobility of the implant, it has been suggested to convert from a supraperiosteal to a subperiosteal dissection laterally, 1 cm to 1.5 cm[40] or 2 cm[34] to 3 cm[11,28] lateral to the midline. This provides stability laterally while theoretically avoiding bone resorption centrally.

■ POSTOPERATIVE CARE

Minimal care is required postoperatively. The dressing, in place for 3–5 days, minimizes swelling and bruising and is a reminder to the patient that surgery did take place because postoperative pain is often not significant. Pain may be greater for a larger implant due to distention of the periosteum.

Trauma, such as that which may be encountered with an active child, could result in displacement. A soft diet should be followed to minimize muscle motion.

■ PITFALLS AND THEIR MANAGEMENT

Complications

Marginal mandibular nerve injury

If the elevator levers upward off bone into overlying soft tissue, the marginal mandibular nerve is at risk of injury. This may occur if its angle of entry is restricted by too small an incision. A larger incision will assist in keeping the elevator on bone as it follows the curvature of the mandible posteriorly.

A 'false tunnel'[20] created in this way may allow placement of an implant tail into it resulting in nerve compression. Figure 30.10A illustrates a case in which marginal mandibular nerve injury was clinically demonstrated by weakness of the left lip depressors and inability to pull the ipsilateral lip downward and laterally. Nerve stimulation testing revealed the nerve to be functional (thus intact), rather than having been severed and non-functional. CT scan documented the position of the left limb of the implant to be inferior to the mandible laterally, and not in contact with bone but rather in the soft tissue in proximity to the marginal mandibular nerve (Fig. 30.10B).

The implant was subsequently removed, the lateral limbs shortened by trimming the implant with curved scissors, and repositioned entirely on bone. A larger incision was used to allow the elevator to better follow the curvature of this patient's narrow mandible, improve visualization of the pocket and allow easier insertion of the implant. Following this revision, the patient exercised the lip depressors and nerve stimulation was performed. Complete recovery of the injured nerve occurred in 2 months.

Mental nerve injury

Short-term dysesthesias may be experienced by 20—30% of patients.[11] This may occur from operative trauma to the mental nerve by direct contact or cautery, or indirectly by traction on the nerve or by swelling around the nerve within the non-expandable subperiosteal pocket, or by hematoma. If complete anesthesia exists, or if dysesthesia (unilaterally or bilaterally) is present 2 weeks[20] to 3 weeks[13] postoperatively, and is not resolving or improving, removal should be considered. Prior to removal, if any questions about the position of the implant remains, a 3-dimensional model can be made from a CT scan to show the position of the implant relative to the mental foramen. This may document impingement on the mental nerve, and if so, should be followed by surgical removal of the implant. Prior to immediate replacement, the surgeon should develop the pocket inferiorly to allow the implant to descend and settle. If the CT shows a properly positioned implant at the inferior mandibular border still with impingement on a low foramen, as in a vertically short mandible,[17] the implant should be modified by trimming its superior border laterally under the position of the nerve. This should be performed by 4 weeks. Permanent loss of sensation may occur if impingement is allowed to persist for 8 weeks or more.[13] If impingement is not present on CT or if the above revisions do not restore sensation, the nerve may have been severed, although this is rare. Extended implants increase the risk to the mental nerve, as central implants are not as long. Central implants reside medial to the foramina, not inferior and lateral to the nerve as extended implants do (Fig. 30.6).

Overcorrection

As noted above, no mathematical formulas exist to correctly choose implant size in every patient. For example, a chin implant may meet the vertical plane established by Gonzalez-Ulloa, but it may still appear overcorrected in the formula of Riedel. Consideration of ethnicity and relationships with the nose, lips, and neck may influence the decision.

Another factor that makes precise measures difficult is that the soft tissue response is not 1 : 1. For a chin implant, the ratio is reported to be from 0.66 : 1,[22] to 0.8 : 1.[15] For example, at a soft tissue ratio of 0.66 : 1 an implant with a 0.8 cm anterior projection will provide approximately 0.52 cm of projection[22] because of redistribution and circumferential displacement of soft tissues, as well as

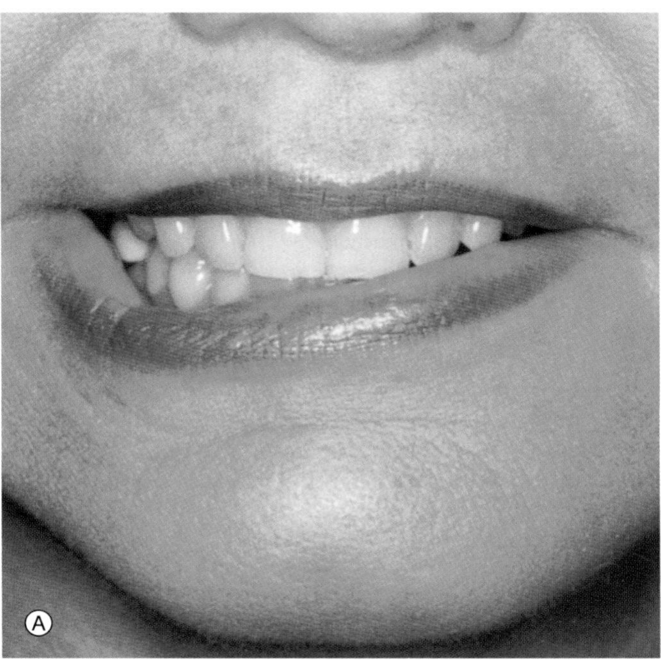

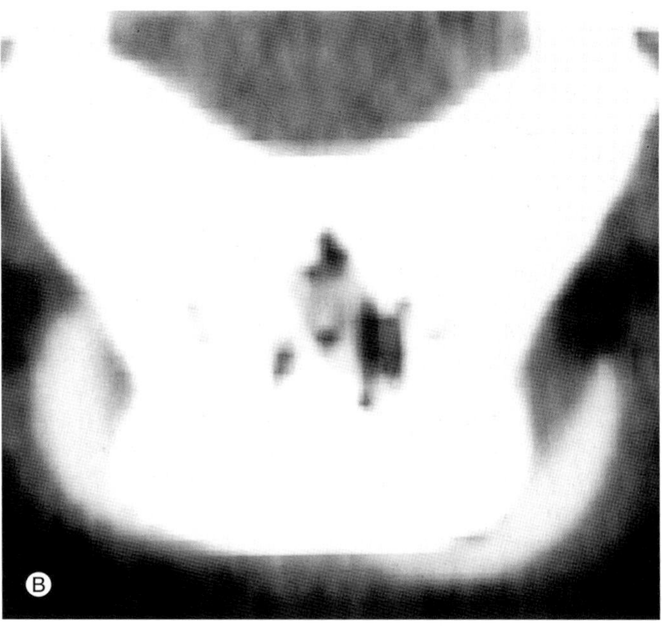

Figure 30.10 (A) Left-sided injury to marginal mandibular nerve results in inability of lip depressors to pull lip downward and laterally when smiling. (B) CT scan showing left limb of implant displaced inferiorly and laterally in the soft tissues away from bone, impinging upon the marginal mandibular nerve.

posterior settling into bone.[41] Most properly selected patients with microgenia only require a slight increase in volume.[14] The augmentation should not need to exceed 0.5 cm.[22] If a larger implant than size small or medium is required, orthognathic surgery should be offered because of complications arising from too large an implant.[22]

Undercorrection

Undercorrection may be addressed by adding a Glasgold Wafer (Implantech, Ventura, CA) without having to replace the original implant,[12] or replacement with a larger implant.

Removal of implants

If an implant is removed because it is too large, it should be replaced with a smaller implant because of unpredictable distortion of the soft tissue chin pad after removal without replacement.[13,17] Others suggest osseous genioplasty on all patients who require removal of chin implants.[42]

Visible or palpable projections

The borders of implants may be visible or palpable; a firm, non-flexible (acrylic, or hard rubber) central type implant may be too stiff to conform to the curvature of the mandible, causing projection laterally. Larger central implants are more likely to do so (Fig. 30.11). Serial cuts made on the back of a stiff, non-conforming implant have been described to allow the implant to conform to the bony arch.[30] An articulated chin implant is also manufactured to accomplish the same thing (Allied Biomedical Corporation, Goose Creek, SC).

An implant may be visible in a patient with very thin skin. This would be more likely with supraperiosteal dissection (Fig. 30.11); subperiosteal placement entirely, or at least laterally, should minimize this possibility, by holding the implant in a more compact space over bone.

Softer flexible, extended implants with thin tapered tails help implants conform to the shape of the mandible and almost imperceptibly blend with bone inferiorly and laterally, where the skin is more thin and the implant potentially more visible.

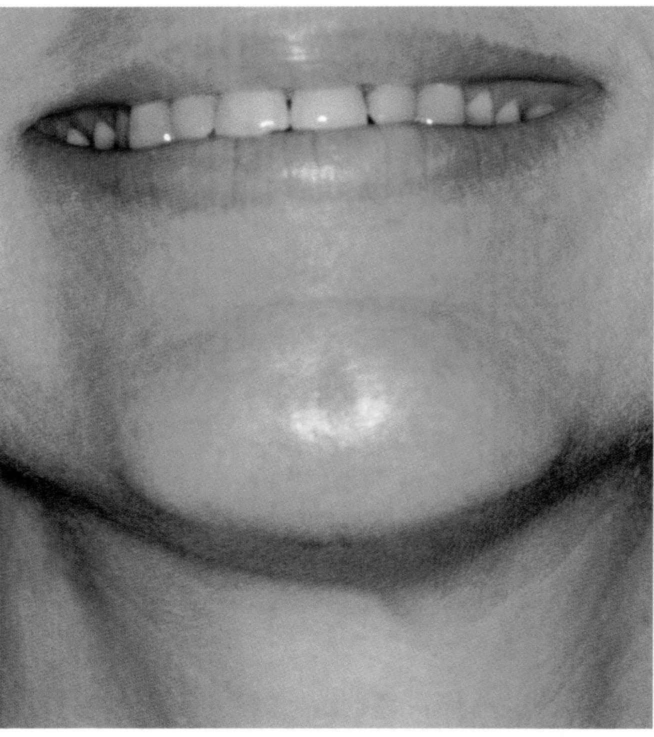

Figure 30.11 Visible borders in a patient with thin skin who was augmented with a large, non-conforming, non-tapered, central implant placed above the periosteum. Also note accentuation of pre-jowl sulcus.

Bone resorption

First reported in 1969[43] bone resorption was radiographically documented in 12 of 14 patients. A subsequent study of 85 asymptomatic patients revealed 47 to have bone resorption.[44] Common to these groups of patients reported in the 1960s and 1970s was subperiosteal placement.

There is evidence that the placement above or below the periosteum does not make a difference in bone resorption,[45] and that when implants are properly placed over the thick cortical bone of the inferior mandible, bone resorption is asymptomatic and of minor concern. Loss of correction has not been noted with bone resorption,[44,46] which is self-limiting, occurring during the first 6–12 months[22,47] and stabilizing after 2 years. Bone resorption is a problem if the implant is resting over the thin alveolar bone overlying dental roots.[29] Erosion though this bone can damage the roots of the teeth and cause premature loss. Local symptoms, such as toothache, require radiographic evaluation.[48] This positioning can result from cephalad migration of the implant, more likely with the intraoral approach because of difficulty stabilizing the implant to the inferior mandible.

Increased pressure of an implant on bone resulting in bone resorption can occur with too large and/or hard an implant as a result of mentalis muscle action. Extended implants spread the pressure on the bone over a much wider area, 9–12 cm versus 3–4 cm for a central implant, presumably reducing the incidence of bone resorption.[28] This pressure effect is increased in patients with more mandibular retrusion or severe microgenia, secondary to more tensing of the mentalis muscle to create good lip seal. A clinical sign of this potential problem is labial incompetence[29] (Fig. 30.12A). In these patients, lip seal is accomplished by mentalis muscle strain leading to skin dimpling (fasciculation) in the chin. This also occurs during speech and swallowing. These patients should be followed clinically and radiographically for signs of dental root impingement[49] which, if discovered, suggests bone resorption resulting from cephalad migration and/or original cephalad positioning and requires implant removal. Silastic implants should be avoided in these patients. Rather, they should be offered correction using orthognathic surgical techniques.

In properly selected patients with mild microgenia, no chin dimpling, or labial incompetence, with implants properly positioned over the lower, central, thick, hard mentum, bone resorption is asymptomatic, self-limiting, may help stabilize the implant as it settles into bone,[29] and does not require removal.

Migration/malposition

Improper position of an implant may be secondary to incorrect surgical positioning of the implant, or to subsequent migration. Displacement of silicone implants occurs in less than 0.5%.[31] The implant should rest over the thick bone at the inferior mandibular border, laterally

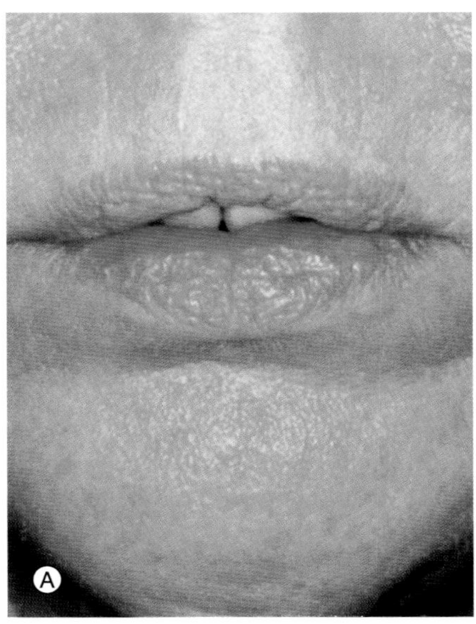
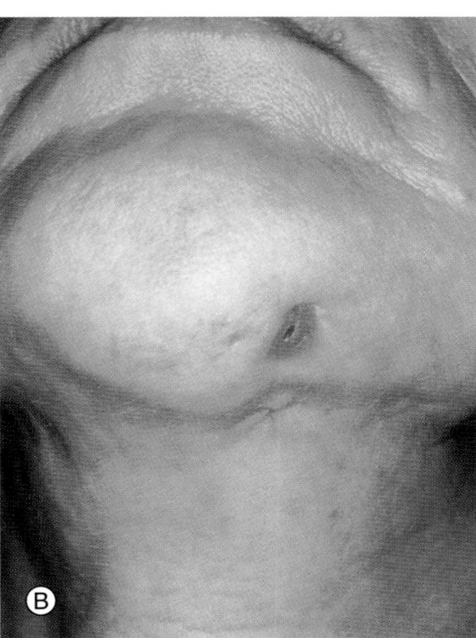

Figure 30.12 (A) Labial incompetence. (B) Fistula. Infection, possibly from poor dental hygiene, or mobility secondary to labial incompetence, resulted 1 year postoperatively in a draining fistula. This patient had an extended silicone implant placed subperiosteally, through the submental route.

extending beneath the mental foramina. The lateral extensions and mental nerves help stabilize the lateral limbs.[20] Stabilization can be achieved by subperiosteal placement of the implant[20] either entirely or laterally.[11,34,40] Suture may be used to secure the implant, preventing migration and cephalad slippage,[13,34] one on each side of the midline[11,12,14] or three sutures 1 cm apart.[20] Screw fixation may also be used to accomplish stabilization.[18,35]

Mentalis hyperactivity in patients with labial incompetence may also contribute to migration.

Some surgeons choose porous implants such as Mersiline mesh (Ethicon, Sommerville, NJ) for tissue ingrowth and stability.[33] Gore-Tex (WL Gore and Associates, Flagstaff, AZ) has pore sizes up to 30 microns allowing limited fibrous tissue ingrowth,[34,35,40] and early stabilization,[18] though still requiring suture stabilization.[34]

Infection

Infection with silicone implants has been reported to be rare, at 0.7%[31] (Fig. 30.12B). The intraoral procedure had a higher infection rate in one report.[50] The implant material has been suggested to play a role because with porous materials, such as Gore-Tex and Medpor, tissue, blood, and bacteria can enter the implant, through the pores, whereas this is not the case with Silastic.[38,51.52] Mobility may predispose to infection.[46] 'Micromotion' may lead to chronic inflammation which in turn can result in secondary bacterial seeding.[35]

Infection may manifest as cellulitis, abscess, or fistula. A 3–4 week trial of oral antibiotics or a brief course of intravenous antibiotics may be tried.[46] Porous implants are less likely than silastic to be salvaged in this way.[15,38] If infection persists, the implant should be removed. In a retrospective study of 480 implants, 0.62% of patients required removal because of infection.[30] If an implant must be removed because of infection, a reinsertion delay of 3 months,[37] 6 months, or 12 months[38,46,48] should be observed.

Infection may be avoided with the use of perioperative antibiotics, removal of glove powder, or by soaking the implants and sizers in an antibiotic solution of gentamicin[11] or cephazolin[20] and using this solution to irrigate the pocket. Irrigation also assists in removing any blood or tissue debris. Avoidance of hematoma[38] and use of sterile technique are important.

Late infections are usually from seeding from another source, such as a dental infection[31,46,53] or dental procedure.[46] Because many patients will not think to tell their surgeon about their dental appointments, it has been suggested that patients reveal the presence of an implant to their dentist prior to dental procedures,[20,46] and patients with chin implants should be given prophylactic antibiotics 12–24 hours before a dental procedure, even cleaning.[51]

Extrusion

Extrusion of silicone implants is uncommon, affecting fewer than 0.5% of cases,[31] but does occur. It is not secondary to allergic or foreign body reactions.[37] A pocket that is too small may cause a pressure point on skin or oral mucosa; an implant that is too large for the pocket, especially if placed intraorally, may increase tension on the incision and result in extrusion.[17,38]

Infection,[53] trauma,[38] hematoma,[48] or the sharp edges of a hand-carved silicone implant are additional etiologies.

Hematoma

Hematoma is also uncommon.[22] The subperiosteal plane is relatively avascular and should be less likely than the supraperiosteal dissection to develop this complication. Most bleeding is encountered at the incision site. The mental artery exits the mental foramen with the nerve; this neurovascular bundle is to be carefully avoided. Intraoperative hemostasis is achieved with the use of epinephrine (adrenaline) 1 in 100 000 to 1 in 200 000 in the local infiltrate, electrocautery, including directly on bleeding from bone,[46] and blood pressure control. Preoperatively, avoidance of the numerous agents that predispose to bleeding (aspirin, anticoagulants, herbal products, and foods) and attention to hypertension are required.

To prevent hematoma postoperatively, a compression dressing for at least 3–5 days, pain control, rest, avoidance of trauma, gentle mastication with soft diet, maintenance of normal blood pressure and control of nausea and vomiting[51] are essential.

Necrosis

The compression dressing must not be placed too tightly as this has been reported to cause ischemia and necrosis of overlying skin;[48] tape should be applied with little tension. Pressure necrosis may result from a large implant placed intraorally exerting tension on the closure, resulting in extrusion.[17]

Asymmetry

Asymmetry may result from early postoperative edema,[38,48] hematoma, malpositioning during placement, migration postoperatively, or unappreciated preoperative asymmetry. It can be avoided by adequately preparing the pocket, stabilizing the implant, visualizing the midline marker on the implant aligned with the patient's midline, and recognizing and addressing with the patient preoperative asymmetry.

If unrecognized, preexisting asymmetry can be exaggerated by the addition of an implant, which may be a cause of patient dissatisfaction if not discussed preoperatively. The patient should be told that asymmetries will often persist and are difficult to correct with implants.

If asymmetry is noted postoperatively, preoperative photographs should be reviewed, and edema, infection, hematoma, folding of a lateral limb and migration must be considered and addressed. To correct minor asymmetries, an implant may be carved or a Glasgold Wafer[12] (Implantech, Ventura, CA) modified and added. Significant bony asymmetry should be referred for orthognathic surgery.

Changes in pre-existing characteristics

Changes in pre-existing characteristics may also occur. A central cleft or dimple may be changed by alloplastic augmentation.[28] If a new dimple is desired, this may not be achievable by placing clefts in the implant because the overlying soft tissue may be too thick and stretched to conform to a depression in the implant.

Dentures

Dentures may create excess pressure by resting on the implant in the labial sulcus. Edentulous patients have a shorter vertical mandibular height, and implants placed intraorally may be positioned higher on the mandible. If this occurs, the implant should be trimmed superiorly or repositioned inferiorly. The edge of dentures may also place pressure on an intraoral incision and lead to possible pressure necrosis.

Speech and smile alterations

Swelling and disruption of the muscles of the chin may cause temporary changes in smiling and speech. The central portion of the lower lip may not function properly due to disruption of the mentalis muscle, more common with the intraoral approach.[42] The lip depressors originate along the oblique line at the inferior mandibular border; dissection at this point, distention by the implant, or edema may cause temporary dysfunction. This, along with alteration in sensation, may cause slight speech impediment. These problems usually resolve in 2–4 weeks as muscles reattach to the capsule that forms around the implant.[37] Other problems may be caused by disinsertion of muscles, including disfigurement.[42]

Avoidance of pitfalls

- Failure to offer or perform chin augmentation resulting from lack of proper preoperative analysis
- Nerve injury (marginal mandibular or mental nerve) due to lack of knowledge of anatomy or poor technique
- Permanent nerve damage if impingement upon nerve not recognized early and corrected
- Overcorrection due to inadequate preoperative analysis
- Bone resorption resulting in dental root injury if implant placed too high
- Migration if implant not stabilized by sutures or subperiosteal placement, or if displaced by unrecognized mentalis muscle hyperactivity in patients with labial incompetence
- Infection from unrecognized dental source or later infection from dental procedure
- Asymmetry secondary to improper placement or unrecognized preoperative asymmetry

SUMMARY

Chin augmentation with silicone implants produces pleasing aesthetic results by contributing to facial balance and harmony, while not appearing 'surgical' or artificial. It can be performed independently or with complimentary procedures, enhancing the outcome of these procedures in a subtle manner (Figs 30.13–30.17).

Properly performed on appropriate patients, chin implants have minimal morbidity and provide great patient satisfaction.

The surgeon who offers and performs a chin implant has provided the patient with a long-term predictable procedure. This can only be accomplished after a thorough profile analysis with the patient's head posed in the Frankfort plane. Chin augmentation with silastic implants significantly improves the results of neck sculpting and face lifts, as well as liposuction of the neck.

With diligent attention to surgical technique, including creating a subperiosteal pocket and stabilizing the implant with sutures, complications can be minimized, and corrected when they do occur, typically in less than 1% of patients.

Profile enhancements with chin implants accomplish a natural look and feel while providing permanent improvement in facial balance.

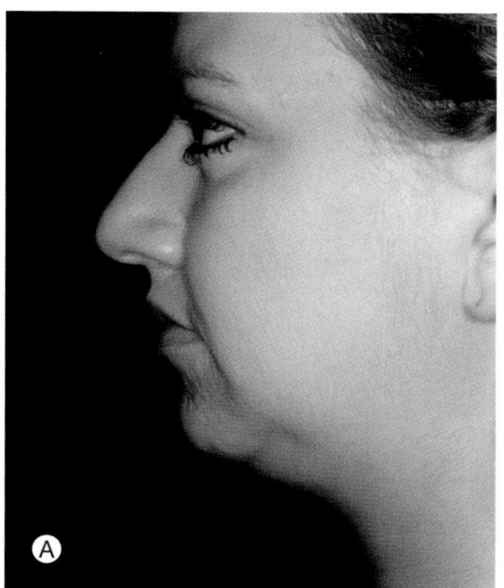

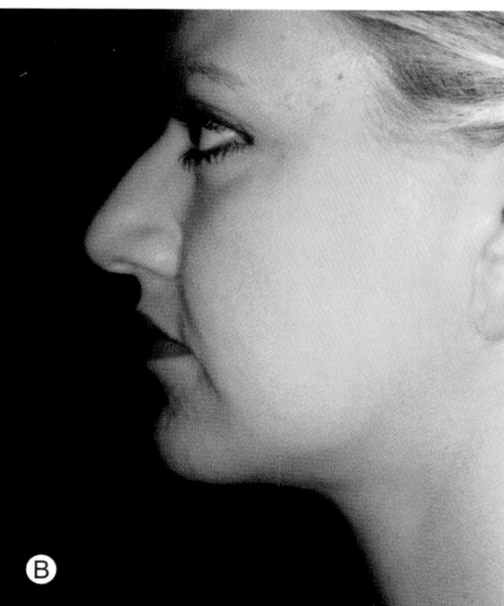

Figure 30.13 Patient (A) before and (B) after submental liposuction and chin augmentation.

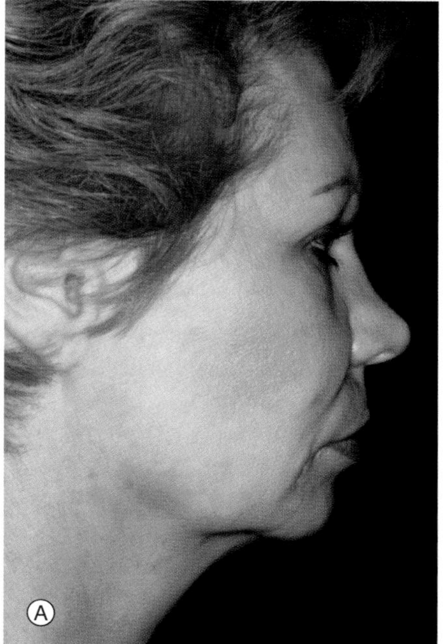

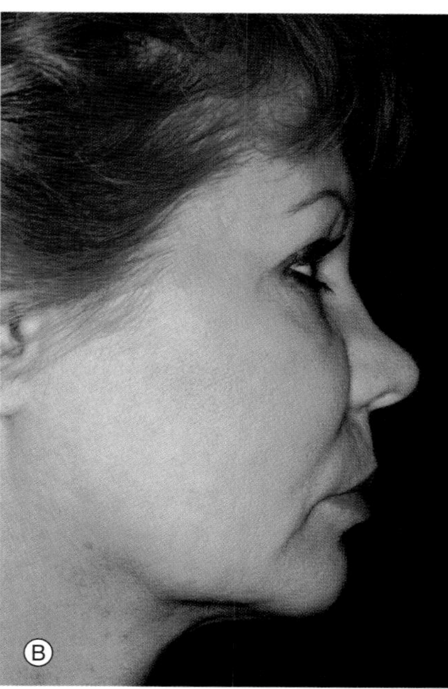

Figure 30.14 Patient (A) before and (B) after submental liposuction and chin augmentation, and fat grafting to mid-face and cheeks.

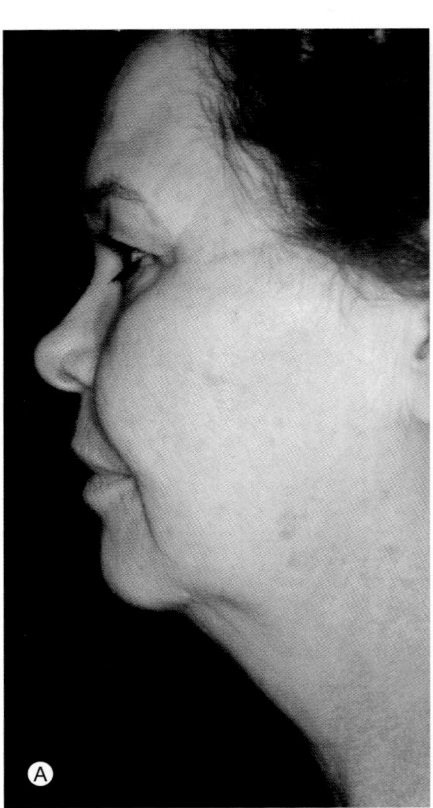

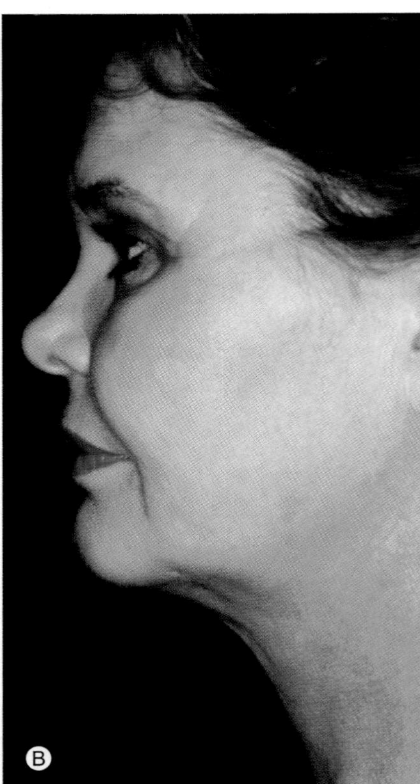

Figure 30.15 Patient (A) before and (B) after medium-depth chemical peel, upper blepharoplasty, submental liposuction, and chin augmentation.

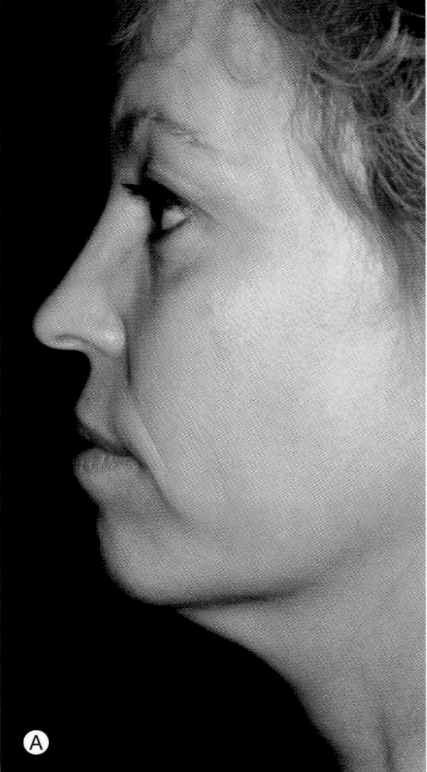

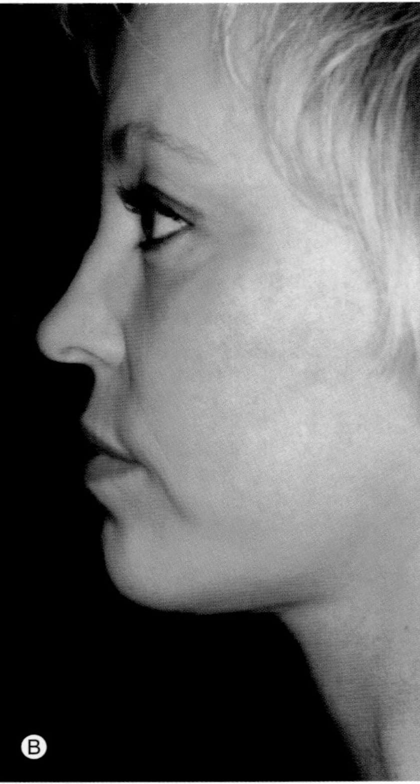

Figure 30.16 Patient (A) before and (B) after upper blepharoplasty, medium-depth full face peel with deep periorbital peel, face lift, and chin augmentation.

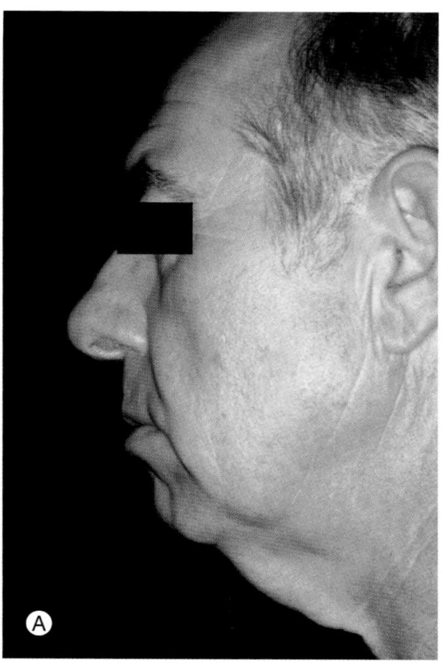

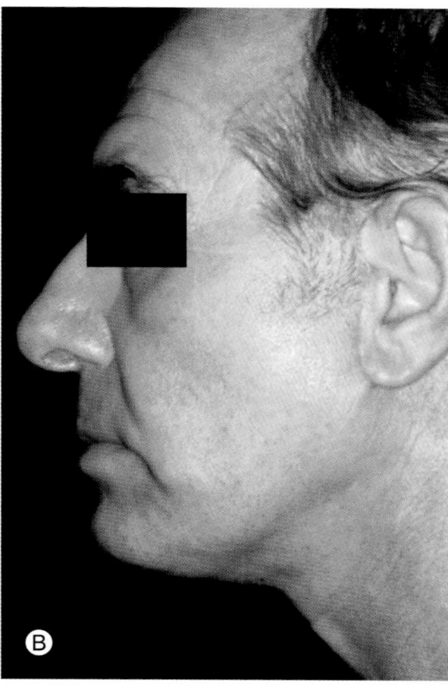

Figure 30.17 Patient (A) before and (B) following upper blepharoplasty, face lift, and chin augmentation.

■ REFERENCES

1. Etcoff N. Survival of the prettiest. The science of beauty. New York: Doubleday; 1999;75.
2. Farkas LG, Sohm P, Kolar JC, Katic MJ, Munro IR. Inclinations of the facial profile: art versus reality. Plast Reconstr Surg 1985; 75:509–519.
3. Tolleth H. Aesthetics and plastic surgery. In: Terino EO, Flowers RS, eds. The art of alloplastic facial contouring. St Louis: Mosby; 2000; 3–11.
4. Gonzalez-Ulloa M. Quantitative principles in cosmetic surgery of the face (profileplasty). Plast Reconstr Surg 1962; 29:186–198.
5. Gonzalez-Ulloa M. A quantum method for the appreciation of the morphology of the face. Plast Reconstr Surg 1964; 34:241–246.
6. Gonzalez-Ulloa M, Stevens E. The role of chin correction in profileplasty. Plast Reconstr Surg 1968; 41:477–486.
7. Borman H, Ozgur F. A simple instrument to define the Frankfurt horizontal plane for soft tissue measurements of the face. Plast Reconstr Surg 1998; 102:580–581.
8. Ricketts RM, Schulhof RJ, Bagha L. Orientation—sella-nasion or Frankfort horizontal. Am J Orthod 1976; 69:648–654.
9. Manuscript criteria and information: Instructions for authors. Arch Facial Plast Surg 2003; 5:132. Available online: http://www.archfacial.com (last accessed 1 June 2004).
10. Nassif PS, Kokoska MS. Aesthetic facial analysis. Facial Plast Surg Clin North Am 1999; 7:1–15.
11. Mittelman H. Augmentation of the chin and prejowl sulcus. In: Terino EO, Flowers RS, eds. The art of alloplastic facial contouring. St Louis: Mosby; 2000; 167–181.
12. Glasgold AI, Glasgold MJ. Mentoplasty. Facial Plast Surg Clin North Am. 1994; 2:285–299.
13. Zide BM, Pfeifer TM, Longaker MT. Chin surgery: I. Augmentation—the allures and the alerts. Plast Reconstr Surg 1999; 104:1843–1853.
14. Szachowicz E, Kridel RWH. Adjunctive measures to rhinoplasty. Otolaryngol Clin North Am 1987; 20:895–912.
15. Guyuron B. Genioplasty. In: Goldwyn RM, Cohen MN, eds. The unfavorable result in plastic surgery. Avoidance and treatment. 3rd edn. Philadelphia: Lippincott Williams and Wilkins; 2001; 1036–1042.
16. Brennan HG, Parkes ML. Submentoplasty: classification and theoretical outline of management. Arch Otolaryngol 1972; 95:24–29.
17. McCarthy JG, Kawamoto H, Grayson BH, et al. Surgery of the jaws. In: McCarthy JG, ed. Plastic surgery. Philadelphia: WB Saunders; 1990; 1188–1474.
18. Choe KS, Stucki-McCormick SU. Chin augmentation. Facial Plast Surg 2000; 16:45–54.
19. Auletta MJ, Grekin R. Local anesthesia for dermatologic surgery. New York: Churchill Livingstone; 1990; 62–63.
20. Terino EO. Alloplastic contouring in the premandible-jawline lower third facial aesthetic unit. In: Terino EO, Flowers RS, eds. The art of alloplastic facial contouring. St Louis: Mosby; 2000:153–165.
21. Tebo HG, Telford IR. An analysis of the relative positions of the mental foramen. Anat Rec 1950; 106:254–255.
22. LaTrenta GS. Facial contouring. In: Rees TD, LaTrenta GS, eds. Aesthetic plastic surgery 2nd edn. Philadelphia: WB Saunders; 1994:784–889.
23. Zide BM, McCarthy J. The mentalis muscle: an essential component of chin and lower lip position. Plast Reconstr Surg 1989; 83:413–420.
24. Baker OC, Conley J. Avoiding facial nerve injuries in rhytidectomy. Plast Reconstr Surg 1979; 64:781–795.
25. Bannister LH, Berry MM, Williams PL, et al, eds. Gray's anatomy, 38th edn. New York: Churchill-Livingstone; 1995; 578.
26. Mittelman H. The anatomy of the aging mandible and its importance to face lift surgery. Facial Plast Surg Clin of North Am 1994; 2:301–311.
27. Carney JM. Chin implants. In: Cutaneous surgery. Philadelphia: WB Saunders; 1994:626–643.
28. Flowers RS. Alloplastic augmentation of the anterior mandible. Clin Plast Surg 1991; 18:107–138.
29. Matarasso A, Elias AC, Elias RL. Labial incompetence: a marker for progressive bone resorption in silastic chin augmentation. Plast Reconstr Surg 1996; 98:1007–1014.
30. Mahler D. Chin augmentation—a retrospective study. Ann Plast Surg 1982; 8:468–473.
31. Rubin JP, Yaremchuk MJ. Morbidity and facial implants. In: Terino EO, Flowers RS, eds. The art of alloplastic facial contouring. St Louis: Mosby; 2000; 273–286.
32. Newman J, Dolsky RL, Mai, ST Submental liposuction extraction with hard chin augmentation. Arch Otolaryngol 1984; 110:454–459.
33. Gross EJ, Hamilton MM, Ackermann K, Perkins SW. Mersilene chin augmentation. A 14-year experience. Arch Facial Plast Surg 1999; 1:183–189.
34. Romo T, Baskin JZ, Sclafini AP. Augmentation of the cheeks, chin and pre-jowl sulcus, and nasolabial fold. Facial Plast Surg 2001; 17:67–77.
35. Friedman CD, Constantino PD, Sajjandian A. Alloplastic materials for facial skeletal augmentation. Facial Plast Surg Clin NA 1999; 7:95–103.
36. Binder WJ, Kamer FM, Parker ML. Mentoplasty—a clinical analysis of alloplastic implants. Laryngoscope 1981; 91:383–391.
37. Smith EM. Silicone: its chemistry and biocompatibility. In: Terino EO, Flowers RS, eds. The art of alloplastic facial contouring. St Louis: Mosby; 2000; 241–250.
38. Terino EO. Alloplastic facial contouring. In: Goldwyn RM, Cohen MN, eds. The unfavorable result in plastic surgery. Avoidance and

treatment, 3rd ed. Philadelphia: Lippincott Williams and Wilkins; 2001;1011–1031.
39. Stambaugh KI. Chin augmentation. An important adjunctive procedure to rhinoplasty. Arch Otolaryngol Head Neck Surg 1992; 118:682–686.
40. Sykes JM, Strong EB. Mentoplasty. Facial Plast Surg Clin North Am. 1999; 7:85–94.
41. Vuyk HD. Augmentation mentoplasty with solid silicone. Clin Otolaryngol 1996; 21:106–118.
42. Cohen SR, Mardach OL, Kawamoto HK. Chin disfigurement following removal of alloplastic chin implants. Plast Reconstr Surg 1991; 88:62–66.
43. Robinson M, Shuken R. Bone resorption under plastic chin implants. J Oral Surg 1969; 27: 116–118.
44. Friedland JA, Coccaro PJ, Converse JM. Retrospective cephalometric analysis of mandibular bone absorption under silicone rubber chin implants. Plast Reconstr Surg 1976; 57:144–151.
45. Pearson DC, Sherris DA. Resorption beneath silastic mandibular implants: effects of placement and pressure. Arch Facial Plast Surg 1999; 1:261–264.
46. Daw JL. Alloplastic facial contouring. In: Goldwyn RM, Cohen MN, eds: The unfavorable result in plastic surgery. Avoidance and treatment. 3rd ed. Philadelphia: Lippincott Williams and Wilkins; 2001:1032–1035.
47. Spira M. Editorial addendum. Plast Reconstr Surg 1973; 51:174.
48. Snyder GB. Augmentation mentoplasty. In: Goldwyn RM, ed. The unfavorable result in plastic surgery: avoidance and treatment, 2nd ed. Boston: Little Brown; 1984: 651–668.
49. Friedland JA. Discussion: labial incompetence: a marker for progressive bone resorption in silastic chin augmentation. Plast Reconstr Surg 1996; 98:1015.
50. Beckhuis GJ. Augmentation mentoplasty using polyamide mesh. Laryngoscope 1976; 86:1600–1605.
51. Terino EO. Chin and mandibular augmentation. In: Peck GC. Complications and problems in aesthetic plastic surgery. New York: Gower; 1992; 6:1–31.
52. Reed EH, Smith RG. Genioplasty: a case for alloplastic chin augmentation. J Oral Maxillofac Surg 2000; 58:788–793.
53. Hoffman S. Loss of a silastic chin implant following a dental infection. Ann Plast Surg 1981; 7:484–486.

31 Use of Botulinum Toxin Type A in Facial Rejuvenation

Alastair Carruthers MD and Jean Carruthers MD

Summary box

- Botulinum toxin A (BTX-A) is one of the seven serotypes of acetylcholine-blocking neurotoxin produced by *Clostridium botulinum;* at recommended doses it does not produce significant systemic effects.
- It is supplied as a freeze-dried powder for reconstitution to the required therapeutic concentration.
- Since its introduction for cosmetic use in the 1990s BTX-A injection has become increasingly popular as a safe and efficient, albeit temporary, method of facial rejuvenation.
- The best-known indications are dynamic lines in the upper, middle, and lower face and neck, however BTX-A also has a role in the correction of facial asymmetry and as a non-surgical approach to masseteric hypertrophy.
- BTX-A is used routinely as an adjunct to surgery, soft tissue augmentation, laser resurfacing and broadband light therapy.
- Contraindications to BTX-A include all neuromuscular disorders that could intensify its effects as well, of course, as pregnancy.
- Complications are few and usually related to poor injection technique.
- There have been no reported long-term adverse effects for cosmetic uses of BTX-A.

Historical vignette

- The pure crystalline form of BTX-A was isolated in 1946, and its mechanism of action was identified in the 1950s[1].
- Dr Alan Scott of the Smith-Kettlewell Eye Research Foundation began to investigate BTX-A in the treatment of strabismus in monkeys in the 1960s; his research over the ensuing 20 years led to the development of BTX-A for human treatment.
- The Food and Drug Administration (FDA) approved BTX-A for strabismus and blepharospasm in 1989, and for cervical dystonia in 2000.
- We began using BTX-A in 1983; in 1987 we observed improvement in the appearance of glabellar lines in patients treated for blepharospasm, and in 1992 we published the first report of BTX-A for cosmetic use[2] (other published reports of aesthetic benefits in patients treated for facial dystonias appeared around this time).[3,4]
- BTX-A (Botox Cosmetic) was approved by the FDA in 2002 for the treatment of glabellar lines, and its use in cosmetic problems caused by muscular overactivity in the face and neck continues to expand.

INTRODUCTION

Since the introduction of botulinum toxin type A (BTX-A) for cosmetic use in the early 1990s, the popularity of BTX-A injections has grown exponentially. The simplicity of the treatment and its safety and efficacy in facial rejuvenation have led to the widespread integration of BTX-A into the practice of cosmetic dermatology, and BTX-A injections are now among the most commonly performed cosmetic procedures. As clinical use increases and becomes more sophisticated it is important that clinicians are instructed in the appropriate application of this powerful neurotoxin.

In this chapter we provide an overview of the cosmetic use of BTX-A in the face and neck, covering preoperative considerations, injection techniques, optimizing outcomes, postoperative care, and complications.

Botulinum neurotoxins

Seven distinct serotypes of botulinum neurotoxin (BTX-A to BTX-G) are produced by the bacterium *Clostridium botulinum*. BTX serotypes differ slightly in their mechanism of action and clinical effect, but all block neuromuscular transmission by binding to receptor sites on motor nerve terminals and inhibiting acetylcholine release.[5] Intramuscular injection of BTXs at therapeutic doses produces temporary chemodenervation of the muscle, yielding localized reduction in muscle activity. In patients without existing neuromuscular dysfunction, injection at recommended doses does not induce systemic clinical effects.

Sources

In North America, two commercial toxin formulations are currently available: Botox and Botox Cosmetic (BTX-A; Allergan Inc, Irvine, CA) and Myobloc (BTX-B, Elan Pharmaceuticals, San Diego, CA). Botox Cosmetic is the only botulinum toxin approved for cosmetic use in North America, but Dysport (BTX-A, Ipsen Ltd, Maidenhead, UK) is available in Europe and is under review for licensing by the FDA. Each toxin preparation differs with respect to C. *botulinum* strain, potency, and manufacturing process. Botox, Myobloc, and Dysport each have unique biological behaviors and clinical effects, and the doses for these products are not interchangeable. The bulk of our clinical experience lies with Botox. Unless otherwise specified, all references to BTX-A in this chapter refer to the Botox or Botox Cosmetic formulations.

Pharmacology and mechanism of action

BTX acts by selectively blocking the regulated exocytosis of acetylcholine, causing profound, transitory muscular paralysis.[6] BTX-A and BTX-B are 150 kD di-chain polypeptides composed of heavy and light chains linked by disulfide bonds,[5] and both serotypes form differing neurotoxin-protein complexes (900 and 700 kD, respectively) during biosynthesis.[7] Following successful binding of the heavy chain to the motor nerve terminal, the toxin is internalized via receptor-mediated endocytosis, a process in which the plasma membrane of the nerve cell invaginates around the toxin receptor complex, forming a toxin-containing vesicle inside the nerve terminal. The neurotoxin molecule is released into the cytoplasm and cleaved into the heavy and light chains. The light chain of BTX-A cleaves a 25 kD synaptosome-associated protein (SNAP-25), a protein integral to the successful docking and release of acetylcholine from vesicles situated within nerve endings. The light chain of BTX-B cleaves vesicle-associated membrane protein (VAMP or synaptobrevin). The variation in clinical effect reported between BTX-A and BTX-B may be partly due to these differences.

Understanding of the cellular recovery process following BTX injection is incomplete. Collateral sprouting of active terminal buds in proximity to the parent terminal coincides with initial recovery of muscle contraction following administration of BTX-A and BTX-B. However, research suggests that these new terminal buds are transitory and are eventually eliminated, with neurotransmission ultimately restored at the original nerve ending.[6]

Comparative efficacy of BTX preparations

The mouse lethality assay (MLA), in which 1 unit is defined as the murine LD_{50} of intraperitoneal-injected BTX, is the standard for assessing BTX potency. The potencies of 1 unit of Botox, Dysport, and Myobloc differ markedly in humans, though the reasons for this are unclear. Research suggests that the Botox to Dysport potency ratio is between 1 : 2 and 1 : 6,[8,9] while the Botox to Myobloc potency ratio has been described as 1 : 50 to 1 : 100.[10,11] Despite these suggested ratios, no precise dosage conversion factors exist.

The clinical efficacy and safety of BTX-A have been well documented.[2,12] Compared to the literature on BTX-A, studies concerning cosmetic use of BTX-B are relatively few, but the reports that do exist suggest important differences between the two subtypes. BTX-B has a faster onset but a shorter duration of action and diffuses more widely than BTX-A, and is associated with greater pain and other side effects compared to BTX-A.[13–18] BTX-A is generally associated with greater therapeutic success, improved duration of effect, and fewer side effects.

Storage and reconstitution

Each vial of Botox Cosmetic contains 100 mouse units of vacuum-dried C. *botulinum* type A neurotoxin complex. The product should be stored in a freezer at or below –5 °C or in a refrigerator between 2 °C and 8 °C. Freezing BTX-A after reconstitution is neither recommended nor required.

The appropriate volume of diluent is chosen based on the desired concentration of the injection solution. Higher doses of BTX-A administered in smaller volumes (50 or 100 units/ml) keep the effects more localized and enable precise delivery of the toxin with little diffusion, while smaller doses in larger volumes (5–10 units/ml) may generate more widespread effects.[19,20] We find it most efficient to apply low-volume, concentrated toxin (100 units/ml), although good results have been reported using dilutions as high as 10 units/ml to smooth 'crow's feet' and the brow area.[21]

Manufacturer guidelines recommend that the product be reconstituted with sterile, non-preserved 0.09% saline solution and that the vial be discarded after 4 hours.[5] However, it has been reported that the product retains efficacy for up to 6 weeks following reconstitution.[22,23] Furthermore, reconstitution with preserved saline has been shown to reduce pain on injection[24] and does not impair the stability of BTX-A.[22,25]

Myobloc is available in 0.5-ml, 10-ml, and 20-ml vials containing a liquid formulation of BTX-B 5000 units/ml, saline, human serum albumin, and sodium succinate, and does not require reconstitution. The pH of the formulation is approximately 5.6, explaining the stinging sensation reported on injection. If saline is to be added, this should be done in the syringe to avoid overfilling the vials. Unopened Myobloc is stable for months or years and once opened the labeling is similar to BTX-A.[26]

Dysport is a lyophilized product available in vials containing 500 units of BTX-A, as well as sodium chloride, lactose, and human serum albumin. The difference in effectiveness between Dysport and Botox may be partly explained by the smaller amount of albumin present in Dysport. The product should be transported at ambient temperature and stored at 2–8 °C. Guidelines for its reconstitution and use are similar to those for Botox.[27]

■ PREOPERATIVE PREPARATION

Contraindications and precautions

Contraindications include the presence of any neuromuscular disorder that could intensify the effect of the drug, such as myasthenia gravis, Eaton-Lambert syndrome, myopathies, or amyotrophic lateral sclerosis; infection or inflammation at the injection site; or a known hypersensitivity to any of the product contents. Caution should be exercised in disorders that produce a depletion of acetylcholine, or when BTX-A is used with aminoglycosides or other drugs that interfere with neuromuscular transmission.[5] The safety of BTX-A in pregnant or nursing women has not been studied.

BTX-A is most effective in reducing dynamic facial lines caused by underlying muscle pull rather than by age-related loss of dermal elasticity in patients aged 20–45 years. Patients with marked facial lentigines, telangiectasia, and telangiectatic matting with fine rhytides and diminished skin texture may not achieve a satisfactory response to BTX-A alone.[28] The general appearance of fatigue, frustration, and age in such patients often persists after treatment.[29]

Patient assessment and education

Successful cosmetic treatment with BTX-A depends in large part on careful assessment and education of the patient. In addition to explaining the procedure, the time course of clinical effects, the need for retreatment after 3–6 months, and possible side effects, the clinician should endeavor to learn the patient's motivation for treatment and expectations regarding outcome. A patient with unrealistic expectations is likely to be dissatisfied with the results, regardless of whether the clinician deems the procedure successful. A thorough history of prior cosmetic interventions and patient satisfaction with these procedures can be highly useful in this regard. The patient should be informed about what to expect following injection, and safety concerns should be discussed.

Documentation

Preoperative, intraoperative, and postoperative documentation of the facial anatomy should be undertaken, paying particular attention to atypical features. Digital photography (see Chapter 6) represents an excellent medium for documentation as it provides the ability to capture both still and moving images, the latter being particularly valuable in demonstrating the dynamic effects of BTX-A treatment. In addition, the archiving and reproduction capabilities of digital photography far outstrip those of conventional photography.

■ TECHNIQUES

Injection techniques

General technique

Individual patient characteristics are key to successful treatment, and are determined through standardized color photographs of the target region both when muscles are at rest and during maximal contraction. For the beginner, marking the area to be injected while the patient is seated upright will yield the most accurate delineation of natural muscle movement and corresponding facial rhytides.

The desired dose of BTX-A is drawn into the syringe and the air expressed. Our preference is for the *Becton-Dickinson Ultra-Fine II* short-needled 0.3-ml insulin syringe. Its integrated 30-gauge, silicon-coated needle minimizes patient discomfort and drug waste compared to syringes with a needle hub.[30] The needle dulls after approximately six injections and so only up to that number of cutaneous penetrations should be planned with each needle/syringe. We use a bottle-opener to carefully remove the rubber stopper so that the injecting needle does not get dulled by piercing the stopper. In our experience, pain associated with injections can be minimized by reconstituting with preserved saline, infusing slowly with a 30-gauge needle, and injecting small volumes of relatively concentrated solution. Standard precautions of sterility and skin preparation should be followed.

The upper face

Although the first reports of BTX application in the face were published in 1990, clinical experimentation began during the late 1980s by clinicians impressed with the simplicity of BTX injection, its safety, and its striking benefits. To date, treatment of the upper face has produced the greatest wealth of clinical experience with BTX-A.

Glabellar rhytides

Clinical benefits of BTX-A treatment for glabellar rhytides are reported as lasting 3–4 months in the majority of patients, although in some the clinical effect may persist for 6–8 months. Of course, this depends on the method of assessment of the effect produced. Comparison with pretreatment photographs shows reduced ability to use mimetic muscles with the same power as prior to BTX treatment which typically lasts 20–28 weeks.[31,32] The smoothing of the brow may last even longer. Individual patient characteristics such as the type of brow arch, brow asymmetry, whether the brow is ptotic or crosses the orbital rim, and the amount of regional muscle mass are important factors in determining doses and injection sites (Fig. 31.1). Probably due to its greater muscle bulk, the male brow typically requires doses of 60 or 80 units BTX-A to yield reduction in glabellar lines; in contrast, paresis can be induced in women with doses of 30 or 40 units.[31,32] When treating men, we halve the volume of saline used to reconstitute the vial. This provides a simple method of reducing the injected volume while doubling the dose. We use an initial dose of 30 units and 60 units for women and men, respectively. If this does not produce the desired response, we then titrate the dose to 40 units and 80 units in women and men, respectively.

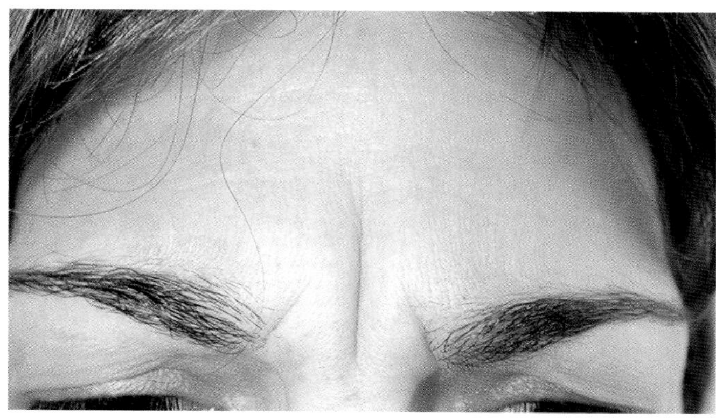

Figure 31.1 An individual with deep lines requiring a higher initial dose of botulinum toxin type A.

With the patient seated, chin down, and head slightly lower than the clinician's, the needle is inserted just above the eyebrow, directly above the caruncle of the inner canthus. Regardless of eyebrow position, the injection site is always above the bony supraorbital ridge. The supratrochlear vessels are located immediately medial to the injection site and bleeding may occur; one should therefore select a site where it is safe to apply postinjection pressure.

After injecting, the needle is slowly withdrawn (with its tip kept superficially beneath the skin), repositioned, and advanced superiorly and superficially to at least 1 cm above the previous injection site in the orbicularis oculi, where an additional dose of toxin is injected. To obtain a balanced appearance, the procedure is repeated on the opposite side of the brow. We also inject into the procerus in the midline, at a point below a line joining the brows and above the crossing point of the 'X' formed by joining the medial eyebrow to the contralateral inner canthus. Finally, in patients with horizontal brows, we inject into a point 1 cm above the supraorbital rim in the mid-pupillary line (Fig. 31.2).

Patients are instructed to remain vertical and to frown as much as possible for 2–3 hours immediately following treatment (while the toxin is binding) but are warned not to manipulate the treated area. Patients return for a follow-up examination 2–3 weeks after treatment, at which time we perform 'touch-up' injections, if necessary. Filling agents may be considered in individuals with persistent deep furrows at follow-up (see BTX-A as Adjunctive Therapy, page 508). In patients with deep glabellar frown lines, subsequent injections at 3- to 4-month intervals over a period of 1 year will maintain muscle paralysis and allow the furrows to drop out.[33]

Horizontal forehead lines

BTX-A injected into the forehead diminishes the appearance of undesirable horizontal forehead lines for a period of 4–6 months.[34] Caution must be exercised when treating horizontal lines, as excessive weakening of the frontalis muscle without weakening of the depressors will result in unopposed action of the depressors, producing a lowering of the brow and an angry expression. A conservative approach to BTX-A injections will ensure that some function remains intact. Injection sites must be kept well above the brow to avoid ptosis or a complete lack of expressiveness. Patients with a narrow brow (defined as less than 12 cm between the temporal fusion lines at mid-brow level) receive fewer injections (four sites, compared to five) and lower doses than patients with broader brows.

In our experience, a total of 48 units injected in the procerus, frontalis, lateral orbicularis oculi, and depressor muscles produces the greatest improvement in horizontal rhytides and a satisfactory duration of response (Fig. 31.3). It is important to remember, however, that adverse effects are dose-related.[34]

Brow shaping

A thorough knowledge and understanding of the action of BTX-A in the glabellar region can be used to good effect in altering the shape of the brows in patients who desire a more aesthetically pleasing appearance.

Brow elevation

Brow elevation following treatment of the glabellar lines has been reported in several publications,[35–37] and we have demonstrated lateral and mid-pupil elevation as a beneficial result of 30 and 40 units BTX-A in the glabellar region.[31] We initially believed this to be due to the action of the toxin on the medial (corrugator supercilii, procerus, and the medial portion of the orbicularis oculi) and lateral (the lateral portion of the orbicularis oculi) brow depressors. A more thorough analysis revealed that a total of 10 units BTX-A injected in the glabella produced mild, medial brow

Glabellar injection sites

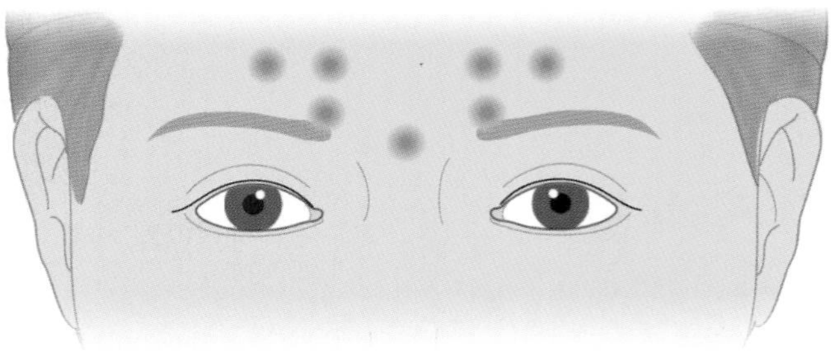

Figure 31.2 Glabellar injection sites.

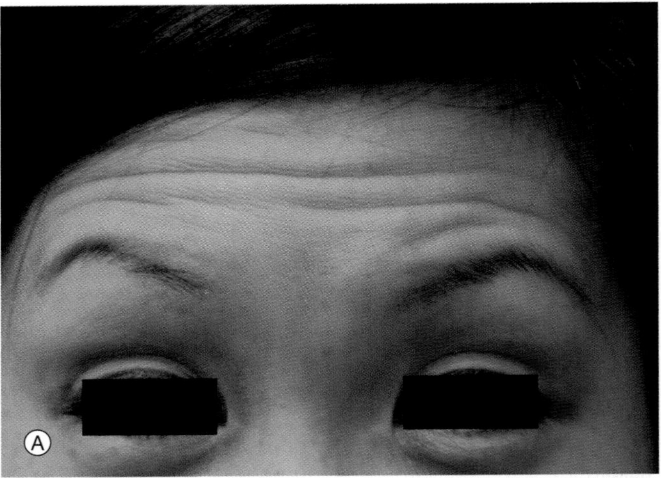

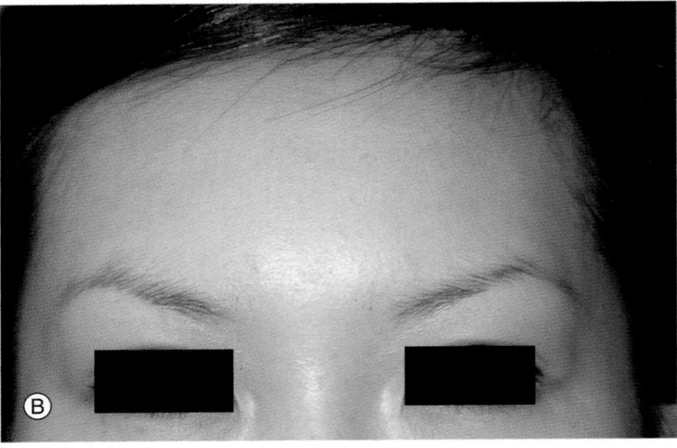

Figure 31.3 Horizontal forehead lines (A) before and (B) after treatment with botulinum toxin type A.

ptosis that disappeared after 2 months.[38] However, 20–40 units produced lateral eyebrow elevation initially, followed by central and medial eyebrow elevation that peaked at 12 weeks but was still significantly present at 16 weeks. Peak effect in skeletal muscle usually occurs at 4 weeks; this marks our first experience of peak effect occurring at 12 weeks. Based on the observation that the primary effect is lateral, an area not injected, we now believe that the brow lift is due to partial inactivation of the frontalis and not to the action on the brow depressors. The subsequent central and medial eyebrow elevation could be due to a gradual lift following 'resetting' of the tone in the frontalis muscle.

Eyebrow asymmetry

BTX-A injections into the frontalis muscle can be used to produce greater symmetry of the eyebrows in patients wishing to avoid surgery. The toxin is injected into or overlying the frontalis muscle, approximately 1 cm above the eyebrow. As noted, BTX-A injections for glabellar frown lines can produce mild ptosis of the medial brow, lateral brow elevation, and a more pleasing contour to the eyebrow (Fig. 31.4). Understanding that the lateral, orbital aspect of the orbicularis oculi muscle above the lateral retinaculum serves as an antagonist muscle to the lateral frontalis muscle will aid clinicians in improving the shape and position of the eyebrows.[39]

The mid-face and lower face

Although the greatest clinical experience with the cosmetic use of BTX-A lies in the upper face, recent years have seen a dramatic increase in its use in the mid-face and lower face. These wider applications are pushing BTX-A away from being simply a clinical procedure and are re-defining it as an 'art.' As with the upper face, individual patient features and musculature demand an expert approach, and these more advanced procedures should only be performed by clinicians with a large base of clinical experience as well as a thorough understanding of facial anatomy (both dynamic and resting) and vasculature. Poor technique in these procedures can result in severe impairment of muscular function and expression, and for this reason the use of electromyographic (EMG) guidance is recommended in some patients.[40]

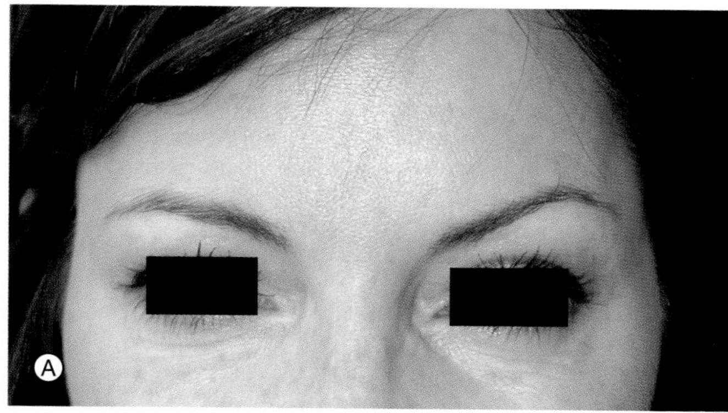

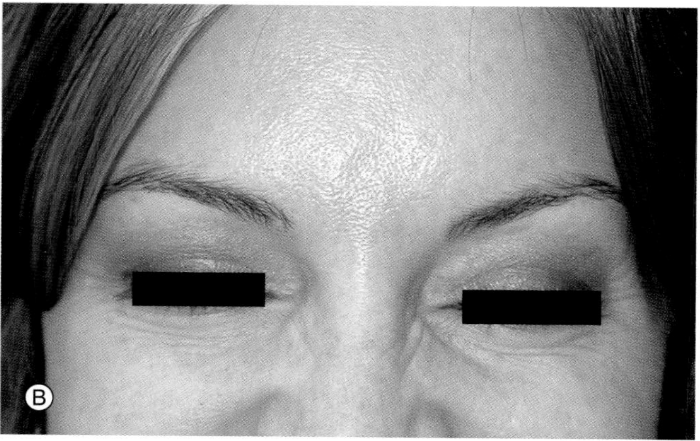

Figure 31.4 Correction of eyebrow asymmetry (A) before and (B) after botulinum toxin type A.

Crow's feet

BTX-A lessens the appearance of crow's feet rhytides, even in severely photodamaged skin, by relaxing or weakening (rather than paralyzing) the orbicularis oculi. Two to three injection sites lateral to the lateral orbital rim are generally used,[4,21,40,41] with equal doses of toxin (approximately 4–7 units per site and 12–21 units per side) injected into each site. Recommendations for optimal dosage in the lateral orbital region vary. A recent dose-ranging study found no significant difference in efficacy between 6 units per side and 18 units per side.[41] Total dose ranges used by others include 5–15 units[42] and 4–5 units per eye over two or three injection sites.[21] Our practice is to inject 12–15 units per side, distributed equally over two to four sites. We recommend using as few and as superficial injections as possible[40] to minimize bruising.

To identify the injection sites, have the patient smile maximally and note the center of the crow's feet. The first injection site is in the center of the area of maximal wrinkling, approximately 1 cm lateral to the lateral orbital rim. The second and third injection sites are approximately 1–1.5 cm above and below the first injection site, respectively (Fig. 31.5). Crow's feet are distributed equally above and below the lateral canthus in some individuals, while in others, crow's feet appear primarily below the lateral canthus. In the latter case, the injection sites may be in a line that angles from anteroinferior to superoposterior. Irrespective of distribution, the most anterior injection should be placed lateral to a line drawn vertically from the lateral canthus. The injection should not be performed while the subject is still smiling, as the toxin may then affect the ipsilateral zygomaticus complex, causing ptosis of

Injection sites for crow's feet

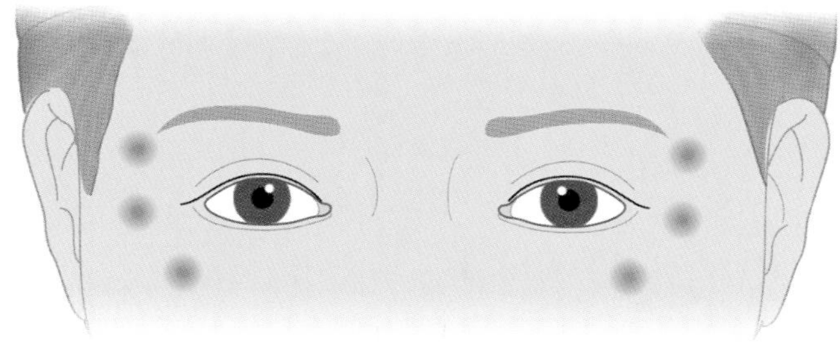

Figure 31.5 Injection sites for treatment of crow's feet.

the upper lip. Results from the first injection session persist for approximately 3 months. A duration of greater than 4 months has been reported following subsequent treatments[41] (Fig. 31.6).

Perioral rhytides

Overactivity of the orbicularis oris causes vertical perioral rhytides radiating outward from the vermilion border (Fig. 31.7). The goal in this instance is to weaken the orbicularis oris without causing a paresis that could interfere with speech and suction. Small doses of BTX-A (1–2 units per lip quadrant) are usually sufficient, especially when used in combination with a soft-tissue augmenting agent. The dilution is increased and a total dose of 6 units is applied to eight injection sites (0.75 units in 0.3 ml per injection), carefully measuring the sites to balance on either side of the columella or the lateral nasal ala.

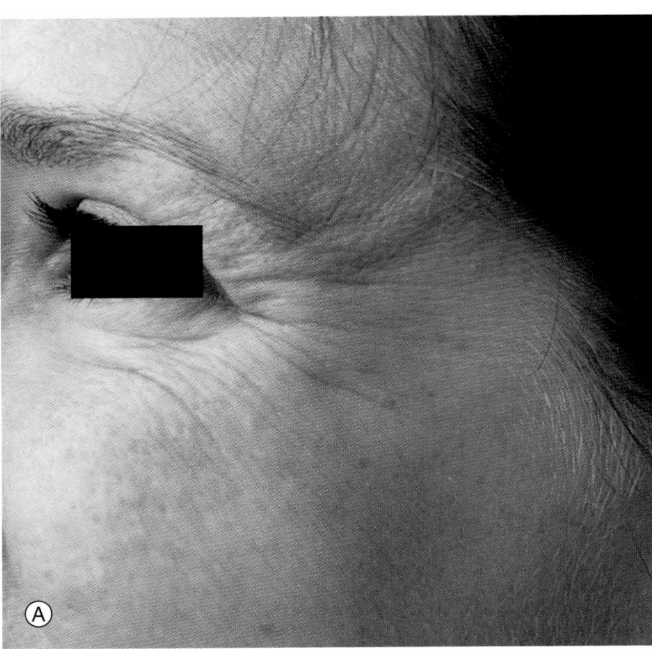

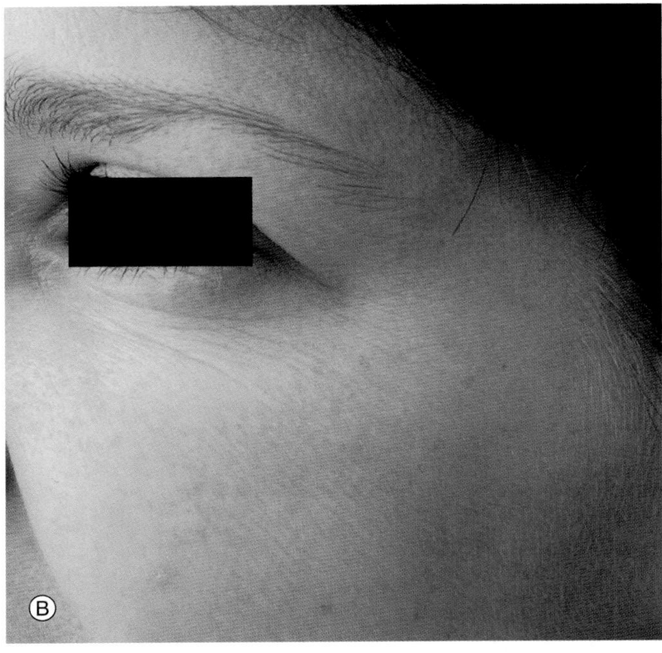

Figure 31.6 Crow's feet (A) before and (B) after treatment with botulinum toxin type A.

Hypertrophic orbicularis

Smiling can transiently diminish the perceived size of the palpebral aperture, particularly in Asian patients. Our experience shows that application of 2 units into the lower pretarsal orbicularis will relax the palpebral aperture, both at rest and while smiling.[40] Mean palpebral aperture increases of 1.8 mm (at rest) and 2.9 mm (at full smile) have been reported after subdermal injections of 2 units, delivered 3 mm inferior to the lower pretarsal orbicularis, and three, 4-unit injections placed 1.5 cm from the lateral canthus, with 1 cm between injection sites.[43]

Nasalis

BTX-A injected anterior to the nasofacial groove on the lateral wall of the nose can significantly soften the appearance of 'bunny lines' (radial rhytides that fan obliquely across the radix of the nose). The toxin should be applied well above the angular vein. Caution should be used to avoid injecting the nasofacial groove, as this can affect the levator labii superioris and levator labii superioris alequae nasi. Gentle massage of the area following injection will help diffuse the toxin.

Injecting the lower nasalis is also beneficial in patients with repeated nasal flare caused by involuntary dilatation of the nostrils. In these cases, the toxin is injected in the lower nasalis fibers, which drape over the lateral nasal ala.

Nasolabial folds

Patients desiring elongation of a naturally short upper lip can be treated with 1 unit BTX-A applied to each lip elevator complex in the nasofacial groove. This will elongate the upper lip muscles, but will also collapse the upper aspect of the nasolabial fold and flatten the mid-face. Weakening the lip levator, zygomaticus, and risorius muscles may not be desirable in every patient. Take care to ensure that patients fully understand the aesthetic result of the procedure and its long duration of effect (± 6 months).

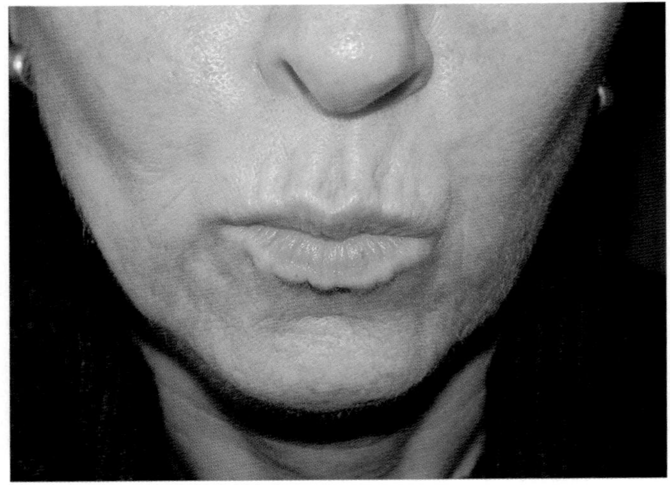

Figure 31.7 Perioral rhytides.

Depressor anguli oris

The depressor anguli oris (DAO) extends inferiorly from the modiolus to attach into the inferior margin of the mandible on the lateral aspect of the chin. The DAO is a cosmetically important muscle: contraction causes a downward turn to the corner of the mouth, creating a negative appearance. Since the DAO overlies the depressor labii inferioris, asymmetrical paresis usually results from direct injections. To avoid this, we inject 3–5 units at the level of the mandible but at its posterior margin, close to the anterior margin of the masseter. This produces significant weakening, rather than paralysis, of the muscle (Fig. 31.8).

Melomental folds

Melomental folds—deep folds of skin that extend from the depressed corner of the mouth to the lateral mentum—have traditionally been treated with soft-tissue augmentation alone. However, soft-tissue augmentation in combination with BTX-A injected into the DAO will extend the duration of soft-tissue augmentation and obviate the repeated molding and contortion of the augmenting agent.

Mental crease

The mental crease can be weakened by injecting mentalis anterior to the point of the chin. As with the perioral area, the aim of treatment is to weaken, rather than paralyze, the muscle. This is achieved by injecting 3–5 units into each side of the midline under the point of the chin, just anterior to the bony mentum, rather than injecting centrally. Do not inject at the level of the mental crease, as this will weaken the lower lip depressors and orbicularis oris and cause serious adverse effects that may endure for 6 months or more, depending on the dose.

'Peau d'orange' chin

A 'peau d'orange' appearance in the chin occurs due to loss of subcutaneous fat and dermal collagen, and is evident when the mentalis and depressor labii muscles are used in speech that requires co-contraction of the orbicularis oris (Fig. 31.9). Traditionally treated using soft-tissue augmentation and laser resurfacing, 'peau d'orange' chin can be softened by soft-tissue augmentation and BTX-A in the mentalis, or by BTX-A injection alone in patients who do not require augmentation.

Mouth frown

BTX-A does not act on muscles in isolation. The effect of the toxin on one muscle often has an effect—positive or negative—on another. 'Mouth frown,' a permanent downward angulation of the lateral corners of the mouth caused by the action of the DAO and the upward motion of the mentalis, is a good example of this. Attempting to treat mouth frown by injecting the DAO or mentalis alone may yield successful results in certain patients, but we have found this approach to be ineffective or associated with unacceptable side effects in many individuals and we currently inject both muscles simultaneously. In women we use 3 units of BTX-A into each DAO and each side of the mentalis, for a total of 12 units, which produces a subtle weakening effect. We recommend that this procedure only be performed in individuals who have experienced BTX-A injection elsewhere in the face. Careful patient counseling is required, and photographic documentation of the response to treatment, including any adverse effects, is necessary.

The neck

Chemodenervation with BTX-A can yield good cosmetic effects in the aging neck, reducing the appearance of necklace lines and platysmal bands.

Necklace lines

Necklace lines are horizontal lines of skin indentation caused by subcutaneous muscular apaneurotic system attachments. The simplest treatment method is to inject along the lines with 1–2 units at each site in the deep intradermal plane. Use deep dermal injections, taking care to avoid the deeper venous perforators that may bleed, and the underlying muscles of deglutition, which are cholinergic and may be affected. We recommend injecting no more than 10–20 units per treatment session, and massaging the area gently after injection to prevent bruising.

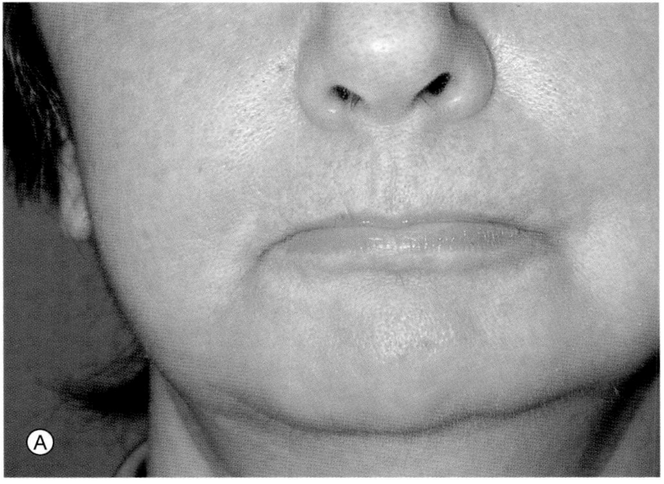

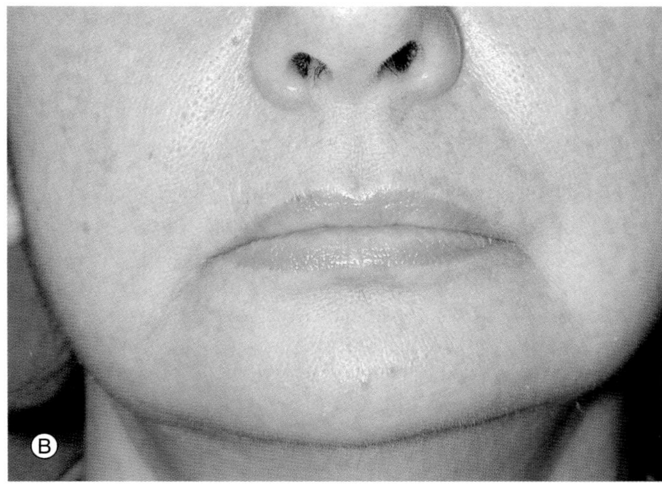

Figure 31.8 Depressor anguli oris (A) before and (B) after treatment with botulinum toxin type A.

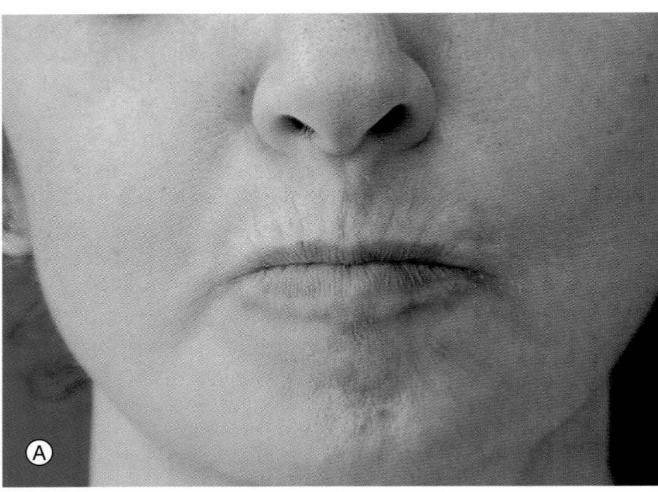

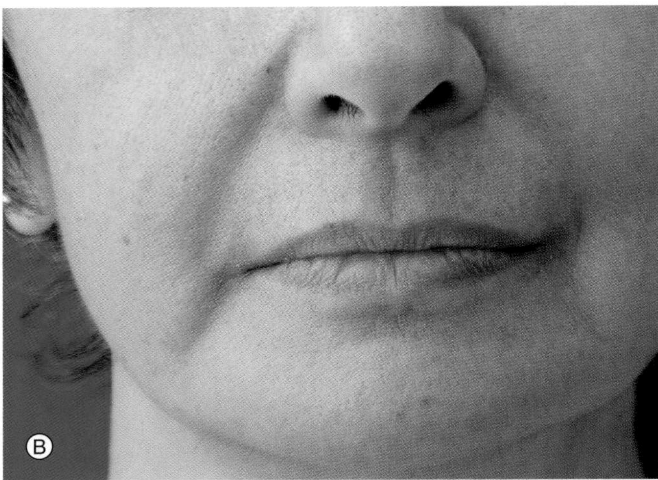

Figure 31.9 'Peau d'orange' chin (A) before and (B) after treatment with botulinum toxin type A.

Platysmal bands

While traditional rhytidectomy surgery remains the gold standard for the aging neck, good results have been reported for BTX-A in 44 patients with platysmal bands.[44] It must be stressed, however, that BTX-A can worsen the appearance of platysmal bands in patients with accompanying jowl formation and bone resorption; careful patient selection is therefore especially important. Patients with obvious platysmal bands, good cervical skin elasticity, and minimal fat descent are good candidates for BTX-A. Particular care must be taken when injecting the neck, as the vertically oriented platysmal bands are external to muscles of deglutition and neck flexion. We recommend using no more than 30–40 units per treatment, as higher doses can cause profound dysphagia.[40]

Facial asymmetry

Facial asymmetry due to muscular causes can be successfully treated using BTX-A. Repeated clonic and tonic facial movements associated with hemifacial spasm, for example, distort the facial midline toward the hyperfunctional side. The midline can be returned to a central position by using BTX-A to relax the hyperfunctional zygomaticus, risorius, and masseter. Similarly, hypofunctional asymmetry seen following paresis of the VIIth cranial nerve requires injection in the normofunctional side of 1–2 units in the zygomaticus, risorius, and orbicularis, and 5–10 units in the masseter. Asymmetry of jaw movement can be corrected by intraoral injection of 10–15 units BTX-A into the internal pterygoid.

BTX-A is also beneficial in treating asymmetry due to surgical causes. Surgical or traumatic cutting of the orbicularis oris or risorius muscle, causing unopposed action of the corresponding muscles in the normally innervated side, can result in decentration of the mouth. Toxin applied in the overdynamic risorius, immediately lateral to the lateral corner of the mouth and in the mid-pupillary line, will return the mouth to a central position when the face is at rest. Similarly, in patients with congenital or acquired weakness of the DAO, resulting in the inability to depress the corner of one side of the mouth, chemodenervation of the corresponding muscle will restore functional and aesthetic balance.

Masseteric hypertrophy

BTX-A for contouring in the lower face may represent a simple alternative to surgical shaping of the mandible and has the advantage of a short recovery period. Most of the literature is from small series,[45,46] though a larger study showed that 25–30 units BTX-A injected in five to six sites evenly at the prominent portions of the mandibular angle produced a gradual reduction in masseter thickness (average 1.5–2.9 mm reduction).[47] The clinical effect persisted from 6–7 months following injection, and side effects (mastication difficulty, muscle pain, and verbal difficulty during speech) lasted from 1–4 weeks.

BTX-A as adjunctive therapy

While BTX-A is highly effective in the treatment of facial lines caused by hyperactivity of underlying musculature, it is not effective as monotherapy for non-dynamic rhytides. It is generally recognized that treatment of lentigines, telangiectasias, and pore-size components of facial aging requires additional agents. BTX-A adjunctive to surgery, soft-tissue augmentation, laser resurfacing, and broadband light therapy has become an integral aspect of facial rejuvenation.

Surgery

BTX-A can be used to relax the facial muscles prior to surgery, reducing their action and facilitating tissue manipulation. This may enable greater surgical correction or better concealment of incisions. In addition, it has been reported that intraoperative or postoperative BTX-A prevents or slows the return of the wrinkles by reducing the action of the responsible muscles.[19]

A variety of BTX-A surgical applications have been reported in the literature. Preoperative relaxation of the muscular brow depressor complex with BTX-A 1 week prior to brow-lift surgery may allow for a greater brow elevation, while postoperative BTX-A may help prolong the benefits of surgery by relaxing the muscles working to re-establish the depressed brow.[19] Stabilization of brow musculature is important to achieving a predictable final brow position, since cosmetic outcomes for surgical brow lifts may be variable based on postoperative healing.[48]

BTX-A treatment concurrent with periorbital rhytidectomy improves and increases the longevity of the surgical results. Pre-treatment of the crow's feet with BTX-A relaxes the muscles, facilitating greater accuracy in estimating the amount of skin to be resected during surgery and better placement of the incision.[49] During repair of lower eyelid ectropion and 'roundeye,' the use of BTX-A transiently weakens the lateral fibers of the orbicularis, which can pull on the medial side of the temporal incision and lead to dehiscence after surgery.[19]

Soft-tissue augmentation

BTX-A is used routinely as adjunctive therapy with soft-tissue augmentation to increase the effect and duration of results. BTX-A often eliminates or reduces the muscular activity responsible for wrinkle formation, improves the response, and increases the longevity of the filling agent.[39]

In a prospective, randomized study of 38 patients with moderate-to-severe glabellar rhytides, BTX-A plus non-animal stabilized hyaluronic acid (NASHA) yielded a better response both at rest and on maximum frown than NASHA (Restylane) alone.[50] Combination therapy also produced a longer duration of response: the median time for return to pre-injection furrow status occurred at 18 weeks in the NASHA alone or BTX-A alone groups, compared to 32 weeks in patients treated with BTX-A plus NASHA.

Applied in conjunction with soft-tissue augmentation, BTX-A may decrease the amount of filling agent required. Our procedure is to inject BTX-A first, wait 2–4 weeks for BTX-A to soften the muscle contractions, and then inject the filling agent to correct the remaining lines.

Laser resurfacing

BTX-A in combination with laser resurfacing yields superior outcomes and greater duration of cosmetic effect. While laser treatment acts on static facial lines and stimulates collagen production, BTX-A prevents the recurrence of dynamic lines. Furthermore, the adjunctive use of BTX-A aids the healing of newly resurfaced skin long enough to encourage more permanent eradication of wrinkles. To allow sufficient time for BTX-A to prevent muscle movement during resurfacing, the toxin should be given up to 2 or 3 weeks prior to laser resurfacing and at least 1 week before.[51,52]

Compared to laser resurfacing alone, regular post-operative BTX-A injections given every 6–12 months prolong the effects of resurfacing, especially for the improvement of forehead, glabellar, and canthal rhytides.[51] West and Alster found an enhanced and longer-lasting improvement of forehead, glabellar, and canthal rhytides in patients treated with postoperative BTX-A injections in conjunction with carbon dioxide laser resurfacing compared to those receiving laser resurfacing alone.[53] Lowe et al. found that BTX-A injections in conjunction with ablative resurfacing in the treatment of crow's feet resulted in significantly higher treatment success rates compared with laser alone.[54]

Broadband light therapy

Both BTX-A and broadband light (BBL) therapy are non-invasive procedures associated with brief recovery time and little epidermal wounding. Although combined BTX-A and BBL therapy has not been thoroughly investigated, early results suggest that the combination may work in concert to treat facial aging.[29] In the first prospective, randomized study of BTX-A and BBL therapy (intense pulsed light) in 30 patients with moderate to severe crow's feet, patients in the BTX-A plus BBL group demonstrated better response at rest and on maximum smile compared to BBL alone. The combination therapy group also showed a slightly improved response to treatment of associated lentigines, telangiectasia, pore size, and facial skin texture compared to BBL alone, and a 15% global aesthetic improvement compared to BBL alone. These results are promising for patients with extensive facial aging and photodamage.

■ POSTOPERATIVE CARE

Careful postoperative instructions to patients will help minimize unwanted effects and ensure the best cosmetic outcome. Patients are instructed to remain vertical during the period immediately following injection, and are strictly advised not to rub, press, or otherwise manipulate the treated area. During the 2–3 hours following treatment, while the toxin is binding, patients are instructed to exercise the facial muscles as much as possible by performing a range of facial expressions. A follow-up appointment 2–3 weeks after treatment will enable the clinician to assess both response and patient satisfaction, and to perform touch-up injections as required. The theoretical possibility of an immunological response dictates that caution be used in re-injecting; we recommend that touch-up injections be given no sooner than 2 weeks following initial treatment.

■ PITFALLS AND THEIR MANAGEMENT

Avoidance of pitfalls

- In the upper face avoid use of low concentrations (large volumes) which encourage spread of toxin (causing brow ptosis) and diffusion into the orbital septum (causing upper eyelid ptosis) as well as shorter duration.
- Do not inject at or under the mid-brow or within 1 cm above the central bony orbital rim, to avoid bruising, diplopia, ectropion, upper lid ptosis or a drooping lateral lower lid.
- When planning infraorbital orbicularis injection, exclude patients who have scleral show pretreatment or dry eye; the result may be an exacerbation rather than an improvement.
- In the lower face, start with low and superficially placed injections to avoid drooling, asymmetry and other adverse events.
- When injecting depressor anguli oris, avoid areas too close to the mouth to avoid incompetent mouth and other complications, and remember that patients who use perioral muscles with intensity are poor candidates for this injection.
- Advise patients to remain upright and not manipulate the injected area for 2 hours after treatment, to reduce spread of the toxin outside the target area.

Cosmetic treatment with BTX-A is exceedingly safe. Adverse effects associated with injections include transient swelling or bruising at the injection site, mild headache, and flu-like symptoms. A conservative approach in most patients is supported by the observation that smaller doses of BTX-A are less likely to cause problems than larger doses. The complications associated with BTX-A in cosmetic treatment are few and [many are] anecdotal, and are related to poor injection technique. There have been no reported long-term adverse effects or health hazards for any cosmetic indication.[55]

Upper face complications

The most serious complications in the upper face—brow and lid ptosis and asymmetrical changes to the appearance of the eyebrows—can be avoided in most cases through careful patient selection and proper injection technique.

Brow ptosis

Brow ptosis is related to poor injection technique and occurs when the injected toxin affects the frontalis during glabellar or brow treatment. A higher concentration of toxin enables more accurate placement, greater duration of effect, and fewer side effects. Lower concentrations encourage the spread of toxin, and there is an area of denervation associated with each point of injection due to toxin spread of about 1–1.5 cm (diameter 2–3 cm). Patients must be instructed to remain upright, to strictly avoid rubbing or manipulating the injected area for 2 hours following treatment, and to exercise the treated muscles as much as possible during the first 4 hours.[55]

Brow ptosis creates an extremely negative appearance and can persist for up to 3 months. It is avoided by proper selection of patients (BTX-A is most effective in younger patients aged between 20 years and 45 years) and preinjection of the brow depressors if necessary (in patients with low-set brows or mild brow ptosis, and those over the age of 50 years).[55] Clinicians should remember that the brow shape can be modified, and diminished expressiveness may follow injection of the frontalis lateral to the mid-pupillary line. Inject above the lowest fold produced when the patient elevates the frontalis and limit the treatment of forehead lines to the portion 3 cm or more above the brow. Injecting the glabella and the whole forehead in one session is more likely to produce brow ptosis.[55] Apraclonidine (Iopidine (Alcon, Ft Worth, TX) 0.5%), alpha-adrenergic agonist ophthalmic eye drops that stimulate Müller's muscle, can be used to correct mild brow ptosis. It is important to note that allergic contact dermatitis can occur with the use of apraclonidine.

'Mr Spock' eyebrow

Inappropriate injection of the lateral fibers of the frontalis muscle can cause the untreated lateral fibers of the frontalis to pull upward on the brow, producing a questioning or 'cockeyed' appearance. Correction can be achieved by injecting BTX into the fibers of the lateral forehead exerting the upward pull. Only a small amount of BTX-A is required; overcompensation can lead to an irreversible and unsightly hooded brow that partially covers the eye.[55]

Upper eyelid ptosis

Upper eyelid ptosis occurs when the toxin diffuses through the orbital septum, affecting the upper eyelid levator muscle, and is most commonly seen following treatment of the glabellar complex. Ptosis can appear as early as 48 hours or as late as 14 days after injection and may last from 2–12 weeks.[55] As with brow ptosis, eyelid ptosis is associated with poor injection technique. Avoid large injection volumes, accurately place injections no closer than 1 cm above the central bony orbital rim, and advise patients to remain upright and not to manipulate the injected area for several hours after injection. Do not inject at or under the mid-brow.[55] As with brow ptosis, eyelid ptosis can be treated with apraclonidine, which lifts the lid by 1–2 mm and compensates for the weakness of the levator palpebrae superioris. One or two drops three times a day can be continued until the ptosis resolves.

Periorbital complications

Reported complications of BTX-A treatment in the periorbital area include bruising, diplopia, ectropion, or a drooping lateral lower eyelid and an asymmetrical smile (caused by the spread of toxin to the zygomaticus major). Inject laterally at least 1 cm outside the bony orbit or 1.5 cm lateral to the lateral canthus and do not inject close to the inferior margin of the zygoma. Injecting superficially in a wheal or a series of continuous blebs can reduce ecchymoses. Blood vessels can be avoided by placing each injection at the advancing border of the previous injection.

Injecting the infraorbital orbicularis can produce significant benefit in younger individuals, but the reverse may occasionally be true, especially in older patients. Poor candidates for infraorbital orbicularis injection include patients who exhibit a significant degree of scleral show before treatment; those who have previously undergone significant surgery beneath the eye; those who have a large amount of redundant skin below the eye; or those who have a slow snap test of the lower eyelid, indicating increased lid laxity.[55] Most patients injected in the infraorbital orbicularis are female, and clinically significant dry eyes represent a major problem in this group. Asking patients about dry eye symptoms (whether they experience dry eyes during air travel) may help identify individuals who will experience an exacerbation of these symptoms with weakening of the infraorbital orbicularis oculi. If in doubt, a Schirmer's test should be performed.

Lower face and cervical complications

Complications in the lower face include effects on muscle function and facial expression and are usually caused by overzealous use of large doses of BTX-A.[55] The potential for complications such as drooling and asymmetry can be reduced by starting with low doses and injecting more superficially rather than deeply. Injection symmetry will help ensure uniform postinjection muscle movement. Improper technique when injecting the DAO can result in a flaccid cheek, incompetent mouth, or asymmetric smile; to limit these complications, avoid areas too close to the mouth, injection into the mental fold, and interaction with the orbicularis oris. Singers, certain musicians, or other patients who use their perioral muscles with intensity, are poor candidates for injection in the DAO. Large doses (>100 units) of BTX-A in the platysma have yielded reports of dysphagia and weakness of the neck flexors.

Immunogenicity

Botulinum toxins are proteins capable of producing neutralizing antibodies and eliciting an immune response, causing patients to cease responding to treatment.[19] Individuals demonstrating initial response who subsequently fail to respond completely are termed 'secondary non-responders' and are considered to have neutralizing antibodies to BTX. Data on the rate of neutralizing antibody formation are sparse, and the factors responsible for formation of neutralizing antibodies have not been well characterized.[5] However, the total protein concentration and number of units injected are critical in determining potential immunogenicity. More frequent injections, or those with higher doses of BTX-A may lead to a greater incidence of antibody formation.[5] The protein concentration in current lots of BOTOX is significantly lower than that of previous lots and the antigenicity is reduced compared to the original product. Secondary lack of effectiveness to BTX-A due to the development of immunologic resistance is exceedingly rare in patients receiving cosmetic treatment. A much more common degree of resistance is seen with the need for increased doses, though this is probably not caused by immunologic mechanisms.

■ SUMMARY

BTX-A is safe and effective as primary therapy for correction of dynamic facial lines and is beneficial as adjunctive therapy in the treatment of non-dynamic elements of facial aging. Careful patient selection, a sound understanding of facial soft-tissue anatomy, and good injection technique in combination with the use of the lowest effective dose will maximize the clinical effect of BTX-A therapy while minimizing the possibility of complications. While BTX-A is not a replacement for surgery, skin resurfacing, or soft-tissue augmentation, it represents a compelling clinical tool capable of yielding highly satisfactory cosmetic results in the face and neck. We anticipate that its use will continue to expand and become more refined as clinical experience grows.

■ REFERENCES

1. Schantz EJ. Botulinum toxin: the story of its development for the treatment of human disease. Persp Biol Med 1997; 40:317–327.
2. Carruthers JD, Carruthers JA. Treatment of glabellar frown lines with C. *botulinum*-A exotoxin. J Dermatol Surg Oncol 1992; 18:17–21.
3. Borodic GE. Botulinum A toxin for (expressionistic) ptosis overcorrection after frontalis sling. Opthal Plast Reconstr Surg 1992; 8:137–142.
4. Blitzer A, Brin MF, Keen MS, et al. Botulinum toxin for the treatment of hyper-functional lines of the face. Arch Otolaryngol Head Neck Surg 1993; 9:1018–1022.
5. Allergen Inc. Product monograph: BOTOX Cosmetic (botulinum toxin type A for injection) purified neurotoxin complex. Markham, Ontario: Allergan Inc; 2001.
6. Meunier FA, Schiavo G, Molgo J. Botulinum neurotoxins: From paralysis to recovery of functional neuromuscular transmission. J Physiol Paris 2002; 96:105–113.
7. Sakaguchi G. Clostridium botulinum toxins. Pharmacol Ther 1982; 19:165–194.
8. Nussgens Z, Roggenkamper P. Comparison of two botulinum-toxin preparations in the treatment of essential blepharospasm. Graefes Arch Clin Exp Ophthalmol 1997; 235:197–199.
9. Odergren T, Hjaltason H, Kaakkola S, et al. A double blind, randomised, parallel group study to investigate the dose equivalence of Dysport and Botox in the treatment of cervical dystonia. J Neurol Neurosurg Psychiatry 1998; 64:6–12.
10. Brashear A, Lew MF, Dykstra DD, et al. Safety and efficacy of NeuroBloc (botulinum toxin type B) in type A-responsive cervical dystonia. Neurology 1999; 53:1439–1446.
11. Brin MF, Lew MF, Adler CH, et al. Safety and efficacy of NeuroBloc (botulinum toxin type B) in type A-resistant cervical dystonia. Neurology 1999; 53:1431–1438.
12. Carruthers JA, Lowe NJ, Menter MA, et al. A multicentre, double-blind, randomized, placebo-controlled study of efficacy and safety of botulinum toxin type A in the treatment of glabellar lines. J Am Acad Dermatol 2002; 46:840–849.
13. Ramirez AL, Reeck J, Maas CS. Botulinum toxin type B (MYOBLOC) in the management of hyperkinetic facial lines. Otolaryngol Head Neck Surg 2002; 126:459–467.
14. Sadick NS. Botulinum toxin type B (MYOBLOC) for glabellar wrinkles: A prospective open-label response study. Dermatol Surg 2003; 29:501–507.
15. Sadick NS. Prospective open-label study of botulinum toxin type B (MYOBLOC) at doses of 2400 and 3000 units for the treatment of glabellar wrinkles. Dermatol Surg 2003; 29:501–507.
16. Alster TS, Lupton JR. Botulinum toxin type B for dynamic glabellar rhytides refractory to botulinum toxin type A. Dermatol Surg 2003; 29:516–518.
17. Lowe N, Lask G, Yamauchi P. Efficacy and safety of botulinum toxins A and B for the reduction of glabellar rhytides in female subjects. Presented at the American Academy of Dermatology 2002 Winter Meeting, 22–27 Feb 2002, New Orleans, LA.
18. Matarasso SL. Comparison of botulinum toxin types A and B: A bilateral and double-blind randomized evaluation in the treatment of canthal rhytides. Dermatol Surg 2003; 29:7–13.
19. Carruthers A, Carruthers J. Botulinum toxin type A: History and current cosmetic use in the upper face. Semin Cutan Med Surg 2001; 20:71–84.
20. Carruthers A, Carruthers J. Dose dilution and duration of effect of botulinum toxin type A (BTX-A) for the treatment of glabellar rhytides. Presented at the American Academy of Dermatology 2002 Winter Meeting; 22–27 Feb 2002; New Orleans, LA.
21. Garcia A, Fulton JE Jr. Cosmetic denervation of the muscles of facial expression with botulinum toxin: A dose–response study. Dermatol Surg 1996; 22:39–43.
22. Klein AW. Dilution and storage of botulinum toxin. Dermatol Surg 1998; 24:1179–1180.
23. Hexsel DM, Trindade de Almeida A, Rutowitsch M, et al. Multicenter, double-blind study of the efficacy of injections with botulinum toxin type A reconstituted up to 6 consecutive weeks before application. Dermatol Surg 2003; 29:523–529.
24. Alam M, Dover JS, Arndt KA. Pain associated with injection of botulinum A exotoxin reconstituted using isotonic sodium chloride with and without preservative: A double-blind, randomized controlled trial. Arch Dermatol 2002; 138:510–514.
25. Huang W, Foster JA, Rogachefsky AS. Pharmacology of botulinum toxin. J Am Acad Dermatol 2000; 43:249–259.
26. Package insert. MYOBLOC (botulinum toxin type B) injectable solution. Elan Pharmaceuticals Inc, San Diego, CA.
27. Package insert. Dysport: Clostridium botulinum Type A toxin-haemagglutinin complex. Ipsen Limited, Maidenhead, Berkshire, UK.
28. Pribitkin EA, Greco TM, Goode RL, Keane WM. Patient selection in the treatment of glabellar wrinkles with botulinum type A injection. Arch Otolaryngol Head Neck Surg 1997; 123:321–326.
29. Carruthers J, Carruthers A. The effect of full face broadband light treatments alone and in combination with bilateral crow's feet BTX-A chemodenervation. Dermatol Surg 2004; 30:355–366.
30. Flynn TC, Carruthers A, Carruthers J. Surgical pearl: The use of the Ultra-Fine II short needle 0.3-cc insulin syringe for botulinum toxin injections. J Am Acad Dermatol 2002; 46:931–933.
31. Carruthers A, Carruthers J, Said S. Dose-ranging study of botulinum toxin type A in the treatment of glabellar lines. Presented at the 20th World Congress of Dermatology, 1–5 July 2002, Paris, France.
32. Carruthers A, Carruthers J. Botulinum toxin Type A for treating glabellar lines in men: A dose-ranging study. Presented at the 20th World Congress of Dermatology, 1–5 July 2002, Paris, France.
33. Carruthers A, Kiene K, Carruthers J. Botulinum A exotoxin use in clinical dermatology. J Am Acad Dermatol 1996; 34:788–797.

34. Carruthers A, Carruthers J, Cohen J. Dose dependence, duration of response and efficacy and safety of botulinum toxin Type A for the treatment of horizontal forehead rhytides. Presented at the American Academy of Dermatology 2002 Winter Meeting, 22–27 Feb 2002, New Orleans, LA.
35. Huilgol SC, Carruthers A, Carruthers JDA. Raising eyebrows with botulinum toxin. Dermatol Surg 2000; 25:373–376.
36. Ahn MS, Catten M, Maas CS. Temporal brow lift using botulinum toxin A. Plast Reconstruct Surg 2000; 105:1129–1135.
37. Huang W, Rogachefsky AS, Foster JA. Brow lift with botulinum toxin. Dermatol Surg 2000; 26:55–60.
38. Carruthers A, Carruthers J. Glabella BTX-A injection and eyebrow height: A further photographic analysis. Presented at the Annual Meeting of the American Academy of Dermatology, 21–26 March 2003, San Francisco, CA.
39. Fagien S, Brandt FS. Primary and adjunctive use of botulinum toxin type A (BOTOX) in facial aesthetic surgery: Beyond the glabella. Clin Plast Surg 2001; 28:127–148.
40. Carruthers J, Carruthers A. BOTOX use in the mid and lower face and neck. Semin Cutan Med Surg 2001; 20:85–92.
41. Lowe NJ, Lask G, Yamauchi P, et al. Bilateral, double-blind, randomized comparison of 3 doses of botulinum toxin type A and placebo in patients with crow's feet. J Am Acad Dermatol 2002; 47:834–840.
42. Keen M, Kopelman JE, Aviv JE, et al. Botulinum toxin: A novel method to remove periorbital wrinkles. Facial Plast Surg 1994; 10:141–146.
43. Flynn TC, Carruthers JA, Carruthers JA. Botulinum-A toxin treatment of the lower eyelid improves infraorbital rhytides and widens the eye. Dermatol Surg 2001; 27:703–708.
44. Kane MA. Nonsurgical treatment of platysmal bands with injection of botulinum toxin A. Plast Reconstr Surg 1999; 103:656–663.
45. To EW, Ahuja AT, Ho WS, et al. A prospective study of the effect of botulinum toxin A on masseteric muscle hypertrophy with ultrasonographic and electromyographic measurement. Br J Plast Surg 2001; 54:197–200.
46. von Lindern JJ, Niederhagen B, Appel T, Berge S, Reich RH. Type A botulinum toxin for the treatment of hypertrophy of the masseter and temporal muscle: An alternative treatment. Plast Reconstr Surg 2001; 107:327–332.
47. Park MY, Ahn KY, Jung DS. Botulinum toxin type A treatment for contouring of the lower face. Dermatol Surg 2003; 29:477–483.
48. Dyer WK, Yung RT. Botulinum toxin-assisted brow lift. Facial Plast Surg 2000; 8:343.
49. Guerrissi JO. Intraoperative injection of botulinum toxin A into orbicularis oculi muscle for the treatment of crow's feet. Plast Reconstr Surg 2000; 105:2219–2228.
50. Carruthers J, Carruthers A. A prospective, randomized, parallel group study analyzing the effect of BTX-A (BOTOX) and non animal sourced hyaluronic acid (NASHA, Restylane) in combination compared to NASHA (Restylane) alone in severe glabellar rhytides in adult female subjects. Dermatol Surg 2003; 29:802–809.
51. Carruthers J, Carruthers A, Zelichowska A. The power of combined therapies: BOTOX and ablative facial laser resurfacing. Am J Cosmet Surg 2000; 17:129–131.
52. Carruthers J, Carruthers A. Combining botulinum toxin injection and laser resurfacing for facial rhytides. In: Coleman WP, Lawrence N (eds). Skin Resurfacing. Baltimore: Williams and Wilkins; 1998; 235–243.
53. West TB, Alster TS. Effect of botulinum toxin type A on movement-associated rhytides following CO_2 laser resurfacing. Dermatol Surg 1999; 25:259–261.
54. Lowe N, Lask G, Yamauchi P, Moore D, Patnaik R. Botulinum toxin type A (BTX-A) and ablative laser resurfacing (erbium:YAG): A comparison of efficacy and safety of combination therapy vs. ablative laser resurfacing alone for the treatment of crow's feet. Presented at the American Academy of Dermatology 2002 Summer Meeting, 31 July to 4 August 2002, New York, NY.
55. Klein AW. Complications and adverse reactions with the use of botulinum toxin. Dermatol Surg 2003; 29:549–556.

32 Liposuction

Naomi Lawrence MD and Janie M Leonhardt MD

Summary box

- Tumescent anesthesia using lidocaine and epinephrine (adrenaline) allows the removal of large volumes of fat with minimal blood loss and postoperative morbidity.
- A preconsultation questionnaire standardizes the medical history and focuses the consultation on issues that are crucial to the success of the liposuction.
- Most bleeding disorders and any medications that prolong bleeding time are a contraindication to liposuction.
- Liposuction is not a method for losing weight, but can create a more aesthetic figure, and improve functionality and glucose control at an individual's current weight.
- Continuous blood pressure monitoring, cardiac monitoring with pulse oximetry and the availability of supplemental oxygen should be in place for procedures removing more than 100 ml of aspirate.
- Following liposuction around 12% of patients undergo a touch-up procedure. If a patient gains weight, the liposuctioned area will resist weight gain, which may cause fat to accumulate in a new area.

INTRODUCTION

Liposuction with local anesthesia had its inception in 1987 with the publication of the seminal paper by Jeffery Klein on tumescent anesthesia.[1] Before this, adipose deposits had been removed by en bloc resection in combination with skin excision and scraped out through small incisions.[2,3]

A father-and-son team of Italian cosmetic surgeons, Arpad and Georgio Fischer, introduced the suction technique for the removal of fat.[4,5] The Fischers also introduced the use of a blunt cannula and criss-cross tunneling. Illouz, a gynecologist, is credited for popularizing liposuction by using the Fischer's technique with the Karmen cannula—a widely available, reasonably priced, suction pump that was developed for abortion procedures.[6] Illouz is also responsible for the original 'wet technique' in which a hypotonic saline solution with hyaluronidase was injected into the fat. He theorized that the hyaluronidase would lyse the fat cells and make aspiration easier.[6,7] A French plastic surgeon named Fournier is considered one of the main pioneers in liposuction and an enthusiastic teacher of his technique. He reviewed the field of fat transfer, and promoted syringe rather than machine liposuction.[8]

Although the term 'wet technique' liposuction had been introduced in Europe, the predominant form of liposuction in the USA was the dry technique using minimal local anesthesia; under general anesthesia significant blood loss was not uncommon with this approach.

When Klein introduced tumescent anesthesia in 1987, it revolutionized the technique among dermatologic surgeons and cosmetic surgeons at large. The safe limits of lidocaine by tumescent anesthesia were outlined by Klein, Lillis and later Ostad.[9–12] Liposuction with local anesthesia allows the removal of large volumes of fat with minimal blood loss or postoperative morbidity, excellent cosmesis, and a remarkable safety profile.

PREOPERATIVE PREPARATION

Consultation

The consultation starts on the phone when the receptionist books the appointment. It is important that the person who answers the phone is knowledgeable about the procedure so they can obtain some initial information, to determine whether the person calling is a candidate for liposuction. If their health, or physical characteristics, or their expectations clearly make them a poor candidate, it is best to find out before they come in. If the receptionist is too busy to spend time with a potential liposuction candidate, we transfer the call to the cosmetic consultant. The time spent on the phone is rewarded with good quality consultations. It is not unusual for patients to tell us that they booked the consultation with our office because we gave them more information on the telephone than any other office they called. A thorough consultation takes at least 30 minutes and more often an hour. We use a preconsultation questionnaire (Fig. 32.1). This helps in a number of ways:

Liposuction questionnaire

Patient name:.. Date:

....

1. Do you have any medical allergies? Yes No

....

....

....

....

Describe reaction

....

....

....

....

2. Are you on any medication or hormones? Yes No

....

....

....

....

3. Do you take any over the counter medications on a regular basis? Yes No
(Aspirin, antihistamines, etc.)

....

....

....

....

4. Do you have any of the following medical problems?

Heart disease	Yes	No	Asthma	Yes	No
High blood pressure	Yes	No	Lung disease	Yes	No
Diabetes	Yes	No	Liver disease	Yes	No
Bleeding problems	Yes	No	Kidney disease	Yes	No
Pulmonary embolus	Yes	No	Immune suppression	Yes	No
Hepatitis	Yes	No	Artificial joints or heart valves	Yes	No
Thrombophlebitis (vein inflammation)	Yes	No			

– 1 –

Figure 32.1 Liposuction questionnaire. Developed by Naomi Lawrence.

If you have answered yes to any of the above, please describe your condition, or any medical disorder you may have that is not listed:

....

....

....

....

....

Who is your primary care physician?

....

5. What is your height? .... What is your weight? ....

6. Which of the following best describes your weight pattern? Please circle below.
    a. I have maintained the same weight for many years. It rarely varies.
    b. I usually stay within 5 to 10 pounds of my stated weight.
    c. My weight tends to fluctuate 20 pounds or more.
    d. I have recently lost .... pounds to achieve my present weight.
    e. Other:

....

7. Which of the following best describes your exercise habits?
    a. I do not exercise on a regular basis.
    b. I do a 30 minute workout 2 to 3 times a week.
    c. I do a 30 minute or greater workout 4 or more times a week.
    d. My occupation involves daily exercise (i.e. aerobics instructor); or I am involved in intense training (Triathlete, marathon runner).

8. Place a check by all areas that you are interested in having evaluated for possible liposuction. Circle the area that bothers you most.

.... Face	.... Waist	.... Buttock
.... Neck	.... Flanks	.... Outer thigh
.... Arms	.... Abdomen	.... Knees
.... Back	.... Hips	.... Calves and ankles
		.... Inner thigh

Other: ....

– 2 –

Figure 32.1, *continued*.

9. Check those statements that best reflect your expectations of liposuction.

   .... I am overweight and am looking to liposuction as an alternative to diet and exercise.

   .... I expect to lose weight through liposuction.

   .... I expect immediate results after liposuction.

   .... I am mostly interested in getting rid of cellulite

   .... I am near my ideal weight (or overweight) and would like to reduce a localized area to make my figure more proportional.

   .... I exercise regularly but have a couple of areas that seem resistant to diet and exercise.

– 3 –

Figure 32.1, *continued*.

the questionnaire standardizes the intake of medical history and focuses the consultation on the issues that we know are crucial to the success of the liposuction.

Medical and surgical history

Liposuction is an elective cosmetic procedure, best done on healthy patients. Patients should be screened carefully for any medical conditions that would put them at increased risk of surgical complications. Most physicians feel that cosmetic procedures should be limited to patients who fall into American Surgical Association class I or II (rarely Class III) (see Table 32.1) It is important to have a low threshold to request medical clearance or speak to the primary care physician because patients sometimes downplay the severity of their medical condition, because of their desire for the procedure. We routinely request medical clearance in all patients over 60 years old, or in those with a cardiac history, history of hypertension, or diabetes. As lidocaine is metabolized by the liver, be concerned about any patient with potential impairment of liver function such as hepatitis C, chronic active hepatitis B, alcoholic liver disease, previous treatment with chemotherapy and antiretroviral therapy (for HIV).[13–15]

People with immunosuppression, such as those who are HIV positive, those with diabetes, or on chronic immunosuppressive medications, are at increased risk of infection. In these patients one must consider the risk–benefit ratio and confer with the specialist monitoring their care. Patients are also screened for increased risk of thromboembolism as evidenced by a prior history of thrombophlebitis, deep venous thrombosis, or pulmonary embolism, protein C or protein S deficiency, high-dose estrogen therapy, and tobacco use.[16]

Medical allergies

It is very important to elicit any history of medical allergies as well as usage of medications that could potentially interact unfavorably with the drugs given during the procedure. In many practices patients are given a preoperative dose of antibiotics that have good coverage against *Staphylococcus aureus*. In the authors' practice patients are given 1 g of intravenous Ancef (Watson Laboratories Inc, Corona, CA). If they are allergic to penicillin or cephalosporins, they are given oral clindamycin to start the night before the procedure. Allergy to latex is important to note so the surgeon and assistants are sure to wear latex-free gloves and use latex-free dressings. Most medical tubing is now latex free and does not pose a problem.

The two major drugs given in the tumescent fluid are lidocaine and epinephrine (adrenaline). Allergy to lidocaine is extremely rare and is a contraindication to the procedure. Most patients that claim allergy to lidocaine are actually allergic to the preservative methylparaben in the anesthetic.[17] If the patient claims to be allergic to lidocaine we advocate referral to an allergist for testing. If the allergy is only to the preservative, preservative-free lidocaine is available in the form of Xylocaine-MPF (Astra USA Inc Westborough, MA). People who are allergic to ester anesthetics should also have preservative-free lidocaine, because the ester metabolite *p*-aminobenzoic acid (PABA) is the allergen which cross reacts with the metabolite of methylparaben.[17]

Epinephrine (adrenaline), which is added to the fluid as a vasoconstrictor to decrease bleeding, is an endogenous catecholamine to which allergy is not possible. Some patients are more sensitive to its effects, particularly when it is administered in a highly vascular area such as the oral mucosa during dental work. These patients may describe episodes of palpitations in the past. However, even in this group of patients it is rare to find someone with such symptoms following tumescent anesthesia for liposuction because this compartment (the adipose) is relatively less vascular. When seen, tachycardia due to the epinephrine (adrenaline) in the tumescent infusion is probably due to a hypersensitive conduction system in the patient.[18] For us, this is extremely rare now that we have decreased the epinephrine (adrenaline) dose to 0.65 mg per liter bag in the tumescent fluid, and give Clonidine 0.1 mg to every patient with a blood pressure of 100/70 or greater.[18]

Table 32.1 ASA surgical risk classifications

I. Normal healthy patients
II. Mild systemic disease and no functional limitation
III. Moderate to severe disease that results in some functional limitation
IV. Severe systemic disease that is a constant threat to life and functionally incapacitating
V. Moribund and not expected to survive 24 hours with or without surgery

Reprinted from Butterwick KJ, Liposuction: consultation and preoperative considerations. In: Narins R, ed. Safe liposuction and fat transfer. New York; 2003, by courtesy of Marcel Dekker Inc.

Surgical history

The patient's history of surgical abdominal procedures is very important if they are being evaluated for abdominal liposuction. Special attention should be paid to any surgeries complicated by dehiscence, hernia, infection, or subsequent adhesions that might leave an incomplete rectus abdominus muscle layer over the peritoneum. If this history is suspicious one can obtain medical records, or reports, or radiologic studies, and discuss the matter with the patient's surgeon. Other important information is the age of the scars—older scars are soft and pliable and can be suctioned *through*, but newer scars should be suctioned *around*. Any history of keloids or hypertrophic scars should be discussed thoroughly as multiple incisions for cannula insertion are necessary.

Most bleeding disorders are a contraindication to liposuction. We highlight five questions by putting them on a separate page of the questionnaire to identify patients with potential bleeding abnormalities (Fig. 32.2). Screening blood work should include platelet count and prothrombin/thromboplastin time but this will not uncover all bleeding disorders (such as von Willebrand's disease); therefore a thorough history is essential.

Medication history

The medication history must be complete and the patient should be queried about hormone replacement, herbal supplements, over-the-counter medications as well as

Liposuction questionnaire

1. Do you have abnormal or heavy periods?

....

2. Do you have recurrent nose bleeds?

....

3. Have you had persistent bleeding after tooth extraction?

....

4. Do you have a history of anemia (low blood count)?

....

5. Do you have a history of easy bruising?

....

6. Do you have any family members with abnormal bleeding?

....

Figure 32.2 Liposuction questionnaire. Developed by Naomi Lawrence.

prescription drugs. As mentioned previously, high-dose estrogen can put a woman in a higher risk category for thromboembolism, particularly if she is a smoker, or is within the first year of therapy with high-dose estrogen.[19–21] Drife chronicles the history of oral contraceptives and the risk for venous thromboembolism.[22] In the 1960s thromboembolic risk was linked to taking higher doses of daily estrogen, which led to production of pills with reduced estrogen. In 1995, three case-controlled studies linked the risk of venous thromboembolism to the type of progestogen, rather than the dose of estrogen. Nevertheless, it appears that these newer progestogens do not increase the risk of venous thromboembolism beyond the 3-fold to 6-fold already delineated in the past.[23] The issue of high-dose estrogen oral contraceptives was recently addressed by Butterwick.[23] She concluded that current standard of care was to allow patients to remain on low-dose oral contraceptives as the risk of thrombosis from these agents is extremely low.

Any medications that prolong bleeding time are contra-indicated with liposuction. These include prescription medications such as warfarin or clopidogrel bisulfate, and over-the-counter medications such as aspirin and non-steroidal anti-inflammatory drugs (NSAIDS). The anti-platelet effects are irreversible and last 10–14 days on aspirin and 7–10 days on non-steroidal drugs. Patients should be instructed to check all over-the-counter medications with the physician's office in the 2 weeks before surgery as many have 'hidden' aspirin or non-steroidal ingredients. If the patient inadvertently takes these medications, the liposuction is postponed.

Patients are also given a full list of herbal supplements that can prolong the bleeding time (see Table 32.2) and asked to refrain from taking them for 2 weeks before the surgery. Lidocaine is metabolized by the liver enzyme cytochrome p450 (CYP450). There are a number of drugs which induce this enzyme system or act as competitive inhibitors (see Tables 32.3, 32.4). Competitive inhibition can decrease the metabolism of lidocaine, causing an increase in blood levels of lidocaine, and thereby potentiating its toxicity. Lidocaine can safely be given at 55 mg/kg in a patient on no such medications. When a patient is taking one of these medications the physician can either request that they discontinue the medication, or decrease the maximum dose of lidocaine used; however, there are no clear guidelines documenting how this should be done. The antidepressant fluoxetine (Prozac, Eli Lilly, Indianapolis, IN) has metabolites that last approximately 2 months after administration has ceased. For this reason we often decrease the maximum dose and perform the liposuction in two or more sessions.

Diet and exercise

Our questionnaire focuses on two other key areas: diet and exercise history. Dieting has long been an area rife with controversy. There are several areas of concern when evaluating a patient's dieting and weight history. Weight cycling—repeated weight loss and weight gain—is a common pattern for many people who struggle with their weight.[24] When looking at predictors of weight loss maintenance, those who diet frequently show significantly more weight regain than those who diet less frequently.[25] Skender et al.[26] compared the 2-year weight loss trend in three groups: diet only, a combination of diet and exercise, and exercise only. They found that the combination group lost the most weight but the exercise-only group maintained weight loss best. The diet-only group regained weight to 0.9 kg above baseline.[26]

If the potential liposuction candidate has recently lost weight on a very-low-calorie diet and liposuction is done at this point in their weight cycle, subsequent weight regain can have a negative impact on the result. The type of diet that the liposuction candidate has been on is also important information. Diets with a behavioral modification component have a higher degree of success.[27] Diets that are very low in calories and fat have a low rate of success in maintenance as they can cause the metabolism to slow down to conserve energy, leaving the dieter hungry all the time.[28] When the dieter returns to eating normally, regain of weight can be very quick. Diets with high protein and fat, and low carbohydrates (such as the Atkins diet)[29] push the body into burning fat rather than carbohydrates for energy, which expends more energy.[29–31] In addition, the dieter is more satiated, and is more likely to maintain weight loss.

The exercise history is important as it affects basal metabolic rate, maintenance of weight loss, and overall health of the patient. Additionally, muscle tone impacts on body contour in a number of areas where we commonly perform liposuction.[32] The physician can get a sense of the type of workout the patient is currently doing during the preoperative consultation. As the physician does a good physical exam, she can instruct the patient on what areas could be improved by increasing muscle tone, such as the upper arms in women, where there can be excess adipose, skin laxity and poor muscle tone, which contribute equally to the problem. In our experience, many women concentrate on aerobic exercise to burn calories, and neglect weight training to build and tone muscle. It is important to remind them that weight training is essential for a more sculpted appearance to the upper arms.

Conversely, some women have good muscle tone in the upper arms, but are looking for individual muscle definition, as is common in men. Because even the thinnest women have a higher body fat composition than men, this look is usually only attainable if they bring their body fat composition to an extremely low, often dangerous, level; this can give them a cachectic appearance in the face, upper chest, and neck. The buttocks and abdomen are other areas where muscle tone positively impacts overall contour. While muscle tone and extramuscular fat are the primary predictors of buttock contour, abdominal fullness may also involve intra-abdominal fat rectus abdominus diastasis (usually in multiparous women) and a ventral hernia.

Expectations

An entire section of the questionnaire is devoted to exploring patient perceptions of liposuction and their goals in regard to their body and this particular procedure. They usually have very realistic expectations. During the consultation, explore the patient's goals and make sure that they are congruent with what liposuction can accomplish. Liposuction is not a weight-loss procedure, so people considering this procedure for weight loss are not good candidates.

Table 32.2 Herbs that may cause bleeding or thrombosis

Herbal Compound	Effect	Constituent(s)
Agrimony	Coagulant	Vitamin K
Alfalfa	Anticoagulant; coagulant	Coumarin; vitamin K
Angelica	Anticoagulant; antiplatelet	Coumarin
Anise	Anticoagulant (excessive doses)	Coumarin
Arnica	Anticoagulant	Coumarin
Asafoetida	Anticoagulant	Coumaric
Aspen	Antiplatelet	—
Black cohosh	Antiplatelet	Salicylate
Bogbean	Bleeding risk	Unknown
Boldo	Anticoagulant	Coumarin
Borage seed oil	Anticoagulant	Enzyme
Bromelain	Anticoagulant	Enzyme
Capsicum	Antiplatelet	Capsaicinoid
Celery	Antiplatelet	Apigenin (coumarin)
Clove	Antiplatelet	Eugenol
Danshen	Anticoagulant	Procatechualdehyde 3,4-dihydroxyphenyl-lactic acid
Dong Quai	Anticoagulant; antiplatelet	Coumarin
European mistletoe	Coagulant	Coumarin
Fenugreek	Anticoagulant	Coumarin
Feverfew	Antiplatelet (crude extract)	—
Fish oils	Antiplatelet; prostacyclin synthesis; vasodilatation; reduced platelets and adhesiveness; prolonged bleeding time	—
Fucus	Anticoagulant; increased risk of bleeding	—
Garlic	Inhibition of platelet aggregation; increased risk of bleeding (excessive doses)	—
Ginger	Anticoagulant; increased risk of bleeding	—
Ginkgo	Inhibition of platelet aggregation; decrease in blood viscosity	—
Ginseng	Anticoagulant; antiplatelet	—
Goldenseal	Coagulant	Berberine
Horse chestnut	Anticoagulant	Aesculin (coumarin)
Horseradish	Anticoagulant	Coumarin
Licorice	Antiplatelet	Coumarin
Meadowsweet	Anticoagulant	Salicylate
Northern prickly ash	Anticoagulant	Coumarin
Onion	Antiplatelet	Unknown
Papain	Bleeding risk	Unknown
Passionflower	Anticoagulant	Coumarin
Pau D'Arco	Anticoagulant	Lapachol
Plantain	Coagulant	Vitamin K
Poplar	Antiplatelet	Salicin
Quassia	Anticoagulant	Coumarin
Red clover	Anticoagulant	Coumarin
Roman chamomile	Anticoagulant	Coumarin
Safflower	Anticoagulant	Safflower yellow
Southern prickly ash	Anticoagulant	Coumarin
Stinging nettle	Coagulant	Vitamin K
Sweet clover	Anticoagulant	Dicumarol
Sweet vernal grass	Anticoagulant	Coumarin
Tonka bean	Anticoagulant	Coumarin
Turmeric	Antiplatelet	Curcumin
Vitamin E	Inhibition of platelet aggregation and adhesion; interference with vitamin-K-dependent clotting factor (large doses)	—
Wild carrot	Anticoagulant	Coumarin
Wild lettuce	Anticoagulant	Coumarin
Willow bark	Antiplatelet	Salicylate
Yarrow	Coagulant	Achilleine

With permission from Shiffman MA, Am J Cosmet Surg 2001; 18:131–132.

An elegant study done by Ozgur et al. in 1998 looked at three groups: patients seeking aesthetic surgery (AG), patients seeking reconstructive surgery (RG), and a control group (CG) of non-surgery seekers from the normal population. Each group consisted of 100 people, and all 300 were asked to complete a sociodemographic questionnaire, the life-satisfaction index (LSI), a self-esteem inventory (SEI), and a body-image inventory (BII). The LSI and BII were not significantly different between the three groups.[33] The SEI was significantly better in the AG than the RG. This confirms what we see in practice—that patients seeking cosmetic procedures generally do not have low satisfaction with their life or distorted body images.

Ten years ago the ideal candidate was described as a person with an ideal body weight but with a small disproportionate adiposity, causing contour deformity. Most liposuction surgeons now have a broader definition of 'ideal' because we have seen overweight patients (not morbidly obese) with disproportionate adipose distribution and insulin-dependent diabetics benefit greatly from liposuction. Good candidates are not seeking to lose weight, but to create a more aesthetic figure, and improve functionality and glucose control at their current weight. Often, this group of patients is so inspired by the results of liposuction that they go on to lose weight through diet and exercise.

During the consultation it is very important to help patients to shape their expectations of the results of liposuction. In all areas this result is limited by the pre-existing bony structure, the texture and quality of the skin, the tone and build of muscle, and adipose in the areas that are not amenable to liposuction. For example, in the neck subplatysmal fat, platysmal banding and excessive skin laxity can lead to a less than optimal result. Many patients will choose a less invasive procedure such as liposuction over a face lift procedure because they prefer less morbidity. It is important that they understand the components that will not be corrected by liposuction alone. Patients are usually very accepting of the remaining imperfections if they are counseled in advance of the procedure.

Table 32.3 CYP450 3A4 inhibitors affecting lidocaine metabolism

Acetazolamide	Naringenin (grapefruit juice)
Alprazolam	Nefazodone
Amiodarone	Nelfinavir
Anastrozole	Nevirapine
Cannabinoids	Nicardipine
Cimetidine	Nifedipine
Clarithromycin	Norfloxacin
Ciclosporin	Norfluoxetine
Danazol	Omeprazole
Diazepam	Paroxetine
Diltiazem	Quinidine
Erythromycin	Remacemide
Felodipine	Ritonavir
Fluconazole	Saquinavir
Fluoxetine	Sertindole
Fluvoxamine	Sertraline
Indinavir	Stiripentol
Isoniazid	Terfenadine
Itraconazole	Triazolam
Ketoconazole	Troglitazone
Metronidazole	Troleandomycin
Mibefradil	Verapamil
Miconazole	Zafirlukast
Midazolam	Zileuton

With permission from Klein JA, Cytochrome P450 3A4 metabolism and lidocaine metabolism. In: Klein JA, ed. Tumescent technique: Tumescent anesthesia and microcannular liposuction. St Louis: Mosby; 2000:133.

■ TECHNICAL ASPECTS

Physical examination

A thorough physical examination of the liposuction candidate is important in the initial consultation to evaluate suitability for the procedure. The patient should change into a gown and stand for the examination. The physician should discretely examine the fatty prominences, first concentrating on areas that the patient wishes to have treated, and then assessing general body proportions. The areas of fatty prominence should be gently pinched between the thumb and forefinger to assess the subcutaneous fat. Asking the patient to contract underlying musculature will aid in a complete evaluation. For each area there are certain maneuvers which help to isolate subcutaneous fatty tissue, and which allow assessment of the degree to which the area is accessible to the liposuction cannula. Flexion of the gluteus muscle is a particularly important maneuver in the buttock region where muscular laxity and protrusion can contribute to the overall prominence of the buttock region, including 'saddle bags' (the area of the lateral thigh below the trochanteric fossa).[34]

Inherent skin features should also be noted in the liposuction candidate. The presence of striae distensae, cellulite, and actinic damage, as well as the evaluation of the skin tone and elasticity, should be noted in the chart and brought to the attention of the patient. Complete examination should include pulling the skin away from the patient's body and observing elastic recoil. The patient should be made aware that striae and cellulite will not improve with the procedure and that loss of skin tone and elasticity and the presence of actinic damage can reduce the best result available, due to a reduction in the retraction and remodeling that can be obtained.[35] However, in the experience of many liposuction experts, even patients with poor skin elasticity often achieve worthwhile results. Patients should also be made aware that postoperative skin

Table 32.4 CYP450 3A4 megabolic substrates

Alfentanil	Dexamethasone	Methadone	Sildenafil
Alprazolam	Dextromethorphan	Methylprednisolone	Simvastatin
Amitriptyline	Donepezil	Midazolam	Tacrolimus
Amlodipine	Erythromycin	Nicardipine	Tamoxifen
Astemizole	Estrogens	Nimodipine	Terfenadine
Atorvastatin	Felodipine	Nisoldipine	Testosterone
Carbamazepine	Fentanyl	Pentoxifylline	Tetracycline
Cerivastatin	Flurazepam	Pravastatin	Theophylline
Chloramphenicol	Fluvastatin	Prednisone	Thyroxine
Cisapride	Imipramine	Progestins	Valproic acid
Clomipramine	Isradipine	Propafenone	Warfarin
Clozapine	Losartan	Rifabutin	Zileuton
Ciclosporin	Lovastatin	Rifampin	Zonisamide

With permission from Klein JA, Cytochrome P450 3A4 metabolism and lidocaine metabolism. In: Klein JA, ed. Tumescent technique: Tumescent anesthesia and microcannular liposuction. St Louis: Mosby; 2000:135.

redundancy may occur in the setting of a loss of elasticity in the lower abdomen and that surgical correction may be necessary following liposuction. Careful examination of surgical scars should be performed, and inquiries made into the age of any scars, particularly in the abdominal area, to evaluate for the presence of underlying hernias and fibrous adhesions.

Evaluation of body proportions, shape, and symmetry is important for two reasons. Bony and muscular asymmetry (especially scoliosis) can contribute to a poor end-result and must be brought to the attention of the patient during the consultation. In addition, suction of a localized area, for example the hips or waist of a patient with 'saddle bag' thigh deformities, can accentuate the unsuctioned deformity. Therefore, it is important to discuss these issues and together plan a procedure that will leave a proportional and symmetric appearance. This may mean extending the procedure to regions that the patient had not planned on treating initially.

Photographs should be obtained during physical examination of the consultation. These serve to aid in education of the patient for procedure planning, as well as to document the patient's preoperative appearance. Postoperative photographs should also be obtained to document the final result of the procedure.

Surgical suite and set-up

An optimal surgical suite and equipment can enhance surgical outcomes by providing a safe and comfortable environment for the patient, the staff, and the physician. The surgical suite should be large enough to accommodate an electric or pneumatic table with vertical mobility, suction machinery, and liposuction equipment (intravenous pole, infusion pump, and Mayo stand) with easy access by the physician and staff to all sides of the patient.[36] In addition to equipment for the procedure, items to enhance the comfort of the patient should be available; these include a well-padded surgical table, sterile towels for draping the patient during the procedure, and the POPP (Gaymar Industries Inc, Orchard Park, NY) distilled-water warming blanket, which is placed underneath the sterile waterproof cover on the table.[37] Sterility should be maintained and is achieved through the use of sterile instrument trays, gowns, gloves, towels, and waterproof disposable fabric for the table. The physician and staff should wear masks and surgical hair caps and must adhere strictly to sterile technique during the procedure.

According to the guidelines of care for liposuction set forth by the task force on liposuction of the American Academy of Dermatology, all liposuction surgeons and designated operating-room staff should have training in the management of acute cardiac emergencies. Baseline vital signs, including blood pressure and heart rate, should be taken preoperatively and postoperatively. For procedures removing more than 100 ml of aspirate, there should be the capability for continuous blood pressure monitoring, cardiac monitoring with pulse oximetry, and supplemental oxygen should be available. A plan for medical emergencies should also be established.[38]

A number of additional pieces of equipment are necessary to perform liposuction, including the aspiration pump, liposuction cannulae, and the infusion pump. The mechanical aspiration pump is an electrically powered machine designed to create negative pressure and collect the fatty tissue throughout the procedure. There are a variety of machines available for purchase, and those with a closed collection system, overflow trap, and disposable air filter with efficient and uninterrupted suction are ideal.[36]

Liposuction cannulae may be comprised of stainless steel, aluminum, deldrin, or brass.[37] The shape, diameter, hole placement, and size determine the ease of fat removal, as well as the relative injury to the tissue. Cannulae with several holes and large-diameter tapered end (usually 3 mm) holes placed distally on the tip are more aggressive and allow for easier fat removal, along with increased potential for bleeding and trauma to the tissue (for example, Capistrano, Pinto, Cobra, Becker and Eliminator cannulae (Wells Johnson Company, Tucson, AZ)) (Fig. 32.3A). Cannulae that have smaller diameters (of up to 3 mm), blunted ends, fewer holes, and holes that are placed more proximally and away from the tip are less aggressive and gentler to tissue (e.g. Klein, Fournier, Standard cannulae (Wells Johnson Company, Tucson, AZ)) (Fig. 32.3B).

Most liposuction surgeons choose cannulae with various sizes and match both the type of tip and diameter to the procedure at hand. In fibrous areas, it is best to start with a cannula that has an aggressive tip and small diameter. As the case progresses and fibrous adhesions are diminished, a less aggressive cannula with a larger diameter can be used. Finally, in areas where the fat is soft, such as the inner thigh, less aggressive, smaller cannulae should be used to avoid oversuction. According to the American Academy of Dermatology liposuction guidelines, a cannula for liposuction should be no larger than 4.5 mm in diameter; however, most liposuction cannulae are 2–3 mm in size or less.[38] Various mechanical pumps are available for infusing tumescent solution. Those with variable speed settings are preferable. The apparatus is prepared by connecting the bag of tumescent solution to intravenous tubing, which is threaded through the power pump and connected directly to the infusion cannula or needle.

In addition to the above equipment, a sterile field is established on a Mayo stand at the patient's head. On the stand are the infusion and suction cannulae, sterile tubing, syringes with 1% lidocaine with or without epinephrine (adrenaline), a #11 blade, gauze, and towel clamps to secure tubing and drapes in place.

Procedure

As with any procedure, a review of the surgical plan with the patient is necessary before beginning. Patients are given lorazepam 1–2 mg (Ativan, Mylan Pharmaceuticals Inc, Morgantown, WV)—which does not compete for the enzyme cytochrome P450—to take on the night before surgery and on the morning of surgery. Therefore, all verification of the patient's understanding must take place at the preoperative visit. Clonidine 0.1 mg (an α-adrenergic antagonist) is administered by mouth on the day of the procedure (given a resting blood pressure of more than 100/70) to prevent epinephrine (adrenaline)-induced tachycardia and to aid in relaxation of the patient. On the day of the procedure, a negative urine pregnancy test should be confirmed in all premenopausal women. An intravenous line is placed in the patient's arm with an antibiotic such as

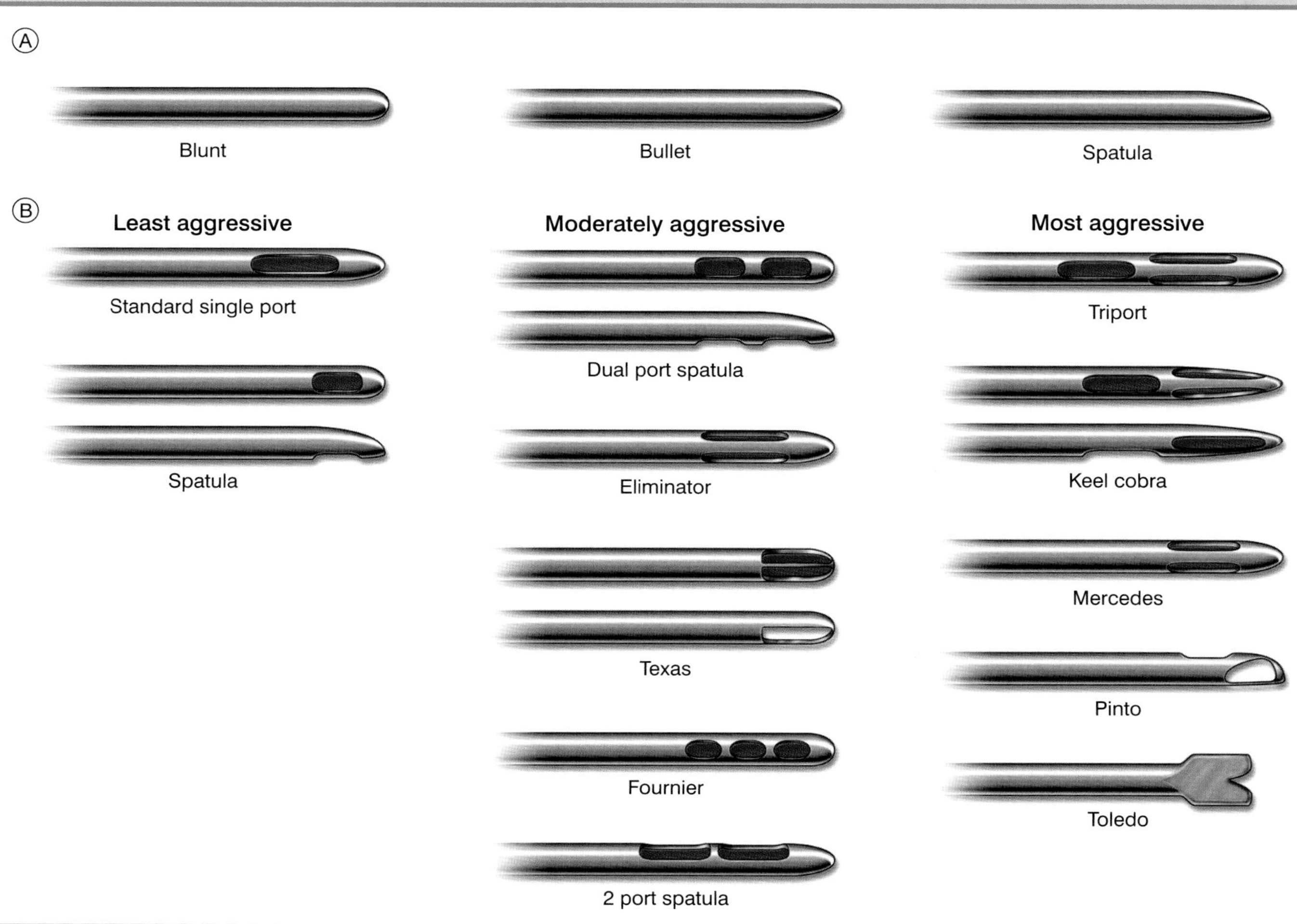

Figure 32.3 (A) Basic tip configurations and (B) tip styles. Adapted with permission from Bernstein G, Instruments for liposuction. In: Coleman WP, Lillis P, eds. Dermatologic clinics, volume 17. Philadelphia: WB Saunders, 1999; 743.

cefazolin (Ancef, Watson Laboratories Inc, Corona, CA), for example, administered before the procedure starts. A formal surgical scrub should take place for those in contact with the patient during the procedure (see Chapter 2). The patient should be scrubbed with Betadine (Becton, Dickinson & Co, Franklin Lakes, NJ) or Hibiclens sponges (Regent Medical, Norcross, GA) with extension of the field well beyond the area to be suctioned to ensure proper disinfection. The patient is then helped into sterile undergarments for the procedure. Markings should be placed with a sterile pen including insertion sites and areas to be treated. The patient is then assisted onto the sterile draped table with care taken not to contaminate the field. With the physician and staff gowned and gloved, the procedure may begin.

Tumescent anesthesia

Tumescent solution should be prepared on the day of the procedure by licensed medical personnel only. The preferred vehicle is 0.9% sodium chloride (normal saline) available in 1-liter or 500-ml bags. The anesthetic is lidocaine, available in 1% or 2% solution. It is prudent for an office performing liposuction to always prepare bags from either 1% or 2% lidocaine to maintain uniformity of preparation and minimize error. Epinephrine (adrenaline) and sodium bicarbonate are added to the solution to aid in vasoconstriction and acidic buffering respectively. A conservative dosage guideline for a maximum lidocaine dose in tumescent anesthesia is 35–45 mg/kg.[39] Doses as high as 55 mg/kg have been shown to be safe.[40] Lower doses of lidocaine (35 mg/kg) are given when the patient is taking a medication that interferes with the cytochrome P450 (CYP), specifically the CYP3A4 isoenzyme, responsible for clearance of lidocaine.[39] In particularly petite people, lidocaine concentrations in the range from 0.05% to 0.75% are used most of the time as total dose is limited by weight. Higher concentrations of lidocaine (0.1%) are generally used for more sensitive areas such as the periumbilical area and the waist and chest.[41] Elsewhere, a concentration of 0.05% is usually sufficient to provide adequate anesthesia for the procedure. The total amount of tumescent fluid required for an anticipated procedure can be estimated using general guidelines (Table 32.5) aided by experience and dictated by the area being treated. Epinephrine (adrenaline) is added to the solution at a concentration of 1 in 1 000 000 (1 mg of 1 in 1000 epinephrine (adrenaline) to a 1 liter solution of saline). Lower doses are effective, and in

Table 32.5 Tumescent infiltration: estimated time and volume

Anatomic Area	Small Patient (min/ml)	Large Patient (min/ml)
Outer thighs	15/600	25/1400
Inferolateral buttocks	4/200	6/400
Inner thighs	15/800	25/1600
Inner knees	5/200	10/400
Hips	15/600	25/1200
Waist	10/300	20/600
Flanks/postaxilla	15/400	25/800
Buttocks	15/400	20/900
Abdomen	30/1400	60/2800
Arms	20/500	30/1000
Male breasts	15/400	30/1000
Male flanks	15/600	25/1000

Time and volume according to patient tolerance. For bilateral symmetric areas, use double the indicated time per side. Physician may prefer to manually infiltrate chin, cheeks, jowls, and breasts, which require special techniques.
With permission from Klein JA, ed. Tumescent technique: Tumescent anesthesia and microcannular liposuction. St Louis: Mosby; 2000; 228.

our office 0.65 mg of 1 in 1000 epinephrine (adrenaline) is added to a 1 liter bag of saline with excellent vasoconstriction and potentially less risk of tachycardia. Finally, bicarbonate is also added in the amount of 10 mEq in 1 liter of solution. The preferred concentration of sodium bicarbonate (NaHCO3) is 8.4% solution, which contains 1 mEq/ml. Before mixing, the saline should be warmed to enhance the comfort of the patient during the infusion process. Heating can be accomplished with a reliable microwave, taking great care that the infusion fluid does not reach a potentially injurious temperature (usually 1 minute is appropriate for a liter bag, but this varies according to machinery and altitude). The lidocaine, bicarbonate, and epinephrine (adrenaline) are added to the saline after warming.

Tumescent anesthesia is administered once the patient is relaxed and comfortable on the operating table. Insertion sites should be marked and then anesthetized with buffered 1% lidocaine with epinephrine (adrenaline), usually at a dilution of 1 in 100 000. Incisions are created with a #11 blade through the dermis to allow for entry of the blunt-tipped infusion cannula into the subcutaneous tissue. The infusion cannula should be inserted and the infusion pump turned on at a rate appropriate for the site being infused. The infusion rate should be less than 100 ml per minute to minimize patient discomfort. If using the Klein infiltration system (Wells Johnson Company, Tucson, AZ), rates in the range of 2–3 are generally well tolerated in minimally sedated patients.[42] Gentle advancement of the cannula should be preceded by infusion of the tumescent solution. In smaller areas, such as the neck, cheeks, and the arms, a lower rate is required to prevent overinfusion and compression of vital structures. Anesthesia should be performed in a fanned approach from each entry site with care taken not to stretch the entry sites. It is always preferable to make additional entry sites rather than to cause large wounds in an attempt to reach the outermost portions of the surgical field. If the patient experiences significant pain with the infusion process, slowing the rate of the infusion can help to make the pain more bearable.[43] The endpoint of infusion is best appreciated by palpating the edges of the field, which become firm and indurated when adequately infused. Within minutes, the area infused will begin to blanch due to epinephrine (adrenaline)-induced vasoconstriction.

Once anesthesia is complete, and after allowing 15–20 minutes for the full epinephrine (adrenaline) vasoconstriction effect, suction may begin. Suction should be performed through the insertion sites. More aggressive, thinner cannulae may be used first to break up fibrous septae and create tunnels making for easier removal of fat subsequently with larger (usually 3 mm) less aggressive cannulae. Suction movement should be in a linear and vertical manner with little horizontal movement of the cannula in the creation of subcutaneous tunnels. The cannula should be directed so that the apertures for suction are facing away from the dermis. Deep and superficial tunneling should be performed as the physician's free hand or 'smart hand' monitors the placement of the cannula tip so as to avoid extending beyond the anesthetized regions.

At first during the suctioning, the area is tense from infusion. As suctioning progresses, the area becomes more flaccid and it helps to use several techniques to stabilize the tissue so that the surgeon is sure to suction at a consistent plane. One helpful maneuver is to have an assistant flatten the region by gently placing countertraction on the skin, while the surgeon continues suction guided by their free hand. It is also helpful for the assistant to gently grasp the flaccid skin adjacent to the suction area of focus and roll in such a way as to flatten the suction region for the surgeon. The endpoint of suctioning is determined by a number of factors. When a tunnel is empty, the aspirate may be notably devoid of suctionable fat and become increasingly bloody with further suctioning. When this occurs, the cannula should be repositioned and suction should be stopped in this area. Pockets of fat should be sought out and removed by placing the cannula (with the suction apparatus off) into tunnels and gently pulling back and up against the dermis. Pockets of fat may become more pronounced with this maneuver, and further suctioning of these well-defined areas helps to create a more even result. The procedure should be planned so that the total volume of fat removed does not exceed 4500 ml in a single operative session according to formal guidelines.[38] This is usually the equivalent of 6000–8000 ml of total aspirate, assuming 50–60% of aspirate is fat. If a patient possesses areas of treatment where the estimated fat aspirate is greater than 4500 ml, treatments should be planned over multiple visits.

■ OPTIMIZING OUTCOMES

Abdomen

The shape of the abdomen is affected by a number of factors including fatty deposition (underneath or overlying the rectus abdominus), muscle laxity, antecedent abdominal surgery, and inherent cutaneous features including scars, striae, and elasticity. Again, the initial physical examination and consultation should serve to identify the overall shape of the person, the presence of hernias, scars, a history of previous liposuction or laparoscopy (which can make subsequent liposuction more difficult due to fibrous adhesions), and to set realistic expectations for the procedure and its outcome. Liposuction achieves excellent results when performed in a young, nulliparous woman with toned musculature where skin elasticity is optimal, and fatty deposition localizes in the lower abdomen. While most patients presenting for liposuction of the abdomen do not fall into this category, worthwhile results still may be achieved, sparing the patient from a procedure such as an abdominoplasty which has a much longer recovery period and higher risk profile.

The overall shape of the person should be examined in the preoperative physical examination. There is a spectrum of body types, each requiring different areas of focus ranging from liposuction of the lower abdomen alone to that of the upper hips, abdomen, waist, and back. Narins divides abdominal liposuction patients into five groups based on fat distribution (Table 32.6).

Table 32.6 Five groups of patients: abdominal liposuction

1. Liposuction: lower abdomen
2. Liposuction: upper and lower abdomen
3. Liposuction: hourglass abdomen; upper and lower abdomen, hips, waist, and back
4. Liposuction and skin excision: mini-abdominoplasty with or with umbilical translocation
5. Complete abdominoplasty

Reprinted from Narins R, Abdomen, hourglass abdomen, flanks and modified abdominoplasty. In: Narins R, ed. Safe liposuction and fat transfer. New York; 2003, by courtesy of Marcel Dekker Inc.

The lower abdomen patients are typically those with a thin body habitus and a localized fatty deposition of the lower abdomen.[44] They tend to respond very well to liposuction with excellent patient satisfaction.

Those requiring liposuction of both the upper and lower abdomen must be carefully evaluated; this group may also be relatively thin, so suction of the lower abdomen alone may leave a prominent and possibly overhanging upper abdomen. It is therefore imperative to do both areas to avoid an unsightly disproportionate appearance. People who require liposuction of the upper and lower abdomen, and the hips, waist, and back tend to be older postmenopausal women, or those on hormone replacement therapy with a history of weight gain.

Men may also require a similar procedure as fat deposits of the abdominal area are usually accompanied by fat excess of the chest, flanks, and back as well (Fig. 32.4A–B). It is important to note that men with protuberant abdomens are not always good candidates for abdominal liposuction because much of the fat deposition may be behind the rectus abdominus and is therefore unsuctionable.

The fourth group of patients demonstrates atrophic, stretched skin resulting from pregnancy, advancing age, and 'yo yo' weight gain and loss.[44] While more extensive liposuction is needed, it often provides satisfactory improvement. As such, it is prudent to wait 3–4 months after the initial liposuction procedure to re-evaluate the patient for possible future abdominoplasty.[39]

The patient should be marked while standing to accentuate the larger areas of fatty deposition (which

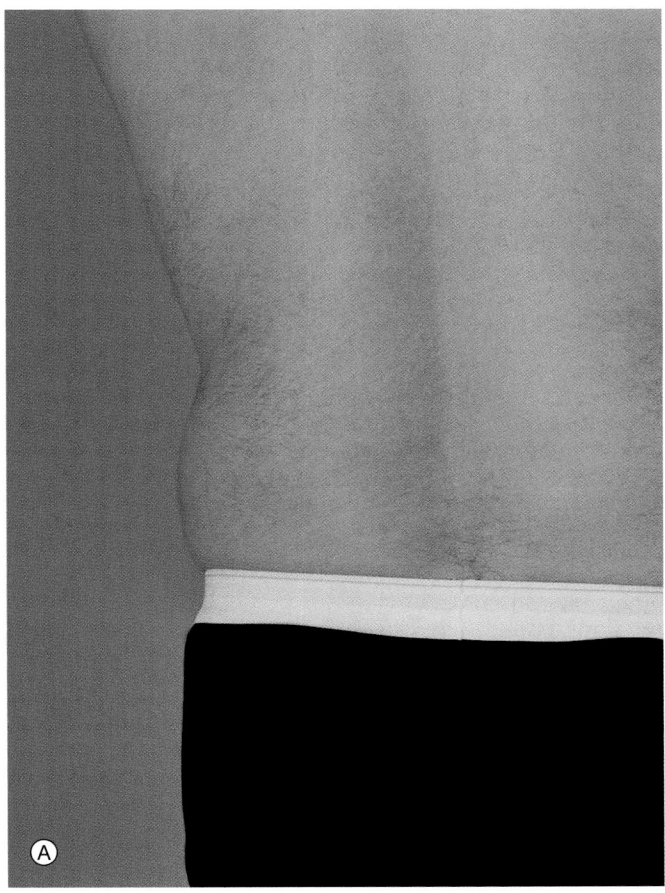

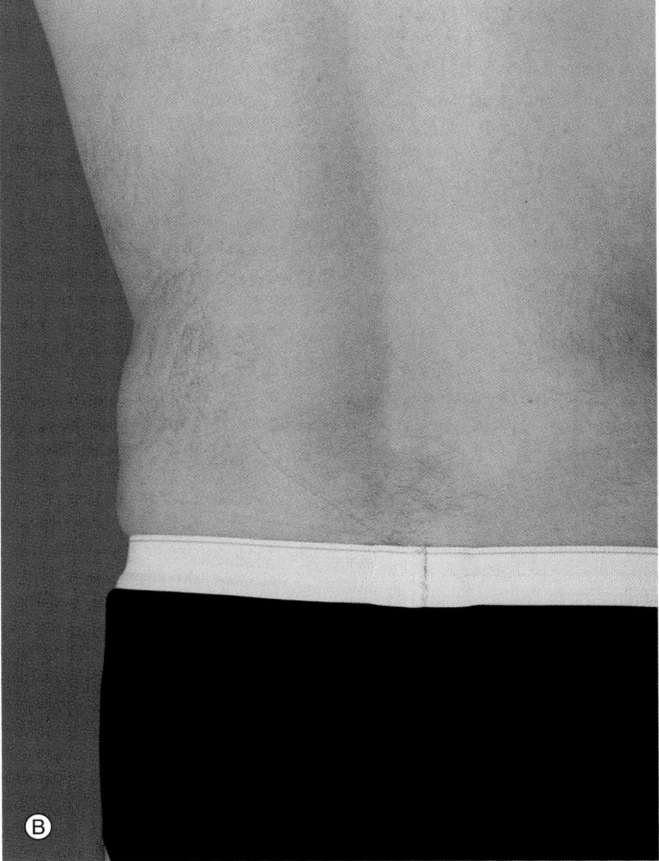

Figure 32.4 Flanks (A) before liposuction and (B) after liposuction.

should be outlined and detailed). Incision sites are typically made, with two or three in the suprapubic region, one at the umbilicus, and two on the lateral portions of the abdominal fat depositions. The upper abdomen and periumbilical regions tend to be more tender, and it is helpful to use 0.1% lidocaine to infuse these areas. The patients should be lying on their back on the surgical table for this procedure. As the patient is awake throughout, it is helpful to bring the legs into a slightly flexed position at times during the procedure to make grasping the abdominal skin easier. Towards the end of the procedure, it is helpful to have the patient examined for fatty pockets while lying on both lateral decubitus positions, as pockets of fat that appear flattened in a supine position become more apparent as they fall away from the rectus muscle. The goal of abdominal liposuction should be to reduce the deeper fatty layers while maintaining a superficial, even layer of fat attached to the skin. Oversuction may lead to dimpling of the skin, uneven fatty depositions, and even dermal necrosis[39] (Figs 32.5A–B, 32.6A–B)

Hips, outer thighs, and buttocks

Evaluation of a patient for liposuction in these regions requires a three-dimensional approach. If isolated treatment occurs to only one of these areas, a disproportionate appearance of enlargement may occur in the unsuctioned areas. For the hips, outer thighs, and buttocks it is important to take note of underlying musculature, cellulite, and inelastic skin. None of these imperfections can be improved with liposuction. It is important to discuss with the patient what their ideal shape would be, as cultural and personal preferences vary.

Positioning is key in preventing oversuctioning and resultant lipotrop. For the hips, the patient should be in the lateral decubitus position. For liposuction of the outer thighs, the patient should also be in the lateral decubitus position with a surgical pillow placed between the legs, which rotates the femur anterior-medially with the toes pointed inward, mimicking a standing position.[34] Again, the importance of positioning is to prevent oversuctioning, which is a potential problem in these areas because the fat tends to be less fibrous. Additionally, anatomical landmarks such as the trochanteric process create a pseudobulge of the lateral thigh in certain positions, which can misguide the unprepared or inexperienced surgeon. The end result of suctioning should be a region that is flat—never concave. Subcutaneous fat tunnels may not be emptied, in contrast to the abdomen where empty tunnels are helpful in determining suction endpoints. Suctioning should be equal on both sides and care should be taken to monitor amounts of fat removed relative to proportions of each side.

Liposuction of the buttock must be done carefully, with special consideration made to the inferolateral gluteal crease, where a 'banana roll' comprised of a defined infragluteal fat pocket may worsen or lead to a ptotic buttock with oversuction. It is advised by some authors to avoid suction of the 'banana roll' altogether or to suction superficially to avoid trauma to the infragluteal ligaments (Luschke's ligament).[34] As always, the physical examination must focus on bony and muscular prominences and asymmetry. Realistic expectations should be set, as liposuction will not improve bony asymmetry, the presence of large or asymmetrical muscle masses, or skin laxity. Conservative buttock suction is recommended with removal of no more than 30–50% of fat from the middle and deep fat layers. Superficial suctioning of the buttocks should be avoided as it may result in undesirable dimpling[34] (Fig. 32.7A–B)

The medial thigh and knee

The medial thigh and knee are often considered together because most women have fat that extends from one region into the other. Excess fatty deposition here is rarely found in men. Once again, a potential pitfall in this area is oversuctioning. The fat in these regions is much less fibrous than in other regions and suctioning can quickly lead to overcorrection defects. Positioning is important when treating the inner thighs, and the patient should be placed in the lateral decubitus position with the resting, superior thigh flexed into a 'high step' position. It is helpful to place a brick-shaped surgical pillow underneath this thigh to assist in patient comfort, and to place the legs in a more anatomic position optimal for liposuction of the inferior extended leg.[39] Careful observation must be made in the marking phase of the procedure as the fatty deposits of the medial thigh often encompass the anterior, medial, and posterior thigh, and therefore, must be approached in a three-dimensional manner. If circumferential thigh liposuction is needed, this is usually recommended as a serial procedure, as significant lymphostasis may result if the entire circumference of the thigh is treated at once.[39]

Liposuction of the knee can create a more attractive, defined appearance, and is often performed along with liposuction of the medial thigh. A supine or lateral decubitus position is preferred with treatment of the inferior extended leg, as a flexed knee can move the medial knee fat pads posteriorly and obscure them. Avoid aggressive suctioning in this area because injury may occur to lymphatic vessels creating a seroma, sensory nerve injury, or damage dermal vasculature leaving a persistent reticulated hyperpigmentation.[39]

Arms

Liposuction of the arms is typically done in women who present with laxity of the proximal arm musculature and pendulous fatty prominence. This is best appreciated when the arms are abducted at 90° from the body. Gentle liposuction of the medial and posterior (or extensor) arm with avoidance of the anterior flexural surface can create a proportionate, attractive improvement. Oversuctioning must be avoided. The goal is to create an even, proportionate appearance, not to remove as much fat as possible. As skin redundancy is usually a significant contributing factor to the patient's overall appearance, the patient should be prepared for decreased convexity of the arms rather than complete recontouring. Excessive tumescent infusion should be avoided, as there is a small risk of developing a 'compartment syndrome' where a functional tourniquet develops distal to the infused region, due to fluid compression of neural, vascular, and lymphatic structures.[39] At least two positions should be used to gain access to the regions of the arms that are to be treated. Two helpful positions include the entire arm laying flat, palm

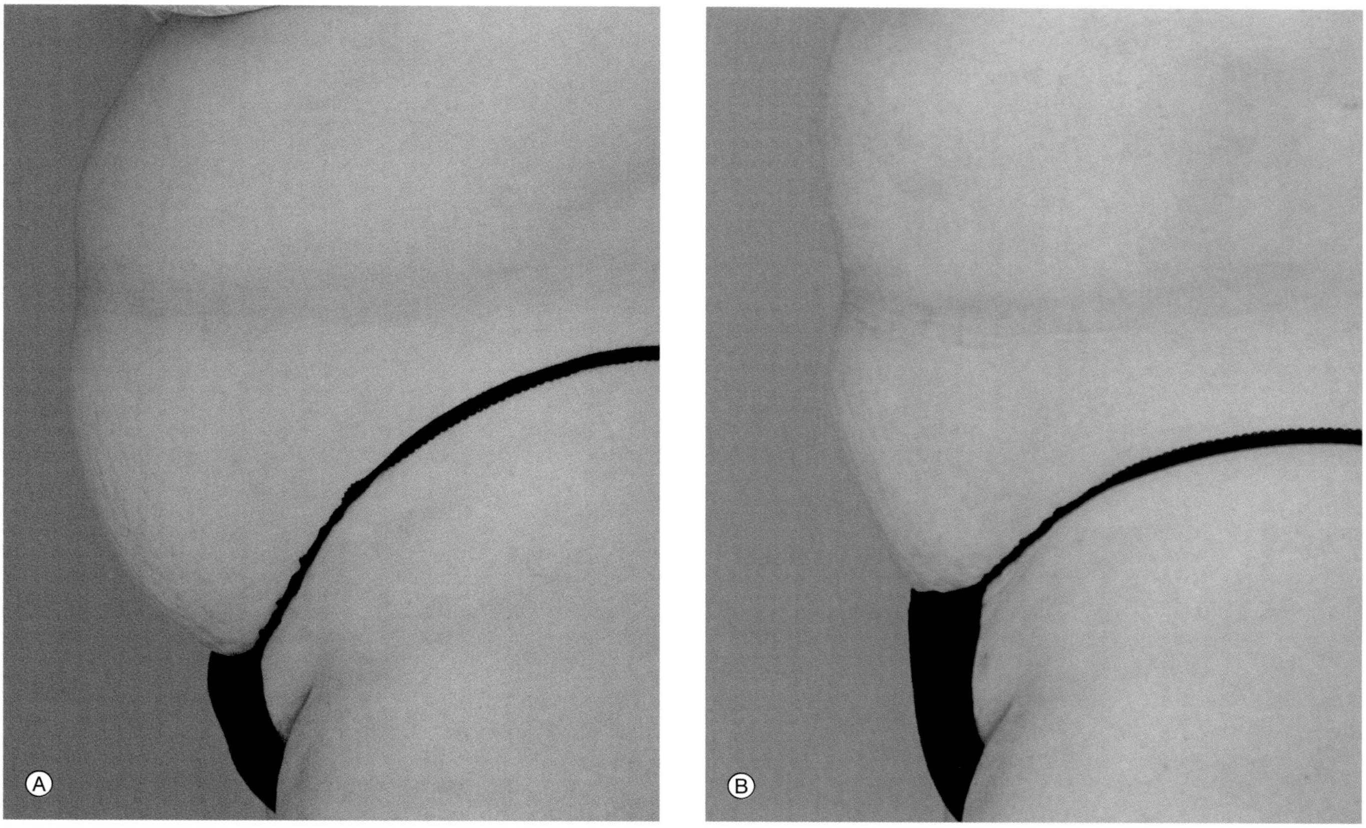

Figure 32.5 Abdomen (A) before liposuction and (B) 1 year after liposuction.

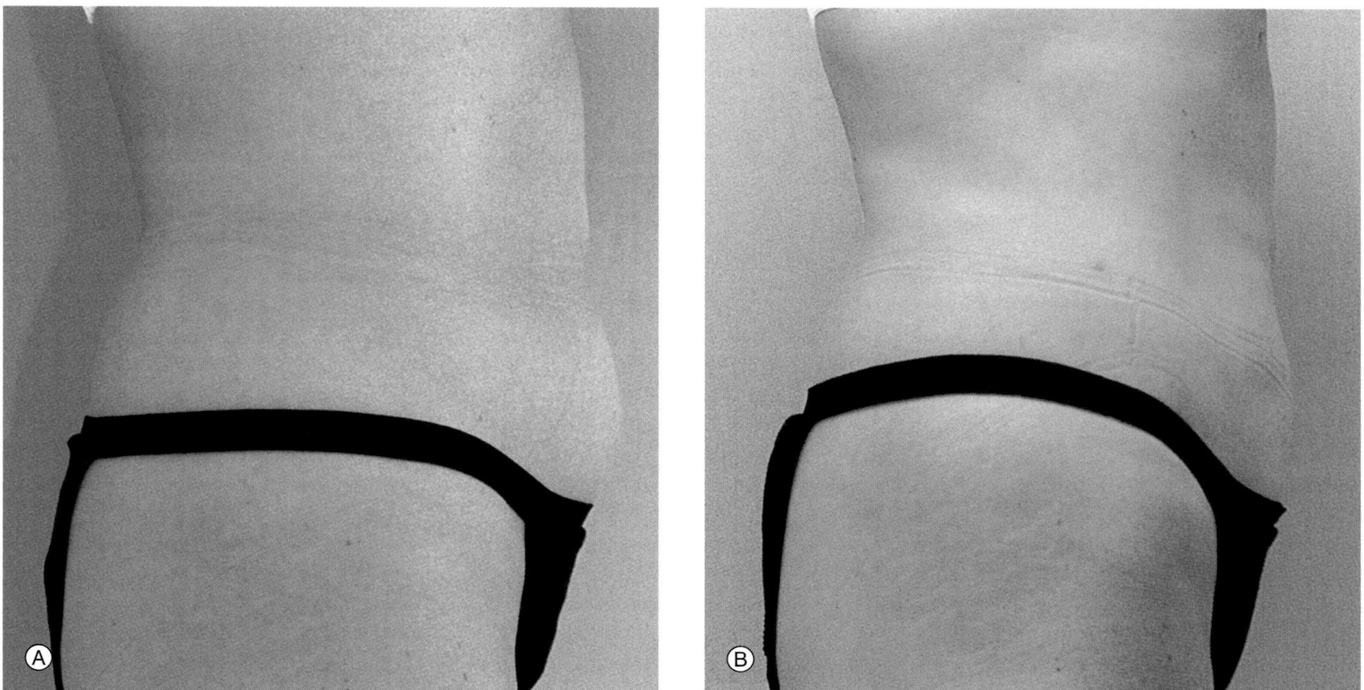

Figure 32.6 Abdomen and waist (A) before liposuction and (B) 3.5 months after liposuction.

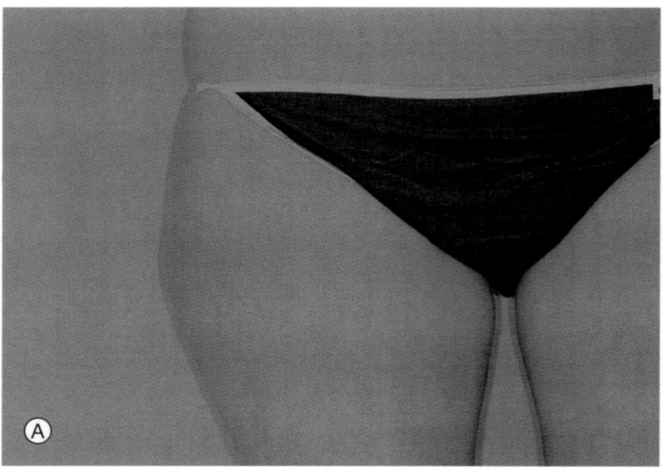

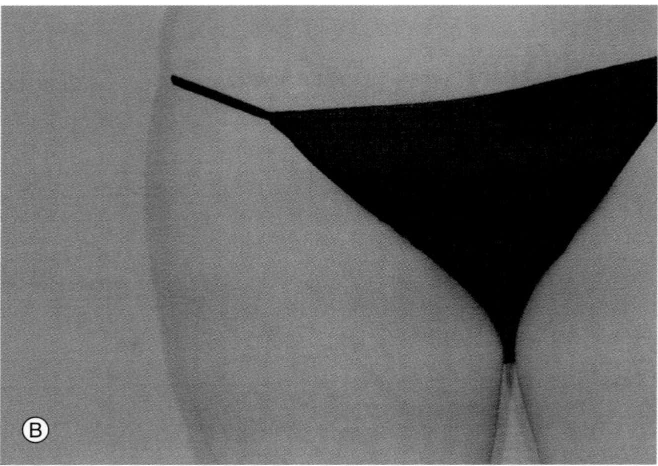

Figure 32.7 Outer thigh (A) before liposuction and (B) after liposuction.

down, over the hips with the body in a lateral decubitus position to maximally expose the posterior portion of the arm. The other position that is often helpful is for the patient to be supine or in a lateral decubitus position with the hand brought behind the head, the forearm flexed, and the elbow pointing away from the face, to expose the posterior portion of the arm.[39] Liposuction of the axilla should be avoided as a number of important neurovascular structures, including the brachial plexus, traverse this area. It is often helpful to combine liposuction of the arms with suctioning of the anterior axillary fat pad, which can become prominent with age. For this, the patient should be lying supine with the forearm flexed at an 90-degree angle and the arm abducted and lying flat on the bed. Even suctioning of this area is important to avoid unnatural creases and folds.[39]

Neck and jowls

Liposuction of the neck (see Chapter 43) and jowls is both safe and successful in rejuvenation of these regions, giving redefinition of the cervicomental angle and jawline. Patient selection is paramount because concomitant or adjuvant procedures such as platysma plication, subcutaneous musculoaponeurotic system (SMAS) plication, carbon dioxide laser resurfacing, chin implants, and a full-face lift are sometimes necessary to achieve optimal results. An aged appearance in this region is due to a multitude of factors including ptosis of fatty tissue and decreased elastic tissue resulting in a loss of the neck sling function, allowing the anterior margins of the platysma to slide forward and the submental and submandibular fat to bulge.[45] Fullness in the region can be due to redundant skin, muscle, or a low or anteriorly positioned hyoid bone (making for an obtuse cervicomental angle). Patients with low-set or anteriorly placed hyoid bones are much less likely to benefit from neck liposuction alone. During the physical examination, one should note hyoid positioning (which should ideally be at the level of the C3–C4 vertebrae), the jowls, and the submental fat. The ideal candidate has full jowls with retained skin elasticity, a high-set hyoid bone, and a palpable submental fat pad.[46] As in other areas evaluated for liposuction, having the patient flex underlying musculature can aid in determining how much of the skin laxity is due to overlying subcutaneous fat versus fat located underneath the musculature. Asking the patient to show their lower teeth can accentuate platysmal bands and help identify patients who would benefit from platysmal plication. It is important to identify the position of the submandibular salivary glands as ptotic glands can mimic jowls and cannot be treated by liposuction.[46]

As with all procedures, expectations for results and recovery must be set well in advance. With liposuction of the neck, patients should be warned that the area may retain a firm, indurated, uneven appearance for up to 8 months following the procedure, particularly after large lipectomies with more dramatic preoperative skin laxity.[47] Male skin often takes longer to retract than female skin, and the less elasticity retained, the less optimal the result.[46] For marking the neck liposuction patient, the following boundaries should be noted: the mandibular border, the jowls, submental fat pad, anterior borders of the sternocleidomastoid, platysmal bands, and the thyroid cartilage.[46] Marking should always be performed with the patient seated in an upright position looking straight ahead. The optimal position for the patient during this procedure is with the head gently extended posteriorly, and the chin raised with a supportive small pillow for neck support. Tumescent fluid can be infused with a 25-gauge 1.5-inch needle into the submental area, jowl, neck, and lateral cheeks. Care must be taken not to overinfuse the buccal region as intraoral airway occlusion can occur.[46] Following infiltration, it is preferable to wait for 20 minutes as this results in adequate vasoconstriction, anesthesia, and diffusion of tumescent fluid (detumescence), which allows easier handling of tissues during the procedure.[39]

Liposuction entry sites are typically placed in the submental crease at the mid-pupillary line, just below or lateral to the jowls. If extensive lateral neck fat is present two additional entry points are placed just behind the earlobes, in a neck crease. Suctioning should begin in the plane of fat just above the platysma muscle, with subsequent suction more superficially with small (1.5–2 mm suction cannulae).[46] It is crucial to avoid plunging the cannula through the platysma with resulting perforation, below the cervical fascia. This is a concern particularly in

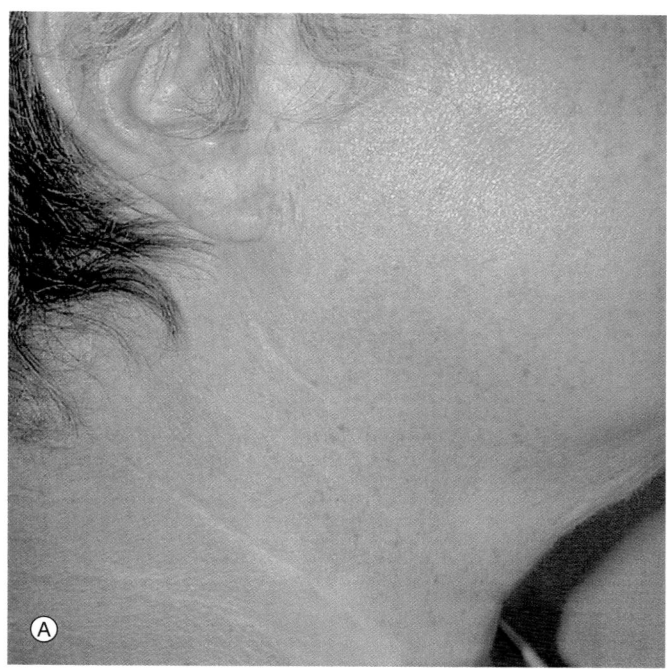

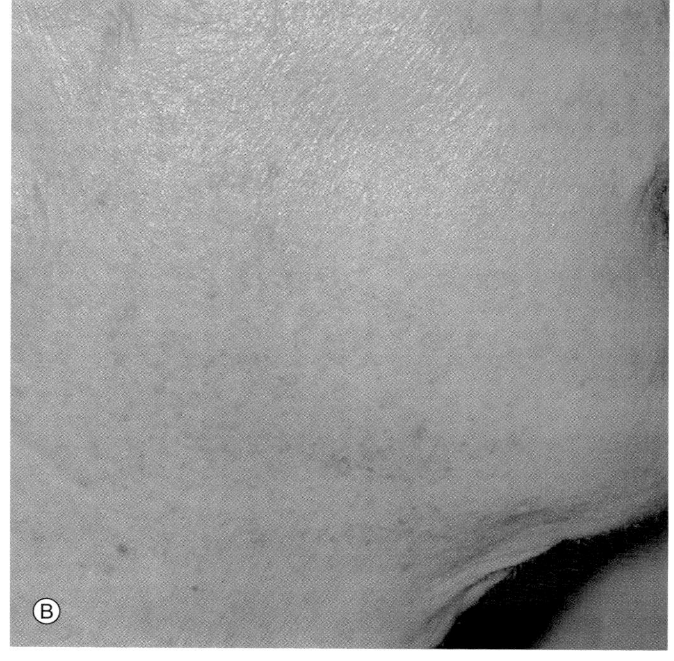

Figure 32.8 Neck (A) before liposuction and (B) after liposuction.

older people who often present with platysmal atrophy (see Chapter 1).[48] Take care to avoid trauma to the marginal mandibular branch of the facial nerve as it drops below the angle of mandible in the hyperextended neck and crosses over the mandible at the anterior border of the massetter muscle. When the patient's head is extended, the nerve may be located as far as two fingerbreadths from the posterior mandibular border and become more superficial and more susceptible to injury.[46] It is prudent to use the suction cannula to elevate the subcutaneous fat away from underlying structures during suctioning to avoid injury in these areas. Avoid oversuctioning of the cheeks and jowl–cheek margin, as undesirable dimpling or hollowing may occur.[46] Suctioning lateral to the anterior border of the sternocleidomastoid should be avoided as there are numerous vital structures traversing in this area.

The most common postoperative deformities following liposuction in this region are submental depressions or nodules and platysmal band deformities. These deformities tend to occur in those patients with mild preoperative bands, redundant cervical skin, and submental obesity.[49] Surgical correction of this occurrence may be necessary. (Fig. 32.8A–B)

Male chest

Before undertaking breast liposuction in men, take a thorough history and carry out a physical examination, paying special attention to palpation of the gynecomastia and regional lymph nodes. Some authors recommend palpation of the testes to examine for the possibility of testicular tumors.[50] Although rare, breast malignancy does occur in men, and an asymmetric, irregular, firm, or fixed mass warrants a mammogram or biopsy.[50] Possible etiologies for male breast enlargement include fatty deposition, glandular deposition, medications (estrogens, spironolactone, digitalis, diazepam, phenytoin, and clomiphene), alcoholism, hypogonadism, and testicular and adrenocorticosteroid-secreting tumors.[39]

The male breast is one of the more vascular regions on which liposuction may be performed. Bleeding is minimized by the tumescent technique, and by taking great care not to traumatize the underlying pectoralis muscle during either infiltration or suction. The male breast is also one of the most fibrous regions on which liposuction is performed, varying greatly in the content of glandular tissue and fatty tissue. This creates a challenge for the liposuction surgeon during the procedure and an inherent unpredictability in the results as fatty tissue is easily contoured by liposuction, while glandular tissue is not.[50,51] Patients should expect about a 50% improvement.[39] Persistent glandular tissue may necessitate excision, and the possibility of this must be conveyed to the patient before undergoing the procedure.[39]

Tumescent anesthesia can be done with an infusion cannula, or a 25-gauge needle.[39] Incision sites are placed along the periphery of the breast and in the inframammary crease to allow for complete infiltration and suction in a criss-cross pattern. Following infusion of tumescent solution, it is helpful to wait 20 minutes before suctioning to allow for complete fluid dispersion and improved vasoconstriction.[51] Suction is typically begun with microcannulae, allowing for easier passage through the tissue. Klein recommends beginning with a 16-gauge Capistrano cannula (HK Surgical, Oceanside, CA) for initially tunneling with progression to usage of the larger 14-gauge microcannula.[39] Even the subareolar breast tissue may be gently suctioned with the use of a short (5-cm or 7.5-cm) 16-gauge Capistrano cannula.[39]

As with other liposuction procedures, open drainage of insertion sites is recommended with proper compression. This serves to minimize postoperative ecchymosis and hematomas.[39]

Female breast

Traditional reduction mammoplasty is a major surgical procedure which requires general anesthesia. It also has a significant risk for infection, seroma, hematoma, scarring, skin loss, and fat necrosis.[52,53] The procedure requires an inverted T-shaped incision from the areola to the inframammary crease, leaving an unattractive scar. Liposuction has been used adjunctively to remove adipose from the anterior axillary fold and chest wall.[52,54] Although liposuction of the male chest has been successfully used for years, liposuction of the female breast is a relatively new procedure, and as the sole method of reduction has only been described in a small number of papers.[52,54–56]

Most physicians recommend women with moderate breast enlargement as candidates as there is a concern that extreme nipple ptosis and excess skin of gigantomastia would not adequately respond to liposuction alone. Currently a personal or family history of breast cancer is considered a contraindication. A screening preoperative mammogram should be preformed at baseline and repeated 6 months after liposuction. As this is a new indication the best parameters have not been fully realized. A measurement of preoperative breast mass, either through scale or volume displacement, should be performed preoperatively. This gives the surgeon some indication as to how much fat to remove if they consider a percentage reduction.

The patient should be positioned supine with the ipsilateral arm behind the head or with the arm posteriorly displaced to bring the breast flat against the chest wall. The breast is thoroughly tumesced with anesthesia (0.1–0.125% lidocaine is preferable). Kaminer recommends two incisions in the lateral axillary line and one in the mid-inframammary crease. The suctioning is concentrated in the deep to mid-plane of the lateral and inferior quadrants. Less is taken from the upper quadrants as this flattens naturally with age. The surgeon suctions the predetermined amount, based on the desired reduction. Correlation between the volume of fat removed and the reduction in cup size is an area for further study. At this point most are advocating removal of small amounts (about one third of the measured volume) at one session, and a serial approach for further reduction. Breast reduction by liposuction alone is a promising new area for liposuction surgeons.

■ POSTOPERATIVE CARE

Immediate postoperative period

Immediately after the liposuction, decisions must be made whether to suture insertion points, and whether to use a drain. As a rule of thumb, dependent insertion sites ought to be left open to drain, and a vacuum suction drain should be utilized for large abdominal cases (at least 2000 ml fat removed) or where copious bleeding is noted intraoperatively. Thereafter, patients are brought to a standing position gradually to prevent orthostatic hypotension. Excess fluid is expressed by compressing the areas with a towel. This is ideally performed in a shower if one is readily available in the surgical suite. A seat should be available because the patient may experience a vasovagal reaction. The patient is then cleaned off with sterile sponges or cloth. Absorbent pads (such as sanitary napkins or HK pads) are placed over the incision sites and held in place with tape or a tubular elastic retainer (Surgilast; Glenwood Inc, Tenafly, NJ).

The patient is assisted into the girdle and the appropriate binder is placed over the girdle for the abdomen and neck areas. Klein advocates a technique of bimodal compression—i.e. heavy compression in the first 24 hours to facilitate drainage and then mild compression for two to four days.[57] According to Klein, the traditional approach of prolonged (2–4 weeks) heavy compression can result in post-traumatic edema. Klein postulates that excessive compression can impair subcutaneous lymphatic drainage, impeding lymphatic uptake of large osmotically active molecules.

In the first 24 hours, application of ice is helpful—crushed ice in a bag, or frozen peas, wrapped in a thin towel and applied over the girdle. Cold therapy causes vasoconstriction, which decreases exudate of blood and inflammatory cells in the injured tissue.[58–60] The decrease in temperature depresses the local metabolic rate, lowering the tissue requirement for oxygen. This makes the injured tissue more resistant to further damage through hypoxemia.[61,62] Finally, cooling tissue provides an analgesic effect by decreasing the excitability of the free nerve endings and depressing nerve impulse conductors.[58,63] To prevent cold injury the patient should be instructed to apply the ice in cycles of 10–20 minutes of cold followed by 10-minute breaks.[64,65]

The incision sites should be treated with moist occlusion as soon as the drainage has ceased. A spot Band-Aid is preferable to a strip Band-Aid as the adhesive that completely surrounds the central non-stick pad provides a more complete seal.

■ PITFALLS AND THEIR MANAGEMENT

During the course of the procedure the patient may complain of one or two areas that are hypersensitive even if they are well infused. The pitfalls of liposuction are summarized in Table 32.7.

The surgeon can try one of several measures to overcome this. The first to try is to approach the area from another entry site. Sometimes the discomfort is due to a pull on certain fibrous septae that can be changed by direction of suction. A decrease in cannula diameter can also eliminate the problem. The areas can be re-infused with tumescent fluid (can increase concentration of lidocaine). If the area is small the surgeon can directly inject 5–6 ml of 1% lidocaine with epinephrine (adrenaline) into it. Finally, a small amount of intravenous pain medication (25 mg of fentanyl (Durogesic; Jansen Pharmaceutic, Titusville, NJ) can get the surgeon past the problem area.

Occasional ventricular ectopy can be present in some patients and is often undiagnosed before the procedure as the patients are not symptomatic. If known to be present, the patient should be referred to a cardiologist for control of the ectopy prior to surgery. Although this is a rare occurrence, it can necessitate canceling the procedure.

Vasovagal reaction is always possible with any procedure and is managed with supportive care (Trendelenberg position, cool packs, oxygen). Klein recommends 0.3 mg atropine given intravenously.[66] Prophylaxis for people predisposed to vasovagal reactions can be given preoperatively, as well as atropine.

Table 32.7 Pitfalls of liposuction

Intraoperative	Immediate Postoperative	Long Term
Discomfort: 'hot spots' (reinfuse, consider administration of intravenous pain medicine)	Infection (consider prophylactic antibiotics)	Less than optimal reduction of target area (consider 'touch-up' after 1 year)
Bigeminy: ventricular ectopy; epinephrine (adrenaline) hypersensitivity	Poor healing of insertion sites (monitor for proper technique)	Weight gain (exercise and diet control)
Vasovagal: Trendelenberg position and support (consider atropine)	Decreased skin sensation and dysesthesias (improves with time)	
Tachycardia: if blood pressure greater than 100/70 mmHg [give] clonidine	Irregularity in target area (set expectation with 'touch-up' in mind)	
	Seroma: compression (leave dependent insertion sites open; consider short-term drain)	

Tachycardia secondary to epinephrine (adrenaline) in the infusion can be virtually eliminated by two measures: first, by decreasing the epinephrine (adrenaline) from 1 mg to 0.65 mg in each bag of local anesthetic; and, second, by giving 0.1 mg clonidine to all patients with blood pressure over 100/70 preoperatively.

Infection is a rare complication of tumescent liposuction. Klein postulates that this is due to the bacteriostatic properties of lidocaine.[66] It is treated with oral or intravenous antibiotics depending on the severity of the infection and the presence of systemic symptoms. The cannula entrance sites should heal in 7–10 days with appropriate technique. The most common cause for poor healing is through non-compliance with wearing Band-Aids over the sites after drainage stops. The written postoperative instructions must be very clear on this point as leaving the sites unoccluded delays healing and results in less than optimal scarring. During the surgery it is important not to stretch or excessively traumatize the entrance sites. It is always better to make a new or larger entrance site if necessary to reach a remote area or accommodate a larger cannula. Patients should be warned that entrance sites, like any healing wound, can develop hyperpigmentation at 2–3 months. Treatment with hydroquinone 4% or mequinol 2% (with or without tretinoin) will successfully reverse this over several weeks.

For the experienced liposuction surgeon, less than optimal fat reduction of the target area occurs in a few circumstances. Sometimes the surgeon incorrectly assesses the amount of fat in the subcutaneous layer. This is probably more likely to happen with the abdomen than any other area. Less than complete suctioning of an area can also occur because the patient is not tolerant of the procedure and the usual measures failed to make them comfortable, or an unusually bloody aspirate causes premature termination of suctioning.

Butterwick studied the number of touch-up procedures done in a large liposuction practice. She found that over a 2-year period 12.3% of 954 liposuction procedures had a touch-up procedure.[67] Men and women had an equal number of touch-up procedures. The most common areas for touch-up were the neck and abdomen. These were also the most commonly treated sites. The highest incidence of touch-ups were done on the back, chest, and ankles. The weight pattern after liposuction may play a role as 47% of these patients had increased weight.

It is important when approaching the issue of touch-up to set reasonable expectations with the patient. Some patients are looking for a level of perfection—a completely seamless contour—that is simply not achievable for most. If a touch-up procedure is anticipated we prefer that they wait a year before proceeding as subcutaneous fibrosis will continually remodel and an area that may appear to be uneven at first may smooth out. It is important that the surgeon appreciates the abnormality that the patient wants corrected. It is a mistake to resuction an area because the patient demands it. If there is no correctable problem, there is no endpoint for the procedure. The patient that complains of perceived deformities that are not clinically evident is rarely pleased with touch-up procedures. It is best to deal with this patient directly and not get caught up in a cycle of procedures.

It is very common for a patient to notice another area of adiposity once their target area is corrected. The best way to prepare them for this is to discuss it preoperatively. We try to make note and point out during the physical examination what areas might appear disproportionate once the target area is reduced. This has to be done carefully as it is important for the patient not to feel pressured to add additional areas. Once patients are made aware of this phenomenon, they are much more reasonable when they notice disproportionate adjacent areas postoperatively. If the remaining areas bother them enough, they schedule additional liposuction.

Long-term outcome

Early in the screening for liposuction procedures, we spend a considerable amount of time learning about patients' past weight patterns, diet, and exercise history. We discourage any candidates that have a chronic weight cycling pattern, or have recently lost more than 9 kg on a very-low-calorie diet, but have not maintained that loss for at least 6 months. The biggest pitfall in the long-term result for liposuction is subsequent weight gain. If a patient gains weight after liposuction, the area liposuctioned will resist weight gain and this may cause fat to accumulate in a new area (including one not amenable to liposuction—that is, deep to muscle), or to distribute unevenly. In the first scenario the enlargement of a new area is sometimes a welcomed event. Yun et al. retrospectively reviewed 73 liposuction cases and found breast enlargement in 34%.[68] Although these patients on average lost about 3.2 kg, a high percentage of the group reporting breast enlargement had weight gain. In a patient with a small abdomen that was fine-tuned with liposuction, even a small weight gain can increase abdominal girth by increasing fat deep to the rectus, and negate the results of the liposuction. The neck and the abdomen have fatty areas deep to muscle that can enlarge with weight regain. In the second scenario, patients are often happier with evenly distributed weight gain than they were with a disproportionate adiposity.

■ SUMMARY

Liposuction with local (tumescent) anesthesia is a procedure that was originated and developed by dermatologic surgeons. It is a procedure with excellent longevity of results and high patient satisfaction. Studies by Bernstein, Hanke, Coleman, and Housmen of dermatologic liposuction have repeatedly shown that it is an extremely safe and effective procedure.[69–72] Tumescent liposuction should be considered as an option in appropriate patients desiring a more sculptured physical appearance.

■ REFERENCES

1. Klein JA. The tumescent technique for liposuction surgery. Am J Cosmet Surg 1987; 4:263–267.
2. Pitanguy I. Trochanteric lipodystrophy. Plast Reconstr Surg 1964; 34:280–283.
3. Schrudde J. Lipexheresis liposuction for body contouring. In Grazer F, ed. Clinics in plastic surgery, volume 11. Philadelphia: WB Saunders 1984; 445–456.
4. Fischer G. Liposculpture: The 'correct' history of liposuction, part I. J Dermatol Surg Oncol 1990; 16:1087–1089.
5. Fischer A, Fischer G. First surgical treatment for molding body's cellulite with three 5-mm incisions. Bull Int Acad Cosmet Surg 1976; 3:35.
6. Illouz Y. Body contouring by lipolysis; A 5-year experience with over 3000 cases. Plast Reconstr Surg 1983; 72:591–597.
7. Grazer F. Suction assisted lipectomy, suction lipectomy, lipolysis, lipexheresis. Plast Reconstr Surg 1983:72:620–623.
8. Fournier P. Body sculpturing through syringe liposuction and autologous fat re-injection. Corona del Mar: Samuel Rolf International, 1987.
9. Klein JA. Tumescent technique for regional anesthesia permits lidocaine doses of 35–55 mg/kg for liposuction. Peak plasma are diminished and delayed 12 hours. J Dermatol Surg Oncol 1990; 16:248–263.
10. Lillis PJ. The tumescent technique for liposuction surgery. In Lillis PJ, ed. Dermatology clinics, volume 8. Philadelphia: WB Saunders 1990; 439–450.
11. Lillis PJ. Liposuction surgery under local anesthesia. Limited blood loss and minimal lidocaine absorption. J Dermatol Surg Oncol 1988; 14:1145–1148.
12. Ostad A, Kageyama N, Moy RL. Tumescent anesthesia with a lidocaine dose of 55 mg/kg is safe for liposuction. Dermatol Surg 1996; 22:921–927.
13. Butterwick J. Liposuction. consultation and preoperative considerations. In: Narins RS, ed. Safe liposuction and fat transfer. New York: Marcel Dekker 2003; 41–67.
14. Kelley L. Lipotoxic at low lidocaine levels. World Congress on Liposuction, Detroit, Michigan, 2000.
15. Currier JS, Havlir DV. Complications of HIV disease and antiretroviral therapy. Int AIDS Society USA 2000; 2:16–20.
16. Klein JA. Thrombosis and embolism. In: Klein JA, ed. Tumescent technique, tumescent anesthesia and microcannular liposuction. St Louis: Mosby 2000; 67–78.
17. Eggleston ST, Lush LW. Understanding allergic reactions to local anesthetics. Ann Pharmacother 1996; 30:851–857.
18. Klein JA. Ancillary pharmacology. In: Klein JA, ed. Tumescent technique. St Louis: Mosby 2000; 196–209.
19. Brown S, Cropfield O. The case for a lower dose pill. Assessing the impact of estrogen dose. ORGYN 1995; 2:36–39.
20. Peverill RE. Hormone therapy and venous thromboembolism. Best Pract Res Clin Endocrinol Metab 2003; 17:149–164.
21. Lidegard O, Edstrom B, Kreiner S. Oral contraceptives and venous thromboembolism. A five-year national case–control study. Contraception 2002; 65:187–196.
22. Drife J. Oral contraception and the risk of thromboembolism. What does it mean to clinicians and their patients? Drug Safety 2002; 25:893–902.
23. Butterwick KJ. Should dermatologic surgeons discontinue hormonal therapy before tumescent liposuction? Dermatol Surg 2002; 28:1184–1187.
24. Brownell KD, Rodin J. Medical, metabolic, and psychological effects of weight cycling. Arch Intern Med 1994; 154:1325–1330.
25. Pasman WJ, Saris WH, Westerterp-Plantenga MS. Predictors of weight maintenance. Obes Res 1999; 7:43–50.
26. Skender ML, Goodrick GK, Del Junco DJ, et al. Comparison of two-year weight loss trends in behavioral treatments of obesity; diet, exercise, and combination interventions. J Am Diet Assoc 1996; 96:342–346.
27. Wing RR, Greeno CG. Behavioral and psychosocial aspects of obesity and its treatment. Bailliére's Clin Endocrinol Metab 1994; 8:689–703.
28. McCargar LJ. Can diet and exercise really change metabolism? Medscap Women Health 1996; 1:5.
29. Atkins RC. Dr Atkins' new diet revolution. New York: HarperCollins 2002.
30. Rabast U, Schonborn J, Kasper H. Dietetic treatment of obesity with low and high carbohydrate diets. Comparative studies and clinical results. Int J Obes 1979; 3:201–211.
31. Rabast U, Vornberger KH, Ehl M. Loss of weight, sodium and water in obese persons consuming a high or low carbohydrate diet. Ann Nutr Metab1981; 25:341–349.
32. McInnis KJ. Exercise and obesity. Coron Artery Dis 2000; 11:111–116.
33. Ozgur F, Tuncali D, Guker Gursu K. Life satisfaction, self-esteem, and body image. a psychosocial evaluation of aesthetic and reconstructive surgery candidates. Aesthetic Plast Surg. 1998 22:412–419.
34. Cox SE. Violin hips, outer thighs, and buttocks. In: Narins RS, ed. Safe liposuction and fat transfer. New York: Marcel Dekker 2003; 121–148.
35. Butterwick KJ. Liposuction: Consultation and preoperative considerations. In: Narins RS, ed. Safe liposuction and fat transfer. New York: Marcel Dekker 2003; 41–67.
36. Monheit GD. The surgical suite for the liposuction surgeon. In: Narins RS, ed. Safe liposuction and fat transfer. New York: Marcel Dekker 2003; 19–28.
37. Bernstein G. Instrumentation for liposuction. Dermatol Clin 1999;14: 735–749.
38. Coleman WP, Glogau RG, Klein JA et al. Guidelines of care for liposuction. J Am Acad Dermatol 2001; 45:438–47.
39. Klein JA. Tumescent technique. Tumescent anesthesia and microcannular liposuction. St Louis: Mosby 2000.
40. Ostad A, Kageyama N, Moy R. Tumescent anesthesia with a lidocaine dose of 55 mg/kg is safe for liposuction. Dermatol Surg 1995; 22: 921–927.
41. Jacob, CI, Kaminer MS. Tumescent anesthesia. In: Narins RS, ed. Safe liposuction and fat transfer. New York: Marcel Dekker 2003; 29–40.
42. Narins RS, Coleman WP. Minimizing pain for liposuction anesthesia. Dermatol Surg 1997; 23:1137–1140.
43. Narins RS, Coleman WP IIIrd. Minimizing pain for liposuction anesthesia. Dermatol Surg 1997; 23:1137–1140.
44. Narins RS. Abdomen, hourglass abdomen, flanks, and modified abdominoplasy. In Narins RS, ed. Safe liposuction and fat transfer. New York: Marcel Dekker 2003; 95–119.
45. Kamer FM, Binder WJ. Avoiding depressions in submental lipectomy. The Laryngoscope 1980; 90:1396–1400.
46. Jacob CI, Kaminer MS. Surgical approaches to the aging neck. In Narins RS, ed. Safe liposuction and fat transfer. New York: Marcel Dekker 2003; 197–214.
47. Goddio AS. Suction lipectomy. The gold triangle at the neck. Aesth Plast Surg 1992; 16:27–32.
48. Adamson PA, Cormier R, Tropper G, McGraw B. Cervicofacial liposuction. Results and controversies. J Otolaryngol 1990; 19:267–273.

49. Kamer FM, Minoli JJ. Postoperative platysmal band deformity. A pitfall of submental liposuction. Arch Otolaryngol Head Neck Surg 1993; 119:193–196.
50. Samdal F, Kleppe G, Amland PR, Abyholm. Surgical treatment of gynecomastia. Scan J Plast Reconstr Hand Surg 1994; 28:123–130.
51. Bermant M. Gynecomastia-dynamic technique. In Narins RS, ed. Safe liposuction and fat transfer. New York: Marcel Dekker 2003: 215–234.
52. Gray LN. Liposuction breast reduction. Aesthetic Plast Surg 1998; 22:159–162.
53. Short K, Ringler SL, Bengston BP, Hunstad JP, Henry E. Reduction mammoplasty. A safe and effective outpatient procedure. Aesthetic Plastic Surg 1996; 20:513.
54. Matarasso A, Courtiss EH. Suction mammoplasty; the use of suction lipectomy to reduce large breasts. Plast Reconstr Surg 1991; 87:709–717.
55. Kaminer MS. Breast liposuction in liposuction course. American Academy of Dermatology meeting, San Francisco, 22 March 2003.
56. Pon K, van Laborde S, Kaminer MS. Case report of breast reduction by liposuction. Cosmet Dermatol 2002; 16:51–54.
57. Klein JA. Postliposuction care. Open drainage and bimodal compression In: Klein JA, ed. Tumescent technique. St Louis: Mosby 2000; 281–293.
58. Landry GL, Gomez JE. Management of soft tissue injuries. Adolesc Med 1991; 2:125–140.
59. Knight KL. Cryotherapy: Theory, technique, and physiology. Chattanooga: Chattanooga Corp, 1985; pp. 53–55 and 67–70.
60. Farry PJ, Prentice NG, Hunter AC, et al. Ice treatment of injured ligaments. An experimental model. NZ J Med 1980; 91:12–14.
61. El Hawary R, Stanish WD, Curwin SL. Rehabilitation of tendon injuries in sport. Sports Med 1997; 24:347–358.
62. Knight ATC. Cold as a modifier of sports-induced inflammation. In: Leadbetter WB, Buckwalter JA, Gordon SL, eds. Sports-induced inflammation. Clinical and basic science concepts. Parkridge: American Academy of Orthopedic Surgeons 1990: 463–478.
63. Kellett J. Acute soft tissue injuries—a review of the literature. Med Sci Sports Exerc 1986; 18:489–500.
64. Karunakara RG, Lephart SM, Pincivero DM. Changes in forearm blood flow during single and intermittent cold application. J Orthop Sports Phys Ther 1999; 29:177–180.
65. Drez D, Faust DC, Evan JP. Cryotherapy and nerve palsy. Am J Sports Med 1981; 9:256–257.
66. Klein JA. Miscellaneous complications. In: Klein JA, ed. Tumescent technique. Tumescent anesthesia and microcannular liposuction. New York: Mosby 2000; 43–60.
67. Lawrence L, Butterwick KJ. Immediate and long-term postoperative care and touch-ups. In Narins RS. Safe liposuction and fat transfer. New York: Marcel Dekker 2003; 329–341.
68. Yun PL, Bruck M, Felsenfeld L, Katz BE. Breast enlargement observed after power liposuction. A retrospective review. Dermatol Surg 2003; 129:165–167.
69. Bernstein G, Hanke CW. Safety of liposuction. A review of 9478 cases performed by dermatologists. J Dermatol Surg Oncol 1988 14:1112–1114.
70. Hanke CW, Bullock S, Bernstein G. Current status of tumescent liposuction in the United States. Dermatol Surg 1996; 22:595–598.
71. Coleman WP IIIrd, Hanke CS, Lillis P, Bernstein G, Narins R. Does the location of the surgery or the specialty of the physician affect malpractice claims in liposuction? Dermatol Surg 1999; 25:343–347.
72. Housman TS, Lawrence N, Mellen BG, et al. The safety of liposuction. results of a national survey. Dermatol Surg 2002; 39:971–978.

33 Autologous Fat Transfer: Evolving Concepts and Techniques

Kimberly J Butterwick MD

Summary box

- There is increasing demand for fat transfer as a means of facial volume restoration in cosmetic rejuvenation—not just as a corrective technique for soft tissue defects and rhytids but to correct the atrophy due to the aging process.
- Recently the emphasis has shifted from overcorrection to transfer of small volumes of fat, on the basis of improved understanding of the process of neovascularization and fat as a living graft.
- Autologous fat is usually harvested by gentle syringe aspiration and concentrated by centrifugation prior to reinjection into subcutaneous fat or muscle.
- Fat autograft muscle injection (FAMI) follows the patient's anatomical landmarks by placing fat within or adjacent to facial muscles.
- Potential complications of all fat transfer techniques include nodule formation due to overcorrection, fat necrosis, infection, and vascular occlusion, most of which can be avoided by careful, sterile technique.
- Data on long-term outcome is scarce and is largely based on two dimensional photography. Further research on outcome and factors affecting survival of adipocytes is needed and will necessitate finding an improved means of objective measurement.

INTRODUCTION

Fat augmentation is a popular and effective method for restoring volume to facial and body defects utilizing a variety of techniques. In many regards, fat fulfills the criteria as the ideal filling substance. It is readily available in most patients, inexpensive, non-allergenic, has no potential for infectious disease transmission, and has high patient acceptance. How well fat fulfills other key criteria of an ideal filler, such as predictability and persistence of correction over time, is controversial. This chapter will examine the evolving concepts in fat transplantation and the debates regarding the optimal techniques for achieving long-term results.

Historical Vignette

The history of fat transfer dates back to 1893 in an oft-quoted report by Neuber involving transfer of 1 cm pieces of fat from the arm to facial depressions caused by tuberculosis.[1] Lexer utilized fat for facial hemiatrophy and malar augmentation in 1910[2] and Bruning was the first to report injecting fat through a needle in 1919.[3] It was not until the 1950s that a report appeared regarding retention of transplanted fat, in which Peer noted a 40–50% retention at 1 year.[4]

In the late 1970s and early 1980s an increased interest in fat transplantation techniques was stimulated by advancements in liposuction by Illouz.[5] Fat could now be extracted by suction rather than the older methods of excision. Fat grafting was still an open or semi-open procedure until Fournier's inadvertant discovery in 1985 that fat could be extracted with a syringe and needle.[6] The popularity of fat transfer subsequently grew and provoked further inquiry into optimal techniques for harvesting, processing, and injection of fat for achieving adipocyte survival and longevity of results. The literature of the 1980s abounds with anecdotal and empirical reports regarding fat cell viability, but few if any controlled studies. Some reported dissatisfaction with transient results.[7]

The 1990s brought a second, even more explosive surge of interest in liposuction, with an 8-fold rise in the number of procedures performed in the United States from 1990–1999.[8] This growth was due in large part to Klein's introduction of the tumescent technique, allowing this procedure to be performed less invasively under local anesthesia with minimal postoperative downtime and unparalleled patient safety.[9] The increase in liposuction procedures fueled an increased interest in using the fat for correction of soft tissue defects and furrows. The 1990s also gave rise to an aging 'baby boomer' population with an increased demand for non-surgical rejuvenating procedures, including fat augmentation.[10]

New trends

Concepts and techniques regarding fat transfer changed during this period. One of the most significant changes in technique has been a shift from overcorrecting to transferring small volumes of fat.[11] This reflects a transition in the concept of fat as a temporary resorbed filler to fat as a living graft. In the 1980s and early 1990s it was not uncommon for large volumes of fat to be placed with deforming overcorrection of 50% or more.[12–14] It was reasoned that all the fat was absorbed and that overcorrection would result in more fibrosis. The rate of resorption of these volumes was often variable, unpredictable, and asymmetric.

The survival theory postulates that following transfer to the recipient site, the transplanted fat becomes ischemic. Some cells die and others survive as intact adipocytes or preadipocytes until a blood supply is established from the periphery. In the late 1980s, Coleman championed the survival theory of fat grafting and developed a method he called Lipostructure™.[15] He advocated placing small parcels of fat with repetitive passes into multiple new tissue planes, reasoning that a blood supply was more easily established. Gentle atraumatic handling of the fat cells was required for survival of the cells. Others reported improved longevity with smaller injection volumes and less traumatic harvesting and processing.[16] In 1994, Carpeneda validated these empiric findings when he compared viability of fat cylinders of different diameters. He found that smaller injected volumes, less than 3 mm in diameter, had optimal viability. At 2 months, viable fat cells were noted only in the peripheral zone of larger grafts having diameters of 3.5 mm or more.[17] The core of larger grafts had undergone necrosis due to lack of vascularization. In a recent review of the literature, small volume transfer versus overcorrection was the common denominator in studies reporting good longevity of fat.[18]

During the 1990s and into the 21st century we have also seen an expansion in the indications for fat transfer. In the 1980s fat was typically injected directly under rhytides or soft tissue defects. A relatively new concept in rejuvenation of the aging face is replacement of volume, not simply under specific rhytides and furrows, but for full-face volume restoration. It has been increasingly recognized among aesthetic surgeons that rhytidectomy alone does not necessarily rejuvenate a patient's appearance. Berman thoughtfully challenges the traditional concepts of rejuvenation, that the taut skin achieved through rhytidectomy may not equate with a youthful appearance.[19] He and others recognize the need to correct the atrophy of hard and soft tissues that occurs with age to achieve a truly rejuvenated appearance (Fig. 33.1).[19,20–22] It has also been pointed out that rhytidectomy may cause soft tissues to thin out even more, resulting in accelerated aging and a skeletonized appearance.[20] In addition to atrophic changes in soft tissues, remodeling of the craniofacial skeleton is now recognized to occur throughout life and impart further changes to the overlying soft tissue.[22–27] These concepts of aging diverge from the traditional view, that facial aging is a result of gravity-induced ptosis. Restoring volume to the aged face is now becoming an integral part of facial rejuvenation in addition to—or in some cases instead of—more conventional methods. In order to restore full facial volume, larger quantities in the range of 20–100 ml or more are required. Such quantities are not currently feasible with synthetic fillers primarily due to expense of numerous syringes and the temporary nature of most synthetic fillers. Autologous fat is the natural choice for volume correction of this degree. The challenge is the same, whether filling a furrow with fat or replacing full facial volume. How do we achieve optimal longevity of transferred fat?

Controversies in procedure

Autologous fat transfer is a multistep procedure. A review of the literature reveals that the proper method of performing every step of the procedure has been the subject of debate. At issue is the survival of the adipocyte

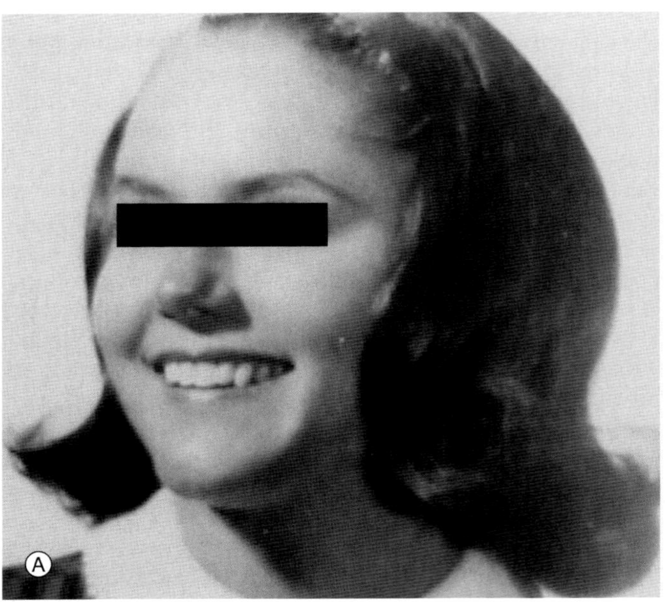

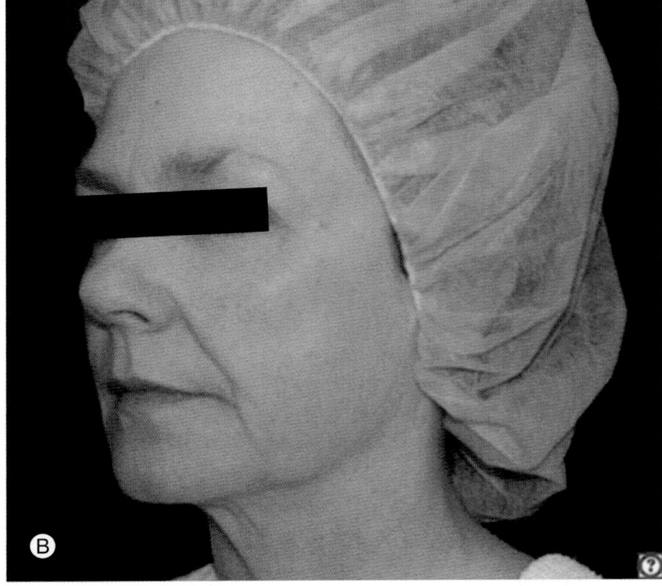

Figure 33.1 30-year facial volume loss.

and what factors have a positive or negative impact on survival (Table 33.1).

Each of these factors has been examined to some degree but definitive answers are lacking. Although the literature is replete with anecdotal reports, there are few objective studies. The difficulty in establishing consensus is a reflection of the difficulty in measuring outcome. There is no practical method to objectively document results. Transferred fat can not be labeled or distinguished from recipient site fat cells with a distinct histologic marker. Successive imaging with magnetic resonance or ultrasonography are expensive and expose the patient to unnecessary radiation. Measuring outcome is further complicated by variable rates of aging over time and changes in weight over time. We must therefore rely on photographic results until a better means of assessing outcome is available.

■ PREOPERATIVE PREPARATION

A preoperative history and physical examination are performed to screen for serious medical conditions, concomitant infections, bleeding diatheses, medications, and allergies. Medications containing aspirin and non-steroidal anti-inflammatory agents are discontinued 2 weeks before surgery. Vitamin E and certain herbal formulations should be discontinued before surgery. Prophylactic oral antibiotic therapy is started the night before the procedure: cephalexin 500 mg orally twice daily for 7 days, or minocycline 100 mg orally once or twice daily for penicillin-allergic patients. To minimize potential bruising, mephyton may be prescribed. The choice for the donor site is discussed with patients in advance. Benefits and risks are reviewed, as well as the postoperative sequelae. It is important to inform patients of expected downtime in advance.

■ TECHNICAL ASPECTS

Harvesting

Donor site

The optimal donor site has not been unequivocally established. Many choose the outer thigh as the ideal site due to its non-fibrous nature and relative avascularity. The rationale is that the least vascularized tissue will best survive the initial hypoxic period after transfer. Hudson found that adipocytes from the buttock and outer thigh areas are the largest and have the greatest lipogenic activity.[28] Ullman injected fat from various sites into nude mice and found the outer thigh fat to have the lowest resorption rate.[29] In any given patient, availability of fat is certainly a factor. Indeed, many patients desiring improvement of a gaunt facial appearance have very little body fat and one must obtain fat wherever possible. Areas that are diet-resistant such as the knee are often recommended in that, theoretically at least, the transplanted cells will be stable whether the patient gains or loses weight over time.

Table 33.1 Controversial factors in fat cell survival

Choice of harvesting site
Degree of negative pressure during harvesting
Diameter and type of harvesting cannula
Exposure of fat cells to air, blood, or lidocaine
Centrifugation of the fat
Rinsing the fat
Vascularity and mobility of recipient site
Diameter and type of injecting cannula or needle
Freezing fat for later use

Use of lidocaine

Some studies indicate that lidocaine has a negative effect on fat cell viability. This has been shown both with lidocaine 1.0% and diluted lidocaine 0.1%.[30,31] The effect could be removed by rinsing with saline. Despite these findings, lidocaine is widely used for donor site anesthesia. Differing dilutions of tumescent anesthesia have been recommended with or without epinephrine (adrenaline). Amar recommends infiltrating Klein's solution much like a ring block around the core of fat to be harvested in order to minimize contact with lidocaine. A few authors recommend the use of Ringer's lactate rather than normal saline, reasoning that glucose-containing solution may enhance fat cell viability.[11]

Harvesting technique

Utilizing an enzymatic assay of fat cell damage, Lalikos et al. showed that harvesting by suction versus direct excision of fat did not increase apparent damage to the fat cell.[32] Other studies have also indicated that fat cells harvested by syringe, machine aspiration, or direct excision all appear to have similar viability. Suction aspiration at low level negative pressure did not appear to rupture cells in two studies, although partial breakage was seen at negative pressures of 700 mmHg and higher.

Syringe aspiration with low negative pressures is most often recommended (Fig. 33.2). Those advocating the gentlest handling suggest 10-ml syringes to minimize vacuum pressures with the plunger held back no more than 2–3 ml.[11,12,15] Other experienced surgeons report harvesting with larger 20–60-ml syringes without harming the fat cells, as documented with cell culture for up to 2 months.[33] Although various cannulae and needles have been recommended, Shiffman compared harvesting and reinjection with 2.5–3.0-mm cannulae or an 18-gauge needle. None of these caused disruption of fat

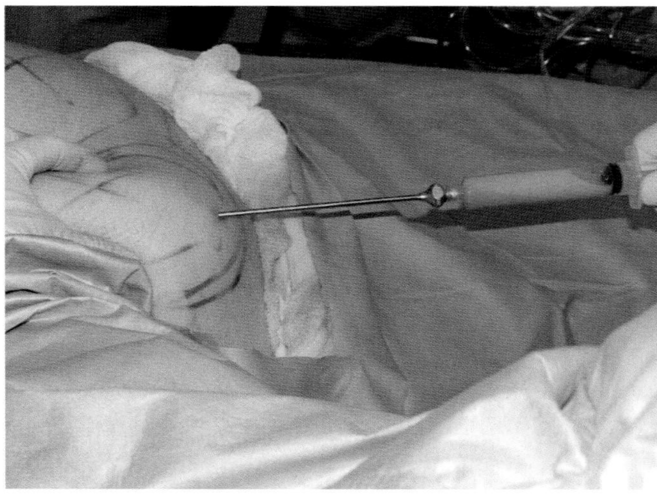

Figure 33.2 Gentle harvesting with a 10 ml syringe held back with 1–2 ml pressure.

cells histologically.[34]

Processing the fat

Once the fat is harvested, the next issue is whether or not it requires further processing before injection. All would agree on the first step, which is to stand the syringes upright for a period of 15–60 minutes to allow separation into supranatant and infranatant fractions (Fig. 33.3). The infranatant fluid is then drained off the bottom and the oil fraction on top is often decanted off. In Griffen's survey of experienced cosmetic surgeons, 62% wash the fat with saline or Ringer's lactate to remove lidocaine or blood.[35] Lidocaine has been shown to effect fat cell growth in culture and blood is thought to stimulate phagocytosis of fat cells.[36] In Sommer's review, all authors agreed that blood in transplanted fat accelerates degradation of transplanted fat.[18]

Rather than rinse, many surgeons prefer to centrifuge the fat. Centrifugation has been shown to separate fat cells from blood products, proteases, free lipids, and lipases which may degrade freshly grafted adipocytes.[37] Various speeds and time intervals for centrifugation have been recommended. Histologically, fat cells centrifuged for 10–60 seconds at 3600 r.p.m. show no evidence of cell damage although cells centrifuged for 15 minutes have been shown to have distorted morphology.[34,38] Whether or not centrifugation removes lidocaine has not been demonstrated. Centrifugation does concentrate fat cells resulting in a larger number of cells per ml of volume transferred (Fig. 33.4). When 10 ml of fat is centrifuged at 3600 r.p.m. for 3 minutes, there is a volume loss of approximately 30–40% (Fig. 33.5). In one of the few controlled studies, a double-blind comparison of fat transfer to the dorsum of the hands with centrifuged versus non-centrifuged fat, improved longevity and aesthetic results were observed with the centrifuged fat at the 3-month and 5-month follow-up visits in 100% of patients (Fig. 33.6).[39] The author now routinely utilizes centrifuged fat in essentially all cases. Fulton uses centrifuged fat for facial correction, but prefers non-centrifuged fat for larger volume transfers into breasts, biceps, or buttocks—areas in which lumpiness has been noted with centrifuged fat.[11] One must use sterilized canisters or sleeves within the centrifuge, as *Pseudomonas* and other pathogens have been cultured from the centrifuge.[40]

Injection techniques

The most common placement for transplanted fat is within the subcutaneous fat.[16,41,42] The suggested degree of overcorrection has decreased through the years from 50% to 30% and now to minimal or no overcorrection.[4,11,41,42] Smaller volumes of fat are thought to improve graft survival as previously mentioned. Small volumes also reduce downtime for patients because postoperative edema, as a general rule, is directly proportional to the amount transferred.[43,44] Retrograde injection with gentle pressure is performed to minimize injecting a large bolus of fat and to reduce the rare risk of intravascular injection. The cannula is inserted and advanced to the most distal site. Fat is then injected as the cannula is withdrawn and small parcels of fat are placed. The recommended syringe size for transfer varies from

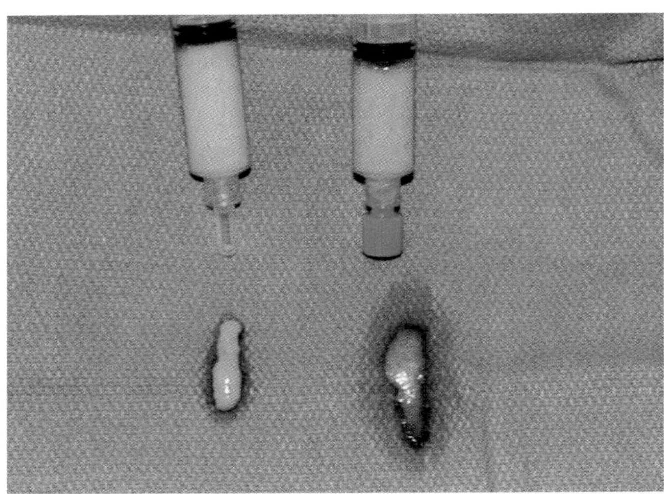

Figure 33.4 Centrifuged fat on left appears more concentrated and cohesive on injection than non-centrifuged fat.

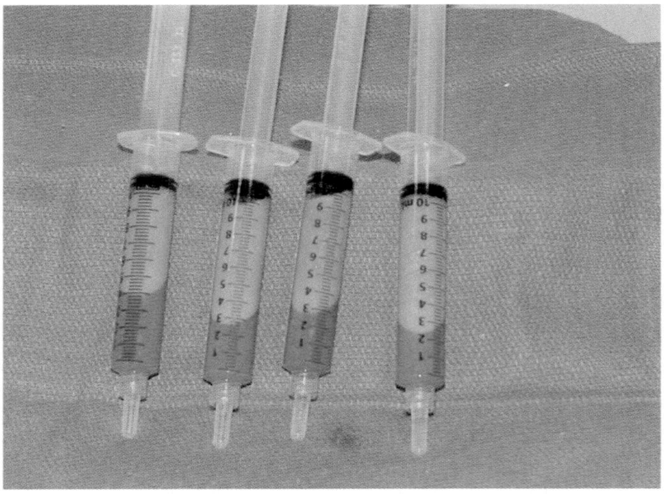

Figure 33.3 Syringes held upright for 10 minutes separate into supranatant and infranatant fractions.

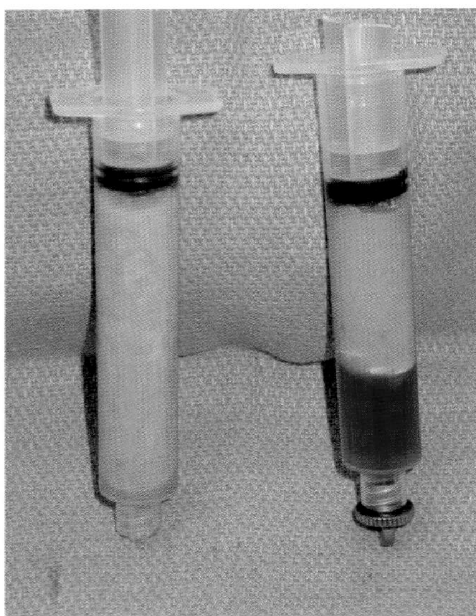

Figure 33.5 Before and after centrifugation at 3600 r.p.m. for 3 minutes. Note 30% volume loss.

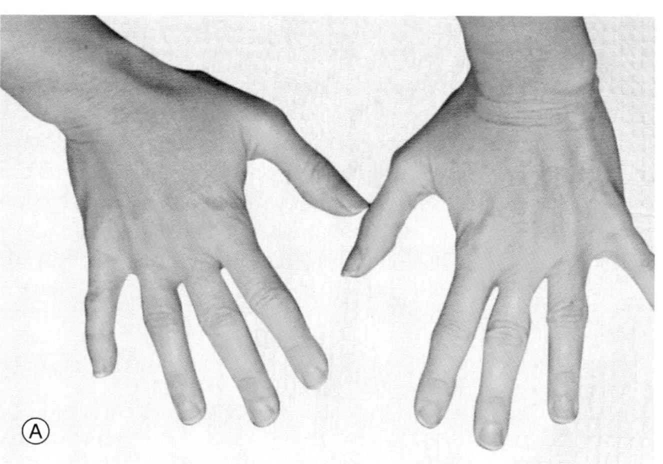

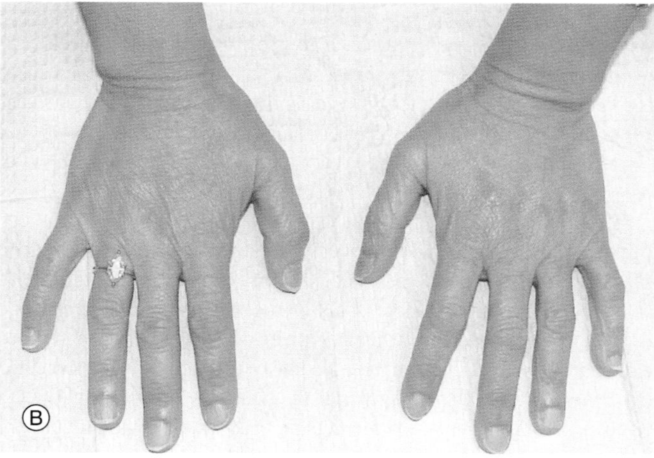

Figure 33.6 (A) Before and (B) 12 months after long-term survival of the fat in the dorsum of the hands. Note improved result on patient's left with centrifuged versus non-centrifuged fat.

10 ml[34,44] to 3 ml[11,41] to 1 ml.[15,37,45] The author prefers the 1-ml syringe as less pressure is required to empty it and the size of the fat particles is smaller (Fig. 33.7). When transferring to smaller syringes, a female-to-female adapter is available and allows transfer without exposure to air. Prolonged air exposure has been demonstrated to negatively impact fat cell viability.[46] A 10-ml syringe rack is useful for placing and securing the upright syringes (Fig. 33.8).

Both blunt-tipped cannulae and 14–25-gauge needles have been advocated for transfer.[47] Some studies have suggested the minimum diameter size of the injection instrument be no smaller than 18-gauge to prevent damage to the fat cell.[48,49] In Shiffman's study, injection with smaller diameter 20-gauge and 22-gauge needles caused damage to adipocytes as evidenced by histologic changes in cellular and nuclear morphology.[34] Blunt-tipped cannula reduce the risk of bleeding and the rare risk of intravascular injection. However, it is argued they pass through tissue with more friction and trauma, which may cause increased bleeding and inflammation in the recipient site.

Indications for fat augmentation

The most common indications for fat augmentation of the face include the nasolabial fold, the marionette fold, and the lips. Other indications for fat transfer of the face include augmentation of the chin, cheeks, malar area, and chin. Body areas are sometimes augmented with fat such as the buttocks, biceps, calf, and breast. Fat augmentation of the breast is a controversial area given that calcifications may develop postoperatively.[50–52]

Although these calcifications have been shown to differ radiographically from those caused by breast cancer, the areas could require biopsy, causing undo morbidity for the patient.[51] Rejuvenation of the dorsum of the hands is another indication for fat augmentation. Generally, 10 ml or less are placed in each hand, although Coleman recommends 20–30 ml per hand.[53] Defects from disease or trauma are also commonly treated with fat augmentation. Acne scars, linear morphea, lupus profundus or erythematosus, and cellulite are other indications for fat augmentation.

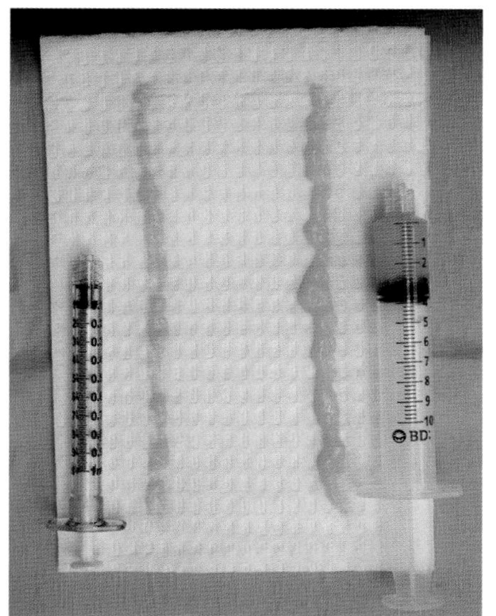

Figure 33.7 Fat particles are smaller when injected through a 1-ml syringe versus a 10-ml syringe with similar injection pressures.

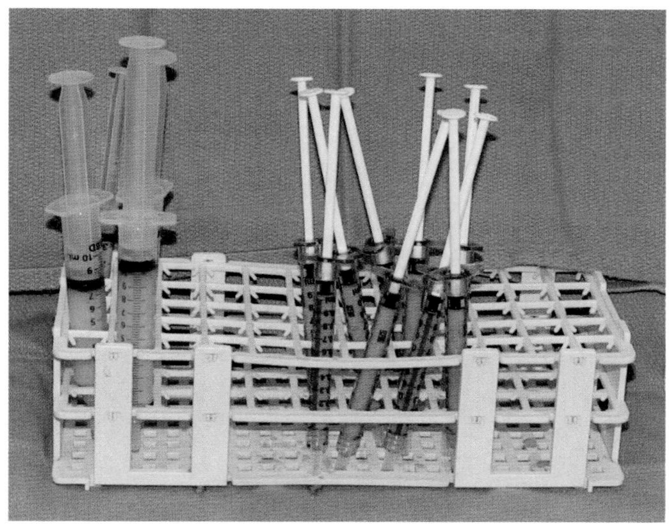

Figure 33.8 Syringe rack for securing upright 1-ml and 10-ml syringes.

In the past decade, cosmetic surgeons have also begun to restore soft tissue volume, not simply under the rhytide or defect, but for full-face volume correction. Newer approaches for restructuring the face include Lipostructure™,[15] panfacial rebalancing,[35] and FAMI (fat autograft muscle injection).[21]

Lipostructure™

Sidney Coleman was one of the first to champion the placement of small 'parcels' of fat in order to facilitate neovascularization. He was also one of the first to advocate full-face three-dimensional enhancement of youthful contours, which he termed Lipostructure™. His method involves an intricate layering of minute quantities of fat within multiple tissue planes, not only in the subcutaneous plane but also adjacent to bone, fascia and muscle. Each droplet of fat is placed 'within 1.5 mm of living vascularized tissue'. Typically, 30 or 40 passes are required to empty a 1-ml syringe with a blunt-tipped 17-gauge or 18-gauge cannula. Quantities injected for a full face often exceed 100 ml. Because the fat is viewed as a living graft, it is handled gently with atraumatic harvesting, no rinsing, and brief centrifugation for 30 seconds.

Coleman reports long-term results with his method in the order of years. 'Before and after' photographs suggest that Lipostructure™ [15] may replace the need for rhytidectomy. The single most significant drawback to this method is the marked edema seen for weeks or months postoperatively. The benefit of dramatic panfacial correction must be weighed against the extended recovery period for the patient.

Facial rebalancing

In order to circumvent prolonged edema for the patient, Donofrio modified Coleman's procedure with a method of 'fat rebalancing,' also involving the entire face but with repeated smaller procedures (6–12) over a 1–2-year period.[37] Fresh fat is utilized the first time, but in most patients frozen fat is injected on subsequent visits. The entire face is treated with smaller total quantities (approximately 20–30 ml), which reduces the downtime for patients to 1–10 days, depending on the extent of the procedure. Fat is processed atraumatically and injected with blunt-tipped cannulae with the intricate, repetitive pass, layered method recommended by Coleman. Fat is placed exclusively in the subcutaneous space. Donofrio focuses not only on replacing fat, but also addresses areas of fat hypertrophy that are found in the aging face.[22] Microliposuction of the jowls and other areas is typically performed during the fat transfer procedure for aesthetic rebalancing (Fig. 33.9).

Fat autograft muscle injection (FAMI)

Most cosmetic surgeons agree that an abundantly vascularized recipient site for transplanted fat will result in optimal survival of the fat, an opinion confirmed by several histologic studies.[12,17,35,54] French anatomist and plastic surgeon, Roger Amar, has incorporated this principle into a new technique, in which fat is injected into or immediately adjacent to the muscles of facial expression, and which he coined FAMI. The concept of FAMI was inspired by a study in 1996 by Guerrosantos, in which he demonstrated 5-year survival of fat in rat muscle.[55] Muscle thickness continued to increase for 6 months following fat grafting. The FAMI technique involves full-face volume correction following the landmarks of the patient's own anatomy, namely the origin and insertion of various muscle groups. Volumes placed range from approximately 20 ml to 70 ml utilizing a set of blunt-tipped cannulae which are curved and angled to conform to the skeletal contours of the face (Fig. 33.10). There is less apparent trauma than methods using repetitive passes: a 1 ml syringe is emptied in one to three passes. The fat is placed along vectors which parallel blood supply, minimizing trauma to the vessels. Patients are able to return to work in 3–7 days depending on volumes placed. Amar has reported longevity of 3–5 years with this method.[56]

FAMI can be performed as a full-face volume correction or for localized volume loss such as the lips, tear-trough deformity, chin, or perioral regions. It is ideal after

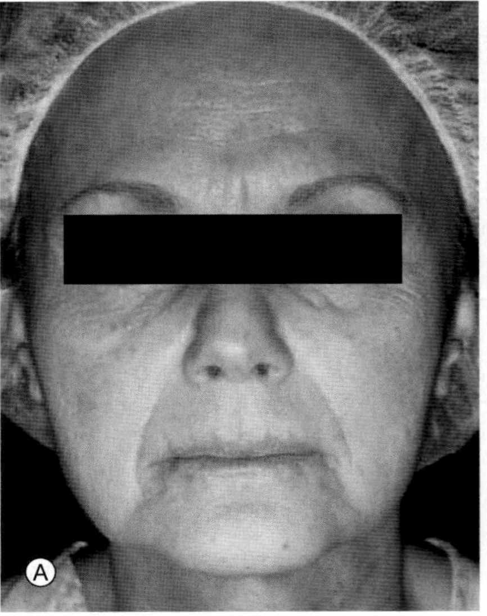

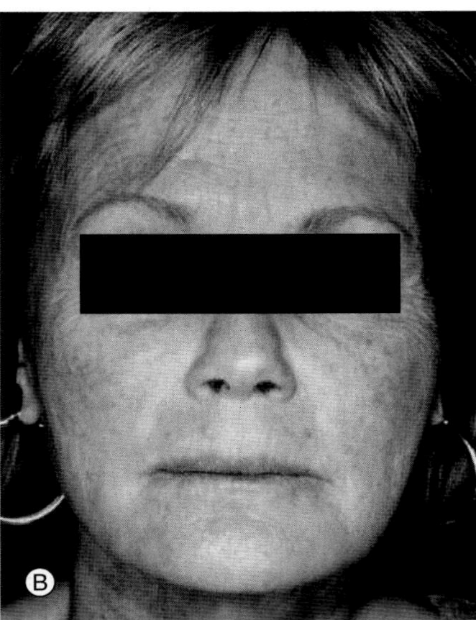

Figure 33.9 (A) Before and (B) after facial rebalancing. Courtesy of L Donofrio.

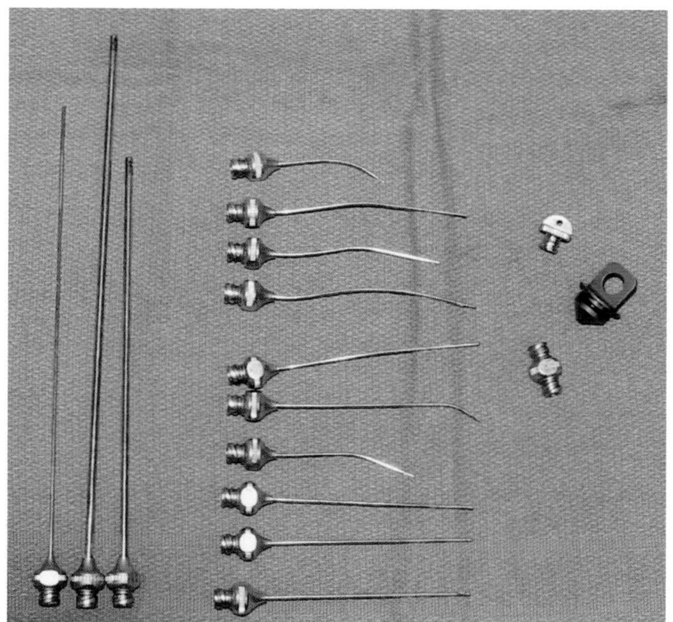

Figure 33.10 FAMI injection cannulae are curved and angled to conform to musculoskeletal contours.

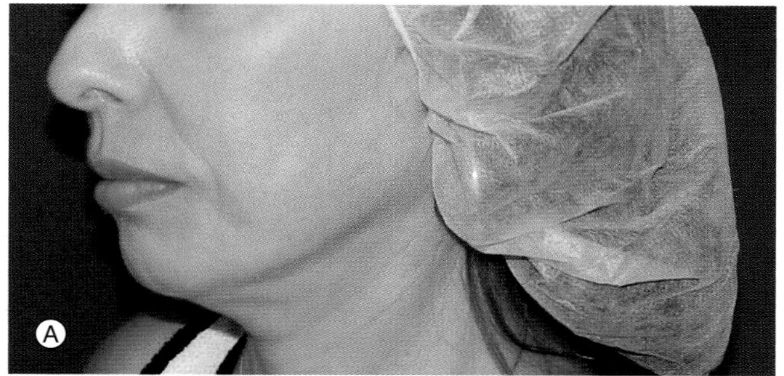

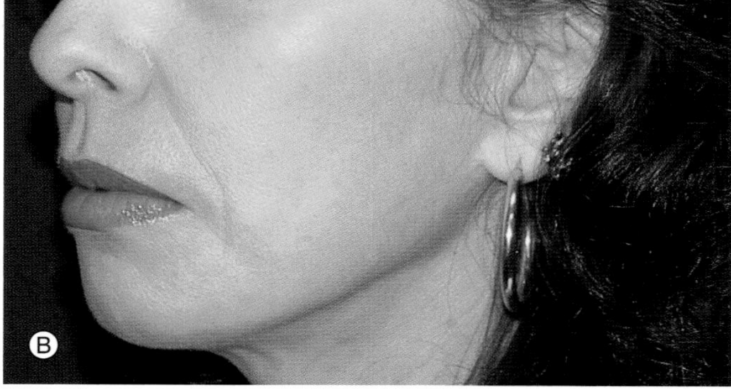

Figure 33.11 (A) Before and (B) after lower face FAMI with 9.7 ml injected and concomitant liposuction of the neck. Note improved chin height and mandibular border.

rhytidectomy in patients with thin, overly taut skin. It is also indicated in conjunction with liposuction of the neck for replacing volume of the chin, mandibular border, prejowl notching, and lower perioral regions[57] (Fig. 33.11). Patients are asked to bring a photograph of themselves taken 10–20 years before the consultation in order to appreciate the volumes that have been lost. In restoring the muscle sling of the face, the overlying skin drapes in the smooth, uninterrupted contours of youth.

Table 33.2 Facial muscles commonly injected in FAMI

Muscle	Plane
Frontalis	Superficial
Procerus	Superficial
Corrugator	Deep
Orbicularis oculi	Superficial
Zygomaticus minor	Superficial
Levator labii superioris alaeque nasi	Mid
Levator labii superioris	Mid
Levator anguli oris	Deep
Zygomaticus major	Mid
Depressor labii inferioris	Mid
Depressor anguli oris	Mid
Mentalis	Deep
Buccinator	Deep
Risorius	Mid
Platysma	Mid
Orbicularis oris	Mid

Amar's harvesting and processing techniques include utilizing the medial knee as his preferred donor site, and processing of the fat with centrifugation at 3600 r.p.m. for 3 minutes. Injection into the muscles is based on anatomic knowledge of the origin, insertion, and plane of each muscle to be injected as well as familiarity with the bony landmarks of the skull[58–60] (Table 33.2; Fig. 33.12). Specific injection cannulae have been developed for various muscle groups, allowing for smooth passage of the cannula. The cannula is directed to the origin or insertion of the muscle and the fat is injected in a retrograde fashion with low injection pressure (Figs 33.13, 33.14). There are three ways the surgeon determines that he is injecting in the muscle. For certain muscles, the bundle can be palpated as the enveloping fascia is filled. Other muscles are very thin, not palpable, and the surgeon must rely on bony anatomic landmarks to inject as close as possible to the muscle. With some muscle groups, a loss of resistance is the clue that the cannula has penetrated the fascia and is within the muscle. Anesthesia for this procedure is achieved with nerve blocks, supplemented with oral or intravenous sedation depending on individual patient requirements.

The postoperative course of FAMI is unremarkable. There is essentially no pain and usually little bruising which may not appear until the second or third day. Edema is the most significant symptom and patients need to be warned in advance or they will be concerned that too much fat has been placed (Fig. 33.15). The recovery period will depend on the quantities placed. With a full-face correction of 70 ml, the patient may require 7–10 days of downtime. In a preliminary report, the author utilized 20–30 ml on average for partial face corrections with good results[61] (Fig. 33.16).This lower total volume replacement reduces the downtime to 3–5 days. Complications of this technique have not been reported except for the usual postoperative sequelae of bruising, edema, and temporary palpable lumpiness, which is not generally visible. Potential complications are discussed below.

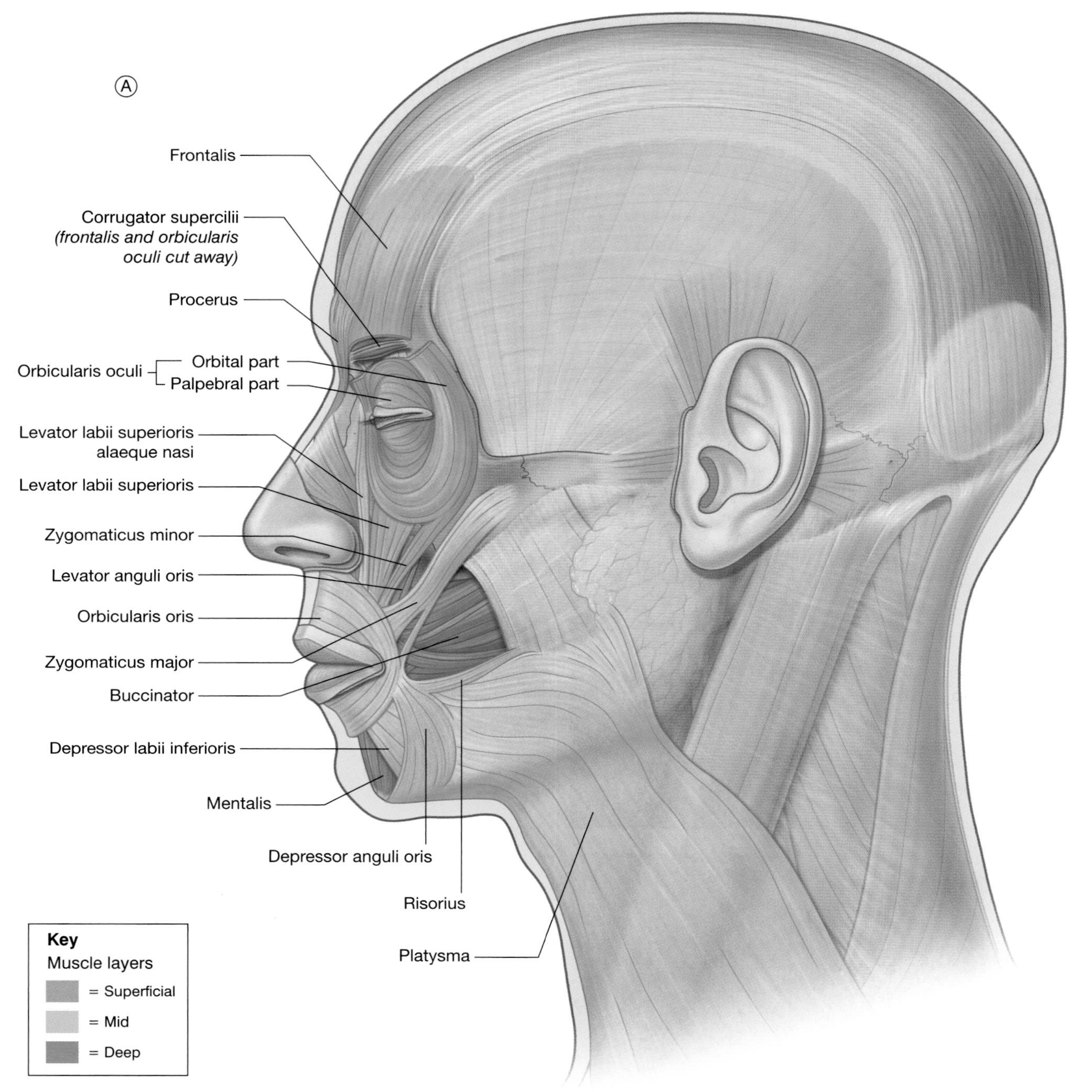

Figure 33.12 Muscles of facial expression. (A) Side view.

■ OPTIMIZING OUTCOMES

The optimal results will be determined by proper placement and by survival of the fat cells.

Longevity

The literature contains few objective studies regarding the longevity of transplanted fat. Horl demonstrated a 49% volume loss at 3 months, 55% loss at 6 months, and negligible loss between 9 and 12 months utilizing magnetic resonance imaging of fat transplants.[62] Ultrasound imaging has been utilized to demonstrate long-term correction up to 1 year in patients with defects due to disease processes.[63,64] Sadick et al. used a marker of fatty acid composition that was specific to the donor site.[65] He was able to demonstrate a 1-year persistence of that marker in the recipient site in one of six patients. In the other five, the donor site marker was undetectable. He speculated that perhaps recipient site factors caused conversion of the donor site marker to the fatty acid composition of the recipient site.

Facial muscles commonly injected in FAMI continued

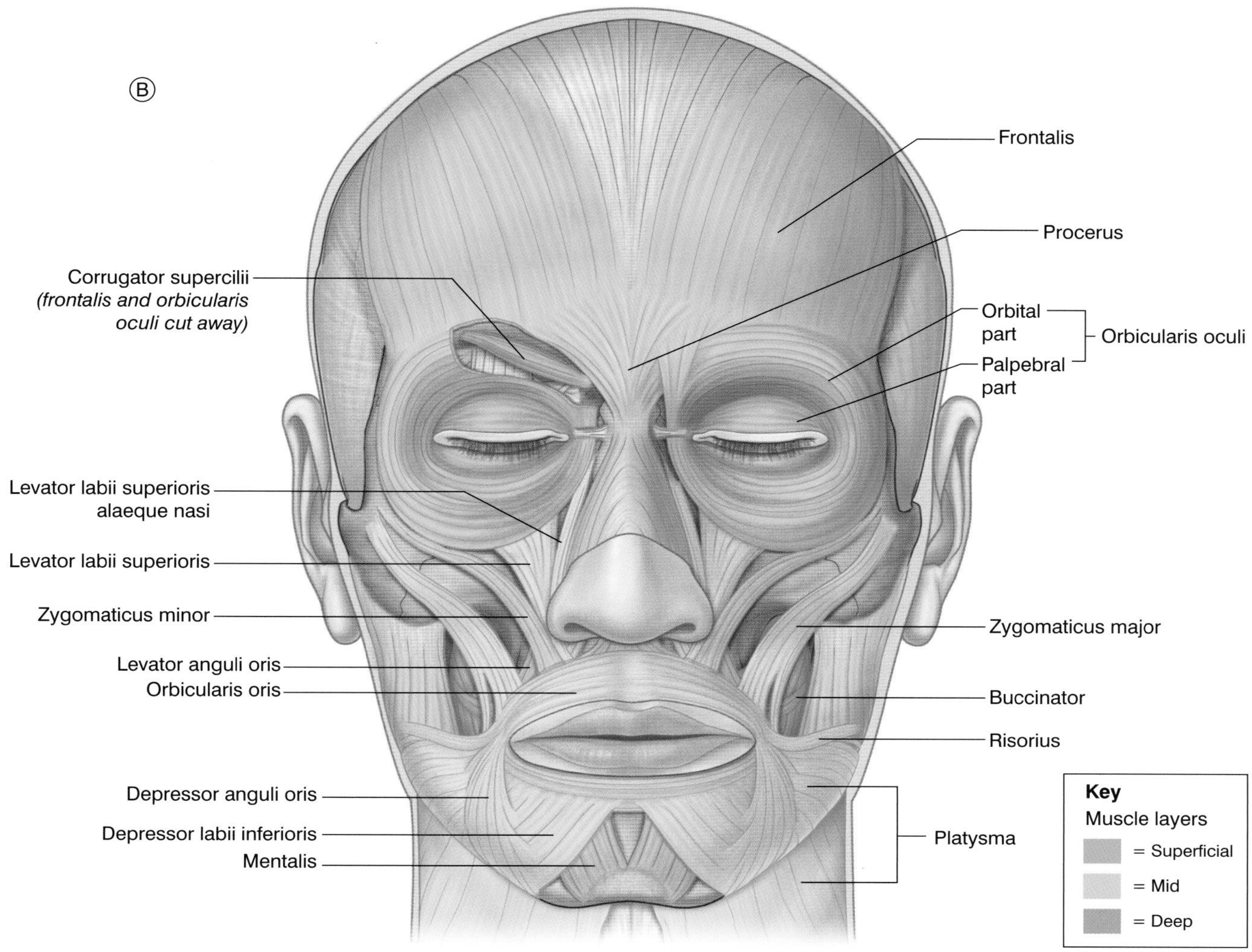

(B)

Frontalis
Procerus
Corrugator supercilii (frontalis and orbicularis oculi cut away)
Orbital part
Palpebral part
Orbicularis oculi
Levator labii superioris alaeque nasi
Levator labii superioris
Zygomaticus minor
Zygomaticus major
Levator anguli oris
Orbicularis oris
Buccinator
Risorius
Depressor anguli oris
Depressor labii inferioris
Mentalis
Platysma

Key
Muscle layers
= Superficial
= Mid
= Deep

Figure 33.12, continued Muscles of facial expression. (B) Front view.

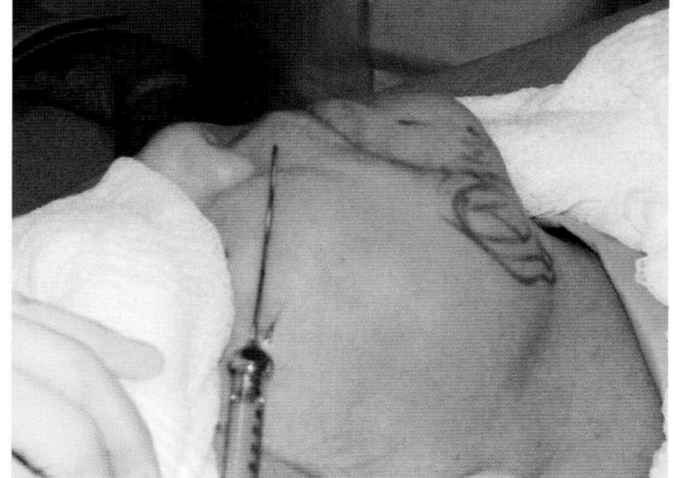

Figure 33.13 Injection of the zygomaticus minor with cannula #4.

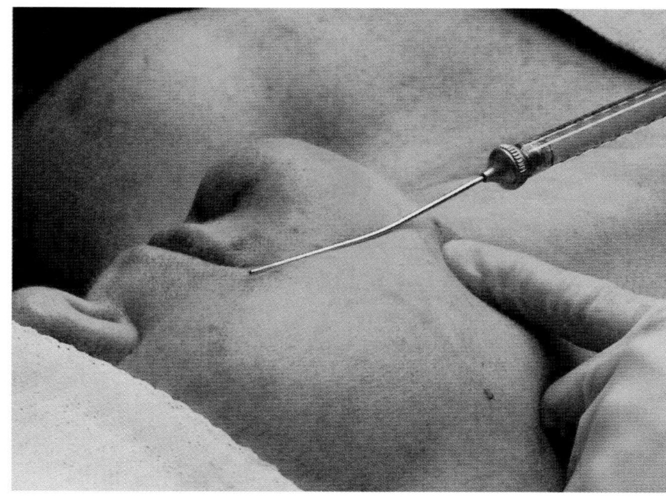

Figure 33.14 Injection of the depressor anguli oris with cannula #5.

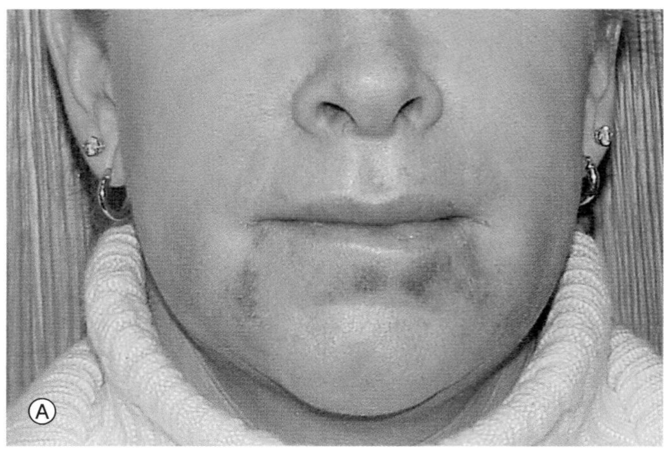

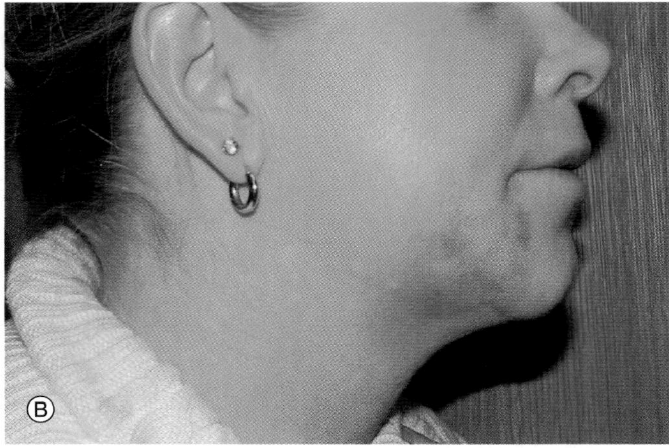

Figure 33.15 Postoperative edema on day 3 after FAMI of lower face with 30.3 ml injected.

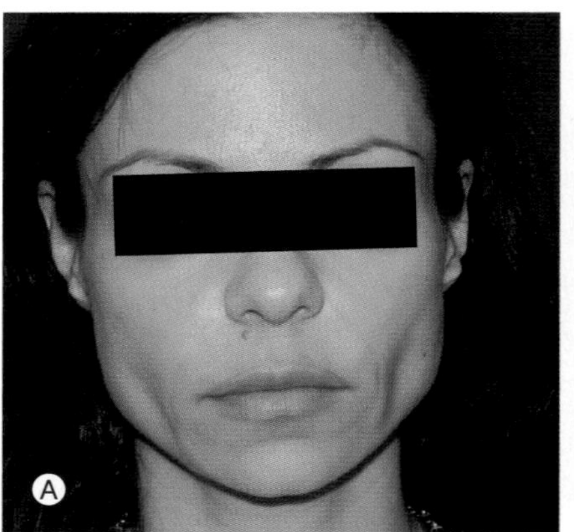

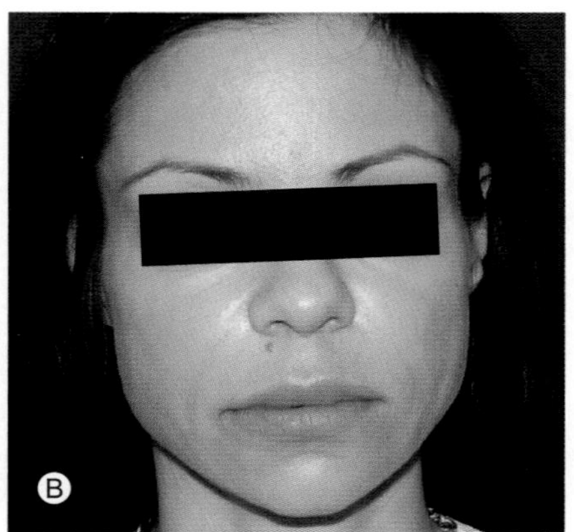

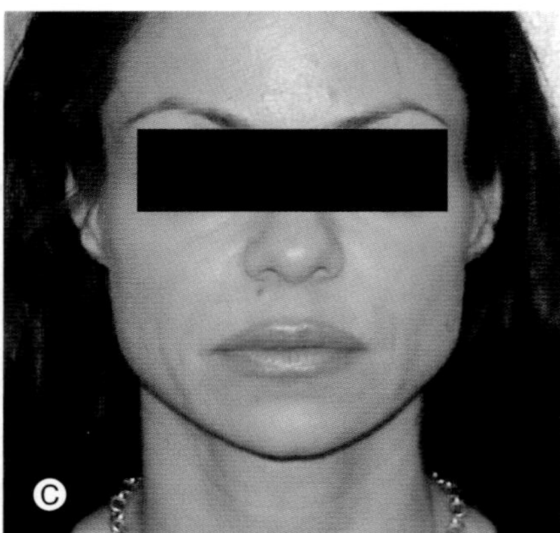

Figure 33.16 (A) Before, (B) 5 weeks after, and (C) 8 months after partial face FAMI with 24.7 ml.

Animal studies have shown long-term survival of autologous fat. Nguyen found persistence of transplanted fat in rats at 9 months when fat was injected into the muscle.[66] Fat injected into the subcutaneous plane was completely absorbed. Guerrosantos reported 5-year survival of fat when injected into rat muscle.[55]

Studies based on photographic results and physician assessment have reported long-term results varying from 'disappointing' to many years.[7,11,41,42,44,67–70] Some have noted the longest survival when the recipient site is relatively immobile, such as the fixed scars of linear morphea,[13] the forehead,[16] the infraorbital area,[11] or the backs of the hands[71,72] (see Fig. 33.6). The most mobile area of the face—the lips—has been least responsive to long-term correction in other reports.[11,49] Eremia found that longevity was related to recipient site.[49] Good to excellent results were seen at 5–8 months for the nasolabial and melolabial folds and poor results were observed in the lip and glabella. Perez notes more permanent results in younger patients.[69] Based on the limited objective data, animal studies, and empirical results from experienced cosmetic surgeons, one can conclude that long-term fat survival is achievable. Further studies are ongoing to define the factors resulting in optimal survival.

Touch-up procedures

Many recommend touch-up procedures for optimal results. There are several reasons that touch-up procedures are performed. With the use of small volumes for fat transfer versus overcorrection, one treatment session may not be adequate to achieve optimal volume restoration. In addition, the patient may not have enough down time to undergo placement of more than 30 ml, yet have a deficit of 100 ml or more. There is also variable longevity of transplanted fat from months to years due to incompletely understood factors. Ongoing aging and/or weight loss of patients further contribute to the need to replace additional fat after the initial session (Fig. 33.17). Lastly, patients are often reluctant to have too much volume placed, particularly in the lips, but when they see the initial results, realize they would like an even fuller look.

Use of frozen fat

Frozen fat is commonly utilized in clinical practice for augmentations and touch-up procedures with apparently pleasing results.[37,44,70] However, it is argued that freezing fat affects its viability. It is certainly efficacious to use frozen fat for touch-up procedures rather than reharvest in a sterile

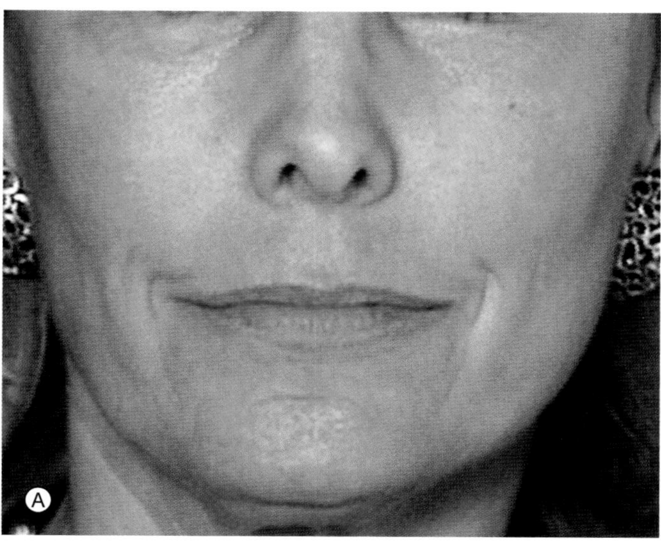

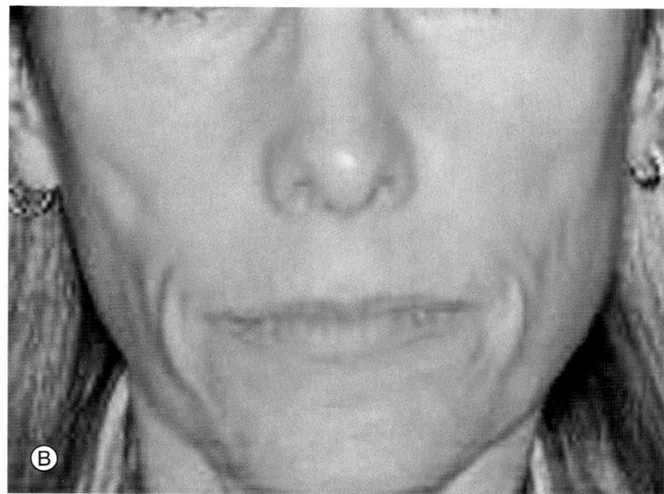

Figure 33.17 Dramatic facial volume changes due to weight loss of only 10–15 pounds (4.54–6.81 kg) such as this will significantly affect longevity of fat augmentation.

fashion. Few studies have addressed this question. Histologic studies have shown frozen and thawed adipocytes that are identical to those of normal tissue.[73] Takasu reported long-term retention of fat that had been frozen for up to 7 years.[73] Shoshani et al. compared frozen fat versus fresh fat injected into nude mice.[74] Assessments by clinical observation, weight and volume measurement, and histologic parameters demonstrated successful take at 15 weeks in both groups with no statistically significant difference in volume at 15 weeks. In a side-by-side comparison study of fresh versus frozen fat injected to the dorsum of the hands, it was found that frozen fat lasted as long or longer at 3-month and 5-month intervals.[75] Indeed, aesthetically, the hand with the frozen fat was preferred at the 3-month and 5-month follow-up (Fig. 33.18). The frozen fat was preferred initially as well in a majority of patients because there was less postoperative edema of the hand. However, other studies reject the use of frozen fat. Lawrence found no viable adipocytes in frozen aspirates measured by cell culture.[76] Research regarding the viability of frozen fat is ongoing and clearly needed.

Figure 33.18 Fresh fat (patient's left) versus frozen fat (patient's right) in dorsum of hands. Equal or better results seen with frozen fat at 5 months.

Author's protocol

With so many techniques and opinions, it may be confusing for the novice in fat augmentation to know how to begin. Data has been presented in this chapter to help the new surgeon weigh the merits of the various methods. The author has experience in many different techniques and has found the FAMI technique a logical, learnable procedure with predictable results.

A typical protocol in the author's practice is to have one larger session of FAMI with 30–40 ml of fresh fat expecting down time of 5–7 days. This is followed by one to three touch-up sessions, at intervals of 4–6 months, of less than 10 ml of frozen fat. These smaller sessions heal over the weekend (Table 33.3). Variations from this protocol include injection sessions monthly or every other month for 1–2 years with frozen fat for gradual sequential augmentation.[37] Others repeat the entire initial session every few years as needed with fresh fat.[15] Fournier advocates periodic injections every few years to keep pace with the aging process.[70] He also regularly uses frozen fat as needed for touch-up procedures.

Table 33.3 Author's protocol for FAMI
Sterile prep and drape
Donor site anesthesia with Klein's tumescent formula
Nerve blocks of the face
Gentle harvesting with 10-ml syringes
Syringes held upright and infranatant fluid discarded
Full 10-ml syringe centrifuged at 3600 r.p.m. for 3 minutes
Oil and infranatant fractions discarded
Transfer to 1-ml syringes
Inject cephalad to caudad each muscle group, bilaterally
Post operative checks at 24 hours and 1 week
Evaluate for touch-up session at 4–6 and 8–10 months postoperatively
Touch up injections with <10 ml of frozen fat prn

■ PITFALLS AND THEIR MANAGEMENT

The complication rate is low with all fat augmentation techniques.

Avoidance of pitfalls

- Avoid overcorrection due to injection of a large bolus of fat; as the infraorbital area is most prone to overcorrection, this area is best done by the experienced surgeon using only minute quantities with low injection pressure.
- Screen patients preoperatively for infection, especially in facial areas, and treat prior to surgery. Use antibiotic prophylaxis in all patients and use sterile technique in all steps of the procedure.
- Avoid intravascular penetration by using blunt-tipped cannula, retrograde injection after withdrawal to assure one is not intravascular, and minimal injection pressure with 1-cc syringes.

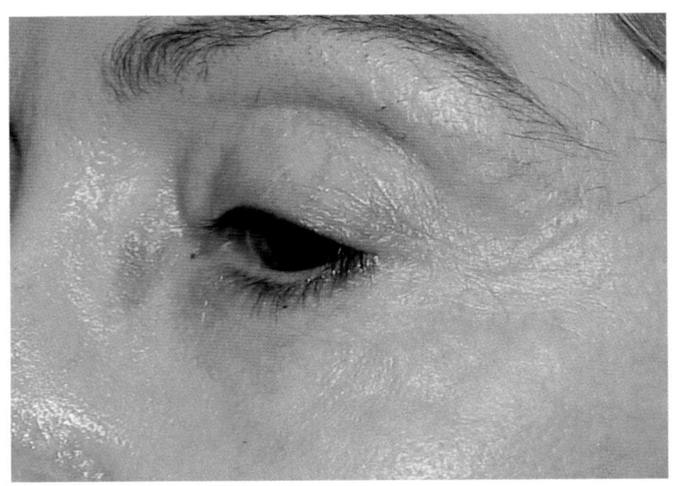

Figure 33.19 Overcorrection in infraorbital region with numerous small visible nodules.

Overcorrection is probably the most common complication, particularly in the infraorbital area. Visible, superficial nodules may develop with overcorrection of this area, or from injecting too large a bolus of fat too superficially (Fig. 33.19). Caution is advised in this area if it is to be injected at all. Experienced surgeons recommend that very minute quantities are injected in the periorbital area with each pass of a 1-ml syringe.[45,77] Overcorrection may be difficult to treat. Low-dose steroid injection, repeated massage, and excision have been suggested treatments.[45,77]

Other complications are sometimes seen after fat augmentation. Fat hypertrophy may follow weight gain after fat augmentation, and may require surgical revision.[78] The symmetry with the FAMI technique appears to mitigate this problem (Fig. 33.20). Fat necrosis may occur on occasion resulting in extrusion of fat. Infection is another potential complication. Patients need to be screened adequately for concomitant, recurrent, or chronic infections, particularly of adjacent facial areas such as sinus, dental or ocular regions.[79] These infections need to be adequately treated before undergoing the procedure. The use of prophylactic antibiotics is generally recommended in all patients. Fat augmentation should be carried out as a sterile procedure. The centrifuge has been the source of infection with *Pseudomonas*.[40] Sterile centrifuge sleeves should be utilized, as well as sterile instruments (Fig. 33.21). There have also been reports of infection with *Staphylococcus*, *Streptococcus*, and *Mycobacterium*.[40,41,45,79]

The most serious potential complication of fat augmentation is vascular occlusion caused by inadvertent intravascular injection. Blindness has been reported following fat injections of the glabellar lines.[80,81] Middle cerebral artery occlusion and ocular fat embolism have also been reported following fat injection of the face.[82,83] Occlusion or emboli are rare complications. Reports have indicated sharp instrumentation and 10-ml syringes with high injection pressures were utilized.[83] Use of blunt-tipped

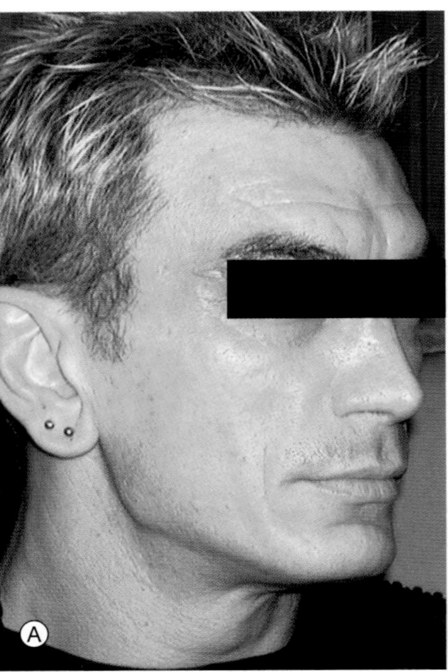

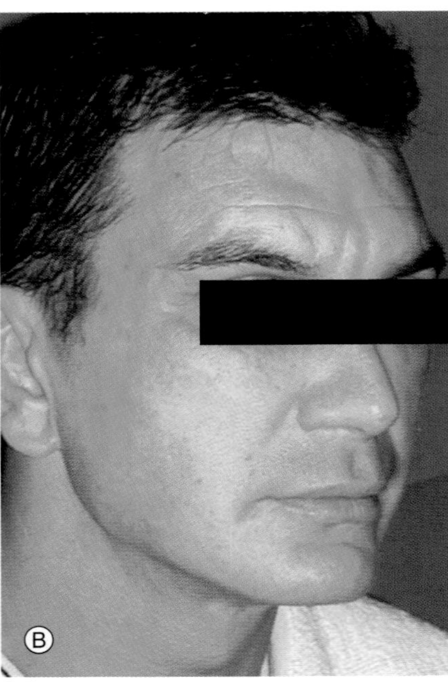

Figure 33.20 (A) Before and (B) 2 years after full-face FAMI in a 39-year-old man. The patient's face is symmetric despite a 10 lb (4.5 kg) weight gain. Courtesy of R Amar.

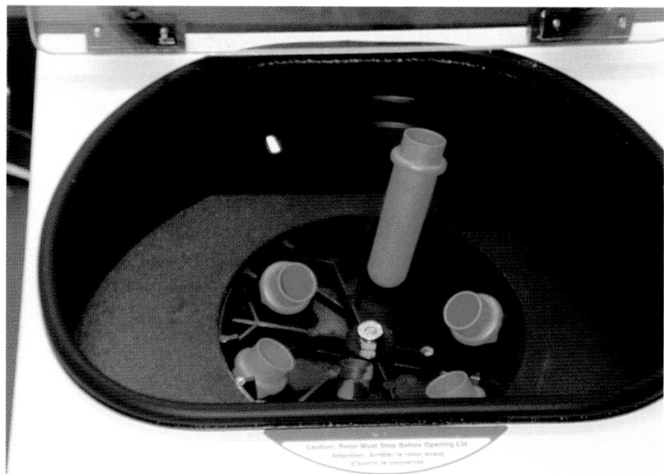

Figure 33.21 Removable centrifuge sleeves should be sterilized for each case.

cannulae will minimize the risk of vascular penetration as well as initial withdrawal of the plunger to assure one is not intravascular. Retrograde fill, 1-ml syringes, and low injection pressures further reduce the risk of intravascular injection. When evidence of vascular compromise is seen on the skin with dramatic blanching, Wexler advises placing the patient in Trendelenberg, applying nitroglycerin paste, and massaging the area until the flush of the skin returns.[84] A potential complication of intramuscular injection is dysfunction of facial muscles. Although not reported by Amar, weakness of facial muscles of mastication has been observed when fat is injected intramuscularly.[85] The masseter muscle is not injected in the FAMI procedure. In addition, the curved and angled cannula of FAMI most likely minimize injury to the muscle.

■ SUMMARY

Fat augmentation has been practiced for decades with good reason. It is safe, relatively inexpensive, and readily available. Now that cosmetic surgeons are recognizing that facial aging is not simply due to gravity but rather to atrophy of tissues, the use of fat for volume restoration is becoming even more popular. Newer techniques of Lipostructure™,[15] facial fat rebalancing, and FAMI, are targeted to achieve true full-face three-dimensional rejuvenation.

We are lacking an effective, practical means of objectively measuring outcome. Without this, we will not be able to answer basic questions of optimal harvesting site, processing technique, and most effective injection technique. Histologic and animal studies suggest there is greater potential for revascularization with small volumes of fat thereby enhancing survival. Limited data suggests centrifugation contributes to long-term results. Gentle handling and cannula size of more than 18-gauge seem to be important to survival. Scientific research is emerging to address these issues. Further research will also elucidate the role of preadipocytes or stem cells in adipose tissue.

These are exciting times to be performing fat augmentation. It is a dynamic, expanding field offering the cosmetic surgeon a creative outlet and the patient gratifying results.

■ REFERENCES

1. Neuber F. Fat transplantation. Chir Kongr Verhandl Dsch Gesellch Chir 1893; 20:66.
2. Lexer E. Correccion de los pechos dedulos (Mastoptose) por medio de la implantacion de grasa. San Sebastian Guipuzcoa Media 1921; 63:13. (Translated in Hinderer UT, del Rio JL. Erich Lexer's mammoplasty. Aesthetic Plast Surg 1992; 16:101–107.
3. Bruning P. Cited by Newman J, Ftaiha Z. The biographical history of fat transplant surgery. Am J Cosmet Surg 1987; 4:85.
4. Peer LA. Loss of weight and volume in human fat grafts. Plast Reconstr Surg 1950; 5:217–230.
5. Illouz YG. The fat cell 'graft,' a new technique to fill depressions. Plast Reconstr Surg 1986; 78:122–123.
6. Fournier PF. Facial recontouring with fat grafting. Dermatol Clin 1990; 8:523–537.
7. Fredricks S: Transplantation of purified autologous fat: A three year follow-up is disappointing. Plast Reconstr Surg 1991; 87:228 (discussion).
8. Leever N. Cosmetic surgery—a comparison of its growth in the 1990s. Available at www.cosmeticsurgery.org (compiled for the American Academy of Cosmetic Surgery).
9. Klein JA. Tumescent technique for regional anesthesia permits lidocaine doses of 35 mg/kg for liposuction. J Dermatol Surg Oncol 1990; 16:248–263.
10. Cosmetic Dermatology STATS. Statistics courtesy of American Society for Aesthetic Plastic Surgery. Dermatol Times, April 2003; S24–S25.
11. Fulton JE, Suarez M, Silverton K, Barnes T. Small volume fat transfer. Dermatol Surg 1998; 24:857–865.
12. Niechajev I, Sevuk O. Long-term results of fat transplantation: Clinical and histological studies. Plast Reconstr Surg 1994; 94:496–506.
13. Pinski K, Roenigk H. Autologous fat transfer. Long-term follow-up. J Dermatol Surg Oncol 1992; 18:179–184.
14. Chajchir A, Benzaquen I. Fat-grafting injection for soft-tissue augmentation. Plast Reconstr Surg 1989; 85:921–934.
15. Coleman SR. Facial recontouring with Lipostructure. Clin Plast Surg 1997; 24:347–367.
16. Pinski KS. Fat transplantation and autologous collagen: A decade of experience. Am J Cosmet Surg 1999; 16:217–224.
17. Carpaneda CA, Ribeiro MT. Study of the histological alterations and viability of the adipose graft in humans. Aesth Plast Surg 1993; 17:43–47.
18. Sommer B, Sattler G. Current concepts of fat graft survival: Histology of aspirated adipose tissue and review of the literature. Dermatol Surg 2000; 26:1159–1166.
19. Berman M. The aging face: A different perspective on pathology and treatment. Am J Cosmet Surg 1998; 15:167–172.
20. Guerrerosantos J. Simultaneous rhytidoplasty and lipoinjection: A comprehensive aesthetic surgical strategy. Plast Reconstr Surg 1998; 102:191–198.
21. Amar RE. Microinfiltration adipocytaire (MIA) auniveau de la face, ou restructuration tissulaire par greffe de tissue adipeux. Ann Chirp Last Aesthet 1999; 44:593–608.
22. Donofrio LM. Fat distribution: A morphologic study of the aging face. Dermatol Surg 2000; 26:1107–1112.
23. Pessa J, Desvigne L, Lambros V, Nimerick J, Sugunan B, Zadoo V. Changes in ocular globe-to-orbital rim position with age: Implications for aesthetic blepharoplasty of the lower eyelids. Aesth Plast Surg 1999; 23:337–342.
24. Pessa J. An algorithm of facial aging. Verification of Lambros's theory by three-dimensional stereolithography, with reference to the pathogenesis of mid facial aging, scleral show, and the lateral suborbital trough deformity. Plast Reconstr Surg 2000; 106:479–488.
25. Haffner C, Pessa J, Zadoo V, Garza J. A technique for three-dimensional cephalometric analysis as an aid in evaluating changes in the craniofacial skeleton. Angle Orthod. 1999; 69:345–348.
26. Zadoo V, Pessa J. Biological arches and changes to the curvilinear form of the aging maxilla. Plast Reconstr Surg 2000; 106:460–468.
27. Pessa J, Chen Y. Curve analysis of the aging orbital aperture. Plast Reconstr Surg 2002; 109:751–755.
28. Hudson DA, Lambert EV, Block CE. Site selection for auto-transplantation. Some observations. Aesth Plast Surg 1990; 14:195.
29. Ullman Y, Hyams M, Ramon Y, et al. Enhancing the survival of aspirated human fat injected into nude mice. Plast Reconstr Surg 1998; 101:1940–1944.

30. Alexander RW, Maring TS, Aghabo T. Autologous fat grafting: A study of residual intracellular adipocyte lidocaine concentrations after serial rinsing with normal saline. Am J Cosmet Surg 1999; 16:123–126.
31. Moore J, Kolaczynski JW, Morales LM, et al. Viability of fat obtained by syringe suction lipectomy: Effects of local anesthesia with lidocaine. Aesth Plast Surg 1995; 19:335–339.
32. Lalikos J, Ya-Qi L, Roth T, Doyle J, Matory W, Lawrence W. Biochemical assessment of cellular damage after adipocyte harvest. J Surg Res 1997; 70:95–100.
33. Jones JK, Lyles ME. The viability of human adipocytes after closed-syringe liposuction harvest. Am J Cosmet Surg 1997; 14:275–279.
34. Shiffman MA, Mirrafati S. Fat transfer techniques: The effect of harvest and transfer methods on adipocyte viability and review of the literature. Dermatol Surg 2001; 27:819–826.
35. Griffin EI. Results of fat transfer survey: Criteria and interpretation. American Academy of Dermatology Annual Meeting, March 21, 1999, New Orleans, LA.
36. Johnson JG. Body contouring by microinjection of autogenous fat. Am J Cosm Surg 1987; 16:248–262.
37. Donofrio LM. Structural autologous lipoaugmentation: A pan-facial technique. Dermatol Surg 2000; 26:1129–1134.
38. Chajchir A, Benzaquen I, Moretti E. Comparative experimental study of autologous adipose tissue processed by different techniques. Aesthetic Plast Surg 1993; 17:113–115.
39. Butterwick KJ. Lipoaugmentation for the aging hands: A comparison of the longevity and aesthetic results of centrifuged vs non-centrifuged fat. Dermatol Surg 2002; 28:987–991.
40. Finder K. Personal communication. January 2001.
41. Hernandez-Perez E, Lozano-Guarin JC. Fat grafting: Techniques and uses in different anatomic areas. Am J Cosmet Surg 1999; 16:197–204.
42. Perez MI. Autologous fat transplantation: Past and current practice. Cosmet Dermatol 1999; June:7–13.
43. Coleman WP III. Fat transplantation. Dermatol Clin 1999; 17:891–898.
44. Markey AC, Glogau RG. Autologous fat grafting: Comparison of techniques. Dermatol Surg 2000; 26:1135–1144.
45. Berman M. Rejuvenation of the upper eyelid complex with autologous fat transplantation. Dermatol Surg 2000; 26:1113–1116.
46. Agris J. Autologous fat transplantation: A 3-year study. Am. J. Cosmet Surg 1987; 4:95–102.
47. Sadick N. Fat viability studies. In: Narins R, ed. Safe liposuction and fat transfer, 10th edn. New York: Marcel Dekker; 2003;527–544.
48. Shiffman MA. Effect of various methods of fat harvesting and reinjection. Am J Cosmet Surg 2000; 17:91–97.
49. Eremia S, Newman N. Long-term follow-up after autologous fat grafting: Analysis of results from 116 patients followed at least 12 months after receiving the last of a minimum of two treatments. Dermatol Surg 2000; 26:1148–1158.
50. Fulton J. Stabilization of fat transfer to the breast with autologous platelet gel. Int J Cosmet Surg 1999; 7:60–65.
51. Bircoll M. Autologous fat transplantation: An evaluation of microcalcification and fat cell survivability following (AFT) cosmetic breast augmentation. Amer J Cos Surg 1988; 5:283–288.
52. Shiffman MA. History of breast augmentation with fat. In: Autologous fat transplantation. New York: Marcel Dekker 2001;199–206.
53. Coleman SR. Hand rejuvenation with structural fat grafting. Plast Reconstr Surg 2002; 110:1731–1744.
54. Baran CN, Celebiogiu S, Sensoz O, Ulusoy G, Civelek B, Ortak T. The behavior of fat grafts in recipient areas with enhanced vascularity. Plast Reconstr Surg 2002; 109:1646–1651.
55. GuerreroSantos J, Gonzalez-Mendoza A, Masmela Y, Gonzalez MA, Deos M, Diaz P. Long-term survival of free fat grafts in muscle; An experimental study in rats. Aesthetic Plast Surg 1996; 20:403–408.
56. Amar RE. Fat autograft muscle injection. Presented at Association of Cosmetic Surgery Annual Meeting, February 2001; San Diego, CA.
57. Butterwick KJ. Enhancement of the results of neck liposuction with the FAMI technique. J Drugs Dermatol 2003; 2:487–493.
58. Salasche SJ, Bernstein G, Senkarik M. Muscles of facial expression. In: Salasche SJ, Bernstein G (eds). Surgical anatomy of the skin. Norwalk: Appleton & Lance 1988; 69–87.
59. Gray H. The facial muscles. In: Gross CM, eds. Anatomy of the human body, 107th ed. Philadelphia: Lea & Febiger; 1969; 382–390.
60. Rose J, Lemke B, Lucarelle M, et al. Anatomy of facial recipient sites for autologous fat transfer. Am J Cosmet Surg 2003; 20:17–25.
61. Butterwick KJ, Lack E. Facial volume restoration with fat autograft muscle injection (FAMI): Preliminary experience with a new technique. Dermatol Surg 2003; 29:1019–1026.
62. Horl HW, Feller AM, Biemer E. Technique for liposuction fat reimplantation and long-term volume evaluation by magnetic resonance imaging. Ann Plast Surg 1991; 26:248.
63. Goldman R, Carmargo CP, Goldman B. Fat transplantation and facial contour. Ann J Cosmet Surg 1998; 15:41–44.
64. Glogau RG. Microlipoinjection. Arch Dermatol 1988; 124:1340.
65. Saddick NS, Hudgins LC. Fatty acid analysis of transplanted adipose tissue. Arch Dermatol 2001; 137:723–727.
66. Nguyen A, Pasyk KA, Bouvier TN, Hassett CA, Argents LC. Discussion: Comparative study of survival of autologous adipose tissue taken and transplanted by different techniques. Plast Reconstr Surg 1990; 85:378–386.
67. Kaminer MS, Omura NE. Editorial—Autologous fat transplantation. Arch Dermatol 2001; 137:812–814.
68. Chajchir A, Benzaquen I, Wexler E. Suction curettage lipectomy. Aesthetic Plast Surg 1983; 7:195–202.
69. Perez M. Update on autologous fat transplantation. Cosmet Derm 2002; 15:36–40.
70. Fournier PF. Fat grafting: My technique. Dermatol Surg 2000; 26:1117–1128.
71. Aboudib JHC Jr, deCastro CC, Gradel J. Hand rejuvenescence by fat filling. Ann Plast Surg 1992; 28:559–564.
72. Abrams HL, Lauber JS. Hand rejuvenation: The state of the art. Dermatol Clin 1990; 8:553–561.
73. Takasu K, Takasu S. Long-term frozen fat transplantation. Int J Cosmet Surg 1999; 7:33–38.
74. Shoshani O, Ullmann Y, Shupak A, et al. The role of frozen storage in preserving adipose tissue obtained by suction-assisted lipectomy for repeated fat injection procedures. Dermatol Surg 2001; 27:645–647.
75. Butterwick KJ. Fresh versus frozen fat: a comparison of the longevity and aesthetic results for lipoaugmentation of the aging hands. Annual meeting of the American Society of Dermatologic Surgery. 2002; Chicago, IL.
76. Lawrence N. The science of fat transplantation. Advanced Cosmetic Seminar. Annual meeting of the American Society of Dermatologic Surgery; October 2002, Chicago, IL.
77. Donofrio L. Technique of periorbital lipoaugmentation. Dermatol Surg 2003; 29:92–98.
78. Miller J, Popp J. Fat hypertrophy after autologous fat transfer. Ophthalmic Plast Reconstr Surg 2002; 18:228–231.
79. Obagi S. Autologous fat augmentation and periorbital laser resurfacing complicated by abscess formation. Am J Cosmet Surg 2003; 20:155–157.
80. Dreizen NG, Framm L. Sudden unilateral visual loss after autologous fat injection into the glabellar area. Am J Ophthalmol 1989; 107:85–87.
81. Teimourian B. Blindness following fat injections. Plast Reconstr Surg 1988; 80:361.
82. Feinendegen D, Baumgartner R, Schroth G, Mattle H, Tschopp H. Middle cerebral artery occlusion and ocular fat embolism after autologous fat injection the face. J Neurol 1998; 245:53–54.
83. Coleman SR. Avoidance of arterial occlusion from injection of soft tissue fillers. Aesthetic Surg J 2002; 22:555–557.
84. Wexler P. Tissue augmentation. Present and future. American Academy of Dermatology Annual meeting. March 2000, San Francisco, CA.
85. Coleman S. Complications of fat grafts and structural fillers. In: Techniques in minimally invasive aesthetic surgery. Los Angeles; 2002.

34 Follicular Unit Hair Transplantation

Robert M Bernstein MD

Summary box

- Follicular unit transplantation (FUT) is a method of hair restoration surgery that relocates hair in follicular units, its naturally occurring groupings. The small size of the units allows for tremendous versatility in their placement, the creation of hair patterns closely mimicking nature and transplant procedures large enough that a full restoration can often be achieved in just two sessions.
- Follicular unit transplantation requires large numbers of grafts, so it is important to accurately assess patients' donor reserves in the initial planning. Densitometry enables the physician to estimate the total number of movable hairs, the size of the individual follicular units, and the degree of miniaturization in both the donor and recipient areas; scalp laxity assessment is also crucial to the surgical planning.
- Great care should be taken to screen for patients who are too young or whose hair loss may be diffuse and involve the donor area.
- Identifying androgenetic alopecia often proves more difficult in women as other medical conditions must be considered. Options for medical treatment are more limited in women and many experience diffuse hair loss, a relative contraindication to surgery.
- Determining the right size and location of the donor strip prevents problems such as widened and/or visible scars; the follicular units obtained from donor strips are delicate structures, and careful dissection, gentle handling, and adequate hydration are essential to their survival.
- In order to dissect and place the thousands of grafts often required in FUT, the surgical team must be proficient in stereomicroscopic dissection and insertion techniques—skills that can take a year or more to develop.
- Follicular unit transplantation requires an astute aesthetic sense for optimal hairline design, correct angling and distribution of grafts and the establishment of a master plan that anticipates further hair loss and is consistent with the long-term goals of the patient.

INTRODUCTION

Within the past decade, follicular unit transplantation (FUT) has transformed hair transplantation from a cosmetically unpredictable procedure to one that can produce consistently natural results. The key to its effectiveness lies in the fact that scalp hair tends to grow in tiny bundles, called 'follicular units,' rather than individually.[1] By working with these naturally occurring units, instead of larger or smaller grafts, FUT creates as natural a look as possible while minimizing the transplant wound size and accelerating postoperative healing. A recently developed refinement—follicular unit extraction—promises to eliminate, for select candidates, the procedure's most invasive aspect: the surgical removal of a strip of tissue from which the units are harvested.[2]

Follicular units are made up of one to four terminal hairs, one to two vellus hairs, their associated sebaceous glands, neurovascular plexus, an erector pilorum muscle, and a circumferential band of adventitial collagen, the perifolliculum.[3] The tendency of scalp hair to grow in this way, rather than as single hairs, can be most easily demonstrated by clipping the hair to approximately 1 mm in length and then viewing it with a densitometer (Fig. 34.1) at × 30 magnification in a 10-mm field.[4] What this also reveals is that these compact units are surrounded by significant amounts of non-hair-bearing scalp (Fig. 34.2).[5] Including this extra skin in the dissection—as do transplants with larger grafts, such as plugs and mini-grafts—requires a larger recipient wound, as well as risking visible scarring in the skin around the grafts and distortions of the growing hair.

In FUT these naturally occurring units are used exclusively. The FUT procedure takes advantage of the anatomic proximity of the hairs within each unit to:

- keep the recipient site wound size to a minimum
- virtually eliminate any skin surface change in the recipient area
- facilitate postoperative healing
- enable grafts to be placed very close together

- permit large numbers of grafts to be safely transplanted in a single session (because of the small recipient wound size).[1,6]

The ability to insert up to four hairs in a tiny recipient site is especially valuable cosmetically and has been instrumental in eliminating the see-through quality of micrografting. In the end, what this means is that the transplanted hair will look natural, given that as the transplant surgeon makes the right aesthetic decisions about graft placement, angling, and distribution.[7,8]

The higher precision of FUT as compared to mini-micrografting is especially obvious when methods of harvesting the grafts are compared. In FUT, once a strip of donor tissue has been removed, follicular units are taken out intact through careful stereomicroscopic dissection, avoiding injury to the follicles.[9,11] The grafts in mini-micrografting, on the other hand, may or may not correspond to individual follicular units. They are cut from the donor strip according to the number of hairs they contain (optimally one to six, but often more) and/or the size of tissue required to fit into a given recipient site—a process known as 'grafts cut to size.' Often the dissection is performed without magnification, and it is also common for the donor tissue to be removed with a multibladed knife, rather than as a single strip, causing significant destruction of follicles. Because the grafts may be too large to fit into a slit incision, an excision (where recipient tissue is removed, such as with a small punch) is sometimes needed. In contrast, the recipient sites used for FUT always consist of small incisional slits.

In a new procedure called follicular unit extraction (FUE),[2] the need for a donor strip is eliminated entirely. In this procedure, individual follicular units are removed (extracted) directly from the donor area through a small circular incision with, or without, microdissection. Although this procedure obviates the need for a linear strip, it has limitations, particularly in the inability to efficiently utilize all the tissue in the mid-portion of the permanent zone. As of this writing, most surgeons performing FUE have used it for select patients only. A brief description of this procedure will be included in the section on donor harvest under Techniques.

The purpose of this chapter is to elaborate on the basic technical skills and aesthetic judgments involved in FUT. It should be taken as a framework for physicians interested in learning the procedure, not an exhaustive review of the various surgical techniques used in FUT or of other hair restoration methods. The chapter will not cover mini-micrografting (which is still widely practiced),[12] the combining of large and small grafts,[13] laser hair transplantation,[14,15] scalp reductions,[16,17] scalp lifts,[18] or flaps.[19] These procedures have been detailed in many excellent publications, as well as in two comprehensive textbooks.[20,12]

When learning FUT, the importance of hands-on experience and beginning with small sessions until skills develop cannot be overemphasized. Having a well-trained team of assistants is also important to a successful outcome, particularly for those procedures involving a large number of grafts.

Although simple in concept, FUT has many nuances and complexities. Those wishing to perform FUT in their clinical practice are encouraged to join the International Society of Hair Restoration Surgery (ISHRS) and attend its annual meeting, to subscribe to *Hair Transplant Forum International* (the trade publication for hair restoration surgeons), and to follow relevant medical literature. Although it is an independent board, certification by the American Board of Hair Restoration Surgery (ABHRS) indicates a basic competency in the field and requires 3 years of clinical experience and passing both oral and written examinations. The process of preparing for ABHRS certification is a worthwhile endeavor and recommended for those serious about surgical hair restoration.

Historical Vignette

Reports of successful hair transplants appeared as early as 1930 in Japanese literature, beginning with Sasagawa's hair-shaft insertion procedure[21] and then Okuda's success in pioneering 2-mm to 4-mm punches for the treatment of various alopecias of the scalp, eyebrows, and moustache. Okuda made the important observation that using smaller punches in the recipient area improved cosmetic results.[22]

By 1943, Tamura had treated 137 cases of non-androgenetic alopecia of various etiologies using techniques very similar to modern day hair transplantation.[23] For instance, he harvested donor grafts by making an elliptical incision that was sutured closed, prepared recipient sites with a thick needle, stored grafts in physiologic saline, and observed postoperative telogen effluvium. Most significantly, Tamura demonstrated that single-hair grafting resulted in growth practically indistinguishable from naturally grown hair—and much more natural looking than transplants using larger grafts. But it took several decades before western surgeons would apply Tamura's insights to their hair restoration procedures.

The first hair transplant in the United States was performed by Dr Norman Orentreich in 1952 with grafts measuring 6–8 mm in diameter,[24] significantly larger than those of either Tamura or Okuda. At first, incredulous editors rejected Orentreich's work, not believing that hair transplantation was even possible. He finally found a publisher in 1959, in the *Annals of the New York Academy of Science*. The paper laid out the concept of 'donor dominance'—the idea that grafts continue to show the characteristics of the donor site after they have been transplanted to a new site. This remains the basic tenet of all hair transplantation surgery. Yet while donor dominance insured that transplanted hair could grow, it did not guarantee that the results would look natural.

Not until 40 years later would transplants in the United States start to produce consistently natural-looking results and promise predictable cosmetic improvements in most patients. It was a slow evolution, but the large grafts used throughout the 1960s and 1970s eventually gave way to mini-grafts in the 1980s[4] and mini-micrografting in the early 1990s.[25] The stage was then set for follicular unit transplantation. First appearing in the medical literature in 1995[1] it quickly emerged as the standard in hair restoration—supplanting mini-micrografting in the treatment of androgenetic alopecia and rendering other well-established procedures such as scalp reductions, scalp lifts, and flaps virtually obsolete.

So swift was the ascent of FUT that the two standard textbooks on surgical hair restoration, published in 1995[20] and 1996,[12] as well as the most comprehensive text on trichology, published in 1997,[26] make not one mention of the terms 'follicular unit' or 'follicular unit transplantation'. At the 1996 meeting of the International Society of Hair Restoration Surgeons, three 7-minute presentations on the procedure were given; but at the 2002 meeting, FUT was the subject of entire seminars and workshops and suffused every aspect of the week-long gathering.

The follicular unit was first defined by Headington in his landmark 1984 paper entitled 'Transverse microscopic anatomy of the human scalp.'[3] Follicular unit transplantation had its origins in the microscopic dissection techniques of Dr Limmer in 1988 that was described in his paper 'Elliptical donor stereoscopically assisted micrografting as an approach to further refinement in hair transplantation' in 1994.[9] The term 'follicular unit' was introduced into the hair transplant literature by Bernstein and Rassman in 1995. The conceptual framework for FUT was mapped out by these authors in the 1995 publication 'Follicular transplantation'[1] and in the paired articles 'Follicular transplantation: patient evaluation and surgical planning' and 'The aesthetics of follicular transplantation' in 1997.[7,8]

The name 'follicular unit transplantation' was formalized by a group of hair restoration surgeons in a 1998 publication in *Dermatologic Surgery*.[10] In this paper, the procedure was precisely defined and included the two basic techniques, single-strip harvesting and stereomicroscopic dissection, as integral parts of the procedure. However, because follicular units can now be harvested directly from the donor area without the necessity of a strip incision (using follicular unit extraction[2]) the original definition has become too restrictive.

The term follicular unit transplantation should now be used to encompass all hair restoration procedures that utilize naturally occurring individual follicular units exclusively in the surgery, regardless of how these units are harvested. The caveat, of course, is that the harvesting technique must always maintain the follicular unit's integrity.

■ PREOPERATIVE PREPARATION

Patient evaluation and surgical planning

Diagnosis and classification of androgenetic alopecia

The diagnosis of androgenetic alopecia in men is usually straightforward. It is made by observing a 'patterned' distribution of hair loss and confirmed by the presence of miniaturized hairs in the areas of thinning. The diagnosis is supported by both the inexorable progression of the hair loss according to a recognizable pattern and a history of baldness in the family.[27] In women, the diagnosis is more complex because the most common presentation, a diffuse pattern, can be mimicked by a host of non-androgenetic etiologies.

Miniaturization—the progressive diminution of the hair shaft's diameter and length in response to androgens—can be most readily observed with a densitometer,[12] a handheld instrument that magnifies a small area of the scalp where the hair has been clipped to about 1 mm. One type, the Rassman densitometer,[4] magnifies by × 30 in a visual field of 10 mm^2, making it easy to spot miniaturization and calculate hair density (Figs 34.1–34.3).

When describing hair loss, particularly in the early phases, it is preferable to think in terms of changes in volume rather than density. Density is simply the number of hairs per unit area, whereas volume reflects both hair shaft diameter as well as the absolute numbers of hairs.[28] The earliest sign of hair loss, that of miniaturization, results in volume changes caused by the individual hair decreasing in size without a decrease in their number. Only in more advanced balding will the actual number of hairs start to decrease.[1]

The Norwood classification of male hair loss, published in 1975, remains the most widely used.[29] It defines two major

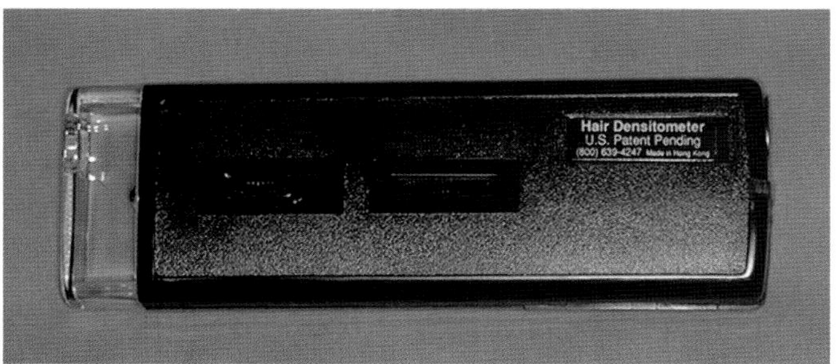

Figure 34.1 Hair densitometer.

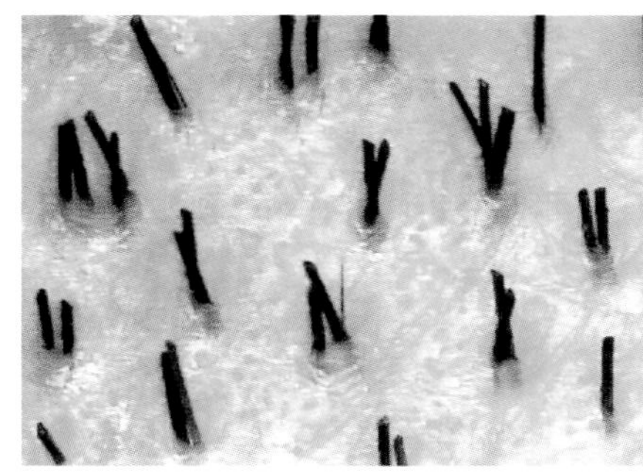

Figure 34.2 Natural hair groupings as seen through a densitometer (magnification × 30).

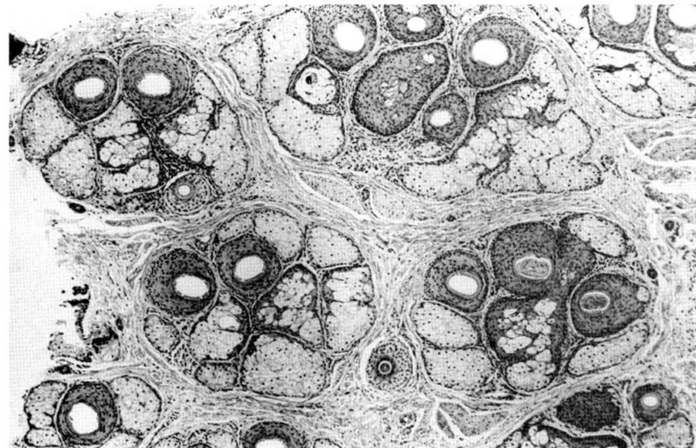

Figure 34.3 Histological view of follicular units corresponding to the natural hair groups observed on the scalp surface. Transverse section taken at the level of sebaceous glands (hematoxylin and eosin; original magnification × 40).[6]

patterns and several less common types (Fig. 34.4). In the regular Norwood pattern, two areas of hair loss—a bitemporal recession and thinning crown—gradually enlarge and coalesce until the entire front, top, and crown (vertex) of the scalp are bald. The less common pattern, Norwood class A, is characterized by a distinctly anterior-to-posterior progression, usually resulting in baldness on the front and top of the scalp, but more limited loss in the crown. In both patterns, the sides and back tend to resist androgenetic changes, though the sides may exhibit significant thinning in senile alopecia.

Two other types of genetic hair loss not emphasized in the literature, diffuse patterned and diffuse unpatterned alopecia, pose the greatest challenge both for diagnosis and patient management. A thorough familiarity with all of these patterns is essential for diagnosing androgenetic alopecia and planning FUT (Table 34.1).

Diffuse patterned alopecia (DPA) is an androgenetic alopecia manifested as diffuse thinning in the front, top, and vertex, with a stable permanent zone. In DPA, the entire top of the scalp gradually miniaturizes without passing through the typical Norwood stages. Diffuse unpatterned alopecia (DUPA) is also androgenetic but lacks a stable permanent zone and affects men much less often than DPA. DUPA tends to advance faster than DPA and eventuates in a horseshoe pattern resembling the Norwood class VII. However, unlike the Norwood class VII, the DUPA horseshoe can look almost transparent due to the low density of the back and sides. Differentiating between DPA and DUPA is very important because DPA patients often make good transplant candidates, whereas DUPA patients almost never do, as they inevitably suffer extensive hair loss without a stable zone for harvesting.[7]

There are five early signs of DUPA:

- A rapid decrease in hair volume (as distinguished from density) and a change in hair texture at an early age, often in the teens.
- The maintenance of an adolescent hair pattern and persistent frontal hairline in spite of dramatic volume change.
- A see-through donor area, which is greatly accentuated when the hair is lifted up.
- Significant miniaturization of the donor area (more than 35%).
- A donor density of less than 1.5 hairs per mm^2. (Densitometry's acute sensitivity in detecting early DUPA certainly justifies its routine use in the evaluation of hair loss.)

If a diagnosis of DUPA is even remotely suspected, any decisions regarding surgical hair restoration should be postponed. The possibility of missing a DUPA diagnosis is one of the most powerful arguments against performing hair transplantation at an early age.

Both DPA and DUPA occur in women, but—in contrast to men—DUPA proves far more common. As with men, women with DUPA do not make good transplant candidates (except possibly when donor hair is used solely to soften the frontal edge of a wig). Indeed, the higher DUPA incidence in women explains why a smaller proportion of women than men qualify as transplant candidates. Interestingly, the most common classification used for women, the Ludwig Classification, does not differentiate between DPA and DUPA.[30]

It is important to emphasize that because a wide variety of medical conditions can produce diffuse hair loss, a non-androgenetic differential must be considered in all unpatterned alopecias. This is particularly relevant in evaluating women in whom unpatterned hair loss is the rule rather than the exception (Table 34.2). The following

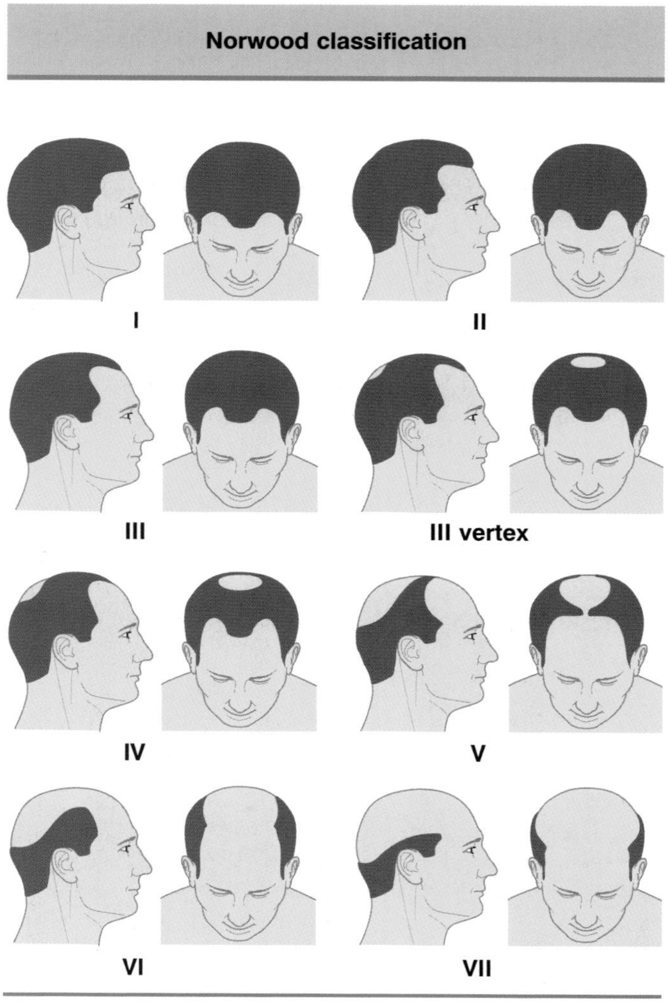

Norwood classification

I

II

III

III vertex

IV

V

VI

VII

Figure 34.4 Norwood classification.[28]

Table 34.1 Classification of androgenetic alopecia

Norwood classes	Regular classes I to VII Type A variant (IIa to Va) Variations: persistent frontal forelock; persistent frontal hairline
Diffuse androgenic alopecias	Diffuse patterned alopecia (DPA) Diffuse unpatterned alopecia (DUPA)
Senile alopecia	

Table 34.2 Non-androgenetic causes of diffuse hair loss in women

Anemia
Endocrine diseases (especially thyroid)
Connective tissue disease
Obstetric/gynecologic conditions (e.g. postpartum, polycystic ovarian disease)
Weight loss (esp. crash diets)
Emotional and physical stress (e.g. surgery, anesthesia)
Medications: oral contraceptives, thyroid drugs, antihypertensives (especially β-blockers), psychotropics, anticoagulants, antilipemics, gout therapy, prednisone, excessive vitamin A or tryptophan use

Table 34.3 Surgical patient selection for androgenetic alopecia

Age: 23–25 years or older
Inadequate response to medication after 1 year
Significant hair loss: Norwood class III or greater
Diffuse patterned alopecia (DUPA) has been ruled out
Non-androgenetic causes of hair loss have been ruled out*
No medical contraindications to surgery (drug sensitivities, keloids, connective tissue disease)†
Reasonable patient expectations

**Many non-androgenetic causes of hair loss can be treated with hair transplantation.*
†Some are relative contraindications.

laboratory tests are often useful when a non-androgenetic cause for diffuse hair loss is suspected: chemistry screen, complete blood count, serum iron, total ion-binding capacity, triiodothyronine, thyroxine, thyroid-stimulating hormone, antinuclear antibody, and serologic test for syphilis.

In women, diffuse or patterned hair loss may be a sign of excessive androgen production. A further medical evaluation is indicated when the hair loss is associated with any of the following: cystic acne, irregular menses, hirsuitism, virilization, infertility, or galactorrhea. Serum levels of DHEA-sulfate, androstenedione, total and free testosterone, and prolactin can serve as a useful screen.[31]

When the diagnosis of androgenetic alopecia is uncertain, further diagnostic information can be gleaned from a hair-pull test for telogen effluvium, a potassium hydroxide mount and culture for fungus, a microscopic examination of the hair bulb and shaft, and a scalp biopsy (sectioned horizontally).[32] But a dermatologic consultation is warranted whenever the diagnosis of hair loss is unclear.

Who is a candidate for hair transplantation?

In all cosmetic procedures, a successful outcome depends on proper patient selection (Table 34.3). In surgical hair restoration, proper timing is also crucial. The only reason for performing a transplant sooner rather than later is for its cosmetic benefit; there are no medical or surgical advantages to transplanting at an early age. The popular rationale that transplants should be performed at a young age so that 'no one will notice' does not make sense: if there is nothing to notice after the transplant matures, why perform it in the first place? FUTs heal so quickly and the hair growth is so gradual that, once the short postoperative period ends, the process is almost always undetectable.

Patients seeking hair transplantation while still in their early 20s invariably wish to have their adolescent hairline and original density restored. Since neither of these goals can be achieved surgically without compromising the patient's future appearance, the procedure should not be performed at this age. It should be explained that hair transplantation is a procedure that moves—rather than creates—new hair, so that it can never increase overall hair volume. And, in the face of decreasing total volume over time, the pattern of the transplanted hair must take into account this decreased total hair mass. In other words, patients who will have significant balding need to have built-in temporal recession, and possibly a crown that is significantly thinner than the surrounding hair, for the transplant to look natural over time. Unfortunately, neither of these is generally acceptable to a young man in his early 20s.

Another reason to postpone transplants for those under 25 years, or with only limited hair loss, is to give medications—particularly finasteride—adequate time to work. As patients may continue to show regrowth for up to 2 years after treatment is initiated, they should in general take finasteride at least this long before surgery is considered. It is inappropriate, therefore, to start younger patients on finasteride and schedule surgery at the same time. Fortunately, finasteride works best in younger patients, and especially those with large areas of miniaturized scalp rather than areas that are totally bald. On the other hand, for older patients who would be taking finasteride to maintain rather than regrow hair, and for those whose advanced state of hair loss makes results from finasteride unlikely, the medication may be prescribed concomitantly with surgery (see Preoperative Preparation).

With the availability of finasteride, medication plays an increasingly important role in the management of androgenetic hair loss. Although the incidence is small (2%), the stigma of possible sexual side effects has turned many against this drug. Some also consider surgery a more conservative form of treatment than the potential lifetime use of a drug. Because of these concerns, and the often palpable desire of panicked patients to rush to surgery, the physician should take time to thoroughly discuss the pros and cons of medical therapy.

In the Norwood Classification, class I represents a normal adolescent pattern and class II a normal non-balding adult. Therefore, as a minimum, patients should qualify as class III before transplants are contemplated. Early class III patients will often benefit from medication alone, so this should be considered first. On the other end of the spectrum, extensive balding need not make a patient unsuitable for surgery, if the donor zone is stable (miniaturization of less than 20%) and the patient's expectations are commensurate with his or her available donor supply. As long as the patient is in good health there is no upper age limit. In fact, older patients tend to have the most reasonable expectations and often make the best candidates.

There are few absolute medical contraindications to surgical hair restoration, particularly because it is an outpatient procedure not requiring general anesthesia. Relative contraindications include: bleeding disorders, immunodeficiency, unstable arrhythmias, chronic obstructive pulmonary disease, sensitivity to local anesthetics or epinephrine (adrenaline), a history of keloid formation or connective tissue disease, and major psychiatric disorders. When in doubt about the patient's medical condition it is always best to get medical clearance from their primary physician. Patients should be able to tolerate being in the surgical chair for a good part of the day; consequently, back and neck problems as well as claustrophobia can sometimes make the procedure problematic. Special care should be taken when evaluating patients with significant psychiatric problems, particularly depression. In such cases, a psychiatrist or psychologist should participate in the decision-making process.

Possibly the most difficult part of the consultation is managing patients' expectations. It is almost a cliché to say that they must have 'reasonable expectations', but ensuring this is the essence of the evaluation. The surgeon cannot stress strongly enough that, because transplants move rather than create hair, the resulting density will be significantly less than in the original site. It is also important to emphasize that it is the patient's own hair, from the sides and back of his or her head, that will be transplanted. And the final result can be best described with reference to the texture, color, curl, and other qualities of their existing hair. But in addition to a thorough discussion, it is also helpful to provide prospective patients with printed material and photos, and to make past patients available for them to meet.

Assessing the patient's donor supply

The main factors in determining total donor reserves are donor density, scalp laxity, and size of the donor area.

Donor density

The number of follicular units in the mid-portion of the donor area of a normal Caucasian man who has not had surgery is approximately one per mm^2.[8] In the first procedure, therefore, the donor area should yield approximately one follicular graft per mm^2 of scalp, provided there is no significant wastage during surgery. The average yield declines when longer strips are taken because density decreases towards the sides. In some people, density varies dramatically throughout the donor area, but this is the exception rather than the rule.

Since the number of follicular units per unit area stays relatively constant, donor density is an indication of the average number of hairs per graft. For example, if a patient has a density of two hairs per mm^2, the donor area will generally contain one follicular unit per mm^2 and the grafts will consist of a combination of one-, two- and three-hair units, with the average being two hairs per graft. With a density of 2.3 hairs per mm^2, there will still be one follicular unit per mm^2, so the same number of grafts will be harvested per unit donor area, but the grafts will have an average of 2.3 hairs per mm^2 and consist of a mix of fewer one-hair units and a larger percentage of three- and four-hair units.[8]

Follicular unit density varies according to race, therefore the number of grafts obtained per unit area of donor tissue will exhibit racial variability and must be accounted for in the surgical planning.[8]

If the scalp has been stretched from previous transplants, scalp reductions, or scalp lifts, the follicular units will be spaced further apart, making it necessary to actually measure the density of follicular units to accurately estimate the number of grafts obtainable from the strip (as the density of follicular units will now be less than one per mm^2).

Donor scarring from previous surgeries will also significantly diminish the donor yield. All donor harvests, no matter how perfectly executed, entail some loss of hair. In addition, the angle of the hair surrounding the scar will be altered slightly, creating more transection in any subsequent harvest.

A person can lose a substantial amount of hair volume—either due to actual loss of hair or to miniaturization—before it becomes noticeable. When the hair is blonde or white it takes longer for thinning to show, while it is evident sooner for those with black hair and white skin. For those with average density and average hair attributes, approximately half of the hair in the donor area may be moved without a significant change in appearance.

Scalp laxity

Scalp laxity is an important factor in determining total available donor hair. In those with loose scalps, harvesting the donor strip merely removes some scalp redundancy while only slightly affecting density (hairs per mm^2). With tight scalps, however, each procedure stretches the skin, measurably decreasing density. The limitations of a tight scalp are usually not apparent in the initial surgery, but in subsequent procedures it can become much harder to perform a non-tension closure or, in the face of decreased density, to harvest a significant amount of hair. Therefore, the long-term goals of those with tight scalps must reflect a more limited donor supply.

At the same time, patients with very loose scalps tend to heal with widened scars and so often make poor candidates for procedures using a linear incision. Some, in fact, may have undiagnosed connective tissue disease.[33] Follicular unit extraction should be considered in cases of very loose and very tight scalps.[2]

Donor dimensions

The mid-portion of the harvestable donor zone generally lies over the occipital protuberance and extends to within 3 cm of the temple hairline on either side. This distance is approximately 32–34 cm. Recession at the temples can signal extensive balding and portends a limited donor supply. The height of the permanent zone can vary markedly from person to person and should be carefully measured. Hair should be harvested only where it is stable, that is, where it lacks significant miniaturization. An often overlooked sign is the 'ascending' hairline, characterized by miniaturization in the lower margin of the permanent zone. Both receding temples and an ascending posterior hairline indicate a shrinking donor zone and mandate conservative surgical planning.

Planning the first hair transplant session

Ideally, the main goals of the first transplant session should be:

- to establish the frontal hairline and frame the face
- to provide coverage to all bald areas of the scalp, from the frontal hairline back to the vertex transition point[34]
- to create sufficient density so that the results will look natural after one session, though additional sessions may be desired.[7]

These goals may not be achievable with a small or inexperienced surgical team, but should be the ultimate aim of those performing hair restoration surgery. In this author's opinion, there is little medical or aesthetic justification for performing the surgery in arbitrarily small sessions. It is preferable that each procedure cover the entire area of hair loss intended to be treated and be designed to 'stand alone.'[7,8]

In an alternate approach to surgical planning, the objective is to achieve final density in a one-pass procedure by creating high density in smaller area and then transplanting another area in a subsequent session. This is accomplished in part by using very small recipient sites, limiting graft size to three hairs and using the stick-and-place method, in which grafts are inserted as soon as the recipient sites are made.[35]

As the number of grafts placed per unit area (density) rises, so too does the risk of vascular compromise that may result in suboptimal graft growth. Technical problems of popping that may cause the grafts to become desiccated or that exposes the grafts to mechanical injury on reinsertion, also become more likely. Proper patient selection and technical expertise help avoid such problems, but the risks are increased nevertheless. It certainly behoves those with more limited experience to be conservative in this aspect of the procedure.

Because the blood supply to the scalp is extensively collateralized,[36] the risk of vascular compromise is related more to the density of grafts in a specific area and the size of the recipient wounds, than the absolute numbers of grafts placed. For this reason, the transplantation of a large number of grafts over a broad area does not seem to pose the same problems as producing very high densities. In addition, popping becomes less of a technical issue when the same number of grafts are placed over a larger area. However, transplanting large number of grafts (in 'mega-sessions') poses its own challenges, such as increasing the time the grafts remain outside the body, requiring more staff, contributing to patient and staff fatigue, and creating organizational issues. As with dense packing, the use of very large sessions should be reserved for only the most experienced surgical teams.

Though the amount of hair needed to cover the front and top of the patient's scalp will vary, an attempt should be made to achieve this coverage, if only lightly, in the first session. Crown coverage should not be a goal of the first session unless the patient has an above-average donor supply; if it is attempted in the first session the patient's options will be more limited and the chances for an aesthetically balanced transplant may be permanently compromised.

Table 34.4 offers general guidelines as to the number of follicular units recommended for the first hair transplant procedure.

Table 34.4 Number of grafts in first follicular unit transplant session

Norwood Class	Follicular Units	Total Units with Crown
III	800–1000 +	—
III Vertex	800–1000 +	1100–1300 +
IIIa	1300–1600 +	—
IV	1100–1400 +	1500–1800 +
IVa	1700–2100 +	—
V	1500–1800 +	1900–2400 +
Va	2000–2400 +	—
VI	2000–2400 +	2400 +
VII	2000–2400 +	—

Planning a second session

Timing of the second session

Transplanted hair sheds around 2–6 weeks after the procedure, and the first signs of new growth occur on average in approximately 10 weeks, though the onset can vary considerably, taking as long as 4–6 months or more. Hair gradually increases in both thickness and length, so that the initial growth is often not indicative of the final result. In less than 5% of patients, hair grows unabated after surgery, without shedding.

One should generally wait 8–12 months to best appreciate the cosmetic impact of the procedure. During this time, the continued increase in the hair's diameter and length strikingly alters the patient's appearance. Once the hair reaches styling length, both the patient and physician can make aesthetic judgments about the distribution of additional grafts.

It will also be advantageous to delay the second procedure to maximize the donor harvest. Although each procedure results in a potentially tighter scalp, some of the preoperative donor laxity returns in the months following the surgery. The major change will occur during the first month as the edema and inflammation subside. However, further loosening will occur as the scalp stretches over the next 12 months.

In the uncommon event of telogen effluvium occurring in the donor area, the telogen follicles may not be easily identifiable in the dissection. Since recovery in the donor area may take up to a year, it is essential that patients wait until complete re-growth has taken place before a second session is performed. In rare cases, if the closure is too tight, the effluvium may eventuate in permanent hair loss.

Goals for the second session

The main goals of the second session are:

- to add density to areas transplanted in the first session
- to refine the hairline
- to follow the progression of the hair loss (if necessary)
- to extend the transplant into the crown (when appropriate).

In general, most patients require two sessions to achieve adequate density. The hairline often can benefit from a little tweaking to make the leading edge softer and more irregular. Placing the hairline too low is a common mistake, but so is placing it too high, something often done with the intention of bringing it down on the second session, once the patient can see how it looks. It is better to try to get the hairline position right in the first session; lowering it later often leaves the leading edge too thin.

The decision regarding crown coverage is important because it is the least visible of the balding regions, but can potentially occupy a very large surface area, producing an almost inexhaustible demand upon the donor supply.

If extensive balding appears likely and the patient has a modest donor supply, the crown should be treated as an extension of the top, rather than an isolated region, to ensure that the patient will not be short of hair if the intervening bridge between the front and crown were to require additional grafts. Unless the patient's history, age, and physical examination indicate limited balding, it is particularly important to avoid creating high density in the crown, as subsequent balding could leave an isolated island of hair.

A useful alternative to covering the crown with transplanted hair is to halt the transplant at the vertex transition point.[34,37] The patient can then groom the hair back to conceal the non-transplanted area. This is recommended when direct crown coverage is not realistic or it is too early in the balding process to determine whether significant crown coverage will be possible in the future. Another advantage of sparing, or lightly covering, the crown is that donor reserves may be saved to address further diminution of the lateral donor fringe.

Subsequent transplant sessions

The surgeon should make every attempt to accomplish the restoration in as few sessions as possible, rather than putting patients through an unnecessarily protracted course of multiple surgeries that can mar both their donor area and lifestyle. A second session is especially problematic for actively balding people; therefore, when they are experiencing an accelerated phase of hair loss, medical therapy should be encouraged and in general surgery should be postponed.

The number of grafts required to achieve patient satisfaction varies widely due to the great variability in hair characteristics. Moreover, because hair loss patterns form a continuum while the Norwood classes are discrete, even the transplant size necessary for each class can vary significantly. Table 34.5 shows the approximate number of follicular unit grafts necessary for a complete restoration, without and with crown coverage.

Table 34.5 Total number of follicular unit grafts for complete restoration

Norwood class	Follicular Units	Total Units with Crown
III	900–1500	—
III Vertex	900–1500	1300–2000
IIIa	1400–2200	—
IV	1200–2000	1700–3000
IVa	1800–3600	—
V	1700–3000	2100–4000
Va	2400–4400	—
VI	2200–4600	3000–5600
VII	2200–4800	4000–6600

The patient

Doctors commonly place patients on finasteride before surgery to minimize the chance of postsurgical effluvium. Although there are no scientific studies confirming that it is effective in doing this, it would seem that if the goal is to prevent postsurgical shedding, the medication should be prescribed at least several months before the procedure. If, however, the intent is to postpone or obviate the need for surgery, then it should be taken for a minimum of 1 year.

Patients using topical minoxidil are advised to discontinue its use several days before surgery (because of its vasodilator properties) and wait until a week after the procedure before resuming (to avoid the irritating effects of the alcohol in the 2% solution or the propylene glycol in the 5% solution). Although we suggest minoxidil in combination with finasteride for patients with early hair loss, we generally do not recommend its use after a hair transplant, unless it is being used in an area other than that which was transplanted (such as the crown). We feel that minoxidil has little added value for the average post-transplant patient. We do, however, encourage the continued use of finasteride to help retard further balding. Those who do not plan to use minoxidil after surgery should discontinue it immediately, so that any of its beneficial effects may be reversed by the time of surgery.

Patients are advised to avoid products that are used to thicken the hair or stain the scalp for 3 days before the procedure, as these often take several days to completely wash out of the scalp. Their presence during surgery can decrease visibility and make placing more difficult. All hair systems should be removed before surgery and be replaced with, or converted to, a clip-on system. The front edge of the piece can be kept in place with a stiffening rod, without the need for glue or tape. However, any form of attachment at or near the frontal hairline risks dislodging grafts. Patients are encouraged to permanently discontinue the system after the procedure, but those who feel the need to use them until their hair grows in should wait at least 5 days postoperatively.

Systemic antibiotics are not indicated for clean surgical wounds in healthy patients, so their routine use in hair transplantation is not necessary; however, many doctors—perhaps the majority—do routinely use them. Because there are no specific guidelines for antibiotic prophylaxis in hair transplantation for patients with a history of endocarditis or mitral valve prolapse, the decision to use them must be based on the individual patient's risk factors. This topic is covered in a recent review.[38]

The other preoperative instructions are relatively straightforward and will depend to some degree on the preferences of the operating surgeon. Patients should be notified well in advance of the procedure date regarding the need to discontinue certain medications, to stop smoking and abstain from alcohol before surgery. Table 34.6 is a summary of the main preoperative instructions.

All patients undergoing hair transplantation should be treated with universal precautions. Although there is no consensus on the need to perform routine blood tests

Table 34.6 Preoperative instructions

Continue medications currently prescribed by your physician, particularly those for high blood pressure. Those taking broad β-blockers (such as propranolol) should switch to select β-blockers, as the former may interact with epinephrine (adrenaline). This should be done under a doctor's supervision.
Discontinue topical minoxidil and avoid products used to thicken the hair or stain the scalp 3 days before the procedure.
In order to minimize bleeding, avoid the following before surgery: aspirin or other anti-inflammatory medications (1–2 weeks), vitamin B or vitamin E (1 week), or alcoholic beverages (3 days). Do not drink coffee or any other caffeinated beverages on the day of your procedure as these substances will increase your sensitivity to medications such as adrenaline.
Do not smoke tobacco products for at least 24 hours before your procedure and at least 1–2 weeks after. Smoking will slow down healing and heighten the chances of wound infection and scarring.
On the morning of your procedure take a bath or shower and wash your hair thoroughly using a surgical scrub (contains 3% chloroxylenol). If possible, leave your hair long in the back and on the sides to cover the sutures.
Wear clothes that do not need to be pulled on over your head; this will help keep your bandage in place and avoid any damage to your grafts immediately after surgery.
Eat breakfast the morning of your procedure. If you are scheduled for surgery in the afternoon, have a light lunch before you arrive.
Because you may be receiving medications during the procedure that can make you drowsy, you cannot drive home following the surgery. If you must drive or take public transportation, please let your doctor know ahead of time.

before the procedure, the following tests provide an additional level of safety:

- complete blood count
- hepatitis B surface antigen and antibody
- hepatitis C antibody
- HIV screen.

One should obtain medical clearance for HIV-positive patients to make sure that they are immunocompetent enough to withstand a potential series of procedures. With the hepatitis antigen-positive patient, there is a concern about active disease and one should inform the patient's primary physician of any positive screening. Other tests, such as a platelet count and prothrombin and thromboplastin times are performed only if warranted by the history and physical.

The surgical consent form should be given to patients to read at their leisure well in advance of the procedure and should be signed before any medications that can cause drowsiness or impair judgment have been given. The exact time of signing should be indicated. The major elements of the consent form are listed in Table 34.7.

On the morning of the surgery the patient should shower using a chlorhexadine surgical scrub as shampoo. Though it does not sterilize the scalp, the chlorhexadine binds to the stratum corneum, decreasing transient and pathogenic microorganisms and resident skin flora. Caution is advised as it can be toxic to the middle ear and irritating to the eyes. After showering, the patient should dress in comfortable clothes and wear a button-up shirt.

Table 34.7 Elements of consent form for hair transplant

Nature of the procedure, with specific reference to its cosmetic nature
Indications for surgery
Risks: reactions to anesthetics; allergic reactions; sterile folliculitis, infection; cyst formation at graft site; scarring in donor area; hair loss related to the procedure; hair texture changes; failure of transplanted hair to grow; numbness; paresthesia; temporary swelling or bruising
Benefits
Alternatives: doing nothing, change hair styles (e.g. lightening or keeping hair very short); medical therapy; another form of hair restoration surgery (e.g. mini-micrografting); wearing a hairpiece
Results are not guaranteed
Consent for photograph as part of the medical record
Caution about driving under the influence of medication
Statement that the above are understood and all questions have been answered
Signature of the patient with date and time (before the administration of drugs), countersigned by the operating physician and witnessed by a staff member

■ THE OPERATING ROOM

Follicular unit transplantation is typically performed in an outpatient office setting. The guidelines of care for office surgical facilities delineated by the American Academy of Dermatology should be reviewed before setting up facilities.[39,40] Though major complications occur only rarely, protocols should be in place to handle emergencies such as hypersensitivity reactions or anaphylaxis, stroke, seizures, arrhythmias, acute myocardial infarction, and hypertensive crisis. At the very least, specific arrangements should be made with a local Emergency Medical Services (EMS) facility to take care of distressed patients.[41]

The medical staff should be comfortable dealing with problems such as bleeding, syncope, petit mal episodes and anxiety reactions. The medical staff should be certified in cardiopulmonary resuscitation, and at least some in advanced cardiac life support. The amount of in-office emergency equipment will depend on staff capability and training, and proximity to an EMS unit. Basic equipment includes portable oxygen, an automated defribrillator, intravenous setup, and oral or nasopharyngeal airway.[41]

Because of the scalp's abundant vascular supply and relative resistance to infection, it is common practice for doctors' technique to be aseptic, rather than sterile. And because the scalp is not usually shaved and prepped, strict sterile technique is not practical. However, at least until the donor area is sutured closed, a sterile environment should be maintained. This issue is discussed in greater detail by Sebben and Davis.[42,43]

The single most important instrument for FUT is the dissecting stereomicroscope,[9,44] which is available with either a binocular view or with LCD screen. Each member of the surgical team performing the dissection should have one. Experienced teams generally require one staff member per 500 to 750 grafts (for graft dissection and placing), so that a typical 2000-graft procedure would necessitate three or four staff members in addition to the physician, though this will vary considerably among practices. Less-experienced teams may require more people. The staff's other responsibilities, as well as possible absenteeism, must also be taken into account.

Regular operating-room tables are generally inadequate. Rather, the tables must be contoured and provide some lumbar support when patients are sitting. They also need to be low to the ground, with the seat not more than 56 cm from the floor, so the staff can work comfortably around the head while the patient is seated.

Equally important are comfortable working areas for the staff. Dissecting tables with a bull nose, rather than squared edge, are easier on their arms, and adjustable seating saves them from bending over to look into the microscopes (Fig. 34.5). The long duration of the surgery makes meticulous attention to ergonomic issues all the more crucial.[45] Bright fluorescent ceiling lighting is preferable to surgical operating-room lights because it generates less heat. We use high-intensity surgical lights only for working on the donor area, as they can be angled to illuminate the posterior scalp of the seated patient.[46]

The Petri dishes containing grafts pending placement should be kept on a stable, wall-mounted surface to keep them from being inadvertently knocked over (Fig. 34.6). The typical operating room Mayo stand is not stable enough.[47] Normal saline is the most frequently used holding solution for grafts, but we prefer the more physiologic lactated Ringer's. Limmer has shown a high survival rate for grafts kept in chilled saline for up to 8 hours.[48] More exotic solutions with potential graft-sustaining properties have been developed, but they are not widely used.[49,50]

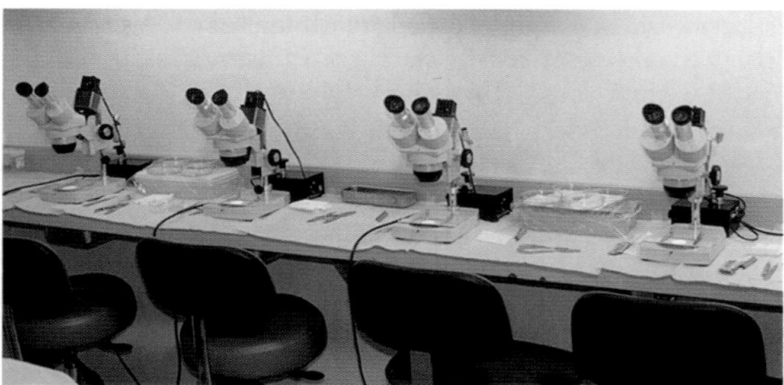

Figure 34.5 Dissecting stereomicroscopes on cutting table.

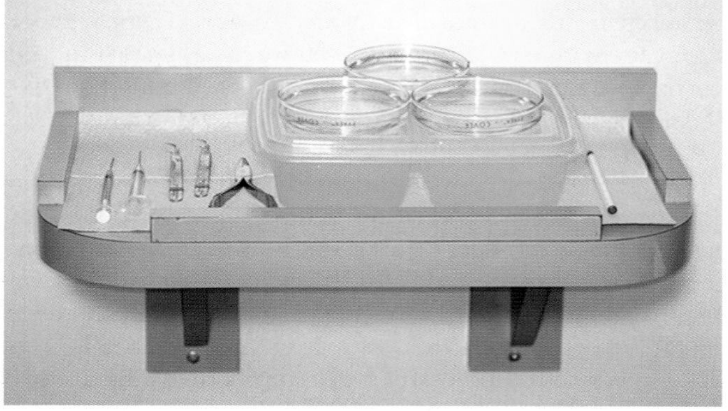

Figure 34.6 Wall-mounted placing stand for ice blocks, grafts, and instruments.[47]

Grafts should be refrigerated most of the time they are outside the body. Approximately 1 hour before placement, we remove a portion of the grafts from refrigeration and put them into Petri dishes which are resting on ice packs that maintain the Ringer's solution at 59 °C. This is set on a wall-mounted stand conveniently located at the head of the operating chair.

It is preferable to have all the dissection performed in the operating room. In addition, a small refrigerator used solely for graft storage should be located in each room. Performing all the dissection and storing the grafts in the same room eliminates the risk of inadvertently placing grafts in the wrong patient. Although obvious, this is particularly important in a busy practice where more than one person is being operated on per day. The minimum room size for a physician and five staff members to work comfortably is approximately 15.5 square meters.

In advance of the procedure, it is helpful to set up complete surgical trays, including the local anesthetic mixtures predrawn into syringes. This serves a number of purposes: it makes it easier to keep track of how much anesthetic is used in each part of the procedure, helps to ensure that safe dose limits are not exceeded[51] and minimizes the risk of needle-stick injury, because the preparation takes place before the operating room begins to bustle.

Local anesthesia is administered with a ring-block consisting of lidocaine, bupivacaine, and epinephrine (adrenaline) buffered with sodium bicarbonate. Lidocaine, the major component, is used for its safety and quick onset. Bupivacaine is added to increase the duration of anesthesia, but in smaller quantities to limit its potential cardiac toxicity.[52] Epinephrine (adrenaline) increases the anesthetic duration while decreasing its toxicity and providing some hemostasis, though its vasoconstrictive action is relatively short-lived. Bicarbonate is added to bring the acidic pH of the epinephrine (adrenaline)-containing solution closer to 7.4, lessening its sting.[53] This is particularly useful for injections at the hairline, where the scalp tends to be most sensitive. Though mentioned elsewhere in this text, it is worth repeating that the combined use of epinephrine (adrenaline) and broad β-blockers (e.g. propranolol) can result in potentially life-threatening reactions.[54]

The anesthetic solution used for a typical 2000-graft session is listed in Table 34.8. The anesthetic is drawn into 13 5-ml syringes then fitted with 27-gauge needles. The tumescent mixture consists of three 10-ml syringes with 25-gauge needles. These quantities are preprinted on the operative report and circled as each syringe is used. If patients require additional anesthesia, they are re-evaluated and then the medication drawn up and dose recorded.

■ TECHNIQUES

On arriving at the office, patients sign the consent form (which was given to them well in advance). The surgical plan is reviewed and any last-minute questions answered. Next, density is checked to confirm the measurement taken at the initial consultation; if the number differs or it appears that density varies in the donor area, multiple measurements are taken. Scalp laxity is also reassessed and recorded on the operative report.

Patients proceed to change into a cotton surgical gown and have their picture taken with a digital camera against a

Table 34.8 Anesthetic mixture

Ring Block Component	Concentration	Amount in Mixture
Lidocaine	0.5%	≈ 60%
Bupivacaine	0.025%	≈ 40%
Sodium bicarbonate[a]	8.4%	1:10
Epinephrine	–	1:200 000
Volume[b]	**Initial Quantity**	**Boost**
Donor area	20 cc	10 cc
Recipient area	25 cc	10 cc
Tumescent mixture for donor harvest Component	**Concentration**	**Amount in Mixture**
Lidocaine	0.17%	≈ 100%
Epinephrine	–	1:600 000
Volume[b]	**Quantity**	
Donor area	30cc	

[a]*Used prn.*
[b]*Volume of mixture typically used in 2000-graft session.*

light-blue background. Then the hairline and other important landmarks, such as the vertex transition point and crown swirl, are marked in Gentian violet and shown to the patient using two mirrors. If the patient approves of the hairline design, additional pictures are taken, this time of the marked scalp, usually from the front and aerial views. Three-quarter and close-up photos are sometimes taken to illustrate particular cosmetic issues. Occasionally pictures are taken during and after the operation for teaching purposes. All photos are kept as part of patients' permanent medical record.

Typical patients are premedicated with oral diazepam 15 mg, oral dicloxacillin 1000 mg (with a second dose of 500 mg 6 hours into the procedure) and an intramuscular injection of methylprednisolone 80 mg (i.e. 40 mg in each arm). The premedication is optional.

Donor harvest

In preparation for the donor harvest, patients are seated upright on the operating table. The hair in the donor area—that covering the donor strip plus the 0.5 cm beyond its perimeter—is then cut to 1–2 mm using electric clippers (the extra 0.5 cm to facilitate suturing). The trimmings are thoroughly vacuumed away and the hair above the strip is held back with tape, fully exposing the donor area. A gauze headband is placed around the patient's head just below the clipped area and sterile drapes are taped to the headband.

In the first session, in a patient with average scalp laxity, we generally harvest a donor strip that is 1 cm wide. In calculating the length, we use the general rule of 100 follicular units per cm^2.[6] For example, if 1500 follicular unit grafts are planned, the strip would measure 18 cm in length (15 cm plus 3 cm for tapering). African and occasionally Asian people have a lower follicular unit density and a strip of this dimension will yield a lower number of follicular unit grafts. However, the length should not be increased; rather the session should be planned using fewer grafts.[8]

Local anesthesia

A ring-block is established using an anesthetic mixture of lidocaine, bupivacaine and epinephrine (adrenaline) (Table 34.8). The anesthetic solution is injected into the deep subcutaneous fat layer approximately 1 cm below the lower portion of the clipped area and extending several centimeters past it on either side.

Approximately 0.75 ml of anesthesia are used per centimeter of donor area, so that a 25-cm-long incision would require slightly less than 20 ml of anesthetic solution. It is important to avoid injecting into the muscle, as epinephrine (adrenaline) will cause vasodilatation (due to the action on β_2-receptors), quickly dissipating the local effects of the anesthetic and increasing its toxicity.[55]

The ring-block takes approximately 15 minutes to induce anesthesia. As soon as the donor-area skin becomes numb, tumescent anesthesia is administered by injecting larger quantities of a more dilute lidocaine epinephrine (adrenaline) solution into the mid-fat to make the area firm. The tumescence serves six purposes: to widen the distance from the follicles residing in the upper fat to the nerves and larger blood vessels lying just above the fascia; to increase the rigidity of the donor area; to decrease follicular transection; to decrease bleeding; to produce more uniform anesthesia; and to reduce the amount of anesthetic required.

Tumescence can be achieved using a dilute solution of epinephrine (adrenaline) and lidocaine (Table 34.8) in somewhat higher concentrations than used in liposuction surgery, as this will provide additional anesthesia that is particularly important in repeat procedures, or for patients with significant donor scaring.[56] In situations where there is scarring, direct cutaneous innervation to the donor area from the occipital branches can be blocked so that innervation to the donor area arrives in a rostral–caudal direction, rendering inferiorly placed ring-block anesthesia ineffective. At times, when there is an excessive amount of donor scarring even the tumescence is inadequate, and the initial ring-block mixture must be injected above or directly into the scarred area to make it numb.

Follicular Unit Extraction

Follicular Unit Extraction (FUE)[2] is a conceptually simple procedure, where individual follicular units are harvested through a small circular incision created by a trephine or similar instrument. The punch cuts into the reticular dermis and the remainder of the follicular unit is literally extracted from the scalp. The advantage of this procedure is that it obviates the need for a linear incision. Difficulties lie in the intrinsic variability of each patient with respect to the ease of extraction, the increased risk of follicular transection compared to other techniques, and the organizational limitations of not being able to have multiple persons (more than two) working in parallel, as with microscopic dissection.

FUE is appropriate for patients who have limited hair loss and who want to wear their hair so short that a linear donor scar might become visible. The procedure is also useful in patients who have healed poorly, or who have very tight scalps. An important application of this technique is to camouflage a linear donor scar from a prior hair transplant procedure.[2]

FUE's main limitation is that it is less efficient in harvesting hair than follicular unit transplantation performed with strip harvesting. In FUT, all the hair from the optimal (central) part of the donor region can be removed and transplanted, and the resulting defect is sewn closed. In contrast, the FUE defects remain open to heal by second intention with significant amounts of intervening hair left behind and, therefore, a much larger region must be accessed to harvest the necessary amount of donor hair.

With FUE, the second intention healing causes microscopic fibrotic changes in the donor area, distorting adjacent follicular units and making subsequent sessions more difficult. As mentioned, transection during the harvest is greater than stereo-microscopically controlled FUT. Taken together, these factors limit the total amount of hair that can be accessed through FUE rendering it a less robust procedure than Follicular Unit Transplantation. In a procedure where a finite donor supply is the main constraint, inefficient use of donor tissue poses a significant problem. Table 34.9 summarizes the pros and cons of this follicular unit extraction.

The ability to perform FUE with minimal transection varies significantly among patients. Because of this, a test measuring the ease of extraction (the FOX Test)[2] should be performed prior to recommending the procedure. Patients undergoing follicular unit transplantation should also be tested for follicular unit extraction at the time of surgery, in case the latter procedure is needed (or desired) at a future date. It is encouraging that follicular unit extraction techniques continue to improve.

Strip excision

The ideal position for the donor incision is in the mid-portion of the permanent zone lying at the level of the external occipital protuberance. A 1-cm-wide donor strip is excised using two parallel blades set 1.2 cm apart. (The extra 2 mm accounts for the skin stretched from the tumescence.) A convenient harvesting device is the Rassman handle that is loaded with two #10 blades. The handle holds the blades at an angle of 30°, making them parallel to the emergent hair.[1] The handle should hold the blades in a pre-angled position; otherwise, in following the angle of the hair, the surgeon may cut superficially with the upper blade while too deep into the scalp with the lower (Fig. 34.7). Once the main parallel portion of the incision is complete, a single scalpel blade is used to taper the ends into an ellipse. In general, the length of each tapered end should measure at least one and half times the width of the strip, so that the ends lie flat (Fig. 34.8).

Alternatively, the entire excision can be performed with a long free-hand ellipse after the skin is marked.[9] This allows the angle of the blade to be adjusted as each edge is cut. On the other hand, this technique makes it harder to keep the width uniform, which is necessary for predictable graft yields. Cutting the second edge also becomes more difficult because the rigidity of the tumescence is lost. The first incision renders the second wound edge mobile and there is more distortion of the wound edge and hair follicles

Table 34.9 Pros and cons of follicular unit extraction

Pros	Cons
No linear scar	Requires multiple sessions to equal the size of a single follicular unit transplantation procedure
Useful when the patient wants (or needs) to wear the hair styled back from the face and with the sides very short	Takes longer to perform and is more expensive than follicular unit transplantation
Provides an alternative when the scalp is too tight for a primary closure or when the patient heals with widened scars	Risks the eventual loss of transplanted grafts by harvesting from outside the 'sweet spot' of permanent hair in the donor zone
Ideal for camouflaging donor scars that cannot be excised	After large numbers of grafts are harvested, fine stippled scars may become visible due to thinning of donor area
Makes it possible to harvest non-scalp hair (e.g. beard or body hair)	Scarring and distortion of follicles may make further harvesting by follicular unit extraction difficult
	Maximum possible yield lower than with follicular unit transplantation

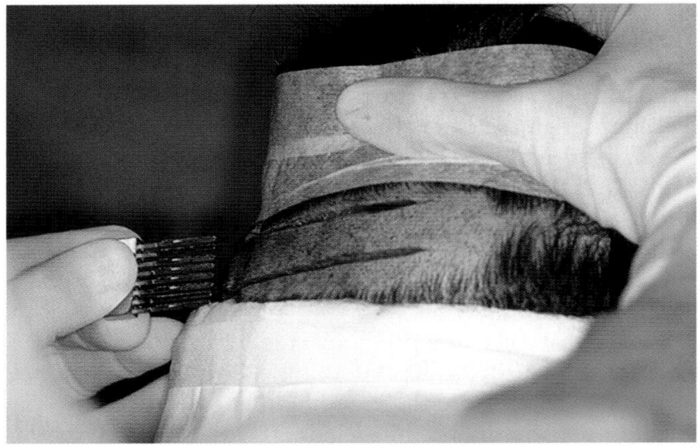

Figure 34.7 Donor-strip harvesting using two parallel blades on a Rassman handle pre-angled at 30° to allow both blades to lie flush against the scalp.

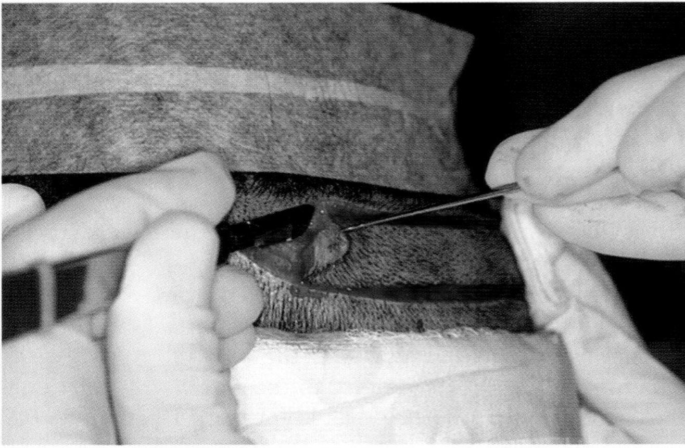

Figure 34.8 Dissection at the tapered corner of the strip in a mid-subcutaneous plane, just below the follicles.

due to the relative elasticity of the dermis compared to the epidermis and fat.

Donor closure

Once the strip is removed it is immediately placed into a chilled Ringer's lactate solution. The donor wound is sutured with a running 5-0 suture made of poliglecaprone 25,[57] although a wide variety of suture materials and techniques are available.[58,59] Absorbable sutures can be placed very close to the wound edge, so close that they are quickly buried after the procedure making removal difficult. Placing sutures close to the wound edge minimizes entrapment of follicles and avoids strangulation if there is significant postoperative edema. To further limit damage to follicles, the sutures should be placed approximately 4.5 mm apart and the suture should be advanced on the surface, rather than under the skin (as in traditional surgery), as this will minimize the amount of suture in contact with the follicles (Fig. 34.9).

The needle should be passed through the full thickness of the dermis and exit the wound edge just below it (at the level of the bulbs) without incorporating any significant amount of subcutaneous tissue. The needle track must be kept parallel to, and within 1.5 mm of the wound edge (Fig. 34.10). Particular attention should be paid to placing the needle parallel to the upper wound edge where the angle is very acute. Basic guidelines for using poliglecaprone 25 sutures can be found in Table 34.10.

If staples are used to close the wound edges, it is important to be certain that the wound edges are flush before the staples are applied. The edges can be approximated by grasping the lower edge with a skin hook and using rat-toothed forceps to hold and slightly evert the upper edge (this requires the help of an assistant). The staples should then be placed approximately 0.6 cm apart (Fig. 34.11). Staples have virtually no tissue reactivity, but they make flush apposition of wound edges difficult and can be uncomfortable and painful to remove. In the balance we prefer absorbable sutures, though staples may be better for some patients with high density and very loose scalps.[57]

Graft dissection

Once the donor strip is removed, it is immediately placed into lactated Ringer's solution and passed to the head member of the surgical team stationed at a stereomicroscope (Fig. 34.12). The strip dimensions are measured and recorded. The next step is performed under strict stereomicroscopic control in a process called 'slivering.'[10,35]

In one method of slivering, the donor strip is placed on its side, on a wooden tongue-depressor blade (soaked in

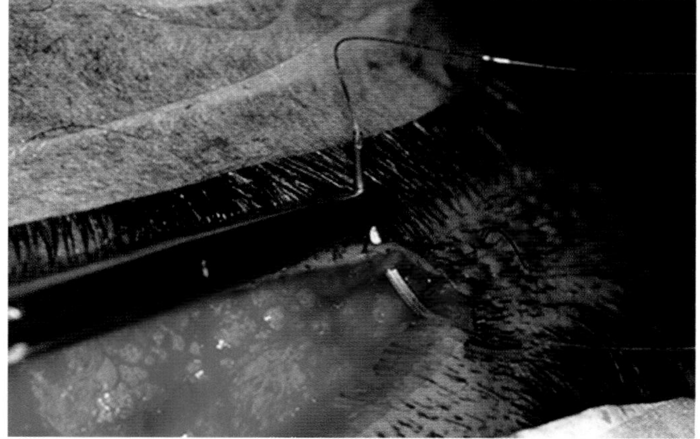

Figure 34.9 Suturing the donor area using absorbable sutures. Note the needle track is parallel and very close to the wound edges.[57]

Suturing technique for sewing donor scalp

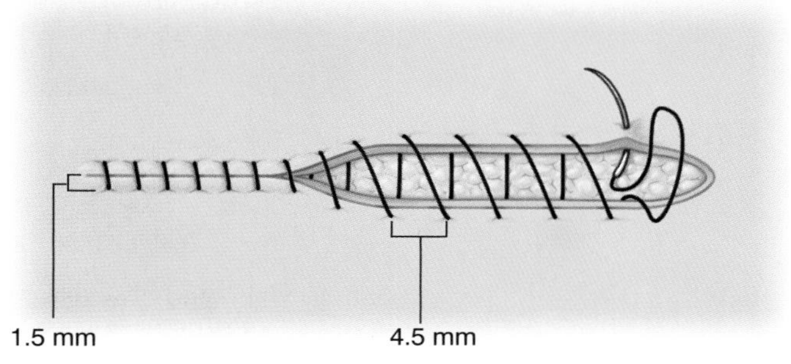

Figure 34.10 Schematic of the suturing technique recommended for sewing the donor scalp. The spacing between loops is 4.5 mm.[57]

Table 34.10 Guidelines for use of poliglecaprone 25 sutures

Plan width of donor strip so that there is little or no tension on closure
Use tumescent anesthesia to harvest donor strip in mid-fat
Use sutures no heavier than 5-0
Use a simple running stitch, advancing each loop on the skin surface
Keep needle parallel to and within 1.5 mm of wound edge
Incorporate epidermis and dermis only
Use 4.5 mm spacing between loops

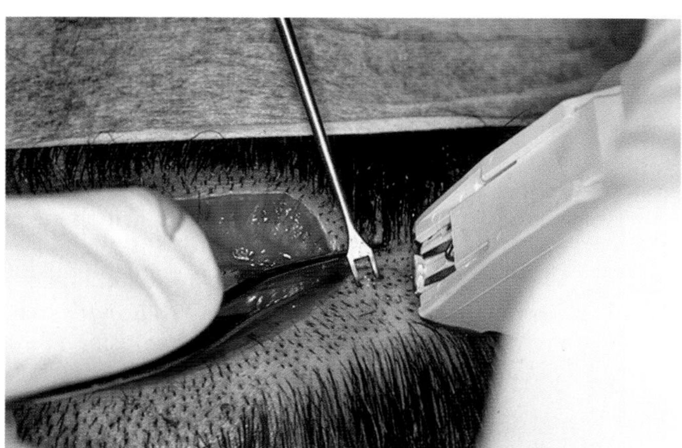

Figure 34.11 Stapling technique illustrating very controlled apposition of wound edges, using skin hooks for the lower edge, and forceps to evert the upper.[57]

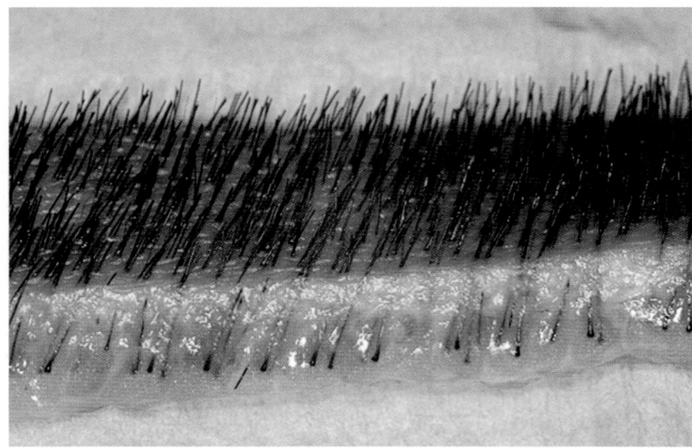

Figure 34.12 Close-up view of a donor strip showing the natural hair groupings at the surface, the slightly curved path of the hair through the dermis, and the random distribution of bulbs in the fat. It is this unique anatomy that makes stereomicroscopic dissection essential in preventing follicular transection.

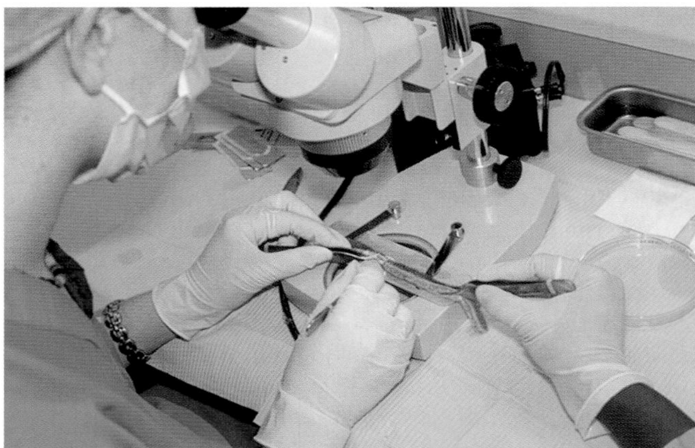

Figure 34.13 'Slivering' the donor strip into sections.

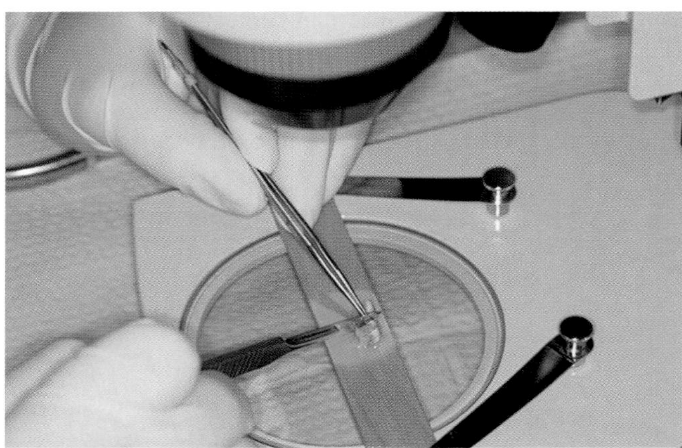

Figure 34.14 Stereomicroscopic dissection of one section into smaller pieces.

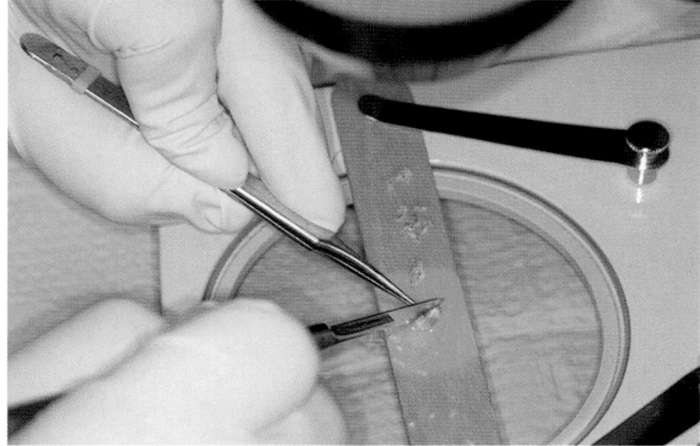

Figure 34.15 The final step of the dissection: generating individual follicular units.

Ringer's) with the hair pointing away from the dissector and the convex surface of the strip facing upward. For a right-handed person performing dissection, the left end of the strip is held with rat-toothed forceps in the dissector's left hand. An assistant applies tension to the strip, holding it a few centimeters away from the area being cut with rat-toothed forceps held in the right hand. Using a Personna #10 blade on a #3 blade handle held in the right hand, the dissector begins to cut the strip into 2–2.5 mm wide sections, by guiding the blade between follicular units using a one-directional fillet-like movement from the epidermal side to the subcutaneous surface. A back-and-forth sawing motion should be avoided as it will increase the risk of transection (Figs 34.13, 34.14). The pieces generated are then passed along to the other members of the surgical team who complete the dissection. In the last step, the individual pieces are placed on their sides, stabilized with straight jeweler's forceps, and then dissected under the stereomicroscope with a scalpel into individual follicular units of one to four hairs (Figs 34.15, 34.16).

Next, the units are sorted according to the number of hairs they contain into separate Petri dishes held on ice blocks and filled with Ringer's lactate (Fig. 34.17). When a substantial number of grafts (several hundred) have been dissected, they are put into more secure plastic specimen containers and refrigerated.

An alternate slivering method involves dissecting the donor strip into slivers as wide as one follicular unit, approximately 1 mm. The units are then isolated from the very thin strip. The key to either method is that every step is performed under stereomicroscopic control, which keeps the units intact and avoids follicular transection. It is also vital that all the pieces of the strip remain in chilled Ringer's lactate except when they are being cut. While under the microscope, they should be kept well-hydrated using 10-ml syringes containing Ringer's lactate, kept by each cutting surface.

Recipient sites

The way recipient sites are prepared determines the critical aesthetic factors of the transplant: the angle at which the new hair grows, its distribution, its density, and how natural the hair will look as it emerges from the scalp. A thorough discussion of site creation is beyond the scope of this chapter, but the four basic elements will be briefly reviewed. These are recipient site size, hair direction, site density, and graft distribution, and they are covered in greater detail in Bernstein and Rassman.[8]

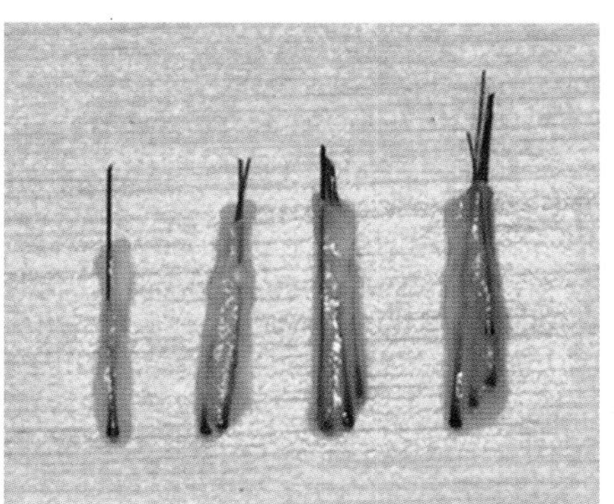

Figure 34.16 Dissected one-hair, two-hair, three-hair, and four-hair follicular units.

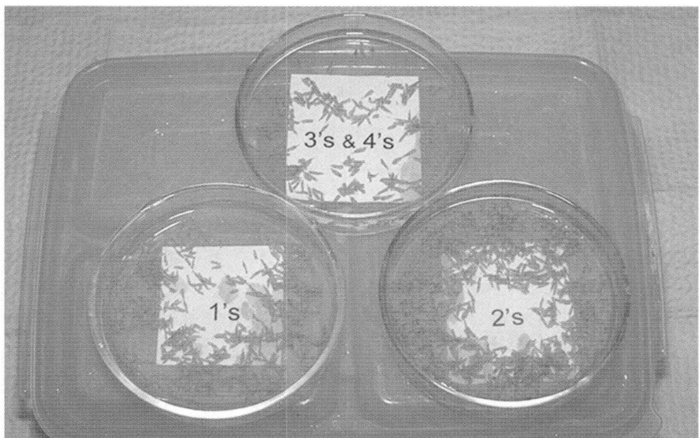

Figure 34.17 Petri dishes with one-hair to four-hair follicular units immersed in Ringer's lactate.

Recipient site sizes and orientation

The sites should provide a snug fit for the graft: just large enough to accommodate a follicular unit, but not so small that insertion is difficult or traumatic.[1] Numerous instruments have been developed to create recipient sites. The main aspect to consider in choosing one is its diameter.[60] Although there are many viable options, the following are used by many practitioners:

- a 19- or 20-gauge hypodermic needle for one-hair and thin two-hair follicular unit grafts
- an 18-gauge needle for thick two-hair and all three- and four-hair follicular unit grafts

These needles can be fitted on 3-ml syringes for ease of use, obviating expensive handles. Some physicians advocate smaller recipient sites, but this may require dividing four-hair follicular units—a technique that this author does not recommend.[35] For very fine hair, or in special situations like transplanting eyebrows, a 20-gauge (or finer) needle can be used.

Most instruments used to make sites create tiny slits as they cut through the skin and these slits can have either a coronal (horizontal) or sagittal (vertical) orientation. The purported advantages of coronal incisions are: a more natural appearance (since the original orientation of most follicular units seems to be coronal); a fuller look; and less tendency of the growing hair to elevate in the vertical plane. The purported advantages of a sagittal orientation are:

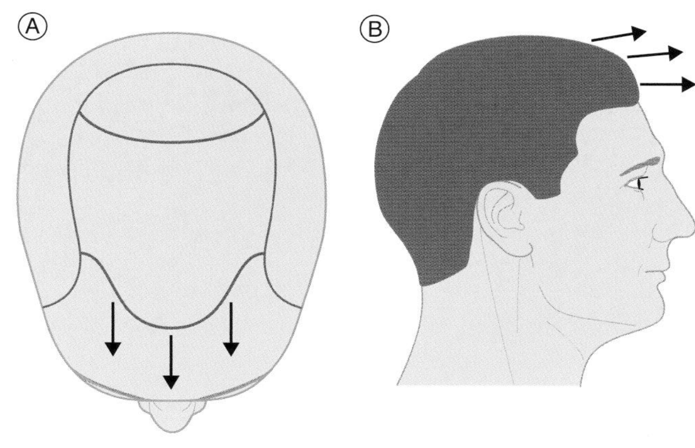

Figure 34.18 Normal hair direction. (A) Top view and (B) side view.[8]

greater visibility of sites; ease of graft placement; less trauma to existing hair; and less lateral (radial) splay of hair.

Hair direction

Hair should be placed into the scalp at the angle it originally grew in, not in the direction that it is to be groomed. In general, hair anterior to the vertex transition point should point forward, with the angle becoming more acute as it reaches the anterior hairline, where it is essentially horizontal to the ground (regardless of the slope of the forehead). The direction of hair in the frontal hairline points forward, rather than growing radially, and only deviates significantly from this as it approaches the temples (Fig. 34.18).[8]

Recipient site density

The average non-balding scalp has 100 follicular units per cm^2. Approximately 50% may be lost before there is any noticeable thinning. It would be wasteful, therefore, for more than 50% to be replaced—especially because transplants are always performed in the face of diminished total hair volume. We generally recommend transplanting up to 25 follicular units per cm^2 into the frontal area of a balding scalp in the first session. If the larger three-hair and four-hair units are placed in select areas, more than 25% of the initial density can be achieved in one pass. With two procedures the ideal transplant density can be achieved in many patients.[8]

Some physicians advocate a 'one-pass' procedure to achieve the final density.[35] Although this may be appropriate for some patients, the increased incidence of graft popping and desiccation, insertion injury, and possible vascular compromise may lead to poor growth. For very bald patients, very dense packing does not allow coverage of an entire bald area. Moreover, transplants of more than 2500–3000 follicular units often necessitate that the grafts be out of the body so long that their survival may be diminished. It is this author's view that covering the entire bald area and then increasing density in a subsequent session is a better goal for most patients.

Distribution

For simplicity, the area of the scalp subject to androgenetic change can be divided into three regions: the frontal region that includes the frontal hairline; the top or mid-scalp; and the vertex or crown. The vertex transition point separates the top of the scalp from the crown (Fig. 34.19).[34] As most social interaction takes place face to face, and people generally view themselves from the front, the overall impact of the transplant is defined by the position of the frontal hairline and density of the frontal region of the scalp.

For most patients who are moderately or extensively bald, or are destined to be, the limitations of the donor supply make restoring the entire bald scalp to ideal density impossible. Consequently, creating the greatest density in the front part of the scalp produces the best cosmetic result. This 'forward weighting' can be accomplished by putting recipient sites closer together, placing larger follicular units (i.e. those with three and four hairs) in those sites, or by doing both.

In general, recipient site density should be the highest in the front part of the scalp and gradually tapered toward the crown. In contrast, the largest follicular units should be placed in the forelock region of the scalp. This overlapping distribution of sites and follicular unit grafts may be visualized in Figure 34.20. It is explained in greater detail in Bernstein and Rassman.[8] The pattern serves two functions: it creates a natural central-forelock density without the need for spacing sites closer towards the mid-scalp (where the blood supply can most easily be compromised) and ensures the most natural look by placing the larger follicular units in a forward-central position, but away from the frontal hairline. Density in the forelock area brings about a 'patterned look' and avoids the diffuse thinning that often results when small grafts are evenly distributed over the scalp.

Practically every patient has enough donor hair to provide at least light coverage extending to the vertex transition point. This is a natural stopping point because, even if the crown continues to enlarge, transplants performed to this point will still look natural without additional surgery. Transplants should be extended past the vertex transition point into the crown only when there is adequate hair to create a swirl and follow the hair loss if the balding progresses. The indications for transplanting the crown are discussed in detail in Bernstein and Rassman.[7]

The distribution of grafts in the first transplant session should, in general, be symmetric. However, once the first transplant has had a chance to grow and the patient is willing to commit to styling his hair in a specific pattern, 'side weighting' should be considered. This is accomplished either by placing a greater proportion of the grafts on the parted side of the scalp, using larger follicular units on that side, or doing both. It results in increased fullness when one's hair is combed to the side. In situations where there is a great imbalance in the supply/demand ratio, such as after scalp reductions or old plug procedures, a more exaggerated form of 'side weighting' should be considered. In this case the follicular unit grafts are concentrated on the front and part side of the scalp, but widely scattered in the top and back (Fig. 34.21).[8]

The number of follicular unit grafts required in the first and subsequent transplant sessions, with and without crown coverage, can be found in Tables 34.4 and 34.5.

When the follicular units are completely dissected and grouped in Petri dishes they are placed at the head of the

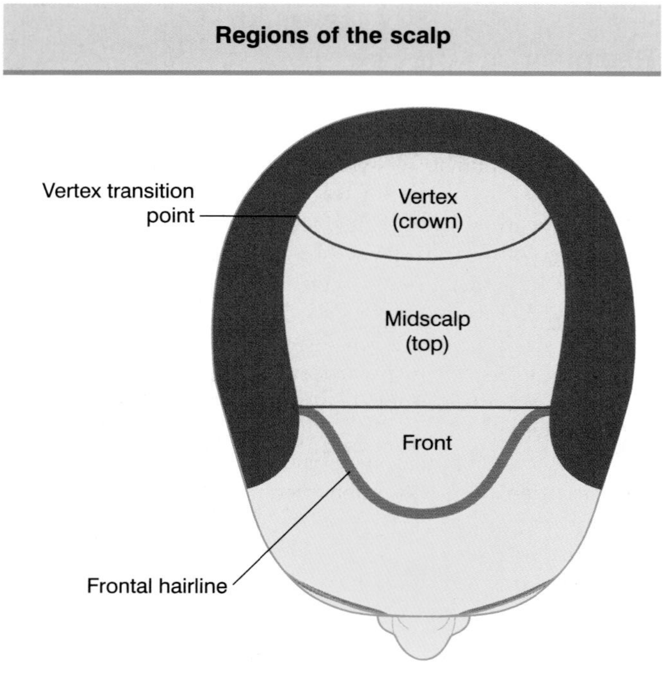

Regions of the scalp

Figure 34.19 Regions of the scalp.

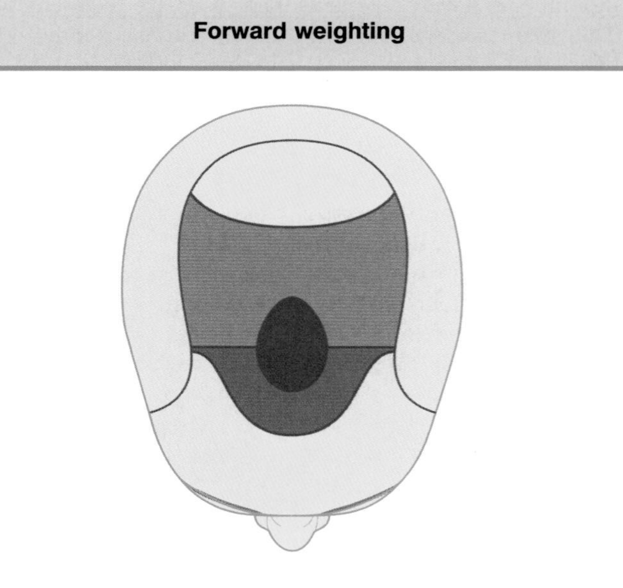

Figure 34.20 Schematic of 'forward weighting,' achieved by close placement of recipient sites (shaded dark grey), and central density, accomplished by placing larger follicular units in the forelock area (dark brown oval).

operating table on ice blocks. Graft placement, carried out in a front-to-back pattern, begins at the frontal hairline with one-hair follicular units. In a typical transplant, approximately 250 one-hair units are used for the leading edge of the frontal hairline, immediately followed by two-hair grafts. Three-hair to four-hair units are concentrated in the forelock area (Fig. 34.22), while toward the back and sides the pattern is reversed so that the three-hair and four-hair units are always central to the one-hair and two-hair units.

Approximately 20–30 grafts are transferred at one time from the dish to the index finger, held on the finger in a droplet of Ringer's solution. The grafts are inserted using curved jeweler's forceps. Each graft should be carefully grasped by the fat at its bottom or at its edge, not at the germinative center. In the two-handed technique, gauze—held between the free fingers of the hand holding the grafts—is used to keep the partially inserted grafts in place as the forceps are repositioned higher along the length of the graft, to facilitate the last phase of insertion.

In an alternative method, termed 'stick and place', the grafts are inserted at the same time that the recipient sites are made.[35] In this technique, the needle that is used to make the recipient hole can also serve as a 'shoehorn' to help guide the graft into the site. The advantage of this method is that it eliminates the possibility that sites may be left unfilled or that two grafts may be placed into one site (piggybacking). It also moves the surgery along faster, since the staff does not need to wait for the surgeon to make the sites and they do not need to search for the ones that are empty.

On the other hand, there is more bleeding when sites are made concomitantly with graft placement (decreasing visibility) and there is an increased risk of the grafts popping and then drying out on the surface of the scalp. In addition, the staff must make judgments regarding the angling and distribution of the sites they are creating at a time when they must also be focusing on the technical aspects of graft insertion. This leaves many of the aesthetic decisions in the hands of the technicians, who are actively engaged in stick and place, rather than with the physician who could take a more strategic view of the procedure.

Side weighting

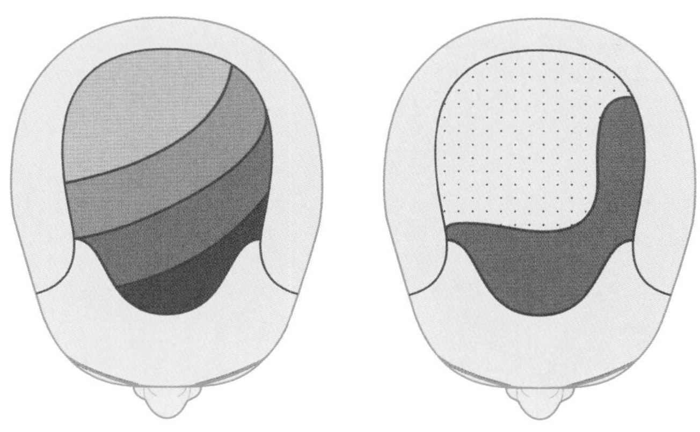

Figure 34.21 Left shows schematic view of left-to-right 'side weighting.' Right shows extreme side weighting employed when the donor supply is severely diminished.

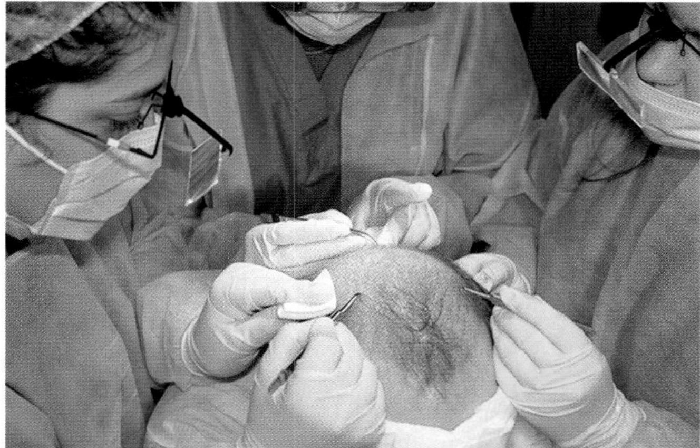

Figure 34.22 Staff using loop magnification and curved jeweler's forceps to place follicular unit grafts into pre-made recipient sites.

Patient disposition

After graft insertion is complete, the scalp is cleaned with distilled water, bacitracin zinc ointment is applied to the sutures and a head-band type pressure dressing is placed over the donor area. The transplanted area is covered with a surgeon's cap. Prior to leaving, patients are given verbal and printed postoperative instructions, a neck pillow and medications for sleep and pain (Table 34.11). Patients leave the office wearing a bandana covering the cap and the headband. It is worth stressing that patients given sedatives or pain medication do not drive after surgery.

Table 34.11 Common medications in hair transplant

Class	Medication	Use
Topical antibacterials	Hibiclens	Preoperative
Systemic antibiotics	Dicloxacillin, cephalosporin	Intraoperative prophylaxis*
Sedatives/hypnotics	Diazepam, aprazolam	Intraoperative sedation
Corticosteroids	Betamethasone	Postoperative swelling
Topical antibiotics	Bacitracin ointment	Postoperative care, donor area
Opiates	Hydrocodone	PRN, postoperative pain
Antihiccup agents	Chlorpromazine	PRN, hiccups
Analgesics	Nitrous oxide[55]	PRN during injections†
Wound healing promoters	Copper-peptide	Postoperative healing†
Hair growth promoters	Finasteride, minoxidil	Pre and postoperative*

**See text.*
†Not used in our practice.

■ OPTIMIZING OUTCOMES

Transition zones

A soft natural hairline is the hallmark of an optimal transplant. However, careful observation of a normal frontal hairline reveals that there is no actual 'line,' but rather an irregular, slightly asymmetric 'transition zone' or gradation of follicular units of increasing size and density. This is what should be replicated in the transplant (Fig. 34.23A–B). Transition zones are not limited to the frontal hairline; they must be recreated wherever the edge of the transplanted area is visible. In Figure 34.23C, one notes that transition zones have been created at the frontal hairline, sides and vertex transition point leading to the crown.

Although there are an infinite number of ways to create a transition zone at the frontal hairline, the placement of approximately 50–100 single follicular units in front of a band of staggered single units, one to three rows deep, will usually achieve the appropriate softness. This should be followed by two-, three- and eventually four-hair units, but the larger units should be more centrally located (Fig. 34.23B). With finer hair, larger units may be placed closer to the hairline. It is important to limit the depth of the single hair units, or the zone will appear too thin.

Visibility

Pre-making all the recipient sites before graft insertion helps to control bleeding and limits the need for epinephrine (adrenaline) (Fig. 34.23C). It initiates the 'extrinsic pathway' so that coagulation can begin before the grafts are introduced and allows for easy cleaning of the recipient area of any blood or coagulum, without the risk of dislodging grafts. It also makes it possible to place sites close together without a concern for grafts in adjacent sites from popping. Most importantly, it provides maximum visibility in the placing phase of the procedure.[46]

If the initial sites are scattered, they tend to cause the cutaneous vasculature of the scalp to 'clamp down', increasing visibility for subsequent passes and allowing the skipped areas to be filled in. When pre-marking sites, the logistics of matching the number of sites to the number of grafts can be solved by making 'projections' of the anticipated number of grafts while the dissection is still in progress.

Recipient site influences

Some hair characteristics, such as waviness, are governed by the recipient site. When individual follicular units are placed into very small wounds, there is little fibrotic reaction to the grafts and the recipient area can exert its influences on hair growth. In Figure 34.24, note the delicate wave produced by the recipient scalp. It sometimes takes a year or more for the hair character to return to normal.

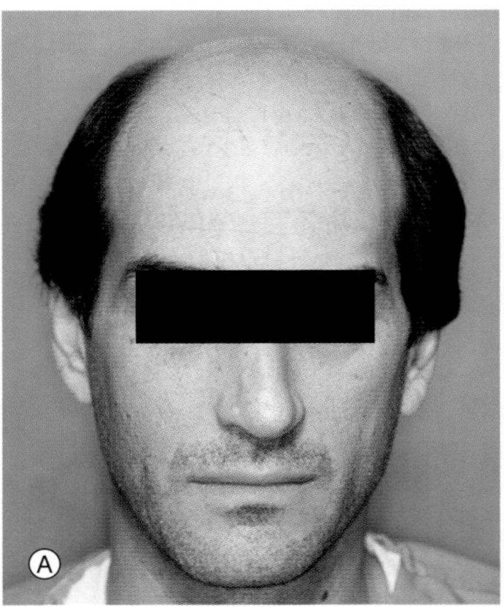

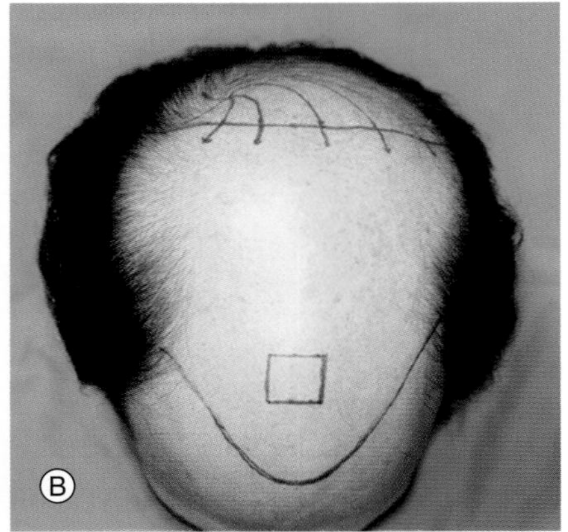

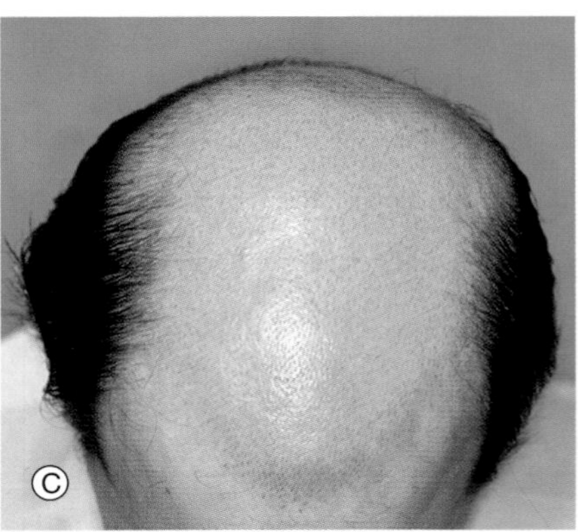

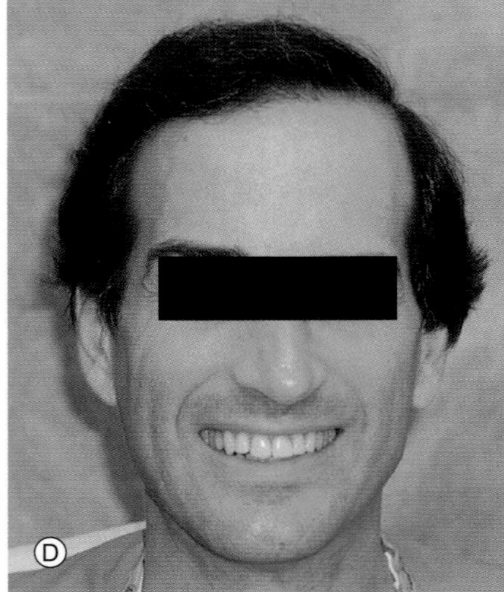

Figure 34.23 (A) Before and (D) 1 year after two sessions totaling 4295 follicular unit grafts. (B) Preoperative markings of the planned procedure. (C) First session just before placement, showing the distribution of 2355 recipient sites.

Hair direction

When the hair is planted at the frontal hairline in its natural forward-pointing direction, combing it back causes it to bow, giving it the appearance of fullness. A common mistake is to point the hair in the direction that the patient plans to comb their hair; this makes the hair lie flat and bodiless when groomed. On the other hand, as the frontal hairline approaches the temples, the hair direction should be abruptly changed, so that it is angled downward and lying very flat on the scalp. Perfect integration of the frontal hairline with hair on the sides and temples is essential if the transplant is to look completely natural (Fig. 34.25).

Hairline placement

If it is to look natural throughout the patient's life, the transplanted hairline must simulate that of a mature adult. In the adolescent male, the frontal hairline touches the top crease of the brow when the eyebrows are raised (that is, the hair begins at the upper border of the frontalis muscle). In a mature adult, the mid-portion of the frontal hairline rests approximately one finger-breadth (1.5–2 cm) above the brow crease. Although the degree of temple recession can vary dramatically in the normal adult hairline, the mid-part of the frontal hairline is crucial in framing the face.[1,8] Significant bitemporal recession was built into the restoration of the patient in Figure 34.26, yet the forward-placed mid-portion sets his facial features in the correct proportions.

Forelock integration

A persistent frontal forelock poses an interesting dilemma. When hair is transplanted around the forelock, the patient may be left with a gap in his frontal hairline if the forelock eventually disappears. On the other hand, it is wasteful to add hair to a forelock with adequate density that may persist for years. The solution is to check for miniaturization with a densitometer. The patient in

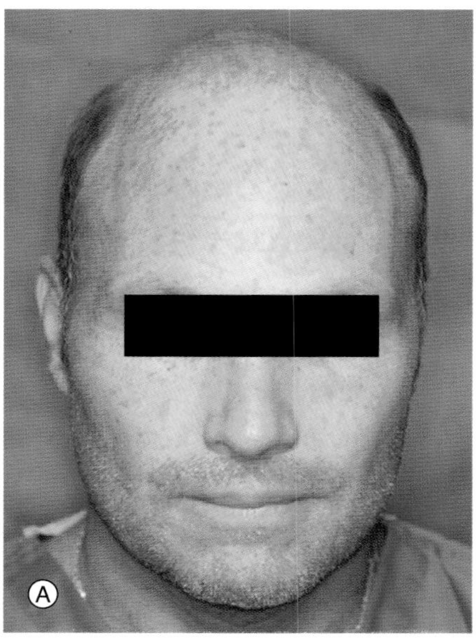

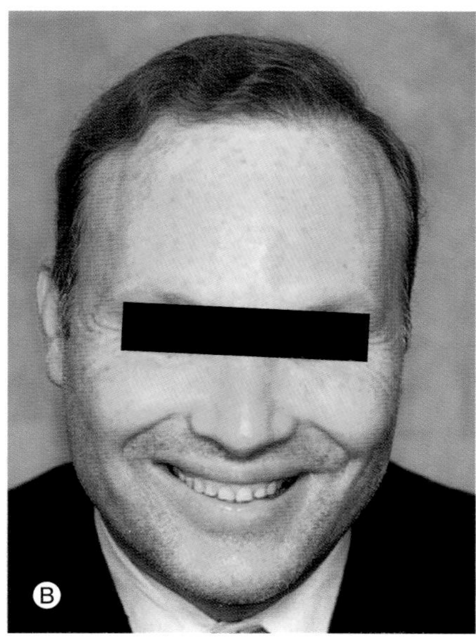

Figure 34.24 Norwood class VI, with very fine, blonde hair, and a donor density of 2.5 hairs per mm^2. (A) Before and (B) 1 year after two sessions of 2678 and 1836 follicular unit grafts.

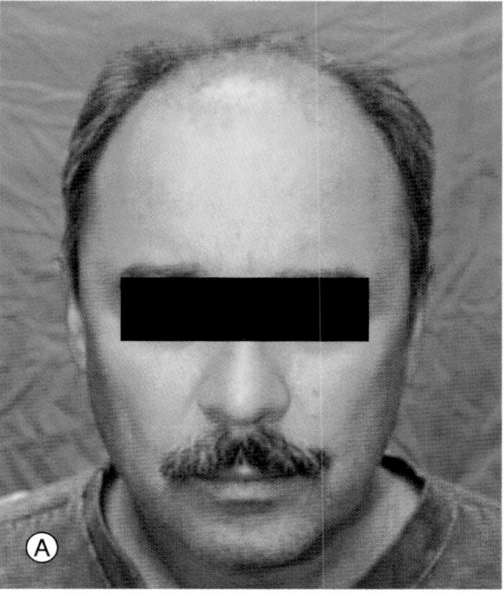

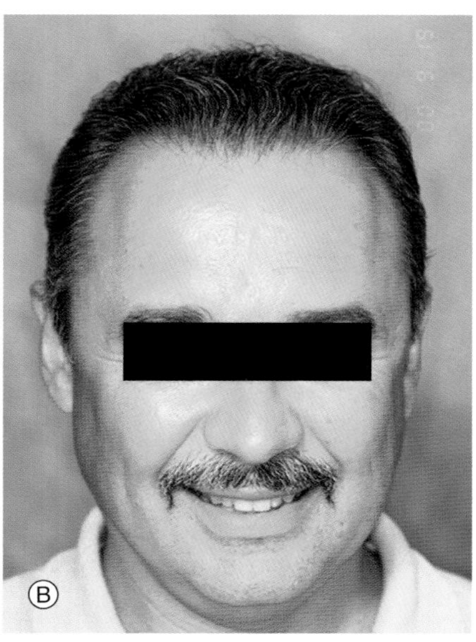

Figure 34.25 Early Norwood class VI. (A) Before and (B) 1 year after one session of 2520 follicular unit grafts.

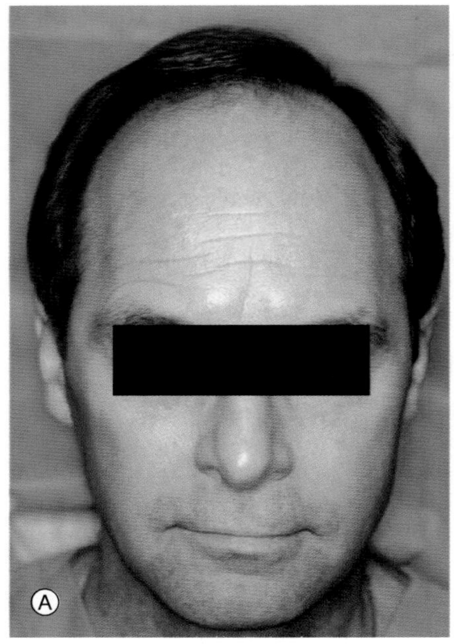

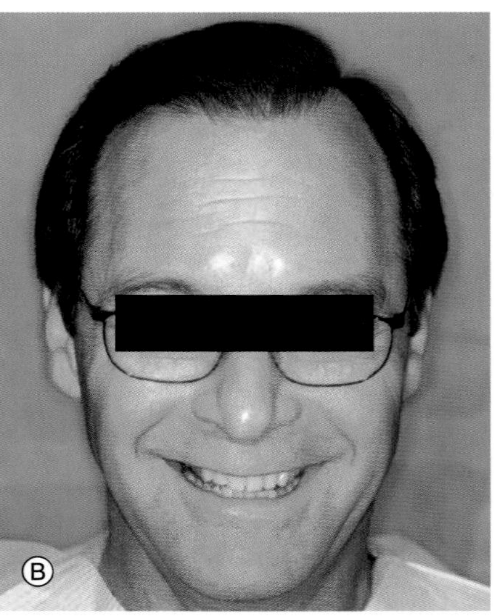

Figure 34.26 Early Norwood class V. (A) Before and (B) 1 year following two sessions of 2105 and 1665 follicular unit grafts.

Figure 34.27 had miniaturization in his forelock greater than 50%, suggesting that it would not be stable over time. Two sessions were used to integrate transplanted hair into the resident terminal hair of the forelock, producing a central density that will be permanent.

Optimizing density

One of the beauties of FUT is the ability to sort the three-hair and four-hair units and place them in the forelock area, creating a density significantly greater than if the grafts were evenly distributed. This is possible because the compactness of the follicular unit allows four-hair grafts to be placed into very small sites.[6,8] In certain instances, follicular units may contain more than four hairs, and adjacent follicular units are occasionally so close together that they can fit into a small recipient site.[61,62] However, as long as these 'grouped grafts' are placed in a central location and the recipient wounds are kept small, this technique can add density without risking an unnatural look. It is important to keep in mind that ultimate density depends on the absolute number of hairs moved rather than the size of the grafts.[63] Using grafts larger than follicular units always risks that the transplant may look unnatural. The patient in Figure 34.28 achieved a very dramatic frontal density in two sessions using the technique of follicular unit sorting.

Creating camouflage

A sizable part of many practices involves repairing transplants performed with older techniques. FUT is ideal for this because of the small size of follicular units and high hair count.[64,65] Often fixing a 'pluggy' look requires graft excision (with reimplantation) before the actual transplant. However, the patient in Figure 34.29 had a row of plugs set far enough back from his frontal hairline that camouflage with follicular units alone was sufficient for the repair.

Automation

Short of cloning follicular units in a Petri dish, the future in FUT optimization lies in the development of automated devices that can harvest the donor strip, isolate individual follicular units, create recipient sites, and insert grafts—all without the risk of human variability or error. A number of creative instruments have been designed toward this end, but thus far their success has been limited.[66–69] Much of the difficulty lies in the inherent variability of the human scalp and the follicular unit itself. The full automation of a procedure that is labor intensive, organizationally complex, and dependent on the aesthetic judgment of the surgeon remains a formidable challenge.

■ POSTOPERATIVE CARE

Patients are called at home the day after the procedure and seen in our office 1 week postoperatively. They come in again 10 months later to assess growth, have their pictures taken, and to discuss the possibility of additional surgery. Those with questions or concerns are seen as frequently as needed. Table 34.12 summarizes typical postoperative instructions.

■ PITFALLS AND THEIR MANAGEMENT

A number of problems arising in hair transplant surgery have been well described in the literature. Table 34.13 summarizes them, along with their most likely cause (though some etiologies may be multifactorial) and methods for preventing and managing them should they occur.[12,70,71]

Although FUT eliminates many of the shortcomings of the older techniques, such as a 'pluggy' look, a 'moth-eaten' donor area, or midline scalp reduction scars, poor aesthetic judgment and techniques that compromise graft growth can still lead to problems. Perhaps because FUT requires large numbers of grafts (using a significant portion of the donor

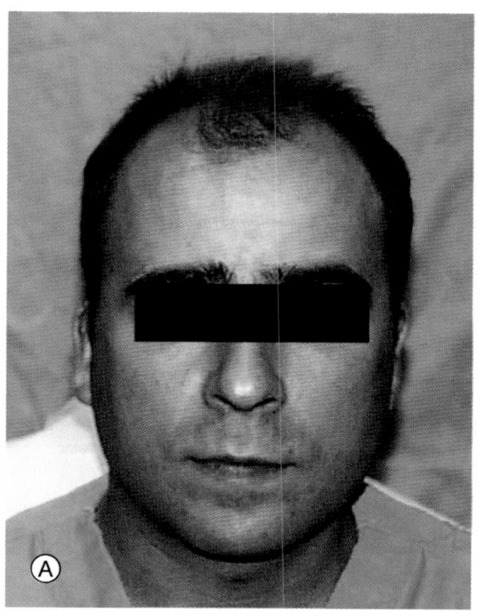

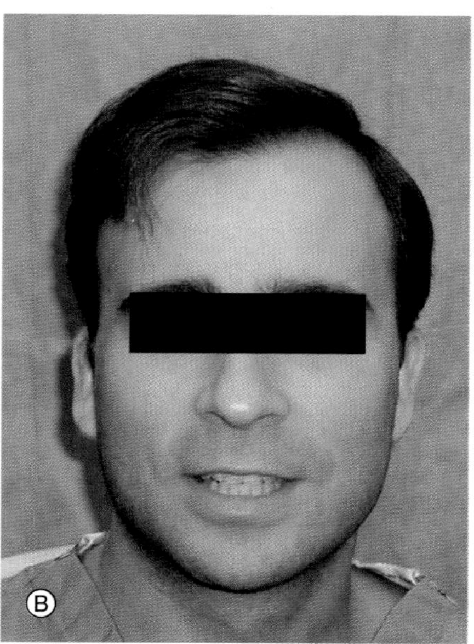

Figure 34.27 Norwood class V. (A) Before procedure. (B) Integrating hair with a persistent frontal forelock (1 year following two sessions of 2133 and 1171 follicular unit grafts).

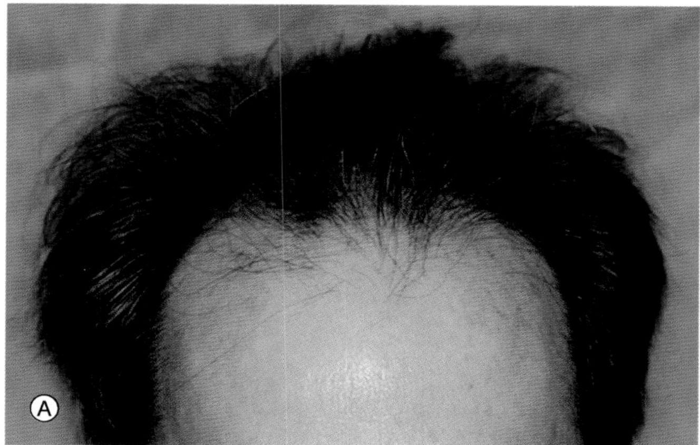

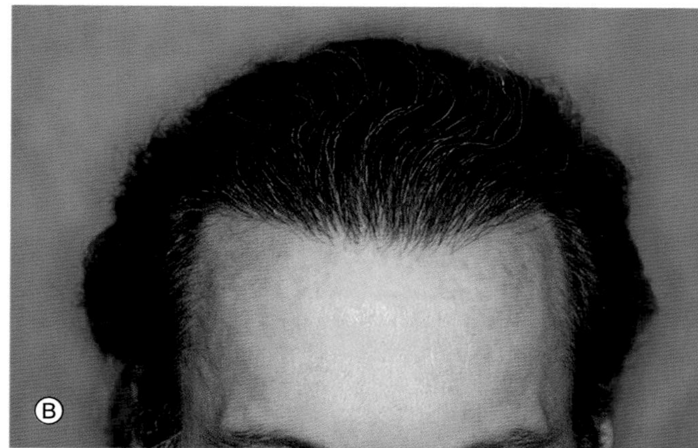

Figure 34.28 46-year-old early Norwood class IVa with wavy medium-coarse hair. (A) Before transplant. (B) After two sessions of 2085 and 1438 follicular unit grafts.

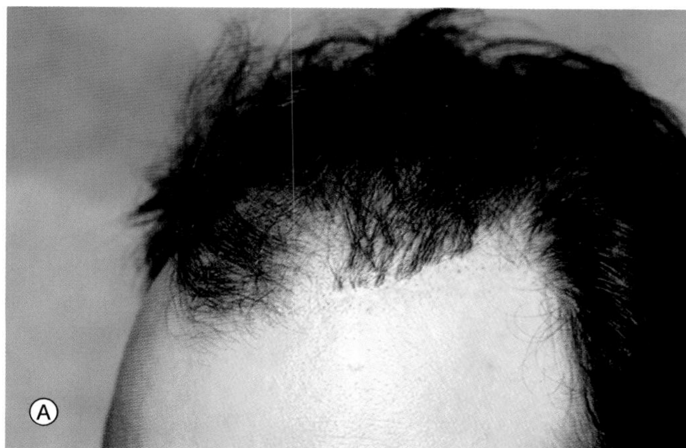

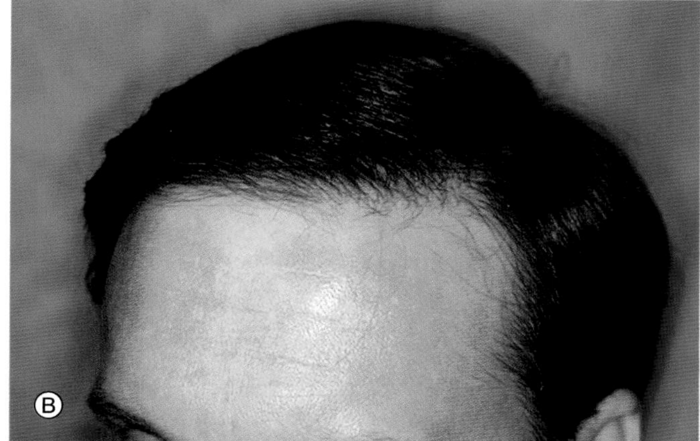

Figure 34.29 (A) Before transplant, showing large grafts forming a literal wall of plugs. (B) Camouflage from one session of 1818 follicular units.

Table 34.12 Summary of instructions following follicular unit transplantation	
Care of transplanted area	Shampoo every 3–4 hours the day following surgery and then twice daily until the 1-week postoperative visit. Be especially careful when cleaning the transplanted site in the first few days so that the grafts will not be dislodged. However, a thorough but gentle rinsing of the recipient area will minimize crusting and make the transplant less noticeable. When shampooing and rinsing the transplanted area, be gentle for the first 2 weeks following surgery. Do not rub, pick, or scratch, as this may dislodge grafts.
Care of sutured area and non-transplanted parts of scalp	Gently wash the sutured area with your fingertips using a copper peptide-containing shampoo. Shower water may hit the sutured area in the back of your scalp directly. You may use a hair dryer set on warm, but not hot. Do not use any scalp or hair-coloring agents for at least 2 weeks after your procedure.
Postoperative medications	After your procedure, you will be given sleeping medication and medication for pain. Itching: You may experience some itching either in the transplanted area or sutured area following your procedure. Hydrocortisone ointment may be applied locally to the areas that itch as needed, up to four times a day. Swelling: You will be given an injection of cortisone during your procedure to decrease swelling after surgery. If there is significant swelling, it usually occurs around the second to fifth postoperative day and should not be cause for concern. It resolves by itself after a few days and does not require any special treatment. Cool, wet dressings may be placed over the swollen area, but make sure they do not touch the grafts. Bleeding: Before you leave the office, all bleeding will be controlled. Rarely some bleeding may occur after the procedure. If this happens, apply firm continuous pressure on the area. If you are unable to contact us through our pager, go to the nearest emergency room and show our instructions to the physician on duty. Exercise, alcohol, smoking and other restrictions: Avoid direct trauma to the head for 2 weeks after the procedure, and abstain from sexual intercourse, alcohol use, and smoking for 3 days after the procedure. After 2 weeks, you may resume your normal daily activities. However, be careful not to stretch the donor area until instructed by your physician. Sun: Avoid unprotected exposure to sunlight for 3 months. Wear a hat when you are going to be outside or use a strong sunscreen with an SPF factor (sun protection factor) of 30+. Infection: Redness, swelling and slight tenderness are to be expected for the first few days after a procedure. Persistent swelling, pain, or tenderness in the sutured area may be a sign of infection. Fever and/or chills are indications of infection as well. There also may be a discharge or pus in the suture line. If any of these conditions should occur, please contact the office. Numbness: Scalp numbness, tingling or similar sensations may occur temporarily. This generally disappears within a few weeks to months, as nerve endings re-grow.
Hair-loss medications	Minoxidil 5%: If you plan to continue this medication, resume it 1 to 2 weeks after the procedure. Finasteride 1 mg: This medication should not be discontinued for the surgery.

area at one time), because so many staff members are involved in the process, and because some of the problems of small-graft procedures are very difficult to correct, improperly performed follicular unit transplantation can sometimes pose a greater risk to patients than traditional grafting. The risk is compounded by the fact that many physicians perceive FUT as a safe, risk-free procedure and describe it to patients as such.

The remainder of this section will focus on some of the most common mistakes made by FUT practitioners, particularly in the areas of planning, transplant design, and handling large numbers of small grafts. These problems and how they may be avoided are summarized in Table 34.14.

Operating on patients that are too young or before medical therapy

Patents in their early 20s have their flat adolescent hairline and original density fresh in their memory. A transplant designed with enough frontal and temporal recession to look good for one's entire life will rarely satisfy a younger patient. Creating a density that suits a younger person will not leave enough hair in reserve if there is further loss. In addition, at this age the extent of future balding is difficult to even reasonably anticipate. For these reasons, surgery should rarely be considered in patients with androgenetic alopecia who are younger than 25 years old.

Often doctors begin medical therapy and schedule surgery at the same time. However, if there is a possibility that using a medication, such as finasteride, can make transplantation unnecessary, then the medication should be used for at least a year before any decision on surgery is reached. Medication should be the first line of therapy for all younger patients with androgenetic alopecia, regardless of the degree of their hair loss.

Failing to identify low donor density before surgery

Earlier in this chapter (Patient Evaluation and Surgical Planning) the importance of assessing patient's donor supply with densitometry was stressed. A low donor density, generally less than 1.5 hairs per mm^2, usually indicates that donor supply is insufficient to create adequate density or coverage, rendering the procedure inadvisable. An exception might be an older person with very conservative goals. High miniaturization in the donor area, particularly in a person under the age of 30, suggests diffuse unpatterned hair loss (DUPA), which is a contraindication to surgery.[7]

Transplanting patients with low donor density will also risk a visible scar if the hair is worn short. FUE is not appropriate in such cases, because it further limits the total available hair. In fact, because the contrast between bald and non-balding scalp in patients with low donor density is naturally low, their best option tends to be wearing their hair short, to decrease the contrast further (rather than having surgery).

Table 34.13 Problems of follicular unit hair transplantation and their management

Problem	Cause	Prevention	Treatment
Syncope	Anxiety, vasovagal reaction	Premedicate with diazepam or atropine, administer local anesthesia with patient lying flat	Lie patient supine and elevate legs
Anxiety, palpitations	β_1- and α-adrenergic effects of epinephrine (adrenaline)	Administer epinephrine slowly, premedicate with diazepam	Patience (the half-life of epinephrine is short); lidocaine for arrhythmias
Hypertension, bradycardia	Epinephrine (adrenaline) interaction with β-blocker	Use selective β_1-blockers	α-adrenergic blockers; treat as cardiac emergency
Agitation, confusion, perioral numbness	Lidocaine toxicity	Use more dilute anesthetic mixture, use ring blocks rather than local infiltration	Intravenous fluids, oxygen, ventilate, Diazepam; treat as cardiac emergency
Pruritus, urticaria, angioedema	Allergic reaction or anaphylaxis to drugs or food	Careful history	Oxygen, epinephrine (adrenaline) subcutaneously
Excessive bleeding	Elevated blood pressure, non-steroidal anti-inflammatory agents	Discontinue antiplatelet agents before surgery, continue antihypertensive medications on day of surgery, pulse oximetry	Operate with patient seated; with elevated blood pressure, consider antihypertensives
Postoperative edema	Surgical trauma, buffered anesthetic	Keep recipient sites small, preoperative and post-operative systemic corticosteroids	Head elevation, additional postoperative corticosteroids
Sterile folliculitis	Growing hair trapped by epidermal overgrowth	Keep grafts slightly elevated	Resolves spontaneously; incision and drainage if persistent
Cyst formation at graft site	Foreign body reaction to imbedded graft	Avoid piggybacking one graft over another in the same site	Incision and drainage, topical and/or systemic antibiotics
Bacterial folliculitis	Picking, scratching, poor hygiene, secondary to infected sterile folliculitis or cyst	Frequent postoperative showering, topical corticosteroids for pruritus	Topical and systemic antibiotics
Infected donor wound	Suture bites too large or tight; with postoperative edema, causes vascular compromise	Harvest a narrower donor strip under less tension, change suturing technique	Systemic antibiotics; if severe, leave portion of donor area to heal by second intention
Widened scar in donor area	Donor strip too wide or placed too low, patient tendency to heal with stretched scar	Careful history, conservative donor strip located at level of occipital protuberance	Excision ± (can worsen scar), follicular unit extraction
Raised donor scar	History of keloids, racial susceptibility, incision placed too low	Careful history, patient selection, test biopsy	Intralesional corticosteroids
Persistent numbness or paresthesias in the back of the scalp	Transection of branches of the occipital nerves	Limit donor depth to deep subcutaneous layer, use tumescent anesthesia	Subsides spontaneously if the cut nerve branches were small
Hiccups	Possible injury to C2-C4 indirectly stimulating the vagus or diaphragmatic nerves	Limit donor depth to deep subcutaneous layer, use tumescent anesthesia	Chlorpromazine
Hair texture changes	Trauma to grafts, sebaceous glands removed in dissection	Careful atraumatic dissection and placing, avoid trimming follicular units too close	Usually resolves spontaneously
Skin texture changes	Recipient wounds too large	Make wounds no larger than the equivalent size of a 19-gauge needle at the frontal hairline	Add coverage with one- and two-hair follicular units at the frontal hairline using very small sites
Hair loss in recipient area related to the procedure	Telogen effluvium[75]	Possibly effective: small surgical wounds, limit epinephrine, pretreat with finasteride	Terminal non-miniaturized hair should return spontaneously, finasteride
Hair loss in donor area	Strangulation of follicles by sutures, transection of follicles during harvest	Narrower donor strip, meticulous suturing techniques	Follicular unit transplantation, follicular unit extraction, local excision
Failure of transplanted hair to grow	Desiccation,[74] crush injury,[72] transection,[73,76,77] grafts out of the body too long[48]	Keep grafts well hydrated in an isotonic solution, careful microscopic dissection and handling	None

Table 34.14 Twelve common pitfalls in follicular unit transplantation

1. Operating on patients that are too young or prior to medical therapy
2. Failing to identify low donor density prior to surgery
3. Failing to identify a tight scalp
4. Harvesting a donor strip that is too wide
5. Placing the donor incision too low or too high
6. Using a multi-bladed knife
7. Crushing grafts during insertion
8. Allowing grafts to dry
9. Placing the frontal hairline too far forward
10. Creating a hairline that is too broad
11. Angling hair in the wrong direction
12. Attempting to cover an area that is too large

Failing to identify a tight scalp

Assessing scalp laxity is an underappreciated aspect of the patient evaluation, probably because it is difficult to quantify. However, a tight scalp severely limits the total amount of harvestable donor hair and can constitute a contraindication to surgery, except when patients have extremely conservative goals or are expected to experience only limited balding. The constraints that poor scalp laxity impose generally manifest themselves after the first transplant session. Though laxity should be judged in the preoperative evaluation, the intraoperative assessment, made while suturing, is most accurate in predicting future difficulties. Therefore, every operative report should include a record of the ease of closure and intraoperative suture tension.[7]

Harvesting a donor strip that is too wide

In large sessions, it can be tempting to take a slightly wider donor strip in order to conserve on length. A strip that is 25 cm by 1 cm, for instance, can be shortened by 6 cm if widened by just 3 mm—and yield the same amount of hair. However, a wide strip puts unnecessary tension on the donor closure and is probably the most common cause of widened scars. If larger sessions are appropriate, and the scalp lacks adequate mobility, the surgeon should consider a longer incision rather than a wider one.

If a wide donor strip has been identified as the likely cause of a stretched scar, it is advisable to wait at least 8 months, to give the scar a chance to mature and regain some of its original laxity. When the next excision is made the strip should measure at least 3–6 mm narrower than the previous one. Attempts to remove the entire width or length of the old scar invariably lead to a recurrence, or worsening, of the old scar. To facilitate healing, the new excision should extend to the patient's hair-bearing edge, and be shorter than the old incision.

Unfortunately, attempts to re-excise scars commonly result in either no improvement or an even wider defect. For this reason, we have been using follicular unit extraction to place hair directly into the scar as our primary treatment.

Placing the donor incision too low

The location of the donor incision greatly affects scalp mobility. The ideal position for it is in the mid-portion of the permanent zone that lies, in most people, at the level of the external occipital protuberance and the superior nuchal line. The muscles of the neck insert into the inferior portion of this ridge, so an incision below this anatomic landmark will be impacted by the muscle movement directly beneath it. A stretched scar in this location is extremely difficult to repair because re-excision, even with undermining and layered closure, tends to heal with a wider scar. To compound the problem, one is more likely to cut through fascia with a low donor incision; and once the fascia has been violated, the risk of widening the scar rises considerably.[36]

In addition to the slightly greater risk of a widened scar, the main problems of harvesting hair too high are lack of permanence of the transplanted hair (because it may be subject to androgenic alopecia) and future visibility of the scar if the donor fringe narrows further. Incisions made too high are best left untreated, unless the scar is wide and poor surgical technique has been identified as the cause. The temptation to transplant permanent donor hair into a high scar should be resisted, as progressive balding would isolate the hair-bearing scar, presenting new cosmetic problems.

Interestingly, in the case of young patients with traumatic scars and hair-loss patterns that are still unclear, follicular unit extraction can function as a hedge against this risk. If the hair is harvested from the immediate vicinity of the scar, any future balding will affect the transplanted hair in the scar at the same rate as the hair surrounding it.

Using a multibladed knife

In order to save time, doctors performing large transplants may use a multibladed knife (one with three or more blades) for harvesting donor tissue. The resulting presliced multiple thin strips are much easier to work with than a single intact strip. Unfortunately, harvesting this way causes unacceptable levels of follicular transection while destroying the naturally occurring follicular unit and is therefore incompatible with FUT.[10]

Crushing grafts during insertion

Proper placing technique necessitates the use of forceps to grasp the graft by the fat below the bulb or by the dermis alongside the hair shaft in order to avoid damaging the germinative components of the follicle. Though placers often exercise enormous care while initially grasping the graft, there is a tendency to become rougher when repositioning the forceps for further inserting, replacing a popped graft or transferring grafts from the holding solution to the fingers. As follicular units and other small grafts are particularly susceptible to crush injury, improper handling can more than negate the benefits of careful stereo-microscopic dissection.[72,73]

Allowing grafts to dry

An elegant study using electron microscopy has shown that desiccation is by far the most significant form of injury to grafts and makes them much more susceptible to other forms of injury, such a mechanical trauma and warming. Grafts should therefore be kept well-hydrated with chilled isotonic solution (such as Ringer's lactate) from the moment the tissue is harvested until the time they are reinserted into the scalp.[74]

Placing the frontal hairline too far forward (too low)

Despite the fact that individual follicular units at the hairline in themselves look natural, their proper placement is no less important than in traditional grafting. The frontal hairline should be placed no lower than 1.5 cm above the upper brow crease.[1,8] Particularly if the underlying skin is normal, follicular units placed too low can be removed with an alexandrite (755 nm) or diode (800 nm, 810 nm) laser. Electrolysis is more difficult and time-consuming with transplanted follicles, but should also be considered. Punch excision is too imprecise for very small grafts and risks scarring.

Creating a hairline that is too broad

Since significant temporal recession is characteristic of a normal adult man's hairline, a broad, flat transplanted hairline will not age well and can cause cosmetic problems if baldness becomes extensive. The treatment is the same as with low hairlines, but it should be noted that if grafts larger than follicular units were used, and/or if there is scarring of the recipient skin, punch excision with reutilization of the hair may be indicated.

Angling hair in the wrong direction

As noted earlier, in the front and top part of the scalp, hair grows in a distinctly forward direction, changing to a radial pattern as it approaches the crown. It emerges from the scalp at an acute angle, with the hair lying practically flush to the skin at the temples.

There has been a tendency among some hair restoration surgeons to transplant grafts perpendicular to the skin—probably due to the fact that the mechanics of the old plug procedures made sharp angling technically difficult. The cosmetic consequence of this is most apparent at the frontal hairline. When the hair is perpendicular, the viewer's eye is guided to the base of the hair shaft where it inserts into the skin; conversely, when hair is transplanted in its natural, forward-pointing position, it is bowed by grooming and the eye settles on the body of the hair shaft.

When grafts at the frontal hairline are transplanted in a radial direction, combing the hair in any style becomes problematic and invariably results in an unhappy patient. As with low or broad hairlines, hair that is angled in the wrong direction, particularly in the frontal hairline, should be removed.

Attempting to cover an area that is too large

Attempting to cover an area greater than the donor supply can adequately fill may leave cosmetically important areas thin or untransplanted. Note that, in general, the first region to bald is the area where you should be *most* hesitant to transplant. Recession at the temples and thinning in the crown are usually the earliest manifestations of baldness, but they are acceptable, especially as patients age, so these areas may be left untransplanted. The central forelock region, however, is generally late to bald, but when balding occurs the patient loses the frame to his face and its restoration becomes essential.[7]

Whether or not these areas need coverage at the time of the initial transplant, an adequate amount of hair must always be reserved for critical areas, such as the forelock and top of the scalp. If donor reserves are limited, the transplantation of less critical areas should be postponed or avoided all together.[7]

■ SUMMARY

Developed within the past decade, follicular unit transplantation has emerged as both the standard and the cutting edge in surgical hair restoration. In conserving donor hair, achieving optimal coverage, and creating a natural look, FUT represents a considerable advance over earlier methods of hair restoration. Appropriately, it also demands considerably more from its practitioners. Surgical teams must develop the skill and stamina for the delicate handling of large numbers of follicular unit grafts, while surgeons must cultivate a keen aesthetic sensibility with regard to transplant design and graft placement.

In view of the psychological aspects of hair loss, follicular unit transplantation requires a thorough preoperative assessment to understand the patient's expectations, a careful examination to determine if surgery is appropriate and, most importantly, the establishment of realistic goals. If the surgical route is chosen, meticulous attention to detail is required in every aspect of the procedure so that these goals may be realized. It is a daunting task for the hair restoration surgeon and surgical team to develop the necessary expertise for perfecting follicular unit transplantation; but when they do their work can benefit patients for their lifetime.

■ REFERENCES

1. Bernstein RM, Rassman WR, Szaniawski W, Halperin A. Follicular transplantation. Int J Aesthetic Rest Surg 1995; 3:119–132.
2. Rassman WR, Bernstein RM, McClellan R, Jones R, et al. Follicular unit extraction: minimally invasive surgery for hair transplantation. Dermatol Surg 2002; 28:720–727.
3. Headington JT. Transverse microscopic anatomy of the human scalp. Arch Dermatol 1984; 120:449–456.
4. Rassman WR, Pomerantz, MA. The art and science of minigrafting. Int J Aesthetic Rest Surg 1993; 1:27–36.
5. Limmer B. Thoughts on the extensive micrografting technique in hair transplantation. Hair Transplant Forum Int 1996; 6:16–18.
6. Bernstein RM, Rassman WR. The logic of follicular unit transplantation. Dermatol Clin 1999; 17:277–295.
7. Bernstein RM, Rassman WR. Follicular transplantation: patient evaluation and surgical planning. Dermatol Surg 1997; 23:771–784.
8. Bernstein RM, Rassman WR. The aesthetics of follicular transplantation. Dermatol Surg 1997; 23:785–799.
9. Limmer BL. Elliptical donor stereoscopically assisted micrografting as an approach to further refinement in hair transplantation. Dermatol Surg 1994; 20:789–793.
10. Bernstein RM, Rassman WR, Seager D, Shapiro R, et al. Standardizing the classification and description of follicular unit transplantation and mini-micrografting techniques. Dermatol Surg 1998; 24:957–963.
11. Seager D. Binocular stereoscopic dissecting microscopes: should we use them? Hair Transplant Forum Int 1996; 6:2–5.
12. Stough DB, Haber RS, eds. Hair replacement: surgical and medical. St Louis: Mosby; 1996.
13. Unger WP. Different grafts for different purposes. Am J Cosmet Surg 1997; 14:177–183.

14. Unger WP. Laser hair transplanting 1997. Am J Cosmet Surg 1997; 14:143–148.
15. Bernstein RM, Rassman WR. Laser hair transplantation: is it really state of the art? Lasers in Surg Med 1996; 19:233–235.
16. Norwood OT. Scalp reductions: are they necessary? Hair Transplant Forum Int 1993; 3:1–7.
17. Bernstein RM. Are scalp reductions still indicated? Hair Transplant Forum Int 1996; 6:12–13.
18. Swinehart JM, Brandy DA. Scalp lifting: anatomic and technical considerations. J Dermatol Surg Oncol 1994; 20:600–612.
19. Epstein JS, Kabaker SS. Scalp flaps in the treatment of baldness: long-term results. Dermatol Surg 1996; 22:45–50.
20. Unger WP. Hair transplantation. New York: Marcel Dekker; 1995.
21. Sasagawa M. Hair transplantation. Jpn J Dermatol 1930; 30:473 (in Japanese).
22. Okuda S. Clinical and experimental studies of transplantation of living hairs. Jpn J Dermatol Urol 1939; 46:135–138 (in Japanese).
23. Tamura H. Pubic hair transplantation. Jpn J Dermatol 1943; 53:76 (in Japanese).
24. Orentreich N. Autographs in alopecias and other selected dermatologic conditions. Ann NY Acad Sci 1959; 83:463–479.
25. Rassman WR, Carson S. Micrografting in extensive quantities; the ideal hair restoration procedure. Dermatol Surg 1995; 21:306–311.
26. Camacho F, Montagna W. Trichology: Diseases of the pilosebaceus follicle. Madrid: Aula Medica; 1997.
27. Kuster W, Happle R. The inheritance of common baldness: two B or not two B? J Am Acad Dermatol 1984; 11:921–926.
28. Bernstein RM. Measurements in hair restoration. Hair Transplant Forum Int 1998; 8:27.
29. Norwood OT. Male pattern baldness: classification and incidence. So Med J 1975; 68:1359–1365.
30. Ludwig E. Classification of the types of androgenetic alopecia (common baldness) occurring in the female sex. Br J Dermatol 1977; 97:247–254.
31. Olsen EA. Female pattern hair loss. J Am Acad Dermatol 2001; 45:S70–S80.
32. Chartier MB, Hoss DM, Grant-Kels JM. Approach to the adult female patient with diffuse non-scarring alopecia. J Am Acad Dermatol 2002; 47:809–818.
33. Bernstein RM, Rassman WR. The scalp laxity paradox. Hair Transplant Forum Int 2002; 12:9–10.
34. Beehner M. Nomenclature proposal for the zones and landmarks of the balding scalp. Dermatol Surg 2001; 27:375–380.
35. Seager, D. The 'one-pass hair transplant'—a six-year perspective. Hair Transplant Forum Int 2003; 12:176–178; 194–196.
36. Salasche SJ, Bernstein G, Senkarik M. Surgical anatomy of the skin. Norwalk, CT: Appleton & Lange; 1988:151–162.
37. Beehner M. Where is thy crown, your majesty? Hair Transplant Forum Int 1998; 8:18–19.
38. Haas A, Grekin R. Antibiotic prophylaxis in dermatologic surgery. J Am Acad Dermatol 1995; 32:155–176.
39. Drake LA, Ceilley RI, Cornelison RL, et al. Guidelines of care for office surgical facilities, part I. J Am Acad Dermatol 1992; 26:763–765.
40. Drake LA, Ceilley RI, Cornelison RL, et al. Guidelines of care for office surgical facilities, part II. Self-assessment checklist. J Am Acad Dermatol 1995; 33:265–270.
41. Fader DJ, Johnson TM. Medical issues and emergencies in the dermatology office. J Am Acad Dermatol 1997; 36:1–16.
42. Sebben, JE. Survey of sterile technique used by dermatologic surgeons. J Am Acad Dermatol 1988; 18:1107–1112.
43. Sebben, JE. Sterile technique in dermatologic surgery: what is enough? J Dermatol Surg Oncol 1988; 14:487–489.
44. Bernstein RM, Rassman WR. Dissecting microscope versus magnifying loupes with transillumination in the preparation of follicular unit grafts: a bilateral controlled study. Dermatol Surg 1998; 24:875–880.
45. Blugerman G, Schavelzon D. Ergonomics applied to hair restoration. Hair Transplant Forum Int 1996; 6:1–14.
46. Bernstein RM, Rassman WR. Limiting epinephrine (adrenaline) in large hair transplant sessions. Hair Transplant Forum Int 2000; 10:39–42.
47. Bernstein RM, Rassman WR. Wall mounted placing stand. Hair Transplant Forum Int 1997; 7:17–18.
48. Limmer BL. Micrograft survival. In: Stough DB, Haber, RS, eds. Hair replacement: surgical and medical. St Louis: Mosby; 1996:147–149.
49. Raposio E, Cella A, Panarese P, et al. Power boosting the grafts in hair transplantation surgery. Evaluation of a new storage medium. Dermatol Surg 1998;24:1342-1346.
50. Krugluger W, Moser K, Hugeneck J, Laciak K, Moser C. New storage buffers for micrografts enhance graft survival and clinical outcome in hair restoration surgery. Hair Transplant Forum Int 2003; 13:325; 333–334; 343.
51. Grekin R, Auletta M. Local anesthesia in dermatologic surgery. Am Acad Dermatol 1988; 19:599–614.
52. McCaughey W. Adverse effects of local anesthetics. Drug Safety 1992; 7:178–189.
53. Skidmore R, Patterson J, Tomsick R. Local anesthetics. Dermatol Surg 1996; 22:520
54. Foster C, Aston S. Propranolol-epinephrine (adrenaline) interaction: a potential disaster. Plast Reconstr Surg 1983; 72:74–78.
55. Goodman AG, Gillman LS. The pharmacological basis of therapeutics, 7th edn. New York: Macmillan; 1985:151–159.
56. Bernstein RM, Rassman WR. Hemostasis with minimal epinephrine. Hair Transplant Forum Int 1999; 9:153.
57. Bernstein RM, Rassman WR, Rashid N: A new suture for hair transplantation: Poliglecaprone 25. Dermatol Surg 2001; 27:5–11.
58. Bennett RG. Selection of wound closure materials. J Am Acad Dermatol 1988; 18:619–637.
59. Moy RL, Waldman B, Hein DW. A review of sutures and suturing techniques. J Dermatol Surg Oncol 1992; 18:785–795.
60. Arnold J. Mini-blades and a mini-blade handle for hair transplantation. Am J Cosm Surg 1997; 14:195–200.
61. Seager D. Dense hair transplantation from sparse donor area—introducing the 'follicular family unit.' Hair Transplant Forum Int 1998; 8:21–23.
62. Tykocinski A. A one-year study of using exclusively 'follicular grouping grafts' in specific areas to increase hair density and volume during FUT. Hair Transplant Forum Int 2003; 13:366; 369–700.
63. Limmer BL. The density issue in hair transplantation. Dermatol Surg 1997; 23:747–750.
64. Bernstein RM, Rassman WR, Rashid N, Shiell R. The art of repair in surgical hair restoration—part I: basic repair strategies. Dermatol Surg 2002; 28:783–794.
65. Bernstein RM, Rassman WR, Rashid N, Shiell R. The art of repair in surgical hair restoration—part II: the tactics of repair. Dermatol Surg 2002; 28:873–893.
66. Choi YC, Kim JC. Single hair transplantation using Choi hair transplanter. J Dermatol Surg Oncol 1992; 18:945–948.
67. Rassman WR, Bernstein RM. Rapid Fire Hair Implanter Carousel: A new surgical instrument for the automation of hair transplantation. Dermatol Surg 1998; 24: 623–627.
68. Boudjema P. A new hair graft implanter: the hair implanter pen. Hair Transplant Forum Int 1998; 8:1–4.
69. Rassman WR, Bernstein RM. The automation of hair transplantation: past, present, and future. In: Harahap M, ed. Innovative techniques in skin surgery. New York: Marcel Dekker; 2002:489–502.
70. Meza DP. Complications in hair restoration surgery. Hair Transplant Forum Int 2000; 10:145.
71. Fader DJ, Johnson TM. Medical issues and emergencies in the dermatology office. J Am Acad Dermatol 1997; 36:1–16.
72. Greco J. The H-factor in micrografting procedures. Hair Transplant Forum Int 1996; 6:8–9.
73. Cooley J, Vogel J. Loss of the dermal papilla during graft dissection and placement: another cause of X-factor? Hair Transplant Forum Int 1997; 7:20–21.
74. Gandelman M, Mota AL, Abrahamsohn PA, De Oliveri SF. Light and electron microscopic analysis of controlled injury to follicular unit grafts. Dermatol Surg 2000; 26:31.
75. Headington JE. Telogen effluvium: new concepts and review. Arch Dermatol 1993; 129:356–363.
76. Limmer BL, Razmi R, Davis T, Stevens C. Relating hair growth theory and experimental evidence to practical hair transplantation. Am J Cosmet Surg 1994; 11:305–310.
77. Bernstein RM. Blind graft production: value at what cost? Hair Transplant Forum Int 1998; 8:28–29.
78. Bernstein RM, Rassman WR. Follicular unit graft yield using three different techniques. Hair Transplant Forum Int 2001; 11:1; 11–13.
79. Marritt E, Dzubow L. The isolated frontal forelock. Dermatol Surg 1995; 21:523–538.
80. Weber P, Weber R, Dzubow L. Sedation for dermatologic surgery. J Am Acad Dermatol 1989; 20:815–826.

35 Laser Hair Removal

Sandy S Tsao MD and George J Hruza MD

Summary box

- Lasers and light sources can provide temporary hair reduction for all individuals.
- At present permanent hair reduction is possible only in individuals with pigmented terminal hairs.
- Proper patient selection is vital to ensure effective treatment with minimal side-effects.
- A thorough knowledge of laser–tissue interactions is mandatory to minimize side-effects.
- Treatment outcome is optimized by understanding the attributes of specific laser and light systems.
- Close follow-up care is necessary to provide optimum patient outcome.

INTRODUCTION

Excessive and unwanted body hair is a common frustration for many individuals, and despite the many etiologies, the desire for permanent removal remains universal. Before the development of lasers and light sources, treatments for the removal of unwanted hair were tedious, generally temporary in nature and often associated with significant side-effects. The ability to selectively target and destroy hair follicles with lasers and light sources has revolutionized the ability to eliminate unwanted hair temporarily and permanently in many individuals. As laser technology advances, the ability to treat individuals of all skin types and all hair colors broadens.

Proper patient selection and laser and light source selection are key to the success of laser treatment. An understanding of hair anatomy, growth and physiology, together with a thorough understanding of laser–tissue interactions, in particular within the context of designing optimal laser parameters for effective laser hair removal, must be acquired before using lasers for hair removal.

Hair anatomy

The hair follicle is a complex, hormonally regulated structure with a cyclical growth pattern. Each follicle is formed through an interaction between dermal and epidermal components.

In the pregerm stage, there is an accumulation of basal cells and associated mesenchymal cells, which form the primitive hair germ. A solid column of epidermal cells progressively penetrates into the dermis to form a rudimentary hair follicle. The broad tip becomes concave and encloses the dermal papilla, which is a neurovascular structure that supplies the cells of the rapidly dividing proliferating matrix forming the hair shaft.

Two swellings appear at the posterior edge of the follicle, with the upper swelling representing the future sebaceous gland and the lower bulge representing the site of attachment of the arrector pili muscle. The hair emerges from the surface at an angle such that the arrector pili muscle and bulge are on the deeper aspect of the follicle.

The first hair follicles are formed at the end of the second and beginning of the third month of gestation in the eyebrow, upper lip, and chin regions, with further hair growth in a cephalad to caudal direction during the fourth to fifth months of gestation. No further follicular neogenesis occurs after birth.[1]

The hair follicle is divided into three anatomical units: infundibulum, isthmus, and inferior segment (Fig. 35.1). The infundibulum includes the region from the hair follicle orifice to the sebaceous duct entrance. The isthmus includes the region between the entrance of the sebaceous duct and the arrector pili muscle. The inferior segment extends from the insertion of the arrector pili muscle to the base of the follicle, including the hair bulb.

The hair bulb is composed of matrix cells interspersed with melanocytes. The matrix cells differentiate along separate pathways and form, from the outside inward, the outer root sheath, the three layers of the inner root sheath

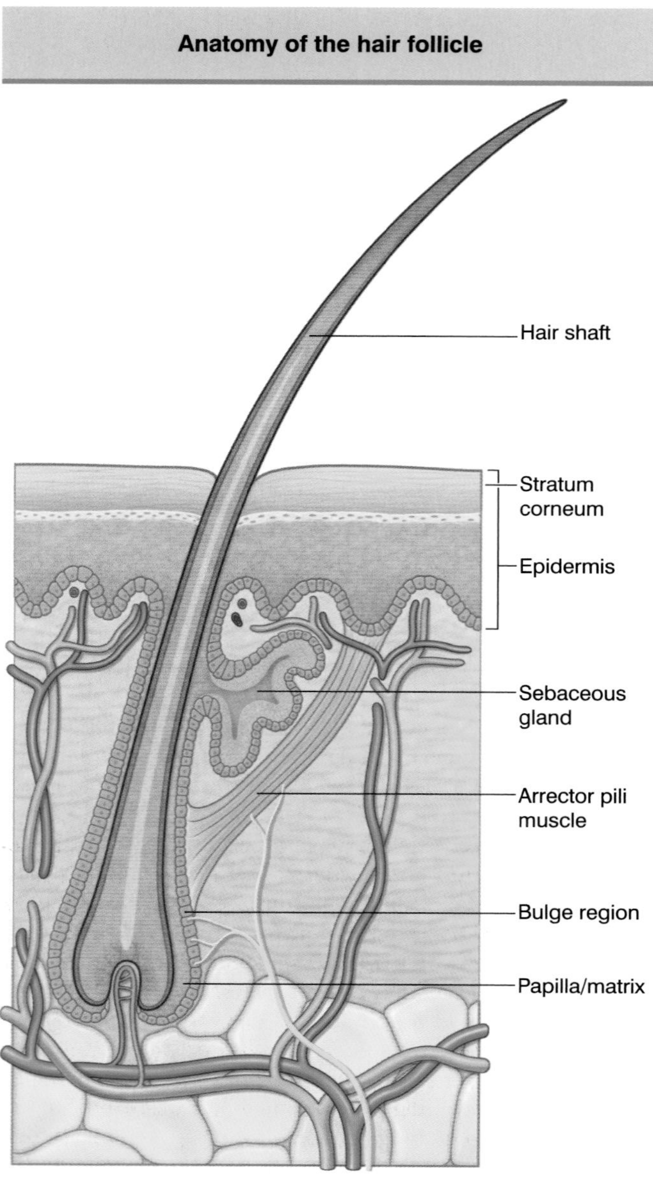

Figure 35.1 Anatomy of a hair follicle.

(Henle, Huxley, and cuticle), and the three layers of the hair shaft itself (cuticle of the hair shaft, cortex, and medulla).

Hair growth

Each hair follicle consists of a permanent and nonpermanent part, with the lowermost aspect of the permanent part at the level of the insertion of the arrector pili muscle (the follicular bulge).

All hair undergoes intrinsic cyclical growth, consisting of three phases (Fig. 35.2). In periods of active growth (anagen) the rapidly developing bulbar matrix cells differentiate into the hair shaft and inner root sheath, both of which migrate outward as the hair lengthens. Anagen bulbs are 2–7 mm below the skin surface. A transition period follows in which the bulbar part of the hair follicle, including matrical melanocytes, is almost totally degraded through apoptosis (catagen). The follicle decreases to approximately one third of its former length, with its lowermost part coming to lie at the level of attachment of the dermal papilla. A resting period (telogen) phase ensues. With new regrowth in early anagen, new epithelial cell division occurs near the arrector pili insertion, a new matrix develops, and hair growth resumes.

The hair follicle is self-renewing, with a population of stem cells capable of regenerating the follicle within or near the hair bulb matrix. Another population of slow-cycling stem cells has been defined in the follicular bulge arising off the outer root sheath at the site of arrector pili muscle attachment, approximately 1 mm below the skin surface. This region represents the lower end of the permanent part of the hair follicle. It is postulated that during late telogen to early anagen, these follicular bulge stem cells are activated by dermal papillary signals to proliferate briefly to form more differentiated follicular cells before returning to their noncycling state in mid-anagen.[2]

The duration of each of these growth phases varies according to the body site (Table 35.1). Body sites with long hair (e.g. scalp) have a prolonged anagen phase, whereas areas with short hair (e.g. female upper lip) have short anagen and prolonged telogen phases. The duration of anagen growth of the upper lip is typically 16 weeks, catagen 1 week, and telogen 6 weeks. The duration of anagen growth on the scalp is generally 150 weeks, catagen 1–3 weeks, and telogen 12 weeks. The rate of hair growth is approximately 0.44 mm/day on the scalp and 0.27 mm/day for the beard region. Seasonal variation does exist, with a higher rate of growth during the summer months and slower growth during the winter months. This variability correlates with fluctuations in androgen levels, with higher levels of testosterone noted during the summer. Any method of hair treatment that induces telogen can produce a prolonged absence of hair growth that may not represent permanent hair loss. It is critical in the management of patients with excess hair growth to understand the variability of these growth phases to provide effective treatment and follow-up expectations with predictable outcomes.

Hair type

Hair can be classified according to its texture and length, with the three main types being defined as lanugo, vellus, and terminal hairs. Hair features, such as the amount of pigment and hair shaft diameter increase from lanugo to terminal hairs. Hair diameter is determined by the size of the papilla and hair bulb. Lanugo hairs are soft, fine hairs that cover a fetus and are shed before or shortly after birth. Vellus hairs are nonpigmented, with a diameter of 30 μm or less. Secondary vellus hairs represent miniaturized or hypoplastic terminal hairs and have the same diameter as vellus hairs, but are pigmented. Terminal hair shafts range from 200 to 300 μm in cross-sectional diameter. Both vellus and terminal hairs go through all stages of follicular growth, but the duration of anagen is much shorter for vellus hairs. The type of hair produced by an individual follicle may change, as observed by the replacement of vellus by terminal hairs at puberty or the conversion of terminal to secondary vellus hairs with androgenetic alopecia. Vellus hair bulbs extend to a depth of less than 1 mm into the skin, whereas telogen

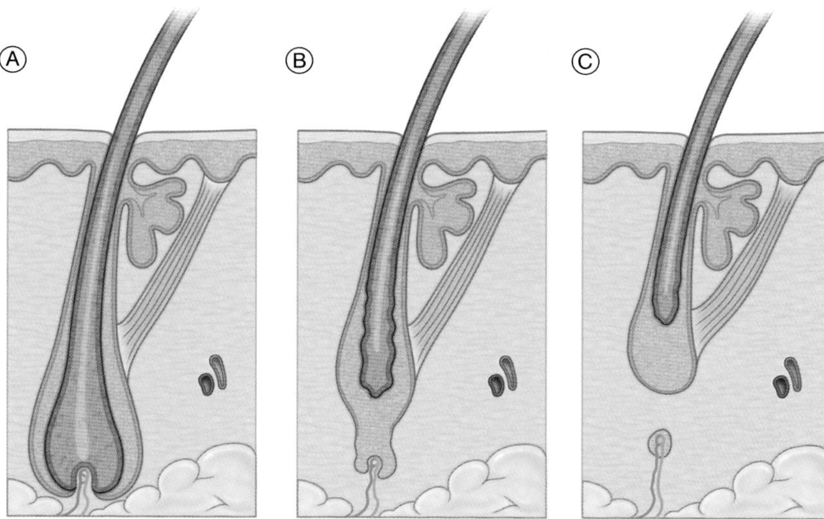

Figure 35.2 Stages of hair growth. (A) Anagen; (B) Catagen; (C) Telogen.

Table 35.1 Hair growth table

Body site	Telogen duration (months)	Anagen duration (months)
Upper lip	1–2	3–4
Axillae	3–4	3–6
Pubic area	3–4	3–6
Lower limbs	5–6	4–5
Scalp	3–4	35–40

hair bulbs may extend 2–7 mm into the skin. The bulge maintains a constant depth throughout the hair cycle.[3]

Hair color

Hair color is genetically determined and is dependent on the amount of pigment in the hair shaft.[4] Follicular melanocytes produce two types of melanin—eumelanin, a brown–black pigment; and pheomelanin, a red pigment. They are biologically related and share a common metabolic pathway, in which dopaquinone is a key intermediate. Pheomelanin absorption is 30 times lower than eumelanin at 694 nm and is poorly absorbed at wavelengths longer than 700 nm.[5] Melanocytes occur in the upper part of the hair bulb and outer root sheath of the infundibulum with a 1 : 5 ratio of melanocytes to keratinocytes. Melanogenesis is halted during catagen and reinitiated during early anagen. Pigment transfer is halted during telogen, resulting in an unpigmented telogen bulb. Hair varies in its type of melanin—black and brown hair contains ellipsoidal heavily melanized eumelanosomes; red hair contains spherical pheomelanosomes; blond hair contains incompletely melanized melanosomes or fewer melanosomes; gray hair producing follicles contain few melanocytes, with poorly melanized melanosomes; while white hair producing follicles contain no dopa-positive melanocytes.

Classification of excess hair

The removal of unwanted hair is a daily challenge for many men and women. Two main groups of individuals seek hair removal—individuals with increased hair in undesirable locations secondary to an underlying medical condition or genetic predisposition, and individuals with hair in areas considered to be normal in density and distribution, but for social, emotional or other reasons is not desired.

Individuals with increased hair density are classified as having hypertrichosis or hirsutism. Hypertrichosis is defined as localized or excessive hair at any body site in a male or female and may develop as a result of a drug interaction to certain medications such as cyclosporine, phenytoin, and anabolic steroids. Internal malignancy, trauma, malnutrition, patients with a hair-bearing skin graft, endocrine disturbance, and a genetic or ethnic predisposition have also been implicated.[6]

Excessive terminal hair growth in androgen-dependent areas, including the upper lip, chin, chest, lower abdomen, and thighs is classified as hirsutism. Other cutaneous signs that may be associated with hirsutism include acne, acanthosis nigricans, striae distensae, and androgenetic alopecia. Systemic signs of virilization such as a voice deepening, hypertension, increased muscle bulk, and clitoromegaly may indicate a hyperandrogenic state, such as polycystic ovarian syndrome, 21-hydroxylase-deficient non-classic adrenal hyperplasia, insulin-resistant acanthosis nigricans, androgen drug intake or an androgen-secreting neoplasm.[6] Appropriate laboratory tests, include tests for free testosterone, and dehydroepiandrosterone sulfate (DHEA-S) should be obtained to exclude elevated androgen levels as a cause of hirsutism.

Traditional treatment modalities

Numerous treatment modalities exist for the removal of hair. Temporary hair removal is obtained by shaving, tweezing, bleaching, waxing, and employing chemical depilatories.

Though inexpensive and easy to perform, many women loathe shaving because of the masculine connotations associated with the procedure or the mistaken belief that shaving will coarsen hair or make it grow faster.[6] Tweezing and waxing provide temporary hair loss for several weeks; however, these techniques are painful and may result in undesired side-effects such as postinflammatory hyperpigmentation, ingrown hairs, folliculitis, and scarring. Bleaching provides a lightening of treated hairs, masquerading their presence. This technique is most effective for light-skinned individuals. Chemical depilatories commonly contain thioglycolates that dissolve hairs by disrupting disulfide bonds. The resultant hair removal includes some of the hair shaft below the skin surface.[7] Although effective for temporary hair removal, they are messy to use and can provide significant irritation, especially when used on the face.

Antiandrogenic medications, including oral contraceptives for hormonal suppression, and spironolactone, flutamide, and cyproterone acetate for peripheral androgen blockade have been employed for the treatment of hirsutism with variable success. They provide only partial and temporary hair loss and are associated with significant side-effects, which warrant monthly monitoring.

Attempts to delay hair growth have been performed. There are three ways to slow down hair growth—decrease the anagen phase, delay the onset of anagen, or prolong the telogen phase. To date, pharmacological prolongation of the telogen phase or anagen onset is not possible. It is, however, possible to decrease the anagen phase. Eflornithine hydrochloride 13.9% cream (Vaniqa, Bristol-Myers Squibb) was approved by the Food and Drug Administration (FDA) in August 2000 as the first topical prescription treatment for the reduction of unwanted facial hair in women. It acts as an irreversible inhibitor of ornithine decarboxylase (ODC), an enzyme that is critical for the biosynthesis of cationic polyamines, which are necessary for cell growth. ODC is abundantly expressed in the proliferating bulb cells of anagen follicles. When ODC is decreased, anagen is reduced with subsequent hair growth delay. The mean percutaneous absorption for eflornithine 13.9% cream is less than 1%. It is not metabolized and is excreted unchanged in the urine.[8] Two multicenter, double-blind, vehicle-controlled, randomized studies were carried out, with twice daily application of the creams for 24 weeks, followed by 8 weeks of no treatment, to the chin and upper lip. Statistically and clinically significant hair growth delay was noted in the eflornithine group when compared to the vehicle. Hair growth was noted to approach pretreatment levels within 8 weeks of treatment withdrawal.[9] Applied twice daily, eflornithine hydrochloride 13.9% cream is effective in slowing facial hair regrowth temporarily and may complement other hair removal methods. Skin-related side-effects include stinging, burning, tingling, acne, and folliculitis at the treatment site. It is classified as a pregnancy category C agent.[8]

For several decades electrolysis was the only available means of achieving safe, permanent hair removal. Two types of electrolysis have been employed for hair removal: galvanic electrolysis and thermolysis. During galvanic electrolysis, a needle carrying direct electric current is inserted into each individual hair follicle. The current destroys the follicle by producing sodium hydroxide within the follicle. Thermolysis generates a high-frequency alternating current through a needle inserted into the follicle, which destroys the hair follicle through heat production.[10] Both forms of electrolysis can provide permanent hair removal. However, the process is tedious, time consuming, costly, painful, and can result in postinflammatory hyperpigmentation, hypopigmentation, and ice pick scarring; and the results are variable, with efficacy of 30–40% for destroying individual hair follicles. It is not a practical means of hair removal for individuals with extensive hair or large areas to treat.

■ PREOPERATIVE PREPARATION

Preoperative preparation for laser hair removal requires a pretreatment consultative visit to determine eligibility. A thorough history and physical examination are paramount for treatment success. Patient and physician expectations must be fully defined before treatment initiation. Treatment risks and benefits must be thoroughly reviewed and understood.

A review of a patient's past medical history should include the presence of any underlying medical conditions (Table 35.2). Even though no scientific evidence exists to suggest that laser hair removal penetrates deep enough to injure a fetus, the treatment of a pregnant woman is best avoided in our litigious society. The presence of any underlying conditions that may cause hirsutism requires further workup before laser treatment. A past history of herpes simplex virus at or near the treatment site requires prophylactic antiviral therapy. A history of keloids or hypertrophic scar formation may preclude the use of lasers for hair removal. Documentation of past hair removal treatment modalities, including method, frequency, date of last treatment, and response is essential. Treatment should be avoided in patients taking photosensitizing medications or isotretinoin within the previous 6 months, past or current use of gold therapy, underlying photosensitizing conditions such as lupus erythematosus, or koebnerizing conditions such as psoriasis.

Fitzpatrick skin phototype classification is used to assist in the determination of eligibility (Table 35.3). The ideal candidate for laser hair removal is fair-skinned (skin types I and II) with dark terminal hair. Less ideal are patients with darker skin (skin types III and VI) and dark hair. Patients with blond, gray, red, or white hair need to be aware that it is unlikely that laser treatment will result in permanent hair removal. Patients with skin types V and VI have an increased risk for side-effects, and as such may not be optimal candidates for laser hair removal.

Absence or presence of a tan should be noted. If an active tan is present or there is recent sun exposure, laser treat-

Table 35.2 Pertinent history in patient selection for laser hair removal

Underlying endocrine disorders
Hypertrophic or keloidal scarring
Intake of isotretinoin within the past month
Koebnerizing dermatologic disorder
Herpes simplex infection
Recurrent skin infection
Gold therapy
Recent suntan or exposure to tanning booths

Table 35.3 Fitzpatrick skin phototype

Skin type	Sunburn and tanning history
I	Extremely fair skin – always burns, never tans
II	Fair skin – always burns, sometimes tans
III	Medium skin – sometimes burns, always tans
IV	Olive skin – rarely burns, always tans
V	Moderately pigmented brown skin – never burns, always tans
VI	Markedly pigmented black skin – never burns, always tans

ment should be postponed up to 6 weeks, depending on the degree of tan, to allow the tan to lighten to minimize potential side-effects. Patients are instructed to avoid excessive sun exposure for a month before and during the entire treatment course. Documentation of existing tattoos, nevi, and scars within treatment areas is critical in managing treatment outcome. Patients with numerous lentigines should be aware that laser hair removal might result in permanent removal of these freckles.

Patients must fully understand the risks and benefits of treatment, as well as the long-term results. Patients should be aware that laser hair removal offers a method to significantly delay hair growth. After multiple treatments, the treatment areas will have less hair growth and finer hair growth.[11] Temporary hair loss is achievable for all patients. Hair loss in patients with blond, red, gray, or white hair can be maintained by treatment at approximately 3-month intervals. Long-term hair reduction is strongly correlated with hair color, skin color, and tolerated fluence.[12] In general, a 20–30% hair loss has been observed with each treatment when effective fluences can be used in patients with fair skin and dark hair.[13] With the use of lower fluences, as are needed for Fitzpatrick skin types III or greater, the percentage of hair loss is decreased, and complete permanent hair removal is unlikely. Treatment risks for all patients include blistering, ulceration, scar formation, folliculitis or acne flare, hyperpigmentation, hypopigmentation, increased hair growth, poor-to-no response, and recurrence. These risks should be addressed before each treatment and informed consent obtained.

Pretreatment instructions include strict sun avoidance for 6 weeks before treatment and daily use of a broad-spectrum sunscreen throughout the treatment course. A bleaching cream such as 4% hydroquinone with or without 0.025% retinoic acid and 2% hydrocortisone can be prescribed for patients with Fitzpatrick skin types III or greater and for patients with a recent sun exposure. Side-effects after treatment have been reported to be reduced with the pretreatment use of sunscreens and bleaching creams.[14] Plucking, waxing, and electrolysis are to be avoided to maintain an intact hair shaft. Shaving, bleaching, and depilatory creams may be used.

■ TECHNIQUES

Several components are necessary to selectively damage a hair follicle with a laser or light source, including a chromophore in the follicle, a laser or light source that selectively targets the chromophore, and appropriate parameters that selectively damage the hair follicle. At present, it is understood that it is necessary to damage stem cells in the bulge area at the interface of the outer root sheath and the connective tissue sheath, or irreversibly damage a hair follicle at the level of the dermis by replacing it with connective tissue.[15] Damage to the bulb area is also likely to be critical.

Laser hair removal was first applied nonspecifically for the removal of hair from flaps and grafts[16] and to treat trichiasis. Most recently, laser-assisted hair removal has been based on the principle of selective photothermolysis—confining thermal injury to the targeted chromophore.[17] This selective thermal destruction by light occurs when energy is delivered at a wavelength of light well absorbed by the hair follicle within a time period less than or equal to the thermal relaxation time (TRT) of the follicle. When the proper pulse duration, wavelength, and energy fluence are used, selective damage to the hair follicle occurs. During laser treatment, thermal damage must be confined to the hair follicle alone to avoid nonspecific tissue injury.

Chromophores

The endogenous chromophore targeted for selective destruction of hair follicles is melanin, although water has also been used as a chromophore with minimal success to date (Table 35.4). Melanin is in the hair shaft, the outer root sheath of the infundibulum, and the matrix area.[18] It functions as a natural chromophore over a wide range of wavelengths, up to 1 100 nm[19] (Fig. 35.3). Most lasers and noncoherent light sources with cut-off filters used for hair removal deliver energy at red or near infrared wavelengths, which target melanin within the hair follicle. The amount and type of melanin within the follicle determines the amount of follicular damage possible. Red and near infrared wavelengths are poorly absorbed by competing chromophores such as hemoglobin and are able to penetrate into the deep dermis.

Exogenous chromophores have been employed when hairs lack significant pigment as a target. The first FDA-approved method of laser hair removal employed the use of a Q-switched neodymium:yttrium aluminum garnet (Nd:YAG) laser with topically applied carbon particles suspended in mineral oil massaged into hair follicles.[20] Even though this method did not provide permanent hair removal, the concept has been expanded to include the use of other exogenous chromophores. Liposomal targeting of melanin to hair follicles has been achieved in the scalp and the ability to color hair with melanin has been demonstrated.[21] A topical melanin-encapsulated liposomal spray has been FDA-approved to enhance the effects of lasers in nonpigmented hair (Meladine, Creative Technologies Inc, Chesapeake, VA). It contains water, glycerol, melanin, natural soy lecithin, and 2-phenoxyethanol, is odorless and nontoxic, and requires refrigeration when opened. It must be applied twice daily to the treatment site(s) up to 4–6 weeks in advance of treatment, with six to eight coatings used with each application. Its long-term efficacy for permanent hair removal has not been documented in formal studies to date.

Site-specific microsphere targeting of both hydrophilic and lipophilic particles may also be used. A particle bead size between 3 and 7 μm in diameter is necessary for optimal deposition within the hair follicle, with larger and

Table 35.4 Chromophores for hair removal with lasers and light sources

Endogenous	Exogenous
Melanin	Aminolevulinic acid Carbon particles Meladine

Absorption spectrum of various substances

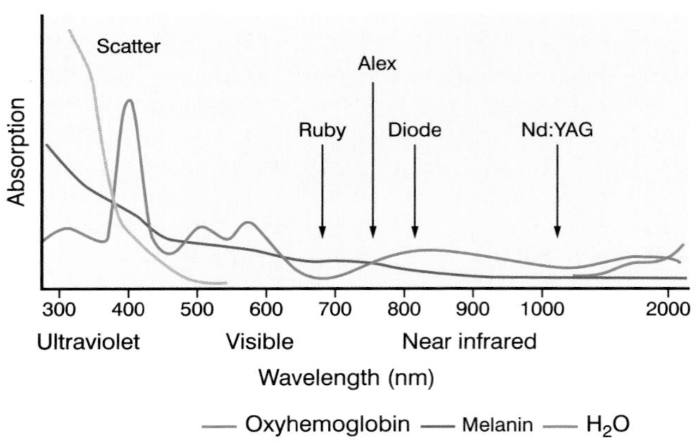

Figure 35.3 Absorption spectrum of various substances. Laser targeting of these substances is wavelength dependent.

smaller particles depositing preferentially in the stratum corneum and skin surface. Methylene blue has been demonstrated to selectively deposit within pilosebaceous units using 5 μm porous nylon microspheres[22] in hairless rats. Human applications derived from this work will be beneficial in the treatment of nonpigmented hair.

Light can also be used to photochemically activate an exogenously administered or induced photosensitizer within hair follicles, a technique known as photodynamic therapy. Aminolevulinic acid (ALA) is the most commonly used drug. When applied topically, ALA is absorbed by hair follicles over several hours and converted to the photosensitizing compound protoporphyrin IX. Red light near 635 nm is then applied to the surface, activating protoporphyrin IX, resulting in singlet oxygen production and follicular cell destruction. PDT has been reported to induce temporary hair loss for 3 months, depending on the ALA concentration used and light dose applied. An advantage of PDT is that hair color and skin color[23] are not important variables for treatment success.

Optimal target

Bulbar stem cells were originally thought to be the key follicular target for laser hair removal. With the discovery of stem cells in the bulge area,[15] it is likely that both the bulge and bulb are important for permanent hair follicle destruction.

The influence of hair cycle growth on laser-induced hair removal is not completely understood. The depth and pigmentation of the bulb are dependent on the hair cycle stage. Telogen hair bulbs are unpigmented and thus not active targets for light absorption. Melanogenesis resumes during early anagen. At this stage the bulb is more superficial in the dermis in close proximity to the bulge and the bulge stem cells are actively dividing. It is at this stage that cells are more susceptible to injury. As anagen progresses, the bulb and papillae descend into the deep dermis and subcutis, and the bulge cells become quiescent. It is therefore believed that follicles in early anagen are more responsive to laser and light treatment. Attempts to synchronize hair growth to early anagen by waxing 6–8 weeks before laser hair removal have demonstrated only a modest increase in permanent hair reduction.[24]

Wavelength

Most present strategies for laser hair removal employ the use of visible and near infrared light, with wavelengths between 600 and 1064 nm (see Fig. 35.3). Melanin is the dominant chromophore at these wavelengths, with an optical window between 600 and 1100 nm. Shorter wavelengths are associated with increased light scatter, limiting beam penetration. Using longer wavelengths of light, 800 nm or greater, allows deeper penetration into the skin. The ratio of energy deposited in the dermis compared to the epidermis is greater because of this increased penetration. At longer wavelengths, higher fluences are required for follicular destruction as a result of decreased melanin absorption.

The optimal wavelength for hair removal is dependent on the color contrast between the epidermis and hair shaft (Table 35.5). Individuals with light skin and dark hair can tolerate all wavelengths of light with minimal risk of epidermal damage. The use of a shorter wavelength (694 nm, 755 nm) is well tolerated in these individuals. For darker skin and dark hair, longer wavelengths (800 nm and greater) are essential for epidermal protection. Red and red–brown hair absorbs 800 nm to 1100 nm light poorly, thus requiring shorter wavelengths. Blond, white, and gray hairs require the shortest wavelength possible (694 nm) to allow for maximum melanin absorption.

Pulse duration

Q-switched lasers produce instantaneous hair shaft vaporization and a photoacoustic effect through the delivery of very short pulses. Separation of the shaft from the surrounding tissue and alteration of the optical thermal properties of the shaft led to a compromise in further laser energy absorption and less effective treatment. When longer pulse durations are used, more efficient heat transfer occurs. The most selective damage is obtained when the pulse duration is equal to or less than the TRT of the hair follicle, which is estimated to be 40–100 ms for terminal hairs with a diameter of 200–300 μm[25] (Table 35.6). In addition, the pulse duration should exceed the TRT of the epidermis (estimated to be 3–10 ms) to minimize epidermal damage. The optimal pulse duration for permanent hair reduction while minimizing epidermal injury is between 10 and 50 ms. Longer pulse widths allow for higher tolerated fluences for all skin types (see Table 35.5).

Altshuler et al[26] have proposed an expanded theory of selective photothermolysis to take into consideration the variability in heat absorption between the high heat absorbing, melanin-bearing structures including the hair shaft and matrix cells, and the bulge and bulb, both containing stem cells, which are the targets for follicular destruction, but lacking sufficient chromophore for heat absorption. These weakly absorbing targets have to be damaged by heat diffusion from the highly pigmented, strongly absorbing regions. The delay between chromophore heating and distant target heating is referred to as thermal damage time (TDT) and is the time required to irreversibly damage the target with sparing of the surrounding tissue. The TDT may be significantly longer than the TRT of the target. Pulse widths within or below the TDT may allow for maximal efficacy as well as optimized epidermal cooling. With laser hair removal, the chromophore is melanin within the hair follicle, whereas the ultimate target is the follicular stem cell, which is located in the bulb or bulge. The time required to transfer heat from the hair follicle to the bulb or bulge is referred to as the TDT.

Table 35.5 Optimal wavelength for hair removal

Hair color	Fitzpatrick skin type	Wavelength (nm)
Brown	I, II	694, 755, 800
Brown, black	III, IV, V	800, 1064
Red, gray	I, II	694, 755
Blond, white	I, II	694

Table 35.6 Thermal relaxation time for various follicular structures

Structures	TRT (ms)
Whole epidermis	10
Hair shaft, mid-dermis	3–5
Epidermal basal layer	0.1
Hair follicle, mid dermis	40–100
Individual melanosome	0.001
Hair bulb	20–40

Spot size

Optical scattering by dermal collagen causes light to diffuse as it penetrates into the dermis. Photons that are scattered out of the beam are essentially wasted because they do not carry enough thermal energy to cause significant thermal damage.[27] A larger spot size (>9 mm) (Fig. 35.4) allows for a greater likelihood that photons will be scattered back into the incident collimated beam with resultant beam broadening. This greater photon density results in deeper energy penetration. A larger spot size also allows for faster administration of treatment. Note that even for large spot sizes, there are edge effects, with variability in treatment success based on the location of the spot. Areas near the edge of the beam receive less fluence. Slight overlapping of treatment pulses helps to reduce this occurrence.

Fluence

Temporary hair removal is possible with all devices at any fluence (Table 35.7). A critical threshold fluence is needed to obtain long-term hair removal.[12] Because there is evidence that sublethal laser doses induce catagen and telogen, it may be possible to synchronize follicular growth to some degree using lower fluences. Once the follicles are in early anagen, larger fluences with longer pulse durations could be used to destroy the follicle.

Cooling

For many skin types, the threshold light energy required to maximally damage the hair follicle for permanent hair removal also produces maximum melanin absorption by the

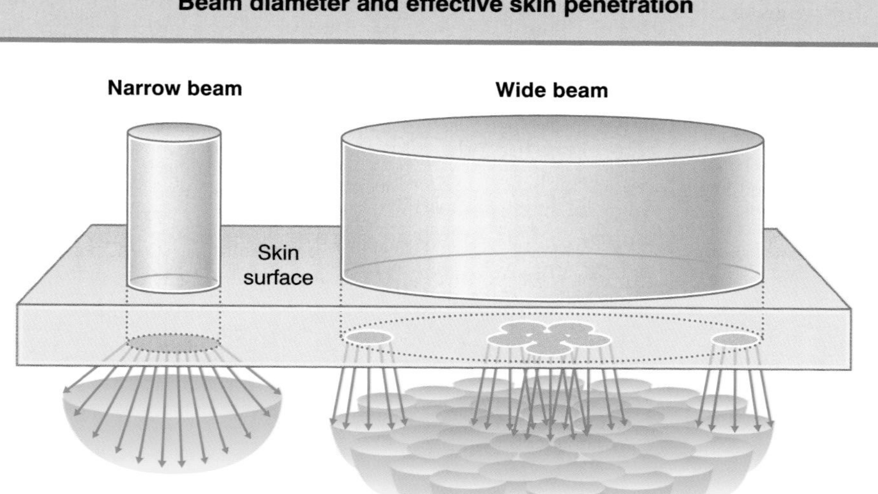

Figure 35.4 Effect of beam diameter on effective laser penetration. Optical scattering by dermal collagen causes light to diffuse as it penetrates into the dermis. A larger spot size allows for a greater likelihood that photons will be scattered back into the incident collimated beam with resultant beam broadening at any given depth and greater energy delivery.

Table 35.7 Fluences for minimal side-effect profile

Fitzpatrick skin type	Pulse duration (J/cm²)		
	30 ms	100 ms	200 ms
I	>60	>60	>60
II	>45	>60	>60
III	>45	>60	>60
IV	<30	<45	<45
V	<15	<30	<45
VI	Cannot safely treat	<15	<15

Figure 35.5 Effect of epidermal cooling. Areas treated using similar fluences and pulse durations, with and without cooling. No epidermal damage is noted with pretreatment cooling. Postoperative vesiculation is noted without cooling. (Courtesy of C Dierickx.)

epidermis with resultant injury to the overlying skin. This precludes the use of higher fluences in darker skinned individuals, which limits the possibility of permanent hair reduction. To minimize this occurrence, selective epidermal cooling is employed—a component that is especially critical in the treatment of darker skinned individuals (Fig. 35.5).

Five types of cooling systems have been devised in conjunction with laser hair removal.

- Passive cooling with an aqueous gel.
- Active contact cooling with water encased in a glass housing.
- Active contact cooling with water encased in a sapphire housing.
- Dynamic active cooling with a cryogen spray.
- Forced air cooling.

The use of a water-based gel works to hydrate the stratum corneum, improving the thermal conductivity at the skin surface. The effect is temporary with only a small amount of heat extracted because the temperature is not maintained. A sapphire window circulates water at approximately 2–6 °C, resulting in expedient heat extraction. This allows for rapid movement of the laser handpiece with adequate cooling. Applying the window for more than 0.5 seconds may result in undesirable levels of bulbar and shaft cooling. The index of refraction obtained with the sapphire window optimizes laser–tissue coupling with reduced backscatter. Water surface condensation may result in beam attenuation with the use of either a sapphire or glass window.

Evaporative cooling systems typically employ a cryogen spray delivered before the laser pulse. This generates greater epidermal protection with less inadvertent dermal cooling. An FDA-approved cryogen uses tetrafluoroethane as a surface cooling agent, with a boiling point of –26.2 °C. It is nontoxic, nonflammable and environmentally safe.[28] Irregularities in cryogen droplet size may lead to variable cooling. A cryogen film left on the skin surface may result in laser light attenuation as a result of increased surface reflection and scattering. Measurement of laser light attenuation following cryogen spray cooling has been examined. A minimum average transmittance value of approximately 97% was measured using a 30 ms spurt duration and 30 ms delay, thus showing negligible light attenuation at the two wavelengths studied.[29] A lack of laser–tissue coupling may increase backscatter with the technique.

Forced air cooling with air at –5 °C, or colder, effectively reduces the epidermal temperature, thus protecting the epidermis, reducing the pain of treatment, and eliminating the noxious odor of singed hair.

The epidermal protection afforded by the use of surface cooling allows for increased tolerated fluences for all skin types.

Histology

Biopsies obtained immediately after laser treatment demonstrate selective thermal damage to pigmented hair follicles, with vaporization of hair shafts and apoptosis of follicular epithelial cells. Patients with permanent hair loss demonstrate a reduction in the number of terminal hairs and an increase in vellus-like hairs without fibrosis[30] (Fig. 35.6). These findings most closely resemble the histological picture of androgenetic alopecia.

Specific laser systems

The first laser-assisted hair removal device was marketed in 1996. The FDA has since approved numerous laser and light sources for this use (Table 35.8).

Ruby laser

The normal mode ruby laser (694 nm) was the first laser employed that demonstrated both temporary and permanent hair reduction. Grossman et al[25] reported selective injury to hair follicles using the long-pulsed ruby laser in 13 patients with fair skin and brown or black hair. Treatment sites were shave or wax-epilated before delivery of a single laser treatment using a 6-mm spot size, fluences of 20–60 J/cm² and pulses of 0.27-ms duration. Hair growth delay lasting 1–3 months was noted in all patients. Biopsies immediately after treatment showed selective thermal damage to pigmented hair follicles. Long-term follow-up of seven of the 13 patients after 1 or 2 years revealed permanent hair loss only in the shaved areas at all fluences.[30] Skin sites treated at the highest fluence (60 J/cm²) revealed the greatest hair loss.

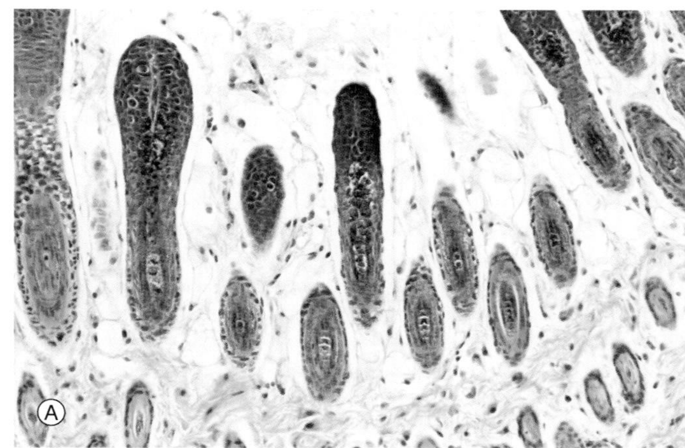

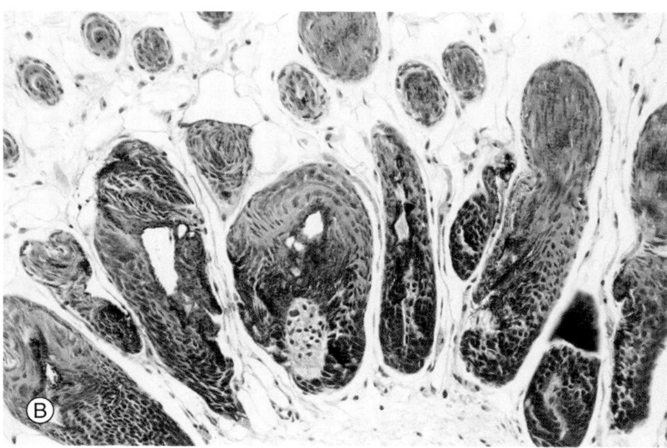

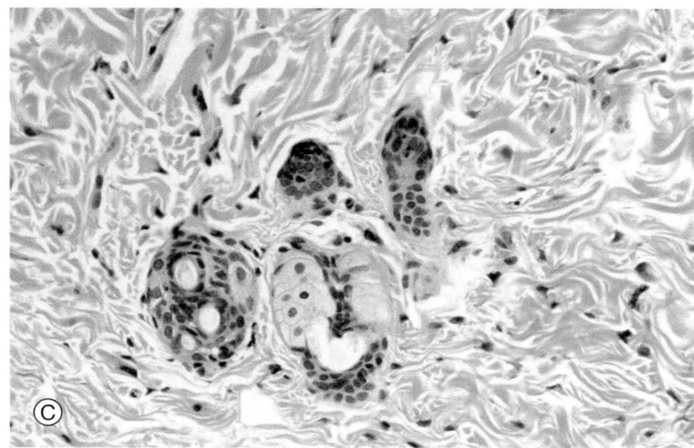

Figure 35.6 Skin biopsies of a hair follicle using a normal mode ruby laser. (A) Pretreatment. Intact follicles penetrate deeply into the deep dermis and subcutis. (B) Immediately following treatment. Thermal damage to the follicles is observed, with hair shaft vaporization and follicular cell apoptosis noted. (C) 6 months after treatment. A reduction in terminal hairs and an increase in vellus-like hairs are seen. No fibrosis is observed. Hematoxylin and eosin stain, original magnification ×32. (Courtesy of T Flotte.)

Although the ruby laser is an effective method of hair removal, there are significant dose-related side-effects. High epidermal melanin absorption may result in epidermal injury, manifested as acute vesiculation, crusting, or pigmentary change. Even though these changes may be observed with any laser system, they are more commonly observed with the ruby laser. Use of the ruby laser should be avoided in patients with a history of persistent postinflammatory hyperpigmentation, darkly tanned skin, or skin type darker than Fitzpatrick type III. A relative disadvantage is that the two commercially available ruby lasers (Epilaser, Palomar Medical, Lexington, MA; Epitouch, Lumenis, Israel) each have a slow pulse repetition rate, making it time-consuming to treat large body sites.

Alexandrite laser

Several long-pulsed alexandrite lasers (755 nm) are available for hair removal. These include the Apogee series (Cynosure, Chelmsford, MA), Epicare (Light Age), and Gentlelase (Candela, Wayland, MA). The longer wavelength allows for a slightly greater depth of penetration. There is also a lower risk of epidermal damage because of the slightly lower melanin absorption at this wavelength. McDaniel et al. showed a 40–50% hair reduction at 6 months after one treatment with the variable-pulsed alexandrite laser.[31] Nanni and Alster demonstrated equivalent long-term hair removal with the long-pulsed alexandrite laser at pulse durations of 5, 10, and 20 ms. Longer pulse durations provided more effective epidermal protection.[32]

Diode laser

The introduction of diode lasers (800–810 nm) further expanded the laser hair removal market because they are less costly to produce, reliable, and compact in size. Advantages of the diode laser include longer pulse durations and longer wavelength, allowing for the treatment of Fitzpatrick skin type III and IV patients because there is less epidermal melanin absorption. Long-term results (>12 months) suggest that the pulsed, 800 nm diode laser is as effective as the long-pulsed ruby laser in the removal of dark, terminal hair.[33,34]

Nd:YAG laser

Long-pulsed 1064 nm Nd:YAG lasers have deeply penetrating wavelengths. Reduced melanin absorption at this wavelength requires the use of higher fluences for adequate follicle injury. This laser is not as effective in treating patients with lighter hair. It is a safe treatment option for patients with Fitzpatrick skin types III to V.[35] Q-switched Nd:YAG lasers are available for hair removal. Although capable of treating darker skin types and inducing delayed regrowth, these systems do not produce long-term hair removal.

Intense pulsed light

Intense-pulsed (nonlaser) light sources (IPL) that emit noncoherent, multiwavelength light are being used for hair removal. The output spectrum extends across the 500–1000 nm range. Filters are placed to allow more selective treatment. Shorter wavelengths are blocked for Fitzpatrick skin types III and darker to avoid excessive

Table 35.8 Lasers and light sources for hair removal

Laser/light source	Wavelength (nm)	System name	Pulse duration (ms)	Fluence (J/cm²)	Spot size (mm)	Other features
Long-pulse ruby	694	Epilaser (Palomar, Burlington, MA)	3	10–40	7,10	Epiwan
		Epitouch (Sharplan, Allendale, NJ)	1.2	10–40	3–6	Dual mode, may also be Q-switched
Long-pulse alexandrite	755	Apogee 5500,6200,9300 (Cynosure, Chelmsford, MA)	5–40	50	10, 12.5, 15	Smartcool cold air
		Arion (Cynosure)	1–15	5–140	60 × 65	Skin cooling (air)
		EpiCare SP,LP,LPX,2H,4H (Light Age, Somerset, NJ)	3–300	12–100	7, 9, 12, 15 15	Smartscreen user interface
		GentleLASE plus (Candela, Wayland, MA)	3	10–100	10, 12, 18	Dynamic cooling
		Photogenica LPIR (Cynosure)	5, 10, 20	25–40	7, 10	Cooling tip available
Diode	800–810	Apex 800 (Iridex, Mountainview, CA)	5–100	5–60	1–5, 10	Adjustable handpiece
		F1 Diode (Opusmed, Montreal, Canada)	10–100	10–40	5, 7, 10	Air cooling
		Lightsheer ET,ST,XC (Lumenis, Santa Clara, MA)	5–400	10–100	9 × 9, 12 × 12	Chilltip handpiece
		SLP100 (Palomar)	50–1000 ns	Up to 575		Three contact cooling handpieces
Nd:YAG	1064	Acclaim7000; SmartEpil II (Cynosure)	0.4–300	16–300	2, 5, 5, 7, 10	Smartcool cold air
		Coolglide Classic, Excel, XEI, Vantage (Cutera, Brisbane, CA)	0.1–300	10–300	Multiple	
		Gentle YAG (Candela)	3	10–100	10, 12	
		Lyra (Laserscope, San Jose, CA)	20–100	5–900	1–5, 10	Adjustable handpiece
		Mydon (Wavelight, Erlangen, Germany)	20–200	15–50	60 × 65, 3	Air or contact cooling
		Profile (Sciton, Palo Alto, CA)	0.1–200	4–400	Scanner up to 31 × 31	Contact cooling
		Softlight (Telsar, Wood River, IL)	12–18	2–3		Q-switched; patented carbon lotion
Intense-pulsed light source	525–1200	Estelux Y,R,Rs, Medilux Y,R (Palomar)	10–100	Up to 15–30	16 × 46, 12 × 28	
	400–1200	PhotoLight (Cynosure)	5–50	3–30	46 × 18, 46 × 10	
	550–900	Prolite (Alderm Irvine, CA)		10–50	10 × 20, 20 × 25	
	510–1200	Quadra Q4 (DermaMed, Lenni, PA)	48	10–20		Closed cooling system
	400–1200	Spectraclear (Symedex LLC, Minneapolis, MN)	34	10–50	55 × 22	Five small area adapters
Fluorescent pulsed light	615–920	OmniLight (Medical Bio Care, Newport Beach, CA)	2–500	Up to 45		
Photothermal	400–1200	Skin Station (Radiancy, Orangeburg, NY)	35	3–10	22 × 55	
Optical energy combined w/RF electrical energy	580–980	Aurora DS, DSR (Syneron, Richmond Hill, Canada)	Up to 100	10–45 optical; 5–25 J/cm³ RF	8 × 12	Contact cooling
Diode combined w/RF electrical energy	800	Polaris DS (Syneron)	Up to 100	Up to 25 optical, up to 20 J/cm³ RF	8 × 12	Contact cooling

W/RF, with radiofrequency.

epidermal heating. Shorter wavelengths are used for Fitzpatrick skin types I and II for maximal energy delivery.[36] A disadvantage of IPL systems is that most devices use large rectangular spots, creating difficulty in the treatment of convex or concave hair-bearing areas.

Microwave technology

A microwave-based hair removal system (Microwave Delivery System, MW Medical, Scottsdale, AZ) has been FDA approved for hair removal in all body sites except the face. Pulses of microwave energy are delivered to the skin in conjunction with a coolant spray. No published data are available to assess the efficacy of this technology.

Treatment delivery

Treatment can be initiated after a consultative appointment has been performed and the risks and benefits of laser hair removal reviewed. An oral antiviral medication is initiated 24 hours before the laser procedure and continued for a total of 7 days in patients with a history of herpes simplex virus near the laser treatment site. Each patient signs an informed consent on the day of service. Preoperative pictures are recommended to monitor patient progress.

To minimize treatment discomfort, a topical anesthetic cream may be applied. We recommend LMX 4 (4% lidocaine cream) or LMX 5 (5% lidocaine cream) (Ferndale Laboratories, Ferndale, MI), an over-the-counter mixture to be applied 30–45 minutes before the procedure without occlusion. Alternatively, EMLA (eutectic mixture of 2.5% lidocaine/2.5% prilocaine) (Astra Pharmaceuticals, Westboro, MA) is applied 1 to 1.5 hours before the procedure under plastic wrap occlusion. Each cream should be applied as a thick layer to the entire treatment site to maximize efficacy. The anesthetic cream is removed immediately before laser treatment.

Patients are instructed to clip or shave the treatment site 1 day before treatment. Shaving may be performed by the staff immediately before treatment if patients are reluctant to shave. The hair should be cut to approximately 1 mm in length to minimize plume and prevent hair char and subsequent epidermal damage. All make-up should be removed before treatment to allow for maximum laser energy delivery and to minimize light scatter.

Patients are positioned comfortably on a surgical table to permit maximum accessibility to the targeted surfaces. All staff and the patient must wear protective glasses or goggles with a minimum optical density of 5 specific for the wavelength of light being used. A polarizing headlamp with magnifying loupe may be used (Seymour light, Syris Scientific, Gray, ME) for improved visibility of treatment sites. The plume generated by vaporized hair shafts has a sulfur smell and in large quantities can be irritating to the respiratory tract not to mention bothersome to the patient because of malodor. Use of a smoke evacuator and good room ventilation is recommended except with the cold air blowing system, which disperses the odor from the area. If the device is not equipped with a cooling device, an ice-cold cooling gel is generously applied before laser treatment for epidermal cooling. With dynamic cooling, short bursts of cryogen are emitted before the delivery of the laser pulse. With contact cooling, the chilled handpiece is applied firmly to the skin before pulse delivery.

Laser parameters are tailored to each patient and each device to ensure maximum efficacy with minimal side-effects. The highest tolerated fluence and the largest spot size should be used to obtain the best results. Mild traction on the skin with slight pressure may help to provide uniform illumination and prevent capillary blood flow, which may interfere with light transmission to the hair follicles. Applying gentle skin traction decreases the relative depth of the bulb and bulge relative to the skin surface.

The treated skin is monitored for a 5-minute interval after initiation of treatment for the desired erythema and perifollicular edema. If any whitening, vesiculation, or forced epidermal separation (positive Nikolsky's sign) is noted, the fluence must be decreased and repeat monitoring observed at the lower energy. In general, the treatment fluence should be at 75% of the Nikolsky's sign threshold fluence. Treatment sites bearing tattoos should not be treated to avoid alteration of the tattoo pigment. With direct contact cooling systems the laser handpiece should be wiped clean every 10–20 pulses to remove debris. The laser handpiece must be disinfected with Virex II (Johnson Wax Professional, Sturtevant, WI) or a similar agent between patients to minimize contamination.

■ OPTIMIZING OUTCOMES

The optimal candidate for laser hair removal is the individual with fair skin (skin types I or II) and dark terminal hair because maximal follicular pigment is vital for permanent hair reduction and minimal epidermal pigment is desired to minimize side-effects (Fig. 35.7). Individuals with red, gray, or white hair may lack sufficient follicular melanin to allow for permanent hair reduction. Individuals with darker skin present with an increased risk of side-effects at any given energy, although longer wavelengths offer some degree of protection of epidermal melanin.

To achieve maximum benefit, an appropriate wavelength, pulse duration, and fluence must be tailored to each individual. Using the highest tolerated fluence and largest spot size allows for more effective hair removal.

The complicating factor in selecting follicular melanin as the target for laser hair removal is that melanin is also found in the epidermis. With laser treatment, epidermal damage may occur as a result of absorptive interference by epidermal melanin. Darker skinned individuals (Fitzpatrick skin types III to V) benefit from longer pulse durations (>30 ms) because this allows for the simultaneous cooling of the band of melanin at the dermoepidermal junction, and more time for heat extraction from the skin surface (Fig. 35.8). This reduces the risk of epidermal injury. Cooling allows higher fluences to be used for more permanent hair removal. Patients with a Fitzpatrick skin type III or greater should not be treated with a long-pulsed ruby laser to minimize side-effects. The alexandrite and long-pulsed Nd:YAG lasers and IPL sources operating at near infrared wavelengths and long pulse durations have been safely used to treat these patients. Patients with an active tan should not be treated.

A laser test spot should be considered for any patient in whom there is a concern about the potential for side-effects. This test spot should be performed within or adjacent to the proposed treatment site if possible. The treatment site

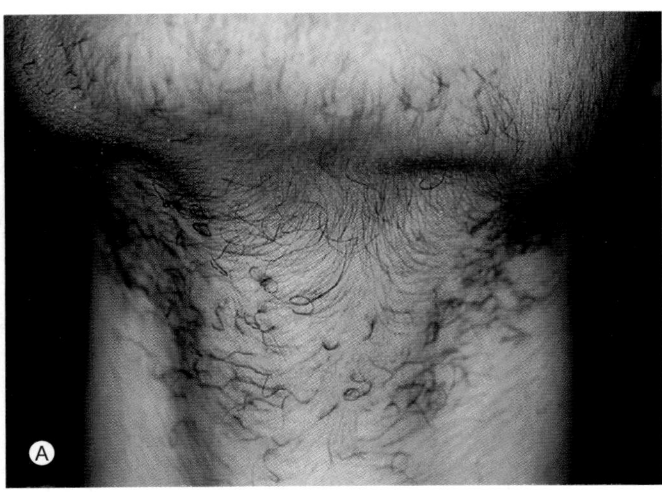

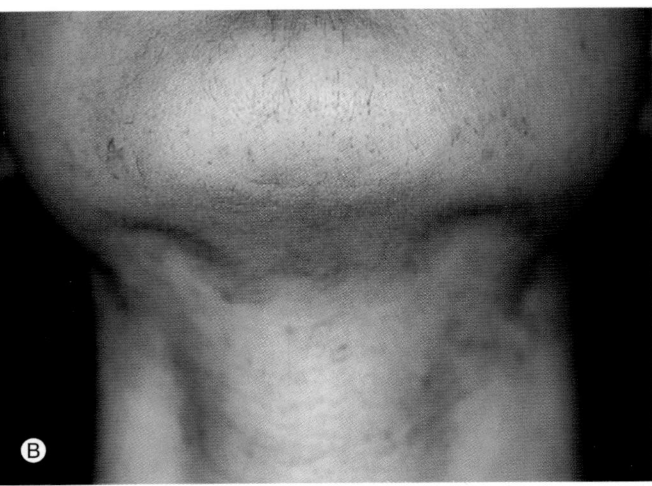

Figure 35.7 Laser hair removal. (A) Pretreatment, neck area of a patient with Fitzpatrick skin type II. (B) Noted hair reduction after three treatments using an 800 nm diode laser, 20 ms pulse duration, 42 J/cm² and contact cooling.

should be observed immediately and 1 week after treatment to assess for any adverse reaction. Treatment can be initiated at the 1-week follow-up visit if no side-effects are noted.

It is best to avoid the treatment of vellus hairs, in particular of the jawline because new hair growth may be induced as a result of sublethal laser doses, with resultant induction of terminal hair.[37] This has been reported to occur more commonly in females of Mediterranean descent. For highly dense hair-bearing areas, such as the back and chest, it is imperative to use lower fluences to prevent non-selective damage through excessive heat diffusion. Appropriate laser safety precautions must be followed (see Chapter 37).

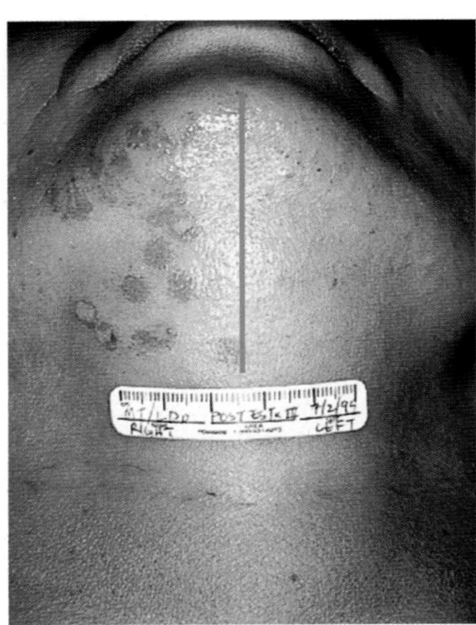

Figure 35.8 Epidermal protection using longer pulsed durations in the treatment of Fitzpatrick skin type V patient. The patient's right submental area was treated with an Nd:YAG laser using a 30 ms pulse duration and 30 J/cm² with immediate vesiculation and skin sloughing. The patient's left submental area was treated using a 100 ms pulse duration and 30 J/cm² without complication. (Courtesy of E Battle.)

■ POSTOPERATIVE CARE

Laser-treated sites generally demonstrate perifollicular edema lasting up to 48 hours, and erythema, which may persist for up to 1 week. Ice is applied to the treatment sites immediately on treatment completion to minimize these effects and reduce postoperative discomfort. If the erythema persists beyond 10 days, a low to mid-potency corticosteroid cream may be applied twice daily until the redness subsides. Infrequently perifollicular crusting lasting 7–10 days may occur. Twice daily application of topical petrolatum or topical antibiotic ointment is recommended until the scabbing has completely resolved. Any trauma such as picking or scratching of the area must be avoided. Purpura is rarely observed, resolving over 2 weeks when noted. Analgesics are generally not required unless extensive areas are treated.

Patients should be informed that the treated hair will continue to 'grow' for 1–2 weeks after treatment, until each hair is expelled from the skin surface. Patients can shave, tweeze, or wax these treated hairs to expedite their removal once all inflammation has resolved. Depending on the treatment site, patients will note hair regrowth of those hairs not in anagen during treatment within 2–6 weeks thereafter.

Strict photoprotection is stressed for the duration of the treatment course. Treatment is to be avoided if an active tan is noted. Patients are instructed to complete their antiviral medication, when appropriate. Treatment intervals are site-dependent. In general, treatments are spaced every 6–8 weeks for the face, axillae, and bikini areas where regrowth is faster, and every 12–16 weeks for legs, chest, arms and back where regrowth is slower.

■ PITFALLS AND THEIR MANAGEMENT

Pitfalls and their management

- Adverse reactions may occur—patients should be made aware of what to expect postoperatively and instructed to notify the office as soon as possible if an adverse reaction occurs.
- Potential pigmentary changes include postinflammatory and temporary or permanent hypopigmentation. They generally resolve slowly over months to years. Strict sun avoidance is mandatory. Twice daily application of a bleaching cream to hyperpigmented areas helps lighten the affected sites.
- Hair thinning is common, with an associated fading and lightening of the hair color.[38] Conversion of vellus hairs to terminal hairs may also occur. Use of the highest tolerated fluence minimizes these occurrences.
- Temporary or permanent leukotrichia after IPL and laser hair removal therapy is avoided by using sufficient fluences to induce germinative cell death concurrently with melanocyte death.
- If patients are properly selected during the consultation, few adverse events should be observed. Patients should be made aware of what to expect postoperatively and instructed to notify the office as soon as possible if an adverse reaction develops to allow for proper management and follow-up.

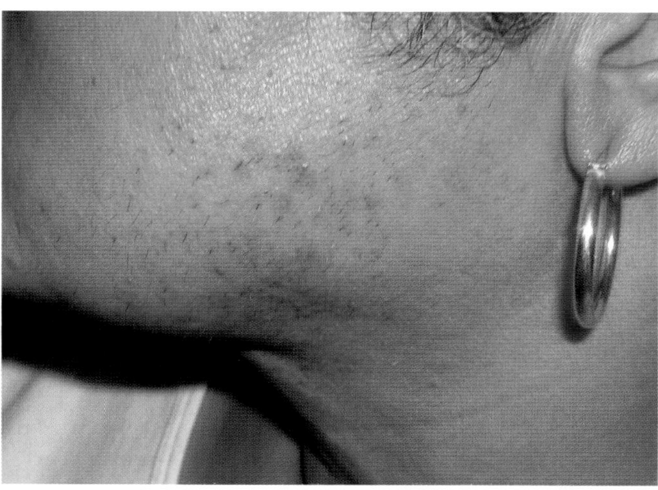

Figure 35.9 Transient hypopigmentation 4 weeks after treatment.

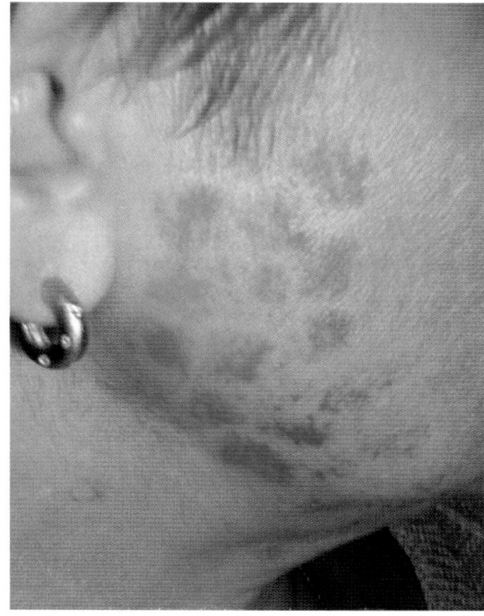

Figure 35.10 Transient blistering and hyperpigmentation 2 days after treatment. The patient was treated with a long-pulsed Nd:YAG laser, 100 ms, 20 J/cm^2.

Pigmentary changes that can occur include post-inflammatory hyperpigmentation and temporary or permanent hypopigmentation (Figs 35.9, 35.10). This occurs most frequently in patients who do not avoid sun exposure before or after treatment and in patients with Fitzpatrick skin type III or greater. These pigmentary changes generally resolve slowly over time, but may take months to years for full resolution. Strict sun avoidance is mandatory to avoid further tanning of the affected sites. Twice daily application of a bleaching cream to hyperpigmented areas helps to lighten the affected sites. Patients must be aware that topical hydroquinone creams rarely cause an irritant dermatitis with long-term use. Blistering may occur, requiring localized wound care and use of a mid-potency corticosteroid cream. Scar formation is extremely rare.

Hair thinning is frequently observed, with an associated fading and lightening of the hair color.[38] This may represent partial rather than complete destruction of germinative cells at the bulge and bulb regions. Hair growth induced by laser hair removal has also been reported[37] This is especially seen in people with darker skin types, possibly due to sublethal fluences used that paradoxically increase hair growth. Conversion of vellus hairs to terminal hairs may also occur in this setting. Use of the highest tolerated fluence minimizes these occurrences. On the other hand, significant pain needs to be tended to and may be a warning that fluences are unduly high and causing tissue destruction.

Temporary or permanent leukotrichia may develop following IPL and laser hair removal therapy. This likely represents the destruction of the melanocytes within the hair follicles without destruction of the germinative cells. Temporary leukotrichia may represent a temporary arrest in melanin synthesis by damaged, but viable melanocytes. The melanocytes may become functional after a while, leading to the restoration of hair color. Hair color restoration occurs more frequently in younger patients, whose melanocytes may be less susceptible to permanent thermal damage. In patients with permanent depigmentation of their treated hair, permanent melanocyte destruction may occur. Permanent leukotrichia was reported in 29 of 770 patients of skin types I–IV treated primarily for unwanted facial and submental hair using a noncoherent IPL system with a 650 nm flashlamp filter. The white hairs were found to be as thick as the pretreatment black hairs.[39] The use of sufficient fluences to induce germinative cell death concurrently with melanocyte death is critical in avoiding this side-effect.

■ SUMMARY

Numerous laser and light sources are available for the rapid, safe, and effective hair removal. Temporary hair removal can be achieved with all systems regardless of hair color. Numerous published studies have confirmed the long-term efficacy of laser and flashlamp technology. The ability to achieve longlasting hair removal depends on hair color, skin type, and treatment fluence. Uniform permanent hair reduction has proven difficult, probably because of the broad distribution of pluripotential cells, as well as the hardiness of the hair follicle. To date, no laser specific parameters provide predictable permanent hair follicle destruction. The number of treatments needed to obtain complete permanent hair removal for different anatomic sites varies and is unknown. The benefits of this technology have largely been limited to patients with fair skin and dark hair. Studies using devices with longer wavelengths, longer pulse durations, and epidermal cooling have shown that it is possible to safely and effectively treat darker skinned individuals. The remaining challenge is to develop a means to eliminate light and nonpigmented hair. Advancing technologies and broadening understanding of follicular biology and growth will allow for improved means of hair removal.

The treatment of blond, red, white, and gray hair may be possible with the use of combined IPL and radiofrequency devices such as the Aurora (Syneron, Israel) by directing the radiofrequency current to the hair follicle through heating of the follicle with the IPL. Heating reduces impedance, resulting in concentration of the radiofrequency to the follicular target. In addition, the hair shaft with its low water content and high impedance encourages the electrical current to become concentrated around the hair shaft in the hair follicle resulting in further localized follicular heating. Another alternative is the use of photodynamic therapy. In a pilot study, ALA combined with red light photodynamic therapy has shown promise in hair reduction. Using ALA eliminates the need for pigment in the hair follicle.

■ REFERENCES

1. Pinkus H. Embryology of hair. New York: Academic Press; 1958.
2. Lavker RM, Miller S, Wilson C, et al. Hair follicle stem cells: their location, role in hair cycle, and involvement in skin tumor formation. J Invest Dermatol 1993; 101:16S–26S.
3. Headington JT. Transverse microscopic anatomy of the human scalp: a basis for a morphometric approach to disorders of the hair follicle. Arch Dermatol 1984; 120:449–456.
4. Cesarini J. Hair melanin and color. In: Orfanos C, Happle R, eds. Hair and hair diseases. Berlin: Springer–Verlag; 1990.
5. Menon IA, Persad S, Haberman HF, et al. A comparative study of the physical and chemical properties of melanins isolated from human black and red hair. J Invest Dermatol 1983; 80:202–206.
6. Kvedar J, Gibson M, Kruskinsi P. Hirsutism: evaluation and treatment. J Am Acad Dermatol 1985; 12:215–225.
7. Richards RN, Uy M, Meharg GE. Temporary hair removal in patients with hirsutism: a clinical study. Cutis 1990; 45:199–202.
8. Malhotra B, Noveck R, Behr D, Palmsano M. Percutaneous absorption and pharmacokinetics of eflornithine HCl 13.9% cream in women with unwanted facial hair. J Clin Pharmacol 2001; 41:972–978.
9. Schrode K. Randomized double blind vehicle controlled safety and efficacy evaluation of eflornithine 15% cream in the treatment of women with excessive facial hair. Paper presented at American Academy of Dermatology Annual Meeting, 2000; San Francisco, California.
10. Richards RN, Meharg GE. Electrolysis: observations from 13 years and 140 000 hours of experience. J Am Acad Dermatol 1995; 33:662–666.
11. Lin DT, Dierickx CC, Campos VB, et al. Reduction of regrowing hair shaft size and pigmentation after ruby and diode laser treatment. Arch Dermatol Res 2000; 292:60–67.
12. Dierickx CC, Grossman MC, Farinelli WA, et al. Long-pulsed ruby laser hair removal. Lasers Surg Med 1997; S10:167.
13. Descamps V, Valance A, Edlinger C, et al. Association of human herpes virus 6 infection with drug reaction with eosinophilia and systemic symptoms. Arch Dermatol 2001; 137:301–304.
14. Marchell NL, Alster TS. Evaluation of temporary and permanent hair removal methods. J Aesth Dermatol Cosmet Dermatol Surg 1999; 1:3–12.
15. Sun T, Cotsarelis G, Lavker RM. Hair follicle stem cells: the bulge activation hypothesis. J Invest Dermatol 1991; 96(suppl 5):77S–78S.
16. Finkelstein LH, Blatstein LM. Epilation of hair-bearing urethral grafts using the neodymium:YAG surgical laser. J Urol 1991; 146:840–842.
17. Anderson RR, Parrish JA. Selective photothermolysis: precise microsurgery by selective absorption of pulsed radiation. Science 1983; 220:524–527.
18. Ross E, Laden Z, Kreindel M, et al. Theoretical considerations in laser hair removal. Dermatol Clin 1999; 17:333–355.
19. Anderson RR, Parrish JA. The optics of human skin. J Invest Dermatol 1981; 77:13–19.
20. Nanni CA, Alster TS. Optimizing treatment parameters for hair removal using a topical carbon-based solution and 1064 nm Q-switched neodymium:YAG laser energy. Arch Dermatol 1997; 133:1546–1549.
21. Hoffman RM. Topical liposome targeting of dyes, melanins, genes and proteins selectively to hair follicles. J Drug Targeting 1997; 3:27–74.
22. Mordon S, Sumian C, Devoisselle JM. Site-specific methylene blue delivery to pilosebaceous structures using highly porous nylon microspheres: an experimental evaluation. Lasers Surg Med 2003; 33:119–125.
23. Grossman M, Wimberly J, Dwyer P, et al. PDT for hirsutism. Lasers Surg Med 1997; 7(suppl):44.
24. Lehrer MS, Crawford GH, Gelfand JM, et al. Effect of wax epilation before hair removal with a long-pulsed alexandrite laser: a pilot study. Dermatol Surg 2003; 29:218–123.
25. Grossman M, Dierickx C, Farinelli W, et al. Damage to hair follicles by normal-mode ruby laser pulses. J Am Acad Dermatol 1996; 35: 889–894.
26. Altshuler GB, Anderson RR, Manstein D, et al. Extended theory of selective photothermolysis. Lasers Surg Med 2001; 29:416–432.
27. Duque V, Dierickx C, Lin D, et al. Long-pulsed ruby laser for hair removal: comparisons between different spot size, temperatures, and interval between first and second treatment. Lasers Surg Med 1998; 10(suppl):39.
28. Nelson JS, Milner TE, Anvari B, et al. Dynamic epidermal cooling during pulsed laser treatment of portwine stain: a new methodology with preliminary clinical evaluation. Arch Dermatol 1997; 131: 695–700.
29. Edris A, Choi B, Aguilar G, et al. Measurements of laser light attenuation following cryogen spray cooling spurt termination. Lasers Surg Med 2003; 32:143–147.
30. Dierickx C, Grossman M, Farinelli WA. Permanent hair removal by normal-mode ruby laser. Arch Dermatol 1998; 134:837–842.
31. McDaniel DH, Lord J, Ask K, et al. A review and report of the use of the long-pulsed alexandrite laser for hair reduction of the upper lip, leg, back and bikini region. Dermatol Surg 1999; 25:425–430.
32. Nanni CA, Alster TS. Long pulsed alexandrite laser assisted hair removal at 5, 10 and 20 millisecond pulse durations. Lasers Surg Med 1999; 24:332–337.
33. Dierickx CC, Grossman MC, Farinelli WA, et al. Comparison between a long-pulsed ruby laser and a pulsed infrared laser system. Lasers Surg Med 1998; S10:199.
34. Grossman MC, Dierickx CC, Quintana A, et al. Removal of excess body hair with an 800 nm pulsed diode laser. Lasers Surg Med 1998; 10 (suppl):42.
35. Alster TS, Bryan H, Williams CN. Long-pulsed Nd:YAG laser-assisted hair removal in pigmented skin: a clinical and histologic evaluation. Arch Dermatol 2001; 137:885–889.
36. Gold MH, Bell MW, Foster TD, et al. Long-term epilation using the Epilight broad band, intense pulsed light hair removal system. Dermatol Surg 1997; 23:909–913.
37. Hirsch R, Farinelli WA, Dover JS, et al. Hair growth induced by laser hair removal. Paper presented at American Society for Laser Medicine and Surgery, 2003; Anaheim, California.
38. Dierickx CC, Grossman MC, Farinelli WA, et al. Hair removal by a pulsed, infrared laser system. Lasers Surg Med 1998; 10 (suppl):198.
39. Radmaneshi M, Mostaghimi M, Yousefi I, et al. Leukotrichia developed following application of intense pulsed light for hair removal. Dermatol Surg 2002; 28:772–574.

36 Microdermabrasion and Dermabrasion

James M Spencer MD MS and Christopher B Harmon MD

Summary box

- Microdermabrasion is the second most widely performed cosmetic procedure in the US and is commonly offered at spas and beauty salons.
- Microdermabrasion is widely used to treat photodamage, dyschromias, acne, scars, and stretch marks.
- Available studies indicate that changes in the epidermis and dermis can be objectively measured after microdermabrasion, and that patients and physicians alike perceive a clinical benefit.
- Mechanical dermabrasion with a rotating diamond fraise or wire brush is one of the most effective means for resurfacing a variety of skin defects and blemishes.
- The most common indication for dermabrasion is facial acne scars.

INTRODUCTION

Traditional dermabrasion utilizes a wire brush or diamond fraise on a rotary hand engine to mechanically remove tissue and has been widely utilized since its development in the 1950s. This technique can produce outstanding results, but it creates a significant wound that can require weeks to heal, and aerosolizes blood into the operating room during the procedure. It is quite operator-dependent and requires hands-on learning and significant experience. Scarring, dyspigmentation, and infection are potential complications of any deep abrasion procedure.

An abrasion or resurfacing procedure that is bloodfree, safer, and with less healing time has been a goal for many practitioners. In 1985, Marini and Lo,[1] working in Italy, developed microdermabrasion as an abrasive resurfacing technique that would fulfill these goals.

Microdermabrasion

Microdermabrasion has been widely utilized to treat photodamage, dyschromias, acne, scars, and stretch marks. Despite the widespread use of microdermabrasion, surprisingly little is known about its clinical efficacy.

The first paper on microdermabrasion in the medical literature appeared in 1995. Tsai et al.[2] treated 41 patients with different types of scars (including acne, traumatic, varicella, and burn scars) with microdermabrasion. These investigators used an aggressive vacuum setting of 76 mmHg and performed multiple treatments. The authors reported 'good to excellent' clinical improvement after a mean of 9.1 treatments; acne scars required a mean of 15.2 treatments for improvement. Mild postinflammatory hyperpigmentation was the only side-effect. A limitation of this study was the lack of objective evaluation of efficacy. The outcome was measured solely by the physician's subjective visual evaluation. The human eye has a remarkable sensitivity to mild aesthetic improvements, thus we can see if someone 'looks better.' However, objectively quantifying an aesthetic judgment is difficult and is a problem in attempting to scientifically evaluate novel cosmetic treatments. Several recent papers have tried to solve this problem.

Shim et al.[3] combined the patient's and physician's subjective evaluation with histology. Fourteen patients with photoaging were treated once every 2 weeks at a mild vacuum setting for a total of six to seven treatments. Eleven of the 14 patients also had comedomal acne or milia, and three had acne scarring. Following the series of treatments, patients completed a questionnaire to evaluate their perception of the procedure. Overall, patients were pleased with the treatment, reporting a perceived benefit in overall complexion, skin roughness, and mottled pigmentation. They did not perceive an improvement in fine wrinkles, comedomal acne, or milia. An unblinded physician investigator subjectively evaluated before and after photographs of the three patients with acne scars. The acne scars were treated much more aggressively than the photodamage patients, usually with more than 20 passes each session. One patient was considered to have 'good' improvement, one 'fair' improvement, and one no improvement.

This study also includes some limited histologic evaluation. First, a single piece of excised abdominal skin was treated with 20 passes of microdermabrasion at settings of

–12 inHg, then immediately processed and evaluated histologically. Permanent sections were prepared and stained with H&E. Surprisingly little abrasion was seen, with only partial ablation of the stratum corneum and compaction of the remaining stratum corneum. No viable epidermis was affected. They performed in vivo histologic evaluation of three patients. The dorsal forearm was treated once every 2 weeks for a total of six treatments. Ten passes were performed at each session at a setting of –16 inHg. Following completion of six treatments, after-treatment biopsies were compared to before-treatment biopsies. In these three subjects, six microdermabrasion treatments produced thickening of the epidermis with no change in the stratum corneum. Fontana–Masson staining revealed a more regular distribution of melanosomes and less melanization of the epidermis. There was an increase in elastin content in two of the three subjects, and no consistent change in mucin or collagen content of the papillary dermis.

This study supports the observation that both patients and physicians perceive a benefit to microdermabrasion. In clinical use, the authors report pinpoint bleeding, petechiae and even purpura when 20 passes are performed on acne scars. This implies that injury, in the form of suction or abrasion proceeds to the papillary dermis where the blood vessels are located. In this study, when 20 passes were performed on an excised piece of skin, the level of abrasion did not go past the stratum corneum. Suction injury may be the cause of pinpoint bleeding in the absence of epidermal and dermal abrasion. It is unclear whether this effect correlates with outcomes.

Freedman et al.[4] evaluated the histologic changes in ten patients who received a series of six microdermabrasion treatments. The posterior auricular area was biopsied before treatment, after three treatments, and after six treatments. There was thickening of both the epidermis and papillary dermis after three and six treatments. There was flattening of the rete pegs, and normalization of the stratum corneum, as compared to controls. In the dermis, collagen fibers showed hyalinization with thicker, horizontally-oriented collagen bundles that were more tightly packed when compared to controls. An improvement in the appearance of the elastic fibers was noted, as well as increased dermal inflammatory activity.

Hernandez-Perez et al.[5] confirmed most of these observations in a study of seven patients with facial photodamage who received five weekly microdermabrasion treatments of three passes each. The subjective evaluation of the appearance of the skin was assessed by recording the patient's, nurse's, and physician's evaluation of the degree of skin oiliness, porosity, sebaceousness, fine wrinkling, and overall appearance (oily skin, dilated pores, thick skin, fine wrinkles, and general appearance). As in other reports, patients and operators alike perceived a benefit with microdermabrasion. Patients and clinicians (doctors and nurses) alike reported subjective improvement in all parameters assessed. All patients underwent biopsies of the left malar region before and after treatment. Investigators reported an increase in epidermal thickness, as seen in other papers, and additionally, an improvement in the polarity of epidermal cells and a decrease in basal cell liquefaction. There were dermal changes, including a decrease in solar elastosis, and what is described as a slight improvement in the degree of dermal telangiectasias, edema, and inflammation.

These studies used different microdermabrasion equipment with different vacuum settings and treatment protocols, and yet come to the same general conclusions. Taken together, these studies suggest that the following.

- Most patients are somewhat pleased with the results of a series of microdermabrasion treatments.
- Physicians perceive at least some degree of benefit.
- Very subtle histologic changes are noted in the epidermis and the dermis following a series of treatments.

One puzzle from these studies is the finding by Shim et al.[3] that when a single piece of excised abdominal skin was treated with 20 passes of microdermabrasion, then immediately examined histologically, almost no abrasion was seen. In fact, much of the stratum corneum was left intact. How then, are histologic changes in the dermis produced?

Tan et al.[6] used subjective and objective measures to shed some light on this question. First, two patients received four microdermabrasion passes at an aggressive setting of 60–65 mmHg to one forearm with biopsies both before treatment and immediately after treatment. In both patients, aggressive microdermabrasion produced only thinning of the stratum corneum, with no abrasion of the viable epidermis. However, dermal changes, which included dermal edema, vasodilatation, and perivascular inflammation, were noted. Clinically, the treated areas developed significant erythema and overall improvement which lasted a week (Fig. 36.1). The authors speculated that these changes were unlikely to result from the impact of the aluminum oxide crystals (abrasion) and more likely to result from the effects of suction on dermal vasculature.

The same investigators also treated ten subjects with facial photodamage with weekly microdermabrasion for five to six sessions. The vacuum line was set to a moderate level as per the manufacturer, and each patient received four passes per session (30 mmHg). One week after the last treatment session, most patients subjectively reported at least a mild improvement in the appearance of the skin. Similarly, blinded physician evaluators also subjectively rated pre and post photographs as showing at least a mild improvement in most patients.

For objective measurement, the investigators utilized a sebumeter to quantify surface sebum levels, silicone replicas to measure skin topography (i.e. wrinkling), and an advanced cutometer to measure skin biomechanical properties (i.e. skin integrity). Sebumeter readings showed a significant decrease in surface sebum levels immediately following each treatment. However, this effect was gone by one week. Silicone impressions revealed a temporary increase in skin roughness and a mild flattening of some wrinkles immediately after treatment, consistent with abrasion of the stratum corneum. This effect had disappeared 1 week after treatment and maybe earlier since this was the earliest postoperative evaluation after the day of treatment. However, in the two patients who showed the greatest increase in surface roughness immediately after treatment, a significant decrease in skin roughness was seen 1 week after the final session. The biomechanical analysis of the skin by cutometer revealed the most interesting findings. The device used was a BTC 2000 (SRLI, Nashville, TN). This device applies suction to the skin through a

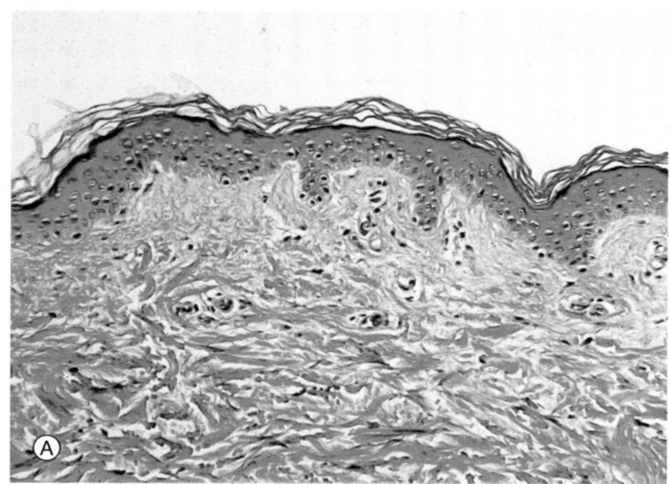

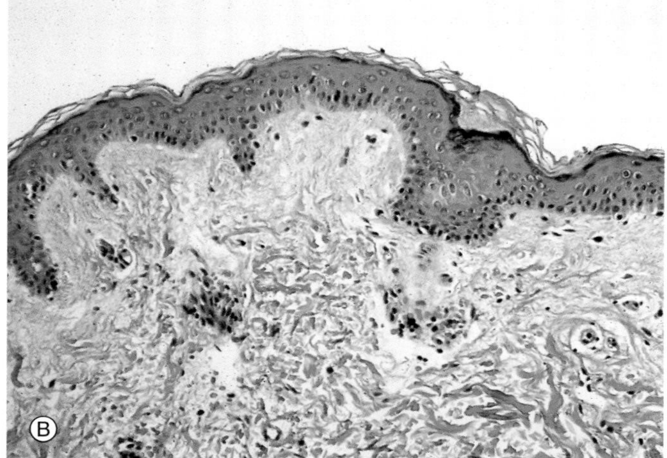

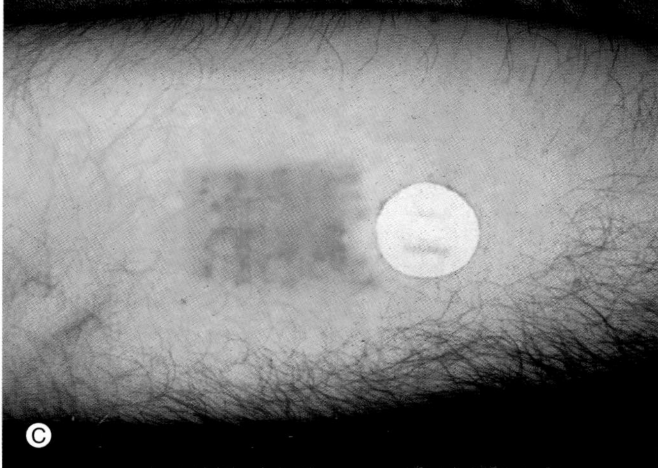

Figure 36.1 (A) Normal skin of the forearm before microdermabrasion. (B) The same area after four passes of microdermabrasion at an aggressive setting. Only the stratum corneum is abraded: there is no abrasion of viable epidermis. (C) The treated area showing marked erythema that persisted for 1 week. Despite a lack of any true abrasion, a visible clinical response is readily noted.

plastic tube. Infrared light is utilized to measure how much the skin moves over a range of negative pressures. Once the suction is released, the device also measures the return to presuction position. Skin elasticity, stiffness, and compliance can thus be calculated. It was found there was a significant decrease in skin stiffness and increase in skin compliance on the cheek throughout the study. This effect persisted 1 week after the final session. This is consistent with increased edema and hydration of the skin. One can think of this as a stiff, dry sponge becoming soft and compliant as it is hydrated. This finding is consistent with the edema and vasodilatation seen from the forearm biopsies. Two patients agreed to preauricular biopsies before and 1 week after the final treatment. There was an increase in orthokeratosis, mild flattening of the rete ridges, and most significantly, persistent dermal edema, vascular ectasia, and perivascular inflammation extending to the upper reticular dermis.

These results indicate that microdermabrasion can produce persistent dermal edema, vasodilatation, and perivascular inflammation with essentially no abrasion or wound formation. This edema makes the skin plumper and softer. It is unlikely that abrasion from the crystal impact produces this effect, but rather that this occurs due to the suction itself.

Objective confirmation of a biologic effect due to microdermabrasion from a wholly different perspective was provided by Rajan and Grimes.[7] In this study, epidermal barrier function was assessed by measuring transepidermal water loss (TEWL), stratum corneum hydration, skin surface pH, and sebum content. Patients were treated with conventional aluminum oxide microdermabrasion on one side of the face, and a similar device using sodium chloride as an abrasive on the other side. TEWL scores increased on both sides 24 hours after the procedure, suggesting disruption of barrier function. However, TEWL scores decreased when measured after 7 days, suggesting an improvement in barrier function. Stratum corneum hydration increased on both sides 24 hours after the procedure, and stayed increased on the sodium chloride side at 7 days. There was no sustained change in surface pH or sebum content. This study suggests microdermabrasion produces changes in epidermal barrier function which are sustained for at least 7 days, and the authors speculated these changes could be responsible for the perceived clinical benefit.

Like microdermabrasion, 20% glycolic acid peels are considered low risk with little downtime but are mildly effective as a treatment for facial rejuvenation. In an unblinded, subjective study of ten patients comparing a series of microdermabrasion treatments to a series of 20% glycolic acid treatments, seven out of ten patients preferred the glycolic acid peels.[8]

The sum of the available studies are that subtle changes in the epidermis and dermis can be objectively measured after microdermabrasion, and that patients and physicians alike may perceive a slight clinical benefit.

Dermabrasion

Mechanical dermabrasion with a rotating diamond fraise or wire brush continues to offer one of the most effective means of resurfacing a number of skin defects and blemishes. Initially described by Paul Kurtin in 1953,[9,10] the technique of dermabrasive surgery continues to be refined and articulated among a host of other new resurfacing treatments including chemical peels, ablative and nonablative laser resurfacing and radiofrequency treatments. A broadening understanding and appreciation of the advantages and specific applications of the nonthermal, sculpting nature of dermabrasive injury uniquely places this mode of resurfacing alongside and in combination with many of the other resurfacing options. This section will address the specific clinical situations for which dermabrasion is uniquely indicated in the context of other resurfacing options.

Today, as well as in the initial series of patients presented at the Mount Sinai Hospital by Paul Kurtin,[9] the most common indication for dermabrasion continues to be facial acne scars.[11] Specifically, deep-shouldered acne scars that do not disappear by simply stretching the skin can be sculpted and recontoured by a nonthermal resurfacing dermabrasive procedure. These punched-out scars frequently present along with stretchable or distensible scars over the cheeks and forehead. Dermabrasion as a 'sculpting' procedure can be combined with carbon dioxide (CO_2) laser as a 'tightening' procedure to address both types of acne scars within the same surgical setting. Not uncommonly, patients with extensive acne scars may also require surgical excision, punch grafting,[12,13] and/or subcision to treat full-thickness defects that extend into the subcutaneous tissue.[12,14] Such surgical procedures should be performed 6–8 weeks or more before dermabrasive or laser resurfacing.[15]

Like acne scars, deep rhytides, especially around the mouth, usually occur in the context of more diffuse photodamage over the entire face. The CO_2 laser and to a lesser extent, the erbium:yttrium aluminum garnet (erbium: YAG) laser, will tighten and smooth superficial acne scars and rhytids.[16] Dermabrasion is a helpful resurfacing adjunct for sculpting the elevated ridges of wrinkles that persist despite two to three passes with an ablative laser. Furthermore dermabrasion removes the thermal coagulum left after the heat-induced injury of CO_2 lasers, thereby promoting healing and reducing postoperative erythema.

Rhinophyma responds well to dermabrasion. The nodules of rhinophyma can be debulked and the shape of the nose re-contoured with dermabrasion. The sebaceous nature of rhinophymatous tissue allows a significant volume of excessive growth on the nasal tip to be removed with minimal risk of scarring. Initially it is difficult to debulk these large nodules with a pulsed or scanned CO_2 laser alone. Mechanical dermabrasion can efficiently remove the build-up of connective tissue and sebaceous glands, after which the natural shape of the nasal bulb and ala can be restored with one or two CO_2 passes, which will symmetrically contract the overlying dermis.

Epidermal nevi, seborrheic keratoses, syringomas, angiofibromas, and trichoepitheliomas can be dermabraded with good results, as described by Roenigk.[17] Similarly decorative tattoos can be abraded followed by the application of 1% Gentian violet directly to the abraded surface and dressed with Adaptic gauze (Johnson & Johnson, New Brunswick, NJ). The Gentian violet is thought to promote the removal of tattoo pigment by stimulating phagocytes to carry away the abraded pigment.[18] Deeply placed tattoo pigment, which can be resistant to the selective photothermolysis of alexandrite, neodymium:YAG, and Q-switched ruby lasers can often be removed with this technique. However, in nonfacial sites the risk of hypopigmentation is significant.

Traumatic and surgical scars can also be greatly improved with programmed dermabrasion performed as early as 6–8 weeks following injury or surgery.[15,19] Dermabrasion has been shown to be more effective than 5-fluorouracil in removing precancerous actinic keratoses.[20] In fact, superficial basal cell carcinoma and squamous cell carcinoma in situ can also be treated with dermabrasion with reasonable outcomes.

■ HISTORICAL VIGNETTE

Since ancient times it has been appreciated that producing a partial-thickness wound on the skin results in healing with new skin that has an enhanced cosmetic appearance. The ancient Egyptians used salt, alabaster, and animal oils as an abrasive, whereas a mixture of urine and pumice was used in India. When ancient Egyptian women bathed in sour milk, they were in fact performing a light chemical peel with lactic acid. In Turkey, fire was used to lightly singe the skin in an effort to perform a thermal exfoliation, a technique that finds modern expression in laser resurfacing.

Over the past century, the ancient idea of creating a controlled partial-thickness abrasion for cosmetic enhancement of the skin has been refined and widely accepted in medical practice. In general, the deeper the wound created (to a point), the greater the cosmetic benefit. Skin can be removed to the level of the midreticular dermis and heals with improved appearance. Wounding deeper than this level results in scar formation. Partial-thickness wounds can be created with acids (which produce a controlled chemical burn wound) and lasers (which vaporize tissue thermally), and by mechanical removal of tissue by dermabrasion.

MICRODERMABRASION

TECHNIQUE

Microdermabrasion has quickly become one of the most popular cosmetic procedures performed. The American Academy of Cosmetic Surgery estimates it is the second most widely performed cosmetic procedure, with injection of botulinum toxin being first. The procedure is essentially painless, quick, easy to perform, and has few associated risks. Compared to lasers, these devices are inexpensive. From a regulatory point of view, resurfacing can be purchased and utilized by anyone. As such, this treatment is commonly offered at spas and beauty salons. When first introduced to the US, it was presented as an improvement to the already existing technique, namely dermabrasion.

The FDA classified microdermabrasion devices as type I devices (i.e. non-life sustaining). This classification does not require the manufacturer to establish performance standards, but rather only to follow good manufacturing practice guidelines. Microdermabrasion devices also received an exempt status from the FDA, releasing it to be sold without the completion of clinical trials. Therefore, it was not necessary to demonstrate the device was effective before bringing it to market. It has since become very popular, with over 36 models currently available.

When originally developed, microdermabrasion employed aluminum oxide crystals, which are sharp-edged and hard, as an abrasive. In this technique, aluminum oxide crystals are whisked by the skin in a closed circuit. One line in the handpiece blows aluminium oxide crystals onto the skin while the other line acts as a vacuum to pull crystals and tissue debris away from the skin and into the waste receptable. This same vacuum is what serves to suction skin into the device. In most machines, the operator controls only the vacuum line, measured in millimeters of mercury (mmHg), which indirectly affects the forward flow of the crystals. The operator passes the handpiece over the skin, and the speed with which the handpiece is moved (contact time) as well as the number of times the skin is treated (passes) will affect the outcome.

Although the clinical benefits of microdermabrasion are modest, the procedure's simplicity and safety suggest it will remain a popular treatment. Following treatment, mild erythema is present, but quickly resolves making it a popular lunch-time procedure with no real down-time. Overly aggressive treatment can produce purpura, but this should resolve without scarring. Corneal abrasions from the crystals are possible, so eye protection is indicated. Chronic exposure of the operator to aluminum oxide has been raised as a possible safety concern. There has been inconclusive evidence that chronic exposure to aluminum (but not aluminum oxide) may be associated with impaired cognition and the development of Alzheimer's disease.[21–23] This possible link applies to workers chronically exposed to metallic aluminum, such as aluminum miners or factory workers, and not those who work with aluminum oxide. Aluminum oxide has enjoyed a long experience with human use as a dental abrasive and in joint replacements. It is an inert ceramic, that is insoluble in water. Therefore, it cannot enter the blood and be carried to the brain. Inhalation is a potential route of exposure, raising the possibility of pulmonary fibrosis. However, the particle size of aluminum oxide used for microdermabrasion is quite regular at approximately 100 mm, and particles larger than 50 mm are unlikely to reach the alveoli. Furthermore, the crystals are quite heavy, and quickly drop to the floor when sprayed into the air. The Occupational Safety and Health Administration (OSHA) considers aluminum oxide to be a nuisance dust that is not considered to stimulate a biologic response. OSHA does recommend limiting total exposure to 10-15 mg/m^3 unless respiratory protection is worn.[24] As such, it is prudent for the operator to wear a mask when performing microdermabrasion.

In response to these theoretic safety concerns, alternative abrasives have been developed for microdermabrasion equipment. Both sodium chloride and sodium bicarbonate have been utilized. However, in the devices initially developed, both these materials tended to clog the vacuum line. Since then, devices utilizing sodium chloride or bicarbonate as an abrasive have been developed that work without a vacuum line. These devices employ 'positive pressure' only, meaning the crystals are blown forward into the handpiece. It is unclear how effective these devices will be without the suction component, which seems to provoke so much of the dermal change in the original devices. Ongoing studies are needed to elucidate upon this.

POSTOPERATIVE CARE DERMABRASION

PREOPERATIVE PREPARATION

Preoperative photographs should be taken from standardized camera angles: directly in front of the patient, right and left lateral views, and right and left 45° angle views. The events before and during surgery and the postoperative routine of dressing changes should be reviewed in detail to prepare patients and their caregivers for dermabrasive surgery.

A comprehensive resurfacing evaluation includes three main components: discussion of the patient's goals and objectives within the bounds of reasonable surgical outcomes; careful examination of the skin and its defects, as well as a complete medical history; and review of the advantages and disadvantages of a variety of available resurfacing options. In our experience, cosmetic patients undergoing dermabrasive surgery should expect 30–50% improvement in the appearance of deep acne scars and adynamic rhytides. Realistic outcome expectations can be aided by reviewing before and after photographs.

In examining the patient's skin, careful attention should be given to the Fitzpatrick skin type, the sebaceous quality of the skin, and the presence of hypertrophic scarring, vascular malformations, or pigmentary alterations. Distensible acne scars and dynamic rhytides that disappear by stretching are best treated with tissue tightening procedures such as ablative and even nonablative laser resurfacing treatments. On the other hand, sharp shoulder scars of chicken pox or acne and deep nondistensible rhytides require sculpting and re-contouring by mechanical dermabrasion. Some surgeons will opt to use the erbium:YAG laser for sculpting. Many patients will have a combination of defects that require more than one method of resurfacing for optimal results. For full-thickness defects, surgical excision punch grafting and/or dermal grafts should be performed at least 6–8 weeks before resurfacing. Other surgical procedures requiring extensive undermining such as face lifts, can be carried out at the same time as resurfacing if the resurfacing treatment is superficial, especially over the undermined areas. Many surgeons prefer to wait 6 months after resurfacing to perform face lifts and vice versa.

Patients with a history of impetigo require a nasal swab to screen for *Staphylococcus aureus* colonization. These patients should receive prophylactic antibiotics (cephalexin 1–2 g daily for 10–14 days); otherwise patients undergoing dermabrasion do not need prophylactic antibiotics. On the other hand, all patients undergoing ablative resurfacing including dermabrasion require prophylactic antiviral medication until fully epithelialized (i.e. valaciclovir 1 g daily for 7–14 days or famciclovir 500 mg daily for 7–14 days). In our experience, most herpetic infections occur 7–9 days after resurfacing surgery, and as such we recommend that the antiviral prophylaxis should be continued for 14 days.

Delayed re-epithelialization and hypertrophic scarring have been reported in patients undergoing dermabrasion during or shortly after isotretinoin therapy. Therefore dermabrasion should be postponed 6–12 months after a course of isotretinoin. The isotretinoin molecule is thought to have an adverse effect on the wound healing role of epidermal cells and fibroblasts in abraded skin.[25–28] Alternately, topical tretinoin cream when applied daily for 2–3 weeks before dermabrasion has been shown to reduce the time required for re-epithelialization.

A test spot dermabrasion is recommended in patients with a history of keloids or koebnerizing condition such as psoriasis, lichen planus, vitiligo, or pyoderma gangrenosum. An atopic diathesis or immunosuppression may cause delayed wound healing or an increased risk of postoperative infection. Baseline laboratory work should include a complete blood count, chemistry profile, hepatitis panel, and screening for HIV. Patients with viral hepatitis and HIV infections also have an increased risk for delayed wound healing and postoperative infection. Because of the aerosolized viral particles produced by dermabrasion, all healthcare personnel should observe universal precautions in performing dermabrasion.

The areas to be abraded should be outlined preoperatively with Gentian violet while the patient is sitting. For full face procedures a line drawn one to two fingerbreadths below the angle of the mandible should extend from earlobe to earlobe in a symmetric fashion. This allows the transition zone from the nonabraded skin on the neck to the abraded facial skin to be hidden in the shadow of the jawline. Similarly, partial abrasions (e.g. around the mouth, nose) should follow the lines of facial cosmetic subunits.

Use of cryoanesthesia and spray refrigerants has been controversial because of their potential to produce injury and scarring in the skin, but they are helpful in that they provide a firm surface upon which to work. Refrigerants containing freon-12 (–30 to –60 °C) produce excessive cold injury and scarring.[20,29,30] The refrigerant most commonly used today is freon-114 (Frigiderm, Delasco Dermatologic Lab & Supply Inc, Council Bluffs, IA). A 10-second spray time will freeze acne scars and rhytides in position so that they can be sculpted.

Tumescent anesthesia with a 0.05–0.1% lidocaine solution can be used to anesthetize the entire face for dermabrasion as well as CO_2 or erbium:YAG laser resurfacing.[31,32] Before infiltrating the cheeks, central facial nerve blocks (mental, infraorbital, and supraorbital nerves) can be performed (see Chapter 3). The blocks will provide anesthesia without hemostasis of the central face. The lateral cheeks and forehead can then be infiltrated with a 25-gauge spinal needle from a single entry point just in front of the preauricular crease. Thereafter, the central face can be tumesced if indicated for hemostasis. If this is not required, supplemental injections will still be necessary if the full face is to be treated around the oral commissures medial and lateral canthi, eyelids, mid-chin, mid-upper lip/nose. This is most efficiently carried out using a 30-gauge 1 inch needle attached to a 10-mL syringe. A volume of 250–350 mL of tumescent solution is adequate for the entire face. The infiltrate should be placed in a superficial plane just beneath and into the dermis so that complete blanching is produced. Complete anesthesia allows the procedure to be much less traumatic for the patient and the surgeon. The use of spray refrigerants on tumescent tissue should be carried out with caution. The vasoconstriction of the tumescent anesthesia extends the length of time that the skin remains frozen. A 10-second spray time should be reduced to 5 seconds.

Diazepam (5–10 mg orally) is given 30 minutes before surgery along with meperidine hydrochloride (50–75 mg intramuscularly) and hydroxyzine hydrochloride (25 mg intramuscularly) to reduce the discomfort of placing the nerve blocks and infiltrating the tumescent anesthesia. Preoperative patient anxiety and intraoperative patient discomfort can be further reduced by flurazepam (15–30 mg orally), zolpidem tartrate (5–10 orally mg orally) or zaleplon (5–10 mg orally) taken the night before surgery as well as when the patient is sleeping in a full face dressing after surgery. If patients experience claustrophobia with a full face dressing, diazepam (5–10 mg sublingually) can be

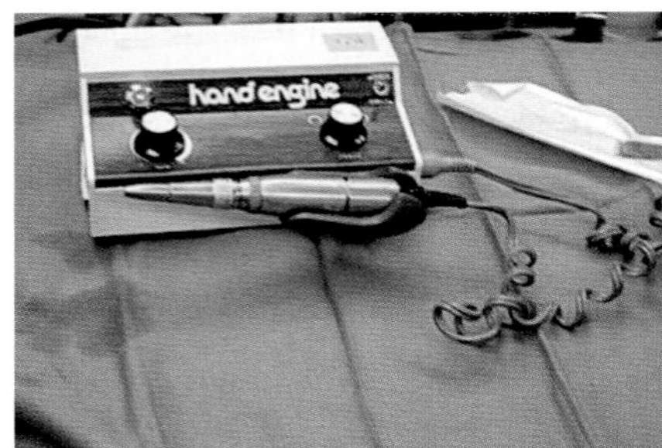

Figure 36.2 Bell hand engine 18 000–20 000 RPMs.

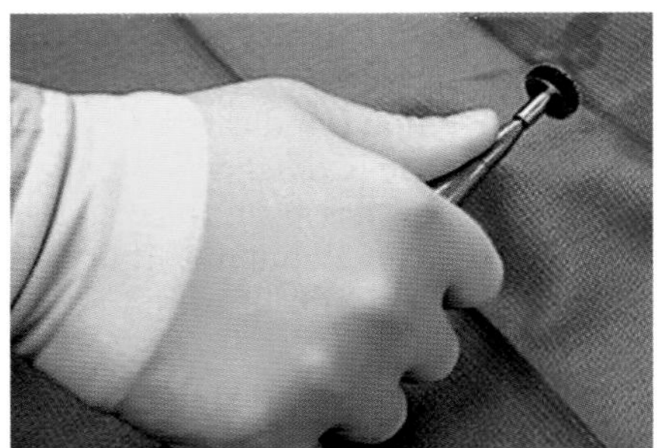

Figure 36.3 Proper hand position with the thumb stabilizing the neck of the abrader and the forefingers around the body of the engine.

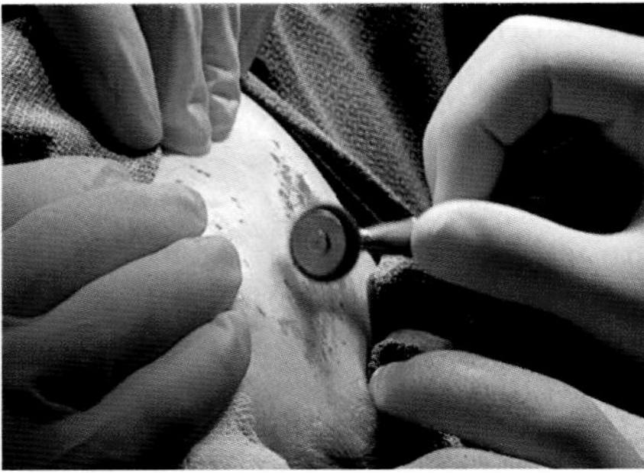

Figure 36.4 Arciform strokes are performed by pulling the hand engine perpendicular to the direction of the rotating endpiece.

helpful, especially when used prophylactically in those with a history of anxiety.

■ TECHNIQUE

A variety of hand engines can be used in dermabrasive surgery. Manufacturers such as Osada, Bell, Ellis, and Schumann produce battery powered and electrical units that rotate at 15 000–30 000 rpm (Figs 36.2–36.4). Many hand engines can also power dermatomal and osteotomal attachments. For resurfacing treatments, the abrading endpiece may be a serrated wheel, diamond fraise or wire brush. Fraises are available in a variety of sizes, shapes and grades of coarseness. Cone-shaped fraises are ideal for confined areas around the nose, mouth and eyelids. Broader surfaces on the forehead and cheeks are best resurfaced with wheel shaped fraises or the wire brush. There are excellent reviews by Yarbrough and Alt on the technique of wire brush and diamond fraise surgery.[33,34] Generally the extra coarse fraise is more forgiving than the wire brush (Fig. 36.5). The bristles of the wire brush are angled such that clockwise rotation cuts more deeply in the skin whereas counterclockwise rotation brushes the bristles over the surface of the skin more gently.

The body of the hand engine is held with the forefingers and the neck of the dermabrader is stabilized with the thumb. The abrading endpiece is passed over the skin in arciform strokes perpendicular to the direction of endpiece

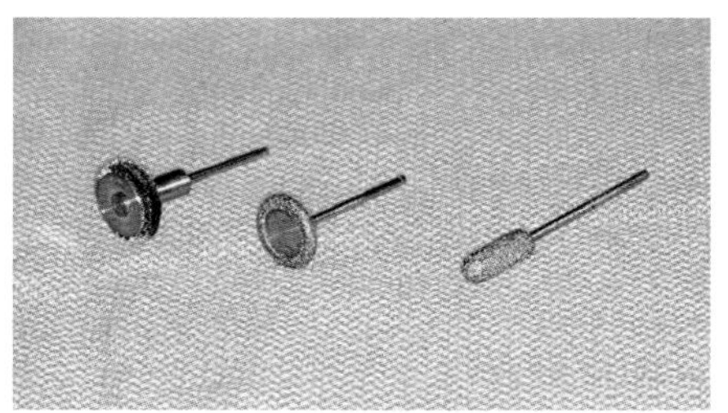

Figure 36.5 Abrasive endpieces: wire brush (left), diamond fraise (middle), pear-shaped or cone fraise (right).

rotation. To abrade, the hand engine is pulled rather than pushed over the skin surface. The outer peel of an orange or grapefruit provides a good surface upon which to develop a feel for using a handheld dermabrader. During surgery, the patient is supine and the skin surface being abraded should be parallel to the floor so that the surgeon's hand can move freely back and forth without obstruction.

Direction of rotation is only important when a wire brush is used. For deep resurfacing of acne scarring on the mid-cheek, traumatic or surgical scars, or debulking large nodules of rhinophyma, clockwise rotation is more efficient and requires a frozen or tightly tumesced surface upon which to abrade. Counterclockwise rotation is more easily controlled in that the brushing action of the bristles is less likely to gouge the skin or grab the free edge of the lip or nose. In fact, wire brush dermabrasion with counterclockwise rotation as well as fraise surgery can be performed without the use of spray refrigerants. In performing full face procedures it is not uncommon to alternate between the fraise and the wire brush as well as between the direction of rotation of the wire brush endpiece from clockwise to counterclockwise.

For full face procedures, it is best to start abrading along the jawline or the preauricular area and progress toward the center of the face and nose. This allows bleeding from the abraded areas to flow away from the skin being abraded. Three-point retraction of the skin produced by the two hands of the assistant and the nondominant hand of the surgeon stabilizes the area being abraded. When using spray refrigerant, the scar or rhytid should be frozen in its unstretched position, then three-point retraction is applied while abrading.

The depth of abrasion can be monitored by closely observing the abraded surface. As the epidermis is removed the papillary dermis appears as a glistening white surface. Corn rows of pinpoint bleeding can be seen as the vascular loops of the rete pegs are interrupted. As the depth of abrasions proceeds further into the dermis the points of bleeding become larger.[35] The yellow globules of sebaceous glands are seen with deep abrasion of acne scars in the mid cheek or rhinophyma of the nose. The hemostasis of tumescent anesthesia reduces the visibility of points of bleeding as does the diamond fraise so this cannot be used as a sole endpoint. Nevertheless, these surgical landmarks together provide a reliable means of following the depth of abrasion. The dermal fibrosis produced by acne scars will crumble and become friable with abrasion. The peripheral margin of the abraded regions should be feathered to create a natural looking transition zone. The arciform strokes should be parallel to the border of the abraded areas to avoid jagged stop and start streaks, much like coloring with crayons in a direction parallel with a borderline rather than perpendicular to it.

■ POSTOPERATIVE CARE

Upon completion of a full face dermabrasion procedure, most of the abraded areas are no longer bleeding. However the application of gauze soaked with 1% lidocaine with epinephrine (adrenaline) 1 : 100 000 completes hemostasis and soothes any postoperative stinging. Postoperative edema can be reduced by intramuscular triamcinolone acetonide 40 mg given immediately postoperatively. Propoxyphene N-100 pills (100 mg) every 4–6 hours as needed eliminates postoperative stinging or discomfort.

The abraded surface is dressed with a semipermeable dressing (i.e. Vigilon (CR Bard, Murray Hill, NJ), 2nd Skin (Spenco Medical, Waco, TX)), which is held in place with paper tape and backed with nonadherent pads and gauze. Surgilast netting (Western Medical Ltd, Tenafly, NJ) secures the mask and is much less bulky than Kling wrap or ACE bandages and contours to the face. The patient returns to the office for the full face dressing to be changed every day for 5 days. With the use of full face dressings, patients experience very little postoperative discomfort. Antiviral prophylaxis is continued for 14 days and antibiotics or antifungal medications are only necessary in the event of a rare secondary infection.

Close and meticulous attention to the sequential events of wound healing during the postoperative course will allow for the early detection and intervention of any postoperative complications. The development of pain with or without erosions is the sine qua non for a postoperative herpetic infection. The herpes virus requires viable epidermal cells in which to propagate, therefore this infectious complication is usually seen 5–10 days after surgery. The pain is usually accompanied by punched out ulcerations or erosions in the new skin which may or may not heal with residual scarring (Fig. 36.6). Antiviral medication (valaciclovir 1 g three times daily for 7 days or famciclovir 500 mg three times daily for 7 days) is necessary to treat these lesions.

Superinfection by bacteria or fungi is much less common following dermabrasion (Fig. 36.7). Daily dressing changes with careful debridement contribute to the low incidence of secondary infections. Like the herpetic outbreaks, bacterial or fungal infections will present as painful, nonhealing erosions. Consequently any painful or nonhealing erosions should be presumed to be herpetic and treated with zoster

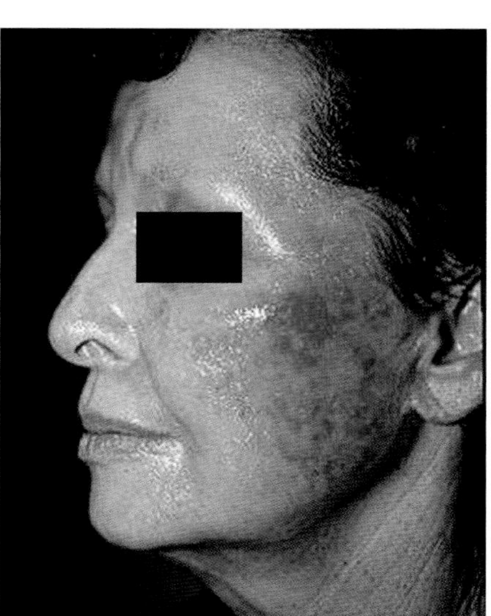

Figure 36.6 Viral infections present as painful punched out lesions 7–10 days following surgery after epithelialization is complete.

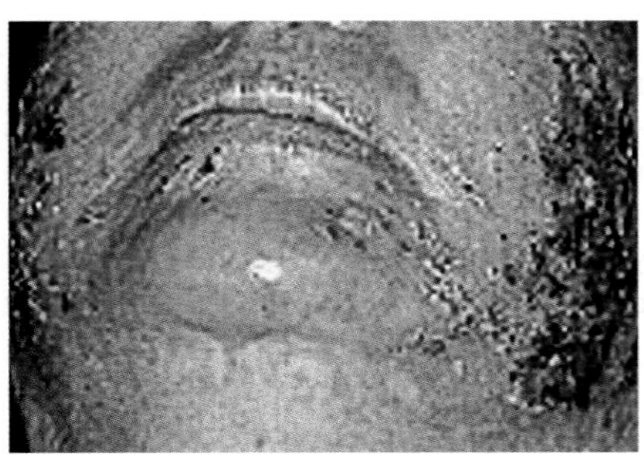

Figure 36.7 Bacterial infections present with crusting at postoperative day 3 or 4.

doses of antiviral medications, but cultures for bacteria and fungus should also be performed. Appropriate systemic antibiotics or antifungal medications as directed by the culture results will clear these lesions.

The presence of bright erythema after the first 2–3 postoperative weeks is the first sign of early scar formation and should be treated with topical high-potency steroid ointment or Cordran tape (Oclassen Pharmaceuticals Inc, San Rafael, CA) applied once or twice daily. These areas should be followed every 1–2 weeks so that pulsed dye laser intervention can be employed, which has been shown to decrease erythema and scar induration.[36] Intralesional steroid injections (5–40 mg/mL triamcinolone acetonide) can be given if any induration, elevation, or hypertrophy develops. Early and aggressive management of scar formation will prevent progression to scar contracture and disfigurement. Small focal areas of hypopigmentation are usually the final outcome of successful aggressive scar management.

The patient returns to the office daily for 3–5 days to have this mask dressing changed. After the first 48 hours there is a significant decrease in the amount of transudate and oozing such that the nonadherent pads and gauze are no longer needed. With each visit, crusting, coagulum, and fibrin build-up are debrided. Following 3–5 days of wearing a full face mask, an open wound care technique can be employed with topical petrolatum ointment. The ointment should be reapplied three to four times daily until re-epithelization is complete.

The open wound produced by dermabrasion heals by the well described mechanism of second intention wound healing. Re-epithelialization occurs as new cells migrate in a 'leap-frog' fashion from the skin appendages and the periphery of the wound over the denuded surface. Typically, regions rich in sebaceous glands such as the nose and mid-cheek re-epithelize more quickly than the more peripheral skin over the bony prominences of the forehead, malar cheek, and mandible. Clinically, the pink new skin can be seen as it replaces the eroded surface.

During the remodeling phase of wound healing, fibroblasts lay down new collagen fibers in an organized fashion parallel to the surface the skin (see Chapter 7). The initial deposition of fibronectin and type III collagen fibers is replaced by type I collagen fibers as stromal re-organization proceeds. In dermabrasive wounding, the collagen fibers align parallel to lines of tension before intermolecular cross-linkages are complete. This is believed to produce a smoother contour than was present in the original scar. Similarly the re-establishment of a more normal epidermis after the abrasion of scars is facilitated by alterations in the extracellular formation of integrins and tenascin. Following dermabrasion, increased integrin expression may promote cellular migration while tenascin mitigates the epithelial mesenchymal interaction of wound healing.[37] As wound healing progresses, intradermal edema continues to dissipate for up to 3 months. After the edema has resolved, rhytides and depressed scars may appear to have returned. However as the remodeling phase of wound healing continues, new collagen is laid down parallel to the surface of the skin, with continuing improvement of skin surface irregularities and depressions for 6–12 months following surgery. Consequently, it is best to wait 1 year before considering retreatments.

Re-epithelialization is usually complete within 7–10 days following surgery. The application of tretinoin cream 0.05% to the skin several weeks before the dermabrasion has been shown to decrease the time required for re-epithelialization.[38] Additionally the use of semipermeable dressings has reduced the time for re-epithelialization by up to 40% compared to open techniques of wound care. These dressings maintain a critical plane of humidity which enhances epithelial cell migration.[39]

Patients can reapply make-up once re-epithelialization is complete. Green and yellow-based foundations are especially well-suited for camouflaging the ensuing postoperative erythema. Typically the bright red color of new epithelium fades to pink and returns to normal skin tone within 2–3 months. It is during this period of postoperative erythema that complete sun avoidance is required. Despite compliance with this request, most patients will develop some degree of transient postinflammatory hyperpigmentation over the malar prominences and jawline. This darkening reliably responds to topical hydroquinone and tretinoin cream applied either separately or together once to twice daily. This bleaching regimen is tolerated with minimal irritation beginning the third or fourth week after surgery and continued for 4–8 weeks or until the hyperpigmentation resolves.

Permanent pigmentary alteration, which is seen as a loss of normal skin tone, occurs in 20–30% of patients. Skin types III and IV are more likely to develop this complication than light-skinned patients (types I and II) or dark-toned individuals (types V and VI). The mechanism for this loss of pigment is not completely understood but is thought to be caused by a loss of normal melanocytic function. Some progress in re-establishing skin tone as been made with the 308 nm excimer laser.[40]

Another postoperative sequela, known as pseudohypopigmentation, is seen when a normally repigmented abraded skin is seen to have a different tone and appearance than adjacent nonabraded skin. For example, the lentigines and telangiectasias of the nonabraded area contrast with the smooth, even pigmentation of the dermabraded skin. This disparity can be reduced by combination procedures such as superficial- or medium-depth chemical peels of the nonabraded areas to blend treated and nontreated sites. There has also been great progress seen with the use of nonablative lasers and intense pulse light sources in treating the hyperpigmentation and telangiectasias of photodamaged skin. These serve as alternatives to chemical peeling to minimize color mismatch of dermabraded and nondermabraded skin.

Increased milia formation is an expected postoperative sequela, and best treated by gentle extraction after sturdy epithelium has developed (usually after 1 week). Care must be taken not to cause excessive trauma of this fragile skin, which could result in scarring. Acne flares following dermabrasive surgery are usually due to the occlusive nature of the postoperative wound care. These can be managed with routine acne regimes utilizing topical medications (usually tolerated 2 weeks following treatment) and oral antibiotics. Ultimately both these postoperative events—milia and acne flares—are transient and patient reassurance is very helpful.

Optimizing outcomes

- Discuss patient's goals and objectives within the bounds of reasonable surgical outcomes.
- Carefully examine skin and its defects and obtain a complete medical history.
- Review the advantages and disadvantages of a variety of available resurfacing options.
- Encourage realistic outcome expectations by reviewing before and after photographs.
- Review the events before and during surgery and the postoperative routine of dressing changes to prepare patients and their caretakers for dermabrasive surgery.

PITFALLS AND THEIR MANAGEMENT

Pitfalls and their management

- Postoperative infections – prescribe prophylactic antibiotics to patients with a history of impetigo and prophylactic antiviral medication to patients with a history of herpetic infections.
- Postoperative herpetic infection – prescribe antiviral medications.
- Delayed re-epithelialization and hypertrophic scarring in patients during or shortly after isotretinoin therapy – postpone dermabrasion for 6–12 months after a course of isotretinoin.
- Scar formation – treat bright erythema after the first 2–3 postoperative weeks with topical high-potency corticosteroid ointment or Cordran tape (Oclassen) applied once or twice daily and follow every 1–2 weeks so that pulsed dye laser intervention and intralesional corticosteroids can be given if necessary.
- Permanent pigmentary alteration – 308 nm excimer laser has shown some progress in re-establishing skin tone in these patients.
- Pseudohypopigmentation – can be reduced by combination procedures such as superficial- or medium-depth chemical peels of the nonabraded areas to blend treated and nontreated sites.
- Increased milia formation – best treated by gentle extraction once sturdy epithelium has developed (usually after 1 week).
- Acne flares – manage with routine acne regimens.

Dermabrasion

A test spot dermabrasion is recommended in patients with a history of keloids and/or koebnerizing conditions such as psoriasis, lichen planus, or pyoderma gangrenosum.

An atopic diathesis or immunosuppression may cause delayed wound healing or an increased risk of postoperative infection. Patients with viral hepatitis and HIV infections are also at increased risk for delayed wound healing and postoperative infection. Because of the aerosolized viral particles produced by dermabrasion, all healthcare personnel should observe universal precautions in performing dermabrasion.

The development of pain with or without erosions is the sine qua non for a postoperative herpetic infection. Superinfection by bacteria or fungi are much less common following dermabrasion. Daily dressing changes with careful debridement contribute to the low incidence of secondary infections.

SUMMARY

Microdermabrasion was developed as a blood-free and safer technique with less healing time than dermabrasion. It is painless, quick, easy to perform, and has few associated risks. Microdermabrasion has been widely used to treat photodamage, dyschromias, acne, scars, and stretch marks, but surprisingly little is known about its clinical efficacy. Microdermabrasion has clearly found a place in cosmetic practice. It is a mild treatment producing minimal results. Its benefits include safety, ease of use, and no down-time for the patient. However, the clinical benefits of treatment are subtle and it is important to make this clear to patients so that reasonable expectations are set. The available literature principally examines the effectiveness of microdermabrasion on photoaging. Further investigation is needed to understand the long-term benefits, if any, of this treatment for aging skin as well as for other indications including acne, dyspigmentation, and stretch marks.

In this era of ever expanding resurfacing treatments, dermabrasive resurfacing continues to offer a uniquely effective approach for a well-defined subset of defects. Specifically, sharp-shouldered scars of acne and varicella, as well as adynamic, deep rhytides can be efficiently improved by nonthermal mechanical dermabrasion. Similarly, traumatic and surgical scars and rhinophyma can be beautifully recontoured with the diamond fraise or wire brush endpieces. As with any resurfacing procedure, careful attention to surgical technique and close monitoring of patients during the postoperative period will improve surgical outcomes and decrease the rate of complications.

REFERENCES

1. Hopping S. The power peel: its emergence and future in cosmetic surgery. Int J Cosmet Surg 1999; 6:98–100.
2. Tsai R, Wang C, Chan H. Aluminum oxide crystal microdermabrasion: a new technique for treating facial scarring. Dermatol Surg 1995; 21:531–542.
3. Shim EK, Barnette D, Hughes K, et al. Microdermabrasion: a clinical and histopathologic study. Dermatol Surg 2001; 27:524–530.
4. Freedman BM, Rueda-Pedraza E, Waddell SP. The epidermal and dermal changes associated with microdermabrasion. Dermatol Surg 2001; 27:1031–1034.
5. Hernandez-Perez E, Ibiett EV. Gross and microscopic findings in patients undergoing microdermabrasion for facial rejuvenation. Dermatol Surg 2001; 27:637–640.
6. Tan MH, Spencer JM, Pires LM, et al. The evaluation of aluminum oxide crystal microdermabrasion for photodamage. Dermatol Surg 2001; 27:943–949.

7. Rajan P, Grimes PE. Skin barrier changes induced by aluminum oxide and sodium chloride microdermabrasion. Dermatol Surg 2002; 28:390–393.
8. Alam M, Omura NE, Dover JS, et al. Glycolic acid peels compared to microdermabrasion: a right-left controlled trial of efficacy and patient satisfaction. Dermatol Surg 2002; 28:475–479.
9. Kurtin A. Surgical planing of the skin. Arch Dermatol Syphilol 1953; 68:389.
10. Robbins N. Dr. Abner Kurtin, father of ambulatory dermabrasion. J Dermatol Surg Oncol 1988; 14:425–431.
11. Orentreich D, Orentreich N. Acne scar revision update. Dermatol Clin 1987; 5:359–368.
12. Johnson WC: Treatment of pitted scars: punch transplant technique. J Dermatol Surg Oncol 1986; 12:260–265.
13. Solotoff SA. Treatment for pitted acne scarring—postauricular punch grafts followed by dermabrasion. J Dermatol Surg Oncol 1986; 12:1079–1084.
14. Orentreich DS, Orentreich N. Subcutaneous incisionless (subcision) surgery for the correction of depressed scars and wrinkles. Dermatol Surg 1995; 21:543–549.
15. Yarborough JM Jr. Ablation of facial scars by programmed dermabrasion. J Dermatol Surg Oncol 1988; 14:292–294.
16. Alster TS, West TB. Resurfacing of atrophic facial acne scars with a high-energy, pulsed carbon dioxide laser. Dermatol Surg 1996; 22:151–154; discussion 154–155.
17. Roenigk HH Jr. Dermabrasion for miscellaneous cutaneous lesions (exclusive of scarring from acne). J Dermatol Surg Oncol 1977; 3: 322–328.
18. Clabaugh WA. Tattoo removal by superficial dermabrasion. Five-year experience. Plast Reconstr Surg 1975;55:401–405.
19. Coleman WP 3rd, Yarborough JM, Mandy SH. Dermabrasion for prophylaxis and treatment of actinic keratoses. Dermatol Surg 1996; 22:17–21.
20. Hanke CW, O'Brian JJ, Solow EB. Laboratory evaluation of skin refrigerants used in dermabrasion. J Dermatol Surg Oncol 1985; 11:45–49.
21. Rifat SL, Eastwood MR, McLachlan DR, et al. Effect of exposure of miners to aluminum powder. Lancet 1996; 336:1162–1165.
22. McLachlan DR. Aluminum and Alzheimer's disease. Neurobiol Aging 1986; 7:525–532.
23. Candy JM, Oakley AE, Klinowski J, et al. Aluminosilicates and senile plaque formation in Alzheimer's disease. Lancet 1986; 1:354–357.
24. Sittig M. Aluminum and aluminum oxide. In: Sittig M, ed. Handbook of toxic and hazardous chemicals and carcinogens, vol 1, 3rd edn. Park Ridge, NJ: Noyes Publications 1991; 175–177.
25. Rubenstein R, Roenigk HH Jr, Stegman SJ, Hanke CW. Atypical keloids after dermabrasion of patients taking isotretinoin. J Am Acad Dermatol 1986; 15:280–285.
26. Roenigk HH Jr, Pinski JB, Robinson JK, Hanke CW. Acne, retinoids, and dermabrasion. J Dermatol Surg Oncol 1985; 11:396–398.
27. Katz BE, MacFarlane DF. Atypical facial scarring after isotretinoin therapy in a patient with previous dermabrasion. J Am Acad Dermatol 1994; 30:852–853.
28. Roenigk HH Jr, Pinski JB, Robinson JK, Hanke CW. Acne, retinoids, and dermabrasion. J Dermatol Surg Oncol 1985; 11:396–398.
29. Hanke CW, O'Brian JJ. A histologic evaluation of the effects of skin refrigerants in an animal model. J Dermatol Surg Oncol 1987; 13:664–669.
30. Hanke CW, Roenigk HH Jr, Pinksi JB. Complications of dermabrasion resulting from excessively cold skin refrigeration. J Dermatol Surg Oncol 1985; 11:896–900.
31. Coleman WP 3rd, Klein JA. Use of the tumescent technique for scalp surgery, dermabrasion, and soft tissue reconstruction. J Dermatol Surg Oncol 1992; 18:130–135.
32. Goodman G. Dermabrasion using tumescent anesthesia. J Dermatol Surg Oncol 1994; 20:802–807.
33. Alt TH. Technical aids for dermabrasion. J Dermatol Surg Oncol 1987; 13:638–648.
34. Yarborough JM Jr. Dermabrasion by wire brush. J Dermatol Surg Oncol 1987; 13:610–615.
35. Burks JW, Thomas CC. Wire brush surgery. Springfield, IL: Charles C Thomas; 1956.
36. Alster T. Laser scar revision: comparison study of 585-nm pulsed dye laser with and without intralesional corticosteroids. Dermatol Surg 2003; 29:25–29.
37. Harmon CB, Zelickson BD, Roenigk RK, et al. Dermabrasive scar revision—an immunohistochemical and ultrastructural evaluation. Dermatol Surg 1995; 21:503–508.
38. Mandy SH. Tretinoin in the preoperative and postoperative management of dermabrasion. J Am Acad Dermatol 1986; 15:878–879, 888–889.
39. Pinski JB. Dressings for dermabrasion: occlusive dressings and wound healing. Cutis 1986; 37:471.
40. Grimes PE, Bhawan J, Kim J, Chiu M, Lask G. Laser resurfacing-induced hypopigmentation: histologic alterations and repigmentation with topical photochemotherapy. Dermatol Surg 2001; 27:515–520.

37 Laser Treatment of Tattoos and Pigmented Lesions

Vivek Iyengar MD, Kenneth A Arndt MD, and Thomas E Rohrer MD

Summary box

- Various lasers and light sources effectively treat pigmented lesions and tattoos with minimal down-time and superior cosmetic outcomes.
- Q-switched lasers with extremely short pulse durations are best suited for the selective destruction of commonly encountered pigmented lesions.
- Intense pulsed light sources can improve pigmentary and vascular components of photodamaged skin.
- 'Titrating' the fluence for each individual patient based on observed clinical end-points will result in optimal outcomes.
- Strict safety measures including the use of protective eyewear are essential.

INTRODUCTION

Most lasers used in dermatology today are based on the principles of selective photothermolysis.[1] Light energy is preferentially absorbed by a target chromophore and transferred into heat energy in a time shorter than the target's thermal relaxation time (the time required for the target to lose 50% of heat). Different chromophores in the skin, such as melanin in pigmented lesions, oxyhemoglobin in vascular lesions, and water in all cells, preferentially absorb certain wavelengths of light. By designing a laser to produce a wavelength of light that is better absorbed by the target chromophore (the structure you are attempting to destroy) than the surrounding tissue, it is possible to selectively heat that chromophore to the point of irreversible damage. By limiting the time the laser is fired into the chromophore (the pulse duration), it is possible to contain the damage to the selected chromophore. If the laser pulse duration is too long (greater than the chromophore's thermal relaxation time), the heat produced in the chromophore will have time to spread to surrounding structures and cause nonselective damage. This may lead to scarring. Choosing an appropriate wavelength and pulse duration make it possible to selectively heat and destroy certain chromophores in the skin without damaging surrounding structures. In this manner, vascular lesions, pigmented lesions, hair, and superficial skin may all be selectively targeted and destroyed.

By inducing selective damage to the melanosome through the use of laser radiation a number of commonly encountered pigmented lesions can be treated with excellent cosmetic outcomes. A number of lasers and light sources are available to treat tattoos and pigmented lesions (Table 37.1). They may be categorized as pigment nonselective, somewhat pigment selective, and highly selective for pigment removal based on the wavelength of light emitted (Fig. 37.1). Pigment nonselective lasers such as the carbon dioxide and erbium:yttrium aluminum garnet (Er:YAG) lasers can eliminate epidermal pigment by removing the entire epidermis and its associated melanocytic structures as a secondary event. Continuous wave lasers such as the argon (488,514 nm), copper vapor (511,578 nm), and krypton lasers (521,530 nm) can somewhat selectively remove epidermal pigment. However, as a result of the inability to reliably provide confined thermal injury these lasers may have a higher risk than necessary.

Short-pulsed pigmented lesion lasers safely and reliably treat both epidermal and dermal pigmented lesions. In addition, the recent use of intense light sources with polychromatic light ranging from 515 to 1200 nm with filters to cut off light below a predetermined wavelength have demonstrated success in the reduction of superficial pigmentation.[1,2]

The chromophore targets in lentigines, and most pigmented lesions, are tiny melanosomes.[3] The estimated thermal relaxation time of a melanosome is approximately 250–1000 nsec.[4] Therefore, lasers with very short pulse durations, in the nanosecond domain, are ideally suited for the task. In fact, lasers with pulse duration in the picosecond domain are now being tested. With pulse durations this short, local pressure waves are created with each pulse as a result of the rapid rise in temperature. These pressure waves, or shock waves, produce much of the damage associated with these lasers. This is termed the photoacoustic or photomechanical effect.[5] The tissue being

Table 37.1 Lasers used in the treatment of pigmented lesions

Device	Manufacturer	Laser type	Wavelength (nm)	Pulse duration	Spot size (mm)	Maximum rate (Hz)
TatuLAZR	Candela (Wayland, MA)	Pulsed dye	510	400 ns	3–5	1
Aura	Laserscope (San Jose, CA)	KTP	532	1–50 ms	1–4	10
Spectrum RD-1200	Spectrum (Palomar, Burlington, MA)	QS ruby	694	28 ns	5, 6.5	0.8
EpiTouch	Lumenis (Santa Clara, MA)	QS ruby	694	25 ns	5	0.8
RubyStar	Aesculap Meditec (Jena, Germany)	QS ruby	694	40 ns	1.5,3,4	1
AlexLAZR	Candela	QS alexandrite	755	50 ns	2,3,4	5
HT 10	Cynosure (Chelmsford, MA)	QS alexandrite	755	45–75 ns	2,4	10
VersaPulse VPC	Lumenis	FD Nd:YAG	532	2–50 ms	2–10	6
		QS FD Nd:YAG	532	4 ns	2–6	10
		QS Nd:YAG	1064	5 ns	2–6	10
		QS alexandrite	755	45 ns	2–6	10
Medlite CG	Continuum (Santa Clara, CA)	QS FD Nd:YAG	532	5–7 ns	2,3,4,6	10
		QS Nd:YAG	1064	5–7 ns	3,4,6,8	10
Quantum	Lumenis	IPL (Flashlamp)	515–1200 nm	0.5–25 ms	8×15,8×35	1 pulse/ 8 seconds
SkinStation	Radiancy (Orangeburg, NY)	Flashlamp		35 ms	22×57	1 pulse/ 8 seconds
EsteLux	Palomar	Flashlamp				

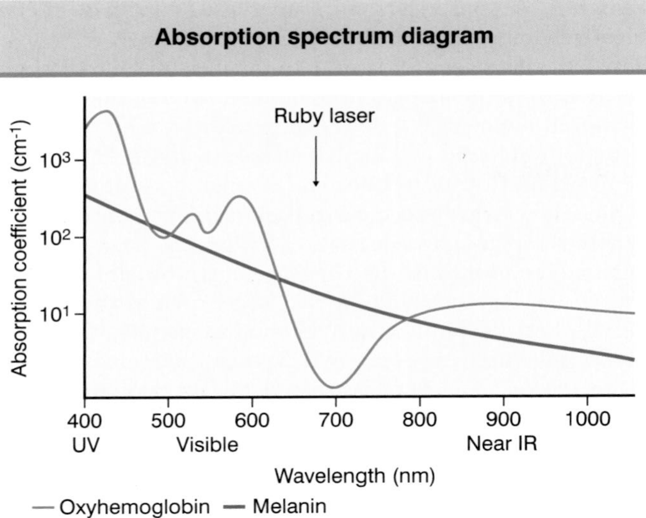

Figure 37.1 Absorption spectrum diagram.

treated usually temporarily turns white in color. This response relates to melanosome rupture seen on electron microscopy,[6] and is thus a likely consequence of this phenomenon. The exact cause of the white color remains unknown. However, it is hypothesized that it is caused by gas bubble formation, which intensely scatters light. The composition of these bubbles is another subject of debate and they may result from water vapor, nitrogen, or other gases. Regardless of its scientific cause, the whitening serves as a useful clinical end-point relating to melanosome or tattoo ink rupture.[7]

The fate of tattoo ink particles after laser irradiation remains unclear. Possibilities include direct fragmentation of ink particles, release of ink into the extracellular dermal space, partial elimination of ink in a scale crust when present, re-phagocytosis of laser-altered residual tattoo ink particles, and increased ink elimination via the lymphatics.[7]

Ideal wavelengths to treat pigmented lesions would be those with greater absorption by melanin than by oxyhemoglobin. The absorption of melanin decreases over the range of wavelengths between 200 and 2000 nm.[8] Therefore longer wavelengths penetrate deeper, but are absorbed less by melanin. A variety of lasers have been used to successfully treat pigmented lesions. Given that the pigment in lentigines is very superficial, pigmented lasers with shorter wavelengths, such as pulsed dye (510 nm), Q-switched potassium titanyl phosphate (KTP) (532 nm) Nd:YAG and Q-switched ruby (694 nm) are typically used. Longer wavelength pigmented lasers including the Q-switched diode (800 nm), and Q-switched Nd:YAG (1064 nm) are used for lesions where the pigment is located in the dermis such as nevus of Ota and tattoos. Q-switched refers to 'quality-switched', describing the ability of the laser unit to store large amounts of energy in the laser cavity through the use of an optical shutter. When the laser fires, the shutter is then able to release a high-powered pulse with an extremely short pulse duration, in the nanosecond range. Q-switched alexandrite (755 nm) lasers, with an intermediate wavelength, may be used for both superficial and deep pigment.

A laser successfully used in the treatment of superficial pigment is the variable-pulsed 532-nm (KTP) Nd:YAG laser. This laser may be used to treat superficial vascular lesions as well as superficial pigmented lesions.[9] The shorter wavelength only allows for limited penetration depth of the laser radiation and is thus not optimal for the treatment of dermal pigmented lesions or deeper vascular lesions.

Longer pulse width ruby, alexandrite, and Nd:YAG lasers, predominantly used for hair removal, have the same wavelengths as the Q-switched versions used in the treatment of pigmented lesions. However, they operate in a non-Q-switched mode resulting in laser energy delivery over a longer time interval—milliseconds rather than nanoseconds. The longer pulse width creates somewhat less confined thermal damage, but with higher energies and less epidermal cooling than used during hair removal, they are capable of removing some pigmented lesions in the epidermis. The longer pulse widths also allow for higher fluences so that larger structures such as hair follicles and nests of pigmented cells may be targeted. Their use in the treatment of congenital and acquired nevi remains under investigation.

■ HISTORY

The first described use of laser irradiation in the treatment of skin pigmentation was in 1963. At that time, Dr Leon Goldman et al. demonstrated selective absorption of ruby laser energy with a 0.5-ms pulse width in pigmented lesions of the skin.[10] Subsequently, they demonstrated even greater success with a Q-switched ruby laser with a 50-nanosecond pulse width. However, the selectivity of the Q-switched lasers for pigmented lesions was not appreciated until 20–30 years later. As such, during this 'unenlightened' period nonselective continuous wave devices such as the carbon dioxide and argon lasers were employed. The description of the principle of selective photothermolysis by Anderson and Parrish in 1983[1] predicted that thermal confinement will occur in the melanosome or tattoo particle over a range of wavelengths when the laser pulse width is less than 1 microsecond. Subsequently, with thermal relaxation times predicted in the nanosecond range for melanosomes and tattoo particles, Q-switched lasers with nanosecond pulse widths were developed. These lasers demonstrated remarkable efficacy in the selective destruction of melanosomes and tattoo pigment.[8,11,12]

■ PREOPERATIVE PREPARATION

Patient evaluation

Before treatment, a thorough medical history should be taken. In particular, if there is any history of poor wound healing, postinflammatory hyperpigmentation, bleeding disorders, or isotretinoin use in the preceding 6 months proceed with extra caution. In addition, pigmented lesions should be properly diagnosed before laser treatment. If there is any question as to the character of a lesion, a biopsy should be performed in order to assure that a given lesion has no significant atypia or malignant potential. Furthermore, biopsies may be helpful in determining the depth of pigment present (i.e. epidermal versus dermal) and possibly the type of pigment in a lesion possibly caused by foreign body implantation. Finally, patients should be counseled appropriately with regard to having realistic expectations in that multiple treatments may be necessary and that all lesions may not clear completely.

Safety

Of primary concern in the use of pigmented lesion lasers (as with other laser devices) is ocular safety. Retinal injury is the primary hazard and protective goggles must be worn by all personnel in the room. The 'light' from these lasers is out of the visible range and is deeply penetrating and of great intensity. Hence, these lasers are potentially even more dangerous than visible light lasers. The patient must have appropriate eyewear and the placement of intraocular metal eye shields should be considered when treatment is in the immediate periocular area. Furthermore, reflective surfaces and windows should be covered, no flammable materials should be present, and access to the procedure room should be limited during laser treatment.

Q-switched lasers, and especially the Q-switched 1064-nm Nd:YAG laser, can cause some tissue and blood splatter. As such, universal precautions and the use of the protective plastic cone to attach to the handpiece should be employed to prevent splatter onto the actual lens. Alternatively, a clear film (i.e. Second Skin (Spenco Medical, Waco, TX), Tegaderm (3M Healthcare, St Paul, MN)) may be placed on the skin over the treatment area to eliminate outward splatter. However, it must be noted that this technique results in a slightly reduced laser light transmission and may increase the risk of ocular injury as a result of reflection from the surface of the dressing. When using this technique, an additional 0.5–1.0 J/cm^2 is required to achieve equivalent target absorption.

Of paramount importance in the preoperative preparation of the patient is thorough removal of all make-up, creams, topical anesthetics, sunblocks, etc. These products can hinder the delivery of laser energy to the target and may contain ingredients with the potential to ignite. Furthermore, the use of alcohol in cleaning the area must be followed by assurance that alcohol is not present on the surface of the skin at the time of laser energy delivery because alcohol is also a potential source for flash fire development.

Anesthesia

Typically, neither infiltrative nor topical anesthesia is required for the vast majority of treatments using laser or light source energy in the treatment of pigmented lesions. However, one must take into account the location, size, and depth of the lesion as well as the individual pain threshold of the patient. In our practice, neither topical nor infiltrative anesthesia is routinely employed in the treatment of lentigines and photodamage with either the intense pulsed light source or Q-switched lasers. For the treatment of larger tattoos, lesions containing large amounts of dermal pigment such as nevus of Ota, or when ablative lasers are used, infiltrative local anesthesia infiltration or regional nerve blocks are at times employed.

■ TECHNIQUES

Epidermal lesions

Q-switched ruby (694 nm) lasers, Q-switched alexandrite (755 nm) lasers, 532-nm lasers, short pulsed dye (510 nm) lasers, and intense pulse light devices have all demonstrated efficacy in the treatment of various epidermal lesions including lentigines, café au lait macules (CALMS), and ephelides.[1,2,9,11,13,14] In addition, intense pulsed light and 532 nm ms pulsed lasers have demonstrated benefit for 'background' pigmentation from photodamage. Q-switched laser has been shown to be superior to both 35% trichloroacetic acid and cryotherapy in the treatment of lentigines.[15,16] Shorter wavelength lasers are generally well suited for the treatment of epidermal lesions as a result of their high absorption by melanin and limited depth of penetration (Fig. 37.2). However, their efficacy in the

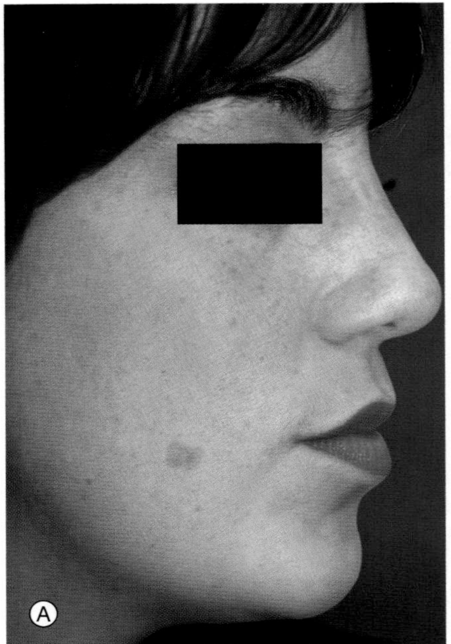
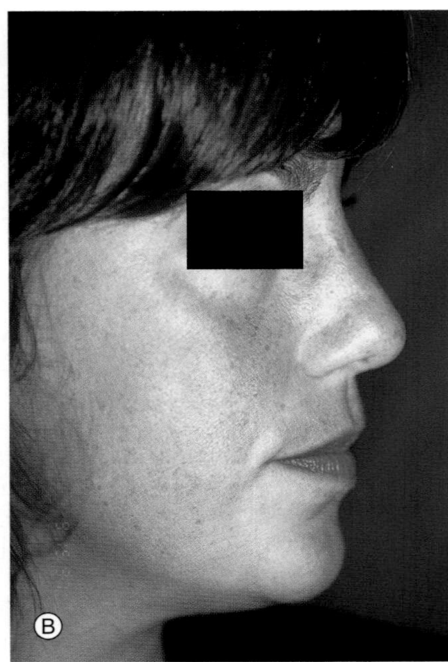

Figure 37.2 Solar lentigines of the right lower cheek (A) before and (B) after one treatment with 532 nm KTP laser.

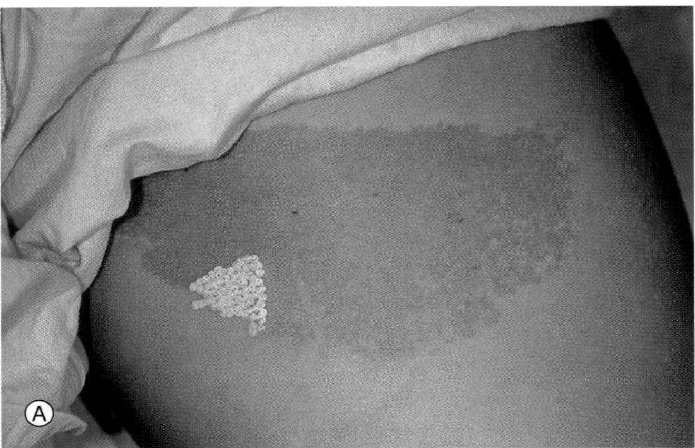
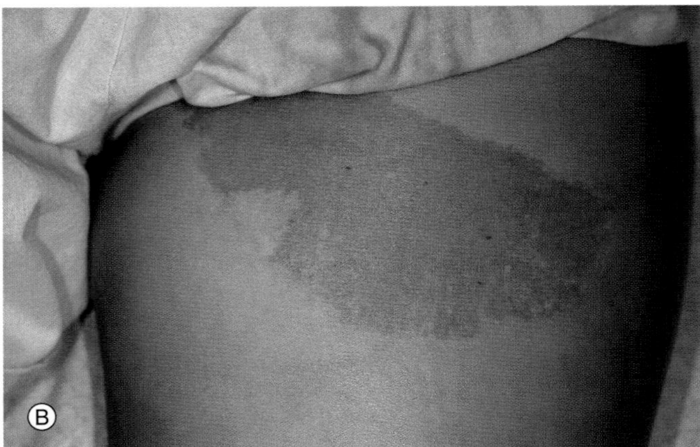

Figure 37.3 Café au lait macule on the left thigh (A) immediately after and (B) 2 months following a test spot with a 755 nm alexandrite laser with a 50 ns pulse duration.

treatment of dermal pigmented lesions is limited because of this limited penetration depth. Conversely, the longer wavelength lasers such as the 1064-nm Q-switched Nd:YAG while providing better penetration depth for dermal lesions falls off in its absorption of melanin and thus is perhaps slightly less effective than shorter wavelength Q-switched lasers in the treatment of epidermal pigment.

Q-switched lasers and 510-nm pulsed-dye lasers are reliably effective in the treatment of some flat seborrheic keratoses. Slightly thicker seborrheic keratoses however, usually require adjunctive cryotherapy.

The response of CALMs and ephelides to laser treatment is often unpredictable (Fig. 37.3). Multiple treatments may result in clearance and some lightening but recurrence is common. Furthermore, transient hyperpigmentation in the treatment of CALMs in darker skin phototypes can be problematic. Recently, some have described the use of Er:YAG superficial resurfacing of CALMs for better longer term clearance.[17]

Intense pulsed light

Unlike laser devices with a collimated beam at a specific wavelength, intense pulsed light devices emit a broad wavelength of energy from a flashlamp with cut-off filters to allow for some wavelength selectivity. Thus, by providing light energy over broader wavelengths, one advantage this may have over other devices is the intense pulsed light's ability to improve the vascular component of photodamage along with the pigmentary changes with one device. In our practice, we find that photodamaged patients with both mild and subtle vascular and pigmentary changes are the best candidates for treatment with the intense pulsed light devices. We prefer to treat patients with more significant and larger lentigines with a more selective Q-switched laser device or trichloroacetic acid peel. Photodamaged patients with a predominantly vascular component are treated with variable pulse-width pulsed dye (595 nm), or long pulse width KTP (532 nm) lasers for those with wispy isolated telangiectasias.

Dermal pigmented lesions and tattoos

The advent of Q-switched lasers revolutionized the treatment of dermal melanocytosis and tattoos. Before this development, only nonselective treatments such as dermabrasion, excision, cryosurgery, and other procedures were available. Q-switched alexandrite (755 nm) and Nd:YAG (1064 nm) are typically the most effective for deeper dermal pigment and tattoos.

Nevus of Ota histologically demonstrates dendritic melanocytes in the papillary and reticular dermis. It is most common in Asian populations, occurring in Caucasians at lower incidence rates. Clearance of 70% or more is reported in patients treated at least five times with the Q-switched ruby laser[15] (Fig. 37.4). Successful treatment of nevus of Ota has also been demonstrated with Q-switched alexandrite and Q-switched 1064-nm Nd:YAG lasers.[16,18] No comparative trials between Q-switched lasers in the treatment of this disorder appear in the literature.

Treatment of melanocytic nevi with Q-switched lasers remains controversial. In-vitro studies of melanoma cells have shown ultrastructural changes with subsequent alterations in cellular migration.[19] Furthermore, benign lesions that recur after laser irradiation may demonstrate increased atypia.[20] However, no study thus far has demonstrated malignant transformation of nevomelanocytic cells irradiated with Q-switched lasers.[21] In addition, some have postulated that laser treatment of nevi may decrease malignancy risk by eliminating a pool of potentially malignancy transforming cells.[22] The authors do not routinely treat melanocytic nevi with laser irradiation. However, with careful patient and lesion selection, treatment successes are attainable. If there is any doubt with regard to lesion diagnosis, a biopsy must be performed. Furthermore, patients with a personal or family history of melanoma should not be treated in this manner. When treating nevi, multiple treatments and a high rate of recurrence are typical, with thicker lesions being more resistant to treatment. Congenital nevi with nests residing deeper in the dermis and around adnexa are particularly difficult to treat with laser therapy. One group of investigators has obtained impressive clearance with non Q-switched lasers with pulse widths in the millisecond domain.[23] The wider pulse width allows for less selective thermal damage and perhaps better delivery of energy to entire nests rather than to individual pigmented cells. Current investigation is elucidating the role of longer pulse width alexandrite and ruby lasers used primarily in hair removal for the treatment of nevi.

Other dermal pigmented lesions commonly encountered include melasma, periorbital pigmentation, and medication-induced pigmentation. The treatment of melasma remains difficult. Cessation of offending medications, sun protection, and the use of topical bleaching agents in conjunction with peeling agents and/or corticosteroids are the gold standard. Q-switched laser treatment often paradoxically increases dermal melanophages and is generally not recommended for the treatment of melasma or postinflammatory pigmentation. Periorbital pigmentation may result from dermal melanin deposition, chronic dermatitis, chronic edema, or prominent superficial blood vessels. When secondary to dermal melanin deposition, Q-switched laser has been shown to be effective.[24] However, responses are less predictable. Numerous medications may cause unusual skin pigmentation. The most commonly encountered in dermatology is minocycline-induced pigmentation. In this condition, pigment within dermal macrophages typically stains positively for melanin and occasionally iron.[25] Although pigmentation typically resolves with cessation of therapy, a long delay may occur before total resolution. As such, treatment with Q-switched lasers is reported to be effective and may be warranted.[26,27]

Tattoos

In amateur tattoos, pigment is typically present in lower concentrations and located in various levels of the dermis. In contrast, in professional tattoos dense pigment is typically implanted at the junction of the papillary and reticular dermis.[28] Commonly used pigments in professional tattoos include cinnabar and cadmium red (red), cadmium sulfide (yellow), chromium salts (green), cobalt salts (dark blue), titanium dioxide (white), and iron oxide (red–brown). Unfortunately, no regulation exists at the state and federal level with regard to standards in the composition or amount of pigment deposited at the time of tattoo placement. As a result, the response to laser treatment of professional tattoos is often difficult to predict. Q-switched lasers lighten the majority of tattoos, but clearance is related to density, color, and composition of the

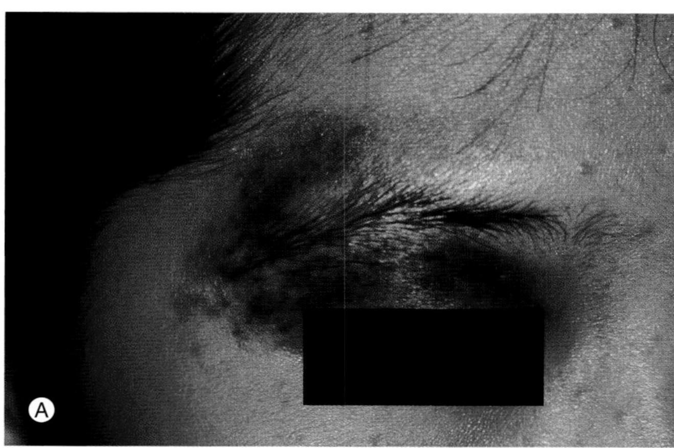

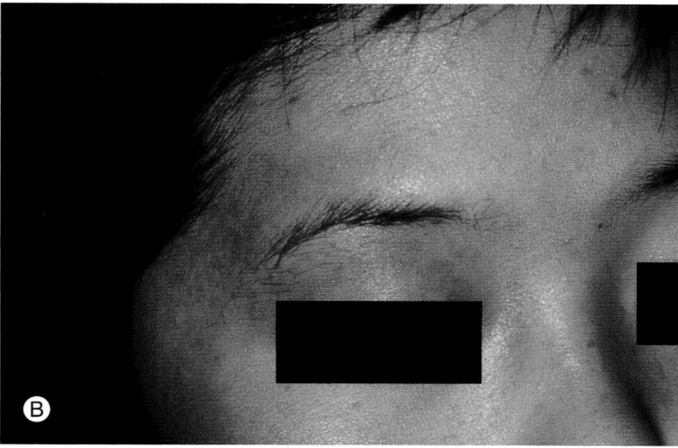

Figure 37.4 Nevus of Ota (A) before and (B) after five treatments. Photo courtesy of Dr Tadashi Tezuka.

tattoo. Typically, amateur dark uniformly colored tattoos clear with some reliability after three to five treatments (Fig. 37.5). Professional multicolored tattoos do not respond predictably and may not clear completely even after more than ten treatments (Fig. 37.6). Tattoos with red, yellow, and orange are particularly difficult to completely clear with most tattoo lasers. Older tattoos, especially those that have started to fade slightly on their own, tend to clear in fewer treatments than the more densely pigmented new tattoos. Furthermore, tattoos on distal extremities tend to be more resistant to treatment as a result of decreased lymphatic drainage.[29]

■ OPTIMIZING OUTCOMES

Epidermal lesions

As outlined previously, preoperative considerations are of the utmost importance. Typically, anesthesia is not required. The skin surface of areas to be treated should be thoroughly cleaned to ensure the absence of any creams, make-ups, etc. The laser must be calibrated before operation and the handpiece should be held perpendicular to the skin with an attached plastic cone or guide on the skin to ensure proper delivery of laser energy to the desired point. The parameters selected depend on laser type, skin phototype of the patient, and melanin content of the target lesion. Table 37.2 outlines common treatment parameters for various epidermal pigmented lesions. Generally, lower fluences are used for darker lesions with abundant target chromophore. The target endpoint is uniform, but faint, whitening without epidermal disruption (Fig. 37.7). If the fluence is too low, whitening may be imperceptible. With higher fluences, solid whitening with epidermal disruption and pinpoint bleeding may occur. At fluences less than threshold, paradoxical hyperpigmentation may occur as a result of melanocyte stimulation. Excessive fluences can result in a thermal burn with tissue sloughing, prolonged wound healing, hypopigmentation, hyperpigmentation, scarring, and textural changes. For darker phototypes, lower fluences with test spots should be employed. Similarly, patients with a tan should postpone treatment because of the higher risk of spotty pigmentation abnormalities, which may persist for months. Typically, treatments are spaced 4–6 weeks apart. Lentigines often require only one to two treatments, while CALMs or ephelides may require multiple treatments.

Treatment of CALMs with Er:YAG resurfacing typically requires only one treatment with a fluence sufficient for complete removal of the epidermis. However, treatment

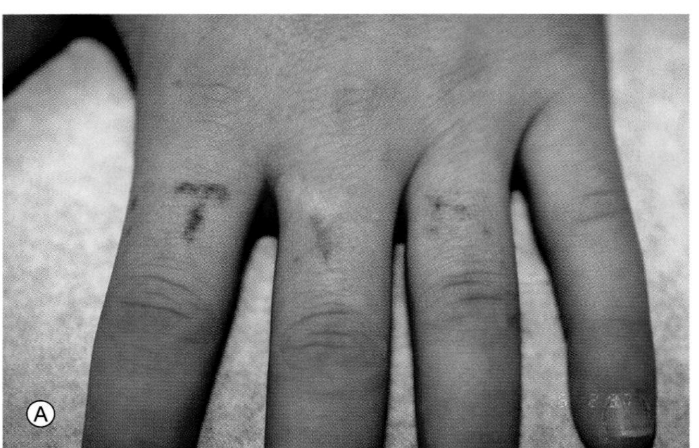

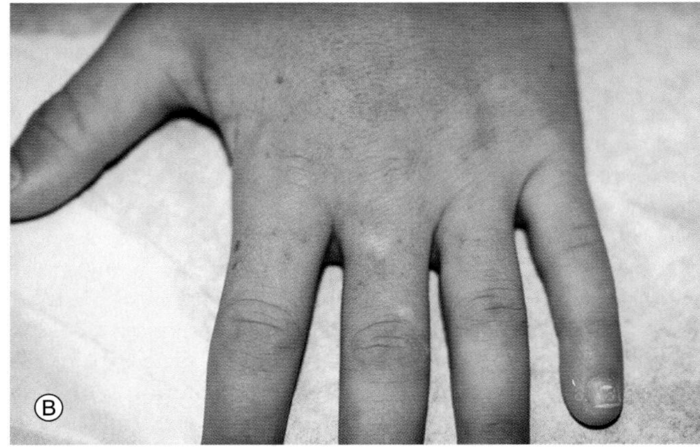

Figure 37.5 Amateur black India ink tattoo (A) before and (B) after two treatments using a 755 nm alexandrite laser with a 50 nsec pulse duration. Note the clearing of amateur tattoo with only two treatments.

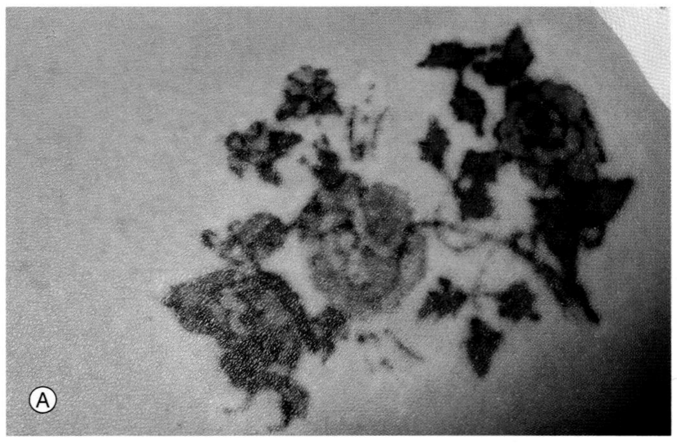

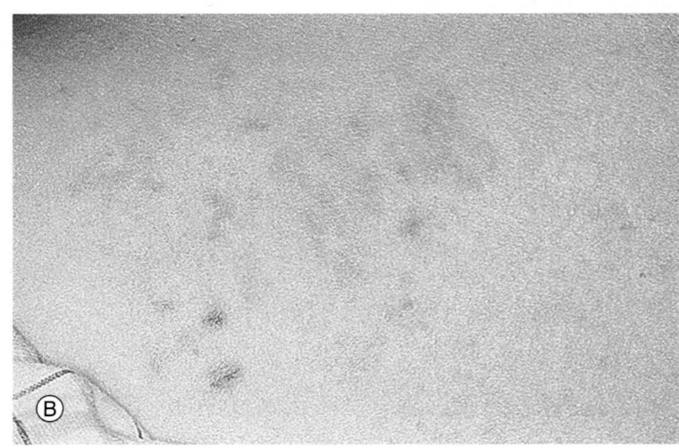

Figure 37.6 Multicolor tattoo (A) before and (B) after ten treatments.

Table 37.2 Standard treatment parameters for pigmented lesions and tattoos

Lesion	Laser	Spot size (mm)	Fluence (J/cm²)	Retreatment
Lentigines	QS ruby	6.5	2.0–4.0	4–8 weeks
	QS Nd:YAG (532 nm)	3	0.7–1.0	
	QS alexandrite	4	4.0–6.0	
	Pulsed dye (510 nm)	3	2.5	
CALMS	QS ruby	6.5	3.0–4.5	4–8 weeks
	QS Nd:YAG (532 nm)	3	1.0–1.5	
	QS alexandrite	4	4.0–6.0	
	Pulsed dye (510 nm)	5	2.0–3.5	
	Er: YAG	3–7	5.0–10	
Becker's nevus	QS Ruby	6.5	3.0–4.5	4–8 weeks
	QS Nd:YAG (532 nm)	3	1.5–1.8	
	QS Nd:YAG (1064 nm)	3	4.0–5.0	
	QS alexandrite	3	4.0–9.0	
Nevus spilus	QS ruby	6.5	3.0–4.5	4–8 weeks
	QS Nd:YAG (532 nm)	3	1.5–2.0	
	QS Nd:YAG (1064 nm)	3	4.0–4.4	
	QS alexandrite	3	6.0–9.0	
Nevus of Ota	QS ruby	6.5	5.0–6.0	6–12 weeks
	QS Nd:YAG (1064 nm)	3	4.0–5.0	
	QS alexandrite	3	6.0–9.0	
Tattoos	QS ruby	5	7.0–10.0	6–12 weeks
	QS ruby	6.5	3.0–6.0	
	QS Nd:YAG (532 nm)	3	2.0–3.5	
	QS Nd:YAG (1064 nm)	3	4.0–8.0	
	QS alexandrite	3	6.0–9.0	
	Pulsed dye (510 nm)	3–5	2.5–3.5	

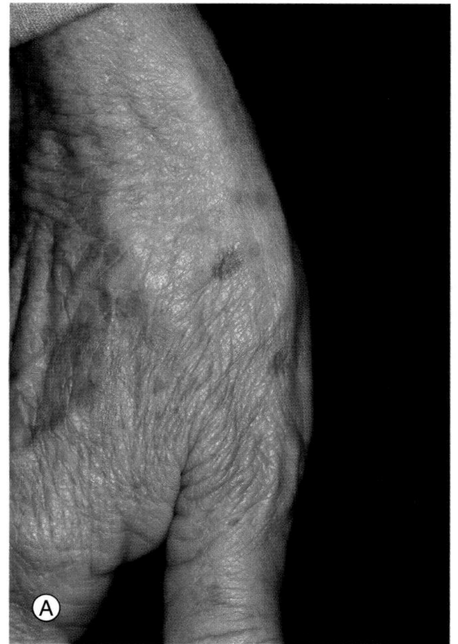

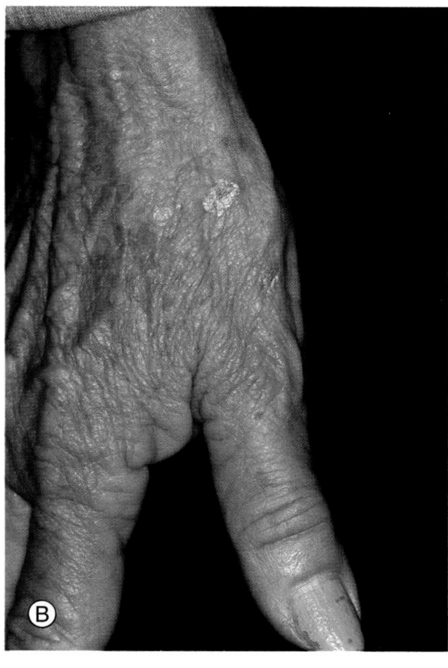

Figure 37.7 Immediate whitening of epidermal pigment following treatment with a Q-switched 694 nm ruby laser (A) before and (B) after treatment.

does carry a higher risk of scarring than treatment with more selective Q-switched lasers. If Er:YAG resurfacing lasers are used to treat CALMs, infiltrative anesthesia is necessary. Many patients are more comfortable with the use of preoperative topical anesthesia.

Intense pulsed light

Unlike treatment with laser devices in which 'specific' lesions are treated, patients undergoing intense pulsed light treatments typically have the entire face or large subunits treated. Similar to treatment with lasers, the practitioner must be certain to wipe all topical anesthesia, creams, make-up, etc., from the treated surface before starting treatment. All personnel in the room must wear protective goggles. In addition, the practitioner must take special precautions to ensure that the contact cooling device is placed in the 'on' position while treating.

Unlike Q-switched lasers, cooling is vitally important to minimize the risk of significant epidermal injury. To ensure proper cooling, a coolant medium (e.g. ultrasound gel) should be applied liberally to the area to be treated. The handpiece in then placed in direct contact with the coolant medium on the skin surface and the area is treated with slightly overlapping pulses with the handpiece. Areas may be single, double, or triple pulsed according to the user's discretion. At least six treatment sessions spaced 4–6 weeks apart are recommended to achieve optimal results. One of the benefits of this series of treatments is the improvement in vascular telangiectasia and skin texture. The practitioner should take extra care to turn off the cooling device and wipe the handpiece clean of any residual coolant gel when not in 'treatment mode'. If not, the gel may freeze and harden on the handpiece.

Dermal lesions and tattoos

Like epidermal lesions, isolated dermal lesions typically do not require the use of anesthetic. However, larger areas, such as nevus of Ota, may require a topical anesthetic or the use of nerve blocks for patient comfort. For local tissue infiltration around the eyes, a mixture of equal parts 2% lidocaine with 1 : 100 000 epinephrine and 0.5% bupivacaine, with the addition of 75 U of hyaluronidase can facilitate tissue diffusion and provide longlasting anesthesia.

As with epidermal lesions, the surface to be treated must be thoroughly cleansed to ensure the removal of any creams, make-up, etc. that may interfere with the transmission of laser energy. The laser must be calibrated before operation and the handpiece should be held perpendicular to the skin with an attached plastic cone or guide on the skin to ensure proper delivery of laser energy to the desired point. The parameters selected depend on laser type, skin phototype of the patient, and melanin content of the target lesion. Generally, higher fluences are employed for dermal lesions than for epidermal lesions. Uniform whitening is the desired endpoint after treatment with an approximately 10% overlap (Fig. 37.8). Fluences that are too low may cause a paradoxical hyperpigmentation, whereas excessive fluences may result in epidermal sloughing, prolonged wound healing, pigmentary abnormality, and scarring. Patients with darker phototypes require the use of lower fluences and are probably best treated with longer wavelength lasers such as the 1064-nm Nd:YAG. The 1064-nm wavelength with its decreased melanin absorption and deeper penetration may allow for sparing of epidermal melanocytes. Although no Q-switched systems available commercially presently incorporate a cooling device, the use of a cooling device helps protect the epidermis and dermoepidermal junction and may provide safer treatment of dermal pigmented lesions, especially in patients with darker skin types.

Multiple treatment sessions spaced 6–8 weeks apart are typical. Because the clearing of dermal pigment is in large part a function of phagocytosis, clearing is slow and gradual. Patients continue to see lightening of their lesions for many months following treatment.

Tattoos

For smaller tattoos, anesthesia is generally not required. However, infiltrative anesthesia with a 30-gauge 1-inch needle utilizing a fanning technique is preferred for larger tattoos. Preoperative skin preparation and technique are essentially the same as that for dermal lesions with slight overlap of pulses to avoid untreated fragments of tattoo. When pulses are spaced too far apart, the treated tattoo often takes on a 'honeycomb' appearance, which is cosmetically less appealing than the original tattoo.

Treatment with the highest possible fluence is generally recommended. Lesions should be treated with one to two pulses to determine the tissue response. The desired response is immediate, bright tissue whitening (see Fig. 37.8). Epidermal disruption or bleeding represents excessive fluence and should be adjusted accordingly. However, some pinpoint bleeding is acceptable. For tattoos with darker, dense pigment, lower fluences are recommended for initial treatments. As the pigment lightens, higher fluences can be used. In darker skin patients the 1064-nm Nd:YAG laser is recommended for blue or black pigment as a result of the longer wavelength and lower melanin selectivity sparing epidermal melanin.[30] Additionally, a cooling device may be used to help protect the epidermis and dermoepidermal junction. Similar to dermal pigmented lesions, pigment may

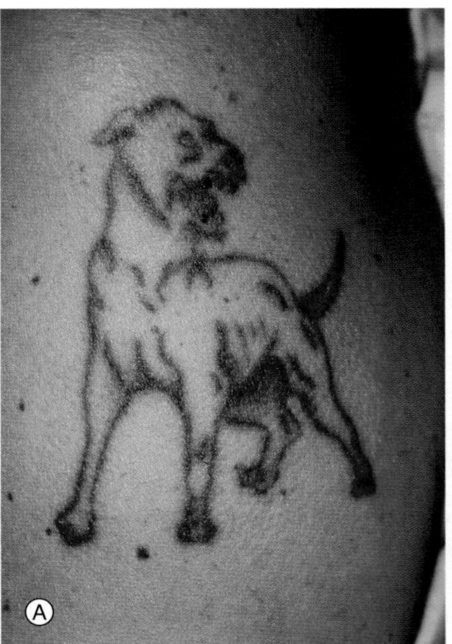

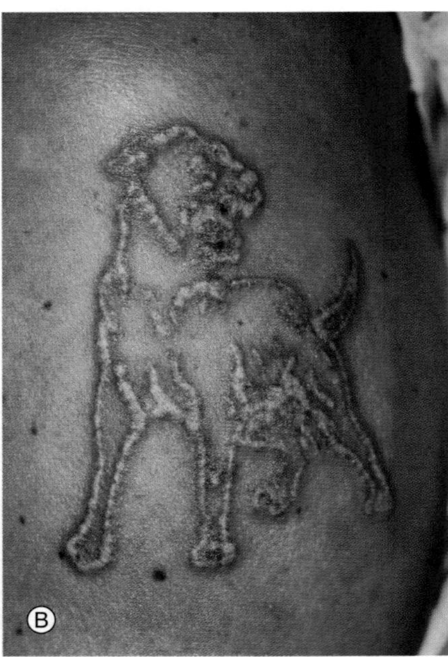

Figure 37.8 Immediate whitening and some mild pinpoint bleeding of tattoo following treatment using a 755 nm alexandrite laser with a 50 nsec pulse duration.

lighten for several months following treatment, with treatment intervals typically 6–8 weeks apart.

No laser is capable of single-handedly eliminating all tattoo colors. Q-switched ruby[8] and alexandrite lasers[31] are best for black, blue, and green pigments, whereas Q-switched Nd:YAG (1064 nm)[32] is best for blue and black, but not green pigments. Shorter wavelength lasers such as the 510-nm pulsed dye[33] and Q-switched 532-nm Nd:YAG[28] are best for red and yellow pigments.

Practitioners should be wary of treating cosmetic tattoos with shades of white, red, orange, tan, or brown as is often seen in permanent lip lining. These tattoos when treated with Q-switched lasers are at risk of immediate irreversible darkening of the pigment as a result of reduction in the iron oxide (conversion of ferric oxide to ferrous oxide) or titanium dioxide contained in these pigments. If this occurs, the therapeutic armamentarium includes multiple additional treatments, resurfacing, and often surgical excision. Recently, reports of multiple treatments with single pass resurfacing laser have demonstrated success in treating these tattoos with minimal risk of pigment darkening.[34,35] Alternatively, cosmetic tattoos around the vermilion border may be treated cautiously with a carbon dioxide and or Er:YAG resurfacing laser. In addition to partially or completely removing the cosmetic tattoo pigment, the perioral rhytides may be significantly improved (Fig. 37.9).

■ POSTOPERATIVE CARE AND COMPLICATIONS

Postoperatively, cool compresses, emollient application, and/or the use of occlusive dressings (i.e. Vigilon [C R Bard, Murray Hill, NJ], Second Skin) can provide some pain relief. The whitening caused by laser irradiation typically fades within 20–30 minutes. Some patients may develop an urticarial reaction with edema and pruritus, which will subside within the hour but can be treated with oral antihistamines. Treated areas may appear darker and develop crusting in the first 7–10 days after treatment. Patients should be instructed to gently clean treated areas daily, apply occlusive emollient ointments to hasten healing, and allow crusts to slough on their own. Furthermore, patients need to avoid excessive sun exposure and apply appropriate sunscreens. Patients treated with the 532-nm Nd:YAG or 510-nm pulsed dye lasers may develop purpura for 7–10 days as a result of the significant absorption of hemoglobin at these wavelengths.

Given the more aggressive nature of the treatment of dermal lesions and tattoos versus epidermal lesions, postoperative changes are more pronounced. The whitening may fade after 20 minutes and erythema and edema should be expected. In addition, surface crusting typically occurs and then resolves in 7–10 days. Vesiculation may occur with shorter wavelength Q-switched laser treatment of tattoos, but typically heals without scarring or textural changes. However, the development of blistering in the treatment of dermal lesions typically indicates the use of excessive fluences.

Ice-packs, cool compresses, and hydro-occlusive dressings will reduce postoperative stinging and pain. Daily cleansing of treated areas with soap and water and frequent application of occlusive ointments are recommended.

Because treatment of dermal lesions and tattoos is more aggressive than that of epidermal lesions, complications, and in particular, pigmentary and textural changes are more likely. Patients should also be counseled with regard to sun protection and avoidance to minimize the risk of unwanted hypo and/or hyperpigmentation. Although the risk of scarring and permanent hypopigmentation is very low, the risk is slightly higher when treating tattoos. Factors that may increase risk include excessive fluences using small spot sizes, tattoos containing 'double ink,'[35] pulse stacking, too frequent treatment, and treatment of tattoos in areas more prone to scar such as the ankle, deltoid, and chest areas. In addition, textural changes that may be present but camouflaged before laser treatment may become more apparent after treatment. The use of preoperative photographs may be helpful and essential in this regard.

Patients with CALMs treated with Er:YAG resurfacing may have an occlusive dressing placed on the wound for the first few days postoperatively. Subsequently, daily cleaning, soaks to minimize crusting, and frequent application of

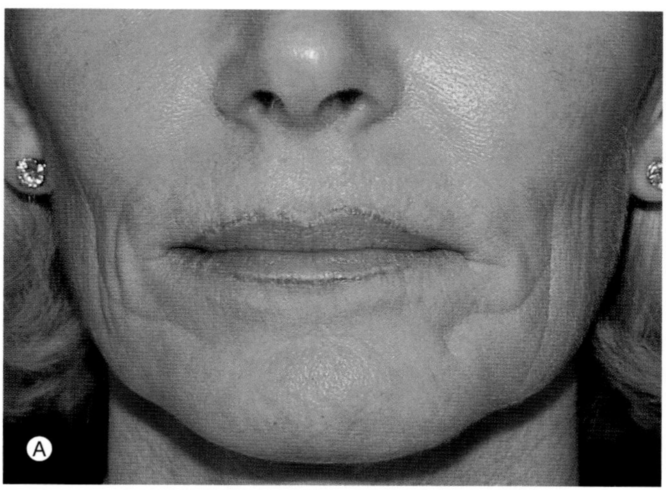

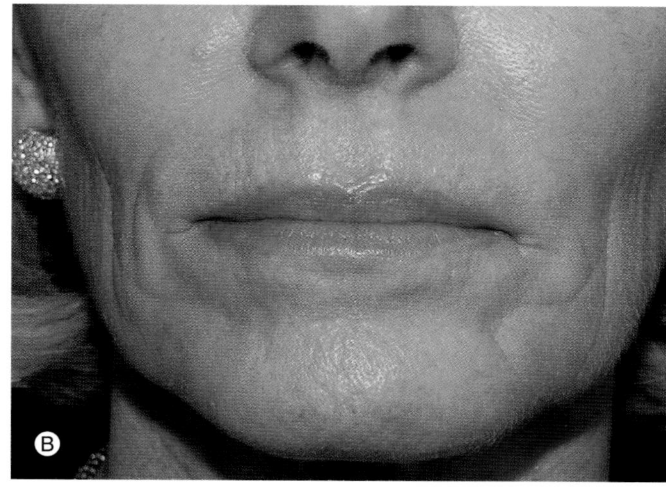

Figure 37.9 Cosmetic tattoo of the vermilion border (A) before and (B) 4 weeks after treatment with a combined carbon dioxide and Er:YAG laser resurfacing procedure.

occlusive emollients is required. After re-epithelialization, erythema may persist for some time, which may require prolonged patient reassurance.

In those patients treated with intense pulsed light devices, postoperative reactions as described are less pronounced. As such, daily emollient application is usually unnecessary. However, patients often require multiple treatments to achieve the desired result. Nevertheless, some patients may develop some mild postoperative erythema and burning, which can be soothed with cool compresses.

Pitfalls and their management

- Patients should be counseled with regard to sun protection and avoidance to minimize the risk of unwanted hypo or hyperpigmentation.
- The development of blistering in the treatment of dermal lesions typically indicates the use of excessive fluences.
- Postoperative stinging and pain can be reduced with the use of ice-packs, cool compresses, hydro-occlusive dressings, daily cleansing of treated areas with soap and water, and frequent application of occlusive ointments.
- Patients treated with intense pulsed light devices, often require multiple treatments to achieve the desired result. They may develop some mild postoperative erythema and burning, which can be soothed with cool compresses.

SUMMARY

Various pigmented lesions and tattoos can be safely and effectively treated with laser irradiation with superior cosmetic outcomes when compared with standard nonselective therapies. Proper patient selection and preoperative safety are essential. 'Titrating' laser fluences to desired immediate clinical endpoints will result in optimal results while minimizing untoward effects. The advent of nonlaser flashlamp devices has enabled the practitioner to treat both the vascular and pigmented component of photodamage simultaneously. Future directions may include the use of combinations of devices, longer pulse widths for larger pigmented structures, and the addition of photodynamic therapy.

REFERENCES

1. Anderseon RR, Parrish JA. Selective photothermolysis: precise microsurgery by selective absorption of pulsed irradiation. Science 1983; 220:524.
2. Weiss RA, Goldman MP, Weiss MA. Treatment of poikiloderma of Civatte with an intense pulsed light source. Derm Surg 2000; 26:823–828.
3. Polla LL, Margolis RJ, Dover JS, et al. Melanosomes are a primary target of Q-switched ruby laser irradiation in guinea pig skin. J Invest Dermatol 1987; 89:281.
4. Murphy GF, Shepard RS, Paul BS, et al. Organelle-specific injury to melanin-containing cells in human skin by pulsed laser irradiation. Lab Invest 1983; 49:680.
5. Ara G, Anderson RR, Mandel KG, et al. Irradiation of pigmented melanoma cells with high intensity pulsed radiation generates acoustic waves and kills cells. Lasers Surg Med 1990; 10:52.
6. Watanabe S, Anderson RR, Brorson S, et al. Comparative studies of femtosecond to microsecond laser pulses on selective pigmented cell injury in skin. Photochem Photobiol 1991; 53:757.
7. Anderson RR. Laser–tissue interactions. In: Goldman MP, Fitzpatrick RE, eds. Cutaneous laser surgery: the art and science of selective photothermolysis. St Louis: Mosby 1994; 14–15.
8. Taylor CR, Gange RW, Dover JS, et al. Treatment of tattoos by Q-switched ruby laser: a dose-response study. Arch Dermatol 1990; 126:893–99.
9. Lee MW. Combination 532nm and 1064nm lasers for noninvasive skin rejuvenation and toning. Arch Dermatol 2003; 139:1265–1276.
10. Goldman L, Blaney DJ, Kindel DJ, Franke EK. Effect of the laser beam on the skin: preliminary report. J Invest Dermatol 1963; 40:121–122.
11. Taylor CR, Anderson RR. Treatment of benign pigmented epidermal lesions by Q-switched ruby laser. Int J Dermatol 1993; 32:908–912.
12. Reid WH, Miller ID, Murphy MJ, et al. Q-switched ruby laser treatment of tattoos: a 9-year experience. Br J Plast Surg 1990; 43:663–669.
13. Kilmer SL, Wheeland RG, Goldberg DJ, Anderson RR. Treatment of epidermal pigmented lesions with the frequency doubled Q-switched Nd:YAG laser. Arch Dermatol 1994; 130:1515–1519.
14. Fitzpatrick RE, Golman MP, Ruiz-Esparza J. Laser treatment of benign pigmented epidermal lesions using a 300 nsecond pulse and 510 nm wavelength. J Dermatol Surg Oncol 1993; 18:341–347.
15. Watanabe S, Takahashi H. Treatment of nevus of Ota with the Q-switched ruby laser. N Engl J Med 1994; 331:1745–1750.
16. Alster TS, Williams CM. Treatment of nevus of Ota by the Q-switched alexandrite laser. Dermatol Surg 1995; 21:592–596.
17. Alora MB, Arndt KA. Treatment of a café-au-lait macule with the erbium:YAG laser. J Am Acad Dermatol 2001; 45:566–568.
18. Tse Y, Levine VJ, McClain SA, Ashinoff R. The removal of cutaneous pigmented lesions with the Q-switched ruby laser and the Q-switched neodymium:yttrium-aluminum-garnet laser. J Dermatol Surg Oncol 1994; 20:795–800.
19. van Leeuwen RL, Dekker SW, Byers HR, et al. Modulation of alpha 4 beta 1 and alpha 5 beta 1 integrin expression: heterogeneous effects of Q-switched ruby, Nd:YAG, and alexandrite lasers on melanoma cells in vitro. Lasers Surg Med 1996; 18:63–71.
20. Dummer R, Kempf W, Burg G. Pseudo-melanoma after laser therapy. Dermatology 1998; 197:71–73.
21. Grevelink JM, van Leeuwen RL, Anderson RR, Byers R. Clinical and histological responses of congenital melanocytic nevi after single treatment with Q-switched lasers. Arch Dermatol 1997; 133:349–353.
22. Waldorf HA, Kauvar ANB, Geronemus RG. Treatment of small and medium congenital nevi with the Q-switched ruby laser. Arch Dermatol 1996; 132:301–304.
23. Ueda S, Imamaya S. Normal-mode ruby laser for treating congenital nevi. Arch Dermatol 1997; 133:355–359.
24. Lowe NJ, Wider JM, Shorr N, et al. Infraorbital pigmented skin: preliminary observations of laser therapy. Dermatol Surg 1995; 21:767–770.
25. Argenyi ZB, Finelli L, Bergfeld WF, et al. Minocycline-related cutaneous hyperpigmentation as demonstrated by light microscopy, electron microscopy and X-ray energy spectroscopy. J Cutan Pathol 1987; 14:176–180.
26. Tsao H, Dover JS. Treatment of minocycline-induced hyperpigmentation resolves after treatment with the Q-switched ruby laser. Arch Dermatol 1996; 132:1250–1251.
27. Wilde JL, English JC, Finley EM. Minocycline-induced hyperpigmentation: treatment with the neodymium:YAG laser. Arch Dermatol 1997; 133:1344–1346.
28. Taylor CR, Anderson RR, Gange RW, et al. Light and electron microscopic analysis of tattoos treated by Q-switched ruby laser. J Invest Dermatol 1991; 97:131–136.
29. Fitzpatrick RE, Goldman MP. Tattoo removal using the alexandrite laser. Arch Dermatol 1994; 130:1508–1514.
30. Grevelink JM, Duke D, van Leeuwen RL, et al. Laser treatment of tattoos in darkly pigmented patients: efficacy and side effects. J Am Acad Dermatol 1996; 34:653–656.
31. Kilmer SL, Anderson RR. Clinical use of the Q-switched ruby and the Q-switched Nd:YAG (1064nm and 532 nm) lasers for the treatment of tattoos. J Dermatol Surg Oncol 1993; 19:330–338.

32. Kilmer SL, Lee MS, Grevelink JM, et al. The Q-switched Nd:YAG laser effectively treats tattoos: a controlled, dose–response study. Arch Dermatol 1993; 129:971–978.

33. Grekin RC, Shelton RM, Geisse JK, Frieden I. 510-nm pigmented lesion dye laser: its characteristics and clinical uses. J Dermatol Surg Oncol 1993; 19:380–387.

34. Mafong EA, Kauvar AN, Geronemus RG. Surgical pearl: removal of cosmetic lip-liner tattoo with the pulsed carbon dioxide laser. J Am Acad Dermatol 2003; 48:271–272.

35. Alora MBT, Arndt KA, Taylor CR. Scarring following Q-switched laser treatment of 'double tattoos.' Arch Dermatol 2000; 136:269–270.

38 Laser Skin Resurfacing: Ablative and Non-ablative

Tina S Alster MD and Elizabeth L Tanzi MD

Summary box

- Many aspects of cutaneous photodamage are amenable to treatment with a variety of ablative and non-ablative lasers and light sources.
- Ablative laser skin resurfacing offers the most substantial clinical improvement; but is associated with several weeks of postoperative recovery.
- Severe side effects and complications after ablative laser skin resurfacing can be minimized by careful patient selection, proper surgical technique, and meticulous postoperative care.
- Non-ablative laser skin remodeling is a good alternative for patients who desire modest improvement of photodamaged skin without significant post-treatment recovery.
- Good candidates for non-ablative laser and light-source treatments are patients with mild-to-moderate photodamage and rhytides and realistic clinical expectations.
- With ongoing advancements in laser technology and techniques, more improved clinical outcomes with minimal postoperative recovery will be realized.

INTRODUCTION

Years of damaging UV light exposure manifests clinically as a sallow complexion with roughened surface texture, and variable degrees of dyspigmentation, telangiectasias, wrinkling, and skin laxity.[1,2] Histologically, these extrinsic aging effects are usually limited to the epidermis and upper papillary dermis and are therefore amenable to treatment with a variety of ablative and non-ablative lasers and light-sources.[3]

The armamentarium of lasers and light-based sources available to treat cutaneous photodamage is larger than ever before (Table 38.1). The most appropriate technique will depend upon the severity of photodamage and rhytides, the expertise of the laser surgeon, and the expectations and lifestyle of the individual patient.

Historical Vignette

Although dermatologic laser surgery is nearly four decades old, the field was revolutionized in 1983 when Anderson and Parrish elucidated the principles of selective photothermolysis.[4] This basic theory of laser-tissue interaction explains how selective tissue destruction is possible. In order to effect precise thermal destruction of target tissue without unwanted conduction of heat to surrounding structures, the proper laser wavelength must be selected for preferential absorption by the intended tissue chromophore. Furthermore, the pulse duration of laser emission must be shorter than the thermal relaxation time of the target–thermal relaxation time (T_R) being defined as the amount of time necessary for the targeted structure to cool to one-half of its peak temperature immediately after laser irradiation. The delivered fluence (energy density) must also be sufficiently high to cause the desired degree of thermal injury to the skin. Thus, the laser wavelength, pulse duration, and fluence each must be carefully chosen to achieve maximal target ablation while minimizing surrounding tissue damage.

The first system developed for cutaneous laser resurfacing was the carbon dioxide laser, which was

Table 38.1 Lasers and light sources for photorejuvenation

	Laser Type	Wavelength
Ablative	Carbon dioxide (pulsed)	10 600 nm
	Erbium:YAG (pulsed)	2490 nm
Non-ablative	Pulsed dye	585–595 nm
	Nd:YAG (Q-switched; normal mode)	1064 nm
	Nd:YAG, long-pulsed	1320 nm
	Diode, long-pulsed	1450 nm
	Erbium:glass	1540 nm
	Intense pulsed light source	515–1200 nm

Nd, neodymium; Q-switched, quality-switched; YAG, yttrium–aluminum–garnet.

approved by the Food and Drug Administration (FDA) in 1996. The earliest systems were continuous-wave (CW) lasers, which were effective for gross lesional destruction.[5,6] However, these systems could not reliably ablate fine layers of tissue because of prolonged tissue dwell times and production of unacceptably high rates of scarring and pigmentary alteration.[7–9] The unpredictable nature of these lasers prevented their widespread use in facial resurfacing procedures. With the subsequent development of high-energy, pulsed lasers it became possible to safely apply higher energy densities with exposure times that were shorter than the thermal relaxation time of water-containing tissue, thus lowering the risk of thermal injury to surrounding non-targeted structures.[3,10]

The short-pulsed erbium:yttrium–aluminum–garnet (Er:YAG) laser was approved by the FDA in 1996 for cutaneous resurfacing. It was introduced as an alternative to carbon dioxide skin resurfacing in an attempt to minimize the recovery period and limit side effects while maintaining clinical benefit.

In an attempt to limit the prolonged postoperative recovery period associated with ablative laser skin resurfacing and in response to growing public interest in minimally-invasive treatment modalities, non-ablative laser and light source technology was developed. Rapid advances in this technology have produced several lasers and light-based sources capable of improving fine facial rhytides, dyspigmentation, and telangiectasia associated with cutaneous photodamage.

■ ABLATIVE LASER SKIN RESURFACING

Preoperative preparation

The ideal patient for ablative cutaneous laser resurfacing is one with a fair complexion (skin phototype I or II), cutaneous lesions that are amenable to treatment with a resurfacing laser, and realistic expectations of the resurfacing procedure. Adequate preoperative patient evaluation and education are absolute essentials to avoid pitfalls and optimize the clinical outcome. Proper patient selection is paramount as ablative laser resurfacing can be complicated by a prolonged postoperative recovery, pigmentary alterations, or unexpected scarring. The patient's emotional ability to tolerate an extended convalescence is an important factor in determining the most appropriate choice of laser. Although carbon dioxide lasers or modulated Er:YAG lasers will produce the most dramatic results, some patients may be unable to tolerate the intensive recovery period. For patients unable or unwilling to tolerate extended postoperative healing, a short-pulsed Er:YAG laser or application of non-ablative laser procedures may be more suitable choices.

Currently, there is no consensus among laser experts regarding the most appropriate preoperative regimen for ablative laser skin resurfacing patients. The use of topical retinoic acid compounds, hydroquinone bleaching agents, or α-hydroxy acids for several weeks before ablative cutaneous resurfacing has been touted as a means of speeding recovery and decreasing the incidence of postinflammatory hyperpigmentation.[11] Topical tretinoin enhances penetration of chemicals through the skin and has been shown to accelerate postoperative re-epithelialization after dermabrasion or deep chemical peels.[12] However, because ablative laser-induced wounds are intrinsically different from those created by physically destructive methods, laser skin penetration is not typically affected by the topical application of any of these medications. In addition, being that postinflammatory hyperpigmentation is relatively common after ablative cutaneous laser resurfacing, many laser surgeons originally believed that the prophylactic use of topical bleaching agents would reduce the incidence of this side effect, but investigators subsequently demonstrated that the preoperative use of topical tretinoin, hydroquinone, or glycolic acid had no effect on the incidence of postablative laser hyperpigmentation.[13]

Due to the moist, de-epithelialized state of ablative laser-resurfaced skin and the possibility of bacterial contamination and overgrowth, many laser surgeons advocate oral antibiotic prophylaxis, however, this practice remains controversial due to the results of a controlled study that demonstrated no significant change in post-laser resurfacing infection rate in patients treated with prophylactic antibiotics.[14]

■ TECHNICAL ASPECTS

Carbon dioxide laser

The Ultrapulse 5000 (Lumenis Corp, Yokeam, Israel), one of the first high-energy, pulsed-laser systems developed, emits individual carbon dioxide pulses (ranging 600 μs to 1 ms) with peak energy densities of 500 mJ, whereas the SilkTouch (Lumenis Corp, Yokeam, Israel), another high-energy pulsed laser system, is a continuous-wave carbon dioxide system with a microprocessor scanner that continuously moves the laser beam so that light does not dwell on any one area for more than 1 ms. The peak fluences delivered per pulse or scan range from 4–5 J/cm^2, which are the energy densities necessary for complete tissue vaporization.[7,15–17] Studies with these and other pulsed and scanned carbon dioxide laser systems have shown that after a typical skin resurfacing procedure, water-containing tissue is vaporized to a depth of approximately 20–60 μm, producing a zone of thermal damage ranging from 20–150 μm.[7,16,18–20]

The depth of ablation is directly correlated with the number of passes performed and usually is restricted to the epidermis and upper papillary dermis.[21] However, stacking of laser pulses by treating an area with multiple passes in rapid succession or by using a high overlap setting on a scanning device leads to excessive thermal injury with subsequent increased risk of scarring.[22,23] An ablative plateau is reached, with less effective tissue ablation and accumulation of thermal injury. This effect is most likely caused by reduced tissue water content after initial desiccation, resulting in less selective absorption of energy.[23] The complete removal of partially desiccated tissue and avoidance of pulse stacking is paramount to prevention of excessive thermal accumulation with any laser system.

The objective of ablative laser skin resurfacing is to vaporize tissue to the papillary dermis. Limiting the depth of penetration decreases the risk for scarring and permanent pigmentary alteration. When choosing treatment parameters, the surgeon must consider factors such as the anatomic location to be resurfaced, the skin phototype of the patient, and previous treatments delivered to the area.[15,24] In general, areas with thinner skin (e.g. periorbital) require fewer laser passes and non-facial (e.g. neck, chest) laser resurfacing should be avoided due to the relative paucity of pilosebaceous units in these areas.[24] To reduce the risk of excessive thermal injury, partially desiccated tissue should be removed manually with wet gauze after each laser pass to expose the underlying dermis.[23]

The clinical and histologic benefits of cutaneous laser resurfacing are numerous. With the carbon dioxide laser, most studies have shown at least a 50% improvement over baseline in overall skin tone and wrinkle severity (Fig. 38.1a–b).[10,25–29] The biggest advantages associated with carbon dioxide laser skin resurfacing are the excellent tissue contraction, hemostasis, prolonged neocollagenesis and collagen remodeling that it provides. Histologic examination of laser-treated skin demonstrates replacement of epidermal cellular atypia and dyplasia with normal, healthy epidermal cells from adjacent follicular adnexal structures.[7,19] The most profound effects occur in the papillary dermis, where coagulation of disorganized masses of actinically induced elastotic material are replaced with normal compact collagen bundles arranged in parallel to the skin's surface.[30,31] Immediately after carbon dioxide laser treatment, a normal inflammatory response is initiated, with granulation tissue formation, neovascularization, and increased production of macrophages and fibroblasts.[19]

Persistent collagen shrinkage and dermal remodeling are responsible for much of the continued clinical benefits observed after carbon dioxide resurfacing and are influenced by several factors.[32,33] Thermal effects of laser irradiation of skin produce collagen fiber contraction at temperatures ranging from 55 °C to 62 °C through disruption of inter-peptide bonds resulting in a conformational change to the collagen's basic triple helical structure.[34,35] The collagen molecule is thereby shortened to approximately one third of its normal length. The laser-induced shrinkage of collagen fibers may act as the contracted scaffold for neocollagenesis, leading to subsequent production of the newly shortened form. In turn, fibroblasts that migrate into laser wounds after resurfacing may up-regulate the expression of immune modulating factors that serve to enhance continued collagen shrinkage.[36]

The carbon dioxide resurfacing laser is a most effective tool for improving photo-induced facial rhytides; however, dynamic rhytides are not as amenable to laser treatment. Many patients experience recurrence of movement-associated rhytides (particularly in the glabellar region) within 6–12 months postoperatively. Thus, cosmetic denervation with intramuscular injections of botulinum toxin type A is often used concomitantly with laser resurfacing to provide prolonged clinical improvement.[37]

Absolute contraindications to carbon dioxide laser skin resurfacing include active bacterial, viral, or fungal infection or an inflammatory skin condition involving the skin areas to be treated. Isotretinoin use within the preceding 6–12-month period or history of keloids also are considered contraindications to carbon dioxide laser treatment because of the unpredictable tissue healing response and greater risk for scarring.[38,39]

In an attempt to address many of the difficulties associated with the use of multiple-pass carbon dioxide laser skin resurfacing, refinements in surgical technique have been developed. In 1997, a minimally traumatic single-pass carbon dioxide laser resurfacing procedure was described that resulted in faster re-epithelialization and an improved side effect profile than reported after use of the multiple-pass technique.[40] Rather than remove partially desiccated tissue (as is typical with multiple-pass procedures), the lased skin is left intact to serve as a biologic wound dressing. Additional laser passes can then be applied focally only in areas of more extensive involvement in order to limit unnecessary thermal and mechanical trauma to less involved skin. Subsequent reports have substantiated the improved side effect profile of this less aggressive procedure.[41–43]

Erbium:yttrium–aluminum–garnet laser

The Er:YAG laser is a more precise ablative tool than the carbon dioxide laser and emits 2940 nm wavelength light that corresponds to the 3000 nm absorption peak of water. The absorption coefficient of the Er:YAG is 12 800 cm^{-1}

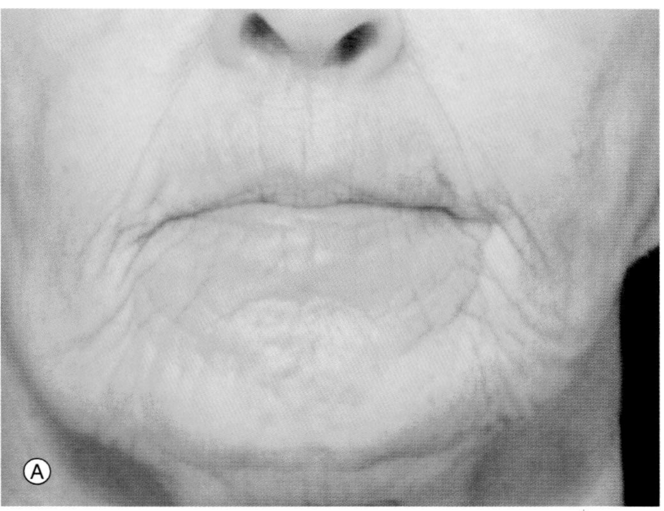

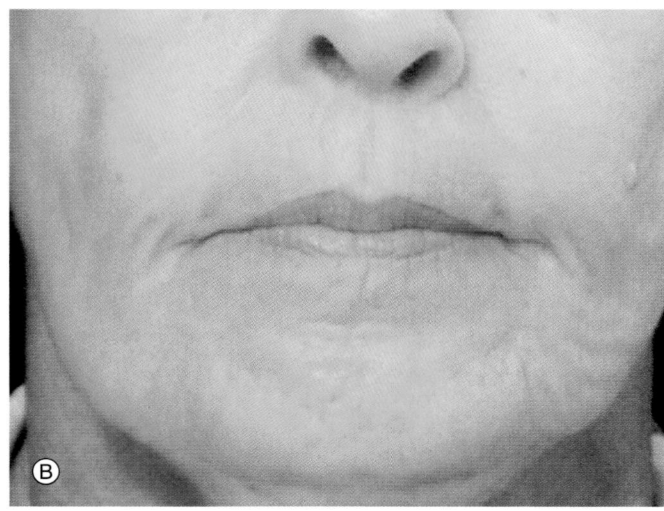

Figure 38.1 Perioral rhytides (A) before and (B) several months after carbon dioxide laser skin resurfacing.

(compared with 800 cm^{-1} for the carbon dioxide laser), making it 12 to 18 times more efficiently absorbed by water-containing tissue than is the carbon dioxide laser.[44] The pulse duration (mean 250 μs) is also much shorter than the carbon dioxide laser, resulting in decreased thermal diffusion, less effective hemostasis, and increased intraoperative bleeding which often hampers deeper dermal treatment. Because of limited thermal skin injury, the amount of collagen contraction is also reduced with Er:YAG treatment (1–4%) compared to that observed with carbon dioxide laser irradiation.[11,45]

The erbium laser's efficient rate of absorption, short exposure duration, and direct relationship between fluence delivered and amount of tissue ablated leads to 2–4 μm of tissue vaporization per J/cm^2, producing a shallow level of tissue ablation. Much narrower zones of thermal necrosis, averaging only 20–50 μm, are therefore produced.[44,46–48] Laser-induced ejection of desiccated tissue from the target site produces a distinctive popping sound. Thermal energy is confined to the selected tissue, with minimal collateral thermal damage. Because little tissue necrosis is produced with each pass of the laser, manual removal of desiccated tissue is often unnecessary.

The short-pulsed erbium laser fluences used most often range from 5–15 J/cm^2, depending on the degree of photodamage and anatomic location. When lower fluences are used, it is often necessary to perform multiple passes to ablate the entire epidermis. The ablation depth with the short-pulsed Er:YAG does not diminish with successive passes, because the amount of thermal necrosis is minimal with each pass. It takes three to four times as many passes with the short-pulsed Er:YAG laser to achieve similar depths of penetration as with one pass of the carbon dioxide laser at typical treatment parameters.[3,11] To ablate the entire epidermis with the short-pulsed Er:YAG laser at 5 J/cm^2, at least two or three passes must be used which increases the possibility of uneven tissue penetration. Deeper dermal lesions or areas of the face with extreme photodamage and extensive dermal elastosis may require up to nine or ten passes of the short-pulsed Er:YAG laser, whereas the carbon dioxide laser would effect similar levels of tissue ablation in two or three passes.[7,16,44]

Pinpoint bleeding caused by inadequate hemostasis and tissue color change with multiple Er:YAG passes can impede adequate clinical assessment of wound depth. Irradiated areas whiten immediately after treatment and then quickly fade. These factors render it far more difficult for the surgeon to determine treatment endpoints and thus requires extensive knowledge of laser–tissue interaction.

Conditions amenable to short-pulsed Er:YAG laser resurfacing include superficial epidermal or dermal lesions, mild photodamage and subtle dyspigmentation. The major advantage of short-pulsed Er:YAG laser treatment is its shorter recovery period. Re-epithelialization is completed within an average of 5.5 days, compared with 8.5 days for multiple-pass carbon dioxide procedures.[16,46] Postoperative pain and duration of erythema are reduced after short-pulsed Er:YAG laser resurfacing, with postoperative erythema resolving within 3–4 weeks. Because there is less thermal injury and trauma to the skin, the risk of pigmentary disturbance is also decreased, making the short-pulsed Er:YAG laser a good alternative in patients with darker skin phototypes.[3,49] The major disadvantages of the short-pulsed Er:YAG laser are its limited ability to effect significant collagen shrinkage and its failure to induce new and continued collagen formation postoperatively.[3,46,50] The final clinical result is typically less impressive than that produced by carbon dioxide laser skin resurfacing for deeper rhytides. However, for mild photodamage, improvement of approximately 50% is typical (Fig. 38.2A–B). Although clinical and histologic effects are much less impressive than those produced with the carbon dioxide laser, short-pulsed Er:YAG laser skin resurfacing still affords modest improvement of photodamaged skin with a shorter recovery time.[15,46]

To address the limitations of the short-pulsed Er:YAG laser, modulated Er:YAG lasers systems were developed to improve hemostasis and increase the amount of collagen shrinkage and remodeling effected. The Er:YAG-carbon dioxide hybrid laser system delivers both ablative Er:YAG and coagulative carbon dioxide laser pulses. The Er:YAG component generates fluences up to 28 J/cm^2 with a 350 μsec pulse duration, while excellent hemostasis is provided by the carbon dioxide component which can be

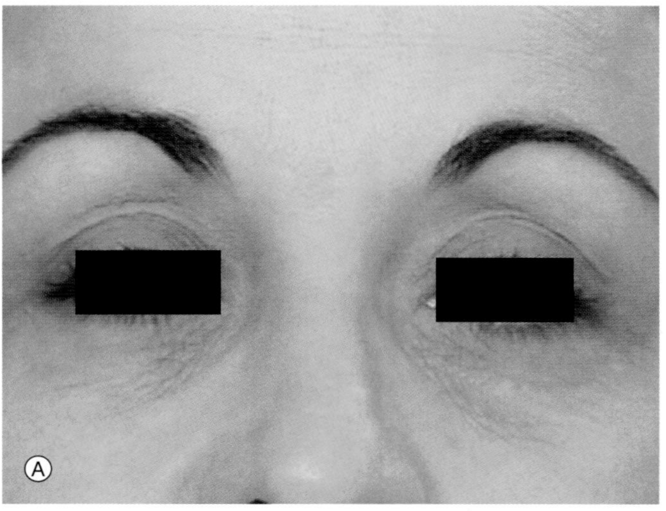

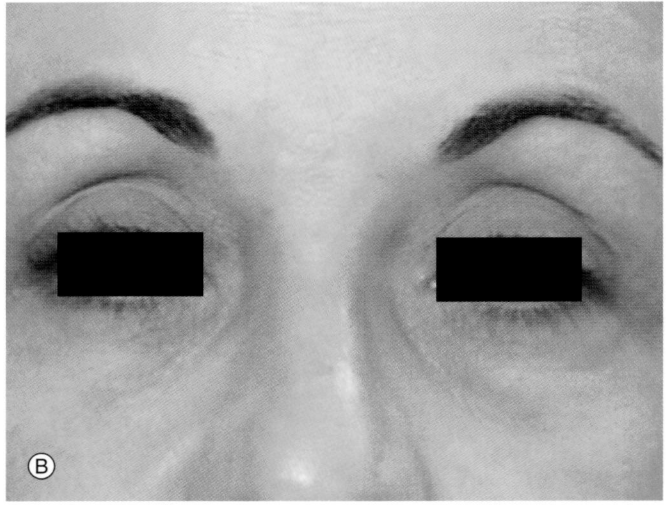

Figure 38.2 Periorbital rhytides and infraorbital hyperpigmentation (A) before and (B) several months after erbium laser skin resurfacing.

programmed to deliver 1–100 msec pulses at 1–10 W power. Zones of thermal necrosis measuring as much as 50 μm have been observed depending on the treatment parameters used and significant increase in collagen thickness has been noted 3 months after four passes with this hybrid technology.[51] Another modulated Er:YAG device is a dual-mode Er:YAG laser that emits a combination of short (200–300 μsec) pulses and long coagulative pulses to achieve tissue ablation depths of up to 200 μm per pass. The output from the two Er:YAG laser heads are combined into a single stream in a process called optical multiplexing.[52] The desired depth of ablation and coagulation can be programmed by the laser surgeon into the touch-screen control panel. Several investigators have studied the histologic effects of dual-mode Er:YAG laser resurfacing and found a close correlation between the programmed and actual measured depths of ablation.[53,54] The actual zones of thermal injury correlate well to the first pass with decreasing coagulative efficiency on subsequent passes. The variable-pulsed Er:YAG laser system delivers pulse durations ranging from 500 μsec to 10 msec. Shorter pulse durations are used for tissue ablation and longer pulses are used to effect coagulation and zones of thermal injury similar to the carbon dioxide laser.[52,55]

Since the modulated Er:YAG lasers were developed to produce a greater thermal effect and tissue contraction than their short-pulsed predecessors, investigators compared collagen tightening induced by the carbon dioxide laser with that of the carbon dioxide–Er:YAG hybrid laser system.[56] Intraoperative contraction of approximately 43% was produced after three passes of the carbon dioxide laser, compared with 12% contraction following Er:YAG irradiation. At 4 weeks, however, the carbon dioxide and Er:YAG laser treated sites were contracted to the same degree, highlighting the different mechanisms of tissue tightening observed after laser treatment. Immediate thermal-induced collagen tightening was the predominant response seen after carbon dioxide irradiation, whereas modulated Er:YAG laser resurfacing did not produce immediate intraoperative contraction but instead induced slow collagen tightening.[52,56]

■ OPTIMIZING OUTCOMES

Carbon dioxide laser skin resurfacing

Side effects associated with carbon dioxide laser skin resurfacing vary and are related to the expertise of the laser surgeon, the body area treated, and the skin phototype of the patient (Table 38.2). Certain tissue reactions, such as erythema and edema, are expected in the immediate postoperative period and are not considered adverse events. Erythema can be intense and may persist for several months after the procedure. The degree of erythema correlates directly with the depth of ablation and the number of laser passes performed.[3,57] It may also be aggravated by underlying rosacea or dermatitis. Postoperative erythema resolves spontaneously but can be reduced with the application of topical ascorbic acid which may serve to decrease the degree of inflammation.[58,59] Its use should be reserved for at least 4 weeks after the procedure in order to avoid irritation. Similarly, other topical agents such as retinoic acid derivatives, glycolic acid, fragrance-containing or chemical-containing cosmetics and sunscreens should be strictly avoided in the early postoperative period until substantial healing has occurred.[57]

Adequate preoperative patient evaluation and education are absolute essentials to avoid the pitfalls discussed below and optimize the clinical outcome.

Mild side effects of laser resurfacing include milia formation and acne exacerbation, which may be caused by the use of occlusive dressings and ointments used during the postoperative period, particularly in patients who are prone to acne.[22,24,57,60] Milia and acne usually resolve spontaneously as healing progresses and the application of thick emollient creams and occlusive dressings ceases. Oral antibiotics may be prescribed for acne flares that do not respond to topical preparations.[29,57,60] Contact allergies, irritant or allergic, can also develop from various topical medications, soaps, and moisturizers used postoperatively. Most of these reactions are irritant in nature due to decreased barrier function of the newly resurfaced skin.[57,61]

Wound infections associated with ablative laser resurfacing include *Staphylococcus*, *Pseudomonas*, or cutaneous candidiasis and should be treated aggressively with an appropriate systemic antibiotic or antifungal agent.[62] However, the use of prophylactic antibiotics remains controversial.[14] The most common infectious complication is a reactivation of labial herpes simplex virus (HSV), most likely caused by the thermal tissue injury and epidermal disruption produced by the laser.[22,57] Any patient undergoing full-face or perioral ablative resurfacing should receive antiviral prophylaxis, even if a history of HSV is denied. It is impossible to predict who will develop HSV reactivation, because a negative cold sore history is an unreliable method to determine risk, as many patients do not remember having had an outbreak or are asymptomatic HSV carriers. After carbon dioxide resurfacing, approximately 7% of patients develop a localized or disseminated form of HSV.[57] These infections develop within the first

Table 38.2 Side effects and complications of ablative laser skin resurfacing

Expected Side Effects	Complications		
	Mild	***Moderate***	***Severe***
Erythema Edema Pruritus	Extended erythema Milia Acne Contact dermatitis	Infection (bacterial, viral, fungal) Hyperpigmentation	Hypopigmentation Hypertrophic scarring Ectropion

postoperative week and can present as erosions without intact vesicles because of the denuded condition of newly lased skin. Even with appropriate prophylaxis, a herpetic outbreak still can occur in up to 10% of patients and must be treated aggressively.[15] Oral antiviral agents, such as acyclovir, famciclovir, and valacyclovir are effective agents against HSV infection, although severe (disseminated) cases may require intravenous therapy. Patients should begin prophylaxis by the day of surgery and continue for 7–10 days postoperatively.

The most severe complications associated with ablative cutaneous laser resurfacing include hypertrophic scar and ectropion formation.[22,57] Although the risk of scarring has been significantly reduced with the newer pulsed systems (compared to the continuous wave lasers), inadvertent pulse stacking or scan overlapping, as well as incomplete removal of desiccated tissue between laser passes can cause excessive thermal injury that could increase the development of fibrosis. Focal areas of bright erythema, with pruritus, particularly along the mandible, may signal impending scar formation.[24,63] Ultrapotent (class I) topical corticosteroid preparations should be applied to decrease the inflammatory response. A pulsed dye laser also can be used to improve the appearance and symptoms of laser-induced burn scars.[63]

Ectropion of the lower eyelid after periorbital laser skin resurfacing is rarely seen but, if encountered, usually requires surgical correction.[24] It is more likely to occur in patients who have had previous lower blepharoplasty or other surgical manipulation of the periorbital region. Preoperative examination is essential to determine eyelid laxity and skin elasticity. If the infraorbital skin does not return briskly to its normal resting position after a manual downward pull (snap test), then ablative laser resurfacing near the lower eyelid margin should be avoided. In general, lower fluences and fewer laser passes should be applied in the periorbital area to decrease the risk of lid eversion.

Hyperpigmentation is one of the more common side effects of cutaneous laser resurfacing and occurs to some degree in all patients with darker skin tones (Fig. 38.3).[24,57] The reaction is transient, but its resolution can be hastened with the postoperative use of a variety of topical agents, including hydroquinone, retinoic, azeleic, and glycolic acid. Regular sunscreen use is also important during the healing process to prevent further skin darkening. The prophylactic use of these products preoperatively, however, has not been shown to decrease the incidence of post-treatment hyperpigmentation.[13] Postoperative hypopigmentation is often not observed for several months and is particularly difficult because of its tendency to be intractable to treatment. The use of an excimer laser or topical photochemotherapy to stimulate repigmentation has proven successful in some patients.[64,65]

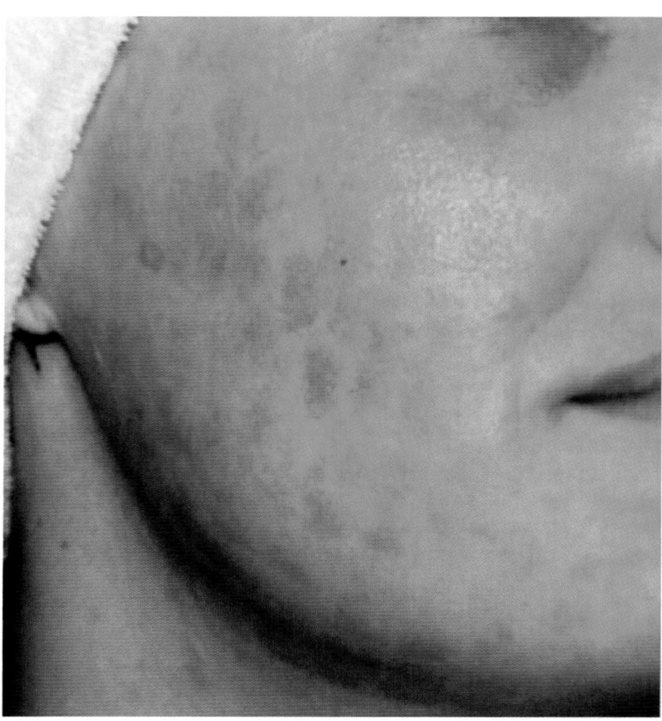

Figure 38.3 Post-treatment hyperpigmentation is often observed 3–4 weeks after carbon dioxide laser skin resurfacing. Its resolution can be hastened by the topical application of hydroquinone and/or glycolic, retinoic, and ascorbic acids.

Erbium:YAG laser skin resurfacing

Side effects and complications following Er:YAG laser resurfacing are similar to those observed after carbon dioxide laser skin resurfacing, although they differ in respect to duration, incidence, and severity.[49,66,67] Although greater postoperative erythema is seen after modulated Er:YAG laser treatment than is usually produced with a short-pulsed Er:YAG system, the side effect profile and recovery period after modulated Er:YAG laser skin resurfacing remain more favorable than after multiple-pass carbon dioxide laser treatment. In an extended evaluation of 50 patients, investigators reported complete re-epithelialization in an average of 5 days after dual-mode Er:YAG laser skin resurfacing with only three patients having prolonged erythema beyond 4 weeks.[67] In a split-face comparison of 16 patients after pulsed carbon dioxide and variable-pulsed Er:YAG laser skin resurfacing, other investigators reported decreased erythema, less edema, and faster healing on the Er:YAG laser-treated facial half.[68]

Postinflammatory hyperpigmentation is not uncommon after any cutaneous laser resurfacing procedure. While hyperpigmentation following modulated Er:YAG laser skin resurfacing (mean 10.4 weeks) can last longer than after treatment with a short-pulsed Er:YAG laser, it is not as persistent as that observed after multiple-pass carbon dioxide laser resurfacing (mean 16 weeks).[67] However, when comparing the most current trends in ablative cutaneous laser resurfacing—*single*-pass carbon dioxide versus multiple-pass, long-pulsed Er:YAG laser skin resurfacing—postoperative healing times and complication profiles are comparable, even in patients with darker skin phototypes. In a retrospective review and analysis of 100 consecutive patients, Tanzi and Alster[43] showed average time to re-epithelialization was 5.5 days with single-pass carbon dioxide and 5.1 days with long-pulsed Er:YAG laser resurfacing. Postoperative erythema was observed in all patients, lasting an average of 4.5 weeks after single-pass carbon dioxide laser treatment and 3.6 weeks after long-pulsed Er:YAG laser treatment. Hyperpigmentation was seen in 46% of patients treated with single-pass carbon dioxide and 42% of patients treated with the long-pulsed

Er:YAG laser (average duration 12.7 weeks and 11.4 weeks, respectively). Delayed-onset permanent hypopigmentation —a serious complication that has been observed several months after multiple-pass carbon dioxide laser skin resurfacing—has not yet been seen following single-pass treatment. To date, only three cases of hypopigmentation after modulated Er:YAG laser skin resurfacing have been reported.[69,70] Since it is possible for hypopigmentation to present several years postoperatively, clinical studies are ongoing to determine its true incidence following either single-pass carbon dioxide or modulated Er:YAG laser skin resurfacing.

■ POSTOPERATIVE CARE

Wound care during the immediate postoperative period is vital to the successful recovery of ablative laser-resurfaced skin. During the re-epithelialization process, an open- or closed-wound technique can be prescribed. Partial-thickness cutaneous wounds heal more efficiently and with a much reduced risk of scarring when maintained in a moist environment because the presence of a dry crust or scab impedes keratinocyte migration.[71] Although there is consensus on this principle by laser surgeons, disagreement exists regarding the optimal dressing for the laser-ablated wound. The 'open' technique involves frequent application of thick healing ointment to the de-epithelialized skin surface; whereas occlusive or semi-occlusive dressings are placed directly on the lased skin in the 'closed' technique. While the open technique facilitates easy wound visualization, the closed technique requires less patient involvement and may also decrease postoperative pain. Proposed advantages of closed dressings include increased patient comfort, decreased erythema and edema, increased rate of re-epithelialization, and decreased patient involvement in wound management.[71,72] On the other hand, additional expense and a higher risk of infection have been associated with the use of these dressings.[3,60,62]

In addition to the prescribed wound care, ice pack application and anti-inflammatory medications should be used during this time. Furthermore, pain medication is particularly important for ablative laser-resurfaced patients during the first few postoperative days.

■ PITFALLS AND THEIR MANAGEMENT

Proper patient selection

While a variety of epidermal and dermal signs of facial photodamage are amenable to laser skin resurfacing, suspicious growths should be biopsied for histologic examination prior to laser irradiation.

Has the patient ever had the areas treated before?

Ablative laser resurfacing may unmask hypopigmentation or fibrosis produce by prior dermabrasion, cryosurgery, or phenol peels. In addition, the presence of fibrosis may limit the vaporization potential of ablative lasers, thereby decreasing clinical efficacy. Patients who have had prior lower blepharoplasties (using an external approach) are at greater risk of ectropion formation after infraorbital ablative skin resurfacing.

What is the patient's skin phototype?

Pale skin tones have a lower incidence of undesirable postoperative hyperpigmentation compared to patients with dark skin tones after ablative laser skin resurfacing.

Does the patient have a history of herpes labialis?

Reactivation and/or dissemination of prior herpes simplex infection can occur with laser resurfacing. The de-epithelialized skin is also particularly susceptible to primary inoculation by herpes simplex virus, therefore all patients should be treated with prophylactic antiviral medication prior to ablative laser skin resurfacing.

Does the patient have an autoimmune disease or other immunologic deficiency?

Because the postoperative course associated with ablative skin resurfacing is prolonged, intact immunologic function and collagen repair mechanisms are necessary to optimize the tissue-healing response. In addition to possible delayed wound healing, patients with scleroderma, lupus erythematosus, and vitiligo may also exhibit worsening of their conditions after ablative skin resurfacing.

Are there other dermatologic conditions present which could potentially spread after treatment?

Psoriasis, verrucae, and molluscum contagiosum are but a few conditions that could conceivably undergo Koebnerization after ablative laser skin resurfacing. Thus, the skin should be carefully inspected to rule out the presence of these and other inflammatory or infectious cutaneous lesions so that the final clinical result is optimized.

Is the patient taking any medications that are contraindicated?

Concomitant isotretinoin use could potentially lead to an increased risk of postoperative hypertrophic scar formation due to its detrimental effect on wound healing and collagenesis. Because the alteration in healing is idiosyncratic, a safe interval between the use of oral retinoids and ablative laser skin resurfacing is difficult to calculate; however, most practitioners delay the treatment for at least 6–12 months after cessation of the drug.

Does the patient have a tendency to form hypertrophic scars or keloids?

Patients with a propensity to scar will be at greater risk of scar formation after laser resurfacing, independent of the laser's selectivity and the operator's expertise.

Is the patient prone to acne breakouts?

Complete control of acne eruptions should be obtained prior to ablative laser skin resurfacing with appropriate topical or systemic antibiotics. Occlusive ointments used in the immediate postoperative period may induce acne and complicate the postoperative course.

Does the patient have realistic expectations of the procedure and will he/she be compliant with postoperative instructions?

Patients who believe that every rhytide will be removed with the ablative laser resurfacing procedure are not good treatment candidates. Furthermore, those who can not physically or emotionally handle the prolonged postoperative course should also be dissuaded from pursuing ablative laser skin resurfacing procedures.

■ SUMMARY

Ablative laser skin resurfacing has revolutionized the approach to photodamaged facial skin. Technology and techniques continue to evolve, further enhancing the ability to achieve substantial clinical improvement of rhytides and dyspigmentation with reduced postoperative morbidity. Utilizing proper technique and treatment parameters, excellent clinical results can be obtained with any one or combination of carbon dioxide and Er:YAG laser systems available. Therefore, the best choice of laser ultimately depends on the operator's expertise, clinical indication, and individual patient characteristics. Regardless of the type of ablative resurfacing laser used, the importance of careful postoperative follow-up cannot be overemphasized.

■ NON-ABLATIVE LASER SKIN REMODELING

Preoperative preparation

Proper patient selection is critical to the success of non-ablative laser skin remodeling. Patients with mild-to-moderate facial photodamage with realistic expectations of treatment are the best candidates for non-ablative procedures. Patients seeking immediate improvement in photodamaged skin or those who desire a dramatic result may be less than satisfied with the overall clinical outcome.

For patients with a strong history of herpes labialis, prophylactic oral antiviral medications should be considered when treating the perioral skin. Reactivation of prior herpes simplex infection can occur after non-ablative laser skin remodeling due to the intense heat produced by the laser or light source.

Prior to non-ablative laser procedures, sun exposure should be avoided, particularly when using shorter-wavelength systems such as the pulsed dye laser or intense pulsed-light source. Unwanted absorption of irradiation by activated epidermal melanocytes can increase the risk of side effects, including crusting, blistering, and dyspigmentation.

■ TECHNICAL ASPECTS

Many of the non-ablative laser systems currently in use emit light within the infrared portion of the electromagnetic spectrum (1000–1500 nm). At these wavelengths, absorption by superficial water-containing tissue is relatively weak, thereby effecting deeper tissue penetration.[73] Since non-ablative remodeling involves creation of a dermal wound without epidermal injury, all of these laser systems employ unique methods to ensure epidermal preservation during treatment. These methods typically include contact cooling hand-pieces or dynamic cryogen devices capable of delivering variable duration spray spurts either before, during, and/or after laser irradiation. Since laser beam penetration and dermal wounding must be targeted to the relatively superficial portion of the dermis, contact cooling devices that theoretically lead to excessive dermal cooling may affect the level or degree of energy deposition in the skin. As such, there remains no general consensus concerning which method of cooling is most efficacious during treatment.

In general, treatment of facial photodamage with non-ablative technology does not produce results comparable to those of ablative carbon dioxide and Er:YAG lasers; however, many patients are willing to accept modest clinical improvement in exchange for fewer associated risks and shorter recovery times.

Pulsed dye laser

Clinical studies have demonstrated the ability of 585 nm and 595 nm pulsed dye laser (PDL) to reduce mild facial rhytides with few side effects.[74] The most common side effects of PDL treatment include mild edema, purpura, and transient postinflammatory hyperpigmentation. Although increased extracellular matrix proteins and types I and III collagen and procollagen have been detected following PDL treatment, the exact mechanism whereby wrinkle improvement is effected remains unknown.[75] One theory states that vascular endothelial cells damaged by the yellow laser light release mediators that stimulate fibroblasts to produce new collagen fibers.[76]

Intense pulsed light source

Several investigators have shown successful rejuvenation of photodamaged skin after intense pulsed light (IPL) treatment.[77,78] The IPL source emits a broad, continuous spectrum of light in the range of 515 nm to 1200 nm. Cut-off filters are used to eliminate shorter wavelengths depending on the clinical application, with shorter filters favoring heating of melanin and hemoglobin. Bitter[78] showed improvement in wrinkling, skin coarseness, irregular pigmentation, pore size, and telangiectasia in the majority of 49 patients treated with a series of IPL treatments (fluences 30–50 J/cm^2). In a retrospective review of 80 patients with skin phototypes I-IV, Weiss and colleagues[79] reported signs of photoaging, including telangiectasias and mottled pigmentation of the face, neck, and chest, improved by a series of IPL treatments. While substantial clinical improvement of dyspigmentation and telangiectasia associated with cutaneous photodamage is often seen, neocollagenesis and dermal collagen remodeling with subsequent improvement in rhytides following IPL treatment has been more modest. The effect on dermal collagen is thought to be induced by heat diffusion from the vasculature with subsequent release of inflammatory mediators stimulated by vessel heating.[80]

1064 nm Q-switched Neodymium:YAG Laser

The 1064 nm quality(Q)-switched (QS) neodymium:YAG laser was the first mid-infrared laser system used for non-ablative remodeling. Although absorption of energy by tissue water is relatively weak at the 1064 nm wavelength, it was possible to achieve dermal penetrative depths that could potentially induce neocollagenesis. The nanosecond range pulse duration of the QS Nd:YAG laser was also determined to limit significant thermal diffusion to surrounding structures, thereby making it suitable for non-ablative rejuvenation.

In 1997, Goldberg and Whitworth[81] published their experience using a 1064 nm Nd:YAG laser for facial rhytide reduction. Eleven patients (skin phototypes I, II) with mild to moderate periorbital or perioral rhytides underwent treatment on one side of the face with a QS Nd:YAG laser at a fluence of 5.5 J/cm^2 (3 mm spot size) and carbon dioxide laser ablation on the contralateral side for comparison purposes. Pinpoint bleeding was used as the clinical endpoint of treatment on the QS Nd:YAG laser-treated facial half. Not unexpectedly, all of the carbon dioxide-laser irradiated sites demonstrated significant rhytide improvement at the end of the study. On the QS Nd:YAG laser-treated side, however, only three patients demonstrated improvement. These three patients had also developed prolonged post-treatment erythema (lasting up to one month)—suggesting that the amount of dermal wounding (with subsequent collagen remodeling) was directly related to the degree of cutaneous injury. Another study using the QS Nd:YAG laser for rhytide reduction in 61 patients (242 sites) was conducted using a topical carbon solution for improved optical penetration of the 1064 nm light.[82] Patients underwent a series of three monthly treatment sessions with a QS Nd:YAG laser at a fluence of 2.5 J/cm2, 7 mm spot size, and pulse duration 6–20 ns. At least slight improvement was seen in 97% of class I rhytides and 86% of the class II rhytides. Side effects of treatment were mild and limited, including transient erythema, purpura, and postinflammatory hyperpigmentation.

A long-pulsed Nd:YAG laser has also been used for photorejuvenation. Lee[83] evaluated a combination technique using a long-pulsed 1064 Nd:YAG laser and long-pulsed 532 nm potassium-titanyl-phosphate (KTP) laser, both separately and combined, for non-invasive photo-rejuvenation in 150 patients, skin phototypes I through V. Patients treated with the combined laser approach showed at least 70% improvement in erythema and pigmentation and 30–40% improvement in fine rhytides. In the patient groups treated with monotherapy, patient satisfaction was greater with KTP laser treatment than with long-pulsed Nd:YAG laser treatment primarily due to a reduction in dyspigmentation and telangiectasias.

1320 nm Nd:YAG laser

A 1320 nm Nd:YAG laser was the first commercially available system marketed solely for the purpose of non-ablative laser skin remodeling. The 1320 nm wavelength is associated with a high scattering coefficient that allows for dispersion of laser irradiation throughout the dermis. The latest model is capable of delivering energy densities up to 24 J/cm^2 with a pulse duration of 350 μs through a 10-mm spot size hand-piece. The 1320 nm Nd:YAG laser hand-piece contains three portals: the laser beam itself, a thermal feedback sensor that registers skin surface temperature, and a dynamic cryogen spray apparatus used for epidermal cooling. When skin surface temperatures are maintained at 40–45 °C dermal temperatures reach 60–65 °C during laser irradiation, thereby effecting collagen contraction and neocollagenesis. In order to prevent unwanted sequelae (e.g. blistering) from excessive heat production, it is imperative that epidermal temperatures be kept lower than 50 °C. A series of three or more treatment sessions are scheduled at regular intervals (typically once a month) for maximum mitigation of fine rhytides.[73] Side effects of treatment are generally mild and include transient erythema and edema.

Menaker et al.[84] reported effective rhytide reduction in an early study using a prototype 1320 nm Nd:YAG laser. Ten patients with periocular rhytides received three consecutive laser treatments at bi-weekly intervals. Three 300 μs pulses were delivered at 100 Hz and fluence of 32 J/cm^2 with a 5-mm spot size hand-piece. Epidermal protection was achieved with application of a 20 ms cooling spray after a 10 ms preset delay. Patients were evaluated at 1 and 3 months after treatment. Although four of the ten patients showed clinical improvement in rhytide severity by end-study, these findings were not statistically significant. Similarly, the slight homogenization of collagen noted on histology at 1 and 3 months following treatment was not statistically significant and inconsistent with the clinical findings.

In another study, Kelly et al.[85] treated 35 patients with mild, moderate, and severe rhytides using a 1320 nm Nd:YAG laser. Three treatments were delivered at 2-week intervals using fluences ranging 28–36 J/cm^2 with a 5 mm spot size. Cryogen spray cooling was applied in 20–40 ms spurts with 10 ms delays. Patients were evaluated at 12 and 24 weeks following treatment with statistically significant improvement noted in all clinical grades after 12 weeks. Only the most severe rhytides; however, showed persistent improvement 24 weeks following treatment.

Goldberg devised two similar studies to examine the effectiveness of the 1320 nm Nd:YAG laser for the treatment of facial rhytides. In the first study, ten patients with skin types I–II and class I–II rhytides in the periorbital, perioral, and cheek areas were treated.[86] Four treatments were administered over a 16-week period using fluences of 28–38 J/cm^2 with a 30% overlap and a 5 mm spot size. One or two laser passes were applied to achieve the treatment endpoint of mild erythema. Skin surface temperatures were limited to 40–48 °C using the aforementioned dynamic cooling spray in order to provide epidermal protection, whilst effecting dermal temperatures ranging 60–70 °C. Six months following treatment, two patients showed no clinical improvement, six showed 'some' improvement, and two showed 'substantial' improvement. This study emphasized several key points in non-ablative laser resurfacing. It suggested a thermal feedback sensor is best used intraoperatively with this technology in order for appropriate treatment fluences to be selected based upon the individual patient's cutaneous temperature, thereby maximizing dermal temperatures that effectively lead to collagen reformation. Furthermore, longer follow-up periods are usually required to fully appreciate the effect of serial treatment sessions on dermal collagen stimulation. In the second study, ten patients underwent full-face treatments with the 1320 nm Nd:YAG laser at 3–4-week intervals.[87] As with the first study, treatment results were inconsistent—four patients showed no improvement, four showed some improvement, and two showed substantial improvement in facial rhytides and overall skin tone.

Others also studied the 1320 nm Nd:YAG laser for treatment of facial rhytides in ten women.[88] Full-face treatment was administered to three patients, whereas two patients had periorbital treatment, and five patients received perioral treatment. Laser fluences of 30–35 J/cm^2 were delivered in triple 300 μs pulses at a repetition rate of 100 Hz. Dynamic cryogen spray cooling was used with a 30 ms spurt and a 40 ms delay between cryogen spurt and laser irradiation. A thermal sensor was also used to maintain peak surface temperatures in the range of 42–45 °C in order to avoid excessive tissue heating. Treatments were administered twice a week over a period of 4 weeks, for a total of eight treatment sessions. Only two out of ten patients expressed satisfaction with their final result despite clinician evaluations showing significant improvement in five of ten patients and fair improvements in another three. Moreover, there was no correlation between histologic changes and the degree of subjective clinical improvement as judged by the patients.

A more recent study by Fatemi et al.[89] demonstrated that the 1320 nm Nd:YAG laser produced mild subclinical epidermal injury that could potentially lead to enhanced skin texture and new papillary collagen synthesis by stimulation of cytokines and other inflammatory mediators. Thus, the long-term histologic improvement seen in photodamaged skin may not be based solely on direct laser heating of collagen, but by further stimulation of cytokine release by heating the superficial vasculature. In addition, the histologic findings suggested that multiple passes with fluence and cooling adjusted to a T_{max} of 45–48 °C can yield improved clinical results, as compared to those specimens in which epidermal temperatures above 45 °C were not achieved.

1450 nm diode

The 1450 nm mid-infrared wavelength diode laser targets dermal water and penetrates the skin to an approximate depth of 500 μm. This low-power laser system achieves peak powers in the 10–15 W range with relatively long pulse durations of 150–250 ms. Because of these long exposure times, epidermal cooling must be delivered in sequence during the application of laser energy in order to avoid excessive thermal build-up within the superficial layers of the skin.

Goldberg et al.[90] reported on the effects of 1450 nm diode laser irradiation in 20 patients with class I-II rhytides. Two to four treatment sessions were delivered with 6 months follow-up evaluation. Patients were treated with laser and cryogen spray cooling on one facial half and cryogen spray cooling alone on the contralateral side. On the laser-treated facial halves, seven did not demonstrate any improvement, ten showed mild improvement, and three had moderate improvement. None of the sites treated with cryogen alone showed any improvement after 6 months. Side effects of treatment were mild and included transient erythema, edematous papules, and one case of postinflammatory hyperpigmentation persisting for 6 months. The authors concluded that the 1450 nm diode laser was effective for treatment of mild to moderately severe facial rhytides with minimal morbidity. Additionally, their study demonstrated that non-ablative laser treatment alone was responsible for the clinical improvements and that the non-specific injury induced by cryogen spray cooling could not effect the changes seen.

Hardaway and colleagues[91] demonstrated statistically significant mean wrinkle improvement of 2.3 (range 0–4, with 4 representing severe wrinkling) at baseline to 1.8 at 6 months following a series of three 1450 nm diode laser treatments. They concluded that although the 1450 nm diode laser is capable of targeting dermal collagen and stimulating fibrosis, clinical improvement of rhytides was mild and did not correlate well with the degree of histologic change noted in previous studies.

In a controlled clinical and histologic study, Tanzi and Alster[92] demonstrated improvement in mild to moderate perioral or periorbital rhytides in 25 patients treated with four consecutive 1450 nm diode laser treatments. Peak clinical improvement was seen 6 months after the series of laser treatments. The periorbital area was more responsive to laser treatment than the perioral area—a finding consistent with results obtained using other non-ablative laser systems (Fig. 38.4A–B).[92] Side effects were limited to transient erythema, edema, and postinflammatory hyper-

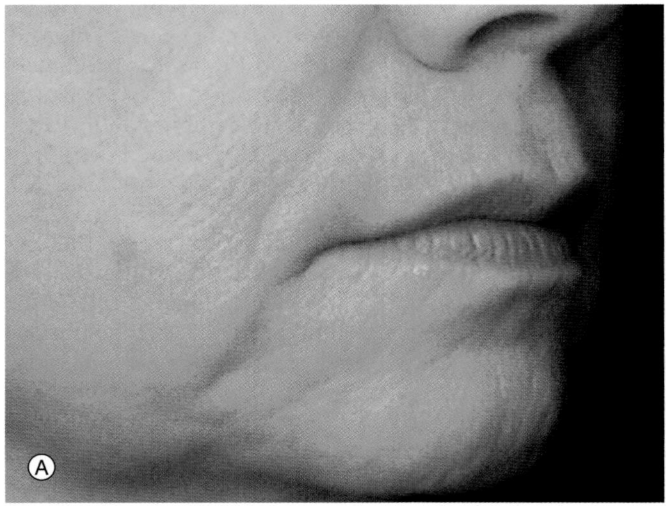

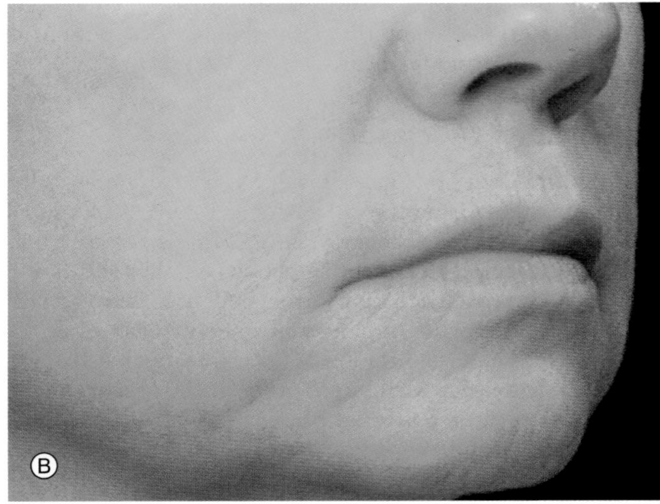

Figure 38.4 Facial rhytides (A) before and (B) 6 months after a series of 3-monthly 1450 nm long-pulsed diode laser treatments

pigmentation. In a separate controlled study performed by the same group, 20 patients with transverse neck lines received three consecutive monthly treatments using a long-pulsed 1450 nm diode laser.[93] Modest improvements in appearance and texture of the transverse neck lines was reported, as measured by blinded clinical assessments and through three-dimensional *in vivo* microtopography (PRIMOS Imaging System; GFM, Germany). Mean fluences of 11.6 J/cm^2 were used with a 6 mm spot size and 50 msec total cryogen.

1540 nm Erbium:glass laser

The 1540 nm erbium-doped phosphate glass laser is another mid-infrared range laser that has also been used for amelioration of fine facial rhytides and atrophic facial scars. Similar to other infrared laser systems, the erbium:glass laser targets intracellular water and penetrates tissue to a depth of 0.4–2 mm.[73] The 1540 nm wavelength has the least amount of melanin absorption compared with the 1320 nm and 1450 nm laser systems—a potential advantage of this system when treating tanned or darker-skinned patients. Mordon et al.[94] studied the 1540 nm erbium:glass laser on hairless rat abdominal skin with pulse train irradiation (1.1 J, 3 Hz, 30 pulses) and varying cooling temperatures (+5 °C, 0 °C, –5 °C). Biopsies were obtained after 1, 3, and 7 days following treatment, and demonstrated fibroblast proliferation and new collagen synthesis as early as the third day. The authors concluded that this laser system held promise for treating facial rhytides because of its high water absorption and reduced scattering effect allowing light energy deposition to remain in the upper dermis where most solar elastosis is evident.

Ross et al.[95] used the 1540 nm erbium:glass laser with a sapphire cooling hand-piece to treat the preauricular skin of nine patients. A 5 mm collimated beam was used to deliver fluences of 400–1200 mJ/cm^2. Epidermal necrosis and scar formation were noted at the highest pulse energies. Several key points were illustrated by this study; namely, that denatured collagen located deep in the dermis (more than 600 μm) is associated with granuloma formation, and that the peaks of heating and cooling with non-ablative laser remodeling are in proximity, by necessity, since maximum wrinkle reduction may be achieved by a zone of thermal injury 100–400 μm beneath the skin surface.

Lupton et al.[96] reported their use of a 1540 nm erbium:glass laser to treat 24 patients with fine periorbital and perioral rhytides. Patients underwent a series of three treatments on a monthly basis using a 4 mm spot size, 10 J/cm^2 fluence, and 3.5 ms pulse duration. Epidermal protection was achieved with concomitant application of a contact sapphire lens cooled to 5 °C. Histologic specimens demonstrated increased dermal fibroplasia at 6 months following the series of laser treatments. Average clinical scores were improved at 1 and 6 months following the third treatment session with slightly better results observed in the periorbital regions. Side effects of treatment were mild and included transient erythema and edema.

More recently, Fournier and colleagues[97] treated 42 patients (skin phototypes I–IV) with five consecutive 1540 nm diode laser treatments at 6-week intervals. Patients were evaluated using clinical data, patient satisfaction surveys, digital photography, ultrasound imaging, and profilometry data from silicone imprints. The majority of patients demonstrated modest improvement in objective and subjective measurements which remained stable throughout the 14-month evaluation period.

Non-ablative radiofrequency

A novel radiofrequency device (ThermaCool TC; Thermage Inc, Hayward, CA) has also been studied for deep dermal heating with subsequent tightening of photodamaged skin. Unlike a laser in which light energy is converted into heat, the radiofrequency device generates electric current which produces heat through resistance in the dermis. The energy is delivered to the patient through a sophisticated hand-piece and treatment tip with a coupling membrane, which allows for uniform delivery of heat over the entire treatment area. Epidermal protection is provided by simultaneous cryogen cooling within the contact treatment tip. Using this technique, a reverse thermal gradient is generated. The depth of heat penetration is dependent upon the size and specifics of the detachable treatment tip and can be changed according to the clinical application. Preliminary animal studies demonstrated selective dermal heating at the levels of the papillary dermis and as deep as the subcutaneous fat could be achieved.[80] Ruiz-Esparza and Gomez[98] reported facial tissue tightening in 14 of 15 patients 3 months after a single radiofrequency treatment with minimal side effects. Ongoing research trials are currently taking place at several centers to determine the most appropriate clinical indications and best treatment parameters for this innovative radiofrequency technology.[99]

■ OPTIMIZING OUTCOMES

Rarely, postoperative hyperpigmentation can develop several weeks after non-ablative skin remodeling and is more likely to be experienced by patients with darker skin tones. In some cases, investigators demonstrated an association of post-treatment hyperpigmentation with excess intraoperative epidermal cryogen cooling.[92] Although always transient, topical bleaching agents and light glycolic acid peels can hasten the resolution of postinflammatory hyperpigmentation.

In the weeks following a series of non-ablative laser procedures, follow-up visits can help identify patient concerns and increase the overall satisfaction with treatment. Clinical improvements after a series of non-ablative laser procedures may take weeks to realize, thus reassurance by the laser surgeon regarding the patient's progress can be particularly important.

■ POSTOPERATIVE CARE

Since the epidermis remains intact following non-ablative laser skin remodeling, postoperative care is minimal. Some patients experience mild erythema and edema lasting less than 24 hours.

■ PITFALLS AND THEIR MANAGEMENT

Is the amount of photodamage amenable to non-ablative laser skin remodeling?

Patients with mild-to-moderate facial photodamage are the best candidates for non-ablative procedures. Patients with severe rhytides and skin laxity may be disappointed with the overall clinical outcome.

Does the patient have a history of herpes labialis?

Reactivation of prior herpes simplex infection can occur with perioral non-ablative laser skin remodeling due to the intense heat produced by the laser. Patients with a strong history of herpes simplex labialis may require prophylactic oral antiviral medication to avoid an outbreak.

What is the patient's skin phototype?

Although the majority of current non-ablative systems used are within the mid-infrared range of the electromagnetic spectrum and not avidly absorbed by epidermal melanin, patients with darker skin phototypes may develop postinflammatory hyperpigmentation after non-ablative laser treatment. This temporary reaction most likely develops following inflammation created by concomitant cryogen-spray epidermal cooling.

Does the patient have realistic expectations of non-ablative laser skin remodeling?

Patients seeking immediate improvement after a single non-ablative treatment are not good candidates as clinical improvement occurs after multiple sequential treatment sessions (usually three to five) and is often delayed 3–6 months after the final non-ablative laser procedure. Moreover, patients seeking dramatic results following non-ablative laser skin techniques should be dissuaded from treatment as clinical improvement may be subtle.

■ SUMMARY

For those patients who desire a less aggressive approach to photorejuvenation than ablative laser skin resurfacing, non-ablative dermal remodeling represents a viable alternative for patients willing to accept modest clinical improvement in exchange for ease of treatment and a favorable side-effect profile. Treatments are typically delivered at monthly intervals with final clinical results taking several months after laser irradiation to be realized. Although clinical outcomes with these non-ablative systems are not yet comparable with those of ablative carbon dioxide or Er:YAG lasers, they do improve overall skin texture, tone and elasticity—subjective findings often difficult to represent in photographs. None of the non-ablative laser systems has yet emerged as being clearly superior—each produces similar degrees of improvement in dermal pathology after multiple sessions at standard treatment parameters. With continued research efforts focused on non-ablative laser skin remodeling, it is possible that further refinements and advances in this technology will more closely approximate the effects of ablative laser treatment without its associated complications and risks.

■ REFERENCES

1. Taylor CR, Stern RS, Leyden JJ, Gilchrest BA. Photoaging/photodamage and photoprotection. J Am Acad Dermatol 1990; 22:1–15.
2. Lavker RM. Cutaneous aging: chronological versus photoaging. In Gilchrest BA, ed. Photodamage. Cambridge, MA: Blackwell Science 1995; 123–135.
3. Alster TS. Cutaneous resurfacing with CO_2 and erbium:YAG lasers: preoperative, intraoperative, and postoperative consideration. Plast Reconstr Surg 1999; 103:619–632.
4. Anderson RR, Parrish JA. Selective photothermolysis: precise microsurgery by selective absorption of pulsed radiation. Science 1983; 22:524–527.
5. Shapshay SM, Strong MS, Anastasi GW, Vaughan CW. Removal of rhinophyma with the CO_2 laser. A preliminary report. Arch Otolaryngol 1980; 106:257–259.
6. Dufresne RG, Garrett AB, Bailin PL, et al. CO_2 laser treatment of chronic actinic cheilitis. J Am Acad Dermatol 1988; 19:876–878.
7. Alster TS, Kauvar ANB, Geronemus RG. Histology of high-energy pulsed CO_2 laser resurfacing. Semin Cutan Med Surg 1996; 15:189–193.
8. Tanzi EL, Lupton JR, Alster TS. Review of lasers in dermatology: four decades of progress. J Am Acad Dermatol 2003; 49:1–31.
9. Lanzafame RJ, Naim JO, Rogers DW, Hinshaw JR. Comparisons of continuous-wave, chop wave, and superpulsed laser wounds. Lasers Surg Med 1988; 8:119–124.
10. Alster TS, Garg S. Treatment of facial rhytides with a high-energy pulsed CO_2 laser. Plast Reconstr Surg 1996; 98:791–794.
11. Alster TS: Preoperative preparation for CO_2 laser resurfacing. In Coleman WP, Lawrence N, eds. Skin resurfacing. Baltimore: Williams & Wilkins; 1998:171–179.
12. Hevia O, Nemeth AJ, Taylor JR. Tretinoin accelerates healing after trichloroacetic acid chemical peel. Arch Dermatol 1991; 127:678–682.
13. West TB, Alster TS. Effect of pretreatment on the incidence of hyperpigmentation following cutaneous CO_2 laser resurfacing. Dermatol Surg 1999; 25:15–17.
14. Walia S, Alster TS. Cutaneous CO_2 laser resurfacing infection rate with and without prophylactic antibiotics. Dermatol Surg 1999; 25:857–861.
15. Alster TS, Lupton JR. An overview of cutaneous laser resurfacing. Clin Plast Surg 2001; 28:37–52.
16. Alster TS, Nanni CA, Williams CM. Comparison of four CO_2 resurfacing lasers: a clinical and histopathologic evaluation. Dermatol Surg 1999; 25:153–159.
17. Walsh JT, Deutsch TF. Pulsed CO_2 laser tissue ablation: measurement of the ablation rate. Lasers Surg Med 1988; 8:264–275.
18. Fitzpatrick RE, Ruiz-Esparza J, Goldman MP. The depth of thermal necrosis using the CO_2 laser: a comparison of the superpulsed mode and conventional mode. J Dermatol Surg Oncol 1991; 17:340–344.
19. Stuzin JM, Baker TJ, Baker TM, et al. Histologic effects of the high-energy pulsed CO_2 laser on photo-aged facial skin. Plast Reconstr Surg 1997; 99:2036–2050.
20. Walsh JT, Flotte TJ, Anderson RR, et al. Pulsed CO_2 laser tissue ablation: effect of tissue type and pulse duration on thermal damage. Lasers Surg Med 1988; 8:108–118.
21. Rubach BW, Schoenrock LD. Histological and clinical evaluation of facial resurfacing using a CO_2 laser with the computer pattern generator. Arch Otolaryngol Head Neck Surg 1997; 123:929–934.
22. Bernstein LJ, Kauvar ANB, Grossman MC, et al. The short- and long-term side effects of CO_2 laser resurfacing. Dermatol Surg 1997; 23:519–525.
23. Fitzpatrick RE, Smith SR, Sriprachya-anunt S. Depth of vaporization and the effect of pulse stacking with a high-energy, pulsed CO_2 laser. J Am Acad Dermatol 1999; 40:615–622.
24. Alster TS, Lupton JR. Prevention and treatment of side effects and complications of cutaneous laser resurfacing. Plast Reconst Surg 2002; 109:308–316.
25. Lowe NJ, Lask G, Griffin ME, et al. Skin resurfacing with the ultrapulse CO_2 laser: observations on 100 patients. Dermatol Surg 1995; 21:1025–1029.
26. Alster TS. Comparison of two high-energy, pulsed CO_2 lasers in the treatment of periorbital rhytides. Dermatol Surg 1996; 22:541–545.
27. Apfelberg DB. Ultrapulse CO_2 laser with CPG scanner for full-face resurfacing of rhytides, photoaging, and acne scars. Plast Reconstr Surg 1997; 99:1817–1825.
28. Lask G, Keller G, Lowe NJ, et al. Laser skin resurfacing with the SilkTouch flashscanner for facial rhytides. Dermatol Surg 1995; 21:1021–1024.
29. Waldorf HA, Kauvar ANB, Geronemus RG. Skin resurfacing of fine to deep rhytides using a char-free CO_2 laser in 47 patients. Dermatol Surg 1995; 21:940–946.

30. Ratner D, Viron A, Puvion-Dutilleul F, et al. Pilot ultrastructural evaluation of human preauricular skin before and after high-energy pulsed CO_2 laser treatment. Arch Dermatol 1998; 134:582–587.
31. Ratner D, Tse Y, Marchell N, et al. Cutaneous laser resurfacing. J Am Acad Dermatol 1999; 41:365–389.
32. Fulton JE, Barnes T. Collagen shrinkage (selective dermoplasty) with the high-energy pulsed carbon dioxide laser. Dermatol Surg 1998; 24:37–41.
33. Ross E, Naseef G, Skrobal M, et al. In vivo dermal collagen shrinkage and remodeling following CO_2 laser resurfacing. Lasers Surg Med 1996; 18:38.
34. Flor PJ, Spurr OK. Melting equilibrium for collagen fibers under stress: elasticity in the amorphous state. J Amer Chem Soc 1960; 83:1308.
35. Flor PJ, Weaver ES. Helix coil transition in dilute aqueous collagen solutions. J Am Chem Soc 1989; 82:4518.
36. Alster TS. Commentary on: Increased smooth muscle actin, factor XIII a, and vimentin-positive cells in the papillary dermis of CO_2 laser-debrided porcine skin. Dermatol Surg 1998; 24:155.
37. West TB, Alster TS. Effect of botulinum toxin type A on movement-associated rhytides following carbon dioxide laser resurfacing. Dermatol Surg 1999; 25:259–261.
38. Katz BE, MacFarlane DF. Atypical facial scarring after isotretinoin therapy in a patient with a previous dermabrasion. J Am Acad Dermatol 1994; 30:852–853.
39. Roegnik HH, Pinski JB, Robinson K, et al. Acne, retinoids, and dermabrasion. J Dermatol Surg Oncol 1985; 11:396–398.
40. David L, Ruiz-Esparza J. Fast healing after laser skin resurfacing: the minimal mechanical trauma technique. Dermatol Surg 1997; 23:359–361.
41. Ruiz-Esparza J, Gomez JMB. Long-term effects of one general pass laser resurfacing: a look at dermal tightening and skin quality. Dermatol Surg 1999; 25:169–174.
42. Alster TS, Hirsch RJ. Single-pass CO_2 laser skin resurfacing of light and dark skin: extended experience with 52 patients. J Cosmet Laser Ther 2003; 5:39–42
43. Tanzi EL, Alster TS. Single-pass CO_2 versus multiple-pass Er:YAG laser skin resurfacing: a comparison of postoperative wound healing and side-effect rates. Dermatol Surg 2003; 29:80–84.
44. Walsh JT, Flotte TJ, Deutsch TF. Er:YAG laser ablation of tissue: effect of pulse duration and tissue type on thermal damage. Lasers Surg Med 1989; 9:327–337.
45. Ross EV, Anderson RR. The erbium laser in skin resurfacing. In Alster TS, Apfelberg DB, eds. Cosmetic laser surgery, 2nd edn. New York: John Wiley; 1999:57–84.
46. Alster TS. Clinical and histologic evaluation of six erbium:YAG lasers for cutaneous resurfacing. Lasers Surg Med 1999; 24:87–92.
47. Hibst R, Kaufmann R. Effects of laser parameters on pulsed Er:YAG laser ablation. Lasers Med Science 1991; 6:391–397.
48. Hohenleutner U, Hohenleutner S, Baumler W, et al. Fast and effective skin ablation with an Er:YAG laser: determination of ablation rates and thermal damage zones. Lasers Surg Med 1997; 20:242–247.
49. Alster TS, Lupton JR. Erbium:YAG cutaneous laser resurfacing. Dermatol Clin 2001; 19:453–466.
50. Khatri KA, Ross EV, Grevelink JM, et al. Comparison of erbium:YAG and carbon dioxide lasers in resurfacing of facial rhytides. Arch Dermatol 1999; 135:391–397.
51. Goldman MP, Marchell N, Fitzpatrick RE. Laser skin resurfacing of the face with a combined CO_2/Er:YAG laser. Dermatol Surg 2000; 26:102–104.
52. Sapijaszko MJA, Zachary CB. Er:YAG laser skin resurfacing. Dermatol Clin 2002; 20:87–96.
53. Pozner JM, Goldberg DJ. Histologic effect of a variable pulsed Er:YAG laser. Dermatol Surg 2000; 26:733–736.
54. Ross EV, McKinlay JR, Sajben FP, et al. Use of a novel erbium laser in a Yucatan minipig: a study of residual thermal damage (RTD), ablation, and wound healing as a function of pulse duration. Lasers Surg Med 1999; 15:17.
55. Newman JB, Lord JL, Ash K, et al. Variable pulse erbium:YAG laser skin resurfacing of perioral rhytides and side-by-side comparison with carbon dioxide laser. Lasers Surg Med 1998; 24:1303–1307.
56. Fitzpatrick RE, Rostan EF, Marchell N. Collagen tightening induced by carbon dioxide laser versus erbium:YAG laser. Lasers Surg Med 2000; 27:395–403.
57. Nanni CA, Alster TS. Complications of carbon dioxide laser resurfacing: an evaluation of 500 patients. Dermatol Surg 1998; 24:315–320.
58. Alster TS, West TB. Effect of topical vitamin C on postoperative carbon dioxide resurfacing erythema. Dermatol Surg 1998; 24:331–334.
59. McDaniel DH, Ash K, Lord J, et al. Accelerated laser resurfacing wound healing using a triad of topical antioxidants. Dermatol Surg 1998; 24:661–664.
60. Horton S, Alster TS. Preoperative and postoperative considerations for cutaneous laser resurfacing. Cutis 1999; 64:399–406.
61. Fisher AA. Lasers and allergic contact dermatitis to topical antibiotics, with particular reference to bacitracin. Cutis 1996; 58:252–254.
62. Sriprachya-anunt S, Fitzpatrick RE, Goldman MP, et al. Infections complicating pulsed carbon dioxide laser resurfacing for photo-aged facial skin. Dermatol Surg 1997; 23:527–536.
63. Alster TS, Nanni CA. Pulsed-dye laser treatment of hypertrophic burn scars. Plast Reconstr Surg 1998; 102:2190–2195.
64. Friedman PM, Geronemus RG. Use of the 308-nm excimer laser for postresurfacing leukoderma. Arch Dermatol 2001; 137:824–825.
65. Grimes PE, Bhawan J, Kim J, et al. Laser resurfacing-induced hypopigmentation: histologic alteration and repigmentation with topical photochemotherapy. Dermatol Surg 2001; 27:515–520.
66. Rohrer TE. Erbium:YAG laser resurfacing-experience of the first 200 cases. Aesthet Dermatol Cosmet Surg 1999; 1:19–30.
67. Tanzi EL, Alster TS. Side effects and complications of variable-pulsed erbium:yttrium–aluminum–garnet laser skin resurfacing: extended experience with 50 patients. Plast Reconstr Surg 2003; 111: 1524–1529.
68. Rostan EF, Fitzpatrick RE, Goldman MP. Laser resurfacing with a long pulse erbium:YAG laser compared to the 950 ms pulsed carbon dioxide laser. Lasers Surg Med 2001; 29:136–141.
69. Ross VE, Miller C, Meehan K, et al. One-pass carbon dioxide versus multiple-pass Er:YAG laser resurfacing in the treatment of rhytides: a comparison side-by-side study of pulsed carbon dioxide and Er:YAG lasers. Dermatol Surg 2001; 27:709–715.
70. Zachary CB. Modulating the Er:YAG laser. Lasers Surg Med 2002; 26:223–226.
71. Tanzi EL, Alster TS. Effect of a semiocclusive silicone-based dressing after ablative laser resurfacing of facial skin. Cosmetic Dermatol 2003; 16:13–16.
72. Batra RS, Ort RJ, Jacob C, et al. Evaluation of a silicone occlusive dressing after laser skin resurfacing. Arch Dermatol 2001; 137:1317–1321.
73. Alster TS, Lupton JR. Are all infrared lasers equally effective in skin rejuvenation. Sem Cutan Med Surg 2002; 21:274–279.
74. Zelickson B, Kilmer S, Bernstein E, el al. Pulsed dye laser therapy for sun damaged skin. Lasers Surg Med 1999; 25:229–236.
75. Zelickson B, Kist D. Effect of pulse dye laser and intense pulsed light source on the dermal extracellular matrix remodeling. Lasers Surg Med 2000; 12:68.
76. Bjerring P, Clement M, Heickendorff L, et al. Selective non-ablative wrinkle reduction by laser. J Cutan Laser Ther 2000; 2:9–15.
77. Goldberg DJ, Cutler KB. Non-ablative treatment of rhytides with intense pulsed light. Lasers Surg Med 2000; 26:196–200.
78. Bitter PH. Non-invasive rejuvenation of photodamaged skin using serial, full-face intense pulsed light treatments. Dermatol Surg 2000; 26:835–843.
79. Weiss RA, Weiss MA, Beasley KL. Rejuvenation of photoaged skin: 5 years results with intense pulsed light of the face, neck, and chest. Dermatol Surg 2002; 28:1115–1119.
80. Hardaway CA, Ross EV. Non-ablative laser skin remodeling. Dermatol Clin 2002; 20:97–111.
81. Goldberg DJ, Whitworth J. Laser skin resurfacing with the Q-switched Nd:YAG laser. Dermatol Surg 1997; 23: 903–907.
82. Goldberg DJ, Metzler C. Skin resurfacing utilizing a low-fluence Nd:YAG laser. J Cutan Laser Ther 1999; 1: 23–27.
83. Lee MW. Combination visible and infrared lasers for skin rejuvenation. Semin Cutan Med Surg 2002; 21:288–300.
84. Menaker GM, Wrone DA, Williams RM, et al. Treatment of facial rhytids with a non-ablative laser: A clinical and histologic study. Dermatol Surg 1999; 25: 440–444.
85. Kelly KM, Nelson S, Lask GP, et al. Cryogen spray cooling in combination with non-ablative laser treatment of facial rhytides. Arch Dermatol 1999; 135: 691–694.
86. Goldberg DJ. Non-ablative subsurface remodeling: Clinical and histologic evaluation of a 1320 nm Nd:YAG laser. J Cutan Laser Ther 1999; 1: 153–157.

87. Goldberg DJ. Full-face non-ablative dermal remodeling with a 1320 nm Nd:YAG laser. Dermatol Surg 2000; 26: 915–918.
88. Trelles MA, Allones I, Luna R. Facial rejuvenation with a non-ablative 1320 nm Nd:YAG laser. A preliminary clinical and histologic evaluation. Dermatol Surg 2001; 27: 111–116.
89. Fatemi A, Weiss MA, Weiss RA. Short-term histologic effects of non-ablative resurfacing: Results with a dynamically cooled millisecond-domain 1320 nm Nd:YAG laser. Dermatol Surg 2002; 28: 172–176.
90. Goldberg DJ, Rogachefsky AS, Silapunt S. Non-ablative laser treatment of facial rhytides: A comparison of 1450 nm diode laser treatment with dynamic cooling as opposed to treatment with dynamic cooling alone. Lasers Surg Med 2002; 30: 79–81.
91. Hardaway CA, Ross EV, Paithankar DY. Non-ablative cutaneous remodeling with a 1.45 micron mid-infrared diode laser: phase II. J Cosmet Laser Ther 2002; 4:9–14.
92. Tanzi EL, Williams CM, Alster TS. Treatment of facial rhytides with a non-ablative 1450-nm diode laser: a controlled clinical and histologic study. Dermatol Surg 2003; 29:124–129.
93. Tanzi EL, Alster TS. The treatment of transverse neck lines with a non-ablative 1450 nm diode laser. Dermatol Surg 2004 (in press).
94. Mordon S, Capon A, Creusy C, et al. In vivo experimental evaluation of non-ablative skin remodeling using a 1.54 μm laser with surface cooling. Lasers Surg Med 2000; 27:1–9.
95. Ross EV, Sajben FP, Hsia J, et al. Non-ablative skin remodeling: selective dermal heating with a mid-infrared laser and contact cooling combination. Lasers Surg Med 2000; 26:186–195.
96. Lupton JR, Williams CM, Alster TS. Non-ablative laser skin resurfacing using a 1540 nm erbium:glass laser: A clinical and histologic analysis. Dermatol Surg 2002; 28:833–835.
97. Fournier N, Dahan S, Barneon G, et al. Non-ablative remodeling: a 14-month clinical ultrasound imaging and profilometric evaluation of a 1540 nm Er:glass laser. Dermatol Surg 2002; 28:926–931.
98. Ruiz-Esparza J, Gomez JB. The medical face lift: a non-invasive, non-surgical approach to tissue tightening in facial skin using non-ablative radiofrequency. Dermatol Surg 2003; 29:325–332.
99. Alster TS, Tanzi EL. Improvement of neck and cheek laxity with a non-ablative radiofrequency device: a lifting experience. Dermatol Surg 2004; 30: 503–507.

39 Laser and Light Treatment of Acquired and Congenital Vascular Lesions

Arielle NB Kauvar MD and Agneta Troilius MD PhD

Summary box

- Laser light is emitted as a single discrete wavelength.
- The photobiologic effects of laser or light on skin result from absorption and excitation.
- Longer pulse durations minimize photomechanical injury and reduce post-treatment purpura.
- Longer wavelengths provide deeper penetration into the skin and enable treatment of larger diameter and deeper blood vessels.
- Cooling the skin before, during and after laser pulse impact reduces tissue injury, while cooling the skin before and after laser exposure can reduce pain and swelling.
- Lasers can be used to treat a wide range of lesions, including port-wine stains, hemangiomas, telangiectasias, rosacea, angiokeratomas, warts and scars.

INTRODUCTION

The development and refinement of laser technology provided, for the first time, an acceptable and effective means of treatment for many congenital and acquired cutaneous vascular disorders. Early efforts in the 1970s and 1980s centered around investigating the argon and other continuous and quasicontinuous wave lasers for port-wine stains (PWS), hemangiomas, and telangiectasia.[1–4] These laser treatments often produced excellent lightening or clearance of the lesions, but with an unacceptable rate of scarring and pigmentary alteration. Macular lesions and pale, immature PWS were at highest risk for these complications.

The formulation of the theory of selective photothermolysis, and its application to the development of the pulsed dye laser in the 1980s, revolutionized the treatment of cutaneous vascular lesions. The principles of selective photothermolysis describe the requirements for lasers or light energy to produce selective heating and destruction of a targeted skin lesion, such as a blood vessel, without damaging nearby structures.[5] The pulsed dye laser quickly emerged as the gold standard of treatment for PWS, hemangiomas, and facial telangiectasia. Laser treatment produced excellent clinical efficacy with an incidence of scarring less than 1%, even after multiple, repetitive treatments.[6,7] A deeper understanding of the complex laser–tissue interactions and advancements in laser technology have further refined laser therapy over the past decade.

Lasers and light devices now being applied to the treatment of cutaneous vascular lesions include the potassium titanyl phosphate (KTP), pulsed dye, alexandrite, diode, and neodymium:yttrium aluminum garnet (Nd:YAG) lasers, as well as intense pulsed light (IPL).

Principles of laser–tissue interaction

Electromagnetic radiation

The term laser is an acronym for **L**ight **A**mplification by the **S**timulated **E**mission of **R**adiation. Albert Einstein introduced the concept of stimulated light emission in 1917 when he proposed that a photon of electromagnetic energy can stimulate emission of an equivalent photon from atoms or molecules that are in an excited state.[8] Laser light is emitted as a single discrete wavelength, which is determined by the laser medium which may be a solid (e.g. alexandrite crystal), liquid (pulsed dye), or gas (carbon dioxide). All the effects of light on tissue begin with the absorption of electromagnetic radiation. The photobiologic effects of lasers or light on skin result from absorption and excitation. When discussing electromagnetic radiation, energy is measured in units of joules (J). The amount of energy that is delivered per unit area is the fluence (or dose) and is measured in joules (J/cm^2). Power is the rate at which energy is delivered, and is measured in watts (W). By definition, one watt is one joule per second (W = J/sec).

Selective photothermolysis

Anderson and Parrish inaugurated a new era in the application of lasers to cutaneous disease with their development of the concept of selective photothermolysis in 1983. The term selective photothermolysis describes the production of site-specific, thermally mediated injury of microscopic, pigmented tissue targets by selectively absorbed pulses of radiation.

Three requirements must be met to achieve selective photothermolysis. First, the wavelength of light must be preferentially absorbed by the desired target structures, and must be capable of penetrating the tissue sufficiently to reach that structure. Light deposits energy only in sites of absorption. Atoms or molecules that absorb energy from light are termed chromophores. The major chromophores in skin are hemoglobin, melanin, and water.[9,10] When targeting a vascular lesion, the wavelength of light chosen should be well absorbed by hemoglobin and poorly absorbed by melanin. When light is absorbed by these structures, heat is produced and contained in these structures.

The second requirement for selective photothermolysis is that the pulse duration or laser exposure time is less than or equal to the time necessary for cooling of the target structures. The goal is to selectively heat these structures without allowing diffusion of thermal energy to the surrounding tissue structures, which could result in damage to epidermal and dermal components, and result in scarring. When selective photothermolysis is achieved light is absorbed by the structure, and heat is produced and contained within the structure. Selective heating of the target is produced when the energy is deposited at a rate faster than the rate for cooling of the target structure. Heat is dissipated by conduction and radiative transfer as soon as it is created.

The final requirement for selective photothermolysis is that sufficient fluence (or energy density) is used to reach a damaging temperature in the target.

Wavelength

The wavelength of light chosen must be capable of reaching the target structure. For a given wavelength, the optical penetration into skin depends on absorption and scattering.[11] For wavelengths in the ultraviolet to near infrared spectrum, absorption and scattering are stronger for shorter wavelengths. In the dermis, collagen fibers produce strong wavelength-dependent scattering. Light penetration into dermis is primarily determined by this scattering. The most penetrating wavelengths are in the 650–1200 nm red and near infrared region. The least penetrating wavelengths are in the far ultraviolet, where protein absorption dominates, and the far infrared, where water absorption dominates. The depth of penetration therefore gradually increases with longer wavelengths (Fig. 39.1).

To target vascular lesions, the wavelength of light chosen must be preferentially absorbed by blood vessels. Blood absorption is dominated by oxyhemoglobin and reduced hemoglobin absorption.[12] Hemoglobin is present at high concentrations within blood vessels. Oxyhemoglobin has major absorption peaks at 418, 542, and 577 nm, in the blue, green, and yellow wavelengths (Fig. 39.2). Melanin normally occurs in the epidermis and hair follicles, and absorbs broadly across the visible light spectrum. Despite strong absorption by blood in the blue band (418 nm), wavelengths in this region are less desirable because of limited penetration and interference by melanin absorption. The yellow band (577 nm) of oxyhemoglobin absorption was initially chosen for targeting superficial small vessels

Longer wavelengths penetrate skin more deeply

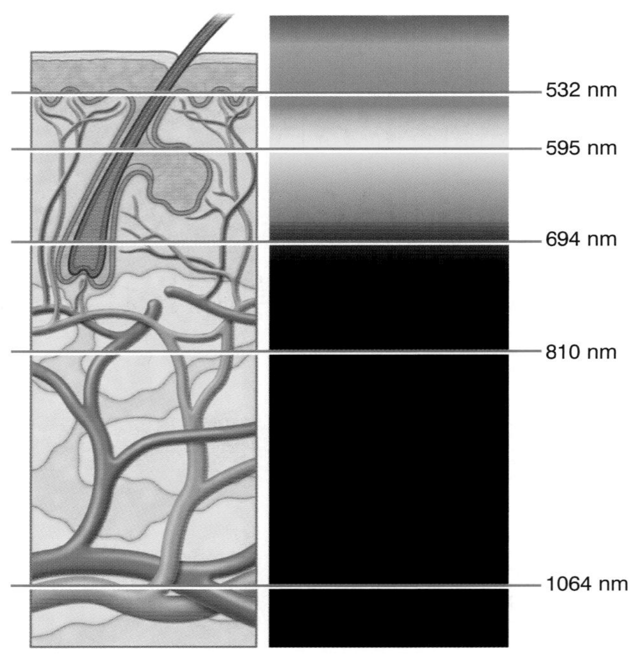

Figure 39.1 For a constant laser spot size and fluence, longer wavelengths penetrate skin more deeply.

Absorption spectra: major chromophores

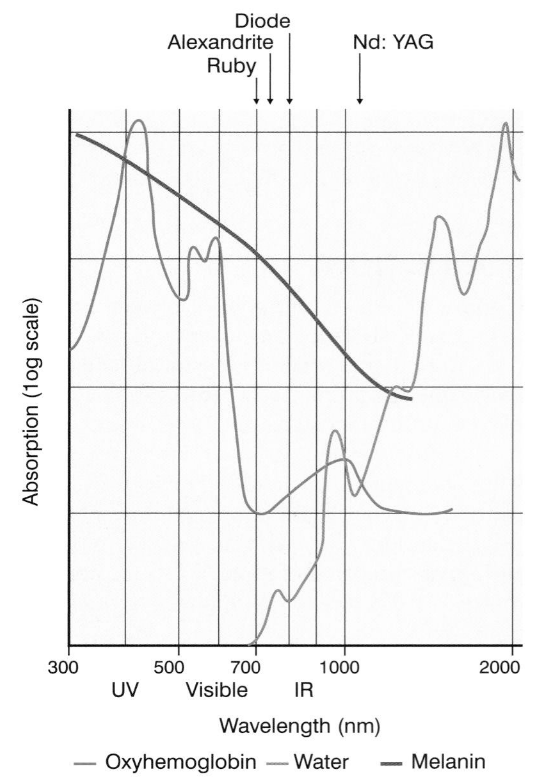

Figure 39.2 Absorption spectra for the three major chromophores—oxyhemoglobin, water, and melanin.

using the flashlamp-pumped pulsed dye laser.[13] The wavelength of this laser was subsequently increased to 585 nm and later 595 nm to provide increased depth of penetration into tissue. Pulsed KTP lasers emit at 532 nm in the green light spectrum. Green light is absorbed by hemoglobin approximately as well as yellow light and has roughly the equivalent depth of penetration through fair skin.

There is also a broad oxyhemoglobin band beyond 900 nm that provides preferential hemoglobin absorption, with minimal interference with melanin, and much greater depth of penetration. Lasers in the near infrared region have recently been applied to the treatment of cutaneous vascular lesions, and include the alexandrite (755 nm), diode (800 nm), and Nd:YAG (1064 nm) lasers. IPL sources use high-intensity pulsed flashlamps that produce broadband emission from 515–1100 nm. The broad emission spectrum provides absorption by oxygenated and deoxygenated hemoglobin and deep penetration into the skin for larger diameter, more deeply situated vessels (Table 39.1).

Pulse duration and thermal relaxation time

An important concept underlying selective photothermolysis is that the exposure time or pulse duration of the laser determines the confinement of heat and extent of thermal injury produced in tissue.[11,14–17] The thermal relaxation time (TRT) refers to the time needed for significant cooling of the microscopic tissue target. Maximal thermal confinement occurs when the laser exposure time is less than the thermal relaxation time.

The cooling of microscopic tissue structures is determined by heat conduction. Conduction is the transfer of heat between two interacting systems, and is driven by a temperature gradient between the systems. The thermal relaxation time for heat conduction is proportional to the square of the object size. It is approximated by the formula $TRT = d^2/4\kappa$, where (d) is the diameter of the object or thickness of the tissue layer and (κ) is the thermal diffusivity. Thermal diffusivity is a material property that expresses the ability of heat to diffuse. The cooling time of an object depends on its shape owing to differences in volume and surface area. In general, for a given thickness of tissue, spheres cool faster than cylinders, which cool faster than planes. Smaller objects cool more quickly than larger objects. For objects comprised of the same shape and material, an object half the size cools in one-quarter of the time and an object one tenth the size cools in one hundredth the time.

Spot size

The optical penetration of laser light is determined in part by the beam diameter (or spot size).[18,19] With smaller spot sizes, a greater fraction of photons scatter outside the beam area and are rendered ineffective. Larger spots allow more photons to remain within the diameter of the incident beam of light. The increased scattering within the beam diameter produces higher fluences at a given depth within tissue. The ratio of dermal to epidermal damage increases as the spot size increases. Treatment fluences are therefore decreased with larger spots compared to smaller spot sizes. A 7 and 10 mm spot size require only $\frac{1}{2}$ to $\frac{2}{3}$ the fluence for a 5 mm spot with the 585 nm pulsed dye laser.

Fluence and epidermal protection

Sufficient fluence must be supplied to produce irreversible damage to the target when targeting dermal blood vessels. Increasing the fluence produces more effective photocoagulation, but may lead to an increase in side-effects. Absorption by epidermal melanin and heat transfer from dermal targets can result in inadvertent epidermal injury. Ideally, the epidermis should remain unaffected to prevent adverse clinical outcomes. Recently developed skin cooling methods minimize tissue injury by extracting heat from the epidermis.[20–25]

Cooling the skin, before, during, and after laser pulse impact reduces tissue injury. Cooling the skin before and after laser exposure tends to reduce pain and swelling. Cooling the skin during laser treatment decreases epidermal heating. Skin cooling devices extract heat from the epidermis by means of conduction. Cold ice cubes may be applied to the skin before or after treatment. During laser treatment, the application of a cold gel or a liquid medium provides a more conductive material than air, and increases heat dissipation. Cold sapphire laser tips extract even more heat than cold gels or liquids (Fig. 39.3). Excellent heat extraction from the epidermis is also provided by the application of a liquid cryogen spray during laser treatment (Fig. 39.4).

Vascular lesion removal by selective photothermolysis

Since the development of the first pulsed dye laser, newer developments in laser technology and a deeper under-

Table 39.1 Lasers and light sources for vascular lesions

Laser/light source	Wavelength (nm)	Pulse duration (msec)
Pulsed KTP	532	1–200
Pulsed dye	585	0.45
Long-pulsed dye	585, 590, 595, 600	1.5–40
Long-pulsed alexandrite	755	3–20
Diodes	800, 810, 930	1–250
Long-pulsed Nd:YAG	1064	1–100
Intense pulsed light source	515–1200	0.5–30

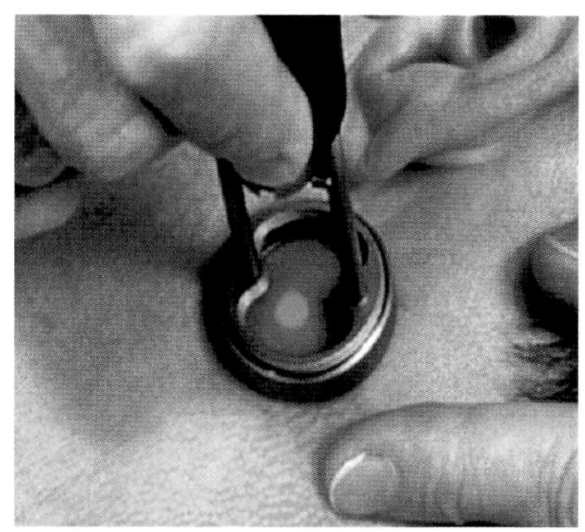

Figure 39.3 Water-cooled sapphire laser chill tip on a pulsed KTP laser. (Courtesy of Lumenis, Inc.)

Dynamic cooling device

Laser beam

Epidermis

Dermis

Blood vessel

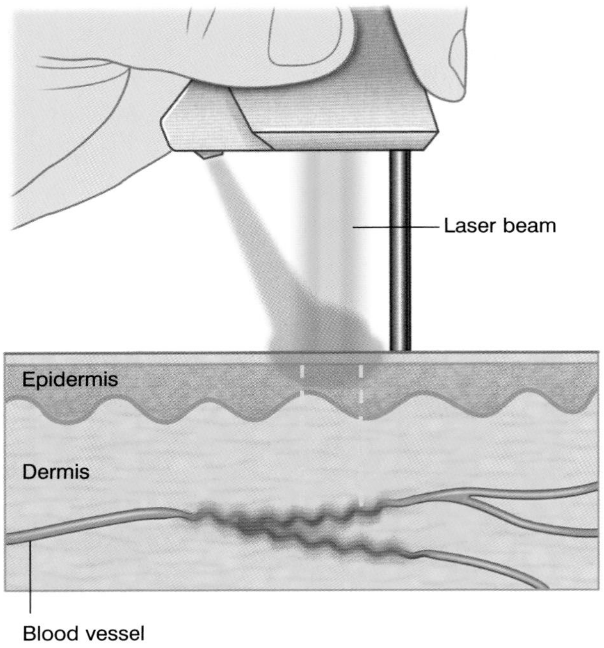

Figure 39.4 The Dynamic Cooling Device (DCD) provides a brief spurt of cryogen that selectively cools the epidermis during Vbeam® laser application. (Courtesy of Candela Laser Corp, Wayland, MA.)

Table 39.2 Pulsed KTP lasers

Name	Aura	Versapulse	Diolite
Manufacturer	Laserscope, San Jose, CA	Coherent/ Lumenis, Palo Alto, CA	Iridex, Mountainview, CA
Wavelength (nm)	532	532	532
Pulse duration (msec)	1–50	2–50	1–100
Maximum fluence (J/cm²)	1–999	0.2–38	0.1–950
Cooling	Contact	Contact	

standing of laser–tissue interactions have led to improved treatment responses with greater margins of safety. A wide variety of laser and light systems are now used for vascular lesions (Tables 39.2–39.8).

The theoretical formulation of selective photothermolysis predicted that a 577 nm, 1 msec pulse duration was ideal for immature PWS.[26] For vessels 10–50 µm in diameter the thermal relaxation time should be 0.1–10 msec, with an average of 1.2 msec.[14] Pickering et al.[27] demonstrated that exposure times of 0.1–0.3 msec are required to irreversibly damage 100-µm diameter vessels with wall thicknesses of 3–6 µm. In early studies, shorter pulse durations of 1–20 µsec were tested at a wavelength of 577 nm in normal human and animal skin.[28,29] Laser treatment produced

Table 39.3 Pulsed dye lasers

Laser	SPTL-1B	Cbeam	Photogenica V
Manufacturer	Candela, Wayland, MA	Candela, Wayland, MA	Cynosure, Chelmsford, MA
Wavelength (µm)	585	585	585
Pulse duration (msec)	0.45	0.45	0.45
Maximum fluence (J/cm²)	10	16	10
Cooling		Cryogen	Air

selective vascular injury, but extensive vessel rupture and hemorrhage resulted from erythrocyte explosion.[30] This was consistent with mechanical rupture of blood vessels from vaporization of blood. The pulse duration of the pulsed dye laser was then lengthened to maximize thermal coagulation of vessels and minimize vaporization injury. Longer pulse durations minimized the hemorrhage, but required higher threshold fluences to achieve vessel coagulation.[31] Based on these studies, a 400-µsec, 577-nm pulsed dye laser was developed and produced excellent clinical lightening with a low risk of scarring in pediatric and adult patients.[32,33]

The wavelength of the pulsed dye laser was subsequently increased to 585 nm which provided similar vascular selectivity and doubled the depth of penetration in tissue.[32,34] Extensive clinical experience with the 585-nm, 400-µsec pulsed dye laser demonstrated excellent clearing of PWS with a high safety profile in infants, children and adults.[35–40] Clinically, this laser produces transient blue–black purpura as a result of hemorrhage and a delayed vasculitis. Histologic examination shows selective intravascular and perivascular coagulation necrosis with epidermal injury in fair skin.[40] In the 1990s, newer pulsed dye lasers were developed with pulse durations greater than 1 msec because the 0.5-msec pulse width was theoretically too short for most PWS, and produced disfiguring purpura for as long as 10 days following treatment. Dierickx et al.[41] performed a landmark in-vivo study of PWS thermal relaxation time in 1995, and experimentally demonstrated that the thermal relaxation time for vessels approximately 60 µm in diameter was between 1 and 10 msec.

Millisecond-duration pulsed KTP lasers were introduced in the 1990s. Pulsed KTP lasers emit at 532 nm in the green light spectrum. KTP crystals are convenient to work with and highly reliable. The 532-nm KTP light is absorbed by hemoglobin approximately as well as 585-nm light, and has roughly the equivalent depth of penetration through fair skin. With pulse durations in the 1–200-nm range, purpura is precluded by the more uniform heating of blood vessels. Most of the available laser systems use grouped nanosecond-domain Q-switched pulses to produce millisecond exposure times.

The longer pulse durations minimize photomechanical injury and clinically reduce post-treatment purpura. Pulse durations of more than 1 msec produce gentle vaporization of blood. Rather than producing explosive vessel rupture, evacuation of blood from the vessel produces an empty,

Table 39.4 Long-pulsed dye lasers

Laser	Sclerolaser/Scleroplus	VBeam	Photogenica VLS	V-Star Photogenica
Manufacturer	Candela, Wayland, MA	Candela, Wayland, MA	Cynosure, Chelmsford, MA	Cynosure, Chelmsford, MA
Wavelength (nm)	585–600	595	585–600	585/595
Pulse duration (msec)	1.5	0.45–40	0.45–1.5	0.5–40
Maximum fluence (J/cm^2)	20	25	10	40
Cooling	Cryogen	Cryogen	Air	Air

Table 39.5 Long-pulsed alexandrite lasers

Laser	GentleLase	Apogee	Arion Wavelight
Manufacturer	Candela, Wayland, MA	Cynosure, Chelmsford, MA	Cynosure, Chelmsford, MA
Wavelength (nm)	755	755	755
Pulse duration (msec)	3	5–40	1–50
Maximum fluence (J/cm^2)	100	50	5–70
Cooling	Cryogen	Air	Air

Table 39.6 Diode lasers

Laser	MedioStar	Apogee	SkinPulse	Apex	Light Sheer	EpiStar	SLP 1000	MedArt 435
Manufacturer	Asclepion-Meditec, Jena Germany	Cynosure, Chelmsford, MA	Dornier, Munich, Germany	Iridex, Mountainview, CA	Lumenis, Santa Clara, CA	Nidek, Fremont CA	Palomar, Burlington	ASAH Medico, Hvidovre, Denmark
Wavelength (nm)	810	800	940	800	800	810	810	810
Pulse duration (msec)	5–30	50–500	10–Continuous	5–100	5–100	200	50–100	100
Maximum fluence (J/cm^2)	64	50	600	5–60	10–60		179	168
Cooling	Contact	Air		Contact	Contact		Contact	Contact

Table 39.7 Long-pulsed Nd:YAG lasers

Laser	CoolGlide/Vantage	Gentle YAG	Varia	Lyra	Image	Mydon
Manufacturer	Altus Burlingame, CA	Candela, Wayland, MA	ICN, Costa Mesa, CA	Laserscope, San Jose, CA	Sciton, Palo Alto, CA	Wavelight, Erlangen, Germany
Wavelength (nm)	1064	1064	1064	1064	1064	1064
Pulse duration (msec)	0.1–300	3–20	0.3–200	10–100	5–200	20–140
Maximum fluence (J/cm^2)	300	10–120	500	200	10–400	15–400
Cooling	Contact	Cryogen	Cryogen/Contact	Contact	Contact/Air	Contact/Air

thermally coagulated blood vessel.[42] Lengthening the pulse duration of the pulsed dye laser to 1.5 msec significantly reduced the intensity and duration of purpura. Studies of adult PWS with a 595-nm, 1.5-msec pulsed dye laser demonstrated reduced purpura compared to the 585-nm, 450-μsec laser.[43] Lengthening the pulse duration also minimizes epidermal damage. Melanosomes are less efficiently heated with longer pulses; they cool rapidly during laser pulse delivery because of their small size.

Longer wavelengths provide deeper penetration into the skin and enable treatment of larger diameter and deeper blood vessels. The absorption coefficient of blood decreases with increasing wavelengths beyond 577 nm. However, highly selective microvascular injury can be achieved by increasing the fluence to produce the same heating of the blood vessels. Longer wavelength pulsed dye lasers at 595 nm work well for treating larger vessels (0.1–1-mm diameter), PWS, and telangiectasias, as long as higher fluences are used. Pigment cell injury is minimized by the use of longer pulse durations (1.5 msec) and active or passive skin surface cooling.

IPL systems[44] are high-intensity flashlamps that emit a broad spectrum of polychromatic light from 515–1200 nm. Cut-off filters are used to match the spectrum of delivered

Light source	Quantum	Vasculight	Estelux/Medilux	Ellipse Flex	Aurora DS/Aurora SR
Manufacturer	Lumenis, Santa Clara, CA	Lumenis, Santa Clara, CA	Palomar, Burlington, MA	Danish Dermatologic Development, Hoersholm, Denmark	Syneron Yokneam, Israel
Wavelength (nm)	515–1200	515–1200	500–1200	550–950	680–980/580–980
Pulse duration (msec)	2–7	0.5–2.5	10–100		7–100
Maximum fluence (J/cm^2)	45	90	4–12/30		10–30
Cooling	Contact	Contact			Contact
Frequency of RF					1

Table 39.8 Intense pulsed light sources

Table 39.9 Clinical applications for vascular lasers and light sources

Capillary malformations	Infantile PWS Macular PWS in adults Hypertrophic PWS in adults
Hemangiomas	Superficial hemangiomas Subcutaneous hemangiomas Compound hemangiomas Involuting hemangiomas
Venous malformations	Blue rubber bleb nevi
Telangiectasias	Spider angiomas Actinic telangiectasia CREST syndrome Essential telangiectasia
Hereditary hemorrhagic telangiectasia	
Radiation dermatitis	
Rosacea	
Facial erythema	Associated with rosacea Flushing and blushing
Cherry angiomas	
Venous lakes	
Poikiloderma of Civatte	
Other lesions treated with vascular lasers	Angiokeratomas Glomus tumors Pyogenic granulomas Adenoma sebacea Hypertrophic and erythematous scars Striae distensae Warts

Table 39.10 Mulliken and Glowacki's classification of congenital vascular anomalies

Tumors (arise by endothelial hyperplasia)	Malformations (arise by dysmorphogenesis, normal endothelial turnover)
Hemangioma	Capillary Lymphatic Venous Arteriovenous Combined

light to the required depth of optical penetration and to maximize absorption by the targeted chromophores. By filtering out shorter visible wavelengths, deeper or larger diameter blood vessels are more effectively targeted. The pulses are delivered as single or multiple synchronized pulses with exposure times of 0.5–80 msec. The pulse duration is matched to the thermal relaxation time of the vessels being treated. The interpulse delays allow cooling of the epidermis and smaller vessels while heat is retained in the larger vessels.

Most recently, the near-infrared wavelengths have been applied to the treatment of vascular lesions. Alexandrite (755 nm), diode (800, 940 nm), and Nd:YAG (1064 nm) lasers rely on the broad oxyhemoglobin absorption band in the 800–1000-nm spectrum, and provide greater depth of penetration. These larger lasers and light sources are being used to treat larger vessel vascular anomalies, as well as larger leg veins (1–5-mm diameter).

PRACTICAL APPLICATIONS

The clinical applications for vascular lasers and light sources are listed in Table 39.9.

Port-wine stains

Port-wine stains are congenital capillary malformations (Table 39.10) that occur in 0.3–0.5% of live births, grow commensurately with the child, and never regress.[45] There are no differences in vessel number, but there is an altered or even absent neural modulation of the vascular plexus[46] with a decrease in both sympathetic and sensory nerve innervation of the papillary plexus.[47] PWS begins as flat pink cutaneous patches, predominantly located on the head or neck. Most PWS are isolated lesions, but they may be associated with complicated syndromes requiring prompt diagnosis and intervention. The most common of these syndromes are Sturge–Weber[48] and Klippel–Trenaunay.[49] PWS is characterized histologically by ectatic vascular channels with normal turnover of endothelial cells. It is usually present at birth and grows proportionately with the individual. With age a PWS darkens in color and becomes increasingly nodular.

By the fifth decade of life, up to 65% of patients develop hypertrophy or nodularity of the lesion, and these changes are associated with a risk of spontaneous bleeding or hemorrhage, with injury to the site. Hypertrophy of lesions in the periorbital region may obstruct vision and in the perioral and nasal region may interfere with eating or breathing.[50] Soft tissue and skeletal hypertrophy occurs in some facial PWS, and may require surgical correction or orthodontic treatment.[51] A PWS can have profound psychosocial consequences; many patients report low self-esteem and difficulties in their personal and professional relationships attributed to their vascular lesions.

With the documentation of psychosocial morbidity associated with PWS, especially with increasing age, some groups have conducted studies of the potential benefits of early laser treatments of the cutaneous lesions. Troilius et al. report a study evaluating 231 young patients with PWS before and after laser treatments for psychosocial consequences.[52] Most patients were in the treatment process and answered questions about their feelings before treatment retrospectively. Troilius et al. reported that 75% of respondents found that their PWS had a negative impact on their lives, 47% suffered low self-esteem, 28% reported that their PWS made school life more difficult, and 76% of families thought that the patient was negatively impacted by the PWS.

All these symptoms, however, decreased significantly after successful laser treatment. Patients reported better social relationships, fewer problems with the opposite sex, and fewer negative reactions from peers. Based on these results, Troilius et al. advocate treatment of PWS as early as possible to avoid the high psychosocial morbidity associated with the lesion.[53] Treatment of PWS can prevent many of these complications. The preponderance of evidence suggests that treatment early in life is not only safe, but enables more rapid clearing. The greater lesional clearance observed in children can be attributed to thinner skin thickness (allowing better laser penetration), smaller vessel diameter, and smaller lesional surface area.

Pulsed dye laser treatment of PWS

The safety and efficacy of the pulsed dye laser for the treatment of PWS in children and adults has been well established in the literature. Gradual clearing of PWS is produced with successive laser treatments, usually performed at 4–6-week intervals. Early studies demonstrated 75% or more lightening in approximately 36–44% of adult patients with PWS, and at least 50% lesional lightening in 75% of pediatric patients after a total of four treatments.[30–34,54] With the pulsed dye laser, damage to vascular tissue is so selective that there is inconsequential absorption by melanin in fair-skinned individuals. Epidermal damage is, therefore, rarely seen following pulsed dye laser treatment, and the laser can be safely used in skin types I to IV (Fig. 39.5). In a study of 500 patients, atrophic scarring was reported in less than 0.1% of patients, spongiotic dermatitis in 0.04%, hyperpigmentation in 1%, and hypopigmentation in 2.6% of patients.[6] Treatment of darker skin is not performed because the higher density of melanin results in decreased vascular absorption and the possibility of epidermal damage.[55] Newer studies of cryogen cooling techniques suggest that safe treatment of darker skin phototypes may be possible in the near future.[56]

Advances in pulsed dye laser include the use of larger spot sizes, longer wavelengths, and longer pulse durations. Kauvar and associates have shown that the use of larger 7 and 10-mm spot sizes improves PWS treatment.[57,58] Increased clearance is achieved at lower fluences, purpura is reduced, and there is less post-treatment reticulation of the skin. Longer wavelengths and longer pulse durations improve PWS clearance. In a side-by-side comparison study, Kauvar et al. found increased clearance of PWS in patients treated with a 595-nm, 1.5-msec pulsed dye laser when compared to a 585-nm, 450-μsec pulsed dye laser.[59] The longer wavelengths provide more deeply penetrating light to target deeper vessels. The longer pulse durations enable more even heating of larger diameter vessels, which minimizes post-treatment purpura.

Another advance in the laser treatment of PWS has been the addition of skin cooling methods. Nelson et al. demonstrated that selective cooling of the epidermis could be achieved while maintaining the temperature of the laser-heated dermal blood vessels by applying millisecond duration cryogen spurts preceding each laser pulse.[21] The use of cryogen spray in conjunction with the 585-nm, 450-μsec pulsed dye laser, decreased patient discomfort during treatment without compromising efficacy.[60] Kauvar et al. examined the use of cryogen spray in conjunction with a 595-nm, 1.5-msec pulsed dye laser, and found an overall decrease in healing time from 9.5 to 5 days with reduced edema, erythema, and crusting.[61] This study also demonstrated that a laser fluence of 10 J/cm^2 could be safely administered in infants, children, and adults because of the epidermal protection afforded by the skin cooling.

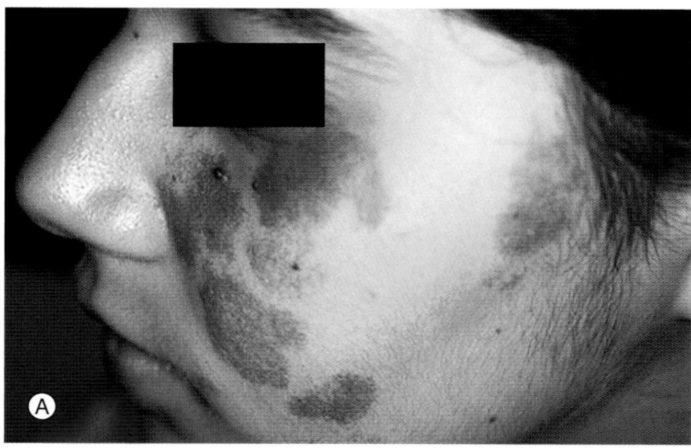

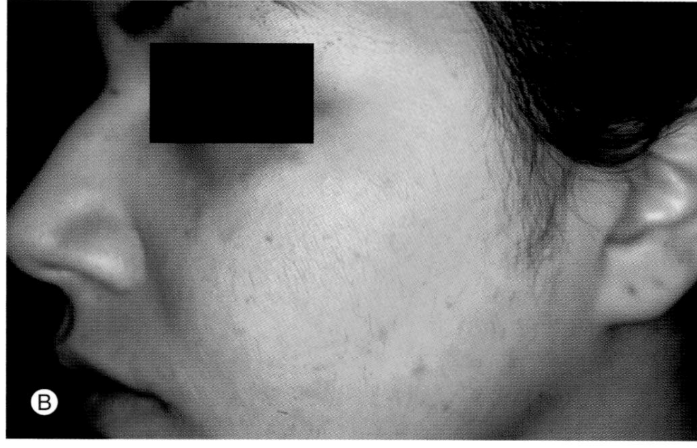

Figure 39.5 Port-wine stain (A) before and (B) after several pulsed dye laser treatments.

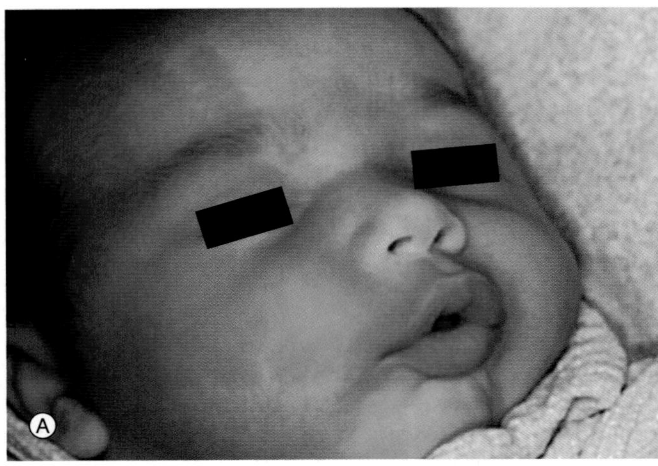

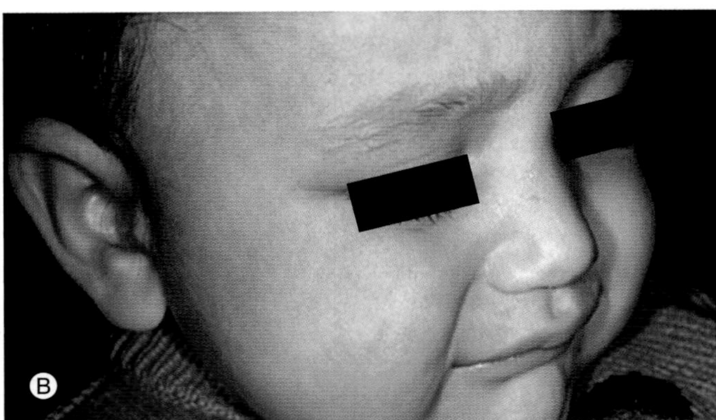

Figure 39.6 Infantile port-wine stain (A) before and (B) after four treatments with a 595 nm, 1.5-msec pulsed dye laser. (Reprinted with permission Arch Derm 2000; 136:942.)

Based on these results, studies were undertaken evaluating higher fluences (up to 15 J/cm^2) in the treatment of PWS in infants and adults with a 595-nm, 1.5-msec pulsed dye laser (Fig. 39.6). Dramatic clearing of PWS was achieved in fewer treatments with the safe use of higher laser fluences afforded by the cryogen spray cooling used to protect the epidermis.[62,63]

Factors affecting pulsed dye laser treatment response for PWS

The response of a PWS to pulsed dye laser treatment depends, in part, on its size, anatomical location, and the types of vessels that comprise the lesion. Among PWS located on the head and neck, lesions present in the central facial area or in a V2 dermatomal distribution respond more slowly than PWS located elsewhere on the head and neck.[64] PWS located on the extremities respond more slowly to laser therapy than lesions on the trunk, and lesions on the distal extremities respond the slowest.[65] In a study of 91 consecutive patients, Nguyen et al.[66] found that with pulsed dye laser treatment, the mean decrease in lesion size was greatest for the smaller lesions: a 67% decrease for lesions less than 20 cm^2, compared to a 23% decrease for lesions over 40 cm^2. In a histological study, Fikerstrand et al.[67] showed that lesions with a poor response to a 585-nm, 450-µsec dye laser had small vessels. Moderate responses were observed for PWS with deeper and larger vessels. The best response was seen in superficially located, larger diameter vessels.

Vessel morphology correlated with PWS color.[68] Pink lesions had the smallest diameter vessels, and purple, the largest. Red lesions were comprised of more superficially located vessels than pink or purple ones. Red color predicted a good response, whereas pink color predicted a poor response to laser therapy. Using videomicroscopy, Motley et al.[69] demonstrated two types of vascular ectasia within PWS. One type showed ectasia localized to the capillary loops, and the other was composed of ring-like, dilated, ectatic vessels in the superficial horizontal plexus. The first type correlated with a poor response to pulsed dye laser treatment, and the second type correlated with a good response. Kauvar and Geronemus showed that even slowly responsive PWS continues to clear with repetitive pulsed dye laser treatment with no increased risk of adverse effects.[70]

Several studies of pulsed dye laser treatment for PWS during infancy indicate that not only is early treatment safe, but more rapid clearance is possible. In a study of 35 children aged 3 months to 14 years of age, Tan et al. found that children less than 7 years old required fewer treatment sessions than older children for PWS clearance.[71] A study of 73 children reported that patients between 3 months and 6 years of age showed increased lightening of their PWS after one treatment compared with patients between 7 and 14 years of age.[40] Pulsed dye laser treatment of PWS in 83 children resulted in complete clearance in 32% of children who began treatment before 1 year of age compared to 18% of children treated after 1 year of age.[72] Alster and Wilson reported 87% PWS clearance in patients under 2 years of age and 73% in patients 16 years of age and older.[73] Similarly, a study of 133 patients found the highest percentage of good and excellent results in those aged 0–10 years.[74] In contrast, a study by Van der Horst et al.[75] found no difference in treatment results between age groups. However, in this study, only partial treatment of PWS lesions was performed during each treatment session, and treatment intervals were long.[76] The greater success of the pulsed dye laser treatment in infants and young children can be attributed to decreased skin thickness allowing better laser penetration, smaller vessel diameter, and smaller lesional surface area.

Treatment technique—pulsed dye laser

Treatment of PWS with the 585-nm, 0.45-msec laser is usually performed with the largest spot size available to prevent reticulation. Typical treatment fluences are 5.0–7.0 J/cm^2 with a 7-mm spot and 5.0–6.0 J/cm^2 with a 10-mm spot size, depending on the age of the patient and thickness of the lesion. Using the 595-nm, 1.5-msec pulsed dye lasers in conjunction with cryogen spray cooling, fluences of 8.0–11.0 J/cm^2 are used with a 7-mm spot size, and fluences of 5.0–7.5 J/cm^2 are used with the 10-mm spot in infants and children. The Dynamic Cooling Device (DCD, Candela, Wayland, MA) is generally used with a 30-msec spray and a 30-msec delay. For adults with hypertrophic lesions, fluences up to 13 J/cm^2 can be used with a 7-mm spot size and fluences up to 7.5 J/cm^2 with a 10-mm spot size, in conjunction with cryogen cooling.

Determination of the appropriate fluence and DCD parameters should be assessed with test sites performed during the initial evaluation. A test endpoint of graying indicates the use of too high a fluence resulting in epidermal disruption. If tissue graying results, the skin should be immediately cooled with ice packs to avoid epidermal necrosis, crusting, and the possibility of scarring. Treatment should be performed with the lowest possible fluence that produces purpura without tissue graying or whitening. When skin cooling is employed during laser therapy, the patient is observed for several minutes after treatment to visualize the final tissue reaction, which may be delayed with the use of skin cooling devices.

Immediately after treatment with the 585-nm, 0.45-msec pulsed dye laser, intense purpura develops for approximately 7–10 days. At equivalent fluences, the intensity and duration of purpura are significantly lower using pulse durations of 1.5 msec. If crusting occurs, patients are instructed to apply a topical antibiotic ointment daily until it resolves. Following the resolution of purpura, lesional lightening takes place over a period of 4–8 weeks, when repeat treatments are performed. The subsequent treatment session should be delayed until all traces of reactive erythema have subsided.

The development of various skin cooling methods has obviated the necessity for local or general anesthesia in most cases. With the exception of young children, most infants, teenagers and adults tolerate the treatment well with the use of a topical anesthetic cream such as EMLA or LMX 4 (Ferndale Laboratories Inc, Ferndale, MI). The topical anesthetic creams should be carefully washed off several minutes before laser treatment to avoid interference with the transmission of the laser light. The topical anesthetic creams have maximal limits based on patient weight, and these are provided in the manufacturer's drug information. When general anesthesia is used care must be taken to avoid leakage of flammable anesthetics in the operating field, which can promote the ignition of a fire on hair-bearing skin by the pulsed dye laser[77] (see page 641). Endotracheal tubes and laryngeal masks provide better seals than face masks and are preferred for this purpose. As an added measure of precaution, the airway tube and mouth region should also be covered with wet drapes.

IPL treatment of PWS

IPL devices are broadband filtered xenon flashlamps that work based on the principles of selective photothermolysis. The emission spectrum of 515–1200 nm is adjusted with the use of a series of cut-off filters, and the pulse duration ranges from approximately 0.5 to 100 msec, depending on the technology. The first commercial system, Photoderm VL (Lumenis, Yokneam, Israel) became available in 1994, and has been used to treat vascular anamolies. Another, IPL Technology (Danish Dermatologic Development [DDD] Hoersholm, Denmark) with a dual mode light filtering has also been used to treat PWS. Many other IPL systems have recently been developed, and the appropriate parameters for congenital vascular lesions are being developed. The IPL has been used successfully to treat PWS (Fig. 39.7),[78–80] but pulsed dye laser remains the treatment of choice.

IPL technology has also been used to treat pulsed dye laser-resistant PWS. In the study by Bjerring and associates seven of 15 patients achieved over 50% lesional lightening after four IPL treatments. Most of these patients had lesions involving the V2 dermatome (medial cheek and nose), which are relatively more difficult to lighten. Six of seven of these patients showed over 75% clearance of their PWS. A 550–950-nm filter was used with 8–30-msec pulse durations and fluences of 13–22 J/cm^2 to achieve tissue purpura. The 530–750-nm filter can also be used with

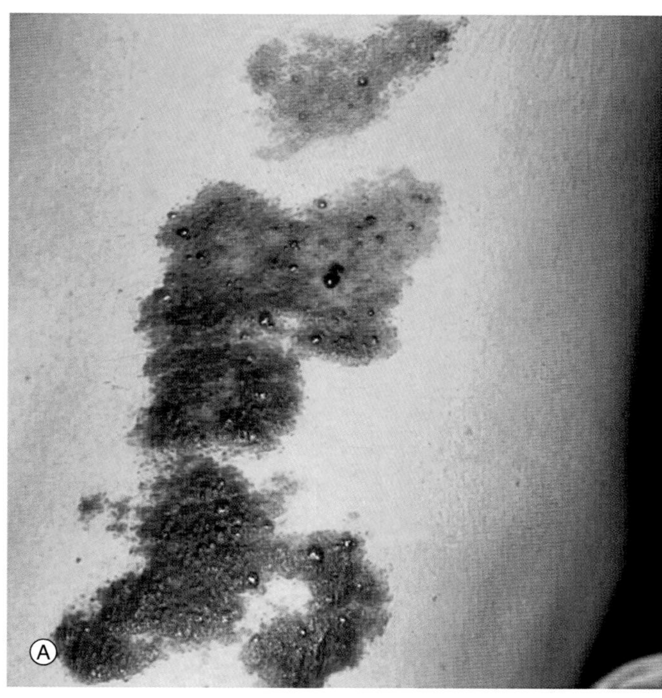

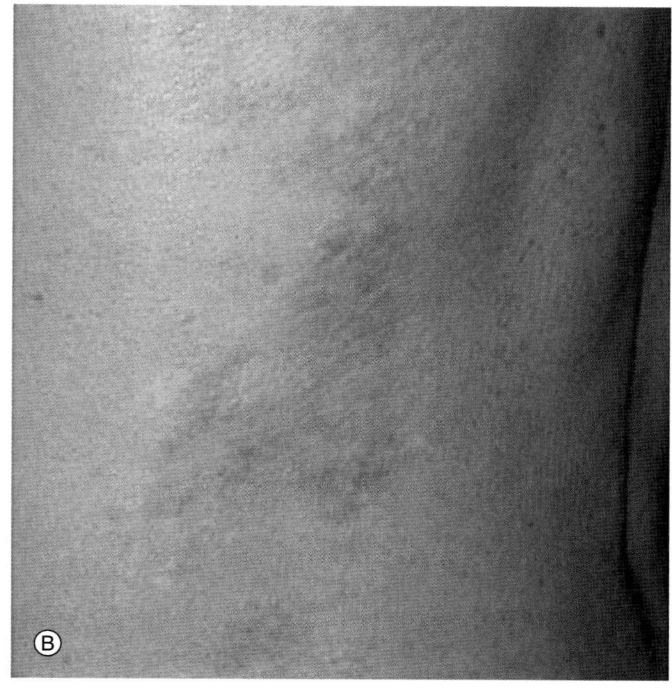

Figure 39.7 Port-wine stain (A) before and (B) after five treatments with an IPL.

double 2.5-msec pulses, with a 10-msec delay and fluence of 8–10 J/cm^2. Epidermal cooling was not required. Treatment resulted in immediate erythema and edema, and occasional crusting. Hypopigmentation was observed in three patients, hyperpigmentation in one patient, and epidermal atrophy in one patient.

Other laser treatment for PWS

A variety of other laser types offer vascular selectivity and may be applicable to the treatment of PWS. The KTP laser provides relatively equivalent absorption and depth of penetration as the pulsed dyed laser, and can be used for PWS with proper cooling and technique.[81] The 1064-nm Nd:YAG lasers provide enhanced tissue penetration, and when used with high fluences and short-millisecond pulsed durations, may have a role in the treatment of deeper, ectatic lesions. A recent pilot study demonstrated excellent clearance of PWS with a 3-msec alexandrite laser used in conjunction with cryogen cooling.[82]

Hemangiomas

Hemangiomas are common benign vascular lesions of childhood and are present at birth in 2–3% of newborns,[83] up to 12% of infants by 1 year of age, and up to 22% of preterm infants weighing less than 1000 g.[84] Hemangiomas have a female to male preponderance of 3 : 1.85 and 60–70% are localized to the head and neck. Hemangiomas are differentiated from other vascular malformations such as PWS, venous malformations, and arteriovenous and lymphatic malformations, by their rapid proliferation (see Table 39.10).[85–87] Histologically, hemangiomas are characterized by endothelial hyperplasia. They initially appear as white or pink macules, or telangiectasia with surrounding vasoconstriction, and then undergo a period of rapid proliferation out of proportion to the growth of the infant during the first year of life. They can increase rapidly in both height and lateral spread, sometimes reaching gigantic proportions. After approximately 1 year, hemangiomas undergo a slow period of involution that takes 5–10 years. Involution may not be complete, and approximately 50% of patients are left with residual telangiectasia, redundant fibrofatty tissue, and epidermal atrophy.[88,89]

Hemangiomas are further classified by their depth in tissue and extent of involvement.[87,90] Superficial hemangiomas appear as bright red vascular papules or plaques when fully developed. Deep hemangiomas appear as a bluish colored nodule within the skin and have only a subcutaneous component without the superficial red plaque. Compound hemangiomas have both a superficial and a deep component. Hemangiomas may also be focal or diffuse. Focal lesions present as solitary masses and represent 85% of lesions. They appear to occur along the lines of embryological fusion. Diffuse lesions are segmental in distribution. They usually present as superficial or compound lesions and carry a high risk of ulceration. Although hemangiomas regress during childhood, involution is usually incomplete, and lesions persist in 35–50% of children who begin school. Laser therapy, often in conjunction with other modalities, is useful in treating these lesions during both the proliferation and involution periods.

The natural history of an individual hemangioma is variable and unpredictable. Patients with hemangiomas require close observation, and for complicated or aggressive lesions, patients are best served by multidisciplinary evaluation and treatment. Lasers are often used as monotherapy for superficial or thin, mixed-type, and involuting hemangiomas. They are also used adjunctively with intralesional or systemic treatments for more complicated lesions. While the majority of hemangiomas undergo spontaneous regression, up to 50% of lesions persist in school-age children, and 15% of children have residual skin changes. Pulsed dye lasers prevent lesional enlargement, promote involution, induce re-epithelialization of ulcerations, and reduce the vascular ectasia.

Laser treatment of proliferating hemangiomas

Since the study of Sherwood and Tan[91] reporting complete resolution of a superficial hemangioma after several treatments, other authors have reported similar results. Ashinoff and Geronemus[92] treated a series of ten children with superficial and deeper hemangiomas. Superficial and involuting lesions responded well, but results were mixed for thick proliferating lesions. Similar results were found by others[93,94] treating with a 585-nm pulsed dye laser and a 5-mm spot. Garden et al.[95] found that the thicker the lesion the less the response, and thin lesions less that 1 mm in height responded best. Waner et al.[96] induced early involution of superficial proliferating hemangiomas with up to six pulsed dye laser treatments. Barlow et al.[97] achieved some decrease in the thickness of mixed-type proliferating lesions. In a more recent study of 225 hemangiomas using a pulsed dye laser, Poetke et al.[98] found that superficial hemangiomas involuted more completely than mixed-type hemangiomas. Mixed-type hemangiomas lightened but persisted. Hemangiomas treated early in the prodromal phase of growth responded better than those treated during active proliferation; 13 of 74 initially flat, superficial hemangiomas showed proliferation of the subcutaneous component. All these studies were performed with a 585-nm, 300–450-msec pulsed dye laser.

As with PWS, recent improvements in pulsed dye laser technology have led to improved results for hemangiomas. Longer wavelengths, millisecond pulse durations, and the addition of skin cooling improve treatment efficacy (Fig. 39.8). Lou et al.[99] showed faster clearing of hemangiomas with a 595-nm, 1.5-msec pulsed dye laser compared to historical controls using the 585-nm, 450-msec laser. Chang et al.[100] found that the 595-nm, 1.5-msec laser used in conjunction with cryogen cooling produced more improvement in lesion volume and texture and required fewer treatments compared to the 585-nm, 450-msec laser. The addition of cryogen cooling enabled the safe use of light doses of 9–10 J/cm^2 compared to 5.5–8 J/cm^2 used with the 585 nm laser. The IPL device, emitting a range of visible to near-infrared wavelengths, has been used successfully to treat hemangiomas. The long-pulsed 755-nm alexandrite and 1064-nm Nd:YAG lasers are likely to provide improved results for thicker hemangiomas because of their more deeply penetrating wavelengths.

Laser treatment of ulcerated hemangiomas

Ulceration is the most common complication of hemangiomas.[101,102] Ulceration usually occurs during the first few weeks of life or during periods of rapid proliferation. Approximately 12% of focal lesions and 65%

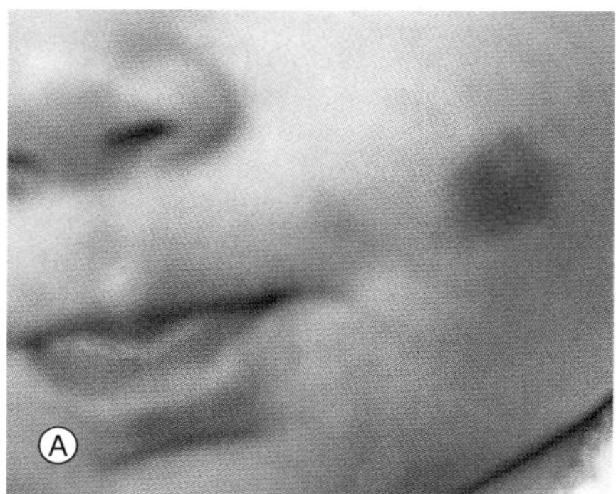

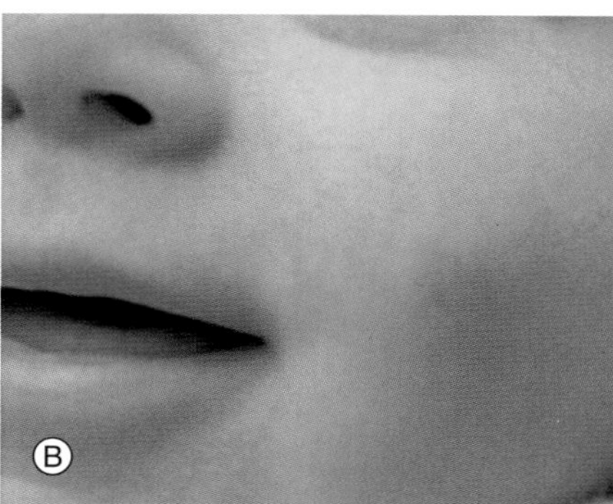

Figure 39.8 Proliferating mixed-type hemangioma (a) before and (b) after eight treatments with a 595-nm, 1.5 msec pulsed dye laser used with cryogen cooling.

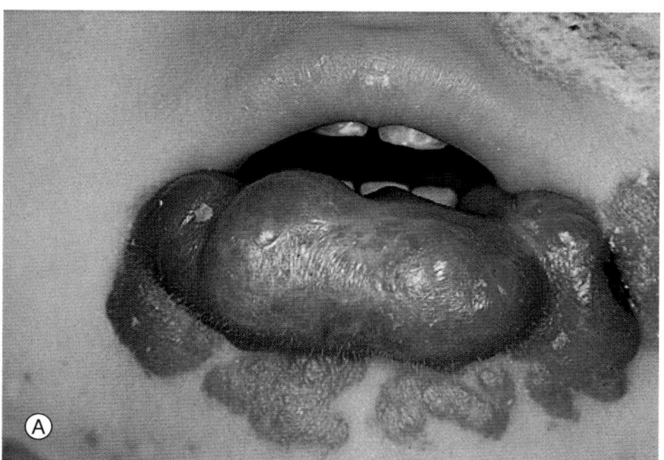

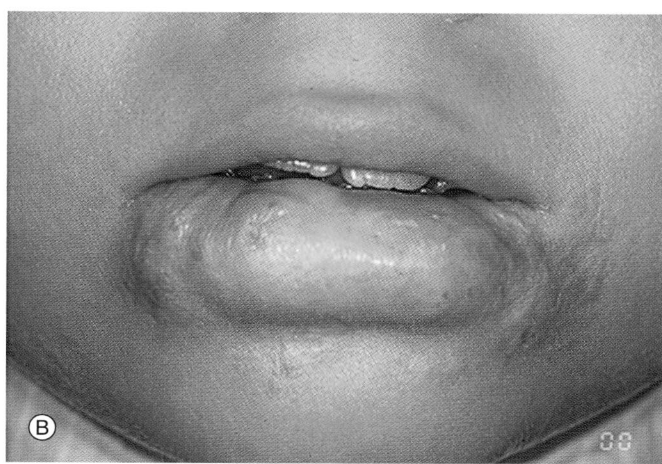

Figure 39.9 Segmental ulcerating hemangioma. (A) No response to systemic corticosteroids. (B) A response occurs after treatment with alfa interferon and pulsed dye laser.

of diffuse or segmental hemangiomas ulcerate. Ulcers may heal and reappear, and always result in a scar. Ulcerations may be painful, particularly in the anogenital region. Ulcerated hemangiomas are managed with multiple modalities, including local wound care, topical and systemic antibiotics, systemic corticosteroids and pulsed dye laser therapy.[103] Ulcers respond well to pulsed dye laser treatment if the ulceration is limited and the hemangioma is not undergoing rapid proliferation (Fig. 39.9). Laser treatment induces rapid re-epithelialization, decreases pain, and accelerates involution.[94,104,105] Despite the general success using pulsed dye laser therapy for ulcerated lesions, there have been several reported cases of laser treatment leading to ulceration in segmental hemangiomas treated early in the growth phase. Systemic corticosteroids are therefore recommended for this group of hemangiomas when they ulcerate.[103]

Laser treatment of compound or deep hemangiomas

Pulsed dye lasers have little effect on the subcutaneous component of hemangiomas because of their limited depth of penetration. Interstitial laser therapy has been successfully used by several groups to shrink large hemangiomas.[98,106,107] A 600-μm quartz fiber coupled to a near-infrared diode or Nd:YAG laser is introduced into the substance of a hemangioma percutaneously or transmucosally (Fig. 39.10).

Low-intensity light (1–2 W) is delivered to the interstitium of the lesion for a period of 500–1000 seconds to achieve photocoagulation. Because a 15-mm zone of coagulation is expected around the emission point of the fiber, epidermal damage remains a risk. This can be minimized by ultrasound-guided placement of the fiber or cooling of the skin surface with ice.

Laser treatment of involuting hemangiomas

Residual vascular ectasia often persists during involution along with residual fibrofatty tissue, hypopigmentation, and atrophic scarring. In addition to the pulsed dye lasers, pulsed KTP lasers and the IPL can be used to treat these skin changes. Carbon dioxide lasers, and long- and short-pulsed ER:YAG lasers, produce excellent improvement in the atrophic scarring and textural change that accompany involution.[108] These lasers ablate the epidermis and superficial dermis, and produce intra-operative collagen shrinkage.[109–112] Re-epithelialization is accompanied by the production of a new layer of collagen that undergoes remodeling for a period of 12–18 months.[109,110] The textural changes improve and the scarring is diminished

Telangiectasia

Most patients seek treatment for facial telangiectasia because of cosmetic concerns. Techniques used to treat facial

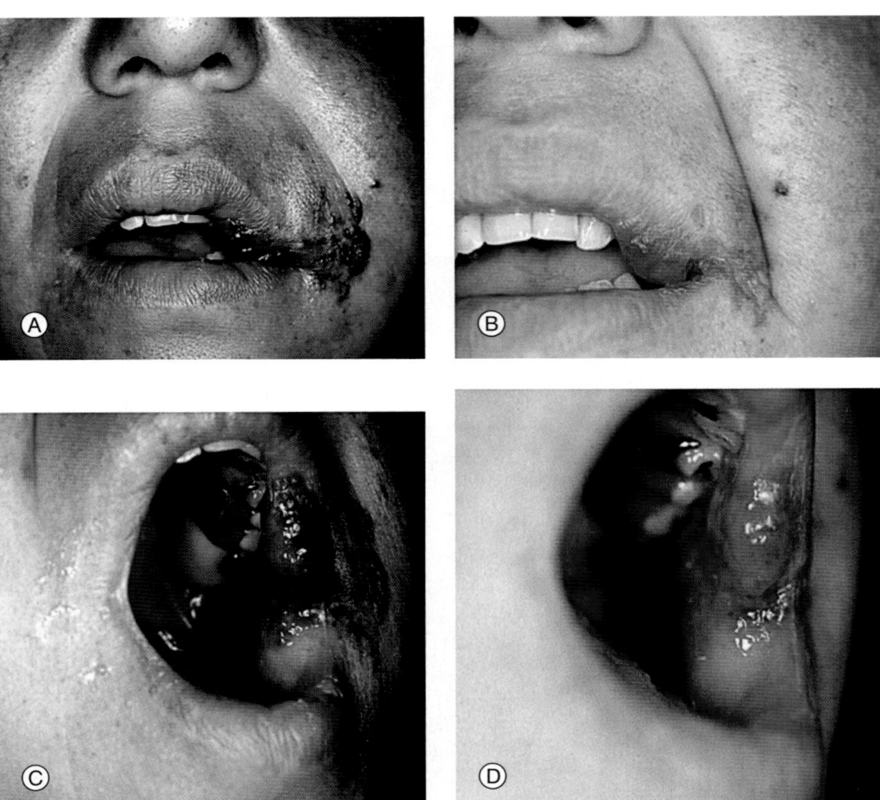

Figure 39.10 Swelling venous malformation of the (A)–(B) cheek and (C)–(D) lip before and after ethanol injections and three long-pulsed Nd:YAG laser 532-nm treatments with high fluences and cooling (Versapulse Help G, Coherent/Lumenis, Palo Alto, CA).

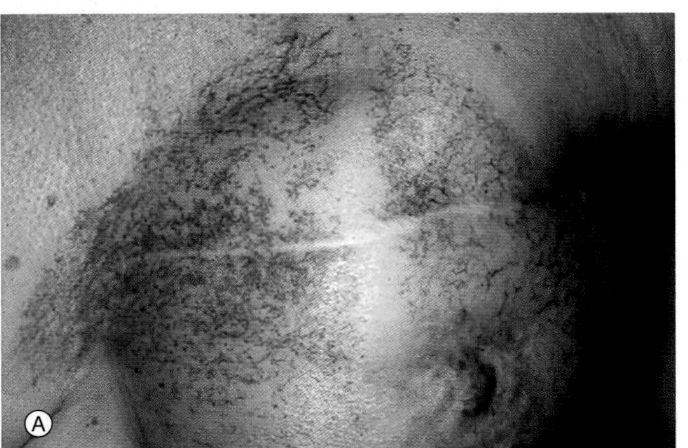

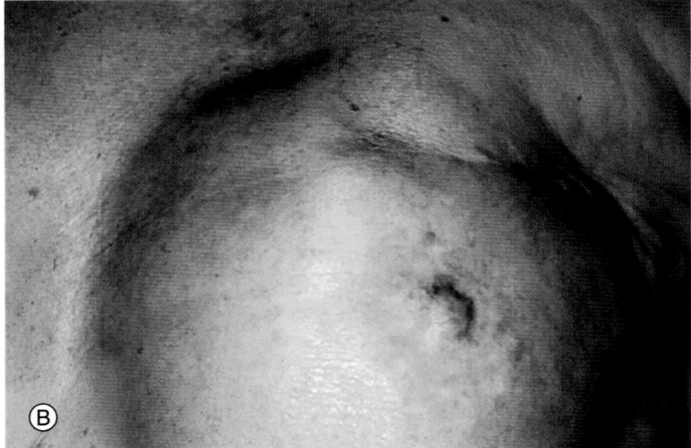

Figure 39.11 Radiation dermatitis (A) before and (B) after three pulsed dye laser treatments at fluences of 3–4 J/cm^2.

telangiectasia have included electrosurgery, sclerotherapy, and treatment with continuous wave and quasicontinuous wave lasers, but these methods may produce textural and pigmentary irregularities. The development of pulsed lasers and light sources enabled efficient, effective, and low-risk treatment of these common skin lesions.

Telangiectases are capillaries, venules, or arterioles that measure 0.1–1.0 mm in diameter and are visible as superficial cutaneous vessels. Facial telangiectases are common, and in fair-skinned individuals they are often associated with rosacea or actinic damage. Other etiologies include collagen vascular disease, genetic disorders, hormonal disorders, primary cutaneous disease, and radiation dermatitis (Fig. 39.11). Spider angiomas are telangiectases with a central feeding arteriole, typically appearing in preschool and school-aged children, with a peak incidence between the ages of 7 and 10 years.

A wide variety of vascular laser systems produce excellent clearance of facial telangiectases. The 585- and 595-nm pulsed dye lasers with 0.45- and 1.5-msec pulse durations produce excellent results in one or two treatment sessions, but induce purpura lasting 7–14 days.[113] Treatment is performed by applying contiguous laser pulses with approximately 10% overlap. The newer, millisecond duration pulsed dye lasers, used at 6–10 msec, clear facial telangiectases without purpura production (Fig. 39.12). Effective treatment usually requires stacking of three to four laser pulses with an endpoint of vessel blanching or

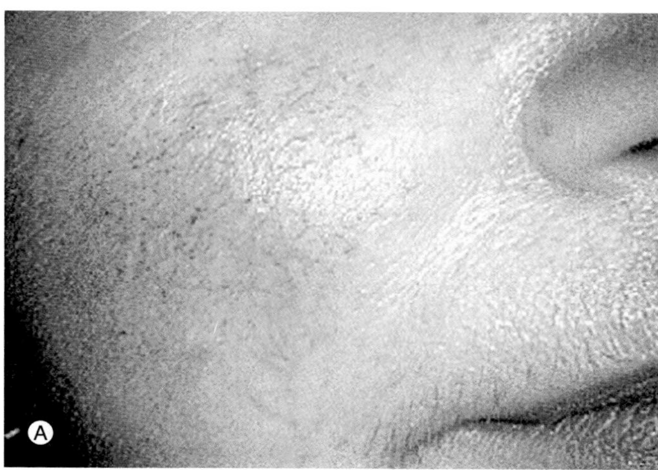

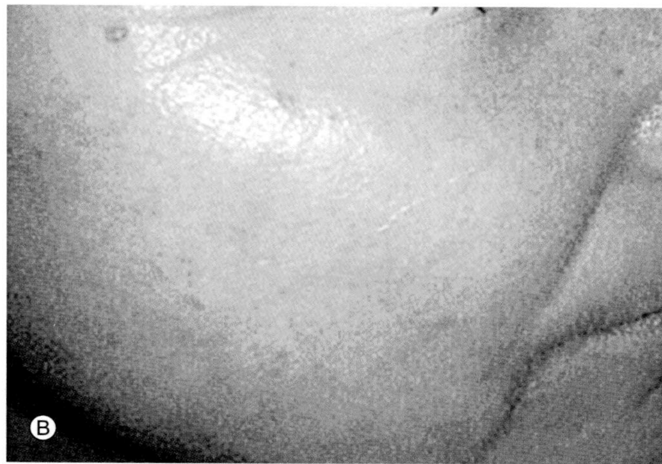

Figure 39.12 Rosacea-associated telangiectasia (A) before and (B) after treatment with a 595 nm pulsed dye laser using a 20 msec pulse duration. (Courtesy of Giuseppe Scarcella MD and Candela Laser Corp.)

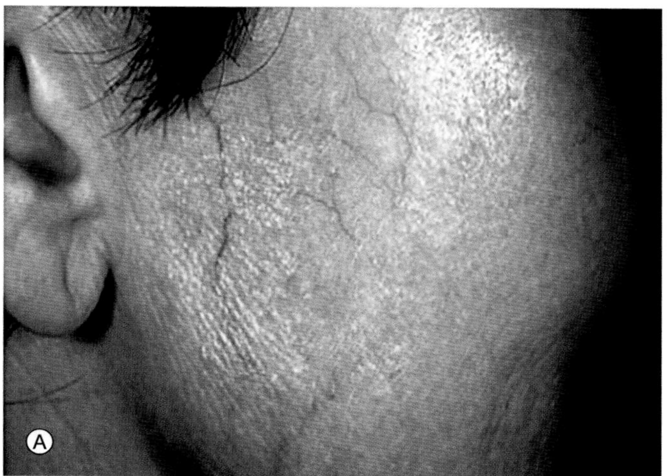

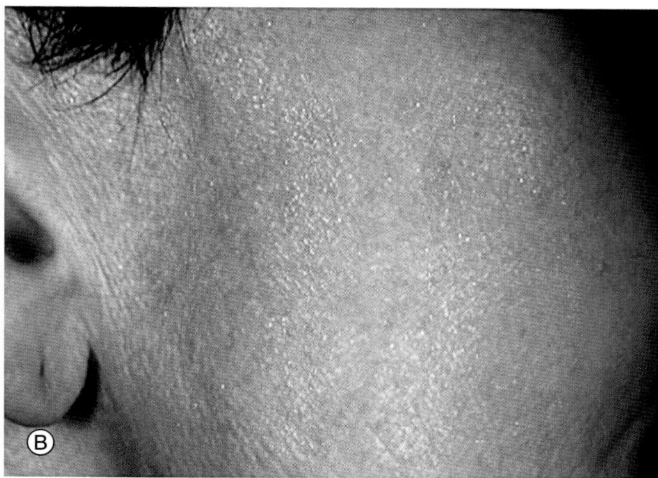

Figure 39.13 Facial venulectasia (A) before and (B) after one treatment with a long-pulsed Nd:YAG laser. (Courtesy of Altus Laser Corp.)

transient thrombosis.[114] The 532-nm KTP laser produces excellent results for the treatment of facial telangiectasia in one to three treatment sessions.[115,116] Contiguous laser pulses are applied directly over the vessels, with additional pulses, if necessary, to achieve visible vessel blanching. Treatment parameters used for telangiectases are pulse durations of 15–40 msec with spot sizes of 2–4 mm and fluences of 10–16 J/cm^2. Some of the KTP systems are equipped with cooled sapphire handpieces that enable easy gliding of the laser tip over the skin, when used with cold gel, and relatively painless treatment.

Long-pulsed Nd:YAG lasers (Fig. 39.13), used with spot sizes of 1–3 mm and fluences of 120–250 J/cm^2 also produce excellent results for facial telangiectases without purpura production.[117,118] With the use of higher fluences, proper skin cooling and avoidance of pulse stacking are necessary to prevent epidermal damage, particularly around the nasal ala. The long pulsed Nd:YAG lasers are particularly useful for the treatment of the larger caliber paranasal vessels that often require multiple, repetitive treatments with the shorter wavelength lasers (Fig. 39.14).

Venulectasia, commonly seen on the lateral cheeks following rhytidectomy, often usually clear in one treatment session. Visible facial veins have also been treated with Nd:YAG lasers, but extreme caution must be exercised to avoid laser exposure within the orbital rim with this deeply penetrating wavelength. The IPL devices also clear facial telangiectases, but multiple treatment sessions may be necessary.[119] In most patients, adequate clearance of facial telangiectases is achieved in an average of two treatment sessions using the 530–750 nm filter with a 14 msec pulse duration and fluences of 12–14 J/cm^2 (Agneta Troilius MD, personal observation). This can also be shown with telangiectases on the body (Fig. 39.15).

Facial erythema

Facial erythema with or without associated telangiectasia is a common cosmetic concern. The erythema is usually a manifestation of rosacea or a flushing or blushing disorder. Effective treatment can be achieved with the pulsed dye, pulsed KTP, and pulsed Nd:YAG lasers, and IPL sources, using large spot sizes to avoid reticulation.[120,121] Purpura-

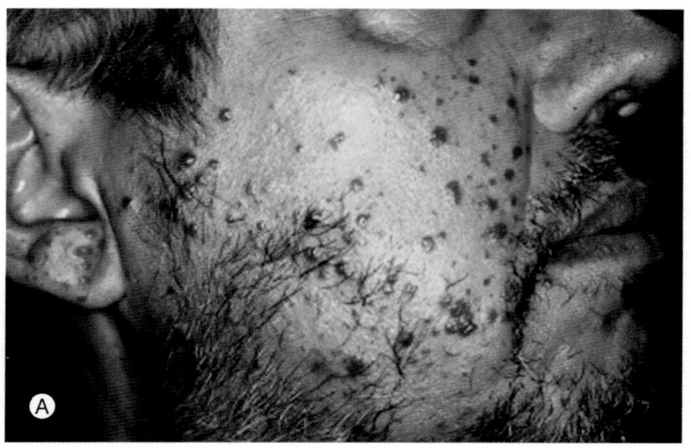

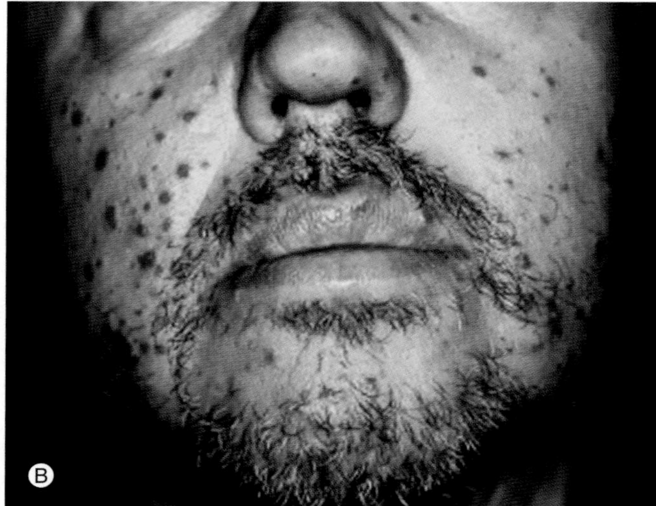

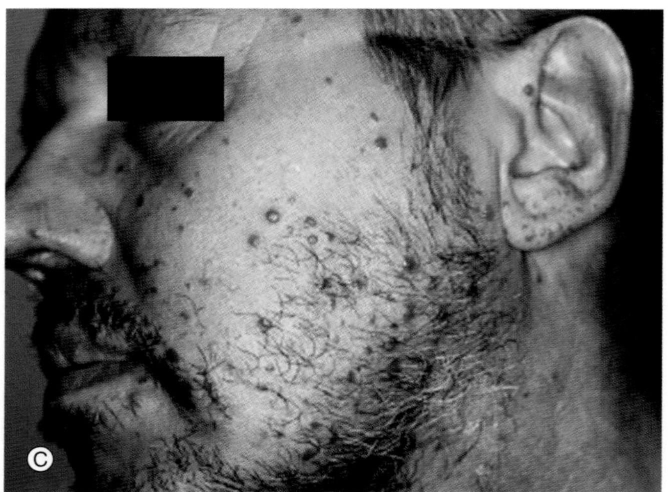

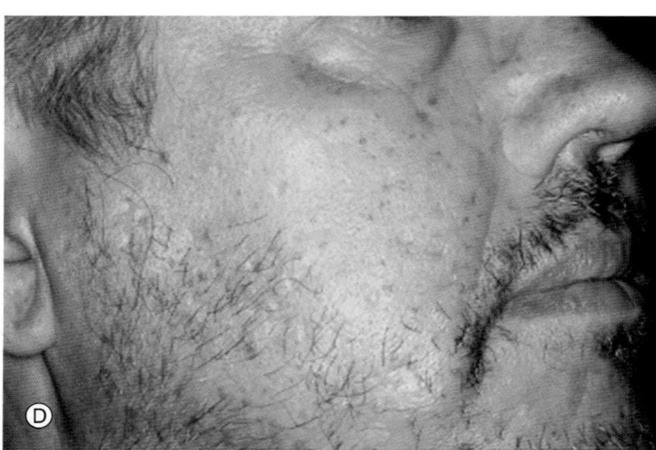

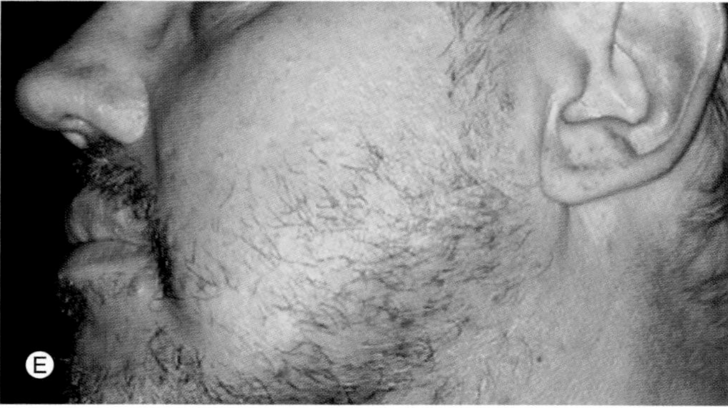

Figure 39.14 Spontaneously bleeding Osler-Rendu-Weber syndrome (hereditary hemorrhagic telangiectasia) (A–C) before and (D–E) after treatment with 532 nm Versapulse Help G, 4 mm spot, 30 ms, and 18 J with cooling.

free treatment is possible with all these laser systems, including the newer pulsed dye lasers used with 6–10-msec pulse durations, and the IPL devices. Multiple treatment sessions (two to six) may be necessary to achieve good clinical results. An improvement in associated symptoms such as warmth and burning usually accompanies the reduction in erythema.

The pulsed dye lasers are used with a 10 mm spot. Fluences of 4.0–5.0 J/cm^2 are used with the 585-nm, 0.45-msec laser. Fluences of 6.0–7.5 J/cm^2 are used with the 595-nm laser with pulse durations of 1.5–6.0 msec. The longer pulse durations do not produce purpura, but require two to three laser passes for equivalent efficacy. The KTP and Nd:YAG lasers are used with millisecond duration pulses, larger spot sizes, and a painting technique for this purpose.

Poikiloderma

Poikiloderma is treatable with lasers and light sources. Poikiloderma of Civatte is relatively common in fair-skinned, actinically-damaged individuals. Clinically, poikiloderma appears as a combination of telangiectasia, irregular pigmentation, and atrophic changes. The treatment of this diffuse condition is best accomplished using the pulsed dye lasers (Fig. 39.16) or IPL devices with large spot sizes to

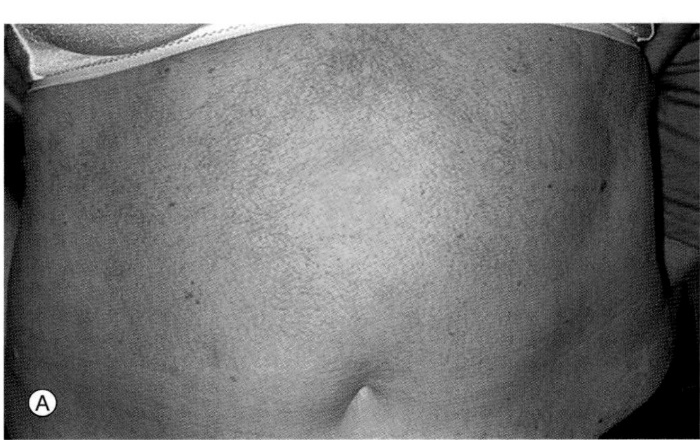

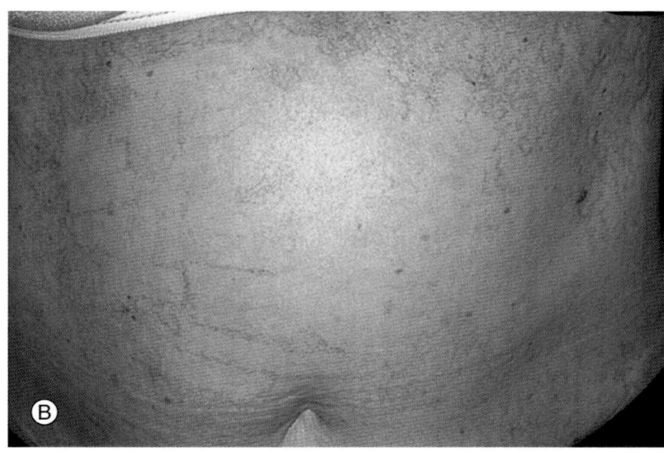

Figure 39.15 General essential telangiectases on the body before (A) and after (B) one IPL (Ellipse, Danish Dermatologic Development, Hoersholm, Denmark) treatment with 530–750 nm, 13 J, and 14 ms. Leftover telangiectases are seen where there had been no overlapping of the crystals.

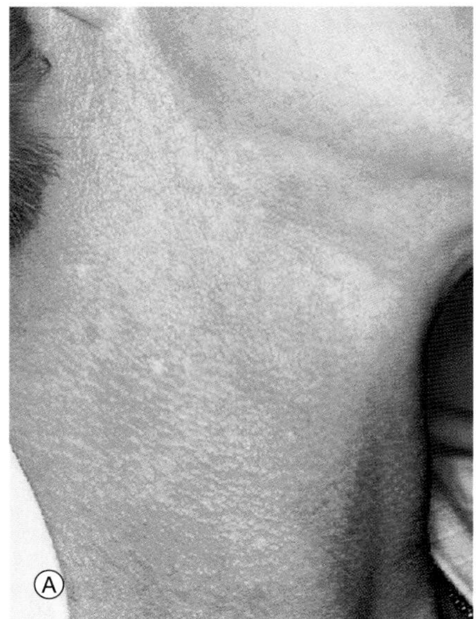

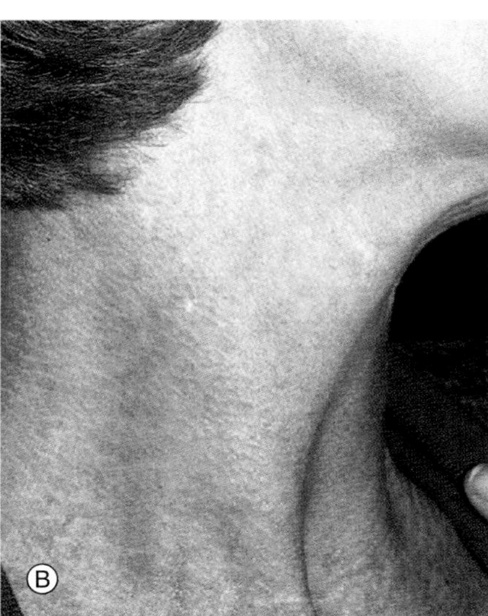

Figure 39.16 Poikiloderma of Civatte (A) before and (B) after treatment with a 10-msec pulsed dye laser used with cryogen cooling. (Courtesy of Stephen Eubanks and Candela Laser Corp.)

avoid reticulation.[44,122,123] Overly aggressive treatment with any laser or light source can produce atrophy and hypopigmentation. Treatment should not be performed on individuals with suntanned skin because this will increase the risk of epidermal damage and hypopigmentation; treatment should be delayed for a minimum of 4 weeks following sun exposure.

Compared to the treatment of telangiectasia, fluences should be lowered by approximately 25–30% to avoid adverse effects. The 585 nm, 0.45-msec pulsed dye laser is used with a 7-mm spot and fluence of 5–6 J/cm^2 or 10 mm spot and fluences of 3–4 J/cm^2. The 595-nm, 1.5-msec laser with cryogen cooling is used with a 10-mm spot and fluence of 5–6 J/cm^2. Treatment of poikiloderma using the 6–10-msec pulsed dye lasers appears to achieve equivalent results to the shorter pulsed systems without the development of purpura. Contiguous laser pulses are applied with minimal overlap. The Lumenis IPL is used with a 515–550-nm cut-off filter, double pulses of 2–4 msec, and a fluence of 20–24 J/cm^2 with a thin layer of a gel applied to the skin surface. The DDD IPL system is used with a 530–750-nm filter, a single 14-msec pulse and a fluence of 12–14 J/cm^2 with good results. Erythema and edema may be present for 2–3 days after treatment. The axis of the rectangular spot should be alternated with each treatment to reduce the risk of reticulation.

Hypertrophic and erythematous scars

Pulsed dye laser therapy can be used to improve erythematous and hypertrophic scars. Clinical response rates are from 57% to 83%.[124–126] The pulsed dye laser reduces erythema by eliminating the underlying dilated microvasculature. Scar height and skin surface texture changes are improved, presumably by altering collagen production (Fig. 39.17). Multiple treatment sessions are often necessary, particularly with thicker scars, and adjunctive treatment with intralesional corticosteroid injections is useful. The best results are

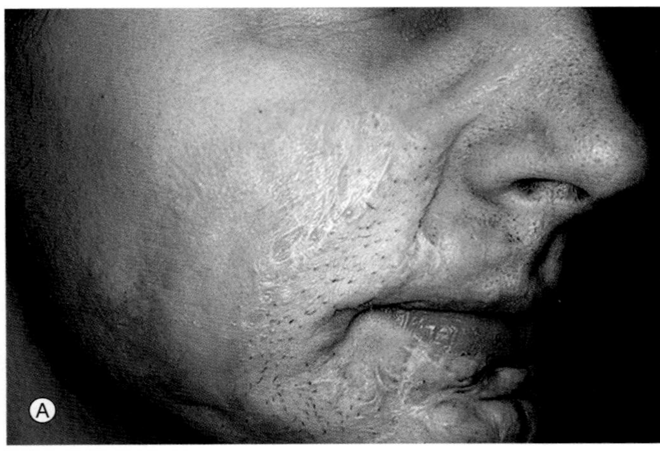

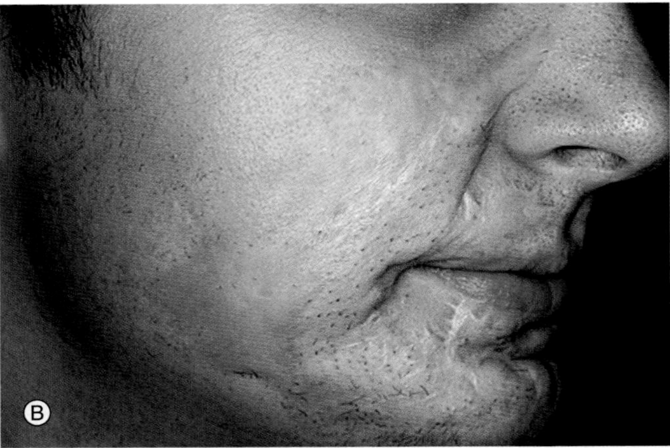

Figure 39.17 Scarring after a severe chemical burn (A) before and (B) after one carbon dioxide skin resurfacing (Ultrapulse, Santa Clara, CA) and three pulsed dye laser treatments with low fluences (SPTL 1B, Candela, Wayland, MA).

achieved using the 585 or 595 lasers with a 10-mm spot sizes and fluences of 4–5 J/cm^2 without skin cooling and 5–7 J/cm^2 with skin cooling. Treatment intervals are typically 6–8 weeks in duration.

Striae distensae

Low-fluence pulsed dye laser therapy also improves the appearance of striae.[127] Striae rubra shows the best response, and can sometimes be entirely eliminated with early laser intervention. The skin textural irregularities in striae alba can be improved with pulsed dye laser treatment and other nonablative lasers and light sources. The mechanism of improvement is presumed to be via fibroblast activation and induction of collagen production. Treatment fluences are used just at or below the purpura threshold – 3.5–4.5 J/cm^2 are used with the 585-nm, 0.45-msec pulsed dye laser with a 10 mm spot. The 595-nm, 1.5-msec laser is used with a 10-mm spot fluence of 5.0–5.5 J/cm^2, in conjunction with cryogen cooling. Pulses are applied in a contiguous pattern. Three to five treatment sessions are usually required, and are performed at 6–8-week intervals. Vascular treatment improves textural irregularities in striae, but has no effect on the hypopigmentation. Treatment is therefore only useful in individuals with type I or II skin, where the textural changes predominate rather than the dyspigmentation. Excimer lasers and narrow band UVB light sources have been used to repigment striae, but upwards of ten treatments are required, and the results are shortlived.

Warts

Pulsed dye lasers effectively treat cutaneous lesions of human papillomavirus, including condyloma acuminata, plantar warts, periungual warts, flat warts, and verrucae vulgaris.[128] The mechanism of improvement appears to be via thermal alteration of the virally-infected tissue.[129] Laser treatment appears to be more effective than conventional wart therapy, and carries a minimal risk of scarring, even when used for deep plantar warts, and subungual and periungual lesions. Treatments are performed using the 585- or 595-nm pulsed dye laser at 0.45 or 1.5 msec using a 5- or 7-mm spot at fluences of 6.0–9.0 J/cm^2 without cooling, following paring of hyperkeratotic lesions. Recalcitiant warts require three to four repetitive treatments at 3–4-week intervals. Uncomplicated warts usually respond in one session.

■ PREOPERATIVE PREPARATION

Anesthesia

Vascular lasers and light sources produce a brief stinging or burning sensation. Most patients tolerate treatment with minimal anesthesia requirements. Cumulative laser pulses may produce increasing discomfort in some patients. Young children or adults with larger lesions may require topical anesthetics, such as EMLA (a eutectic mixture of prilocaine and lidocaine), LMX 4 (Ferndale Laboratories Inc), or Betacaine (Theraderm, Tampa, FL). Topical anesthetic preparations should be washed off several minutes before treatment to reduce vasoconstriction and avoid interference with light transmission. Local anesthesia with lidocaine or nerve blocks was often used in the past for the treatment of facial PWS, but is generally unnecessary with the availability of epidermal cooling methods and topical anesthetic preparations. Intravenous sedation or general anesthesia is usually reserved for children who require immobilization or highly anxious patients with extensive lesions.

■ TECHNIQUES AND POSTOPERATIVE CARE

Laser and IPL safety procedures

The treatment room should be free of all reflective surfaces, and windows should be covered. The door must bear a 'laser-in-use' label and be locked from within. Flammable anesthetic gases or materials may not be present. All personnel in the treatment room and the patient must wear laser surgery glasses that specifically absorb the wavelength being used. Treatment around the eyes requires intraocular metal eye shields, which are placed after instillation of an ophthalmic topical anesthetic agent. The IPL should not be used to treat within the orbital rim, and the beam should always be directed away from the orbit when treating in the eye region.

The pulsed dye laser is capable of igniting a fire in the presence of oxygen and nitrous oxide. Leakage of gases from the edge of the face mask has been reported to ignite the hairs.[77,130] The safest way to deliver inhalational anesthetics is by endotracheal intubation or by using a laryngeal mask airway which fits over and seals the larynx. Wet drapes are placed around the mouth area and tubing, and the surrounding hair-bearing skin is lubricated with a nonflammable ointment such as Surgilube (Fougera, Melville, NY).

Pulsed dye lasers

The pulsed dye laser is used with short pulse durations (0.45 and 1.5 msec) to treat PWS. Test areas are performed in areas representative of the entire lesion using several fluences to determine the parameters with the best therapeutic responses, and are evaluated after 4–6 weeks. Beam profiles vary among the different manufacturers of the pulsed dye laser, and laser fluences should be chosen accordingly. Larger spot sizes produce greater efficacy and reduce the potential for reticulation between treatment sessions. Using the chosen fluence, pulses are applied contiguously or with minimal overlap. Treatment fluences can be increased with the use of air cooling and cryogen cooling devices that are equipped with these systems.

Shorter pulse durations (<3 msec) produce an immediate ashen-gray color with laser impact. Gradually, the color turns to purplish red. The pupura is most intense with the 0.45-msec pulse duration and requires approximately 10 days for resolution. At 1.5 msec, the purpura usually resolves within 1 week.

With the use of epidermal cooling techniques, blistering or crusting is a rare event. If crusting occurs, a topical antibiotic ointment is applied twice daily until it resolves. When prolonged purpura or crusting does occur, subsequent treatment fluences should be lowered accordingly.

At pulse durations greater that 6 msec, purpura is not produced. Laser pulse impact results in urticarial papules that resolve over several hours. Head elevation and the application of ice packs immediately after laser treatment help reduce swelling. Most vascular lesions require multiple treatment sessions. PWS and hemangiomas may require multiple laser treatments. Small telangiectases usually clear after one treatment, but larger vessels may require two or more treatments. High-flow spider angiomas may require several treatments, and may recur months later. Treatment results are assessed at 4–6 weeks after treatment and repeat treatment is performed if necessary.

Sunscreen with a sun protection factor (SPF) greater than 15 should be used before treatment if the patient is at risk of developing a sun tan. Suntanned individuals should not be treated because of the risk of epidermal absorption of energy and the subsequent development of hypopigmentation. Sunscreen with a SPF over 15 should be used for 4 weeks following treatment to prevent the development of postinflammatory hyperpigmentation.

Pulsed dye laser light at wavelengths of 585–600 nm is well absorbed by melanin. Suntanned patients and individuals with skin types V and VI should not be treated with these wavelengths because of the risk of epidermal damage and the possibility of a poor clinical response as a result of shielding of the laser light by epidermal melanin. Individuals with skin type IV and the absence of a sun tan can be safely treated with higher fluences and skin cooling.

Pulsed KTP lasers

Facial telangiectasias and erythema respond well to millisecond-duration KTP lasers. The spot sizes and fluences used vary depending on the size of the vessel. Individual vessels are best traced with the laser beam, applying contiguous or minimally overlapping pulses. Facial erythema is treated using large spot sizes (4–10 mm) with a painting technique. Pulse stacking should be avoided because of the risk of epidermal damage. Patients with suntans or skin types V and VI cannot be treated with this wavelength because of its strong absorption by melanin.

Anesthesia is rarely required for these procedures. ELMA or LMX 4 or 5 may be used for those patients sensitive to pain. Lasers that are equipped with a sapphire chill tip require direct contact with the skin, but only minimal pressure is applied to avoid blanching of the vessels. A thin layer of gel applied to the skin surface prevents fogging of the lens and facilitates movement of the handpiece over the skin. Treatment of nonplanar surfaces of the face such as the nasal ala and alar crease requires extreme care to maintain skin contact with the chilled handpiece.

Following treatment, there may be erythema and urticarial edema of the treated skin lasting up to 24 hours. Cool dressings, ice, and the application of a mid-potency topical corticosteroid immediately after treatment will reduce the redness and swelling. Crusting develops infrequently, but may occur with overly aggressive therapy, treatment with improper cooling techniques, or treatment of tanned skin. When crusting occurs, a topical antibiotic ointment should be applied twice daily until it resolves. Sunscreen should be used for 4–6 weeks after laser treatment.

Scarring rarely occurs, but may result from excessive fluence, overlapping of laser pulses, or inadequate skin cooling, which results in nonselective thermal damage to the epidermis or dermis.

Pulsed Nd:YAG lasers

Several new Nd:YAG lasers are now available that use high fluences and millisecond pulse durations. The Nd:YAG laser can be used with large spot sizes (usually 10 mm) in a painting technique for the treatment of facial erythema. Individual telangiectases are treated with smaller spot sizes (1–3 mm) and high fluences (>100 J/cm^2). Larger paranasal and preauricular telangiectases and venulectases, which may not clear with green and yellow light, respond well to this wavelength because of its great depth of penetration. Extreme caution must be exercised when treating vessels in the periorbital region with the 1064 nm wavelength. Internal metal ocular shields are used and treatment is limited to outside the orbital rim.

Anesthesia is usually not required, but treatment of larger caliber vessels may be more painful. The use of topical anesthetic creams such as EMLA or LMX 4 or 5 may be necessary.

Nonspecific thermal damage leading to scarring may result from treating with excessive fluence or overlapping of laser pulses. The nasal ala and alar crease are difficult anatomic areas to treat. Proper skin cooling techniques are required, whether it is cryogen spray or contact cooling. When a chilled sapphire handpiece is being used, a thin layer of gel is applied to the skin surface and there should be good contact with the cooling plate.

Erythema and urticarial edema develop after treatment and last up to 24 hours. Cold dressings or ice, and the application of a mid-potency corticosteroid immediately after treatment will minimize these changes. Antibiotic ointment should be applied twice daily if crusting develops. Sun protection is required for 4–6 weeks after treatment.

Intense pulsed light sources

IPL devices deliver noncoherent, pulsed white light from 515 to 1200 nm, with multiple pulse modes and fluences ranging from 3 to 90 J/cm^2, through a large rectangular footprint. The range of wavelengths delivered can be altered with a series of cut-off filters to correspond with the patient's skin type and lesion depth.

Shorter wavelength filters (515 nm) and the single pulse mode are used on skin type I with fine, superficial vessels. Larger and deeper vessels are treated with longer cut-off filters (570 or 590 nm) and double or triple pulse modes. Longer wavelengths and longer interpulse delays are used for darker skin types.

A thick layer of cool water gel is applied to the skin surface. The light guide is gently placed over the skin on top of a 1–2-mm layer of gel. Test spots with increasing fluences should be performed carefully inspecting for signs of epidermal damage until the desired endpoint of faint erythema is achieved. The individual pulses are applied contiguously with minimal overlap. A second pass may be performed with the axis of the light guide perpendicular to the first pass, to avoid reticulation.

Reactive erythema and edema develop for 24 hours after treatment. Cold dressings, ice, and the application of a mid-potency corticosteroid reduce the burning, erythema, and edema. As with the laser devices, suntanned individuals should not be treated, and sunscreen with an SPF over 15 should be used for 4 weeks before and after light treatment.

■ SUMMARY

Appropriate treatment begins with the correct diagnosis. Parameters must be set according to the type of lesion being treated. Vessel size and depth, blood flow, skin type, melanin, recent suntan, natural behavior, recurrence rate and autoimmune disease are just a few parameters that one has to assess when treating vascular lesions with lasers or IPL. In future we need to find ways to treat deeper vascular lesions with less risk of scarring.

■ REFERENCES

1. Dixon JA, Huether SE, Rotering SH. Hypertrophic scarring in argon of port-wine stains. Plast Reconstr Surg 1984; 73:771–779.
2. Hobby LW. Argon laser treatment of superficial vascular lesions in children. Lasers Surg Med 1986; 6:16.
3. Brauner GJ, Schliftman A. Laser surgery for children. J Dermatol Surg Oncol 1987; 13:178.
4. Brauner G, Schliftman A, Cosman B. Evaluation of argon laser surgery in children under 13 years of age. Plast Reconstr Surg 1991; 87:37.
5. Anderson RR, Parrish JA. Selective Photothermolysis: precise microsurgery by selective absorption of pulsed radiation. Science 1993; 220:524–527.
6. Levine VJ, Geronemus RG. Adverse effects associated with the 577- and 585-nanometer pulsed dye laser in the treatment of cutaneous vascular lesions: a study of 500 patients. J Am Acad Dermatol 1995; 32:613–617.
7. Geronemus R, Kauvar A. Pulsed dye laser treatment of hemangiomas. Plast Reconstr Surg 1996; 97:1302–1303.
8. Einstein A. Zur Quantentheorie der Strahlung. Physiol Z 1917; 18:121–8.
9. Van Gemert MJ, Jacques SL, Sterenborg HJ, Star WM. Skin Optics, IEEE Trans Biomed Eng 1989; 36:1146.
10. Anderson RR, Parrish JA. The optics of human skin. J Invest Dermatol 1981; 77:13.
11. Anderson R. Laser-tissue interactions. In: Goldman M, Fitzpatrick R, eds, Cutaneus laser surgery: the art and science of selective photothermolysis. St Louis: Mosby; 1994.
12. Van Germert MJ, Henning JP. A model approach to laser coagulation of dermal vascular lesions, Arch Dermatol Res 1981; 270:429.
13. Anderson RR Parrish JA. Microvasculature can be selectively damaged using dye lasers: a basic theory and experimental evidence in human skin, Lasers Surg Med 1981; 1:263.
14. Garden JM, Tan OT, Kerschmann R, et al. Effect of dye laser pulse duration on selective cutaneous vascular injury. J Invest Dermatol 1986; 87:653.
15. Garden JM, Polla LL, Tan OT. The treatment of port-wine stains by the pulsed dye laser: analysis of pulse duration and long-term therapy, Arch Dermatol 1988; 124:889.
16. Morelli JG, Tan OT, Garden J, et al. Tunable dye laser (577 nm) Treatment of PWS. Lasers Surg Med 1986; 6:94.
17. Dierickx CC, Casparian JM, Venugopalan V, Farinelli WA, Anderson RR. Thermal relaxation of port wine stain vessels probed in vivo: the need for 1–10-msec laser pulse treatment. J Invest Dermatol 1995; 105:709–14.
18. Keijzer M, Pickering JW, van Germert MJ. Laser beam diameter for port wine stain treatment. Lasers Surg Med 1991; 11:601.
19. Ross E, Farinelli W, Skrobal M, Anderson R. Spot size effects on purpura threshold with the pulsed dye laser (Abstract). Lasers Surg Med 1995; 7(suppl):54.
20. Grossman MC, Dierickx C, Farinelli W. Damage to hair follicles by normal-mode ruby laser pulses. J Am Acad Dermatol 1996; 35:889.
21. Nelson JS, Milner TE, Anvari B, et al. Dynamic epidermal cooling in conjunction with laser induced photothermolysis of port wine stain blood vessels. Lasers Surg Med 1996; 19:224.
22. Anvari B, Milner TE, Tanenbaum BS, et al. Selective cooling of biological tissues: application for thermally medicated therapeutic procedures. Phys Med Biol 40:241, 1995.
23. Anvari B, Tanenbaum BS, Milner TE, et al. A theoretical study of the thermal response of skin to cryogen spray cooling and pulse laser irritation: implication for treatment of port wine stain birthmarks. Phys Med Biol 1995; 40:1451. (Published erratum in Phys Med Biol 1996; 41:1245.)
24. Chess C, Chess Q. Cool laser optics treatment of large telangiectasia of the lower extremities. J Dermatol Surg Oncol 1993; 19:74.
25. Greve B, Hammeres S, Raulin C. The effect of cold air cooling on 585 nm pulsed dye laser treatment of port wine stains. Dermatol Surg 2001; 27:633–636,
26. Anderson RR, Parrish JA, Microvasculature can be selectively damaged using dye lasers: a basic theory and experimental evidence in human skin. Lasers Surg Med 1981; 1:263.
27. Pickering JW, Botler Ph, Ring BJ, et al. Thermal profiles of blood vessels heating by laser. Australas Phys Eng Sci Med 1989; 12:11–15.
28. Paul BS, Anderson RR, Jarve J, Parrish JA. The effect of temperature and other factors on selective microvascular damage caused by pulsed dye laser. J Invest Dermatol 1983; 83:333
29. Garden JM, Tan OT, Kerschmann R, et al. Effect of dye laser pulse duration on selective cutaneous vascular injury. J Invest Dermatol 1986; 87:653
30. Garden JM, Polla LL, Tan OT. The treatment of port-wine stains by the pulsed dye laser: analysis of pulse duration and long-term therapy. Arch Dermatol 1988; 124:889.

31. Morelli JG, Tan OT, Garden J, et al. Tunable dye laser (577 nm) treatment of port-wine stains. Lasers Surg Med 1986; 6:94.

32. Tan OT, Morrison P, Kurban AK. 585 nm for the treatment of port-wine stains. Plast Reconstr Surg 1990; 86:1112.

33. Tan OT, Murray S, Kurban AK. Action spectrum of vascular specific injury using pulsed irradiation. J Invest Dermatol 1989; 92:868.

34. Tong AK, Tan OT, Boll J, et al. Ultrastructure: effects of melanin pigment on target specificity using a pulsed dye laser (577 nm). J Invest Dermatol 1987; 88:747.

35. Alster TS, Wilson F. Treatment of port-wine stains with the flashlamp-pumped pulsed dye laser: extended clinical experience in children and adults. Ann Plast Surg 1994; 32:478–484.

36. Ashinoff R, Geronemus RG. Flashlamp-pumped pulsed dye laser for port wine stains in infancy: Earlier versus later treatment. J Am Acad Dermatol 1991; 24:467–472.

37. Garden JM, Polla LL, Tan OT. The treatment of PWS by the pulsed dye laser. Arch Dermatol 1988; 124:889–896.

38. Goldman MP, Fitzpatarick RE, Ruiz–Esparza J. Treatment of PWS (capillary malformation) with the flashlamp-pumped pulsed dye laser. J Pediatr 1993; 122:71–77.

39. Tan OT, Stafford TJ. Treatment of port-wine stains at 577 nm: clinical results. Med Instr 1987; 21:218–221.

40. Reyes BA, Geronemus R. Treatment of port-wine stains during childhood with the flashlamp–pumped pulsed dye laser. J Am Acad Dermatol 1990; 23:1142–1148.

41. Dierickx CC, Casparian JM, Venugoplan V, et al. Thermal relaxation of port–wine stain vessels probed in vivo: the need for 1–10 millisecond laser pulse treatment. J Invest Dermatol 1995; 105:709.

42. Dierickx C, Farinelli W, Anderson R. Clinical and histologic response of blood vessels to long (msec) laser pulses (Abstract). Lasers Surg Med Suppl 1996; 6:48.

43. Kauvar ANB. Long–pulse, high energy pulsed dye laser treatment of PWS and hemangiomas. Lasers Surg Med 1997; 9(suppl):36.

44. Raulin C, Greve B, Grema H. IPL technology: A review. Lasers Surg Med 2003; 32:78–87.

45. Jacobs A, Walton RG. The incidence of birthmarks in the neonate. Pediatrics 1976; 58:218–222.

46. Smoller BR, Rosen S. Port-wine stains: a disease of altered neural modulation of blood vessels. Archer Dermatol 1986; 122:177–179.

47. Rydh M, Malm M, Jernbeck J, et al. Ectatic blood vessels in port wine stains lack innervations. Possible role in pathogenesis. Plast Reconstr Surg 1991; 87:419–442.

48. Enjolras O, Riche MC, Merland JJ. Facial port-wine stains and Sturge-Weber syndrome. Pediatrics 1985; 76:48–51.

49. Fishman SJ, Mulliken JB. Vascular anomalies: a primer for pediatricians. Pediatr Clin N Am 1998; 45:1455–1477.

50. Geronemus RG, Ashinoff R. The medical necessity of evaluation and treatment of port-wine stains. J Dermatol Surg Oncol 1991; 17:76–79.

51. Enjolras O, Mulliken JB. The current management of vascular birthmarks. Pediatr Dermatol 1993; 10:311–333.

52. Troilius A, Wrangsjo B, Ljunggren B. Potential psychological benefits from early treatment of port-wine stains in children. Br J Dermatol 1998; 139:59–65.

53. Troilius A, Wrangsjo B, Ljunggken B. Patients with port wine stains and their psychosocial reactions after photothermolytic treatment. Dermatol Surg 2000; 26:190–196.

54. Tan OT, Sherwood K, Gilchrest BA. Treatment of children with PWS using the flashlamp-pulsed tunable dye laser. N Engl J Med 1989; 320:416–421.

55. Ashinoff R, Geronemus RG. Treatment of a port-wine stain in a black patient with the pulsed dye laser. J Dermatol Surg Oncol 1992; 18:147.

56. Aguilar G, Diaz SH, Lavernia EJ, Nelson JS. Cryogen spray cooling efficiency: improvement of port wine stain laser therapy through multiple intermittent cryogen spurts and laser pulses. Lasers Surg Med 2002; 31:27–35.

57. Ashinoff R, Geronemus RG. Capillary hemangiomas and treatment with the flashlamp-pumped pulsed dye laser. Arch Dermatol 1991; 127:202–205.

58. Bernstein LJ, Grossman MC, Kauvar ANB, Geronemus RG. The effect of 10 mm versus 5 mm and 7 mm on pulsed dye laser treatment of PWS and hemangiomas. Lasers Surg Med 1996; 8(suppl):32.

59. Kauvar ANB. Long-pulse, high energy pulsed dye laser treatment of PWS and hemangiomas. Lasers Surg Med 1997; 9(suppl):36.

60. Waldorf HA, Alster TS, McMillan K, Kauvar ANB, Geronemus RG, Nelson JS. Effect of dynamic cooling on 585–nm pulsed dye laser treatment of port-wine stain birthmarks. Dermatol Surg 1997; 23:657–662.

61. Kauvar ANB, Grossman MC, Bernstein LJ, Kovacs SO, Quintana AT, Geronemus RG. The effects of cryogen spray cooling on pulsed dye laser treatment of vascular lesions. Lasers Surg Med 1998; 10(suppl):211.

62. Geronemus R, Quintana A, Lou W, Kauvar ANB. High fluence modified pulsed dye laser photocoagulation with dynamic cooling of port wine stains in infancy. Arch Dermatol 2000; 136:942–943.

63. Kauvar ANB, Lou WW, Zelickson B. Effect of cryogen spray cooling on 595-nm, 1.5-msec pulsed dye laser treatment of port wine stains. Laser Surg Med 2000; (suppl 12):24.

64. Renfro L, Geronemus RG. Anatomical differences of port-wine stains in response to treatment with the pulsed dye laser. Arch Dermatol 1993; 129:182–188.

65. Kauvar ANB, Renfro LR, Geronemus RG. Anatomical differences of PWS located in the trunk and extremities in response to treatment with the pulsed dye laser. Laser Surg Med 1994; 14:47.

66. Nguyen CM, Yohn JJ, Huff C, et al. Facial port wine stains in childhood: prediction of the rate of improvement as it functions of the age of the patient, size and location of the port wine stain and the number of treatments with the pulsed dye (585 nm) laser. Br J Dermatol 1998; 138:821–825.

67. Fikerstrand EJ, Svaasand LO, Kopstad G, et al. Laser treatment of port wine stains: therapeutic outcome in relation to morphological parameters. Br J Dermatol 1996; 134:1039–1043.

68. Fikerstrand EJ, Svaasand LO, Kopstad G, et al. Photothermally induced vessel-wall necrosis after pulsed dye laser treatment; lack of responses in port-wine stains with small sized or deeply located vessels. J Invest Dermatol 1996; 107:671–675.

69. Motley RJ, Lanigan SW, Katugampola GA. Videomicroscopy predicts outcome in treatment of port wine stains. Arch Dermatol 1992; 133:921–922.

70. Kauvar ANB, Geronemus RG, McDaniel DH. Pulsed dye laser treatments improve persistent port-wine stains. Dermatol Surg 1995; 21:515–521

71. Tan OT, Sherwood K, Gilchrest BA. Treatment of children with port-wine stains using the flashlamp-pulsed tunable dye laser. N Engl J Med 1989; 320:416–421.

72. Morelli JG, Weston WL. Pulsed dye laser treatment of port-wine stains in children. In: Tan OT, ed. Management and treatment of benign cutaneous vascular lesions. Philadelphia: Lea & Febiger; 1992.

73. Alster TS, Wilson F. Treatment of port-wine stains with the flashlamp–pumped dye laser: extended clinical experience in children and adults. Ann Plast Surg 1994; 32:474.

74. Fitzpatrick RE, Lowe NJ, Goldman MP, Borden H, Behr KL, Ruiz-Esparza J. Flashlamp-pumped pulsed dye laser treatment of port-wine stains. J Dermatol Surg Oncol 1994; 20:743–748.

75. Van der Horst CM, Koster PHL, de Borgie CAJM, Bossuyt PMM, van Gemert MJC. Effect of the timing of treatment of port-wine stains with the flash-lamp-pumped pulsed-dye laser. New Engl J Med 1998; 338:1028–1033.

76. Sherwood KA, Tan OT. Treatment of a capillary hemangioma with the flashlamp pumped dye laser. J Am Acad Dermatol 1990; 22:136–137.

77. Waldorf HA, Kauvar ANB, Geronemous RG. Remote fire with the pulse dye laser: risk and prevention. J Am Acad Dermatol 1996; 34:503–506.

78. Bjerring P, Christiansen K, Troilius A. Intense pulse light source for the treatment of dye laser resistant port wine stains. J Cosmetic Laser Ther 2003; 5:7–13.

79. Raulin C, Gerve B, Gvema H. IPL technology: a review. Laser Surg Med 2003; 32:78–87.

80. Raulin C, Schroeter CA, Wess RA, et al. Treatment of port wine stains with a non coherent pulsed light source. A retrospective study. Arch Dermatol 1999; 135:679–683.

81. Chowdhury MM, Harris S, Lanigan SW. Potassium titanyl phosphate laser treatment of resistant port wine stains. Br J Dermatol 2001 144:814–817.

82. Chotzen VA, McClaren M, Kilmer SL. Treatment of bulky congenital vascular malformations with long pulsed lasers. Laser Surg Med 2002; 14(suppl):231.

83. Jacobs AH, Walton RG. The incidence of birthmarks in the neonate. Pediatrics 1976; 58:218–222.

84. Amir J, Metzker A, Krikler R, Reisner SH. Strawberry hemangiomas in preterm infants. Pediatr Dermatol 1986; 3:331–332.

85. Finn MC, Glowacki J, Mulliken JB. Congenital vascular lesions: clinical application of a new classification. J Pediatr Surg 1983; 18:894–899.

86. Mulliken JB, Glowacki J. Hemangiomas and vascular malformations in infants and children: a classification based on endothelial characteristics. Plast Reconstr Surg 1982; 69:412–420.

87. Finn M, Glowacki J, Mulliken JB. Congenital vascular lesions: clinical approach of a new classification. J Pediatr Surg 1983; 18:894.

88. Waner M, Suen JY. The natural history of hemangiomas. In: Waner M, Suen JY, eds. Hemangiomas and vascular malformations of the head and neck. New York: John Wiley & Sons 1999; 13–45.

89. Waner M, Suen JY. A classification of congenital vascular lesions. In: Waner M, Suen JY, eds. Hemangiomas and vascular malformations of the head and neck. New York: John Wiley & Sons 1999; 1–12.

90. Dixon JA, Huether SE, Rotering SH. Hypertrophic scarring in argon laser treatment of port-wine stains. Plast Reconstr Surg 1984; 73:771–779.

91. Sherwood KA, Tan OT. Treatment of a capillary hemangioma with the flashlamp pumped dye lasers. J Am Acad Dermatol 1990; 22:136–137.

92. Ashinoff R, Geronemus RG. Capillary hemangiomas and treatment with the flashlamp-pumped pulsed dye laser. Arch Dermatol 1991; 127:202–205.

93. Landthaler M, Hohenleutner U, El-Raheem Ta. Laser therapy of childhood hemangiomas. Br J Dermatol 1995; 133:275–281.

94. Scheepers JH, Quaba AA. Does the pulsed tunable dye laser have a role in the management of infantile hemangiomas? Observations based on 3 years' experience. Plast Reconstr Surg 1995; 95:305–312.

95. Garden JM, Bakus AD, Paller AS. Treatment of cutaneous hemangiomas by the flashlamp-pumped pulsed dye laser: prospective analysis. J Pediatr 1992; 120:555–560.

96. Waner M, Dinehart S, Mallory SB, Suen JY. Laser photocoagulation of superficial proliferating hemangiomas. J Dermatol Surg Oncol 1994; 20:1–4.

97. Barlow RJ, Walker NPJ, Markey AC. Treatment of proliferative hemangiomas with the 585 nm pulsed dye laser. Br J Dermatol 1996; 134:700–704.

98. Poetke M, Philipp C, Berlien HP. Flashlamp-pumped pulsed dye laser for hemangiomas in infancy; treatment of superficial vs mixed hemangiomas. Arch Dermatol 2000; 136;628–632.

99. Lou WW, Kauvar ANB, Geronemus R. Treatment of hemangiomas with 595nm, 1.5 millisecond pulsed dye laser (Scleroplus laser, Candela, Wayland, MA). Laser Surg Med 2000; (suppl 12):25.

100. Chang CJ, Kelly KM, Nelson JS. Cryogen spray cooling and pulsed dye laser treatment of cutaneous hemangiomas. Ann Plast Surg 2001; 46:577–583.

101. Margileth AM and Museles M. Cutaneous hemangiomas in children: diagnosis and conservative management. JAMA 1965; 194:523–526.

102. Esterly NB. Cutaneous hemangiomas, vascular stains and malformations, and associated syndromes. Curr Probl Pediatr 1996; 26:3–39.

103. Kim HJ, Colombo M, Frieden I. ulcerated hemangiomas: clinical characteristics and response to therapy. J Am Acad Dermatol 2001; 44:962–972.

104. Morelli; JG, Tan OT, Weston WL. Treatment of ulcerated hemangiomas with the pulsed turnable dye laser. Am J Dis Child 1991; 145:1062–1064.

105. Morelli JG, Tan OT, Yohn JJ, Weston Wl. Treatment of ulcerated hemangiomas in infancy. Arch Pediatr Adolesc Med 1994; 148:1104–1105.

106. Mathewson K, Coleridge-Smith P, O'Sullivan J, Northfield T, Brown S. Biological effects of intrahepatic neodymium:yttrium-aluminum-garnet laser photocoagulation in rats. Gastroenterology 1987; 93:550–557.

107. Berlien HP, Muller G, Waldschmidt J. Lasers in pediatric surgery. In: Angerpointer TA, Gauderer MWL, Hecker WCH, et al, eds. Progress in pediatric surgery. New York: Springer–Verlag 1990; 6–22.

108. Waner M. Laser resurfacing and the treatment of involuting hemangiomas (Abstract). Lasers Surg Med 1996; 8(suppl):40.

109. Alster TS. Cutaneous resurfacing with CO_2 and erbium: YAG lasers: preoperative, intraoperative, and postoperative considerations. Plast Reconstr Surg 1999; 103:619–632.

110. Kauvar ANB, Waldorf H, Geronemus RG. Char free tissue ablation: a comparative histopathological analysis of new carbon dioxide laser systems. Dermatol Surg 1996; 22:343–348.

111. Kauvar ANB, Geronemus R. Histology of laser resurfacing. Dermatol Clin 1997; 15:459–169.

112. Kauvar ANB. Laser skin resurfacing: perspectives at the millennium. Dermatol Surg 2000; 26:174–177.

113. West TB, Alster TS. Comparison of the long-pulsed dye and KTP lasers in the treatment of facial and leg telangiectasia. Dermatol Surg 1998; 24:221–226.

114. Iyengar V, Chatrath V. Rohrer TE. Does pulse stacking improve results for treatment with variable pulsed dye lasers? Lasers Surg Med 2003; (suppl 15):80.

115. Adrian RM, Taughetti EA. Long pulse 532 nm laser treatment of facial telangiectasia. Dermatol Surg 1998; 24:71–74

116. Goldsberg DJ, Meine JG. Treatment of facial telangiectases with the diode-pumped frequency-doubled Q-switched Nd:YAG laser. Dermatol Surg 1998; 24:828–832.

117. Eremia S, Li CY. Treatment of face veins with a cryogen spray variable pulse width 1064 nm Nd:YAG laser: a prospective study of 17 patients. Dermatol Surg 2002; 28:220–223.

118. Major A, Brazzin B, Compolmi P, et al. Nd:YAG 1064 nm laser in the treatment of facial and leg telangiectasias. J Eur Acad Dermatol Venereol 2001; 15:559–565.

119. Bierring P, Christiansen K, Troilius A. Intense pulsed light source for treatment of facial telangiectasias. J Cosmet Laser Ther 2001; 3:169–173.

120. Angermeier MC. Treatment of facial vascular lesions with intense pulsed light. J Cutan Laser Ther 1999; 1:95–100.

121. Lowe NJ, Behr KL, Fitzpatrick R, et al. Flashlamp pumped dye laser for rosacea-associated telangiectasia and erythema. J Dermatol Surg Oncol 1991; 17:522–525.

122. Wheeland RG, Applebaum J. Flashlamp-pumped pulsed dye laser therapy for poikiloderma of Civatte. J Dermatol Surg Oncol 1990; 16:12–16.

123. Weiss RA, Goldman MP, Weiss MA. Treatment of poikiloderma of Civatte with an intensed pulsed light source. Dermatol Surg 2000; 26:823–827.

124. Alster TS, Kurban, A K, Grove GL, et al. Alteration of argon laser-induced scars by the pulsed dye laser. Lasers Surg Med 1993; 13:368–373.

125. Alster TS . Improvement of erythematous and hyypertrophic scars by the 585 nm flashlamp–pumped pulsed dye laser. Ann Plast Surg 1994; 32:186–190.

126. Alster TS, Williams CM. Improvement of hypertrophic and keloidal median sternotomy scars by the 585 nm flashlamp-pumped pulsed dye laser: a controlled study. Lancet 1995; 345:1198–1200.

127. McDaniel DH, Ash K, Zukowski M. Treatment of stretch marks with the 585 nm flashlamp-pumped pulsed dye laser. Dermatol Surg 1996; 22:332–337.

128. Kauvar ANB, Geronemus RG, McDaniel DH. Pulsed dye laser treatment of warts. Arch Fam Med 1995; 4:1035–1040.

129. Ross EV, McDaniel DH, Anderson RR, Kauvar ANB, Geronemus RG. Pulsed dye (585 nm) treatment of warts: a comparison of single versus multiple pulse techniques examining clinical response, fast infrared thermal camera measurements, and light electron microscopy. Lasers Surg Med 1995;(suppl 7):59.

130. Fretkin S, Beeson WH, Hanke CW. Ignition potential of the 585 nm pulsed dye laser. Dermatol Surg 1996; 22; 699–702.

40 Endovenous Ablation Techniques with Ambulatory Phlebectomy for Varicose Veins

Mitchel P Goldman MD and Robert A Weiss MD

Summary box

- Reflux from valvular incompetence in the great saphenous vein (GSV) or lesser saphenous vein must be eliminated along with treating distal or branch varicose veins.
- Failure to treat proximal incompetence results in vein recurrence.
- Endoluminal radiofrequency (RF) or infrared laser energy can effectively seal and eliminate abnormal saphenous veins.
- Ambulatory phlebectomy (AP) is performed on distal or branch varicose veins in combination with endovenous techniques.
- Tumescent anesthesia is effective and necessary for both AP and endoluminal RF and laser closure.

Historical vignette

- Ambulatory phlebectomy first described by dermatologist Robert Muller in the 1950s
- 1966—Ambulatory phlebectomy is introduced to the French Society of Phlebology by Dr Muller
- 1990—Tumescent anesthesia introduced for AP (Goldman and Weiss)
- 1996—Ambulatory phlebectomy is added to American College of Phlebology core curriculum
- 1998—Ambulatory phlebectomy is added to American Society for Dermatologic Surgery curriculum
- 1998—First clinical trials of endoluminal RF closure
- 1999—First clinical trials of endoluminal laser closure

INTRODUCTION

Dermatologic surgery in the 21st century has evolved into a minimally invasive subspecialty. Procedures once performed under general anesthesia, those in which large incisions are made to remove diseased tissue, are being replaced by techniques that allow the treatment of damaged organ systems to occur with small incisions under local anesthesia. This chapter discusses two methods whereby a patient's damaged and improperly functioning axial (saphenous) vein is treated without requiring its removal—endovenous closure through the thermal action of RF or a number of infrared laser wavelengths.[1]

The first attempt to minimize surgery for varicose vein disease was ligation of a GSV and distal varicose veins treated with either sclerotherapy or AP. This simple technique was demonstrated to result in a high degree of recurrence secondary to re-anastomosis through hemodynamically significant perforator veins present, extending from the knee to the groin which were not eliminated during the surgical procedure.[1–5] Evidence has shown that for maximal improvement in abnormal venous hemodynamics and resolution of symptoms, complete removal of the GSV from the saphenofemoral junction (SFJ) to the knee is required after ligating the SFJ.[5] This surgical procedure is most often performed under general anesthesia with patients usually requiring up to 6 weeks to return to normal activities.

Two methods of endovenous ablation have evolved. One utilizes RF energy delivered through a specially designed endovenous electrode to accomplish controlled heating of the vessel wall, causing vein shrinkage or occlusion by contraction of venous wall collagen. With worldwide clinical experience on over 50 000 patients since 1998 (data on file at VNUS Medical, San Jose, CA), this technique has been added to the armamentarium of ways to eliminate saphenous venous reflux (also known as axial or truncal reflux). Along with development of RF closure, endoluminal laser delivery has followed closely as a technique to effectively close axial veins through dispersed thermal damage, collagen contraction of the vessel wall with subsequent thrombosis and resorption of the damaged vein. Endovenous occlusion techniques are less invasive alternatives to saphenofemoral ligation or stripping. They are typically performed under local anesthesia with patients returning to normal activities within 24–48 hours. Ambulatory phlebectomy may be required as an adjunctive procedure to eliminate branch varicosities.

Although the concept of endovenous elimination of reflux is not new, previous approaches have relied on electrocoagulation of blood. This resulted in thrombus occluding the vein with a high potential for recanalization of thrombus. The concept of application of RF directly to tissue, rather than blood has been effectively applied to ablate abnormal conduction pathways for arrhythmias.[1] This concept was conceived for the treatment of varicose veins because venous occlusion with RF by the mechanism of venous blood coagulation has been previously reported, but was not very successful.[6,7] Another technique that preceded the modern application of RF to vein walls is endovascular diathermic vessel occlusion, in which a spider-shaped intravascular electrode produced venous occlusion by electrocoagulation with minimal perivascular damage.[8]

■ PREOPERATIVE PREPARATION

Doppler ultrasound

Historically, the handheld Doppler ultrasound is the main tool used to detect reverse flow or reflux in the superficial venous system. Smaller and less expensive duplex ultrasound units are slowly replacing handheld Doppler units as the primary tool. Optimal frequencies for examining superficial vessels (1–2 cm below the skin) are 8–10 MHz, whereas deeper vessels require a lower frequency of 4–5 MHz. Blood flow in the venous system is very slow and intermittent; it is mainly pulsed by calf muscle contraction. To generate an audible signal of flow, a maneuver such as manual compression of the calf (simulating a muscle contraction) must be performed by the examiner. When compression is released, gravitational hydrostatic pressure causes reverse flow to cease within 0.5–1.0 seconds when valves are competent, but a long flow sound is audible when valves are incompetent.

The Doppler examination is usually performed with the patient standing or sitting, because gravitational hydrostatic pressure enhances the volume and velocity of retrograde flow and makes it easier to detect. To perform this test, the nondominant hand gently squeezes the leg well below (distal compression) or above (proximal compression) the point of auscultation, while the dominant hand holds the Doppler transducer lightly against the skin. Under normal circumstances, flow should be heard only during active distal compression. Flow that is heard during proximal compression or immediately after the release of distal compression is retrograde flow—a clear sign of incompetent valves. This technique is best demonstrated in a hands-on workshop.

Duplex ultrasound

Duplex ultrasound is a dual mode diagnostic tool that allows a timed pulse echo to be superimposed with the continuous wave Doppler. This allows one to 'see' the anatomy in two dimensions while superimposing the Doppler flow sounds as a visual color marker. Reflux can then be shown visually rather than purely audibly as with the handheld. The site of origin of reflux can be pinpointed. Duplex is very useful to guide placement of access sheaths before endovenous treatment by direct visualization of the vein entry point.

Structures that absorb, transmit, or scatter ultrasonic waves appear as dark areas, while structures that reflect the waves back to the transducer appear as white areas in the image. Therefore a needle placed in the vessel appears as brightly white. Vessel walls reflect ultrasound, while blood flowing in a vessel absorbs and scatters ultrasound in all directions, thus the normal vessel appears as a dark-filled white-walled structure.

Reflux is diagnosed by placing the transducer over the vessel in a longitudinal plane and observing the Doppler signal in the vessels while (with the free hand) the distal leg is momentarily compressed and released to increase the cephalad movement of blood. Functional valves permit flow only in the antegrade direction, but normal vessels can demonstrate brief retrograde flow due to slow closing of valves. Retrograde flow of greater than 1 second duration is considered to be pathologic reflux, and reflux that lasts more than 2 seconds is hemodynamically significant. A Valsalva maneuver is a valuable way to demonstrate incompetence of the terminal valve at the SFJ.

In the longitudinal view, the origin of the GSV is identified as it courses off the common femoral vein (Fig. 40.1). Two valves can be visualized in the proximal GSV. The first is the terminal valve, which lies at the vein origin. Distal augmentation or Valsalva for Doppler flow reveals competence or incompetence of this valve. The second valve, about 2 cm below the subterminal valve, is examined in the same fashion. Major tributaries that empty into the region of the SFJ can be identified here. These include the circumflex, pudendal, epigastric, and others. Most commonly seen is the epigastric because of its size and position in the same plane as the termination of the GSV. Once incompetence of the GSV has been demonstrated with reverse flow, the patient is a candidate for an endovenous ablation technique.

■ TECHNIQUES AND POSTOPERATIVE CARE

Radiofrequency

Directing RF energy into tissue to cause its destruction is potentially safer and more controllable than other mechanisms. Delivered in continuous or sinusoidal wave mode, there is no stimulation of neuromuscular cells using a high frequency between 200 and 3000 kHz. For vein treatment, 500 kHz is typically utilized. The mechanism by which RF current heats tissue is resistive (or ohmic) heating of a narrow rim (<1 mm) of tissue that is in direct contact with the electrode. If tissue is heated above 100 °C, it begins to boil, so the optimal target temperature is 70–90 °C.[9] By carefully regulating the degree of heating or watts with microprocessor control, subtle gradations of either controlled collagen contraction or total thermocoagulation of the vein wall can be achieved.

When the RF catheter is pulled through the vein while feedback-controlled with a thermocouple, the surgeon can heat the vein wall to a specified temperature. This is a relatively safe process because the temperature increase remains localized in a narrow rim around the active electrode. This requires close, stable contact between the active electrode and the vessel wall. By limiting temperature to

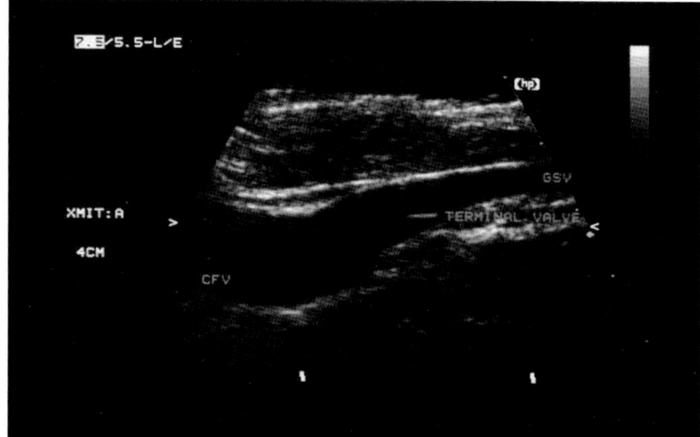

Figure 40.1 Appearance of the SFJ in longitudinal view using duplex ultrasound. The position of the valve at the SFJ is shown by the arrow. (CFV, common femoral vein; GSV, great saphenous vein.)

85–90 °C, boiling, vaporization and carbonization of the tissues is avoided and debris does not accumulate on the electrode tips.[10] Using thermography, it has been demonstrated that heating the electrodes to a target temperature of 85 °C results in a rapid drop-off to approximately 65 °C about 1 mm away from the electrode tip.

An additional safety factor is that electrode-mediated RF vessel wall ablation is a self-limiting process. As shrinkage and compaction of tissue occurs, there is a decrease in impedance that decreases heat generation.[11] Alternatively if clot builds up on the electrodes, blood is heated instead of tissue, and there is a marked rise in impedance (resistance to RF). The RF generator can be programmed to rapidly shutdown when impedance rises, thus ensuring minimal heating of blood but efficient heating of the vein wall.

Recent technological advances include the introduction of specific application electrodes and accompanying microprocessor controlled systems to precisely monitor the electrical and thermal effects applied to the venous system. The primary device is the Closure catheter (VNUS Medical Technologies, San Jose, CA). Bipolar electrodes are placed in contact with the vein wall. When the vein wall contracts the electrodes fold up within the vein, which allows maximal physical contraction (Fig. 40.2). Selective insulation of the electrodes results in a preferential delivery of the RF energy to the vein wall and minimal heating of the blood within the vessel. Animal experiments demonstrate endothelial denudation along with denaturation of media and intramural collagen with a subsequent fibrotic seal of the vein lumen (Fig. 40.3).

Five years of clinical experience suggest that the Closure procedure is very effective at occluding saphenous veins and abolishing reflux. This observation is supported by numerous studies following patients treated with either a percutaneous approach or with a vein cut-down allowing access of the Closure catheter to treat the proximal GSV with phlebectomy of the distal GSV and tributaries.

RF closure standard technique

Several studies have detailed the outcome of RF endovenous occlusion.[12–15] In multicenter studies involving up to 324 patients with up to 2-year follow-up, the vein occlusion rate at 1-year examination was 91.6% from nine centers and

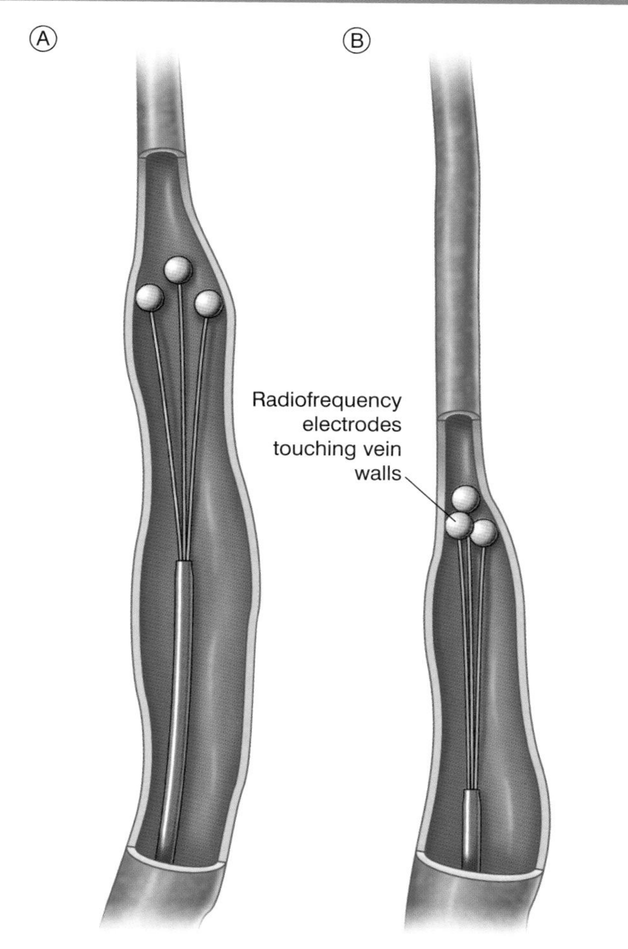

Figure 40.2 Design of the radiofrequency catheter. (Modified with permission from VNUS Medical, San Jose, CA.)

81.9% from 14 centers; 49 patients were followed up at 2 years with duplex scans and showed a 89.8% closure rate. There was a 3% incidence of paresthesia which could be reduced to 1.6% when treatment was confined to the thigh rather than extended below the knee. Two limbs (0.8%) developed scarring from skin burns and three patients developed a deep venous thrombosis (DVT), with one embolism. The reason for the increase in adverse effects appears to be the use of general anesthesia without tumescent anesthesia by most of the surgeons.

Sybrandy and Wittens from Rotterdam reported 1-year follow-up of 26 patients treated with VNUS Closure.[16] They reported five patients with postoperative paresthesia of the saphenous nerve and one with a cutaneous burn, resulting in an overall complication rate of 23%. They concluded that reduction of complications is possible by limiting treatment below the knee. A total of 88% of their patients had a totally occluded GSV. The probable reason for the increase in adverse effects was their use of a spinal anesthesia instead of the recommended tumescent anesthesia. In addition they treated patients from the ankle proximally, which exposed the GSV within the calf to heat from the RF catheter.

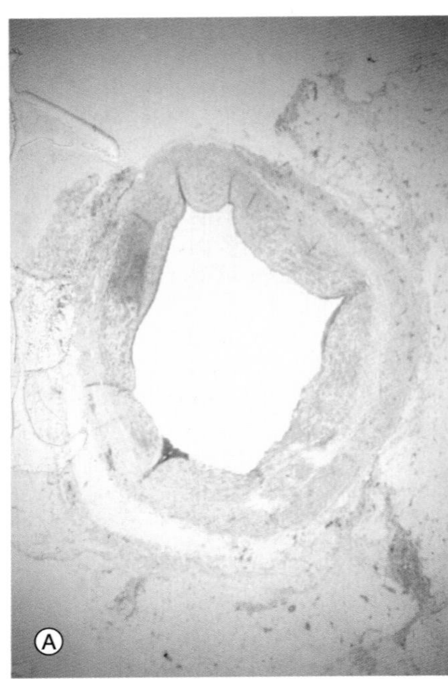

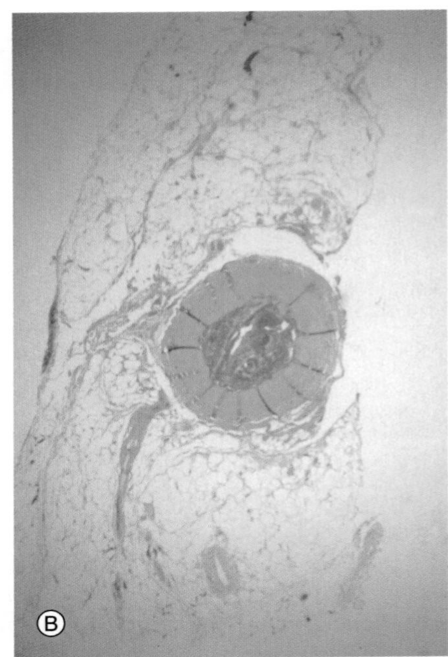

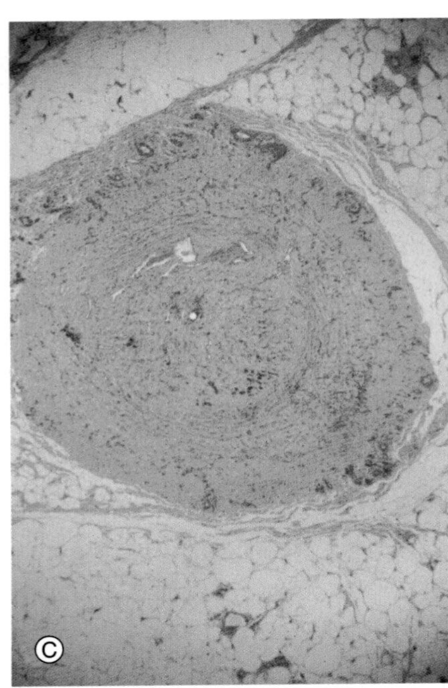

Figure 40.3 Histology of radiofrequency occlusion of sheep saphenous vein. (A) Before treatment. (B) Acute histologic features of radiofrequency occlusion. (C) At 6 weeks demonstrating fibrous cord with no recanalization. (Hematoxylin and eosin 100×.) (Courtesy of VNUS Medical, San Jose, CA.)

Another report describes two episodes of DVT in 29 patients treated with the RF Closure.[17] The surgeons treated the patients with a groin incision and passage of the catheter from the groin downward. The authors do not report the type of anesthesia used or the length of vein treated. It is presumed that patients were not ambulatory and treated under general anesthesia.

We conclude from these reports and our experience that the most important factors in minimizing side-effects are the use of tumescent anesthesia and immediate ambulation. General anesthesia is the most significant risk factor in developing DVT and the failure to use tumescent local anesthesia the major risk factor for developing skin burns. It is also advisable to limit RF treatment to the GSV segment above the knee to minimize the risk of paresthesia resulting from injury to the saphenous nerve. In our experience, using tumescent anesthesia in every case and using the technique on nonsedated patients, only two patients have developed focal numbness 4 cm in diameter on the lower medial leg. Numbness resolved within 6 months in both patients. No skin injury or thrombus has been observed in any of our patients.

For clinical symptoms, the RF endovenous occlusion procedure rapidly reduces patient pain, fatigue, and aching correlating with a reduction in CEAP (clinical, etiological, anatomical, pathophysiological) clinical class for symptoms and clinical severity of disease (Table 40.1). When patients have had surgical stripping of the opposite leg, the degree of pain, tenderness, and bruising have been far greater on the leg treated by stripping. Early side-effects of the Closure technique (during the first year of implementation) included thrombus extension from the proximal GSV in 0.8%, with one case of pulmonary embolus; skin burn (before the tumescent anesthesia technique) in 2.5%; clinical phlebitis at 6 weeks in 5.7%; temporary quarter-sized areas of paresthesia in 18% with most of these occurring immediately above the knee and resolving within 6 months to 1 year.

Table 40.1 CEAP class description with findings after endovenous RF occlusions

CEAP clinical class	Description
0	Asymptomatic
1	Telangiectasia
2	Varicose veins
3	Edema
4	Skin changes
5	Healed venous ulcer
6	Venous ulcer

Mean CEAP Class of Closure study population

	Before treatment	6 weeks	6 months
	2.0	0.5	0.5
	3.0	0.5	0.3
	4.0	2.3	1.4
Total	2.4	0.8	0.6

With more experience and proper technique including the use of tumescent anesthesia, the incidence of these complications has become negligible. Endovenous RF occlusion compares favorably to traditional surgery of ligation and stripping of similar size saphenous veins. The side-effects of DVT and nerve injury are far lower than traditional ligation and stripping.

Our experience at 5 years indicates a 92% long-term effectiveness rate. This is a more favorable outcome on varicose veins than traditional surgery. Patients remain symptom-free and the remnants of the GSV are not visible under duplex ultrasound. Furthermore, results observed at 6 months are indicative of the long-term results. We typically see resolution of all the major tributaries at the SFJ except for the superficial epigastric, which continues to empty superiorly into the common femoral vein. We believe that there is a high margin of safety by maintaining flow through this tributary. The high flow rate appears to diminish the possibility of extension of any thrombus (in the unlikely event that this would occur) from the GSV. In our personal experience, thrombus has not been observed.[15]

RF closure with ligation and/or AP

Closure combined with AP can be very effective in eliminating saphenous reflux along with varicose tributaries. Our experience with over 100 patients with RF combined with AP confirms this. The technique of RF plus AP and ligation is initiated by AP in the mid-thigh to expose the GSV.[18] For preparation, varicose veins are marked with the patient standing and again with the patient lying down in the operative position using transillumination.[19] After appropriate marking, the area surrounding the GSV and distal tributaries to be treated is infiltrated with 0.1% lidocaine tumescent anesthesia (see also Chapter 3). The amount of tumescent fluid ranges from 400 to 800 mL with a typical lidocaine dose of 4–8 mg/kg. The GSV can be accessed through a 2–3-mm incision in the medial mid-thigh usually 20 cm inferior to the SFJ or can be cannulated by duplex ultrasound guidance in the lower third of the thigh. The GSV is then treated with VNUS Closure and the varicose tributaries removed with a standard AP technique. A ligature is placed on the exposed portion of the GSV. Ninety-five percent of all patients can resume all pre-operative activities within 24 hours. Approximately 90% of patients experience elimination of leg pain and fatigue.

Technique of closure without phlebectomy

The patient undergoes the same diagnostic process as previously outlined. Presently, patients with reflux in the greater or lesser saphenous vein are candidates if the vein size does not exceed 1.6 mm. Reflux may originate at the junction itself and this region may be safely treated. After eliciting a detailed history as with all the other venous procedures, and describing alternative procedures such as ligation and stripping in detail, the patient signs the appropriate consent form (Fig. 40.4).

The procedure begins with the vein to be treated marked on the skin using duplex ultrasound. An appropriate entry point is selected. This is usually just below where reflux is no longer seen in the GSV or where the vein becomes too small to cannulate with a 16-gauge introducer set. For most patients in our series this is at a point just above or below the knee along the course of the GSV. Before proceeding; the patient's feet are wrapped in warm material or socks to minimize vasoconstriction, a heating pad is placed under the thigh and a small amount of 2% nitroglycerin ointment (Nitro-Bid, E Fougera & Co, Melville, NY) is rubbed onto the intended entry point to minimize vasoconstriction during the initial cannulation process.

The patient is then prepped and draped, after which 0.1 mL of 1% lidocaine without epinephrine (adrenaline) is injected at the pre-marked site. It is important that the patient experience no pain during cannulation because the perception of pain will cause an immediate and rapid contraction of the saphenous vein. It may not be possible to continue without a venous cut-down after a contraction occurs.

To place the sheath, a guidewire must be first inserted through the 16-gauge needle initially inserted into the skin. The guidewire is passed approximately 5 cm into the GSV. The sheath is then threaded along the guidewire, piercing the skin; its progress is followed by duplex until it is seen firmly placed within the lumen of the GSV. After establishing the intraluminal placement of the sheath, the guidewire is carefully withdrawn.

Once the sealed sheath is placed into the vein, the Closure catheter is then inserted. Others prefer initializing entry via a venous cut-down or pulling of the vein close to the surface with a phlebectomy hook.

The Closure catheter, with a diluted heparin solution or normal saline running slowly through a central lumen, is now advanced through the sheath. Its progress up the GSV is monitored by duplex. If the catheter gets hung-up on a valve or slight bend of the GSV no additional force is used or perforation will occur. Rather the catheter is twisted or external pressure is applied to the leg to change the shape of the GSV. Sometimes the patient must rotate the leg.

Once the Closure catheter is in place, tumescent anesthesia (consisting of 0.1–0.2% lidocaine neutralized to pH 7 with sodium bicarbonate) is injected between the skin and the cannulated GSV. Duplex monitoring of the anesthesia injection is recommended to ensure that the tumescent fluid is injected into the perivenous space and that the fascial planes are pushed away from the vein (Fig. 40.5).

The final check of the position of the catheter is made with duplex ultrasound. The tip is positioned with the electrodes deployed. The tips of the electrodes are placed so that they align 1 cm below the base of the terminal valve cusps. Once positioned, an impedance and temperature check is performed to make sure the catheter is functioning properly. Impedance of the vein wall should be between 200 and 350 ohms and the thermocouple should transmit a baseline temperature of 28–35 °C. The temperature may be substantially lower than body temperature as a result of the perivenous tumescent anesthesia.

The RF is then applied; the physician monitors the temperature and impedance. Within 15 seconds the target temperature of 85 °C should be reached. If this does not occur, the catheter has been mistakenly advanced too far into the common femoral vein. Impedance would most likely rise quickly and the RF generator shut down automatically.

After the target temperature is achieved, one waits 30 seconds and then the slow withdrawal of the catheter begins. The first 4 cm are treated over 3 minutes but then the catheter is advanced at a rate of 2.5 cm/minute. If the patient experiences a sudden sharp pain the catheter is pulled 1 mm past that point quickly to minimize the possibility of nerve injury. If a sharp drop in temperature occurs during pullback, this most likely represents a large branch point or perforator and the catheter is temporarily held in place for 5–10 seconds until 85 °C is reached again.

When the catheter has been pulled back to the introducer sheath site, impedance will suddenly rise and the RF generator will cut off. Duplex ultrasound of the SFJ should reveal no flow except the superficial epigastric emptying into the common femoral vein. The GSV should be more echogenic with thicker appearing walls. If flow is seen in the GSV, the procedure may be repeated assuming the Closure catheter can be advanced past the treated distal segment. If one cannot pass the catheter easily no repeat treatment is performed because vein perforation would be the most likely outcome of such an attempt.

Consent form for vein Closure^{TM} procedure

PATIENT NAME:.. **DATE:**..

____ **A) AUTHORIZATION FOR VEIN SURGERY**

I hereby authorize.. to perform the Endovenous Ablation procedure on my veins for the purpose of attempting to improve the symptomatology and/or appearance of my legs.

____ **B) ALTERNATIVES**

I understand that alternative treatments for varicose veins exist, including conservative treatments (elastic stockings), sclerotherapy (injection of sclerosing agents into diseased veins), ambulatory phlebectomy (pulling out a short segment of vein) and stripping and vein ligation.

____ **C) RISKS**

The nature of the procedure to be performed has been explained to me, and I understand that among the known risks are bruising, swelling of the leg, and pain. I am aware that in addition to the minor risks specifically described above, there are other risks that may accompany any surgical procedure, such as loss of blood, infection, and inflammation in the venous systems with formation of a thrombus (clot), postoperative bleeding, and nerve trauma that may lead to temporary numbness.

____ **D) ANESTHESIA**

I consent to the local anesthesia, to be administered by.. . I am aware that risks are involved with the administration of local anesthesia, such as allergic or toxic reactions to the anesthetic and cardiac arrest.

____ **E) PROPOSED TREATMENT RESULTS**

I know that the practice of medicine and surgery is not an exact science, and, therefore, reputable practitioners cannot guarantee results. No guarantee or assurance has been given by anyone as to the results that may be obtained. I have had sufficient opportunity to discuss my condition and proposed treatment with the doctor, and all of my questions have been answered to my satisfaction. I believe that I have adequate knowledge on which to base an informed consent to the proposed treatment. I hereby authorize the doctor to perform any other treatment that may be deemed necessary should he/she encounter an unhealthy or unforeseen condition during the course of the procedure. After the endovenous ablation procedure, sclerotherapy can begin at your 6 week follow-up visit. The cost of the endovenous ablation procedure includes <u>one</u> sclerotherapy treatment of veins which are directly related to the vein that is treated with endovenous ablation. Any further treatments or treatment of leg veins which are not related to the vein being treated with endovenous ablation will be charged at the regular practice fee for sclerotherapy. Repeat endovenous ablation procedures using modified parameters may need to be done at the discretion of the doctor.

____ **F) COOPERATION**

I agree to keep the doctor and staff informed of any changes in my permanent address, and I agree to cooperate with them in my after-care. I agree to keep my follow-up appointments at 1 week, 6 weeks, 6 months, and 1 year.

____ **G) PHOTOGRAPHS**

I consent to be photographed before, during, and after the treatment. I understand that these photographs shall remain the property of the doctor and may be published in scientific journals, presented in scientific meeting sessions and/or shown for scientific reasons.

____ **H) INFORMED CONSENT**

I certify that I have read and understand the above consent for surgery. It has been explained to me and I fully understand the inherent potential risks, complications, and results of both the surgical procedure and the anesthetic to be administered. I accept all responsibility for these or any other complications that may arise or result during the surgical procedure(s) to be performed at my request according to this consent and surgical permit.

PLEASE INITIAL EACH PARAGRAPH AND SIGN BELOW

Patient signature .... Date ....

Witness ....

Figure 40.4 Consent form for vein Closure^{TM} procedure.

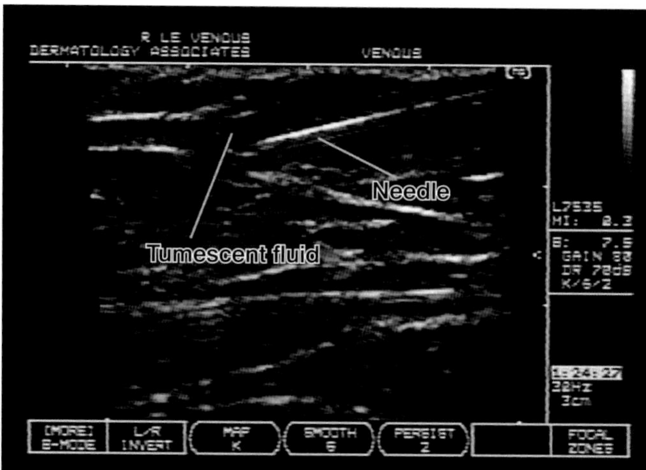

Figure 40.5 Duplex image of tumescent fluid around the GSV.

Technique for closure with AP

After establishing incompetence of the SFJ with duplex and/or Doppler examinations, the patient is asked to stand and the locations of all varicose veins are highlighted with a marking pen. The location of the GSV (which is usually not visible) is marked with either Doppler or duplex control. The patient then lies on the examining table in the operative position and all varicose veins are transilluminated and marked with another marking pen. Confirmation of the location of the GSV in the mid thigh is obtained in the operative position with duplex or Doppler.

The patient is then taken to the operating theater, the leg is prepped with a standard sterile prep and sterile drapes are placed, allowing exposure of the varicose veins including the SFJ and medial thigh. The table is placed in the 30° Trendelenburg position. Tumescent anesthesia is then given as previously described through a 21-gauge spinal needle. Intravenous midazolam (2–3 mg) is sometimes given through a heplock to alleviate patient apprehension. Tumescent anesthesia is given along the entire course of the varicose veins as well as around the GSV both above the facial sheath as well as circumferentially around the GSV within its facial sheath. Typically 750–1000 mL of 0.1% lidocaine with 1 : 100 000 epinephrine (adrenaline) is used averaging between 5–10 mg/kg of lidocaine.

A 2–3-mm incision is then made with a number 11 blade medial to the GSV in the mid-thigh typically 20 cm distal to the SFJ. A number three or number 4 Muller hook is used to grasp the GSV and bring it through the incision. This 'blind' retrieval of the GSV is usually accomplished in less than 1 minute. Hemostats are placed across the exposed GSV and it is ligated. The proximal portion is then opened with two-toothed hemostats. The Closure catheter is then placed into the vein and its tip positioned to within 1–2 cm of the SFJ. Correct tip placement is confirmed by measuring the length of the catheter and with duplex ultrasound. A slow heparin drip is then started and the catheter withdrawn slowly as described above.

After the entire proximal GSV is treated, the distal stump is sometimes ligated with a 3–0 Vicryl suture (Ethicon Inc, Johnson & Johnson Co, Somerville, NJ). The distal GSV and varicose veins are then removed through a series of 2-mm incisions with a standard AP technique.

At the conclusion of the surgery, the entire leg is wrapped in a short stretch compression bandage with copious padding over the varicose veins removed through phlebectomy. No incisions are closed with sutures. The open 2-mm incisions allow for drainage of the anesthetic solution over 24 hours, minimizing bruising. The patient is seen the next day and the compression bandage is removed. The leg is checked for hematoma or other adverse sequelae. All incisions are covered with antibacterial ointment and an adhesive dressing and a 30–40-mmHg graduated stocking is applied.

Postoperative care

Class 2 compression hosiery is worn for 3 days with the percutaneous Closure technique and 7–14 days with the Closure plus phlebectomy technique. Patients will note some bruising from the tumescent anesthesia but very little from RF alone. Anesthesia of the treated portion of the leg may persist for 8–24 hours. To gain experience, we recommend that for the initial cases, one re-evaluates the treated veins at 3 days by duplex ultrasound. This will allow a correlation of results with the pullback rate or any difficulty encountered during the procedure. Once comfortable with the procedure, the physician may want to see the patient for a duplex ultrasound follow-up study at 6 weeks. At that time, any open segments can be treated by duplex-guided sclerotherapy. It has been our experience that when closed at 6 weeks, the GSV will remain closed, fibrosed, and almost indistinguishable from surrounding tissue at 6 months in all cases. Symptom reduction is rapid, with many patients experiencing relief at 3 days, but some not until 6 weeks. Clinical improvement in appearance of varicosities is typically seen within 6 weeks as well (Fig. 40.6). Patient instructions after the Closure technique are very straightforward and include 3 days of compression. All patients are provided with an instruction sheet (Fig. 40.7).

Endoluminal laser ablation

Endovenous laser treatment (EVLT^{TM}) allows delivery of laser energy directly into the blood vessel lumen to produce endothelial and vein wall damage with subsequent fibrosis. It is presumed that destruction of the GSV with laser is a function of thermal destruction. The target for lasers with 810, 940, 980, and 1064-nm wavelengths is intravascular red blood cell absorption of laser energy. The newest wavelength to be studied is 1320-nm, which has allowed the targeting of water only, rather than hemoglobin. The extent of thermal injury to tissue is strongly dependent on the amount and duration of heat the tissue is exposed to. Therefore for the hemoglobin-dependent wavelengths, the amount of residual blood in the vein following tumescent anesthesia is important. However, it is impossible to standardize this.

Moritz and Henriques investigated the time–temperature response for tissue exposed to up to 70 °C.[20] They found that skin can withstand temperature rises for very short exposure times and that the response appears to be logarithmic as the exposure times become shorter. For example, an increase in body temperature to 58 °C will produce cell destruction if the exposure is longer than

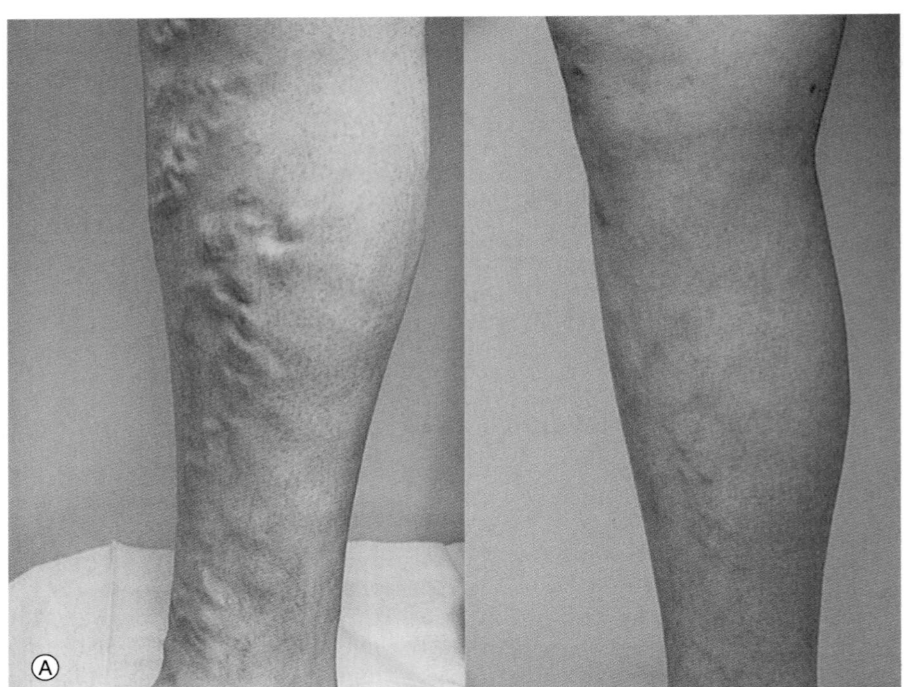

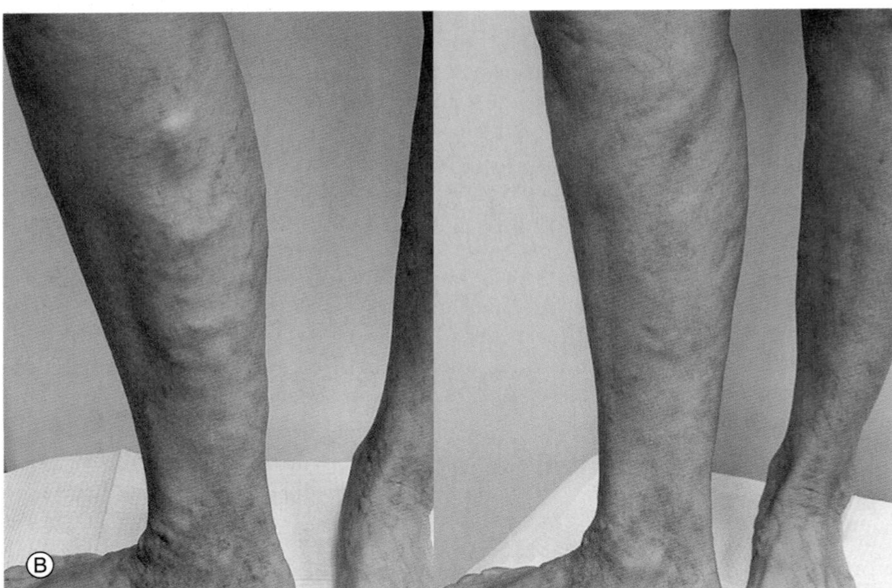

Figure 40.6 (A)–(B) Two cases of right lower leg VNUS Closure (before and after treatment).

10 seconds. Tissues, however, can withstand temperatures up to 70 °C if the duration of the exposure is maintained for less than 1 second. Thus, any tissue injury from brief exposure to temperatures less than 50 °C would be expected to be reversible.

One in-vitro study model has predicted that thermal gas production by laser heating of blood in a 6-mm tube results in 6 mm of thermal damage.[21] These authors used a 940-nm diode laser with multiple 15-J, 1-second pulses to treat the GSV. A median of 80 pulses (range 22–116) were applied along the treated vein every 5–7 -mm. Histologic examination of one excised vein demonstrated thermal damage along the entire treated vein with evidence of perforations at the point of laser application described as 'explosive-like' photodisruption of the vein wall. This produced the homogeneous thrombotic occlusion of the vessel. Because a 940-nm laser beam can only penetrate 0.3-mm in blood,[22] the formation of steam bubbles is the probable mechanism of action. The lack of significant heating of perivenous tissues probably explains the low complication rate.

Initial reports have shown that this technique with an 810-nm diode laser has excellent short-term efficacy in the treatment of the incompetent GSV, with 96% or higher occlusion at 9 months with a less than 1% incidence of transient paresthesia.[23,24] Although most patients experience some degree of postoperative ecchymosis and discomfort, no other major or minor complications have been reported. Our observation has been that postoperative pain and ecchymosis are highest in hemoglobin-dependent wavelengths. Radiofrequency

Postoperative instructions for closure

1. Keep bandage and stockings on until bedtime
If your toes turn blue or feel numb loosen the bandage
If symptoms persist, call the doctor immediately

2. You can resume normal activities today
(walking is okay)

3. You can resume exercising in 3 days
(no weights with the legs for 1 week)

4. You can take a shower tomorrow morning but
no hot baths for 1 week

5. Wear your support hose for 3 days, from first thing in the morning (ideally, take a quick 5-1 minute shower and then put them on before doing the rest of your morning ritual), until last thing at night

6. Schedule the next follow-up visit in 6 weeks

7. Bruising, local swelling and some tenderness are normal after surgery, but please feel free to call the office if you have any questions

Figure 40.7 Postoperative patient instructions for Closure.

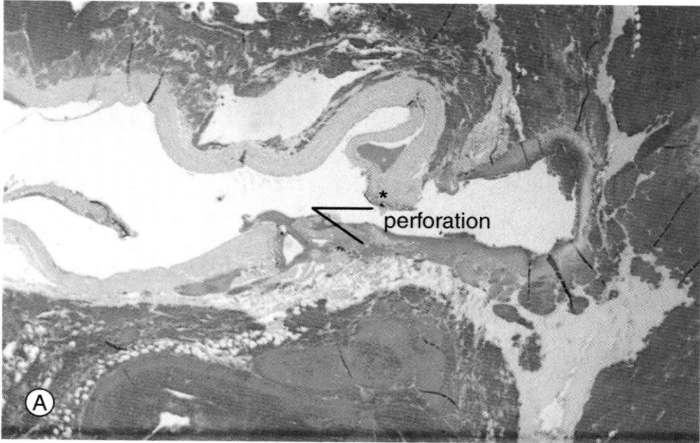

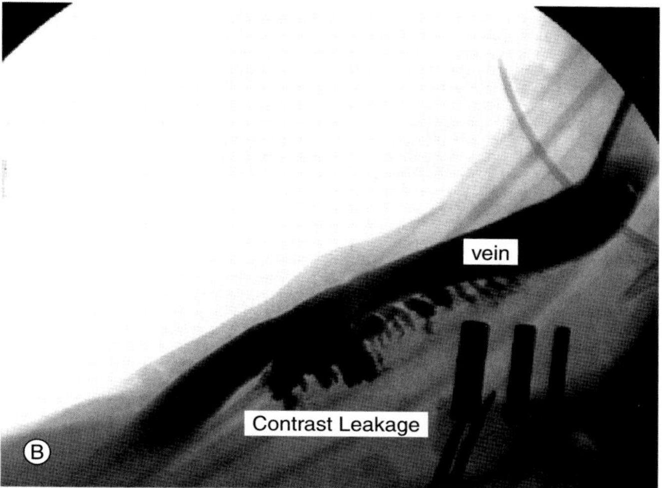

Figure 40.8 Perforation caused by 810 nm diode laser in goat jugular vein. (A) Hematoxylin and eosin. Perforation shown by arrowhead. 20×. (B) Appearance under fluoroscopy intraoperative injection of contrast material showing leakage through multiple vein perforations.

and 1320-nm laser, which target water and transmit thermal energy more directly to the vein wall, result in little postoperative discomfort. Our patients treated with EVLT with an 810-nm diode laser have shown a significant incidence of post-treatment purpura and tenderness. Most of our patients treated with 810-nm laser do not return to complete functional normality for 2–3 days as opposed to the 1 day 'down-time' with RF Closure or 1320-nm endovenous laser of the GSV. Because the anesthetic and access techniques for the two procedures are identical, we believe that nonspecific perivascular thermal damage is the probable cause for this increased tenderness. Recent studies suggested that pulsed 810 nm diode laser treatment increases the risk for perforation of the vein as opposed to continuous treatment[25] (Fig. 40.8). This has been proposed as a reason for the increased symptoms with EVLT vs RF treatment.[21] In our experience attempts at modifications including reduced fluence and treating with continuous laser emission versus pulsed laser emission have not resulted in a reduction of patient postoperative symptoms using the 810-nm diode laser (Fig. 40.9).

It has been hypothesized that a longer wavelength, such as 940-nm, will penetrate deeper into the vein wall with resulting increased efficacy. A report of 280 patients with 350 treated limbs with 18 months of follow-up demonstrated complete closure in 96%.[26] Twenty vein segments were examined histologically. When veins were treated with 1-second duration pulses at 12 J, perforations were not present. When the fluence was increased to 15 J with 1.2- and 1.3-second pulses, microperforations did occur and were said to be self-sealing. The authors suggest that their use of tumescent anesthesia as well as the above-mentioned laser parameters are responsible for the lack of significant perforations and enhanced efficacy.

Several studies have evaluated a 1064-nm neodymium: yttrium aluminum garnet (Nd:YAG) endoluminal laser. In one study, the lateral saphenous goat vein was used.[27] Occlusion was more likely when fluence exceeded 84 J/cm^2. More importantly, treated vessels were not perforated even with a fluence of 224 J/cm^2. A diffusing fiber was also used to obtain circumferential damage.

A clinical study using an endoluminal 1064-nm Nd:YAG laser in the treatment of incompetent GSV in 151 men and women with 252 treated limbs was also reported.[28] Ligation was also performed at the SFJ, which did not allow for a determination of the efficacy of GSV laser ablation. Spinal anesthesia was used and the laser was used at 10–15 watts of energy with 10-second pulses with manual retraction of

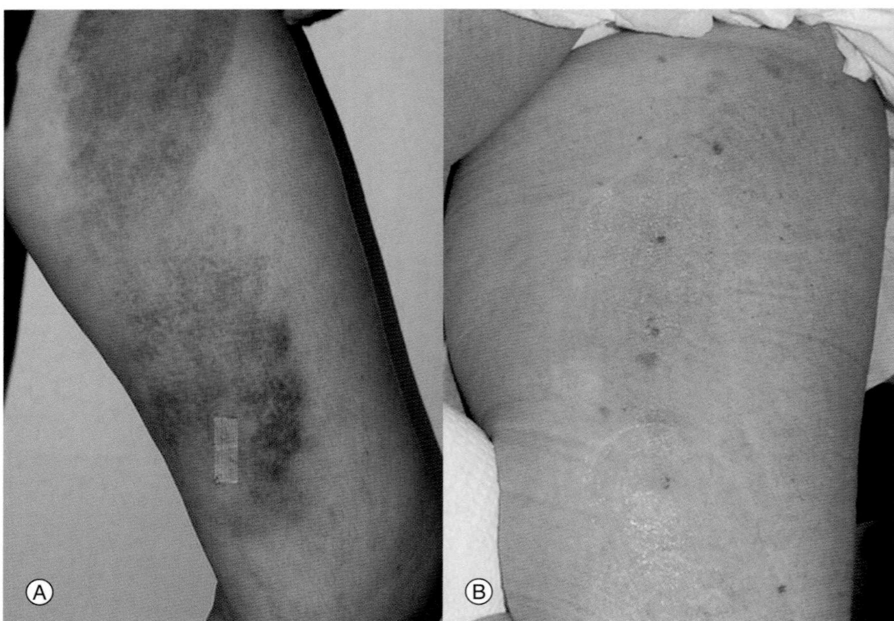

Figure 40.9 Clinical appearance on postoperative day 1. (a) 810 nm diode continuous laser application, not pulsed. (b) 1320 nm Nd:YAG continuous laser application.

the laser fiber at a rate of 6 cm/minute. Skin overlying the treated vein was cooled with cold water. The side-effects were notable with superficial burns in 4.8% of patients, paresthesia in 36.5%, superficial phlebitis is 1.6%, and localized hematomas in 0.8%.

In an attempt to bypass absorption of hemoglobin we have explored the 1320-nm wavelength for endoluminal use. At this wavelength, tissue water is the target and the presence of red blood cells within the vessels is not required as for the other wavelengths. We also utilize a mechanical catheter drawback system and a diffusing laser fiber to provide uniform heating of the vessel. Studies in the porcine GSV demonstrate full thickness thermal damage at 5 W with the 1320-nm laser and 20 W with the 1064-nm laser.[29] Clinical studies have demonstrated 98% efficacy without evidence of vessel perforation with the use of the 1320-nm Nd:YAG intravascular laser in 140 patients with a 16–18-month follow-up (at the time of this writing). Clinical results as well as postoperative adverse sequelae are identical to those seen with VNUS Closure treatment.

Technique for endovenous occlusion using endoluminal laser

The patient is evaluated and marked in an identical manner as with RF Closure of the GSV. Anesthesia is given along the vein in an identical manner as with RF Closure. The only difference between the two procedures is that with EVLT a 600-μm laser fiber is inserted into the vein within a protective sheath so that only the distal 2–3-mm of laser fiber exits from the sheath. A helium neon aiming beam that is continuously illuminated when the laser is on ensures that the laser fiber is outside of the sheath. If the laser fiber retracts within the sheath thermal melting of the sheath occurs and plastic breakdown products may be released into the vein (Fig. 40.10). A Steri-strip (3M, St Paul, MN) is placed on the fiber to mark the length at which 1 cm of the laser fiber protrudes from the sheath to prevent this from occurring. An additional safety factor is the visualization of the helium neon aiming beam because this is not visualized when the laser fiberoptic is withdrawn into the sheath.

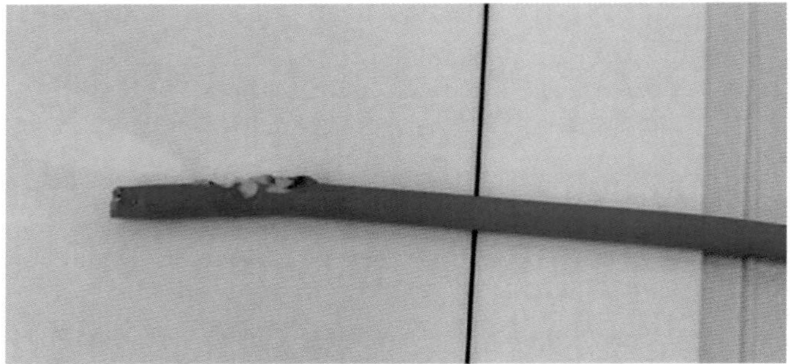

Figure 40.10 Plastic sheath burn caused by 810 nm diode fiber withdrawn while firing into the sheath.

Correct placement of the laser fiber tip 2-cm distal to the SFJ is confirmed through direct visualization with duplex ultrasound and secondarily by laser fiber measurement and viewing the He:Ne aiming beam through the skin. To minimize risks of perforation and bruising, we advocate using the laser in a continuous firing mode with withdrawal at a rate of 1 cm/second. Typical fluence used is 12–14 J/cm^2. Endovenous laser treatment is stopped when the distal tip of the fiber reaches a point 1–3 cm from the vein entry site. This can be confirmed with direct visualization of the red aiming beam through the skin. Total laser application time is recorded. Repeat ultrasound of the saphenous vein is performed confirming successful treatment. When the terminal portion of the vein (immediately adjacent to the point of entry) is treated, the catheter/sheath and the fiber are withdrawn and manual pressure is applied to the puncture site. If clinically indicated, AP and/or sclerotherapy of the tributaries are performed.

Pitfalls and their management

- If tissue is heated above 100 °C it begins to boil so the optimal target temperature is 70–90 °C. With careful regulation of the degree of heating, subtle gradations of controlled collagen coagulation or total thermocoagulation of the vein wall can be achieved.
- Blood is heated instead of tissue if clots build up on the electrodes, leading to a rise in impedance. The RF generator can be programmed to rapidly shutdown when this occurs ensuring minimal heating of blood but efficient heating of the vein wall.
- Use of general anesthesia without tumescent anesthesia leads to adverse effects. Tumescent anesthesia provides a safety heatsink around the vessel, which is essential for safe endovenous treatments.

SUMMARY

A new technique for endovenous occlusion using RF ablation catheters or endoluminal laser delivered by fiberoptics offers a less invasive alternative to traditional ligation and stripping. Initial clinical experience in several hundred patients shows a high degree of success with minimal side-effects, most of which can be prevented or minimized with minor modifications of the technique. The use of AP for associated branch varicosities makes these techniques even more successful. With over 50 000 RF procedures and thousands of laser procedures performed with over a 90% success rate, these techniques are rapidly replacing traditional venous surgery.

REFERENCES

1. McMullin GM, Coleridge Smith PD, Scurr JH. Objective assessment of high ligation without stripping the long saphenous vein. Br J Surg 1991; 78:1139–1142.
2. Jakobsen BH. The value of different forms of treatment for varicose veins. Br J Surg 1979; 66:182–184.
3. Munn SR, Morton JB, MacBeth WAAG, McLeish AR. To strip or not to strip the long saphenous vein? A varicose vein trial. Br J Surg 1981; 68:426–428.
4. Rutherford RB, Sawyer JD, Jones DN. The fate of residual saphenous vein after partial removal or ligation. J Vasc Surg 1990; 12:422–428.
5. Sarin S, Scurr JH, Coleridge Smith PD. Assessment of stripping the long saphenous vein in the treatment of primary varicose veins. Br J Surg 1992; 79:889–893.
6. Gradman WS. Venoscopic obliteration of variceal tributaries using monopolar electrocautery. J Dermatol Surg Onc 1994; 20:482–485.
7. Van Cleef JF. La 'nouvelle electrocoagulation' en phlebologie. Phlebologie (Fr) 1987; 40:423–426.
8. Cragg AH, Galliani CA, Rysavy JA, Castaneda-Zuniga WR, Amplatz K. Endovascular diathermic vessel occlusion. Radiology 1982; 144:303–308.
9. Haines DE. The biophysics of radiofrequency catheter ablation in the heart: the importance of temperature monitoring. Pacing Clin Electrophysiol 1993; 16:586–591.
10. Haines DE, Verow AF. Observations on electrode–tissue interface temperature and effect on electrical impedance during radiofrequency ablation of ventricular myocardium. Circulation 1990; 82:1034–1038.
11. Lavergne T, Sebag C, Ollitrault J, et al. [Radiofrequency ablation: physical bases and principles]. Arch Mal Coeur Vaiss 1996; 89 Spec No 1:57–63.
12. Chandler JG, Pichot O, Sessa C, Schuller-Petrovic S, Osse FJ, Bergan JJ. Defining the role of extended saphenofemoral junction ligation: A prospective comparative study [In Process Citation]. J Vasc Surg 2000; 32:941–953.
13. Manfrini S, Gasbarro V, Danielsson G, et al. Endovenous management of saphenous vein reflux. Endovenous Reflux Management Study Group. J Vasc Surg 2000; 32:330–342.
14. Merchant RF, Depalma RG, Kabnick LS. Endovascular obliteration of saphenous reflux: a multicenter study. J Vasc Surg 2002; 35: 1190–1196.
15. Weiss RA, Weiss MA. Controlled radiofrequency endovenous occlusion using a unique radiofrequency catheter under duplex guidance to eliminate saphenous varicose vein reflux: a 2-year follow-up. Dermatol Surg 2002; 28:38–42.
16. Sybrandy JE, Wittens CH. Initial experiences in endovenous treatment of saphenous vein reflux. J Vasc Surg 2002; 36:1207–1212.
17. Komenaka IK, Nguyen ET. Is there an increased risk for DVT with the VNUS closure procedure? J Vasc Surg 2002; 36:1311.
18. Goldman MP. Closure of the greater saphenous vein with endoluminal radiofrequency thermal heating of the vein wall in combination with ambulatory phlebectomy: preliminary 6-month follow-up. Dermatol Surg 2000; 26:452–456.
19. Weiss RA, Goldman MP. Transillumination mapping prior to ambulatory phlebectomy. Dermatol Surg 1998; 24:447–450.
20. Moritz AR, Henriques EC. Studies of thermal injury II: The relative importance of time and surface temperature in the causation of cutaneous bums. S Am J Pathol 1947; 23:695–720.
21. Proebstle TM, Lehr HA, Kargl A, et al. Endovenous treatment of the greater saphenous vein with a 940 nm diode laser: thrombotic occlusion after endoluminal thermal damage by laser-generated steam bubbles. J Vasc Surg 2002; 35:729–736.
22. Roggan A, Friebel M, Dorschel K, et al. Optical properties of circulating human blood in the wavelength range 400–2500 nm. J Biomed Opt 1999; 50:523–529.
23. Min RJ, Zimmet SE, Isaacs MN, Forrestal MD. Endovenous laser treatment of the incompetent greater saphenous vein. J Vasc Interv Radiol 2001; 12:1167–1171.
24. Navarro L, Min RJ, Bone C. Endovenous laser: a new minimally invasive method of treatment for varicose veins—preliminary observations using an 810 nm diode laser. Dermatol Surg 2001; 27:117–122.
25. Weiss RA. Comparison of endovenous radiofrequency versus 810 nm diode laser occlusion of large veins in an animal model. Dermatol Surg 2002; 28:56–61.
26. Bush RG. Regarding 'Endovenous treatment of the greater saphenous vein with a 940 nm diode laser: thrombolytic occlusion after endoluminal thermal damage by laser-generated steam bubbles'. J Vasc Surg 2003; 37:242.
27. Parente EJ, Rosenblatt M. Endovenous laser treatment to promote venous occlusion. Lasers Surg Med 2003; 33:115–118.
28. Chang CJ, Chua JJ. Endovenous laser photocoagulation (EVLP) for varicose veins. Lasers Surg Med 2002; 31:257–262.
29. Goldman MP, Detwiler SP. Endovenous 1064 nm and 1320 nm Nd:YAG laser treatment of the porcine greater saphenous vein. Cosmetic Dermatol 2003; 16:25–28.

41 Minimum Incision Face Lift

Robert C Langdon MD, Gerhard Sattler MD, and C William Hanke MD MPH

Summary box

- In most parts of the face and neck, a component of the subcutaneous musculoaponeurotic system (SMAS) lies just deep to the subcutaneous fat.
- SMAS elevation by plication with skeletal anchoring provides stable correction of lower face and neck ptosis.
- Tumescent anesthesia greatly reduces postoperative morbidity in face lift surgery.
- The structure at greatest risk of injury in face lift surgery is the temporal branch of the facial nerve.
- Liposuction of neck and jowls and platysmaplasty are important components of face lift surgery.
- Mid-face ptosis can be corrected by suture suspension of the malar fat pads.

INTRODUCTION

Facial aging occurs through three mechanisms: photoaging, gravitational aging, and volumetric aging. Photoaging is the result of sun damage and affects primarily the skin; it probably does not occur to a significant degree in tissues deeper than the dermis. Gravitational aging is manifested by stretching and sagging of soft tissues, especially those of the superficial musculoaponeurotic system (SMAS). Volumetric aging is manifested by atrophy of soft tissues (primarily fat and muscle) and of bone. Soft tissue atrophy is most evident in the anterior face and cheeks and can produce cheek hollowing in the lateral maxillary area. In advanced age, bony atrophy results in recession of the mandible. Volumetric aging has an unknown etiology.

The most direct solution to gravitational aging is lifting surgery. The goal of a face lift (rhytidectomy) is to elevate sagging soft tissue along vectors that reverse the effect of gravity on those tissues. The most common surgical lifting procedure (a SMAS lift) elevates the SMAS of the neck and lateral cheeks.

This chapter will describe a minimum incision (short scar) rhytidectomy that can be performed under tumescent local anesthesia. First there will be a review of the anatomy of the neck, lower face, and mid-face regions and a discussion of how face lift surgery can correct gravitational aging of these structures. This will be followed by a discussion of the variations of face lift surgery and how different techniques have been devised to improve results, especially in the mid-face. In the minimal incision technique preferred by the author, tumescent local anesthetic solution is infused throughout the operative field. The tumescent anesthetic solution can be administered in a nearly painless fashion, which enables the use of minimal perioperative sedation. The tumescent anesthetic facilitates surgical dissection in the subcutaneous plane and also enhances hemostasis. The prolonged vasoconstriction that results from the use of the tumescent anesthetic results in minimal postoperative ecchymosis and edema, which greatly accelerates the patient's recovery.

Pre-excision of juxta-auricular skin (in an 'S' configuration) increases visibility of the operative field and facilitates undermining in the supra-SMAS plane. Undermining as far medial as the malar fat pad enables use of a suspension suture to elevate the pad. Malar fat pad suspension is a safe and effective way to improve mid-face aging, including correction of deep nasolabial folds and of infraorbital hollowing. SMAS plication is achieved with purse string sutures that take multiple bites into the SMAS and are stably anchored in the periosteal tissue of the posterior zygomatic arch. Because of the skeletal anchoring of these sutures, significant tension can be applied to the SMAS plication. Upon SMAS plication the 'S' form skin excision can be closed in a predictable way using key sutures and minimizing the need for additional skin removal and dog-ear repairs.

Anatomy relevant to face lift surgery

Safe and effective face lift surgery requires a thorough understanding of facial anatomy, especially that pertaining to the SMAS and its retaining ligaments, the platysma and other superficial muscles of expression, and motor nerve branches. If dissections are successfully confined to supra-

SMAS planes, blood vessels and sensory nerves are of less significance to the surgeon.

The SMAS is a complex mesenchymal tissue system that is most broadly defined as the superficial muscles of facial expression, fascial planes that are continuous with these muscles, and myriad septal attachments between these fascial planes and the dermis. Through the cutaneous attachments of the superficial facial musculature and of the fascial planes of the SMAS, contractions of the muscles are conveyed to the skin, resulting in facial expression. In most parts of the face and neck, a component of the SMAS lies just deep to the subcutaneous fat. The SMAS includes the platysma muscle in the neck and a robust fascia in the lateral cheek area. The fascial components of the SMAS are continuous with, or envelope, the superficial muscles of expression, including the platysma, orbicularis oculi, risorius, and zygomatic muscles.

In the anterior face, the superficial fascia level is continuous through the galea, frontalis, orbicularis oculi, SMAS and platysma. More laterally, in the temple region, the superficial fascia manifests as the superficial temporal fascia (also called temperoparietal fascia). This superficial fascia merges with deep temporalis fascia at the zygomatic arch and is discontinuous with the SMAS, which converges on the zygomatic arch from below.[1]

The SMAS is attached to dermis above and to bone below via two distinct retaining ligaments: the zygomatic (also referred to as 'McGregor's patch') and mandibular ligaments.[2] In addition, there are several ligamentous attachments between SMAS and dermis, including those in the masseteric, preauricular, and infra-auricular areas (Fig. 41.1).[2,3] In a supra-SMAS dissection for rhytidectomy, many of these retaining ligaments are encountered and divided. Many of them surround perforating vessels and small sensory nerve branches. The vessels generally require bipolar cautery for hemostasis; the nerves tend to regenerate postoperatively with restoration of sensation in the cheek region.

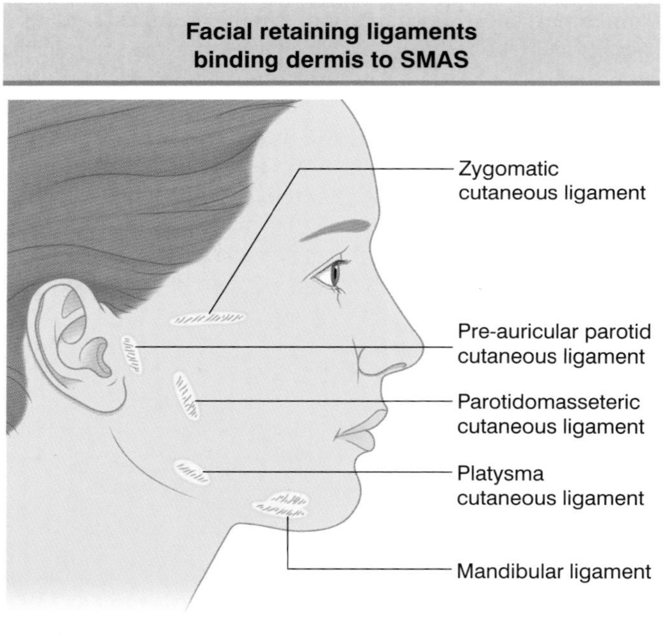

Figure 41.1 Facial retaining ligaments. All of these ligaments bind the dermis to the SMAS. The zygomatic and mandibular positioning ligaments also provide firm attachments between SMAS and bone. Skin mobility is increased if the dermal attachments of these ligaments are partially or completely severed during rhytidectomy. Adapted from Ozdemir R, et al. Anatomicohistologic study of the retaining ligaments of the face and use in face lift: retaining ligament correction and SMAS plication. Plast Reconstr Surg 2002; 110: 1134–1147 with permission.

The most important structure at risk of damage during face lift surgery is the facial nerve (Fig. 41.2). The nerve is deep to the parotid gland at its foramen and begins its branching deep to the gland. Inferior to the zygomatic arch, the facial nerve branches travel below the SMAS and innervate the muscles of facial expression via the underside of the muscles. In a typical SMAS lift, in which undermining is done superficial to the SMAS, all of these lower branches of the facial nerve are protected from injury by the SMAS itself.

The facial nerve branches at greatest risk during rhytidectomy are the temporal branches, which lie within the superficial temporal fascia at and cephalad to the zygomatic arch (see Fig. 41.2). Great care must be taken to undermine at a level superficial to this fascia (preferably within the subcutaneous fat) over and cephalad to the zygomatic arch. If the zygomatic arch or the zygoma bone is to be used as an anchor point for SMAS or malar fat pad elevation, the distribution of temporal branch rami as they cross the zygomatic arch must be considered. In a study in which 35 cadaver hemifaces were dissected, the most posterior ramus of the facial nerve temporal branches crossed the zygomatic arch on average at a point 1.8 cm anterior to the auricle.[4] The most anterior ramus of the temporal branch crossed the zygomatic arch on average at a point 2.0 cm posterior to the anterior origin of the arch.

Surgery that tightens the SMAS in a superior direction results in an en bloc elevation of facial soft tissues at and superficial to the SMAS. Elevated tissues include subcutaneous fat and skin, which is attached to SMAS via the aforementioned retaining ligaments.[2] The robust fascia of the lateral cheek SMAS can withstand significant tension and is the ideal soft tissue layer for suture placement to mediate lifting. In contrast, the dermis has much less tensile strength and will stretch to produce a spread scar if sutured under too much tension.

Variations on rhytidectomy

Four major variables characterize face lift surgeries. These are:

- the anatomic plane(s) of dissection or undermining
- the method of tightening the tissue plane(s) to be lifted
- the point of fixation or anchoring of the tightened tissue plane(s)
- the vectors along which the tissue planes are tightened.

Face lift operations involve undermining along one or more tissue planes and resuspension of tissue planes to reverse gravitational sagging. Face lifts can be classified according to the depth of the plane of dissection. The most superficial plane is subcutaneous (supra-SMAS). The next level is sub-

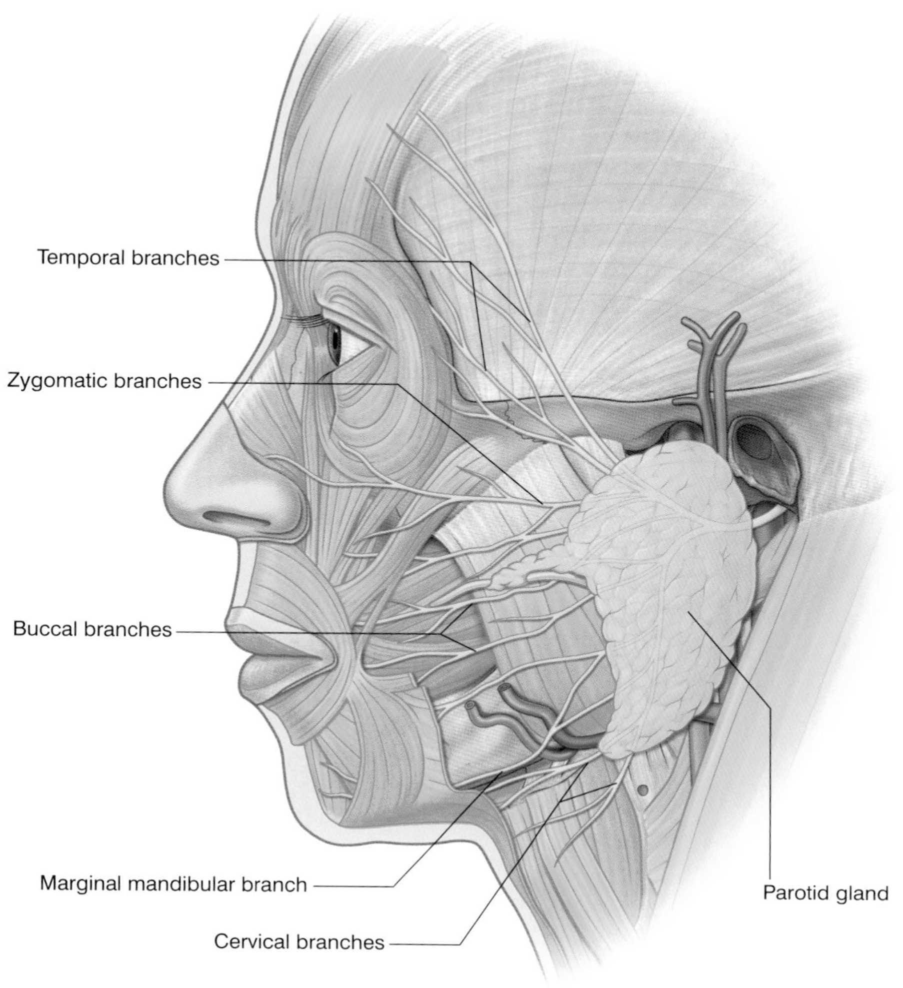

Figure 41.2 Branches of the facial nerve. Caudal to the zygomatic arch, all facial nerve branches lie beneath the parotid gland and SMAS, and are protected from injury if undermining is done superficial to these structures. Superficial to the zygomatic arch and in the temple region, the temporal branches run within the superficial temporal fascia. (For additional information, see Figs 1.14 and 1.15.)

SMAS; deeper still is subperiosteal dissection. The deeper-level face lifts are designed to provide a greater degree of structural lifting to fascia and superficial musculature. Deep-plane dissection generally includes release of the deep retaining ligaments that bind the SMAS to the underlying skeleton. These are the zygomatic and mandibular ligaments.[2] In theory, releasing these deep attachments affords greater mobility of the more anterior facial musculature and greater improvement of the mid-face, especially the nasolabial folds. There is considerable disagreement as to the long-term efficacy of deeper plane face lifts.[5–7]

Recent anatomic studies have shown that in the mid-face (defined as the cheek medial to a line drawn from the malar prominence to the modiolus (Fig. 41.3)), ptosis of supra-SMAS tissues is largely responsible for the stigmata of aging.[8,9] The malar fat pad is a roughly triangular accumulation of subcutaneous fat that lies over the maxilla (Fig. 41.3). Its superolateral corner extends into the malar area and its lower apex is near the modiolus. Gravitational descent of the malar fat pad results in deepening of the nasolabial fold, infraorbital hollowing and lowering and flattening of the youthful convexity of the mid-face. Cadaver dissection studies of the mid-face region have indicated that suspension of superficial tissues (such as skin or subcutaneous fat) affords superior correction of mid-face ptosis.[8]

Hoefflin advocates a supra-SMAS dissection that extends widely enough to enable release of all retaining ligaments between SMAS and dermis.[10] Undermining is immediately superficial to platysma and SMAS so that all fat superficial to the fascia remains attached to skin. Suspending only this thick skin/fat flap (without the SMAS) is effective in correcting ptosis of the central face and jowls.

In a SMAS lift, the SMAS layer can be tightened by either plication, imbrication, or SMAS-ectomy. Plication is the simplest method and is performed by suturing the SMAS to itself in order to shorten its expanse. With plication the SMAS is not incised. Imbrication involves incising and raising a SMAS flap by undermining, then excising excess SMAS and suturing the free edge to a less mobile structure in order to anchor it. SMAS-ectomy is

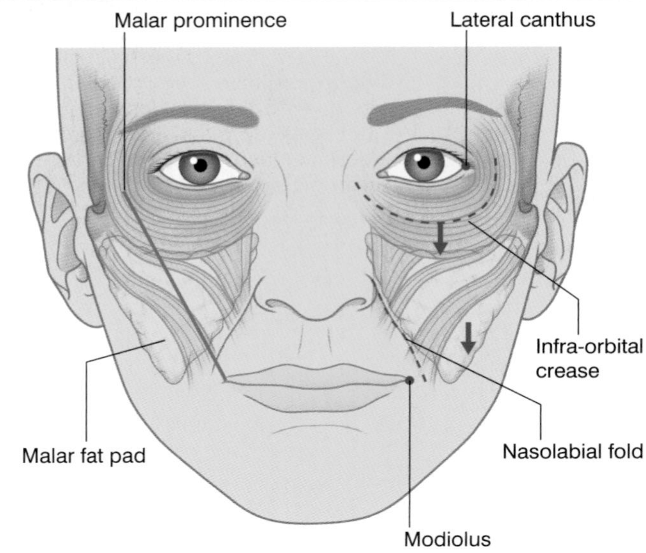

Figure 41.3 The mid-face and the malar fat pad. The mid-face region lies medial to a line drawn from the malar prominence to the modiolus (red line). Gravitational aging of this region results from the descent of the malar fat pad, a roughly triangular shaped accumulation of relatively fibrous subcutaneous fat. Adapted from Owsley JQ, Zweifler M. Midface lift of the malar fat pad; technical advances. Plast Reconstr Surg 2002; 110: 674–685 with permission.

similar to imbrication but without any undermining; the cut edges of SMAS are simply reapproximated.

When the SMAS is mobilized by either plication or imbrication, it must be anchored to a relatively immobile point of fixture to maintain a stable tightening. In general, the SMAS itself is relatively stable in the lateral cheek areas (preauricular and infra-auricular). The mastoid periosteum is a stable fixation point that can be used to secure platysma.[11,12] Skeletal fixation can also be achieved by suturing SMAS to the periosteum of the zygoma[13] or of the lateral zygomatic arch.[14]

PREOPERATIVE PREPARATION

As with any major surgery, patients must avoid any prescription or over-the-counter medications that can predispose to bleeding. Aspirin should be discontinued 2 weeks prior to surgery. Vitamin E should be avoided starting one week before surgery. Because several over-the-counter herbal preparations can inhibit hemostasis, it is best to discontinue all herbal supplements 1 week preoperatively.

Patients who smoke should discontinue smoking at least 2 weeks prior to surgery and not resume for at least 2 weeks postoperatively. Smoking causes peripheral vasoconstriction, which can compromise revascularization of the face lift skin flap and result in distal flap necrosis.

Preoperative laboratory evaluation should include bleeding parameters such as prothrombin and partial thromboplastin times, complete blood count (including platelets), and blood chemistries.

TECHNIQUES

In the surgical technique described herein, tumescent local anesthetic solution is instilled in the subcutaneous tissue of the cheeks and neck. Complete anesthesia as well as significant vasoconstriction is provided to the entire operative field. If necessary, liposuction of the neck and jowls and platysmaplasty are performed. Rhytidectomy begins with pre-excision of most of the skin to be removed from the preauricular and infra-auricular areas in a specific pattern that will facilitate final closure. Next, subcutaneous dissection of the cheek and neck is performed at a level superficial to the SMAS and platysma. Optional maneuvers include release of mandibular ligaments, blunt undermining beneath the malar fat pads, and suture suspension of malar and jowl fat pads. A permanent suture is anchored to periosteal tissue of the posterior zygomatic arch and used in a purse string style to plicate the platysma of the lateral neck in a superior vector and the lateral cheek SMAS in a superolateral vector. Finally, excess skin is trimmed and the skin is closed.

After informed consent is obtained, preoperative photographs are taken with the patient sitting upright. Five poses are used with the camera angle in the same horizontal plane as the patient's face; these include frontal, left and right oblique, and left and right lateral views of the entire face and neck. The oblique angle is standardized so that the anterior nasion and inner canthus are aligned. Three additional low angle photos are taken from the frontal and oblique views (see Fig. 6.2).

Next, a small area of hair in the lower sideburn area (within the skin to be excised) is shaved with a barber-style (electric) shaver. Then, skin markings are made after the skin is degreased with acetone (Fig. 41.4) The S-form excision in the sideburn, preauricular, and infra-auricular area will remove an amount of skin that approximates that which would be redundant after plication of the platysma and SMAS. The preoperative markings for this S-form moiety must be carefully done. This excision should not be so wide that it results in excessive skin removal and a difficult final skin closure.

Additional skin markings (see Fig. 41.4) include demarcation of the mandibular border and the medial border of the sternocleidomastoid muscles; these serve as guides for neck liposuction. The jowl fat pad is delineated by the labial–mandibular sulcus medially and by the palpable edge of the fat pad laterally. In the mid-face, the nasolabial and tear trough furrows are marked. The latter structure denotes the cutaneous attachment of the orbitomalar septum.[15] This structure lies between the arcus marginalis (at the inferior orbital rim) and the dermis and is somewhat impermeable to the passage of fluid. To avoid lower eyelid edema, the orbitomalar septum should not be traversed during surgery. The tear-trough marking serves as an aid to avoiding violation of the septum during mid-face surgery.

A radial mark approximately 7 cm from the tragus and a horizontal line at the level of the lateral canthus denote the extent of subcutaneous undermining. A line along the vector from the corner of the mouth toward the superior aspect of the tragus will serve as a guide to the direction of lateral SMAS plication. A similar line perpendicular to the nasolabial furrow, or slightly more vertical, denotes the vector for suspension of the malar fat pad.

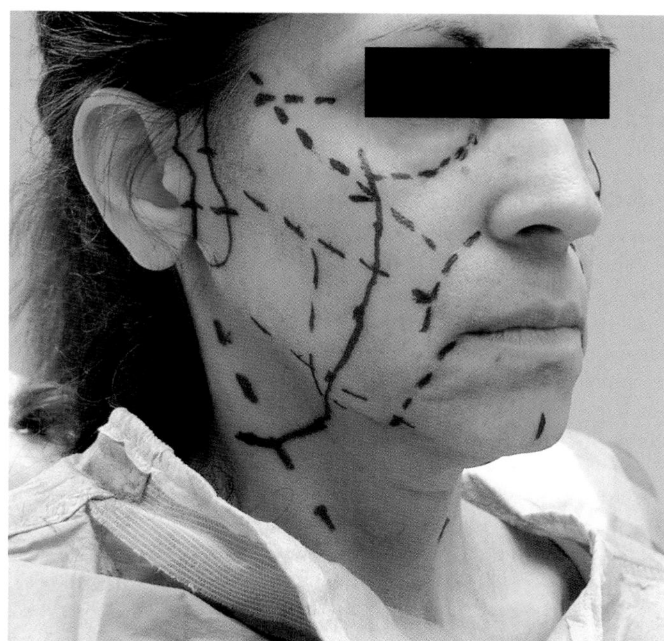

Figure 41.4 Presurgical markings. Patient marked for liposuction of neck and jowls, S-lift minimum incision face lift and mid-face lift via malar fat pad suspension suture. The S-form moiety that denotes skin to be excised from the juxta-auricular area is marked with a solid line. The solid line on the cheek and neck marks a 7-cm radius from the tragus and is used as a guide for the extent of subcutaneous undermining. Dashed lines denote anatomic features including the tear trough, the nasolabial fold, the labiomandibular fold (prejowl sulcus), the inferior border of the mandible, and the anterior border of the sternocleidomastoid muscle. The tear trough line indicates the cutaneous insertion of the orbitomalar septum. Two dashed lines indicate the vectors for malar fat pad suspension and superolateral SMAS plication. The dashed line on the temple at the level of the lateral canthus denotes the approximate cephalad limit of subcutaneous undermining. Not marked is the vertical vector for SMAS plication.

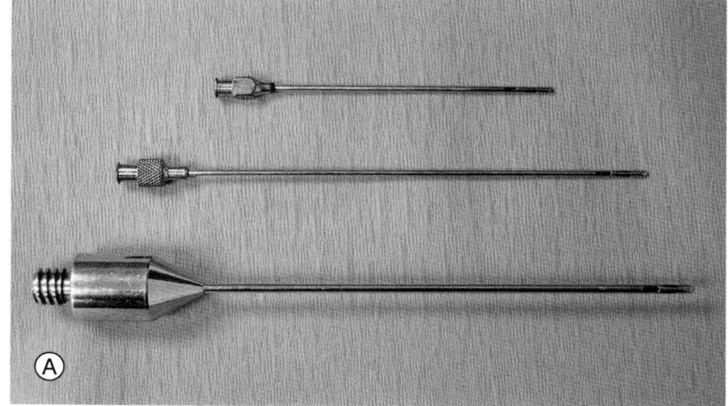

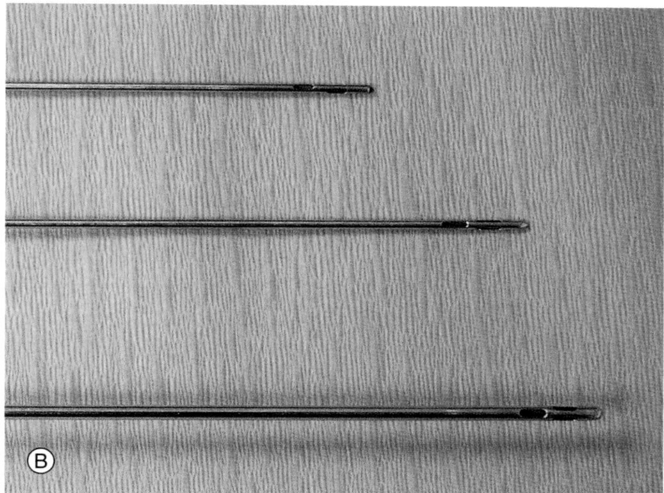

Figure 41.5 (A) Cannulae used for liposuction of neck and jowls. (B) All are tri-port (accelerator) design. The larger 3-mm diameter cannula is used for machine-assisted liposuction of the neck. The smaller 18-gauge cannulae are used for syringe liposuction of the jowls.

Blood pressure is checked. If systolic pressure is above 110 mmHg and/or diastolic pressure is greater than 70 mmHg, a single dose of clonidine 0.1 mg is given orally. Next, sedation is administered with midazolam 2.5–5.0 mg and hydroxyzine 25 mg, both intramuscularly. Arterial oxygen saturation is monitored by pulse oximetry.

Tumescent local anesthetic solution composed of 0.2% lidocaine, epinephrine (adrenaline) 1 in 250 000 and sodium bicarbonate 10 mEq/L is administered subcutaneously throughout the anterior neck extending to 3 cm lateral to the medial border of the sternocleidomastoid muscle. Included in the area of anesthesia are the mastoid and postauricular areas and the jowls. The medial jowl, including the area of the mandibular ligament, is anesthetized (see Figs 41.1 and 41.4).

Liposuction of the anterior neck and jowls is performed using five incisions.[16] From a single submental and two infralobular incisions, the neck is liposuctioned using a 3-mm accelerator (tri-port) cannula (Fig. 41.5A–B). The entire submental area below the mandibular border and extending to the medial (anterior) border of the sternocleidomastoid muscle is treated. A partial suctioning (from an infralobular incision) is done over the belly of the sternocleidomastoid muscle to taper into the untreated lateral neck. (Tapering prevents a potential 'shelf' between treated and untreated areas.) Treating the neck from three incisions enables 'criss-crossing' and more thorough fat removal. In the submental area the cannula is 'turned up' so that the ports are directed toward the under surface of the skin. This last maneuver facilitates postoperative skin contraction in the central neck.

The jowls are suctioned manually using a 10-ml syringe and a 14-gauge mini-accelerator (tri-port) cannula (see Fig. 41.5a–b) (Byron, Tucson, AZ) from an infralobular and an ipsilateral infrajowl incision. This area is treated conservatively in order to avoid over-resection. The aspirate is allowed to separate in the syringe to enable quantitation of supernatant fat and to assure consistency of aspirate volume between the left and right jowls.

If midline platysma plication is necessary, an incision (approximately 3 cm long) is made in the submental crease. Under direct headlight visualization, a dissection is carried out onto the anterior neck in the supra-platysmal plane to a distance of 6–8 cm from the incision. Undermining is performed using Metzenbaum scissors. Most septal attachments between platysma and skin are divided. Larger blood vessels are avoided and small bleeding vessels are coagulated by bipolar cautery. The anterior platysma borders are plicated using the corset technique.[17] A running suture of 3-0 Ethibond (Ethicon, Somerville, NJ) is used to approximate the two muscle edges, beginning just caudal to the incision and continuing to a distance of 4 cm down the neck. Bites into the muscle are taken approximately 3–4 mm from the medial edge. The running suture is continued in the reverse (cephalad) direction with larger bites (approximately 6–8 mm on each side) in order to increase the medial pull on the platysma muscles. The running suture terminates at its origin near the submental incision. The knot is buried on the underside of the approximated muscle edges. After complete hemostasis of the undermined tissue is confirmed, the skin is closed in a bilayered interrupted fashion with buried dermal sutures of 5-0 Vicryl (Ethicon) and surface sutures of 5-0 Prolene (Ethicon).

After completion of neck treatments, additional tumescent anesthetic solution is instilled in the cheek area. A 10-ml syringe with a 27-gauge needle is used to inject anesthetic in the area of skin marked for excision in the preauricular, infra-auricular and sideburn areas. Approximately 20 ml is injected in these areas, mostly into the subcutaneous fat. The lateral cheeks are anesthetized up to and beyond the previously marked 7-cm radius using a 22-gauge spinal needle and a 30-ml syringe (Fig. 41.6). The immediate subcutaneous fat layer of the cheeks is gently tumesced with care taken to include the entire subcutaneous space. (Discontinuous distribution of tumescent solution within the operative field will result in incomplete anesthesia.) Approximately 100 ml is used per cheek. The upper border of the operative field is the level of the lateral canthus in the lower temple (see Fig. 41.4). The maxillary area (including the malar fat pad) is included down to and over (beneath) the nasolabial fold. Additional anesthesia to the maxillary area can be provided by a nerve block of the infraorbital nerve using 0.5% bupivacaine with epinephrine (adrenaline) 1 in 200 000.

Rhytidectomy is performed beginning with excision of the juxta-auricular S-form skin moiety. In the hair-bearing sideburn area the incision is made parallel to the hair follicles. The incision follows the supratragal notch (Fig. 41.7) and descends just anterior to the tragus in the preauricular sulcus (Fig. 41.7). In most patients the mark adjacent to the ear is within an existing skin fold. The skin incision is carried into the subcutaneous fat with care taken to stay superficial (well above the SMAS) in the superior portion of the excision cephalad to the inferior border of the zygomatic arch. (The temporal branches of the facial nerve run within the SMAS layer superficial and cephalad to the zygomatic arch). Inferior to the zygomatic arch (over the parotid gland) the incision is extended well into subcutaneous fat. Excision of the skin moiety is completed using 12.7-cm Supercut scissors to divide the subcutaneous tissue from the underlying SMAS. Inferior to the zygomatic arch the division is done just superficial to the SMAS. Superior to the arch the division is more superficial and is immediately deep to the hair follicles of the lower sideburn.

Subcutaneous undermining of the lateral cheek/lateral neck skin flap is accomplished using 12.7-cm and 17.8-cm Metzenbaum scissors. Over the parotid gland the undermining is done deep to the subcutaneous fat, directly superficial to the SMAS. Deep undermining in the lateral part of the flap produces a thick flap that includes the subcutaneous fat. A thicker distal flap will be better vascularized, decreasing the risk of vascular compromise (and subsequent flap necrosis) postoperatively. In the infralobular lateral neck area, the undermining is done immediately superficial to platysma. If liposuction of the neck was performed, the lateral neck dissection will connect with the 'tunnels' created by liposuction. Care must be taken to assure that the neck undermining is done

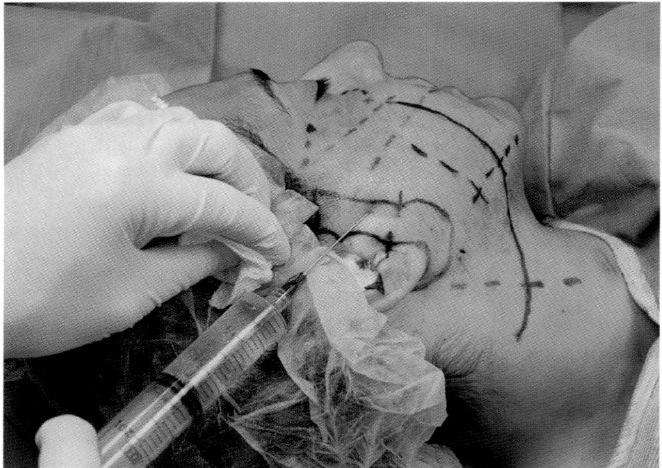

Figure 41.6 Injection of tumescent anesthetic solution in the cheek area. A 30-ml syringe and a 7.6-cm 22-gauge needle are used to inject anesthetic solution subcutaneously throughout the surgical field.

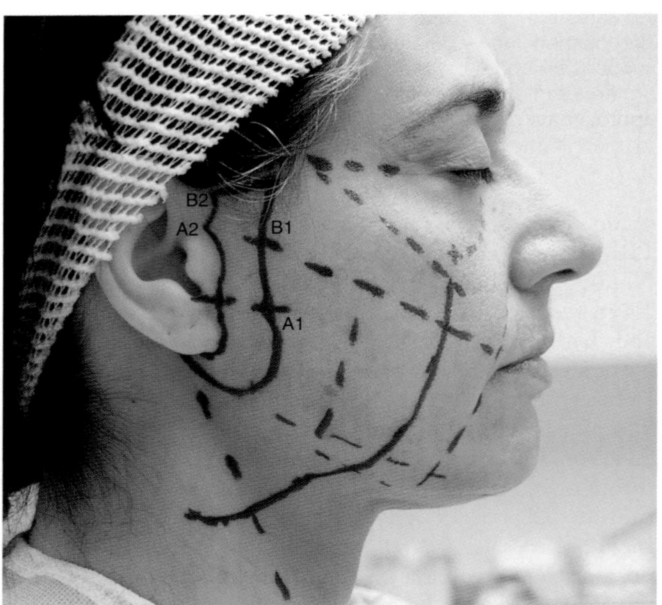

Figure 41.7 S-form juxta-auricular skin marking. The marking outlines skin to be excised at the beginning of rhytidectomy. The line follows the preauricular sulcus anterior to the tragus. Horizontal lines are drawn at the levels of the superior and inferior edges of the tragus. A notch just superior to the tragus is outlined (at point A2); this notch is reflected in the anterior line of the S-form marking at the level of the inferior edge of the tragus (at point A1). The key suture for skin closure approximates point A1 to point A2. Thus, the vertical elevation of the cheek flap is equivalent to the height of the tragus. This patient is also marked for liposuction of the neck and jowls.

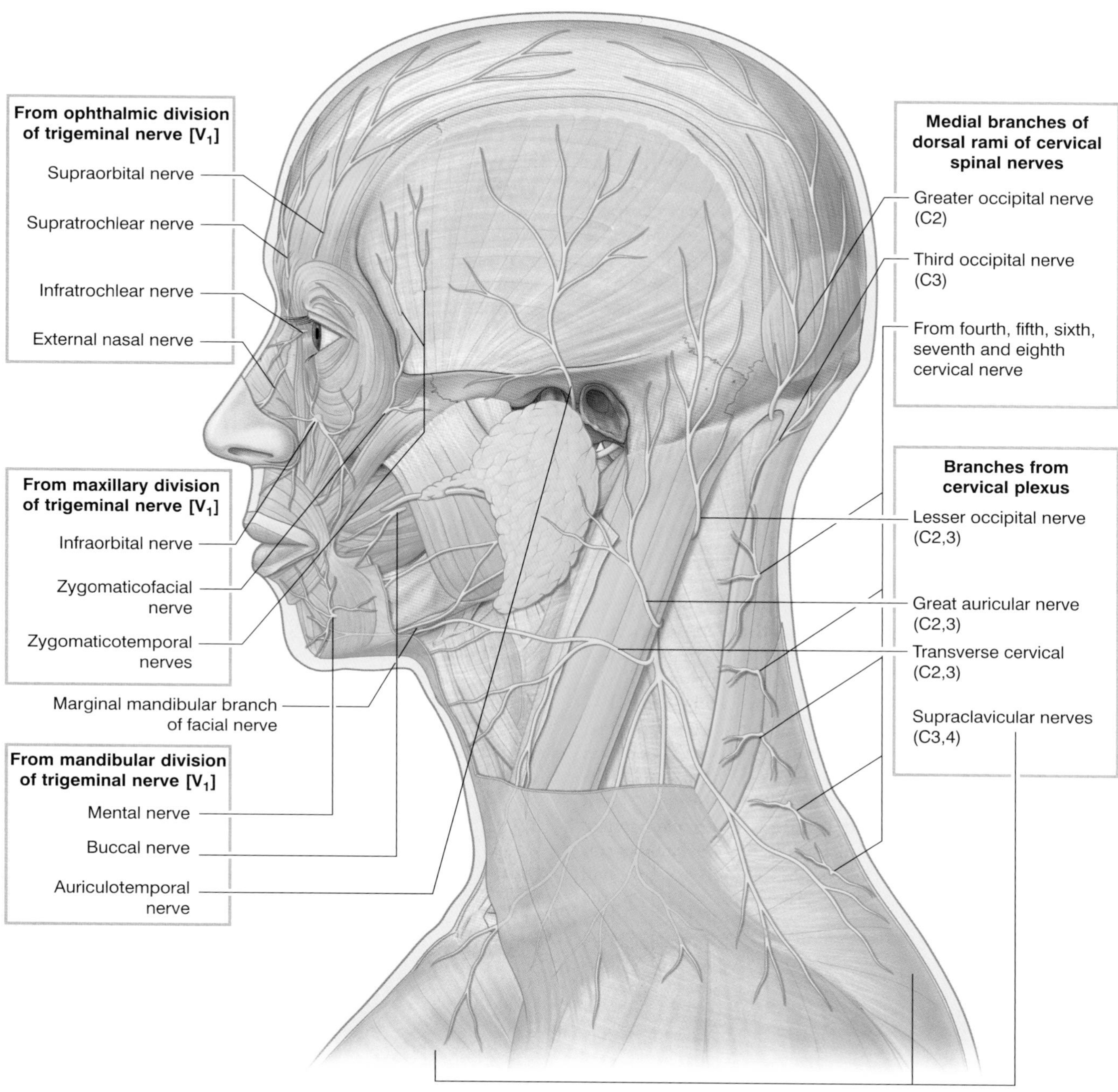

Figure 41.8 Sensory nerves of the neck and cheek. The great auricular nerve lies on the sternocleidomastoid muscle, and is at risk of injury if undermining in the lateral neck is done deep to the platysma. Adapted from Standring S, et al. Gray's anatomy, 39th edn. Edinburgh: Churchill Livingstone, 2005.

superficial to the platysma in order to avoid damage to the great auricular nerve, which lies directly on the belly of the sternocleidomastoid muscle (Fig. 41.8), or to the marginal mandibular nerve (see Fig. 41.2). Both of these nerves lie deep to the platysma. The dissection should extend somewhat postauricularly onto the mastoid fascia. The mastoid area lacks significant subcutaneous tissue; in this area undermining essentially separates the deep dermis from the mastoid fascia.

Undermining of the cheek should extend to 7 cm from the tragus, but generally it is not necessary to undermine into the temple cephalad to the level of the lateral canthus. Increased difficulty will be encountered when dissecting through the parotidomasseteric and zygomatic retaining ligaments (see Fig. 41.1). These retaining ligaments attach the SMAS to the overlying dermis and are composed of relatively thick collagenous tissue. Frequently, bleeding is encountered when these ligaments are divided because they usually surround communicating blood vessels. This bleeding may necessitate bipolar cautery to achieve hemostasis. Medial to the parotid gland, the distal branches of the facial nerve are no longer protected by the overlying gland, and the undermining should be done somewhat more superficially (within subcutaneous fat) to assure a supra-SMAS level of dissection and to lessen the risk of damage to these nerve branches. If liposuction of the jowl area was previously performed, the medial dissection will communicate with the 'tunnels' created earlier. Hemostasis should be periodically reassessed by direct visualization of the undermined flap, with bipolar cautery used as necessary.

After dissection of the cheek flap is complete, a periosteal elevator can be used to partially release the mandibular retaining ligament (Fig. 41.9). Release of this ligament (between SMAS and dermis) will improve lateral mobility of the overlying skin in the jowl area. The periosteal elevator can also be used to blindly undermine the malar fat pad to the level of and slightly beyond the nasolabial fold. Undermining the malar fat pad will increase its mobility if a suture suspension of the fat pad is performed subsequently. The undermining should be done just superficial to the zygomatic and lip levator muscles, beneath the malar fat. Care should be taken to avoid traversing the orbitomalar septum, the dermal attachment of which is manifested by the tear trough (that was previously marked).[15]

To suspend the malar fat pad, a suture of 3-0 Ethibond (Ethicon, Somerville, NJ) is placed in the deep portion of the superolateral corner of the pad. The malar fat is relatively fibrous and is capable of holding a suture.[18,19] The integrity of this suture should be tested by pulling on it. The pull should be in a direction perpendicular to the nasolabial fold or slightly more vertical to this vector. If too much skin dimpling is produced, the suture should be reinserted at a deeper level in the fat pad. After this suture has been satisfactorily placed, the needle is cut off to enable passage along a subcutaneous tract to its anchor point behind the temporal hairline.

To prepare the anchor point for the malar suspension suture, a small incision (10–15 mm long) is made just behind the temporal hairline and parallel to the nasolabial fold (Fig. 41.10). A hemostat is used to bluntly separate subcutaneous tissue to expose the superficial temporal fascia, which will appear as a glistening white layer. This fascia is then divided using iris scissors. The closed scissors are used to puncture the superficial fascia; the scissor tips are then spread apart to divide the fascia progressively until the deep temporalis fascia is reached. The deep fascia appears striated and remains fixed when the superficial tissues (superficial temporal fascia, subcutaneous fat and skin) are moved by finger traction.

After the deep temporalis fascia is definitively identified, a 'suture passer,' such as a long, small caliber cannula (for example, a 14-gauge or 16-gauge liposuction cannula) is passed within the subcutaneous fat layer from the temporal incision toward the point beneath the rhytidectomy flap at which the suture was passed through the malar fat pad. Both ends of the suture are then passed in and out of the ports of the cannula and the cannula is withdrawn in a cephalad direction to pass the suture to the temporal incision site. Tension will be applied to the suspension suture after completion of SMAS plication.

A similar suspension suture of 3-0 Ethibond can also be placed deep in the jowl fat pad. This suspension suture can be considered in those patients who have very prominent jowls with deep labial–mandibular furrows. The vector of suspension should be perpendicular to the labial–mandibular furrow, generally parallel to the mandibular border. The integrity of this suture should also be tested. Gentle tension should flatten the jowls but not cause undue skin dimpling. The needle should be left on the suture to enable later placement in lateral cheek SMAS after the SMAS plication sutures are tightened and tied off.

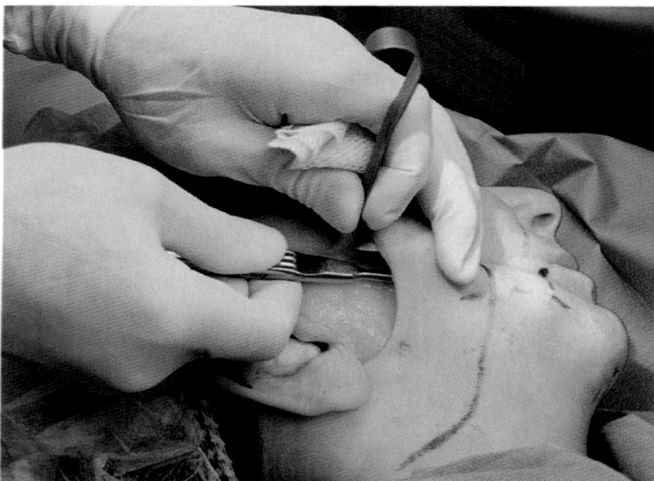

Figure 41.9 Use of periosteal elevator to partially release the mandibular retaining ligament. The ligament attaches the dermis to the underlying SMAS and bone. The instrument is advanced beyond the undermined area (demarcated by the solid blue line) at the subcutaneous level and is used to weaken the ligament.

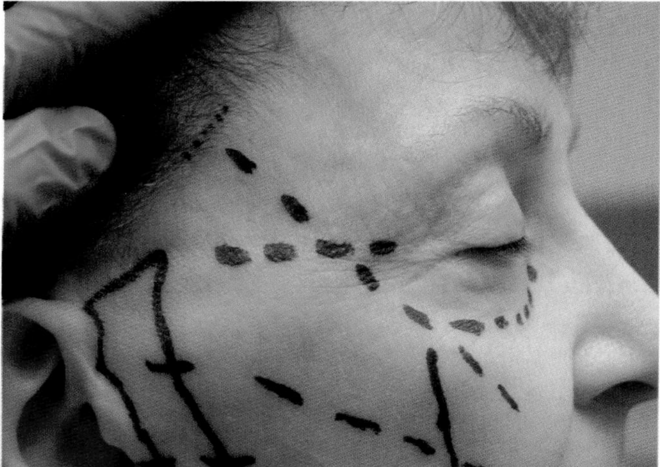

Figure 41.10 Markings for malar suspension suture. The fine dotted line just behind the temporal hair line marks the incision for the anchor point for the malar suspension suture. The suture will be anchored to the deep temporalis fascia. The oblique dotted line demarcates the subcutaneous course of the suspension suture between the malar fat pad and the anchor point. Also marked is the tear trough, the cutaneous insertion of the orbitomalar septum. To minimize postoperative edema, the suspension suture should not violate this septum.

The SMAS plication begins with passage of a suture of 2-0 Ethibond through the dense periosteal tissue of the posterior zygomatic arch. This suture can be placed either horizontally or vertically in the area of the arch anterior to the superficial temporal vessels (usually visible) and posterior to a point on the arch that is 1.8 cm anterior to the auricle. Posterior placement of this suture minimizes the risk of injuring the most posterior ramus of the temporal branch of the facial nerve (see Fig. 41.2). Vertical placement of this anchoring suture decreases the risk of injury to the most posterior ramus of the temporal branch of the facial nerve. Horizontal placement may provide a more secure anchor, however. After placement of this plicating suture, its integrity should be tested by pulling up on both ends; the patient's head should easily be lifted.

The SMAS plication suture is run directly caudal toward the lateral neck by taking intermittent bites through the SMAS to create a purse string. The low point of this suture should be 4.0 cm below the caudal edge of the tragus (measured with a ruler or scalpel handle). At its nadir, a horizontal bite is taken through the platysma and the suture is carried in an anterior direction so that it is slightly flared at its base (Fig. 41.11). The suture continues in a cephalad direction toward its origin, with the final bite taken approximately 4 mm from the suture origin. This first plication suture is then tied with a degree of tension to the surgeon's choosing. More tension will cinch the purse string to a greater extent and will provide more vertical lift to the lateral platysma. The degree of tension to apply to this suture is the only variable that determines the amount of platysma elevation; care should be taken to use comparable tension on both sides of the face. To hold this suture in place, after the first double overhand throw, an assistant should clamp down on the knot using a smooth (non-serrated) needle holder. The surgeon then completes one throw of the knot in the opposite direction to complete a square knot, which is tightened simultaneously with the assistant's release and withdrawal of the needle holder. Three additional throws in alternating opposite directions are made to further secure the knot. The suture is not cut; rather it is used to create the second loop for lateral SMAS plication.

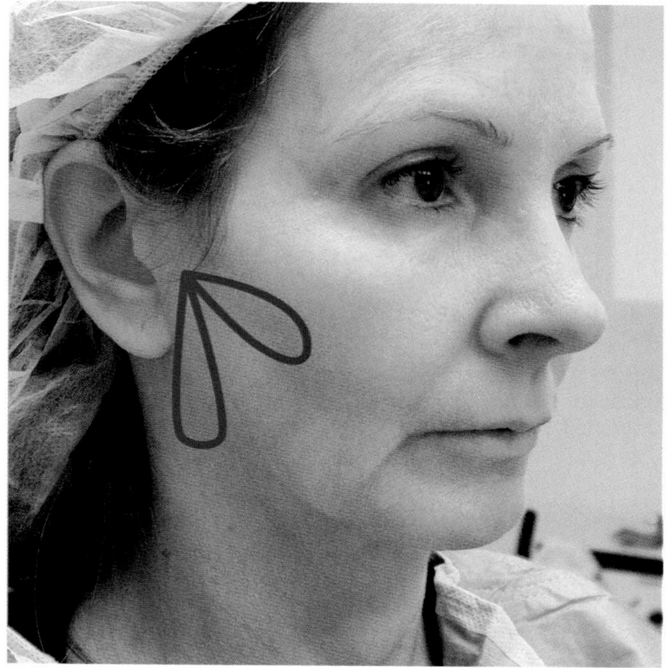

Figure 41.11 Location of the purse string SMAS plication sutures. An initial bite through the periosteum of the posterior zygomatic arch anchors the suture. The vertical plication is accomplished by taking multiple additional bites through the SMAS in a caudal direction to a nadir 4 cm caudal to the tragus, then completing the loop by returning to a point approximately 4 mm from the origin of the suture. The suture is then tied under tension to accomplish lifting of the SMAS, but the suture is not yet cut. Next, the suture is used to plicate the lateral cheek SMAS in a superolateral direction. Again, a loop (usually with a radius of 4 cm) is created by taking multiple bites through the SMAS. This second purse string suture terminates near the origin of the first suture and is tied off to the end of the suture opposite the needle.

The lateral cheek SMAS is plicated by extending the purse string suture, from its anchored origin on the posterior zygomatic arch, in an oblique direction oriented along a vector that runs from the corner of the mouth toward the superior tragus (see Fig. 41.11); this vector is also marked in Figure 41.4. If a more vertical direction of the SMAS plication is desired, this vector can be adjusted accordingly. This second plication loop is somewhat oval in shape, with the direction of the oval following the desired vector. As before, multiple bites are taken through the SMAS to create a purse string, and the suture is cinched to the desired degree of tension, then tied off as before and cut. No more than five alternating throws should be used in the knot in order to decrease its postoperative palpability. The net effect of these two SMAS plication loops is the en bloc elevation of superficial cheek and neck tissues in a superolateral direction. The undermined cheek flap is advanced by the SMAS plication and the edges of the original preauricular skin excision are largely approximated.

Next, the malar fat pad suspension suture is anchored, tightened, and tied off. To anchor the suture to the deep temporalis fascia, one of the ends is threaded through a one half circle Ferguson needle (Fig. 41.12). The needle is passed through the fascia at the site of the incision just

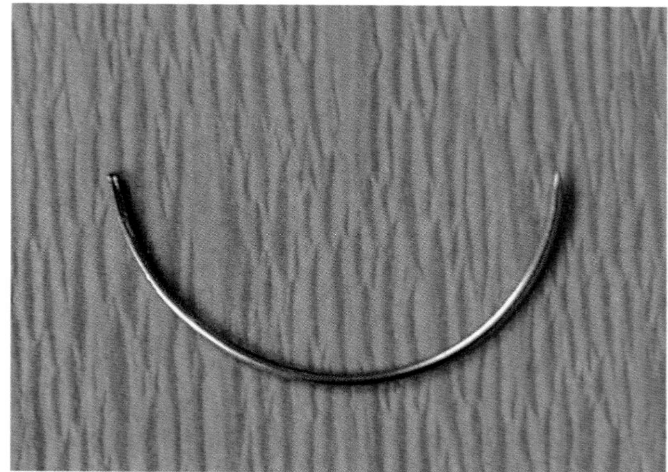

Figure 41.12 Half circle Ferguson needle. This reusable needle is used to place the malar suspension suture through the deep temporalis fascia at the anchor point.

lateral to the temporal hairline. This bite of fascia is oriented perpendicular to the direction of the suspension suture. After placement of the suture, the needle is removed and the two ends of the suture are tied with the desired tension to elevate the malar fat pad. Tension should be limited because too much tension may result in a visible skin dimple (postoperatively) superficial to the site at which the suture is passed through the malar fat pad.

If a suspension suture was placed earlier in the jowl fat pad, it should now be passed through lateral cheek SMAS along a vector perpendicular to the labial–mandibular furrow. Sufficient (but not excessive) tension should be applied to this suture to partially flatten the jowl. Any skin dimpling caused by this suspension suture should be effaced upon skin flap advancement to close the juxta-auricular excision. A test skin closure will verify that the appropriate tension has been applied to the jowl suspension suture, which can then be tied off.

Attention is now directed toward skin closure with trimming of redundant skin and dog-ear repair as needed. Sutures of 3-0 Vicryl are used for dermal-to-dermal buried closure. The first buried key suture is placed to approximate the point on the flap labeled A1 (see Fig. 41.7), on the anterior side of the S-form skin excision (at the level of the inferior tragus) to the point marked A2 on the posterior side of the excision (at the level of the superior tragus) (see Fig. 41.7). Generally, point B1 is then approximated to point B2.

Depending on the amount of superior pull applied to the platysma of the lateral neck by the first (vertical) plication suture, there may be redundant skin inferior to the ear that should be trimmed (Fig. 41.13). To measure the redundant skin, an instrument designed by Pitanguy (Fig. 41.14) (SSR Inc, Oyster Bay, NY) may be used. The V-shaped moiety on the lower arm of the instrument is held in position at the juxta-auricular edge of the wound, while the free margin of cervical skin is pulled up under mild tension, over the lower arm of the instrument (Fig. 41.15). To mark the point on the flap to be excised, the instrument is then clamped down, creating a visible indentation in the skin of the flap.

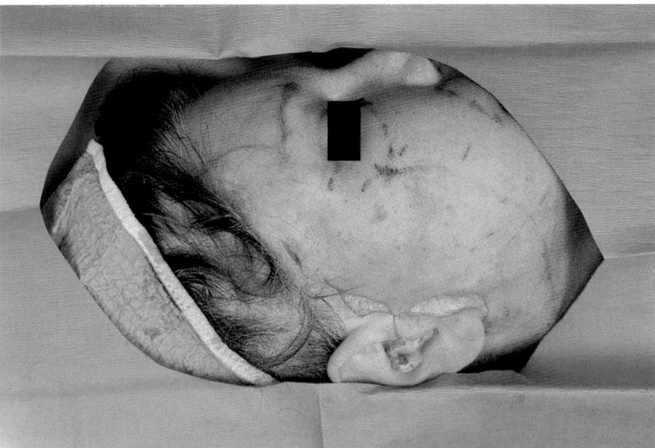

Figure 41.13 Skin closure after placement of the key suture. This dermal suture approximates the notch on the anterior edge of the preauricular skin excision, at the level of the inferior edge of the tragus, with the corresponding notch on the posterior edge of the incision at the level of the superior edge of the tragus.

Supercut scissors can then be used to make a curvilinear excision of redundant skin along the free edge of the flap. After additional buried sutures of 3-0 Vicryl are placed, dog-ear repairs may be required at either or both poles of the skin closure. At the inferior pole, the dog-ear should be excised in the area of postauricular skin overlying the mastoid fascia, preferably hidden near or behind the inferior ear lobe. Over the mastoid fascia there is no subcutaneous fat; the dermis lies directly on the fascia. Finally, cutaneous interrupted sutures of 5-0 Prolene are placed to complete the skin closure.

■ OPTIMIZING OUTCOMES

The great majority of patients benefit from liposuction of neck and jowls performed at the time of face lift. Aggressive liposuction of the neck will result in significant skin contraction that synergizes with lateral platysma tightening from face lift. In the authors' experience, turning the cannula ports 'upward' toward the underside of the dermis is a safe method for increasing postoperative skin contraction. An aggressive 'window wiper' transverse motion of the cannula, in order to sever all attachments between dermis and platysma, should be avoided.[16] Even those patients with moderate amounts of submental fat will have improved results if neck liposuction is performed

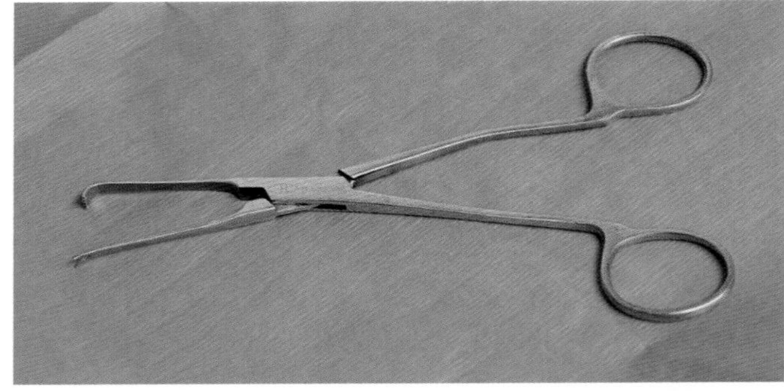

Figure 41.14 Pitanguy flap demarcator. This instrument is useful for estimating the amount of additional skin to be trimmed from the cervicofacial flap on skin closure.

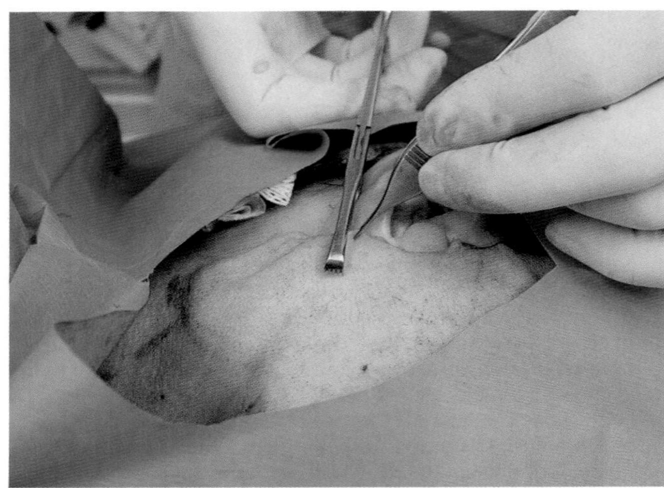

Figure 41.15 Use of Pitanguy flap demarcator to estimate redundant skin to be trimmed on skin closure.

along with face lift. Liposuction of the jowls will reduce the convexity of the jowl but should be done conservatively to avoid a postoperative depression. For most patients, 5 ml or less of supernatant fat should be removed from each jowl.

Platysma plication via corset platysmaplasty should be performed in any patient who has prominent platysmal bands or in any patient who expresses concern over even relatively mild platysmal bands. Platysmaplasty should also be considered in patients with less conspicuous bands but who also demonstrate visible animation of the medial platysma while talking or making facial expressions. Cinching the platysma muscles in the midline via platysmaplasty can enhance the tightening of the neck by face lift via a hammock or sling effect conveyed by the superolateral pull of the SMAS/platysma plication.

In those patients with chin recession, augmentation can be provided by a chin implant (see Chapter 30). Before closure of the submental skin incision, an alloplastic implant can be placed subperiosteally along the anterior surface of the lower edge of the mandible.

Several features of the described face lift procedure are standardized. One such feature is the extent of subcutaneous undermining (approximately 7 cm from the tragus). This distance can be increased as needed to enable better access to the mid-face. Moderately extensive skin undermining allows for more vigorous platysma and SMAS plication because the free skin flap can be directed independent of the SMAS in order to avoid distortion.

Also standardized are the radii of the two purse string SMAS plication sutures. These radii should be measured so that they are identical on both sides of the face. The only variable that determines the actual degree of plication is the tension under which the sutures are tied. Although this tension is appreciated subjectively, equal amounts should be applied on opposite sides of the face. Robust purse string plication of the SMAS can result in significant bunching of the fascia. To smooth the contour, excess fat can be trimmed off the fascia using Metzenbaum scissors. Such trimming should be done cautiously in the area near the zygomatic arch because of the presence of facial nerve branches within the fascia.

■ POSTOPERATIVE CARE

Generally, no drain is needed. Parenteral corticosteroids to reduce postoperative edema are generally not necessary. A head wrap (Design Veronique, Richmond, CA), as is used after cervical liposuction, is placed. Gauze squares of 7.6 × 7.6 cm are placed between the secured skin flap and the head wrap to increase compression over the flap (Fig. 41.16). The level of compression should be mild to moderate so as not to compromise vascular sufficiency of the flap. Postoperative medications include an oral antibiotic (usually cephalexin 500 mg twice daily for 5 days) and an analgesic to be used if needed (e.g. Vicodin). The head wrap dressing should be left on overnight. The patient is generally seen 1 day after surgery and at 7 days for suture removal.

■ PITFALLS AND THEIR MANAGEMENT

The preoperative marking of the juxta-auricular S-form skin excision should be carefully done. The amount of SMAS laxity should be assessed to aid in determining the width of this marking. After SMAS plication, the skin edges should be largely approximated so that dermal sutures can be placed under only mild tension. If too much skin is excised initially, it may be difficult to re-approximate the skin edges after SMAS plication. It is best to be conservative with the initial skin removal; excess skin can always be trimmed at the time of skin closure.

The S-form skin excision should include the subcutaneous fat but should not violate the SMAS. The fat is deeper caudal to the zygomatic arch. Superficial and cephalad to the arch, the skin excision must be done carefully to avoid injury to the superficial temporal vessels and to the most posterior ramus of the temporal branch of the facial nerve (which lies within the superficial temporal fascia).

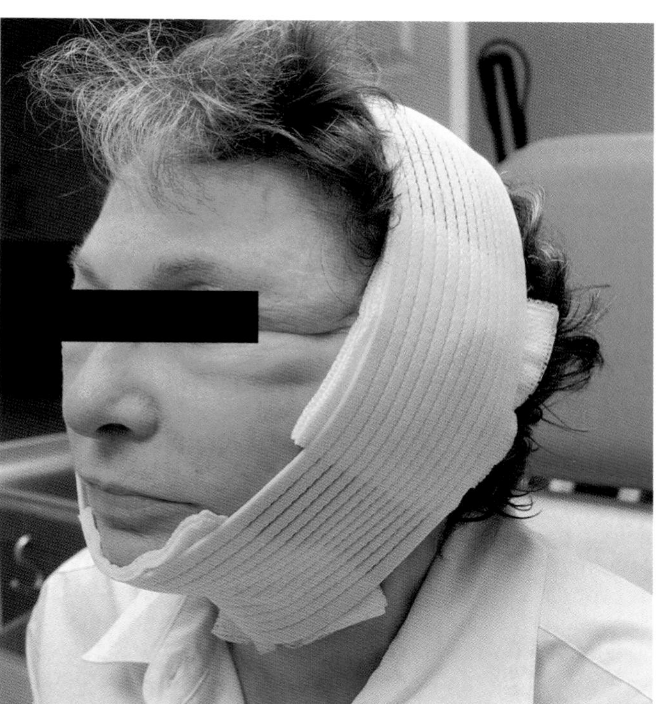

Figure 41.16 Cervicofacial head wrap. This elastic band is placed postoperatively and is worn at least 23 hours per day for 3 days. The wrap provides gentle compression.

Avoidance of pitfalls

- Be conservative with initial skin removal to avoid problems with skin reapproximation.
- Stay superficial to the platysma to avoid injury to the great auricular or marginal mandibular nerves.
- Use bipolar cautery to secure hemostasis.
- Warn smokers to cease smoking for 2 weeks before and after surgery because of the danger of flap necrosis.
- Take care to avoid disrupting the orbitomalar septum, which may result in significant postoperative edema.
- Exercise caution when trimming excess skin upon closure to avoid undue skin tension, which may result in wide scars or 'pixie ear'.

While undermining onto the neck, one must take care to stay superficial to the platysma. Patients who have undergone liposuction of the neck on a previous date may present with considerable subcutaneous fibrosis in this area. This fibrosis can increase the difficulty of undermining and also increase the risk of inadvertently entering the subplatysmal plane. Over the sternocleidomastoid muscle, the great auricular nerve is vulnerable to injury if the plane of dissection goes deep to the platysma. Similarly, the marginal mandibular nerve may be injured by sub-SMAS dissection in the vicinity of the inferior jowl. Metzenbaum scissors can be used to undermine without cutting by advancing the blunt tips of the scissors through subcutaneous fat, then spreading the tips. Some septal attachments between the SMAS and dermis must be cut; this should be done under direct visualization as provided by magnifying loupes and a headlamp (see Table 41.1).

The most feared complication of face lift surgery is hematoma. The vasoconstriction afforded by tumescent anesthesia greatly reduces intra-operative bleeding, but meticulous hemostasis is required to prevent postoperative bleeding. Bipolar cautery is essential to achieve adequate hemostasis. Non-stick bipolar forceps will stay clean of debris (see Table 41.1).

At the end of surgery, the patient should be inspected for evidence of active bleeding. Localized swelling with bruising mandates removal of sutures, identification of the bleeding vessel, and bipolar cautery.

Patients who smoke are at significant risk of flap necrosis postoperatively. If a smoker fails to adhere to the admonition of discontinuing smoking for 2 weeks prior to and after surgery, the vasoconstrictive and toxic effects of cigarette smoke may cause necrosis of the distal part of the flap. Incipient necrosis manifests as a dusky color near the suture line. A healthy flap is pink in color and refills quickly after pressure diascopy. If examination suggests poor revascularization, topical nitroglycerin may be of help as a vasodilator and may forestall necrosis.[20] Oral pentoxifylline may also be of benefit.[20] Necrosis will likely result in a wide scar adjacent to the suture line. This scar can be removed by simple linear excision at a later date.

Undermining in the infraorbital area should be done caudal to the orbitomalar septum.[19] Disrupting this septum can result in significant postoperative edema in the lower eyelid area. The dermal attachment of the septum is denoted by the tear trough (see Fig. 41.4); the inferolateral extent of the septum is generally at a point 2.5–3.0 cm caudal to the lateral canthus.[15,19]

Upon skin closure, excess skin should be trimmed cautiously to avoid removing too much. Tension on the dermal sutures should be mild. Too much tension can result in a wide scar or, at the caudal border of the ear lobule, a ‘pixie ear’ deformity in which downward tension obliterates the normal sulcus between the lobule and the skin of the mastoid area.

■ SUMMARY

The minimal incision rhytidectomy described herein can result in significant improvement in gravitational facial aging, especially if combined with liposuction of neck and jowls, platysmaplasty, and suspension of the malar fat pads. Tumescent local anesthesia, if properly administered, enables the use of very low dose perioperative sedation. Vasoconstriction provided by the tumescent anesthetic provides excellent hemostasis and reduces postoperative bruising and swelling, thus speeding patients’ recovery.

A well-planned juxta-auricular skin excision improves visibility beneath the flap during undermining and simplifies skin closure. Undermining to a moderate distance onto the cheek allows re-draping of the skin flap independently of the SMAS. A periosteal elevator can be used to release the mandibular ligament and the malar fat pad without the need to extend subcutaneous undermining to these areas. Release of the mandibular ligament weakens the cutaneous attachment medial to the jowl and improves the mobility of the jowl upon SMAS plication and skin closure. A suspension suture through the jowl fat pad can further

Table 41.1 Instruments used in minimum incision face lift

Item	Source	Comments
18-gauge mini-accelerator cannulae with luer lock attachment	Byron Medical, Tucson, AZ	These cannulae can be attached to a 10-ml syringe for controlled liposuction of the jowls[16]
SuperCut iris scissors	SSR Inc, Oyster Bay, NY	Useful for excising and trimming skin
Metzenbaum scissors (5 inch, 7 inch)	Miltex Inc, York, PA	Used for undermining
Converse blade retractors (sizes 3 and 4)	Miltex Inc, York, PA	Used for retracting face-lift flap
Mini rake retractor (4 prong)	Van Sickle Surgical Instruments, Bedford, TX	Used for retracting face-lift flap
Periosteal elevators (4 mm, 6 mm, 10 mm)	Implantech, Ventura, CA	Used for release of mandibular ligament and malar fat pad; also useful for sub-periosteal undermining in endoscopic forehead lift and for placement of chin implants
Ferguson needles, half circle	Miltex Inc, York, PA	Used to pass suspension suture through deep temporalis fascia
Non-stick bipolar forceps	Silverglide Surgical Technologies, Boulder, CO	Resistant to accumulating tissue debris during use
Pitanguy flap demarcator	SSR Inc, Oyster Bay, NY	Used to mark excess skin for excision from distal edge of a skin flap
Surgitel micro-mini fiberoptic head-light system	General Scientific Corp, Ann Arbor, MI	Light weight, provides very good illumination of surgical field

correct jowl ptosis. Ptosis of the malar fat pad, the primary cause of gravitational aging of the mid-face, can be lessened by suspension sutures placed in the fat pad and anchored in the deep temporalis fascia behind the temporal hair line.

Superior plication of the lateral platysma and superolateral plication of lateral cheek SMAS can be achieved with purse string sutures through these structures that are anchored in the periosteal tissue of the posterior zygomatic arch. The periosteal anchor is very stable and allows for the application of significant tension to these plication sutures. Enough tension can be applied to provide appreciable lift without the need for release of deep retaining ligaments between bone and SMAS.

The patients depicted in Figures 41.17A–B and 41.18A–B demonstrate the results of the minimum incision face lift described in this chapter.

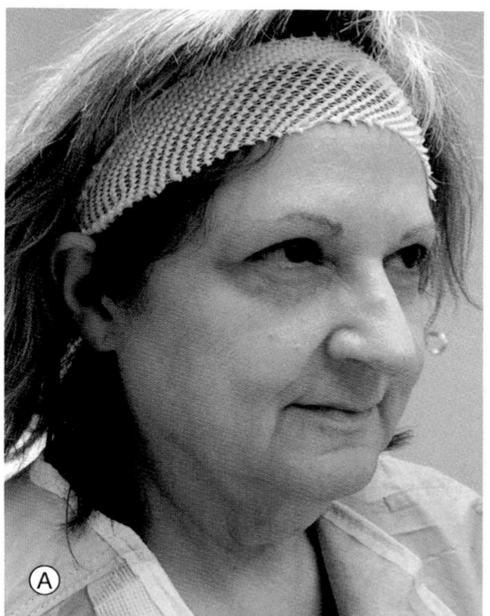

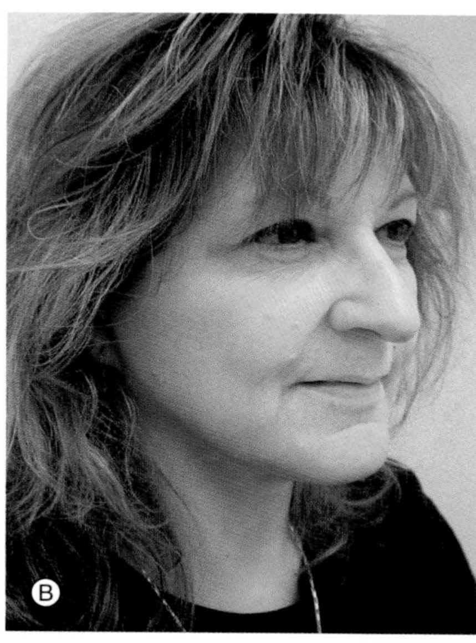

Figure 41.17 This 61-year-old patient is shown (A) before and (B) after liposuction of neck and jowls, corset platysmaplasty and S-lift minimum incision face lift with suture suspension of malar fat pads.

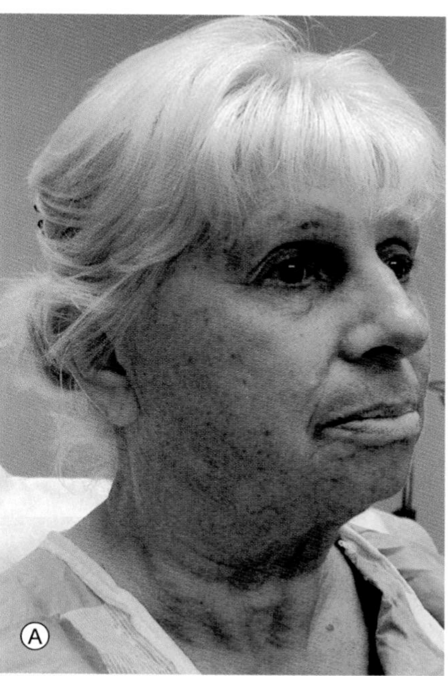

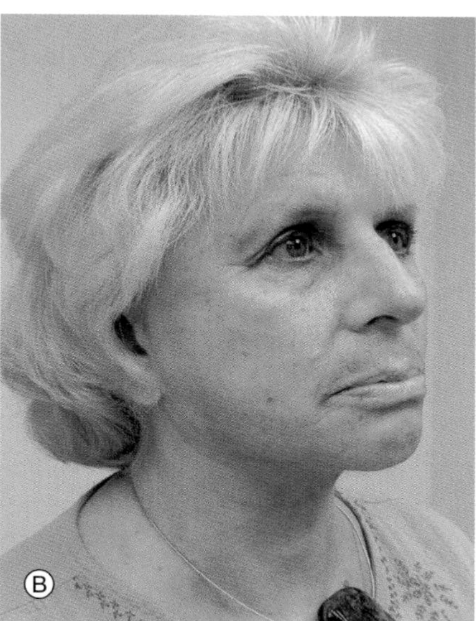

Figure 41.18 This 62-year-old patient is shown (A) before and (B) after liposuction of neck and jowls, corset platysmaplasty, chin implant, and S-lift minimum incision face lift with suture suspension of malar fat pads.

FACIAL SOFT TISSUE LIFTING USING APTOS THREADS

INTRODUCTION AND HISTORY

Facelifts and lipotransfer are standard treatments for facial aging due to gravitational effects and soft tissue atrophy. Correction of facial ptosis with Aptos threads (PromoItalia Wellness Research, Rome, Italy) is a minimally-invasive alternative that was initially reported by Sulamanidze, et al. in 2000.[21,22]

INDICATIONS

Indications for soft tissue lifting with Aptos threads include malar fat pad ptosis, mandibular/submandibular ptosis, and eyebrow ptosis. Aptos threads can be used in combination with other treatments such as liposuction of the neck, subcision of nasolabial folds, and various filling agents.

TECHNIQUE

Aptos threads, produced in Russia and Italy, are comprised of polypropylene. The threads have multiple microhooks on the surface (Fig. 41.19). The microhooks are oriented in one direction on one half of the length of the thread. The microhooks are oriented in the opposite direction on the other half of the thread. This structure causes the thread to anchor itself in tissue resulting in the desired lifting effect. The areas to be treated are marked and injected with local anesthesia (Fig. 41.20). The threads are placed in the subcutaneous tissue using a 16-gauge or 20-gauge flexible metal cannula as a guide. The skin overlying the cannula is "pinched" thereby placing the threads in proper position. The cannula is then withdrawn leaving the thread in place.

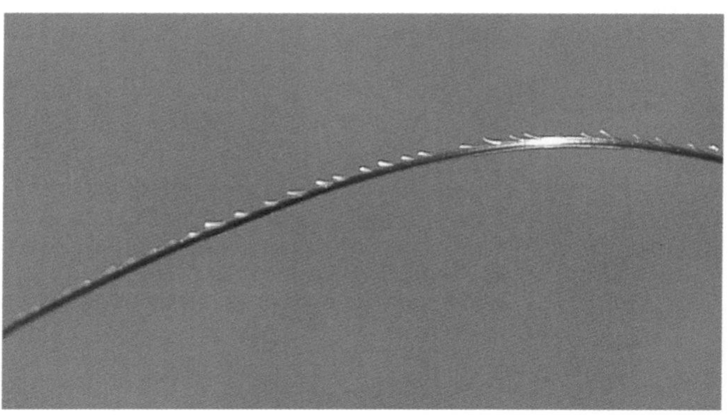

Figure 41.19 Aptos threads are made of polypropylene and contain multiple microhooks. (With permission from Gerhard Sattler MD)

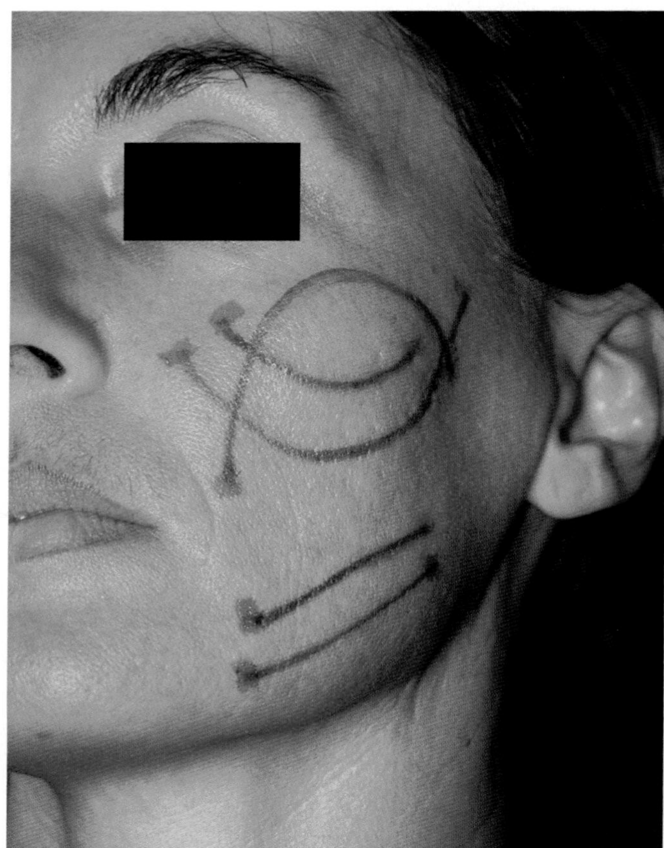

Figure 41.20 Preoperative marking for classic positioning of Aptos threads. (With permission from Gerhard Sattler MD)

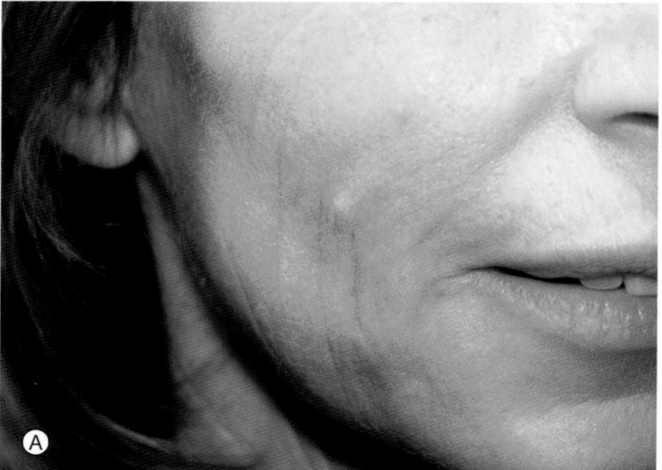

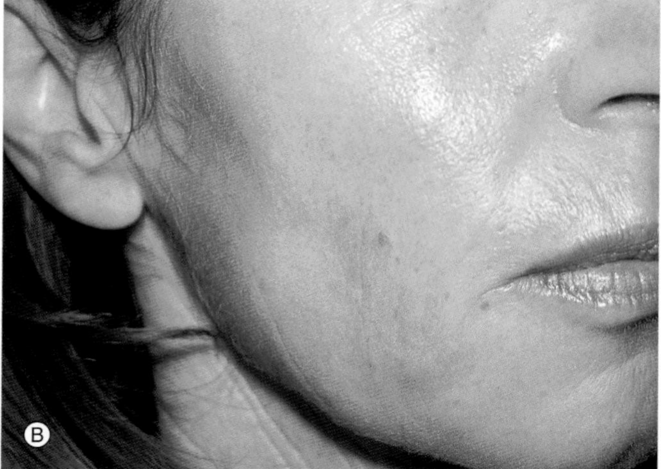

Figure 41.21 (A) Preoperative: typical vertically-oriented facial rhytids are present on the cheek (preoperative). (B) Postoperative: rhytids on the cheek demonstrate improvement following treatment with Aptos threads. (With permission from Gerhard Sattler MD)

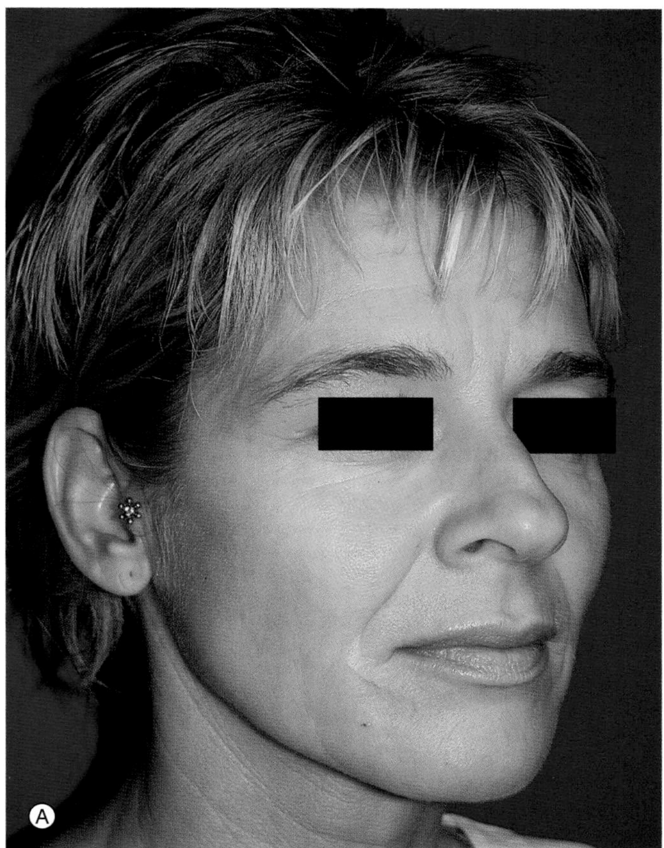

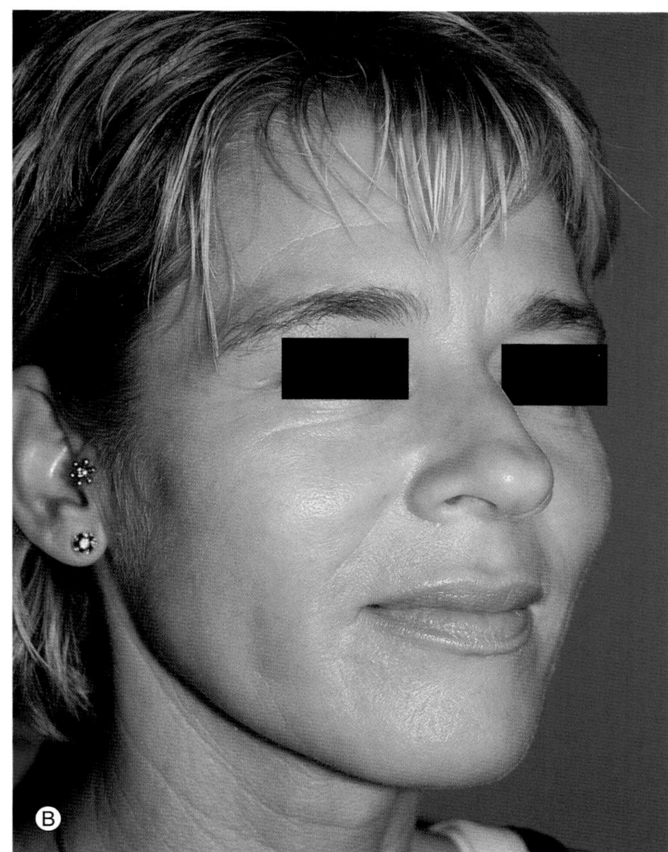

Figure 41.22 (A) Preoperative: deep nasolabial folds are a manifestation of aging changes due to facial ptosis. (B) Postoperative: the nasolabial folds have been improved following elevation of the ptotic malar fat pad with Aptos threads. (With permission from Gerhard Sattler MD)

The redundant portion of the threads are cut off and the ends are buried in the subcutaneous tissue. Both sides of the face are treated as identically as possible.

RESULTS AND COMPLICATIONS

Minimal swelling of treated areas is present postoperatively. Fibrosis develops around the threads over 4–6 weeks. Patients are generally pleased with the results and the minimally-invasive nature of the procedure (Figs 41.21 and 41.22). We have treated 100 patients with Aptos threads to date. Complications have been minimal and occasional, and include asymmetric placement, asymmetric bulging, inflammatory dermal papules (from improperly buried threads), and movement of threads due to different numbers of microhooks on one side of the face compared to the other. Removal of threads is occasionally necessary and is easily accomplished. Other authors have begun to report their experience.[23,24]

■ REFERENCES

1. Gosain AK, Yousif NJ, Madiedo G, et al. Surgical anatomy of the SMAS: a reinvestigation. Plast Reconstr Surg 1993; 92:1254–1263.
2. Furnas DW. The retaining ligaments of the cheek. Plast Reconstr Surg 1989; 83:11–16.
3. Özdemir R, Kilinç H, Ünlü E, et al. Anatomicohistologic study of the retaining ligaments of the face and use in face lift: retaining ligament correction and SMAS plication. Plast Reconstr Surg 2002; 110:1134–1149.
4. Bernstein L, Nelson RH. Surgical anatomy of the extraparotid distribution of the facial nerve. Arch Otolaryngol 1984; 110:177–183.
5. Hamra ST. A study of the long-term effect of malar fat repositioning in face lift surgery: short-term success but long-term failure. Plast Reconstr Surg 2002; 110:940–951.
6. Mendelson BC. A study of the long-term effect of malar fat repositioning in face lift surgery: short-term success but long-term failure. Plast Reconstr Surg 2002; 110:952–955 (discussion).
7. Hester TR. A study of the long-term effect of malar fat repositioning in face lift surgery: short-term success but long-term failure. Plast Reconstr Surg 2002; 110:956–959 (discussion).
8. Yousif NJ, Gosain A, Matloub HS, et al. The nasolabial fold: an anatomic and histologic reappraisal. Plast Reconstr Surg 1994; 93:60–69.
9. Gosain AK, Amarante MTJ, Hyde JS, et al. A dynamic analysis of changes in the nasolabial fold using magnetic resonance imaging: implications for facial rejuvenation and facial animation surgery. Plast Reconstr Surg 1996; 98:622–636.
10. Hoefflin SM. The extended supraplatysmal plane (ESP) face lift. Plast Reconstr Surg 1998; 101:494–503.
11. Baker DC. Lateral SMAS-ectomy. Plast Reconstr Surg 1997; 100:509–513.
12. Baker DC. Minimal incision rhytidectomy (short scar face lift) with lateral SMAS-ectomy: evolution and application. Aesth Surg J 2001; 21:14–26.
13. Mendelson, BC. SMAS fixation to the facial skeleton: rationale and results. Plast Reconstr Surg 1997; 100:1834–1842.
14. Saylan Z. Purse string-formed plication of the SMAS with fixation to the zygomatic bone. Plast Reconstr Surg 2002; 110:667–671.
15. Pessa JE, Garza JR. The malar septum: the anatomic basis of malar mounds and malar edema. Aesth Surg J 1997; 17:11–17.
16. Langdon RC. Liposuction of neck and jowls: five-incision method combining machine-assisted and syringe aspiration. Dermatol Surg 2000; 26:388–391.

17. Feldman JJ. Corset platysmaplasty. Plast Reconstr Surg 1990; 85:333–343.
18. Sasaki GH, Cohen AT. Meloplication of the malar fat pads by percutaneous cable-suture technique for mid-face rejuvenation: outcome study 392 cases, 6 years' experience. Plast Reconstr Surg 2002; 110:635–654.
19. Owsley JQ, Zweifler M. Mid-face lift of the malar fat pad: technical advances. Plast Reconstr Surg 2002; 110:674–685.
20. Karacaoglan N, Akbas H. Effect of parenteral pentoxifylline and topical nitroglycerin on skin flap survival. Otolaryngol Head Neck Surg 1999; 120:272–4.
21. Sulamanidze MA, Fournier PF, Paikidze TG, Sulamanidze GM. Removal of facial soft tissue ptosis with special threads. Dermatol Surg 2000; 28:367–71.
22. Sulamanidze MA, Shiffman MA, Paikidze TG, et al. Facial lifting with aptos threads. Int J Cosm Surg Aesthet Dermatol. 2001; 4:275–80.
23. Sandhofer M, Sandhofer-Novak R, Blugerman G, Sattler G. Aptos-Lifting: Eine minimal invasive Methode zur Gesichtsrejuvenation. Aesthet Dermatol 2003; 1:10-17.
24. Lycka B, Bazan C, Poletti E, Treen B. The emerging technique of the antiptosis subdermal suspension thread. Dermatol Surg 2004; 30:41–44.

42 Blepharoplasty and Brow Lift

Brent R Moody MD and Paul J Weber MD

Summary box

- Blepharoplasty and brow lifting are common functional and cosmetic surgical procedures that are well within the scope of the dermatologic surgeon's practice.
- Appropriate preoperative evaluation and counseling help to ensure appropriate patient selection. Referral to an ophthalmic surgeon may be warranted in questionable cases.
- Upper and lower eyelid blepharoplasty can be performed as distinct procedures or can be combined in the same surgical setting. Brow lifting can be performed concomitantly. If blepharoplasty and brow lifting are to be combined, upper eyelid skin should be conservatively removed.
- Blepharoplasty can be performed as an office-based procedure with local anesthetic.
- Brow lifting should be considered whenever brow ptosis is present.

INTRODUCTION

Blepharoplasty is a popular cosmetic surgical procedure. A conservative estimate is that over 250 000 blepharoplasties were performed in the United States in 2002. Brow lifting is less commonly performed than blepharoplasty but still remains a popular procedure.[1] Blepharoplasty and brow lifting are performed by surgeons of different training backgrounds. Dermatologic surgeons, oculoplastic surgeons, otorhinolaryngologists, oral and maxillofacial surgeons and plastic surgeons all perform the procedures and contribute to the surgical literature. Most blepharoplasties are performed to achieve aesthetic improvement of the periocular face. However, the surgical techniques of cosmetic blepharoplasty apply to functional lid surgery as well. Upper blepharoplasty may seek to restore a full visual field in the patient with extreme dermatochalasis or be necessary to repair defects from injury or tumor extirpation. Excess upper eyelid skin may serve as a donor site for full-thickness skin grafts. Much like blepharoplasty, brow lifting has roles in both cosmetic and functional surgery. The primary functional role of brow lifting is for the patient with significant brow ptosis from injury or aging.

The goal of this chapter is to provide the reader with a thorough understanding of the surgical anatomy and principles involved with eyelid and brow surgery. While no single standard or cookbook approach exists for any surgical procedure, certain concepts and techniques have withstood the test of time and are generally accepted.

Key anatomic considerations

A thorough knowledge of orbital anatomy allows the surgeon to customize the surgical approach for any patient, avoid complications, and obtain the desired outcome. The surgeon should have a working knowledge of surface anatomy as well as all dissected tissue planes and structures involved. Figure 42.1 demonstrates germane surface anatomy landmarks. Figure 42.2 illustrates key cross-sectional anatomic structures of the upper and lower lids. Surgeons should make special note of the inferior oblique (Fig. 42.3) and inferior rectus muscles, as these extraocular muscles can be injured during lower lid blepharoplasty.[2,3] Likewise, the trochlea and superior oblique muscle tendon may be injured during upper blepharoplasty.[4] Figure 42.4 shows the locations of the fat pads that are frequently modified during cosmetic blepharoplasty, as well as the canthal tendons and inferior oblique muscle.

Make note of the lacrimal gland laterally as well as the canthal tendons. The nasal (medial) upper fat pad is usually white in color, in contrast to the yellow preaponeurotic fat pad.[5] Immediately beneath the preaponeurotic fat pad lies the levator aponeurosis. The lower lid rectractors—the capsulopalpebral fascia (CPF)—illustrated in Figure 42.2 should also be noted as injury and scarring to this structure can lead to lower eyelid retraction.

Blepharoplasty

Patients will present to the surgeon desiring either a cosmetic enhancement or functional improvement in their

Surface anatomy of the eye

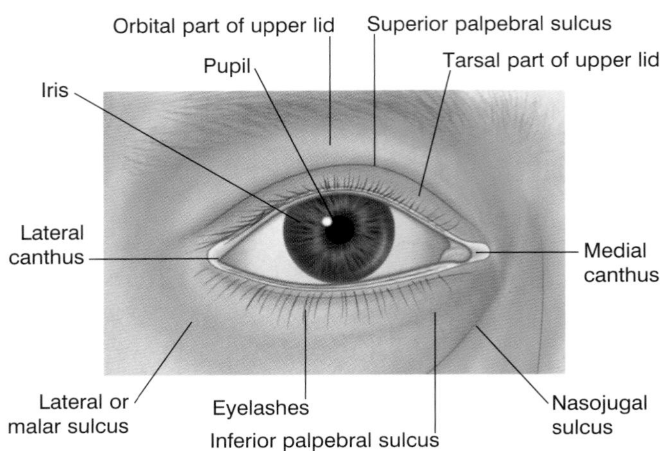

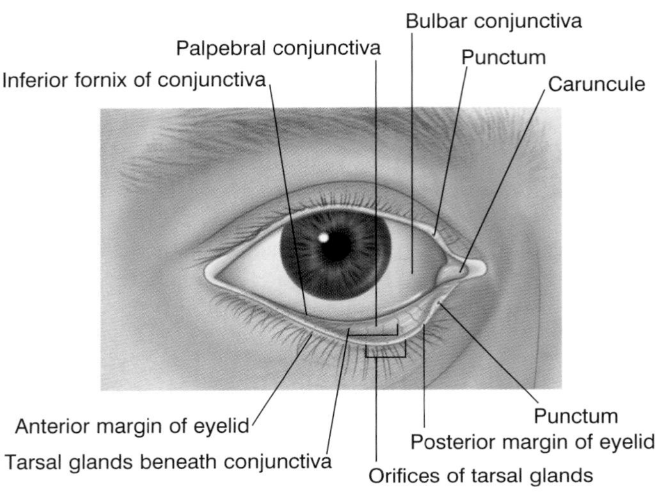

Figure 42.1 Superficial periocular anatomy.

eyelids or brow region. The preoperative evaluation should include a thorough discussion of the risks and benefits of the planned procedure. People seeking cosmetic enhancement often need additional preoperative counseling and guidance to ensure that realistic expectations are set. When interviewing and evaluating patients, it may be best to use open-ended questions such as 'what do you wish to improve?' This interview process is optimized when patients contemplate and articulate their own goals for surgery. Ask patients to bring old photos; these may help the surgeon determine what they want the postoperative result to approximate. A hand-held mirror allows patients to look at their face as a cotton-tipped applicator is used to hold up excess skin. The surgeon should be wary of the patient who asks what should be done. The surgeon may advise what can be done with an acceptable probability of success. Ultimately, patients must decide if what is possible is congruent with their aesthetic goals. Most patients will present with some combination of brow or lid ptosis, excess skin, or prominent fat pads. Blepharoplasty and brow lifting may address these concerns.

After the patient's goals for surgery have been defined, the obligation of the surgeon is to evaluate the patient thoroughly. The first step is to define the problem or problems and ensure that the planned procedure can address them. A patient with significant lid ptosis will not likely be well served if only a blepharoplasty is performed and the underlying ptotic lid is not addressed. In a patient with significant dermatochalasis and mild ptosis simply pointing out the drooping of the eyelid preoperatively will be important. Similarly, a patient with excess lower lid skin may require more than simple fat pad removal through a transconjunctival approach.

It is helpful to develop standardized preoperative evaluation sheets. A sample patient questionnaire is presented in Figure 42.5. A sample physician template is presented in Figure 42.6. The use of the template requires the surgeon to demonstrate conscious consideration of each aspect of the evaluation and avoid omissions. While the value of routine preoperative ophthalmic evaluation has been questioned, the authors require it of each patient, as an adjuvant to our evaluation.[6] Particular attention is paid to signs or symptoms of thyroid ophthalmopathy, dry eyes (Schirmer's test), and lid laxity. Standard laboratory evaluation includes hematologic and coagulation profiles (complete blood count with platelets, prothrombin and partial thromboplastin times), a blood chemistry profile, and a thyroid panel.

Tests for lower-lid laxity are paramount in the preoperative evaluation because scleral show or frank ectropion are possible after lower lid blepharoplasty. Two tests that should be routinely performed are the distraction test and the snap test. The distraction test is performed by pulling the lower lid anteriorly away from the globe. If greater than 7 mm of lid excursion occurs, lower-lid horizontal laxity is present. In the snap test, the lower lid is pulled inferiorly. If the lid does not spontaneously return to the normal position prior to the next blink, the test is positive, indicating lower-lid laxity. The snap test is a test of orbicularis oculi tone. Lower-lid laxity is not a contraindication to surgery, but rather an indication that a lid-tightening procedure may be needed.[7] Figure 42.7 illustrates the snap and distraction tests.

An evaluation for lid ptosis is also warranted. Some cases of ptosis are obvious, whereas others are relatively subtle. The preferred test for ptosis is measurement of the marginal reflex distance (MRD). The MRD describes the position of the eyelids relative to the mid-pupillary line. MRD can be performed by measuring the relationship in millimeters from the margin of the upper eyelid to a penlight reflex in the pupil. A normal MRD is 4 mm. While an exact measurement is not necessary, the relationship of the light reflex to the lower eyelid is important to note. It should be symmetric between the eyelids and may be an indication of globe malposition if asymmetric. The patient with globe malposition should be evaluated by an ophthalmic surgeon as this condition may be associated with an orbital tumor or thyroid ophthalmopathy. Lower scleral show may be an indication of eyelid laxity. Mild ptosis is manifested by an upper MRD of 1.5–2 mm; moderate ptosis by an MRD of 0.5 mm; and severe ptosis by an MRD of –0.5 mm. Figure 42.8 illustrates the MRD and palpebral fissure measurements. An assessment of levator function is also required. Levator function can be

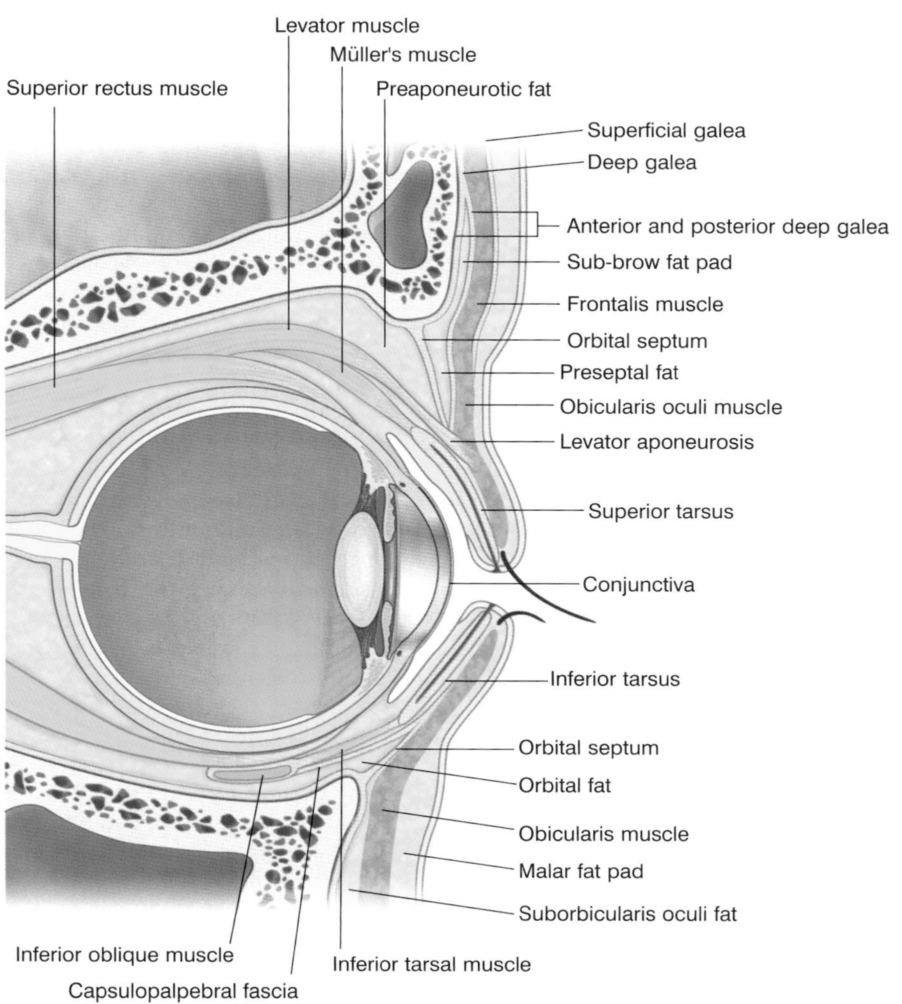

Figure 42.2 Cross-sectional anatomy of upper and lower eyelids.

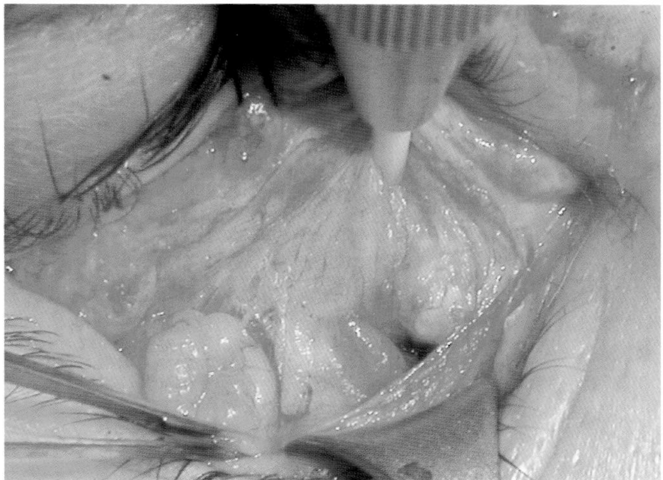

Figure 42.3 Inferior oblique muscle from surgeon's view during lower eyelid transconjunctival blepharoplasty. The inferior oblique muscle may prolapse with the orbital fat and can be visualized between the central and medial fat pads. The muscle is superior to the Desmarres lid retractor. Courtesy of John B Holds MD and Valerie Vick MD.

tested by measuring upper eyelid excursion when the patient moves the eyes from maximal downgaze to maximal upgaze with a fixed brow position. A full discussion of the evaluation and management of ptosis may be found in various references. Blepharoplasty surgeons should be familiar with the etiology of adult ptosis. The surgeon may also consider consultation from an ophthalmologist. Most cases of adult acquired ptosis are involutional and can be corrected with levator aponeurosis advancement at the time of blepharoplasty.[8,9]

After devising a surgical plan, the surgeon must make every effort to maximize the possibility of success. As discussed later, bleeding is a rare but serious complication of blepharoplasty. All anticoagulants must be stopped prior to surgery. If a patient has a medical condition that requires uninterrupted anticoagulants, proceeding with surgery should be seriously reconsidered. Herbal supplements and some vitamins may increase the tendency for bleeding and many common over-the-counter medications contain aspirin or non-steroidal anti-inflammatory drugs. Blepharoplasty surgeons should maintain an updated list of such products.[10] Blood pressure under good control helps to minimize bleeding complications.

Upper and lower eyelid fat pads and tendons

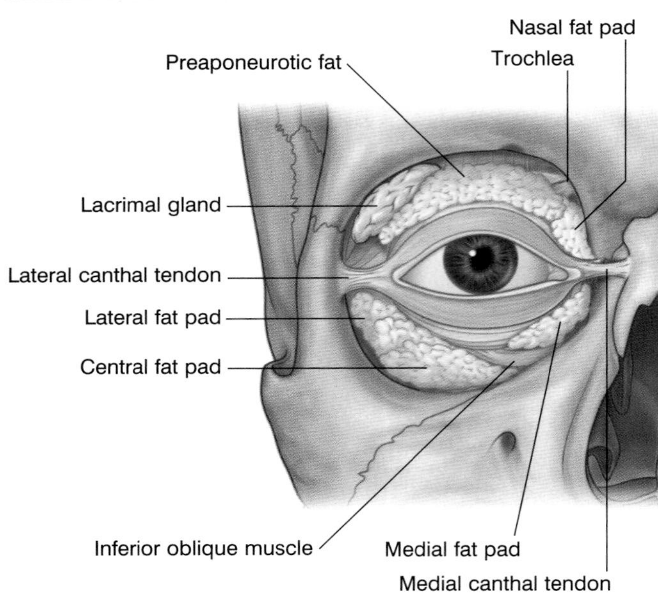

Figure 42.4 Upper and lower eyelid fat pads and tendons.

Brow lifting

The preoperative evaluation of the brow lifting patient is similar to that of the blepharoplasty patient. A detailed ocular history is performed, just as in blepharoplasty. Attention is paid to symptoms of dry eye and a Schirmer test is performed. Special attention should be paid to the brow position in relationship to the orbital rim. The male brow typically is relatively flat and rests at the level of the orbital rim. The female brow will generally arch laterally with its apex at the lateral canthus.[11] As age-related changes occur, the position of the brow will descend. Frequently, patients will present with an eyelid complaint, when in fact brow ptosis is a significant factor in their problem. Patients will employ unconscious constant frontalis muscle contraction to overcome brow ptosis. This phenomenon should be recognized and explained to the patient. Many patients who would benefit from a combined brow lift and blepharoplasty elect blepharoplasty alone. They do so to minimize surgical cost and morbidity. These patients need to firmly understand the limitations of blepharoplasty and acknowledge that a blepharoplasty alone should be considered a compromise solution.

If the operative plan includes general anesthesia or significant sedation, an assessment of the patient's overall health must be taken into consideration.

■ TECHNIQUES

Upper-eyelid blepharoplasty

The fundamental purpose of upper-lid blepharoplasty is to remove redundant skin and muscle from the upper lid (Figs 42.9–42.16). Fat is removed in variable amounts.

Skin marking

Experienced surgeons may expertly mark most planned skin excisions by visual inspection alone. However, the neophyte surgeon benefits from a more systematic approach to eyelid marking. The upper eyelid crease is marked either with a full line of surgical marking ink or, most preferably, by a series of dots. Determination of the upper lid crease is facilitated by the patient slowly looking up and down. The planned excision is then marked, paying attention to crease symmetry between the two eyelids. In women, the planned excision is approximately 8–10 mm above the lash line (8 mm medially, 10 mm centrally, 9 mm laterally) and 10–15 mm below the eyebrow. In men, the excision should be 6–8 mm above the lash line and 15–20 mm below the eyebrow. Figure 42.9 illustrates suggested skin markings for upper-eyelid blepharoplasty.

After marking, the patient should assume an upright position to recheck the surgical markings. Alternatively, the patient can be initially marked while sitting. Pinch testing the planned resection with non-toothed forceps helps ensure an appropriate surgical plan, leaving enough skin to allow complete eyelid closure. The amount of skin removed must be customized for each patient and desired outcome. A conservative approach should minimize the risk of over resection of skin.[11] The goal of surgery is to create a symmetric result, which may necessitate asymmetric removal of skin, muscle, and fat. Again note that concurrent brow lifting will require a more conservative skin excision.

Anesthesia and skin preparation and drape

Depending upon the patient, upper blepharoplasty may be performed as an office-based procedure entirely under local anesthetic. The addition of oral or intravenous sedation may enhance patient comfort, but is not required. Commercially available lidocaine 2% with epinephrine (adrenaline) 1 in 100 000 is the preferred initial anesthetic injection and is buffered to decrease patient discomfort. The initial anesthetic may be followed with a 50/50 mixture of lidocaine 2% and bupivacaine 0.5% with epinephrine (adrenaline). The authors do not routinely use hyaluronidase, as there is a small risk of allergic reaction, and the lack of hyaluronidase does not hamper the efficacy of the surgery.

Approximately 1–1.5 ml of anesthetic is injected subcutaneously into each lid. We use a 3-ml syringe and 30-gauge needle. Gentle pressure can be applied to the lid to minimize the risk of hematoma formation.[11] Ten minutes are allowed to lapse to achieve maximum vasoconstriction from the epinephrine (adrenaline).

A sterile surgeon's bonnet cap covers and controls the patient's hair. To allow for visualization of the entire face during surgery, no drapes are placed over the face. The entire surgical field, including the exposed face is then prepped. Sterile drapes are then placed around the patient's face and head.

Skin and muscle excision

Using a surgical blade, electrosurgical needle, or carbon dioxide laser, the skin and underlying orbicularis oculi are incised (Fig. 42.10). Once the initial incisions have been made, the skin-muscle flap can be excised with scissors, a #15 scalpel blade, electrosurgical needle, or carbon dioxide laser (Fig. 42.11). The choice of instrumentation is based

Blepharoplasty questionnaire

1

Date of your last eye exam: ....

Name and address of the physician who performed the examination: ....

....

CIRCLE THE ANSWERS; USE OTHER SIDE OF PAGE FOR LONGER ANSWERS PLEASE

No Yes 1. Do you wear glasses or contact lenses? (circle which)

No Yes 2. Do you have any history of glaucoma or other eye disease?

No Yes 3. Have you had any injuries or surgery to the eyes or lids? Explain:

....

....

No Yes 4. Do you have frequent irritations to the eyes themselves or the skin of the lids?

No Yes 5. Do you now take or have you taken medications or drops for the eyes? Explain:

....

....

No Yes 6. Are you bothered by dry eyes?

No Yes 7. Do your eyes tear excessively?

No Yes 8. Do you now have or have you ever had visual problems with one or both eyes? Explain:

....

....

No Yes 9. Are there any other problems we have not asked about that you feel we should know?

....

No Yes 10. On looking in a mirror, do you notice any differences between the right and left eyes?

....

No Yes 11. Do you notice any intermittent or cyclical swelling of the eyes? How often are the cycles?

....

Figure 42.5 Blepharoplasty questionnaire. With permission from Weber PJ, Oleson GB, Moody BR. Evaluation documentation in cosmetic oculoplastic surgery. Int J Cosmetic Surg 2000; 2:41.

Blepharoplasty questionnaire (continued)

2

Patient Name:.. Date:...

No Yes 12. Are you pleased with the appearance of your eyebrows? If not, why?

(Please refer to the diagram below) What do you believe are the problem areas of your eyes (as far as appearance is concerned) indicate by circling.

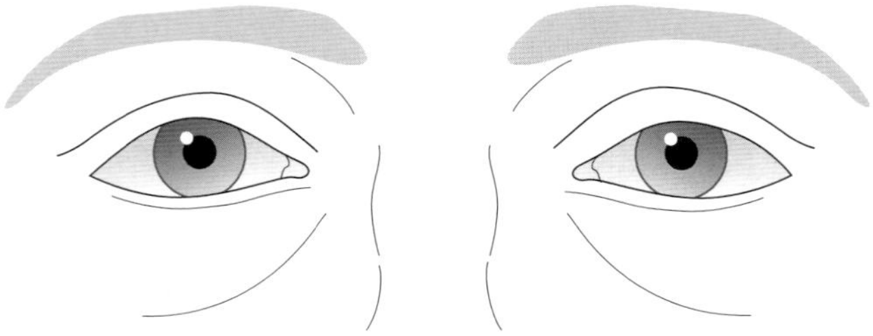

Which of the following seven items regarding your eyes would you like to be changed: (circle):

Color texture fine wrinkles "bagginess" coarse wrinkles thin skin crow's feet

How many years younger do you wish your eyes to look? (circle) 20 10 5 or (appropriate for my age)

Please read the following and carry out the instructions:

Cover your RIGHT eye and read THIS sentence with your LEFT eye only.

Are you able to read it comfortably?....... with glasses (Y or N)....... without glasses (Y or N)

Cover your LEFT eye and read THIS sentence with your RIGHT eye only....... with glasses...... without glasses.

If there is any difference in your vision please indicate:

..........Both eyes same (approximately)....... Right eye stronger....... Left eye stronger

I signify that the information provided above is correct to the best of my knowledge:

X.. ....

(signature) (date)

Figure 42.5, continued.

Blepharoplasty examination

Patient Name: .... Date: 1

EYEBROW: Hair density: 0 + ++ +++ Symmetry: Ⓡ vs. Ⓛ
Brow insertion (at or above) orbital rim (circle):...
Segmental brow ptosis? If yes, what is the lift necessary (mm)?
Ⓡ lat( ) Ⓡ mid( ) Ⓡ nasal( ) Δ Ⓛ nasal( ) Ⓛ mid( ) Ⓛ lat( )
(+/–) High forehead; (+/–) receding hairline; (+/–) sparse scalp hair

LACRIMAL GLAND: + or –, Ⓡ or Ⓛ
( ) Visible temporal fullness; ( ) lid double eversion;
( ) Visible on digital globe pressure; Schirmer test in mm Ⓡ ( ) vs. Ⓛ ( ) (+/–) anesthetized

VISUAL ACUITY: With contacts or glasses in: ( ) 20/20 Ⓡ, ( ) 20/20 Ⓛ
Ophthalmologist or optometrist (circle): ....
Refraction: Ⓡ:........... /........... Ⓛ:........... /........... Exam date:...

OTHER: ( ) Ⓡ Ⓛ ( ) Bell's phenomenon
PERRLA: + or – (circle)
Pigment or tattoo at lid margins: upper....... lower lids.......

( ) Round facies; ( ) hypertrichosis; ( ) thinned eyebrows;
( ) protuberant globes; ( ) sweating

PTOSIS LIDS: (Lid margin coverage of limbus)
MRD upper lid: Ⓡ Ⓛ
MRD lower lid: Ⓡ Ⓛ

PTOSIS grade: ( ) Ⓡ middle Δ Ⓛ middle( )

MRD Upper
Normal 4mm
Mild ptosis 1.5–2mm
Moderate ptosis 0.5mm
Severe ptosis -0.5mm

LEVATOR function: ( ) Ⓡ middle Δ Ⓛ middle( )mm excursion
Upper lid from far upgaze to downgaze with the eyebrow fixed over three trials (normal = 12–16 mm; good = 8–12; fair = 5–7; poor ≤ 4mm)

VISUAL FIELDS: (2–3" from examiner, opposite eye occluded)

(untouched) ____________|________ ____________|________
– Ⓡ nasal Ⓛ nasal –

(brows only elevated) ____________|________ ____________|________
– Ⓡ nasal Ⓛ nasal –

(lids and brows elevated) ____________|________ ____________|________
– Ⓡ nasal Ⓛ nasal –

Vertical palpebral fissure (N = 8–10mm) ( ) Ⓡ middle Δ Ⓛ middle( )
Horizontal fissure (mm) ( ) ⟨A⟩ ( )

UPPER LIDS: Skin thickness of upper lid (circle): very thin, thin, normal, thick

Figure 42.6 Blepharoplasty examination. Modified with permission from Weber PJ, Oleson GB, Moody BR. Evaluation documentation in cosmetic oculoplastic surgery. Int J Cosmetic Surg 2000; 2:41.

2

Patient Name: .... Date: ....

XS-skin (mm): XS-skin (mm):Ⓡlateral( )Ⓡmiddle( )Ⓡnasal( )△Ⓛnasal( )Ⓛmiddle( )Ⓛlat( )

UPPER LIDS (cont'd): Natural crease height (by pulling up on lower eyebrow) in mm:
Ⓡlat( )Ⓡmid( )Ⓡnasal( )△Ⓛnasal( )Ⓛmid( )Ⓛlat( )
Estimated excision (mm necessary) upper lid SKIN:
Muller's muscle/epi. Test: neosynephrine response ( )Ⓡ middle△Ⓛmiddle( )

FATTY pockets (eyes closed tightly, gentle pressure on globes, 0, +, or ++):
uppers: Ⓡlat( )Ⓡmid( )Ⓡnasal( )△Ⓛnasal( )Ⓛmid( )Ⓛlat( )
lowers: Ⓡlat( )Ⓡmid( )Ⓡnasal( )△Ⓛnasal( )Ⓛmid( )Ⓛlat( )

LOWER lids: 'Bags on bags' (orbicularis festooning), 0 / + / ++ ( )Ⓡ middle△Ⓛ middle( )
If + and not longstanding: Allergy: ....
Renal: .... Thyroid: ....
Scleral 'show' (mm):
uppers ( )Ⓡmiddle△Ⓛmiddle( ); lowers ( )Ⓡmid△Ⓛmid( )
Eyelid edema/erythema: ( )Ⓡmiddle△Ⓛmiddle( )
Tattoo or pigment? ....
Hypertrophic orbicularis muscle: ( ) middle middle( )
Hypoplasia of maxilla, malar eminences? Y / N, if 'yes' discuss: ....

HORIZONTAL TONE / LAXITY: 'Snap-back test' (w/o blinking) 0/ +/ ++........... seconds : ( )Ⓡmiddle△Ⓛ middle( )
(Orbicularis 'cheating' = with .... # of blinks) .... #: ( )Ⓡmiddle△Ⓛ middle( )

TENZEL 'Snap-back' (laxity gradation: 'mild' = no 'show', slowly back; 'mod' = >1 mm 'show', 2–3 blinks for return; 'marked' ≥ 1mm of 'show' and/or ectropion)

MARGIN DISTRACTION ('Pull test' 6–8 mm = lax) ( )Ⓡmiddle△Ⓛmiddle( )

LATERAL CANTHAL TENDON: Lateral canthal 'web': 0 , + , ++ ( )Ⓡmiddle△Ⓛmiddle( )
Distance between lateral orbital rim and canthus in mm (N << 1 fingerbreadth)

MEDIAL CANTHAL TENDON: Abn., if able to be pulled to medial limbus: ( )Ⓡ△Ⓛ( )
(Tenzel: abn., if pulled ≥ 3mm from med canthus): ( )Ⓡ△Ⓛ( )

OTHER: ....

Pt. Anxiety level (0 (lowest) – 5 (high)):...........; Unreasonable expectations or 'perfectionist': ....
Appears: ( ) unkempt ( ) hygiene; 'dry eyes'....................... ; 'scars' ....
Thyroid symptoms:.............................. ; Who desires blepharoplasty?...
Underlying concerns: ( ) social; ( ) business; ( ) other...
Brow aches .... ; eye 'fatigue'..................... ; visual field loss ....
bleeding history...........; ASA products............; arthritis...........; hypertension...
FH ptosis:...........; child pictures if ptotic?...
Daily history of varying ptosis (myasthenia gravis): ....
Previous eye surgery (cataract, retina, trauma, neovascularizing diseases, etc.) ....
Blepharochalasis (at puberty, bouts of allergic edema, +FH) ....

Figure 42.6, continued.

Snap and distraction tests

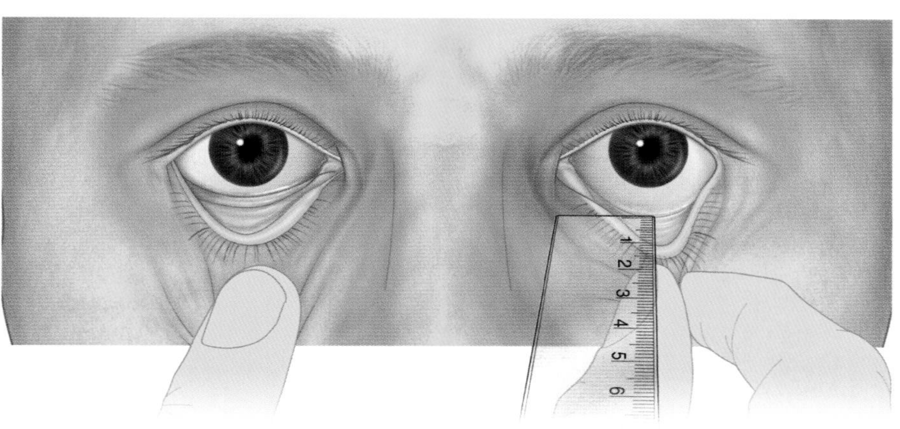

Figure 42.7 The snap and distraction tests, utilized to assess lower-eyelid tone.

Marginal reflex distance and palpebral fissure

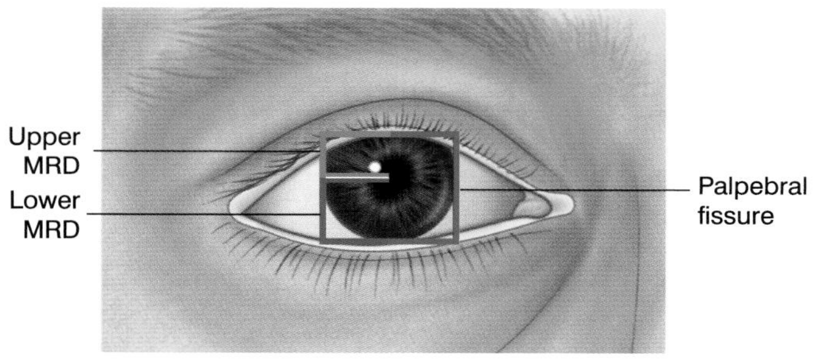

Figure 42.8 Measurement of the marginal reflex distance (MRD) and palpebral fissure.

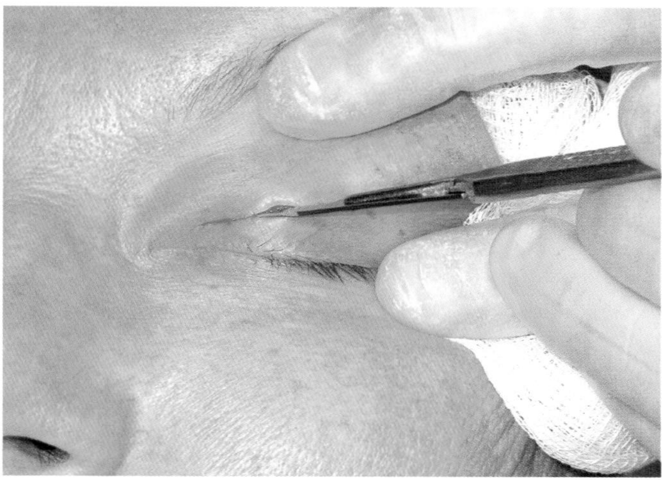

Figure 42.10 Upper blepharoplasty. Incising the skin flap. Courtesy of John B Holds MD and Valerie Vick MD.

Skin markings for upper blepharoplasty

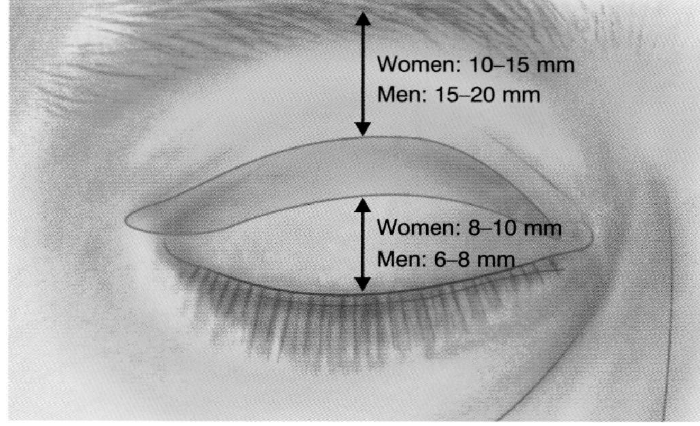

Figure 42.9 Skin markings for upper blepharoplasty.

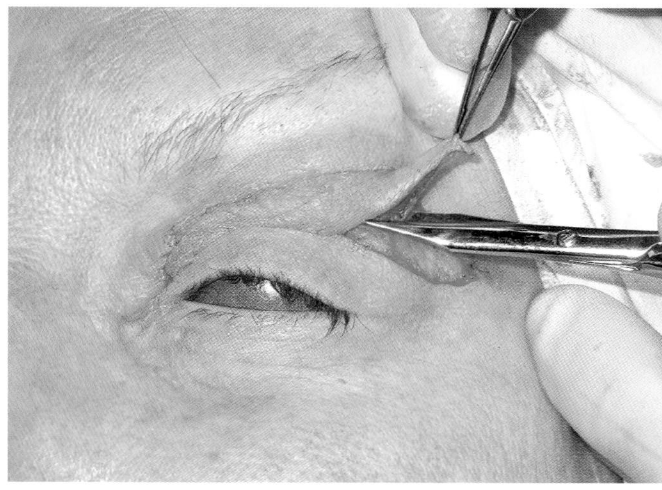

Figure 42.11 Upper blepharoplasty. Dissection of the skin-muscle flap. Optimal plane of dissection is below orbicularis muscle but above the orbital septum. Courtesy of John B Holds MD and Valerie Vick MD.

upon surgeon preference and practice. If no fat pad extraction is planned, the orbital septum is left intact and skin closure is performed. When fat pad extraction is planned, the orbital septum is opened. Some surgeons advocate that septal incision occurs with the skin-muscle flap while others feel that this should be a separate step in the procedure.[11,12] Remaining standing cutaneous cones at the lateral aspect of the excision can be removed by extending the excision into a crow's foot line. In patients with marked tissue redundancy at the medial aspect of the excision, a Burow's triangle of skin can be removed, or W-plasty performed. Care must be taken to avoid extending the excision much beyond the medial punctum as a medial canthal web can result.[13] If it is necessary to extend the medial excision beyond the punctum, a slight upturning of the excision will help prevent webbing (personal communication, J.B. Holds, August 2003). Sutures can be placed to fixate the eyelid crease prior to skin closure.

Fat pad extraction

The amount of fat to be removed is based primarily on two concepts: how much fat should be removed to achieve the desired aesthetic result and how much fat can be removed based upon the patient's fat pad anatomy. The correct amount of fat extraction is the lesser of these two quantities. Overly aggressive fat removal can result in a hollowed appearance to the upper lid. This concept helps determine how much fat should be removed. How much fat can be removed is determined by the amount of fat that prolapses after opening the septum and teasing it out. Fat should never be placed under significant traction as there is a risk of vascular injury.[12,13]

If the septum has not been opened as part of the skin muscle flap, it may now be incised (Fig. 42.12). Identification of the orbital septum is based upon the visible fibrous strands within the septum.[11] Additionally, gentle traction with forceps will confirm the septum's attachment to the orbital rim. The septum can be opened in two ways. The entire septum can be opened as a single incision over both nasal and central fat pads. Alternatively, separate incisions can be made over the medial and central fad pads.[4] The former is a simpler technique and advocated by most surgeons.[11–13] To avoid injuring the levator muscle, the septum may be opened midway between the upper tarsus and orbital rim.[14]

Once the septum has been opened, fat pad dissection can begin. The yellowish preaponeurotic fat will usually be evident. Additional local anesthetic is injected into the fat pads (Fig. 42.13). Monopolar electrosurgical needle usage in the retroseptal planes can be painful in the awake patient. If the patient does not tolerate the use of the monopolar electrosurgery, bipolar, or disposable hand-held cautery may be employed. The preaponeurotic fat is excised first, then attention is paid to the nasal fat pad. The capsule of the whiter nasal fat is opened and the fat is teased out. The fat pads, with or without cross-clamping, can be removed with scissors or electrosurgically cut (Figs 42.14 and 42.15). Care must be taken to avoid injury to the trochlea and superior oblique muscle tendon.[4] In the upper lid, the lacrimal gland is in the lateral position and no dissection should be performed laterally.[7] Meticulous hemostasis aids in reducing hemorrhagic complications.

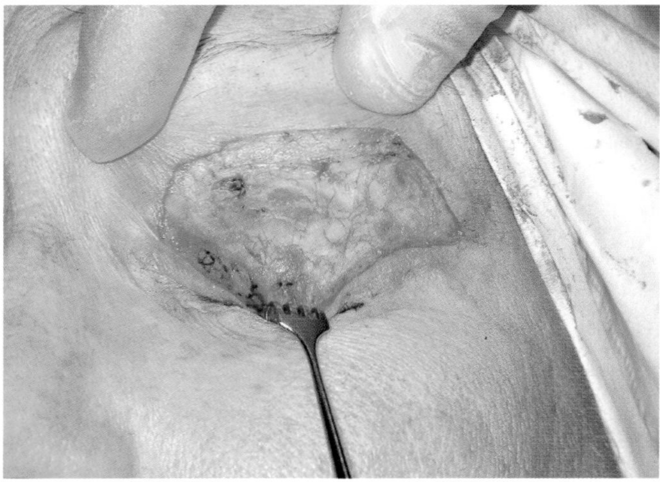

Figure 42.12 Upper blepharoplasty. Demonstration of the orbital septum. Fat can be appreciated below the septum. Courtesy of John B Holds MD and Valerie Vick MD.

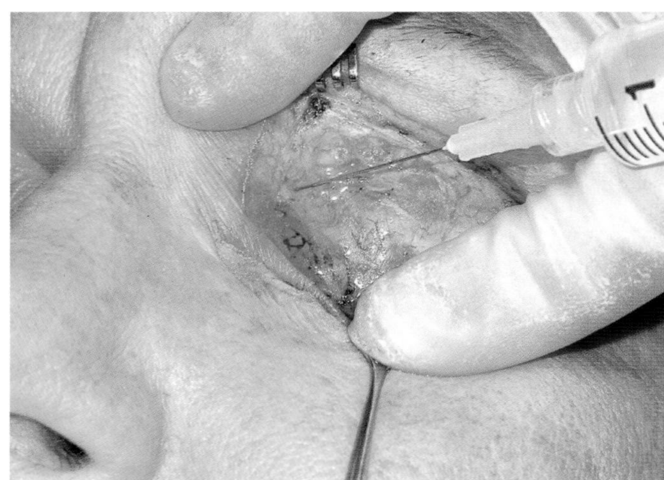

Figure 42.13 Upper blepharoplasty. Reinjecting local anesthetic into the fat pads (in this case the nasal or medial fat pad) prior to removal. Courtesy of John B Holds MD and Valerie Vick MD.

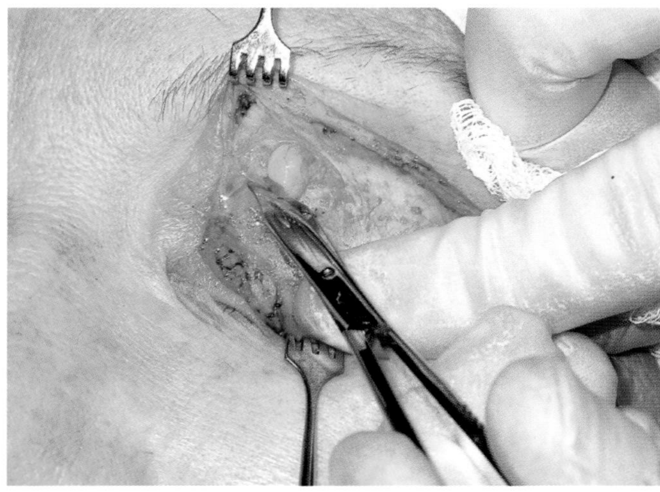

Figure 42.14 Upper blepharoplasty. Opening the orbital septum to reveal orbital fat. Courtesy of John B Holds MD and Valerie Vick MD.

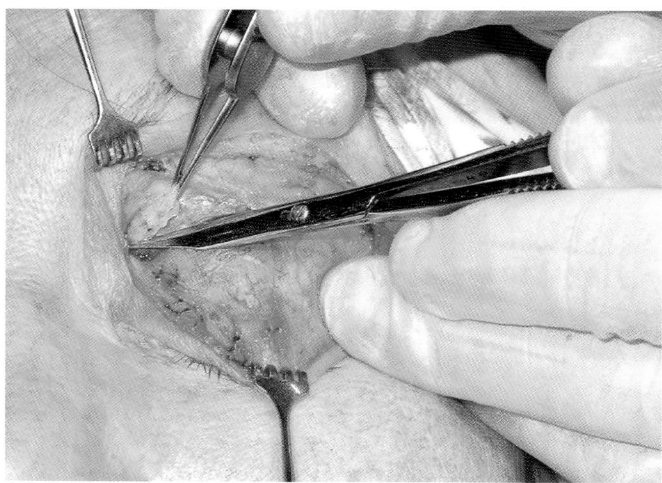

Figure 42.15 Upper blepharoplasty. Removal of orbital fat. When removing fat with scissor technique it may be helpful to cross clamp and treat the fat with bipolar electrocautery to minimize bleeding. Courtesy of John B Holds MD and Valerie Vick MD.

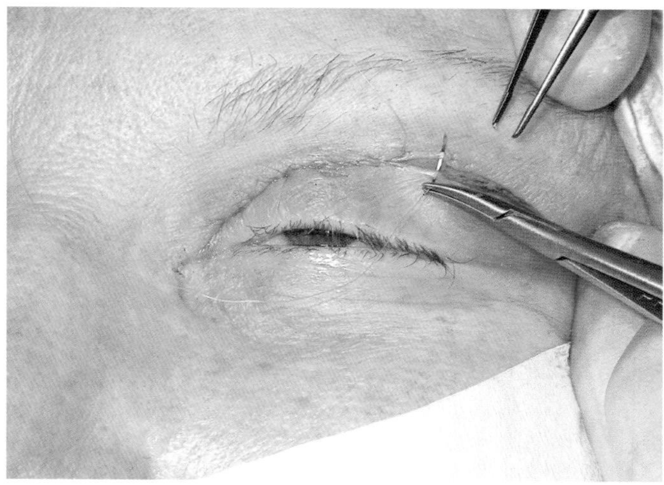

Figure 42.16 Upper blepharoplasty. Closing skin. Care should be taken to precisely align the wound edges to assure epidermis-to-epidermis apposition. Courtesy of John B Holds MD and Valerie Vick MD.

Skin closure

It has been suggested that women, who comprise most blepharoplasty patients, prefer a re-formation of the skin crease, while men do not.[12] If the skin crease is to be re-formed, a suture is passed from the lower incision skin edge through muscle to levator aponeurosis and then to the upper incision muscle and skin. The number of required sutures usually ranges from one to six.[11,12] The patient should be examined in the sitting position and final lid position checked. If the surgeon is satisfied with the result, skin closure is performed (Fig. 42.16). The orbital septum does not require closure.[11]

Advanced considerations of upper blepharoplasty

There are numerous advanced surgical techniques that can be employed during upper blepharoplasty. A trans-blepharoplasty browpexy can improve mild brow ptosis.[11,15] Patients with prominent nasal fat pads but little skin and muscle redundancy may benefit from a transconjunctival upper blepharoplasty approach.[16,17] Finally, the aesthetic appeal of the volume depleting effects of skin, muscle, and fat removal has been questioned.[18] This should serve to remind the surgeon of the paramount importance of adequate preoperative counseling.

Lower-eyelid blepharoplasty

Lower-eyelid blepharoplasty may be performed alone or in combination with upper eyelid surgery. Unlike upper blepharoplasty, it is unlikely that a lower blepharoplasty—as a stand-alone procedure—will be performed solely for functional reasons. In a recent review, one surgeon found that he performed transconjunctival blepharoplasty slightly more frequently than the transcutaneous approach.[19] The transconjunctival approach essentially addresses fat pad herniation. Many experienced surgeons have abandoned the transcutaneous lower blepharoplasty. If there is lower-lid laxity, a simultaneous lid-tightening procedure can be performed. The presence of excess skin and muscle usually requires the use of the transcutaneous approach alone, or a skin excision in combination with the transconjunctival approach.

Transconjunctival lower-lid blepharoplasty

(Figs 42.17–42.20)

Skin marking

This step is optional and consists only of identifying and marking the bulging fat pads.

Anesthesia and skin preparation and drape

The procedure may be performed with local anesthesia alone. However, patient comfort may be increased with the use of oral or intravenous sedation. The conjunctiva is anesthetized with topical anesthetic drops. Injection of local anesthetic may take place from both a conjunctival or transcutaneous approach. Skin preparation and drapes are the same as with upper blepharoplasty.

Conjunctival incision

A Jagear plate or corneal shields are used to protect the globe. Traction must be placed on the lid. Temporary sutures, manual traction aided by gauze or a specialized retractor may be used to assist traction. The conjunctival incision is performed 2–3 mm below the inferior tarsal edge (Fig. 42.17). If measured from the eyelid margin, the incision is 5–7 mm below the eyelid margin. A scalpel, scissors, laser, or electrosurgical needle may be employed to perform the incision. The incision is most commonly continuous and runs lateral to medial. Alternatively, we have noted that lower lid fat can be removed through three separate conjunctival incisions, allowing for less disruption of the conjunctiva and lower-lid retractors. The discontinuous approach is best undertaken after the surgeon is comfortable with the traditional continuous incision approach.[16]

Fat pad extraction

Once the conjunctival incision is complete, a preseptal plane of dissection may be established. The surgeon should take great care with a preseptal dissection, as a plane established too close to the skin can lead to scarring and lid

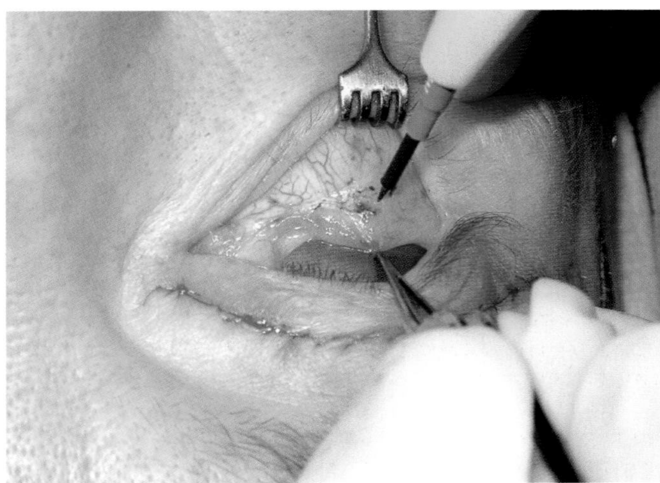

Figure 42.17 Transconjunctival lower blepharoplasty (surgeon's view). Conjunctival incision is 2–3 mm below the tarsal plate. Courtesy of John B Holds MD and Valerie Vick MD.

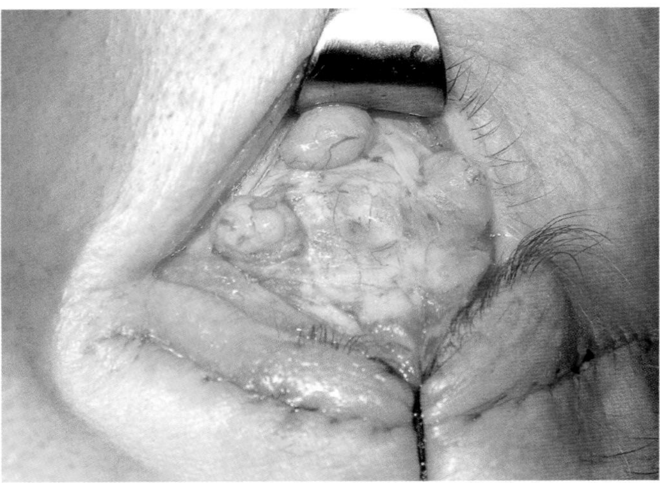

Figure 42.18 Transconjunctival lower blepharoplasty (surgeon's view). Prolapsed fat pads. Courtesy of John B Holds MD and Valerie Vick MD.

retraction. Dissect along this plane to the level of the inferior orbital rim, then open the septum. At this point, additional local anesthetic can be injected into the fat. Identify and modify the nasal and middle fat pads and then progress to the lateral fat pad (Figs 42.18–42.20). Just as with upper blepharoplasty, the fat should be teased out gently. Removal methods are similar to upper lid fat, with scissors, scalpel, laser, or electrosurgical needles being employed.[11] Again, retroseptal application of monopolar electrocautery may be uncomfortable in the unsedated patient. For some surgeons, the lateral fat pad is the most difficult to extirpate. Approaching the right lateral fat pad from the patient's left side, and vice versa, may aid in lateral fat pad visualization and manipulation.[16]

Meticulous hemostasis is required to prevent hemorrhage. Once the septum has been violated, a retro-orbital hemorrhage is possible. Minimization of trauma to the fat pads during removal should decrease hemorrhagic complications. If no lid tightening is required, conjunctival closure can ensue, or the conjunctiva may be left unsutured. The conjunctiva can be left open or closed with as few as one or two soft absorbable sutures, or the entire defect can be closed in a running manner.[11]

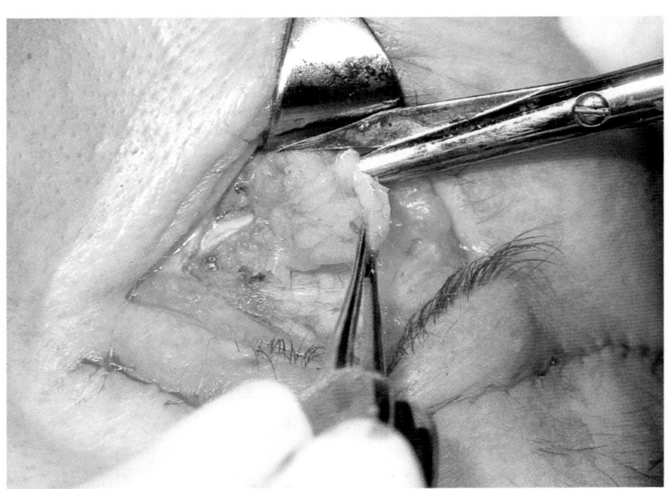

Figure 42.19 Transconjunctival lower blepharoplasty (surgeon's view). Removal of prolapsed fat. When removing fat with scissor technique it may be helpful to cross-clamp and treat the fat with bipolar electrocautery to minimize bleeding. Courtesy of John B Holds MD and Valerie Vick MD.

Transcutaneous lower-eyelid blepharoplasty

The transcutaneous approach to lower blepharoplasty may be utilized in the patient with excess skin-muscle and prolapsed fat pads.

Skin marking

A marking for a subciliary incision 1–3 mm below the lash line is created. The incision will extend from the medial punctum in a curvilinear manner to beyond the lateral canthus. If an upper blepharoplasty is also performed, the planned lower lid incision should be 6–8 mm below the incision from the upper blepharoplasty.[7]

Anesthesia and skin preparation and drape

Anesthesia for trancutaneous lower blepharoplasty is similar to the transconjunctival approach. Topical conjunctival anesthesia is desirable. Local anesthesia may be infiltrated

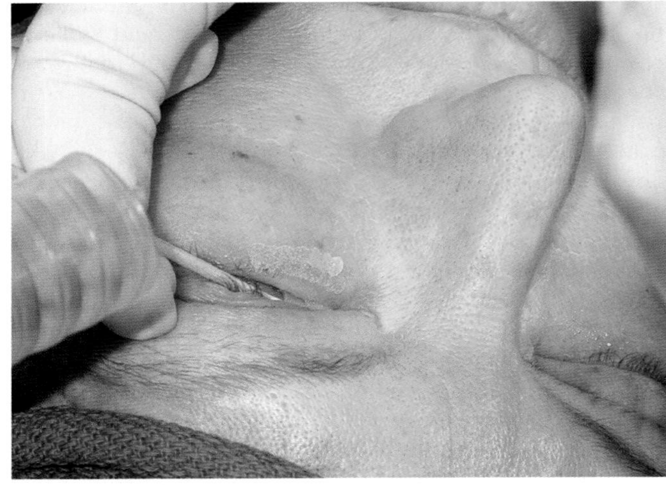

Figure 42.20 Complementing the lower transconjunctival blepharoplasty with laser resurfacing (surgeon's view). Courtesy of John B Holds MD and Valerie Vick MD.

transcutaneously in a subdermal plane. Direct pressure applied after the anesthetic may reduce hematoma formation. Local anesthetic should also be injected transconjunctivally to anesthetize the posterior lamella.

Skin incision

The skin and orbicularis oculi are incised and a skin-muscle flap is created. The dissection of the skin-muscle flap usually extends to the orbital rim.[7,11] The orbital septum is opened and fat pads are identified. Lifting the septum off of the underlying fat pads prior to incising the septum may reduce the risk of severing a vessel within the fat pad.[7]

Fat pad extraction

Fat pad extraction is as previously described. Gentle pressure on the globe will help prolapse the fat. Additional local anesthetic should be injected into the fat prior to removal. If not opened with the septal incision, the fibrous capsule over each fat pad is opened.[11] As described above, the inferior oblique muscle may present with the herniated fat. Great care must be taken to avoid injury to this muscle.

Excise skin and muscle

If no lid-tightening procedure is planned, excess skin and orbicularis muscle are excised. The skin-muscle flap is draped across the lid margin in such a manner as to avoid tension.[12] In general, skin-muscle excision should be conservative (up to 2–3 mm) to avoid lower-lid retraction. If a lid-tightening procedure is performed, more aggressive excision is possible.[11]

Skin closure

Skin closure is performed along the subciliary incision with running suture. Some surgeons add a deep fixation suture, pulling the orbicularis to the periosteum.[11]

Advanced considerations of lower blepharoplasty

For many surgeons, achieving a superior aesthetic and functional outcome is more difficult with lower than upper blepharoplasty.[20] As a result, numerous modifications and enhancements have been proposed. Many of these refinements aid to prevent or correct common postoperative complications of lower blepharoplasty.

Lid retraction, ectropion, and scleral show are postoperative complications that have both aesthetic and functional consequences. The cause of lower-eyelid malposition after surgery may result from a combination of factors. A useful rubric to approach malposition is from an anatomic standpoint. Defects in the anterior lamella (skin and orbicularis) generally lead to ectropion. The lower lid is also subject to retraction if the structures in the middle lamella (orbital septum, orbital fat) or the capsulopalpebral fascia in the posterior lamella are injured. Scarring or adhesions in these structures may result in retraction that requires surgical correction. Care should be taken not to excise, excessively cauterize, or overly traumatize the conjunctiva. Scarring may lead to symblepharon or shortening of the inferior fornix.[21]

As mentioned, appropriate preoperative screening to identify at-risk patients and conservative skin-muscle excision is paramount to preventing lid malposition. Take special note of patients who have hypoplastic malar eminences, or those who have had prior surgery or exhibit lid laxity. Examination of old photos is very important when planning lower-eyelid blepharoplasty. Patients differ in their concept of beauty in this area. People may have a straightened or rounded lower eyelid margin preoperatively. Most patients prefer to retain the overall shape of their eyelid margins.

A simple adjuvant procedure is the muscle to periosteum suspension. This suture provides support to the anterior lamella.[20,22] Other techniques share the common feature of tightening the lower lid. Described approaches include the lateral tarsal strip, lateral canthal tendon plication or resection techniques.[22] These techniques seek to tighten and anchor the posterior lamella.

The management of fat pads in blepharoplasty has undergone a change in recent years. The concept of fat removal has been challenged. It has become recognized that aging includes not only a problem of tissue descent, but also one of involutional changes. Some have advocated that fat pad removal has a negative aesthetic effect by causing a concavity below the tarsal plate. The contour of a child's face with a full lower eyelid–cheek continuum is the rational for the aesthetic concerns of fat removal. Some surgeons are now stressing fat conserving and redistributing approaches to blepharoplasty.[23] Fat transplantation to the lower eyelids has been reported in select patients to achieve a youthful appearance of the lower eyelid. Techniques that plicate the orbital septa[24,25] or resuspend the capsulopalpebral fascia have been proposed as alternatives to fat pad extraction.[26] Electrocautery to tighten lax septa has been reported to be effective in both upper and lower blepharoplasty.[27] In patients with tear trough deformity, repositioning of the orbital fat to blunt the concave appearance of the tear trough may be a successful technique.[28] While there is intuitive appeal to fat sparing techniques, the abandonment of fat extraction in lower lid blepharoplasty is far from being universally accepted.

The surgeon should be aware of the concept of lower eyelid orbicularis oculi hypertrophy. Orbicularis oculi hypertrophy describes the appearance of a thickened pretarsal lower eyelid muscle and overlying skin redundancy. Failure to address this anatomic feature in lower blepharoplasty may result in a hollow lower sulcus and an aesthetically unappealing convexity–concavity deformity. Numerous techniques to manage orbicularis oculi hypertrophy center upon reduction of orbicularis function. Described methods include surgical thinning of the muscle,[29] electrosurgical reductions in muscle function,[30] and chemodenervation with botulinum toxin.

Laser resurfacing, as discussed elsewhere in this text, may be a useful adjuvant procedure to improve skin tone and pigmentary irregularities. Finally, it is noteworthy that some experienced surgeons will always approach lower-lid fat removal from the transconjunctival approach. Redundant lower-lid skin will be excised as needed; this approach avoids excessive manipulation of the anterior lamella.

Brow lifting

Brow lifting, while less commonly performed than blepharoplasty, is an important functional and cosmetic surgical procedure. Brow management is critical in a comprehensive approach to upper-face rejuvenation. There are multiple surgical approaches to brow rejuvenation. These techniques range from minimally invasive office-based procedures to highly invasive surgery requiring systemic anesthesia. We will focus our discussion on traditional brow lifting operations, with a brief discussion of newer, less invasive techniques.

The operative plan may include general anesthesia or significant sedation. Advances in anesthesia have greatly decreased the risk associated with anesthesia. However, the risk–benefit ratio of surgery, particularly cosmetic surgery, must always be considered.

Surgical techniques

The introduction of endoscopic brow lifting has reduced the emphasis placed on direct browplasty techniques. However, the direct approach can be highly successful and should not be ignored. Patients with functional brow ptosis may benefit from a direct approach. Many times these procedures, particularly direct browplasty or mid forehead lift, can be performed with local anesthetic alone. Figure 42.21 illustrates the traditional approaches to direct brow lifting.[11] These techniques are, in essence, excisional surgeries. Standard surgical techniques apply. As with any surgical dissection, the surgeon should keep in mind the location of important nerves. In the mid forehead lift, the plane of dissection is in the subcutaneous tissue. Scarring is unavoidable in these approaches. However, in functional cases, it can be quite acceptable.

The coronal forehead and brow lift has been the gold standard against which other approaches have been compared. The brow–forehead lift is intended to improve brow ptosis as well as diminish rhtyides in the forehead and glabella.[31] The overall surgical plan involves a long coronal or modified anterior hairline incision as demonstrated in Figure 42.21. The forehead is elevated in the subgaleal plane centrally and over the deep temporal fascia laterally. The neurovascular bundles are directly visualized as the dissection approached the supraorbital rim. The midline dissection is carried to the nasal bone.[31]

Muscle resection focuses on the corragator muscles as well as the frontalis muscle. Using a scissor-spread technique within the corragator, the supratrochlear nerve is identified. The corragator can then be resected. Frontalis muscle may be resected between the supraorbital nerves to address glabellar lines. Finally, the forehead flap is redraped and the wound closed.[31]

The endoscopic brow lift, introduced in the early 1990s, gained wide acceptance as an alternative to the coronal brow lift. The endoscopic approach seeks to minimize many of the unfavorable sequelae of the open approach, most notably scalp hypoesthesia, alopecia, an alteration in the hairline, and scarring. The surgical technique for the endoscopic approach is similar to an open approach as the same tissue planes are developed. The endoscope and instruments are introduced through incisions in the frontal scalp. Dissection planes are as described for the open technique. The neurovascular bundles and muscles to be resected are visualized endoscopically.[32]

Numerous fixation methods exist for securing the elevated brow. All seek to secure the forehead and brow in place while fibrosis occurs. Common approaches include screws, bone tunnels, and absorbable-pronged tissue securing devices.

Traditional approaches to brow lifting

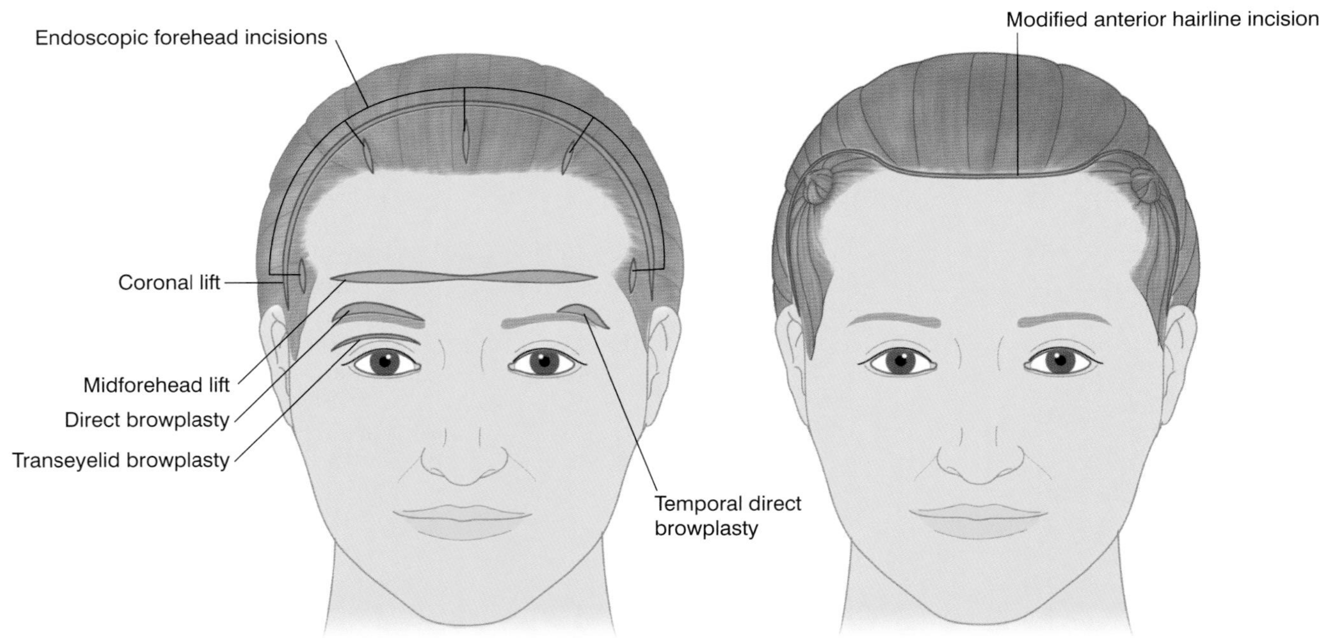

Figure 42.21 Traditional surgical approaches to brow lifting.

Advanced considerations and alternatives to the surgical brow lift

The direct browplasty and mid-forehead lift receive little attention but are valuable techniques in the properly selected patient. Most recent attention has focused on the relative merits of open versus endoscopic surgery. Retrospective reviews have sought to provide insight into this topic. In a study of 84 patients with short-term follow-up (less than 2 years), Puig and LaFerriere detected no significant difference between the approaches when analyzing brow height.[33] A more telling study was performed by Chiu and Baker. They surveyed 21 plastic surgeons who had performed 628 endoscopic brow lifts over a 5-year period. Interesting results included the fact that there was a trend toward less endoscopic but more open brow lifts being performed. Additionally, the surgeons felt that the complications from endoscopic surgery were similar to those of the open technique. While 71% of patients were satisfied after the endoscopic brow lift procedure, only 48% of the surgeons were satisfied with their results 2-years postoperatively. The authors concluded that there is no single superior surgical option for the management of brow ptosis.[34]

Recently, there has been increased interest among patients and surgeons for minimally invasive facial rejuvenation. This is driven by patient desires for limited recovery time. Surgical brow lifting, whether open or endoscopic, typically requires some form of heavy sedation or a general anesthetic. A number of minimally invasive approaches to the management of brow ptosis have been proposed. The concept of using suture material to suspend the brow has considerable appeal. The basic concept is one to place percutaneously a suspending suture from the brow to a fixation point superior to the brow. A number of different materials and techniques have been proposed, but all essentially achieve the same result.[35–37]

A transblepharoplasty browpexy can be a simple brow elevation technique to accompany an upper-lid blepharoplasty. This approach will lift the lateral brow. It is not considered a comprehensive brow-lifting technique—rather it may benefit the patient primarily suffering from lateral brow ptosis.[15]

PITFALLS AND THEIR MANAGEMENT

Avoidance of pitfalls

- Blindness can result from hemorrhage: reduce the risk of perioperative and postoperative bleeding by preoperative evaluation and adjustment of risk factors, and by advising the patient about postoperative activity and warning signs.
- Monitor patients throughout surgery for signs of bradycardia or dysrhythmia, which can be triggered by the oculocardiac reflex, and have a crash cart available.
- Use direct visualization of the inferior oblique muscle to avoid muscle injury.
- Treatment with lubricants and taping lids may help prevent keratoconjunctivitis.
- Conservative skin excision is the best way to avoid lagophthalmos.

Complications from blepharoplasty range from aesthetic to functional to catastrophic. As previously discussed, the lower eyelid is more subject to a poor outcome including retraction and scleral show.

The most serious complication from blepharoplasty is blindness. This rare complication is primarily a result of hemorrhagic complications. Estimates of this complication are in the range of 1 in 40 000. The proposed mechanism of blindness is retrobulbar hemorrhage leading to a compartment syndrome, increased orbital pressure, and optic nerve ischemia. Small retrobulbar hemorrhages occur in around 1 in 2500 cases and usually spontaneously tamponade, without resulting in blindness. Violation of the septum, trauma during fat pad removal, and orbital muscle injury are likely precipitants of retrobulbar hematoma.[12,38,39] Retrobulbar hematoma is usually an early complication, occurring within the first 24 hours postoperatively. However, there exist reports of delayed hematoma occurring 7 days postoperatively.[40]

Prevention of bleeding is paramount. All anticoagulative medications or supplements should be withdrawn in a timely manner perioperatively. Hypertension should be under good control and meticulous hemostasis is mandatory. A history of coagulopathy should be obtained as part of the preoperative evaluation. Limiting postoperative activity and avoiding increases in blood pressure or Valsalva maneuvers (cough, vomit, straining at stooling) are advised. Early recognition and treatment of retrobulbar bleeding may spare vision. Generally, blepharoplasty elicits little pain. Therefore significant pain or visual changes should be emergently evaluated. Visual compromise should be emergently treated, usually with lateral canthotomy and cantholysis. Emergent consultation with an ophthalmic surgeon may be desirable. Approaches to treatment include osmotic agents, topical β-blocker drops, frequent assessment of visual function, and surgical exploration.[38]

Extraocular muscle injury resulting in diplopia is another rare complication of blepharoplasty. The inferior rectus and inferior oblique muscles are the most frequently injured. Diplopia or other ocular motility disturbance may result from local anesthesia, edema, hemorrhage, or minor muscle injury, and is usually transient and observation is all that is required. However, permanent injury can occur and strabismus surgery may be required in rare cases.[41–43] Direct visualization of the inferior oblique muscle can decrease the probability of injury. Cautious upper lid dissection, piecemeal fat removal, and judicious use of electrocautery may help minimize superior oblique tendon injury.[44]

Dry eyes, including frank exposure keratitis, can result from blepharoplasty. Temporary lagophthalmos is common in the immediate postoperative period. Treatment with lubricants and lid taping may help prevent keratoconjunctivitis. Additional manipulations such as downward eyelid massage may help. If lagophthalmos is persistent, surgical interventions may be necessary. Techniques include raising the lower lid via lateral canthoplasty and, as a last resort, full-thickness skin grafts to the upper lid.[45] Conservative skin excision is usually the best way to avoid lagophthalmos. When a brow lift is performed, it is appropriate to decrease the amount of upper lid skin removed. Lower-lid laxity and retraction can also be causes of exposure keratopathy. Initial remedies include massage and aggressive topical lubricants at bedtime. If persistent, surgical intervention may be required.[13]

Recall that signs and symptoms of dry eyes are elicited during the preoperative evaluation. While we still obtain a Schirmer test of basal tear secretion (abnormal is less than 8–10 mm at 5 minutes) preoperatively, some have questioned its predictive value.[46]

The oculocardiac reflex is a trigeminal–vagal arc that can lead to bradycardia or dysrhythmia during ocular manipulation. It has been described in the adult cosmetic blepharoplasty patient. Precipitating events include pressure applied to the globe, traction on extraocular muscles, and fat pad traction. Patients should be continuously monitored, and if a decrease in heart rate is noted, the manipulation should be stopped, which usually reverses the problem quickly. Atropine is the treatment for the oculocardiac induced bradycardia and should be available for administration if heart rate does not spontaneously recover. A crash cart should be available.[47] The authors perform blepharoplasty as either an inpatient or outpatient procedure under local anesthesia with or without oral or intravenous sedation.

■ SUMMARY

Rejuvenation of the upper face involves careful consideration of factors relating to the eyelids and brow. Blepharoplasty and brow lifting are traditional and successful approaches to management of the upper face.

■ REFERENCES

1. American Society of Plastic Surgery. 2002 statistical data. http://www.plasticsurgery.org/public_education/2002statistics.cfm (last accessed June 2004).
2. Ghabrial R, Lisman RD, Kane MA, Milite J, Richards R. Diplopia following transconjunctival blepharoplasty. Plast Reconstr Surg 1998; 102:1219–1225.
3. Mowlavi A, Neumeister MW, Wilhelmi BJ. Lower blepharoplasty using bony anatomical landmarks to identify and avoid injury to the inferior oblique muscle. Plast Reconstr Surg 2002; 110:1318–1322.
4. Wilhelmi BJ, Mowlavi A, Neumeister MW. Upper blepharoplasty with bony anatomical landmarks to avoid injury to the trochlea and superior oblique muscle tendon with fat resection. Plast Reconstr Surg 2001; 108:2137–2140.
5. Sires BS, Saari JC, Garwin GG, Hurst JS, van Kujik FJGM. The color difference in orbital fat. Arch Ophthalmol 2001; 119:868–871.
6. Burke AJ, Wang T. Should formal ophthalmologic evaluation be a preoperative requirement prior to blepharoplasty? Arch Otolaryngol Head Neck Surg 2001; 127:719–722.
7. Chen WP. Oculoplastic surgery: The essentials. New York: Thieme: 2001.
8. Small RG, Sabates NR, Burrows D. The measurement and definition of ptosis. Ophthalm Plast Reconstr Surg 1989; 5:171–175.
9. Holds JB. Ptosis. In: Albert DM, ed. Ophthalmic surgery principles and techniques. Malden, MA: Blackwell Science; 2000.
10. Collins SC, Dufresne RG. Dietary supplements in the setting of Mohs surgery. Dermatol Surg 2002; 6:447–452.
11. Nerad JA. Oculoplastic surgery. St Louis: Mosby; 2001.
12. Levine MR. Manual of oculoplastic surgery. Philadelphia: Butterworth Heinemann; 2003.
13. Campbell JP, Maher EA, Della Rocca RC. Blepharoplasty. In: Della Rocca RC, Bedrossian EH, Arthurs BP, eds. Ophthalmic plastic surgery: Decision making and techniques. New York: McGraw-Hill; 2002.
14. Kanter WR, Wolfort FG. Operative technique. In: Wolfort FG, Kanter WR, eds. Aesthetic Blepharoplasty. Boston: Little Brown; 1995.
15. Zarem HA, Resnick JI, Carr RM, Wootton DG. Browpexy: lateral orbicularis muscle fixation as an adjunct to upper blepharoplasty. Plast Reconstr Surg 1997; 100:1258–1261.
16. Weber PJ, Oleson GB, Moody BR. Visible incision reduction in cosmetic oculoplastic surgery. Int J Cosm Surg Aesth Dermatol 2000; 2:57–70.
17. Guerra AB, Metzinger SE, Black EB. Transconjunctival upper blepharoplasty: a safe and effective addition to facial rejuvenation techniques. Ann Plast Surg 2002; 48:528–533.
18. Fagien S. Advanced rejunerative upper blepharoplasty: enhancing aesthetics of the upper periorbita. Plast Reconstr Surg 2001; 110:278–291.
19. Rizk SS, Matarasso A. Lower eyelid blepharoplasty: analysis of indications and the treatment of 100 patients. Plast Reconstr Surg 2003; 111:1299–1306.
20. Widegrow AD. Blepharoplasty lateral internal suspension suture: Bliss suture. Aesth Plast Surg 1998; 22:130–134.
21. Patipa M. The evaluation and management of lower eyelid retraction following cosmetic surgery. Plast Reconstr Surg 2000; 106:438–453.
22. Mommaerts MY, De Riu G. Prevention of lid retraction after lower lid blepharoplasties: an overview. J Craniomaxillofac Surg 2000; 28:189–200.
23. Eder H. Importance of fat conservation in lower blepharoplasty. Aesth Plast Surg 1997; 21:168–174.
24. Huang T. Reduction of lower palpebral bulge by plicating attenuated orbital septa: a technical modification in cosmetic blepharoplasty. Plast Reconstr Surg 2000; 105:2552–2558.
25. de la Plaza R, Arroyo JM. A New technique for the treatment of palpebral bags. Plast Reconstr Surg 1988; 81:677–685.
26. Parsa FD, Miyashiro MJ, Elahi E, Mirzai TM. Lower eyelid hernia repair for palpebral bags: a comparative study. Plast Reconstr Surg 1998; 102:2459–2465.
27. Choo PH, Rathbun JE. Cautery of the orbital septum during blepharoplasty. Ophthalmol Plast Reconstr Surg 2003; 19:1–4.
28. Goldberg RA. Transconjunctival orbital fat repositioning: transposition of orbital fat pedicles into a subperiosteal pocket. Plast Reconstr Surg 2000; 105:743–748.
29. Bernardi C, Dura S, Amata PL. Treatment of orbicularis oculi hypertrophy in lower lid blepharoplasty. Aesth Plast Surg 1998; 22:349–351.
30. Weber PJ, Wulc AE, Moody BR, Dryden RM, Foster JA. Electrosurgical modification of orbicularis oculi hypertrophy. Ophthal Plast Reconstr Surg 2000; 16:407–416.
31. Aston SJ, Thorne CH. The forehead and brow. In: Rees TD, LaTrenta GS, eds. Aesthetic plastic surgery. Philadelphia: WB Saunders; 1994:732–739.
32. DeCordier BC, de la Torre JI, Al-Hakeem, et al. Endoscopic forehead lift: review of technique, cases, and complications. Plast Reconstr Surg 2002; 110:1558–1568.
33. Puig CM, LaFerriere KA. A retrospective comparison of open and endoscopic brow-lifts. Arch Facial Plast Surg 2002; 4:221–225.
34. Chiu ES, Baker DC. Endoscopic brow lift: a retrospective review of 628 consecutive cases over 5 years. Plast Reconstr Surg 2003; 112:628–633.
35. Graziosi AC, Beer SM. Brow lifting with thread: the technique without undermining using minimum incisions. Aesth Plast Surg 1998; 22:120–125.
36. Sulamanidze MA, Fournier PF, Paikidze TG, Sulamanidze GM. Removal of facial soft tissue ptosis with special threads. Dermatol Surg 2002; 28:367–371.
37. Hernandez-Perez E, Khawaja HA. A percutaneous approach to eyebrow lift: The Salvadorean option. Dermatol Surg 2003; 29:852–855.
38. Wolfort FG, Vaughn TE, Wolfort SF, Nevarre DR. Retrobulbar hematoma and blepharoplasty. Plast Reconstr Surg 1999; 104:2154–2162.
39. Sutcliffe T, Baylis HI, Fett D. Bleeding in cosmetic blepharoplasty: an anatomical approach. Ophthal Plast Reconstr Surg 1985; 1:107–113.
40. Cruz AAV, Ando A, Monteiro CAC, Elias J. Delayed retrobulbar hematoma after blepharoplasty. Ophthal Plast Reconstr Surg 2000; 17:126–130.
41. Ghabrial R, Lisman RD, Kane MA, Milite J, Richards R. Diplopia following transconjunctival blepharoplasty. Plast Reconstr Surg 1998; 102:1219–1225.

42. Syniuta LA, Goldberg RA, Thacker NM, Rosenbaum AL. Acquired strabismus following cosmetic blepharoplasty. Plast Reconstr Surg 2003; 111:2053–2059.

43. Harley RD, Nelson LB, Flanagan JC, Calhoun JH. Ocular motility disturbances following cosmetic blepharoplasty. Arch Ophthal 1986; 104:542–544.

44. Wesley RE, Pollard ZF, McCord CD Jr. Superior oblique paresis after blepharoplasty. Plast Reconstr Surg 1980; 66:283–286.

45. Lyon DB, Raphtis CS. Management of complications of blepharoplasty. Int Ophthal Clin 1997; 37:205–216.

46. McKinney P, Byun M. The value of tear film breakup and Schirmer's tests in preoperative blepharoplasty evaluation. Plast Reconstr Surg 1999; 104:566–569.

47. Matarasso A. The oculocardiac reflex in blepharoplasty surgery. Plast Reconstr Surg 1989; 83:243–247.

43 Rejuvenation of the Neck Using Liposuction and Other Techniques

Carolyn I Jacob MD and Michael S Kaminer MD

Summary box

- Evaluate submental adipose tissue, skin elasticity, and platysma laxity and integrity.
- Neck liposuction is appropriate for those with preplatysmal fat, good skin quality, and decussated platysma.
- Add platysmaplasty for patients with good skin quality but with a nondecussated, lax platysma.
- Patients with poor skin quality may require superficial muscular aponeurotic system (SMAS) plication, platysmaplasty, and skin excision.
- Botulinum toxin is an option for patients with good skin tone and platysma bands during teeth clenching.
- Radiofrequency for tissue tightening of the submentum may be beneficial for select patients.

INTRODUCTION

The effects of age, sun, and adipose redistribution take their toll on the neck as well as the face. It is important to keep this in mind when evaluating a patient with photoaging. The appearance of an aged neck in contrast to a newly resurfaced or lifted face is undesirable and a 'white flag' that one has had surgery. In order to balance the face and neck there are a variety of procedures available. Nonsurgical or surgical rejuvenation of the neck can be performed using botulinum toxin, nonablative laser resurfacing, ablative laser resurfacing, radiofrequency tissue tightening, and liposuction with or without platysma repair or SMAS plication. These therapies can be used alone or in combination depending on the condition of the neck tissues. This chapter will focus on surgical recontouring of the neck using liposuction, platysma repair, and SMAS plication, and will also introduce a new tissue tightening procedure using radiofrequency energy.

With the advent of tumescent liposuction in 1987, liposuction of excess adipose tissue from the submental area, jowls, and neck has become an attractive alternative to the face lift for cervicomental aesthetic surgery. With time, sun damage, and gravity, increased deposition of fatty tissue in the submental area, sagging jowls, and neck skin redundancy with or without banding of the platysma muscle occur. This may give the appearance of excessive weight gain or aging to an otherwise healthy person. The traditional approach to these patients has been face lift surgery, but with tumescent anesthesia, neck liposuction has evolved as a safe procedure to enhance the appearance of the neck and jawline in such individuals. Many variations and additions to neck liposuction have been employed. These include concomitant simple platysma plication, the corset platysma repair, simple platysma plication with carbon dioxide resurfacing of the platysma and dermis ('Weekend alternative to the Facelift'),[1] and a combination of neck liposuction, platysma plication, and SMAS plication.

Platysma repair can improve refinement of the cervicomental angle in addition to eliminating visible bands. The etiology of platysma bands is speculated to be due to stretching and loss of contractility of skin and fat overlying the anterior platysma, plus stretching of the overlying SMAS which normally retracts the muscle.[2] Both of these contractility failures are exacerbated with overuse of the muscles and advancing age. An alternative treatment for early and mild platysma muscle banding is Botulinum toxin A (BTX-A) (Allergan Inc, Irvine, CA) or B (Myobloc) (Elan Corporation, San Diego, CA) injections into the vertical platysma bands. Although quite useful for patients with platysmal show during muscle contraction, BTX-A and B injections provide temporary (3–6 months) improvement and do not help patients with persistent sagging bands.

Those patients with excessive jowling or poor skin elasticity will benefit from concomitant SMAS plication and skin excision with repositioning. For patients with severe elastosis of the face with sagging skin at the temporal and malar areas, a full face lift may be appropriate. However, many patients have aging changes limited to the lower cheek and jowl, which can be greatly improved by SMAS plication and skin excision alone. The advantage of this safe, less invasive and less time consuming procedure performed under local anesthesia, is that it eliminates the risks of intravenous or general anesthesia and gives excellent results with reduced morbidity.

For those patients with mild jowling and submental adipose who do not wish to undergo surgery, there is a non-surgical alternative currently being studied. Radiofrequency as an energy source has been used for years in electrosurgery, but a new device, which uses capacitive coupling and an epidermal coolant has been developed to tighten tissue and regenerate collagen. In addition, this device, marketed as the ThermaCool (Thermage Corporation, Hayward, CA), may reduce unwanted adipose as well.[3] Studies have proven its ability to tighten forehead skin and 'lift' the eyebrows and upper lids,[4] and the device has been used to soften the nasolabial fold, improve cheek contour, and tighten the mandibular line.[5]

History of neck rejuvenation

- 1968 Millard, Pigott, and Hedo describe the submandibular lipectomy for neck enhancement.
- 1971 Cronin and Biggs describe the T–Z plasty for the male 'turkey-gobbler' neck.
- 1978 Illouz develops liposuction.
- 1987 Jeffrey Klein develops tumescent liposuction.
- 1992 Joel Feldman describes the corset platysmaplasty.
- 2001 Carruthers and Carruthers describe the use of botulinum in the mid and lower face and neck.
- 2003 Radiofrequency tissue tightening is used to enhance cervicomental angles.

PATIENT EVALUATION

Choosing appropriate candidates for neck rejuvenation is essential and perhaps one of the most important determinants of the postoperative result. Examination for submental adipose, skin quality, and platysma laxity or prominence during teeth clenching can guide the physician to the appropriate procedure or combination of procedures.

In addition, several analyses of cervicomental esthetics have been performed, and show that patients with ideal neck proportions have cervicomental angles between 90° and 135°.[6–10] The ideal position of the hyoid bone was found to be at the vertebral C3–C4 level, and at a location equal to or higher than the menton (the most inferior point on the mandibular symphysis in the midsagittal plane).[11] These details should be considered when selecting patients for neck liposuction because additional procedures may need to be employed for maximum results. For example, those patients with relatively low-set hyoid bones are less likely to achieve a sharp cervicomental angle because their underlying anatomy will not support it. Hyoid position is an important landmark for muscular attachments and is thus an important determinant of neck angles and contour. Optimal candidates for neck liposuction include those patients with full jowls but otherwise good skin elasticity, patients with high-set hyoid bones, and those with submental fat pads palpable by pinch techniques (Fig. 43.1).

Several maneuvers can be performed to assess submental fat; the patient is asked to clench his/her teeth, which will tighten the platysma muscle and define the fat as pre- or retroplatysmal fat. Preplatysmal fat can be suctioned

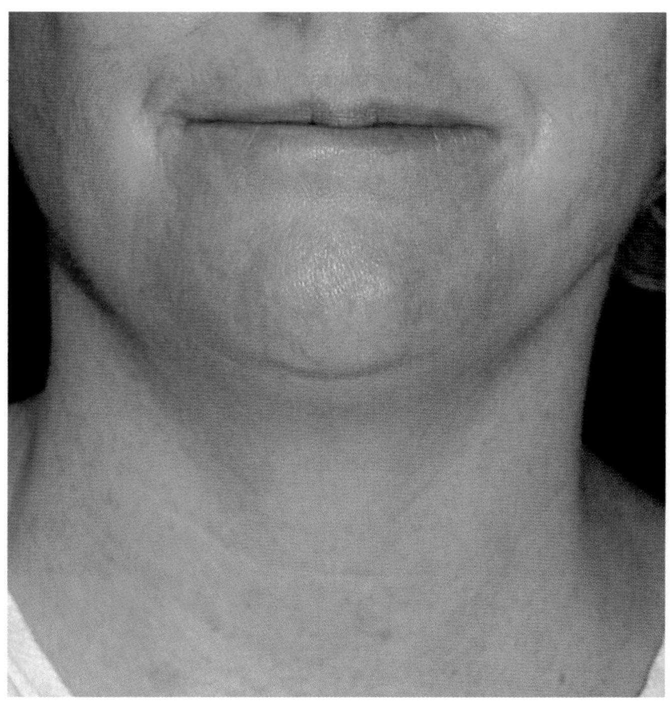

Figure 43.1 Optimal liposuction candidate.

through a small submental incision, but retroplatysmal fat must be excised directly. Asking the patient to place their tongue up against the hard palate will also help the surgeon to identify fat location as more retroplatysmal adipose will protrude. The surgeon should also release the skin as part of a snap test to determine skin elasticity. If the skin feels loose and does not recoil quickly, or if the skin reveals vertical banding at rest, then liposuction alone is unlikely to provide maximal benefit (Fig. 43.2). This type of patient may be a good candidate for a partial SMAS plication and/or platysma repair. The clenched teeth test is also useful to evaluate the platysma location and banding because nondecussating platysma muscle fibers become evident. Patients with prominent platysmal banding should be given the option for platysma repair at the time of liposuction because this will maximize final results (Fig. 43.3).

The surgeon should also evaluate submandibular gland position. Many patients have ptotic submandibular glands which appear as a subcutaneous fullness bilaterally along the inferior midportion of the mandibular ramus. This ptotic gland can resemble jowls, and is important to identify preoperatively. Platysma repair over these glands can improve this ptosis in some patients.

Gender may play a role in patient selection as well. We have found that male neck skin takes longer to retract and re-drape after neck liposuction compared with female neck skin. Whether this is a result of differences in hormones, skin thickness, or volume of fat removed remains unclear. As with all patients, postoperative skin retraction may be suboptimal if preoperative skin elasticity is poor.

Patients with mild jowling, good skin quality, and minimal neck adipose are good candidates for the ThermaCool radiofrequency treatment. Optimal patient selection parameters include patients aged 35–55 years, those with thinner faces, and thin skin.[12] Other factors leading to patient success are still being investigated.

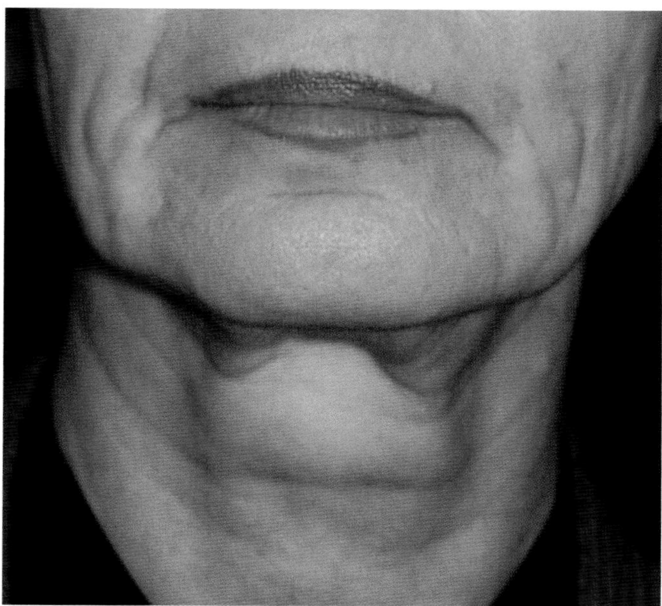

Figure 43.2 Aged neck displaying poor skin quality.

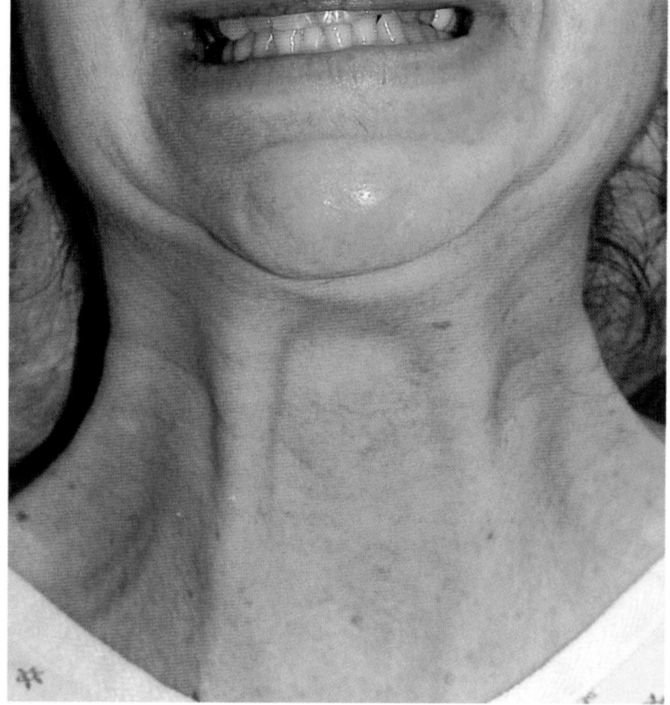

Figure 43.3 Prominent platysmal banding.

■ TECHNIQUES

Liposuction of the neck

The process of neck liposuction involves first marking the mandibular border, jowls, submental fat pad, anterior borders of the sternocleidomastoid muscle, left and right platysma bands (if present), and the thyroid cartilage. This is done with the patient in a seated position (Fig. 43.4). Care must be taken to identify the jowl bilaterally because it will extend slightly below the mandibular ramus. The superior extents of the jowl should be marked as well.

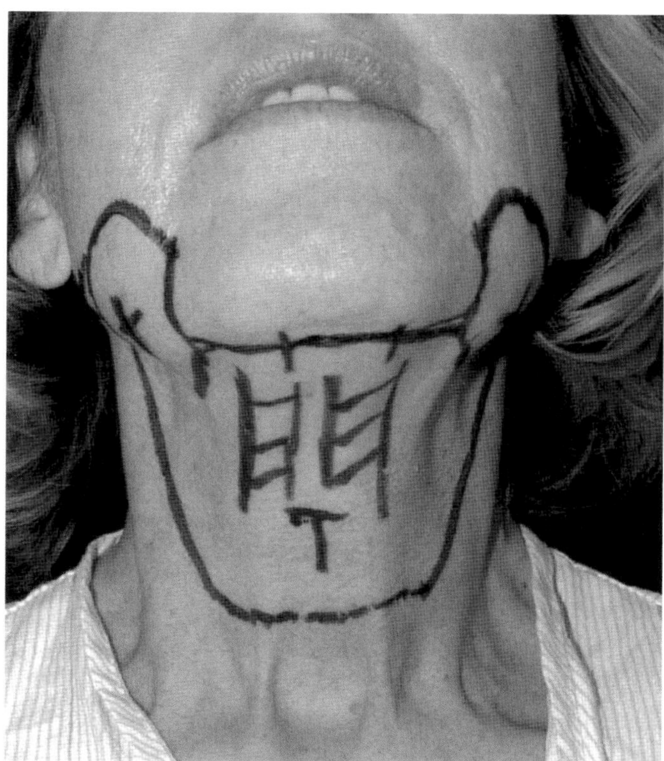

Figure 43.4 Preoperative patient markings.

These guides help to delineate the areas for liposuction, and the top of the 'T' placed at the level of the thyroid cartilage marks the distal extent for plication of the platysma, if necessary. Preoperative marking is essential to define landmarks that will be otherwise distorted after tumescence.

The procedure is performed in a well-equipped ambulatory surgery setting, with appropriate sterile technique, nursing staff assistance and procedure-specific cannulae. The patient's face, neck, and upper shoulders are cleansed thoroughly with povidone-iodine and sterile towels are wrapped around the head. After the patient is prepped and draped in sterile fashion, a small amount of local full strength tumescent (0.1% lidocaine) anesthesia is administered in the submental crease. With a #11 blade, a small 2–3-mm incision site is made in the anesthetized area. The patient's head is gently extended back with the chin raised. A small diameter, 6-inch sprinkler tipped infusion cannula is used to carefully deliver full-strength tumescent (0.1% lidocaine) solution through the submental incision into the immediate subdermal adipose compartment. Before and after tumescence, the patient is asked to purse the lips and clench the lower teeth to check the functioning of the marginal mandibular nerves. Occasionally the anesthesia will inhibit functioning of the nerve which is important to note before proceeding with the liposuction. For the lateral cheeks, a 20-gauge, $3\frac{1}{2}$-inch spinal needle (Becton Dickinson and Co., Franklin Lakes, NJ) is used to create infusion points 2 cm below the tragus. Tumescent solution is infused into the subcutaneous cheek and jowl areas bilaterally. Caution must be exercised during this buccal infiltration because overzealous filling can potentially lead to intraoral airway occlusion. A total of 400–500 mL of tumescent anesthesia is required to anesthetize the average patient's neck, cheeks, and jowls.

Instrument	Manufacturer
3-mm, 6-inch spatula-tipped cannula	Bernsco Surgical Supply, Inc, Seattle, WA
2-mm, 3-inch spatula-tipped cannula	Wells Johnson, Tuscon, AZ
4-mm closed neck dissector	Byron Medical, Tuscon, AZ

Table 43.1 Neck liposuction instruments

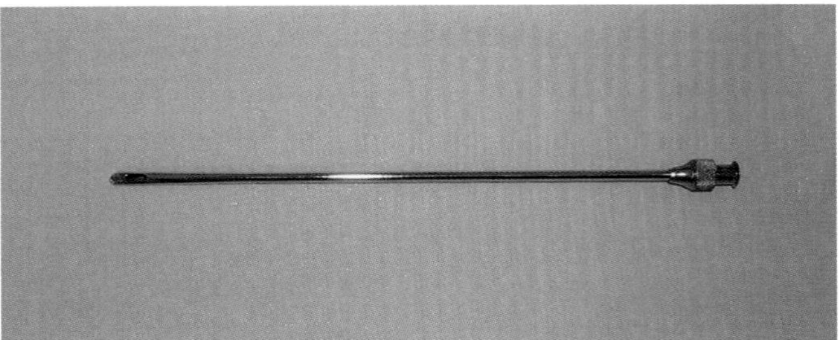

Figure 43.5 3-inch, 2-mm spatula cannula.

After tumescent anesthesia is complete and has been allowed to take effect over a 45-minute time period, a 3-mm spatula-tipped liposuction cannula is used to gently debulk the submental, anterior, and lateral neck adipose tissue via machine suctioning through the submental incision (Aspirator III, Wells Johnson, Tuscon, AZ) (Table 43.1). This is fine-tuned by aspiration using a 2-mm, 3–4-inch spatula-tipped cannula attached to either machine suction or a 5-mL syringe (Fig. 43.5). The syringe method of suction has been evaluated by several surgeons and found to be a precise and controlled method for adipose removal.[13,14] Caution must be used to keep the cannula in the mid to superficial fat and to stay medial to the anterior border of the sternocleidomastoid muscle. This helps to avoid injury to large veins in the area (Fig. 43.6). Suctioning is then continued with the 2-mm spatula-tipped cannula through #11 blade stab incision sites placed along the lateral portion of the jawline. Head extension and lateral rotation provide appropriate positioning for suctioning the cheek, jowl, lateral neck, and jawline. The midplane of jowl suctioning is first identified with syringe-assisted hand suctioning, followed by gentle contouring of the jowl and jawline by machine-assisted liposuction. During suctioning, the operator's free hand is used to identify the mandibular rim and the skin is lifted upwards by the cannula motion to prevent injury to the marginal mandibular nerve. It is important to note that while the patient's head is extended and laterally rotated, the marginal mandibular nerve may drop as much as two fingerbreadths below the mandible, become more superficial, and pose a greater risk for nerve injury (Fig. 43.7). Care is taken to stay in a mid to superficial adipose plane.

At times it can be helpful to briefly turn the cannula opening upwards towards the dermis, particularly in the submental region. While contouring the cheeks and jowls, one must avoid aggressive suctioning of the medial and superior cheeks because this can result in unwanted dimpling or hollowing. This is most likely to occur at the junction of the buccinator and masseter muscles where the parotid duct travels through the buccinator to the oral mucosa. Labiomandibular tethering near the depressor anguli oris may require gentle blunt dissection with the cannula to allow adequate adipose removal and contouring of the jowls. Removal of neck adipose extending to the medial border of the sternocleidomastoid muscles bilaterally and to the thyroid cartilage inferiorly is necessary if the surgeon will be performing platysma repair. After contouring is achieved, a 4-mm closed neck dissector (Byron Medical, Tuscon, AZ) is used to release the superficial submental and anterior neck septa via the submental incision (Fig. 43.8). It is essential to release these tethering fibrous bands to allow smooth redraping of the neck skin. The sharp 'V'-shaped notch of the dissector allows a more thorough and gentle approach than aggressively swiping the area with a blunt cannula. Gentle rasping of the underside of the dermis may also facilitate tightening and adherence of the skin to the underlying muscle, but this concept is anecdotal and unproven. A cannula may then be used in a side-to-side motion to check for full release of the fibrous bands. Figure 43.9 demonstrates the results of a liposuction only procedure.

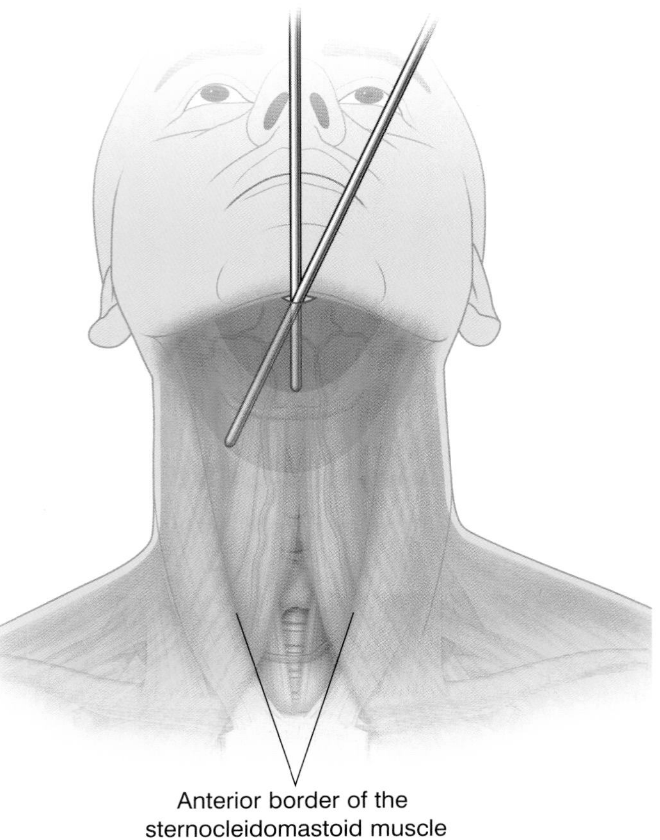

Figure 43.6 Anterior borders of the sternocleidomastoid muscles of the neck define the area of neck suctioning.

Location of the marginal mandibular nerve

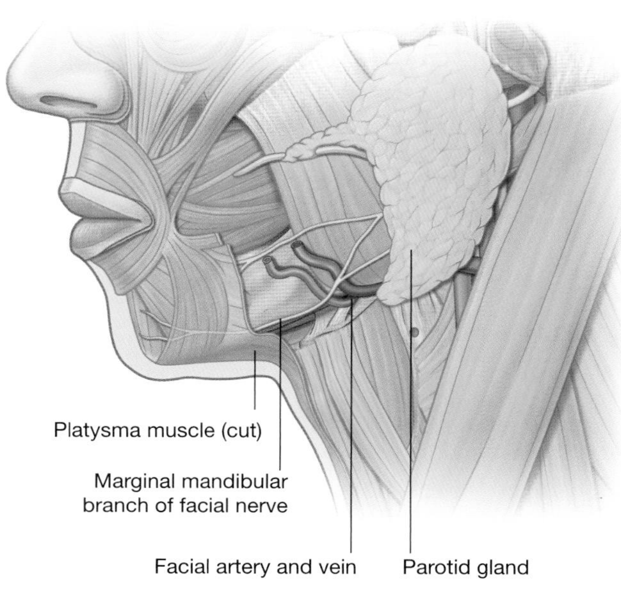

Figure 43.7 Location of the marginal mandibular nerve. (For further information, see Figs 1.14 and 41.1.)

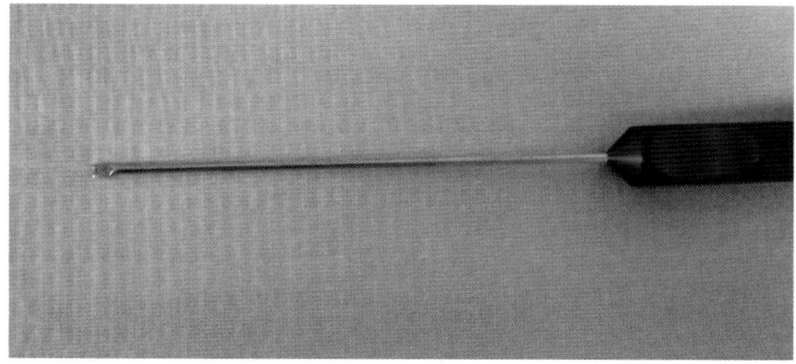

Figure 43.8 Byron closed neck dissector.

Table 43.2 Corset platysma repair instruments

Instrument	Manufacturer
Neck liposuction instruments as in Table 43.1	
Surgical loupes and fiberoptic headlight	SurgiTel Systems, Ann Arbor, MI
Electrocautery pencil with 13-cm straight electrode extension adapter	Surgistat, Valley Labs, Boulder, CO
Deaver retractor	Sklar Instruments, Westchester, PA
Long Metzenbaum scissors	Sklar Instruments, Westchester, PA
7-inch DeBakey atraumatic tissue forceps	Sklar Instruments, Westchester, PA
7-inch Webster smooth needle holder	Sklar Instruments, Westchester, PA

Platysma repair and SMAS plication

In patients who lack decussation of the platysma (crossing of the medial fibers of the platysma), or who have visible platysma bands or laxity of the muscle fibers, plication can be performed. Current methods of platysma repair include bilateral platysma plication, midline platysma plication with transection of distal fibers, and neck lift with skin excision.[15–17] The corset platysmaplasty, originally described by Joel Feldman is an extremely effective and comprehensive anterior approach to platysma tightening and correction of submandibular ptosis[15,18] (Table 43.2).

Simple midline platysma repair with transection

Following liposuction, a 3-cm ellipse is removed encompassing the submental incision site. Gentle lifting of the submental skin for platysmal visualization is performed with a Deaver retractor (Sklar Instruments, Westchester, PA) (Fig. 43.10). After diligent hemostasis using an electrocautery pen equipped with a 13-cm straight electrode extension adapter (Surgistat, Valley Labs, Boulder, CO), the platysma bands are identified using long Metzenbaum

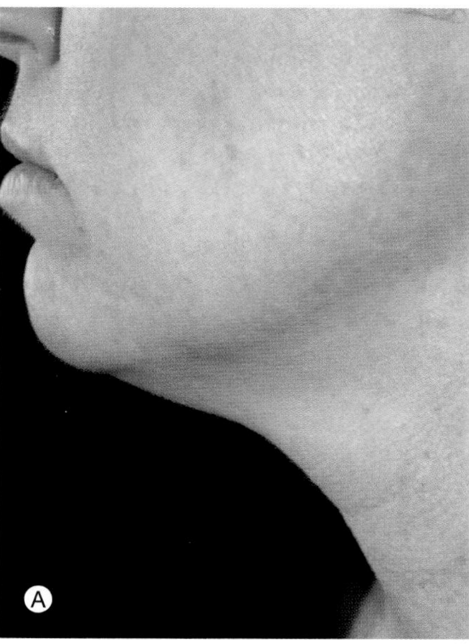

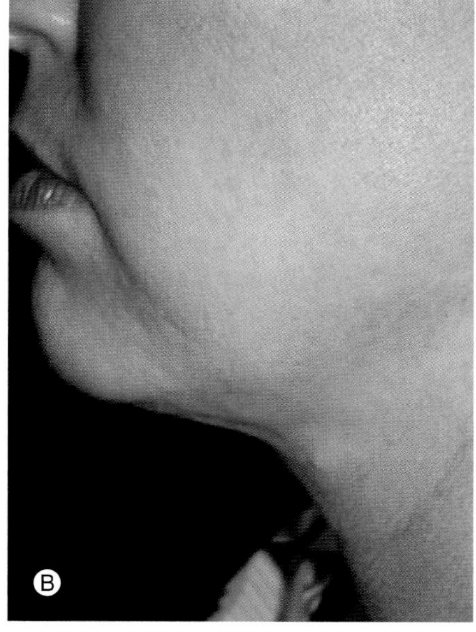

Figure 43.9 (A) Patient preoperatively, side view. (B) Patient postoperatively, side view 3 weeks after neck liposuction alone.

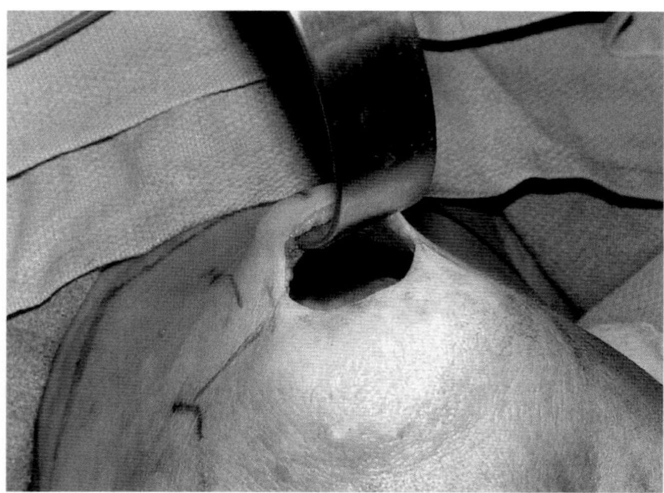

Figure 43.10 Visualization of the platysma using a Deaver retractor. View is from the top of the patient looking down to the chin and submental incision. Black ink markings are noted on the neck.

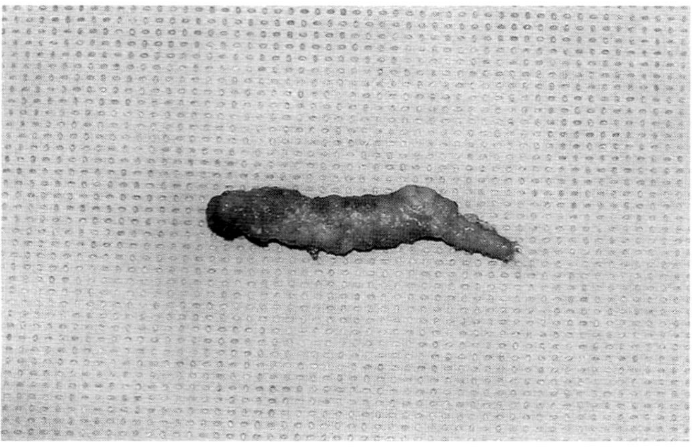

Figure 43.11 Retroplatysmal fat.

scissors (Sklar Instruments, Westchester, PA) and forceps. Platysma repair is performed by approximating the medial portions of the left and right platysma bands with CV-4 Gore-tex (WL Gore & Co., St. Louis, MO) or similar buried sutures. Other authors have used 4–0 polyglactin 910 (Vicryl, Ethicon, Inc., Somerville, NJ) or polyglycolic acid (Dexon, Davis & Geck, Wayne, NJ) sutures with similar results.[18,19] The platysma repair is continued inferiorly to just above the level of the thyroid cartilage. Electrosection is then used to transect the distal portion of the platysma bilaterally from the proximal midline bundle. The skin incision is closed with 5-0 polyglactin 910 and 6-0 polypropylene sutures. The small incision sites on the cheeks and jawline are left for drainage purposes and heal secondarily.

Corset platysma repair

The corset platysma repair is performed following liposuction of the neck, and is begun by creating a 3-cm elliptical incision enveloping the submental crease incision. Surgical loupes (SurgiTel Systems, Ann Arbor, MI) and a fiberoptic headlight are essential to obtain an adequate visual field. A Deaver retractor is used to retract the skin and the medial bands of the platysma are identified and isolated by blunt dissection using long Metzenbaum scissors. Hemostasis is achieved and any further platysma–dermal tethers are removed by electrocautery. The retroplatysmal space is then accessed through a small incision in the fascia overlying the midline platysma. If excess retroplatysmal fat is present superior to the hyoid bone, a small amount (approximately 3 mL) is excised after careful dissection of the superficial fascia (Fig. 43.11). Care is taken to identify, divide, and coagulate any prominent veins when necessary as they may lie in the fat deep to the fascia and the medial platysma edges. The medial borders of the split platysma bands are then identified with blunt and sharp dissection to produce clearly defined borders for suturing the muscle together. Hemostasis is then confirmed. A running 4–0 mersilene (Ethicon, Inc., Somerville, NJ) or 3–0 polydioxanone (PDS) (Ethicon, Inc., Somerville, NJ) suture is used, and with a 7-inch needle holder, a running suture is started at the superior portion of the split platysma bands. Seven-inch DeBakey atraumatic tissue forceps (Sklar Instruments, Westchester, PA) are used to gently grasp the medial edges of the platysma bands, and suturing is continued inferiorly in a running locked fashion as the edges of the right and left platysma muscle are approximated. The running suture proceeds inferiorly towards the thyroid cartilage, making sure that adequate sections (approximately 1 cm) of platysma and overlying fascia are incorporated into each bite. Upon reaching the level of the thyroid cartilage, the running suture is continued in a running reverse direction proximally while plicating the more lateral borders of the platysma muscle over the now sutured medial fibers (Fig. 43.12). This is the corset portion of the repair, and the double-layer plication creates a smooth surface to the midline plication as well as superb muscular apposition and tightening. This 'overplication' produces firm tightening of the anterior platysma and sharpening of the cervicomental angle as well as the jawline. Upon reaching the submental incision site, the suture is tied upon itself in buried knot fashion. During the overplication corset phase of the repair, there is a gratifying part of the procedure where the platysma literally falls onto the underlying hyoid bone as the muscular tightening causes the muscle to assume its natural shape on the neck.

Some patients have prominent submandibular glands as a result of ptosis of the glands inferior to the jawline. These patients benefit from an oblique plication performed on the left and right submandibular area to further tighten the platysma muscle and elevate the ptotic submandibular gland. These lateral platysma bands and associated muscle laxity are less clearly identified, and the lateral positioning makes the approach to their repair challenging through the small submental incision. On each side, small oblique running sutures are placed to a length of 5–8 cm with 4-0 mersilene or 3-0 PDS suture. A locked running suture is first placed from proximal to distal, and then a running 'baseball-type' stitch is performed as the suture is continued from distal to proximal (Fig. 43.13). The suture is then tied upon itself. Finally, in the original description by Feldman, two interlocking sling sutures are performed, one from the right submental platysma fibers to the left mastoid process, and one through the left submental platysma fibers to the right mastoid process. The sutures are interlocked in the submental position. We have not found this portion of the procedure to be necessary in the majority of patients, but it may benefit those patients with extreme platysma laxity or ptotic submandibular glands.

Redraping of the neck and jawline skin occasionally requires further release of the lateral platysma–dermal bands to avoid puckering of the skin at the lateral neckline. Occasionally redundant skin occurs submentally after the plication. Excision of this skin at the level of the submental incision can be performed if the superfluous skin is substantial. Closure of the submental incision is accomplished with 5–0 polyglactin 910 and 6–0 polypropylene sutures (Fig. 43.14).

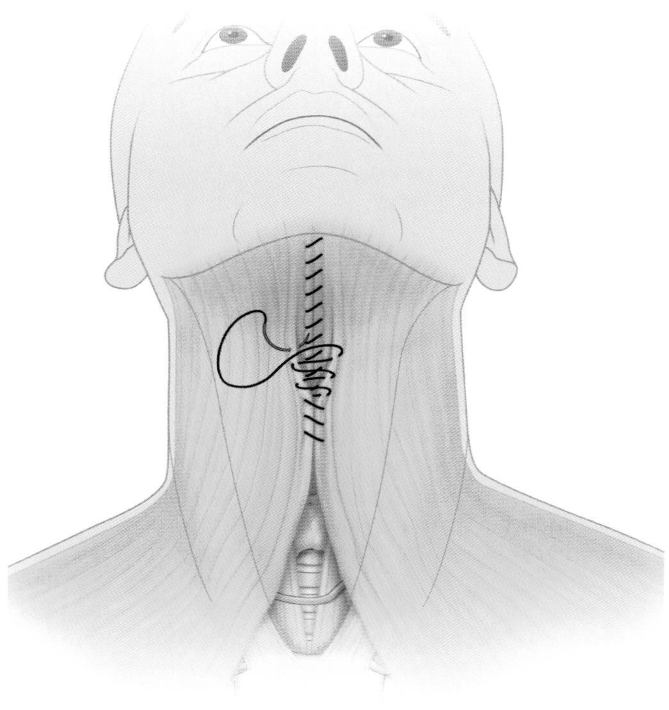

Figure 43.12 Reverse running suture of the corset platysmaplasty.

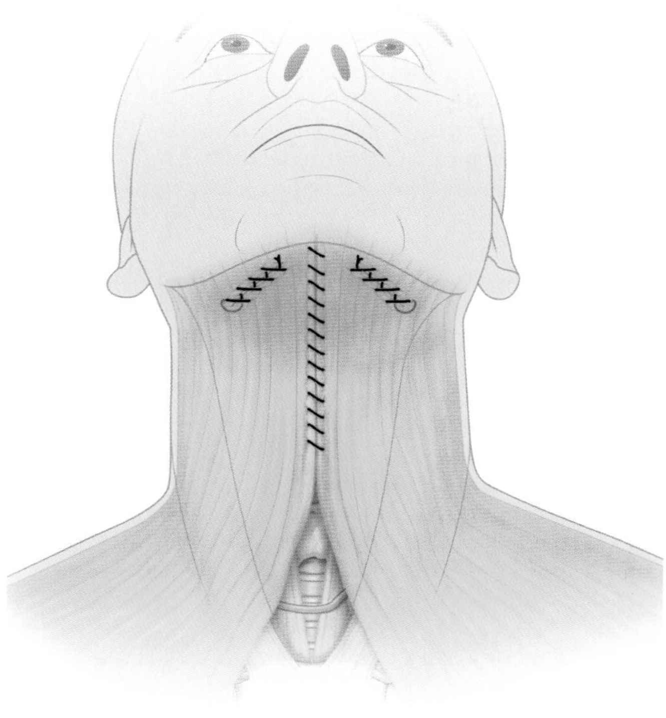

Figure 43.13 Plication over the lateral submental platysma.

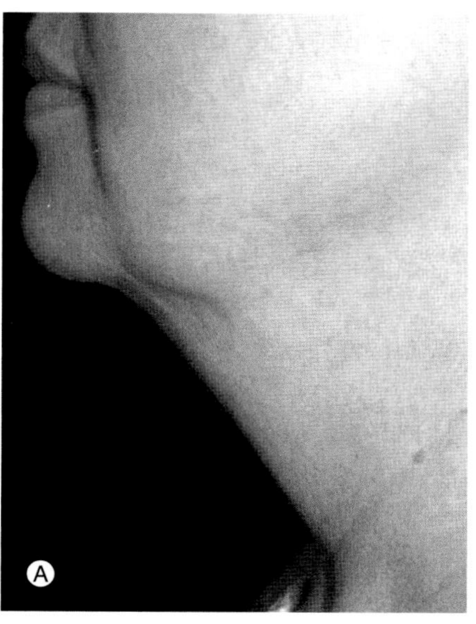

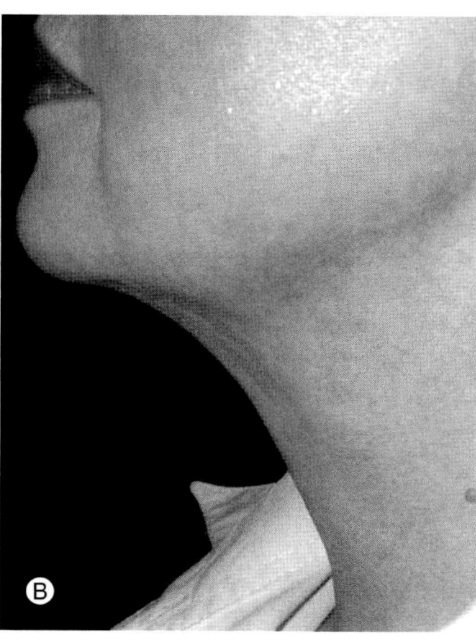

Figure 43.14 (A) Patient preoperatively, side view. (B) Patient postoperatively, side view 2 months after liposuction and platysmaplasty. Note softening of the jowls as well as improved contours of the cervicomental angle.

SMAS plication

In patients with excessive sagging of the jowl and jawline skin, or advanced age and poor skin elasticity, a SMAS plication can be performed in the preauricular zone. Following liposuction and repair of the platysma muscle, lidocaine (1% with 1 : 100 000 epinephrine (adrenaline)) is locally injected along the planned periauricular incision line to an area 5 cm anterior to the ear (in the lateral cheek area in the region to be undermined), as well as in the postauricular sulcus. An incision is made along the inner rim of the tragus (similar to standard face lift incision in this area),[20] extended inferiorly anterior to and under the ear lobe, and then superiorly along the posterior ear sulcus to approximately one-third to one-half the length of the ear. Undermining 3 cm anteriorly from the incision in the mid-subcutaneous plane allows visualization of the SMAS. Suture plication of the SMAS is performed in a superolateral direction and the skin is redraped. SMAS plication is intended to tighten the musculature along the jawline and upper neck. A total of 7–10 sutures are used, with plication extending down from the pretragal region, anterior to the earlobe, and along approximately 3–5 cm of the superior aspect of the sternocleidomastoid muscle. It is essential to place buried knot plication sutures along vectors that optimize jawline definition and enhancement. Redundant pre- and postauricular skin is excised and the edges are reapproximated with 5–0 polyglactin 910 and 6–0 polypropylene sutures.

Postoperatively, conventional bandages, a tape support (3M Medical-Surgical Division, St. Paul, MN), and a five tabbed compression neck liposuction garment (Flex support compression garments, Universal facial garment, Wells Johnson, Co., Tuscon, AZ) are applied and left in place for 24 hours. The bandages are then removed, and the patient is instructed to wear a two tabbed garment (Facial, Chin, Neck Supporter, Cosmetic Surgery Suppliers, Tucker, GA) layered with a chin strap support garment (The Wrap, Byron Medical, Tuscon, AZ) 23–24 hours daily for 1 week, then at least 8 hours a day for the following 3–4 weeks. The use of double-layered postoperative compression garments appears to enhance skin redraping and jawline contouring. Final cosmetic results occur several weeks to months postoperatively because mild edema requires time to resolve, and skin retraction may be slower in the aging neck (Fig. 43.15).

Radiofrequency tissue tightening

Electrical energy has been used for years to coagulate or cut tissue by creation of heat. Recently, a new device has been developed to harness the heat, selectively focusing it in the dermis, while simultaneously providing a coolant to protect the epidermis. With radiofrequency, heat is generated based on tissue's resistance to the movement of electrons within an electric field. This follows the principles of Ohm's law, where impedance in Z (ohms) to the movement of electrons creates heat relative to the amount of current I (amps) and time t (seconds). The resulting energy (joules) is equal to the current squared multiplied by impedance and time ($J = I^2 \times Z \times t$). The device, known as the ThermaCool™ is unique in its ability to provide capacitive coupling of radiofrequency to the skin, creating a uniform electric field (zone of heating) in tissue at controlled depths. The energy is dispersed across a specific treatment tip membrane to create this effect (Fig. 43.16).

The patient's face is cleansed and a thick layer of 5% lidocaine plus prilocaine cream (LMX 5, Ferndale Laboratories, Ferndale, MI) is placed on the areas to be treated. After 1 hour, the cream is removed, and a temporary ink treatment grid is placed along the cheeks, extending from the malar edge superiorly, the nasolabial fold medially, the preauricular area laterally, and the jawline and submentum inferiorly (Fig. 43.17). This treatment area extends approximately 3–4 cm below the mandible. A coupling gel is spread on the treatment area to allow complete contact of the treatment tip with the skin. The device is set at a level of 13.5–15.5 (approximately 110–140 J), and each square of the grid is treated. The patient is asked to rate the sensation of the electrical energy at 0 (no sensation) to 4 (prominent discomfort). Patients are treated at energy levels that correspond to a personal rating of 3 (moderate sensation but tolerable). A dynamic cooling spray delivers precooling, postcooling, and simultaneous cooling during each cycle. Each cycle (firing of the

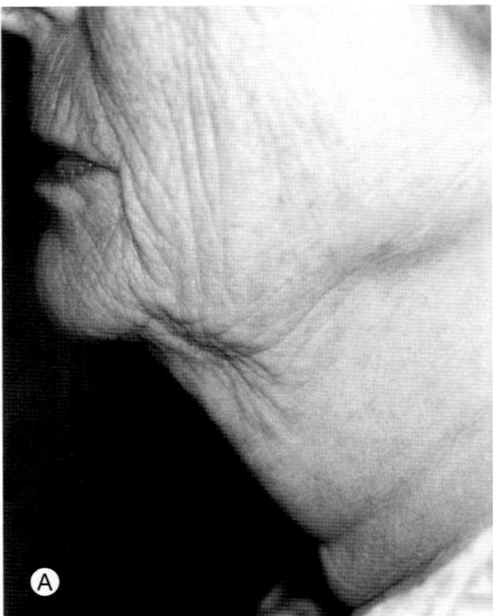

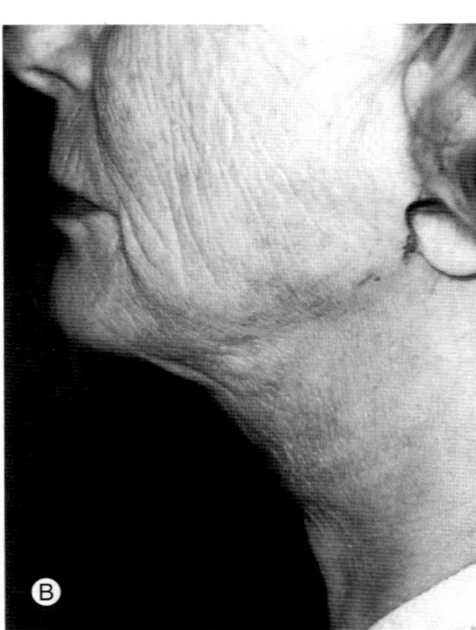

Figure 43.15 (A) Patient preoperatively, side view. (B) Patient side view, 3 weeks postoperative. Liposuction with platysmaplasty and SMAS plication. Although this is a relatively short follow-up, this photo shows the immediate skin tightening achieved with this technique.

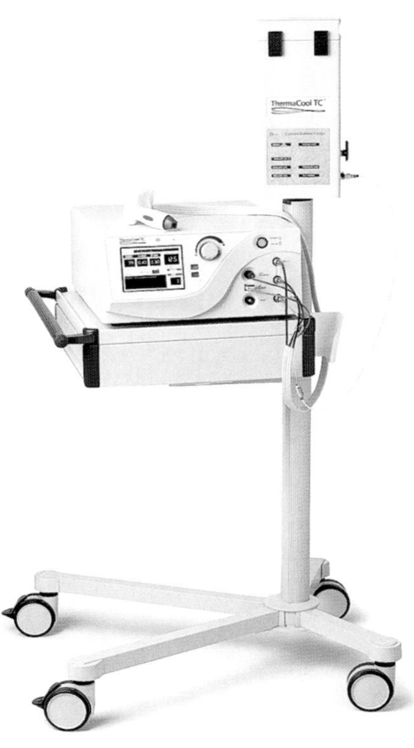

Figure 43.16 The ThermaCool™ radiofrequency device.

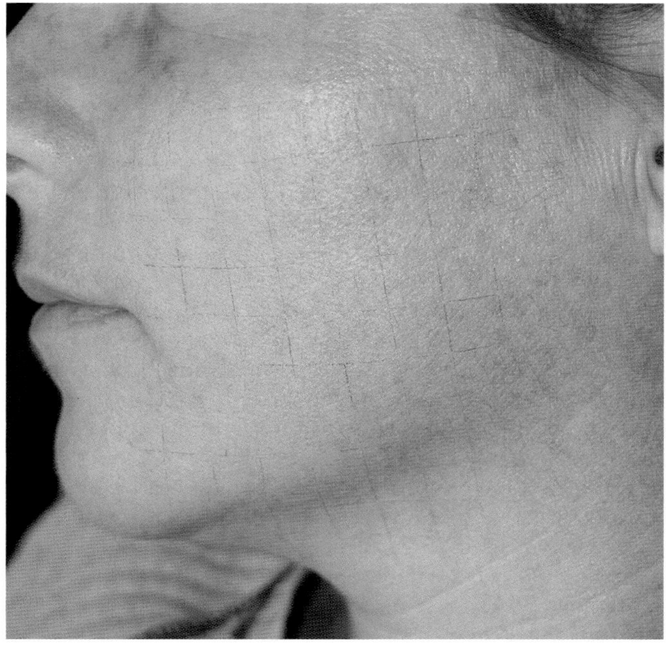

Figure 43.17 Placement of the treatment grid on the cheeks and jawline.

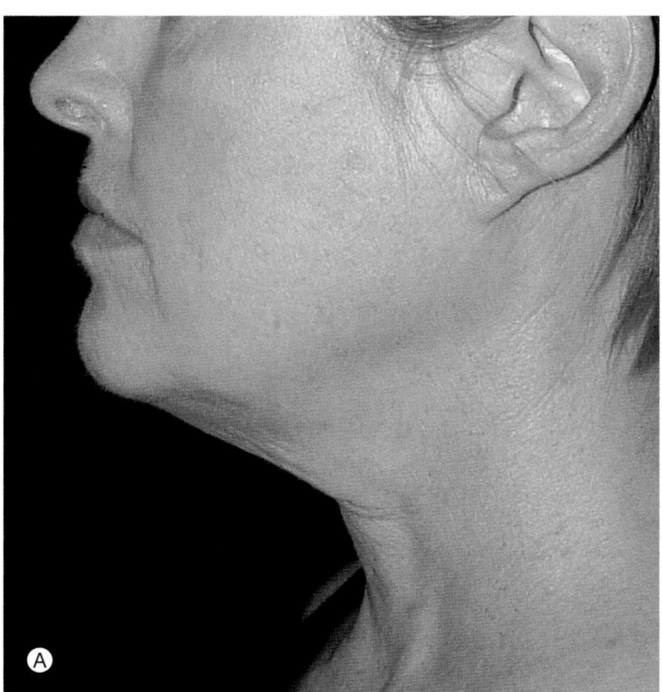

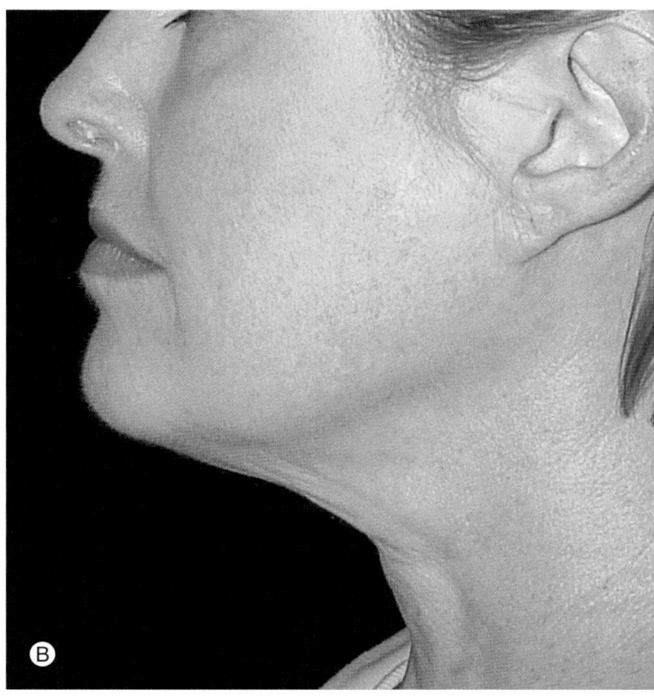

Figure 43.18 (A) Patient before treatment with ThermaCool™. (B) Patient 3 months after treatment with ThermaCool™. Note the improved cervicomental angle.

device) currently takes approximately 6 seconds, and treatment of the cheeks and jawline takes about 45 minutes in total. In a study by Iyer, Suthamjariya, and Fitzpatrick, 70 patients were treated and 70% noted significant improvement in skin laxity and texture 3 months after treatment.[21] Patients may be treated more than once at 8–12-week intervals and may notice further improvement after successive treatments (Fig. 43.18).

■ POSTOPERATIVE CARE

There are two important elements of postoperative care for neck liposuction and/or platysmaplasty: reduction of complications and enhancement of results. Bleeding risks can be reduced through meticulous surgical technique, avoidance of certain medications before and after surgery (nonsteroidal anti-inflammatory drugs, vitamin E), and the use of adequate compression bandages postoperatively. Infection can be minimized with the use of sterile technique and peri- and postoperative antibiotics. Oral cephalosporins are usually sufficient for neck surgery in the non penicillin-allergic patient. Seroma formation can be virtually eliminated through the use of compression bandages and garments for 23 hours a day for 7 days postoperatively.

Results can be enhanced by using carefully applied compression bandages and garments. Skin redraping is an essential component of the healing process, and skin can be guided into place with externally applied bandages. These materials are used to gently hold the skin in place during the healing process, facilitating the skin's attachment to the underlying structures. Failure to adequately compress and support the skin during the important first 7 days postoperatively can produce skin that shows signs of ridging and puckering. If the surgeon sees any signs of skin irregularity during the first postoperative week, it is important to take the time to gently release the skin from the underlying tissue and redrape it in a more neutral position.

Compression garments are worn 23 hours a day for the first postoperative week, then 8–10 hours a day for the next 3–4 weeks. For those patients who suffer from claustrophobia, it may be beneficial to have them try on the garments several weeks before the procedure to make sure they will be able to comply with postoperative instructions.

■ OPTIMIZING OUTCOMES

The most important element of the neck rejuvenation procedure is preoperative patient assessment. The initial evaluation of the patient in many ways determines the ultimate result the patient will receive. If the initial examination is thorough, then the surgeon is able to accurately determine a treatment plan that is appropriate for the patient. If on the other hand the initial evaluation fails to identify, or take into account, certain elements of the patient's anatomy then the ultimate result may be compromised.

For example, if the patient has platysma bands, mild jowl formation, and lax skin with submental ridging at the preoperative examination, the surgeon must form a treatment plan that takes into account all of these elements. Failure to adequately plan for treatment of the submental ridging (via submental skin excision and/or SMAS plication with periauricular skin excision) will likely lead to a paradoxical increase in ridging postoperatively, which will yield both an unhappy patient and surgeon.

An additional factor that at times is minimized during skin surgery is sterile technique. As a result of the invasive nature of the platysma repair procedure, sterile technique is of paramount importance. All surgeons who perform this procedure must have thorough knowledge of the key elements of sterile technique. In addition, the operative suite and ancillary surgical staff must be properly trained in sterile technique. Although minor breaks in sterility can often be overcome during simple skin surgery, infectious complications following surgery to the tissues of the neck can be catastrophic.

■ PITFALLS AND THEIR MANAGEMENT

Pitfalls

- Overaggressive suctioning of the cheeks leading to dimpling
- Seroma formation if proper garments are not worn
- Idiopathic submental nodule formation
- Marginal mandibular nerve injury
- Submental skin ridging and puckering

The neck can be a challenging anatomic region to rejuvenate, and complications are a legitimate concern. There are inherent risks of tumescent neck liposuction, which include bleeding (intraoperative and postoperative), seroma formation, injury to the marginal mandibular nerve, and vertical band formation with poor skin retraction. But, with careful patient selection, surgical neck recontouring can be performed in a safe and efficient manner.

Injury to the marginal mandibular nerve is a known complication of neck surgery. In particular, the nerve is vulnerable to injury as it crosses the mandible in the vicinity of the facial artery and vein, as well as at the posterior angle of the mandible. Injury to the nerve can be avoided by suctioning in the mid-fat over the nerve, and avoiding suctioning that crosses over the mandibular ramus. In instances where injury to the marginal mandibular nerve is the result of liposuction, our experience is that it resolves completely within 2–3 months. The incidence of nerve injury is less than 1–2% of all cases. However, injury to the marginal mandibular nerve can be permanent if the nerve is transected during platysma repair or SMAS plication. It is imperative that the surgeon is familiar with the anatomy of the neck, and is cautious to operate at the level of the mid fat near and below the jawline to prevent injury to the marginal mandibular nerve.

Important measures for maximizing results in neck liposuction include using small (2–3 mm) cannulas, combining hand and machine suctioning, creating sufficient numbers of entry sites for thorough suctioning, releasing submental fibrous subcutaneous bands, and having the patient wear appropriate postoperative garments. Despite proper postoperative care, some patients will develop soft vertical bands or small submental nodules, which resolve with time (usually 6–12 months). Resolution of these may be hastened with the use of ultrasound massage.

■ SUMMARY

Neck liposuction, either alone or in combination with platysma repair and in some cases SMAS plication, can produce excellent recontouring of the aging or obese neck and jawline. Patients with mild submental laxity or excess adipose tissue may benefit from nonsurgical radiofrequency tissue tightening alone or in combination with these procedures. The goal of these procedures is to define the cervicomental angle and jawline. It is important to educate patients regarding duration of healing because the results will continue to improve over several months as the skin tightens and re-drapes over the neck. By carefully utilizing these complimentary procedures in one surgical session, the surgeon can safely and effectively improve neck contours.

■ REFERENCES

1. Cook Jr. WR, Johnson DS. Advanced techniques in liposuction. Semin Cutan Med Surg 1999; 18:139–148.
2. Webster RC, Smith RC, Smith KF. Face lift, part 2: Etiology of platysma cording and its relationship to treatment. Head Neck Surg 1983; 6:590–595.
3. Alster TS, Tanzi EL. Improvement of neck laxity with a nonablative radiofrequency device: a lifting experience. Dermatol Surg 2004; 30:503–507.
4. Fitzpatrick R, Geronemus R, Goldberg DJ, Kaminer MS, Kilmer SL, Ruiz-Esparza J. First multicenter study of a new nonablative radiofrequency device to tighten facial tissue. Radiofrequency controlled tissue rejuvenation. ASLMS, April 9–13, 2003.
5. Ruiz-Esparza J, Gomez JB. The medical face lift: a noninvasive, nonsurgical approach to tissue tightening in facial skin using nonablative radiofrequency. Dermatol Surg 2003; 29:325–332.
6. Marino H, Galeano EJ, Gondolfo EA. Plastic correction of double chin: importance of the position of the hyoid bone. Plast Reconstr Surg 1960; 31:45.
7. Ellenbogen R, Karlin J. Visual criteria for success in restoring the youthful neck. Plast Reconstr Surg 1980; 66:826.
8. Worms F, Isaacson R, Speidel T. Surgical orthodontic treatment planning—profile analysis and mandibular surgery. Angle Orthod 1976; 46:1.
9. Legan H, Burstone C. Soft tissue cephalometric analysis for orthognathic surgery. J Oral Surg 1980; 38:744.
10. Sommerville JM, Sperry TP, BeGole EA. Morphology of the submental and neck region. Int J Adult Orthod Orthognath Surg 1988; 3:97.
11. Moreno A, Bell WH, Zhi-Hao Y. Esthetic contour analysis of the submental cervical region. J Oral Maxillofac Surg 1994; 52:704–713.
12. Kaminer MS, Hsu J. The use of nonablative radiofrequency technology to tighten the lower face and neck. Semin Cutan Med and Surg 2003; 22:115–123.
13. Toledo LS: Syringe liposculpture. Clin Plast Surg 1996; 23:683–693.
14. Hunstad JP: Tumescent and syringe liposculpture: a logical partnership. Aesthetic Plast Surg 1995; 19:321–337.
15. Jacob CI, Berkes BJ, Kaminer MS. Liposuction and surgical recontouring of the neck: a retrospective analysis. Derm Surg 2000; 26:635–632.
16. Knize DM. Limited incision submental lipectomy and platysmaplasty. Plast Reconstr Surg 1998; 101:473–481.
17. Cardoso de Castro C. The changing role of platysma in face lifting. Plast Reconstr Surg 2000; 105:764–775.
18. Feldman JJ. Corset platysmaplasty. Clin Plast Surg 1992; 19:369–382.
19. Kamer FM, Lefkoff LA. Submental surgery: a graduated approach to the aging neck. Arch Otolaryngol Head Neck Surg 1991; 117:40–46.
20. Alt TH. Facelift surgery. In: Elson ML, ed. Evaluation and treatment of the aging face. New York: Springer-Verlag 1995; 110–168.
21. Iyer S, Suthamjariya K, Fitzpatrick RE. Using a radiofrequency energy device to treat the lower face: a treatment paradigm for a nonsurgical facelift. Cosmetic Dermatol 2003; 16:37–40.

PART 4

Special Procedures

44 Keloid Management

Hilary Baldwin MD

Summary box

- Keloids are a hyperproliferative response of connective tissue in response to trauma, appearing most commonly in areas of high skin tension.
- Their etiology and pathogenesis are poorly understood though multiple endocrine factors may play a part, and there is evidence of genetic predisposition.
- In early stages, diagnosis may be difficult, but mature keloids are easily distinguishable from hypertrophic scars.
- Keloids often itch, burn, and cause pain, and in certain locations may cause dysfunction because of restriction of movement.
- Treatment depends on the morphology and location of the keloid, and techniques include corticosteroid therapy, surgical excision, laser surgery, radiation therapy (RT), compression therapy, application of silicon products, interferon injection, imiquimod application, cryotherapy, and 5-fluorouracil (5-FU) therapy.
- Prevention is a major goal in patients with a history of keloids and surgical procedures should be planned with prevention in mind.

INTRODUCTION

Unlike many skin disorders described in textbooks, keloids have been known since ancient times, probably occurring in humans since trauma was first experienced. The first recorded evidence of this is descriptions of keloidal scars that appear in the Smith papyrus (2500 and 3000 BC).[1] The Yoruba tribe of Western Africa recorded their knowledge of keloids in painting and sculpture 10 centuries before modern times.[2] Despite this wealth of ancient knowledge, we have made remarkably little progress since 3000 BC towards understanding why keloids occur. This fundamental ignorance is partially responsible for our current lack of consistently reliable, safe treatment measures. This chapter will briefly review what is known about keloid epidemiology and pathogenesis to gain insight into the development of a rational treatment plan for these unsightly lesions.

Epidemiology

The incidence of keloid formation is a function of the underlying population being studied, and has ranged from a low of 0.09% in England to a high of 16% in Zaire.[3] Such variability is explained by numerous variables such as race, age and trauma frequency and type. In predominantly black and Hispanic populations, incidences between 4.5 and 16% have been reported.[4] Darkly pigmented individuals form keloids 2–19 times more frequently than Caucasians.[5,6] But intensity of pigment alone is not the only factor at work. In Aruba, more children of Polynesian descent form keloids than those of African descent.[7] In Malaysia, the lighter-skinned Chinese are more prone to keloid formation than the darker-skinned Indians and Malays.[8] Although Caucasians form keloids less frequently, those who do may be skin types I and II. These patients are often among the most difficult to treat.

Although keloids can occur at any age, they occur most commonly during and after puberty. New keloid formation is uncommon in the very young, although this may be partly a function of low trauma frequency and severity. However it is also uncommon in the very old, and keloid regression after menopause has been reported.[9,10] Cosman et al. reported a median age of onset of 22.3 years and 22.6 years in women and men, respectively.[11] In an unpublished study of 212 black keloid-formers at Kings County Hospital, we found that ear pierces that resulted in keloids occurred at a median age of 6.4 years after menarche whereas those that did not result in keloid occurred at a median age of 4.25 years before menarche.

Explanations for these findings include the fact that young skin is more taut than the redundant skin in the elderly, and that collagen synthesis occurs at a higher rate in younger patients.[12,13]

There appears to be no gender differences in keloid incidence although there is certainly a reporting bias that makes them seem more common in women. Multiple ear pierces are far more common in women than men, as are the resulting keloids. Additionally, women may more readily seek medical attention for cosmetic improvement.

Etiology

Theories regarding the etiology of keloids abound. The factors that appear to be most significant are some form of skin trauma in an individual with a genetic predisposition for keloids. Other contributing factors may include wound tension and infection as well as endocrine issues (Table 44.1).

Trauma

In most cases, trauma is the primary, if not the only, etiologic factor. Although 'spontaneous' keloids arising in nontraumatized skin have been reported, this author does not believe that such an entity exists. Often the severity of the trauma is so minor as to go unnoticed by the patient. Minor abrasions and burns, insect bites, varicella and zoster, vaccinations, and tattoos can result in significant keloiding. Acne lesions of the anterior chest and deltoid areas often morph imperceptibly into the keloids that they cause. Isotretinoin treatment in these patients prevents additional keloids even when the acne lesions themselves are not readily identifiable. With the exception of ear pierces, deep and significant surgical wounds are actually less likely to keloid than the minor wounds described above.

However, trauma cannot be the only factor. Areas prone to trauma such as the hands and feet rarely keloid. Research has demonstrated a phenotypic difference in the fibroblasts in earlobe keloids when compared to palmar fibroblasts.[14] Immediately adjacent acne lesions often have different outcomes. Women with three or more pierces per earlobe often keloid in only one or two holes despite similar piercing methods and jewelry worn.

Skin tension

With the exception of the earlobes, keloids appear most commonly on areas in which skin tension is the highest, namely the anterior chest, upper back, and deltoid areas. As they progress in these areas, they tend to stretch along skin tension lines forming linear or bow-tie-shaped lesions.

Post-surgical wound tension has been implicated in the literature as a contributing factor in keloid formation.[9,15] Closing a wound against the relaxed skin tension lines results in a wound with twice the tension of one closed along Langer's lines, and may be more likely to result in keloid formation.[16] The loss of tissue that results from surgical excisions may also increase wound tension. Skin grafts may be preferable to primary closure of a tight wound, but the donor wound may also be subject to keloid formation. The use of tissue expanders to stretch the skin preoperatively is perhaps the most sensible option, especially because the pressure applied by the expanding bladder is similar to the pressure that is known to prevent keloid formation postoperatively (see pages 711 and 713).

Wound tension cannot be the only answer considering the high incidence of earlobe keloids following piercing. The only tension on this wound is that of the minor edema that results from the trauma of the pierce. Chronic edema has been reported to increase glycosaminoglycans (GAGs) in the dermis.[17] Because GAGs serve as the lattice upon which collagen deposits, the chronic edema caused by the pierce and subsequent reaction to the presence of a metal foreign body could result in increased incidence of keloid formation.

Table 44.1 Etiologic factors in keloid development

Trauma
Skin tension
Infection—primary infection and wound infections
Endocrine—estrogens and melanocyte stimulating hormone (MSH)
Genetic

Infection

Viral and bacterial infections have been incriminated as etiologic factors. This theory was based on the high incidence of keloids following varicella, zoster, and smallpox infections. Tuberculosis and syphilis were also believed to promote keloid formation.[18,19] There is no evidence to support the supposition that the infectious agents themselves cause keloids. Rather, it is the trauma that they cause in the skin that incites the lesion formation. It is not clear whether the increased trauma and wound tension resulting from a surgical wound infection could also increase the incidence of keloiding.

Endocrine factors

Multiple endocrine factors have been associated with keloid formation, but their actual importance in the etiology of these lesions is unclear. Keloids have been reported to grow more readily or to appear de novo during pregnancy.[9,10] As described above, keloids have been shown to be more common after puberty than before. This was well known by the Yorubas in the 1600s who knew to pierce ears early in life to prevent keloiding. They also perfected ritual keloiding in intricate designs after the age of puberty (Fig. 44.1).

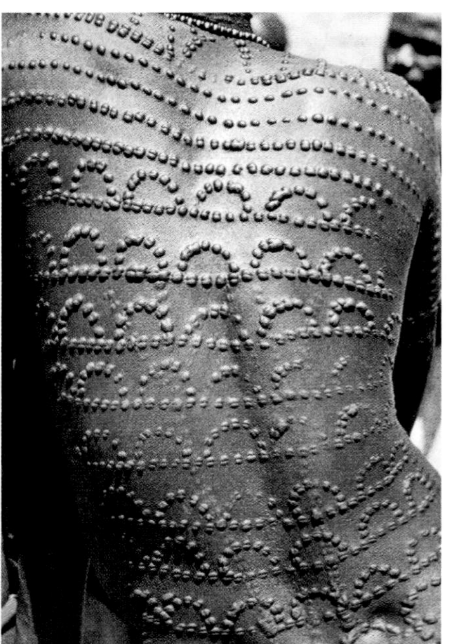

Figure 44.1 Intricate ritual keloiding of the Yoruba tribe.

Melanocyte-stimulating hormone (MSH) has been postulated to play a role in keloid formation. Keloids are more common in patients with hyperpigmentation associated with pregnancy, puberty, and hyperthyroidism.[20] Melanocytes in darker individuals may be more reactive to MSH than in people with lighter skin. This may explain the higher incidence of keloids in darker skinned patients. Additionally, keloids are rare on the melanocyte-poor regions of the palms and soles. An albino patient, even one of African descent, has never been reported to develop a keloid. However, the highly pigmented area of the genitalia is an infrequent site of keloid formation.

Genetic predisposition

Keloids are believed to have a familial predisposition although the pattern of inheritance is unclear.[3,11,21] In our study at King's County Hospital, we found a 32% incidence of first-degree relatives with keloids. However, no study has demonstrated that the familial tendency to keloid is inherited as opposed to being a factor of similarity of skin coloration between family members.

Pathogenesis

The simple answer to the pathogenesis puzzle is that keloid formation is caused by an increase in anabolic activity in the absence of increased catabolism. Why this happens is not known. We know many isolated facts about abnormalities within keloid tissue, but the big picture is not yet complete.

After normal wounding takes place, various signals are sent to the neighboring fibroblasts to fill the hole by increasing production of collagen and GAGs. Upon completion of the job, additional signals are sent to the fibroblasts indicating that they can return to their pre-wound status. Abnormalities in these signals are believed to be partially responsible for keloid growth. In normal wounds, there is regression of connective tissue elements after the third week. In keloid tissue, however, fibroblasts proliferate around the plentiful new and dilated capillaries. Collagen synthesis and GAG synthesis are markedly increased.[22] Cosman et al. found that collagen synthesis is 20 times greater in keloids than in normal skin.[11] The collagen formed is normal in composition. However, there is an increase in the usual ratio of type I to type III.[23] The absolute number of fibroblasts within the entire keloid is not increased, and they appear histologically normal, but the activity of proline hydroxylase is markedly elevated, suggesting that the rate of collagen biosynthesis is increased in a normally-sized fibroblast population.[24,25] Keloidal fibroblasts also appear to resist programmed cell death.[26,27] Defective apoptosis within keloids may be due to a dysfunctional form of p53. This protein is involved in normal fibroblast apoptosis. Interferon may be effective in treating keloids by its enhancement of native p53 function.

Although collagenase is also increased, collagen degradation is not—possibly as a result of an increased deposition of alpha-globulins within the keloid.[24,28] Serum alpha-globulins are known inhibitors of collagenase.[29] Estrogens increase the level of serum alpha-globulins which may help to explain the increased incidence of keloids in pregnant women.[28] Corticosteroids have been shown to reduce the alpha-globulin deposits within keloids.[28] It is theorized that this allows activation of the collagenase, with subsequent breakdown and resorption of the excessive collagen and clinical flattening.

Many other abnormalities have been reported in keloid tissue. However, their role, if any, in the formation of keloids is unclear. Growth factors, such as transforming growth factor-beta and platelet-derived growth factor, are known to play important roles in fibroblast contraction in normal skin.[30] Dysregulation of production or activity of these growth factors may play a role in fibrosis.[30,31] Histamine is found in increased quantities in keloids and has been shown to stimulate fibroblast mitogenesis in keloids. Mast cells are prominent in keloids and are interspersed throughout the dermis rather than being localized around blood vessels as they are in normal skin.[32,33]

Clinical manifestations

The clinical manifestations of keloids are discussed as they pertain to therapeutic options.

Keloids rarely represent a clinical dilemma except in distinguishing them from hypertrophic scars (Table 44.2). This is not merely an academic issue because the lesions respond quite differently to therapy. A mature, aged keloid presents little clinical debate. It is the early, pruritic, red keloid that can be a difficult diagnosis. Hypertrophic scars develop rapidly after surgery, whereas keloids may occur months after the inciting trauma. Ultimately hypertrophic scars will subside with time whereas keloids generally progress until such time as they become stable. They rarely, if ever, regress. Hypertrophic scars achieve a shape that is relative to the size and shape of the preceding trauma, whereas keloids exceed, sometimes greatly, the extent of the initial trauma. Hypertrophic scars are more likely to occur in areas prone to excessive motion, such as those across joints. Keloids are most often found in areas in which there is limited or no motion, such as the chest and back. After appropriate surgery is performed, a hypertrophic scar will often improve whereas a keloid (except perhaps on the earlobe) nearly always recurs unless adjunctive therapy is implemented. The postoperative keloid recurrence is frequently worse than the initial lesion.

Keloids are often symptomatic causing itching, burning, and pain. The sensation of pain can be the result of a lesion that is primarily tender, or because of rubbing of a pedunculated keloid against clothing or furniture. Although cosmetic improvement is the most common reason for

Table 44.2 Clinical features differentiating keloids from hypertrophic scars

Keloids	Hypertrophic scars
Develop slowly over months	Develop rapidly after skin insult
Continue to grow for extended period	Subside with time
Exceed size of initial trauma	Stay within initial wound footprint
Occur in areas with little motion	Occur in areas of motion (i.e. joints)
Recur after therapy	Regress with therapy
Often dome-shaped or pedunculated	Broad and flat-topped

patients to seek dermatologic care for keloids, some patients who seek medical care are concerned primarily or solely with symptoms of itch and pain. Increased symptomatology is also a useful clinical sign of lesion progression because stable, mature keloids are rarely pruritic. Resolution of symptoms during treatment is often rapid and can be used as a guide to treatment success. Once the symptoms are alleviated, the patient may choose to discontinue therapy.

Keloids of the jaw, neck, and anterior chest can also cause dysfunction. Patients with large lesions of the jaw and neck may be unable to fully turn the head from side to side or to extend or flex the neck (Fig. 44.2). Keloids of the mid-chest often pull breast or adipose tissue towards the center of the chest creating the sensation of tightness as well as creating the appearance of cleavage. This is particularly troublesome to male patients. These lesions need not be fully removed to alleviate the dysfunction. Portions of the lesions tethering the skin can be excised to improve mobility, or high-dose corticosteroid injections can be used to intentionally cause atrophy with resultant skin relaxation.

Large keloids of the anterior chest and posterior scalp will often form draining sinus tracts with multiple large, terminal hairs trapped within. Excision of at least the immediate surrounding tissue is usually necessary, but these patients may respond to a short course of oral antibiotics.

Lastly, the morphology and location of the lesion will often dictate the therapeutic plan. Pedunculated lesions, particularly when they occur on soft, mobile skin such as the axilla or earlobe, are amenable to simple excisional surgery (Fig. 44.3). Tight, flat, sessile keloids such as those on the anterior chest are not amenable to surgery and will respond best to injectables (Fig. 44.4). Earlobe keloids come in four varieties—anterior and posterior buttons, wraparound, dumbbell, and lobular. Button keloids can be shaved off in their entirety. Dumbbell keloids have a component within the lobe that must be removed. Lobular keloids are usually recurrent lesions that have now entirely replaced the fatty lobe. Such lesions will require wedge excisions of the entire keloid (see page 711).

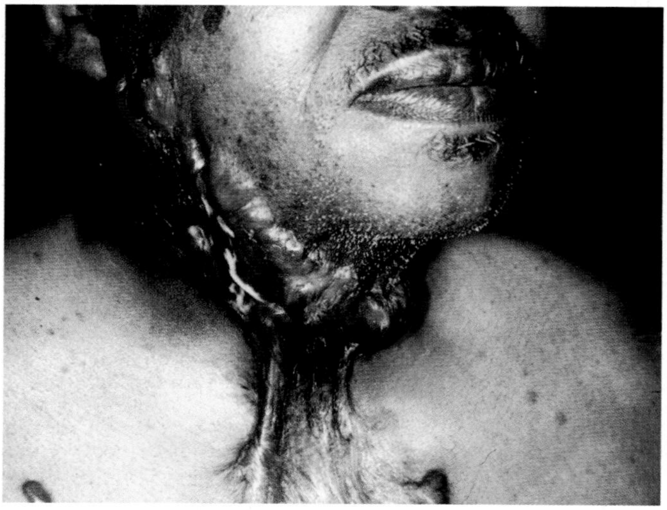

Figure 44.2 Keloid limiting mobility of neck and head.

■ TECHNIQUES

In any medical inquiry, a literature review of available therapy requires attention to study design and validity of conclusions. This is nowhere more evident than in the field of keloid therapy in which one must sift through a vast amount of anecdotal reports and pure conjecture to find a handful of well-performed studies (Table 44.3). The problem begins with the delineation of hypertrophic scars from keloids. Many studies include both entities in the admission criteria yet fail to identify which lesions ultimately respond to therapy. Although it may occasionally be a difficult differential diagnosis, there are plenty of patients to include in these studies whose lesions are clearly diagnosable. Other patient and lesion characteristics are routinely omitted from these studies. Race, patient age, lesion age, symptomatology, lesion size, lesion location, recurrent versus virgin lesion, and lesion morphology (sessile versus pedunculated or dome-shaped) are all important variables that must be included in the patient demographics. Follow-up time should be at least 1 year to allow conclusions to be drawn regarding treatment efficacy. Anyone can remove a keloid; the trick is preventing recurrence.

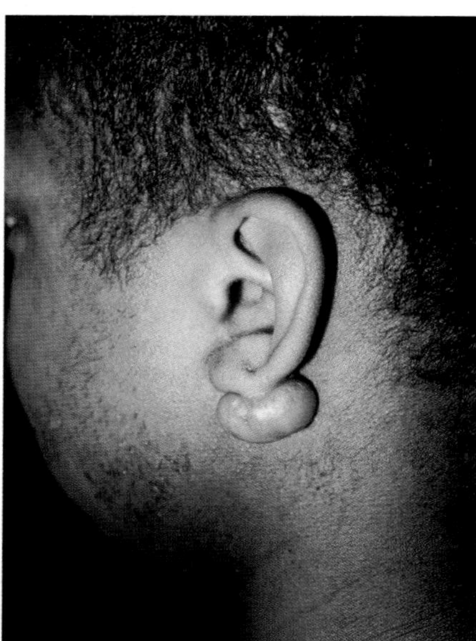

Figure 44.3 Pedunculated keloid of the earlobe.

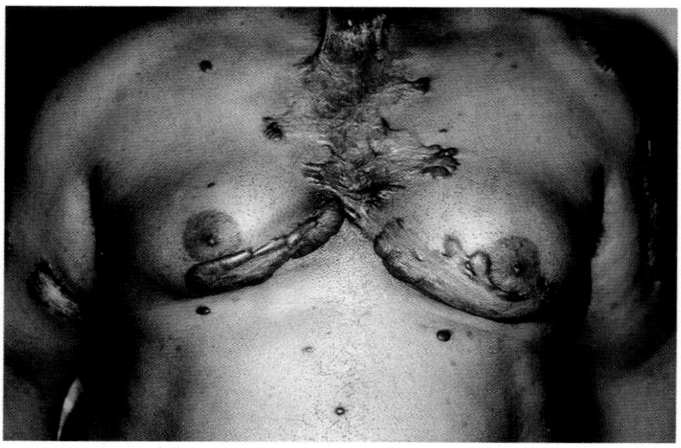

Figure 44.4 Sessile keloids of the chest and arms.

Table 44.3 Keloid characteristics serving as entry criteria for studies

Adequate differentiation between keloids and hypertrophic scars
Patient age and race
Lesion age and symptomatology
Lesion size and location
Lesion status—recurrent versus virgin
Morphology—pedunculated versus sessile
Follow-up time

Table 44.4 Common therapies for keloids

Topical	Corticosteroids
	Retinoids
	Imiquimod
	Mederma
	Vitamin E
Injectable	Corticosteroids
	Interferons
	5-Fluorouracil
	Verapamil
	Bleomycin
Surgical	Surgical debulking or excision
	Laser debulking or excision
Physical	Laser therapy
	Radiation therapy
	Compression therapy
	Silicone sheeting
	Cryotherapy

In a recent review article, Shaffer et al conclude that despite a plethora of papers on the topic of keloids 'there are no definitive treatment protocols'.[34] This is a result of poorly designed and uncontrolled studies in which the endpoint of therapy (cosmesis, function or symptoms) is rarely identified. They further conclude there are adequate data to support efficacy *only* for RT in combination with surgery. Other treatments at this time are still lacking the proof of efficacy that arises only from a well-designed randomized, placebo-controlled trial with adequate patient numbers. Mustoe et al. disagree, concluding that corticosteroid injections and silicone gel sheeting (SGS) are the '… only treatments for which sufficient evidence exists to make evidence-based recommendations'.[35] Bigby, on the other hand, includes SGS (and Mederma, Merz) on a list of offending treatments in his article entitled *Snake oil for the 21st century.*[36] The nature of keloid therapy at this time is such that a comparison of various techniques is not always amenable to double-blinding. But a single technique compared to controls, vehicles, or dummy therapy is possible and existing techniques need to be held to this standard. Shaffer et al. suggest guidelines for future keloid studies.[34]

At the present time, we are using techniques for which definitive data do not exist. Presented below are the techniques that have been reported to be efficacious by several authors (Table 44.4).

Corticosteroids

More because of their ease of administration, low cost, and low risk than because of their efficacy, intralesional corticosteroids alone and in combination are the workhorses of keloid therapy. The effect of corticosteroids on collagen synthesis and degradation is not completely understood. In young keloids, they have been shown to increase the production of collagenase and reduce the collagenase-inhibiting alpha-globulins.[28] Corticosteroid injections postoperatively have been shown to downregulate type I collagen gene expression.[37]

Corticosteroids can be used to treat existing keloids as solo therapy or as a post-surgical adjunct. One of the most successful uses of corticosteroids lies in their use postoperatively to prevent keloid occurrence or recurrence. Although no solid evidence-based literature supports their use in this role, they have become the first-line approach of most physicians dealing with this condition worldwide.

Solo therapy

When used as solo therapy, corticosteroids are most useful for sessile, flat, and broad keloids. They will flatten and soften lesions and relieve symptoms, but will not eradicate the lesion. It is important that the patient realizes that the skin will never look normal, just better. Corticosteroids are unhelpful as solo therapy in pedunculated lesions except to reduce symptoms. Repeated injections into a pedunculated or high, dome-shaped keloid will soften and shrink the keloidal tissue, rendering it a saggy pouch that will eventually need to be excised anyway. An argument can be made, however, that the saggy pouch is more amenable to surgical excision with relaxed closure than the parent lesion.

Corticosteroids often have an impressive initial effect on existing keloids. Patients report improvement in symptomatology within a week. Reduction in firmness occurs more slowly, often appearing after the second or third injection. This minor clinical improvement is almost never noticed by the patient, and should be demonstrated to impress upon him the need for subsequent injections. Ultimately, after many injections, the lesion will appear flatter or smaller. Unfortunately, this response is often temporary and the patient may need to return after several months for repeat treatments. Kiil[38] and Griffith et al.[39] reported recurrences of 50% at 5 years and 11.2% at 4 years respectively. The overall lateral dimensions or 'footprint' of the keloid will never improve with solo therapy. Indeed, lesions often enlarge with therapy. It is useful to inform the patient that the lesion is like modeling clay. As it is flattened, it will become wider. Although this does not always happen, it is a useful analogy and prudent concept to bring into the informed consent before therapy.

Depending on keloid size, shape, age and location, dilutions of triamcinolone acetonide from 10–40 mg/kg can be used. Injections can be repeated every 2–6 weeks, depending on the strength of corticosteroid used and the size of the keloid. The most common cause of corticosteroid failure is the use of too low a dose of corticosteroid. Concentrations less than 10 mg/mL are rarely effective for a mature keloid. Most large mature keloids will require 40 mg/mL. This means that the total area treated in one session will be limited by total safe dose constraints. This author does not inject more than 40 mg per session. Although additional areas may be injected on the following weeks, it is best not to inject the same area with such high doses at less than 2-week intervals. The depot effect of the corticosteroids are such that repeated injections carried out too close together can result in too much thinning too fast, leaving an atrophic area. Hypopigmentation is also more likely in this setting. With subsequent treatments, the strength of the corticosteroid is reduced to fine-tune the ultimate outcome. Treatment schedules used by individual practitioners vary widely with respect to concentration of corticosteroid, volume used, and frequency of injection. Readers should consider the recommended dosing schedules mentioned here to be those that work best in the author's experience, but should be adjusted based on clinical responses in the reader's hands.

Occasionally, mature keloids are so firm that injection is nearly impossible. In this case, injecting through the belly of the keloid from one end to the other with a large bore (23-guage or larger) needle, making multiple parallel tracts can allow small deposits of corticosteroid to remain behind within the needle tracts. Because of the high pressure within the firm keloid, the corticosteroid will start to leak out when the needle is removed. This can be avoided by applying a small drop of cyanoacrylate glue to the hole before injecting and then covering it rapidly with plastic tape immediately upon withdrawal of the needle.

Patients with very firm keloids generally require some form of anesthesia to make the requisite number of tracts. For pain control, topical eutectic mixtures of local anesthetics are not helpful. The pain the patient experiences with these injections is not that of the needle passing through the epidermis. The pain is deeper, and appears to be related to the displacement of the fibrosis by the liquid. This pain is beyond the scope of the topical anesthetics, even after hours of occlusion. They can be used, however, to numb the skin so that painless injections of lidocaine can be given as a ring block around the keloid. The author believes mixing lidocaine with the corticosteroid makes little difference because the pain of the injection is over before the lidocaine takes effect.

Adjunctive therapy

Corticosteroids can be combined with any other treatment modality to improve outcome. Following surgical excision, many authors have shown a reduction in recurrence rates with the addition of postoperative corticosteroids.[40] Combinations with cryotherapy and silicone gel sheets were better than either modality alone.[41–43] Combinations with lasers and interferon alfa have also shown promise.[44]

This author feels that corticosteroids are an important adjunct to all other modalities. Regardless of which modality is used, adjunctive corticosteroids are added to the treatment plan. The treatment plan is the same as for prevention of recurrence (see below).

Prevention of keloid occurrence

As mentioned above, postoperative corticosteroids are crucial adjuncts following surgical keloid removal, and useful adjuncts to any other postoperative treatment plan being followed. Additionally, corticosteroids can be used to prevent keloid formation in a patient who has had previous keloids. This author has the following injection schedule:

- On the day of surgery and then at 2, 4, and 6 weeks out, the wound margins are injected with triamcinolone acetonide 40 mg/mL regardless of the appearance of the wound.
- At 2 months, and every month thereafter, injections are given as clinically necessary. Dosage of the corticosteroids given at each session is determined by the site, size, degree of firmness, and symptoms the patient is experiencing.
- Therapy is best carried out for 1 full year. Most patients who quit before the 1 year mark end up returning for injections in unnecessary recurrences.

Common side-effects of corticosteroid injections include hypopigmentation and skin atrophy. The hypopigmentation can be pronounced and lasts 6–12 months before resolving (Fig. 44.5). Often hypopigmentation accompanies softening of the lesion and can be a marker of clinical success. Both hypopigmentation and atrophy can be reduced by avoiding injecting into the surrounding normal tissue. Care must be taken, especially when injecting very firm keloids, not to suddenly dump large quantities of corticosteroid into the softer surrounding skin. This can easily happen when redirecting the needle and pushing hard on the plunger at the same time. Either redirect or push hard, but not both simultaneously. Skin atrophy is often a necessary consequence of adequate therapy. After treatment, the atrophic surface may appear wrinkled or shiny, and telangiectasias are common. This appearance improves with time and vascular lasers can lessen the telangiectasias. The corticosteroid-treated keloid will never look normal. If the surface is too dark compared with normal skin, hydroquinones can be helpful.

Surgery

Recommended surgical techniques vary according to the size, location, and shape of the keloid. Pedunculated keloids with narrow bases can be excised and closed primarily with little wound tension. Sessile keloids with broad bases are much more difficult to treat surgically. Regardless of lesion morphology, surgical monotherapy results in a high incidence of recurrence (50–100%).[45,46] Surgery must be combined with adjunctive techniques such as RT, corticosteroids, or interferon.

The smallest incision possible is made, extending less than the entire length of the keloid. Any useable epidermis

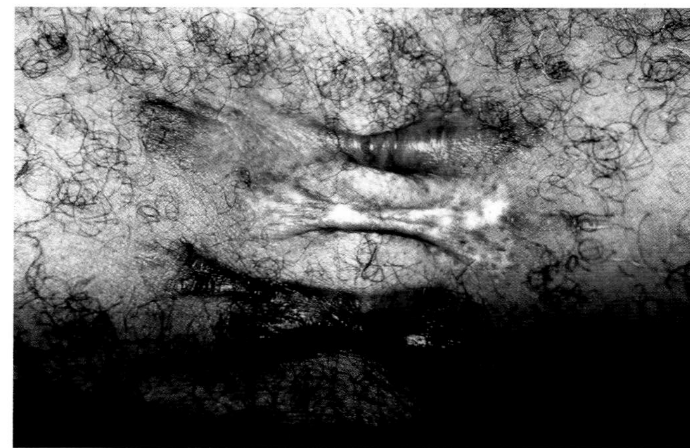

Figure 44.5 Hypopigmentation (central keloid) resulting from corticosteroid injections.

is dissected off the keloid. Unless it would result in gross deformity or loss of function, all the keloid material should be removed. Care should be taken to remove any trapped hairs. Closure is done under the least amount of tension, avoiding buried sutures if possible. Whenever possible monofilament suture should be used to reduce the incidence of wound infection, abscess formation, and inflammation along the suture line. Sutures often need to be left in longer than usual to prevent dehiscence. This is especially true when corticosteroids are injected postoperatively. Surgery followed by grafting alone results in a superior nonrecurrence rate over primary closure (59%).[11] However donor-site keloids are likely. Tissue expanders are probably preferable, and the pressure of the expander may beneficially alter collagen production preoperatively. If the resulting wound is fairly superficial, and the patient is amenable, allowing the wound to heal by second intention often results in a better cosmetic outcome and a lower incidence of recurrence. Some surgeons have recommended that if the lesion is too large to be closed primarily, a rim of keloid tissue should be left behind to act as a splint to prevent excessive central tensile contraction.[47] A full-thickness skin graft is placed on top.

Earlobe keloids

Earlobe keloids deserve to be considered separately. Many authors allude to the reduced rate of keloid recurrence in the earlobe.[48–50] Studies have shown a recurrence rate of only 41% after surgery alone.[51] Studies utilizing both surgery and corticosteroids have shown recurrence rates of 1–3%.[52] With careful aggressive therapy and using multiple adjunctive postoperative modalities, earlobe keloids rarely recur.

Better surgical results on earlobes are probably the result of several factors. First-time earlobe lesions tend to be very discrete, and are easily separated from the surrounding dermis and epidermis. Complete removal of all keloidal tissue is thus easier to accomplish. Most earlobe keloids occur in women who are profoundly motivated to wear earrings again, and are far more compliant than the average keloid patient. The fleshy tissue of the ear makes closure without tension easier to accomplish. Postoperative pressure is easily applied with the use of pressure earrings. These earrings are rather awkward, but the patients find them easy to wear and comfortable. They also make a great covering for postoperative dressings, obviating the need for bulky, and often inadequate pressure dressings.

Earlobe keloids come in four varieties, each of which is approached differently: anterior and posterior buttons, wraparounds dumbbells, and lobular (Figs 44.6–44.10). Anterior and posterior buttons (which are much more common) are most easily removed by a simple shave followed by second intention healing.

So-called dumbbell keloids (anterior and posterior button keloids connected by a smaller core of keloid tissue) are more complicated. In 1983, Salasche and Grabski reported a novel and elegant method for removing dumbbell keloids.[53] In this method, the anterior and posterior portions of the keloid were first dissected away from the earlobe. Then the core within the lobe was dissected from the normal lobular skin, and the entire keloid removed en bloc through the posterior opening. A simpler method that this author prefers is a shave of the anterior and posterior buttons allowing visualization and palpation of the firm tissue remaining within the adipose tissue of the earlobe. The diameter of the core is measured and punched out with a disposable punch at least 1 mm larger than the core itself.

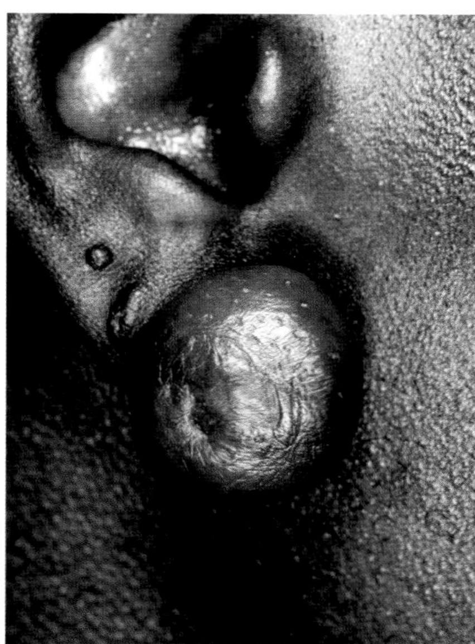

Figure 44.6 Anterior button earlobe keloid.

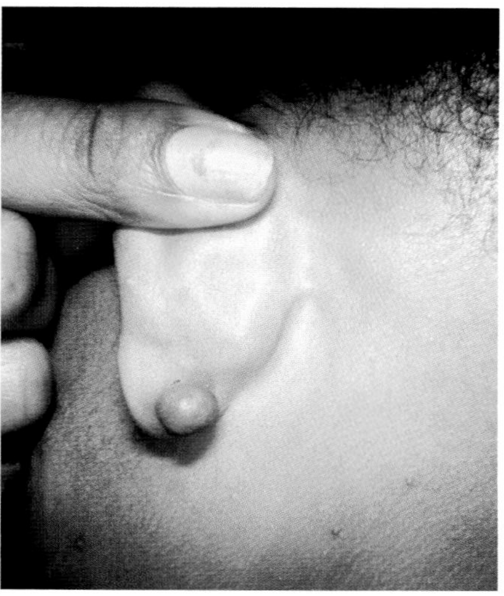

Figure 44.7 Posterior button earlobe keloid.

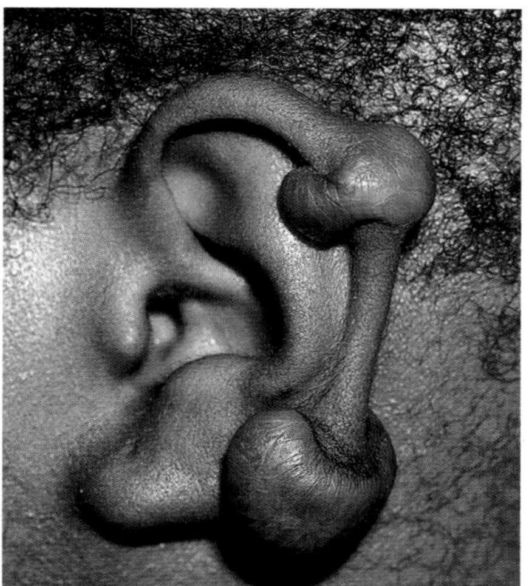

Figure 44.8 Wraparound earlobe keloid.

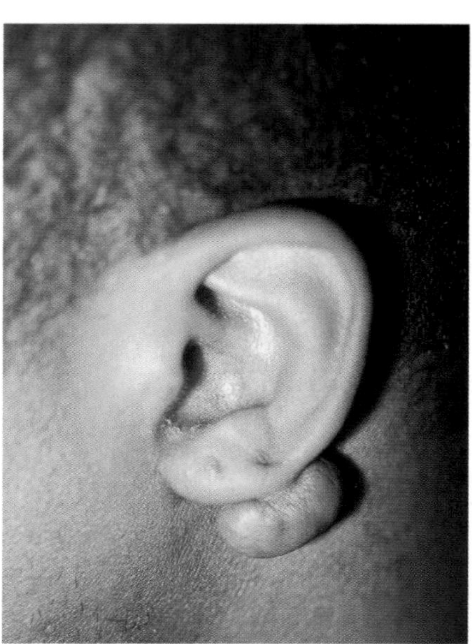

Figure 44.9 Dumbbell earlobe keloid.

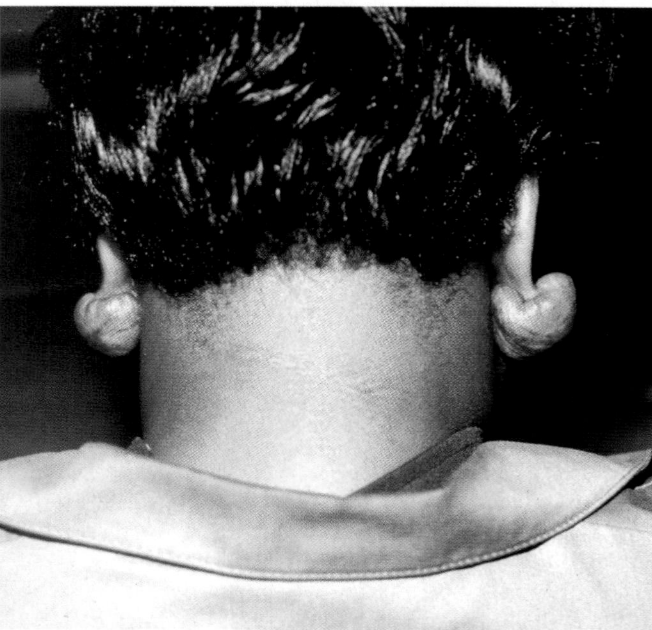

Figure 44.10 Lobular earlobe keloid.

The defect is closed horizontally on the anterior surface of the lobe and vertically on the posterior lobe to prevent a pointed lobe.

Small lobular and wraparound keloids are best excised in a wedge, and closed primarily. Huge lobular keloids and wraparound, multilobular recurrent keloids are the most difficult to manage. Removal of the entire keloid is crucial, but may leave no functioning lobe. A perfectly keloid-free ear is not a successful outcome if earrings are not wearable postoperatively. One option is to sculpt the lobe, removing as much keloid as possible, leaving an earlobe-shaped keloid and relying on postoperative techniques to prevent recurrence. This is not a time for monotherapy or single adjunct therapy. Extensive postoperative treatment with RT and silicone gel and corticosteroid injections and interferon injection and pressure often prevent the regrowth of the keloid. Once the lobe-shaped keloid ages, it becomes stable and functional. Pressure earrings may be necessary for 6–18 months after this technique, but the patients do not seem to mind because they have some adornment on a functioning lobe.

Laser surgery

After initial excitement over the demonstrated ability of the carbon dioxide laser to decrease fibroblast activity in vitro, its use in keloid therapy was a disappointment.[54] Used in the defocused mode, recurrence rate is extremely high. In the focused mode, recurrence rate is similar to that of surgery alone (50–70%).[47] Despite the in-vitro findings, carbon dioxide laser excision appears to have no benefits over cold steel excision except for the technical advantages of increased speed, coagulation of small vessels, and perhaps a lower rate of postoperative discomfort because of the laser's ability to seal off small nerve endings. The neodymium:yttrium aluminum garnet (Nd:YAG) laser has been demonstrated to cause an in-vitro selective bioinhibition of collagen production, but recurrence rates of 53–100% in vivo.[46,55] The combination of ultrapulse carbon dioxide laser and interferon injections was reported by Conejo-Mir.[56] Thirty lesions were treated with 3 million units thrice weekly for 9 weeks, and at 3 years there were recurrences in ten of 14 keloids on the trunk and none of 16 keloids on the ear.

The pulsed dye laser (PDL) has been reported to improve hypertrophic scar symptoms, decrease scar height, and improve skin texture. Alster and West showed a 57–83% improvement with the 585 nm flashpump PDL in sternotomy scars.[57] They noted the importance of starting therapy early for the best results. It has been proposed that the PDL decreases the microvasculature in early keloids and hypertrophic scars resulting in anoxia. Mature keloids are not helped by PDL. Several combination studies have shown that PDL works better in combination with other modalities including corticosteroids, interferon, and carbon dioxide laser.[58,59]

Radiation therapy

The mechanism of action of RT on keloidal tissue is unknown. Its preferential effectiveness in early keloids implies that it may decrease fibroblast collagen synthesis.[60] Alternatively, it may act by decreasing vascular hyperplasia.[59]

Radiation therapy alone is ineffective in existing keloids, although it may resolve the pruritus associated with the lesion.[61,62] In a study of over 300 patients, RT alone at a total dose of 800–2400 rads over 2–5 months was only effective in reducing keloids that were within 6 months of initiation.[62–64] Mature, thicker keloids require excision before RT.[65,66]

For prophylactic treatment of excised keloids and surgical wounds in keloid-prone individuals, X-radiation, electron beam, and interstitial radiation have all been reported to result in similar cure rates (recurrence rates near 20%, which are far superior to other modalities).[67–69] A study of earlobe keloids compared surgery with postoperative kilovoltage RT (recurrence rate of 12.5%) to surgery with postoperative corticosteroids (recurrence rate of 33%).[50] Guix et al reported on 169 patients treated with high-dose-rate brachytherapy in whom only eight patients (4.7%) had recurred at 7 years.[70] They attributed their success rate to the superior deposition of radiation in keloidal tissue rather than normal surrounding skin, a problem seen with low-dose-rate brachytherapy. Escarmant et al. looked at the efficacy of interstitial iridium-192 with 79% cure rate and a 14% incidence of hypopigmentation.[71] Maarouf et al used electron beam in 134 postoperative keloids with a cure rate of 84% at a mean follow-up of 7.2 years.[72] They attributed their success to the superior dose distribution achievable with electron beam over kilovoltage irradiation. Ogawa et al. showed an 18-month 32% recurrence rate in 147 keloids treated with electron beam.[73] Recurrences were more common in areas of high tension (41.1% on the chest, scapula, and suprapubic area) than those without high tension (13.5% on the neck, earlobes, and lower limbs). These authors suggested additional adjunctive therapy in areas with high tension. Wagner et al concurred, finding a higher recurrence rate on the thorax (49%) than the face and neck (2%) following kilovoltage radiation.[74] They added another prognostic factor—keloids resulting from burns had significantly poorer outcomes compared to those after surgery or trauma.

Dosing schedule and fractionation have varied greatly from one study to another, but outcomes are similar. Most authors perform RT on the day of surgery. Several add a second cycle on day 2 or 7. A minimum of 1000 rads administered within the first week appears to be necessary for successful outcome.[75] The cost is variable, often around $1000 depending on the type of radiation and the fractionation. However, the efficacy, especially in recurrent keloids is superior to all other single modalities. Additionally, the short treatment plan required with RT may aid in patient compliance.

Despite its high incidence of success in preventing keloid recurrence, RT is avoided by many clinicians because of concern regarding the possibility of malignancy of the skin or underlying structures. Botwood et al attempted to put these issues into perspective.[76] The major concern about RT comes from the oncology literature and arises from reports of secondary malignancies occurring years after deep radiation. There are only two reported case of post-keloid RT malignancies.[76,77] Both occurred in the breast following chest RT 6 and 23 years previously. The single case report of thyroid cancer occurring after RT to a keloid of the chin was a medullary carcinoma.[77,78] Radiation-induced carcinomas of the thyroid are exclusively papillary carcinomas.[79] Based on dosimetry studies, RT in standard dosages to the ear with proper shielding would expose the ipsilateral thyroid lobe to only 2 rads.[68] Nearly all keloid RT studies, most of them large extensive studies with various types of radiotherapy have shown a 0% carcinogenesis rate. RT is not recommended in children with keloids, or if used, the growth plates must be shielded to prevent retardation of bone growth, which may occur at doses of 400 rads and less.[54] Complications of RT that may commonly be encountered are dyschromias, alopecia, telangiectasias, and cigarette-paper atrophy.

Compression therapy

Compression therapy—applying pressure greater than that of capillary pressure (24 mmHg)—causes a reduction in soft tissue cellularity. Histopathology shows increased interstitial space and collagen bundles that are more widely dispersed.[80]

Pressure alone is ineffective in the treatment of existing keloids. However, dressings that apply more than 24 mmHg, worn 24 hours a day for 4–6 months are often successful in reducing keloid recurrence rates postoperatively. The mechanism of action is not known, but it is theorized that pressure creates hypoxia, resulting in fibroblast degeneration and subsequent collagen degradation. Not all areas are amenable to pressure dressings, which in any event are uncomfortable, hot, and unsightly. Ears are the exception to this rule. Newer pressure earrings have large compression plates and are easily worn all day long. To accommodate the large surface area, the earrings are necessarily broad and bulky. Young patients are often dismayed by the cosmetic appearance of the 'grandma earrings' and most men will not wear them at all in public. The earrings called 'sleepers' are smaller and more acceptable for daytime use even though they have no adornments. Those intended for heavy lobes are always more appropriate postoperatively when the lobe is edematous from the procedure and the healing process. Thin lobe earrings may become necessary as the time goes on to continue consistent pressure.

The most complicated aspect of compression therapy is determining when to discontinue. Pressure can be stopped when the discontinuation does not result in swelling of the affected area. This generally takes 4–6 months, but may occur earlier. It is useful to remind the patient that this noninvasive technique is better used in overkill than underkill.

Kosaka and Kamiishi recently reported an interesting compression device for the more difficult areas.[81] They created a vest into which they sewed the balloon and rubber tubing from a neonatal sphygmomanometer. The balloon was placed over the area to be compressed, and inflated to the desired pressure. They report that it is particularly good for the anterior chest because it fits well over concave and uneven surfaces without the use of tape. There is minimal pain and sweating and the balloon does not displace.

Silicone products

Silicone gel sheeting has been shown in many studies to be efficacious in preventing the development of as well as reducing existing hypertrophic scars and keloids. These studies are often complicated by the absence of blinding and controls, small patient numbers, retrospective design, inadequate follow-up time, and the inclusion of both keloids and hypertrophic scars within the same treatment group. Keeping these confounding factors in mind, these studies have shown that existing keloids may decrease in size by as much as 30% when the gels are applied 24 hours a day consistently for 2 months.[82] Frequently, hyperpigmented lesions also lighten, and erythema is reduced. Lesions also become softer after the use of SGS, and may be more amenable to corticosteroid injections. These dressings are more effective when used preventatively.[82] They have been shown to reduce keloid and hypertrophic scar formation by 70% when used consistently.[83] The mechanism of action of SGS is unknown, but it is known to retard epidermal water loss. The drier silicone agents have been shown to create static electricity which some believe plays a role in its effectiveness. Other, more moist gels do not create static charges. Silicone oil leaches directly from the surface of SGS, and some authors propose that elemental silicone in some way reduces keloidal ground substance. Two recent studies have shown that silicone oil or cream applied directly to keloids or hypertrophic scars are effective when applied under occlusive dressings. No deposition of silicon has been detected in scars resulting from silicone therapy, so it is unclear how an inert element that is not absorbed could influence scar formation.[84] In a controlled, prospective, nonblinded study, SGS was compared to both an occlusive gel dressing without silicone (Duoderm, ConvaTec, Bristol Myers Squibb) and to a control.[85] Both treatment arms showed significant improvement in symptoms, color, induration, linear measurements, and intracicatricial pressure. SGS was not superior to Duoderm, leading the authors to conclude that it was wound hydration, not the presence of silicone that was responsible for clinical improvement.

Interferon injections

As discussed previously, fibroblast activity increases dramatically after wounding. Once the wound is adequately stabilized, signals are sent to the fibroblasts to shut off this excessive production of ground substance and collagen. Interferons are one of these signals. Berman and Duncan reported that short-term intralesional interferon alfa-2b treatment of a keloid resulted in a selective and persistent normalization of keloidal fibroblast collagen, GAG, and collagenase production in vitro and a rapid reduction (41%) in the area of the keloid.[86] Craig showed that the accelerated rate of collagen synthesis in keloid fibroblasts had returned to normal in cells harvested from lesions that were over 2–3 years of age.[87] Interferon is also able to upregulate native p53 that is dysfunctional in keloidal fibroblasts. This might promote the natural cell death of the fibroblasts that are resisting apoptosis.

Both alpha and gamma interferon are available for use. Initial clinical trials with interferon gamma were disappointing and it is no longer being used.[88,89] However several investigators have demonstrated substantial reduction in keloid size and keloid recurrence with interferon alfa.[87,90] Granstein has reported on an unpublished study in which 18 of 19 keloid re-excisions were accomplished without recurrence at 1 year following two postoperative injections of interferon alfa (Granstein, Richard. New York Academy of Science 1996. Personal communication.) Berman reported response in 11 of 12 recurrent keloids of the head and neck after surgical excision and interferon alfa-2b.[90] Berman and Flores reported a recurrence rate of 51.5% following surgery alone, 58.4% after surgery and corticosteroids, and 18.7% when surgery was combined with both interferon and corticosteroid injections.[44] In an as yet unpublished study, we have found that interferon alfa injections can be used to decrease keloid recurrence after earlobe keloid excisions in which keloidal tissue was left behind.

We can predict from the in-vitro findings highlighted above that interferon may work better in young keloids and in keloid prevention than in mature older keloids where the damage has already been done. Clinical investigations have borne this out. Interferon injections do not result in an improvement of existing mature and stable keloids.

Injections of interferon alfa-2b are done on the day of surgery and then 1 week postoperatively directly into the wound. 1 million units per linear centimeter are injected into the wound base and margins. In the case of a wound allowed to heal by second intention, injections are given approximately every square centimeter. This author limits the total dose to 5 million units to prevent significant side-effects.

Side-effects of interferon alfa-2b include a flu-like syndrome, which can usually be reduced or eliminated by the prophylactic use of acetaminophen—1 g is taken 1 hour preoperatively, 3 hours postoperatively, and every 4 hours through the first 24 hours. It is also helpful to time the injections late in the afternoon on a Friday. Most mild febrile reactions will pass unnoticed during sleep, and if ill the patient will not need to miss work on the following day.

Imiquimod application

Imiquimod 5% cream is a topical interferon inducer. Its use in keloid therapy was a logical follow-on to the success with injectable interferon. Berman and Kaufman reported its use postoperatively in an uncontrolled pilot study of 13 keloids removed from 12 patients.[90] Applications were twice daily, beginning on the day of surgery and continuing for 8 weeks. At 24 weeks, none of 11 keloids (10 on the earlobe, one on the back) evaluated had recurred. The authors would have expected between five and seven recurrences at that point. The authors have subsequently reported one recurrence on the back. In a similar ongoing study, we have found a higher recurrence rate in a placebo-controlled, double-blind study of six patients with 12 nonadjacent keloids. On the placebo-treated site, there was a 90–100% recurrence rate. On the imiquimod-treated site, the recurrence rate was 50%. The recurrences in the imiquimod-treated areas occurred later and were easier to treat than placebo-treated recurrences. There were few topical and no systemic side-effects noted in either study. Application of imiquimod to open wounds is rarely irritating. Discontinuation for several days is adequate to control this unlikely side-effect.

More controlled studies need to be performed to assess the effectiveness of this treatment modality. If effective, it would represent a cheaper, less painful method of interferon use. Imiquimod application does not appear to result in an improvement in existing keloids or hypertrophic scars, even when applied under occlusion.

Cryotherapy

Many publications applaud the use of cryotherapy alone and in combination with other products in the treatment of keloids and hypertrophic scars. The proposed mechanism of action is a combination of direct cell damage as well as vascular damage, which leads to further cell anoxia and death. Most authors propose 30-second freeze times repeated 2–3 times per cycle with a 60–75% 'good results' outcome.[91–93] Many papers suggest that younger lesions respond better to treatment than more mature keloids.[92] They do not, however, comment on the method for differentiating hypertrophic scar from young keloid.

Side-effects of cryotherapy include pain and a prolonged healing phase of more than 1 month. The likelihood of hypopigmentation resulting from melanocyte sensitivity to cold makes cryotherapy less applicable in dark-skinned patients.[92] As this is the population most likely to present for therapy, this author finds this technique unhelpful.

Recently, several authors have suggested unique methods of cryosurgery with good results in small numbers of patients. Gupta and Kumar suggested inserting a lumbar puncture needle in one side and out the other side of the keloid.[93] Liquid nitrogen was then passed through the needle utilizing an intravenous infusion set. There were two freeze–thaw cycles of 20–30 seconds each. Patients were treated with between five and ten sessions. Although hypopigmentation was evident in all patients, more than 75% showed flattening. Har-Shai et al. reported a 51.4% reduction in scar volume after only one session of cryotherapy utilizing a cryoprobe to completely freeze the keloid.[94] Other authors have suggested that the combination of cryotherapy and corticosteroids is superior to either modality alone.[41,42] The problem with hypopigmentation remains a major issue in darker-skinned patients.

5-fluorouracil

5-fluorouracil is the mainstay of therapy for Fitzpatrick who has considerable experience with its use.[95,96] There appears to be no study published on this subject. Fitzpatrick reported on his experience in more than 5000 patients with hypertrophic scars and keloids. Small amounts (0.05 mL of 50 mg/mL) were injected at 1-cm intervals along the scar. The total dose per session ranged from 2–50 mg and never exceeded 100 mg. Patients were treated once weekly on average, but as high as thrice weekly for markedly indurated or symptomatic keloids. Fitzpatrick further found that the addition of triamcinolone acetonide (0.1 mL of triamcinolone acetonide10 mg/mL added to 0.9 mL of the 5-FU mixture above) both improved efficacy and decreased the pain of injection.[96] Fitzpatrick found that the younger, more symptomatic scars improved the most.

Like corticosteroids, the mechanism of action appears to be the inhibition of fibroblast proliferation. Unlike corticosteroids, however, Fitzpatrick reports no side-effect of telangiectasia formation. The further addition of PDL therapy to triamcinolone acetonide/5-FU injections was even more successful in Fitzpatrick's hands.[95] He hypothesizes that the PDL causes selective damage of the microvasculature, resulting in a reduction of erythema and improved wound surface texture. Beranek and Masseyeff suggested that the prolonged angiogenesis is the cause of hypertrophic scarring and that an interruption of this process results in lesion improvement.[97]

Miscellaneous therapies

Intralesional verapamil

In vitro, verapamil increases procollagenase synthesis and drives fibroblasts towards extracellular matrix degradation.[98] Its low cost, and good safety profile when used intralesionally lead to its use in keloid therapy. Two studies have shown it to be effective only for early hypertrophic scars.[98,99]

Mederma

Mederma is an onion extract that has been shown to have a wide range of effects in biological systems. It has antioxidant and anti-inflammatory properties demonstrated in many in-vitro studies.[100] However, there is no well-designed study showing any clinical efficacy.

Vitamin E

The use of topical vitamin E on scars is believed to be highly effective by the lay public. There is no evidence that vitamin E improves or prevents hypertrophic scars, and there is clear evidence that it is a common cause of cutaneous side-effects. In one study, it was found to be ineffective in scar improvement and at the same time caused cutaneous adverse reactions in 33% of the patients.[101]

Bleomycin

Espana et al. describe the treatment of 13 patients with bleomycin.[102] 1.5 IU/mL was applied to the surface of the keloid, which was then punctured repeatedly with a 25-gauge needle. A total of between two and five treatments at 1–4-month interval resulted in complete flattening of three of seven keloids, and a thinning of the rest. Side-effects included pain necessitating lidocaine anesthesia and hyperpigmentation in all patients. There were two recurrences at 10 and 12 months.

■ PREVENTION

The first goal of therapy is, of course, prevention. Cosmetic procedures should be discouraged. Necessary surgical procedures should be closed parallel to relaxed skin tension lines with minimal stress (Fig. 44.11).

Skin grafts, tissue expanders, and healing by second intention should be considered to reduce tension. Wounds should be covered with SGS and/or pressure garments. Preventative intralesional corticosteroids should be injected at the time of the procedure and regularly thereafter.

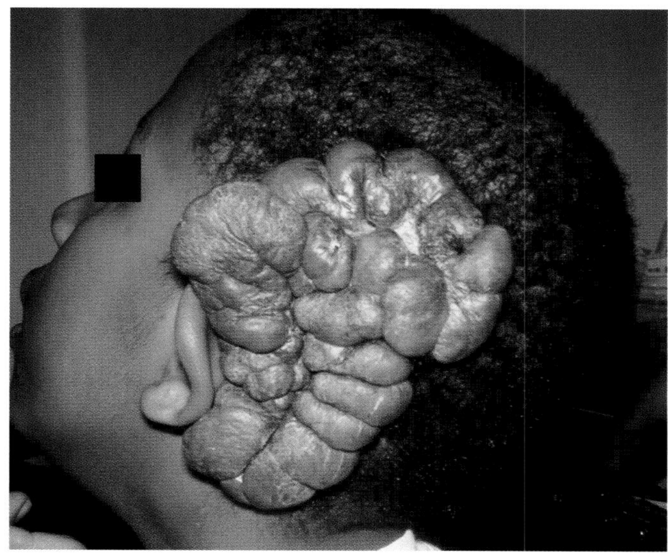

Figure 44.11 Keloid resulting from placement of ventricular shunt.

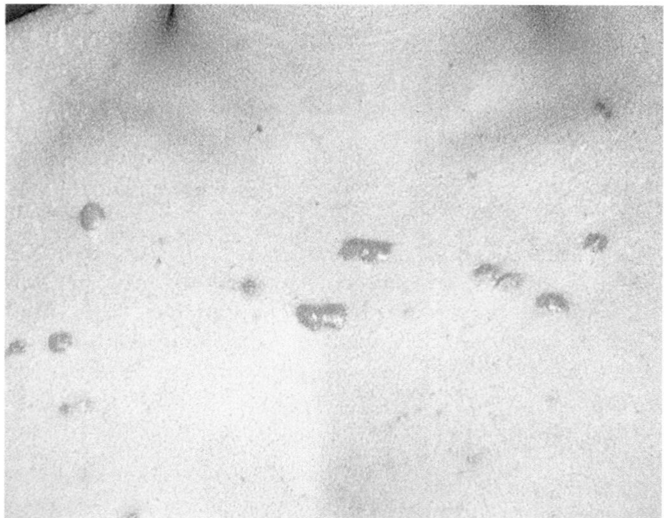

Figure 44.12 Acne merging imperceptibly with keloids.

Intralesional interferon and RT should also be considered. Often this must be coordinated in advance with the patient's general surgeon who may not appreciate interference with the healing wound.

Patients whose acne lesions tend to form keloids must be carefully monitored and treated (Fig. 44.12). They should be educated to present at the first sign of an inflammatory acne lesion for intralesional corticosteroids. Multiple lesions are an indication for oral antibiotics or a trial of isotretinoin.

Optimizing outcomes

- Consider the morphology and location of the lesion carefully when planning therapy for existing keloids.
- Follow up for at least 1 year after therapy to monitor for recurrence.
- For patients with a history of keloids:
  - keep keloid prevention in mind when planning any surgical incision and postoperative care
  - treat viral exanthems aggressively
  - monitor those with acne carefully and institute therapy early if lesions start to form keloids.
- Consider postoperative compression therapy to reduce keloid recurrence rates.
- Consider postoperative corticosteroid injections as an adjunct to prevent recurrence.

Pitfalls and their management

- Educate patients so that their expectations of therapy for keloids are realistic—for example, it is important that they understand that the lesion may become wider with corticosteroid therapy.
- In children, avoid RT for reduction of keloid recurrence— if it must be used, shield growth plates to prevent growth retardation.
- When corticosteroid injection is used, to minimize atrophy and hypopigmentation inject corticosteroid into the lesion rather than the surrounding normal tissue.

Similarly, in dark-skinned individuals with a family history of keloid formation, varicella or zoster should be aggressively treated with antiviral agents.

SUMMARY

Keloids are a challenging problem that have four distinct and equally important features: discomfort, size, color, and dysfunction. All of these issues must be addressed with the patient before embarking on a treatment plan to ensure that what the physician considers to be an optimal treatment goal is shared by the patient. Because therapy is often inadequate and fraught with complications, the patient must be fully prepared for a long treatment course.

The future of keloid therapy rests with our better understanding of the pathogenesis of these fascinating lesions. Keloids can be envisioned as incomplete tumors. They are stuck in a proliferative phase and fail to proceed to the maturation phase. Keloids have several characteristics of malignancy—poor regulation of growth, proliferation beyond the boundaries of the initial insult, and increased collagen synthesis. Yet there has never been a reported case of a keloid becoming malignant. This points to future advances in keloid therapy lying in the direction of an immunologic approach rather than the slash and burn approach we now pursue. Time will tell if interferons or other immune response modifiers will be the magic wand for which our patients are waiting.

REFERENCES

1. Breasted JH. The Edwin Smith surgical papyrus, vol I: Hieroglyphic translation and commentary. Chicago: University of Chicago Press 1930; 403–406.
2. Omo-Dare P. Yoruban contribution to literature on keloids. J Nat Med Assoc 1973; 65:367–406.
3. Bloom D. Heredity of keloids: review of the literature and report of a family with multiple keloids for five generations. New York State J Med 1956; 56:511.
4. Abrahms B, Benedetto A, Humeniuk H. Exuberant keloidal formation. JAOAC Int 1993; 93:863–865.
5. Brenizer A. Keloid formation in the Negro. Ann Surg 1915; 61:87.
6. Fox H. Observations on skin diseases in the American Negro. J Cutan Dis 1908; 26:67.
7. Alhady SM, Sivanantharajah K. Keloids in various races; a review of 175 cases. Plast Reconstr Surg 1969; 44:564.
8. Arnold H, Graver F. Keloids: etiology and management. Arch Dermatol 1959; 80:772.
9. Stucker F, Shaw G. An approach to management of keloids. Arch Otolaryngol Head Neck Surg 1992; 118:63–67.
10. Kelly P. Keloids. Dermatol Clin 1988; 6:413–424.
11. Cosman B, Crikelair G, Ju M, Gaulin J, Lattes R. The surgical treatment of keloids. Plast Reconstr Surg 1961; 27:335–345.
12. Rockwell W, Cohen I, Erlich H. Keloids and hypertrophic scars. A comprehensive review. Plast Reconstr Surg 1989; 84:827–837.
13. Davies D. Scars, hypertrophic scars and keloids. Plast Reconstr Surg 1985; 290:1056–1058.
14. Chipev CC, Simman R, Hatch G, Katz AE, Siegel DM, Simon M. Myofibroblast phenotype and apoptosis in keloid and palmar fibroblasts in vitro. Cell Death Differ. 2000; 7:166–176.
15. Stegman S, Tromovitch T, Glogau R. Treatment of keloids. In: Stegman SJ, eds. Cosmetic dermatologic surgery, 2nd edn. Chicago: Year Book Medical 1990; 201–206.
16. Flint M. The biological basis of Langer's lines. In: Longacre JJ, ed. The ultrastructure of collagen. Springfield: Charles C Thomas 1976; 132–140.
17. Asboe-Hansen G. Hypertrophic scars and keloids; etiology, pathogenesis and dermatologic therapy. Dermatologia 1960; 120:178.

18. Kormoczy B: Enormous keloid (?) on a penis. Br J Plast Surg 1978; 31:268.
19. Garb J, Stone M: Keloids: review of the literature and a report of eighty cases. Am J Surg 1942; 58:315.
20. Johnson T. Now more predictable treatment for keloids. Consultant 1969; 9:35.
21. Addison T. On the keloid of Alibert and on true keloid. Med Clin Trans 1854; 37:27.
22. Absoe-Hansen G. Hormonal effects on connective tissue. Am J Med 1959; 26:470.
23. Abergel R, Pizzurro D, Meeker C, et al. Biochemical composition of the connective tissue in keloids and analysis of collagen metabolism in keloid fibroblast cultures. J Invest Dermatol 1985; 84:384–390.
24. Cohen I, Keiser H, Sjoerdsma A. Collagen synthesis in human keloid patients. Plast Reconstr Surg 1979; 63:689.
25. Craig S, DeBlois G. Schwartz L. Mast cells in human keloid, small intestine and lung by an immunoperoxidase technique using murine monoclonal antibody against tryptase. Am J Pathol 1984; 124:427.
26. Sayah DN, Soo C, Shaw WW, et al. Downregulation of apoptosis-related genes in keloid tissues. J Surg Res 1999; 87:209–216.
27. AkasakaY, Fujita K, Ishikawa Y, et al. Detection of apoptosis in keloids and a comparative study on apoptosis between keloids, hypertrophic scars, normal healed fibrotic scars, and dermatofibroma. Wound Repair Regen 2001; 9:501–506.
28. Diegelmann R, Bryant C, Cohen I. Tissue alphaglobulins in keloid formation. Plast Reconstr Surg 1977; 59; 481.
29. Bauer E, Eisen A, Jeffrey J. Regulation of vertebrate collagenase activity in vivo and in vitro. J Invest Dermatol 1972; 59:50–55.
30. Border W, Noble N. TGF-B. Sci Am Sci Med 1995; 2:68–77.
31. Tan E, Rouda S, Greenbaum S, et al. Acidic and basic fibroblast growth factors down regulate collagen gene expression in keloid fibroblasts. Am J Pathol 1993; 142:463–470.
32. Cohen I, McCoy B, Mohanakumar R, et al. Immunoglobulin, complement and histocompatibility antigen studies in keloid patients. Plast Reconstr Surg 1979; 63:689.
33. Beer T, Baldwin J, West L, Gallagher P, Wright D. Mast cells in pathological and surgical scars. Br J Ophthalmol 1998; 82:691–694.
34. Shaffer J, Taylor S, Cook-Bolden F. Keloidal scars: a review with a critical look at therapeutic options. J Am Acad Dermatol 2002; 46:S63–S97.
35. Mustoe T, Cooter R, Gold M, et al. International clinical recommendations on scar management. Plast Reconstr Surg 2002; 110:560–571.
36. Bigby M. Snake oil for the 21st century. Arch Dermatol 1998; 134:1512–1514.
37. Kauh Y, Rouda S, Mondragon G, et al. Major suppression of pro-alpha 19(1) type I collagen gene expression in the dermis after keloid excision and immediate intrawound injection of triamcinolone acetonide. J Am Acad Dermatol 1997; 37:586–589.
38. Kiil J. Keloids treated with topical injections of triamcinolone acetonide (Kenalog): immediate and long term results. Scand J Plast Reconstr Surg 1977; 11:169–172.
39. Griffith B, Monroe C, McKinney P. A follow-up study on the treatment of keloids with triamcinolone acetonide. Plast Reconstr Surg. 1970; 46:145–150.
40. Chowdri N, Masarat M, Mattoo A, Darzi M. Keloids and hypertrophic scars: results with intraoperative and serial postoperative corticosteroid injection therapy. Aust NZ J Surg 1999:69:655–659.
41. Yosipovitch G, Widijanti Sugene M, Goon A, Chan Y, Goh C. A Comparison of the combined effect of cryotherapy and corticosteroid injections versus corticosteroids and cryotherapy on keloids: a controlled study. J Dermatolog Treat 2001; 12:87–90.
42. Lahiri A, Tsiliboti D, Gaze N. Experience with difficult keloids. Br J Plast Surg 2001; 54:633–635.
43. Akoz T, Gideroglu K, Akan M. Combination of different techniques for the treatment of earlobe keloids. Aesthetic Plast Surg 2002; 26:184–188.
44. Berman B, Flores F. Recurrence rates of excised keloids treated with post operative triamcinolone injections of interferon alpha 2b. J Am Acad Dermatol 1997; 37:755–757.
45. Darzi M, Chowdi, N Kaul S, et al. Evaluation of various methods of treating keloids and hypertrophic scars: a 10-year follow up study. Br J Plast Surg 1992; 45:374–379.
46. Lawrence W. In search of the optimal treatment of keloids: report of a series and a review of the literature. Ann Plast Surg 1991; 27:164–178.
47. Driscoll B. Treating keloids with carbon dioxide lasers. Arch Otolaryngol Head Neck Surg 2001; 127:1145.
48. Kantor G, Wheeland R, Bailin P, Walker N, Ratz, J. Treatment of earlobe keloids with carbon dioxide laser excision: a report of 16 cases. J Dermatol Surg Oncol 1985; 11:1063–1067.
49. Stern J, Lucente F. Carbon dioxide laser excision of earlobe keloids. Arch Otolaryngol Head Neck Surg 1988; 113:1107–1111.
50. Sclafani A, Gordon L, Chadha M, Romo T. Prevention of earlobe keloid recurrence with postoperative corticosteroid injections versus radiation therapy. Dermatol Surg1996; 22:569–574.
51. Cheng LH. Keloid of the earlobe. Laryngoscope 1974; 82:673–681.
52. Rauscher G, Kolmer W. Treatment of recurrent earlobe keloids. Cutis 1996; 38:67–68.
53. Salasche S, Grabski, W. Keloids of the earlobe: a surgical technique. J Derm Surg Oncol 1983:9:552–556.
54. Borok T, Brav M, Sinclair I, Plafker J, LaBirth L. Role of ionizing irradiation for 393 keloids. Int J Radiat Oncol Biol Phys 1988; 15:865–870.
55. Sherman R, Rosenfeld H. Experience with the Nd:YAG laser in the treatment of keloid scars. Ann Plast Surg 1988; 24:231–233.
56. Conejo-Mir. Carbon dioxide laser ablation in association with interferon alfa-2b injections reduces the recurrence of keloids. J Am Acad Dermatol. 1998; 39:1039–1040.
57. Alster T, West T. Treatment of scars: a review. Ann Plast Surg 1997; 39:418–432.
58. Goldman M, Fitzpatrick R. Laser treatment of scars. Dermatol Surg1995; 21:685–687.
59. Connell P, Harland C. Treatment of keloid scars with pulsed dye laser and intralesional steroids. J Cutan Laser Ther 2000; 2:147–159.
60. Doornbos J, Stoffel T, Hass A, et al. The role of kilovoltage irradiation in the treatment of keloids. Int J Radiat Oncol Biol Phys 1990; 18:833–838.
61. Order S, Donaldsen S. Radiation therapy for benign disease. New York: Springer-Verlag; 1990:147–153.
62. Brown J, Bromberg J. Preliminary studies on the effect of time-dose patterns in the treatment of keloids. Radiology 1963; 80:298–302.
63. Edsmyr F, Larsson L, Onyango J, Wanguru S, Wood M. Radiotherapy in the treatment of keloids in East Africa. East Afr Med J 1973; 50:457–461.
64. Garth J, Stone M. Keloids: review of literature and a report of 80 cases. Am J Surg 1942; 58:315–335.
65. Lo T, Seckel B, Salzman F, et al. Single-dose electron beam irradiation in treatment and prevention of keloids and hypertrophic scars. Radiother Oncol 1990; 19:267–272.
66. Ollstein R, Siegel H, Gillooley J, et al. Treatment of keloids by combined surgical excision and immediate post-operative X-ray therapy. Ann Plast Surg 1981; 7:281–285.
67. Layton A, Yip J, Cunliffe W. A comparison of intralesional triamcinolone and cryosurgery in the treatment of acne keloids. Br J Dermatol 1994; 130:498–501.
68. Khumpar D, Murray J, Anscher M. Keloids treated with excision followed by radiation therapy. J Am Acad Dermatol 1994; 31:225–231.
69. Darzi M, Chowdi N, Kaul S, Kahn M. Evaluation of various methods of treating keloids and hypertrophic scars: a 10-year experience. Int J Radiat Oncol Biol Phys 1989; 17:77–80.
70. Guix B, Henriquez I, Andres A, et al. Treatment of keloids by high-dose-rate brachytherapy. Int J Radiat Oncol Biol Phys 2001; 50:167–172.
71. Escarmant P, Zimmerman S, Amar A, et al. The treatment of 783 keloid scars by iridium 192 interstitial radiation after surgical excision. Int J Radiat Oncol Biol Phys 1993; 26:245–251.
72. Maarouf M, Schleicher U, Schmachtenberg, Ammon J. Radiotherapy in the management of keloids. Clinical experience with electron beam irradiation and comparison with X-ray therapy. Strahlenther Onkol 2002; 178:330–335.
73. Ogawa R, Mitsuhashi K, Hyakusoku H, Miyashita T. Postoperative electron-beam irradiation therapy for keloids and hypertrophic scars: retrospective study of 147 cases followed for more than 18 months. Plast Reconstr Surg 2003; 111:547–553.
74. Wagner W, Alfrink M, Micke O, et al. Results of prophylactic irradiation in patients with resected keloids: a retrospective analysis. Acta Oncol 2000; 39:217–220.

75. Urioste S, Arndt K, Dover J. Keloid and hypertrophic scars: review and treatment strategies. Semin Cutan Med Surg 1999:18:159–171.
76. Botwood N, Lewanski C, Lowdell C. The risks of treating keloids with radiotherapy. Br J Radiol 1999; 72:1222–1224.
77. Bilbey J, Muller N, Miller R, Nelemus B. Localised fibrous mesothelioma of pleura following external ionising radiation therapy. Chest 1988; 94:1291–1292.
78. Hoggman S. Radiotherapy for keloids? Ann Plast Surg 1982; 9:265.
79. Sampson R, Kev C, Buschler C, Iijima S. Thyroid carcinoma and radiation. JAMA 1969; 209:65.
80. Davies D. Plastic and reconstructive surgery: scars, hypertrophic scars and keloids. Br Med J 1985; 290:1056–1058.
81. Kosaka M, Kamiishi H. New concept of balloon-compression wear for the treatment of keloids and hypertrophic scars. Plast Reconstr Surg 2001; 108:1454–1455.
82. Gold M. A controlled clinical trial of topical silicone gel sheeting in the treatment of hypertrophic scars and keloids. J Am Acad Dermatol 1994; 30:506–507.
83. Fulton J. Silicone gel sheeting for the prevention and management of evolving hypertrophic and keloid scars. Dermatol Surg 1995; 21:947–951.
84. Ahn S, Monafo W, Mustoe T. Topical silicone gel: a new treatment for hypertrophic scars. Surgery 1989; 106:781–786.
85. Viana de Oliveira G, Nunes T, et al. Silicone versus nonsilicone gel dressings: a controlled trial. Dermatol Surg 2001; 27:721–726.
86. Berman B, Duncan M. Short-term keloid treatment in vivo with human interferon alfa-2b results in a selective and persistent normalization of keloidal fibroblast collagen, glycosaminoglycan and collagenase production in vitro. J Am Acad Dermatol 1989; 21:694.
87. Craig R, Schofield J, Jackson D. Collagen synthesis in normal human skin, normal and hypertrophic scar and keloid. Eur J Clin Invest 1975; 5:69–74.
88. Granstein R, Rook A, Flotte T, et al. Intralesional interferon gamma treatment for keloids and hypertrophic scars. Arch Otolaryngol Head Neck Surg 1990; 118:1159–1162.
89. Berman B, Bieley H. Adjunct therapies of surgical management of keloids. Dermatol Surg 1996; 22:126–130.
90. Berman B, Kaufman J. Pilot study of the effect of postoperative imiquimod 5% cream recurrence rate of excised keloids. J Am Acad Dermatol 2002; 47:S209–S211.
91. Rusciani L, Rossi G, Bono R. Use of cryotherapy in the treatment of keloids. J Dermatol Surg Oncol 1993; 19:529–534.
92. Zouboulis C, Blume U, Buttner P, Orfanos C. Outcomes of cryosurgery in keloids and hypertrophic scars. Arch Dermatol 1993; 129:1146–1151.
93. Gupta S, Kumar B. Intralesional cryosurgery using lumbar puncture and/or hypodermic needles for large, bulky, recalcitrant keloids. Int J Dermatol 1002; 40:349–353.
94. Har-Shai Y, Amar M, Sabo E. Intralesional cryotherapy for enhancing the involution of hypertrophic scars and keloids. Plast Reconstr Surg 2003; 111:1841–1852.
95. Fitzpatrick R. Treatment of inflamed hypertrophic scars using intralesional 5-FU. Dermatol Surg 1999; 25:224–232.
96. Lebwohl M. From the literature. J Am Acad Dermatol. 1999; 42:677.
97. Beranek J, Masseyeff R. Hyperplastic capillaries and their possible involvement in the pathogenesis of fibrosis. Histopathology 1992; 10:543–551.
98. Lee R, Dwong J, Jellema A. The response of burn scars to intralesional verapamil: report of five cases. Arch Surg 1994; 129:107–111.
99. Lawrence W. Treatment of earlobe keloids with surgery plus adjuvant intralesional verapamil and pressure earrings. Ann Plast Surg 1996; 37; 167–169.
100. Phan T, See P, Tran E, et al. Suppression of insulin-like growth factor signaling pathway and collagen expression in keloid-derived fibroblasts by quercetin: a therapeutic potential use in the treatment and/or prevention of keloids. Br J Dermatol 2003; 148:544–552.
101. Baumann L, Spencer J. The effects of topical vitamin E on the cosmetic appearance of scars. Dermatol Surg 1999; 25:311–315.
102. Espana A, Solano T, Quintanilla E. Bleomycin in the treatment of keloids and hypertrophic scars by multiple needle punctures. Dermatol Surg 2001; 27:23–27.

45 Nail Surgery

Eckart Haneke MD PhD and Monica Lawry MD

Summary box

- Nail surgery is delicate and requires in-depth knowledge of the anatomy and biology of the nail, as well as surgical skills and special experience in this particular field.
- Optimal patient preparation, exact planning as to what shall be done, efficient local anesthesia, complete asepsis, and consistent postoperative follow-up usually lead towards a good result.
- Although nail surgery has gained attention in the past few years, standard surgical techniques are often lacking for specific diagnoses and locations within the nail apparatus. Exact case descriptions overcome this disadvantage.

INTRODUCTION

Nail surgery has gained increasing attention over the past few years. Detailed accounts of nail surgery are found in three recent books.[1–3] Nail surgery is aimed at facilitating a diagnosis by performing a skilled biopsy, reducing pain, treating infections, correcting deformities, and removing tumors. Preservation of function and good cosmesis are extremely important. To achieve these goals, an in-depth knowledge of the biology, physiology, normal and pathologic anatomy, histopathology, and particularities of young and old age are essential. Further, nail surgery requires well-developed skills in atraumatic surgery under aseptic conditions using fine instruments, optimal light, often with optical loupes worn on the head or a surgical microscope. Effective local anesthesia and a bloodless field are necessary for most operations.

Surgical anatomy of the nail region

The nail apparatus is an integral part of the tip of the digit. All parts are intimately related to each other forming one functional, sensory, and cosmetic unit. Alterations of one major structure will inevitably have an influence on all the other components.

The tip of the digit is made up of the terminal bony phalanx with the joint and synovial membrane at its proximal end; a fibrous network consisting of ligaments, tendons, and connective tissue strings; blood vessels in a well-defined arrangement and glomus bodies; nerves and receptors, making it an extremely efficient sensory organ; tip and digital pad; and nail unit with matrix, nail bed, nail plate, grooves, and nail folds (Fig. 45.1).

The distal phalanx is widest at its base, has a tapered shaft and its tip carries the processus unguicularis, a horseshoe-shaped rough bone excrescence. Its dorsal aspect is the attachment for the distal nail bed portion and its lateral spines are attachments for the interosseous ligaments. The terminal phalanges of the fingers are considerably longer than those of the toes. The shape of the bone is responsible for the gross shape and size of the nail. Degenerative osteoarthritis causes fingernail overcurvature.

The distal interphalangeal joint is a hinged synovial joint. The base of the distal phalanx fits into the bicondylar surface of the head of the medial phalanx. Strong lateral ligaments prevent dislocation. The extensor tendon widens at its attachment at the base of the distal phalanx covering most of the dorsal aspect of the joint. The flexor tendon widens fan-like and forms the volar base of the joint. The synovial membrane, reinforced by the tendons dorsally and volarly and the lateral collateral ligaments, forms the articular capsule. Ligament extensions expand to the proximal nail bed and to the skin, forming a bone-nail band and a lateral digital band.[3] The blood supply comes mainly from the proper volar arteries, which send branches to the dorsal aspect of the distal phalanx. Here, they form dorsal arcades anastomozing with the respective contralateral artery and sending parallel longitudinal branches in the connective tissue of the nail bed and matrix. Thus, severing an artery on one side is usually compensated by its contralateral counterpart. The venous drainage is much less abundant, although a mainly volar deep and ring-like superficial system exists that has some obliquely arranged anastomoses. Little is known about the lymphatic drainage.

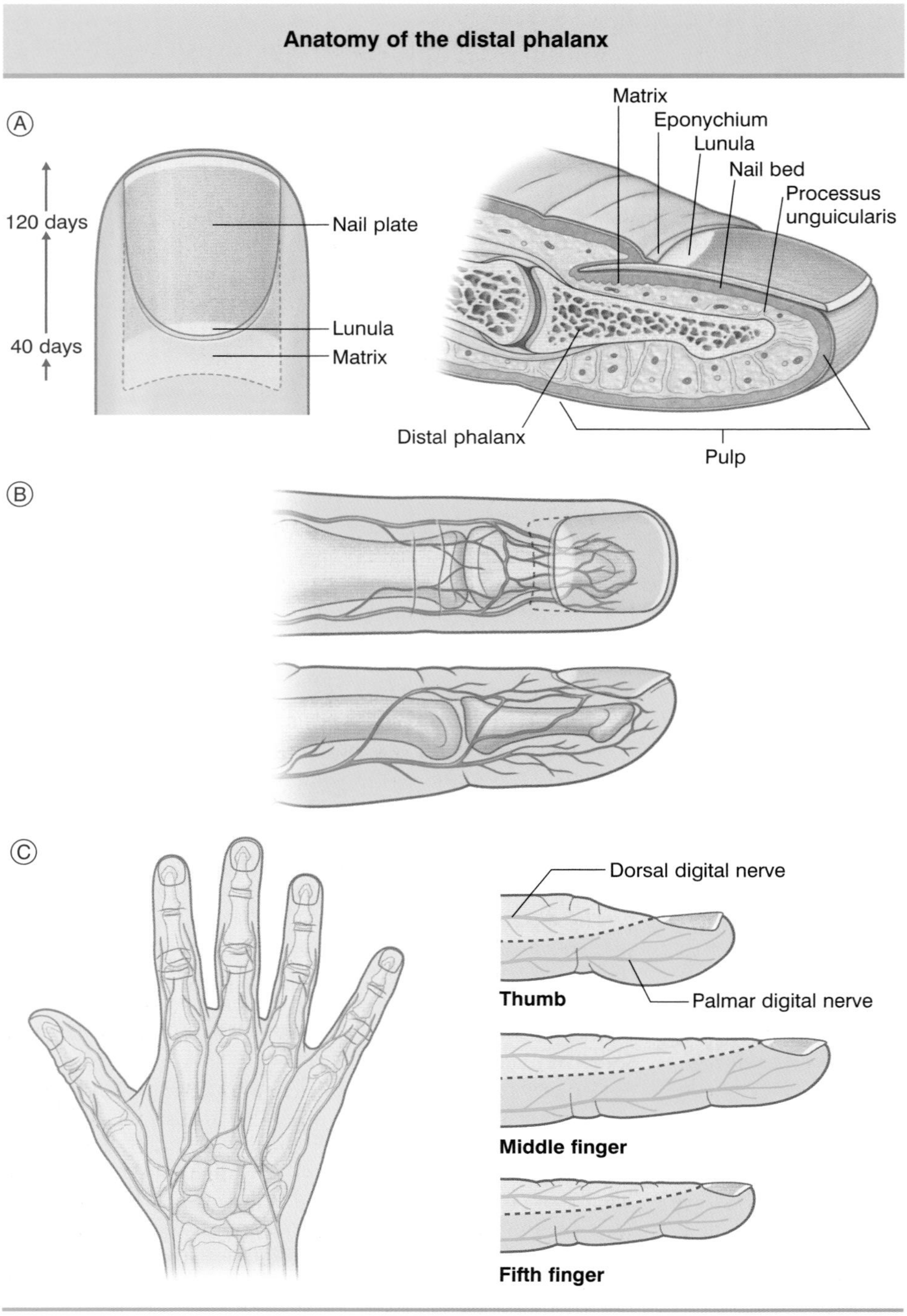

Anatomy of the distal phalanx

Figure 45.1 Anatomy of the distal phalanx. (A) Idealized nail shape and growth rate. (B) Arterial blood supply of the nail. The matrix receives its blood supply from capillary shunts of the tip of the digit. (C) Innervation of the distal phalanges.

The fingers and toes have paired sensory volar and dorsal digital nerves. The dorsal nerves reach the distal phalanx of only the first and fifth digits. The palmar and plantar nerves lie at the side of the flexor tendon and the volar artery. The three branches innervating the distal phalanx divide just distal to the distal interphalangeal joint.

The pulp is the tip of the digit. It consists of two pad spaces with different structure and functions—the distal pulp region representing the extreme tip, and the proximal pulp being the pad. Fine touch is best where these two compartments meet. Wedge-shaped fibrofatty structures anchored at the processus unguicularis make up the bulk of the pulp. It is more mobile against the bone than the tip. Abundant special nerve endings make the pulp one of the most important sensory organs of the body. A dermal network of unmyelinated nerves is responsible for pain and temperature perception. Merkel cells mediate touch sensation. Meissner's corpuscles allow two-point discrimination. Vater–Pacini bodies perceive deep pressure and vibration, but are also associated with glomus bodies. In addition, the pulp contains deeply seated eccrine sweat glands. Its dermatoglyphics are specific for each individual.

The nail unit itself consists of different components, which are interdependent. These are best explained as the germinative component (matrix and nail bed), their product (the nail plate), its sheathing (cuticle, eponychium, and hyponychium), and its framing (proximal and lateral nail grooves and folds, and the supporting connective tissue).

The nail plate is formed by the matrix. A small proximal, large intermediate, and small distal part can be distinguished. The former is at the border between the matrix and the proximal nail fold's undersurface and produces the thin, but very resistant and shiny so-called superficial nail plate. The bulk of the nail is produced by the intermediate matrix, which is also histologically distinctive. Its central distal portion is visible as the lunula. The so-called distal or ventral matrix is the most proximal portion of the nail bed epithelium. The entire nail bed epithelium is firmly attached to the nail plate whereas slight shearing forces easily separate the lower two-thirds of the matrix epithelium from the upper third and the nail plate.

The white color of the matrix contrasts with that of the pink nail bed. Light scattering from the nucleated cells of the keratogenous zone of the matrix and the difference in epithelial thickness and rete ridge arrangement are considered to be the causes for the whitish appearance of the matrix. The nail bed extends from the matrix to the onychodermal band, which is directly proximal to the hyponychium and can be seen as a slightly paler curved band before the free margin of the nail. The nail plate is the product of the matrix. It protects the tip of the digit, allows one to scratch, attack, and defend oneself, enhances the sensory functions of the pulp, and is an extremely versatile tool. Its cosmetic importance cannot be overestimated. Orderly nail formation can be disturbed by impaired blood supply, venous or lymphatic stasis, disease, trauma, and tumors.

The nail folds surround three sides of the nail plate and frame it. The proximal groove is in fact a pocket under the proximal nail fold, whereas the lateral grooves are much less pronounced and flatten distally. The lateral margins of the nail plate are embedded in the lateral grooves. There is a distal groove under the free margin of the nail connecting the hyponychium with the skin of the pulp. When the nail is cut too short, the tip may bulge dorsally and give rise to a distal nail fold which then impedes outgrowth of the nail. The free margin of the proximal nail fold has an acute angle and forms the cuticle which in fact develops because the horny layer of the eponychium, the undersurface of the proximal nail fold (PNF), is pulled out by the growing nail. When the PNF's free margin thickens or the nail stops growing the cuticle gets lost spontaneously. The cuticle is an important structure that seals the nail pocket and prevents pathogens and foreign bodies from entering. The hyponychium seals the connection of the nail bed with the distal groove. It has to be protected from injury by overzealous manicure with sharp instruments.

PREOPERATIVE PREPARATION

Before surgery, a complete personal (and often a family) history and a thorough general examination are crucial to exclude concomitant disorders, genetic traits, and medications potentially posing a risk for nail surgery. Blood glucose levels in patients who have diabetes mellitus have to be well regulated before toenail surgery. Acetylsalicylic acid and other drugs interfering with blood clotting as well as vitamin K antagonists like warfarin have to be adjusted before operation.

A careful examination of the nail is mandatory to make or suggest a diagnosis and to evaluate the extension of the disease and possible related pathologies in the tip of the digit. Clinical examination comprises inspection in a relaxed position, forceful extension and/or flexion and with the pulp pressed on a hard base to visualize circulatory abnormalities, palpation, transillumination, and probing. In addition, radiography or xeroradiography with magnification, magnetic resonance imaging, ultrasound scanning, and sometimes special investigations may be necessary.

Before operation, the hand or foot is scrubbed by the patient with a disinfectant soap the evening before and immediately before surgery. The entire hand or foot is disinfected with a colorless disinfectant. For fingers, a sterile surgical glove is put on to provide a sterile surgical surrounding. A small hole is cut into the tip of the appropriate finger, and rolling the finger up results in an excellent tourniquet. There is also a metallic digit tourniquet with a screw that acts when the screw is tightened. Alternatively, a Penrose drain that is approximately 2.5 cm wide may be used. It is wrapped around the finger starting distally and exsanguinating the digit. When reaching the base of the finger it is held with the finger, the distal part is pulled out leaving about two loops around the finger base. The two ends of the Penrose drain are then clamped together and act as a tourniquet.

Very few special instruments are needed for nail surgery, but most should be as fine as possible, and include a septum elevator, fine skin hooks, pointed curved scissors, small-nosed mosquito hemostats, #11 and #15 scalpel blades, nail clipper, sometimes a bone rongeur, and sturdy straight scissors. The authors prefer sutures that are monofilament nonabsorbable or absorbable 5-0 or 6-0 threads. Fast absorbing chromic is ideal for the matrix. Optical loupes (×3 or ×5) or an operating microscope is a great help for fine operations.

Antibiotic prophylaxis is rarely indicated, but should be considered before surgery, particularly in case of infection. Embedded dirt is removed, starting with hand brushes some days before surgery.

Different types of anesthesia are available for nail surgery, but the proximal digital block is the most versatile and useful for almost all nail operations—2–3 mL of plain 2% lidocaine or prilocaine is used per digit. A 25-gauge or smaller needle minimizes the pain from the pinprick. Ropivacaine 1% is a useful alternative, giving a rapid-onset, long-lasting anesthesia. Alternatives are the distal digital ring block, central local distant digital anesthesia, metacarpal block for neighboring digits, and the transthecal digital block[4–7] (Fig. 45.2). The latter has proved to be extremely valuable for long fingers, avoiding the risk of injuring the neurovascular bundles of the fingers. A wrist block is useful for extensive surgery. Except for children or for psychological reasons in adults, general anesthesia is rarely indicated.

Bleeding may be considerable after releasing the tourniquet. If an artery can be seen during operation this may be ligated using 6-0 resorbable material. However, in most cases this is not possible. To absorb blood a thick padded dressing is usually recommended. This is covered with a non-stick gauze impregnated with antibiotic or povidone-iodine ointment to avoid sticking to the wound.

Splinting of the finger may be indicated after complex nail surgery. The extremity should be elevated during the first 2 days, which considerably reduces postoperative pain. For toenail surgery, the patient should bring a large or open-

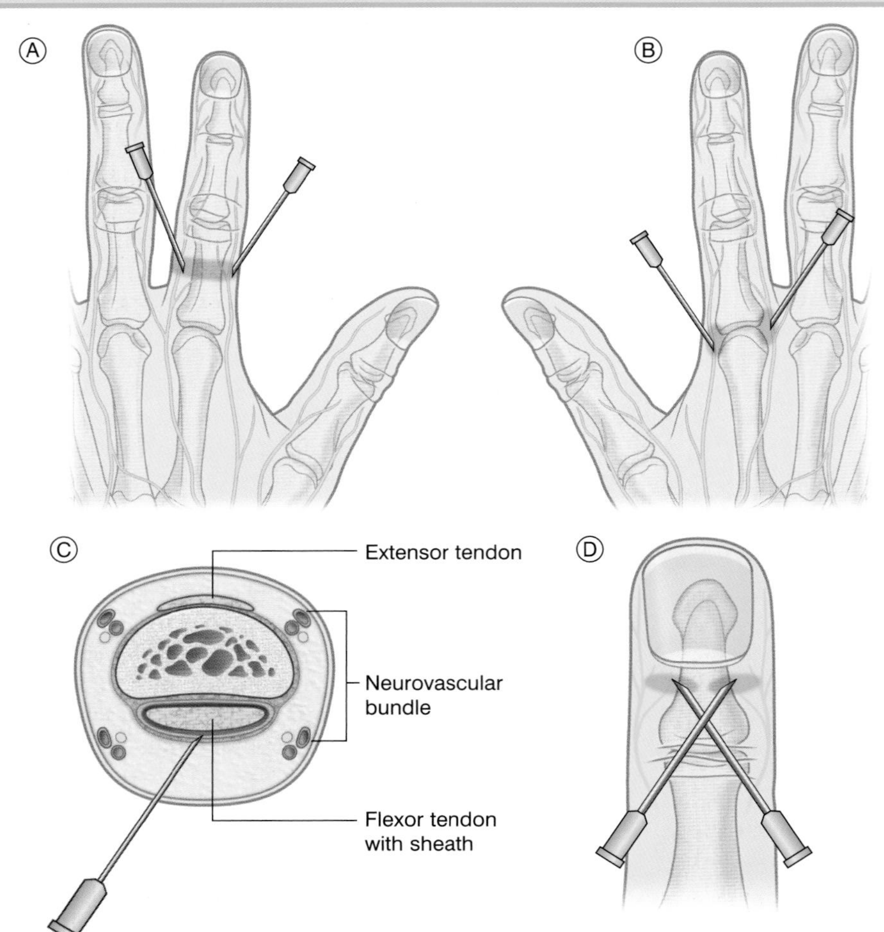

Figure 45.2 Anesthesia for nail operations. (A) Proximal finger block. (B) Metacarpal block. (C) Transthecal block from the volar crease of the metacarpophalangeal joint. (D) Distal wing block with injection points distal of the dorsal interphalangeal joint creases.

toed shoe and remain recumbent. The dressing is first changed after 24–48 hours and then left for several days after sterile procedures. It is changed daily in a warm disinfectant-containing bath in cases of nonsterile surgery, such as for surgery of ingrown toenail with purulent secretion and oozing granulation tissue. Medication for pain has to be given in many cases.

TECHNIQUES

Biopsies of the nail area

Nail diseases are often difficult to diagnose on clinical grounds alone. Blood samples rarely help. Additional imaging techniques are of value in the diagnosis of many tumors and bone alterations. However, the gold standard for nail disease diagnosis is histopathology. This requires a knowledgeable surgeon to take the biopsy, a nail-specific protocol in the laboratory, and an experienced dermatopathologist. The surgeon must be able to suggest special stains for particular diagnoses, but routine hematoxylin and eosin stains should always be supplemented with periodic acid–Schiff (PAS) stain. There is a general rule that the more superficial a nail change is the more proximal the pathogenic process must be—for instance, psoriatic pits derive from the proximal matrix, rough nails of lichen planus from the proximal and intermediate matrix, salmon spots are psoriatic lesions in the nail bed. A nail bed biopsy will therefore be inadequate for most ungual lichen planus cases.

There are several approaches for obtaining material for histopathologic and/or culture examinations (Fig. 45.3).[8]

Nail clippings

Nail clippings should always contain as much subungual keratosis as possible because this is the material that harbors almost all pathogenic fungi. Clippings are often performed for histopathologic examination in onychomycosis and give almost double the rate of positives compared to mycological cultures. In case of proximal subungual onychomycosis, a disk of nail plate is punched out over the onycholytic area without prior anesthesia (Fig. 45.3A) after the digit has been immersed for 5–10 minutes in warm water to soften the nail plate and facilitate punching or cutting through it. In superficial white onychomycosis, a tangential nail plate biopsy taken with a #15 scalpel blade reveals the diagnosis. Pure nail and keratin specimens are not fixed in formalin before processing in the histopathology laboratory.

Lateral longitudinal nail biopsy

The lateral longitudinal nail biopsy (Fig. 45.3B(2)) is appropriate for all diagnostic purposes and reveals the history of many months of the slow-growing nail's pathology, provided

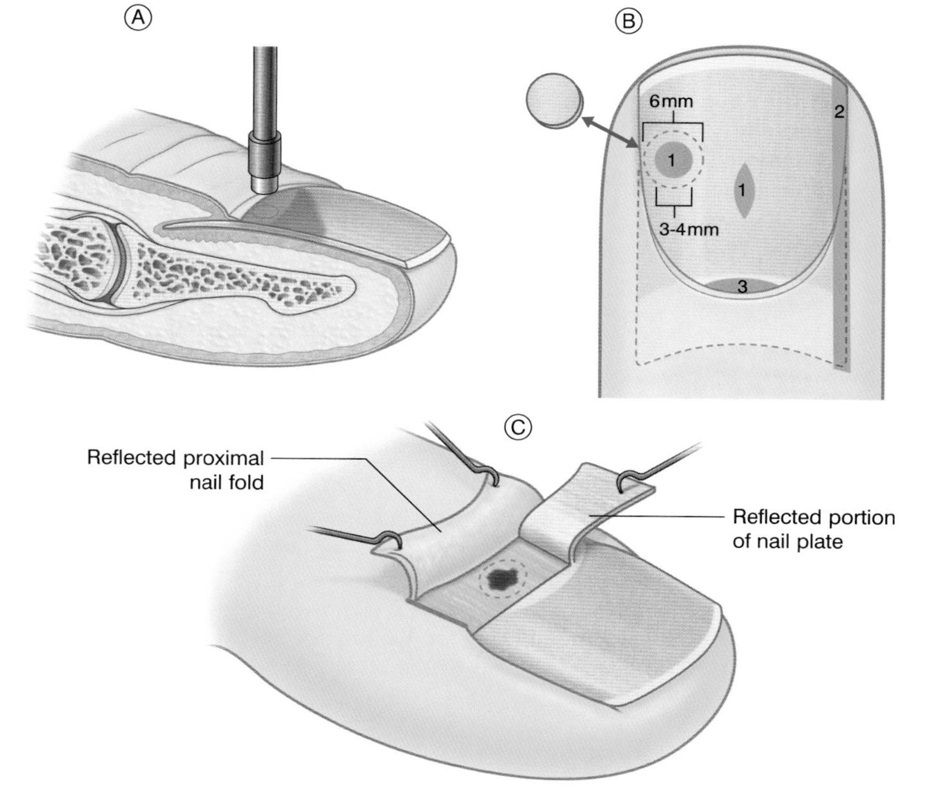

Figure 45.3 Nail biopsies. (A) Punch biopsy from the nail plate in proximal subungual onychomycosis; note that there is usually onycholysis facilitating nail plate biopsy without anesthesia. (B) Nail bed biopsy (1), lateral longitudinal biopsy (2) and fusiform matrix biopsy (3). If a punch biopsy is taken from the nail bed, the disk of nail plate is larger than the specimen from the nail bed and the nail disk is laid back at the end of the operation. (C) Superficial matrix biopsy is taken with the proximal nail fold reflected and the nail plate cut at one side and elevated to visualize the matrix lesion.

the nail pathology is in the lateral portion of the nail apparatus. A straight longitudinal incision starting at the distal crease of the distal interphalangeal joint is carried to the tip about 2 mm centrally from the lateral nail plate margin, and a second incision parallel to the first one along the lateral nail margin in the depth of the nail groove. The slender rectangular block of tissue containing the proximal nail fold, matrix, plate, nail bed, and hyponychium is gently dissected from the underlying bone using curved pointed iris scissors. The lateral aspect of the distal phalanx is mobilized and the defect is sutured with simple sutures through the proximal nail fold and with vertical back sutures in the level of the nail bed, thus elevating the lateral nail wall. This gives the nail a normal appearance after surgery. The biopsy specimen has to be marked by the surgeon to help the technician orient it correctly in the paraffin block. The lateral fold should not be included in this biopsy.

Nail bed biopsies

Nail bed biopsies (Fig. 45.3B(1)) are carried out in a longitudinal fashion. After softening the plate, the biopsy is performed with a #11 scalpel with stabbing motions to minimize trauma while harvesting the tissue specimen. For suturing, the nail bed has to be freed from the surrounding overlying nail plate and mobilized from the underlying bone.[8]

Matrix biopsies

Matrix biopsies are the most important biopsies for most nail diseases. Depending on the position of the proximal nail fold, this may simply be retracted to allow visualization of the area to be biopsied, or bilateral incisions at the junction of the proximal and lateral nail folds are performed, permitting the proximal nail fold to be reflected. A punch biopsy with a maximum diameter of 3 mm does not require a suture because no wound closure is necessary for matrix defects up to 3 mm. This will leave only a narrow longitudinal reddish stripe in the nail distal to the biopsy site. A transverse fusiform or crescentic excision (Fig. 45.3B(3)) is sometimes required for larger lesions. If the nail plate over the matrix lesion is needed, the biopsy is carried through the plate. The nail plate over the matrix is soft, but nevertheless commonly shears off during surgery. If the plate is not necessary for the histopathologic examination, the proximal one-third of the plate is separated and lifted to allow the matrix biopsy. 6-0 resorbable sutures are used for defect closure. These should not be tied too tightly to avoid cutting through the fragile matrix. The nail plate is then laid back and fixed in place by one or two horizontal mattress sutures.

Superficial matrix biopsy

A superficial matrix biopsy (Fig. 45.3C)was developed for the diagnosis of longitudinal melanonychia.[8–10] The proximal end of the pigmented band is localized by separating the nail plate from its overlying proximal nail fold, which is incised at both sides to allow it to be reflected. The plate is then cut transversally at the border between the proximal and middle third so as to be able to detach three-quarters of the proximal third from the matrix and nail bed. This permits the proximal nail plate third to be raised like a trapdoor to expose the pigmented spot in the matrix. A superficial incision is carried around it including a safety margin. Using the shave excision technique, the entire lesion is removed. The nail plate is laid back and fixed to the nail bed and matrix with mattress sutures. Finally, the proximal nail fold is sutured back. Complete matrix re-epithelialization takes place under the protective nail plate, and no postoperative nail dystrophy has been observed in 15 cases so far.[10] We believe that adherence of the superficial layers of the matrix epithelium to the nail plate during detachment may improve healing.

Biopsy of the proximal nail fold

Biopsy of the proximal nail fold is useful for the diagnosis of collagenoses. It may be carried out as a 2-mm punch that does not require suture, or as a narrow wedge with its base being at the free margin of the nail fold. After freeing its undersurface from the nail plate, it can be sutured.

Biopsies from the lateral nail fold

Biopsies from the lateral nail fold are best performed as a narrow spindle that can be sutured directly. Sometimes, a shave biopsy may be adequate.

Any nail biopsy specimen should be evaluated by a skilled dermatopathologist.

Nail avulsion

Nail avulsion represents the most serious iatrogenic trauma to the nail apparatus and must be limited to the few cases where it is indicated. The technique still described in many textbooks of 'minor surgery' uses a sturdy straight hemostat. One branch of its mouth is forcefully inserted laterally under the proximal nail fold, the other branch is run through the hyponychium and under the nail. The nail plate is then grasped and the nail torn out by turning the hemostat. This crude method has had to be abandoned because tearing off the nail bed epithelium causes severe trauma and not infrequently leads to scarring in the nail bed.

Distal nail avulsion

Distal nail avulsion is the classical method of nail avulsion. A blunt instrument, such as a nail or septum elevator with upturned ends, is inserted under the proximal nail fold and then under the nail plate from the hyponychium. With forth-and-back movements from one side to the other to free the nail plate from the overlying proximal nail fold and the nail bed, it can be removed without further trauma. During these maneuvers, the slightly bent blunt tip of the elevator always points to the nail plate (Fig. 45.4A).

Proximal nail avulsion

Proximal nail avulsion is much less traumatic. Using the same instrument, the nail is detached from the proximal nail fold. While leaving its tip in the end of the nail pocket the nail elevator is then turned about 160°, inserted under the proximal edge of the nail and pushed distally to separate the nail from the matrix and nail bed with back-and-forth motions (Fig. 45.4B). The proximal nail avulsion is particularly useful when there is a thick subungual hyperkeratosis (e.g. in onychogryphosis, pachyonychia congenita, and distal subungual onychomycosis) or when the distal groove has disappeared.[11,12]

Nail avulsion alone is almost never a cure by itself. It is seldom indicated except to expose both the matrix and nail bed and allow topical treatment. Repeated nail avulsions frequently cause thickening and overcurvature of the nail plate or even nail dystrophy as a result of scarring of the nail bed or the appearance of a distal nail wall.

Partial nail avulsion

Partial nail avulsion is often more suitable than total avulsion. Removing only the segment of the nail plate involved should be encouraged in onychomycoses. This prevents the development of a distal nail wall. In distal subungual onychomycosis with hyperkeratosis, the heaped-up nail is easily clipped away. In proximal subungual onychomycosis, the affected portion of the nail plate is removed by cutting the

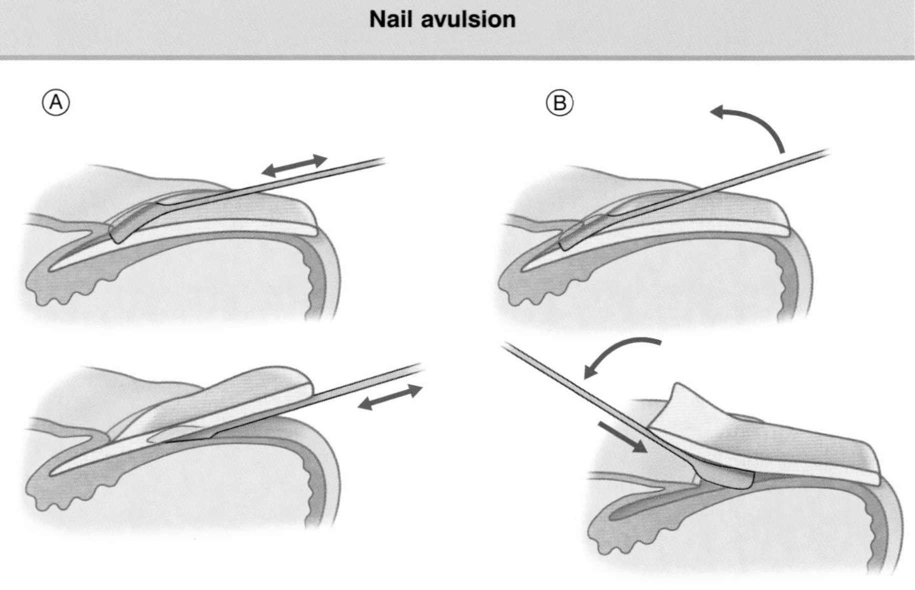

Figure 45.4 Nail avulsion. (A) Distal approach. (B) Proximal nail avulsion.

nail plate transversely with a nail splitter. The distal portion of the nail is left in place, which keeps discomfort to a minimum.[8] Any part of the nail plate can be removed leaving the intact nail plate portion in place.

Matricectomy and nail ablation

Matricectomy is the complete removal of the germinal matrix and nail ablation is definitive extirpation of the entire nail organ (Fig. 45.5).

Matricectomy

Matricectomy may be necessary for some intractable hypertrophic nail conditions (e.g. onychogryphosis). There are several methods, each of which has advantages. Complete surgical excision is performed when the specimen requires histopathologic examination.

The proximal third of the nail is avulsed and laterally directed incisions are performed through the nail fold, which is retracted with small hooks or sutures to expose the entire matrix and allow its lateral horns to be visualized. The nail bed is incised approximately 1–2 mm distally from the lunula border down to the bone from one side to the other. The matrix is dissected from the bone with blunt-tipped scissors along the periosteum and above the extensor tendon until beyond the proximal end of the matrix. The undersurface of the proximal nail fold is de-epithelialized by a tangential excision that meets proximally with the submatrix excision. Finally, the epithelium of the lateral sides and the matrix horns are dissected. The proximal nail fold is laid back with its de-epithelialized ventral surface on the bone covering most of the defect. The rest is left for second intention healing or grafted. If remnants of the matrix horns are left, small nail spicules will grow.

Complete phenolization of the entire nail pocket is an easy-to-perform procedure. Following complete digital exsanguination, liquefied phenol is vigorously rubbed into the epithelium of the matrix, matrix horns, and lateral and dorsal walls of the nail pocket. Three minutes are usually sufficient to cauterize these epithelia. Postoperative morbidity is minimal, but oozing from the wound may persist for 2 or more weeks. Daily baths of the digit are recommended to cleanse the oozing wound and remove scabs and crusts.

Electroradiosurgery is another alternative. The matrix is first curetted and then treated with a spade-like electrode. The power is set at partially rectified current and the electrode is swept from one side to the other about four to six times, with additional electrocautery for the lateral matrix horns.

The carbon dioxide laser may be used instead of electric current. Again, the proximal one-third of the nail is avulsed, and the matrix is vaporized using a defocused beam. The laser light easily reaches into the depth of the matrix horns, making this modality less recurrence-prone.

Total nail ablation

Total nail ablation involves the extirpation of the periungual tissues and the nail. The nail plate may be left in place and serve as a guiding structure during surgery, or be avulsed, in which case it is recommended to stain the matrix with a sterile methylene blue solution and let it dry. This permits the surgeon to observe the level of dissection and removal throughout the entire procedure. An incision is made down to the bone around the tip of the digit, approximately 3–5 mm below the hyponychium, along both lateral aspects of the distal phalanx to the crease of the distal interphalangeal joint and over the dorsal joint crease. Using blunt-tipped scissors, the nail apparatus is dissected from the bone while taking care not to sever the extensor digit tendon. No remnants of the proximal and lateral grooves and the matrix horns must be left. The arteries feeding the nail organ should be ligated. The defect heals by second intention or may be grafted.

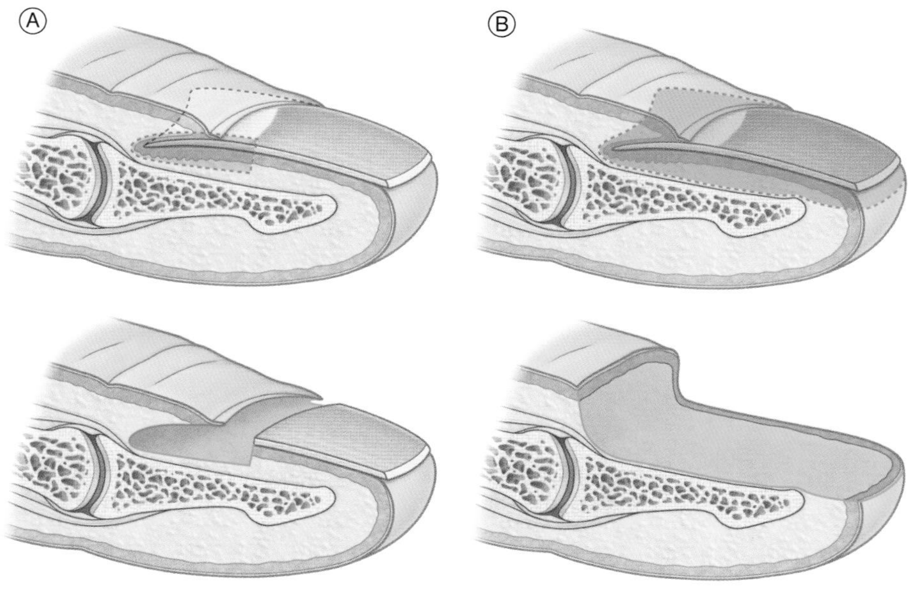

Figure 45.5 (A) Surgical matricectomy. (B) Total nail ablation.

Trauma

Trauma may injure several components of the nail apparatus or even crush the entire tip of the digit. This may, more or less, go unnoticed if there is only a small laceration in the fingertip and a large subungual hematoma is hiding the degree of tissue damage.

For a normal nail, an adequate nail pocket, matrix, and nail bed as well as an intact terminal bony phalanx are required. Hematomas are common signs of trauma and give a hint to the severity of tissue damage. A small hematoma is caused by a small break in the nail bed. Decompression by fenestration of the nail over the hematoma is sufficient. This can be carried out with a small battery-driven drill (Fig. 45.6A), a #11 scalpel blade that is held vertically and rotated until a little hole is made in the plate, or by hot paperclip cautery: A paperclip is unbent and one end is heated with a small flame until it is red, and this is placed on the nail over the hematoma to melt a hole into the plate. Drainage of the hematoma and elevating the extremity will almost immediately alleviate the acute pain.

A large hematoma develops from a significant injury to the nail bed, often associated with a fracture of the distal phalanx. A radiograph is therefore mandatory. The nail plate is removed for appropriate examination of the nail bed and matrix, cleansed, and stored under sterile conditions. Wet gauze is used to clean the nail bed and matrix of blood, but sometimes 3% hydrogen peroxide is needed for cleaning and visualization. A severe crush injury causes numerous lacerations, creating small islands or flaps of matrix. Surgical repair with loupes and fine sutures with 7-0 chromic permits salvage of the nail bed and matrix in these injuries. Amputation of parts or all of the nail matrix is best treated by retrieving the tissue pieces and replacing them as grafts. Nail pocket and matrix are reconstructed in separate layers to avoid the formation of cicatricial pterygium and finally a split nail. The nail plate is trimmed and laid back as a physiological dressing and splint. Drilling a small hole into the plate allows some postoperative drainage.

Approximately 50% of severe nail bed injuries have an accompanying fracture (Fig. 45.6B).[3] Common sequelae of trauma are onycholysis, split nail, pterygium, various nail dystrophies, hook nail, and malalignment. A step formation in the dorsal surface of the terminal phalanx will usually result in a corresponding unevenness of the nail bed or matrix, which may cause a traumatic double nail.[3]

A serious nail matrix and/or nail bed trauma is present if the nail is torn out of its pocket and lies on the proximal nail fold. The nail matrix is fixed to its proximal wound margin by sutures that run through the proximal nail fold. Either the restored nail plate or a thin pliable silicone sheet is placed between the ventral floor and the dorsal roof to prevent scarring between the dorsal and ventral aspects of the nail pocket.[3]

Foreign bodies

Foreign bodies under the nail plate usually cause intense pain, particularly in acute cases. It soon decreases, but increases again after touching the nail. Although often difficult to identify, the foreign body should be removed immediately under local anesthesia, if necessary with partial nail avulsion (Fig. 45.7). Wet antiseptic dressings are applied for 2–3 days. Wooden splinters are notorious for causing

Treatment of subungual hematoma

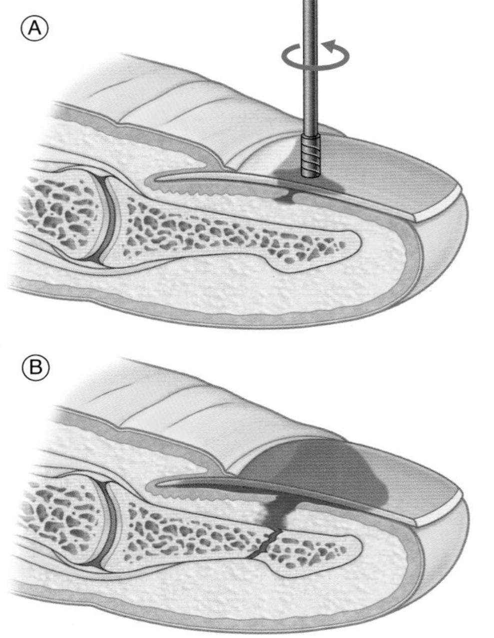

Figure 45.6 Treatment of subungual hematoma. (A) Acute partial subungual hematoma. (B) Total subungual hematoma is commonly associated with a fracture of the terminal phalanx and requires adequate diagnostic procedures and treatment.

Removal of subungual foreign body

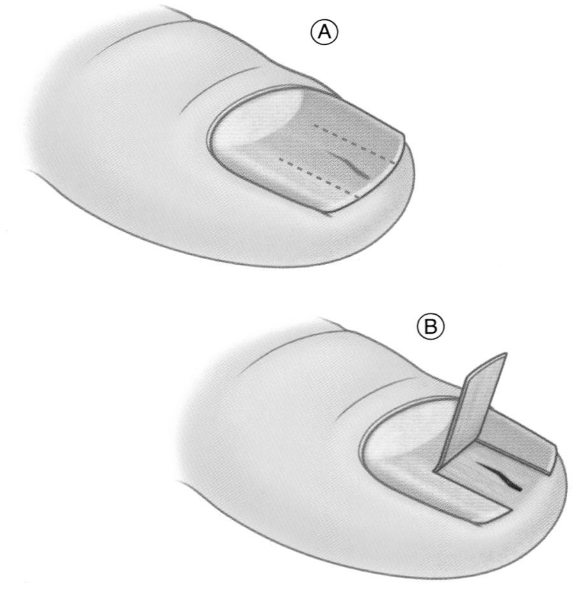

Figure 45.7 Removal of the subungual foreign body. (A) The part of nail plate overlying the foreign body is detached from the nail bed and incisions are made so that this piece can be elevated, which allows access to it. (B) After removal, the nail plate is laid back and fixed with fine stitches, Steri-strips, or an artificial nail kit.

infection if not removed early. A subungual felon may develop after a few days. The nail bed becomes yellow. The pain is pulsating, especially at night. The nail plate is either fenestrated, or partially avulsed. Pain relief is immediate, followed by recovery within a few days.[13]

Onychogryphosis

Onychogryphosis is commonly seen in elderly or debilitated persons. The nail is grotesquely thickened and distorted like a ram's horn and cannot be trimmed by the patient. Conservative management consists of trimming the thickened nail. Subungual keratoses are removed in patients at risk, particularly those with peripheral vascular disease and diabetes mellitus. Periodic clipping of the gryphotic nail is often adequate to keep it under control. This is facilitated by using a warm footbath to soften the thick nail. Treatment of the nail with 40% urea or 50% potassium iodide ointment under occlusion often renders the onychogryphosis softer so that the patient or a podiatrist can trim it with a nail clipper and fine tune it with a nail file.

Nail avulsion offers symptomatic relief of onychogryphosis for some months in most patients, particularly in the elderly in whom the use of a tourniquet may be contraindicated. For permanent eradication, phenolization is the safest and easiest method. A nail elevator is inserted under the proximal nail fold, which is then freed from the nail plate. This procedure almost always shows a very shallow nail pocket. The elevator is then turned 160° and slipped under the nail to separate it from the matrix. The attachment to the nail bed is commonly loose. Bleeding is stopped by applying a tourniquet for 3–4 minutes and liquefied phenol is vigorously rubbed into the matrix and grooves for 2–3 minutes.[14,15] Postoperative pain is minimal, but healing takes between 2 and 4 weeks. During this period, a daily footbath is recommended to remove crusts caused by oozing from the phenolized matrix.

Alternatively, surgical matricectomy is carried out after avulsion of the nail plate. The proximal nail fold is incised at both sides and reflected. Its undersurface is de-epithelialized and the entire matrix resected. This defect is closed with the proximal nail fold flap. To avoid nail spicules after wound healing, care must be taken to include the lateral matrix horns. Keratotic debris may develop after surgery as a 'nail bed nail.'

As noted above, the carbon dioxide laser may be used after avulsion of the onychogrypotic nail to vaporize the nail matrix and bed.

Pachyonychia congenita

Three types of this rare syndrome are known. They are characterized by defects of genes coding for keratins—keratins 6a/16 in pachyonychia congenita of Jadassohn-Lewandowsky, 6b/17 in pachyonychia congenita of Jackson-Lawler. These keratins are present in the nail bed, but not in the matrix. Therefore, the nail plate has a normal structure but overlies, in a horseshoe-like manner, the huge nail bed hyperkeratosis. Vigorous curettage plus electrodesiccation of the matrix and nail bed has been described as the most successful treatment.[16] Healing is by second intention. Phenol cautery is a useful alternative and can be repeated.

Although it is the nail bed that is affected, the entire nail plate apparatus has to be destroyed because the nail plate, formed in an incorrect manner by the matrix, cannot adhere to the pathological nail bed.

Racket fingers

Racket nails are characterized by a short wide nail plate and a lack of lateral nail walls, and radiographically by a short terminal phalanx with a broad base. The thumb is most commonly affected; other fingers and the toes are very rarely involved. Racket nails develop when the epiphysis of the terminal phalanx ossifies prematurely, usually between the ages of 10 and 12 years, so that the longitudinal growth stops while the base of the phalanx continues to broaden. Cosmesis is considerably improved by narrowing the nail plate and creating lateral nail folds. Lateral longitudinal nail biopsies are performed on both sides of the nail as described on page 723. The lateral aspects of the skin over the distal phalanx are mobilized and elevated with vertical back stitches to create lateral nail walls and nail folds (Fig. 45.8). Nail groove epithelium develops by second intention.[17]

Ingrown toenails

Ingrown toenails are common and painful. Their etiology is multifactorial. They are most frequently observed in adolescents and young adults, but may occur in neonates, infants, and the elderly (Table 45.1).[18]

Ingrown toenail in infancy

Three kinds of ingrown toenail occur in infants under 2 years of age (Fig. 45.9).

Distal toenail embedding with normally directed nail

This is commonly inborn and results from a short nail plate that has not yet overgrown the tip of the toe. Quite often,

Table 45.1 Etiology and treatment of ingrown toenails

Type	Etiology	Treatment
Neonatal	Distal nail wall caused by too short a nail plate	Conservative
Infantile		
Hypertrophic lateral lip	Hypertrophic medial nail wall of great toe	Conservative
Congenital malalignment of the great toenail	Lateral deviation of long axis of great toenail	Conservative, surgical
Adolescent	Wide curved nail, narrow nail bed	Surgical
Adult	Thick, hard, (over) curved nail	Surgical
Iatrogenic, post-traumatic	Nail avulsion causes formation of distal nail wall, trauma may break skin in nail fold	Conservative, surgical

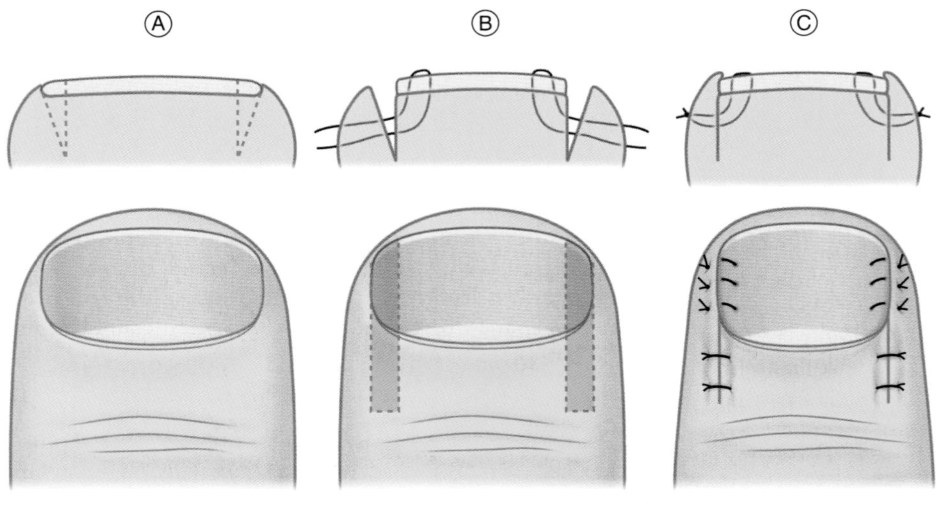

Figure 45.8 Surgical correction of a racket nail—transverse section and dorsal view. (A) Before operation. (B) Incision lines. (C) End of surgery.

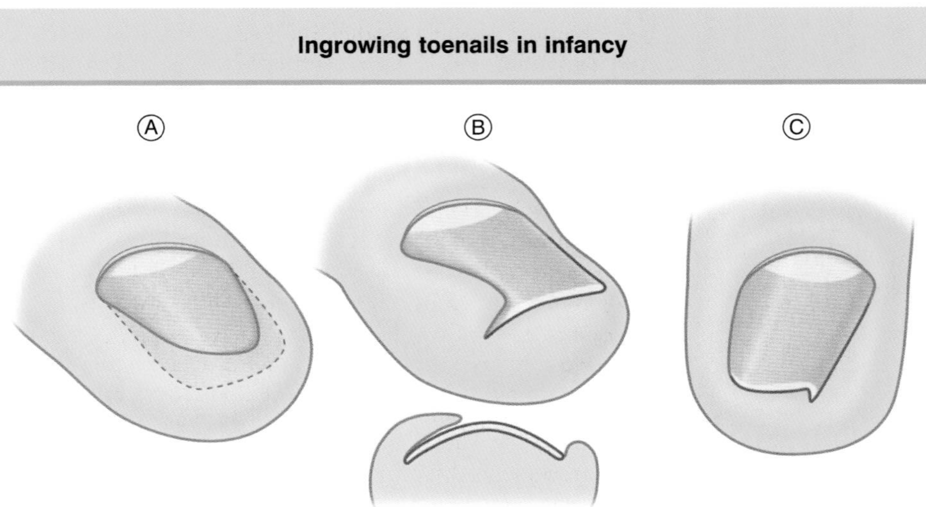

Figure 45.9 Ingrown toenails in infancy. (A) Ingrown toenail in the newborn—there is still a distal nail wall and the lateral nail walls overling the corners of the nail. (B) Hypertrophic lateral lip overlying almost one-third of the nail, surface and end on view. (C) Congenital malalignment of the great toenail—the nail is triangular and oystershell-like, with a sharply bent medial margin.

this condition is associated with lateral nail walls that are directed obliquely and almost meet each other distally (Fig. 45.9A). Conservative management by daily massage with a lubricant ointment after a warm bath is sufficient. Very rarely, permanent improvement is not achieved by 1 year of age and a semicircular soft tissue resection has to be performed in an identical manner as in adults with distally ingrown nails.[17]

Congenital hypertrophic lip of the hallux

Congenital hypertrophic lip of the hallux is characterized by a grossly hypertrophic medial nail fold that may overlie more than one-third of the nail plate (Fig. 45.9B). It usually disappears spontaneously after several months.[19] Its resolution can be accelerated by daily gentle massages from the nail to the medial volar aspect of the toe. This also prevents the accumulation of debris between the nail wall and plate, minimizing maceration and the risk of subsequent infection.

Congenital malalignment of the great toenail

Congenital malalignment of the great toenail[20] was first described under the term of great toe nail dystrophy in infancy. It is characterized by lateral deviation of the longitudinal axis of the great toenail, and sometimes of the entire distal phalanx, with even more pronounced deviation of the nail (Fig. 45.9C). Hypertrophy of the dorsolateral extension of the lateral interphalangeal ligament was thought, at least in part, to be responsible by pulling at the lateral matrix horn and perhaps also at the entire phalanx, explaining the lateral deviation. In addition, the nail is discolored grayish green, has an oystershell-like appearance, and its medial margin is usually bent acutely so that it digs into the flesh; and—most importantly—the malpositioned nail has no attachment with the nail bed. This onycholysis is most important for the prognosis of the condition. If the nail reattaches it will take on a normal appearance, although its axis will remain oblique. Sometimes the distal phalanx is shorter and rounder with a distal nail wall hidden under the malformed nail. The great toe nail will become permanently dystrophic if there is no spontaneous regression during the first years of life. Except for the degree of onycholysis, there is no indicator for spontaneous resolution of this peculiar condition. Surgery is deemed necessary if there is no substantial improvement by the age of 2 years. Under light general anesthesia, proximal toe block anesthesia is performed. A crescentic wedge of soft tissue around the tip is excised and the entire nail apparatus back beyond the matrix is dissected. Care has to be taken not to perforate the nail bed or matrix, particularly at the level of the lateral grooves. The crescent has to be much larger on the medial than on the lateral aspect. The entire nail apparatus is rotated into its correct axis, sometimes with slight overcorrection, and sutured. A small Burow's triangle may be excised dorsally at the start of the medial incision line, facilitating the rotation of the nail flap (Fig. 45.10). Often, the tip of the still cartilaginous terminal phalanx is directed dorsally and is then leveled off. In this case, perioperative antibiotic prophylaxis is recommended. The sutures are removed stepwise after 12–15 days. This operation is successful providing there is still a nail bed–nail plate attachment.[21]

Another treatment approach corrects the hypertrophied dorsal extension of the lateral ligament pulls at the matrix thus causing the deviation. Consequently, it was either cut completely or elongated by Z-like incisions to reduce the pulling action. This hypertrophic part was either completely sectioned or elongated with Z-like incisions to release the tension from the lateral matrix horn.[21] We have seen an immediate response in very young children, but this has to be maintained by special orthopedic measures to keep the nail axis (and probably also the axis of the terminal phalanx) in correct position.

Juvenile ingrown toenail

Hereditary or constitutional imbalance between the width of the nail plate and that of the nail bed[11] and overcurvature of the nail plate[22] are the main causative factors. Additional factors are medial rotation of the toe, thinner nails and thicker nail folds, sweating, convex cutting of the nail, and pointed-toe and high-heeled shoes. They all lead to a relative compression of the tip of the toe so that the distal end of the nail has not enough room to grow and grows into the lateral nail folds.

Treatment of congenital malalignment of the toenail

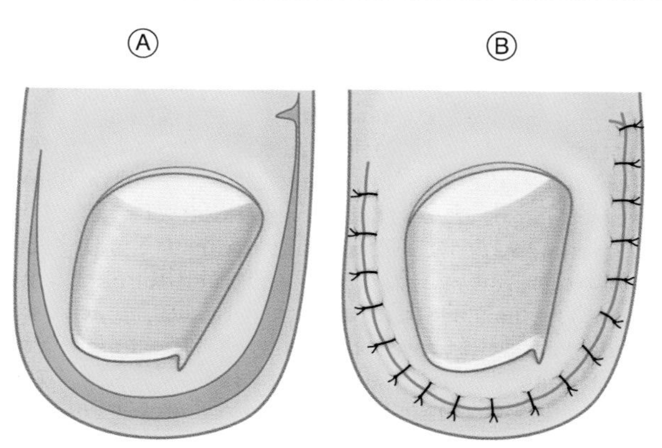

Figure 45.10 Treatment of congenital malalignment of the big toe nail. (A) A crescentic wedge around the distal phalanx is excised and the nail apparatus is dissected from the underlying bone. (B) The nail flap is swung into its correct axis and sutured.

Clinical stages

Clinically, the three stages of juvenile ingrown toenail are as follows.

- Erythema, edema, pain on pressure on the medial, and less frequently on the lateral or both sides. The lateral part of the free edge of the nail digs into the distal part of the nail groove causing pain on pressure and, with time, inflammation. This worsens the condition. The patient tries to remove the offending nail corner by cutting it back as far as possible. However, this induces pain deep in the nail groove and a tiny nail spicule is commonly left behind. With the outgrowth of the nail, this breaks through the epidermis and digs into the tissue, intensifying inflammation and edema.
- Infection and drainage. The ingrown nail acts as a foreign body, keeping the inflammation active and aggravating it. Infection and spontaneous drainage usually follow.
- Granulation tissue and finally lateral nail wall hypertrophy. Granulation tissue is formed, which oozes and produces pus. Over months and sometimes years, the inflamed lateral nail wall and granulation tissue become fibrotic and later sclerotic and may no longer regress to normal size. The patient often habitually cuts the sides of the free nail edge, so aggravating the condition.

Treatment

Treatment for the early stage of juvenile ingrown toenail is conservative. Patient education and compliance are of utmost importance. Well-fitting wide shoes, sandals, or walking bare foot are to be encouraged. Correct trimming of the nails leaving the corners of the free edge long enough so that they cannot dig into the distal part of the lateral groove is crucial. The pliability of the nail can be increased by filing or grinding its central part thinner. Packing of disinfectant-soaked cotton under the lateral edge of the nail alleviates the pressure and pain and allows the wound in the nail groove to heal (Fig. 45.11A). Adhesive tape fixed at the distal portion of the lateral nail fold is pulled obliquely over the plantar surface of the toe giving the nail more space in the groove (Fig. 45.11B). The granulation tissue may be gently cauterized with phenol or silver nitrate. A plastic nail elongation, such as used for cosmetic artificial nails can give support to the periungual soft tissue so that pressure from shoes and during gait will not dislocate it. The orthonyx method with a steel plastic nail brace aims to reduce the overcurvature of the nail. These simple measures should be combined and are often highly effective. However, they have to be performed with skill and require patience.[22]

Gutter treatment has recently gained attention again. Under local anesthesia, the embedded corner of the nail is grasped with a hemostat and freed. A small piece of a plastic tube, for instance from an intravenous drip infusion set, is cut longitudinally and moved over the lateral margin of the nail plate so that it forms a gutter protecting the lateral groove from the pressure of the nail edge (Fig. 45.11C).[23] This gutter is fixed with acrylic glue.[22] A combination with

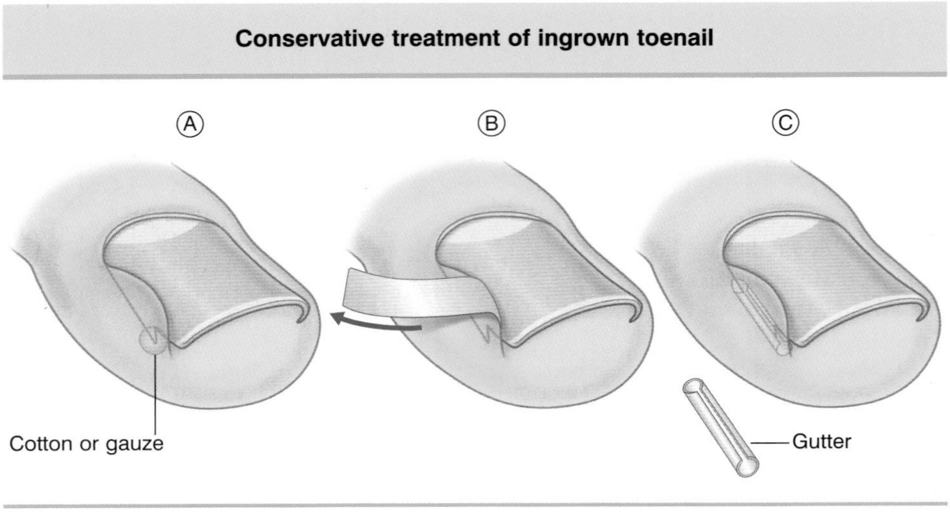

Conservative treatment of ingrown toenail

Ⓐ Ⓑ Ⓒ

Cotton or gauze

Gutter

Figure 45.11 Conservative treatment of adolescent type ingrown toenails. (A) Packing—a whisp of cotton is packed under the ingrowing spicule. (B) Taping—the swollen lateral nail wall is pulled away from the offending nail edge. (C) Gutter treatment—a small tube cut lengthwise is advanced over the lateral nail margin to provide protection for the lateral groove.

the acrylic artificial nail method also allows bathing. Whereas the nail spicule usually found in ingrown nails is left when applying a gutter, it is cut off when only an artificial nail is sculptured.[22] Conservative management requires a high degree of compliance. Recurrences are frequent because the primary cause that led to the development of the ingrown nail is not abolished.

Surgical treatment (Fig. 45.12) is aimed at a definitive cure. Avulsion of the nail alone has recurrence rates of at least 70% and should not be carried out,[15,18,24] not even in association with lateral matrix horn resection. Moreover, when the nail is lacking or too short, the pulp of the hallux tip is pushed dorsally during gait and a distal nail fold forms, which then prevents the nail from regrowing normally. Over 100 years ago, there were more than 75 different methods for operating on ingrown nails. However, most of them have high recurrence rates, for example Emmet's wedge excision, which is obsolete because it leaves mutilated toes and invites recurrences (Fig. 45.12A).

Phenol cautery when carried out correctly, is a simple, effective method with a very low recurrence rate. Using a septum elevator only, the lateral nail strips are freed from the proximal nail fold, nail bed, and matrix, cut longitudinally, and avulsed. This permits access to the lateral matrix horns. Under complete exsanguination achieved with a tourniquet, liquefied phenol (88–90%) is rubbed in vigorously with a cotton-tip applicator for 3 minutes to achieve complete cauterization of the matrix horn epithelium (Figs 45.12C, 45.13). Granulation tissue is ignored because it soon disappears when the offending ingrown nail is removed. Only excessive granulation tissue is gently phenolized. The nail folds can be protected from spillover of phenol with Vaseline. We do not wash the area with alcohol after phenolization is completed because we have never seen any negative effects from the phenol. After cautery, the matrix horns may be rubbed with 40% ferric chloride to stop bleeding after the tourniquet is released. This was also shown to shorten the period of postoperative oozing. Small antibiotic tablets containing a local antibiotic (e.g. Framycetin), a protease, and lidocaine (Leukase-Kegel, Dermapharm, Grünwald, Germany) are put into the small wound cavities. They prevent infection, provide a local anesthetic action, and keep the wounds open so that they can drain. Postoperative pain is minimal because phenol has a local anesthetic action. It is also antiseptic. The matrix epithelium is sloughed off with slight oozing for 2–4 weeks. Daily foot baths with povidone-iodine soap or another disinfective soap solution, such as Hibiscrub (AstraZeneca Pharmaceuticals Inc, Wilmington, DE), prevent infection and accelerate healing.[15,18]

Selective lateral matrix excision requires more surgical skills. After avulsion of the lateral nail strips, an oblique section is performed at both sides of the proximal nail fold and the space of the lateral matrix horns is opened. The lateral matrix horns are then completely dissected from the bone. Because the matrix often reaches far proximally and plantarly, it may be wise to perform an L-shaped or curved incision at the junction of the proximal and lateral nail walls to permit the lateral matrix horns to be better visualized. Inserting a #1 injection needle along the lateral grooves into the tip of the lateral matrix horn and dissecting the matrix around the tip of the needle is even more secure (Fig. 45.12B). The wound cavity is filled with small tapered antibiotic tablets so preventing infection, keeping the space open, and allowing wound secretion. Excess granulation tissue is gently curetted. The nail incisions are closed with two sutures or with Steri-strips (3M, St Paul, MN). Systemic antibiotics are administered only if there is considerable infection.[15] Lateral matrix horn removal by either phenolization or surgical dissection leaves a slightly narrower nail.

A nail bed periosteal flap avoids narrowing the nail. The lateral ingrown strip of nail is avulsed and the lateral groove is incised. The interosseous ligament is resected and the lateral nail wall is de-epithelialized. The lateral portion of the nail bed and matrix are dissected from the phalanx and elevated to allow the de-epithelialized lateral nail wall to be interposed between the bone and the nail bed and matrix flap. They are held in place with 4-0 monofilament mattress sutures. The nail bed is laid back and sutured to the new lateral nail wall. Success rates are high, but postoperative pain and morbidity are higher than after phenol cautery.[24]

Hypertrophy of the lateral nail fold develops in long-standing ingrown nails from chronic inflammation, which in turn may result in hard fibrous tissue. If narrowing the nail plate by phenolization of the lateral matrix horns does not lead to regression after 2–3 months, an elliptical wedge is taken from the lateral aspect of the toe reducing its size and pulling the lateral fold away from the nail (Fig. 45.14).

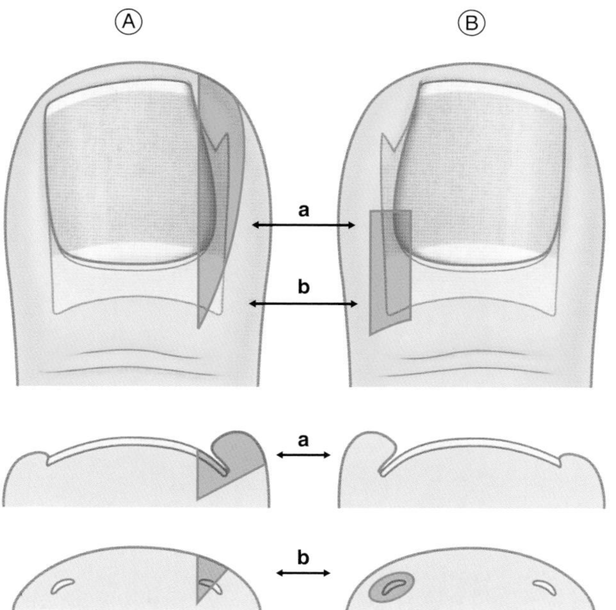

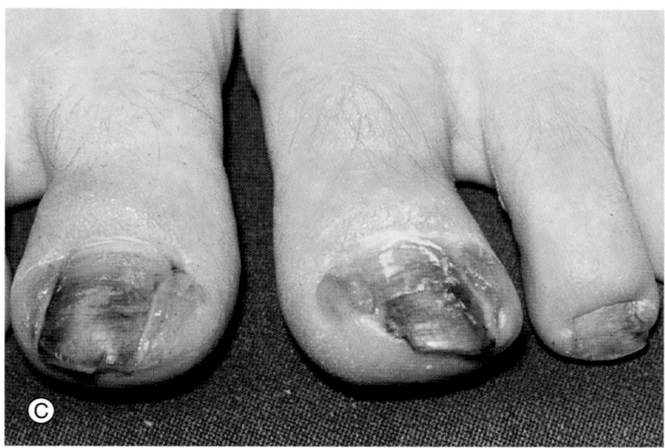

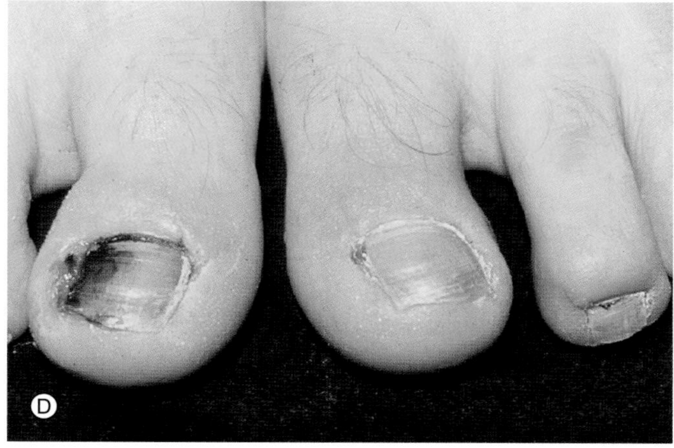

Figure 45.12 Surgical treatment of ingrown toenails. (A) Wedge excision. (B) Selective matrix horn removal. The transverse sections at the level of the proximal nail bed and matrix horn demonstrate the amount of tissue resection and the tip of the matrix horn that is left in place with the wedge excision technique. (C) Ingrown toenails with plenty of granulation tissue. (D) 2 weeks after selective surgical matrix horn resection.

Distal nail embedding

A distal wall is commonly the consequence of avulsion of the big toenail or cutting the big toenail too short over a long period of time. Because of the lack of counterpressure, the tip of the hallux pulp is dislocated dorsally when the foot rolls during walking. When this condition is very longstanding even the dorsal aspect of the processus unguicularis may become hypertrophic. The distal wall impairs the growth of the nail plate, which often becomes thickened, yellowish, and opaque. When the distal wall does not regress from massaging back or pulling back by taping in a distal–plantar direction, an acrylic sculptured nail on the stump nail may enable it to overgrow the distal wall. If this procedure remains ineffective, a fishmouth incision is created parallel to the distal groove around the tip of the toe, starting and ending 3–5 mm proximal to the end of the lateral nail fold. A second incision is then made to yield a crescentic wedge of 4–8 mm width. The dorsal portion is mobilized and an eventual hypertrophy of the dorsal aspect of the processus unguicularis is resected. The distal nail wall disappears when the defect is sutured (Fig. 45.15).[25]

Pincer nails

Pincer nails (tubed nails, trumpet nails) are characterized by transverse overcurvature increasing distally along the longitudinal axis of the nail. The nail edges constrict the nail bed tissue and dig into the lateral grooves. Pain is often surprisingly mild, but can be unbearable. Overcurvature may be partial, with an acute bend of the medial nail plate strip or total, affecting the entire nail. Two varieties of toenail overcurvature can be distinguished:[26]

- Symmetrical involvement—which usually affects several toes, with lateral deviation of the axis of the hallux nails and medial deviation of the lesser toenails. This is probably a genetic trait because it is often seen in other family members.

Matrix horn phenolization for treatment of an ingrown toenail

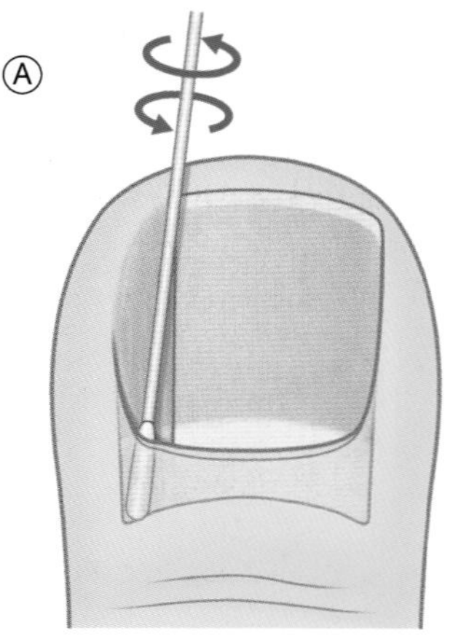

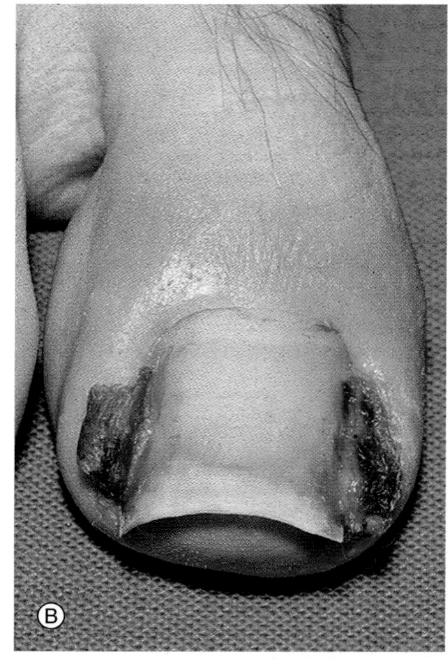

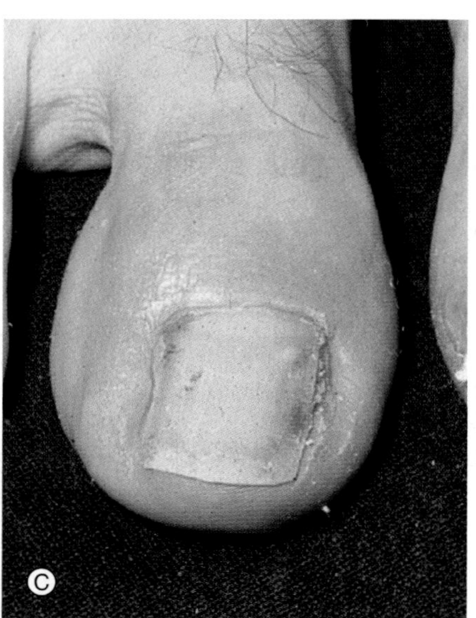

Figure 45.13 Matrix horn phenolization for treatment of an ingrown toenail. (A) Schematic representation of the method—the lateral nail strip is removed and a liquefied phenol is rubbed into the matrix horn with a fine cotton-tip applicator. (B) Ingrown toenail. (C) 6 weeks after selective matrix horn phenolization.

Reduction of hypertrophic fibrotic lateral nail wall

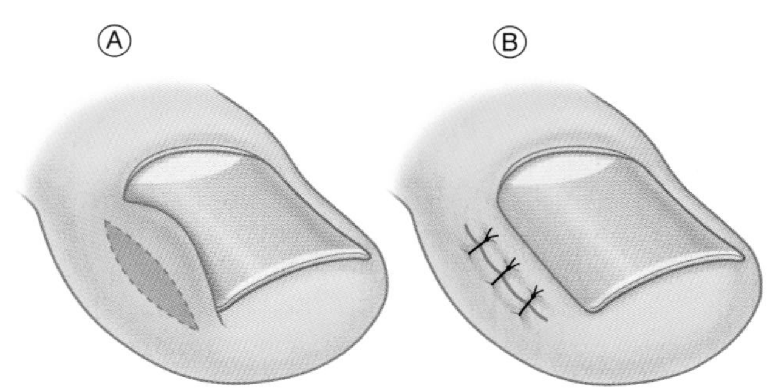

Figure 45.14 Reduction of a hypertrophied lateral nail wall. (A) Incision lines (B) End of operation.

Correction of a distal nail wall

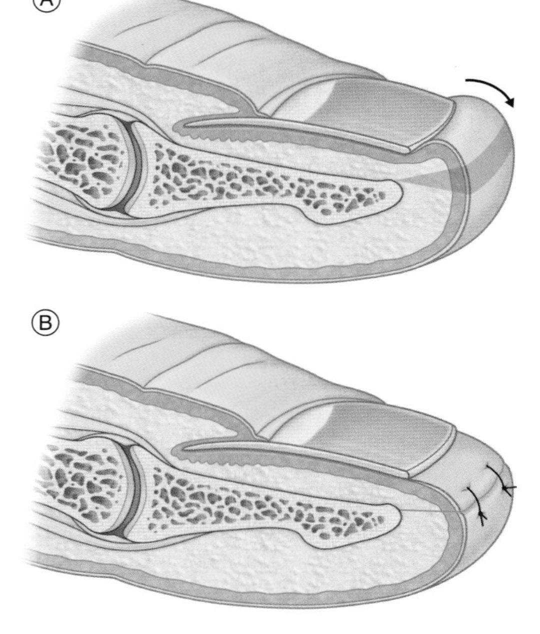

Figure 45.15 Correction of a distal nail wall. (A) Excision of a crescentic wedge. (B) End of operation.

- Asymmetrical involvement— which usually affects only the hallux. The major causes are foot deformities, some dermatoses, and osteoarthritis, especially in the fingers.

Particularly in the genetic form, radiographs show a very wide base of the terminal phalanx, usually with lateral osteophytes, which are often hook-like with their tip showing distally (Fig. 45.16). They are more pronounced on the medial aspect. The entire hallux phalanx is often deviated medially. Hyperostosis is seen on the dorsal tuft of the terminal phalanx as a result of traction from heaped-up nail bed, which is firmly attached to the bone by collagen fibers.[26]

Conservative management consists of clipping down the lateral edge of the nail as proximally as possible, cotton wool packing under the distal edge, grooving the nail plate to make it more pliable, nail braces (orthonyx technique), or application of an artificial nail. Conservative measures have to be maintained almost indefinitely because they have no influence on the pathogenesis of the process.

Surgical treatment is aimed at flattening the nail. After bilateral partial nail avulsion, the lateral matrix horns are cauterized with 90% phenol. If the overcurvature is not too excessive the distal two-thirds of the nail are carefully avulsed. In cases of almost complete tubing of the nail plate, the nail plate is completely avulsed. A median longitudinal incision of the nail bed is carried down to the bone from the lunula border to 3–4 mm beyond the hyponychium. While doing this, the dorsal traction osteophyte is felt. The entire nail bed is dissected from the phalanx. The dorsal tuft together with part of the distal dorsal aspect of the bone is generously removed with a bone rongeur. The nail bed is spread on the bone and sutured with 6-0 polydioxanone (PDS) absorbable sutures. It is kept spread out by using reversed tie-over sutures pulling the lateral nail folds apart. To prevent the sutures from cutting through the lateral folds, thin rubber tubes are placed into the lateral grooves and the suture threads are laid over them (see Fig. 45.16). These sutures are left for 18–21 days to allow the nail bed to adhere to its anatomically restored form.[26]

A number of other techniques are also aimed at flattening the nail. Most are more complicated. However, Rosa's method is very simple. The entire nail bed and approximately the dorsal half of the phalangeal bone are removed. The regrowing flat nail would form a new nail bed. Insertion of a strip of dermis graft under the lateral groove appears to be effective in milder forms, especially of the fingers that result from degenerative osteoarthritis with Heberden's nodes.

Infection

The hand's reaction to infection is dominated by anatomical considerations. Immediate correct diagnosis is crucial. Radiographs identify metallic foreign bodies, bone lesions, fractures, and gas formation.

Acute paronychia

Acute paronychia often follows minor trauma, such as a break in the skin, a splinter, or a prick of a thorn. The most superficial form is bulla repens, a form of bullous impetigo. The blister roof is removed and disinfectant baths are performed twice daily. Antibiotics are rarely necessary. Proximal subungual felon is seen as an abscess in the nail fold or pus accumulation under the nail. It is painful, particularly at night. If it does not improve after 2 days of treatment with penicillinase-resistant antibiotics, surgical treatment is necessary. The proximal one-third of the nail is removed by cutting across with pointed scissors. Non-adherent gauze is laid under the proximal nail fold as a wick. If the infection under the nail is restricted to one side, only this part of the nail is removed. Again, twice daily baths with a disinfectant solution are recommended. It is important to note that the nail matrix of children is

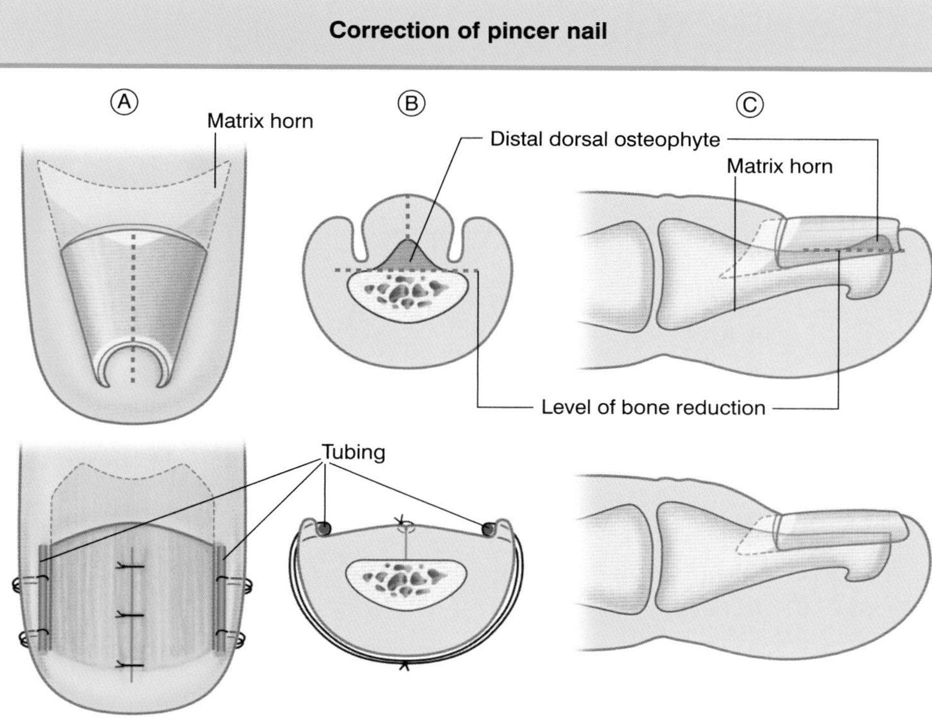

Figure 45.16 Pincer nail operation. (A) Dorsal view. (B) Transverse section. (C) Lateral view. Upper row—before surgery, lower row—after surgery.

particularly sensitive and can be destroyed within 48 hours of acute bacterial infection.

A localized abscess may also be seen adjacent to the cuticle. It is drained by lifting the cuticle and excising the epidermal layer over the infection without anesthesia.

Distal subungual felon is mainly caused by splinter injuries. A small wedge of soft tissue is excised over the yellow lesion and left open for drainage.

Chronic paronychia

Chronic paronychia manifests as a painless swelling with retraction of the perionychial tissue, detachment of the nail from the overlying thickened nail fold, and loss of the cuticle. It often shows subacute flares after variable periods of time. Cultures should be taken from under the proximal nail fold. A sterile loop can be introduced without causing pain, and material for both bacterial and yeast cultures is taken. Using the water jet of an oral irrigator such as Water Pik (Water Pik Inc, Newport Beach, CA) often rinses out a considerable amount of dirt and foreign material. In recalcitrant cases, the thickened nail fold is excised en bloc as a crescent-shaped full thickness specimen with a maximal width of 4 mm. A beveled incision gives excellent results by second intention healing in less than 1 month. For patients with repeated subacute painful flares of chronic paronychia, removal of the base of the nail is recommended.[27]

Subungual infection

Subungual infection is usually characterized by a defined painful area over which the nail has to be fenestrated or a U-shaped piece of the distal nail plate is excised in the region loosened by the pus. The finger is soaked twice daily in antiseptic solutions, such as chlorhexidine, and healing is usually rapid.

Deep infections may affect the bone and cause osteomyelitis.

Tumors of the nail apparatus

The surgical treatment of nail tumors requires knowledge of their histopathology and biological behavior. The approach is dominated mainly by the location within the nail apparatus and whether the tumor is benign or malignant.

Benign tumors

Common warts

Common warts are the most common reactive tumors. They are said to have a natural life span of no more than 3–5 years, but during that time they may be the source of new 'daughter warts.' Treatment must avoid any untoward sequelae, particularly scarring. If conservative treatment with saturated monochloroacetic acid, salicylic acid plaster 60%, daily hot baths, and weekly curettage of the necrotized layers of the warts does not help, careful cryotherapy may be tried. It is repeated at weekly or biweekly intervals until the wart disappears. If this is unsuccessful, needling (or pricking) with bleomycin, usually under finger block anesthesia, often causes the warts to disappear. Carbon dioxide laser vaporization is another option. It has to be stressed that decreasing the size of warts is not sufficient.

Ungual fibrokeratomas

Ungual fibrokeratomas are sausage-like fibrous tumors with a keratotic tip. They may arise from the depth of the nail pocket and grow either directly on the nail plate surface, causing a longitudinal canaliform impression, or in it, forming a longitudinal hollow. When originating from the nail bed they remain subungual, but cause a rim in the nail plate. Fibrokeratomas are best enucleated using a #11 scalpel blade, which is held parallel to the long axis of the lesion and carried around its base down to the bone, from which it is severed with pointed curved scissors (Fig. 45.17). No suture is required. After healing, a normal nail regrows. Subungual fibrokeratomas may require partial nail avulsion, but the plate can be laid back at the end of surgery.

The same kind of treatment is used for multiple Koenen's tumors. Some nail defect may result when too much of the matrix had to be removed. However, it is amazing how much of the nail can regenerate. Patients with Bourneville–Pringle tuberous sclerosis should therefore be encouraged to seek help for their periungual fibromas.

Subungual exostoses

Subungual exostoses are commonly seen on the distal medial aspect of the terminal phalanx of the great toe, but may occur on any other digit. They present as a stone-hard swelling lifting up the nail. Their surface is usually smooth and the stretched epidermis is shiny. A radiograph will not only confirm the diagnosis and determine the extent of the lesion, but also rules out bone fragments from a previous trauma, usually of the finger, that is no longer remembered (Fig. 45.18). A skin incision is made over the exostosis, which is dissected and generously cut off at its base with a nail clipper or bone rongeur. If the lesion is more proximal under the nail plate, the nail plate is partially avulsed to permit access. Sometimes, the skin overlying the exostosis is so overstretched that it has to be excised as a fusiform specimen. Any ulceration of the overlying skin is excised, and perioperative antibiotic prophylaxis is strongly recommended.

Subungual glomus tumors

Subungual glomus tumors are probably the best known nail tumors. Most commonly, they present as a violaceous spot in the proximal nail fold from which a reddish band extends distally to the free nail edge. They stand out by their

Treatment of ungual fibrokeratoma

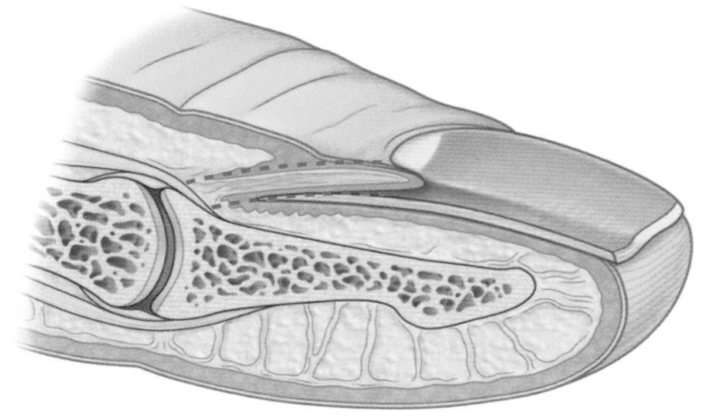

Figure 45.17 Treatment of ungual fibrokeratoma. The incision is carried down to the bone to allow the core of the tumor to be removed.

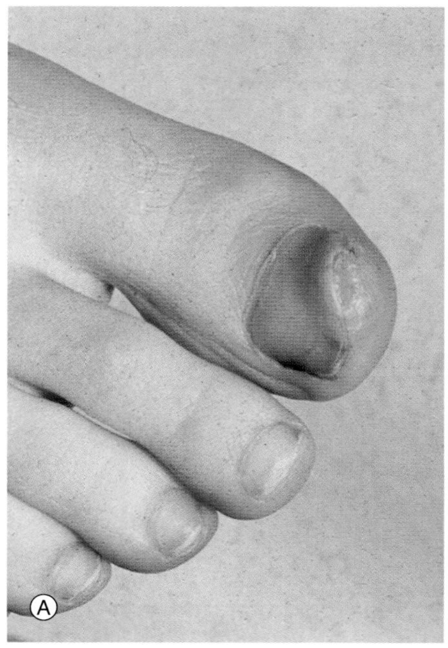

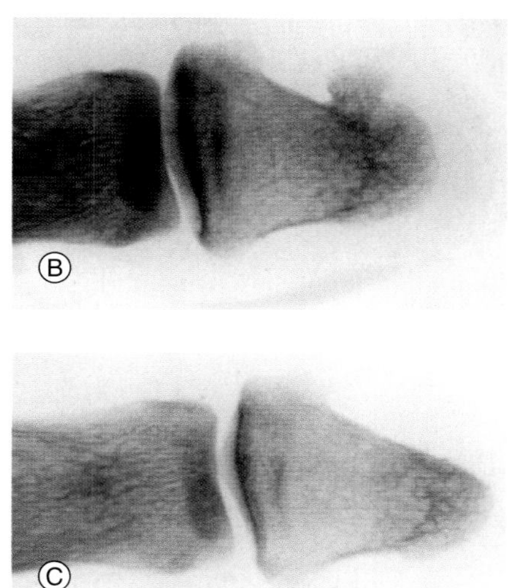

Figure 45.18 (A) Subungual exostosis. (B) Radiograph before and (C) after surgery.

characteristic symptoms: immediate intense pain is elicited by the slightest shock or trauma, probing, or cold, and is alleviated when a pneumatic tourniquet is put around the arm and inflated to over 200 mmHg. Their exact localization may vary from the visually most obvious site, but can be confirmed by probing with a small blunt probe—the site of greatest pain corresponds to their localization. Magnetic resonance imaging is a new and elegant tool for localizing a glomus tumor.

Subungual glomus tumors can usually be readily removed via the lateral aspect of the phalanx when they are in the lateral one-third of the nail bed or matrix. An L-shaped incision is performed and the nail bed is dissected from the bone. The glomus tumor appears as a small, soft, glassy-gray round lesion that is easily distinguished from the white nail bed dermis or the yellow color of the fat. The defect is sutured with 5-0 skin sutures. When centrally located, the tumor is removed after punching a hole into the nail plate and incising the nail bed longitudinally (Fig. 45.19) or the matrix transversally, respectively. The hamartoma is dissected and the defect sutured with 6-0 resorbable material. The nail disk is put back to speed up healing.

Myxoid pseudocysts

Myxoid pseudocysts (dorsal finger cysts) are relatively frequent degenerative lesions that commonly occur in the proximal nail fold, but occasionally also under the matrix. Most commonly, there is a degenerative osteoarthritis of the distal interphalangeal joint. A connection to the distal interphalangeal joint may develop, which is visualized after intra-articular injection of 0.1 mL of sterile methylene blue solution. A U-shaped incision is then carried around the distal and lateral margin of the lesion, the skin is elevated, and the lesion is meticulously dissected; the methylene blue makes the true extent of the lesion easily visible. The stalk to the joint, which appears as a dark-blue spot, is sutured with 6-0 resorbable sutures and the skin is sutured back. If the skin overlying the pseudocyst is too thin to be kept it is removed and a transposition flap is raised to cover the defect (Fig. 45.20). The donor defect rapidly heals by

Removal of subungual glomus tumor

A — Red streak in nail

B — Punched out nail plate

Glomus tumor

Figure 45.19 (A)–(B) Removal of a subungual glomus tumour.

second intention.[28] The finger is splinted in physiological flexion. It has also been recommended to only resect the Heberden's nodes, when present, from the base of the terminal phalanx. A T- or H-shaped incision is made over the joint crease to expose the dorsal aspect of the joint capsule. The bony excrescences are meticulously dissected and removed while hyperextending the joint. The extensor tendon may be weakened by the pathological process as well as by this manipulation, and a cast has therefore been recommended for several weeks.[3] The major complication of any operation at the distal interphalangeal joint is stiffness, which depends on the period of immobilization. We therefore consider that early mobilization should be attempted.

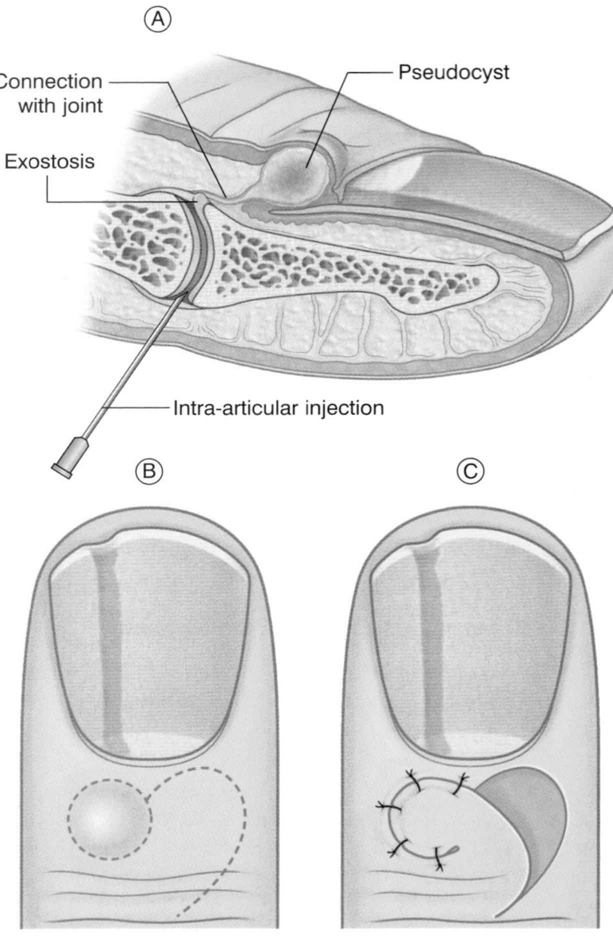

Figure 45.20 Treatment of myxoid pseudocysts of the distal phalanx. (A) Sagittal section through nail unit with myxoid pseudocyst and intra-articular injection of methylene blue. (B) Incision around cyst and marking of a transposition flap. (C) Pseudocyst excised and defect repaired with flap.

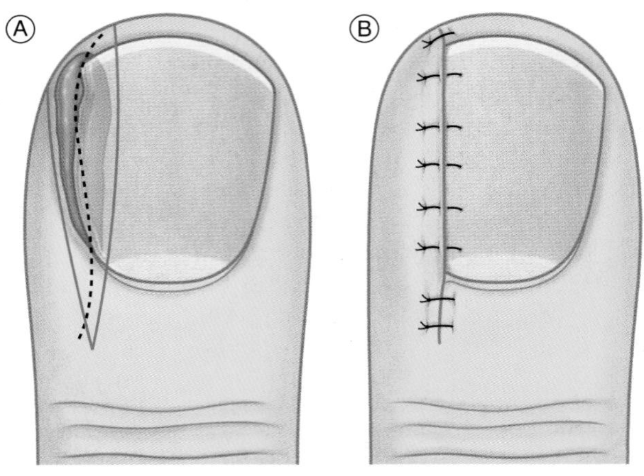

Figure 45.21 Bridge flap for the treatment of laterally positioned Bowen's disease. (A) Tumor defect post Mohs surgery, with additional tissue for excision outlined for development of the flap; relaxing incision at the pulp of the distal phalanx (dotted line). (B) End of operation—the bridge flap covers the defect and vertical mattress sutures elevate the flap over the level of the nail plate recreating a lateral nail fold. The nail is narrower, but cosmetically acceptable.

Malignant nail tumors

Epidermoid carcinoma

Epidermoid carcinoma is the general term now used for both Bowen's disease and squamous cell carcinoma of the nail. It is the second most frequent malignant nail tumor. Clinically, it is usually a warty plaque in the lateral nail groove or on the proximal nail fold extending under and around the nail. In darkly pigmented individuals, longitudinal melanonychia may develop. Ungual Bowen's disease may also mimic fibrokeratoma.[29] Longitudinal leukonychia indicates matrix involvement. Multidigit involvement has been observed. Metastases are very rare. Etiologies are different high-risk human papillomaviruses, chronic radiation exposure, arsenic, and probably as yet unidentified agents. Any warty lesion in the nail organ of an adult should raise suspicion of this particular malignancy. It is excised using Mohs micrographic surgery with immediate three-dimensional margin control. If the defect is no wider than half of the nail, a bridge flap is formed from the lateral aspect of the distal phalanx and sutured to the nail with vertical back sutures, thus creating a new lateral nail wall. A considerably narrower nail, but functionally intact distal phalanx will result (Fig. 45.21). Larger defects may require full-thickness skin grafts or crossfinger flaps.[2,10,30] Amputation is almost never indicated.

Carcinoma cuniculatum

Carcinoma cuniculatum is a variant of verrucous carcinoma and rarely occurs under the nail. It usually presents as a fistulous process that exudes, spontaneously or on pressure, a creamy whitish smelly substance mainly made up of degrading keratinocytes. Although it almost never metastasizes it should be widely excised using Mohs' micrographic surgery.

Other appendageal carcinomas are exceedingly rare in the nail region, especially the 'nail-specific' carcinomas such as malignant proliferating onycholemmal cyst and onycholemmal carcinoma. Microscopically controlled surgery is the treatment of choice.

Ungual melanoma

Ungual melanoma is the most frequent malignant nail neoplasm. Two-thirds to three-quarters are pigmented and most of them begin with a longitudinal melanonychia. Therefore, any melanin-induced longitudinal pigmentation in the nail of an adult fair-complexioned Caucasian should be treated as a potential ungual melanoma and undergo immediate (excisional) biopsy.

Narrow brown streaks in the nail are treated according to their location in the nail—lateral by lateral longitudinal nail biopsy, and median by punch, fusiform biopsy, or shave excision[1,10] (see page 723). Nail biopsy can prevent overtreatment in cases of a benign nevus and potentially fatal undertreatment in cases of malignant melanoma. More detailed information about the diagnostic problems of pigmented nail lesions can be found elsewhere.[31,32]

If there is no doubt about the diagnosis of a melanoma, the lesion must be removed completely. We prefer excision of the entire nail organ with histopathologic margin control (Fig. 45.22). The defect is then closed with a crossfinger flap for the fingers, or with a full-thickness skin or a reversed dermal graft for toes; sometimes, guided second intention healing is used to achieve mechanically resistant tissue under the graft. This recreates a fully functioning distal phalanx with acceptable cosmetic results. Amputation has not been shown to give better survival rates; in contrast, patients treated with conservative surgery have longer disease-free survival times. There is no unanimous opinion concerning sentinel lymph node extirpation for ungual melanoma.

Reconstructive nail surgery

A variety of defects of the nail organ can be repaired, although the problems of brittle or fragile nails are not amenable to surgical modalities.

Defects of the nail folds

Proximal nail fold

The proximal nail fold is not infrequently damaged by a laceration or burn or after tumor removal. For small defects of its median part, a simple technique using two relaxing incisions at either side of the proximal nail fold is used. The defect is transformed to a narrow wedge, the base of which is the cuticle line. The nail plate is separated from the overlying nail fold with a nail elevator. At each junction between the lateral and proximal nail folds, an incision is performed, almost to the distal crease of the distal interphalangeal joint, and the two small flaps are advanced against each other and sutured. The tiny secondary defects are left for second intention healing. Within a relatively short period of time, the scars will become almost invisible. Defects that are wider can be closed with the same technique, but require wider flaps. The fold is detached from the nail plate and two curved incisions are performed from the junction of the lateral and proximal nail folds to form small rotation flaps. To make them freely movable, a tangential incision is made from the level of the nail plate to the flap incision. If the defect is in a lateral position, one relaxing incision is performed through the free nail fold border and another one more laterally to allow for more movement (Fig. 45.23).

Subtotal loss of the proximal nail fold is difficult to repair. Barfod's technique utilizing two narrow distally pedicled flaps was not successful in our hands. The flaps did not unite and although there was no flap necrosis, shrinkage yielded two small stumps.[33] In addition, this technique requires at least two stages and is time consuming and demanding for the patient. Hayes used one distally based, but wider flap and closed the donor defect with a free skin graft.[34] Alsbjörn et al. proposed an incision parallel to the free border of the proximal nail fold, advanced the distal margin and covered the resulting defect with a skin graft.[35] We believe that broad-based rotation flaps from the lateral aspect of the phalanx are safe and can provide more tissue than most of the techniques described, which use slender and relatively long transposition flaps.

Lateral nail fold

The lateral nail fold can be recreated as described above for the lateral longitudinal nail biopsy and racket nail (see Fig. 45.8). Tissue defects are best repaired using adjacent skin from the lateral–volar aspect of the distal phalanx, as already briefly described for the treatment of laterally positioned Bowen's disease (see page 736). An incision is performed about 10 mm volarly that runs parallel to the volar margin of the defect and is slightly longer than it. The skin is undermined at the level of the bone and interosseous ligament, yielding a bipedicled or bridged flap. This is swung into the defect and sutured. If the entire height of the lateral nail fold is absent the flap's dorsal edge is elevated over the level of the nail plate and sutured with vertical mattress sutures to restore it. The donor defect is left for second intention healing. Scarring of the donor site is minimal.

Matrix defects

Nail matrix defects result in nail dystrophy, split nail formation, or a pterygium when scarring has occurred between the ventral bottom (matrix) and dorsal roof (eponychium) of the nail pocket. Double nail formation is caused by a step in the matrix, most commonly after a fracture of the terminal phalanx.

A split in the nail is the result of a narrow, but longitudinal defect in the matrix. Most cases are caused by scars after trauma. The classical split nail repair is excision of the scar and meticulous repair. A narrow strip of nail is avulsed over the split leaving the lateral portions attached to the matrix and nail bed. The proximal nail fold is incised at both sides and retracted, thus revealing the matrix scar, which may reach into the nail bed. This is excised, the edges are cautiously undermined and sutured with 6-0 monofilament absorbable sutures. In the matrix area, the soft nail plate may be taken as a cushion to protect the matrix from the sutures. In the lunula and nail bed area, there is still an area without covering nail left after the avulsion of the nail strip. Using 4-0 nonresorbable material, horizontal mattress sutures are made in the remaining lateral nail plate portions, pulling the sutured matrix and nail bed closely together and supporting the 6-0 matrix and nail bed sutures. This technique gives good results, but a completely normal nail will almost never regrow because even this procedure leaves a narrow longitudinal scar in the matrix (Fig. 45.24).

A wide split and most cases of pterygium cannot be repaired with this excisional technique. A matrix graft has proven to be the treatment of choice. Although it has been recommended to take the graft from the matrix adjacent to the scar, we have found the great toenail to be the superior donor site. Both the damaged and the donor nail are avulsed by the proximal approach. The nail pocket is opened. The matrix defect is superficially excised and, in the case of a pterygium, the depth of the proximal groove recreated. A template for the size of the defect is made and laid on the donor matrix so that a shallow incision can be made to outline the size of the matrix transplant. A color mark is made to facilitate orientation. With a #15 scalpel blade, a very thin slice of matrix is taken; during this procedure, the scalpel blade is seen shining through the matrix graft. It is

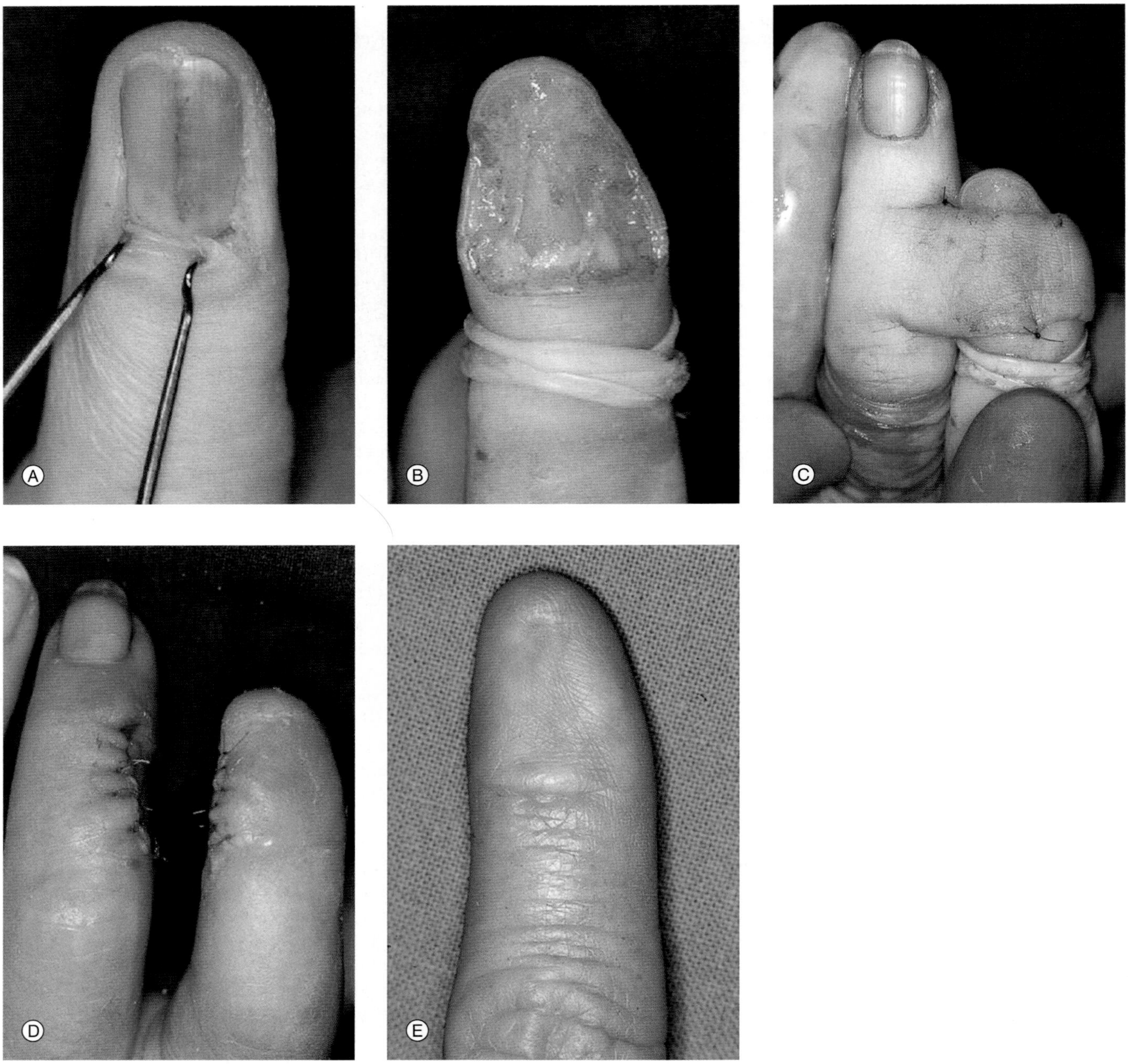

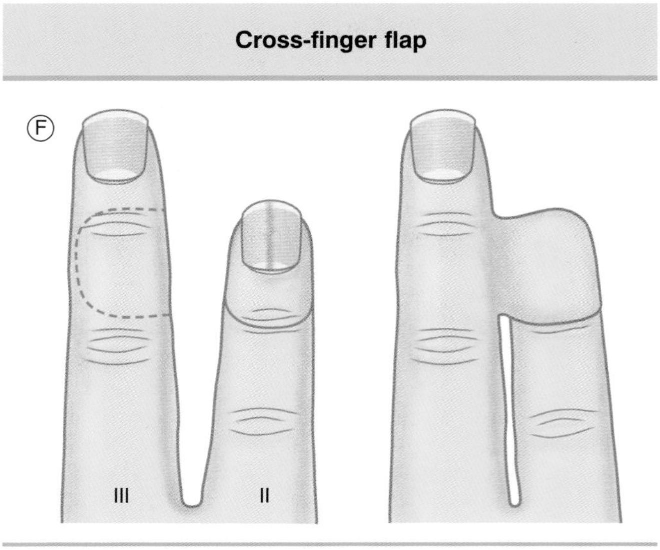

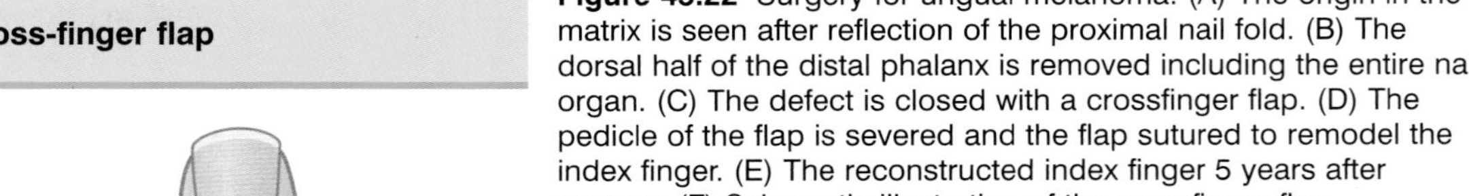

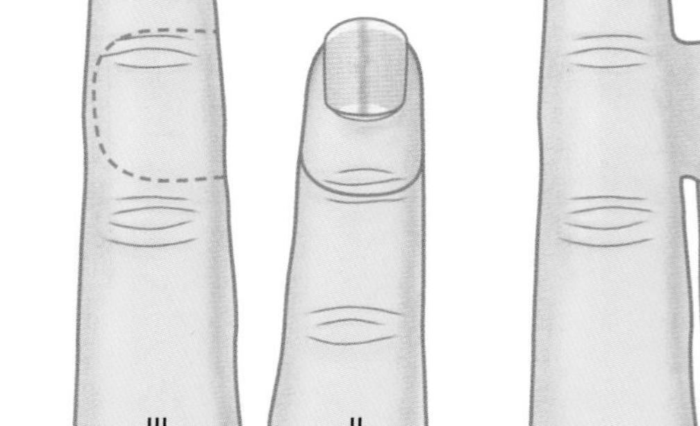

Figure 45.22 Surgery for ungual melanoma. (A) The origin in the matrix is seen after reflection of the proximal nail fold. (B) The dorsal half of the distal phalanx is removed including the entire nail organ. (C) The defect is closed with a crossfinger flap. (D) The pedicle of the flap is severed and the flap sutured to remodel the index finger. (E) The reconstructed index finger 5 years after surgery. (F) Schematic illustration of the crossfinger flap.

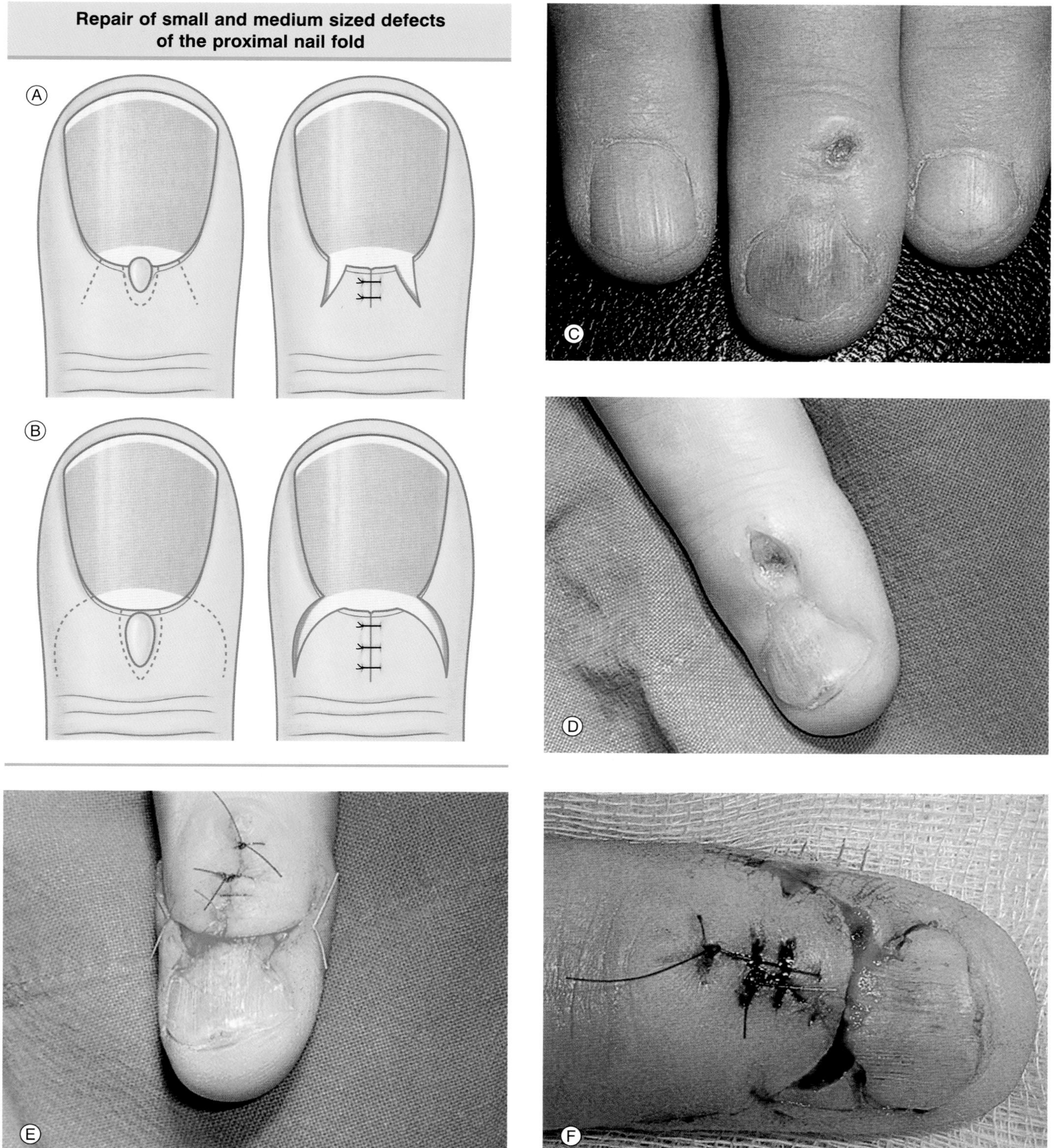

Repair of small and medium sized defects of the proximal nail fold

Figure 45.23 Repair for small- and medium-sized defects of the proximal nail fold. (A) Small tumor in a median position. (B) Medium-sized defect of the proximal nail fold. The small secondary defects are left for second intention healing. (C)–(F) Defect excision and repair after five unsuccessful attempts to remove a myxoid pseudocyst. (C) Defect and recurrence. (D) Excision of the defect. (E) End of operation. (F) 2 days after surgery.

Split nail repair

(A) (B) (C)

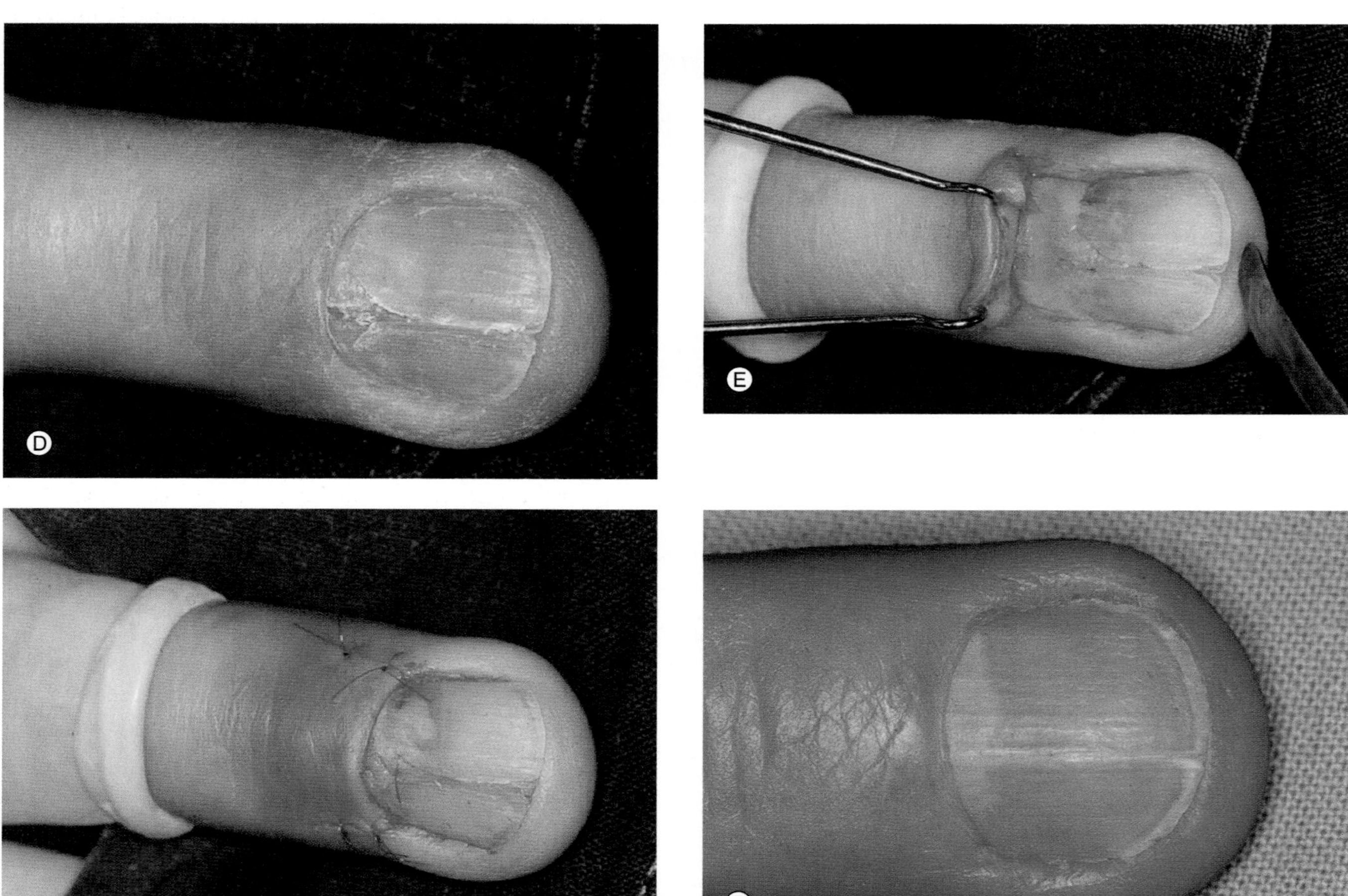

Figure 45.24 Split nail repair. (A) The proximal nail fold is incised at both sides, a strip of nail is avulsed over the matrix and nail bed scar, and the scar is excised. (B) Nail bed and matrix as well as proximal nail fold are sutured. (C) The nail plate is sutured with thick stable stitches. (D) Split nail after car door crash injury. (E) Reflection of the proximal nail fold reveals a scar in the matrix. (F) The scar is excised, the matrix defect is sutured, and the proximal nail fold is sutured back. (G) Considerable improvement 1 year after surgery.

transferred to the original defect and fixed with ophthalmic 7-0 chromic sutures. The color mark ensures that it will be sutured according to the correct growth direction. The great toenail is trimmed so that it fits into the recipient nail pocket where it acts as a physiological dressing and protection and also keeps the bottom and the roof of the nail pocket apart. We prefer to use the split nail plate as a cover for the donor site, but it may not be necessary. Healing is uneventful and without nail dystrophy in the donor nail when the graft is thin enough.

Optimizing outcomes

- Speak with your patient about potential inconveniences after nail surgery, for instance, advising the patient to bring a larger shoe when a toenail will be operated on.
- Meticulous pre- and postoperative care is essential.
- Smoking can be deleterious for nail flaps and other demanding nail surgery.
- Make as correct a diagnosis as possible prior to planning nail surgery.
- Consider a two-step procedure if you are not sure what the diagnosis is.
- Individualize surgical operations according to the diagnosis and extent of the lesion to be operated on.
- Consider Mohs micrographic surgery for malignant lesions.
- Ask an experienced colleague what he or she would recommend – the internet and email offer unique options.

Pitfalls and their management

- Certain general risk factors such as diabetes mellitus, peripheral arterial impairment and immunosuppression increase the risk of infection. These risk factors may potentiate each other. Before doing nail surgery, take a thorough patient history and treat these risk factors as well as possible.
- Interdict smoking even though you cannot expect your patient to really obey – however, you may at least have a chance that he or she will smoke a bit less.
- Elderly patients with dry and scaling feet often have moccasin-type tinea pedis and/or this may be a sign of impaired arterial blood supply.
- Avoid a tourniquet or limit its application time to a minimum whenever you suspect impaired arterial blood supply.
- Pain after nail surgery is common and may sometimes be excruciating. Have the patient elevate the operated extremity for 24 to 48 hours. Pain that develops after 24 to 48 hours is suspicious for an infection, which should be treated as early as possible. Remove the dressing, inspect the wound and perform an antiseptic hand- or footbath to remove crusts from dried wound secretion. Blood is easily and painlessly removed using 3% hydrogen peroxide. If you see reddening and swelling remove stitches overlying the involved area.
- Pain starting after 10 days or longer may be a hint of reflex sympathetic dystrophy that requires intensive treatment to prevent it from becoming chronic.

Proper examination of the patient before nail surgery and correct technique can avoid the commonest complications and rule out high-risk patients.[32]

Bleeding is usually not a problem although it may occur after releasing the tourniquet, which should, however, not be left for longer than 20 minutes; for longer operations, it is released every 15 minutes.

The individual pain threshold is extremely variable. Preoperative sedation is helpful. During surgery, pain is caused by poor anesthesia. The dressing has to be padded to avoid injury. The extremity should be elevated to reduce edema and pain. The foot is raised to 30° and the patient kept recumbent for 48 hours. Pain may be significant, and analgesics are then necessary. The use of ropivacaine for anesthesia or addition of bupivacaine at the completion of the surgery provides longlasting analgesia.

Infection is minimized by adhering to strict antisepsis and atraumatic surgery. However, the subungual space cannot be completely sterilized and antibiotic prophylaxis should be considered if there is any doubt. Postoperative infections include felon, compartmental cellulitis, lymphangitis, and terminal osteomyelitis.

Necrosis, even without overt infection, develops when sutures are too tight and not removed in time.

Permanent residual defects may be caused by the surgery (e.g. after tumors or trauma), or result from one of the complications. However, recurrence is the worst complication in tumor surgery. Defects of a certain size cannot be reconstructed to give a completely normal nail; function of the finger tip is more important than cosmesis in these circumstances.

Stiffening of the distal interphalangeal joint is common. Most patients hold the operated finger stubbornly extended, even though they are told to keep it in physiologic flexion. Prolonged splinting is another cause.

SUMMARY

Once a good knowledge of the nail organ's anatomy, physiology and pathology is present, nail surgery is no longer a difficult task. It requires, however, some imagination because many lesions, particularly nail tumors, will lead to defects and/or situations that are novel. In addition, finely honed surgical skills are mandatory.

Diagnostic nail biopsies for histopathologic examination are the gold standard for making a sound diagnosis. Nail avulsions are very rarely indicated and necessary. Ingrown nails require treatment according to their pathogenesis. Reactive lesions and benign tumors are not rare and can usually be operated with excellent functional and cosmetic results. The treatment of choice for malignant nail tumors is microscopically controlled surgery.

REFERENCES

1. Baran R, Dawber RPR, de Berker DAR, Haneke E, Tosti A. Baran and Dawber's diseases of the nails and their management, 3rd edn. Oxford: Blackwell; 2001:425–514.
2. Dumontier C, ed. L'Ongle. Monographie Soc Franç Chir Main (GEM) Amsterdam: Elsevier 2000; 27:226–235.
3. Krull E, Baran R, Zook E, Haneke E. Nail surgery: a text and atlas. New York: Lippincott Williams & Wilkins; 2001.
4. Chiu DT. Transthecal digital block: flexor tendon sheath used for anesthetic infusion. J Hand Surg 1990; 15:371–377.
5. Harbison S. Transthecal digital block: flexor tendon sheath used for anaesthetic infusion. J Hand Surg 1991; 16:557.
6. Sarhadi NS, Shaw-Dunn J. Transthecal digital nerve block. An anatomical appraisal. J Hand Surg 1998; 23:490–493.
7. Castellanos J, Ramirez C, De Sena L, Bertran C. Transthecal digital block: digital anaesthesia through the sheath of the flexor tendon. J Bone Joint Surg Br 2000; 82:689.
8. Haneke E. Nail surgery. Eur J Dermatol 2000; 10:237–241.
9. Haneke E. Exzisions und Biopsieverfahren. Z Hautkr 1988; 63(suppl):17–19.

10. Haneke E. Operative Therapie akraler und subungualer Melanome. In: Rompel R, Petres J (eds). Operative und onkologische Dermatologie. Fortschritte der operativen und onkologischen Dermatologie. Berlin: Springer; 1999; 15:210–214.
11. Cordero CFA. Ablación ungueal : su uso en la onycomicosis. Dermatol Int 1965; 14:21.
12. Baran R. More on avulsion of nail plate. J Dermatol Surg Oncol 1981; 7:854
13. Andrus CH. Instrument and technique for removal of subungual foreign bodies. Am J Surg 1980; 140:588.
14. Dagnall JC. The history, development and current status of nail matrix phenolisation. Chiropodist 1981; 36:315–324.
15. Haneke E. Surgical treatment of ingrown toenails. Cutis 1986; 37:251–256.
16. Thomsen RJ, Zuehlke RL Beckman BL. Pachyonychia congenita. Surgical management of the nail changes. J Dermatol Surg Oncol 1982; 8:24
17. Haneke E. Behandlung einiger Nagelfehlbildungen. In: Wolff HH, Schmeller W, eds. Fehlbildungen, Nävi, Melanome. Berlin: Springer Verlag; 1985:71–77.
18. Haneke E. Pathogenese-orientierte Behandlung eingewachsener Zehennägel und des angeborenen Nagelschiefstandes bei Kindern. In: Burg G, Hartmann AA, Konz B, eds. Onkologische Dermatologie. Neue Aspekte, altersbedingte Besonderheiten. Fortschritte der operativen und onkologischen Dermatologie. Berlin: Springer; 1992; 7:243–245.
19. Rufli T, von Schultheiss A, Itin P. Congenital hypertrophy of the lateral nail folds of the hallux. Dermatology 1992; 184:296–297.
20. Baran R, Bureau H. Congenital malalignment of the big toe-nail as a cause of ingrowing toe-nail in infancy. Pathology and treatment (a study of thirty cases). Clin Exp Dermatol 1983; 8:619–623.
21. Baran R, Haneke E. Etiology and treatment of nail malalignment. Dermatol Surg 1998; 24:719–721.
22. Arai H, Arai T, Nakajima H, Haneke E. Formable acrylic treatment for ingrowing nail with gutter splint and sculptured nail. J Dermatol 2004; 43:759–765.
23. Wallace WA, Milne DD, Andrew T. Gutter treatment for ingrowing toenails. Br Med J 1973; 2:168–171.
24. Mori H, Umeda T, Nishioka K, Iida H, Aoki K, Yokoyama A. Ingrown nails: a comparison of the nail matrix phenolization method with the elevation of the nail bed-periosteal flap procedure. Dermatol 1998; 25:1–4.
25. Howard WR. Ingrown toenail, its surgical treatment. N Y Med J 1893:579.
26. Haneke E. Etiopathogénie et traitement de l'hypercourbure transversale de l'ongle du gros orteil. J Méd Esth Chir Dermatol 1992; 19:123–127.
27. Baran R. Removal of the proximal nail fold. Why, when, how? J Dermatol Surg Oncol 1986; 12:234–236.
28. Haneke E. Operative therapie der myxoiden Pseudozyste. In: Haneke E, ed. Gegenwärtiger stand der operativen dermatologie. Fortschritte der operativen Dermatologie. Berlin: Springer; 1988:221–227.
29. Haneke E. Epidermoid carcinoma (Bowen's disease) of the nail simulating acquired ungual fibrokeratoma. Skin Cancer 1991; 6:217–221.
30. Haneke E, Bragadini LA, Mainusch O. Enfermedad de Bowen de células claras del aparato ungular. Act Terap Dermatol 1997; 20:311–313.
31. Baran R, Haneke E, Drapé J-L, Zook EG. Tumours of the nail apparatus and adjacent tissues. In: Baran R, Dawber RPR, de Berker DAR, Haneke E, Tosti A. Baran and Dawber's diseases of the nails and their management. 3rd edn. Oxford: Blackwell; 2001:515–630.
32. Haneke E, Baran R. Nail surgery. In: Harahap M, ed. Complications in dermatologic surgery. Springer, Berlin: 1993; 84–91.
33. Barfod B. Reconstruction of the nail fold. Hand 1972; 4:85–87.
34. Hayes CW. One-stage nail fold reconstriction. Hand 1974; 6:74–75.
35. Asbjörn BF, Basse P. Surgical relocation of retracted eponychion. Acta Chir Plast 1991; 33:110–113.

46 Leg Ulcer Management

Carlos A Charles MD, Anna F Falabella MD, and
Adolfo C Fernández-Obregón MD

Summary box

- Most leg ulcers are the result of venous disease, arterial disease, neuropathy, or a combination of these three.
- A careful medical history and thorough physical examination is critical to the diagnosis and management of leg ulcers.
- Compression therapy is the mainstay of venous ulcer treatment.
- Bacterial colonization of chronic wounds may not adversely affect healing and need not be treated as an infection in most situations.
- Moist wound healing is better than dry wound healing.
- Advanced wound bed preparation and appropriate debridement are essential elements of many wound healing approaches.

INTRODUCTION

Leg ulcers result from chronic lower extremity wounds that fail to heal, causing pain and social discomfort. With an ever-increasing aging population, it is estimated that the cost of managing venous ulcers alone, which account for 80% of leg ulcers, is $1 billion per year in the US. The average cost for one patient over a lifetime exceeds $40 000.[1] Leg ulcers may originate from a wide variety of causes (Table 46.1).[2–4] In the vast majority, leg ulcers are the result of venous disease, arterial disease, neuropathy, or a combination of these three. Venous insufficiency is by far the most common cause of leg ulcers. This chapter will attempt to define the most commonly encountered leg ulcers, describe the methods used to evaluate these ulcers, and propose appropriate therapy. An understanding of the principles of treatment of leg ulcers is essential and can help a clinician in applying sound methods to treat the more esoteric ulcers.

Some venous ulcers become chronic wounds after a nonhealing period of 2 months. The term chronic wound is used to define not only nonhealing ulcers of long duration, but also ulcers where many local factors impair healing, including the presence of foreign bodies, tissue maceration, ischemia, or other hemodynamic changes in the microcirculation. An increase in bacterial burden and colonization that can lead to frank infection is often present. Additionally, other factors that may play active roles in nonhealing include malnutrition, diabetes mellitus, renal disease, and hematological or other systemic illnesses. Recent developments in the understanding of wound healing have identified certain clinical settings responsible for the chronic wound. There may be a lack of tissue growth factors, such as platelet-derived growth factors, and transforming growth factor-beta (TGF-β) compared with acute wounds. An imbalance between proteolytic enzymes and their inhibitors can result from overexpression of matrix metalloproteins, resulting in abnormal degradation of the extracellular matrix. Finally, the persistence of senescent fibroblasts that fail to respond to growth factors and other stimulating agents may be important in leading to chronic wounds.[5] Therapies aimed at restoring the normal environment in the wound can set the scene for proper wound healing.

A listing of various types of leg ulcers and their relative frequency is given in Table 46.2,[6,7] which lists specific clinical entities associated with each major category of leg ulcers. An excellent and more complete discussion on the subject of diabetic ulcers can be found in Levin and O'Neal's *The Diabetic Foot*.[8]

Etiology

Venous ulcers

Venous ulcers account for about 80% of all lower leg wounds.[9–11] Although it is known that chronic venous insufficiency is often the cause of venous ulceration, the exact mechanism by which ulcers result is not known, and continues to be the subject of widespread speculation. Gay[12] and Homans[13] made a connection between deep vein damage and ulceration. Under normal ambulatory conditions, the calf muscles serve to pump the blood back up to the heart. Without adequate use of calf muscles, blood that

Table 46.1 Causes of leg ulcers[2–4]

Category	Condition
Venous	Vein thrombosis, venous incompetence, varicose veins, venous stasis, lipodermatosclerosis, complication of sclerotherapy
Arterial	Arterial obstruction, atherosclerosis, thromboangiitis obliterans, cholesterol embolism, arteriovenous malformation, hemangioma, hypertensive ulcer, complication of sclerotherapy
Microcirculation	Diabetic microangiopathy, vasculitis
Neuropathic	Diabetes mellitus, Hansen's disease, tabes dorsalis, syringomyelia, spina bifida, paraplegia, amyotrophic lateral sclerosis, other neuropathic disorders
Hematologic	Sickle cell disease, thalassemia, hereditary spherocytosis, polycythemia vera, leukemia, dysproteinemias, disseminated intravascular coagulation, idiopathic thrombocytopenia, chronic graft versus host disease, acquired homocystinuria, warfarin necrosis, heparin necrosis
Immunologic	Bullous pemphigoid, cicatricial pemphigoid, pemphigus, epidermolysis bullosa acquisita, linear IgA bullous dermatosis, erythema multiforme, allergic contact dermatitis
Infectious	Erythema induratum/nodular vasculitis, mycotic, bacterial, leishmania, herpes
Metabolic	Diabetes mellitus, gout, pretibial myxedema, Gaucher's disease, prolidase deficiency, porphyria cutanea tarda, necrobiosis lipoidica, bullous diabeticorum, diabetic dermopathy, drugs
Renal	Kyrle's disease, reactive perforating collagenosis, calciphylaxis
Nutritional	Scurvy, malnutrition
Genetic diseases	Epidermolysis bullosa, Werner's syndrome, Klinefelter's syndrome
Neoplastic	Basal cell carcinoma, squamous cell carcinoma, keratoacanthoma, malignant melanoma, Kaposi's sarcoma, malignant eccrine poroma, angiosarcoma, cutaneous metastasis, cutaneous lymphoma
Chemical/physical	Caustic agents, decubitus ulcers, thermal injury, mechanical trauma, radiation, frostbite, factitial, Charcot's deformity, chronic osteomyelitis, insect bites, coral and marine life-induced ulcers
Lymphatic disease	Lymphedema, lymphangioma,
Other	Pyoderma gangrenosum, panniculitis, Raynaud's disease

Table 46.2 Types of leg ulcers[6,7]

Ulcer Type	Percentage of presenting ulcers
Venous	80
Arterial	5
Diabetic/neuropathic	2
Pressure	5–20*
Microcirculation	<2
Hematologic	<2
Infectious	<2
Metabolic	<2
Neoplastic	<2
Physical/chemical	<2
Immunologic	<2
Other	<2

**Includes all anatomic locations*

collects in the saphenous venous system and its tributaries cannot make its way swiftly out of the deep veins, and is transmitted instead to the cutaneous vasculature. This all leads to chronic venous hypertension.[14–16] Microcirculatory changes associated with chronic ulcers, diabetes, and repeated bouts of previous vessel damage lead to fibrin cuffs, seen histologically around dermal vessels, which result in impaired cutaneous nutrition, and ultimately ulceration.[17] The action of neutrophils adhering to tissue damaged by ambulatory venous hypertension releases highly reactive substances, which generate free radicals, and subsequently cause tissue injury.[18]

The exact mechanism by which ulcers result from this long series of events is unknown. The 'trap' hypothesis suggests that venous hypertension causes fibrinogen and other macromolecules to leak into the dermis, and trap or bind growth factors, making them unavailable for tissue repair.[19] More recently, the entrapment of activated white cells with their release of activated inflammatory mediators has been thought to play a major role.[20] The 'cuff' hypothesis proposes that the leaked fibrinogen in the dermis polymerizes to form pericapillary fibrin cuffs, forming a barrier to the diffusion of oxygen and other nutrients, and leading to microvascular ischemia.[21] Another theory proposes that dermal fibroblasts from venous ulcers become unresponsive to the action of wound healing mediators and serve to undermine the healing process.[22] It is possible that minor trauma may also play a role in the ulceration process. Up to 50% of patients with chronic venous insufficiency have a history of leg injury.[23] Venous ulcers exude copious drainage—a greenish-yellowish fibrinopurulent adherent exudate may be seen at the base of the ulcer, which may be highly irregular in shape. Superinfection, pain, and malodorous drainage may ensue (Fig. 46.1A).

Chronic lower extremity swelling, often mistaken as originating from cardiac, hepatic, and renal disease leads to varicosities. Erythrocytes extravasate into the dermis under pressure and leave behind hemosiderin deposits in the skin or cayenne pepper purpura. A pruritic rash often appears leading to excoriations and further dermal staining with melanophages as a postinflammatory event. The topical agents used to try to keep it under check often aggravate this venous dermatitis. Further acute inflammation produces a panniculitis, which becomes more sclerotic with time, leading to lipodermatosclerosis (Fig. 46.2). The latter, as proposed by Browse et al., results from high venous pressure leading to endothelial leakage of fibrinogen, resulting in the formation of the pericapillary fibrin cuff and eventual venous ulceration.[17,24] Additionally, dystrophic calcium deposits sometimes develop.

Arterial ulcers

Arterial disease results from the narrowing of the vessel lumen by the accumulation of cholesterol plaques and other tissue debris. The resulting obstruction leads to the development of collateral circulation. Risk factors for arteriosclerotic occlusion are diabetes, smoking, hyperlipidemia, hypertension, obesity, and age.[25–27]

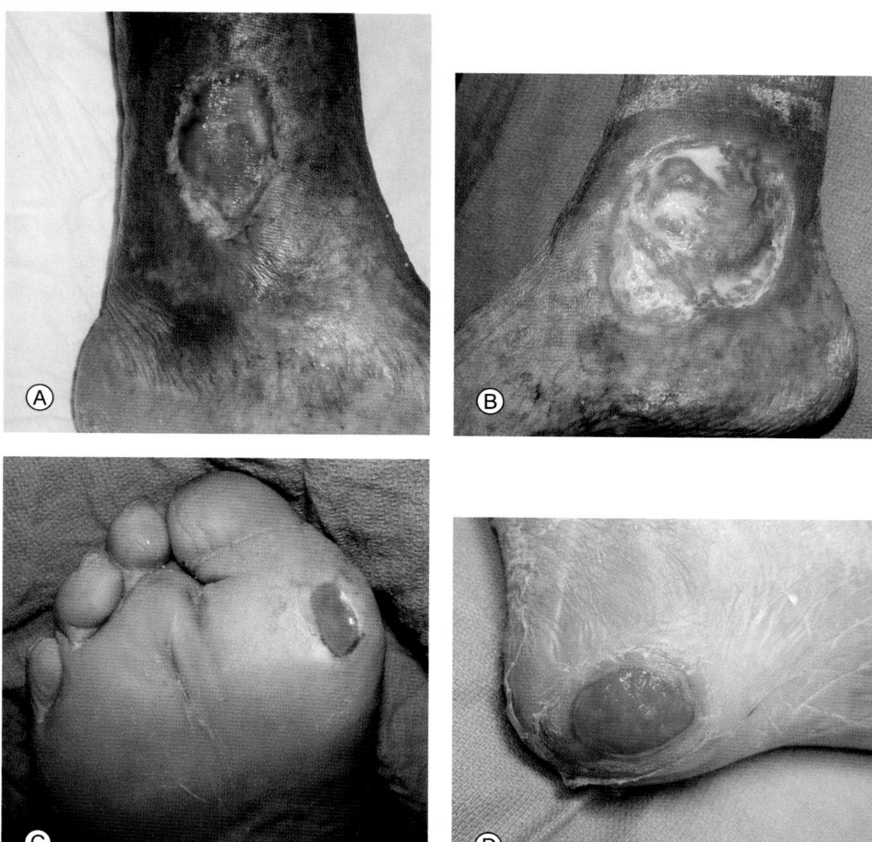

Figure 46.1 The most common leg ulcers. (A) A venous leg ulcer on the medial malleolus of a patient, with characteristic scattered varicosities and hyperpigmentation of the periwound skin. (B) Classic 'punched out' appearance of an arterial ulcer with copious yellow fibrinous exudates and poor granulation tissue. (C) Plantar diabetic foot ulcer. (D) Pressure ulcer overlying the bony prominence of the heel.

Figure 46.2 Diffuse hyperpigmentation associated with the indurated skin characteristic of lipodermatosclerosis.

Arteriosclerotic occlusion usually affects the entire femoropopliteal trajectory including important distal branches (anterior peroneal, anterior tibial, and posterior tibial), and may lead to significant distal damage. It may also affect only small-sized branches, leading to limited skin and subcutaneous tissue infarction. Clinically, patients experience pain or aching in the calves when walking (intermittent claudication), often relieved by rest. Pain tends to be severe and debilitating. On physical examination there may be loss of hair, atrophy, cold surrounding skin, and thickened toenails. Peripheral pulses may be palpable, barely palpable, or absent. Capillary refill time is usually prolonged. Typically, arterial ulcers are located over pressure points, such as the toes and ankles. The ulcer is sharply demarcated with little granulation tissue. It tends to have a punched out appearance (Fig. 46.1B). The wound bed often has a necrotic appearing base. Large occlusions require surgical intervention through revascularization by means of bypasses either using the patient's own veins or artificial vein grafts, or by means of intravascular procedures such as balloon dilatation (percutaneous transluminal angioplasty), sometimes combined with thrombolysis and the placement of stents.

Diabetic ulcers

Diabetes accounts for over 50% of lower extremity amputations in the US. Approximately 85% of all diabetes-related lower extremity amputations are preceded by foot ulcers.[28,29] Ulcers from diabetes occur as neuropathic or ischemic. Although a mixture of each can occur, most patients will exhibit a preponderance of one type. Patients may display other cutaneous markings of diabetes, such as necrobiosis lipoidica diabeticorum, diabetic dermopathy, or diabetic bullae. The most characteristic lesion of the diabetic foot is a mal perforans ulceration (Fig. 46.1C).[30] The neuropathic ulcer is essentially a pressure ulcer resulting from the individual's loss of sensation. It is indistinguishable from the neurotrophic ulcers seen in leprosy, tabes dorsalis, and other neurological syndromes. The ulcer is most characteristically over the pressure points such as the first and fifth metatarsal heads, and the great toes. It is classically well circumscribed, with a surrounding halo of hard callus-like material. The foot involved may have a normal color and even strong arterial pulses. Touch, pressure, and proprioception are diminished or lost. Motor and autonomic nerves may also be involved. Weakening muscles may also lead to toe and foot deformities. Loss of sweating may lead to fissuring and a Charcot foot can develop.

Pressure ulcers

Pressure ulcers have a prevalence of 5–20% in acute care hospitals, and approximately 8% in the domiciliary setting, 15% in nursing homes, and up to 35% in extended care facilities.[31] Immobility is a necessary condition for pressure ulcer development, and therefore, the most significant risk factor. Impaired nutritional states, along with hypoalbuminemia and immobility, can lead to epidermal moisture vapor loss, which causes maceration and then a breakdown of the stratum corneum barrier, rendering the skin more permeable to noxious agents and trauma. Fecal incontinence, and even slight pressure over skin overlying bony prominences, such as the heel or the malleoli of the ankles, can cause enough injury under these conditions to start the process that leads eventually to a pressure ulcer (Fig. 46.1D). Naturally, other causes of pressure ulcers need to be excluded, such as venous stasis, arterial insufficiency, diabetes, neuropathy, vasculitis, systemic lupus erythematosus, drug allergies, neoplasm, sickle cell disease and other hematological abnormalities, polycythemia, pyoderma gangrenosum, bacterial and fungal infections, and trauma.[32]

Inflammatory ulcers

Many diseases can lead to leg ulcers. A broad category that excludes venous, arterial, pressure, and diabetic ulcers as well as the ulcers resulting from neoplasms is the inflammatory ulcer. Kerdel, and Paquette and Falanga offer an excellent review of the subject.[33,34] One major subcategory is the vasculitis ulcer resulting from small vessel thrombi or emboli. Lesions beginning as palpable purpura can lead to vesicles and pustules. The process involving immune complexes, much like an Arthus reaction, sets off the inflammatory cascade, eventuating in the release of vasoactive amines and other mediators. These mediators serve to amplify the process with the deposition of more immune complexes, leading ultimately to an ischemic area, cutaneous necrosis, and ultimately an ulcer.

A group of conditions involve dermal thrombi in the absence of vasculitis. They include thrombotic thrombocytopenia purpura, disseminated intravascular coagulation, cryoglobulinemia, cryofibrinogenemia, purpura fulminans, coumadin necrosis, and the antiphospholipid syndrome (also known as the lupus anticoagulant syndrome). Individuals with this syndrome may or may not have lupus erythematosus. These patients possess antibodies (IgG or IgM) that interfere with the conversion of prothrombin to thrombin. In the laboratory they have a prolonged activated partial thromboplastin time. Some may have a prolongation of the prothrombin time. (The Russel viper venom time, and Exner's test may also be helpful.) The lesions are purpuric, leading to ischemia and ulceration. Livedo reticularis may be seen. There is no frank vasculitis. Lesions are often painful and heal with atrophic scars (atrophie blanche).[33]

Wound repair physiology

The process of normal wound healing can be looked upon as an integration of multiple dynamic, interactive processes involving soluble mediators, formed blood elements and blood cells, an extracellular matrix, and parenchymal cells. In the simplest terms, this process is generally described as occurring in three main phases—inflammation, proliferation and tissue formation, and tissue remodeling. Each phase is characterized by a number of complex intercellular interactions. It is important to note that these phases do not represent separate and distinct events, but are continual and overlapping .

Over the past few years investigators have begun to understand how cells interact between themselves and the extracellular matrix in the wound healing process.[35] The clinical utility of understanding wound healing physiology is potentially far reaching. By understanding the normal processes, investigators and clinicians alike can apply targeted therapeutic modalities in an attempt to achieve wound closure in refractory wounds. The following section briefly reviews the normal physiology of tissue repair and serves as a framework for the information concerning nonhealing leg ulcers and therapeutic modalities for wound management, which will subsequently be described in detail.

Phase 1: inflammation

The first phase of normal wound healing begins immediately after an acute injury, and can last for 24–48 hours. This phase is characterized by the disruption of blood vessels, which leads to a local release of blood cells and blood-borne elements. The main cellular constituent of the inflammatory phase of tissue repair is the platelet, which initiates clotting of the acute wound by both intrinsic and extrinsic pathways. Platelets release a number of chemoattractant factors, which recruit other platelets, leukocytes, endothelial cells, and fibroblasts to the wound area. The inflammatory phase progresses with the addition of neutrophils and macrophages, which acutely debride the wound by scavenging cellular debris and killing bacteria, leading to the second phase of healing (Table 46.3 and Fig. 46.3).

Phase 2: proliferation and tissue formation

The second phase of wound healing is characterized by proliferation and tissue formation and begins approximately 72 hours after injury. This phase can last up to several weeks. In this phase, the keratinocyte plays the primary role in the tissue repair process and undergoes significant changes in morphology and function, allowing for its migration over the wound bed to provide coverage. Additionally, the keratinocyte releases a number of chemokines, which stimulate cellular migration and other key cellular functions, leading to eventual reconstitution of the epidermis and the basement membrane.

The latter segment of the second phase of wound healing is characterized by the formation of granulation tissue. Fibroblasts are instrumental in the reconstitution of the dermal matrix, termed fibroplasia, while endothelial cells play an integral role in the development of new blood vessels, known as angiogenesis. Additionally, the extracellular matrix, with its collection of proteins, growth factors, and enzymes plays an active role in influencing the keratinocytes, fibroblasts, and endothelial cells.

Phase 3: tissue remodeling

The final phase of wound healing, tissue remodeling, begins at the same time as the onset of cellular proliferation and tissue formation. This phase can last several months after the acute injury. This phase is one of gradual physiologic evolution and is characterized by heterogeneous stages of healing throughout the wound; hence, the macromolecular physical composition of the wound margin can vary greatly, both quantitatively and qualitatively with that of the central wound bed. Over the course of this phase, granulation tissue becomes mature scar tissue. Several enzymes are involved in breaking down matrix components, whereas the fibro-

Cytokine	Major source	Target cells and major effects
Epidermal growth factor family		
Epidermal growth factor	Platelets	Pleiotropic—cell motility and proliferation
Transforming growth factor-α (TGF-α)	Macrophages, keratinocytes	Pleiotropic—cell motility and proliferation
Heparin-binding epidermal growth factor	Macrophages	Pleiotropic—cell motility and proliferation
Fibroblast growth factor (FGF) family		
Basic FGF	Macrophages, endothelial cells	Angiogenesis and fibroblast proliferation
Acidic FGF	Macrophages, endothelial cells	Angiogenesis and fibroblast proliferation
Keratinocyte growth factor (KGF)	Fibroblasts	Epidermal cell motility and proliferation
Transforming growth factor-β (TGF-β) family		
TGF-β1 and β2	Platelets, macrophages	Epidermal cell motility, chemotaxis of macrophages and fibroblasts, extracellular matrix synthesis and remodeling
Transforming growth factor β3	Macrophages	Antiscarring effects
Other		
Platelet-derived growth factor (PDGF)	Platelets, macrophages, keratinocytes	Angiogenesis and increased vascular permeability
Vascular endothelial growth factor (VEGF)	Keratinocytes, macrophages	Angiogenesis and increased vascular permeability
Tumor necrosis factor-α	Neutrophils	Pleiotropic expression of growth factors
Interleukin-1	Neutrophils	Pleiotropic expression of growth factors
Insulin-like growth factor I	Fibroblasts, epidermal cells	Re-epithelialization and granulation tissue formation
Colony stimulating factor I	Multiple cells	Macrophage activation and granulation tissue formation

Table 46.3 Cytokines and other factors involved in inflammatory phase of wound healing

With permission from Singer AJ, Clark RA. Cutaneous wound healing. N Engl J Med 1999; 341:738–746.[35]

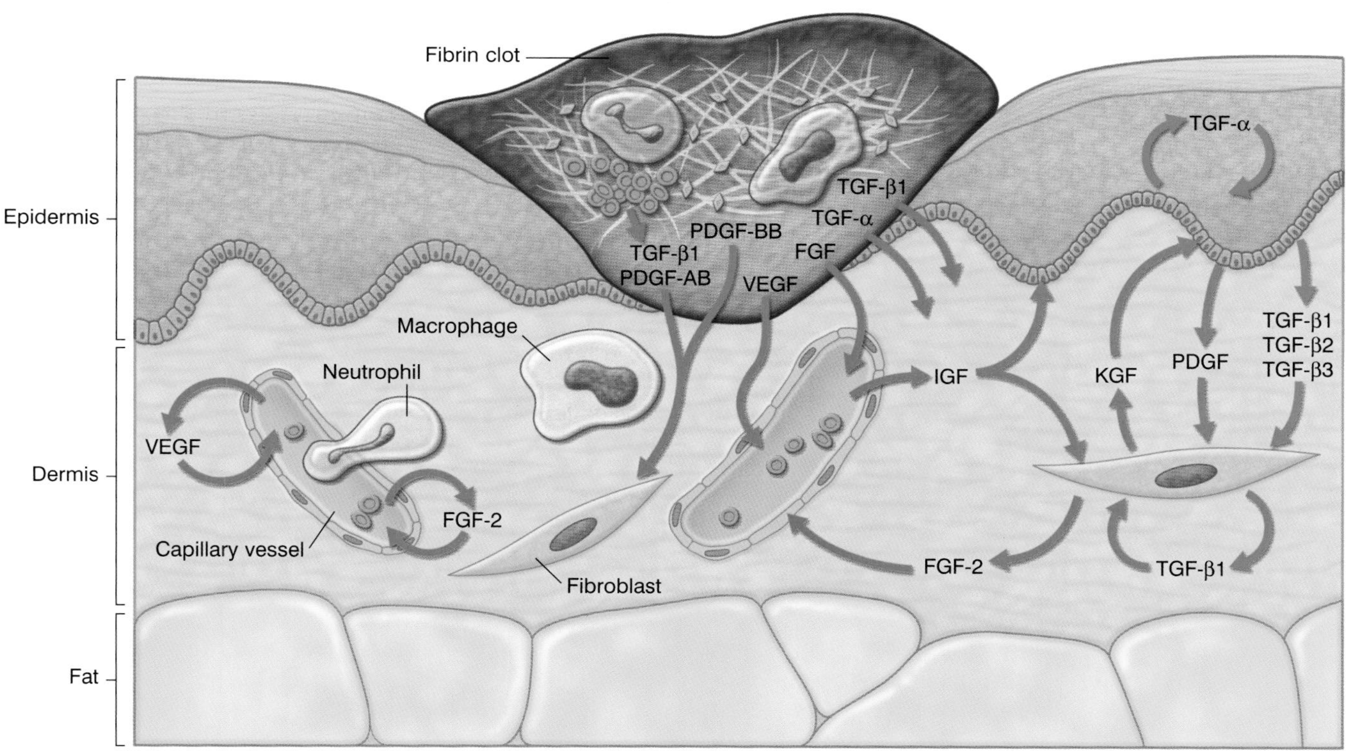

Figure 46.3 A diagrammatic representation of the key events during the inflammatory phase of normal wound healing. (FGF and FGF-2, fibroblast growth factors; IGF, insulin-like growth factor; KGF, keratinocyte growth factor; PDGF, PDGF-AB and -BB, platelet-derived growth factors; TGF-α, -β1, -β2 and -β3, transforming growth factors; VEGF, vascular endothelial growth factor.

blasts produce substances such as fibronectin, hyaluronic acid, proteoglycans, and collagen, to ultimately restore the functional barrier of the skin and increase the tensile strength of the scar. Each of these components plays an important role in the wound healing process. Fibronectin acts as a matrix for cellular migration, as scaffolding for collagen deposition, and as a linkage for myofibroblasts to aid in wound contraction. Hyaluronic acid stimulates wound maturation by promoting cell migration and division.[36] Proteoglycans increase tissue strength, modify collagen deposition, and help to modulate cellular function.[37] Last, collagen is essential for providing structural support and tensile strength, while also playing an important role in the regulation of cellular function. In summary, the tissue-remodeling phase of wound healing is an evolving series of cellular events characterized by extracellular matrix formation, which should result in complete wound maturation and scar formation.

FRAIL (For Recognition of Adult Immobilized Life)

The demographics of the American population are shifting dramatically toward a majority of persons over the age of 65 years. Currently there are almost 34 million Americans aged 65 years or over. This number will grow to over 69 million (20% of the population) by the year 2030. Current average life expectancy for persons living in the US is over 76 years of age.[38]

With a constantly growing aging population, the profile of a newly recognized patient emerges. Many suffer with chronic wounds that fail to progress through an orderly and timely sequence of repair.

To study this population and address their needs, an interdisciplinary group of healthcare professionals from different parts of the country undertook the task of defining 'the FRAIL' patient, and start the process of establishing guidelines for the medical management of these patients. The consensus expressed by the group upheld the belief that the traditionally held endpoint of therapy, the total healing of a wound, may not be appropriate for many of these patients. Palliative measures to keep patients comfortable, pain free, and with wounds that are nonodorous and simple to manage may be just as important, and an acceptable treatment strategy.

Palliative care is a philosophy of care that focuses on providing support for the physical, emotional, social, and spiritual needs of patients. These concepts have value to patients long before death is imminent, or a terminal illness has been diagnosed. Palliative care is best used at the onset of diagnosis and throughout the disease course, and objectives evolve as the disease and patient's preferences change. Palliative care focuses on managing symptoms such as pain, losses to independence, mobility, and degradation of self-image.

The FRAIL Committee report addressed communication and information-sharing techniques, preventive odor management in wounds, and detection and treatment of depression, anxiety, and delirium. As this newly recognized patient population continues to grow, there will be a growing need for specific pharmaceutical products, and medical devices. A plan for continuous education for the public and health professional is needed.[39]

Patients sometimes display a stoic and highly resolved preference to refuse treatment for conditions that deserve aggressive intervention. Not surprisingly, this can include leg ulcers. If left untreated, they can become a chronic source of infection, which can lead to sepsis with the potential for a fatal outcome. Approaching the problem with true concern and compassion is essential, ensuring the dignity of the patient is protected. Understanding a person's right to refuse treatment must be carefully balanced with the proper medical management of the patient. Reasons given for refusing treatment may be based on unfounded fears and concerns, which can be dispelled or minimized once they have been revealed. Very often this illuminating step is all it takes to obtain the patient's cooperation. Psychiatric evaluation may be necessary if the patient is adamant about refusing care. If all else fails, local adult protective services may need to be summoned to assist in the final disposition of the case.

■ PREOPERATIVE PREPARATION

Medical history

Taking a careful medical history is the beginning of evaluating leg ulcers. It is obvious that details surrounding the development of the ulcer with an emphasis on duration, and progression should be determined as well as the presence or absence of pain, and whether certain activities such as walking or leg elevation change the character of pain. Venous ulcer pain is often described as a burning pain. Although pain is generally more common with arterial disease, it may occur in venous ulceration. Ankle swelling may occur. There is often a history of trauma, a family history of phlebitis or varicose veins, and in general a family tendency of thrombophilia.[40]

Race as a factor may be important, as noted in sickle cell disease, hereditary spherocytosis, and thalassemia. Habits such as cigarette smoking may add to the risk of arterial impairment and venous thrombosis. Alcohol abuse, often associated with poor nutrition, may directly affect wound healing. A history of nutritional deficiencies, metabolic disorders, diabetes, hypertension, antiphospholipid syndrome, periarteritis nodosa, pyoderma gangrenosum, atherosclerotic heart disease, and even pregnancy may all serve as aggravating factors. Prior history of collagen vascular disease can lead to vasculitis, which can give rise to an ulcer. The ulcer of pyoderma gangrenosum (Fig. 46.4) may herald or follow inflammatory bowel disease, collagen vascular disease, or a lymphoproliferative disorder. Living or having lived in areas where certain endemic diseases are prevalent, such as Hansen's disease, can predispose the patient to the neurotrophic ulcer on the foot, which can be a late stage manifestation of leprosy.

Travel history to the tropics or semi-arid areas can expose travelers to certain insects, whose bite can lead to myiasis, and the sand fly, which can be responsible for transmitting leishmaniasis. Precipitating factors, such as trauma, are often noted as leading to the development of factitial or neurotrophic ulcers.

Taking a careful medication history is critical for the overall evaluation of any patient. Topical medication can often lead to allergic or irritant contact dermatitis, which can be the initiating event in the formation of a leg ulcer. Antibiotics, such as neomycin, and anesthetics, such as

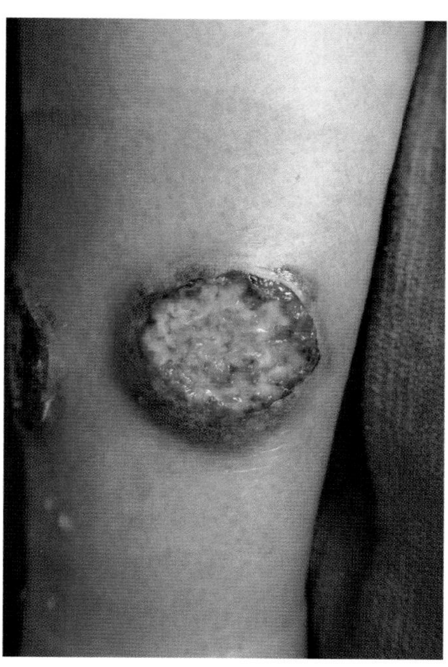

Figure 46.4 Rolled purple-colored edges of a leg ulcer secondary to pyoderma gangrenosum.

benzocaine, and even parabens used as preservatives in widely used topical preparations, can cause an acute eruption.[41]

Oral medication, such as corticosteroids, anticoagulants, antineoplastic agents, cyclosporin A, colchicine, nonsteroidal anti-inflammatory drugs, penicillamine, and salicylates can impair wound healing and contribute indirectly to leg ulcers. With the public's growing awareness of alternative medicines, the popular use of herbal products necessitates physicians to inquire whether these products, regarded by patients as innocent, are being taken orally or being applied in topical preparations.[42–44]

Physical examination

Among the initial impressions, odor may impress the examiner before the patient disrobes or reveals the pathology. The smell may emanate from wound contamination, or may be more specific to the type of ulcer, and severity of infection.

The general appearance should include observation of skin color, dryness, or swelling. Pulses need to be palpated on the skin over the femoral, popliteal, dorsalis pedis, and posterior tibial arteries. Neuropathy should be excluded by a light touch sensation in the great toe. Ulcer size, shape, and border description should be noted. Scars may suggest previous ulcer activity, in support of a chronic problem. Hyperpigmentation and hyperkeratosis along with microvaricosities at the sides of the ankles can be seen in cases of venous dermatitis. Cyanosis and dark colored toes can point to significant arterial deficiency of the distal parts of the extremity. Atrophic changes of the skin will lead to loss of hair and sweat glands, resulting in further skin dryness. Pressure ulcers can be seen over bony prominences, whereas diabetics will have ulcers on the plantar surface of the foot.

Induration and fibrosis of the dermis and underlying tissue can progress to give the lower leg an inverted champagne bottle shape, which is characteristic of chronic venous insufficiency, with a hard doughy to woody texture, known as lipodermatosclerosis. More specific findings are listed in Table 46.4.[40,45,46]

Diagnostic assessment

Although venous disease represents the most common etiology for leg ulceration, a thorough diagnostic assessment must be performed to ensure an accurate diagnosis before initiating treatment. Other common causes for leg ulcers include arterial and neuropathic disease, though the cause of leg ulcers is commonly multifactorial, and may include infectious, inflammatory, malignant, and connective tissue conditions. Simple diagnostic techniques can therefore be performed to help establish a proper diagnosis.

The presence of symptoms such as claudication or rest pain in more severe cases is characteristic of arterial insufficiency. In these patients, the ankle-to-brachial index (ABI), may help in detecting peripheral vascular disease (Fig. 46.5).

Table 46.4 Physical findings in leg ulcers[40,45,46]

Ulcer type	Type of pain	Location	Borders	Surrounding skin	Palpation
Venous	Aching, burning discomfort that increases when the leg is dependent and decreases when the leg is elevated	Medial malleoli; also the lateral and posterior aspect of the leg, close to perforating veins	Shaggy, shallow, irregular, serpiginous border, hemorrhagic edges, granulating	Hemosiderin, lipodermatosclerosis	Interstitial edema and pretibial edema
Arterial—six Ps—pulselessness, pain on paralysis, pallor, polar, punched out defect, pressure sites	Severe cramping pain made worse by elevation and relieved by dependency (claudication)	Pressure sites, bony prominences, toes	Punched-out defect, sharply demarcated border, poor granulation	Hair loss, atrophic shiny skin, leg is cold and pale, painful ulcer	Peripheral pulses absent, capillary refilling time prolonged, change in color with alteration of position
Neuropathic/diabetic	Tingling or burning of various intensity, increasing at night, and diminishing with exercise	Pressure sites, heel, toes, plantar metatarsal area	Punched-out defect, thick surrounding callus, often infected	Nonspecific, painless ulcer	Altered sensation of light touch, vibration, and pinprick

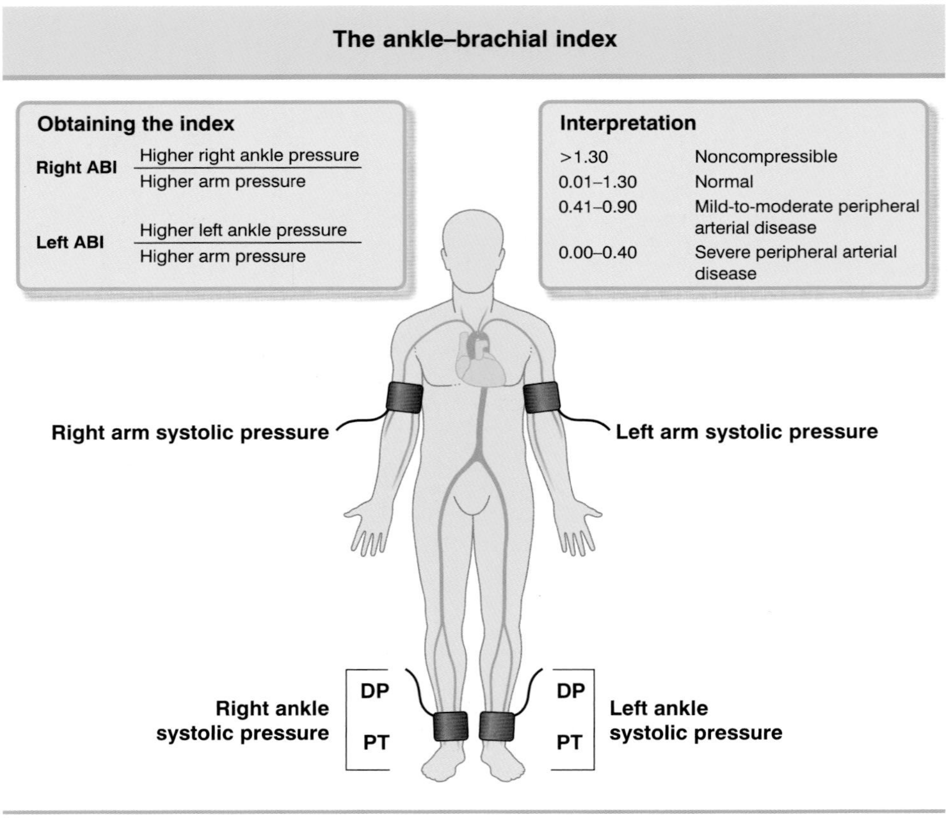

The ankle–brachial index

Obtaining the index

Right ABI = Higher right ankle pressure / Higher arm pressure

Left ABI = Higher left ankle pressure / Higher arm pressure

Interpretation

>1.30	Noncompressible
0.01–1.30	Normal
0.41–0.90	Mild-to-moderate peripheral arterial disease
0.00–0.40	Severe peripheral arterial disease

Right arm systolic pressure

Left arm systolic pressure

Right ankle systolic pressure

DP

PT

Left ankle systolic pressure

DP

PT

Figure 46.5 A diagrammatic representation illustrating important elements in obtaining and interpreting the ankle–brachial index (ABI). DP, dorsalis pedis; PT, posterior tibial.

The lower extremity systolic blood pressure can be measured at the bedside by placing a correctly sized cuff around the calf and inflating it to occlude the pedal arteries. When the pulse sounds are appreciated with Doppler ultrasonography after deflation of the blood pressure cuff, the ankle systolic pressure is obtained. This value is then compared with the highest brachial systolic pressure to determine the ABI. An ABI of 0.97 (see McGee and Boyko)[47] or higher is normal, whereas an ABI of 0.5 or less may indicate severe arterial disease.[48] Values less than 0.97 categorize people with peripheral artery disease with a sensitivity of 96–97% and a specificity of 94–100%.[47] False-positive results may occur in patients who are elderly or diabetic, thus a transcutaneous oxygen measurement may be preferred to assess arterial circulation in these subsets of patients. These assessments are critical because compression therapy, the mainstay noninvasive therapeutic modality for venous ulcers, can lead to worsening of an arterial ulcer, or even gangrene in a patient who has a significantly compromised peripheral arterial circulation.[49]

Infectious organisms may also be of etiological significance for acute or chronic lower extremity ulcers and should be suspected when chronic ulcers do not follow the usual course of healing observed with more common conditions. Tissue culture, particularly to identify fungal or atypical mycobacterial infections may help reveal the cause for nonhealing. Patients with underlying diseases resulting in immunosuppression may be predisposed to ulceration;[50] therefore, the clinician's index of suspicion for infection must be high for these patients.

If osteomyelitis is suspected clinically, radiography, nuclear bone scanning, and bone biopsy should be considered (Table 46.5).[3,51] Although the incidence of osteomyelitis in chronic ulcers is unknown, a prospective trial in diabetic foot ulcers found that probing of sinuses and deep ulcers was a highly sensitive method for detecting bone infection.[49] If bone is palpable at the ulcer base, with no intervening soft tissue, osteomyelitis is probable, and further diagnostic investigation is recommended.

Independent of the suspected cause, a wound present for more than 6 weeks warrants a biopsy to exclude malignancy within the wound.[52] Both basal cell and squamous cell carcinomas can occur in longstanding ulcers. The physical findings of basal cell carcinomas arising from venous ulcers include exuberant granulation tissue rolling onto the wound edges.[53]

Prevention

Although general good health is helpful in preventing leg ulcers, many common-sense issues should be considered. Good nutrition with a high protein intake and vitamin supplementation has been helpful in prevention as well as setting the stage for proper healing. Allman et al. demonstrated that pressure ulcer patients whose protein intake was greater than 590 mmol/day were significantly more likely to improve or to completely heal.[54] Taylor et al. have shown that oral vitamin C at 1000 mg daily plays a role in the healing of pressure ulcers.[55] Proper hygiene and control of urinary incontinence can improve the setting to prevent skin breakdown and avoid the onset of pressure ulcers. Use of pressure-relieving devices can help lighten the weightbearing effect on points over a bony prominence, the site of pressure ulcers. Control of infection is essential to avoid cutaneous damage that can extend ulcers or prevent their healing.

Table 46.5 Laboratory evaluation of leg ulcer patients[3,51]

Item	Reason
Elevated erythrocyte sedimentation rate (ESR)	To help diagnose osteomyelitis or collagen vascular disease
Vitamin A, vitamin C, trace elements, albumin, iron, transferrin, and zinc	To evaluate nutritional state, metabolic abnormality or hematologic disorder
Lupus anticoagulant, VDRL, anticardiolipin antibodies	To rule out the antiphospholipid syndrome
Serum cryoglobulins and plasma cryofibrinogen	Helpful in determining cryoglobulinemia, cryofibrinogenemia, and atrophie blanche
Evaluation of pain—noninvasive tests to determine vascular status—systolic pressure, Doppler flow meter, ABI, photoplethysmography, light reflex rheography, duplex ultrasound	Need to determine presence of arterial disease
Skin biopsy if no change in wound in 3 months	To rule out cutaneous malignancy, which may be easily treatable with excision; also helpful in determining cryoglobulinemia, cryofibrinogenemia, and atrophie blanche
Radiographs, bone scans, indium-labeled leukocyte scans, magnetic resonance imaging, and bone biopsy	To rule out osteomyelitis
Patch tests—sensitizing substances may aggravate the wound and impair healing—items tested should include: neomycin/soframycin/framycetin, bacitracin, gentamicin, quinoline mix, lanolin, formaldehyde, parabens, ethylene diamine, wood alcohol, propylene glycol, balsam of Peru, chinoform, and additives in bandages such as MBT, thiuram, colophony, and anything suspicious for causing dermatitis	To rule out contact dermatitis—identification of sensitizers is vital; withdrawing the offending agent is often sufficient to bring symptomatic relief of itching, pain, and inflammation
Laboratory screening tests for vasculitis	Urine analysis for proteinuria, hematuria; skin biopsy—hematoxylin and eosin, and immunohistopathology; ESR, complete blood count, liver function tests, renal function tests, antinuclear antibody, rheumatoid factor, complement C4, circulating immune complexes, paraproteins, immunoglobulin fractions, antineutrophil cytoplasmic antibodies, serological tests and cultures for underlying infection
Laboratory screening tests for clotting disorders	Activated partial thromboplastin time, prothombin time, thrombin time, Factor V (Leiden) mutation ($^{506}R \rightarrow {}^{506}Q$), Factor II (prothrombin) mutation ($^{20210}G \rightarrow {}^{20210}A$), antithrombin III, protein C and protein S, lupus anticoagulant, anticardiolipin

The best prevention for patients with recurrent venous ulcers is the wearing of a compression garment, which will prevent accumulation of fluid within the lower extremities.[56] Optimal compression is achieved by garments providing 30–40 mmHg. This serves to slow fluid accumulation, which plays such an important role in the pathogenesis of venous ulcers and in the sense of fatigue so frequently expressed by these patients. Measures to increase adherence to the use of compression garments include careful measuring and fitting of the compression stockings, and specific instructions with regard to stocking application. Additionally, patients with comorbidities such as obesity and arthritis, or aged patients may benefit from aids to assist with stocking application.[57] Proper fitting shoes that allow normal heel to toe walking can assist in comfortable walking, which is so essential to get the calf muscle pump to assist in eliminating fluid retention.

For patients with arterial ulcers, the reduction of risk factors responsible for the development of arteriosclerosis is crucial. In addition to age, sex, and race, the major controllable risk factors that should be closely managed include hyperlipidemia, hypertension, diabetes mellitus, and smoking.

Diabetics should avoid going barefoot, indoors or out. They should inspect their feet daily, and pay attention to the interdigital space, using mirrors to facilitate examination. The feet should be washed daily, after testing water temperature with the hand or elbow. Dryness of the skin, and especially the feet, should not go untreated. Women should avoid garters or elastics to hold up stockings and panty girdles that are tight around the legs. The feet should not be exposed to extremes such as very hot sand, water that is very hot, heating pads or hot water bottles, and heaters (including car heaters for long trips). Foot care should be carried out by a professional. Patients should avoid cutting calluses or using physical or chemical agents to reduce them. A podiatrist or other physician should inspect the foot twice a year. Sudden onset of a blister, sore, or puncture should be evaluated immediately by a physician.

For patients not requiring an orthotic or other shoe device to manage deformities and postsurgical care, only comfortable, well-fitting shoes should be used at all times. They should always be worn with socks, and ideally shoes should be changed several times a day. These shoes should have leather uppers that can mold to the shape of the feet. To ensure optimal comfort, new shoes should be bought late in the day. Shoes tried on early in the morning may feel too tight as the day goes by. Sandals and open-toe shoes should be avoided. To ensure integrity of the shoe, shoes should be inspected before wearing, and patients should be encouraged to bring in new shoes for inspection before they begin to wear them. Socks should be 100% cotton or blends of cotton. Wool can be worn, but not by those who get irritation from it. Socks should be free of wear and tear or holes, and should be changed daily.

It is a natural expectation that proper glucose control, proper nutritional diet, and avoidance of smoking are three major essential measures all diabetics must observe.

■ TECHNIQUES

Compression therapy

Graduated compression therapy is the standard first-line therapy of patients with venous leg ulcers. Patients who comply with compression therapy have improved healing rates, and continued compression after healing prevents recurrence.[58] Although most patients tolerate compression without adverse effects, care must be taken in patients with chronic heart failure because compression of the lower extremities can lead to an increase in preload volume and exacerbate their condition.

The exact pressure needed to overcome venous hypertension is not completely known, but an external pressure of 35–40 mmHg at the ankle is required to prevent capillary exudation in legs affected by venous disease.[59] Two types of compression bandages are commonly employed: inelastic and elastic bandages. The prototype rigid bandage is the Unna boot, a moist zinc oxide impregnated paste bandage that hardens to inelasticity.[60] These, rigid, inelastic bandages provide limited pressure at rest, but high pressure with muscle contraction during ambulation. The principal disadvantage of this compression method is that the Unna boot does not accommodate changes in the volume of the leg subsequent to compression and associated edema reduction; furthermore, it has limited absorptive capacity for highly exudative wounds, leading to potential periwound maceration. Thus, Unna boots require frequent reapplication. Rigid bandages such as the Unna boot may be useful to reduce the initial edematous phase commonly associated with venous ulcers.[61]

Alternatively, elastic compression bandages provide continual pressures and conform to the leg, subsequent to changes in leg volume. These elastic compression wraps supply high pressures both during ambulation and at rest. Their major disadvantage is that they require some degree of training for optimal application.[62] Elastic compression bandages are available as single or multilayer systems. A review of the literature with meta-analysis demonstrated that multilayer compression bandages seem to be superior to single-layer bandage systems.[59] A number of multilayer compression systems have been developed and are presently the mainstay of treatment for venous leg ulcers (Table 46.6).

Table 46.6 Compression systems for leg ulcers

Compression system	Brand name	Manufacturer
Unna boots (inelastic bandages)	Gelocast	Beiersdorf (Wilton, CT)
	Unna Flex	ConvaTec (Princeton, NJ)
	Viscopaste PB7	Smith & Nephew (Largo, FL)
	Primer Flexible Unna	Glenwood Inc (Tenafly, NJ)
	Unna Boot Bandage	Dynarex Corp (Brewster, NY)
	Tenderwrap	Kendall (Mansfield, MA)
Elastic bandages	SurePress	ConvaTec (Princeton, NJ)
	SetoPress	Seton Healthcare Group plc (Oldham, UK)
Multilayer bandages	Profore (four-layer)	Smith & Nephew (Largo, FL)
	Dynaflex (three-layer)	Johnson & Johnson (New Brunswick, NJ)
Tubular bandages and compression stockings	Jobst Stockings	Beiersdorf (Wilton, CT)
	TubiGrip	ConvaTec (Princeton, NJ)

The overall standard composition of multilayer compression bandages is as follows—a wool or cotton layer for absorption of exudate and padding, one or two elastic wraps, and a self-adherent wrap to hold all of the layers in place and to maintain the proper position of the bandage on the leg.[63] Multilayer compression systems can be tailored to fit a wide range of ankle circumferences, providing consistent pressures of 40–45 mmHg at the ankle and approximately 17 mmHg below the knee. Although three- or four-layer elastic compression bandages are initially more costly than single-layer bandages, they are cost-effective because they promote faster healing rates.[64] Compression therapy must be used judiciously in patients with concomitant cardiac failure as well as in patients with arterial insufficiency because both these conditions can potentially be exacerbated by lower extremity compression.

Treatment of venous ulcers with compression therapy should continue until the ulcers are healed. Subsequent to complete healing, patients should use graded compression stockings to prevent ulcer recurrence.[65] Specific instructions on the use of compression stockings may help to increase patient compliance. Additionally, aids to assist in the application of compression stocking have been developed. These devices greatly assist elderly, arthritic, or obese patients who can have difficulty in putting on stockings.

Pharmacologic therapy for venous ulcers

A number of medications have been studied for their role in increasing healing rates of venous ulcers. Aspirin has been associated with improved healing speed for venous ulcers. It is believed that aspirin's main mechanism of action here is through its anti-inflammatory action and its action on hemostatic mechanisms.[66] In one study, 20 subjects with chronic venous leg ulcers were randomized to daily enteric-coated aspirin (300 mg) or placebo, with standardized compression bandaging for both groups.[67] After 4 months of treatment, 38% of the patients receiving aspirin demonstrated healing compared with 0% of those receiving placebo ($P < 0.007$). Additionally, 52% of the aspirin-treated group showed a significant reduction in ulcer size compared with 26% of placebo recipients ($P < 0.007$); and reduction in ulcer surface area was significantly better in the aspirin-treated group at 2 ($P < 0.01$) and 4 months ($P < 0.002$) compared with that in the placebo group. Although these findings are promising, a larger sample size must be studied to make definitive conclusions.

Pentoxifylline, a methylxanthine derivative, has also been studied as a pharmacologic adjunct in the treatment of venous ulcers. Its mechanism of action may be due in part to its fibrinolytic properties, its ability to reduce leukocyte adhesion to the endothelium, and its antithrombotic effects.[68,69] The Cochrane Collaboration performed a systematic review on the use of pentoxifylline to treat venous leg ulcers and concluded that pentoxifylline (800 mg three times a day) seems to be an effective adjuvant to compression therapy.[70] The most commonly reported side-effects include indigestion, nausea, and diarrhea.

In terms of topical therapies for venous ulcers, a number of growth factors have been studied and have demonstrated preliminary efficacy. Keratinocyte growth factor-2 (KGF-2), a member of the fibroblast growth factor family in the skin, stimulates normal keratinocyte proliferation. In animal models its topical application has demonstrated increased re-epithelialization and enhanced granulation tissue formation on chronic wounds.[71] Phase IIb trials are presently being conducted to determine the efficacy and safety of KGF-2 in promoting wound healing in humans, and preliminary results from recently completed phase IIa trials are encouraging.[72] Many studies have shown that topical and perilesional injection of granulocyte macrophage-colony stimulating factor (GM-CSF) promotes healing of leg ulcers and is safe.[73,74] Lastly, a randomized trial has reported efficacy with calcitonin gene-related peptide in combination with vasoactive intestinal peptide for the treatment of venous ulcers.[75]

Topically applied high-potency corticosteroids are commonly employed for the treatment of associated venous dermatitis, which is characterized by eczematous changes with redness, scaling, and pruritus. However, one must proceed with caution when treating these symptoms because this eczematous dermatitis is often caused or aggravated by sensitization to the application of topical medications. Furthermore, the prolonged use of high-potency topical steroids should be avoided.[41]

Antimicrobials and the bacterial balance of leg ulcers

Background

The role of microorganisms in leg ulcers and the effects of these microorganisms on the healing process are not completely understood. In an acute wound, which follows the normal phases of healing, the risk of infection is greatest during the first 48–72 hours after injury. Hence, microorganisms detected during this time frame should be considered clinically significant until proven otherwise. Alternatively, chronic leg wounds are commonly at lower risk for infection, except for those in patients with diabetes or compromised immunity. The detection of microorganisms from these wounds typically represents colonization rather than infection.

Diagnosis

The distinction between a wound resulting from injury and one resulting from invasive infection is often not completely clear because both physiologic processes can acutely manifest as inflammation. Additionally, colonizing microorganisms may be identified in wounds resulting from injury. However, simple isolation of colonizing microorganisms from leg ulcers is not always associated with reduced healing rates.[76] In an infected wound the microorganisms invade the healthy tissue and a polymorphonuclear leukocyte response can be demonstrated histologically.[77] Although tissue levels of greater than 10^5 organisms per gram of tissue have been correlated with clinical infection in acute wounds, the specificity and predictive value of this quantification are poor.[78,79]

Both microbiologic studies, such as a swab culture or tissue biopsy for culture, as well as the patient's clinical signs of infection, including edema, erythema, pain, purulent exudate, lymphadenitis, or systemic signs (fever or leukocytosis), must be present to make the diagnosis of active infection. Identifying microorganisms in the culture samples from leg ulcers is not sufficient evidence to demonstrate an active infection that may retard healing. Further research is necessary to strengthen the validity of wound culturing as a predictor for wound infection. Table 46.7 presents a review of the available evidence relating to the clinical validity, benefits, and disadvantages of established methods for wound culturing.

Many factors predispose wounds to infection and influence the manner in which colonized wounds respond, such as advancing patient age, diabetes, compromised immune status, obesity, impaired circulation, malnutrition, and remote infection.[89] Acute wounds are more predisposed to infection than chronic wounds. Additionally, wounds that have not been debrided of necrotic tissue or eschar are more susceptible to infection, thereby emphasizing the importance of wound debridement and thorough wound cleansing.[90]

Antibiotics and antiseptics

The use of topical antibiotics in leg ulcers is controversial because antibiotic-related increased healing rates remain unproven; the potential emergence of resistant organisms with their unnecessary use is a concern.[91,92] Additionally, topical antiseptics have demonstrated cellular toxicities that surpass their bactericidal effects and have been shown to impair wound epithelialization.[93] Of note, however, studies have shown cadexomer iodine preparations are safe and effective as topical applications with antimicrobial properties for wound debridement, stimulation of granulation tissue, and overall wound healing.[94]

Systemic antibiotics used to treat active leg ulcer infections can be divided into five main groups—penicillins, cephalosporins, aminoglycosides, fluoroquinolones, and sulfonamides.[80] Other antibiotics less commonly used in this setting include clindamycin, metronidazole, and trimethoprim.

Many important factors come into play when considering systemic antibiotic therapy for a patient with a leg ulcer. First, the practitioner must fully evaluate the patient to determine the presence of a wound infection. Clinical signs of leg ulcer infection and the overall physical status of the patient, as previously described, must be assessed. The spectrum of coverage provided by the antibiotic should also be considered. Patient-specific factors must be assessed, such as known drug allergies and metabolic impairments, as well as antibiotic-specific parameters, such as the capacity for tissue penetration and the means by which the drug is metabolized. Lastly, antibiotic resistance must be taken into consideration when implementing antibiotic therapy. Methicillin-resistant *Staphylococcus aureus* (MRSA), penicillin-resistant *Streptococcus pneumoniae*, vancomycin-resistant enterococcus, and multidrug-resistant Gram-negative bacilli are the commonly encountered organisms of concern. Therefore, one must be attentive to signs of antibiotic resistance, with particular consideration to the results of laboratory tests, such as wound culture and sensitivity.

Dressings for leg ulcers—moist wound healing

Occlusion refers to the ability of a dressing to reduce the transmission of vapor from the wound surface to the atmosphere.[95] Dressings that achieve this goal have com-

Table 46.7 Wound culturing as a predictor for wound infection

Culture method	Reported clinical validity*	Advantages	Disadvantages
Histologic punch biopsy	Burn biopsy values of ≥ 10^5 as predictors of histologically verified tissue invasion by microorganisms:[81] sensitivity—35.7% (high false-positive rate); specificity—96.1%; positive predictive value—89.7%; negative predictive value—60.9%. Gram stain of burn biopsy culture growth[82]—predictive value—81.9%	• If properly performed identifies only invading bacteria. • Associated with, but not necessarily causes delayed postgraft healing. • Allows quantification of organisms and visualization of the organisms invading viable tissue	• Invasive—may drive bacteria deeper into tissue. • Small sample area. • Processing may compromise some types of bacteria. • Limited access to processing. • Failure to reflect full diversity of microflora.[83] • Invasive tissue damage by biopsy. • Systemic antibiotics may mask local pathogens. • False positives—of all burn wound biopsy cultures ≥ 10^5, harbored true invasive infection
Quantitative swab	In chronic leg ulcers, quantitative swabs were highly correlated with biopsy culture results and validated against ulcer healing:[84] positive predictive value—100% (8/8/) of ulcers with ≥ 10^5 organisms in the swab failed to heal; negative predictive value—60% (3/5) of ulcers with $<10^5$ organisms in the swab healed	• Can sample large areas of wound. • If wound is prewashed before swabbing, swab culture result correlates well with biopsy result[85]	• Samples surface organisms plus those invading healthy tissue. • Potential false-positives as a result of organisms in pools of exudate. • Air between cotton swab fibers can inhibit obligate anaerobe growth
Semiquantitative swab	Swabs correlated with biopsy culture results in infected diabetic foot ulcers:[86] sensitivity—27%; positive predictive value—50%; negative predictive value—50%	• Same advantages as for the quantitative swab	• Same disadvantages as for the quantitative swab, but less accurate
Irrigation–aspiration and needle aspiration	Draining pressure ulcers[87] relative to biopsies for anaerobic bacteria, all four validity measures were 100%; for aerobes: sensitivity—>88%; specificity—>93%; positive predictive value—>93%; negative predictive value—>97%. Anaerobes samples significantly increased clinically measured ulcer inflammation, whereas aerobes did not. In diabetic foot ulcers, aspirate missed isolate in 45% of cases, but found additional isolates in 14% compared with curettage[87]	• Nontraumatic. • Noninvasive. • Large sample area. • High (>91%) retest concordance, indicating no interaction of repeated sampling. • Likelihood of a positive culture increases with large short-bore needles and moving the inserted needle back and forth in the tissue[90]	• Wounds must have drainage. • Reveals only wound surface organisms. • Potential false-positives of organisms in pooled exudate not invading healthy tissue
Curettage	More sensitive and more specific than swab culture and correlates better with deep tissue biopsy than swab or aspirate[88]	• More reliable at harvesting anaerobes. • Yields fewer superficial colonizers	• Invasive tissue damage

** Sensitivity is the percentage of all wound infections successfully predicted by the test. Specificity is the percentage of all wounds not infected that were successfully predicted not to be infected. Positive predictive value is the percentage of all wounds entering the study that were successfully predicted by the test to become infected. Negative predictive value is the percentage of all wounds entering the study that were successfully predicted by the test not to become infected*

Reproduced with permission from McGuckin M, Goldman R, Bolton L, Salcido R. The clinical relevance of microbiology in acute and chronic wounds. Adv Skin Wound Care 2003; 16: 19.[80]

monly been described as 'occlusive' dressings. Studies have demonstrated that a moist wound environment induces acute wounds to re-epithelialize up to 40% faster than air exposed wounds.[96] The beneficial physiologic action extends to the dermis, resulting in a modified inflammatory infiltrate compared to the dermis of air-exposed wounds.[97] The physiological benefit of moist wound healing in chronic wounds is less well understood, but it is believed that these dressings can provide pain relief, decreased pain on wound debridement, and the development of a healthy appearing granulation ulcer bed.[98] Additionally, decreased frequency of changes commonly employed with these dressings maximizes effectiveness.[99]

Conventional wound dressings, such as gauze dressings, do not preserve wound moisture unless they are covered with an impermeable secondary dressing. Primary dressings are those that are in direct contact with the wound bed. Secondary dressings cover the primary dressing and help to maintain it in place. Table 46.8 describes some of the wound dressings used for leg ulcers.

Surgical techniques

Wound bed preparation and debridement

The approach to the treatment of chronic wounds has historically been relatively simple, consisting primarily of

Table 46.8 Wound dressings used for leg ulcers

Type (examples)	Advantages	Disadvantages	Indications
Hydrogels IntraSite Gel, (Smith & Nephew, Largo, FL) Nu-Gel, (Johnson & Johnson, New Brunswick, NJ) Vigilon (Bard Medical, Covington, GA)	Semitransparent, soothing, do not adhere to wounds, absorbent	Require secondary dressing and frequent dressing changes, expensive	Painful, laser, and partial-thickness wounds; after dermabrasion or chemical peel
Alginates Algiderm (Bard Medical) Kaltostat (ConvaTec, Princeton, NJ) Sorbsan (Bertek Pharmaceuticals, Morgantown, WV)	Absorbent, hemostatic, do not adhere to wounds, fewer dressing changes	Require secondary dressing, gel has foul smell	Highly exudative wounds, partial- or full-thickness wounds; after surgery
Hydrocolloids Comfeel (Coloplast, Marietta, GA) DuoDerm (ConvaTec) Restore (Hollister, Libertyville, IL)	Fibrinolytic, enhance angiogenesis, absorbent, create bacterial and physical barrier	Opaque, gel has foul smell, expensive	Partial- or full-thickness wounds, stages 1–4 pressure ulcers
Foams Allevyn (Smith & Nephew) Curafoam (Kendall, Mansfield, MA) Lyofoam (Seton Healthcare Group, Oldham UK)	Absorbent, conform to body contours	Opaque, require secondary dressing, may adhere to wounds, expensive	Partial-thickness exudative wounds, for pressure relief
Films Opsite (Smith & Nephew) Polyskin II (Kendall) Tegaderm (3M, St Paul, MN)	Transparent, create bacterial barrier, adhesive without secondary dressing	May adhere to wounds, can cause fluid collection	Donor sites, superficial burns, partial-thickness wounds with minimal exudate

measures for infection control and the use of gauze dressings for coverage and protection. Wound care has evolved significantly in the past few years, chiefly because of the advent of a number of new technologies for the treatment of chronic wounds. Innovations, such as topically applied growth factors and bioengineered skin products, have brought the concept of advanced wound bed preparation to the forefront. The ability to achieve maximal results from today's advanced wound care products is, however, contingent upon an appropriately prepared wound bed, which is characterized by optimally vascularized granulation tissue with minimal to no wound exudate.[100] Additionally, critical to the successful healing of chronic wounds is the treatment of factors that may impede the wound repair process, such as necrotic and desiccated tissues, impaired vascularization preventing oxygenation, decreased cytokine levels, and the presence of senescent or nonmigratory cells. One active therapeutic intervention for treating all these factors is wound debridement (Fig. 46.6).

Debridement is commonly defined as the process of removing necrotic, devitalized tissue and foreign matter from a wound. Necrotic tissue may have deleterious effects on wound healing by stimulating chronic inflammation, delaying both granulation tissue formation and epithelialization.[101] Wound debridement can be accomplished through several methods including surgical, mechanical, autolytic, enzymatic, and biosurgical.

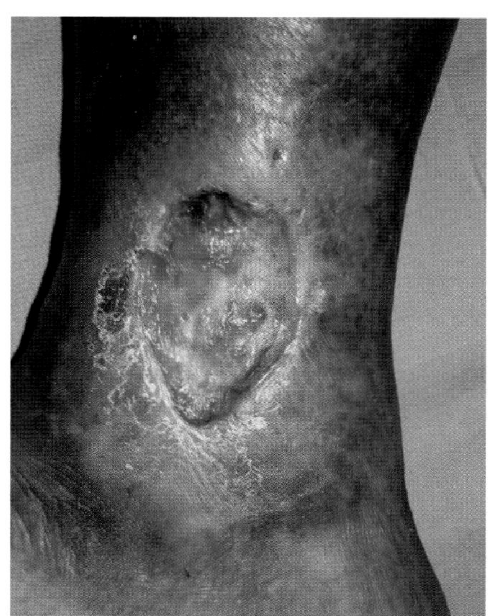

Figure 46.6 A venous leg ulcer with a yellow fibrinous base before surgical debridement.

Removal of bacteria

Necrotic tissue within a chronic wound bed supports the growth of bacterial microorganisms. Although the presence of microbial organisms in a chronic wound is unavoidable and is not necessarily detrimental to the healing process, studies have suggested that significant numbers of bacteria within a wound may impede healing.[102] It is well known that most chronic wounds that heal do so in a polymicrobial environment. However, when bacteria are present in increased numbers or have assumed phenotypes of increased pathogenicity, wound healing may be delayed. The exact number of bacteria required for delayed wound healing is an issue of great controversy, and conventionally, greater than 10^5 colonies per gram of tissue has been associated with reduced healing rates when compared to wounds with fewer bacteria.[103] However, it is unknown whether the bacterial number within wounds is a cause or consequence of impaired healing.

Chronic wounds heavily colonized by bacteria have friable and hemorrhagic granulation tissue with associated decreased tensile strength.[102] In addition to the sheer number of bacteria, the type of bacteria present may also play an important role in delaying healing. Particular bacterial species such as beta-hemolytic streptococci, or certain combinations of species, can be detrimental to the wound healing process, regardless of number.[104] Additionally, recent studies have described the potential role of bacterial biofilms in delaying the wound healing process. Biofilms are aggregates of bacteria and other organisms that are embedded within an exopolysaccharide matrix.[105] Microorganisms within these structures undergo phenotypic changes allowing for increased adherence to the wound bed, increased resistance to antimicrobial agents, and resistance to the host's immune system defense mechanisms.[106] Debridement is performed with the detachment and removal of biofilms from the wound bed.

Many distinct mechanisms have been recognized for the delay of the wound healing process by bacteria. The presence of bacteria within chronic wounds for extended periods of time can lead to a prolonged inflammatory response. Consequently, the release of free oxygen radicals and various lytic enzymes can result in tissue damage.[107] Tissue hypoxia may also occur during the inflammatory response, which may further support bacterial growth. The bacteria may also act directly to impair the healing process by releasing proteases that inactivate growth factors and other cytokines important to the healing process.[108] Lastly, the presence of excessive exudate secondary to increased bacterial burden may impair healing by the degradation of growth factors and matrix proteins, which results in a reduction of cell proliferation.[109] In summary, wound bed debridement can have major effects in the treatment of chronic wounds by effectively decreasing bacterial burden and thereby reducing a number of critical elements that impede the healing process.

Removal of senescent cells

Chronic wounds are populated by senescent (or aged) cells that have significantly decreased proliferation and protein production. Studies have demonstrated that wounds present for a prolonged period of time are characterized by fibroblasts that are less responsive to growth factor stimulation compared to acute or healing wounds. In an in-vitro study conducted on the fibroblasts from the edge of nonhealing venous ulcers, the authors concluded that this population of cells is unresponsive to the action of TGF-β, and that this blunted response may cause faulty deposition of the extracellular matrix needed for re-epithelialization and wound healing.[110] Additionally, senescent fibroblasts have been identified in many different chronic wound models.[111,112] These findings correlate well with studies that have demonstrated that wounds present for an extended period of time are more difficult to heal with standard of care interventions.[113] Wound bed debridement helps to remove senescent fibroblasts, thereby allowing for the growth of younger and more viable cells, which will potentially stimulate healing.

Effects of stimulation of growth factors

Studies have demonstrated that chronic wounds may be deficient in, or have reduced accessibility to, critical growth factors, such as fibroblast growth factor (FGF), platelet-derived growth factor (PDGF), epidermal growth factor (EGF), and TGF-β.[114] Although growth factors may be present, their availability and efficacy may be hindered as a result of abnormal binding to matrix proteins, such as the metalloproteinases.[115] Growth factors present in normal amounts may be ineffective if they are not exposed to properly functioning cells with the proper receptors. Thus, in chronic wounds, dead or necrotic tissue can act as a physical barrier to communication between growth factors and their receptors.[115] Debridement may help to speed the wound healing process by exposing the viable receptors for proper growth factor–receptor interaction. Debridement often results in bleeding of the wound bed tissue, thereby stimulating the chemoattractant and mitogenic effects of blood-borne growth factors, the most important of which are the platelet associated growth factors, including PDGF, TGF-β, and fibronectin.[116] Debridement often precedes the topical application of growth factors in clinical practice. Although not completely proven, debridement in this setting may help to optimize the wound bed for growth factor activity. In fact, a clinical trial demonstrated that patients heal a greater percentage of the time when recombinant human PDGF (rhPDGF) is applied subsequent to surgical debridement in diabetic foot ulcers compared to the application of rhPDGF alone.[108]

Removal of nonmigratory tissue

Chronic wounds often develop a nonmigratory, hyperproliferative edge. This edge, although thickened and hyperproliferative, does not confer any healing properties to the wound because epithelial proliferation and migration are two distinct biologic phenomena.[117] In fact, a hyperproliferative epithelium can often hinder the healing process.

Types of debridement

Several methods for wound debridement have been described. Numerous factors are important when choosing which approach is best for a particular wound. Although some forms of debridement, such as the surgical approach, may act to quickly remove all unwanted necrotic debris in a nonspecific fashion, a more conservative and selective approach may often be desired, such as autolytic or enzymatic debridement.

Surgical/sharp debridement

Surgical debridement is the removal of necrotic or devitalized tissue from the wound bed using a sharp instrument. Most commonly, a scalpel, scissors, curette, or forceps is used (Fig. 46.7). Additionally, sharp debridement with lasers has been described in chronic burn wounds.[118] Large wounds, with a great amount of necrotic debris are particularly good candidates for surgical debridement. Additionally, in cases

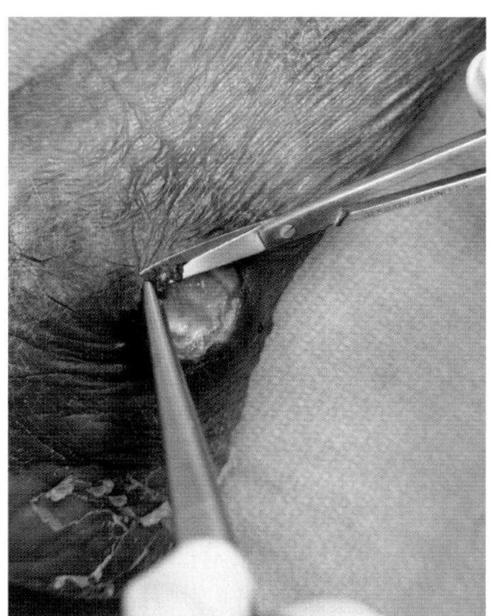

Figure 46.7 Surgical debridement for the removal of periwound nonmigratory tissue using a pair of scissors and forceps.

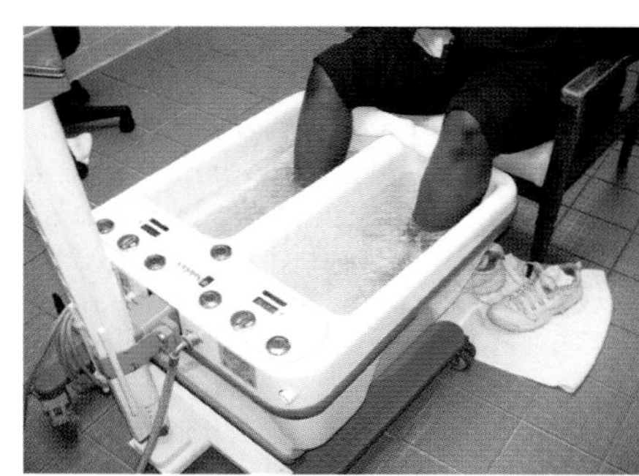

Figure 46.8 Whirlpool bath for the mechanical debridement of leg ulcers.

of fulminant infection, such as sepsis or cellulitis secondary to infected necrotic tissue, surgical debridement is the treatment of choice. Although surgical debridement is rapid, it is also nonselective. Viable tissue lying adjacent to the necrotic tissue may often be excised as well.[119] Controlling patient pain during the procedure is important, and is most commonly managed with topical anesthesia such as lidocaine 2% jelly applied to the wound bed. Postprocedure pain is most commonly managed with analgesics. Only excellent atraumatic surgical technique should be used to avoid damaging the healthy tissue within the wound, so surgical debridement should only be performed by a trained individual.[120] Surgical debridement may be performed either at the bedside or in the operating room, depending on the scale of debridement required. For extensive cases, the use of an operating room may be prudent to limit the risk of secondary infection.

Mechanical debridement

Mechanical debridement can be performed by various methods, including the application of wet-to-dry dressings, whirlpool baths (Fig. 46.8), and high-pressure irrigation.[121] Wet-to-dry debridement is widely used by many wound care practitioners. It is performed by covering the wound with a saline-moistened dressing and allowing it to completely dry. The dressing is subsequently removed, thereby removing the adherent necrotic tissue. This method of debridement is nonselective and can produce considerable patient discomfort because it also lifts away viable tissue within the wound. Wet-to-dry debridement may be the most commonly used technique, but this method of debridement is outdated and should only be used as a last resort. Both high-pressure irrigation and whirlpool baths effectively debride wounds using water; however, overzealous debridement with these methods can lead to periwound maceration. Additionally, there are theoretical concerns that water-borne pathogens could contaminate the wound bed.

Autolytic debridement

Autolytic debridement takes advantage of the body's own enzymes to break down necrotic tissue within the wound. Occlusive and semiocclusive dressings may be used to promote a moist environment to accelerate the autolytic process and allow enhanced contact between the necrotic debris and lysosomal enzymes in the wound.[122] Several moist interactive dressings are available for autolytic debridement including hydrocolloids, hydrogels, alginates, and transparent films. Autolytic debridement has many advantages because it is selective, thereby only removing the necrotic debris, and it causes little or no pain. However, this method of debridement may be slow.

Biosurgical debridement

Biosurgical debridement involves the application of maggots to the wound bed to disinfect and remove necrotic tissue. Wounds best suited for biosurgical debridement include chronic wounds with a great amount of necrotic tissue that have been refractory to other forms of chemical debridement, particularly insensate wounds such as diabetic foot and pressure ulcers.[123] Maggot therapy has also been used before surgical closure or as an alternative to surgical debridement in patients who cannot or choose not to undergo surgery. Sterile maggots are applied directly to the wound and covered with a dressing for approximately 1–3 days. The maggots act to liquefy and ingest the necrotic tissue.[124] Additionally, maggots have the ability to consume bacteria, including antibiotic-resistant strains, which may decrease the patient's risk of developing an infection.[125] Maggots secrete a substance described as a 'healing secretion'.[126] These larval secretions promote the growth of human fibroblasts in vitro, and may augment the effects of debridement for stimulating granulation tissue.[127] Any discomfort experienced by patients from maggot therapy can be treated with analgesics. Furthermore, patients must be comfortable with the notion of applying a living animal to the wound bed. Presently, maggots can be purchased through a variety of European manufacturers and in the US from the laboratory of Ronald A Sherman of the Maggot Therapy Project at http://www.ucihs.uci.edu/com/pathology/sherman/home_pg.htm. Biosurgery with maggot therapy appears to be an effective nonsurgical option for debriding chronic wounds.

Enzymatic and chemical debridement

The enzymatic debridement approach works faster than autolytic debridement, and is more conservative and specific than surgical methods. Several different enzymatic preparations, each with their own unique set of chemical properties, are readily available. The two most commonly used today are the topical preparations of collagenase (such as Collagenase Santyl Ointment, Smith & Nephew,

Largo, FL), and papain–urea (such as Accuzyme, Healthpoint, Fort Worth, TX). The collagenase preparation is composed of a partially purified form of collagenase derived from bacteria. It has the ability to degrade collagen as well as other substrates within the wound bed, with an optimal activity in a pH range of 6–8.[128] Additionally, in-vitro studies have demonstrated its efficacy in degrading elastin, heat denatured porcine skin, and fibrin.[129] The papain-based product is composed of papain, a proteolytic enzyme purified from the papaya fruit, mixed with the chemical agent urea, which acts as an humectant and renders the nonviable proteins within the necrotic tissue more susceptible to the proteolytic action of papain.

Studies have demonstrated the efficacy of the papain–urea combination in heat-denatured degrading porcine skin, with considerable effectiveness against fibrin, which is a common component of necrotic eschar. Both collagenase and papain–urea are considerably more effective against denatured proteins as opposed to proteins in their native state, thereby limiting their adverse effects on the healthy surrounding tissue.

Clinical studies have also been performed to study the relative efficacy of these two products. In a prospective, randomized, parallel group, tricenter, and open-label clinical trial with an evaluation period of 4 weeks in duration, 28 patients were randomly assigned to ulcer treatment with either collagenase ointment ($n = 12$) or papain–urea ointment ($n = 14$). The papain–urea debriding ointment was significantly more effective ($P < 0.0167$) than the collagenase ointment in reducing the amount of necrotic tissue. Additionally, the development of granulation tissue in wounds treated with papain–urea was significantly enhanced as compared to wounds treated with collagenase. Although epithelialization generally correlated with the development of a granulating wound bed, as determined by visual assessment, the general increase in the amount of epithelial tissue associated with the papain–urea-treated wounds did not predict a significantly different rate of reduction in the actual wound area between groups. These findings seem to suggest that the papain–urea-based combination is more effective, but a larger study is required to make any significant conclusions. Of note, neither debriding ointment was associated with any adverse events. Additionally, in the authors' experience, it appears that both papain–urea and collagenase may be slightly more effective when the substrate is solid eschar as opposed to unbound fibrin slough (Fig. 46.9).[130]

Skin grafting

Skin grafting has three major applications in wound care.

- To hasten the wound healing process.
- To improve cosmetic appearance.
- To improve the function of healed wounds.

Skin grafting for the treatment of wounds has been employed for centuries,[131] and although there are no particular indications specifying when skin grafting should be employed, large or nonhealing wounds are cases in which grafting can be considered. In normal individuals, without any underlying pathophysiologic defect, large lower extremity ulcers may require a prolonged period of time to heal. Consequently, it may be impractical to wait for healing by second intention in these wounds and skin grafting may help to accelerate the healing process. Additionally, skin grafting can play an important role in the treatment of all types of hard-to-heal ulcers, such as ulcers secondary to venous insufficiency, diabetes mellitus, and vasculitides.

Split- and full-thickness skin grafts

A split-thickness skin graft, also known as a partial-thickness skin graft, is a portion of skin that contains both epidermis and varying portions of the dermis. A full-thickness skin graft is composed of the epidermis and all of the dermis as well as variable amounts of subcutaneous tissue. Thin grafts, such as split-thickness skin grafts require little revascularization during the healing process and therefore have a greater chance of graft survival than full-thickness grafts. Alternatively, full-thickness grafts are likely to retain the color and texture of the donor skin. Thus, split-thickness skin grafts are more applicable when the desired therapeutic goal is the restoration of function, whereas full-thickness grafts may be more suitable when cosmetic outcome is a central concern.

Split-thickness skin grafts can be divided into three different categories depending on their thickness—thin (0.005–0.012 inch), medium thickness (0.013–0.018 inch), or thick (0.019–0.028 inch). Medium split-thickness grafts provide both optimal graft survival and durability.

The different types of grafts and their physiology are described in more detail in Chapter 23.

Preoperative preparation

Skin grafting of lower extremity ulcers can be performed as either an outpatient or ideally as an inpatient procedure—success rates vary between both approaches among centers.[132] By admitting the patient to the hospital for the procedure the potential for graft take can be optimized by controlling for extraneous factors such as patient ambulation and infection surveillance. Patients are treated preoperatively with strict bed rest, leg elevation, debridement of the wound bed, and antibiotics. With these measures in place, the ulcer bed is commonly ready for grafting by the third treatment day. The combination of antibiotic treatment[133] and leg elevation is important for reducing the bacterial load within the wound bed, thereby optimizing the chance for graft survival.

Patient comfort throughout the procedure can be optimized with the proper premedication regimen. An intramuscular injection of meperidine hydrochloride and hydroxyzine hydrochloride in combination with an oral dose of diazepam 1 hour before the procedure allows for the comfortable administration of the local anesthetic, while also taking advantage of the amnestic effect of the diazepam.

The thigh is usually used as the donor site and is carefully prepared before the procedure. First, it is precisely measured and marked. Both the donor area and the ulcer to be grafted are then thoroughly cleansed with povidone-iodine (Betadine) and rinsed with normal saline. The donor site is subsequently anesthetized with the injection of a local anesthetic. If necessary, surgical debridement of the recipient ulcer bed can then be performed. A curette can be used to obtain a bleeding ulcer base, which is then covered with saline-soaked gauze. The ulcer bed is now ready for grafting.

Preoperative patient education is discussed in Chapter 23.

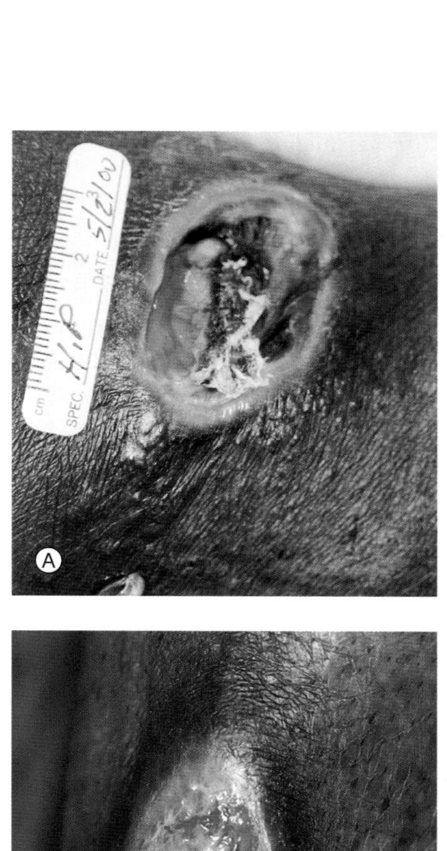

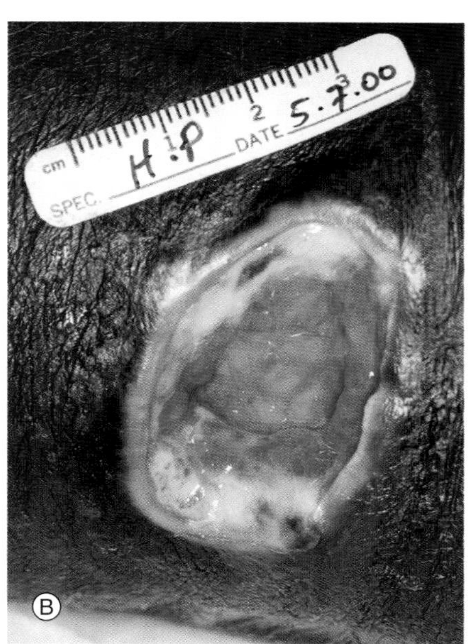

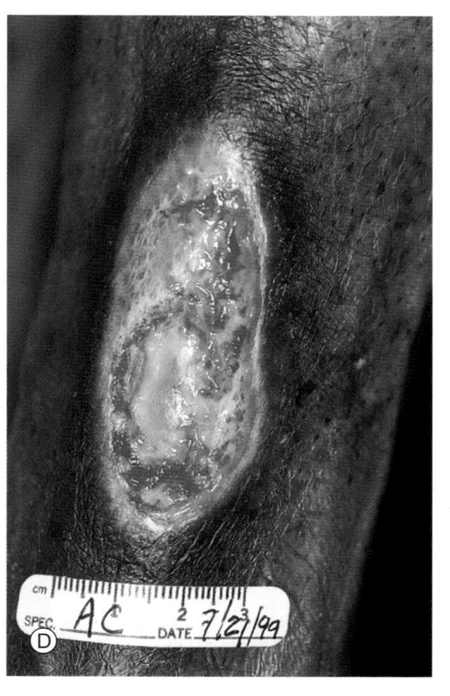

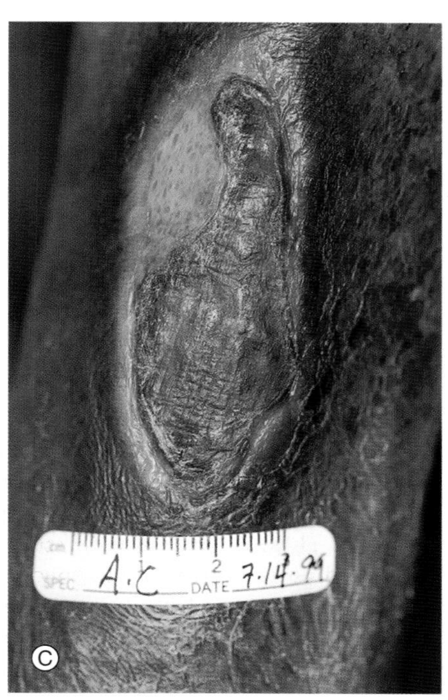

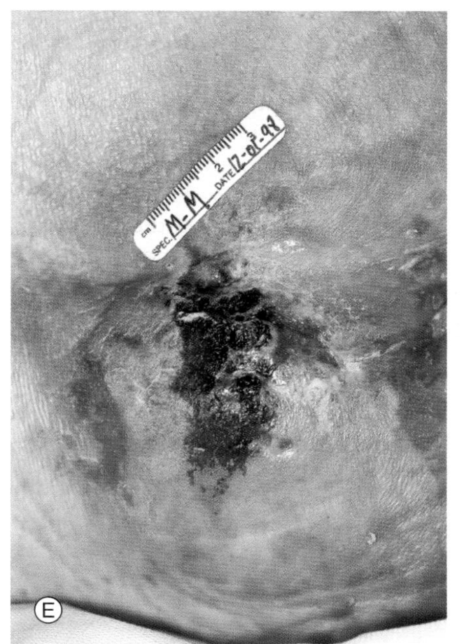

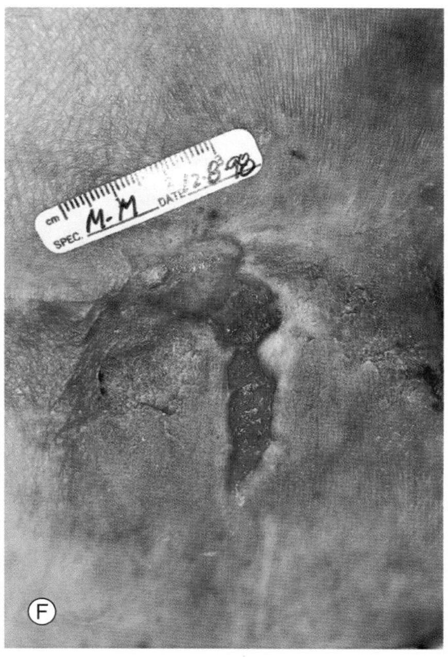

Figure 46.9 Clinical effectiveness of chemical debridement with papain–urea based preparations in three different ulcers. (A)–(B) At day 0 and week 1. (C)–(D) At week 1 and week 2. (E)–(F) At day 0 and week 1.

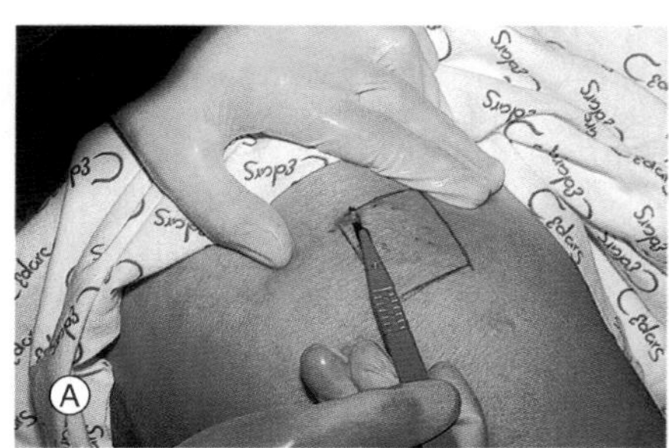
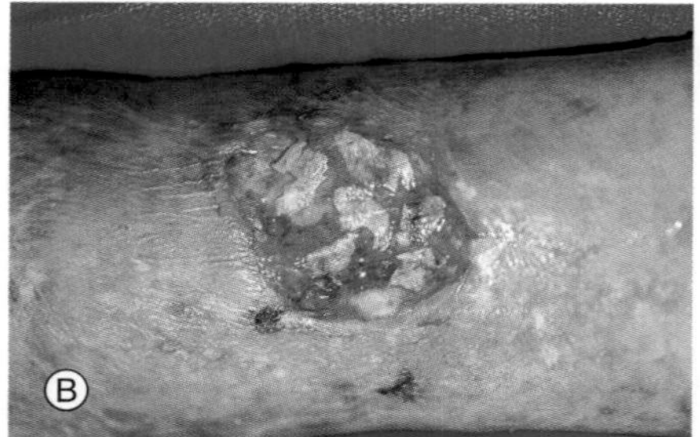
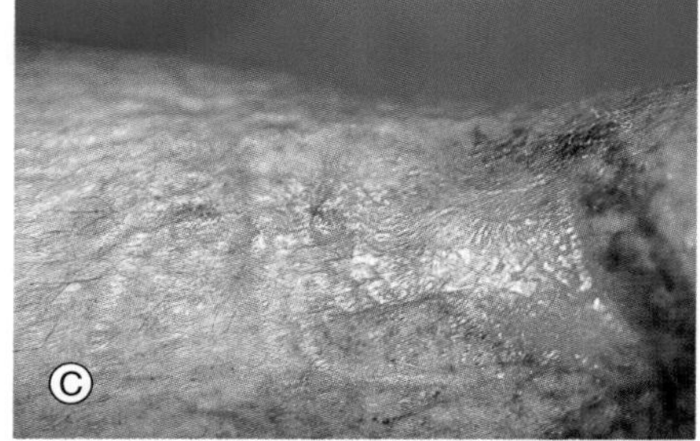

Figure 46.10 (A) The harvesting of pinch grafts from the thigh of a patient using the scalpel technique for the treatment of a chronic ulcer secondary to arterial insufficiency. (B) The appearance of the ulcer bed after pinch grafting. (C) Re-epithelialization of the ulcer approximately 2 months after pinch grafting. (With permission from J Dermatol Surg Oncol 1992 Apr; 18(4):272–283. Blackwell Publishing Ltd.)

Techniques

The various methods for harvesting grafts are described in detail in Chapter 23; here we will concentrate on aspects specific to leg ulcer management. One method is performed freehand and is commonly referred to as 'pinch grafting' (Fig. 46.10). This method, in which small pieces of skin were pinched between the thumb and forefinger and subsequently shaved from the donor site, was first described in 1869.[131] This method has since been modified with the use of various instruments including forceps,[134] skin hooks,[135] and the tip of a needle,[136] or suction[137] to grasp the skin with increased precision. The skin is then shaved with either a scalpel or a double-edged razor blade.[138] This method can also be altered with the use of a punch biopsy instrument for harvesting the tissue. This method, described by Kirsner et al.,[139] uses a 4-mm punch biopsy blade to create a uniform size graft. A thin horizontal slice of tissue is then shaved for transplantation onto the ulcer bed. Much of the ulcer area is covered with multiple grafts; with several millimeters of space maintained between each graft to allow exudate to drain from the wound. Pinch grafting has many advantages—it is a simple to perform office procedure requiring no specialized instruments or complex training. Conversely, pinch grafting is also associated with many drawbacks such as inconsistent graft sizes, relatively poor cosmetic outcome of the donor site, and the need for a lengthy procedure for grafting large ulcers.

Another method for harvesting tissue for split-thickness skin grafts employs the use of a specialized cutting instrument—a dermatome. This instrument is available in both an electrical form or as a manually operated freehand unit. The main advantage of the dermatome is that it can be set at predetermined depths, thereby allowing for consistent thickness between grafts. One additional step that may be implemented in harvesting skin grafts is 'meshing' of the tissue. Meshing is the process of expanding the graft by passing the skin through an electric or manual mesher that creates precisely placed cuts through the graft allowing the solid sheet of tissue to be converted to a net, which covers a far larger area. The combination of using an adjustable dermatome and meshing the skin provides for reliable control of graft thickness, the ability to cover large ulcer areas with speed and efficiency, and the capacity to allow blood and exudate to drain from the wound bed without compromising graft survival (Fig. 46.11). Pinch grafts are usually immobilized by the dressing whereas large split grafts are usually stapled in place.

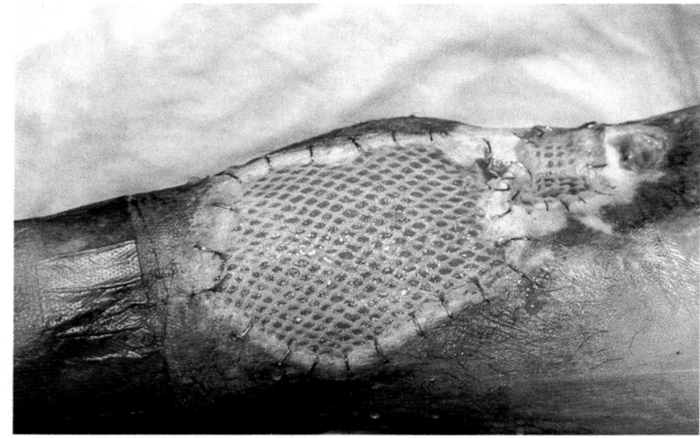

Figure 46.11 The appearance of a meshed split-thickness skin graft on a chronic ulcer. The fenestrations created by the mesher allow fluid to escape from the underlying ulcer bed. (With permission from J Dermatol Surg Oncol 1992 Apr; 18(4):272–283. Blackwell Publishing Ltd.)

Optimizing outcomes

Presently, no formal method for postoperative care of the grafted site has been established. The wound bed can be covered with petroleum-impregnated gauze, super sponges, and gauze bandages, to maintain a moist environment while concomitantly absorbing excess exudate and helping to maintain the proper position of the graft. In venous ulcers, inelastic compression can also be added. The donor site can be treated with the same type of dressing as the graft site; alternatively, a polyurethane occlusive dressing can be applied. Bed rest and leg elevation should be implemented for the first 3 days following grafting. Infection control is accomplished with the maintenance of postoperative systemic antibiotics. Additionally, pain medications are given as needed. The initial dressing change is performed after 2–3 days postoperatively, and daily thereafter. Once the staples are removed on the fifth postoperative day, the patient may begin to ambulate, with continued leg elevation. Ideally, the patient's postoperative care should also be managed as an inpatient, but all these procedures can be easily performed in the outpatient setting as well.

Pitfalls and their management

The most common cause of graft failure is infection of the ulcer bed. Pre- and peri-operative antibiotics and leg elevation are two key preventative measures. Excessive exudate can also lead to graft failure as a result of separation of the

Table 46.9 Bioengineered skin equivalents

Graft type	Type of tissue engineering	Uses
Epidermal grafts		
Cultured epidermal autografts (Epicel, Genzyme Tissue Repair, Cambridge, MA)	Living autologous keratinocyte sheets	Burns, leg ulcers, vitiligo, congenital nevi, epidermolysis bullosa, chronic otorrhea, hypospadias, corneal replacement
Cultured epidermal allografts	Living allogeneic keratinocyte sheets	Leg ulcers, epidermolysis bullosa, burns, dermabrasion, wounds
Dermal replacements		
Alloderm (Life Cell Co., Woodlands, TX)	Nonliving allogeneic acellular extracellular matrix	Surgical wounds, epidermolysis bullosa
Integra (Integra Life Science Corporation, Plainsboro, NJ)	Nonliving extracellular matrix of chondroitin-6-sulfate and silicone backing	Burns
Dermagraft (Smith and Nephew, Largo, FL)	Living allogeneic dermal dermal fibroblasts grown on a degradable scaffold	Diabetic foot ulcers
Composite grafts		
Apligraf (Organogenesis, Canton, MA)	Living allogeneic bilayered construct containing keratinocytes, fibroblasts, and bovine type I collagen	Venous ulcers, epidermolysis bullosa, donor sites, excisional wounds, diabetic foot ulcers

graft from the wound bed. This problem can be controlled by a meticulous approach to postoperative dressing changes, as described above. The postoperative use of occlusive dressings on the graft site has been associated with graft failure because of excessive accumulation of exudate.[139] Alternatively, the use of occlusive dressings at the donor site appears to limit the likelihood of infection. Using very thin split thickness skin grafts can also play an important role in optimizing graft take.

Bullae, of unknown etiology, have been noted to occur at the recipient sites of split-thickness skin grafts.[140] Although the etiology of these bullae is unknown, findings suggest a disease process confined to the skin graft recipient site with ultrastructural and antigenic features identical to those described with recessive dystrophic or immunofluorescence-negative acquired epidermolysis bullosa.[141]

Bioengineered skin equivalents

Over the past three decades, the discipline commonly referred to as tissue engineering or the use of tissue-engineered skin for wound healing has greatly advanced. The concept of cultivating tissues to replace or to stimulate the regeneration of human skin was once merely theoretical, and the only methods for skin regeneration in chronic and acute wounds of diverse etiologies were split- or full-thickness skin grafts as described above, or other surgical interventions such as free tissue transfers, or tissue flaps. Presently, there is a wide range of tissue engineered products approved for use by the US Food and Drug Administration (FDA) and several others currently undergoing testing through well-developed clinical trials.

The advantages to using tissue-engineered products, as opposed to autologous skin grafting are numerous and include the ability to provide tissue therapy without using a donor site and the potential for faster healing with improved cosmetic results.[142] The concept of tissue engineering was first defined in 1987 by the National Science Foundation bioengineering panel as 'the application of the principles and methods of engineering and the life sciences toward the development of biological substitutes to restore, maintain, or improve function.' Although the exact mechanism by which tissue engineered skin products aid in healing acute and chronic wounds is not completely understood, they appear to function by providing the needed matrix materials, cells or cell products, such as growth factors, to stimulate the healing process.[143] Additional clinical studies focusing on genetic modifications of transplanted cells and novel systemic gene product delivery mechanisms are broadening the field of tissue engineering.[144] A complete review of the bioengineered skin equivalents is beyond the scope of this chapter. A brief description of the role of the living allogeneic bilayered skin equivalent known as graftskin (Apligraf, Organogenesis Inc, Canton, MA) in wound healing is given below, and Table 46.9 provides an overview of the numerous products created from cells, extracellular matrix materials, or a combination thereof.

Graftskin as a bioengineered skin equivalent

Graftskin is a living human skin equivalent derived by combining a gel type I bovine collagen with living neonatal allogeneic fibroblasts along with an overlying cornified epidermal layer of neonatal allogeneic keratinocytes. Graftskin closely resembles human skin histologically and is currently the most sophisticated commercially available tissue engineered product. In vivo, Graftskin makes matrix proteins and growth factors; if wounded, Graftskin has the capacity to heal itself.[145] The exact mechanism for Graftskin's efficacy is not completely understood, but Graftskin is thought to stimulate healing from the wound margins or appendage structures. In a study using polymerase chain reaction analysis to determine the longevity of the allogeneic fibroblasts and keratinocytes of Graftskin in venous leg ulcers, investigators found that allogeneic DNA was present in two of eight specimens at 1 month after initial grafting, whereas neither of the two patients showed persistence of the allogeneic DNA at 2 months after initial grafting.[146] Additionally, an acute neonatal epidermolysis bullosa wound failed to show evidence of viable allogeneic

DNA beyond a period of 4 months.[147] These results suggest that allogeneic cells from Graftskin do not survive permanently after grafting and other mechanisms of action are most likely responsible for the efficacy of Graftskin, including cytokine release, and matrix-induced cell migration and activation.

In a prospective, controlled, randomized, multicenter study, significantly more patients achieved complete wound closure of venous ulcers when treated with Graftskin plus compression therapy compared to compression therapy alone (ulcer healing rate of 63 versus 49%). Additionally, patients treated with Graftskin healed more rapidly (61 versus 185 days).[148] These positive findings were again demonstrated in another prospective randomized study by Sabolinski et al.,[149] which also evaluated the efficacy of Graftskin in healing venous ulcers. In this study, the tissue-engineered product was three times more effective than compression therapy alone in achieving complete wound closure at 8 weeks.[150]

Graftskin has also been studied as treatment for acute wounds. A prospective, multicenter, open study of 107 patients with acute, partial-, or full-thickness excisional wounds mostly resulting from excision of skin cancer suggested that Graftskin is safe, useful, and well tolerated.[151] The study found no evidence of clinical or laboratory rejection. Graftskin has also been used successfully in the treatment of the acute and chronic wounds of epidermolysis bullosa.[147,152]

Graftskin has garnered approval by the FDA for the treatment of venous (Fig. 46.12) and diabetic ulcers, and is commercially available. It is shipped in a ready-to-use format and has a shelf life of 5 days. Graftskin has many advantages in that it is easy to use and can be applied in the outpatient setting. Its major disadvantages include its relative cost and short shelf life (5 days).

Subfascial endoscopic perforator surgery (SEPS)

Developments in the surgical management of patients with chronic venous insufficiency (CVI) and venous leg ulcers have recently emerged. Linton and Dodd first described the surgical approach for the ligation of incompetent lower extremity veins in the mid 1940s.[153] This technique, known as the Linton procedure, employed an incision spanning the entire length of the leg to ligate incompetent lower extremity perforator veins. The main disadvantage of this technique was a high incidence of postoperative wound healing complications, which often resulted in prolonged hospital stays and increased costs for caring for patients with CVI.[154] Although abundant evidence was compiled in support of the role of incompetent perforator veins in symptomatic CVI, and many modifications of the open technique were performed, postsurgical patient morbidity limited the acceptance of perforator ligation.[155]

More recently, the techniques for perforator vein ligation have been expanded. The development of an endoscopic approach to subfascial surgery was first described in Germany during the 1980s.[156] In the 1990s these endoscopic techniques were applied to the treatment of CVI. The technique, known as subfascial endoscopic perforator surgery (SEPS), is considerably less invasive than the open Linton technique and decreases the risk of wound healing complications. The goal of the SEPS procedure is to bypass the faulty one-way valves in the perforator veins of the lower extremities in patients with CVI. Access to the lower calf is obtained by placing small incisions in the upper calf, thereby avoiding trauma to lower calf tissue, which may be compromised by lipodermatosclerotic tissue. This tissue in particular demonstrated the greatest postoperative wound healing complications when the Linton procedure was performed.

A clinical classification system for reporting venous disease was developed by a subcommittee of the Society for Vascular Surgery and the International Society for Cardiovascular Surgery in the late 1990s.[157] It describes venous ulcers based on their Clinical picture, Etiology, Anatomic distribution, and Pathophysiology and is known as the CEAP classification system. This classification system is based on objective clinical signs of CVI (Table 46.10). Patients who fulfill the criteria described in classes 4 to 6 are considered candidates for SEPS. The goal of the procedure is to heal existing ulcers or reverse skin changes consistent with lipodermatosclerosis, decrease hemosiderin staining, and to prevent recurrence of venous ulcers secondary to perforator vein incompetence.

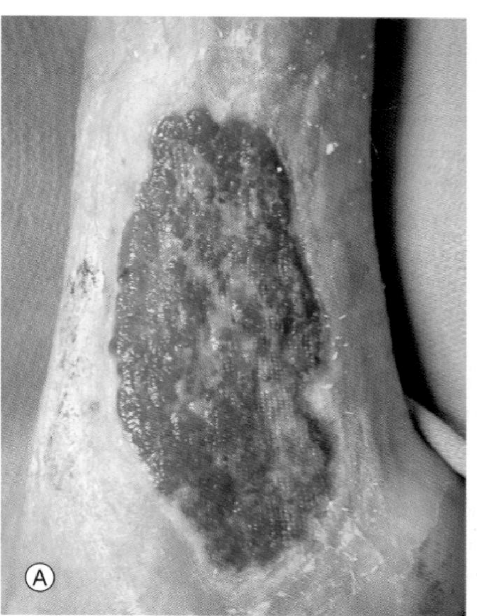

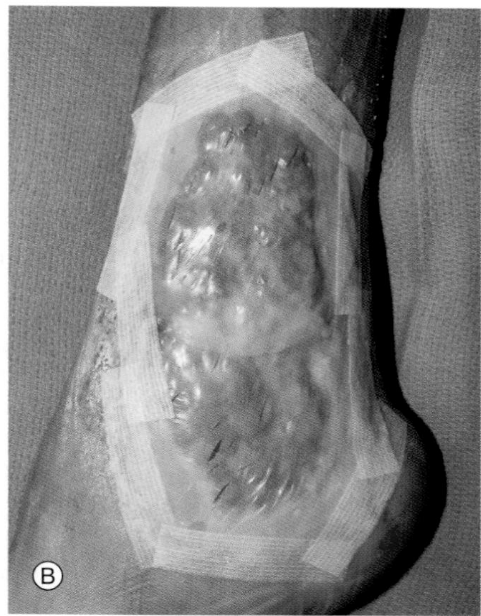

Figure 46.12 Venous leg ulcer (A) before and (B) after treatment with Apligraf bioengineered skin equivalent.

Table 46.10 Objective clinical signs of the CEAP classification system

Clinical stages	Clinical picture
Class 0	No visible signs of venous disease
Class 1	Presence of telangiectasias
Class 2	Visible varicose veins
Class 3	Presence of edema
Class 4	Skin changes, including thickening and increased pigmentation
Class 5	Includes skin changes as in class 4 as well as healed ulcers
Class 6	Active ulceration

The utilization of SEPS in the prevention of venous leg ulcer recurrence has demonstrated some promising results. In a recent study, Murray et al. demonstrated an 85% healing rate for patients with CEAP classification class 6 venous disease within an 8-week period after surgery in 67 patients.[158] The patients were followed-up for a total of 55 months and ulcer healing was demonstrated in 89% of class 6 limbs, while four of 38 ulcerated limbs failed to heal within 3 months. Ulcer recurrence of 23% was demonstrated in 24 months, most commonly in patients with a history of deep venous thrombosis.

Shave therapy for venous ulcers

Ulcers secondary to chronic venous insufficiency are typically surrounded by indurated and hyperpigmented skin in the form of acute or chronic lipodermatosclerosis. Histologically, this area of skin is characterized by clusters of small vessels with prominent endothelial cells and thickened walls, surrounded by several basement membranes, fibrinogen, laminin, and type IV collagen,[159] with the presence of microthrombi. Studies examining the microcirculation by Doppler have demonstrated increased venous blood flow along with decreased transcutaneous and intracutaneous oxygen tension in these diseased areas.[159,160] Additionally, the extent of morphologic and functional abnormalities has been found to correlate with the amount of lipodermatosclerosis.[161] The underlying mechanisms leading from lipodermatosclerosis to venous ulceration have not been completely elucidated, but lipodermatosclerosis has been reported as a poor prognostic factor for healing.[162] Therefore, studies have identified this area of diseased skin as a potential site for therapeutic intervention for patients with chronic venous leg ulcers.

Because extirpation of circumscribed areas of lipodermatosclerosis as well as the venous ulceration has proven beneficial in the treatment of refractory venous ulcers, a surgical procedure known as shave therapy has been employed for the treatment of patients with extensive lipodermatosclerosis and nonhealing ulcers. Briefly, the procedure uses a dermatome to surgically remove all indurated areas beside and underneath the ulcer. The technique excises cutaneous layers superficial to the fascia in a horizontal approach. As layers of skin are removed, the pattern and amount of bleeding are carefully assessed within the indurated area. In the same surgical procedure, meshed split-thickness skin grafts are placed to cover the wound area. Shave therapy can also be combined with saphenectomy or with dissection and ligation of insufficient perforator veins.

One study reported both short-term and long-term results for patients following shave therapy.[163] At 3 months following shave therapy skin grafting, a healing rate of 79% was reported. Additionally, of patients treated in this study, a 1-year, long-term, healing rate of 88% was reported. Only minor adverse events to the procedure were reported at the onset of the trial, and included transient postoperative increases in body temperatures and the need for postoperative blood transfusion in four patients.

In summary, shave therapy seems to be a safe and effective surgical treatment option for patients with recalcitrant venous ulcers and significant lipodermatosclerosis. Although larger trials are still needed to confirm efficacy, short and long-term results are favorable thus far.

Pitfalls and their management

- Chronic wounds can develop malignancies, which will not be diagnosed if not suspected and biopsied.
- It is vital to differentiate between venous, arterial, diabetic, pressure, and immune-modulated inflammatory ulcers to avoid incorrect and ineffective treatments.
- Surgical debridement must be performed by a skilled well-trained operator, otherwise it can result in unnecessary destruction of healthy tissue.
- Thorough pre- and postoperative planning are important to avoid skin graft failure.

■ SUMMARY

Leg ulcers are debilitating, are usually caused by venous insufficiency, and are seen most often in the elderly. They are therefore a major health issue in an aging population. Recent developments in the understanding of wound healing have helped to explain why leg ulcers can become chronic and have assisted in developments in therapy. Compression remains the mainstay of therapy, often with aspirin or pentoxifylline as adjuncts to speed healing. However, chronic wounds may require more intervention. Surgical debridement may be needed, particularly when using advanced wound care products that require debridement as a preparatory step. Skin grafting, SEPS, and shave therapy may be employed. Finally, the use of topical antibiotics remains controversial and antibiotic therapy is often not necessary in the healing of ulcers colonized by bacteria.

We can expect to see future therapeutic developments in leg ulcer therapy in response to improved understanding of the inflammatory processes and wound healing.

■ ACKNOWLEDGMENTS

We would like to express our gratitude to the librarian Mary Hicks, for her invaluable assistance in the literature search. We like to thank Oscar Alvarez PhD for providing technical assistance in the production of the video and for reviewing the manuscript. We thank Gabriel Fernandez-Obregon for his expertise and technical support in the production of the video.

■ REFERENCES

1. Valencia IC, Falabella A, Kirsner RS, Eaglstein WH. Chronic venous insufficiency and venous leg ulceration. J Am Acad Dermatol 2002; 44: 401–421.
2. Choucair MM, Fivenson DP. Leg ulcer diagnosis and management. Dermatol Clin 2001; 19:659–678.
3. Mekkes JR, Loots MAM, Van Der Wal AC, Bos JD. Causes, investigation and treatment of leg ulceration. Br J Dermatol 2003; 148:388–401.
4. Goldman MP. Sclerotherapy treatment of varicose and telangiectatic leg veins. St Louis: Mosby; 1991:239–246.
5. Harding KG, Morris HL, Patel GK. Science, medicine, and the future: healing chronic wounds. Br Med J 2002; 324:160–165.
6. Wiete Westerhof, ed. Leg ulcers: diagnosis and treatment. Amsterdam: Elsevier; 1993.
7. Meehan M. Multisite pressure ulcer prevalence survey. Decubitus 1990; 3:14–17.
8. Bowker JH, Pfeifer MA. Levin and O'Neal's The diabetic foot, 6th edn. St Louis: Mosby; 2001.
9. Burton CS. Management of chronic and problem lower extremity wounds. Derm Clin 1993; 11:767–773.
10. Baker SR, Stacey MC, Jopp-McKay AG, Hoskin SE, Thompson PJ. Epidemiology of chronic venous ulcers. Br J Surg. 1991; 78:864–867.
11. Burton CS. Venous ulcers. Am J Surg. 1994; 167:37S–40S; discussion 40S–41S.
12. Gay J. On varicose diseases of the lower extremities: the Lettsomian Lectures of 1867. London: Churchill Livinstone; 1949.
13. Homans J. The etiology and treatment of varicose ulcer of the leg. Surg Gynecol Obstet 1917; 24:300–311.
14. Bjordal R. Flow and pressure studies in venous insufficiency. Acta Chir Scand 1988; 544(suppl):30–33.
15. McEnroe CS, O'Donnell TF Jr, Mackey WC. Correlation of clinical findings with venous hemodynamics in 386 patients with chronic venous insufficiency. Am J Surg 1988; 156:148–152.
16. Summer DS. Applied physiology in venous problems. In: Bergan JJ, ed. Surgery of the veins. Philadelphia: Grune & Stratton; 1985:3–23.
17. Browse NL, Burnand KG. The cause of venous ulceration. Lancet 1982; 31:243–245.
18. Coleridge Smith PD, Thomas P, Scurr JH, Dormandy JA. Causes of venous ulceration: a new hypothesis. Br Med J (Clin Res Ed) 1988; 18:296:1726–1727.
19. Falanga V, Eaglstein WH. The 'trap' hypothesis of venous ulceration. Lancet 1993; 341:1006–1008.
20. Coleridge Smith PD. Deleterious effects of white cells in the course of skin damage in CVI. Int Angiol 2002; 21(2suppl.1):26–32.
21. Van de Scheur M, Falanga V. Pericapillary fibrin cuffs in venous disease. A reappraisal. Dermatol Surg 1997; 23:955–959.
22. Hasan A, Murata H, Falabella A, et al. Dermal fibroblasts from venous ulcers are unresponsive to the action of transforming growth factor-beta 1. J Dermatol Sci 1997; 16:59–66.
23. Scott TE, LaMorte WW, Gorin DR, Menzoian JO. Risk factors for chronic venous insufficiency: a dual case–control study. J Vasc Surg 1995:22:622–628.
24. Browse NL, Gray L, Jarrett PE, Morland M. Blood and vein-wall fibrinolytic activity in health and vascular disease. Br Med J. 1977; 1:478–481.
25. Leng GC, Davis M, Baker D. Bypass surgery for chronic lower limb ischaemia. Cochrane Database Syst Rev 2000; 3:CD002000.
26. Shaw JE, Boulton AJ. The pathogenesis of diabetic foot problems: an overview. Diabetes. 1997; 46(suppl.2):S58–S61.
27. London NJ, Donnely R. ABC of arterial and venous disease. Ulcerated lower limb. Br Med J 2000; 320:1589–1591.
28. Pecoraro RE, Reiber GE, Burgess EM. Pathways to diabetic limb amputation. Basis for prevention. Diabetes Care 1990; 13:513–521.
29. American Diabetes Association. Consensus Development Conference on Diabetic Foot Wound Care: 7–8 April 1999, Boston, Massachusetts. Diabetes Care 1999; 22:1354–1360.
30. Frykberg RG. Diabetic foot ulcers: pathogenesis and management. Am Fam Physician 2002; 66:1655–1662.
31. Alvarez O. Pressure ulcers: critical considerations in prevention and management. Clinical Material 1991; 8:209–222.
32. Treatment of pressure ulcers: clinical practice guidelines No. 15. AHCPR publication # 95–0652, Dec 1994. Rockville: US Dept of Health and Human Services. Public Health Service Agency for Health Care Policy and Research.
33. Kerdel FA. Inflammatory ulcers. J Dermatol Surg Oncol 1993; 19:772–778.
34. Paquette D, Falanga V. Leg ulcers. Clin Geriatr Med 2002; 18:77–88.
35. Singer AJ, Clark RA. Cutaneous wound healing. N Engl J Med 1999; 341:738–746.
36. Ballard K, Cantor AJ. Treating recalcitrant diabetic wounds with hyaluronic acid: a review of patients. Ostomy Wound Manage 2003; 49:37–49.
37. Gallo RL. Proteoglycans and cutaneous vascular defense and repair. J Investig Dermatol Symp Proc 2000; 5:55–60.
38. American Association of Homes & Services for the Aging and Center for Disease Control & Prevention. National Center for Health Statistics. National Vital Statistics Report, Vol. 47, No. 28. December 13, 1999.Table: Life expectancy for total population: United States. 1997. http://www.aahsa.org/public/agingbkg/htm#graying.
39. Alvarez OM, Meehan M, Ennis W, et al. Chronic wounds: palliative management for the frail population. Wounds 2002; 14(suppl):5S–27S.
40. de Araujo T, Valencia I, Federman DG, Kirsner RS. Managing the patient with venous ulcers. Ann Intern Med 2003; 138:326–334.
41. Siegel DM. Contact sensitivity and recalcitrant wounds. Ostomy Wound Manage 2000; 46(suppl):65–76.
42. Cohen IK, Diegelman DF, Lindbald WJ, eds. Wound healing: biochemical and clinical aspects. Philadelphia: Saunders; 1992.
43. Phillips TJ, Dover JS. Leg ulcers. J Am Acad Dermatol 1991; 25:965–987.
44. Falanga V. Venous ulceration. Dermatol Surg Oncol 1993; 19:764–771.
45. Kanj LF, Phillips TJ. Management of leg ulcers. Fitzpatrick's J Clinical Dermatol 1994; Sept/Oct:60–65.
46. Bowman PH. Hogan DJ. Leg ulcers: a common problem with sometimes uncommon etiologies. Geriatrics 1999; 54:43–54.
47. McGee SR, Boyko EJ. Physical examination and chronic lower-extremity ischemia: a critical review. Arch Intern Med 1998; 158:1357–1364.
48. Barnes RW. Noninvasive diagnostic assessment of peripheral vascular disease. Circulation 1991; 83:120–127.
49. McGuckin M, Stineman M, Goin J, Williams S. Draft guideline: diagnosis and treatment of venous leg ulcers. Ostomy Wound Manage 1996; 42:48,50–52,54.
50. Falabella A, Falanga V. Uncommon causes of ulcers. Clin Plast Surg 1998; 25:467–479.
51. Alazraki N. Imaging diagnosis of osteomyelitis in patients with diabetes mellitus. American College of Radiology ACR Appropriateness Criteria. Radiology 2000; 215(suppl):303–310.
52. Sibbald RG. An approach to leg and foot ulcers: a brief overview. Ostomy Wound Manage 1998; 44:28–32,34–35.
53. Harris B, Eaglstein WH, Falanga V. Basal cell carcinoma arising in venous ulcer and mimicking granulation tissue. J Dermatol Surg Oncol 1993; 19:150–152.
54. Allman RM, Walker JM, Hart MK, Laprade CA, Noel LB, Smith CR. Air-fluidized beds or conventional therapy for pressure sores. A randomized trial. Ann Intern Med 1987; 107:641–648.
55. Taylor TV, Rimmer S, Day B, Butcher J, Dymock IW. Ascorbic acid supplementation in the treatment of pressure sores. Lancet 1974; 2:544–546.
56. Weingarten MS. State-of-the-art treatment of chronic venous disease. Clin Infect Dis 2001; 32:949–954.
57. Cahall E, Spence R. Nursing management of venous ulceration. J Vasc Nurs 1994; 12:48–56.
58. Erickson CA, Lanza DJ, Karp DL, et al. Healing of venous ulcers in an ambulatory care program: the roles of chronic venous insufficiency and patient compliance. J Vasc Surg 1995; 22:629–636.
59. Fletcher A, Cullum N, Sheldon TA. A systematic review of compression treatment for venous leg ulcers. Br Med J 1997; 315:576–80.
60. Margolis DJ, Cohen JH. Management of chronic venous leg ulcers: a literature-guided approach. Clin Dermatol 1994; 12:19–26.
61. Kunimoto BT. Compression therapy: theory and practice. Dermatologic Therapy 1999; 9:63–68.
62. Hansson C, Swanbeck G. Regulating the pressure under compression bandages for venous leg ulcers. Acta Derm Venereol. 1988; 68:245–249.

63. Phillips TJ. Successful methods of treating leg ulcers. The tried and true, plus the novel and new. Postgrad Med 1999; 105:159–161,165–166,173–174.

64. Blair SD, Wright DD, Backhouse CM, Riddle E, McCollum CN. Sustained compression and healing of chronic venous ulcers. Br Med J 1988;297:1159–1161.

65. Weingarten MS. State-of-the-art treatment of chronic venous disease. Clin Infect Dis 2001; 32:949–954.

66. Ibbotson SH, Layton AM, Davies JA, Goodfield MJ. The effect of aspirin on haemostatic activity in the treatment of chronic venous leg ulceration. Br J Dermatol 1995; 132:422–426

67. Layton AM, Ibbotson SH, Davies JA, Goodfield MJ. Randomised trial of oral aspirin for chronic venous leg ulcers. Lancet 1994; 344:164–165.

68. Dale JJ, Ruckley CV, Harper DR, Gibson B, Nelson EA, Prescott RJ. Randomised, double blind placebo controlled trial of pentoxifylline in the treatment of venous leg ulcers. Br Med J 1999; 319:875–878.

69. Falanga V, Fujitani RM, Diaz C, et al. Systemic treatment of venous leg ulcers with high doses of pentoxifylline: efficacy in a randomized, placebo–controlled trial. Wound Repair Regen 1999; 7:208–213.

70. Jull AB, Waters J, Arroll B. Pentoxifylline for treating venous leg ulcers. Cochrane Database Syst Rev. 2002; 1:CD001733.

71. Xia YP, Zhao Y, Marcus J, et al. Effects of keratinocyte growth factor-2 (KGF-2) on wound healing in an ischaemia-impaired rabbit ear model and on scar formation. J Pathol 1999; 188:431–438.

72. Robson MC, Phillips TJ, Falanga V, et al. Randomized trial of topically applied repifermin (recombinant human keratinocyte growth factor-2) to accelerate wound healing in venous ulcers. Wound Repair Regen 2001; 9:347–352.

73. Recombinant human granulocyte-macrophage colony-stimulating factor applied locally in low doses enhances healing and prevents recurrence of chronic venous ulcers. Int J Dermatol 1999; 38:380–386.

74. Randomized, double-blind, placebo-controlled, dose-ranging study of granulocyte-macrophage colony stimulating factor in patients with chronic venous leg ulcers. Wound Repair Regen 1999; 7:17–25.

75. Gherardini G, Gürlek A, Evans GR, et al. Venous ulcers: improved healing by iontophoretic administration of calcitonin gene-related peptide and vasoactive intestinal polypeptide. Plast Reconstr Surg 1998; 101:90–93.

76. Hanssen C, Hobion J, Moler J, Swanbech G. The microbial flora in venous leg ulcers without clinical signs of infection. Acta Derm Venereol (Stockh) 1995; 75:24–30.

77. Bucknall TE. Factors affecting healing. In: Bucknall TE, Ellis H, eds. Wound healing for surgeons. London: Ballière Tindall; 1984:42–74.

78. Pruitt BA Jr. The diagnosis and treatment of infection in the burn patient. Burns Incl Therm Inj 1984; 11:79–91.

79. Robson MC, Lea CE, Dalton JB, Heggers JP. Quantitative bacteriology and delayed wound closure. Surg Forum 1968; 19:501–502.

80. McGuckin M, Goldman R, Bolton L, Salcido R. The clinical relevance of microbiology in acute and chronic wounds. Adv Skin Wound Care 2003; 16:12–23,quiz 24–25.

81. McManus AT, Mason AD Jr, McManus WF, Pruitt BA Jr. A decade of reduced gram-negative infections and mortality associated with improved isolation of burned patients. Arch Surg 1994; 129:1306–1309.

82. Taddonio TE, Thomson PD, Tait MJ, Prasad JK, Feller I. Rapid quantification of bacterial and fungal growth in burn wounds: biopsy homogenate Gram stain versus microbial culture results. Burns Incl Therm Inj 1988; 14:180–184.

83. Davies CE, Wilson MJ, Hill KE, et al. Use of molecular techniques to study microbial diversity in the skin: chronic wounds reevaluated. Wound Repair Regen 2001; 9:332–340.

84. Lookingbill DP, Miller SH, Knowles RC. Bacteriology of chronic leg ulcers. Arch Dermatol 1978; 114:1765–1768.

85. Thomson PD, Smith DJ Jr. What is infection? Am J Surg 1994; 167:7S–11S.

86. Lipsky BA, Pecoraro RE, Wheat LJ. The diabetic foot. Soft tissue and bone infection. Infect Dis Clin North Am 1990; 4:409–432.

87. Ehrenkranz NJ, Alfonso B, Nerenberg D. Irrigation–aspiration for culturing draining decubitus ulcers: correlation of bacteriological findings with a clinical inflammatory scoring index. J Clin Microbiol 1990; 28:2389–2393.

88. Twum–Danso K, Grant C, al–Suleiman SA, et al. Microbiology of postoperative wound infection: a prospective study of 1770 wounds. J Hosp Infect 1992; 21:29–37.

89. Eaglstein WH. Current wound management: a symposium. Clin Dermatol 1984; 2:134–142.

90. Hutchinson JJ, McGuckin M. Occlusive dressings: a microbiologic and clinical review. Am J Infect Control 1990; 18:257–268.

91. Pardes JB, Carson PA, Eaglstein WH, Falanga V. Mupirocin treatment of exudative venous ulcers. J Am Acad Dermatol 1993; 29:497–498.

92. Lineaweaver W, Howard R, Soucy D, et al. Topical antibiotic therapy. Arch Surg 1985; 120:267–270.

93. Geronemous RG, Mertz PM, Eaglstein WH. Wound healing: the effects of topical antimicrobial agents. Arch Dermatol 1979; 115:1311–1314.

94. Gilchrist B, on behalf of the European Tissue Repair Society. Should iodine be reconsidered in wound management? A report of a consensus meeting on the use of iodine in wound care. J Wound Care 1997; 6:148–150.

95. Ovington LG. The well dressed wound: an overview of dressing types. Wounds 1998; 101A–111A.

96. Hinman C, Maibach H. Effect of air exposure and occlusion on experimental human skin wounds. Nature 1962; 200:377–378.

97. Eaglstein WH. Experiences with biosynthetic dressings. J Am Acad Dermatol 1985;12:434–440.

98. Falanga V. Occlusive wound dressings. Why, when, which? Arch Dermatol 1988; 124:872–877.

99. Bello YM, Phillips TJ. Therapeutic dressings. Adv Dermatol 2000; 16:253–272.

100. Falanga V, Brem H. Wound bed preparation for optimal use of advanced therapeutic products. In: Falanga V, ed. Cutaneous wound healing. Boston: Boston University Press 2001; 457–468.

101. O'Meara S, Cullum N, Majid M, Sheldon T. Systematic reviews of wound care management:(3) antimicrobial agents for chronic wounds; (4) diabetic foot ulceration. Health Technol Assess 2000; 4:1–237.

102. Bucknall TE. The effect of local infection upon wound healing: an experimental study. Br J Surg 1980; 67:851–855.

103. Robson MC, Stenberg BD, Heggers JP. Wound healing alterations caused by infection. Clin Plast Surg 1990; 17:485–492.

104. Schuchat A. Group B streptococcus. Lancet 1999; 353:51–56.

105. Harrison–Balestra C, Cazzaniga AL, Davis SC, Mertz PM. A wound-isolated *Pseudomonas aeruginosa* grows a biofilm in vitro within 10 hours and is visualized by light microscopy. Dermatol Surg 2003; 29:631–635.

106. Stewart PS, Costerton JW. Antibiotic resistance of bacteria in biofilms. Lancet 2001; 358:135–138.

107. Laato M, Niinikoski J, Lundberg C, Gerdin B. Inflammatory reaction and blood flow in experimental wounds inoculated with *Staphylococcus aureus*. Eur Surg Res 1988; 20:33.

108. Steed DL, Donohoe D, Webster MW, Lindsley L. Effect of extensive debridement and treatment on the healing of diabetic foot ulcers. Diabetic Ulcer Study Group. J Am Coll Surg 1996; 183:61–64.

109. Falanga V, Grinnell F, Gilchrest B, Maddox YT, Moshell A. Workshop on the pathogenesis of chronic wounds. J Invest Dermatol 1994; 2:125–127.

110. Hasan A, Murata H, Falabella A, et al. Dermal fibroblasts from venous ulcers are unresponsive to the action of transforming growth factor-beta 1. J Dermatol Sci 1997; 16:59–66.

111. Vande Berg JS, Rudolph R, Hollan C, Haywood-Reid PL. Fibroblast senescence in pressure ulcers. Wound Repair Regen 1998; 6:38–49.

112. Mendez MV, Raffetto JD, Phillips T, Menzoian JO, Park HY. The proliferative capacity of neonatal skin fibroblasts is reduced after exposure to venous ulcer wound fluid: a potential mechanism for senescence in venous ulcers. J Vasc Surg 1999; 30:734–743.

113. Margolis DJ, Berlin JA, Strom BL. Which venous leg ulcers will heal with limb compression bandages? Am J Med 2000; 109:15–19.

114. Kirstein MD, Reis ED. Current surgical perspectives in wound healing. Wounds 2001; 13:53–58.

115. Mulder GD, Vande Berg JS. Cellular senescence and matrix metallo-proteinase activity in chronic wounds. Relevance to debridement and new technologies. Am Podiatr Med Assoc 2002; 92:34–37.

116. Gope R. The effect of epidermal growth factor and platelet-derived growth factors on wound healing process. Indian J Med Res 2002; 116:201–206.

117. Decline F, Rousselle P. Keratinocyte migration requires alpha2 beta1 integrin-mediated interaction with the laminin5 gamma2 chain. J Cell Sci 2001; 114:811–823.

118. Reynolds N, Cawrse N, Burge T, Kenealy J. Debridement of a mixed partial and full thickness burn with an erbium:YAG laser. Burns 2003; 29:183–188.
119. Sieggreen MY, Maklebust J. Debridement: choices and challenges. Adv Wound Care 1997; 10:32–37.
120. Attinger CE, Bulan E, Blume PA. Surgical debridement. The key to successful wound healing and reconstruction. Clin Podiatr Med Surg 2000; 17:599–630.
121. Kennedy KL, Tritch DL. Debridement. In: Krasner D, Kane D, eds. Chronic wound care: a clinical source book for healthcare professionals, 2nd edn. Wayne, PA: Health Management Publications 1997; 227–234.
122. Kiernan M. Wet, sloughy and necrotic wound management. Community Nurse 1999; 5:51–52.
123. Thomas S, Andrews A, Jones M. The use of larval therapy in wound management. J Wound Care 1998; 7:521–524.
124. Wollina U, Liebold K, Schmidt WD, Hartmann M, Fassler D. Biosurgery supports granulation and debridement in chronic wounds – clinical data and remittance spectroscopy measurement. Int J Dermatol 2002; 41:635–639.
125. Bonn D. Maggot therapy: an alternative for wound infection. Lancet 2000 30; 356:1174.
126. Livingston SK. The therapeutic active principle of maggots. J Bone Joint Surg 1936; 18:751–756.
127. Prete PE. Growth effects of *Phaenicia sericata* larval extracts on fibroblasts: mechanism for wound healing by maggot therapy. Life Sci 1997; 60:505–510.
128. Silverstein P, Ruzicka FJ, Helmkamp GM Jr, Lincoln RA Jr, Mason AD Jr. In vitro evaluation of enzymatic debridement of burn wound eschar. Surgery. 1973; 73:15–22.
129. Hebda PA, Lo C. The effects of active ingredients of standard debriding agents – papain and collagenase – on digestion of native and denatured collagenous substrates, fibrin and elastin. Wounds 2001; 13:190–194.
130. Alvarez OM, Fernandez–Obregon A, Rogers RS, et al. A prospective, randomized, comparative study of collagenase and papain–urea for pressure ulcer debridement. Wounds 2002; 14:293–301.
131. Hauben DJ, Baruchin A, Mahler A. On the history of the free skin graft. Ann Plast Surg 1982; 9:242–245.
132. Gilmore WA, Wheeland RG. Treatment of ulcers on legs by pinch grafts and a supportive dressing of polyurethane. J Dermatol Surg Oncol 1982; 8:177–183.
133. McGuckin M, Goldman R, Bolton L, Salcido R. The clinical relevance of microbiology in acute and chronic wounds. Adv Skin Wound Care 2003;16:12–23;quiz 24–25.
134. Millard LG, Roberts MM, Gatecliffe M. Chronic leg ulcers treated by the pinch graft method. Br J Dermatol 1977; 97:289–295.
135. Wheeland RG. The technique and current status of pinch grafting. J Dermatol Surg Oncol 1987; 13:873–880.
136. Ceilley RI, Rinek MA, Zuehlke RL. Pinch grafting for chronic ulcers on lower extremities. J Dermatol Surg Oncol 1977; 3:303–309.
137. Camacho F, Noreno JC, Sanchez-Conejo J, Sanchez-Pedreno P. Treatment of venous ulcers by minigrafting epidermal suction. J Dermatol Treat 1989; 1:99–100.
138. Smith JD, Holder WR, Smith EB. Pinch grafts for cutaneous ulcers. South Med J 1971; 64:1166–1171.
139. Kirsner RS, Falanga V. Techniques of split-thickness skin grafting for lower extremity ulcerations. J Dermatol Surg Oncol 1993;19:779–783.
140. Baran R, Juhlin L, Brun P. Bullae in skin grafts. Br J Dermatol 1984; 111:221–225.
141. Epstein A, Hendrick SJ, Sanchez RL, Solomon AR, Fine JD. Persistent subepidermal blistering in split-thickness skin graft sites. Ultrastructural and antigenic features simulating dystrophic or immunofluorescence-negative acquired epidermolysis bullosa. Arch Dermatol 1988; 124:244–249.
142. Eaglstein WH, Iriondo M, Laszlo K. A composite skin substitute (graftskin) for surgical wounds. A clinical experience. Dermatol Surg 1995; 21:839–843.
143. Falanga VJ. Tissue engineering in wound repair. Adv Skin Wound Care 2000; 13(suppl):15–19.
144. Supp DM, Bell SM, Morgan JR, Boyce ST. Genetic modification of cultured skin substitutes by transduction of human keratinocytes and fibroblasts with platelet-derived growth factor-A. Wound Repair Regen 2000; 8:26–35.
145. Falanga V. How to use Apligraf to treat venous ulcers. Skin Aging 1999; 7:30–36.
146. Phillips TJ, Manzoor J, Rojas A, et al. The longevity of a bilayered skin substitute after application to venous ulcers. Arch Dermatol 2002; 138:1079–1081.
147. Falabella AF, Schachner LA, Valencia IC, Eaglstein WH. The use of tissue-engineered skin (Apligraf) to treat a newborn with epidermolysis bullosa. Arch Dermatol 1999; 135:1219–1222.
148. Falanga V, Margolis D, Alvarez O, et al. Rapid healing of venous ulcers and lack of clinical rejection with an allogeneic cultured human skin equivalent. Human Skin Equivalent Investigators Group. Arch Dermatol 1998; 134:293–300.
149. Sabolinski ML, Alvarez O, Auletta M, Mulder G, Parenteau NL. Cultured skin as a 'smart material' for healing wounds: experience in venous ulcers. Biomaterials 1996; 17:311–320.
150. Falanga V. Tissue engineering in wound repair. Adv Skin Wound Care 2000; 13(suppl):15–19.
151. Eaglstein WH, Alvarez OM, Auletta M, et al. Acute excisional wounds treated with a tissue-engineered skin (Apligraf). Dermatol Surg 1999; 25:195–201.
152. Falabella AF, Valencia IC, Eaglstein WH, Schachner LA. Tissue-engineered skin (Apligraf) in the healing of patients with epidermolysis bullosa wounds. Arch Dermatol 2000; 136:1225–1230.
153. Kowallek D, DePalma G. A new approach to an old and vexing problem: subfascial endoscopic perforator surgery. J Vasc Nurs 199; 17:65–70.
154. Kolvenbach R, Ramadan H, Schwierz E. Redone endoscopic perforator surgery: feasibility and failure analysis. J Vasc Surg 1999; 30:720–726.
155. Iafrati M, Welsh H, O'Donnell T. Subfascial endoscopic perforator ligation: an analysis of early clinical outcomes and cost. J Vasc Surg 1997; 25:995–1001.
156. Gloviczki P, Bergan J, Rhodes J, Canton L, Harmsen S, Illstrup D, the North American Study Group. Midterm results of endoscopic perforator vein interruption for chronic venous insufficiency: lessons learned for North American Subfascial Endoscopic Perforator Surgery Registry. J Vasc Surg 1999; 29:489–502.
157. American Venous Forum ad hoc committee. Classification and grading of chronic venous disease in the lower limbs: a consensus statement. J Cardiovasc Surg 1997; 38:437–441.
158. Murray JD, Bergan JJ, Riffenburgh RH. Development of open-scope subfascial perforating vein surgery: lessons learned from the first 67 cases. Ann Vasc Surg 1999;13:372–377.
159. Tronnier M, Schmeller W, Wolff HH. Morphological changes in lipodermatosclerosis and venous ulcers: light microscopy, immunohistochemistry and electron microscopy. Phlebology 1994; 9:48–54.
160. Roszinski S, Schmeller W. Differences between intracutaneous and transcutaneous skin oxygen tension in chronic venous insufficiency. J Cardiovasc Surg (Torino) 1995; 36:407–413.
161. Kirsner RS, Pardes JB, Eaglstein WH, Falanga V. The clinical spectrum of lipodermatosclerosis. J Am Acad Dermatol 1993; 28:623–627.
162. Nemeth AJ, Eaglstein WH, Falanga V. Clinical parameters and transcutaneous oxygen measurements for the prognosis of venous ulcers. J Am Acad Dermatol 1989; 20:186–190.
163. Schmeller W, Gaber Y, Gehl HB. Shave therapy is a simple, effective treatment of persistent venous leg ulcers. J Am Acad Dermatol 1998; 39:232–238

47 Benign Subcutaneous Lesions: Cysts and Lipomas

Jessica J Krant MD MPH and John A Carucci MD PhD

Summary box

- Ensure that the patient is aware of the benign nature of the lesion before surgery, keeping in mind the relative importance of cosmesis in this setting.
- Although most cysts and lipomas are benign, beware of the occult cancer in a cyst wall or malignant lesions simulating benign nodules.
- Consider imaging before surgery for midline lesions, especially of the head, neck, and spinal column.
- Lipoma removal may in some cases be more complex than anticipated.
- The pitfalls to avoid in the management of cysts and lipomas are generally similar and are common to any subcutaneous space-filling lesion.
- Unless trained to manage these specific lesions, it is best to refer patients with sacrococcygeal pilonidal cysts/sinuses to general surgeons experienced in their removal.

■ INTRODUCTION

Because of the generally benign nature of cysts and lipomas, extra consideration must be given to cosmesis relative to the risk–benefit ratio of performing surgery. Although the risks of treating these lesions with surgery are generally low, it is especially important that the patient understands the benign nature of the lesion relative to the medical and cosmetic risks of surgery. Observation may suffice for small, asymptomatic lesions. Cysts may be painful; in some cases they can rupture and cause inflammation or infection. Lipomas, especially of the angiolipoma subtype, may be painful.[1] Both cysts and lipomas may be incompletely removed and may recur. Finally, one must always maintain an index of suspicion regarding the potential for seemingly benign lesions to contain unexpected foci of malignancy, to be malignant tumors, or even to be metastatic nodules.[2–5]

Imaging

The use of soft tissue radiological imaging such as ultrasound,[6] computed tomography (CT),[7] or magnetic resonance imaging (MRI)[8] can be extremely useful in evaluating the nature of subcutaneous lesions before attempting surgery. Some authors suggest that it may be possible to identify abnormal lipomatous tissue,[9] or to identify whether a mass is encapsulated. However, one area in which imaging is of clear medical necessity is in the preoperative evaluation of midline lesions. Nodules, or unusual growths of any kind along the midline of the face, especially at the nasal root, or along the suture lines of the skull, must be evaluated to rule out intracranial extension. Extracranial gliomas, encephaloceles, and dermoid cysts are all potentially problematic.[10] Lesions assumed to be benign lipomas or cysts can occasionally turn out to be extensions of malignant intracranial tumors, such as in the case of intracranial malignant meningioma thought to be a forehead lipoma.[11] Birthmarks along the spinal column above the top of the gluteal cleft are potential markers for spinal dysraphism. Midline lesions should be evaluated by CT scan to identify any underlying bony changes, followed with an MRI and referral to a neurosurgeon if suspicion is high.[12,13]

■ PREOPERATIVE PREPARATION

It is important to identify structures that may be at risk before operating. Marking of the area should be performed before anesthesia to prevent the loss of anatomic landmarks that can occur because of infiltration with local anesthetic. It is helpful with both cysts and lipomas to determine and mark the direction and location of relaxed skin tension lines (RSTL; Fig. 47.1) to assist with later decisions regarding wound closure.[14] Epidermal cysts, other epithelial cysts, and lipomas should all be marked along the palpable outer margin for reference, lest it be lost with anesthesia placement, and with a small dot, line, or ellipse to indicate the planned area of initial incision. One may also consider

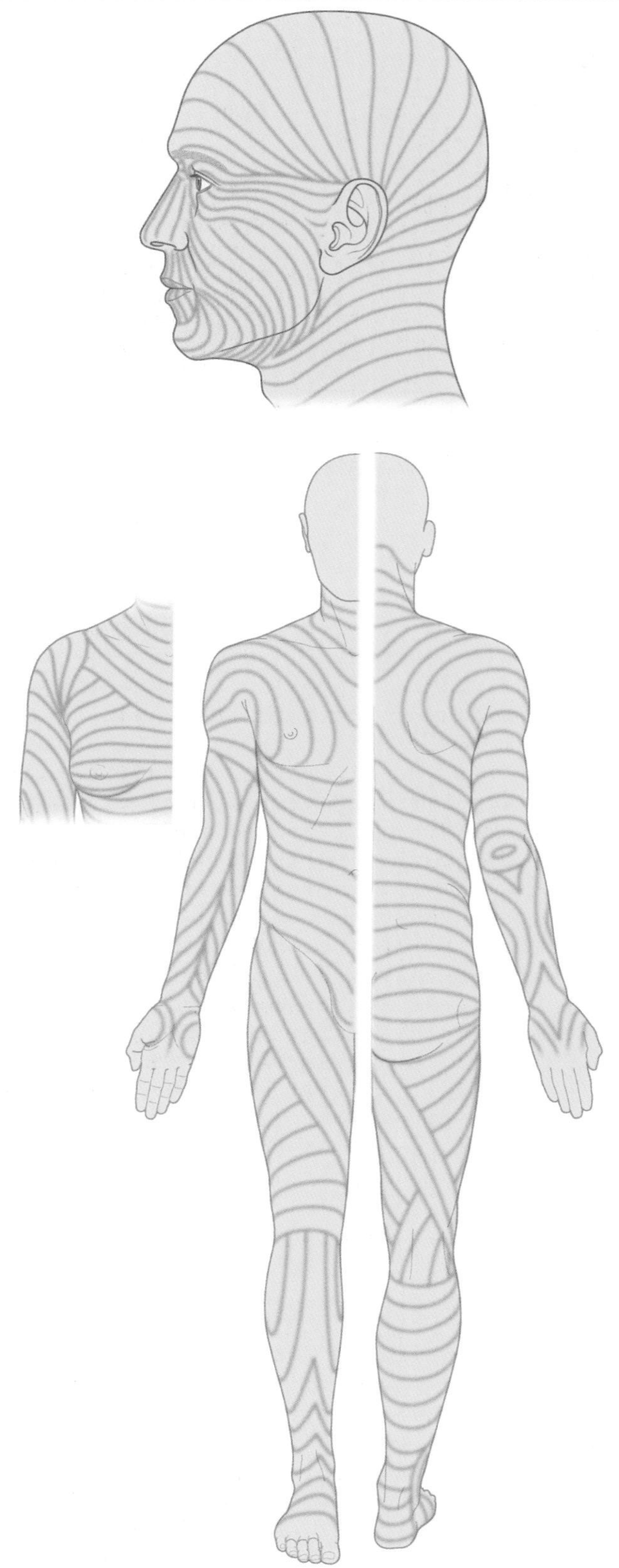

Figure 47.1 Relaxed skin tension lines (RSTLs): incisions made along these lines heal with minimum scarring. The lines shown in more detail on the face and head are Kraissl's lines, generally accepted as being more accurate than earlier descriptions. Differences between the male and female breast are also shown.

approaching the lesion laterally from an incision placed in a cosmetic boundary or within the hairline (Fig. 47.2).[15]

Anesthesia should be placed in a ring pattern around the lesion and beneath it, taking care not to point the needle inward toward the cyst or lipoma and risk rupturing the wall or capsule (Fig. 47.3). An additional small amount of anesthesia can be carefully placed very superficially directly along the incisional marking, to both anesthetize the area and to assist with hydrodissection of the dermis, elevating the skin from the top of the lesion and making it easier to incise the skin and leave the cyst wall or lipoma capsule intact.

Standard sterile surgical preparations are adequate for excision of cysts and lipomas. The surgical tray should include a #15 scalpel blade and handle, toothed forceps, a needle driver, blunt curved dissecting scissors, and suture cutting scissors, as in standard excisions. For cysts and lipomas each tray should also contain skin hooks and Halstead, Hartman Mosquito, or Kelly hemostats of different sizes. Given the subcutaneous location of the growths, hooks are a great help in facilitating visualization of deeper areas during dissection from a small incision site by enhancing retraction of skin edges. Serial placement of hemostat clamps is useful in gently teasing out the abnormal tissue while grasping the lesion. Finally, for space-filling cysts and lipomas, it is important to prevent postsurgical hematoma formation with meticulous hemostasis with electrocautery or suture ligation as needed.

■ TECHNIQUES

CYSTS

'Cyst' is a generic term which encompasses all true epithelial cysts that form in the skin, but is more commonly

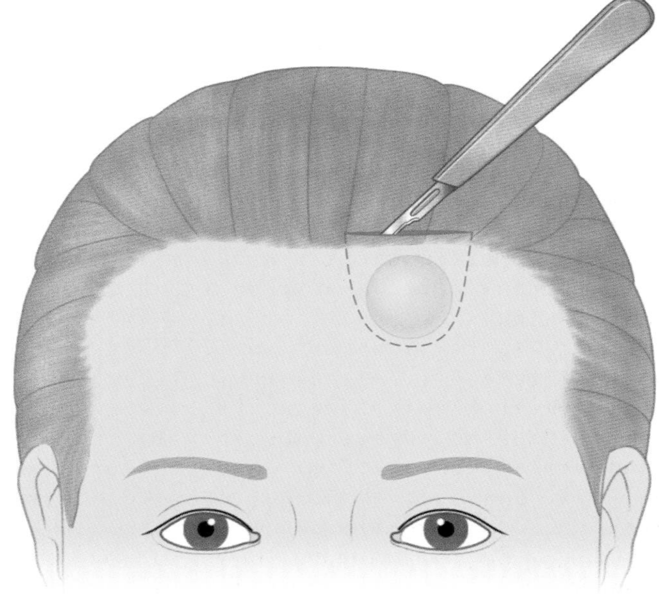

Figure 47.2 Excision planned to hide incision line within hairline or other cosmetic boundary.

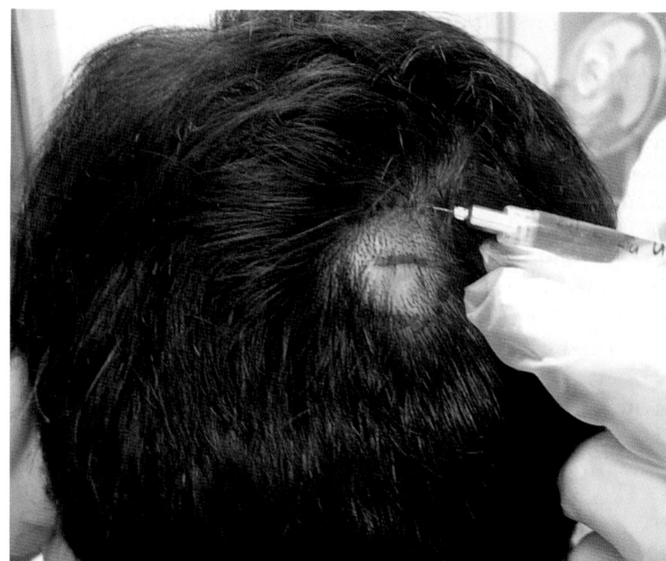
Figure 47.3 Scalp cyst showing marking and anesthesia placement.

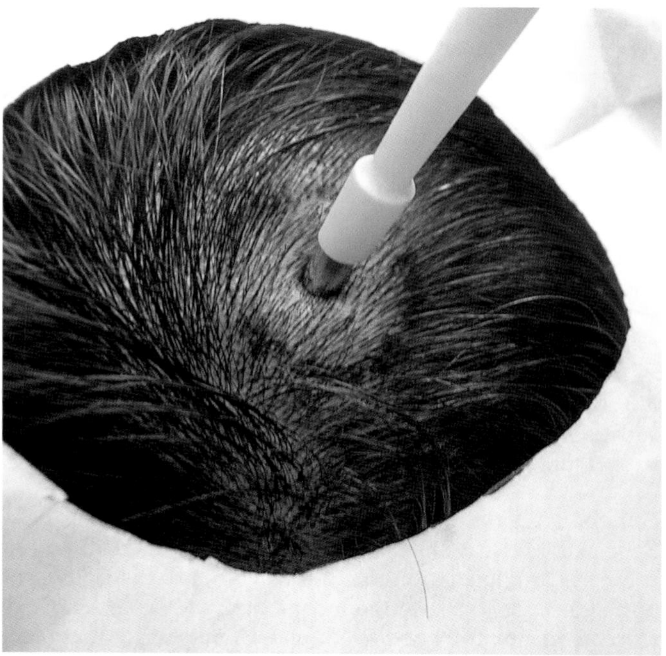
Figure 47.4 Placement of 4 mm punch over cyst for Danna procedure.

taken to imply the most common subtype found within the practice of dermatology: the epidermal cyst. This section reviews the approach toward and surgical treatment of seven types of true epithelial cysts. Selected common pseudocysts, which don't have a true epithelial wall, are briefly addressed.

Epidermal cyst

Also known as epidermoid or infundibular cysts, epidermal cysts are extremely common in clinical practice and most likely represent an epidermal invagination, traumatic implantation, or degenerated follicular structure creating a walled cyst lined with epidermis.[16] Squamous debris is released into the center creating the cheesy, often foul-smelling material that fills cysts and can cause an inflammatory reaction if rupture causes contact with surrounding dermis. A hallmark of these cysts (which can occur anywhere on the body but most commonly are found on the face, neck, back, and genitalia) is the punctum, which is usually visible at the skin surface.

Epidermal cysts are often brought to the attention of the dermatologist only once they have become inflamed or infected. Despite the patient's request for immediate removal, better results are likely to be obtained by waiting until inflammation has subsided. This can be hastened by injection with a small amount of intralesional triamcinolone acetonide (2.5–5 mg/ml, injected until the lesion begins to blanch) with or without empiric oral antibiotics. If the cyst is large and painful, incision and drainage with a large-bore needle or a #11 blade will aid in management along with warm compresses and antibiotics. Culture of purulent exudate should be obtained and antibiotic choice guided accordingly. Empiric antibiotic therapy with a first-generation cephalosporin or antistaphylococcal penicillin is recommended until culture results return. For patients allergic to penicillin, current recommendations favor clindamycin or possibly a newer fluoroquinolone, because of the emergence of macrolide-resistant bacteria.[17] Once the cyst has achieved a quiescent state, one may perform any of several commonly accepted techniques of incisional or excisional surgery.

Removal of an epidermal cyst may be time consuming because of the fragility of the cyst wall and the high degree of fibrosis that can sometimes be found around an aged or previously ruptured, inflamed, or infected cyst. Because of this, there are three basic approaches to consider when attempting removal of a cyst: incision, excision of the cyst alone by gentle dissection around the capsule, and excision of the cyst and surrounding fibrotic dermis as a whole.

Cysts may be removed by incision into, rather than around, the cyst, with partial or total retrieval of the capsule from within. This approach can be useful with cysts (and lipomas) because once the dermis and cyst capsule are invaded through a small slit incision, a small ellipse, or a punch (known as the Danna approach[18], Fig. 47.4), the cyst contents can be gently extruded by even and gradual finger pressure from the outside and the thin intact wall of the cyst can be teased out with a Skeele curette or skin hook slowly afterwards through a smaller opening than that required for excisional surgery. This method is simple if the cyst is small, fresh, not inflamed, and has a rather robust wall.

Perhaps the most common approach to cyst surgery is the traditional excisional approach, the goal of which is to remove intact the entire cyst, thus avoiding contact of the irritating cyst contents with the exposed and vulnerable dermis. With this approach, the surgeon makes a small slit or ellipse (including the cyst punctum if feasible), but instead of puncturing the cyst wall with the incision, gently cuts down until the glistening capsule is visible to the eye, and then slowly and gently dissects the dermis off the wall in all directions until the intact cyst can be extruded or popped out through the surgical opening. For this approach, it is helpful to leave the ellipse of skin attached to the top of the cyst for clasping with a forceps; alternatively a clamp can be used as a handle for grasping the cyst. A good assistant can use skin hooks to lift the dermis off the cyst sides for clear visualization and spreading blunt dissection until the cyst slowly begins to lift out of the cavity and the underside can be dissected or cut away if clear (Fig. 47.5). This method, especially in the case of a cyst with a particularly fragile wall, can be very time consuming. The residual cavity may require trimming and reshaping before closure.

If there has been previous rupture or infection before surgery and the cyst is surrounded by thick fibrosis or scarring, the above two methods will probably not be feasible. The cyst wall will not easily separate and lift out of a small opening using incisional surgery, and dissection of a fibrotic cyst wall can be frustrating to say the least. In cases such as this, en-bloc elliptical excision of the cyst and surrounding fibrotic tissue may be preferable (Fig. 47.6).

Special considerations

Special considerations that arise in the surgical treatment of these space-filling lesions include management of significant postsurgical dead space, redundant skin, the cyst's tendency to recur if not fully removed, and the irritating nature of cyst contents to the exposed dermis. Any spilled cyst contents should be removed by copious irrigation with sterile saline.

Pilar (trichilemmal) cyst

Ten–20% of cysts seen in surgical pathology are pilar or trichilemmal cysts.[10] These are similar to epidermal cysts but form instead when cells histologically similar to the follicular external root sheath create a cyst with trichilemmal keratinization, a thicker wall, and less odorous cyst contents. About 90% of these cysts form on the scalp, the rest on the head and neck, and they have no telltale accompanying epidermal punctum. The thick wall of pilar cysts makes them relatively simple to remove, but their less compressible nature may require longer incision lines in some cases.

Special considerations

The general approach for pilar cysts is the same as that for epidermal cysts; however, in the case of substantial wall thickness, here one may choose to incise the tough cyst wall itself to grasp an edge with a clamp, for easier manipulation of the cyst and dissection of surrounding dermis, again taking care to thoroughly irrigate the wound before closure to ensure no irritating cyst contents remain. In the case of the robust pilar cyst, one may also use increased finger pressure outside the surgical incision area to firmly 'deliver' the cyst through the incision, thus allowing less manipulation of the incised epidermis with forceps and hooks, and

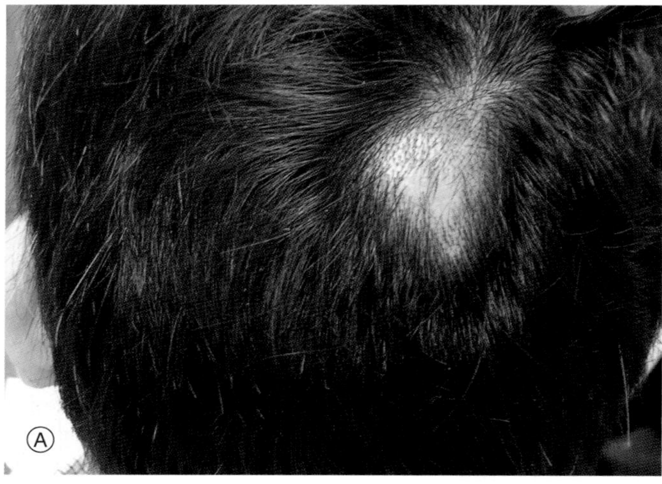

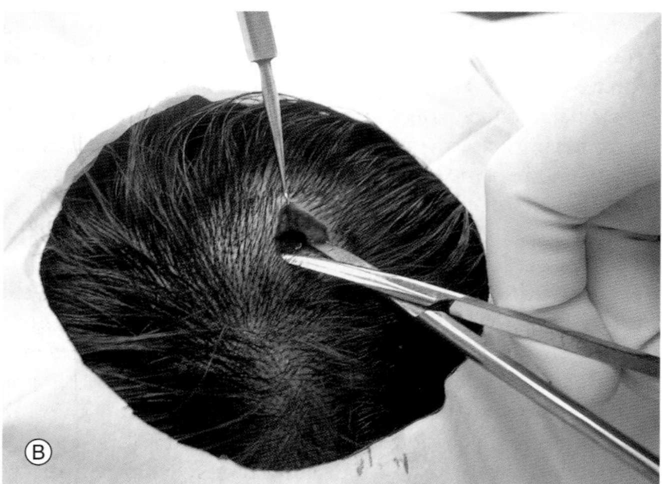

Dissection of cyst

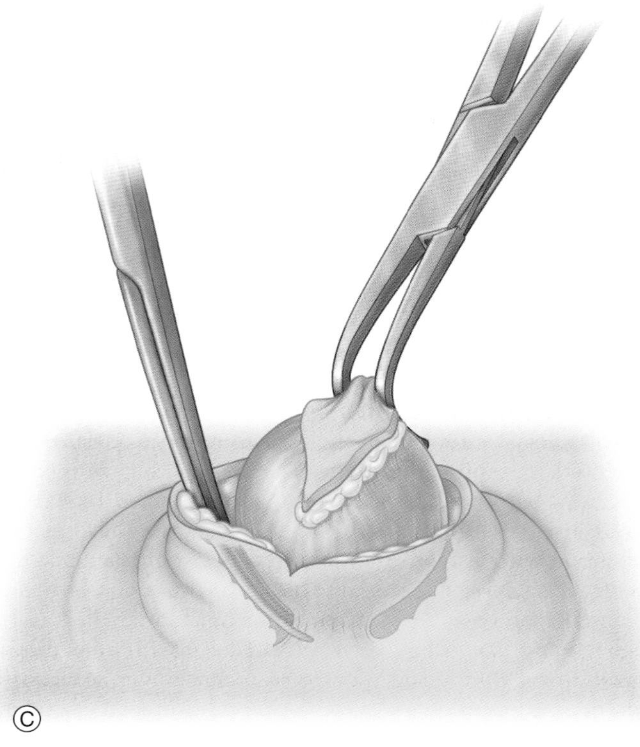

Figure 47.5 Scalp cyst. (A) Localized area of alopecia because of pressure. (B) Surgical dissection of surrounding dermis from cyst wall. (C) Technique for dissection of cyst from wall.

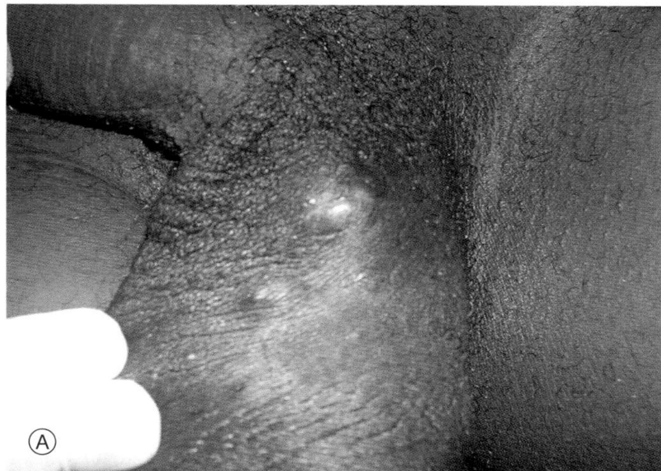

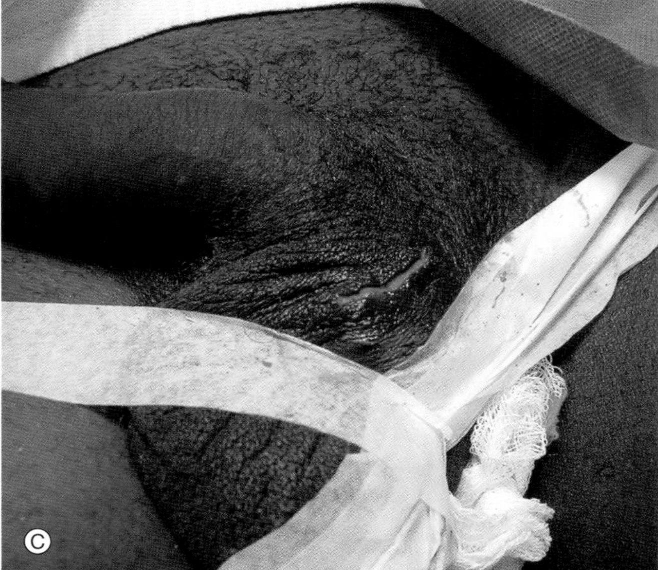

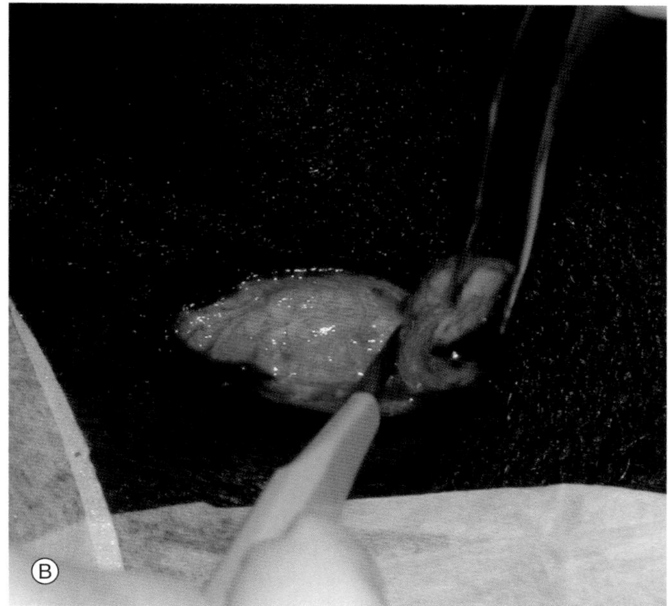

Figure 47.6 Scrotal cysts. (A) Showing puncta. (B) Excision en bloc of fibrosed cyst. (C) After excision, with subcutaneous sutures in place.

then carefully dissect the dermis from underneath with instruments or fingertips, allowing for a relatively quick procedure from beginning to end.[19]

Proliferating trichilemmal cyst

Like the pilar cyst, proliferating trichilemmal cysts (PTCs) form with trichilemmal keratinization, but tend to be more solid than cystic. The surgical approach is similar to that used in removal of pilar cysts. PTCs can be confused with squamous cell carcinoma because of the common presence of cellular atypia.[20] Lopez-Rios et al suggest that wide local excision and long-term follow-up should be considered in these cases given the difficulty of differentiating focally invasive proliferating trichilemmal cysts from squamous cell carcinoma.[21]

Dermoid cyst

Dermoid cysts are similar histopathologically to epidermal cysts except they have no connection with the epidermis above, and therefore no visible punctum. It is believed that they are formed by invagination of epidermis during embryonic development, and thus are more commonly seen in embryonic fusion planes. Because of this, dermoid cysts tend to present at a younger age than epidermal cysts, a factor which can be helpful in determining the need for preoperative imaging.[22] Although dermoid cysts along the orbital rim are often attached to periosteum, they are less likely to invade intracranially than nasal dermoids, which show clinical or radiographic evidence of intracranial extension in 26% of cases, most of which require intracranial and extracranial excision, in a series reported by Rahbar et al.[23] If no intracranial extension is present, dermoid cysts may be excised in a similar way as epidermal cysts, with or without overlying epidermis.

Milium

This type of cyst is a tiny version of the classic epidermal cyst, histologically identical and commonly idiopathic in origin, but often trauma-related. Some believe that there is a relationship with vellus hair follicles.[16] Milia are tiny (1–2 mm) papules that are easily treated with a miniature version of excisional cyst surgery. The milium can be removed with a standard punch biopsy and suture, or removed by pressure, gentle curettage, or by using a comedone extractor or needle tip after a superficial slit is made over the cyst with a blade.

Steatocystoma multiplex

As the name suggests, steatocystoma multiplex is a cyst that usually occurs in aggregates across the chest, proximal arms, and thighs. First present in early childhood, the lesions increase in both size and number during puberty. Steatocystomas are cysts formed from the sebaceous duct lining, and are therefore filled with an oily, yellowish fluid made up of sebum and esters rather than cheesy squamous material.[24] They are difficult to eradicate satisfactorily because of their number, location, and propensity to continue forming.

Special considerations

It may be difficult to optimize cosmesis and effect cure in treating steatocystoma multiplex. Surgical excision of individual lesions, incision and drainage with or without electrodesiccation, curettage, carbon dioxide laser, and cryotherapy[25] all share the unfortunate consequences of less-than-ideal scarring on the chest area. The use of a sharp-tipped cautery needle to puncture the cysts, followed by cyst evacuation and removal of the sac using fine forceps has been described as effective.[26]

Hidrocystoma

Formed from eccrine or apocrine duct or apocrine gland, hidrocystomas are 1–3 mm cysts that are most commonly found around the eyes, and occasionally directly on the lid margin.

Special considerations

Although hidrocystomas are easy to eradicate surgically with incision, removal of cyst wall to prevent recurrence, and a single suture (if necessary), it is important to note that translucent papules around the eyes can also represent small basal cell carcinomas.

Digital myxoid cyst

Unlike the above epithelial cysts, which tend to occur most commonly on the head and neck (and for epidermal cysts, trunk and genitalia), bluish, translucent digital myxoid cysts occur on the fingers and toes, and require special attention. Despite the name 'cyst,' these are not true walled epithelial cysts, but rather pseudocystic formations created either by the extrusion of hyaluronic acid-laden jellylike myxoid contents of synovial joint spaces into nearby dermis, or by de-novo collection of hyaluronic acid produced by locally overproductive fibroblasts at the proximal nail fold, often leading to longitudinal nail plate grooving.[27] Both types can be recurrent and painful. The often undetectable connection with the underlying joint space in the former type (and tendency for multiple, unobserved cysts to be present in the same area) increases the risk of both recurrence and joint infection, and leads some surgeons to refer patients to hand surgery specialists, especially when considering the close proximity of tendons and nerves.

Special considerations

Before attempting surgical removal of a digital myxoid cyst, some advocate first attempting to shrink the myxoid cyst with an injection of triamcinolone 0.1% or simply needle puncturing and releasing the contents repeatedly until it no longer recurs.[28] Alternatively, one may choose to first approach these frequently recurrent lesions with electrodesiccation and gentle curettage of the wall or local cryosurgery[29] rather than time-consuming, meticulous, and possibly unsuccessful scalpel surgery.

For myxoid cysts that are dorsolateral to joint spaces, some authors advocate injection of methylene blue, saline, and hydrogen peroxide into the cyst before surgery to assist in identification of a tenuous connecting stalk and other nearby cyst lobules for thoroughness, followed by dissection of the cyst and removal after raising a rectangular flap from the proximal nail fold, which can be replaced and sutured afterwards.[30] One author suggests that myxoid cysts will resolve with no recurrence if the stalk itself is simply identified and tied off by raising a flap of skin after dye is injected, excising no tissue at all.[31] Others advocate excision of a distal cyst en bloc with the entire proximal nail fold allowing healing by second intention.[27]

A nerve block may be applied at the proximal digit with or without additional local infiltration around the cyst site. Hemostasis during the procedure may be aided by the use of epinephrine (adrenaline) in the anesthetic mix[32] or a digital tourniquet. A sterile glove finger of the appropriate size cut at the tip and rolled back to exsanguinate the digit, or a Penrose drain with gauze padding clamped around the digit have both been used successfully. If using a tourniquet of any type, it is important that it is not left in place for more than 30 minutes at a time, to minimize the risk of necrosis of the distal digit.[33]

Mucous cyst (mucocele)

This cyst, another pseudocyst, is similar conceptually in etiology to the myxoid cyst, except that it most commonly occurs in the mucosal surface of the lower lip, in the buccal mucosa, or rarely, on the tongue. Instead of hyaluronic acid-based myxoid jelly, the cyst contains extravasated sialomucin, often secondary to local trauma. Full-thickness excision is usually not necessary because the cysts resolve easily by cutting away the superficial wall, allowing the contents to drain and allowing healing to take place secondarily, with or without the addition of electrodesiccation to the remaining lining.[22] Some authors have advocated cryotherapy directly to the cyst with no pretreatment.[29] A minimally invasive technique that has been shown to be successful especially in children is the use of micro-marsupialization, in which a 4-0 silk suture is passed through an intact mucocele after the application of topical lidocaine jelly, knotted, and left in place for a week, allowing regression of the lesion.[34]

Pilonidal cyst/pilonidal sinus

Sacrococcygeal pilonidal cysts have been the subject of etiological controversy, but are thought by most now to be acquired lesions caused by the traumatic implantation of broken pieces of hair shaft, rather than being congenital in nature.[35] Pilonidal cysts may also occur in other areas of the body, most notably the hand,[36] but the sacrococcygeal location has proved the most difficult to treat successfully because of the tendency of some lesions to recur and to form deep and unpredictable sinuses in this area that may lead toward the spinal column. Despite the development of promising new procedures to change the shape of the natal cleft and thus prevent hair entrapment,[37] the authors feel that surgical eradication of sacrococcygeal pilonidal cysts and sinus tracts is beyond the scope of this book, and most patients with such lesions should be referred to general surgeons experienced in their removal.

Lipomas

Cutaneous lipomas are usually benign, soft, well-circumscribed, asymptomatic, subcutaneous nodules of mature adipose tissue that represent the most common form of mesenchymal tumor; however, adipose tumors can occur in several different clinical patterns and present divergent histopathological pictures. Familiarity with these is important for the surgeon considering treatment of the patient because it will impact procedural decision-making. Lipomas may be solitary or multiple, may or may not have a well-defined capsule, and in some cases are associated with congenital syndromes. Although usually asymptomatic, they may be painful if larger, deeper, involved with local nerves, or of the angiolipoma subtype. Benign lipomas have been divided into five general subtypes: common lipoma; histopathologic variants (such as angiolipoma, angiomyolipoma, spindle-cell lipoma, pleomorphic lipoma, and benign lipoblastoma); lipomas within nonadipose tissue (such as subfascial or intramuscular lipomas); infiltrating or diffuse lipomas; and hibernomas.[38]

The surgical technique for approaching a lipoma is similar to that for removal of a cyst. After the area is infiltrated and marked and the appropriate instruments are gathered as discussed above, the surgeon makes as small an incision or punch as he or she feels may provide adequate access (Fig. 47.7A). Lipomas are largely compressible (unless subfascial) and may be delivered through a small opening by firm, rocking pressure around the edges once the fibrous bands of attachment are bluntly dissected around the surface of the nodule.[39] The initial linear or elliptical incision should be placed along RSTL when feasible, keeping in mind that a small approach incision can always be extended if necessary. Once the surgeon has gently cut down and visualized the glistening capsule or lobules of abnormal adipose tissue (which may be underneath a layer of normal adipose tissue and thus well-camouflaged), the nodule can be grasped with a clamp if possible, which can then be used to help gently tease the tissue from its bed (Fig. 47.7B). A lipoma sitting within surrounding normal adipose tissue often has larger and somewhat darker yellow-to-orange lobules than the surrounding area, which in some cases may help to differentiate tissue and help identify the endpoint of the procedure.[40] If there is no identifiable capsule to grasp, the surgeon will have to instead rely on assistance and serial clamping, gradually working the tissue out while bluntly dissecting around and underneath to remove the lipoma lobule by lobule, taking care to leave as little to no abnormal tissue behind as possible and thus minimize the risk of recurrence. Dynamic pressure along the outer edges of the palpable lipoma assists its delivery through the incision (Figs 47.7C, 47.8).

■ OPTIMIZING OUTCOMES IN LIPOMA SURGERY

After the surgeon is satisfied that the lipoma is cleared, meticulous hemostasis must be obtained because a dead space will be left after removal of this space-filling lesion, putting it at risk for hematoma or seroma formation. Next, placement of deep sutures is necessary to close the dead space and minimize the risk of both hematoma and a

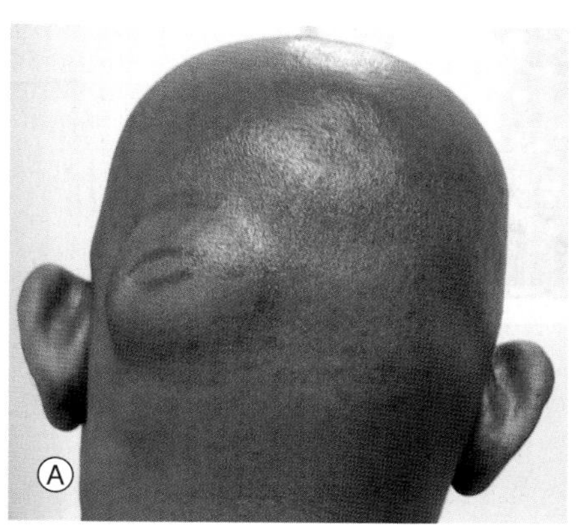

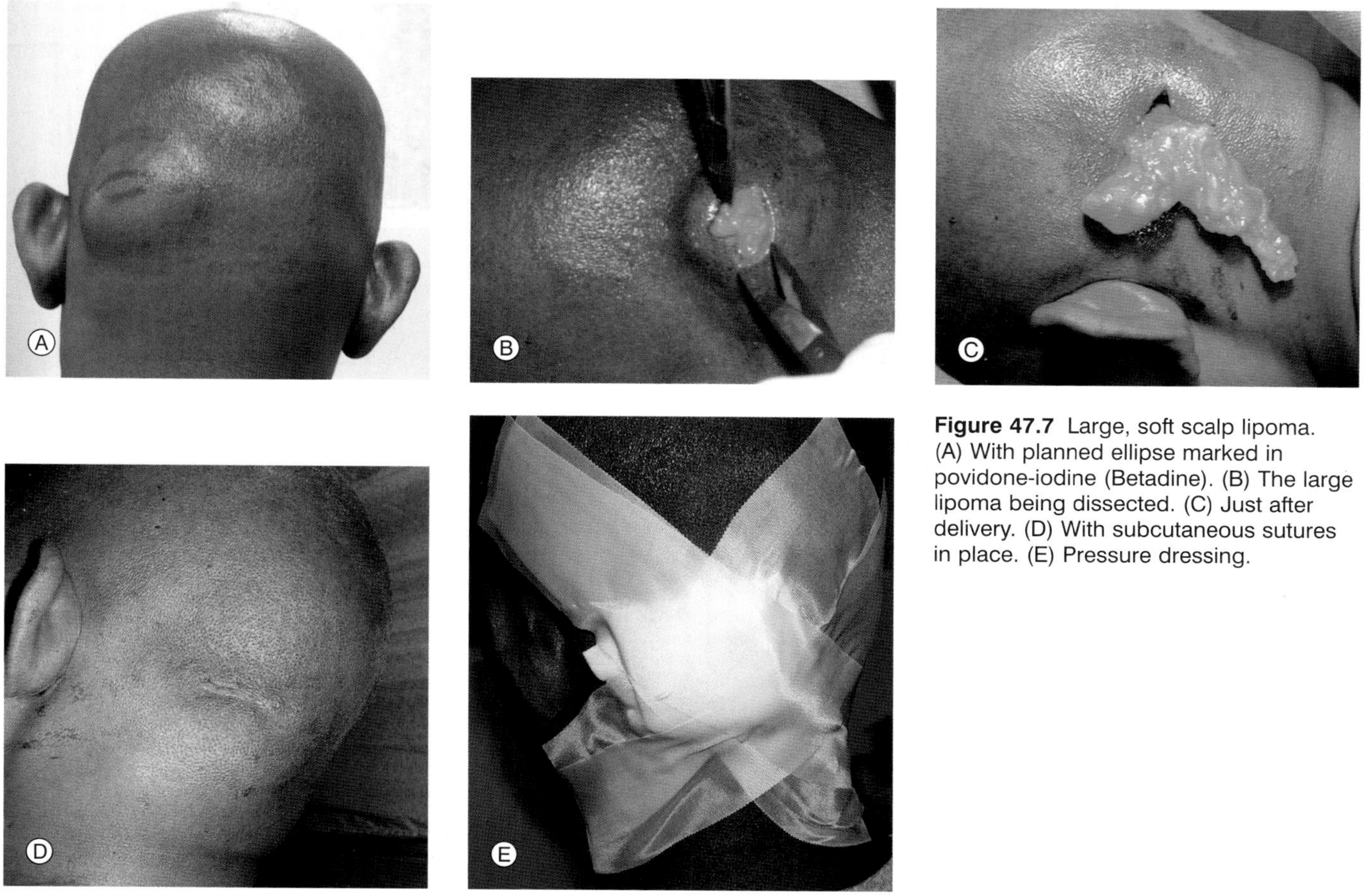

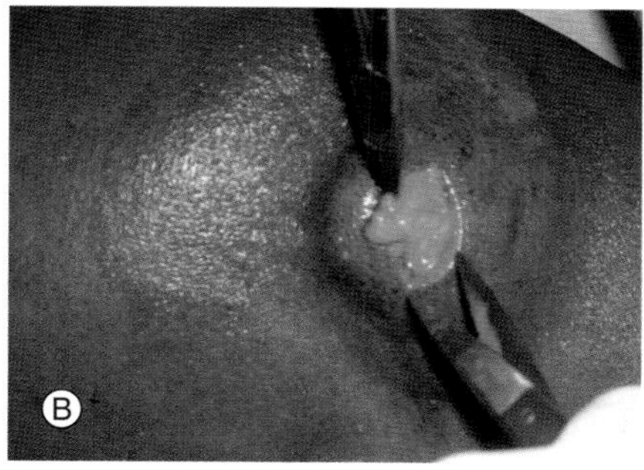

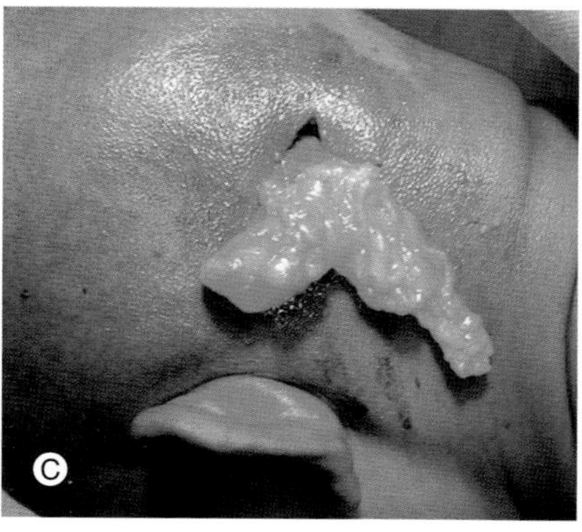

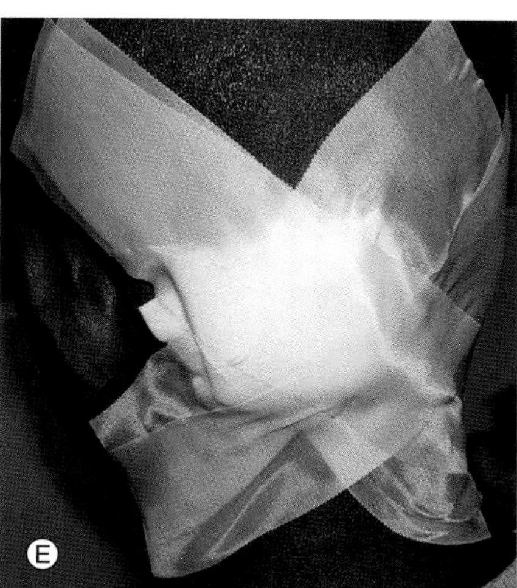

Figure 47.7 Large, soft scalp lipoma. (A) With planned ellipse marked in povidone-iodine (Betadine). (B) The large lipoma being dissected. (C) Just after delivery. (D) With subcutaneous sutures in place. (E) Pressure dressing.

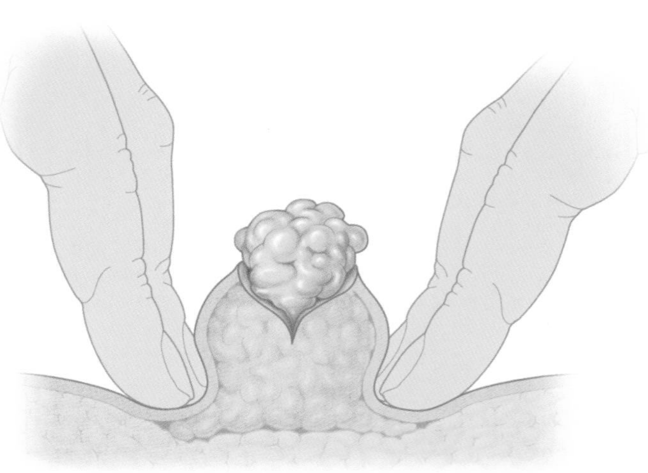

Figure 47.8 Technique for application of firm finger pressure around lipoma (or cyst) to deliver it through incision.

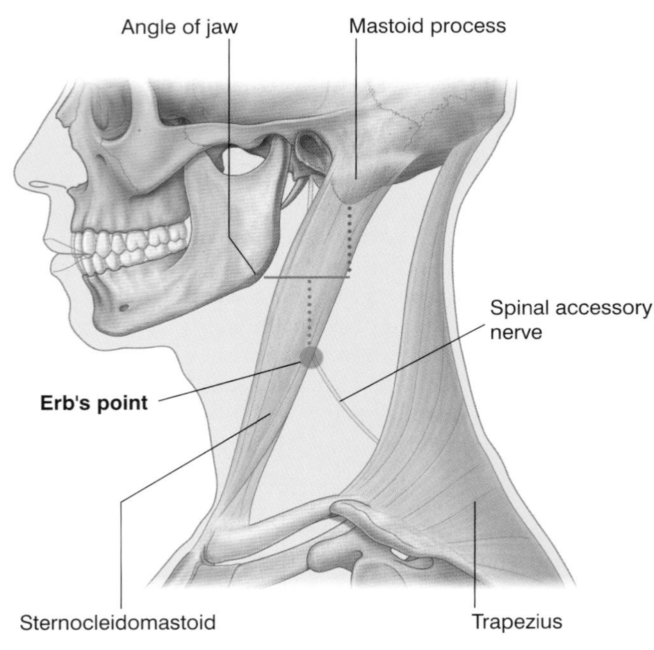

Figure 47.9 Erb's point demonstrated in the posterior triangle of the neck.

surface dell when healing. In some cases, if the lipoma was very deep, a temporary drain may be placed to aid in the first stages of healing. Finally, attention to precise alignment and suture closure of the cutaneous layer is not to be underestimated, remembering that these lesions are generally benign and high value is placed on cosmesis (Fig. 47.7D).

Three areas in lipoma surgery deserve special note to optimize outcomes: anatomic location and level; size, depth, and infiltration; and potential for malignant pathology and recurrence. Most lipomas occur on the proximal limbs, trunk, or distal limbs in the subcutaneous tissue. The surgeon must always be aware of anatomic structures potentially at risk. This is of special importance in several locations, notably, the posterior triangle of the neck where the XIth cranial nerve (spinal accessory nerve) is exposed at the border of the sternocleidomastoid; the hands, feet, and digits; and the forehead and scalp.

Lipomas of the neck and proximal limbs can be tricky because these areas tend to be the most common for deeper penetration of a seemingly cutaneous lesion. In these cases, the tumor must be carefully dissected from surrounding tissues. Damage to the spinal accessory nerve in the posterior triangle of the neck will cause pain, difficulty in shoulder elevation, and scapular winging because of paralysis of the trapezius muscle. The nerve is at high risk because of its superficial location under only skin and fascia in this zone.[41] To avoid injuring this critical nerve, surgeons should note the relationship of the lipoma to the sternocleidomastoid and trapezius muscles and locate Erb's point at the junction of the posterior border of the sternocleidomastoid and a line dropped vertically from the midpoint of a horizontal line drawn between the angle of the jaw and the mastoid process (Fig. 47.9). If the nerve is severed, primary repair within 3 months is optimal.[42]

On the digits and hands, it is common for lipomatous tissue to become involved with local tendons and nerves, and again, one must use extra caution, and should have a low threshold for referral to a hand surgeon.[43] Of note, nodules on the forehead and scalp which at first are diagnosed as cysts, are often found instead to be lipomas in the inter- or intramuscular,[44] or subgaleal plane, firmly sandwiched there above the periosteum (and thus deceivingly immobile and firm to initial palpation).[45] This is important to know, because the surgeon can often save time and prevent excessive tissue damage that might otherwise occur if searching for the tumor too superficially. A very good cosmetic result can often be obtained if a single horizontal incision is made along the RSTL of the forehead, in approaching a subgaleal lipoma here.

Presumed lipomas must be evaluated by a dermatopathologist to identify potential atypical lipomas ('well-differentiated liposarcomas'), which can be resected locally with a margin of normal adipose tissue, or other malignant tumors.[46] Keep in mind that larger, deeper, more infiltrative, recurrent, or faster-growing lipomatous tumors have greater tendency to show malignant patterns.[47] In the case of patients with numerous small and asymptomatic lipomas, it is sometimes helpful for the patient and surgeon to remove at least one or two of the larger, more bothersome lesions and check pathology for reassurance. Finally, even with the best surgical technique, lipomas may recur, and it is important to advise the patient of this risk beforehand.

Liposuction

In the interests of minimizing invasiveness and morbidity and optimizing cosmetic outcome, many reports have appeared in the literature regarding liposuction for removal of fatty tumors. This has been especially true as a proposed option for treating larger lipomas in the pediatric and adult population,[48,49] but has also been shown to be successful as an approach for smaller or medium-sized lipomas.[50] Along with the benefits of minimal scarring, one must keep in mind the same risks of recurrence and of potential malignant pathology in this approach.

■ POSTOPERATIVE CARE

Postoperative care for cysts is the same as for other basic skin surgery, including special attention to a good pressure dressing for the immediate postoperative period to minimize the risk of seroma or hematoma formation.

For lipomas, postoperative wound care is generally the same as for cyst removal, including application of a firm pressure dressing for the immediate postoperative period (Fig. 47.7E).

■ PITFALLS AND THEIR MANAGEMENT

A number of actions can be taken to avoid or minimize the occurrence of pitfalls in surgery for cysts and lipomas.

Pitfalls and their management

- Always send tissue for evaluation by a dermatopathologist.
- Minimize dead space upon closure, and use good pressure dressings.
- Cysts
  - avoid operating on an inflamed or infected cyst
  - ensure that no cyst wall or debris remains in surgical cavity
  - if dissection is not proceeding smoothly because of fibrosis, consider converting to an elliptical excision to remove fibrotic tissue
  - find and remove the punctum if possible—if no punctum is present, the lesion may be a dermoid cyst
  - keep in mind there may be more than one cyst or lobule in a given pocket—search for others before closure.
- Lipomas
  - avoid making the initial incision larger than necessary
  - maintain meticulous hemostasis, especially in larger lipomas
  - identify the abnormal target tissue morphologically or by its capsule to avoid removing healthy tissue
  - note anatomic location of lesion and proceed accordingly, keeping in mind likely depth of lipoma and involvement of local nerves and tendons.

■ SUMMARY

Cysts and lipomas are among the most commonly excised subcutaneous lesions in dermatologic surgery. It is important to keep in mind both the great likelihood of benignity and the small risk of malignancy when approaching patients who complain of these growths, and to adequately review these considerations with the patient before removal. Both types of lesions can in most cases be treated successfully in an office setting by dermatologists.

■ REFERENCES

1. Howard WR, Helwig EB. Angiolipoma. Arch Dermatol 1960; 82:924–931.
2. Theocharous C, Jaworski RC. Squamous cell carcinoma arising in an eccrine hidrocystoma. Pathology 1993; 25:184–186.
3. Dini M, Innocenti A, Romano GF. Basal cell carcinoma arising from epidermoid cyst. Dermatol Surg 2001; 27:585–586.
4. Lopez-Rios F, Rodriguez-Peralto JL, Castano E, Benito A. Squamous cell carcinoma arising in a cutaneous epidermal cyst: case report and literature review. Am J Dermatopathol 1999; 21:174–177.
5. Hermanns-Le T, Jermanns JF, Pierard-Franchimont C, et al. [Let us watch cutaneous cystic lesions. From derision to merit.] Rev Med Liege 2002; 57:314–316.
6. Fornage BD, Tassin GB. Sonographic appearances of superficial soft tissue lipomas. J Clin Ultrasound 1991; 19:215–220.
7. Varma DG, Muchmore JH, Mizushima A. Computed tomography of infiltrating benign lipoma. J Comput Tomogr 1987; 11:45–49.
8. Jabra AA, Taylor GA. MRI evaluation of superficial soft tissue lesions in children. Pediatr Radiol 1993; 23:425–428.
9. Matsumoto K, Hukuda S, Ishizawa M, et al. MRI findings in intramuscular lipomas. Skeletal Radiol 1999; 28:145–152.
10. Freedberg IM, Eisen AZ, Wolff K, et al, eds. Fitzpatrick's dermatology in general medicine, 5th edn. New York: McGraw-Hill; 1999:885–887.
11. Fung MA, Grekin RC, Odom RB. Intracranial malignant meningioma mimicking frontalis-associated lipoma of the forehead. J Am Acad Dermatol 1996; 34:306–307.
12. Drolet B. Birthmarks to worry about. Cutaneous markers of spinal dysraphism. Dermatol Clin 1998; 16:447–453.
13. Kanev PM, Park TS. Dermoids and dermal sinus tracts of the spine. Neurosurg Clin N Am 1995; 6:359–366.
14. Andrews K, Gharami A, Mowlavi A, Goldfarb JN. The youthful forehead: placement of skin incisions in hidden furrows. Dermatol Surg 2000; 26:489–490.
15. Peinert RA, Courtiss EH. Excision from a distance: a technique for removal of benign subcutaneous lesions. Plastic Reconstr Surg 1983 Jul; 72:94–96.
16. Epstein WL, Kligman AM. The pathogenesis of milia and benign tumors of the skin. J Invest Dermatol 1956; 26:1–11.
17. Fung HB, Chang JY, Kuczynski S. A practical guide to the treatment of complicated skin and soft tissue infections. Drugs 2003; 63:1459–1480.
18. Danna JA. A simple treatment for sebaceous cyst. New Orleans Med Surg J 1945; 98.
19. Oliveira AS, Picoto AS, Verde SF, Martins O. A simple method of excising trichilemmal cysts from the scalp. J Dermatol Surg Oncol 1979; 5:625–627.
20. Brownstein MH, Arluk DJ. Proliferating trichilemmal cyst: a simulant of squamous cell carcinoma. Cancer 1981; 48:1207–1214.
21. Lopez-Rios, Rodriguez-Peralto JL, Aguilar A, et al. Proliferating trichilemmal cyst with focal invasion: report of a case and a review of the literature. Am J Dermatopathol 2000; 22:183–187.
22. Bennett RG. Cystic lesions. Fundamentals of cutaneous surgery. St Louis: CV Mosby; 1988:734–757.
23. Rahbar R, Shah P, Mulliken JB, et al. The presentation and management of nasal dermoid: a 30-year experience. Arch Otolaryngol Head Neck Surg 2003; 129:464–471.
24. Lynch FW, Fisher I. Steatocystoma multiplex: an analysis of their contents. J Invest Dermatol 1947; 8:65–67.
25. Notowicz A. Treatment of lesions of steatocystoma multiplex and other epidermal cysts by cryosurgery. J Dermatol Surg Oncol 1980; 6:98–99.
26. Kaya TI, Ikizoglu G, Kokturk A, Tursen U. A simple surgical technique for the treatment of steatocystoma multiplex. Int J Dermatol 2001; 40:785–788.

27. Salasche SJ. Myxoid cysts of the proximal nail fold: a surgical approach. J Dermatol Surg Oncol 1984; 10:35–39.
28. Epstein E. A simple technique for managing digital mucous cysts. Arch Dermatol 1979; 115:1315–1316.
29. Böhler-Sommeregger K, Kutschera-Heinert G. Cryosurgical management of myxoid cysts. J Dermatol Surg Oncol 1988; 14:1405–1408.
30. Goldman JA, Goldman L, Jaffe MS, Richfield DF. Digital mucinous pseudocysts. Arthritis Rheum 1977; 20:997–1002.
31. de Berker D, Lawrence C. Ganglion of the distal interphalangeal joint (myxoid cyst): therapy by identification and repair of the leak of joint fluid. Arch Dermatol 2001; 137:607–610.
32. Wilhelmi BJ, Blackwell SJ, Miller JH, et al. Do not use epinephrine in digital blocks: myth or truth? Plast Reconstr Surg 2001; 107:393–397.
33. Smith IM, Austin OM, Knight SL. A simple and fail safe method for digital tourniquet. J Hand Surg [Br] 2002; 27:363–364.
34. Delbem AC, Cunha RF, Vieira AE, Ribeiro LL. Treatment of mucus retention phenomena in children by the micro-marsupialization technique: case reports. Pediatr Dent 2000; 22:155–158.
35. da Silva JH. Pilonidal cyst: cause and treatment. Dis Colon Rectum 2000; 43:1146–1156.
36. Uysal AC, Alagoz MS, Unlu RE, Sensoz O. Hairdresser's syndrome: a case report of an interdigital pilonidal sinus and review of the literature. Dermatol Surg 2003; 29:288–290.
37. Bascom J, Bascom T. Failed pilonidal surgery: new paradigm and new operation leading to cures. Arch Surg 2002; 137:1146–1150.
38. Enzinger FM, Weiss SW. Benign lipomatous tumors. Soft tissue tumors. St. Louis: CV Mosby; 1988:301–345.
39. Christenson L, Patterson J, Davis D. Surgical pearl: use of the cutaneous punch for the removal of lipomas. J Am Acad Dermatol 2000; 42:675–676.
40. Hardin F. Surgical gem: a simple technique for removing lipomas. J Dermatol Surg Oncol 1982; 8:316–317.
41. Lu L, Haman SP, Ebraheim NA. Vulnerability of the spinal accessory nerve in the posterior triangle of the neck: a cadaveric study. Orthopedics 2002; 25:71–74.
42. Nason RW, Abdulrauf BM, Stranc MF. The anatomy of the accessory nerve and cervical lymph node biopsy. Am J Surg 2000; 180: 241–243.
43. Oster LH, Blair WF, Steyers CM. Large lipomas in the deep palmar space. J Hand Surg 1989; 14:700–703.
44. Ban M, Kitajima Y. Intramuscular lipoma within the temporal muscle. Int J Dermatol 2002; 41:689–90.
45. Zitelli JA. Subgaleal lipomas. Arch Dermatol 1989; 125:384–385.
46. Stewart MG, Schwartz MR, Alford BR. Atypical and malignant lipomatous lesions of the head and neck. Arch Otolaryngol Head Neck Surg 1994; 120:1151–1155.
47. Rydholm A, Berg NO. Size, site and clinical incidence of lipoma: factors in the differential diagnosis of lipoma and sarcoma. Acta Orthop Scand 1983; 54:929–934.
48. Ilhan H, Tokar B. Liposuction of a pediatric giant superficial lipoma. J Pediatr Surg 2002; 37:796–798.
49. Sharma PK, Janniger CK, Schwartz RA. The treatment of atypical lipoma with liposuction. J Dermatol Surg Oncol 1991; 17:332–334.
50. Zitelli JA, Moy RL. The management of lipomas using liposuction. Surg Guide Lines 1988; 3:1–2.

48 Mohs Micrographic Surgery and Cutaneous Oncology

Hubert T Greenway MD and Kurt L Maggio MD

Summary box

- Mohs micrographic surgery is a specialized surgical procedure indicated for basal cell carcinoma, squamous cell carcinoma, melanoma, and other malignancies of the skin and mucous membranes.
- Mohs micrographic surgery provides complete microscopic margin control through the use of horizontal frozen histologic sections of the entire margins of the excised tumor.
- Mohs surgery is cost-effective and provides the highest cure rate for tumors that spread by direct extension.
- Mohs surgery requires a physician trained in surgery and pathology to accurately excise and map tumor extensions.
- Mohs surgery entails a series of precise steps that lead to tumor extirpation and allow for immediate wound repair.
- Mohs surgery has few complications with proper preoperative planning, but can be a time-intensive procedure.

INTRODUCTION

Mohs micrographic surgery is a method of excision that provides complete microscopic control of tumor margins and offers cure rates superior to those of other treatment options. It may be used for any accessible form of cancer, but is most commonly used for cutaneous malignancies, and can be used for benign neoplasms in special situations as well. It is a meticulous technique performed by a physician skilled in cutaneous surgery and pathology, in which horizontal frozen histologic sections of the surgical margins of the excised tumor are generated for the most complete microscopic examination possible. Residual malignant extensions of the margins are mapped and excised selectively until the tumor is removed. It is designed primarily to answer the question 'Is it all out?' as opposed to 'What is it?'[1] Mohs micrographic surgery is usually performed in an outpatient facility over several hours using local anesthesia. The resulting defect is minimized by the procedure's inherent conservation of normal tissue adjacent to the tumor, and may be repaired immediately, allowed to heal by second intention, or undergo delayed reconstruction. Training programs for performing Mohs micrographic surgery are now available throughout the US via a 1- or 2-year fellowship after completion of residency, and in 2003 the Accreditation Council for Graduate Medical Education approved procedural dermatology fellowships in which Mohs surgery is the backbone.

Cutaneous tumors have been successfully treated in a number of ways. These include standard fusiform excision, cryotherapy, radiation therapy, curettage and electrodesiccation, intralesional interferon,[2] topical and intralesional 5-fluorouracil,[3] and ablative laser treatment.[4] Recently, imiquimod, a novel immune response modifier thought to stimulate interferon-α, has been used for cutaneous tumors.[5] These methods can provide excellent results in many circumstances. However, none of them determine that the borders are completely tumor-free and offer the patient the satisfaction of immediately knowing that their tumor has been completely removed. Mohs micrographic surgery offers this information along with a superior cure rate, and is often the method preferred by both patient and physician. Mohs surgery consistently shows the lowest 5-year recurrence rates compared to all other modalities.[6]

Mohs micrographic surgery is predicated on the observation that skin cancers generally grow through direct extension without 'skip' areas. Tumor cells can be found a significant distance from the clinically visible and palpable neoplasm, yet are in continuity with the tumor itself as a result of the tumor's microscopic spread. Thus, the tumor can be traced to its termination by excising it layer by layer and examining the entire margin of each layer under the microscope. Critical in this process is that the skin edge and deep surface are visualized in one plane on the glass slide, and thus the entire margin can be analyzed. A map is constructed for each layer to accurately locate residual

History

- 1930s: Frederic E Mohs, a general surgical trainee, developed a technique of excisional surgery in which a complete margin of skin cancer was plotted in three dimensions[7] and named it 'chemosurgery' because it involved chemical fixation in situ before excision as follows:
  - Zinc chloride (as fixative), combined with stibnite (as permeant) and bloodroot powder *(Sanguinaria canadensis)* (as agglutinant) (Fig. 48.1), was applied to achieve in-vivo tissue fixation while maintaining cytological detail for microscopic evaluation of the excised specimen.
  - One day later the tumor and saucer-shaped specimen containing a narrow margin of normal appearing tissue were excised painlessly in a bloodless surgical field; frozen sections were generated from the specimen with the deep portion and peripheral margin of the excised tissue in a single horizontal plane, and residual tumor was precisely mapped based on the microscopic findings.
  - Overnight, zinc chloride was reapplied (if indicated) and the procedure was repeated to remove another saucer-shaped tissue specimen in the precise location of any residual tumor.
  - The process was repeated until all residual tumor was removed.
  - The wounds were usually left to heal by second intention. Mohs demonstrated significantly higher cure rates than conventional excision, but this technique had limitations, including the time taken (1 day for each surgical layer) and the delay in wound reconstruction as a result of the postoperative fixed tissue slough.
- 1953: Mohs and others demonstrated that the zinc chloride fixation could be replaced by local anesthesia and frozen section processing while still maintaining high cure rates, making the technique simpler and quicker.
- 1985: The official name of this procedure was changed to 'Mohs micrographic surgery' to reflect the shift away from chemical fixation toward a fresh tissue fixation technique, while maintaining reliance on microscopic evaluation of a layer-by-layer pictorial representation of tumor. This allows most tumors to be removed in 1 day, permits immediate wound repair, eliminates preoperative fixative discomfort, and has a cure rate comparable to that of the chemosurgical technique.[8,9] It is now used almost exclusively by most Mohs micrographic surgeons.
- 1986: American College of Chemosurgery, founded by Mohs, renamed American College of Mohs Micrographic Surgery.
- Subsequently: College renamed American College of Mohs Micrographic Surgery and Cutaneous Oncology to reflect changes in the clinical scope of the practice as the procedure enjoyed increasingly widespread application.[10] Other societies around the world have also been formed to increase knowledge about and availability of the Mohs technique.

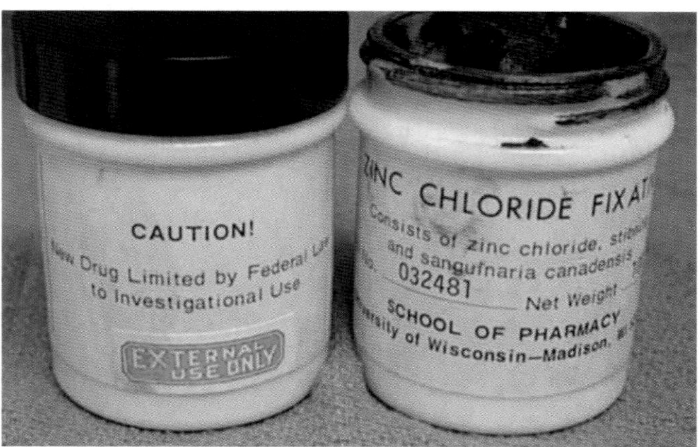

Figure 48.1 Zinc chloride fixative originally used by Dr Mohs in chemosurgery. Note its dark color. A similar bloodroot extract currently commercially available from homeopathic sources for patient self-application ('black salve') is not recommended because of the inherent risks in self-application in an unsupervised setting.

tumor and selectively excise it with the next layer (Fig. 48.2).

Mohs micrographic surgery was conceptualized to address the inadequacy of conventional means of surgical excision with margins. Vertically cut serial sections of an entire excisional specimen require an excessive number of sections to be examined. Step sections, representative vertical sections taken at 2–4-mm intervals, as in the bread-loaf method (Fig. 48.3), are customarily obtained when excisional specimens are sent to the pathology laboratory. However, this method leaves marginal areas between the sections that are not microscopically visualized, and allows examination of less than 1% of the tumor's margin.[11,12] The quadrant method similarly fails to identify residual tumor between sampled areas. Failure to detect subclinical microscopic tumor foci is often responsible for recurrence of the tumor despite 'clear' margins on the pathology report.

There are many advantages of using the Mohs technique.

- First, with its improved method of evaluating the margin, the Mohs technique has significantly improved cure rates. The 5-year cure rate for primary cancers treated by Mohs surgery is 99%, compared with 93% for conventional excision.[13] For recurrent cancers, the 5-year cure rate is 95%, compared with 80% for excision or any other treatment modality.[14]
- Second, Mohs surgery compares favorably in cost-effectiveness to other modalities of treatment of nonmelanoma skin cancer.[15,16]

Mohs surgery is indicated in situations where other treatment modalities have failed. The Mohs technique is used for recurrent tumors or those at high risk for recurrence, those with clinically indistinct margins, and for those tumors that are anatomically located where tissue conservation is important (Table 48.1). It can be used for virtually any neoplasm that spreads by contiguous growth along cutaneous or mucosal surfaces.

One additional advantage of the Mohs technique is that it is tissue sparing. In specific cosmetic or functional areas, this may allow a more cosmetically acceptable or functional

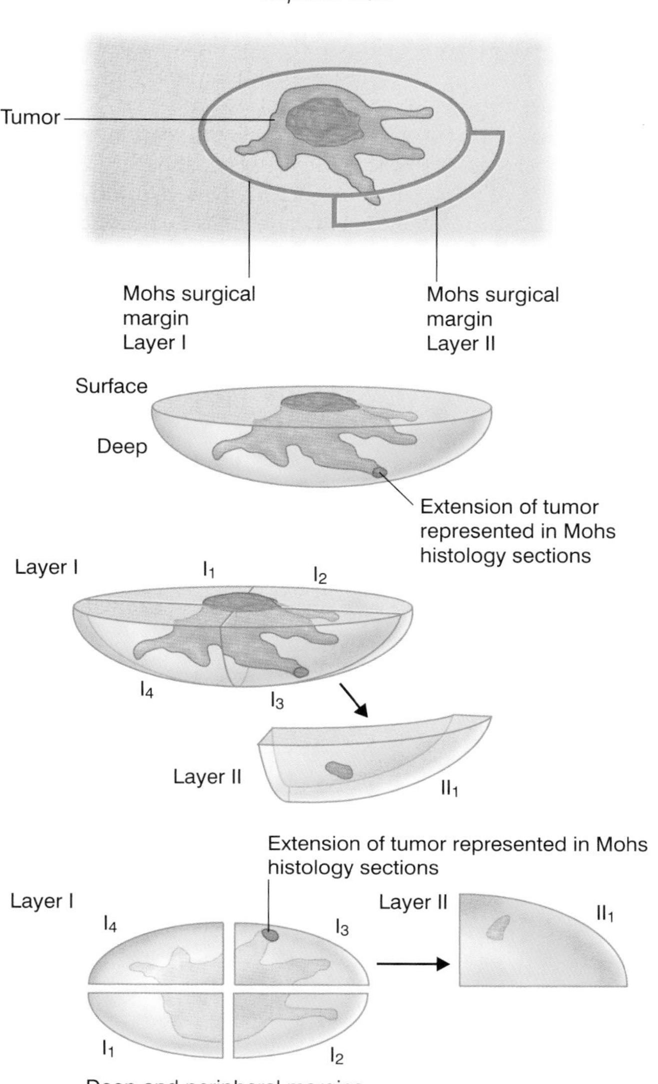

Figure 48.2 Mohs micrographic surgery technique.

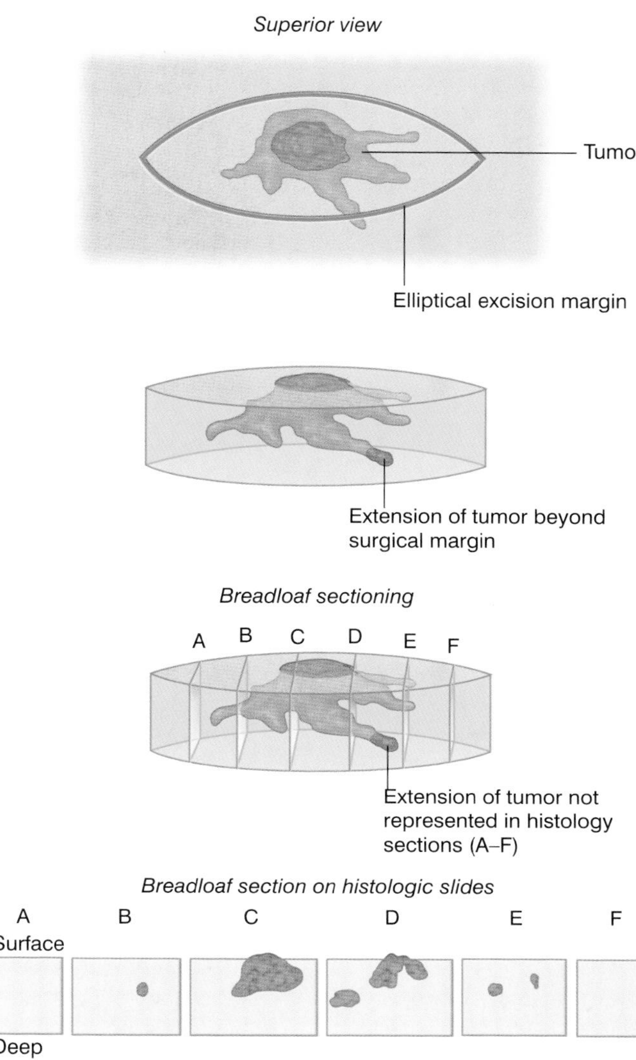

Figure 48.3 Limitation of bread-loaf method of examining the margin of conventional excision. In this example, excisional tip sections A and F are clear of tumor and sections B, C, D, and E demonstrate tumor. No extension to the peripheral margins is detected, and the excision is technically clear on margins. However, this is not an accurate margin assessment. Extension of tumor to the surgical margin between sections D and E is missed because it is not sampled.

result after surgery. Frequently it also can simplify the reconstruction both by tissue conservation within critical cosmetic units as well as by allowing the reconstructing surgeon to be as confident as possible that the entire tumor has been removed.

Mohs surgery is not limited to the skin—treatment of mucosal cancers of the head and neck can benefit from its many advantages.[17]

The face (especially the eyelids, ears, lips, and nose), the digits, the genitalia, and the scalp are specific anatomic locations in which Mohs micrographic surgery can be most helpful in obtaining clear tumor margins while sparing as much uninvolved tissue as possible. These are locations in which tumors can spread along nerves, cartilage, periosteum, bone, and embryonic fusion planes, making them high risk for recurrence.

Mohs micrographic surgery should be considered for virtually all cutaneous malignancies of the face. The face has multiple unique anatomic structures, which must be preserved in reconstruction, making tissue conservation critical. In the US, cutaneous cancers of the face are more common on the left side because of chronic sun exposure in automobiles.[18]

Lesions on the eyelids present special challenges. It was with eyelid tumors that Dr Mohs had his earliest successes with extremely high cure rates.[19] 90% of malignant tumors of the periorbital area are basal cell carcinomas. If the tumor extends to involve the tarsal plate, levator muscle, or lacrimal apparatus, especially the canaliculus, oculoplastic repair is frequently required. Intraocular mucosal spread of basal cell carcinoma has been documented.[20] When operating on the free eyelid margin, layers may be taken

Table 48.1 Indications for Mohs micrographic surgery

Type of tumor	Examples
Recurrent	
Positive margin after simple excision	
At high risk for local recurrence and/or metastasis	Sclerosing(morpheaform), infiltrative, micronodular, metatypical subtypes of basal cell carcinoma
	Perineural basal cell carcinoma or squamous cell carcinoma
	Keratoacanthoma
	Bowen's disease
	Malignant melanoma
	Merkel cell carcinoma
	Dermatofibrosarcoma protuberans
	Atypical fibroxanthoma
	Malignant fibrous histiocytoma
	Microcystic adnexal carcinoma
	Sebaceous carcinoma
	Extramammary Paget's disease
	Angiosarcoma
In an area where tissue conservation is important	Eyelids
	Ears
	Nose
	Lips
	Digits
	Nails
	Genitalia
Facial—in area of embryonic fusion planes	Periorbital, especially medial canthus
	Nasal
	Lips
	Ears
	Retroauricular sulcus
	Melolabial folds
Poorly defined clinical margins	
Perineural spread	
Greater than 2 cm in diameter	
Immunosuppressed patient	
Skin previously treated with ionizing radiation	
Demonstrated biological aggressiveness	

in succession so that the canaliculus is sacrificed only if involved. The postoperative size of medial canthal lesions can be minimized with the Mohs technique, allowing for second intention healing in selected cases. Regardless of the size and extent of the defect, repair of the Mohs defect can commence immediately, saving the patient great anxiety and days of nonproductive time while awaiting repair.

Lesions on the ears may also present significant challenges to the cutaneous surgeon. Making up only 6% of all skin cancers, those that occur on the ear account for a disproportionate number of recurrences. The difficulty in eradication likely stems from the many embryonic fusion planes in the periauricular area. Tumors of the ear may have a predictable pattern of spread. Tumors that arise in the postauricular area tend to spread to the ear itself. Tumors that arise in the preauricular area spread toward the tragus and the medial and superior aspects of the helix. Once at the tragus, the tumor can spread down the external part of the tragus between tragal cartilage and the parotid gland to involve deeper structures such as the facial nerve.[21] Neuropathic pain in this area is frequently an indicator for such involvement. Treatment of tumors involving deep structures, the mastoid, or extending from the concha into the external auditory meatus may require sedation or general anesthesia and consultation with other specialists. Tumors extending beyond the outer third of the ear canal may be difficult to access, requiring specialized surgical expertise and skills. Tumor extirpation can involve significant morbidity to the patient.

The nose is the single most common location for basal cell carcinoma on the entire integument, and also the most common site for recurrence. Like the periauricular area, embryonic fusion planes may offer the path of least resistance and facilitate tumor spread along contiguous anatomical areas. In particular, the alar rim and nasal tip are two areas where tissue conservation is critical and size can affect reconstruction possibilities dramatically. Lesions involving the melolabial folds may be particularly deep and extensive. The Mohs technique should be considered for virtually any malignant neoplasm of the nose.

Tumors of the skin of the upper lip are usually basal cell carcinomas, while those of the cutaneous lower lip are most commonly squamous cell carcinomas. The latter type is highly capable of regional and metastatic spread, especially if over 2 cm in diameter. Larger and more aggressive tumors may require wider excision and lymph node evaluation (i.e. sentinel lymph node mapping), and involvement of a head and neck surgeon may be helpful.

Tumors of the digits may be advanced at the time of presentation. Mohs surgery is useful and often avoids the amputation of a digit, so maintaining function. Treatment of subungual or periungual tumors is particularly challenging to maintain function, avoid infection, and allow for adequate cosmesis. The nail matrix in particular is extremely liable to tissue loss, resulting in visible deformity of the nail plate.

The treatment of tumors of the genitalia may also benefit from Mohs micrographic surgery.[22] Patients may require penectomy for advanced stages of malignancy; Mohs surgery may provide the necessary tissue conservation to avoid this outcome. Larger and more aggressive tumors may require wider margins of excision and regional lymph node examination. The precise location and size of the tumor can greatly influence prognosis. Higher cure rates can be obtained when tumors involve only the glans or prepuce of the penis, and when lesions are less than 1 cm in diameter.

PREOPERATIVE PREPARATION

Patient consultation is provided before the procedure. Critical in this process is the accurate localization of the tumor, which can be obtained using photographs, sketches, and descriptions, often from the referring physician. Physical examination should include contiguous areas and assessment for pre-existing cosmetic and functional deficits. Draining regional lymphatics should be palpated and documented for all patients. Histologic proof of diagnosis is generally required, and the histologic slide is reviewed to confirm the tumor type and pattern. The patient's health history and review of systems should be focused, but comprehensive to minimize complications (Table 48.2). Any history of previous cutaneous procedures (especially those involving the operative site), ultraviolet exposure, and radiation therapy should be elicited. Emphasis on mitigating any bleeding diathesis should be stressed. A detailed

Table 48.2 Preoperative evaluation

Medical/surgical history
Hepatitis
AIDS
Herpes simplex virus
Medications
Vitamins
Nutritional supplements
Allergies to medicines, anesthetics, topical creams, adhesive tape
Immunosuppression
Concurrent malignancies
Concurrent cutaneous disorders
Prosthetic joints and valves
Pacemaker/defibrillator
Bleeding diathesis
Smoking history
Other medical illnesses (e.g. gout)

medication history must include dietary supplement use. In one study, 49% of patients undergoing Mohs surgery reported taking at least one dietary supplement.[23] Patients are instructed to avoid aspirin-containing products, antiplatelet agents, vitamin E, ginkgo biloba, and garlic, which have demonstrated anticoagulation properties. Cessation of warfarin is controversial because of the well-documented risks of abruptly discontinuing therapy perioperatively.[24] It is our practice to consult with the treating physician, if possible, when the patient is on a prescribed aspirin-containing product, antiplatelet agent, or anticoagulant. We are aware of at least one of our patients who experienced a fatal postoperative event after the treating physician stopped medications for the patient's procedure. Good communication between physicians is essential, and even this (as in our case) may not necessarily prevent certain sequelae. Improving hypertensive control and optimizing other medical conditions are important to ensure operative success. Preoperative anxiolytic agents, usually administered sublingually or orally, can be considered in patients with a high level of apprehension. It may be advisable for the patient to come for the procedure after having a light meal and being well-rested and with a family member or friend. Warm layered clothing is advisable in most operating room environments.

The cutaneous surgeon must successfully alleviate the patient's anxieties about their surgery. Many patients present with closely held perceptions about their aesthetic ideal, and some have unrealistic expectations. It may be useful to obtain preoperative digital photographs to document both tumor location and specific anatomic features. A number of patients have researched their cutaneous neoplasm on the internet or by other sources of information, but the cutaneous surgeon should still take this opportunity to educate the patient to ensure the transmission of accurate information. Patient education can take many forms, including websites, morphing software, brochures, pictures, and wax models. However, none are a total replacement for the direct consultation between the physician and patient.

A thorough discussion of risks, benefits, alternatives, and complications of the proposed surgical procedure must take place. Specific alternatives to surgery such as radiation therapy and other modalities of treatment (perhaps even observation) should be discussed. An explanation of the Mohs technique with respect to anesthesia, stages, waiting periods, and repair options should be tailored to the patient's specific case. The possibility of tumor spread to infiltrate contiguous soft tissue and cartilaginous and bony structures should be anticipated and discussed with the patient before or during the operation before proceeding further. The extent of tumor involvement may be assessed by computed tomography (CT), magnetic resonance imaging (MRI), or other diagnostic aids, although a negative test result may be misleading.

The reconstruction of large tumors that infiltrate widely may benefit from the expertise of plastic, oculoplastic, and head and neck surgeons, or other specialists, and their evaluation should be incorporated into the preoperative evaluation of the patient. Medical oncologists may provide useful input and therapeutic options in certain cases. In essence, a team approach may serve the patient best in challenging cases.

■ TECHNIQUE

Before surgery can commence, vital signs, including blood pressure and pulse are recorded, the patient medication history is updated, and informed consent is obtained in writing. The execution of Mohs micrographic surgery requires several precise steps.

First, the site of the tumor is identified with the aid of high-intensity lighting, magnification, and/or Wood's light (Fig. 48.4). Cross-polarized light sources may be helpful in this process. Note that the patient cannot always be counted on to confirm the location with precision. The exact location of the tumor is confirmed and its size is recorded on an anatomic diagram, which functions as a surgical map. A 1–5-mm surgical margin, depending on tumor type, is drawn around the clinically apparent tumor with a surgical marking pen (Fig. 48.5A). Because local anesthesia can distort the anatomy, landmarks and borders

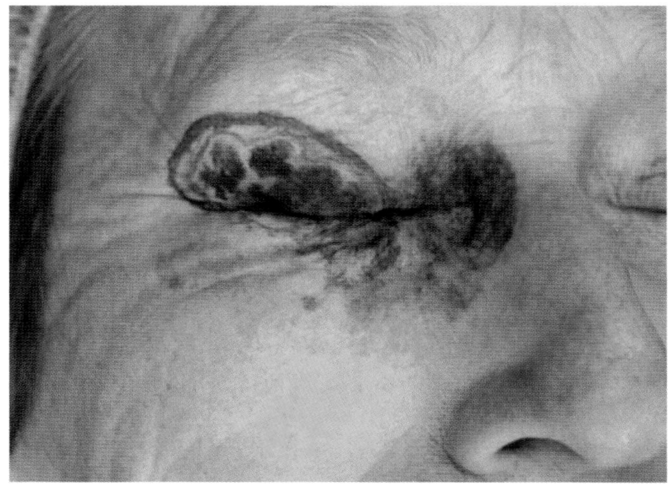

Figure 48.4 Correct selection of tumor site is critical in Mohs micrographic surgery. Correct lighting and magnification are helpful. In this case, a lentigo maligna involving the periorbital region is being excised in a staged fashion. The area for excision as determined by visual inspection is outlined; however, examination using a Wood's light revealed significant subclinical extension of visually evident tumor.

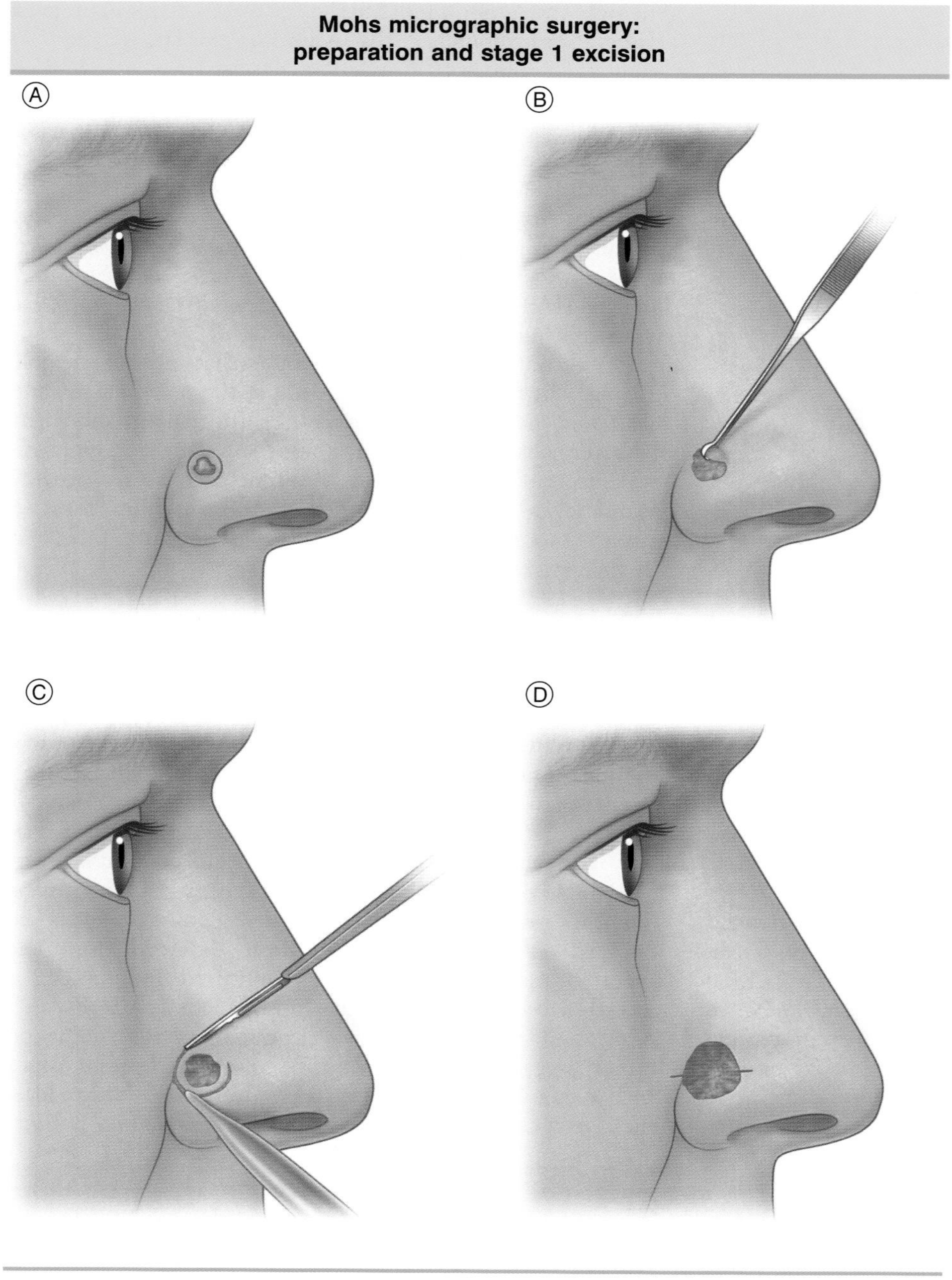

Mohs micrographic surgery: preparation and stage 1 excision

Ⓐ Ⓑ Ⓒ Ⓓ

Figure 48.5 Preparation and excision. (A) Preoperative view of left nasal alar basal cell carcinoma. (B) Debulking with curette. Tumor debulking may be helpful in delineating subclinical extensions of tumor that are not grossly visible. (C) Stage I excision. Note the 30–45° angle of the knife blade and the 2-mm margin of normal-appearing skin around the debulked area. (D) Stage I excision completed with specimen removed. Note scoring of epidermis at medial and lateral margins of operative site corresponding to division of specimen into sections appropriate for processing. Adapted with permission from Grekin RC. Mohs micrographic surgery. In: Robinson JK, Arndt KA, LeBoit PE, Wintroub BU, eds. Atlas of cutaneous surgery. Philadelphia: WB Saunders; 1996.

of cosmetic subunits may also be outlined at this time. The lesion may be photographed preoperatively before or after marking (and at subsequent stages of the procedure as deemed necessary for documentation).

Local anesthesia is obtained with 1 or 2% lidocaine with epinephrine (adrenaline) 1 : 100 000 or 1 : 200 000 in most situations. A slow anesthetic technique is most comfortable, and injecting as the needle is withdrawn is helpful. Topical 20% benzocaine or lidocaine preparations may alleviate the discomfort of the injection. It is advisable to wait several minutes to allow for complete anesthesia and vasoconstriction to occur before proceeding. Occasionally, regional nerve blocks may be helpful for large tumors. This may be supplemented with a longer-acting anesthetic agent such as bupivacaine to enhance patient comfort between layers.

The tumor and surrounding area is then prepped with povidone iodine or chlorhexidine gluconate and draped. If the tumor is large or thick, it may be debulked using a curette or surgical razor blade with or without the use of electrodesiccation (Fig. 48.5B). This may further delineate margins and reduce the number of layers necessary to obtain clear margins. A small specimen of this material may be obtained for a vertical transverse section for documentation and to identify specific tumor growth pattern within the tissue, especially if the biopsy was not definitive. Immediately thereafter, the incision is made along the outlined margin with a scalpel with a #15 or 15c blade and the tumor is sharply excised to an appropriate depth. A #10 blade can be useful for larger tumors overlying thick skin. A saucer-shaped specimen with 30° beveled edges is ideal so that the specimen may be flattened. Flattening means that the bottom and margins can be sectioned by the histotechnician in the same plane. Surgical reference marks are made on the specimen and adjacent tissue with Gentian violet or the scalpel for precise orientation of the specimen before its removal. Once removed, maintaining proper orientation of the specimen is critical to the integrity of the entire procedure. (Figs 48.5C–D, 48.6). Hemostasis is achieved with direct pressure or electrocoagulation, or a handheld battery-operated electrocautery unit if avoidance of electrical interference with implanted devices is required.

A two-dimensional map is then created while the patient is still in the operating suite to document the exact tumor location (Fig. 48.6). It may be helpful to transpose the map onto a digital photograph of the lesion.[25] The specimen is then divided into sections small enough to fit on a microscope slide (0.5–1.5 cm), and its nonepidermal edges are stained to allow proper orientation (Figs 48.6C, 48.7). Two to three colors are used for each specimen to allow for adequate orientation.[26] The number of specimens depends on the size of the tumor, but the numbering sequence of the tissue specimens should be consistent from patient to patient. The clockwise numbering pattern is the one historically and most commonly used, starting at the 1 o'clock position. When large specimens have central portions, the sequence is initiated at the skin edges and then continued into the central portions (Fig. 48.8).

When specimens contain cartilage or bone, or subcutaneous tissue without any skin edge, this should be indicated on the map. At this point, the tissue is handed to the histotechnician for further processing. Patients are advised that each layer may require 1–2 hours, and they may proceed to the waiting area after the placement of a pressure dressing. Occasionally, patients remain in the Mohs operating suite during tissue processing if their mobility is limited or if they require continuous monitoring.

Once in the laboratory, rather than being cut vertically, each specimen is placed bottom-side up on the microtome stage so that horizontal sections can be taken from the deep surface. This process requires many precise steps[27–30] with attention to detail to avoid mapping errors. First the specimen is embedded in optimal cutting temperature (OCT or similar agents) compound (Tissue-Tek, Miles Inc, Diagnostics Division, Elkhart, IN) and a forcep or flat portion of a scalpel handle is used to ensure the specimen is completely flat. If the specimen contains cartilage or fat, this can be more difficult. A variety of devices and maneuvers are available to assist in tissue flattening if the histotechnologist finds them of value.

The tissue is immediately frozen with tetrafluoroethylchloride or liquid nitrogen and then transferred to the cryostat for thorough freezing. (Fig. 48.7C) Obtaining a complete section is critical to prevent errors in tissue interpretation through missing sections. It requires great skill and practice (Fig. 48.7D). Training and certification information are available through several organizations including the American Society for Mohs Histotechnology (Milwaukee, WI). Flattening the specimen, raising its peripheral margins, and cutting through the tissue block with the microtome blade before representative sections are obtained are all helpful techniques to avoid missing skin edges on portion(s) of the microscope slide. Slides are identified and prepared with the patient's name, date, and layer/specimen sequence number, with attention to detail to avoid mapping errors.

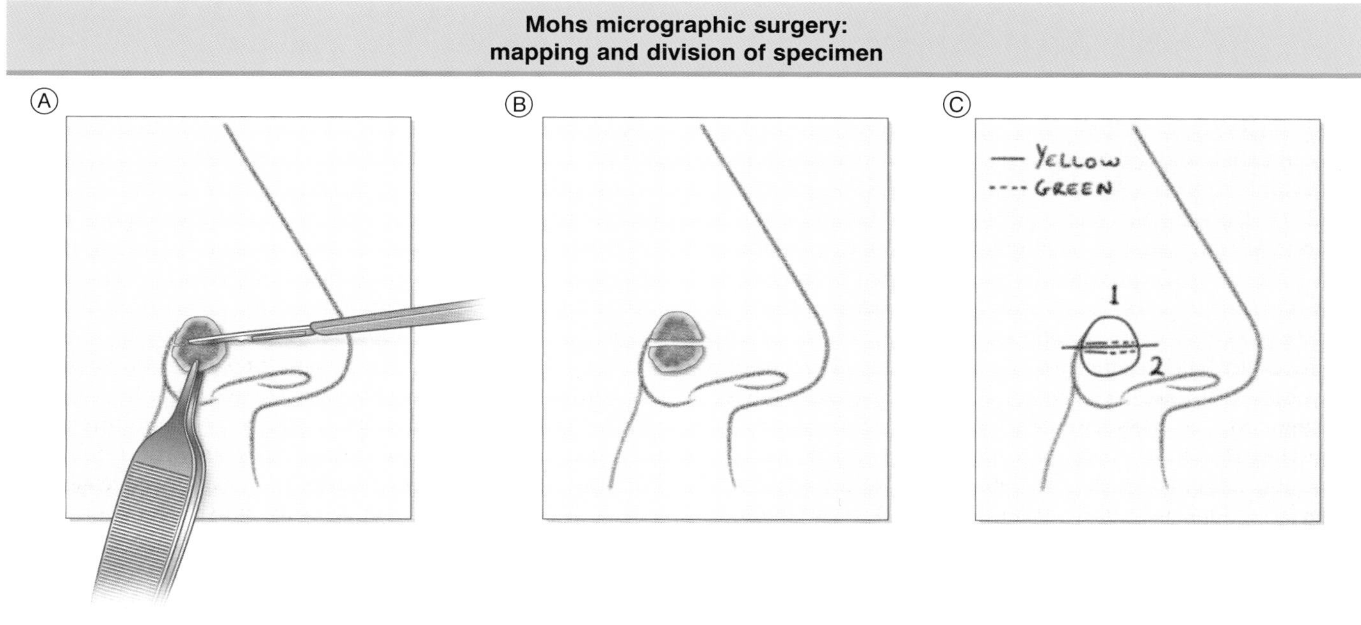

Figure 48.6 Mapping and division of the specimen. (A) Division of specimen using scalpel and forceps. Maintenance of orientation is critical to the procedure. (B) Divided specimen showing orientation. (C) Map orienting tissue specimen and denoting dye-marking of nonepidermal margins. Note that the map is specific to the anatomic area and whether the tumor is on the left or right. Adapted with permission from Grekin RC. Mohs' micrographic surgery. In: Robinson JK, Arndt KA, LeBoit PE, Wintroub BU, eds. Atlas of cutaneous surgery. Philadelphia: WB Saunders; 1996.

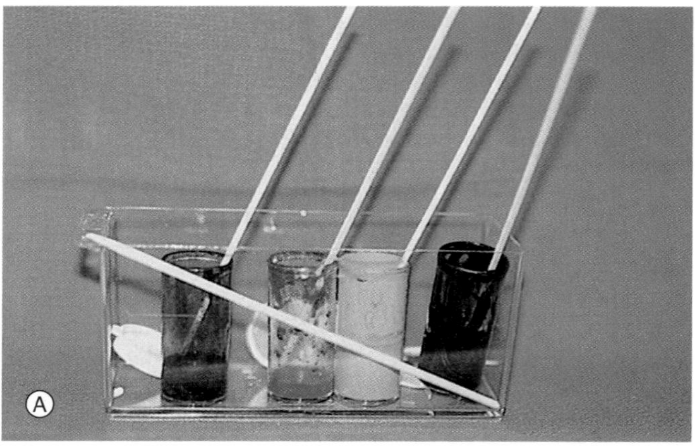

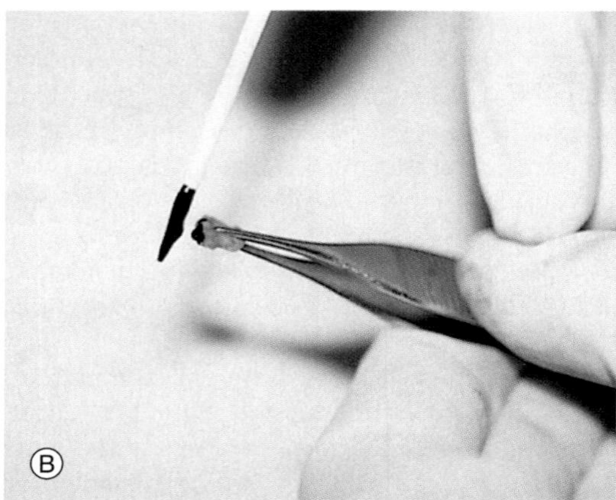

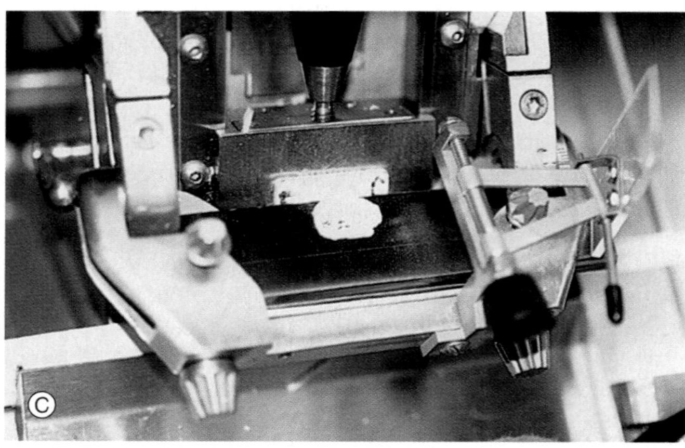

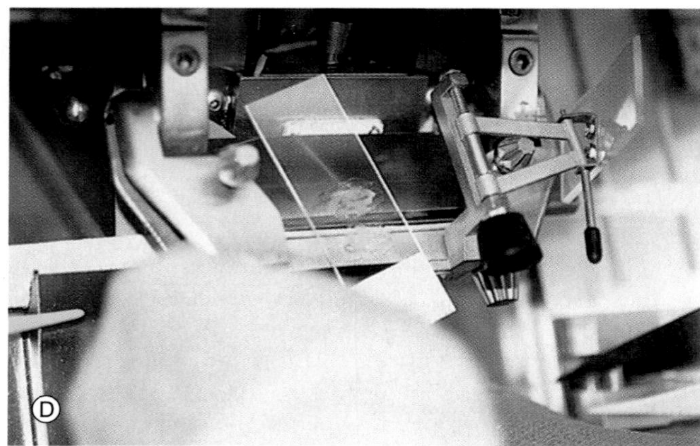

Figure 48.7 Mohs laboratory specimen processing. (A) Tissue dyes. (B) Dye-marking of nonepidermal margins with black ink. (C) Sectioning of frozen specimens. (D) The histotechnician cuts serial sections through specimen block as it passes over the cryostat blade. The thin, cold tissue adheres directly to the room temperature microscope slide applied to it. With permission from Grekin RC. Mohs micrographic surgery. In: Robinson JK, Arndt KA, LeBoit PE, Wintroub BU, eds. Atlas of cutaneous surgery. Philadelphia: WB Saunders; 1996.

The first section obtained is the truest margin and in our practice is placed furthest from the frosted edge of the slide, and then one to three additional sections are obtained at 4–8-μm intervals and placed on the slide sequentially closer to the frosted edge (Fig. 48.9A). The process is repeated for each tissue specimen. Once all tissue has been processed, the slides are stained, usually with hematoxylin and eosin, though toluidine blue is also popular in many practices. In high-volume laboratories, they are placed in an automatic slide stainer such as the Shandon Linistat automated system (Thermo Electron Corporation, Waltham, MA) to decrease processing time by about one-third (Fig. 48.9B). Finally, the slides are rinsed, a clear mounting medium such as Cytoseal-60 (Richard Allen Scientific, Kalamazoo, MI) or similar medium is applied, and cover slips are placed to facilitate microscopic review (Fig. 48.9C).

Most Mohs micrographic surgery laboratories use routine hematoxylin and eosin staining for all specimens. In a comparison study with a cytokeratin marker, Smeets et al. found there was a greater than 99% sensitivity in the identification of basal cell carcinoma with hematoxylin and eosin on Mohs sections.[31] However, adjuvant cytokeratin staining may be useful in selected cases of basal cell carcinomas exhibiting aggressive or poorly circumscribed growth characteristics. Ber-EP4 is one such widely available cytokeratin stain used for this purpose. Toluidine blue can also be used for basal cell carcinomas, favored by some for its optical clarity. Special immunostains can be obtained for other tumor types. However, due to reagent cost, unavailability of automated staining equipment, additional processing time, and additional technician and physician time, the process is impractical for routine use.[32] For melanoma, the use of rapid HMB-45 staining is used by some to increase the accuracy of interpretation of frozen sections. Menaker et al.[33] found that frozen sections using HMB-45 stained consistently with paraffin-embedded permanent sections at each stage of resection in a study of 20 cases of melanoma treated with Mohs micrographic surgery. Albertini et al.[34] found MART-1 to be superior in sensitivity to both HMB-45 and S-100 for frozen sections. Smith et al.[35] found S-100 staining useful for tracking perineural extension of granular cell tumor not evident with hematoxylin and eosin. Harris et al.[36] described the use of carcinoembryonic antigen (CEA) rapid staining in the treatment of extramammary Paget's disease treated by Mohs surgery. Similarly, the CD-34 immunostain has been studied in dermatofibroma sarcoma protuberans. When these stains are used, permanent sections are usually obtained, as in our practice.

Mohs micrographic surgery: specimen markings and sequence numbering

Figure 48.8 Representative numbering sequences of various specimens. A clockwise pattern is most commonly used, with number 1 starting at 1 o'clock. Skin edges are numbered first, followed by interior pieces. Coloured lines represent different tissue dyes. Minimal division of the primary specimen results in less risk of false-positive or false-negative margins. The limiting size of a specimen is a combination of the skill of the histotechnologist and the size of the cryostat specimen object disk and can range from a few millimeters to more than 2 cm in one dimension in some laboratories. Small lesions up to 2 cm in diameter are often halved (A) or trisected (B) if irregularly shaped. Larger lesions may be divided into more pieces (C). If the specimen is too large to contain epithelium on all pieces, single (D) or multiple (E) central specimens might be mapped

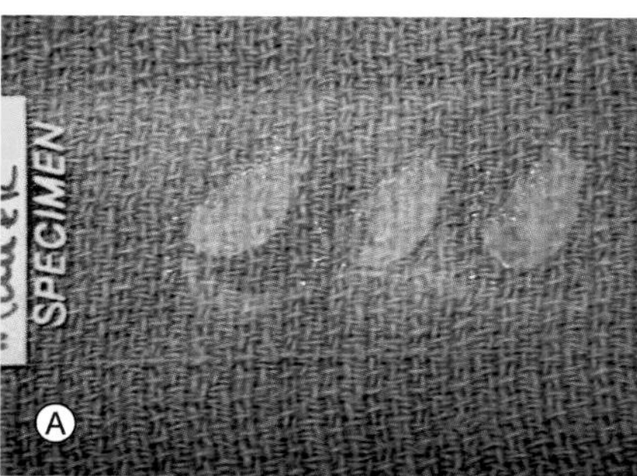

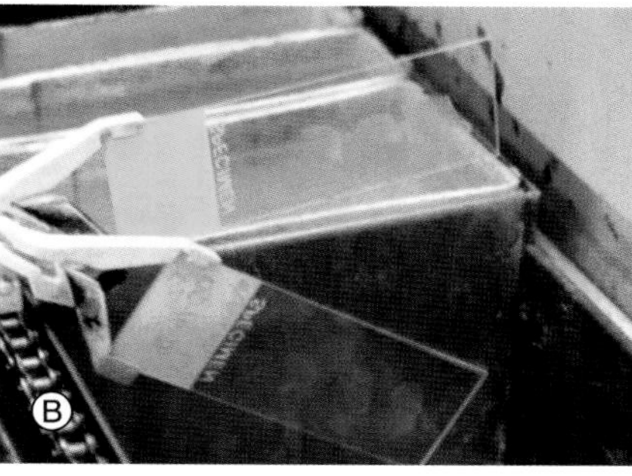

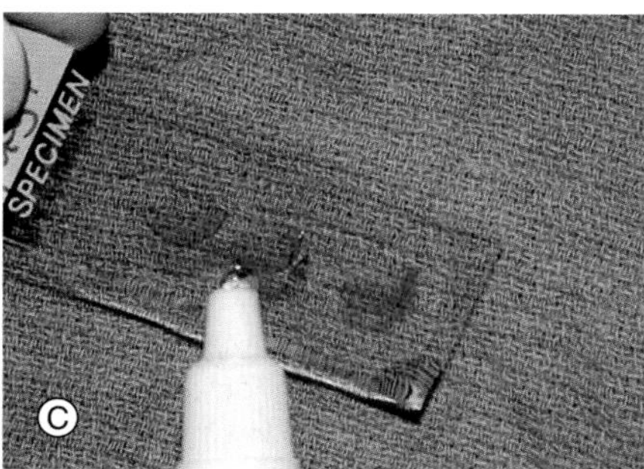

Figure 48.9 Specimen slides. (A) Unstained slide: the first section, representing the true surgical margin, is furthest from the frosted edge of the slide. The histotechnician is able to visually assess for the presence of a complete section. (B) An automatic slide stainer can greatly improve the efficiency of the Mohs laboratory; a large number of slides can be batched to improve patient flow. (C) The slide cover slip has been applied and slides are ready for examination.

Specimen interpretation

At this point, the histotechnician hands the stained slides to the Mohs surgeon for histologic examination. Each microscope slide is examined under light microscopy, carefully noting the slide sequence numbers. Specimens should be superimposed on the Mohs map if there is any uncertainty about the origin or orientation of the specimen. There is a predictable 10–20% tissue shrinkage that occurs during frozen section processing, but any larger size discrepancy (or large holes) should alert the Mohs surgeon that the specimen (and thus the surgical margin) could be incomplete as a result of technical error.[37,38] Technical errors are the most common cause of local recurrences after Mohs surgery.[39]

The vertical specimen is first examined because it may provide more complete information than the biopsy, and may be the only view of the tumor if the first Mohs layer is clear.[5] By examining the slides in numerical order corresponding to the map, residual tumor can be identified and its exact location determined based on the colors of the margins on the slide. It is noted on the map with red marking ink (Fig. 48.10). Additionally, areas of calcification, perineural spread, inflammation, and other incidental skin neoplasms such as actinic and seborrheic keratoses can be identified. Sections need to be carefully examined because rete ridges, hair follicles, and other adnexal structures can look like tumor cells. Dense inflammation may mask small collections of tumor cells. Patients with chronic lymphocytic leukemia and solid organ transplant recipients have a 36% and 13% incidence, respectively, of prominent inflammatory foci on Mohs sections compared with controls (1%), making slide interpretation more difficult.[40] However, the presence of dense inflammation on Mohs sections of basal cell carcinoma does not necessarily obscure the presence of any residual tumor,[41] and may not indicate the need for an additional layer. Similarly, although an intense infiltrate may surround squamous cell carcinoma, any residual tumor can

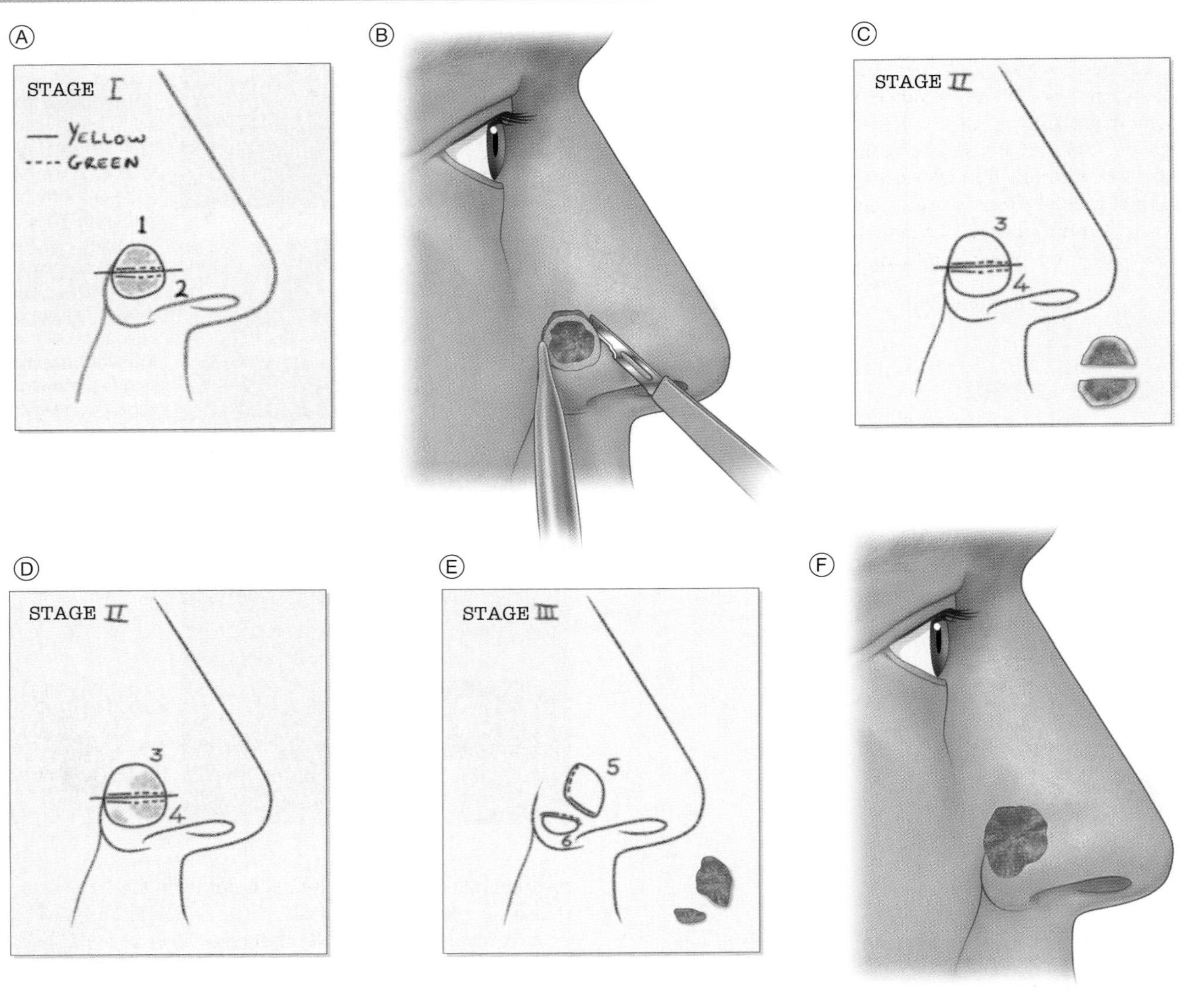

Figure 48.10 Stage II and III excision. (A) Residual tumor in the specimen margins noted by coloring the area red on the map. (B) Excision of stage II includes 2 mm margin of all positive areas. (C) Stage II specimens and map. (D) Residual tumor after stage II noted on map after prepared specimens have been interpreted by the surgeon. (E) Stage III specimens and map. (F) Postoperative defect after stage III. Adapted with permission from Grekin RC. Mohs micrographic surgery. In: Robinson JK, Arndt KA, LeBoit PE, Wintroub BU, eds. Atlas of cutaneous surgery. Philadelphia: WB Saunders; 1996.

be visualized if it is present without the use of special stains.[42] In our practice each case is approached uniquely because we have seen tumor masked by inflammation.

If the pathology on frozen sections is not clear, permanent tissue specimens can be obtained for improved resolution or increased depth of tissue evaluation through levels to trace specific anatomic structures of concern. If any of the specimens examined are missing epidermis, dermis, or subcutaneous tissue, a recut can be obtained after the specimen has been reoriented in the OCT medium. In cases with an extremely large number of specimens, the surgeon may have every other one processed first to give an initial view of the tumor extent.

If residual tumor is identified or a segment of the margin cannot be fully visualized even after recuts have been obtained, the patient is brought back to the operating room for removal of another layer. In this way, the Mohs practitioner functions as both surgeon and pathologist. In a manner similar to the first layer, but avoiding complete re-excision unless all margins are positive, a specimen containing the area of residual tumor and a small amount (2–5 mm) of surrounding tissue is removed after careful marking with Gentian violet (Fig. 48.10). These layers are successively numbered on the Mohs map using Roman numerals. This cycle is repeated until no residual tumor is identified on any slides of a particular layer. Proper interpretation of Mohs micrographic frozen sections is thus critical in the training and practice of the Mohs micrographic surgeon.

Once the tumor has been completely removed, the patient is evaluated for reconstructive options. Cosmetic and functional issues must be considered with each wound before a decision is made to allow second intention healing or cover the wound with a graft or flap. If tumor recurrence is possible, second intention healing or split-thickness skin grafting should be considered. In these situations, flaps are to be avoided because they may mask recurrence. Extensive undermining and tissue advancement, rotation, or transposition may facilitate tumor growth along the path of least resistance. Second intention healing may allow recurrent tumor to be visualized more easily. Similarly, split-thickness skin grafts may allow increased visualization of the defect to detect recurrent tumor.[43] Definitive repair may be delayed to allow for histologic reconfirmation of clear margins at a future time, or to increase the success of a full-thickness skin graft.[44] If tumor recurrence is unlikely, repair can proceed with linear closures, flaps, or grafts.[45–47]

The use of Mohs micrographic surgery provides the maximal assurance that residual tumor cells do not remain in adjacent normal appearing skin and tissue.

■ OPTIMIZING OUTCOMES

Optimizing outcomes

- Ensure appropriate instrumentation and equipment are available (eg specialist instruments for infiltrating tumors that involve deeper structures, curved ophthalmic blades for perioral and perinasal areas).
- Ensure all staff, including nurses and technicians, have specialist Mohs surgery training.
- Use an operating room microscope.
- Recognize potential complications and plan for the unanticipated (e.g. perioperative bleeding or emergencies).

Proper instrumentation, equipment, organization, and set-up in the Mohs surgery area are essential to a successful operative outcome (Figs 48.11, 48.12). Mohs surgery requires a qualified practitioner functioning as both a surgeon and pathologist, as well as a well-trained nursing staff and skilled histotechnician. It also requires patient cooperation in waiting while the time- and labor-intensive layers are performed.

Recognizing potential areas of complication allows the surgeon to be proactive in primary prevention and risk management. Whenever surgery is being performed in the periorbital region, caution must be observed to prevent inadvertent injury to the eye. The eyes can be protected by taping cotton gauze over the eyelids, which also limits the intensity of the operating room lights. If the tumor involves the eyelid margin, a lubricated plastic eye shield may be inserted onto the cornea after topical anesthesia with tetracaine or a similar fast-acting anesthetic solution. The external auditory canal can be protected from undesirable blood by placing gauze into the meatus. Appropriate restraining belts on the operating room table are helpful if the patient is at risk of falling for any reason. A smoke evacuator should be readily available to remove malodorous electrosurgical plume. Suction should always be available in case of unanticipated perioperative bleeding. A plan for handling emergencies or unanticipated events is necessary.

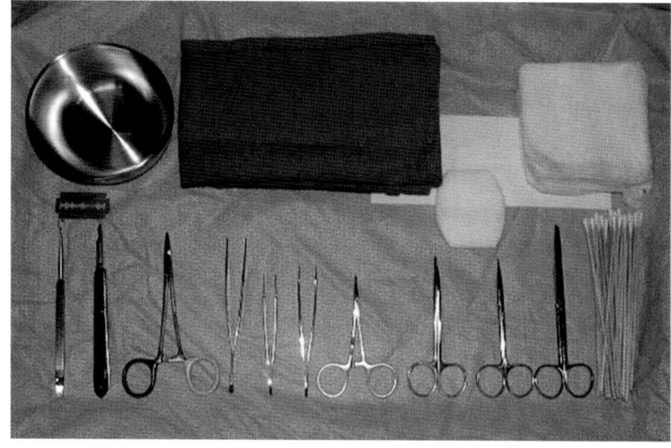

Figure 48.11 Typical patient-specific Mohs tray set-up that functions as both surgery and repair tray. Instruments included in this set, from left to right are 4-mm Fox dermal curette, #3 knife handle with ruler (with #15 blade attached), Webster/Halsy needle holder, Adson Brown forceps 7 × 7, Castro-Viejo fixation forcep with suture platform, Carmault splinter forcep, Hartman mosquito curved hemostat, Kaye scissor (tungsten carbide handle), iris scissor, Deaver (sharp blunt) suture scissors. Also present are a basin for sterile saline, surgical razor blade, sterile towels, one eye pad, 10 sterile 4 × 4 gauze, nonadherent dressing, and 10–20 cotton-tipped applicators.

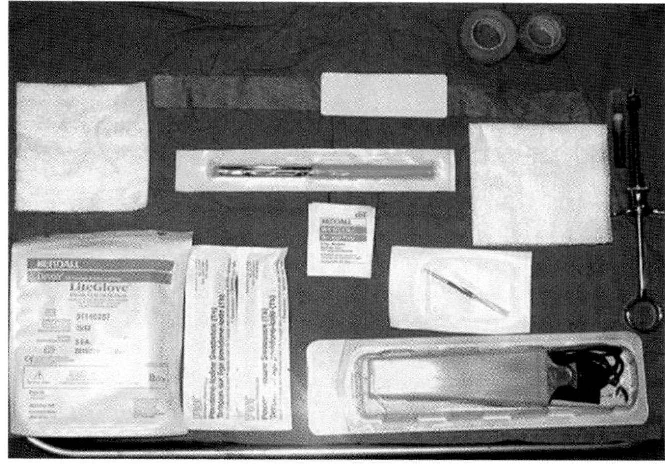

Figure 48.12 Additional supplies recommended for patient-specific Mohs tray. Brown hypoallergenic tape with patient label affixed on which allergies/other warning information can be recorded (i.e. to use battery-operated electrocautery if patient has a pacemaker), alcohol pads, povidone iodine, 4 × 4 gauze, surgical marking pen, surgical light holders, electrosurgical apparatus, and dental syringe.

An efficient outpatient surgical area and laboratory are critical in ensuring overall patient satisfaction.

The removal of infiltrating tumors involving deeper structures requires special instrumentation to harvest the specimen without injuring adjacent structures. A spring-loaded Castro-Viejo needle driver and Westcott scissors are frequently used for periorbital excisions, allowing the cutaneous surgeon superior fine control (Fig. 48.13). In our practice, an operating room microscope may be used to further enhance precision. Ophthalmic mini-blades on cylindrical handles may be useful around the eye as well as for the ear and nose to facilitate making the incision with the desired bevel.[48] Tumors involving perichondrium, periosteum, and the nail can be dissected more easily using a periosteal elevator (Fig. 48.14). For aggressive tumors that involve the skull, facial bones, or sinuses, the deep margin can be cleared by chiseling with a mallet. Bone specimens require decalcification in ethylenediaminetetraacetic acid (EDTA) or similar softening reagent before they are sectioned the next day, necessitating a surgical delay to confirm tumor-free margins. For large tumors, a double-bladed scalpel can be used to allow for maximum tissue conservation and enhance mapping accuracy in peripheral margin control.[49]

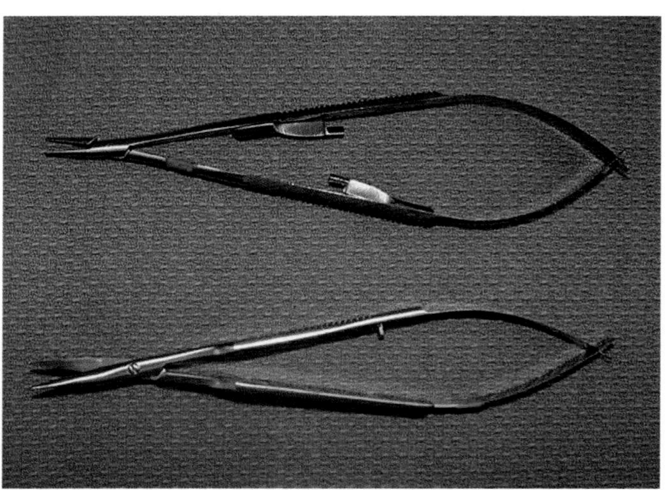

Figure 48.13 Castro-Viejo needle holder (top) with Westcott tenotomy scissors $5\frac{1}{4}$ in can be helpful for excisions around the orbits.

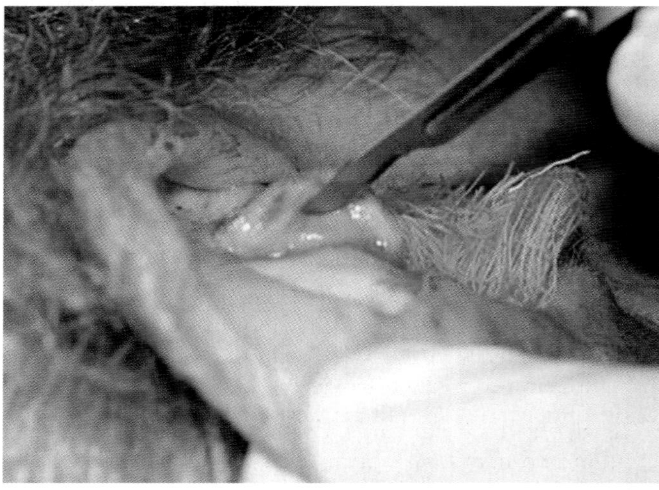

Figure 48.14 Mohs surgery involving the anterior surface of the ear with tumor extension to the perichondrium. Once the cartilage has been exposed, a blunt periosteal elevator instead of the #15 blade may be used to dissect the perichondrium in a bloodless fashion. This will enable the surgeon to obtain a continuous layer without damaging underlying cartilage.

POSTOPERATIVE CARE

Immediately after the procedure, the patient's skin is cleaned of all blood, antiseptic, and markings, and a pressure dressing is secured with skin adhesive, to be left undisturbed for 48 hours in our practice. For difficult facial concavities, such as the melolabial fold, dental rolls may be helpful to secure pressure. Wound care generally consists of cleansing with 3% hydrogen peroxide solution, followed by the application of antibiotic ointment, and then the wound is covered with a nonadherent dressing. This procedure is carried out twice daily. Patients should receive explicit instructions on when and how to call the Mohs surgeon in the event of unexpected problems.

Postoperative pain is usually easily managed after Mohs micrographic surgery. Patients should be instructed to take non-aspirin-containing analgesics for their discomfort. Anatomic locations subject to movement or tension such as the mid-chest, shoulders, and lips may be more likely to be uncomfortable postoperatively. Procedures involving large tumors or patients with low pain thresholds may require narcotic analgesics. Patients experiencing pain several days postoperatively may have a wound infection or hematoma and should be evaluated.

Mohs surgery patients should be seen at least once in the 6-week postoperative period after suture removal to ensure proper wound healing and contraction. Patients may have an unexpected outcome such as a spitting suture, flap tip necrosis, partial graft slough, hypertrophic scar, or other event requiring the surgeon's intervention to optimize the ultimate outcome of the surgical procedure. An additional visit 3 months postoperatively is used to monitor for recurrence and for patient education. Patients should receive regular skin examination, and be aware of their increased risk for additional cutaneous malignancies.

PITFALLS AND THEIR MANAGEMENT

Pitfalls and their management

- Careful preoperative planning minimizes complications.
- Take an anesthetic history to identify allergy to lidocaine, which is rare, but can cause anaphylaxis.
- Monitor patients for procedural or needle anxiety, using sedation if necessary, and take appropriate precautions for fall risk.
- Meticulous surgical technique and patient education help to reduce postoperative infection.
- Assess whether cutaneous and sensory nerves are at risk and take precautionary measures (e.g. injection to tumesce tissue before removal, upward traction, and use of a nerve stimulator with an alarm).
- In the periorbital region take care to avoid direct eye injury—where the eyelid is not directly involved, protect the eyes with taped gauze pads or drapes.
- Advise patients on wound care and give explicit instructions on when to contact the surgeon if unexpected problems occur.

Complications of Mohs micrographic surgery are relatively infrequent. They may be minimized with careful preoperative planning. Cook and Perone, in a prospective study of 1358 cases, had a complication rate of 1.64%, most involving difficulties with hemostasis.[50] Office-based Mohs surgical units provide a safe environment for the patient. A log book should be maintained to detail complications to establish trends and prevent recurrences as far as possible. A complete set of vital signs including blood pressure and pulse should be taken before the procedure.

Of the more serious complications, anaphylaxis to anesthetic agents or other administered medications is the most grave. Use of supplementary oxygen and administration of emergency medical care may be required. Training in Advanced Cardiac Life Support is a required component of fellowship training in Mohs micrographic surgery. Allergy to lidocaine, the most commonly used of the amide local anesthetics, is rare, but can result in anaphylaxis. This agent does not cross-react with the ester class of local anesthetics which are more commonly responsible for untoward effects. When a patient gives a history of 'allergy' to local anesthetics, an episode of epinephrine (adrenaline) sensitivity is most commonly elicited. In these patients and in the elderly with labile hypertension, the concentration of epinephrine used may be reduced while still maintaining the hemostatic effect. Some patients may need an allergy work-up to better characterize their precise sensitivity. Diluting the anesthetic agent with plain 1% lidocaine to achieve an epinephrine concentration of 1 : 300 000 can be used to provide sufficient hemostasis.

Patients may faint because of anxiety about the procedure or a fear of needles. Precautions must be undertaken to avoid the risk of a fall, including patient monitoring and observation, maintaining the surgical table as low as possible to the floor during nonoperative periods, and light patient restraints. Syncopal patients should be placed in the reverse Trendelenburg position. Patients should be encouraged to eat a light meal before surgery to prevent hypoglycemic episodes except when an NPO status is indicated.

Procedural anxiety may be managed first by a caring staff attitude and interactions with comfortable, soothing surroundings, and soft, relaxing music and lighting. A surgeon's expression of confidence in a favorable outcome is also helpful in alleviating anxiety. If anxiety is excessive, the patient may be sedated with an oral or sublingual benzodiazepine, usually diazepam at a dose of 5–10 mg 1 hour preoperatively. Diazepam can reduce blood pressure, so careful monitoring is necessary before further administration. Important causes of patient anxiety are a fear of needles and pain with injection. The patient may recall biopsy-related pain, and fear a commensurate increase in pain with the excision. Slow injections of anesthesia through a small bore needle (30-gauge) are critical. Advancing the needle through previously anesthetized sites and injecting upon withdrawal can greatly minimize discomfort.

Bleeding is the most common complication to be avoided. Despite the use of epinephrine (adrenaline) and meticulous electrocoagulation to aid hemostasis, other measures may be required to limit blood loss. Suture ligation of large transected blood vessels may be necessary, especially of the superficial temporal artery, which is not infrequently encountered in excisions on the temple. If the field is large or bleeding persists despite appropriate hemostatic measures, bovine thrombin or hemostatic gauze (e.g. Seasorb soft alginate dressing, Coloplast Corp, Marietta, GA) may be helpful. Pressure dressings between layers are important to minimize bleeding. Upon repair of the Mohs defect, closure of underlying dead space in layers is critical to prevent hematomas from small arterioles or capillary beds. Postoperatively, pressure dressings for 24–48 hours are helpful. Dental rolls and other bolster materials placed on the skin and secured with tape augmented with skin adhesive (e.g. Mastisol, Ferndale Laboratories Inc, Ferndale, MI) are particularly helpful in the mid-face and periauricular areas.

Infection may develop in the setting of any cutaneous surgery. Tumors treated with Mohs surgery that have required multiple layers to clear or prolonged exposed periods of time may have an increased risk of infection. The risk of infection is also increased if there is abraded or crusted skin and in immunocompromised patients. Patients who allow their wounds to desiccate or lack diligence in their postoperative care are also more likely to develop an infection. Risk can be minimized by meticulous surgical technique, including the removal of hair from the wound, preferably by clipping preoperatively, and ensuring appropriate eversion of skin edges and minimizing dead space. Patients who have a tendency to develop infections postoperatively can be placed on a course of antibiotics, but antibiotics are otherwise not routinely administered prophylactically except for subacute bacterial endocarditis prophylaxis. Total hip and knee replacement patients may need prophylaxis during the initial 90-day inflammatory phase. In our practice we consult with the orthopedic surgeon in this group of patients.

Wound necrosis may occur when the repair places the wound under significant tension. Poor flap design resulting in vascular compromise may result in wound edge necrosis, requiring a portion to heal by second intention. Full-thickness or split-thickness grafts may be lost, again resulting in second intention healing. Sharp wound debridement may be required in some situations where eschar covers the wound.

Large or recurrent tumors in high-risk locations may be so deeply invasive that they may involve cutaneous and sensory nerves. Knowledge of the anatomy will enable the cutaneous surgeon to advise the patient pre- and peri-operatively of the risk of injury and assess for any neurological deficits present. Nerve injury may be avoided in several ways.

- First, an injection of dilute local anesthetic or 0.9% saline can be used to tumesce the tissues immediately before removal of the layer and thus make it unlikely to inadvertently encounter vital structures including nerves.
- Second, gentle traction upward on the tissue as it is dissected minimizes the risk to underlying nerves. A nerve stimulator with auditory alarm may be used in conjunction with the dissection.
- Third, electrocoagulation-induced nerve injury can be minimized in critical locations such as the periorbital area by the use of Teflon-coated bipolar forceps.

Mohs micrographic surgery in the periorbital area must be performed with care to avoid direct eye injury. For surgery of the eyelid, the eye can be anesthetized with two drops of local anesthetic (i.e. tetracaine) and a lubricated plastic corneal shield can be inserted during the procedure. In cases not directly involving the eyelid, the eyes can be protected by taped cotton gauze pads or drapes over the eyelids. This will protect the eyes from inadvertent injury from surgical instruments, and prevent eye irritation by the bright operating room lights.

Management of pitfalls

Unrealistic expectations, poor surgical planning, intervening infection or hematoma, and other factors interfering with healing may result in wound cosmesis that is unacceptable to the patient. Although the main goal of Mohs micrographic surgery is complete extirpation of the tumor, the cosmetic and functional results are frequently of paramount importance to the patient.

Smokers have a higher rate of graft failure and delayed wound healing. Wounds closed under sustained tension frequently develop superficial necrosis, which can adversely affect the cosmetic result. Occasionally a delayed repair is necessary and the ultimate result may not be realized for a year or longer, requiring patience on the part of the physician and patient. Surgical repairs may need refinement in a series of steps for optimal cosmesis and functionality. However, most post-Mohs surgical wounds regain their texture, coloration, and sensation eventually.

Tumors that have extended to a free anatomic margin, such as the eyelid or lip, require additional surgical planning to prevent functional and cosmetic impairment. Ectropion may develop if tension is placed on the lower eyelid free margin. Xerophthalmia and impaired vision may result when the lacrimal apparatus of the eye is compromised. Chondritis may occur when the integrity of the cartilage is disturbed, particularly if perichondrium is lost and second intention healing is used. Air flow through the naris can be compromised when the lateral ala is unsupported after loss of cartilage, requiring composite flap reconstruction. Consultation with other specialists may be helpful pre-, peri- and postoperatively in these situations.

In some situations, complete clearance of the tumor is not achievable, even with the Mohs technique.[51] Occasionally involvement of deep structures means that there is a great risk of functional injury. Sometimes the layers reveal perineural tumor or invasion into bone that cannot be cleared without sacrificing vital structures. In recurrent tumors, unpredictable growth patterns may occur as a result of fibrosis from previous radiation or excision. Tumor may spread far beyond the original site of recurrence along areas of previous surgery that were undermined for previously used flaps or grafts, and on rare occasions may be too extensive to clear completely. In these situations, postoperative radiation therapy is indicated to enhance local cure rates.[52] On occasion, a combined approach is chosen after discussion with the patient midway during the procedure (i.e. between layers). A multidisciplinary approach is helpful in the management of these advanced malignancies.

Radiation therapy can have a primary or adjunctive role in cutaneous malignancy. The Mohs surgeon should be familiar with its capabilities and limitations. Radiation therapy has advanced greatly because of the wide availability of linear accelerators that generate electrons with energy that can be varied so that the physician can treat to different depths (Fig. 48.15). Customization of the beam delivered to the patient through the use of cerrobend cutouts, blocks, contoured aquaplast masks, and lead shielding, and refined dose fractionation schemes that optimize treatment and limit side-effects have also advanced the field (Fig. 48.16). Electron beam radiation penetrates deeply into the tissue, in contrast to the superficial X-ray treatments of the past with their diffuse energy scattering and unpredictable, superficial tissue penetration.

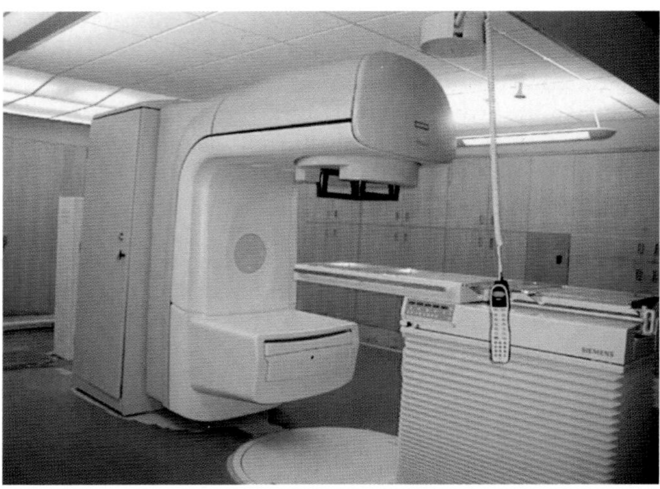

Figure 48.15 Linear accelerator. Typical modern device used for radiation therapy. This requires a large amount of space and a facility with protective shielding to prevent inadvertent exposures.

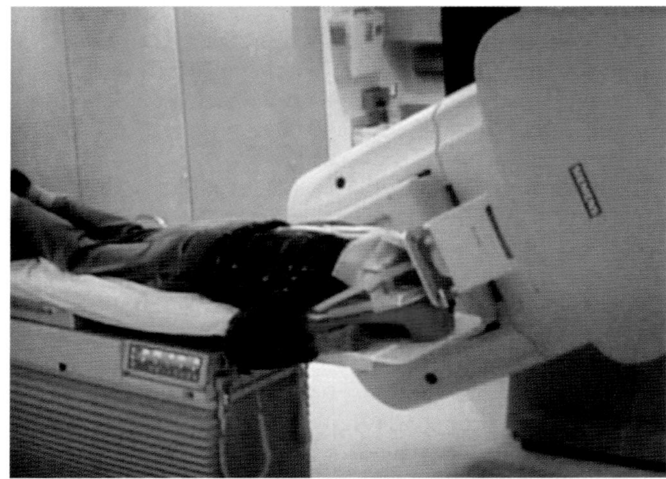

Figure 48.16 Patient treatment with a linear accelerator. Note the specialized patient-specific equipment contoured to the exact anatomical area used to precisely deliver the electron beam. The treatment time is for only several minutes per day; most fractionation regimens involve daily treatment for 4–6 weeks.

■ CUTANEOUS ONCOLOGY

Mohs micrographic surgery has been used most widely and extensively in the extirpation of basal cell and squamous cell carcinomas using the fresh tissue technique. More recently, its use has expanded to include the removal of many other tumor types that have proved challenging to control locally. In most situations, this has involved a permanent tissue technique involving the Mohs technique with slides being generated using formalin fixation. Mohs surgery thus modified by the use of tangential, formalin-fixed, paraffin-embedded histologic specimens, ensures accurate interpretation of histologic specimens while maintaining the tissue conservation of the Mohs technique.[53] There is a resultant delay in the repair, but for many of these tumor types the wait is beneficial for patients, with higher cure rates than with traditional surgical techniques. The rest of this chapter discusses selected tumor types and how Mohs surgery can be used in their treatment.

Basal cell carcinoma

Basal cell carcinoma is the most common malignancy. Tumors are most frequent on the head and neck, where they are more likely to be biologically aggressive and invade vital structures. Brodkin et al. found that of 840 basal cell carcinomas studied, over 90% were on the head and neck.[54] The biologic behavior of a basal cell carcinoma depends on its histologic subtype and clinical features, including its precise anatomic location, size, and duration, and whether it is primary or recurrent. All these factors must be taken into consideration when employing a particular treatment.

Nonsurgical treatment

Nonsurgical treatments of basal cell carcinoma include cryotherapy, radiation therapy, and immunotherapy with topical and intralesional interferon and topical imiquimod.

Cryotherapy with liquid nitrogen is optimally performed with a thermocouple to ensure lesional tissue temperature is –50 °C or below to ensure adequate cellular destruction. Alternatively, clinical assessment of halo thaw times using one of a variety of methods can be used—for an extensive bibliography, see the American Academy of Dermatology Committee on Guidelines of Care for Cryosurgery.[55]

Radiation therapy, when used as a primary modality of treatment, is limited in use because it is often more expensive and inconvenient, and can induce subsequent secondary malignancies within the treatment field.

Greenway et al.[2] demonstrated complete clearance of basal cell carcinoma in eight patients with recombinant α-2 interferon, using a regimen of injections three times per week for 3 weeks without any significant side-effects. Intralesional interferon-α is efficacious in basal cell carcinoma through the upregulation of expression of CD95 on tumor cells, which induces apoptosis, recruitment of $CD4^+$ T cells, and enhanced secretion of cytokines such as interferon gamma and interleukin-2.[56]

Imiquimod, through the upregulation of interferon-α, has emerged as a novel primary treatment for basal cell carcinoma, and it is currently approved for the treatment of superficial basal cell carcinoma. It offers the dual convenience of patient self-treatment using a topical formulation. It appears that once daily topical application for 12 weeks is most efficacious.[57] However, the response rate can vary, with a complete response rate of 87% for superficial basal cell carcinoma, but only 65% for more invasive types.[58] At least one of us (Greenway) is concerned that both physicians and patients may overuse new topical therapies, resulting in an increase of recurrent and residual tumors presenting at a later date.

Mohs surgery may be reserved for those basal cell carcinomas exhibiting one or more indications of biologic aggressiveness. It can also be used for the basal cell nevus syndrome,[59] in which a multiplicity of frequently aggressive tumors creates the need for conservation of the greatest possible amount of normal tissue.

Histologic forms of basal cell carcinoma

The most common histologic forms of basal cell carcinoma are superficial, nodular, ulcerative, metatypical, morpheaform, and infiltrative.

A superficial basal cell carcinoma appears as an erythematous scaly plaque with well-defined borders, and histologically is comprised of small nests of cells with oval and basophilic nuclei with scant cytoplasm along the basal layer of the epidermis. A nodular basal cell carcinoma appears as a translucent papule with telangiectasias, and histologically is comprised of basaloid cells with peripheral palisading of the nuclei and stromal proliferation. An ulcerated basal cell carcinoma appears as a nodular lesion with central ulceration, and histologically contains foci of epidermal ulceration. Metatypical basal cell carcinoma is not distinctive clinically, but histologically contains features of basal cell carcinoma in addition to foci of squamous differentiation resembling squamous cell carcinoma. Morpheaform basal cell carcinoma appears as a yellow-red firm plaque and histologically contains tumor nests and cords enmeshed in a fibrous, sclerotic stroma. Infiltrative basal cell carcinoma is not distinctive clinically, but histologically contains islands of tumor cells with a spiked appearance in narrow cords within a hyalinized stroma.

The more commonly aggressive subtypes of basal cell carcinoma are the ulcerative, metatypical, morpheaform, and infiltrative forms. Recurrent basal cell carcinomas, even if originally of a less aggressive subtype, tend to exhibit one or more of these features. These tumors are frequently found to extend well beyond their clinical margins when on the head and neck. Lateral spread of subclinical disease may be several centimeters beyond that visualized on gross examination. The tumors have an affinity for fascial planes and other natural barriers to tumor growth. They can penetrate to the perichondrium and periosteum and then spread along them widely. Tumor invasion of nerves may also occur, with tumor cells either spreading along the perineurium or directly invading the endoneurium. In 1% of basal cell carcinomas,[60] perineural spread may be several centimeters distant from any involved soft tissues. Perineural spread most commonly involves the supraorbital, infraorbital, and mental nerves. Neurotropic basal cell carcinomas may present with symptoms of pain, paresthesias, or motor loss in the affected nerve distribution.[61] Radiation therapy may be considered as an adjunctive therapy in these situations.

Clinical features

The clinical features of a basal cell carcinoma accurately predict its biological behavior. Many patients are unable to recall or discern when their tumors appeared, making correlation of tumor duration and invasion difficult. However, lesions present for longer periods of time do have a greater chance for deeper invasion into nerves, muscle, cartilage, and bone, and their extirpation can be extensive. In a series of 434 Mohs cases, tumors with perineural invasion required an average of 5.3 Mohs layers for clearance, in contrast to those without perineural invasion, which required only 2.2.[61] Tumors with aggressive histology require more Mohs layers to achieve tumor-free margins.[61] The size of the tumor is also critical in predicting tumor extent. In a large series of 1131 Mohs cases, the most important indicator of extensive subclinical spread in addition to aggressive histology was preoperative size greater than 2.5 cm in diameter.[62] These larger tumors require a wider surgical margin. For tumors with a diameter less than 2 cm, a minimum margin of 4 mm would be expected to clear the tumor in more than 95% of cases.[63] Tumor size is also important for prognosis. In the largest series to date, 5-year cure rates after Mohs surgery for tumors involving the nose decreased commensurately with increased lesion size—for basal cell carcinomas under 1 cm in diameter, 99.9%; for tumors between 1 and 2 cm in diameter, 99.3%; for tumors between 2 and 3 cm in diameter, 98.3%, and for tumors greater than 3 cm in diameter, 84.3%.[1]

Larger tumors in many cases tend to be recurrent tumors, with discontinuity of tumor foci. They may contain intervening scar or radiation changes, which interrupt tumor growth patterns. Recurrent tumors have a much lower cure rate with any form of therapy. Mohs reported a recurrence rate of 7.9% in a large series of recurrent basal cell carcinomas.[1] Robins reported a recurrence rate of 3.4% in a slightly larger series.[64] Recurrences after radiation treatment can be particularly challenging. These tumors, originally with less aggressive histologic features, frequently have morpheaform or metatypical patterns after radiation therapy. In addition, the radiation therapy itself may induce fibrosis and scar formation, enmeshing individual tumor cells and making interpretation of the margins difficult clinically and histologically.

Metastatic basal cell carcinoma occurs in less than 0.5% of cases. The mean time from the appearance of the primary basal cell carcinoma of the skin and distant metastasis is 9 years.[65] Risk factors include tumor invasion into cartilage, bone, skeletal muscle, or parotid gland, previous radiation therapy, and previous treatment with any modality.[65] Anatomic locations on the face, scalp, and genitalia are at higher risk; the ear is the most common site from which metastatic spread occurs.[65] The histologic subtype is not correlated with metastatic diathesis. Metastasis can occur both hematogenously (to lungs, bone, and skin) and through lymphatics. Treatment options include combinations of surgery, radiation, and chemotherapy; of the latter, cisplatin is the most effective agent.[66]

Squamous cell carcinoma

Squamous cell carcinoma is the second most common cutaneous malignancy. It can be treated with multiple modalities, including surgery, cryotherapy, radiation therapy, and intralesional interferon.

Squamous cell carcinomas commonly present as erythematous scaly plaques in sun-damaged locations. They are also seen in areas of previous burn scar or irradiation. The biological behavior depends on many factors, including histologic subtype, anatomic location, duration, previous injury, previous therapy, and immune status of the patient.

Histologically, squamous cell carcinomas consist of irregular proliferating nests of neoplastic keratinocytes arising from the epidermis, with nuclear hyperchromasia, increased mitotic activity, cytoplasmic eosinophilia, and varying degrees of nuclear atypia. Biologically aggressive subtypes include cystic squamous cell carcinoma, adenoid squamous cell carcinoma, clear cell carcinoma, and spindle cell carcinoma. Squamous cell carcinoma presenting as verrucous plaques is referred to as verrucous carcinoma, and demonstrates little epithelial atypia. Bowen's disease (squamous cell carcinoma in situ) presents clinically as ill-defined scaly red patches and demonstrates abnormal keratinocytes confined to the epidermis. Cutaneous horns or other hyperkeratotic lesions may overly squamous cell carcinoma. Squamous cell carcinomas may arise in burns, scars, or other injuries. Tumors arising in immunocompromised patients tend to be more aggressive and have higher metastatic rates.

Squamous cell carcinomas that are more likely to recur or metastasize should be considered for treatment with Mohs micrographic surgery. Preoperatively or concurrently, sentinel node dissection can be performed for the lesions at particular risk for metastatic spread, although most practitioners would consider this additional step to be a research tool and not a standard of care. There is an increased risk for metastatic spread for lesions that are histologically moderately to poorly differentiated, and for facial lesions, particularly temple, nose, lip, periocular, or periauricular lesions. Lesions that are larger than 2 cm in diameter may be more prone to recurrence and metastasis. Squamous cell carcinomas occurring in burn or irradiation scars are also more likely to recur or metastasize, and squamous cell carcinomas demonstrating perineural invasion histologically have an increased risk of recurrence.[66] In our experience, 50% of metastatic cases of squamous cell carcinoma showed perineural spread. There is a risk of neurotropic spread by lesions overlying large sensory or motor nerves, such as the supraorbital, infraorbital, mental, and facial nerve branches. Perineural invasion has been reported in only 11% of squamous cell carcinomas less than 2.5 cm in diameter, but in 64% of those greater than or equal to 2.5 cm.[67] Patients who are immunocompromised tend to have more extensive tumor spread, as do those whose tumors are recurrent. Currently recommended surgical margins for primary cutaneous squamous cell carcinoma are from 4 to 6 mm, depending on the risks delineated above.[68] Mucosal lesions may have extensive subclinical spread; in one study, for 70% of lesions there was microscopically identified tumor 1 cm away from the initial tumor's visible border.[17] As for basal cell carcinoma, tumor spreads to fascial planes and can involve perichondrium and cartilage, and periosteum and bone.

Mohs micrographic surgery for recurrent squamous cell carcinoma can provide local cure rates of 94% or greater.[69] Mohs surgery may also be useful in the treatment of less aggressive forms of disease, including Bowen's disease and verrucous carcinoma, in which tumor-free margins are important to prevent recurrence but metastatic rates are very low. Erythroplasia of Queyrat (squamous cell carcinoma in situ involving the glans penis) and Bowenoid papulosis (squamous cell carcinoma of the penis) may be treated effectively with a variety of modalities, but Mohs surgery may provide the tissue conservation advantage required to preserve vital structures. Mohs surgery for verrucous carcinoma involving the genital and plantar surfaces improves cure rates to as high as 98% compared to 80% for standard surgical excision while avoiding radical surgery.[70] Radiation therapy is contraindicated for verrucous carcinoma because of its propensity to become more aggressive from this treatment.

Therapy for advanced and metastatic squamous cell carcinoma can be difficult. At our institution, a significant proportion of metastatic neck disease arises from squamous cell carcinoma of the skin. Neck dissection can result in significant morbidity for the patient. Surgery and radiation in a combined approach is favored in many cases. In advanced disease, systemic chemotherapy has been used. Sadek et al. reported the use of combination chemotherapy consisting of cisplatin, 5-fluorouracil, and bleomycin. In 14 patients, all with locally recurrent squamous cell carcinoma, and nine patients with nodal involvement, an overall response rate of 79% was achieved.[71] Doxorubicin, retinoids, and interferon have also been used in metastatic disease. Combinations of 13-cis retinoic acid and interferon α-2a have been used with a similar response rate, but dose-related side-effects have significantly limited therapy.[72] An interdisciplinary approach in caring for these patients is required.

Actinic keratoses are precancerous epidermal lesions that are found most frequently on sun-exposed areas. Squamous cell carcinoma may arise within these lesions as the atypical squamous proliferation invades into the dermis, and effective treatment is frequently sought for multiple lesions concurrently. Currently controversy exists regarding the nomenclature for these lesions, because some feel they should be called stage 0 squamous cell carcinoma.[73–82] Surgical approaches include curettage alone, curettage followed by light cautery, and cryotherapy. A variety of nonsurgical modalities of treatment have been used, including topical immune response modifiers, and photodynamic therapy. A chemopreventive strategy was developed in the 1970s using topical 5-fluorouracil after reports that actinic keratoses cleared in patients on intravenous 5-fluorouracil chemotherapy for internal malignancies.[83] There are currently three topical preparations widely available—5% fluorouracil cream, 1% fluorouracil cream, and 0.5% fluorouracil cream in a microsphere preparation. Comparable in efficacy, they cause varying degrees of irritation of perilesional skin that can greatly limit their use. Imiquimod (Aldara, 3M Pharmaceuticals, St Paul, MN) has also been used for the destruction of actinic keratoses, using a two to three times per week application regimen over several months with rest periods according to patient response, but this is also limited by inflammatory response.[84] Photodynamic therapy[85] has shown promise for treating actinic keratoses. Following the administration of a photosensitizer topically, it is selectively accumulated and retained in cancerous lesions. Delta-aminolevulinic acid (Levulan Kerastick, DUSA Pharmaceuticals Inc, Wilmington, MA), a precursor of protoporphyrin IX, is most commonly used as the photosensitizer. It is inactive until irradiated by light. Following administration of light of the appropriate wavelength in the absorption spectrum of the photosensitizer, cellular destruction occurs through the generation of toxic oxygen and other reactive species. This treatment is limited by pain, cost, convenience, and photosensitivity issues, but has demonstrated efficacy and is widely available.

Melanoma

Malignant melanoma, consisting of nests of atypical melanocytes with abnormal morphology, should be considered a systemic disease and remains a serious life-threatening entity. Patients may benefit from a multispecialty evaluation involving a dermatologic and/or Mohs surgeon, medical oncologist, and surgical oncologist. The American Joint Commission on Cancer issued newly revised guidelines for the staging of melanoma in 2003, placing greater emphasis on Breslow depth of spread into the dermis, presence or absence of ulceration in the epidermis, number of involved lymph nodes, nodal macro- or micrometastases, metastases, and measurement of serum lactate dehydrogenase (LDH).[86,87] Melanoma-in-situ and lentigo maligna lesions have atypical melanocytes confined to the epidermis, and thus are not assigned a Breslow depth. Several variants of invasive melanoma have been described, including superficial spreading, nodular, desmoplastic, amelanotic, and acrolentiginous.

Surgical excision with clear margins remains the predominant treatment modality for cutaneous melanoma. Melanoma patients should be staged by assessing for metastatic disease using chest radiography, and CT or MRI scanning when appropriate. Additionally, the recently available positron emission tomography (PET) scan is being used at some centers for staging and follow-up. By imaging glucose metabolism, PET pinpoints areas of increased metabolic activity—an indicator highly correlated with malignant tissue growth.

Before surgical extirpation of a melanoma, additional staging information may be obtained by using the sentinel node biopsy technique. Rapidly increasing in use and availability, the technique provides additional prognostic information for the patient, but has not yet demonstrated any survival benefit. Because the incidence of nodal metastasis greatly increases with Breslow depth, it is normally used for those invasive melanomas intermediate in depth, between 1 and 4 mm. The technique relies on the theory that the sentinel lymph nodes are the first lymph nodes that drain a primary cancer site. Thus, a sentinel lymph node biopsy would be expected to determine the overall status of the regional lymph nodes. The location of the sentinel node is predictable, but not invariable, and can be located contralateral to the tumor. Lymphoscintigraphy using Technetium-99 radiolabeled sulfur colloid injected perilesionally enables precise localization of the sentinel node(s) through the use of a handheld gamma radiation probe. Additionally, a vital blue dye injected perilesionally provides a visual guide because it is taken up by the lymphatics within minutes. Lymph node excision and examination with special stains (i.e. S-100) is then performed in lieu of frozen section to decrease false-negative rates (Figs 48.17–48.20). If positive for nodal disease, a complete nodal basin excision would ordinarily be performed. The technique, usually performed under general anesthesia, has improved the staging accuracy of melanoma.[88] However, it does require additional steps, can lead to surgical delays, and does not always yield a sentinel node. Lymphatic drainage of the head and neck is particularly complex with multiple drainage patterns. Melanomas of the head and neck are thus technically more difficult to evaluate using sentinel node technology,

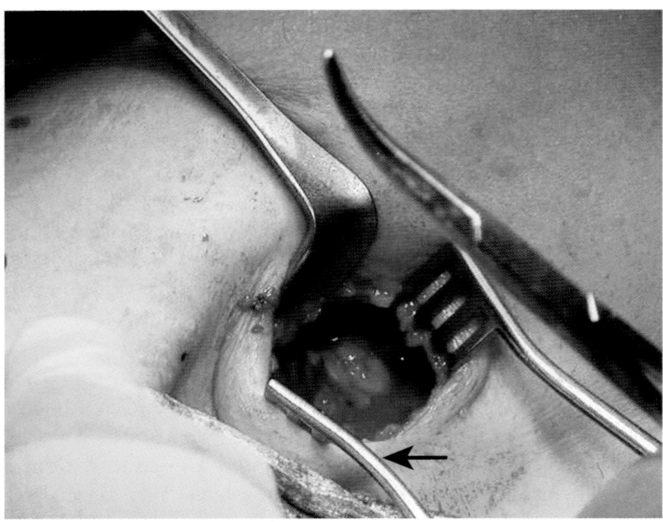

Figure 48.17 A handheld gamma probe (arrow) registers counts in vivo. The lymph node of interest usually has focally significantly elevated counts that register with application of the gamma probe directly to tissue. In addition, the node should be visually blue, having taken up the vital blue dye injected earlier. Negative control (background counts) can be obtained from a distant site, while the lesion injection site is the positive control (maximum counts).

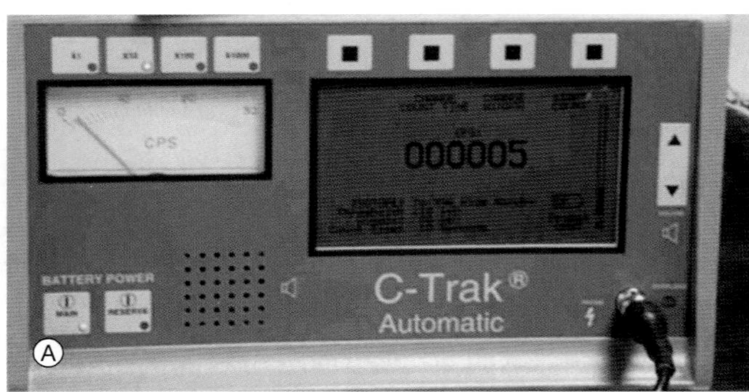

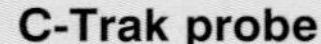

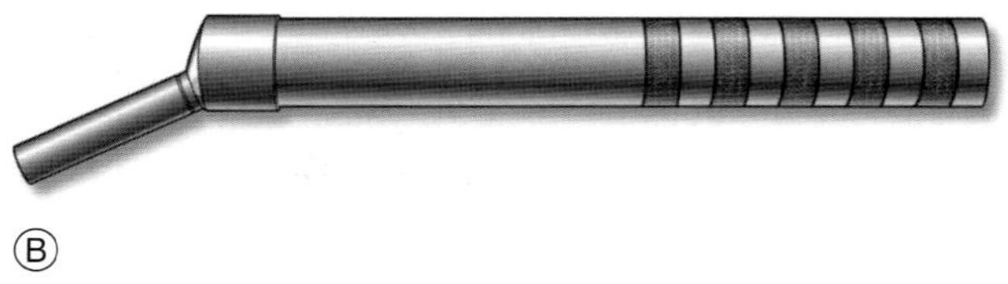

Figure 48.18 (A) C-Trak Surgical Guidance System (Care-Wise Medical Products Corporation, Morgan Hill, CA). (B) Probe.

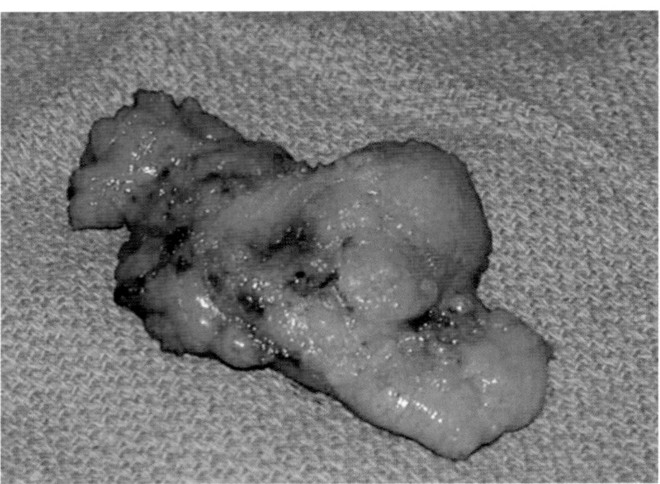

Figure 48.19 Tissue removed during axillary sentinel lymph node dissection. The surgeon confirms the presence of the node visually and by measuring counts with the gamma probe.

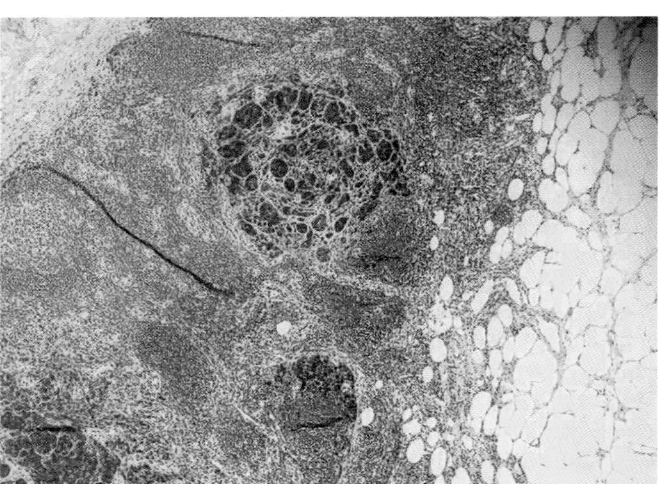

Figure 48.20 S-100 immunostain used on the sentinel node. Note the islands of S-100-positive cells within lymphoid aggregates that may have been missed with routine frozen sections not using immunostains.

particularly if the site is directly overlying a nodal basin. At our institution, sentinel lymph node dissection for head and neck lesions is performed by a head and neck surgeon, and for trunk and extremity lesions by a general surgeon, who often work closely together.

Over the years, as survival data have become refined and focused, recommendations for the margins for width of excision have been steadily reduced from 5 cm to between 1 and 3 cm, depending on Breslow depth, with only 5 mm for melanoma-in-situ.[89,90] Nevertheless, Mohs micrographic surgery can offer a means of achieving clear margins while sparing normal tissue around critical anatomic structures. Reported rates of local control are comparable to standard margin excision. However, the margins required to clear the tumors in 95% of cases have been reported to be 15 mm for melanoma in situ and 26 mm for invasive melanomas.[91] These findings suggest that margins wider than those currently recommended may be required to ensure tumor clearance. Melanoma treatment with this technique requires the Mohs surgeon to be either expert in the histologic interpretation of melanocytic lesions or to adopt the technique to directly involve the dermatopathologist or pathologist in their interpretation. Clinical photographs of gross lesions and sectioned tissue may be helpful in orientation. Excellent technical support is also required, with additional resources to section tissue with the Mohs technique compared to conventional excision.

Histological interpretation of malignant melanoma with the fresh technique may be problematic and has been the source of some controversy. While assessing histologic margins, atypical single melanocytes may be present at the periphery of the obvious invasive portion of the melanoma. Interpretation of the degree of atypia of these melanocytes is difficult and subjective. There are published reports of complete correlation between frozen section tissue margins and permanent section controls,[92] however, for melanoma-in-situ lesions at least, frozen sections alone may be insufficient for margin control.[93]

The use of melanocyte-specific immunohistochemical stains can greatly enhance the accuracy of margin interpretation.[94] Several immunostains that can be used on frozen sections have been studied extensively, including MART-1, S-100, MEL-5, Melan-A (A-103), and HMB-45.[94] Albertini et al. found MART-1 to be superior in sensitivity to both HMB-45 and S-100 for Mohs surgery with the fresh tissue technique. Zalla et al. found Melan-A to be superior in clarity and ease of interpretation of specimens.[94] Positive and negative control specimens from the tumor and distant skin can be used for comparison of staining patterns.[94] Finally, it is critical to review vertical sections of the main portion of the specimen, assessing the presence of and depth of invasion, because this can change the diagnosis (i.e. from melanoma-in-situ to melanoma) and staging of the patient. Some proponents follow in the footsteps of Dr Mohs himself and have found that chemosurgery can be an effective treatment for melanoma,[95] an approach that appears to have an immunologic basis behind it.[96]

Advanced stages of melanoma or unresectable lesions can benefit from cryotherapy, radiation therapy, or immunotherapy, all of which have significant limitations in their efficacy. Topical imiquimod, acting presumably through its effects on interferon-α, has recently been reported to result in clearance of lentigo maligna[97] and cutaneous metastases of melanoma,[98] but insufficient data preclude its recommendation. Intravenous and subcutaneously injected interferon-α regimens, vaccines, and other immunomodulatory treatments have been used. There is now overwhelming evidence that high-dose (20 million units/m^2 intravenously for 4 weeks followed by 10 million units/m^2 subcutaneously three times weekly for 48 weeks) interferon-α improves relapse-free survival after surgery for high-risk melanoma,[99] and strong evidence that it improves overall survival in a select subset of patients.[100] Lower doses of interferon for longer durations, biochemotherapy (concurrent interleukin-2 and interferon α-2b), and vaccines (particularly dendritic cell-based vaccines) are undergoing trials in the treatment of advanced stage melanoma. For a further discussion of melanoma, see Chapter 50.

Merkel cell carcinoma

Mohs micrographic surgery has been used successfully to treat Merkel cell carcinoma, a neuroendocrine tumor of the skin. Clinically, Merkel cell carcinoma is manifest as a skin-colored or bluish nodular lesion that is firm to palpation, which most commonly occurs on the head and neck of elderly men. Histologically, monomorphous sheets of basaloid cells are seen.

Merkel cell carcinoma is an aggressive tumor with reported local recurrence rates of 30%, regional node involvement rates of up to 50%, and metastatic rates of 40%.[101] Survival rates statistically correlate with nodal status. Because of high local recurrence rates after excision, a 3 cm margin is currently recommended for the primary excision of this tumor, but because the tumor occurs on the head and neck in 60% of individuals, this is not always possible without sacrificing vital structures. Mohs surgery successfully limited the required margin to 1.5 cm (1.2 cm on the face and 1.9 cm on the extremities) in one study.[102]

Although the optimal treatment of Merkel cell carcinoma is unknown, radiation therapy is a commonly used adjunct to surgery to improve local control, with several series reporting improved overall survival, relapse-free survival, and disease-free survival with its use.[101,103] The largest series to date, consisting of 45 cases treated with Mohs surgery with and without adjuvant radiation was unable to find such improvement.[104] Adjuvant radiation is recommended for large, recurrent, or incompletely excised tumors which are at high risk for recurrence. In our institution, we have found a combined approach of Mohs surgery and radiation oncology consultation for adjunctive treatment helpful. Brissett et al., based on a retrospective analysis of 22 cases, found that wide local excision and dissection of the lymphatic drainage basin provided the best overall survivial.[105] Adjuvant chemotherapy has been used for metastatic disease, but no chemotherapy protocol has been shown to improve survival. Recent advances in sentinel lymph node technology have been applied to Merkel cell carcinoma, using sentinel lymph node dissection and Mohs surgery simultaneously.[106]

Dermatofibrosarcoma protuberans

Dermatofibrosarcoma protuberans is characteristically a slow-growing, locally aggressive malignant tumor of the skin with a characteristic spindle cell morphology histologically. It is most common on the trunk, upper thighs, and groin, frequently consists of multiple discrete nodular lesions, and clinically may resemble a keloid. Although well-circumscribed, dermatofibrosarcoma protuberans can extend widely from its base. Histologically it frequently invades the fat and tumor-free margins are difficult to obtain with certainty because of its resemblance to normal fibroblasts on hematoxylin and eosin staining. Recurrence rates after wide excision can be as high as 60%, but years may pass before they are noted because of the tumor's slow growth. Metastases are rare.

Mohs surgery has been used to address the subclinical contiguous growth pattern of dermatofibrosarcoma protuberans with micrographically controlled excision.[107] Tumors less than 2 cm in diameter can be cleared with a 1.5-cm surgical margin, whereas larger tumors can be cleared with a 2.5-cm surgical margin.[108] In the world literature, 221 cases have been treated with Mohs surgery, with only five (2.3%) recurrences.[109] Mohs surgery is particularly helpful in conjunction with special immunostains. The presence of scattered dermal spindle cells in the dermis of normal skin makes it difficult to differentiate residual tumor from normal dermis in Mohs layers.[110] Dermatofibrosarcoma protuberans stains positively with CD34,[109] and this can be used to achieve greater accuracy of margin control when used in conjunction with either frozen or permanent section Mohs surgery. Mohs surgery is the treatment of choice for dermatofibrosarcoma protuberans; if immunostains are unavailable, a biopsy of normal skin can be useful as a control to improve histologic accuracy[110] for comparison purposes.

Atypical fibroxanthoma

Atypical fibroxanthoma usually presents as an ulcerated, erythematous nodule or plaque on heavily actinically damaged skin of the head and neck in older men. This fibrohistiocytic tumor with bizarre histology has a favorable prognosis, and metastases are rare. When the tumor does spread, it generally spreads through regional lymphatics. Treatment consists of wide surgical excision with a 1-cm margin. Mohs surgery may be used for large, recurrent tumors or in areas where tissue conservation is important,[111] and can improve cure rates. In a series of five patients with atypical fibroxanthoma treated by Mohs surgery, there were no local recurrences and no metastases after a mean follow-up period of 3 years.[112]

Malignant fibrous histiocytoma

Malignant fibrous histiocytoma, a deeper and more invasive tumor with some shared features of atypical fibroxanthoma, can also be treated successfully with Mohs micrographic surgery. It is a soft tissue sarcoma with a less favorable prognosis than atypical fibroxanthoma. Mohs surgery can improve the cure rate. In a series of 17 patients with malignant fibrous histiocytoma treated by Mohs surgery, there was only one local recurrence and no metastatic disease after a mean follow-up period of 3 years.[112]

Microcystic adnexal carcinoma and other sweat gland neoplasms

Varying in clinical presentation from a flesh colored papule to a firm subcutaneous nodule, microcystic adnexal carcinoma is a rare, locally aggressive malignant tumor that most commonly occurs on the upper lip in middle-aged women.[113] Previous radiation therapy may be an important predisposing factor. The tumor infiltrates deeply by local invasion within the dermis and subcutaneous tissues, and frequently invades skeletal muscle; perineural invasion may be seen. Metastases have not been observed. Histologically, microcystic adnexal carcinoma can resemble basal cell carcinoma and adnexal neoplasms such as desmoplastic trichoepithelioma and syringoma. It contains ductal and glandular structures, keratin cysts, follicular structures, and a desmoplastic stroma. Superficial shave biopsy may not be diagnostic, with many of these features found deep in the dermis.

Microcystic adnexal carcinoma has a high local recurrence rate with standard surgical excision, whereas Mohs surgery has been used successfully. The local recurrence rate by standard excision is almost 50%, whereas that with Mohs surgery is almost 10%.[98] In two recent series of a total of 24 cases with a mean follow-up of 5 years, there were no recurrences.[114,115]

Mohs surgery has also been advocated for the treatment of primary eccrine adenocarcinoma of the skin. Also known as eccrine porocarcinoma, this rare malignant tumor of the eccrine sweat gland displays a tendency for local recurrence, and regional lymphatic spread may occur. The tumor is radioresistant, and skip areas may occur within the tumor nodules.

Primary mucinous carcinoma is another rare sweat gland malignancy with locally aggressive behavior that frequently involves the face for which the Mohs technique results in an improved cure rate and tissue conservation.[116]

Mohs surgery has also been used for benign sweat gland neoplasms, such as the papillary eccrine adenoma. More aggressive lesions on the digits and volar surfaces of the palms and soles are ideal for Mohs surgery, because of the need for tissue conservation and preservation of sensory and motor function.[117]

Sebaceous carcinoma

Sebaceous carcinoma is an aggressive malignant tumor that most frequently occurs on the eyelids, and has a tendency for local invasion and metastases. It is characterized histologically by lobules of atypical sebaceous glands and large cells with mitoses. It has a high local recurrence rate, sometimes requiring orbital exenteration. A pagetoid pattern of intraepithelial tumor spread has been described,[118] making clinical discernment of tumor margins problematic. Mohs surgery has been successfully used for the treatment of this neoplasm.[119] It appears that it does not always spread by direct contiguous extension, and as one would expect there are several reports of recurrences after Mohs surgery. In certain cases with pagetoid spread, because the tumor may be multifocal, it is possible to obtain a tumor-free margin without actually removing the entire tumor. Additionally, recognition of the pagetoid pattern of spread can be difficult with frozen sections; paraffin-embedded sections are recommended.[120] Oil red O stain aids in visualization of the tumor. Some authors have advocated taking an additional Mohs layer after a tumor-free margin has been obtained, citing the presence of multifocal disease or discontinuity on excisional histologic specimens in 6% of cases.[120] Others also recommend conjunctival map biopsies to further delineate tumor involvement.[121]

Extramammary Paget's disease

Extramammary Paget's disease is a rare cutaneous malignancy characterized by scaly red patches that are sometimes pruritic in apocrine-bearing areas such as the axillae and groin. It may be multifocal and usually extends beyond clinically apparent margins. Wide excision is followed by a high recurrence rate as a result of subclinical tumor spread. Mohs surgery has been successfully used for extensive cases of extramammary Paget's disease and tissue sparing of critical anatomic structures can be achieved.[122] Radical excision is not required for most cases, but monitoring for recurrence is important. In the largest case series, two of six cases treated with Mohs surgery recurred locally.[123]

Recently, imiquimod has been shown to have potential value in the treatment of this condition.[124,125]

Angiosarcoma

Angiosarcoma is a rare, highly aggressive malignant neoplasm characterized by a solitary or multicentric violaceous papule or plaque on the head and neck and has a poor prognosis. Surgical management for lesions less than 10 cm in diameter is the treatment of choice.[126] Wide excision results in a high recurrence rate, and treatment is challenging because of extensive subclinical spread beyond the tumor's visible margin. Local control can be achieved with peripheral biopsies to assess tumor extent and Mohs surgery followed by adjunctive radiation therapy.[127]

Other benign and malignant neoplasms

Mohs micrographic surgery is playing an increasingly important role in the surgical management of a wide variety of cutaneous tumors. Rarely encountered tumors such as apocrine adenocarcinoma,[128] malignant cylindroma,[129] syringoid eccrine carcinoma,[130] adenoid cystic carcinoma,[131] leiomyosarcoma,[132] and malignant trichoepithelioma[133] have been successfully treated with the Mohs technique. More recent reports of its use in erosive adenomatosis of the nipple,[134] infantile digital fibroma,[135] spiradenocarcinoma,[136] rhabdomyosarcoma,[137] and granular cell tumor[35] illustrate its versatile application to virtually any neoplasm with contiguous growth characteristics. Clinicians increasingly recognize and value its utility for patients in the management of their malignancies.

■ SUMMARY

Mohs micrographic surgery is a technique with broad applications for malignancies of the skin, soft tissues, and mucous membranes. Through a series of precise, reproducible steps, a high rate of cure can be achieved in a predictable fashion for even the most complex tumors. It has benefited numerous patients immensely. The presently used technique has been modified over the years, with perhaps the most significant advance being the use of the fresh tissue technique. The future for Mohs surgery is bright. Optical coherence tomography or polarized light imaging may be used to determine skin cancer margins and to guide surgical excision during Mohs surgery.[138] Fast confocal reflectance microscopic examinations of excisional material may augment or replace histologic slide reading.[139] Advances in the use of dynamic telepathology may allow the technique to be brought to remote sites, as demonstrated by Nehal et al.[140] In spite of modifications to the technique, the two basic principles guiding Mohs surgery since its inception will remain the same—precise margin control and tissue conservation.

In the field of cutaneous oncology, the use of biological response modifiers, photodynamic therapy, and other innovative treatment modalities is expanding. The future of nonsurgical treatment of cutaneous malignancies is also bright. Recent advances in confocal microscopy enable real-time imaging of skin in vivo. Using this technology, Goldgeier et al.[141] demonstrated that basal cell carcinoma could be noninvasively diagnosed, treated, and cleared with topical imiquimod. Physicians and surgeons as cutaneous oncologists must become familiar with the use, applications, and limitations of these new modalities of treatment that are becoming available.

The opinions or assertions contained herein are the private views of the Authors and are not to be construed as official or as reflecting the views of the Department of the Army or the Department of Defense.

■ REFERENCES

1. Weisberg NK, Becker DS. Potential utility of adjunctive histopathologic evaluation of some tumors treated by Mohs micrographic surgery. Dermatol Surg 2000; 26:1052–1056.
2. Greenway HT, Cornell RC, Tanner DJ, et al. Treatment of basal cell carcinoma with intralesional interferon. J Am Acad Dermatol 1986; 15:437–443.
3. Miller BH, Shavin JS, Cognetta A, et al. Nonsurgical treatment of basal cell carcinomas with intralesional 5-fluorouracil/epinephrine injectable gel. J Am Acad Dermatol 1997; 36:72–77.
4. Wheeland RG, Bailin PL, Ratz JL, et al. Carbon dioxide laser vaporization and curettage in the treatment of large or multiple superficial basal cell carcinomas. J Dermatol Surg Oncol 1987; 13:119–125.
5. Gupta AK, Browne M, Bluhm R. Imiquimod; a review. J Cutan Med Surg 2002; 6:554–560.
6. Thissen MR, Neumann MH, Schouten LJ. A systematic review of treatment modalities for primary basal cell carcinomas. Arch Dermatol 1999; 135:1177–1183.
7. Mohs FE. Chemosurgery, microscopically controlled surgery for skin cancer. Springfield, IL: Charles C Thomas 1978; 1–29.
8. Mohs FE. Cancer of the eyelids. Bull Am Coll Chemosurgery 1970; 3:10–11.
9. Tromovitch TA, Stegman SJ. Microscopically controlled excision of skin tumors: chemosurgery (Mohs): fresh tissue technique. Arch Dermatol 1974; 110:231–232.
10. Mohs FE. Mohs micrographic surgery: a historical perspective. Dermatol Clin 1989; 7:609–611.
11. Rapini RP. Comparison of methods for checking surgical margins. J Am Acad Dermatol 1990; 23:288–294.
12. Abide JM, Nahai F, Bennett RG. The meaning of surgical margins. Plast Reconstr Surg 1984; 73:492–497.
13. Rowe DE, Carroll RJ, Day CL Jr. Long-term recurrence rates in previously untreated primary basal cell carcinoma: implications for patient follow-up. J Dermatol Surg Oncol 1989; 15:315–328.
14. Rowe DE, Carroll RJ, Day CL Jr. Mohs surgery is the treatment of choice for recurrent (previously treated) basal cell carcinoma. J Dermatol Surg Oncol 1989; 15:424–431.
15. Cook J, Zitelli JA. Mohs micrographic surgery: a cost analysis. J Am Acad Dermatol 1998; 39:698–703.
16. Bialy TL, Whalen J, Veledar E, et al. Mohs micrographic surgery vs traditional surgical excision: a cost comparison analysis. Arch Dermatol 2004; 140:736–742.
17. Davidson TM, Haghighi P, Astarita R, et al. Microscopically oriented histologic surgery for head and neck mucosal cancer. Cancer 1987; 60:1856–1861.
18. Scotto J, Fears TR, Fraumeni JF. Incidence of non-melanoma skin cancer in the United States (NIH publication No. 83–2433). Washington, DC: Public Health Service; 1983.
19. Mohs FE. Micrographic surgery for the microscopically controlled excision of eyelid cancers. Arch Ophthalmol 1986; 104:901–909.
20. Fosko SW, Gibney MD, Holds JB. Basal cell carcinoma involving the lacrimal canaliculus. A documented mechanism of tumor spread. Dermatol Surg 1997; 23:203–206.
21. Roenigk RK, Roenigk HH. Dermatologic surgery: principles and practice. 2nd edn. New York: Marcel Dekker Inc 1996; 703–729.
22. Mohs FE, Snow SN, Larson PO. Mohs micrographic surgery for penile tumors. Urol Clin North Am 1992; 19:291–304.
23. Collins SC, Dufresne RG Jr. Dietary supplements in the setting of Mohs surgery. Dermatol Surg 2002; 28:447–452.
24. Alam M, Goldberg LH. Serious adverse vascular events associated with perioperative interruption of antiplatelet and anticoagulant therapy. Dermatol Surg 2002:28:992–998.
25. Lin BB, Taylor RS. Digital photography for mapping Mohs micrographic surgery sections. Dermatol Surg 2001; 27:411–414.
26. Mikhail GR. Mohs Micrographic surgery. Philadelphia; WB Saunders Co 1991; 1–60.
27. Dogan MM, Snow SN, Lo J. Rapid skin edge elevation using the OCT compound droplet technique to obtain horizontal microsections in Mohs micrographic surgery. J Dermatol Surg Oncol 1991; 17:857–860.
28. Motley RJ, Holt PJ. A simple device for optimal tissue preparation for Mohs micrographic surgery. Br J Dermatol 1992; 126:57–59.

29. Leshin B, Cook SR, Frye DW. Cryomold: a device for tissue embedding for Mohs micrographic surgery. J Dermatol Surg Oncol 1991; 17:234–236.

30. Honda NS, Friedman DH. A simple method of tissue embedding for Mohs micrographic surgery. J Dermatol Surg Oncol 1989; 15:502–504.

31. Smeets NW, Stavast-Kooy AJ, Krekels GA, et al. Adjuvant cytokeratin staining in Mohs micrographic surgery for basal cell carcinoma. Dermatol Surg 2003; 29:375–377.

32. Robinson JK. Current histologic preparation methods for Mohs micrographic surgery. Dermatol Surg 2001:27:555–560.

33. Menaker GM, Chiang JK, Taliba B, et al. Rapid HMB-45 staining in Mohs micrographic surgery for melanoma in situ and invasive melanoma. J Am Acad Dermatol 2001:44:833–836.

34. Albertini JG, Elston DM, Libow LF, et al. Mohs micrographic surgery for melanoma: a case series, a comparative study of immunostains, an informative case report, and a unique mapping technique. Dermatol Surg 2002; 28:656–665.

35. Smith SB, Farley MF, Albertini JG, et al. Mohs micrographic surgery for granular cell tumor using S-100 immunostain. Dermatol Surg 2002:1076–1078.

36. Harris DW, Kist DA, Bloom K, Zachary CB. Rapid staining with carcinoembryonic antigen aids limited excision of extramammary Paget's disease treated by Mohs surgery. J Dermatol Surg Oncol 1994; 20:260–264.

37. Grabski WJ, Salasche SJ, McCollough ML, et al. Interpretation of Mohs micrographic frozen sections: a peer review comparison study. J Am Acad Dermatol 1989:670–674.

38. Gardner ES, Sumner WT, Cook JL. Predictable tissue shrinkage during frozen section histopathologic processing for Mohs micrographic surgery. Dermatol Surg 2001; 27:813–818.

39. Hruza GJ. Mohs micrographic surgery local recurrences. J Dermatol Surg Oncol 1994; 20:573–577.

40. Mehrany K, Byrd DR, Roenigk RK, et al. Lymphocytic infiltrates and subclinical epithelial tumor extension in patients with chronic leukemia and solid-organ transplantation. Dermatol Surg 2003; 29:129–134.

41. Katz KH, Helm KF, Billingsley EM, et al. Dense inflammation does not mask residual primary basal cell carcinoma during Mohs micrographic surgery. J Am Acad Dermatol 2001; 45:231–238.

42. Albregts T, Orengo I, Salasche S, et al. Squamous cell carcinoma in a patient with chronic lymphocytic leukemia. An intraoperative diagnostic challenge for the Mohs surgeon. Dermatol Surg 1998; 24:269–272.

43. Shriner DL, Wagner RF, Goldberg DJ. Wound closure techniques: flaps and grafts. In: Demis DJ, ed. Clinical dermatology. Philadelphia: JB Lippincott; 1995.

44. Thibault MJ, Bennett RG. Success of delayed full-thickness skin grafts after Mohs micrographic surgery. J Am Acad Dermatol 1995; 32:1004–1009.

45. Dzubow LM, Zack L. The principle of cosmetic junctions as applied to reconstruction of defects following Mohs surgery. J Dermatol Surg Oncol 1990; 16:353–355.

46. Rudolph R, Miller SH. Reconstruction after Mohs cancer excision. Clin Plast Surg 1993; 20:157–165.

47. Summers BK, Siegle RJ. Facial cutaneous reconstructive surgery: general aesthetic principles. J Am Acad Dermatol 1993; 29:669–681.

48. Shelton RM. The use of a curved ophthalmic blade to facilitate incising Mohs micrographic sections with the desired bevel despite anatomic obstructions. Dermatol Surg 1998; 24:897–899.

49. Moossavi M, Alam M, Ratner D. Use of the double-bladed scalpel in peripheral margin control of dermatofibrosarcoma protuberans. Dermatol Surg 2000; 26:599–601.

50. Cook JL, Perone JB. A prospective evaluation of the incidence of complications associated with Mohs micrographic surgery. Arch Dermatol 2003; 139:143–152.

51. Madani S, Huilgol S, Carruthers A. Unplanned incomplete Mohs micrographic surgery. J Am Acad Dermatol 2000; 42:814–819.

52. Siegle RJ, Houser S, Nag S, et al. Intraoperative radiation therapy and Mohs micrographic surgery on an outpatient basis. Dermatol Surg 1995; 21:975–978.

53. Clayton BD, Leshin B, Hitchcock MG, et al. Utility of rush-paraffin-embedded tangential sections in the management of cutaneous neoplasms. Dermatol Surg 2000; 26:671–678.

54. Brodkin RH, Kopf AW, Andrade R. Basal cell epithelioma and elastosis: a comparison of distribution in the biologic effects of ultra-violet radiation. In: Urbach F, ed. The biologic effects of ultra-violet radiation. Oxford: Pergamon Press; 1969:581.

55. American Academy of Dermatology Committee on Guidelines of Care. Guidelines of care for cryosurgery. J Am Acad Dermatol 1994; 31:648–653.

56. Buechner S, Wernli M, Bachmann F, et al. Intralesional interferon in basal cell carcinoma: how does it work? Recent Results Cancer Res 2002; 160:246–250.

57. Shumack S, Robinson J, Kossard S, et al. Efficacy of topical 5 % imiquimod cream for the treatment of nodular basal cell carcinoma: comparison of dosing regimens. Arch Dermatol 2002; 138: 1165–1171.

58. Sterry W, Ruzicka T, Herrera E, et al. Imiquimod 5% cream for the treatment of superficial and nodular basal cell carcinoma: randomized studies comparing low frequency dosing with and without occlusion. Br J Dermatol 2002; 147:1227–1236.

59. Mohs FE, Jones DL, Koranda FC. Microscopically controlled surgery for carcinomas in patients with nevoid basal cell carcinoma syndrome. Arch Dermatol 1980; 116:777–779.

60. Ratner D, Lowe L, Johnson TM, et al. Perineural spread of basal cell carcinomas treated with Mohs micrographic surgery. Cancer 2000; 88:1605–1613.

61. Orengo IF, Salasche SJ, Fewkes J, et al. Correlation of histologic subtypes of primary basal cell carcinoma and number of Mohs stages required to achieve a tumor-free plane. J Am Acad Dermatol 1997; 37:395–397.

62. Batra RS, Kelley LC. Predictors of extensive subclinical spread in nonmelanoma skin cancer treated with Mohs micrographic surgery. Arch Dermatol 2002; 138:1043–1051.

63. Wolf DJ, Zitelli JA. Surgical margins for basal cell carcinoma. Arch Dermatol 1987; 123:340–344.

64. Robins P, Henkind P, Menn H. Chemosurgery in treatment of cancer of the periorbital area. Trans Am Acad Ophthalmol Otolaryngol 1971; 75:1228–1235.

65. Berlin JM, Warner MR, Bailin PL. Metastatic basal cell carcinoma presenting as unilateral axillary lymphadenopathy: report of a case and review of the literature. Dermatol Surg 2002; 28:1082–1084.

66. Pfeiffer P, Hansen O, Rose C. Systemic cytotoxic therapy of basal cell carcinoma. Review of the literature. Eur J Cancer 1990; 26:73–77.

67. Soo K, Carter RC, O'Brian CJ, et al. Prognostic implications of perineural spread in squamous cell carcinoma of the head and neck. Laryngoscope 1986; 96:1145–1148.

68. Brodland DG, Zitelli JA. Surgical margins for excision of primary cutaneous squamous cell carcinoma. J Am Acad Dermatol 1992; 27:241.

69. Swanson NA. Mohs surgery. Technique, indications, applications and the future. Arch Dermatol 1983; 119:761.

70. Albom MJ, Swanson NA. Mohs micrographic surgery for the treatment of cutaneous neoplasms. In: Friedman RJ, Rigel DS, Kopf AW, et al, eds. Cancer of the skin. Philadelphia: WB Saunders 1991; 484–529.

71. Sadick H, Azli N, Wendling JL. Treatment of advanced squamous cell carcinoma of the skin with cisplatin, 5-fluorouracil, and bleomycin. Cancer 1990, 66:1692–1696.

72. Greenway HT, Abele MK, McKee DL. Medical management of squamous cell carcinoma of the skin. Curr Opin Dermatol 1995; 1:38–43.

73. Ackerman AB. Solar keratosis is squamous cell carcinoma. Arch Dermatol 2003; 139:1216–1217.

74. Ackerman AB. Fill the mind—and exercise it, too! Arch Dermatol 2003; 139:940.

75. Ackerman AB. Opposing views of 2 academies about the nature of solar keratosis. Cutis. 2003; 71:391–395.

76. Heaphy MR Jr, Ackerman AB. The nature of solar keratosis: a critical review in historical perspective. J Am Acad Dermatol 2000; 43:138–150.

77. Brand D, Ackerman AB. Squamous cell carcinoma, not basal cell carcinoma, is the most common cancer in humans. J Am Acad Dermatol 2000; 42:523–526.

78. Cockerell CJ. Pathology and pathobiology of the actinic (solar) keratosis. Br J Dermatol 2003; 149(suppl 66):34–36.

79. Fu W, Cockerell CJ. The actinic (solar) keratosis: a 21st-century perspective. Arch Dermatol 2003; 139:66–70.

80. Evans C, Cockerell CJ. Actinic keratosis: time to call a spade a spade. South Med J 2000; 93:734–736.

81. Cockerell CJ. Histopathology of incipient intraepidermal squamous cell carcinoma ('actinic keratosis'). J Am Acad Dermatol 2000; 42:11–17.

82. Yantsos VA, Conrad N, Zabawski E, Cockerell CJ. Incipient intraepidermal cutaneous squamous cell carcinoma: a proposal for reclassifying and grading solar (actinic) keratoses. Semin Cutan Med Surg 1999; 18:3–14.

83. Omura EF. Skin reaction to systemic 5-FU—a therapeutic bonus. N Engl J Med 1977; 297:946.

84. Stockfleth E, Meyer T, Benninghoff B, et al. A randomized, double-blind, vehicle-controlled study to assess imiquimod cream for the treatment of multiple actinic keratoses. Arch Dermatol 2002; 138:1498–1502.

85. Grapengiesser S, Ericson M, Gudmundsson F, et al. Pain caused by photodynamic therapy of skin cancer. Clin Exp Dermatol 2002; 27:493–497.

86. Balch CM, Soong SJ, Gershenwald JE et al. Prognostic factors analysis of 17,600 melanoma patients; validation of the American Joint Committee on Cancer melanoma staging system. J Clin Oncol 2001; 19:3622–3634.

87. Balch CM, Buraid AD, Atkins MD, et al. A New American Joint Committee on Cancer Staging System for cutaneous melanoma. Cancer 2000; 88:1484–1491.

88. Morton DL, Thompson JF, Essner R, et al. Validation of the accuracy of intraoperative lymphatic mapping and sentinel lymphadenectomy for early-stage melanoma. Ann Surg 1999; 230:453–463.

89. American Academy of Dermatology, Guidelines of care for melanoma, 2002. Schaumberg: American Academy of Dermatology and AAD Association; 2002

90. Veronesi U, Cascinelli N, Adamus J, et al. Thin stage I primary cutaneous malignant melanoma. Comparison of excision with margins of 1 or 3 cm. N Engl J Med 1988; 318:1159–1162 and 1991; 325:292.

91. Carucci JA. Mohs' micrographic surgery for the treatment of melanoma. Dermatol Clin 2002; 20:701–708.

92. Bienert TN, Trotter MJ, Arlette JP. Treatment of cutaneous melanoma of the face by mohs micrographic surgery. J Cutan Med Surg 2003; 7:25–30.

93. Barlow RJ, White CR, Swanson NA. Mohs' micrographic surgery using frozen sections alone may be unsuitable for detecting single atypical melanocytes at the margins of melanoma in situ. Br J Dermatol 2002; 146:290–294.

94. Zalla MJ, Lim KK, Dicaudo DJ, Gagnot MM. Mohs micrographic excision of melanoma using immunostains. Dermatol Surg 2000; 26:771–784.

95. Brooks NA. Fixed-tissue micrographic surgery in the treatment of cutaneous melanoma. An overlooked cancer treatment strategy. J Dermatol Surg Oncol 1992; 18:999–1000.

96. Kalish RS, Wood JA, Siegel DM, Kaye VN, Brooks NA. Experimental rationale for treatment of high-risk human melanoma with zinc chloride fixative paste. Increased resistance to tumor challenge in murine melanoma model. Dermatol Surg 1998; 24:1021–1025.

97. Ahmed I, Berth-Jones J. Imiquimod: a novel treatment for lentigo maligna. Br J Dermatol 2000; 143:843–845.

98. Wolf IH, Smolle J, Binder, B. Topical imiquimod in the treatment of metastatic melanoma to skin. Arch Dermatol 2003; 139:273–276.

99. Sabel M, Sondak V. Is there a role for adjuvant high-dose interferon-alpha-2b in the management of melanoma? Drugs 2003; 63:1053–1058.

100. Kirkwood JM, Ibrahim JG, Sosman JA, et al. High-dose interferon alfa-2b significantly prolongs relapse-free and overall survival compared with the GM2-KLH/QS-21 vaccine in patients with resected stage IIB–III melanoma: results of intergroup trial E1694/S9512/C509801. J Clin Oncol 2001; 19:2370–2380.

101. O'Connor WJ, Roenigk RK, Brodland DG. Merkel cell carcinoma. Comparison of Mohs micrographic surgery and wide excision in eighty-six patients. Dermatol Surg 1997; 23:929–933.

102. Gollard R, Weber R, Kosty MP, et al. Merkel cell carcinoma: review of 22 cases with surgical, pathologic, and therapeutic considerations. Cancer 2000; 88:1842–1851.

103. Herbst A, Haynes HA, Nghiem P. The standard of care for Merkel cell carcinoma should include adjuvant radiation and lymph node surgery. J Am Acad Dermatol 2002; 46:640–642.

104. Boyer JD, Zitelli JA, Brodland DG, et al. Local control of primary Merkel cell carcinoma: review of 45 cases treated with Mohs micrographic surgery with and without adjuvant radiation. J Am Acad Dermatol 2002; 47:885–892.

105. Brissett AE, Olsen KD, Kasperbauer JL, et al. Merkel cell carcinoma of the head and neck: a retrospective case series. Head Neck 2002; 24:982–988.

106. Zeitouni NC, Cheney RT, Delacure MD. Lymphoscintigraphy, sentinel lymph node biopsy, and Mohs micrographic surgery in the treatment of Merkel cell carcinoma. Dermatol Surg 2000; 26:12–18.

107. Ah-Weng A, Marsden JR, Sanders DS, et al. Dermatofibrosarcoma protuberans treated by micrographic surgery. Br J Cancer 2002; 87:1386–1389.

108. Parker TL, Zitelli JA. Surgical margins for excision of dermato-fibrosarcoma protuberans. J Am Acad Dermatol 1995; 32:233–236.

109. Nouri K, Lodha R, Jimenez G, et al. Mohs micrographic surgery for dermatofibromasarcoma protuberans: University of Miami and NYU experience. Dermatol Surg 2002; 28:1060–1064.

110. Massey RA, Tok J, Strippoli BA, et al. A comparison of frozen and paraffin sections in dermatofibrosarcoma protuberans. Dermatol Surg 1998; 24:995–998.

111. Hakim I. Atypical fibroxanthoma. Ann Otol Rhinol Laryngol 2001; 110:985–987.

112. Brown MD, Swanson NA. Treatment of malignant fibrous histiocytoma and atypical fibrous xanthomas with micrographic surgery. J Dermatol Surg Oncol 1989; 15:1287–1292.

113. Callahan EF, Vidimos AT, Bergfeld WF. Microcystic adnexal carcinoma (MAC) of the scalp with extensive pilar differentiation. Dermatol Surg 2002; 28:536–539.

114. Friedman PM, Friedman RH, Jiang SB, et al. Microcystic adnexal carcinoma: collaborative series review and update. J Am Acad Dermatol 1999; 41:225–231.

115. Snow A, Madjar DD, Hardy S, et al. Microcystic adnexal carcinoma: report of 13 cases and review of the literature. Dermatol Surg 2001; 27:401–408.

116. Ortiz KJ, Gaughan MD, Bang RH, Padilla RS, Crooks LA. A case of primary mucinous carcinoma of the scalp treated with Mohs surgery. Dermatol Surg 2002; 28:751–754.

117. Jackson EM, Cook J. Mohs micrographic surgery of a papillary eccrine adenoma. Dermatol Surg 2002; 28:1168–1172.

118. Yount AB, Bylund D, Pratt SG, Greenway HT. Mohs micrographic excision of sebaceous carcinoma of the eyelids. J Dermatol Surg Oncol 1994; 20:523–529.

119. Dixon RS, Mikhail GR, Slater HC. Sebaceous carcinoma of the eyelid. J Am Acad Dermatol 1980; 3:241–243.

120. Snow SN, Larson PO, Lucarelli MJ, et al. Sebaceous carcinoma of the eyelids treated by Mohs micrographic surgery: report of nine cases with review of the literature. Dermatol Surg 2002; 28:623–631.

121. Cook BE Jr, Bartley GB. Treatment options and future prospects for the management of eyelid malignancies: an evidence-based update. Ophthalmology 2001; 108:2088–2098.

122. Wagner RF Jr, Cottel WI. Treatment of extensive extramammary Paget disease of male genitalia with Mohs micrographic surgery. Urology 1988; 31:415–418.

123. Coldiron BM, Goldsmith BA, Robinson JK. Surgical treatment of extramammary Paget's disease. A report of six cases and a reexamination of Mohs micrographic surgery compared with conventional surgical excision. Cancer 1991; 67:933–938.

124. Qian Z, Zeitoun NC, Shieh S, Helm T, Oseroff AR. Successful treatment of extramammary Paget's disease with imiquimod. J Drugs Dermatol 2003; 2:73–76.

125. Zampogna JC, Flowers FP, Roth WI, Hassenein AM. Treatment of primary limited cutaneous extramammary Paget's disease with topical imiquimod monotherapy: two case reports. J Am Acad Dermatol 2002; 47(suppl 4):S229–S235.

126. Goldberg DJ, Kim YA. Angiosarcoma of the scalp treated with Mohs micrographic surgery. J Dermatol Surg Oncol 1993; 19:156–158.

127. Bullen R, Larson PO, Landeck AE, et al. Angiosarcoma of the head and neck managed by a combination of multiple biopsies to determine tumor margin and radiation therapy. Report of three cases and review of the literature. Dermatol Surg 1998; 24:1105–1110.

128. Dhawann SS, Nanda VS, Grekin S, et al. Apocrine adenocarcinoma: case report and review of the literature. J Dermatol Surg Oncol 1990; 16:468–470.

129. Lo JS, Peschen M, Snow SN, et al. Malignant cylindroma of the scalp. J Dermatol Surg Oncol 1991; 17:897–901.

130. Moy RL, Rivkin JE, Lee H, et al. Syringoid eccrine carcinoma. J Am Acad Dermatol 1991; 24:857–860.

131. Chesser RS, Bertler DE, Fitzpatrick JE, et al. Primary cutaneous adenoid cystic carcinoma treated with Mohs micrographic surgery toluidine blue technique. J Dermatol Surg Oncol 1992; 18:175–176.

132. Davidson LL, Frost ML, Hanke CW, et al. Primary leiomyosarcoma of the skin. Case report and review of the literature. J Am Acad Dermatol 1989; 21:1156–1160.

133. Hunt SJ, Abell E. Malignant hair matrix tumor ('malignant trichoepithelioma') arising in the setting of multiple hereditary trichoepithelioma. Am J Dermatopathol 1991; 13:272–281.

134. Lee HJ, Chung KY. Erosive adenomatosis of the nipple: conservation of nipple by Mohs micrographic surgery. J Am Acad Dermatol 2002; 47:578–580.

135. Albertini JG, Welsch MJ, Conger LA, Libow LF, Elston DM. Infantile digital fibroma treated with Mohs micrographic surgery. Dermatol Surg 2002; 28:959–961.

136. Russ BW, Meffert J, Bernert R. Spiradenocarcinoma of the scalp. Cutis 2002; 69:455–458.

137. Hardaway CA, Graham BS, Barnette DJ, et al. Embryonal rhabdomyosarcoma presenting in an adult: a case report and discussion of immunohistochemical staining. Am J Dermatopathol 2003; 25:45–52.

138. Jacques SL, Ramella-Roman JC, Lee K. Imaging skin pathology with polarized light. J Biomed Optics 2002; 7:329–340.

139. Rajadhyaksha M, Menaker G, Flotte T, et al. Confocal examination of nonmelanoma cancers in thick skin excisions to potentially guide Mohs micrographic surgery without frozen histopathology. J Invest Dermatol 2001; 117:1137–1143.

140. Nehal KS, Busam KJ, Halpern AC. Use of dynamic telepathology in Mohs surgery: a feasibility study. Dermatol Surg 2002; 28:422–426.

141. Goldgeier M, Fox CA, Zavislan JM, et al. Noninvasive imaging, treatment, and microscopic confirmation clearance of basal cell carcinoma. Dermatol Surg 2003; 29:205–210.

49 Skin Cancer in the Organ Transplant Patient

Daniel Berg MD FRCPC and Thomas Stasko MD

Summary box

- Increasing success of organ transplantation means that increasing numbers of patients will present to dermatologists for care.
- Organ transplant patients have an increased incidence of skin cancer, most notably squamous cell carcinoma and its precursors.
- Organ transplant patients have more aggressive skin cancers with increased risk of local recurrence, and regional or systemic metastasis.
- High-risk patients and high-risk tumors can be identified and should be followed closely and treated aggressively.
- Dermatologists must take an active role in patient education including teaching skin self-examination and lymph node palpation.
- Treatment of difficult skin cancer involves application of standard modalities as well as consideration of chemoprophylaxis and reduction of immunosuppressive medications.

INTRODUCTION

Organ transplantation has emerged as one of the most dramatic and successful of medical innovations. From humble beginnings in the 1950s, transplantation of kidneys followed by hearts, livers, pancreata, and lungs have become widely available and routinely practised. Detailed information on transplantation in the USA is maintained by the Organ Procurement and Transplantation Network (OPTN), which is administered by The United Network for Organ Sharing (UNOS) under contract with the US Department of Health and Human Services (HHS). Extensive databases are available to the public via their websites (www.unos.org and www.optn.org).

A testament to the success of organ transplantation is the fact that lack of donor organs and large waiting lists are major problems in the field. According to UNOS records, 24 893 organ transplants were performed in the USA in 2002 (Table 49.1). In 2003, UNOS reported approximately 80 000 candidates on the waiting list in the USA for organ transplants. The waiting list increased by 2.7% between 2001 and 2002.[1] The success of transplantation has been due to parallel strides in surgical technique, medical management of complications, and evolving immunosuppressive regimens. National sharing of human leukocyte antigen(HLA)-matched donor kidneys has been an important step forward.[1–3]

The increasing success is highlighted by the example of the kidney. There have been nearly 100 000 renal transplants between 1988 and 1996.[3] Recent studies have shown that in that time the half-life for kidney grafts nearly doubled.[3] Current 5-year survival of patients following living-related or cadaveric renal transplantation is 90% and 80% respectively. Excellent success is also being found in extrarenal transplantation. Five-year patient survival following heart transplantation is now approximately 70%.[1] Over 140 000 solid organ transplant recipients are alive in the USA.[4]

Both the increased numbers of transplants and longer patient survival mean that dermatologists will be seeing more organ transplant recipients in their practices. These patients are at increased risk for a variety of dermatologic

Table 49.1 Organ transplantation in USA in 2002*

Organ transplanted	Number	%
Total	24 893	100
Kidney	14 769	59.3
Liver	5329	21.4
Heart	2154	8.7
Lung	1042	4.2
Kidney and Pancreas	905	3.6
Pancreas	553	2.2
Intestine	108	0.4
Heart and Lung	33	0.1

**Based on OPTN data (http://www.optn.org (last accessed June 2004)).*

conditions including infections and drug-related eruptions. Of most relevance to dermatologic surgeons, transplant recipients have a dramatically increased risk of developing skin cancer. The increased incidence of skin cancer in these patients is compounded by an increased risk of aggressive behavior in those cancers with substantial morbidity and mortality.[4,5] Although the majority of transplant patients with skin cancer can be managed relatively easily, a subset may present with extremely difficult management problems related to overwhelming numbers of and/or highly aggressive skin cancers.

Historical Vignette

- The development of successful organ transplantation has paralleled the advances in immunology, pharmacology, surgery, and critical care which have marked the development of modern medical practice.
- There has been no single watershed event, which made transplantation possible, but rather a culmination of many developments, which led to the current widespread use of the procedure..
- Although the current long-term success of organ transplantation is often attributed to advances in immunosuppression, the development of techniques in surgery, organ preservation and procurement, anesthesia and critical care has also played a vital role. Table 49.2 lists a few of the important milestones in transplantation.

Table 49.2 Progress in transplantation*

Year	Event	Result
1902	Kidney transplant in a dog (Ullman)	Successful
1933	Human kidney allograft transplantation (Voronoy)	Unsuccessful
1939–1945	World War II – dialysis developed	Aided in the progress of kidney transplantation
1946	Human kidney allograft for acute renal failure	Brief period of function
1951	Six human allograft transplants (Hume)	Functioned for up to 6 months without immunosuppression
1953	First living related kidney transplant (Michon)	Unsuccessful
1954	First identical twins kidney transplant	Successful
1958	Use of total body irradiation for immunosuppression	No long term success
1959	6-mercaptopurine (Dameshek & Schwartz)	Successful systemic immunosuppression
1961	Azathioprine available	Less toxic systemic immunosuppression
1962	Use of tissue matching	Increased understanding of rejection
1963	Azathioprine + prednisone	Start of modern era of transplantation
1963	First human liver transplant (Starzl)	Brought transplants to public awareness
1966	First pancreas transplant (Lillehei)	
1967	First heart transplant (Bernard)	
1968	Polyclonal antilymphocyte globulin	Use in induction/acute rejection
1975	Murine monoclonal antibodies	Use in induction/acute rejection
1981	Monoclonal anti CD-3	Use in acute rejection
1983	Cyclosporine A released	Greatly improved graft survival
1989	Tacrolimus	Improved side effect profile over cyclosporine
1991	Mycophenolate mofitil	Improved side effect profile and dosing over azathioprine
1998	Sirolimus	Improved renal function and possible antiproliferative effects

*Adapted from:
Halloran PF, Gourishankar S. Principles and overview of immunosuppression. In: Norman DJ, Turka LA, eds. Primer on transplantation. 2nd ed. Mt Laurel, NJ: American Society of Transplantation 2001; 87–98.
Hamilton D. A history of transplantation. In Morris P, ed. Tissue transplantation. 2nd ed. Edinburgh: Churchill Livingston; 1982.
Crumbly AJ, Bromberg JS, Cofer JB, Rajagopalan PR, Fitts CT. Medical aspects of transplantation. J S Carolina Med Assn 1991; June:313–328.

CURRENT TRENDS IN IMMUNOSUPPRESSION

Pharmacologic immunosuppression aims to block the recipient's immune system from rejecting the graft organ while avoiding the consequences of immunodeficiency, such as infection and malignancy. Ideally, such immunosuppression would be very specifically targeted at only the involved tissue. Unfortunately, even today, most inhibition of the host immune response is non-specific. The process of graft rejection involves the development of T cell-mediated immunity toward allograft antigens and the production of proinflammatory cytokines that also contribute to allograft rejection. Medications currently in use attempt to block this T cell activation and proliferation directly and through cytokine modulation (Fig. 49.1; Table 49.3).

There are at least three distinct applications of immunosuppression associated with successful transplantation: induction, maintenance, and acute rejection.

Induction

At transplantation and during the immediate period after transplantation, the host immune response is very active and the graft, having suffered the injury of transplantation, is very immunogenic. During induction, immunosuppression is usually profound. Corticosteroids are utilized in relatively high doses. In addition a rapid depletion of T cells may be achieved with infused antilymphocyte antibodies such as Muromonab (OKT3), Minnesota antilymphocyte globulin, rabbit antithymocyte globulin, and equine antilymphocyte globulin (Atgam). The interleukin(IL)-2 receptor antagonists, daclizumab and basiliximab, have also had use during induction. At some centers high doses of triple-drug therapy with calcineurin inhibitors, antiproliferatives, and corticosteroids are used for induction.

Maintenance

After several months a partial adaptation occurs between the host and the graft. Partial immunosuppression to keep

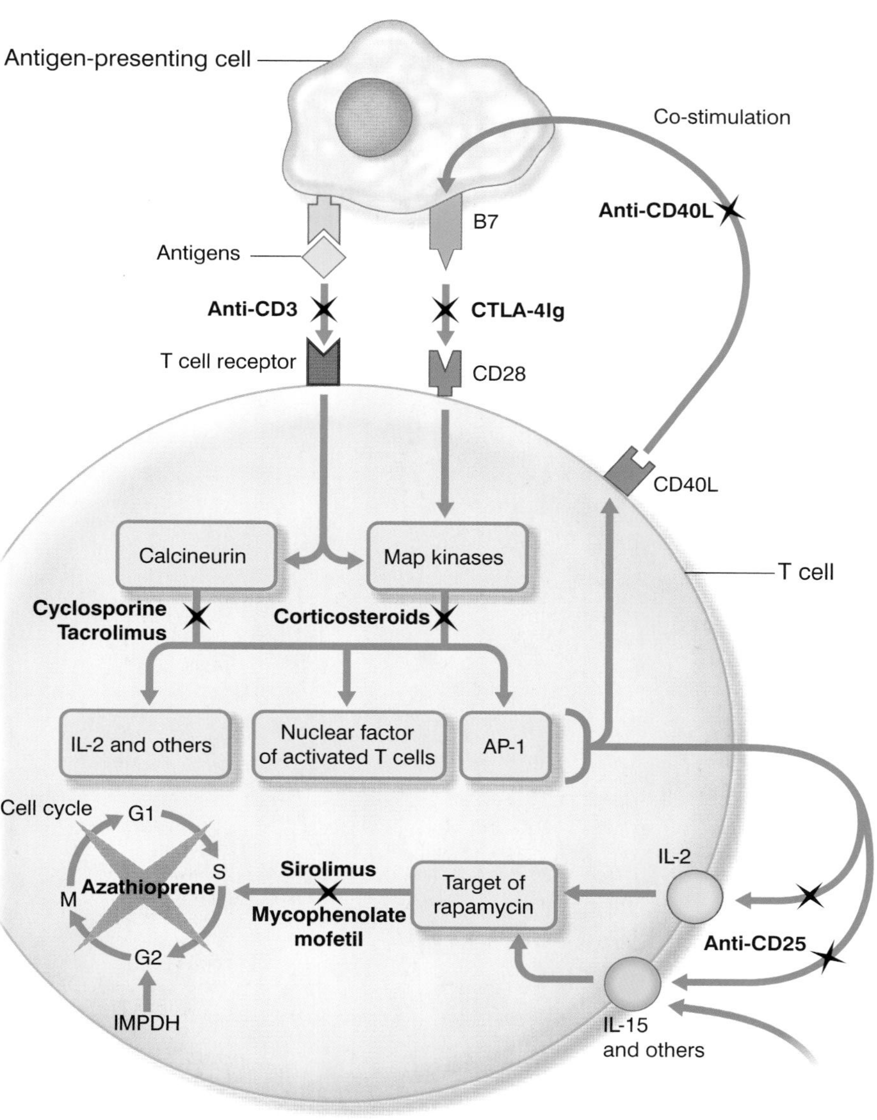

Figure 49.1 Proposed mechanisms of action for immunosuppressive drugs. (Adapted from Halloran PF, Gourishankar S. Principles and overview of immunosuppression. In Norman DJ, Turka LA, eds. Primer on transplantation, 2nd. Mt Laurel NJ: American Society of Transplantation 2001; 87–98.)

rejection at bay but avoid complications such as infection and malignancy is required. Maintenance drugs are usually introduced, if not at the time of transplantation, then within a few weeks. Maintenance therapy usually consists of low-dose corticosteroids, a calcineurin inhibitor (cyclosporine or tacrolimus), and an antiproliferative agent (azathioprine or mycophenolate mofetil) or sirolimus. Patterns of use have changed over the past decade. In recently transplanted patients, most receive mycophenolate mofetil rather than azathioprine and over 50% are placed on tacrolimus rather than cyclosporine (Table 49.4).

Acute rejection

Acute rejection again requires profound immunosuppression. High-dose corticosteroids are often first-line therapy. With severe rejection, increased dosages of calcineurin inhibitors and antiproliferatives are neither effective nor safe. T cell responsiveness can often be abolished for short periods with anti-CD3, or polyclonal antilymphocyte globulin or antithymocyte globulin.

Current investigations seek agents, which will provide specific modulation of graft rejection, without causing global immunosuppression. Biologic therapies targeting specific sites in the immune response cascade have been shown to be effective in rheumatoid arthritis, psoriasis, and other autoimmune diseases. These agents and others directed towards the B7-1 and B7-2 ligands on antigen-presenting cells (CTLA4Ig, CD40, CD11A, IL-15, IL-2), and others are being investigated for use in transplantation. Inhibitors of lymphocyte trafficking also show promise. Lymphocyte activation appears to require costimulation by

Table 49.3 Common immunosuppressive agents*

Class	Mechanism of Action	Pertinent Side Effects
Corticosteroids		
Prednisone	Inhibit macrophage function, cytokine production, adhesion molecule expression, leukocyte migration and trafficking	Cutaneous atrophy Increased risk of infection Impaired wound healing
Calcineurin inhibitors		
Cyclosporine A Tacrolimus	Inhibits interleukin-2 and other proinflammatory cytokine production by T cells Increases transforming growth factor-β production	Increased skin cancer Hyperplasia (gingival, sebaceous, breast, hair) Nephrotoxicity Neurotoxicity
Antiproliferatives		
Azathioprine	Inhibits purine synthesis	Increased skin cancer Bone marrow suppression
Mycophenolate mofetil	Reduces guanosine nucleotide synthesis	Probable increased skin cancer Bone-marrow suppression Gastrointestinal distress
TOR inhibitors		
Sirolimus (rapamycin)	Blocks cytokine-driven T cell activation, proliferation, and maturation Synergistic with cyclosporine	Decreased hemoglobin Decreased platelets Increased triglycerides Delayed wound healing
Protein immunosuppressives		
Polyclonal antilymphocyte antibodies (ATG, ALG)	Depletes lymphoid population	Cytokine release syndrome Increased risk of infection
Murine monoclonal antibodies (OKT3)	Anti-CD3 Opsonization of T cells	Cytokine release syndrome Increased lymphoma
Basiliximab Daclizumab	Binds the interleukin-2 receptor	None known

From: Halloran PF, Gourishankar S. Principles and overview of immunosuppression. In: Norman DJ, Turka LA, eds. Primer on transplantation. 2nd ed. Mt Laurel, NJ: American Society of Transplantation 2001; 87–98.

Table 49.4 Drugs used in first year after renal transplantation in 1992 and 2000

Drug	% of Cases	
	In 1992	*In 2000*
Steroids	100	97
Cyclosporine	96	53
Azathioprine	>90	<10
Tacrolimus	3	52
Mycophenolate mofetil	1	80
Rapamycin	0	16

Data from USA Organ Procurement and Transplantation Network and the Scientific Registry of Transplant Recipients (2003) Annual Report of the USA Scientific Registry of Transplant Recipients and the Organ Procurement and Transplantation Network. Rockville, MD and Richmond, VA: HHS/HRSA/OSP/DOT and UNOS.

two signaling pathways. Inhibition of only one of these two signaling pathways has the potential to induce graft tolerance—the 'holy grail' of transplantation.[6,7]

EPIDEMIOLOGY

All cancers in organ transplant recipients

Early in organ transplantation it was correctly theorized by one of the pioneers, Dr Thomas Starzl, that there might be an increased incidence of malignancies in transplant recipients. Although skin cancer is the most common post-transplant malignancy in these patients, there is a well-documented increase in certain other malignancies. It has been estimated they have an overall increased risk of malignancy of 3- or 4-fold.[8] With the exception of skin cancer, many of the malignancies that are most significantly increased in transplant patients are not the most common tumors in the general population. For example, there is a minimal increase in risk for breast cancer in organ transplant patients.[9] Tumors other than skin cancer that are seen much more frequently in transplant recipients include post-transplant lymphomas, cervical, and anogenital carcinomas, oropharyngeal carcinomas, renal carcinoma, thyroid carcinoma, and various sarcomas.[9] Lymphomas in this setting only infrequently involve the skin, with 70% being B cell in origin and 30% being T cell in origin.[5] Anogenital tumors may present to the dermatologist and may be extensive, appearing as pigmented papular lesions, or mimicking genital warts.[5] Age of onset for these tumors is younger in transplant patients.[10] Dermatologists seeing these patients should have a high index of suspicion for biopsy. Interestingly, several of the malignancies seen more commonly in transplant patients have been linked to viral infections (Table 49.5). Skin cancers are both more numerous and more aggressive, and extracutaneous malignancies also have a more aggressive natural history.[11]

Incidence of skin cancer in organ transplant recipients

Skin cancer is the most common post-transplant malignancy in organ transplant recipients. By far the majority of this increased incidence is accounted for by squamous cell carcinoma. In organ transplant patients, the normal ratio of basal cell carcinoma to squamous cell carcinoma of roughly 4 to 1 is reversed.[4,5] A large number (estimated at 44%) of transplant patients will develop multiple skin cancers.[12] The incidence of skin cancers increases with time since transplant. For example, in Australia one study of renal transplant patients found a cumulative incidence of skin cancer to be 7% after 1 year of immunosuppression, increasing to 45% after 11 years and to 70% after 20 years of immunosuppression.[13] At Oregon Health Sciences University the cumulative risk, based on actuarial survival analysis for development of a basal cell carcinoma or squamous cell carcinoma in heart transplant patients at 1 year, was 3% and increased to 21% and 35% at 5 and 10 years, respectively.[14] Although the trend to increased incidence with time holds true regardless of geography, the magnitude of the incidence increases in locations with more annual sunlight, suggesting the importance of both lighter skin type and UV exposure as important risk factors (Table 49.6). Australian patients have a higher incidence of skin cancer than European patients at all intervals after transplantation. Japanese, Indian, and Egyptian transplant recipients have a very low incidence of skin cancer.[15–17] In 1993, it was considered so unusual in Japan that a renal transplant patient who developed a squamous cell carcinoma was written up as a case report.[18]

Table 49.5 Viral association with increased malignancy in OTR

Malignancy	Associated Virus
Non-Hodgkin lymphoma	Epstein–Barr virus
Carcinoma of the vulva, perineum or cervix	Human papillomavirus
Kaposi sarcoma	Human herpesvirus 8
Cutaneous squamous cell carcinoma	Human papillomavirus

Squamous cell carcinoma

In a Norwegian study of all heart and kidney transplant patients, the increased incidence for squamous cell carcinoma was estimated at 65-fold.[19] A significant number of patients develop multiple squamous cell carcinomas. The percentage of patients who have had a skin cancer increases dramatically with time since transplant and there is geographic variation in the amount of the increase. About 45% of patients reported from Australian studies have a skin cancer within 10 years of transplant,[13,20] whereas patients from the Netherlands, England, or Italy have a 10–15% incidence of skin cancer 10 years on from transplantation.[21–23] Reports on cancer in transplant patients from Japan suggest very little skin cancer in this population.[15,24] The incidence of squamous cell carcinoma appears to be increased two to three times in heart transplant patients compared to age-matched renal transplant patients in most studies.[19,25] This may be due to higher doses of immunosuppression commonly used in heart transplant patients.

Basal cell carcinoma

Because of the lack of population databases for basal cell carcinoma, it is more difficult to quantify the true increased risk of these carcinomas in transplant recipient populations. Nevertheless in one study, the incidence of basal cell carcinoma was 10 times higher than in the general population.[22] This carcinoma is clearly less of a problem than squamous cell carcinoma. About 30–50% of patients with squamous cell carcinoma will also have basal cell carcinoma.[5]

Melanoma

An increased risk of melanoma in transplant recipients is less clearly defined than that of squamous cell carcinoma. Some studies suggest a 2-fold to 3-fold increase in melanoma incidence, but other studies have shown no significant increase.[26–28]

Table 49.6 Geographical variation in skin cancer post transplant

Country	Organ	Percentage with cancer at			Reference
		5 years	*10 years*	*20 years*	
Italy	Kidney and heart	6	11–17		21, 25
Australia	Kidney		45	70	13, 20
	Heart	31	43		
USA	Heart		21	35	14
The Netherlands	Kidney		10	40	22
England	Kidney		14	40	23
Japan	Kidney		Unknown (likely <2%)		15

Other skin cancers

Kaposi's sarcoma is significantly increased in the transplant population[12,19] and 90% of patients with Kaposi's sarcoma have cutaneous or mucosal lesions.[5] Case reports of other skin cancers such as atypical fibroxanthoma and leiomyosarcoma exist in transplant patients, but because of the rarity of these tumors any altered incidence or behavior in transplant patients is difficult to predict. Cutaneous appendageal tumors including sebaceous carcinoma, though still rare, may be increased in these patients.[29] Merkel cell carcinoma is an aggressive tumor in all patients and is probably more common in organ transplant recipients. In a review of 41 cases of Merkel cell carcinoma from the Cincinnati Transplant Tumor Registry it was noted that the ratio of melanoma to Merkel cell carcinoma was 65 to 1 in the general population and 6 to 1 in transplant recipients.[30] The distribution of lesions is similar in transplant patients and the general population; 36% occur on the head and neck.[30] The average age of onset after transplantation of Merkel cell carcinoma is 91 months. Nearly half of patient's with this carcinoma also had other skin cancers.

Unique features of skin cancer in organ transplant recipients

Transplant hand and scalp

Fair-skinned transplant recipients experience a dramatic increase in squamous cell carcinoma and its precursor lesions—actinic keratoses. These hyperkeratotic papules develop in sun-exposed areas. The face, exposed scalp, neck, upper trunk, and the upper extremities are commonly affected but if there has been extensive sun exposure from outdoor activities or sun bathing, other areas such as the lower legs may also be at risk. These lesions are often poorly circumscribed flesh-colored or erythematous macules or papules with an overlying rough, hyperkeratotic scale, which may be minimal, verrucous, or quite protuberant as a cutaneous horn. These keratoses may vary from a few millimeters to a centimeter or more in diameter and may become quite confluent. Sporadic lesions in the non-immunosuppressed population occur most commonly on the face, followed by the dorsal forearms and hands, in a ratio of approximately 9 to 1. In transplant patients, lesions occur more commonly on the hands and forearms than the face with a ration of 4 to 1.[31] On the dorsal forearms and hands, verrucae, actinic keratoses and squamous cell carcinomas on a background of dry skin has been termed 'transplant hand'.[32] Clinically, it is often difficult to distinguish between lesions which on biopsy may be actinic keratosis, verrucae, and squamous cell carcinoma. A similar confluence of lesions may appear on the scalp of organ transplant patients.

Leukoplakia and squamous cell carcinoma of the lower lip

Precancerous and cancerous lesions of the lower lip have been noted to be increased in organ transplant patients. In Norway, squamous cell carcinoma of the lower lip was noted to develop 20 times more frequently in recipients than in the general population.[19] In a comparison with matched controls, King and colleagues found leukoplakia in 13% of organ transplant recipients vs 0.6% in controls; 62% of the lesions in the transplant group showed dysplastic histologic changes and 10% were squamous cell carcinomas (Fig. 49.2). Clinical appearance did not correlate well with histologic findings (Fig. 49.3).[33] Because of the increased risk of metastasis with squamous cell carcinoma of the lower lip, frequent surveillance of this area in transplant patients with early biopsy of lesions is warranted.

■ HISTOLOGY OF SKIN CANCER IN ORGAN TRANSPLANT RECIPIENTS

As previously noted, it can be very difficult to clinically distinguish between warts, actinic keratoses, and squamous cell carcinoma in organ transplant patients. In part, because of this apparent similarity among lesions, distinguishing characteristics of these neoplastic lesions in these patients have been postulated. Architectural features suggestive of viral infection such as symmetry, central pointing with arborization of the epidermal ridge, hyperkeratosis with parakeratotic peaks surmounting the papillae, and ectatic

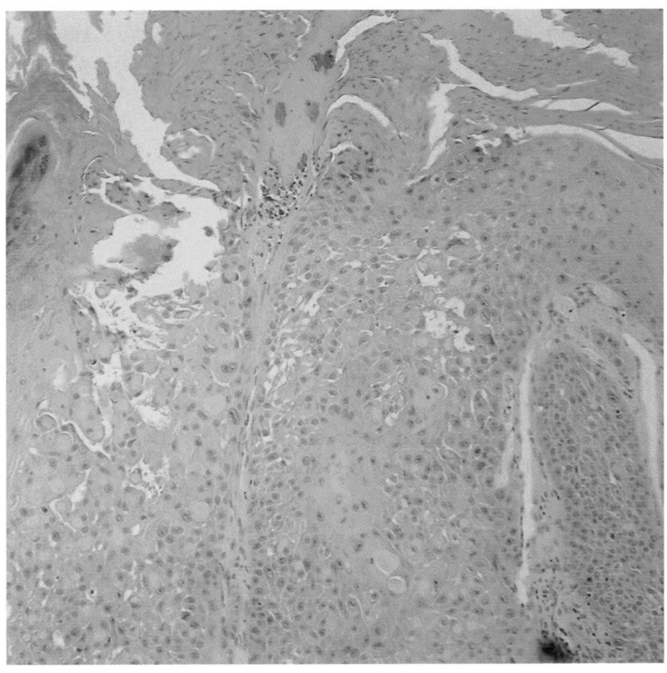

Figure 49.2 Viral features such as symmetry, central pointing arborization of epidermal ridges, hyperkeratosis with parakeratotic peaks, papilliferous or verrucous architecture, ectatic dermal vessels with hemorrhage into the parakeratin, and hypergranulosis are seen in squamous cell carcinomas in organ transplant recipients.

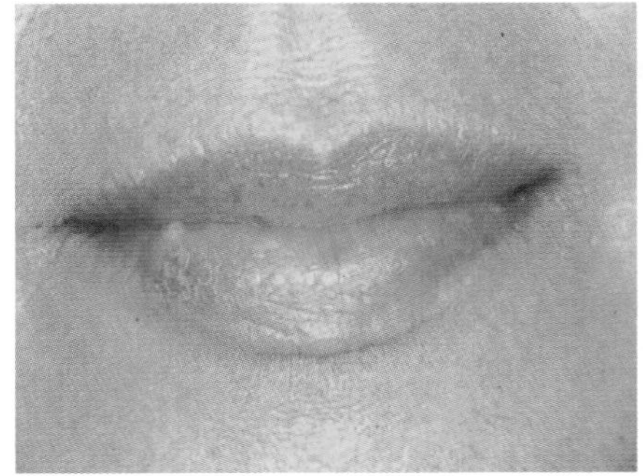

Figure 49.3 Keratotic papule of the right lower lip 20 years after renal transplantation. Histology was an invasive squamous cell carcinoma.

dermal capillaries with hemorrhage into the parakeratin have been noted in lesions of transplant recipients. In addition, even banal-appearing clinical lesions may have marked cytologic changes including eccentric, enlarged and crenated nuclei with perinuclear haloes (see Figure 49.2).[34] Price and colleagues went further in describing subtle but distinct features of cellular atypia which could differentiate lesions removed from transplant patients from those from control patients in 80–90% of cases. These features included Bowenoid changes with a marked degree of cellular atypia, including characteristic multinucleate cells, 'monster' cells (large, dyskeratotic cells with abundant eosinophilic cytoplasm), a vesicular chromatin pattern and abnormal mitoses (Fig. 49.4).[35] Stelow and colleagues agreed that verrucous features were more likely associated with transplant patients, but nuclear atypia and mitoses were not.[36] Glover and colleagues attempted to use 11 similar histologic features to blindly distinguish the squamoproliferative lesions of transplant patients from normal controls and found they could not do so.[37] Boyd and colleagues looked at 16 characteristics in actinic keratoses from these patients and found that bacterial colonization, confluent parakeratosis, hyperkeratosis, increased mitotic activity, and verrucous changes were more prevalent in this group than in controls.[38] The significance and specificity of the histologic features remains unclear, but there is a general belief that squamoproliferative lesions from the recipients frequently exhibit verrucous changes and/or Bowenoid cellular atypia which may not be specific for organ transplant recipients.

■ AGGRESSIVENESS OF SKIN CANCER IN TRANSPLANT RECIPIENTS

Squamous cell carcinoma in transplant patients is characterized by younger age of onset, high incidence of multiple tumors, and increased aggressiveness as characterized by increased risk of local, regional, and distant recurrence (Fig. 49.5).[8]

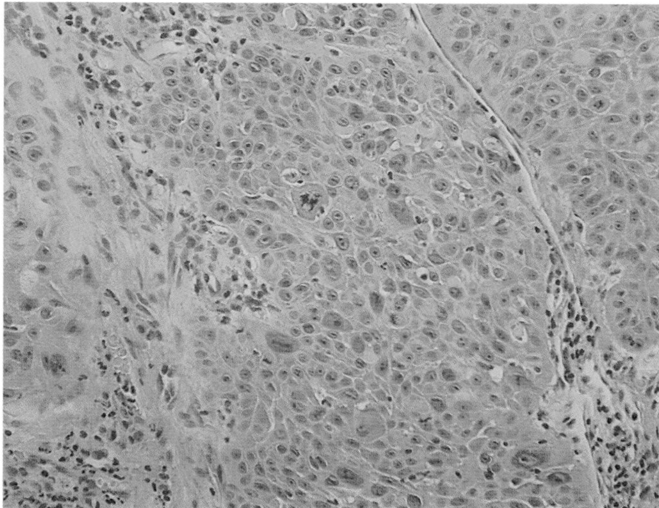

Figure 49.4 Multinucleate epidermal cells, dyskeratotic 'monster' cells with abundant eosinophilic cytoplasm, vesicular chromatin pattern with prominent nucleoli, abnormal mitoses and bowenoid morphology are histologic features of squamous cell carcinomas in organ transplant recipients.

Several recent studies document the aggressiveness of skin cancer, particularly squamous cell carcinoma and melanoma in the transplant population.[20,39] Increased aggressiveness is defined as increased local recurrences, regional and distant metastasis, and deaths from the cancer. In a review of Stanford cardiothoracic transplant patients, about 50% of post-transplant malignancies were skin cancer; 13% of these required extensive management and overall cancer mortality in this group was 55%.[40] In an Australian study, skin cancer accounted for 27% of 41 deaths occurring after the fourth post-transplant year.[20] It appears that young organ transplant patients have a significant risk of aggressive squamous cell carcinoma or melanoma with a 13% lymph node metastasis rate in one study.[41] Finally, patients with a history of skin cancer treated prior to their transplantation seem to be at increased risk of metastasis after the transplant.[42] Skin cancers other than squamous cell carcinoma or melanoma may be more aggressive in transplant recipients as well. In a review of 41 cases of Merkel cell carcinoma from the Cincinnati Transplant Tumor Registry, 68% of patients went on to have lymph node metastases.[30]

Metastatic skin cancer in organ transplant recipients

Metastatic skin cancer may present as in-transit disease, regional nodal disease or systemic disease. In-transit disease is characterized by subcutaneous nodules or papules near the initial tumor (Fig. 49.6). A recent multicenter review of 68 transplant patients with a total of 73 distinct metastatic skin cancers demonstrates a poor clinical outcome once metastasis has occurred.[43] In these patients, the overall 3-year survival rate was 48%. Because of small numbers it was not possible to tell whether survival after metastatic squamous cell carcinoma was different than from other skin cancers like melanoma or Merkel cell carcinoma. Patients with systemic metastases did much more poorly than those with in-transit or regional disease. One-year survival after initial metastasis was 39% in patients with systemic metastases and 89% in patients with in-transit or regional nodal metastases. The mean time from diagnosis of the

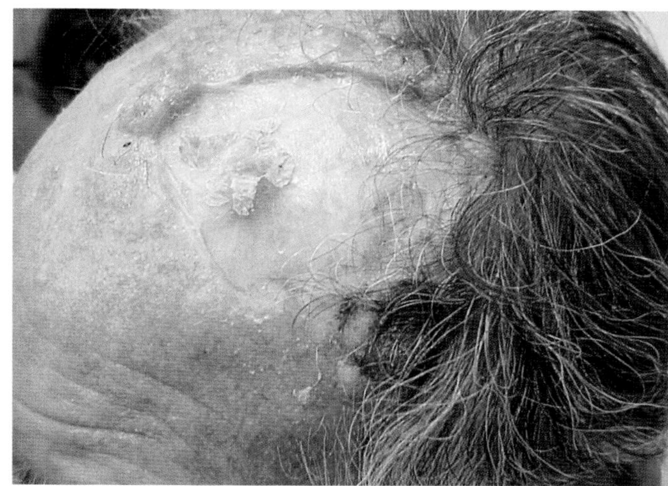

Figure 49.5 Multiple local recurrences of squamous cell carcinoma around previous excision and graft site on forehead.

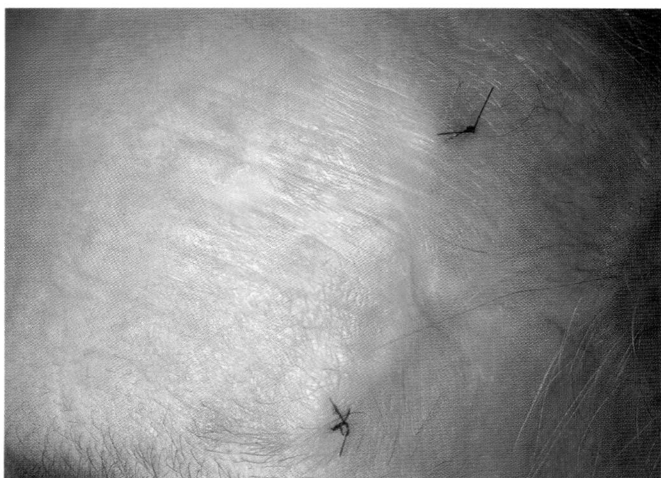

Figure 49.6 In-transit metastasis presenting as a dermal papule inferior to a recurrent squamous cell carcinoma.

primary tumor to metastasis was 1.4 years suggesting the need for close follow-up of transplant patients in whom skin cancers have been diagnosed and treated.

■ PATHOGENESIS OF SKIN CANCER IN ORGAN TRANSPLANT RECIPIENTS

The increased risk of skin cancer in transplant patients may be due to a number of factors. Based on the sun-exposed location of the skin cancers, the increased risk in fair-skinned populations and the increased risk in locations with more sunlight, it is clear that UV light is a major factor in skin cancer for transplant patients and in the general population. The increased risk in these patients may be explained by the fact that the agents used in transplantation may be carcinogenic in themselves. In addition, the chronic immunosuppression may decrease immune surveillance of cancers and may also allow for the facilitation of oncogenic cofactors such as human papillomavirus (HPV) (Fig. 49.7).

Immunosuppressive medications

Immunosuppressive medications used in organ transplantation have undergone major changes in each decade since transplantation first became available. In the past 10 years, significant changes have occurred in the medications used (see Table 49.4). Changes have occurred in induction therapy and treatment of rejection episodes and have involved the use of newer cytotoxic and T cell modulating agents. Because of the mean delay after transplantation of 3 to 8 years before the onset of skin cancer,[5] the impact of currently used regimens is less well-known than that of earlier drugs. Nevertheless, the major changes in the past decade (replacement of azathioprine with mycophenolate mofetil and replacement of cyclosporine with tacrolimus) do not fundamentally alter the mechanism used, and thus are not likely to significantly reduce the load of skin cancers in organ transplant recipients. Promise does exist that newer agents such as rapamycin may have some protective effect against tumors but this remains to be seen.[44,45]

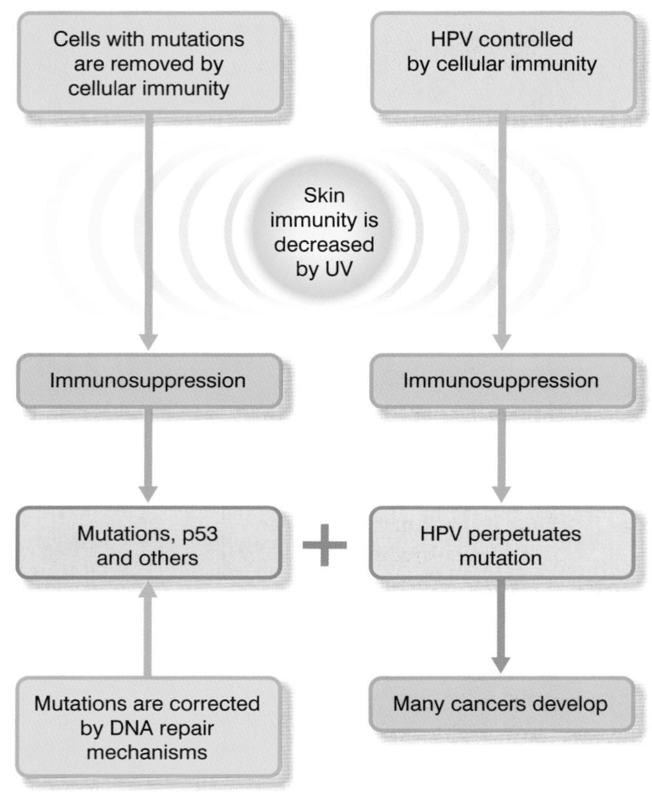

Figure 49.7 There are many influences on the development of cutaneous malignancies in organ transplant recipients.

Evaluation of the medications

Is one drug worse than others?—Animal models

Whether one of the transplant drugs is worse than others remains an interesting and practical question. Mouse models show conflicting data. In one study, albino mice were treated with immunosuppressive agents and exposed to UV light to induce skin tumors. Azathioprine increased tumor number the most, while cyclosporine decreased the time to tumor induction.[46] In another model, UV-induced tumors grew better in mice treated with cyclosporine.[47]

Azathioprine is a known mutagen and photosensitizer.[46,48] Cyclosporine may also play a role in carcinogenesis independent of its immunosuppressive effects. A recent study looking at SCID mice demonstrated induction of cancer progression by cyclosporine (mediated by transforming growth factor-β).[49]

Is one drug worse than others?—Clinical studies

Clinical studies do not easily allow a decision on which immunosuppressive medication contributes the most to skin cancer risk. These studies suffer from difficulties of being retrospective and often compare patient populations from different time periods. Some studies have suggested that cyclosporine may be the worst agent when compared with azathioprine[19,50] or tacrolimus.[51]

Other studies have shown no difference in skin cancer incidence with different drugs.[13,52] Of interest is that early studies before the cyclosporine era were already documenting very high incidences of skin cancer in organ transplant patients.[53] Studies looking at regimens with the newer immunosuppressives, such as tacrolimus, suggest a continuation of the high risk of skin cancer in transplant patients despite the newer protocols.[27] In general, it has been felt that chronic steroids are less important in the induction of skin cancer but they may still play a role.[54] Interestingly, patients themselves choose prednisone when asked which medication they would prefer to reduce.[55]

The combination of data discussed above suggests that the main risk for transplant patients from these drugs is the long-term immunosuppression itself, rather than a specific drug.

Reducing or stopping immunosuppressive agents in the transplant population

In cases of life-threatening cancer, it is possible that reducing or stopping transplant medications may improve the prognosis. In the only study to prospectively evaluate this question, a randomized comparison of high-dose versus low-dose cyclosporine in kidney transplant patients was performed.[56] In 66 months of follow-up there was a significant reduction in cancer in the low-dose group. Although there were more frequent rejection episodes in the low-dose group, overall graft function or survival was not different between groups. Retrospective case review suggests that reduction or discontinuation of immunosuppressives may often cause regression of both squamous cell carcinoma and Kaposi's sarcoma.[57–59] Temporary regression of Merkel cell carcinoma metastasis has been reported with cessation of cyclosporine.[60] It should also be noted that complete discontinuation or dramatic reduction in immunosuppressive agents does not always lead to graft failure.[61]

Despite these data, most transplant physicians in common clinical practice do not lower immunosuppressive agents routinely unless asked to consider it by the patient or dermatologist. This is primarily due to their fears of organ rejection. Armed with the information above, dermatologists should actively address this issue and should consider discussing reduction in immunosuppressive dosages in patients with multiple or life-threatening skin cancer. Communication with transplant physicians is obviously important. This should be considered especially in renal transplant recipients for whom dialysis remains an option in the case of organ failure.

Pathogenic cofactors in skin cancer in organ transplant recipients

Risk factors for skin cancer in transplant recipients include lighter skin types, living in sunnier climates, and prior exposure to UV radiation. These factors strongly suggest that UV radiation is the major modifiable pathogenic factor in transplant patients, as it is in the general population. These patients have an increased incidence of cutaneous warts as well as an increased incidence of tumors with potential viral oncogenic cofactors (see Table 49.5). The oncogenic potential of HPV is well-defined for cervical cancer[62] and there is increasing interest in its possible role as a cofactor in cutaneous cancers, particularly squamous cell carcinoma in organ transplant patients.

Human papillomavirus

There are over 100 types of human papillomavirus (HPV). In the skin they are responsible for warts that are seen in increased numbers in organ transplant patients. The prevalence of HPV has been studied extensively in skin cancers in both these patients and the general population. DNA of multiple HPV types, including those related to epidermodysplasia verruciformis, have been found in cutaneous squamous cell carcinomas in both transplant patients and in non-immunosuppressed patients. The prevalence of HPV DNA is higher in the squamous cell carcinomas of transplant recipients than in the general population, reaching up to 90% in the transplant population.[63,64] Confounding the picture is the fact that a high prevalence of HPV is also found in non-cancerous skin, benign tumors, and normal oral mucosa of both immunosuppressed and immunocompetent people.[4,65] It is clear therefore that HPV presence is only a cofactor in cutaneous carcinogenesis and the presence of HPV DNA is not sufficient to induce skin cancer development. HPV infections are often transient, and it is felt that cell-mediated immunity plays a role in determining whether an infection persists. Interesting information comes from HIV-infected patients who also have both an increased risk of multiple HPV types as well as anogenital and cervical carcinoma.[66] Antiretroviral therapy in those with HIV confers little beneficial effect on regression of cervical disease, and it has been suggested that at least in the HIV population, HPV increases the risk of precancerous high-grade disease but is less important in the final conversion to invasive cancer. Viral proteins E6 and E7 are important in the HPV-16 and HPV-18 induction of carcinoma of the cervix, working to inhibit the product of the tumor suppressor gene, p53. Other mechanisms may be at work in HPV types commonly seen in skin cancer. In the skin of transplant patients, HPV E6 protein inhibits apoptosis both directly and by inhibiting p53, a major pro-apoptotic tumor suppressor protein important in cutaneous basal cell carcinoma and squamous cell carcinoma.[67] In addition, UV light has been shown to upregulate (via p53) cutaneous HPV found in organ transplant patients.[68] It certainly is possible that immunosuppression in organ transplant recipients allows for increased HPV prevalence which inhibits apoptosis, allowing abnormal clones of keratinocytes to persist and continue to receive further mutagenic UV radiation eventually leading to progression to skin cancer.

■ IDENTIFYING RISK FACTORS FOR SKIN CANCER IN TRANSPLANT PATIENTS

The high-risk patient

The immunosuppression inherent to organ transplantation puts all at increased risk for the development of skin cancer. Factors which are associated with the development of squamous cell carcinoma in the general population are also important in organ transplant patients. These factors include:

- a personal history of skin cancer[42] (in Queensland, Australia 76% of renal transplant patients who had experienced skin cancer prior to transplantation developed tumors after transplantation—an average of 16.5 lesions per patient)[13]

- a personal history of actinic keratoses (the number of actinic keratoses is directly related to the development of squamous cell carcinoma)[31]
- fair skin (Fitzpatrick types I–III)[69]
- male gender[70]
- history of chronic sun exposure and/or sun burns[42,71–73]
- older age.[70,74–76]

Other variables more unique to the transplant population also predispose individuals to the development of squamous cell carcinomas:

- time since transplantation and the intensity of immunosuppression[19,56,74,76]
- the type of organ transplanted (cardiac transplants have the greatest risk, followed by renal transplants, followed by liver transplants; organ type may not be an independent variable, but may be related to age at transplantation and immunosuppression regimens)[25,51]
- a history of HPV infection[77,78]
- CD4 lymphocytopenia.[79]

The high-risk lesion

Because of immunosuppression, all squamous cell carcinomas in organ transplant recipients must be considered to be of higher risk for invasion and metastasis. However, as in the general population, certain features indicate higher risk tumors:[80–82]

- advanced age
- additional immunosuppression from lymphoma, chemotherapy, etc.
- size—greater than 0.6 cm, on 'mask' areas of the face, genitalia, hands and feet; greater than 1.0 cm, on cheeks, forehead, neck, and scalp; greater than 2.0 cm, on trunk and extremities
- indistinct clinical borders
- recurrent tumors
- tumors in the field of prior radiation therapy
- rapid growth
- ulceration
- presence of multiple squamous cell carcinoma
- presence of satellite lesions
- deep extension of tumor into the subcutaneous fat
- poor differentiation on histology
- perineural invasion on histology.

■ MANAGEMENT

Education

Education requires instruction on skin cancer risk and detection as well as the need for regular self-examination of the skin, including examination of regional at-risk lymph nodes. Numerous studies of the general population have looked at patients' knowledge of skin cancer and sun-protective behavior as well as interventions to increase both.[83,84] It remains difficult to affect behavior changes in patients, even those at high-risk for skin cancer. Non-compliance with skin self-examination was found to be high even after teaching interventions at the time of removal of a skin cancer.[85] Studies looking specifically at transplant populations have shown a poor knowledge even after teaching at the time of discharge from hospital.[86,87] Only 30% of patients knew why sun protection was necessary.[87] In the UK, only a minority of transplant patients have skin cancer surveillance made available to them.[88] In the pediatric population, only a minority of parents are aware of the need to use sun protection on their child.[89] There is some evidence that regular dermatologic examinations may increase compliance with skin self-exam.[90] It is clear that any education initiative will need to be repeated. More intense interventions are needed than simple instruction by the transplant team at the time of discharge. Dermatologists should not assume that the transplant patient they are seeing has received skin cancer education elsewhere. The active integration of dermatologists into transplant centers may be helpful where possible.[91] Increasing availability of educational materials specifically for transplant patients such as brochures or websites (e.g. those of the International Transplant Skin Cancer Collaborative; www.itscc.org) may also be valuable.

Guidelines for follow-up

Because of the risk of cutaneous malignancy associated with transplantation, ideally all potential recipients should receive a skin cancer-oriented history and physical examination prior to transplantation. If this initial exam detects warts, precancerous, or malignant lesions, treatment should be undertaken prior to transplantation because the intense immunosuppression in the immediate post-transplant period may accelerate the progress of these lesions. At this initial visit, education as to the risk of developing skin cancer should commence. Unfortunately, most patients are seen several years after transplantation, after the development of clinical lesions. Although some opportunities for prevention may have been lost, aggressive education, treatment and follow-up should begin at the first encounter with the transplant patient. Whether seen prior to transplantation or after the development of a squamous cell carcinoma, each transplant recipient should be seen routinely at intervals appropriate to the clinical situation, and must also have the ability to rapidly access care in the face of rapidly developing lesions. Organization of care within a setting designed to provide easy patient access and coordinate care with other involved specialists may provide advantages in some situations.[91] The International Transplant Skin Cancer Collaborative has suggested basic guidelines for follow-up, shown in Table 49.7.

Treatment of squamous cell carcinoma and precursors

Topical medications

Topical medications may have a role to play in chemoprevention and treatment of superficial squamous cell

Table 49.7 ITSCC recommended follow-up intervals for organ transplant recipients*

Patient risk factors	Frequency of skin examination
No risk factors except immunosuppression	Initially, then every 12–24 months
Risk factors but no history of malignant/premalignant lesions	Initially, then every 12 months
Actinic keratoses or warts	Initially, then treatment, then examination every 3–6 months
One basal cell carcinoma	Initially, then treatment, then examination every 3–6 months
One squamous cell carcinoma	Initially, then treatment, then examination every 3–6 months
Multiple non-melanoma skin cancer	Initially, then treatment, then examination every 3 months
High-risk squamous cell carcinoma	Initially, then treatment, then examination every 3 months
Metastatic squamous cell carcinoma	Initially, then treatment, then examination every 1–3 months

**Because of the increasingly high risk of developing skin cancer from the time of transplantation, periodic skin evaluation is recommended throughout the life of the patient.*

carcinoma and its precursors although studies are relatively few. Some data exist to support consideration of topical retinoids. There is a potential role for topical tretinoin in the reduction of actinic keratoses, although studies on transplant patients have not been done. Newer potentially effective topicals for the treatment of actinic keratoses include topical retinoids, such as tazarotene, photodynamic therapy, topical non-steroidal anti-inflammatory drugs (NSAIDs), and the topical immune modifier imiquimod. Of these, imiquimod has been most studied, although proof of its safety and effectiveness in transplant patients awaits further research.[92] Topical 5-fluorouracil for multiple superficial lesions is used widely and should be considered too. Because patients may not tolerate widespread application of this cream, cyclical treatment of smaller areas may allow better compliance. In patients with multiple lesions, this approach allows them some active intervention at home between visits to the physician and may help highlight more concerning lesions by reducing the 'background noise' of actinic keratoses.

Chemoprophylaxis

The primary class of drugs used in cutaneous chemoprophylaxis are retinoids which have been shown to modulate cellular proliferation and apoptosis. Several retinoid receptors (RARα, RARβ, RARγ, and RXRα, RXRβ, RXRγ) are now known to mediate retinoid actions. Both the actions and side effects of retinoids seem to be receptor-specific. Some have hypothesized that RARα upregulation mediates the chemopreventive effect in skin cancer.[93] Selective retinoids that target specific receptors may, in the future, allow more precise targeting of the desired action. Tazarotene and Targretin are examples of new selective retinoids. Neither drug binds RARα and neither has been studied in skin cancer.

Retinoids have been studied in the non-organ transplant population. Early studies showed that high-dose (2 mg/kg) isotretinoin reduced incident skin cancers in xeroderma pigmentosum patients.[94] Toxicity at this high dose led to poor compliance and discontinuation led to a reappearance of the pretreatment phenotype. Subsequent studies looking at 10 mg/day of isotretinoin have shown no efficacy.[95,96] A randomized trial of oral retinol over a median of 4 years showed a small effect on prevention of squamous cell carcinoma but not basal cell carcinoma.[97]

A randomized placebo-controlled trial of acitretin 30 mg/day in 44 renal transplant patients showed a significant decrease in new squamous cell carcinomas over a 6-month period.[98] There was no evidence for adverse effects on renal function. A review of 5 years of acitretin 0.3 mg/kg/day in a similar population suggested as well a significant reduction in new skin cancers with minimal renal side effects.[99] Hyperlipidemia was found in some patients though this is usually easily controlled. Retinoid-associated osteoporosis may be an additional problem in transplant patients on long-term prednisone. The major limiting factor in the use of acitretin is patient intolerance. In one 2-year study, 40% of patients withdrew because of side effects.[100]

Surgical treatment

Warts and keratoses

Treatment of warts in organ transplant recipients may be difficult as the physician cannot depend on the patient's immune responses to help control the HPV infection. As noted, there is evidence that HPV lesions in sun-exposed areas may be implicated in the development of malignant lesions. In addition, lesions may become disfiguring or limit function. As a result treatment should be aggressively undertaken. Treatment may also help limit the spread of the virus and clinical warts. With the exception of therapies which might stimulate systemic immune response (oral cimetidine intralesional interferon), most of the usual treatment modalities for warts are appropriate (Table 49.8).

The development of premalignant lesions should alert the patient and the physician to the need for close surveillance for the development of invasive skin cancers. Individual warts and actinic keratoses are best treated when early and small. The patient should be instructed on self-examination and continued aggressive sun-protection and a periodic follow-up schedule should be established. In addition to topical therapies, individual premalignant lesions can be treated with surgical modalities such as cryosurgery and electrodesiccation and curettage. Diffuse actinic damage with multiple premalignant lesions may also be treated with dermabrasion or carbon dioxide laser ablation. Unfortunately, most of these treatment methods are most effective on non-hyperkeratotic lesions and most transplant patients have hypertrophic keratoses. Dermabrasion or carbon dioxide laser ablation may need to be taken to deeper levels at the site of actinic keratoses with the concomitant increased risk of scarring. In addition, the possible spread of HPV to abraded skin in these patients

Table 49.8 Treatment modalities for warts

Treatment	Comments
Topical keratolytics	Especially useful for palmar/plantar lesions
Cryotherapy	Must be repeated at regular intervals
Electrodesiccation	Useful for thick, recalcitrant lesions
Carbon dioxide laser ablation	Useful for thick, recalcitrant lesions
Intralesional bleomycin	Recalcitrant lesions
Vascular lasers	Must be repeated at regular intervals
Topical retinoids, α-hydroxy acids, topical 5-fluorouracil	May be useful for flat warts
Topical imiquimod	No published data on safety in organ transplant recipients

cannot be ignored. It is often difficult to distinguish premalignant lesions from malignant lesions in transplant patients.[34] Lesions resistant to treatment or atypical in appearance or behavior should be biopsied and the treatment adjusted accordingly.

Squamous cell carcinoma and basal cell carcinoma

Because of the increased incidence and aggressiveness of skin cancer in organ transplant recipients, tumors should be treated at their development in an attempt to reduce the possibility of progression to more invasive disease. However, because the patient may develop numerous lesions in a relatively short period of time, treatment must be individualized to the patient and the tumor. Hopefully, the patient will be seen early, before the appearance of widespread actinic keratoses or invasive tumors. In this circumstance, initial lesions should be treated aggressively with cryosurgery, electrodesiccation and curettage or excision and the threshold for advancement to Mohs micrographic surgery (MMS) should be relatively low. If multiple actinic keratoses are also developing, application of the techniques discussed above should be considered.

Stringent sun protection must be re-emphasized. Communication with the patient's transplant physician about the increasing tumor burden and the possible benefits of decreasing immunosuppression may be undertaken. As multiple tumors develop, small early squamous cell and basal cell carcinomas may still be treated with cryosurgery, electrodesiccation and curettage or excision. When faced with multiple lesions rapidly developing over a short period of time, even relatively large lesions (1–2 cm) that have the clinical appearance of keratoses or keratoacanthoma without significant induration and with histology consistent with well-differentiated squamous cell carcinoma may respond well to aggressive electrodesiccation and curettage or cryosurgery and curettage.[101] Effective communication between the clinician and the dermatopathologist and the clinician's review of the histologic slides will aid in the determination of appropriate treatment. Atypical appearing individual cells including multiple mitotic figures and monster cells do not necessarily portend a poor response to electrodesiccation and curettage in this patient group; however, a loss of differentiation and an infiltrative pattern at the tumor margins may indicate the need for more elaborate treatment with histologic margin control. In general, lesions with the high risk characteristics previously noted should be considered for treatment with Mohs surgery.

For some tumors, the goal of Mohs micrographic surgery in transplant patients may be only to obtain 'relatively' clear margins, rather than the margins of normal skin usually sought. Actinic dysplasia with marked Bowenoid changes and even squamous cell carcinoma in situ may be pervasive in the tissue around an invasive tumor. Within this field of dysplasia, additional small or even microscopic foci of early invasion may be present. In this circumstance, Mohs surgery may be utilized to clear the deep and lateral margins of the invasive tumor, while dysplasia or in situ disease at the peripheral margins may be treated later with other modalities such as electrodesiccation and curettage, cryosurgery, topical 5-fluorouracil or topical imiquimod (Fig. 49.8).

Radiation therapy can be a valuable modality in the primary treatment of skin cancer, especially for inoperable tumors and in patients who would have difficulty tolerating extensive surgery.[102–105] In organ transplant patients, radiation therapy can be difficult secondary to the lack of margin control and the propensity for these patients to develop multiple, often adjacent, tumors which may lie in the radiation field. Verrucous carcinoma histology is a contraindication to radiotherapy in transplant patients as it is in immunocompetent patients.

It is extremely important, in all circumstances, that the patient be routinely examined for evidence of lymph node metastasis. Careful lymph node palpation is adequate in most situations, but imaging with MRI of the appropriate lymph node basins may be useful in large, aggressive lesions, especially of the head and neck. The role of sentinel lymph node dissection (SLND) in the evaluation of high-risk squamous cell carcinoma has not yet been defined. A role may be evolving for its use in the evaluation of high-risk non-cutaneous head and neck squamous cell carcinoma and a recent study[106] found it useful in identifying microscopic nodal metastasis in squamous cell carcinomas greater than 2 cm on the lower lip. Although SLND may be considered

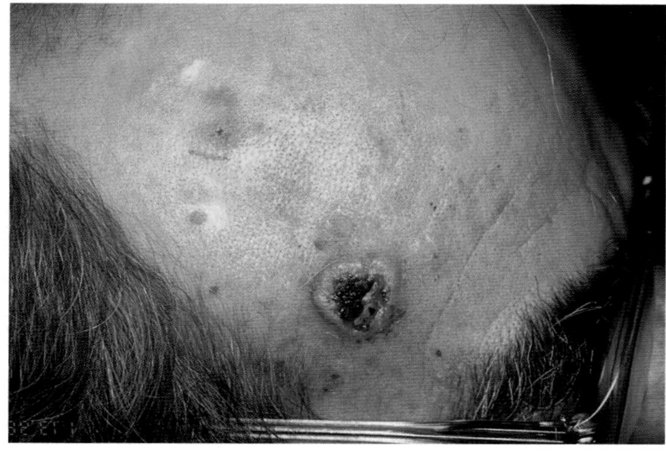

Figure 49.8 Cardiac transplant recipient with a large squamous cell carcinoma, multiple small squamous cell carcinomas/actinic keratoses, and diffuse actinic change of the temple and forehead. The difficulty in obtaining completely clear margins at Mohs surgery for the large lesion is easily appreciated.

in cases of large, deeply invasive squamous cell carcinoma in organ transplant patients, its general use should be reserved for clinical research settings. Palpable lymph nodes should be evaluated with fine needle or open biopsy. Superficial parotidectomy and selective node dissection can be considered for deeply invasive tumors of the pre- and postauricular areas.

A scheme for evaluation and treatment of squamous cell carcinoma in organ transplant recipients is presented in Figure 49.9.

Adjuvant therapies

Adjuvant radiation therapy should be considered for squamous cell carcinomas with particularly aggressive patterns. Radiation therapy may be appropriate when margins clear of invasive tumor are not obtainable or such margins are questionable. In addition, histologic evidence of perineural invasion may require adjuvant radiation therapy.[107–111] In such circumstances the radiation field should widely encompass the area of involvement, the likely direction of perineural spread and possibly the draining lymph node basin(s). A full tumoricidal course of therapy should be administered.

Although protocols for the medical treatment of cutaneous squamous cell carcinoma exist, no highly effective systemic chemotherapy is currently available for extensive primary or metastatic disease. As noted previously, the oral retinoids, isotretinoin, etretinate, and acitretin have shown some success in decreasing the rate of development of new lesions and may be appropriate as adjuvant treatment in patients developing multiple aggressive squamous cell carcinomas. Unfortunately these drugs must be used at dosages that have significant side effects ranging from dry skin and headaches to elevated lipid levels and bony changes of the spine. These drugs must be continued indefinitely. With cessation, the rate of development of new lesions will rapidly return to pretreatment levels. No studies of the long-term safety and efficacy of these drugs in organ transplant patients have been published, but there are individual reports of patients undergoing treatment for several years. Systemic 5-fluorouracil, intravenous or oral, has been purported to be useful in suppressing tumor development and growth in transplant patients and other patients at risk for the development of multiple cutaneous malignancies. No substantial trials have been reported.

Decreasing immunosuppression may result in an improvement for patients with multiple, aggressive or metastatic lesions. Any reduction of immunosuppression must be balanced with the risk of organ rejection.

Treatment of other skin cancers

Melanoma in organ transplant recipients

Because transplant patients may be at increased risk for melanoma, careful attention should be paid to all pigmented lesions. A patient's report of changes in size, color, or texture of a previously existing nevus should be promptly evaluated for melanoma and a biopsy should be considered. As prognosis and treatment are dependent on tumor depth (Breslow measurement), biopsy should usually be taken full-thickness into the subcutaneous fat. Superficial shave biopsy should be avoided, in most circumstances. In general, organ transplant recipients should be treated in the same manner as immunocompetent patients. The treatment of melanoma is based on staging in which tumor thickness, ulceration, and evidence of metastasis are the major determinants. Excision of the tumor is required with margins dependent on tumor depth. Sentinel lymph node biopsy based on lymph node mapping with lymphoscintigraphy and/or dye is now commonly utilized to further evaluate nodal involvement and the need for nodal dissection. Although clinical results indicate a high degree of accuracy with such procedures, the effect on long-term survival is still being determined. Adjuvant therapy for high risk tumors has most recently centered on modulation of the immune system. Interferon-α-2b has been approved for general use in high risk melanoma patients. Experimental protocols have involved the use of adoptive immunotherapy and vaccines. The effect of such therapies in immunosuppressed transplant patients is unclear.

Merkel cell carcinoma in organ transplant recipients

In the largest study of Merkel cell carcinoma in organ transplant recipients, nearly 70% developed metastases and over 50% died of the disease.[30] For this reason early biopsy for diagnosis and aggressive treatment are recommended. Immunostaining and radiologic imaging are beneficial to confirm the diagnosis, exclude metastatic small cell carcinoma of the lung and stage the disease. Wide local excision of the cancer should be undertaken if possible, although Mohs surgery has shown high cure rates in retrospective case series in non-organ transplant patient populations and should be considered if wide local excision is impractical.[112,113] Adjuvant radiation is recommended to the primary site with 3–5 cm margins. Assessment of the regional lymph nodes should be performed with consideration given to sentinel lymph node biopsy at the time of excision if nodes are clinically negative. In clinically node-positive or clinically negative but sentinel-node positive disease, therapeutic lymph node dissection with possible postoperative radiation should be considered for draining nodes. In Merkel cell with clinically and biopsy negative lymph nodes, the role of adjuvant radiation to the regional nodes is not well-defined. Metastatic disease requires medical oncology consultation for chemotherapeutic options although the prognosis for metastatic disease is grim.[114]

Kaposi's sarcoma in organ transplant recipients

Most organ transplant recipients with Kaposi's sarcoma respond favorably to a combination of reduction of immunosuppression and conventional therapies. Conventional therapy for Kaposi's sarcoma ranges from the treatment of individual lesions with cryotherapy, laser therapy, excision, radiation therapy, topical retinoids, and intralesional injection of antineoplastic chemotherapeutic agents or interferon to systemic treatment with cytotoxic chemotherapy, interferon, and zidovudine, either as monotherapies or in combination. Many transplant patients with Kaposi's sarcoma have shown a remarkable response to a simple reduction or withdrawal of immunosuppression.[115–118] In the small number of patients reported, systemic treatment with interferon has been tolerated in transplant patients without loss of graft.[119–121]

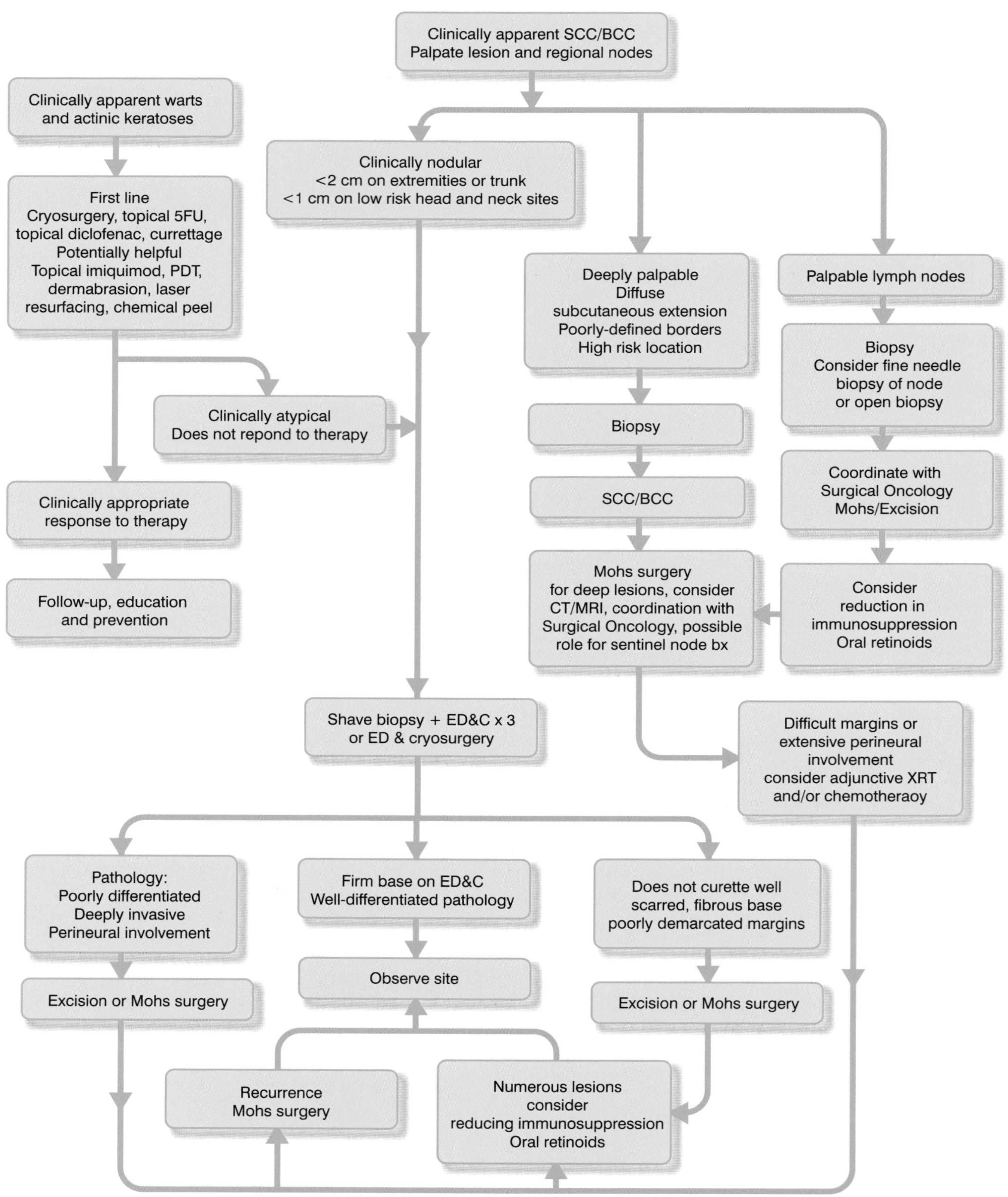

Figure 49.9 The evaluation and treatment of warts, actinic keratoses, squamous cell carcinoma, and basal cell carcinoma in organ transplant recipients.

■ CLINICAL QUESTIONS

Is skin cancer a contraindication to transplantation?

It seems intuitive that an individual with a tumor at high risk of recurrence or metastasis prior to transplantation will still be at risk after transplant. The high levels of immunosuppression necessary for transplantation and the chronic immunosuppression required indefinitely after transplantation probably significantly increase that risk. Although it is established that patients with cutaneous malignancies are at increased risk for additional malignancies, there are no longitudinal studies that detail the course of patients with skin cancer prior to transplantation. Experience in patients with tumors having a poor prognosis in the non-immunosuppressed population, would suggest that these patients are not good candidates for transplantation, at least until a sufficient period of time has passed.

When Conraads and colleagues[122] extensively examined patients prior to cardiac transplantation for pre-existing internal malignancies, 10 of 67 were found to have malignancies. Eight of these 10 were ultimately denied transplantation because of these tumors. These tumors carried significant short-term risk of patient mortality. For internal malignancies with a relatively favorable prognosis, a minimum waiting period of 2 years between treatment and transplantation has been advocated. A 5-year waiting period should be considered for aggressive tumors such as lymphoma, carcinomas of the breast, prostate, or colon, or for large (greater than 5 cm) symptomatic renal carcinomas. A prolonged waiting period is realistic for organs such as the kidney where patients may survive on dialysis and routine waits for organs are long. Candidates for cardiac, pulmonary, or liver transplantation may not survive a 2–5 year waiting period. In these circumstances, proceeding with transplantation may be acceptable if the tumor has been adequately controlled and the prognosis is not extremely poor.[123]

Most institutions do not consider a history of non-melanoma skin cancer in transplantation criteria. Such a policy is appropriate in basal cell carcinoma as the rate of metastasis is extremely low. The majority of squamous cell carcinomas also take a relatively non-aggressive course in the non-immunosuppressed population. However, certain features on page 810 identify higher-risk squamous cell carcinomas. Metastases from squamous cell carcinoma do occur at estimated rates of 1–7%. The overwhelming majority of metastases spread first to the primary nodal basin. The 3-year survival for organ transplant recipients with metastatic squamous cell carcinoma of the skin is 56%.[43] It is estimated that 70% of metastases will occur in the first year after the treatment of the primary and 90% will occur in the first 3 years. Delaying transplantation for 2–3 years in a patient with a history of metastatic squamous cell carcinoma, or with tumors which exhibit multiple high-risk factors for metastasis, may be warranted. Unfortunately, there are no data upon which to base recommendations for the patient who has developed multiple squamous cell carcinoma without metastasis after a first transplant who is now a candidate for retransplantation after a failed organ.

Cutaneous melanoma has a significantly higher risk of metastasis, which is related most accurately to tumor depth and ulceration. Thin melanomas (less than 1 cm) without ulceration have an approximately 95% cure rate. As the risk of metastasis is spread over 15 years or more, there is probably no need to delay transplantation in these patients. Thicker melanomas and tumors with ulceration have a significantly higher rate of metastasis. As most metastases in these patients will occur during the first 3 years after initial diagnosis, a 2–3 year waiting period is appropriate. A similar waiting period will reveal most recurrent or metastatic disease in patients with micrometastasis or limited regional metastasis. Distant metastasis or extensive regional metastasis from melanoma has such a poor prognosis that in most cases transplantation should not be performed unless the patient is disease-free 3–5 years after treatment.

Based on the aggressiveness of Merkel cell carcinoma in organ transplant patients, it appears prudent to delay transplantation for 2–3 years in patients with local disease and to consider denying transplantation in patients with metastastic disease.

Human herpesvirus 8 (HHV-8) has been linked to Kaposi's sarcoma. HHV-8 and Kaposi's sarcoma are increased in organ transplant recipients, especially liver transplant recipients. It has been assumed that the immunosuppression of transplantation would lead to a reactivation of previously treated Kaposi's sarcoma. A recent single case report documented the continued remission of Kaposi's sarcoma after transplantation.[59] Hence, Kaposi's sarcoma is not necessarily a contraindication to transplantation.

Management of multiple scalp lesions

Male organ transplant patients may present with extensive involvement of the scalp with keratotic lesions, which may represent actinic keratoses, in-situ squamous cell carcinoma, or invasive squamous cell carcinoma. The lesions may become confluent and present a diagnostic and therapeutic challenge (Fig. 49.10A). Aggressive attempts at superficial destruction of actinic keratoses with cryotherapy, destructive modalities, and topical agents may be tried but frequent biopsies to rule out invasive disease are necessary. The invasive component of any squamous cell carcinoma should be excised with clear margins although it is often necessary to accept actinic keratosis in the surgical margin. Adjunctive interventions such as reduction in immunosuppressives or institution of acitretin chemoprophylaxis may be used. Once it is clear that the condition is not easily managed as described, consideration should be given to wide local excision of the involved skin with skin grafting (Fig. 49.10B). As noted, vigilance for local nodal involvement is critical (Fig. 49.10C).

Management of multiple hand lesions

Advanced 'transplant hand' with extensive squamous cell carcinomas in organ transplant patients have been successfully treated with excision of the skin from the entire dorsal hand and forearm and replacement with split-thickness skin grafts. The removal must be taken deep enough to remove all deep squamous cell carcinoma. The graft sites, if the donor skin is from sun-protected sites have been reported to remain free from squamous cell carcinoma and keratosis for prolonged periods. There is significant morbidity and rehabilitation associated with the procedure

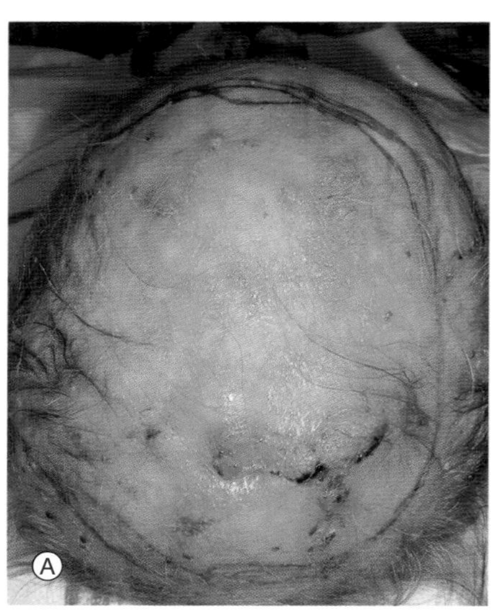

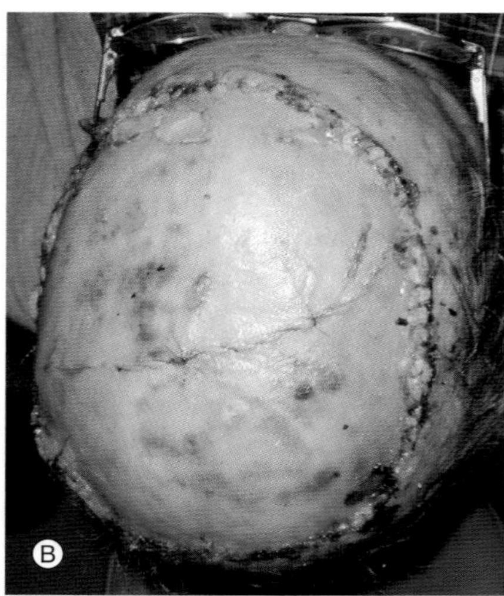

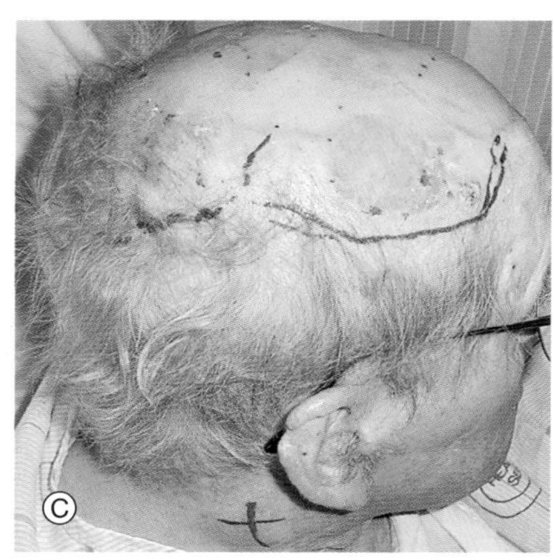

Figure 49.10 (A) Multiple actinic keratoses with recently diagnosed, poorly differentiated squamous cell carcinoma on the scalp in a heart transplant recipient. (B) Immediately after wide excision and split-thickness skin graft. (C) Several weeks later with healed skin graft, multiple involved areas with actinic keratoses, Bowen's, possibly squamous cell carcinoma in the surrounding ungrafted skin, and newly diagnosed metastasis in right occipital lymph node (marked with purple X).

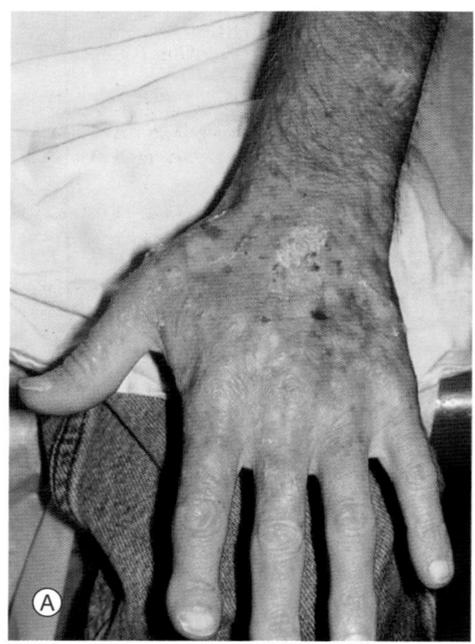

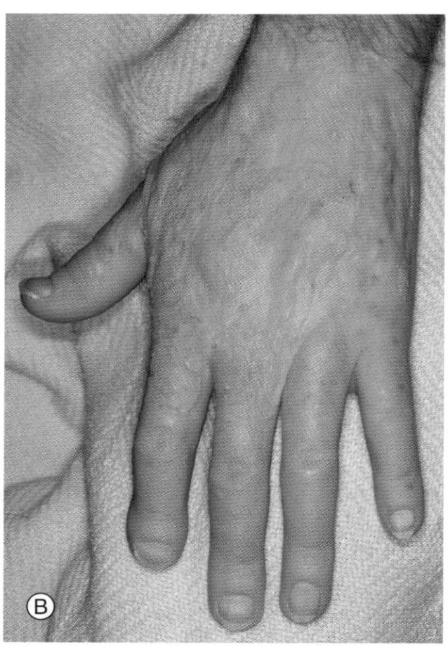

Figure 49.11 (A) 'Transplant hand' with multiple actinic keratoses, squamous cell carcinomas and surgical scars. (B) Appearance of hand after excision of the skin of the dorsum of the hand followed by split-thickness skin graft harvested from the left thigh.

and the graft site has permanent hypesthesia (Fig. 49.11A–B).[124–126]

■ SUMMARY

Because of chronic, non-specific immunosuppression, organ transplant recipients are at markedly increased risk for the development of cutaneous malignancies. Some organ transplant patients will develop multiple malignancies and the risk for metastasis is increased. Cutaneous malignancies are a significant cause of morbidity and mortality in this group. Until more selective immunosuppression is available, understanding the factors which contribute to development of these malignancies, the nature of the malignancies and the state of the host will help the dermatologic surgeon develop strategies to effectively treat organ transplant recipients.

REFERENCES

1. United Network of Organ Sharing (UNOS) 2003 Annual Report of the USA Organ Procurement and Transplantation Network and the Scientific Registry of Transplant Recipients: Transplant Data 1992–2002. Rockville, MD: HHS/HRSA/OSP/DOT; 2004. Available: http://www.optn.org/AR2003/Chapter_I_AR_CD.htm 11 June 2004.
2. Takemoto SK, Terasaki PI, Gjertson DW, Cecka JM. Twelve years' experience with national sharing of HLA-matched cadaveric kidneys for transplantation. N Engl J Med 2000; 343:1078–1084.
3. Hariharan S, Johnson CP, Bresnahan BA, Taranto SE, McIntosh MJ, Stablein D. Improved graft survival after renal transplantation in the United States, 1988–1996. N Engl J Med 2000; 342:605–612.
4. Berg D, Otley CC. Skin cancer in organ transplant recipients: Epidemiology, pathogenesis, and management. J Am Acad Dermatol 2002; 47: 1–17; 18–20.
5. Euvrard S, Kanitakis J, Claudy A. Skin cancers after organ transplantation. N Engl J Med 2003; 348:1681–1691.
6. Halloran PF, Gourishankar S. Historical overview of pharmacology and immunosuppression. In: Norman DJ, Turka LA, eds. Primer on transplantation, 2nd edn. Mount. Laurel, NJ: Am Soc Transplant 2001:73–75.
7. Baran DA, Galin ID, Gass AL. Current practices: immunosuppression induction, maintenance, and rejection regimens in contemporary post heart transplant patient treatment. Curr Opin Cardiol 2002; 17:165–170.
8. Penn I. Post-transplant malignancy: the role of immunosuppression. Drug Safety 2000; 23:101–113.
9. Sheil AG, Disney AP, Mathew TH, Amiss N. De novo malignancy emerges as a major cause of morbidity and late failure in renal transplantation. Transplant Proc 1993; 25:1383–1384.
10. Penn I. Cancers of the anogenital region in renal transplant recipients. Analysis of 65 cases. Cancer 1986; 58:611–616.
11. Barrett WL, First MR, Aron BS, Penn I. Clinical course of malignancies in renal transplant recipients. Cancer 1993; 72:2186–2189.
12. Penn I. Cancers in renal transplant recipients. Adv Ren Replace Ther 2000; 7:147–156.
13. Bouwes Bavinck JN, Hardie DR, Green A, et al. The risk of skin cancer in renal transplant recipients in Queensland, Australia. A follow-up study. Transplantation 1996; 61:715–721.
14. Lampros TD, Cobanoglu A, Parker F, Ratkovec R, Norman DJ, Hershberger R. Squamous and basal cell carcinoma in heart transplant recipients. J Heart Lung Transplant 1998; 17:586–591.
15. Marubayashi S, Tashiro H, Watanabe H, et al. Study on eight patients with malignant tumors after renal transplantation. Hiroshima J Med Sci 2000; 49:17–20.
16. Chugh KS, Sharma SC, Singh V, Sakhuja V, Jha V, Gupta KL. Spectrum of dermatological lesions in renal allograft recipients in a tropical environment. Dermatology 1994; 188:108–112.
17. Bakr MA, Sobh M, el-Agroudy A, et al. Study of malignancy among Egyptian kidney transplant recipients. Transplant Proc 1997; 29:3067–3070.
18. Kimura F, Taoka Y, Asano T, Murai M, Nakamura H. A case of cutaneous squamous cell carcinoma after renal allotransplantation. Nippon Hinyokika Gakkai Zasshi 1993; 84:1127–1129 (in Japanese).
19. Jensen P, Hansen S, Moller B, et al. Skin cancer in kidney and heart transplant recipients and different long-term immunosuppressive therapy regimens. J Am Acad Dermatol 1999; 40:177–186.
20. Ong CS, Keogh AM, Kossard S, Macdonald PS, Spratt PM. Skin cancer in Australian heart transplant recipients. J Am Acad Dermatol 1999; 40:27–34.
21. Naldi L, Fortina AB, Lovati S, et al. Risk of non-melanoma skin cancer in Italian organ transplant recipients. A registry-based study. Transplantation 2000; 70:1479–1484.
22. Hartevelt MM, Bavinck JN, Kootte AM, Vermeer BJ, Vandenbroucke JP. Incidence of skin cancer after renal transplantation in The Netherlands. Transplantation 1990; 49:506–509.
23. London NJ, Farmery SM, Will EJ, Davison AM, Lodge JP. Risk of neoplasia in renal transplant patients. Lancet 1995; 346(8972): 403–406; Erratum, Lancet 1995; 346(8976):714.
24. Kishikawa H, Ichikawa Y, Yazawa K, et al. Malignant neoplasm in kidney transplantation. Int J Urol 1998; 5; 521–525.
25. Fortina AB, Caforio AL, Piaserico S, et al. Skin cancer in heart transplant recipients: frequency and risk factor analysis. J Heart Lung Transplant 2000; 19:249–255.
26. Penn I. Malignant melanoma in organ allograft recipients. Transplantation 1996; 61:274–278.
27. Jain AB, Yee LD, Nalesnik MA, et al. Comparative incidence of de novo non-lymphoid malignancies after liver transplantation under tacrolimus using surveillance epidemiologic end result data. Transplantation 1998; 66:1193–1200.
28. Lindelof B, Sigurgeirsson B, Gabel H, Stern RS. Incidence of skin cancer in 5356 patients following organ transplantation. Br J Dermatol 2000; 143:513–519.
29. Harwood CA, McGregor JM, Swale VJ, et al. High frequency and diversity of cutaneous appendageal tumors in organ transplant recipients. J Am Acad Dermatol 2003; 48:401–8.
30. Penn I, First MR. Merkel's cell carcinoma in organ recipients: report of 41 cases. Transplantation 1999; 68:1717–21.
31. Taylor AE, Shuster S. Skin cancer after renal transplantation: the causal role of azathioprine. Acta Derm Venereol 1992; 72:115–9.
32. Blohme I, Larko O. Skin lesions in renal transplant patients after 10–23 years of immunosuppressive therapy. Acta Derm Venereol 1990; 70:491–494.
33. King GN, Healy CM, Glover MT, et al. Increased prevalence of dysplastic and malignant lip lesions in renal-transplant recipients. New Engl J Med 1995; 332:1052–1057.
34. Blessing K, McLaren KM, Benton EC, et al. Histopathology of skin lesions in renal allograft recipients—an assessment of viral features and dysplasia. Histopathology 1989; 14:129–139.
35. Price ML, Tidman MJ, Fagg NL, Palmer TJ, MacDonald DM. Distinctive epidermal atypia in immunosuppression-associated cutaneous malignancy. Histopathology 1988; 13:89–94.
36. Stelow EB, Skeate R, Wahi MM, Langel D, Jessurun J. Invasive cutaneous verruco-cystic squamous cell carcinoma. A pattern commonly present in transplant recipients. Am J Clin Pathol 2003; 119:807–810.
37. Glover M, Cerio R, Corbett M, Leigh I, Hanby AM. Cutaneous squamoproliferative lesions in renal transplant recipients. Differentiation from lesions in immunocompetent patients. Am J Dermatopathol 1995; 17:551–554.
38. Boyd AS, Stasko T, Cameron GS, Russell M, King LE Jr. Histologic features of actinic keratoses in solid organ transplant recipients and healthy controls. J Am Acad Dermatol 2001; 45:217–221.
39. Euvrard S, Kanitakis J, Pouteil-Noble C, et al. Aggressive squamous cell carcinomas in organ transplant recipients. Transplant Proc 1995; 27:1767–1768.
40. Pollard JD, Hanasono MM, Mikulec AA, Le QT, Terris DJ. Head and neck cancer in cardiothoracic transplant recipients. Laryngoscope 2000; 110:1257–1261.
41. Penn I. Posttransplant malignancies in pediatric organ transplant recipients. Transplant Proc 1994; 26:2763–2765.
42. Penn I. The effect of immunosuppression on pre-existing cancers. Transplantation 1993; 55:742–747.
43. Martinez JC, Otley CC, Stasko T, et al. Defining the clinical course of metastatic skin cancer in organ transplant recipients: a multicenter collaborative study. Arch Dermatol 2003; 139:301–306.
44. Law BK, Chytil A, Dumont N, et al. Rapamycin potentiates transforming growth factor beta-induced growth arrest in non-transformed, oncogene-transformed, and human cancer cells. Mol Cell Biol 2002; 22:8184–8198.
45. DiGiovanna JJ. Retinoid chemoprevention in the high-risk patient. J Am Acad Dermatol 1998; 39:S82–S85.
46. Kelly GE, Meikle W, Sheil AG. Effects of immunosuppressive therapy on the induction of skin tumors by ultraviolet irradiation in hairless mice. Transplantation 1987; 44:429–434.
47. Servilla KS, Burnham DK, Daynes RA. Ability of ciclosporin to promote the growth of transplanted ultraviolet radiation-induced tumors in mice. Transplantation. 1987; 44:291–295.
48. Moore DE, Sik RH, Bilski P, Chignell CF, Reszka KJ. Photochemical sensitization by azathioprine and its metabolites. Part 3. A direct EPR and spin-trapping study of light-induced free radicals from 6-mercaptopurine and its oxidation products. Photochem Photobiol 1994; 60:574–581.
49. Hojo M, Morimoto T, Maluccio M, et al. Cyclosporine induces cancer progression by a cell-autonomous mechanism. Nature 1999; 397(6719):530–534.
50. Schmidt R, Stippel D, Schmitz-Rixen T, Pollok M. Tumors after renal transplantation. Urol Int 1996; 57:21–26.
51. Frezza EE, Fung JJ, van Thiel DH. Non-lymphoid cancer after liver transplantation. Hepatogastroenterology 1997; 44:1172–1181.

52. Blohme I, Larko O. No difference in skin cancer incidence with or without ciclosporine—a 5-year perspective. Transplant Proc 1992; 24:313.
53. Hardie IR, Strong RW, Hartley LC, Woodruff PW, Clunie GJ. Skin cancer in Caucasian renal allograft recipients living in a subtropical climate. Surgery 1980; 87:177–183.
54. Karagas MR, Cushing GL, Greenberg ER, Mott LA, Spencer SK, Nierenberg DW. Non-melanoma skin cancers and glucocorticoid therapy. Br J Cancer 2001; 85:683–686.
55. Prasad GV, Nash MM, McFarlane PA, Zaltzman JS. Renal transplant recipient attitudes toward steroid use and steroid withdrawal. Clin Transplant 2003; 17:135–139.
56. Dantal J, Hourmant M, Cantarovich D, et al. Effect of long-term immunosuppression in kidney-graft recipients on cancer incidence: randomised comparison of two cyclosporin regimens. Lancet 1998; 351(9103)623–628.
57. Otley CC, Coldiron BM, Stasko T, Goldman GD. Decreased skin cancer after cessation of therapy with transplant-associated immunosuppressants. Arch Dermatol 2001; 137:459–463.
58. Duman S, Toz H, Asci G, et al. Successful treatment of post-transplant Kaposi sarcoma by reduction of immunosuppression. Nephrol Dial Transplant 2002; 17:892–896.
59. Euvrard S, Kanitakis J, Bosshard S, et al. No recurrence of post-transplantation Kaposi sarcoma three years after renal retransplantation. Transplantation 2002; 73:297–299.
60. Friedlaender MM, Rubinger D, Rosenbaum E, Amir G, Siguencia E. Temporary regression of Merkel cell carcinoma metastases after cessation of ciclosporine. Transplantation 2002; 73:1849–1850.
61. Ramos HC, Reyes J, Abu-Elmagd K, et al. Weaning of immunosuppression in long-term liver transplant recipients. Transplantation 1995; 59:212–217.
62. Bosch FX, de Sanjose S. Human papillomavirus and cervical cancer-burden and assessment of causality. J Natl Cancer Inst Monographs 2003; 2003(31):3–13.
63. de Villiers EM. Human papillomavirus infections in skin cancers. Biomed Pharmacother 1998; 52:26–33.
64. Harwood CA, Surentheran T, McGregor JM, et al. Human papillomavirus infection and non-melanoma skin cancer in immunosuppressed and immunocompetent individuals. J Med Virol 2000; 61:289–297.
65. Berkhout RJ, Bouwes Bavinck JN, ter Schegget J. Persistence of human papillomavirus DNA in benign and (pre)malignant skin lesions from renal transplant recipients. J Clin Microbiol 2000; 38:2087–2096.
66. Palefsky JM, Holly EA. Immunosuppression and co-infection with HIV. J Natl Cancer Inst Monographs 2003; 2003.31:41–46.
67. Jackson S, Storey A. E6 proteins from diverse cutaneous HPV types inhibit apoptosis in response to UV damage. Oncogene 2000; 19:592–598.
68. Purdie KJ, Pennington J, Proby CM, et al. The promoter of a novel human papillomavirus (HPV77) associated with skin cancer displays UV responsiveness, which is mediated through a consensus p53 binding sequence. EMBO J 1999; 18:5359–5369.
69. Grabbe S, Granstein RD. Mechanisms of ultraviolet radiation carcinogenesis. Chem Immunol 1994; 58:291–313.
70. Mithoefer AB, Supran S, Freeman RB. Risk factors associated with the development of skin cancer after liver transplantation. Liver Transpl 2002; 8:939–944.
71. Ferrandiz C, Fuente MJ, Ribera M, et al. Epidermal dysplasia and neoplasia in kidney transplant recipients. J Am Acad Dermatol 1995; 33:590–596.
72. Liddington M, Richardson AJ, Higgins RM, et al. Skin cancer in renal transplant recipients. Br J Surg 1989; 76:1002–1005.
73. Bavinck JN, De Boer A, Vermeer BJ, et al. Sunlight, keratotic skin lesions and skin cancer in renal transplant recipients. Br J Dermatol 1993; 129; 242–249.
74. Danpanich E, Kasiske BL. Risk factors for cancer in renal transplant recipient. Transplantation 1999; 68:1859–1864.
75. Penn I. Tumors after renal and cardiac transplantation. Hematol Oncol Clin N Am 1993; 7; 431–445.
76. Ramsay HM, Fryer AA, Reece S, Smith AG, Harden PN. Clinical risk factors associated with non-melanoma skin cancer in renal transplant recipients. Am J Kidney Dis 2000; 36:167–176.
77. Shamanin V, zur Hausen H, Lavergne D, et al. Human papillomavirus infections in non-melanoma skin cancers from renal transplant recipients and non-immunosuppressed patients. J Natl Cancer Inst 1996; 88:802–811.
78. Leigh IM, Buchanan JA, Harwood CA, Cerio R, Storey A. Role of human papillomaviruses in cutaneous and oral manifestations of immunosuppression. J Acq Immune Defic Synd 1999; 21:S49–S57.
79. Ducloux D, Carron PL, Rebibou JM, et al. CD4 lymphocytopenia as a risk factor for skin cancers in renal transplant recipients. Transplantation 1998; 65:1270–2.
80. Miller SJ. The National Comprehensive Cancer Network (NCCN) guidelines of care for non-melanoma skin cancers. Dermatol Surg 2000; 26:289–292.
81. Rowe DE, Carroll RJ, Day CL. Prognostic factors for local recurrence, metastasis, and survival rates in squamous cell carcinoma of the skin, ear, and lip. Implications for treatment modality selection. J Am Acad Dermatol 1992; 26:976–990.
82. Euvrard S, Kanitakis J, Pouteil-Noble C, et al. Comparative epidemiologic study of premalignant and malignant epithelial cutaneous lesions developing after kidney and heart transplantation. J Am Acad Dermatol 1995; 33:222–229.
83. Geller AC, Colditz G, Oliveria S, et al. Use of sunscreen, sunburning rates, and tanning bed use among more than 10 000 US children and adolescents. Pediatrics 2002; 109; 1009–1014.
84. Murphy GM. Photoprotection: public campaigns in Ireland and the UK. Br J Dermatol 2002; 146:31–33.
85. Robinson JK. Behavior modification obtained by sun protection education coupled with removal of a skin cancer. Arch Dermatol 1990; 126; 477–481.
86. Cowen EW, Billingsley EM. Awareness of skin cancer by kidney transplant patients. J Am Acad Dermatol 1999; 40:697–701.
87. Seukeran DC, Newstead CG, Cunliffe WJ. The compliance of renal transplant recipients with advice about sun protection measures. Br J Dermatol 1998; 138; 301–303.
88. Harden PN, Reece SM, Fryer AA, Smith AG, Ramsay HM. Skin cancer surveillance in renal transplant recipients: questionnaire survey of current UK practice. BMJ 2001; 323:600–601.
89. Ramrakha-Jones VS. Transplant patients need to be made aware of skin cancer risk. BMJ 2002; 324:296.
90. Robinson JK, Fisher SG, Turrisi RJ. Predictors of skin self-examination performance. Cancer 2002; 95:135–146.
91. Otley CC. Organization of a specialty clinic to optimize the care of organ transplant recipients at risk for skin cancer. Dermatol Surg 2000; 26:709–712.
92. Stockfleth E, Ulrich C, Meyer T, Christophers E. Epithelial malignancies in organ transplant patients: clinical presentation and new methods of treatment. Recent Results Cancer Res 2002; 160:251–258.
93. Hansen LA, Sigman CC, Andreola F, Ross SA, Kelloff GJ, De Luca LM. Retinoids in chemoprevention and differentiation therapy. Carcinogenesis 2000; 21:1271–1279.
94. Kraemer KH, DiGiovanna JJ, Moshell AN, Tarone RE, Peck GL. Prevention of skin cancer in xeroderma pigmentosum with the use of oral isotretinoin. N Engl J Med 1988; 318:1633–1637.
95. Levine N, Moon TE, Cartmel B, et al. Trial of retinol and isotretinoin in skin cancer prevention: a randomized, double-blind, controlled trial. Southwest Skin Cancer Prevention Study Group. Cancer Epidemiol Biomarkers Prev 1997; 6:957–961.
96. Tangrea JA, Edwards BK, Taylor PR, et al. Long-term therapy with low-dose isotretinoin for prevention of basal cell carcinoma: a multicenter clinical trial. Isotretinoin-Basal Cell Carcinoma Study Group. J Natl Cancer Inst 1992; 84:328–332.
97. Moon TE, Levine N, Cartmel B, et al. Effect of retinol in preventing squamous cell skin cancer in moderate-risk subjects: a randomized, double-blind, controlled trial. Southwest Skin Cancer Prevention Study Group. Cancer Epidemiol Biomarkers Prev 1997; 6:949–956.
98. Bavinck JN, Tieben LM, van der Woude FJ, et al. Prevention of skin cancer and reduction of keratotic skin lesions during acitretin therapy in renal transplant recipients: a double-blind, placebo-controlled study. J Clin Oncol 1995; 13:1933–1938.
99. McKenna DB, Murphy GM. Skin cancer chemoprophylaxis in renal transplant recipients: 5 years of experience using low-dose acitretin. Br J Dermatol 1999; 140; 656–660.
100. George R, Weightman W, Russ GR, Bannister KM, Mathew TH. Acitretin for chemoprevention of non-melanoma skin cancers in renal transplant recipients. Australas J Dermatol 2002; 43:269–273.
101. Orengo I, Brown T, Rosen T. Cutaneous neoplasia in organ transplant recipients. Curr Probl Dermatol 1999; 11:127–158.
102. Morrison WH, Garden AS, Ang KK. Radiation therapy for non-melanoma skin carcinomas. Clin Plast Surg 1997; 24:719–729.

103. Fukunaga M, Yokoi K, Miyazawa Y, Harada T, Ushigome S. Penile verrucous carcinoma with anaplastic transformation following. Am J Surg Pathol. 1994 May; 18:501–505.

104. Gilde O, Schultz-Ehrenburg U, Hautkr Z. Biological behavior of epithelioma cuniculatum. 1986; 15:556–558.

105. Swanson NA, Taylor WB. Plantar verrucous carcinoma. Literature review and treatment by the Mohs' chemosurgery technique. Arch Dermatol. 1980; 116;794–797.

106. Altinyollar H, Berberoglu U, Celen O. Lymphatic mapping and sentinel lymph node biopsy in squamous cell carcinoma of the lower lip. Eur J Surg Oncol 2002; 28:72–74.

107. Mendenhall WM, Parsons JT, Mendenhall NP, et al. Carcinoma of the skin of the head and neck with perineural invasion. Head Neck 1989; 11:301–308.

108. McCord MW, Mendenhall WM, Parsons JT, Flowers FP. Skin cancer of the head and neck with incidental microscopic perineural invasion. Int J Radiat Oncol Biol Phys 1999; 43:591–595.

109. McCord MW, Mendenhall WM, Parsons JT, et al. Skin cancer of the head and neck with clinical perineural invasion. Int J Radiat Oncol Biol Phys 2000; 47:89–93.

110. Williams LS, Mancuso AA, Mendenhall WM. Perineural spread of cutaneous squamous and basal cell carcinoma: CT and MR detection and its impact on patient management and prognosis. Int J Radiat Oncol Biol Phys 2001; 49:1061–1069.

111. Mendenhall WM, Amdur RJ, Williams LS, Mancuso AA, Stringer SP, Price Mendenhall N. Carcinoma of the skin of the head and neck with perineural invasion. Head Neck 2002; 24:78–83.

112. Snow SN, Larson PO, Hardy S, et al. Merkel cell carcinoma of the skin and mucosa: Report of 12 cutaneous cases with 2 cases arising from the nasal mucosa. Dermatol Surg 2001; 27:165–170.

113. O'Connor WJ, Roenigk RK, Brodland DG. Merkel cell carcinoma. Comparison of Mohs micrographic surgery and wide excision in eighty-six patients. Dermatol Surg 1997; 23:929–933.

114. Gollard R, Weber R, Kosty MP, Greenway HT, Massullo V, Humberson C. Merkel cell carcinoma: review of 22 cases with surgical, pathologic, and therapeutic considerations. Cancer 2000; 88:1842–1851.

115. Shepherd FA, Maher E, Cardella C, et al. Treatment of Kaposi sarcoma after solid organ transplantation. J Clin Oncol 1997; 15:2371–2377.

116. Montagnino G, Bencini PL, Tarantino A, Caputo R, Ponticelli C. Clinical features and course of Kaposi sarcoma in kidney transplant patients: report of 13 cases. Am J Nephrol 1994; 14:121–126.

117. Aebischer MC, Zala LB, Braathen LR. Kaposi sarcoma as manifestation of immunosuppression in organ transplant recipients. Dermatology 1997; 195:91–92.

118. Hussein MM, Mooij JM, Roujouleh HM. Regression of post-transplant Kaposi sarcoma after discontinuing cyclosporin and giving mycophenolate mofetil instead. Nephrol Dial Transplant 2000; 15:1103–1104.

119. Penn I. Posttransplant malignancy: the role of immunosuppression. Drug Safety 2000; 23:101–113.

120. Besnard V, Euvrard S, Kanitakis J, et al. Kaposi sarcoma after liver transplantation. Dermatology 1996; 193:100–104.

121. Halmos O, Inturri P, Galligioni A, et al. Two cases of Kaposi sarcoma in renal and liver transplant recipients treated with interferon. Clin Transplant 1996; 10:374–378.

122. Conraads VM, Denollet J, Vorlat A, Moulijn AC, Vrints CJ. Screening for solid organ malignancies prior to heart transplantation. Transplantation 2001; 71:1481–1483.

123. Penn I. Evaluation of transplant candidates with pre-existing malignancies. Annals of Transplantation 1997; 2:14–17.

124. Glover MT, Niranjan N, Kwan JT, Leigh IM. Non-melanoma skin cancer in renal transplant recipients: the extent of the problem and a strategy for management. Br J Plast Surg 1994; 47:86–89.

125. Scholtens RE, van Zuuren EJ, Posma AN. Treatment of recurrent squamous cell carcinoma of the hand in immunosuppressed patients. J Hand Surg 1995; 20:73–76.

126. van Zuuren EJ, Posma AN, Scholtens RE, Vermeer BJ, van der Woude FJ, Bouwes Bavinck JN. Resurfacing the back of the hand as treatment and prevention of multiple skin cancers in kidney transplant recipients. J Am Acad Dermatol 1994; 31:760–764.

50 Management of Dysplastic Nevi and Melanomas

Carol L Huang MD, Ashfaq A Marghoob MD, and Allan C Halpern MD

Summary box

- Clinically, atypical moles share many of the features of melanomas.
- Atypical mole syndrome can occur sporadically or can be inherited.
- Both genetics and ultraviolet light exposure may be involved in the phenotypic expression of atypical moles.
- The total number of melanocytic nevi and the presence of atypical moles are independent risk factors for the development of melanoma.
- Patients with even one atypical mole remain at an increased risk for developing melanoma, even after the excision of the lesion.
- Sun avoidance, sun protection, and lifelong skin surveillance are important in the prevention and early detection of melanoma.
- Total body photographs provide a baseline for the detection of often subtle changes in moles during annual skin examinations.
- Any new, changing, or symptomatic pigmented lesion should be examined closely and possibly biopsied.

INTRODUCTION

Clinical features and presentation

Atypical moles or dysplastic nevi—the two terms will be used interchangeably in this chapter—are generally diagnosed on the basis of their clinical and/or histologic features.[1] Clinically, atypical moles share many of the features of malignant melanomas, such as those of the ABCD acronym (Asymmetry, Border irregularity, Color variability, and Diameter > 6 mm) (Fig. 50.1), and on histology have some degree of architectural disorder and cytologic atypia.[2,3] Table 50.1 compares the features of common acquired nevi, atypical nevi, and melanomas.

Dysplastic nevi sometimes have slight border irregularity and often exhibit color variability, with various shades of tans and browns, and sometimes hues of pinks and reds, black, and even white. Blue is usually not seen in atypical moles on clinical examination (Fig. 50.2A), but may be seen on dermoscopy (Fig. 50.2B). The surface of atypical moles is often slightly raised and mamillated, but occasionally may appear papular, nodular, or sessile. A clinical clue in most atypical moles is the presence of a macular lightly pigmented area or 'shoulder' surrounding the centrally elevated portion of the nevus (Fig. 50.3). Atypical moles are often over 6 mm in diameter, but it is not uncommon for them to be smaller. Most atypical moles occur on the trunk[4] (Fig. 50.4); they are less common on the limbs (Fig. 50.5). They are occasionally found in locations usually protected from the sun, such as the buttocks, breasts, scalp, and pubic region[5,6] (Figs 50.6, 50.7). They are almost never on the face.

Approximately 7% of Caucasians have atypical (dysplastic) nevi. Within the US, approximately 4.6 million people are estimated to have at least one atypical mole.[7] Persons with atypical moles exhibit a wide range of phenotypic expressions (Figs 50.8, 50.9). Patients with multiple atypical moles and common nevi have what has come to be known as the atypical mole syndrome or dysplastic nevus syndrome. There are several definitions for atypical mole syndrome (Table 50.2).[5,8–11] In addition, a recent article by Huynh et al. introduced the 'cheetah phenotype' in which the patients do not have clinically atypical moles, but have numerous (>100) dark brown, <4 mm in diameter melanocytic nevi which are uniform in color. These individuals are at increased risk of melanoma[12] (Fig. 50.10).

Atypical mole syndrome can occur sporadically, but in many individuals it appears to be an inherited disorder in which the affected individuals begin to develop atypical nevi during childhood and continue to develop multiple dysplastic nevi over their lifetime. Sporadic expression refers to a person with the atypical mole syndrome who has no relatives in the modified pedigree expressing the trait.

Natural history and progression

The natural history of common acquired moles (melanocytic nevi) is characterized by infrequent occurrence before

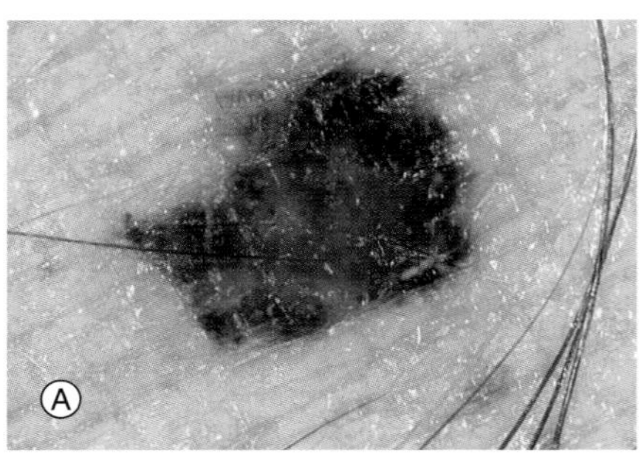

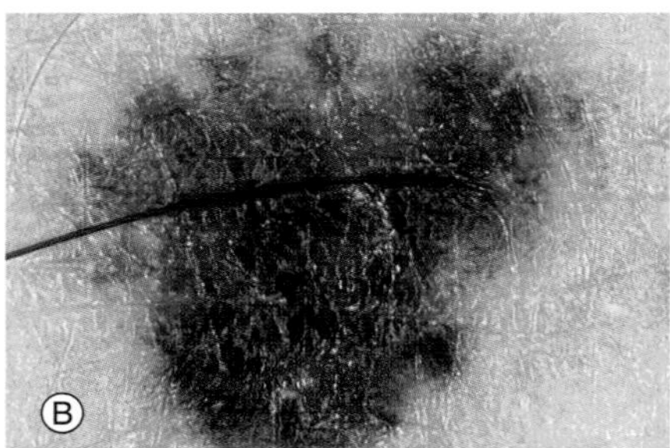

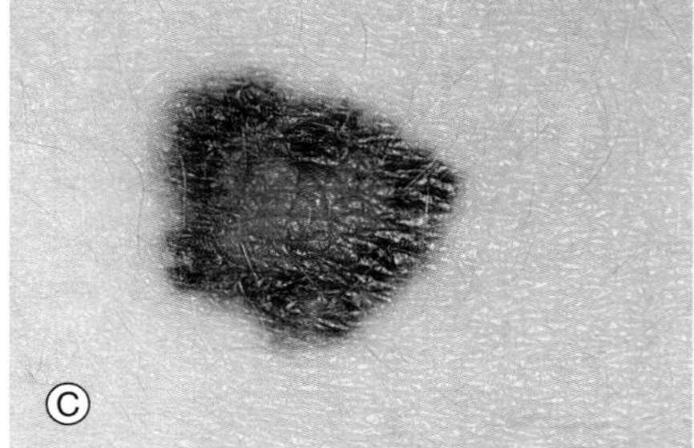

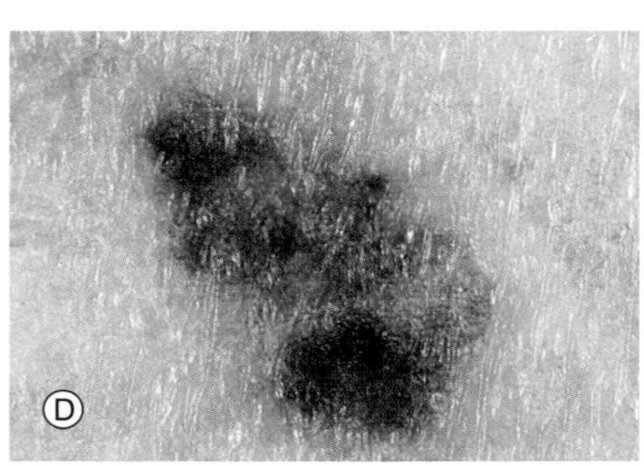

Figure 50.1 Each of the lesions may exhibit more than one of the ABCD features. (A) Asymmetry and variable colors seen in this lesion. (B) Asymmetry and border irregularity. (C) Different colors with shades of dark brown and red. (D) Asymmetric lesion with variable colors and greater than 6 mm in diameter.

Table 50.1 General features of common melanocytic nevi, dysplastic nevi (atypical moles), and melanomas

Feature	Common acquired nevi	Atypical moles	Malignant melanomas
Asymmetry	Symmetric	Variable	Usually asymmetric
Border	Regular	Variable; indistinct	Irregular, often sharp
Color	Uniform tan/brown	Often variegated tan/brown/black/red	Often variegated tan/brown/black/red/white/blue
Diameter	<6 mm	Often >5mm	Often >5 mm
Clinical change	Slow then stable	Slow then stable	Faster (over months)
Surface	Macular or nodular (not both)	Often elevated with peripheral macular 'shoulder'	Macular to nodular

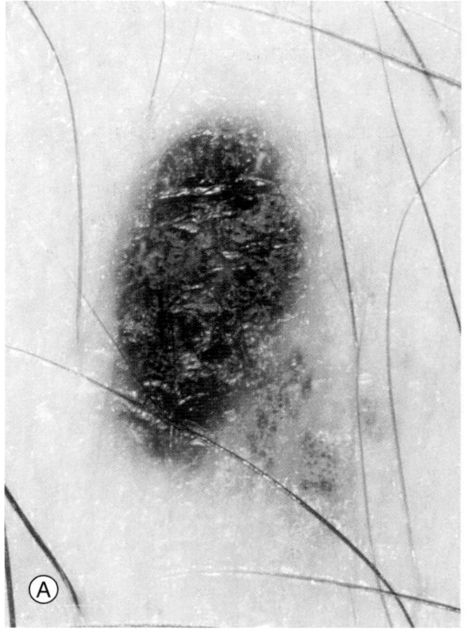

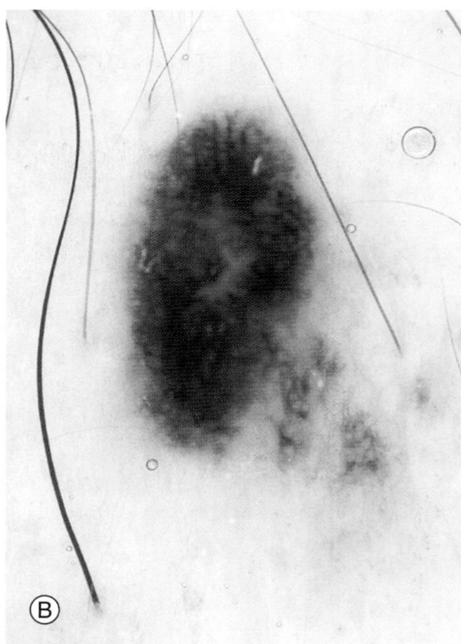

Figure 50.2 Blue color is better appreciated in the dermoscopic image in (B), as compared to the clinical image (A).

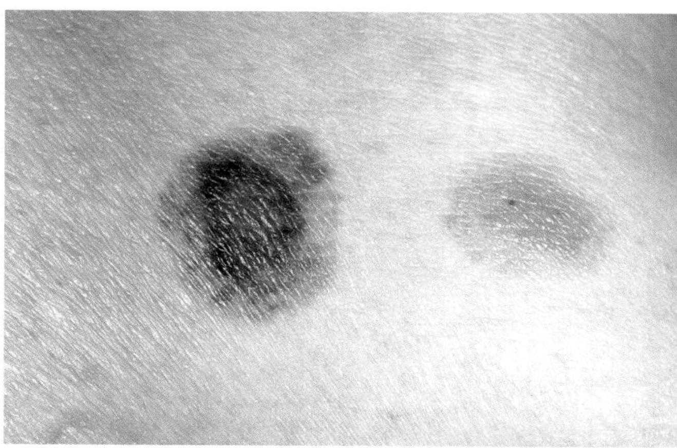

Figure 50.3 The center of the lesions are raised with a macular lightly pigmented periphery.

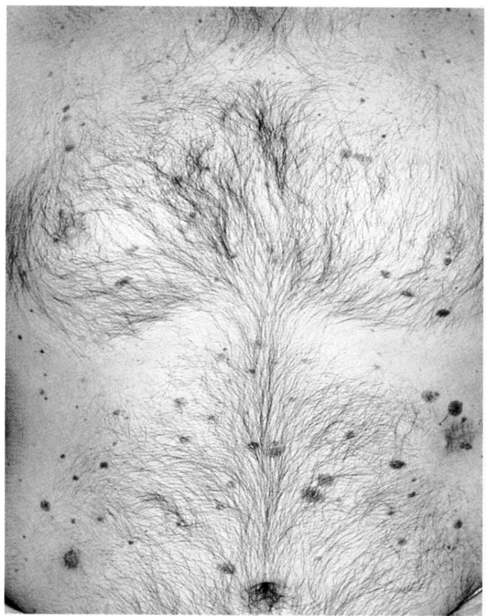

Figure 50.4 Numerous dysplastic nevi on the trunk.

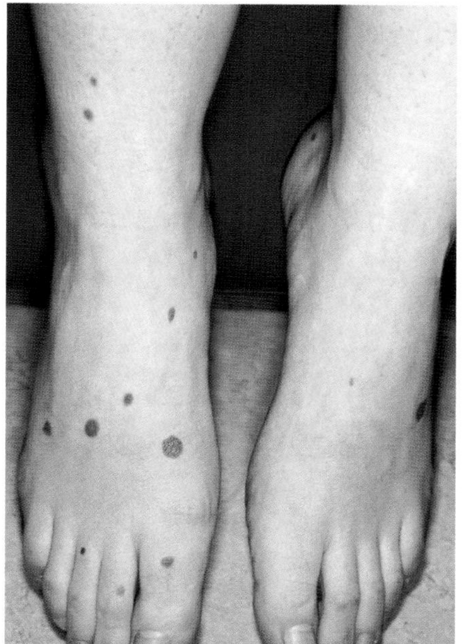

Figure 50.5 Several dysplastic nevi on the right foot.

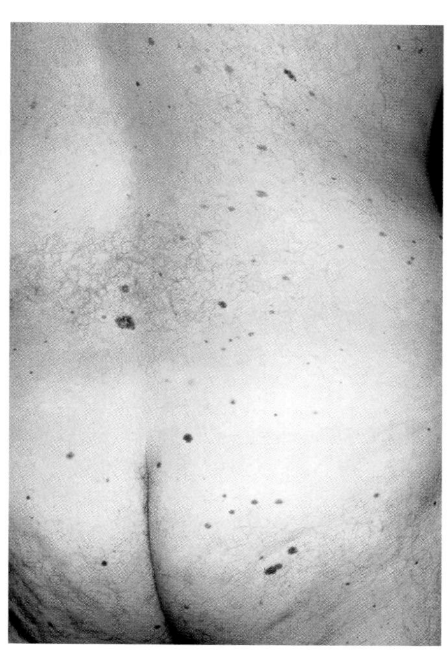

Figure 50.6 Several dysplastic nevi on the sun-protected buttocks.

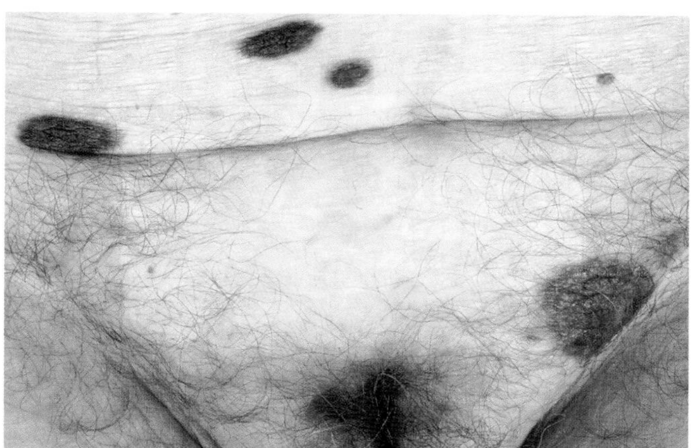

Figure 50.7 Dysplastic nevi on the mons pubis.

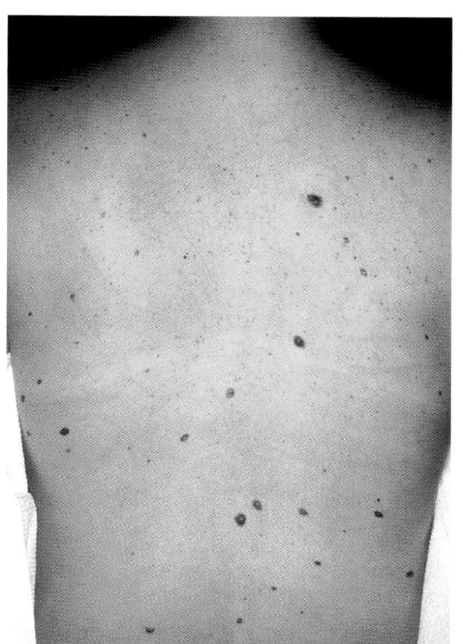

Figure 50.8 A person with fewer dysplastic nevi than shown in Figure 50.9 but within the spectrum of people with dysplastic nevus syndrome.

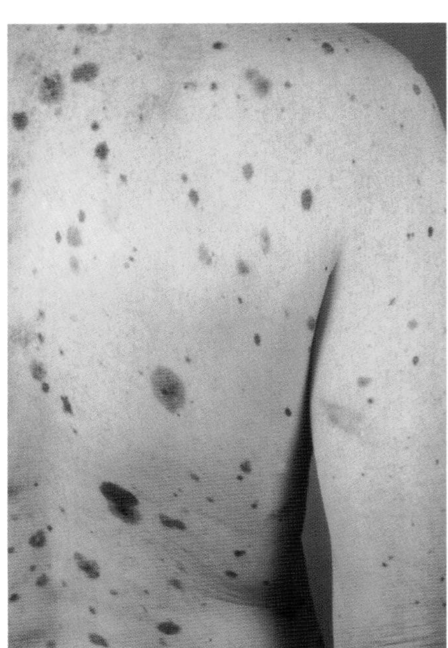

Figure 50.9 This person with numerous, variably sized dysplastic nevi is on the other end of the spectrum (compared with Figure 50.8) of dysplastic nevus syndrome.

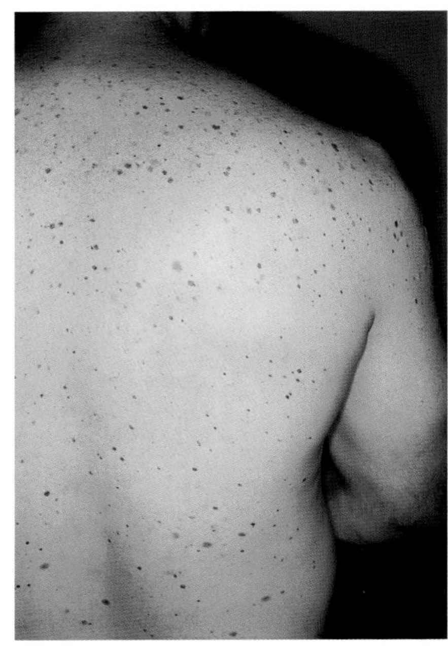

Figure 50.10 'Cheetah phenotype' with numerous, dark brown, uniform nevi.

Table 50.2 Atypical mole syndromes

Syndrome name	Clinical features
Sporadic syndromes	
Atypical mole syndrome[5]	Three or more of the following characteristics 1. Two or more clinically atypical nevi 2. >100 nevi >2mm diameter or >50 nevi if <20 or >50 years of age 3. Nevi abnormally distributed (buttocks or dorsum of foot) 4. Nevi in the anterior scalp 5. Iris pigmented lesion(s)'
Classic' atypical mole syndrome[8]	1. >100 melanocytic nevi 2. One or more nevi >8 mm diameter 3. One or more nevi with atypical features
B-K mole[11]	≥ 10 mm diameter; irregular outline; haphazard mixture of tan, brown, black, and pink; small palpable dermal component
B-K mole syndrome[11]	1. Fewer than 10 B-K moles to more than 100 moles prominent on the upper trunk and extremities, variability of mole size (5–15 mm diameter), outline, and color
Familial syndromes	
Familial atypical mole syndrome[9]	1. Two or more family members with atypical moles 2. One or more family member with melanoma
Familial atypical multiple mole–melanoma syndrome[10]	1. Melanoma in two or more first- or second-degree relatives 2. Many atypical nevi (often more than 50)

1 year of age and a gradual increase in number, peaking in the third decade of life, with a subsequent decrease in the total number of melanocytic nevi with aging.[13–15] Sun exposure has been implicated as a significant factor in the development of melanocytic nevi during childhood, a process termed solar nevogenesis.[16,17] Studies have shown that the anatomic distribution of melanocytic nevi and the frequency with which new nevi appear is in part due to exposure to ultraviolet radiation.[18–23]

The natural progression of atypical melanocytic nevi is somewhat different from that of common melanocytic nevi. Like common acquired melanocytic nevi, atypical moles may first begin to appear during early childhood; however, most will not become fully clinically manifest until puberty.[24] Unlike individuals with common nevi, it is not unusual for persons with atypical nevi to continue to develop new lesions throughout life[1,9] (Fig. 50.11). Both genetics and ultraviolet light exposure may be involved in the phenotypic expression of atypical moles. However, although most acquired nevi develop on skin that receives intermittent sun exposure (i.e. back), it is not uncommon for atypical moles to also develop in relatively sun-protected areas, such as the scalp and groin.[23] Halpern et al. prospectively followed a cohort of 153 dysplastic nevus patients over a minimum of 5 years, and concluded that atypical moles were dynamic in behavior, regardless of the age of the patient.[25] Over 50% of the patients studied had changes within their atypical moles throughout an average follow-up of 89 months. The changes included decreased clinical atypia (35%), the appearance of new atypical moles (33%), increased clinical atypia (15%), and complete disappearance of atypical moles (7%) (Fig. 50.12). One obstacle sometimes encountered in this type of study is the difficulty in absolutely differentiating between common and atypical nevi. Tucker et al. followed 32 families (844 members) with more than two living members with invasive melanoma for 2 to 25 years.[26] Sequential photographs of all

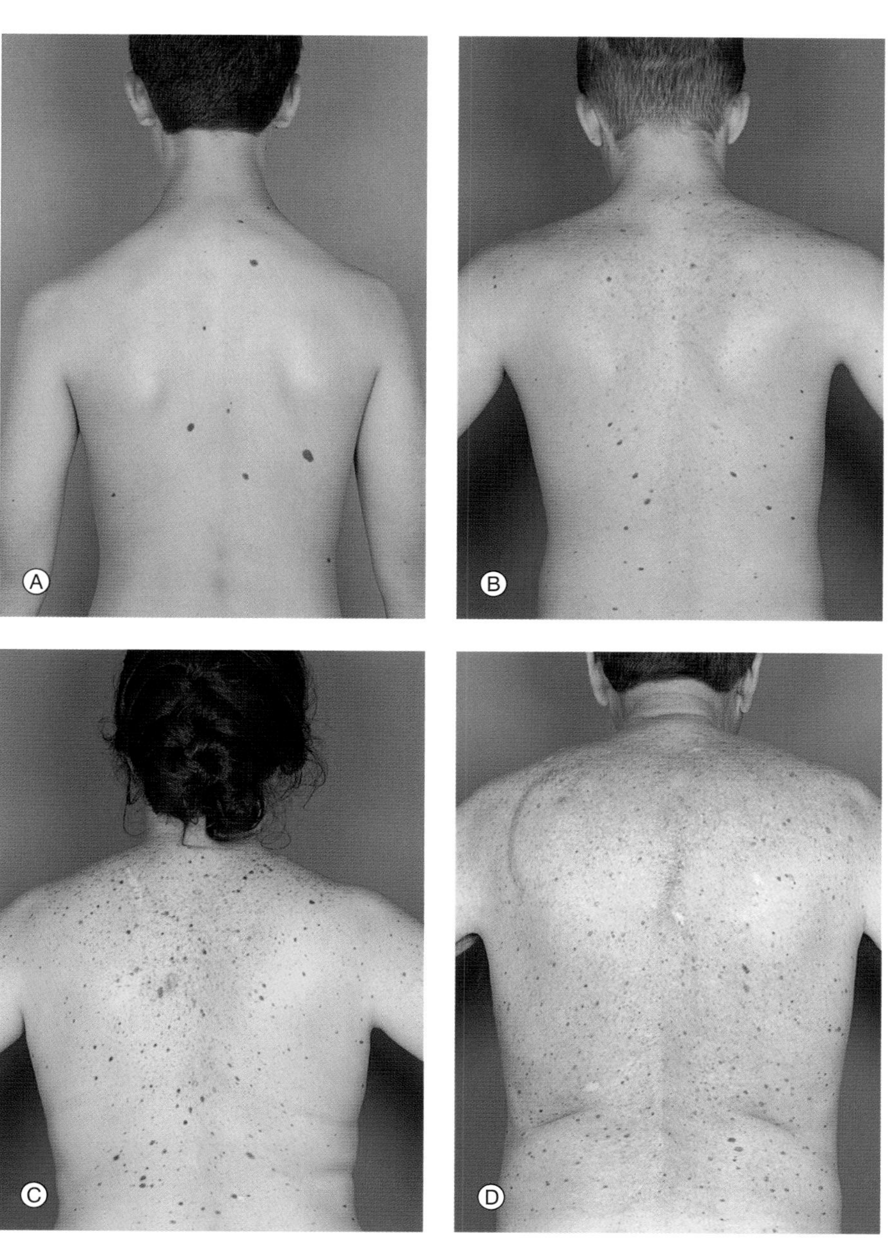

Figure 50.11 (A)–(D) Increasing number of nevi with increasing age.

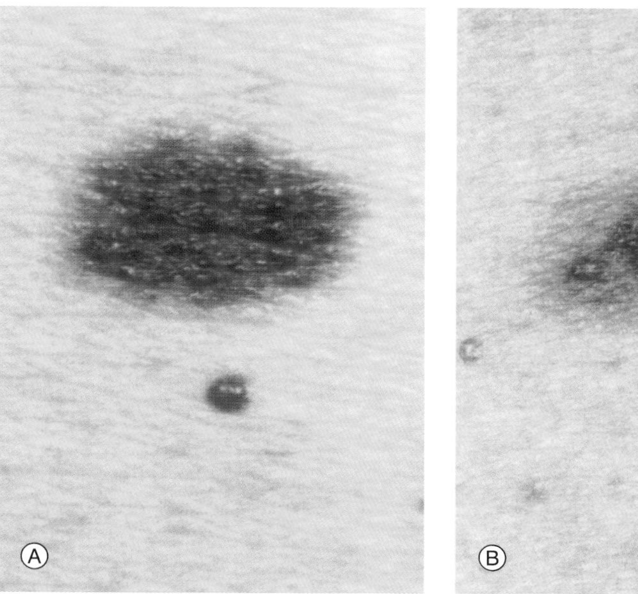

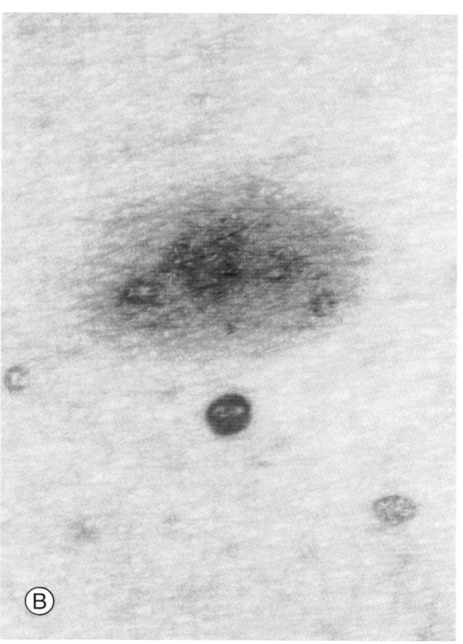

Figure 50.12 (A)–(B) Change in clinical appearance with lightening of color showing regression of this nevus over time.

skin surfaces and the most atypical nevi were taken and followed. A total of 86 new melanomas were found in 37 individuals. Fifty-one were found to have identified precursor lesions, 32 of which were dysplastic nevi. Others occurred in areas without previous known nevi or precursor lesion. Overall, most of the dysplastic nevi remained stable or regressed; a few changed enough to be a cause for concern for melanoma.

Risk of melanoma

Melanocytic nevi are precursors to, and risk markers for, melanomas. Important determinants for the risk of melanoma vary by study. Multiple studies indicate that the total number of melanocytic nevi and the presence of atypical moles are independent risk factors for the development of melanoma[27–35] (Figs 50.13, 50.14).

Many believe that the atypical mole is the most important precursor and risk marker for melanoma. The presence of atypical moles, familial or sporadic, independent of the total number of common nevi, places an individual at high risk for developing melanoma (Fig. 50.15). These melanomas tend to develop at a younger age than melanomas occurring in nonaffected individuals.[24] Melanoma can evolve from a dysplastic nevus (Fig. 50.16), but it can also arise de novo in previously normal skin. The 10-year life-table risk for developing melanoma in a patient with the atypical mole syndrome is estimated to be approximately 12%.[36] In patients with the atypical mole syndrome, the incidence of melanomas arising in association with an atypical mole ranges from 20% to 57%.[37–39] In this population, the incidence of melanoma arising 'de novo' still ranges from 43% to 80%.[40] Importantly, Tucker et al. have demonstrated that a patient with as few as one atypical mole may remain at an increased risk for developing melanoma, even after complete excision of the lesion.[35] Thus, the excision of atypical nevi, is not only impractical, but has a limited impact on melanoma risk. In addition, these individuals are also at increased risk for developing multiple melanomas. In fact, after the diagnosis of a melanoma, approximately 35% of patients with the atypical mole syndrome will develop a subsequent unrelated primary melanoma.[36]

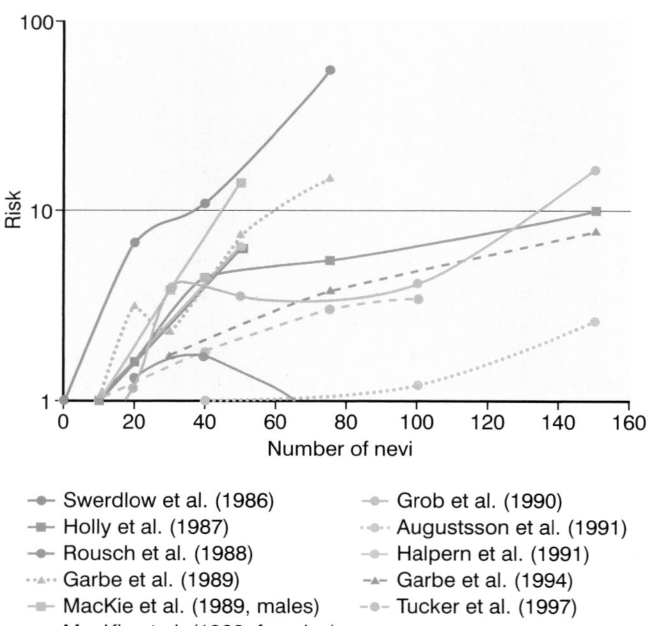

Figure 50.13 Various studies showing the increased risk of melanoma with increasing number of nevi.

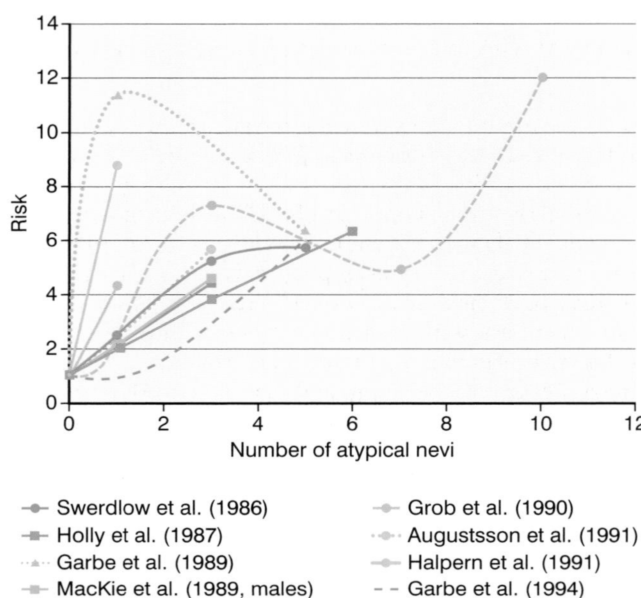

Figure 50.14 Various studies showing the general trend of increased risk of melanoma with increasing number of dysplastic nevi.

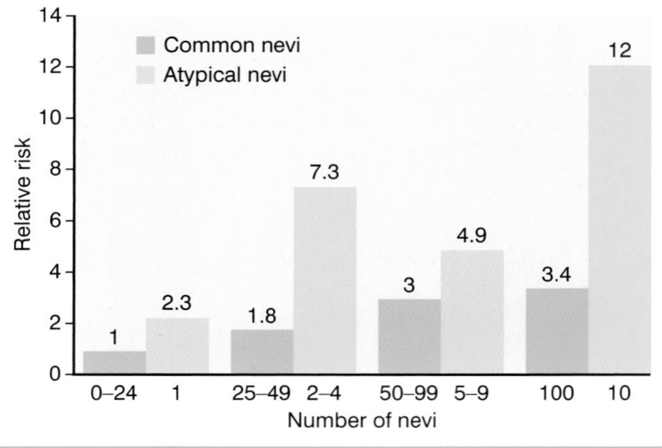

Figure 50.15 Increasing number of common nevi and atypical nevi independently increase the risk of melanoma; individuals with atypical nevi are at greater risk.

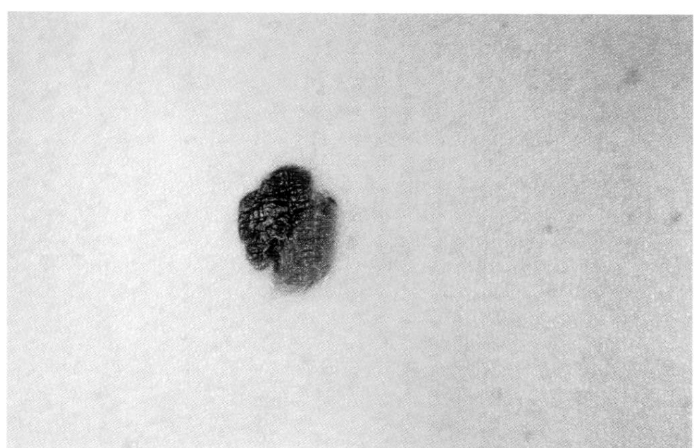

Figure 50.16 Melanoma evolving from a dysplastic nevus.

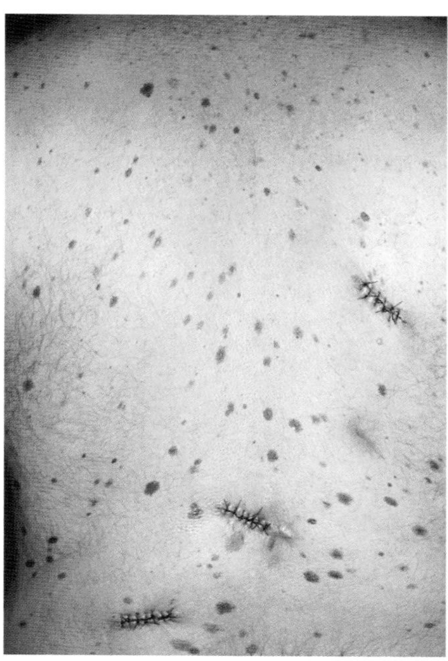

Figure 50.17 Scars on a patient who underwent excision of multiple dysplastic nevi.

Not all patients with atypical mole syndrome are at equal risk for developing melanoma. The magnitude of the risk depends on factors such as the number of nevi, personal or family history of melanoma, and family history of dysplastic nevi. Individuals with large numbers (>50) of common nevi are at increased risk of developing melanoma.[30] Individuals with dysplastic nevi who have at least two blood-related family members with melanoma have a lifetime risk for developing melanoma of greater than 80%.[24]

In studies by MacKie et al. and Garbe et al. the presence of one or two atypical moles was associated with a relative risk for developing melanoma of 2.1 and 11.4, when compared to individuals without atypical moles.[41,42] Individuals with classic atypical mole syndrome are at substantially increased risk for developing melanoma. Marghoob et al. compared the risk of developing melanomas in populations of patients with and without classic atypical mole syndrome.[43] They found a relative risk of 46.7 for patients with the syndrome who do not have a personal or family history of melanoma. The 10-year cumulative risk of developing a newly-diagnosed invasive melanoma was 10.7% for 287 patients who had the classic atypical mole syndrome compared to a 0.62% 10-year cumulative risk for 831 controls. This risk in the controls was similar to that expected in a group matched for age, sex, and duration of follow-up in the general US population. Additionally, patients with 'classic' atypical mole syndrome are at increased risk for the development of a second primary melanoma. Studies have shown that patients with atypical mole syndrome develop multiple melanomas at rates between 13% and 46%, which is higher than the average rate of 8% for patients without atypical mole syndrome.[5,28,30,33,43–52]

Prophylactic excision versus observation

All patients with atypical moles and the atypical mole syndrome should be instructed on the importance of sun avoidance and sun protection. They need to be under lifelong skin cancer surveillance, ideally conducted by a healthcare provider experienced in the evaluation of pigmented lesions. To complement the periodic physician-based skin examinations and to increase the probability of detecting early melanoma it is recommended that these patients perform monthly skin self-examinations.

The prophylactic removal of all atypical moles is not justified because the risk of any given dysplastic nevus developing into a melanoma is small. In addition, many melanomas develop de novo in these patients, not in association with a dysplastic nevus. Thus, the removal of all dysplastic nevi will not eliminate the risk for developing melanoma. Also, many of these patients have hundreds of atypical moles, such that removing all the lesions would be impractical and very disfiguring (Fig. 50.17). The alternative to prophylactic excision is periodic skin examinations with the aim of finding new or changing pigmented lesions that may represent early melanomas. These lesions can be evaluated carefully and biopsied if warranted. As noted above, baseline total body photography can assist in the follow-up examination of these patients.

The use of baseline total body photographs may prove to help not only the physician but also aid the patient at efficiently examining their own skin (Fig. 50.18). Identifying the subtle changes that may occur in an atypical mole is often a challenge. Total body photographs can assist in the detection of individual lesions undergoing change in size, shape, and color within a background of numerous nevi. Photography creates an objective baseline image that can be useful in assessing these changes, and in the detection of early melanoma.[53] In a study with 287 patients each with more than five dysplastic nevi, Kelly et al. showed that photographic surveillance enabled early diagnosis of melanoma.[54] Over half (11/20) of the newly diagnosed melanomas were detected as a result of changes seen during follow-up in comparison with baseline photographs. Another study by Tiersten et al. stated that 11 of the 18 melanomas that they reported in the atypical mole syndrome patients were detected with the aid of total cutaneous photography.[51] Although total cutaneous photography is not mandatory, it may at times aid in the detection of melanomas in their earliest and most curable stages, and perhaps avoid unnecessary excision of unchanging atypical moles.

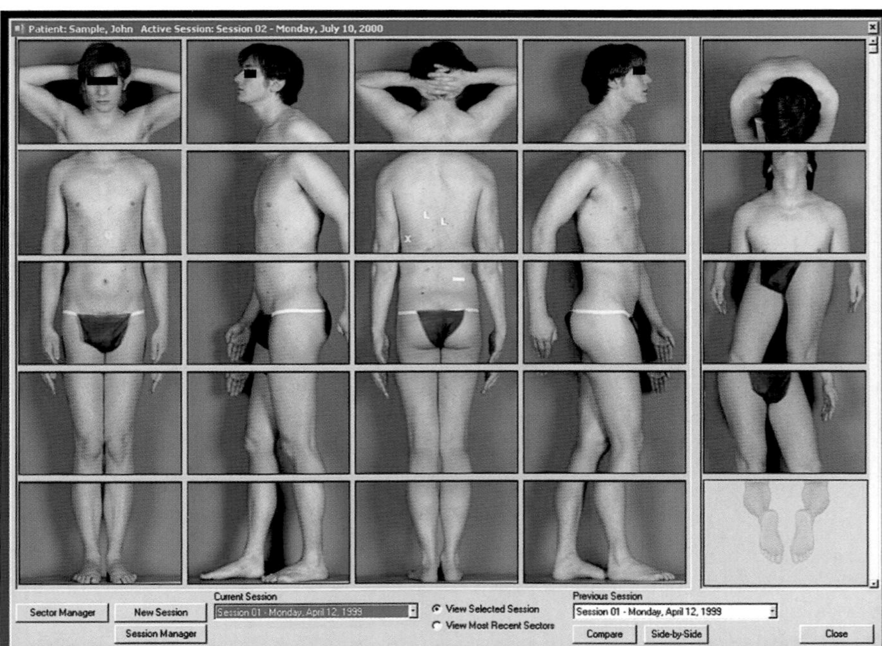

Figure 50.18 An example of total body photography on DermaGraphix, a digital, computerized system. Courtesy of Canfield Imaging Systems, NJ.

■ TECHNICAL ASPECTS

Early detection and prevention

The diagnosis and removal of a melanoma when it is early in its evolution is paramount to ensure a favorable prognosis. Thus, the goal in the management of individuals with atypical moles is to make sure that any evolving melanoma is caught as early as possible. The important elements in the management of patients who have atypical moles are discussed below and listed in Table 50.3.

Table 50.3 Elements for early detection and prevention of melanoma

Periodic routine dermatologic examinations
Regular self-examinations
Ophthalmologic, oral, and genital examinations
Imaging technology
Ultraviolet precautions
Biopsy and histologic evaluation of suspicious lesions

Routine dermatologic examinations

With periodic complete skin examinations, suspicious lesions can be recognized and biopsied earlier. It is important to have the patient undress completely because Rigel et al. determined that patients who had total cutaneous examinations were six times as likely to be diagnosed with melanomas, as individuals who were examined while only partially undressed.[55] Most of these melanomas developed on anatomic locations that would have ordinarily been covered by clothing. Thus, it is recommended that during regular follow-up visits such patients undergo total cutaneous surveillance. Patients with atypical melanocytic nevi have a higher incidence of nevi on the scalp.[5,56] Thus, it is important to routinely examine the patient's scalp. Failure to do so may result in the delayed diagnosis of melanoma[57] (Fig. 50.19). For examination of the scalp, a handheld hair blower is often helpful.[2] Follow-up frequency is a function of individual risk. It is suggested that a person identified as having atypical mole syndrome should have total cutaneous examinations at least once per year. Considering the higher risk for melanoma, persons with a previous personal or family history of melanoma, may be considered for routine follow-up intervals of 3–6 months.

Self-examination

The combination of regular physical examination and self-examination has been shown to be complementary in the early diagnosis of melanoma.[58] In the study by Kelly et al. nearly half (9/20) of melanomas detected were seen by the patients or their partners.[54] One retrospective study concluded that skin self-examination has the potential to reduce melanoma mortality by 63%.[59] Patient education on skin self-examination includes information on the ABCD changes of lesions and instruction on how to perform a thorough total body skin examination. Melanomas may arise de novo or transform from existing nevi.[60] Thus, patients with the atypical mole syndrome should learn to examine their own skins, looking for new and changing lesions, and do so every 1–3 months.[2,45,58,61] Guides on self-examination and on the early signs of melanoma are available from several organizations, including the American Academy of Dermatology, the Skin Cancer Foundation, and the American Cancer Society.

Screening

Although the median age for the development of melanomas in most series is in the early fifties, the average age for developing melanoma in persons with atypical moles

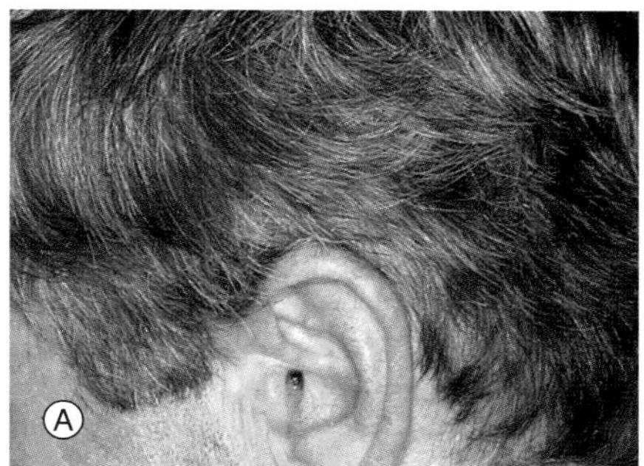

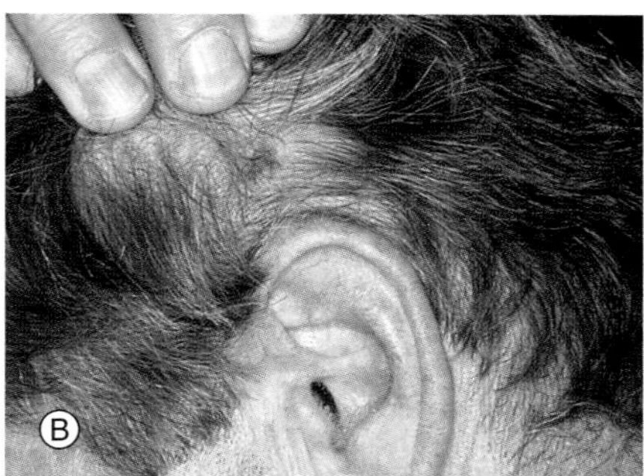

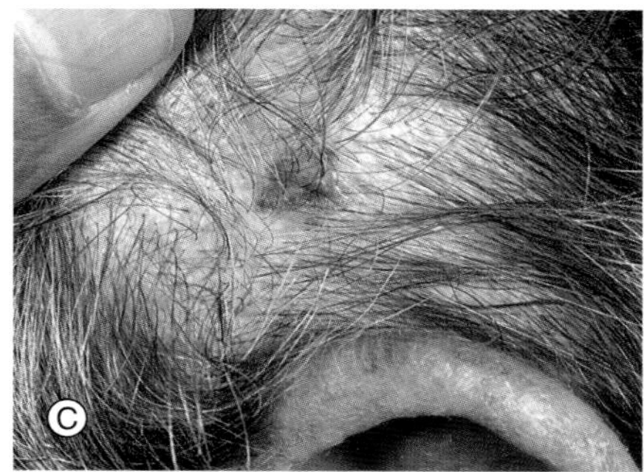

Figure 50.19 A melanoma on the scalp hidden under hair that was detected upon a complete cutaneous examination.

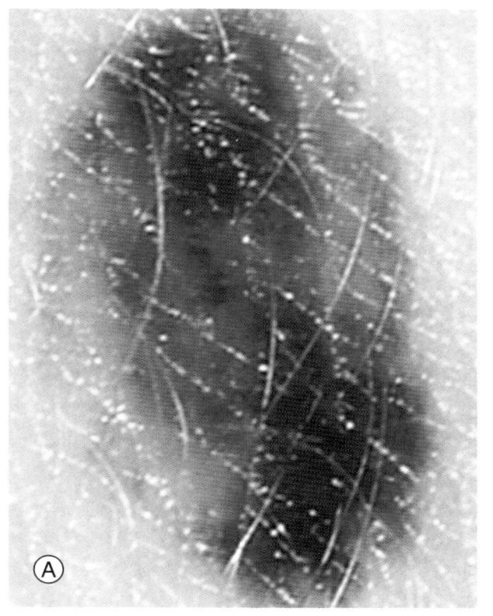

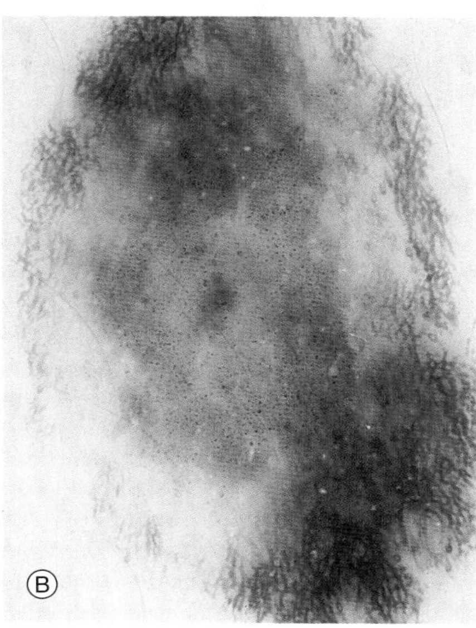

Figure 50.20 (A) Clinical picture of a dysplastic nevus. (B) Dermoscopic image with better visualization of areas of regression.

is much earlier.[9,37,43,46,51] A family history of melanoma and the presence of atypical moles define children at high risk for developing melanoma early in life.[40] The risk begins to increase during puberty.[45] The median age at diagnosis of melanoma may decrease with successive generations in families with melanomas.[62] Additionally, early screening will give the physician the opportunity to educate the patient and his or her family on the importance of lifelong sun protection. Thus, it is suggested that these patients begin receiving regular dermatologic follow-up examinations around puberty.

Many patients with the atypical mole syndrome are unaware that the trait is often familial.[63] Family members with undiagnosed atypical mole syndrome may not be receiving adequate examinations.[63,64] Bergman et al. reported that they diagnosed 12 melanomas by screening a total of 243 family members of patients with the atypical mole syndrome.[65] Therefore, it would seem to be ideal for all family members of the affected individual to have total cutaneous examinations for the presence of atypical moles and melanomas.

Ophthalmologic examination

Individuals with atypical mole syndrome have an increased prevalence of ocular melanocytic nevi and are at increased risk for the development of ocular melanomas.[66–73] In one study 48% of 257 individuals with atypical mole syndrome had ocular nevi, compared to 16% of 264 controls without atypical mole syndrome.[72] Thus, physicians should consider repeated ophthalmologic follow-up for patients with the atypical mole syndrome. These patients should be encouraged to wear UVA and UVB protective sunglasses.[73]

Visual aids

Certain tools are helpful in aiding the naked eye in the evaluation of suspicious lesions. The simplest is a magnifying glass. By enlarging the lesions, details can be better appreciated. A Wood's light can help visualize areas of regression, by enhancing depigmented areas. Dermoscopy (epiluminescence microscopy or skin surface microscopy) is a noninvasive technique utilizing transillumination of a liquid interface (oil, water, or alcohol) coupled with magnification by a dermoscope. It permits visualization of subsurface structures not discernible by the unaided eye by rendering the epidermis more translucent by reducing light reflection, refraction, and diffraction[74,75] (Figs 50.20, 50.21). In experienced hands, dermoscopy is an aid in the diagnosis of some pigmented lesions.[76] Automated dermoscopy systems have been developed to provide objective 'computer-assisted diagnosis' with levels

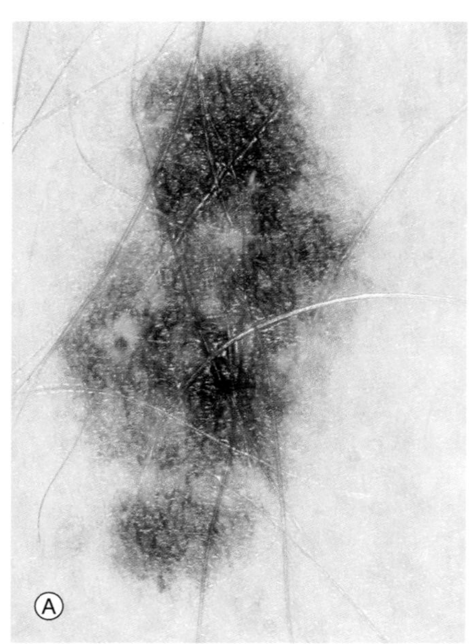

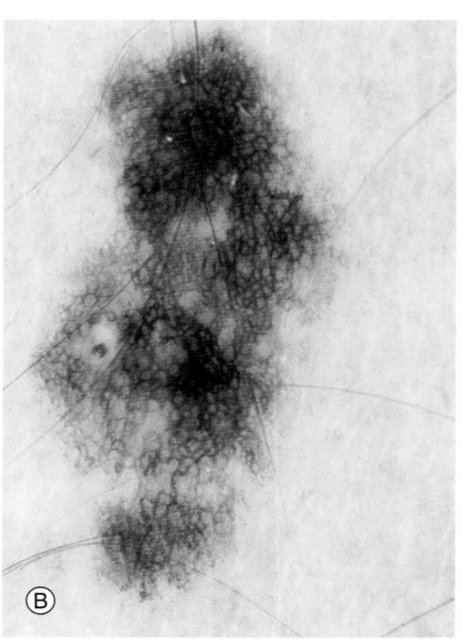

Figure 50.21 (A) Clinical picture of a dysplastic nevus. (B) Dermoscopic image with more well-defined reticulated pigment networks and color contrast.

of sensitivity and specificity approaching or exceeding that of expert dermoscopists.

Sun protection

Sunlight is considered to be an important factor in the pathogenesis of melanocytic nevi and of melanoma.[17–20,77–82] Patients with atypical moles should minimize unnecessary sun exposure and wear sun-protective clothing and sunglasses when outdoors.[83] The use of broad-spectrum (UVA and UVB) sunscreens has been shown to decrease the incidence of solar keratoses and to prevent UVB-induced immuosuppression.[84–86] In a randomized, prospective 3-year study of sunscreen use and development of nevi, white children who used a Sun Protection Factor (SPF) 30 broad-spectrum sunscreen developed fewer nevi compared to the control group who did not receive sunscreen.[87] At this time there is insufficient direct evidence to prove that sunscreen use is helpful in preventing melanomas.[88–91] However, because strong indirect epidemiologic and laboratory data implicate UV in melanoma genesis, the use of sunscreens with an SPF of at least 15 is generally recommended for protection when sun exposure is otherwise unavoidable.[88,92] Sunlamp or tanning bed use may be associated with an increased risk for melanoma and should be assiduously avoided.[93] Because childhood sun exposure is implicated in migration studies and mouse melanoma models as being very important, parents should teach their children about the hazards of the sun and how to protect themselves.[94,95] Recommendations on sun protection are given in Table 50.4.

Examination and possibly biopsy of changing, or symptomatic pigmented lesions

Finally, as part of early detection, any new, changing, or symptomatic pigmented lesions should be examined closely and possibly biopsied. Any lesion that is clinically thought to be a possible melanoma should be biopsied and undergo histopathologic evaluation. The biopsy techniques considered acceptable by the National Institutes of Health (NIH) Consensus Conference (1992) include excision, punch

Table 50.4 Ultraviolet precautions

Precaution	Detail
Minimize sun exposure	Between 10 a.m and 4 p.m
Wear protective clothing in the sun	A wide brimmed hat, long-sleeved shirt, and long pants. Choose tightly-woven materials for greater protection from the sun's rays
Apply a sunscreen when exposure is unavoidable	At least 1 hour before every exposure to the sun, and reapply frequently and liberally, at least every 2 hours while in the sun. Reapply after swimming or sweating heavily. Use broad-spectrum (UVA plus UVB) sunscreen with an SPF of 30 or more
Use a sunscreen	During high altitude activities such as mountain climbing, hiking, or skiing. Also, the sun is stronger near the equator
Do not forget to use sunscreen on overcast days	The sun's rays are as damaging to skin on cloudy, hazy days as they are on bright sunny days
Apply sunscreens every day	Individuals at high risk for skin cancer (outdoor workers, fair-skinned individuals, persons who have already had skin cancer, and persons with the atypical mole syndrome)
Beware of reflective surfaces!	Sand, snow, concrete, and water can reflect more than half the sun's rays onto the skin. Sitting in the shade does not guarantee adequate protection from the sun
Avoid tanning parlors	The ultraviolet light in tanning booths can cause sunburn and premature aging of the skin, and increases the risk for skin cancer
Keep infants out of the sun before 6 months of age	Protect children 6 months of age and older with clothing and sunscreens
Teach children sun protection early	Sun damage occurs with each unprotected sun exposure and accumulates over the course of a lifetime. Childhood behaviors strongly impact lifelong attitudes and behaviors

biopsy, and deep saucerization.[3] If possible, regardless of the procedure chosen, the entire lesion should be removed.[96] This ensures that a small focus of melanoma will not be missed because of sampling error. Evaluation of the overall architecture of the lesions can also be critical to the pathologists' ability to generate the correct diagnosis. For most thin melanomas, the depth of the lesion, as measured from a shave biopsy does not differ from that measured from definitive excision.[97]

Circumstances may arise in which an incisional or partial biopsy may be indicated. It may be difficult to perform an excisional biopsy in certain anatomical locations such as the face, palms, soles, ears, or digits (Fig. 50.22). In such situations, it is acceptable to take a sample of the most concerning portion of the lesions. However, if the histologic diagnosis is benign and the clinical suspicion for melanoma remains, then a repeat biopsy of another portion of the lesion is advisable to ensure adequate sampling. The pathologist should be requested to step-section the specimen. Step-sectioning may help detect a focus of melanoma occurring within an otherwise benign melanocytic neoplasm. Furthermore, by minimizing sampling error, step-sectioning helps to determine the maximum tumor thickness (i.e. Breslow thickness), providing prognostic information. If the physician suspects that there may be a focus of melanoma within a lesion, he or she can mark the area of concern with a suture or dye. The pathologist should be instructed to section through this marked area to ensure that the area of concern is evaluated histologically. If the histologic diagnosis does not fit with clinical suspicion, the physician should seek additional sections or obtain a second opinion.

If the excised lesion is a dysplastic nevus, an excisional biopsy with 2–3 mm margins ensures complete removal of the nevus. It avoids the issues of re-excision of dysplastic nevi in which the pathology report states that the margins are positive. Furthermore, it decreases the potential of dysplastic nevus recurrence, which can be confused with melanoma.[98]

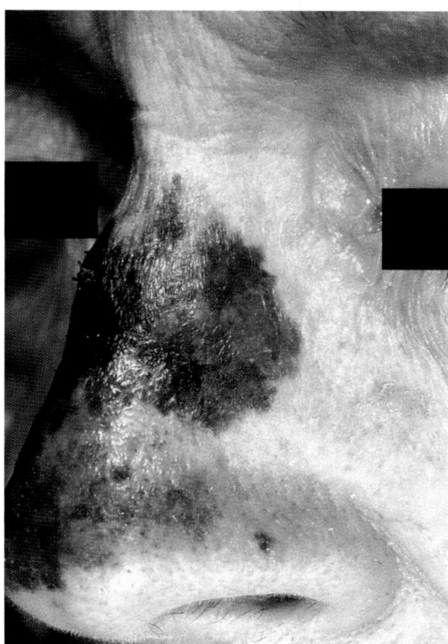

Figure 50.22 A lentigo maligna covering the entire nose. An excisional biopsy or complete surgical treatment would not be feasible.

Chemoprevention

Various topical and systemic agents have been studied for their effects on dysplastic nevi including 5-fluorouracil (5-FU), isotretinoin, and tretinoin. In one case report, all dysplastic nevi treated with 5-FU on a patient responded with inflammation, ulceration, and then disappearance of all lesions.[99] The control was treatment of common nevi, which remained unchanged. Dysplastic nevi treated with topical tretinoin also developed irritation and a decrease in clinical atypia, and in some cases, disappeared.[100,101] Histologic evaluation of treated dysplastic nevi showed disappearance or reversion to banal nevi when compared to untreated nevi or those treated with placebo. In contrast, oral isotretinoin did not change dysplastic nevi.[102] 5-fluorouracil and topical tretinoin seem to have a significant biologic effect on dysplastic nevi, as demonstrated in the small studies and case reports. Additional studies need to be conducted before consideration of their use as treatment of dysplastic nevi.

New agents for the chemoprevention of melanoma are currently being considered. Potential agents include commonly used lipid-lowering medications—lovastatin and gemfibrozil. The statins and fibrates are two classes of medications found on retrospective analysis of cardiology trials to be associated with a decreased incidence of melanoma in large clinical trials with patients being treated for cardiac disease.[103] Another prospective class of medication is the cyclo-oxygenase-2 (COX-2) inhibitors. There is evidence showing that COX-2 is constitutively expressed in melanomas and may be involved in the regulation of melanoma invasion.[104]

Imiquimod, a topical immune response modifier, has been used to treat lentigo maligna melanoma and epidermotropic cutaneous metastases with success and histologic clearance.[105] It stimulates cytokines including interferon (IFN)-α, interleukins (IL)-1, - 6, -8, and -12, and tumor necrosis factor (TNF)-α, which potentiates humoral and cell-mediated immune responses. These are potentially promising therapies that may, with further study, be added to the armamentarium for the chemoprevention and treatment of melanoma.

Management of melanoma

Melanoma is a malignancy derived from the pigment producing cells (melanocytes) and can arise in the skin, mucosa, eye, or the central nervous system. The incidence and mortality rate of melanoma have continued to rise steadily over the past few decades despite a trend toward the diagnosis of earlier disease and advances in immunotherapy. Currently, the lifetime risk of developing melanoma is 1 in 71 and the projected risk by 2010 is that 1 in 50 Americans will develop melanoma in their lifetime.

In 2003, an estimated 54 200 new invasive cases and 37 700 in-situ melanomas will be diagnosed and 7600 people will die from melanoma.[106] It is the deadliest form of skin cancer. An emphasis on prevention and early detection is the key to reducing melanoma morbidity and death.[107] Optimal management of a patient diagnosed with melanoma requires consideration of multiple factors and decisions regarding the management of the primary site, staging procedures, adjuvant therapy, and follow-up. Treatment should be tailored to the needs of each individual patient. This section presents a generalized approach to the surgical management (excision margins) for melanoma, the diagnostic and staging work-up, follow-up recommendations, and adjuvant treatment options.

Diagnosis

Diagnosis of melanoma begins with a biopsy of a suspected lesion (see page 830). Once the diagnosis has been established with histopathologic confirmation, the staging work-up and treatment options are considered, taking into account the prognostic attributes such as thickness of the lesion, location, and overall medical condition of the patient. The new American Joint Committee on Cancer (AJCC) staging classification is listed in Table 50.5.[108] Workup, treatment, and follow-up guidelines take into consideration the stage of the patient's disease.

It is also of great importance to provide psychosocial support for a patient diagnosed with melanoma. It is a serious, potentially fatal cancer that can be a source of great anxiety and fear for the patient and his or her family. Frequent follow-up visits in the period immediately after diagnosis can provide reassurance and comfort from careful surveillance.

Staging

Staging of a melanoma patient begins with a thorough history and physical examination. Accurate staging is important because it can provide the patient with precise prognostic and survival information (Table 50.6). A problem-oriented physical examination should include a complete skin and lymph node examination and assessment of any abnormalities detected on a thorough review of systems. Suspicious signs, symptoms, and physical findings (e.g. in-transit metastases, satellite lesions, and palpable lymph nodes) warrant additional laboratory studies, imaging studies, and possible histological confirmation. The new AJCC staging classification takes into account the status of lymph node involvement for those who undergo lymphatic mapping.

Patients with thin melanomas (<1.0 mm) do not need specific blood work or imaging studies to search for occult metastases. For patients with melanomas over 1.0 mm thickness, baseline laboratory values including complete blood count, lactate dehydrogenase (LDH), liver function tests, and chest radiography have been suggested by some guidelines as part of the initial workup, but have a very low yield.[109] There is no evidence to support the usefulness of these tests, but they are relatively inexpensive and provide a baseline for future reference. Routine imaging studies are not indicated in patients with stage I or II disease. In patients with more advanced stage disease, radiologic imaging and LDH levels may be used to monitor the progression or recurrence of metastatic disease. An elevated LDH level on two separate occasions, at least 24 hours apart, is an indication of metastatic disease based on the new AJCC staging classification, if there are no other obvious causes. It can also be followed as a marker for disease activity. Radiologic and nuclear imaging studies may be useful in the evaluation and guiding the management of stage III and IV patients who have nodal or distant metastatic disease. Computed tomography and, more recently, positron emission tomography, are commonly used to evaluate symptoms or abnormalities noted on follow-up examinations.

In patients who have metastatic melanoma with an unknown primary site, a complete skin examination, including a Wood's light examination should be performed. Wood's light will highlight areas of regression where a melanocytic lesion may have been. Also, an ophthalmologic examination is recommended as well as a gynecologic examination for women.

Table 50.5 New American Joint Committee on Cancer staging

Stage	Description (all sizes are Breslow thicknesses)
0	In situ
IA	≤ 1.0 mm no ulceration
IB	≤ 1.0 mm with ulceration
	1.01–2.0 mm, no ulceration
IIA	1.01–2.0 mm with ulceration
	2.01–4.0 mm, no ulceration
IIB	2.01–4.0 mm with ulceration
	>4.0 mm, no ulceration
IIC	>4.0 mm with ulceration
IIIA	Nonulcerated primary tumor (T1–T4a) with ≤ 3 nodal micrometastases
IIIB	Nonulcerated primary tumor (T1–T4a) with ≤ 3 macrometastases
	Any primary tumor (T1–T4b) with ≤ 3 nodal micrometastases
	Any T with in transit or satellite
IIIC	Any T with ≤ 3 macrometastases
	Any T with ≥ 4 nodes
IV M1a	Distant skin, subcutaneous or nodal metastases with normal LDH
IV M1b	Lung metastasis with normal LDH
IV M1c	All other visceral metastasis with normal LDH or Any distant metastasis with elevated LDH

Table 50.6 Survival data

Stage	1-year survival (%)	5-year survival (%)	10-year survival (%)
IA		95	88
IB		90	80
IIA		78	65
IIB		65	50
IIC		45	32
IIIA		65	60
IIIB		50	40
IIIC		25	20
IV M1a	59	19	16
IV M1b	57	7	3
IV M1c	41	10	6

Stage I, II—worse prognosis with ulceration, increasing thickness, age, axial location, being male
Stage III—worse with increasing number of nodes, macrometastasis, ulceration of primary tumor
Stage IV—depends on site, but differences are minimal—metastases to the lung only has 1-year survival advantage over other visceral metastases

Surgical management

Excisional surgery with margins based on Breslow thickness is the cornerstone of treatment for primary melanoma. All excisions of invasive melanomas should be carried down to deep fat or the fascia layer of the subcutis. The proposed margins from the National Comprehensive Cancer Network (NCCN) are listed in Table 50.7.[109] Margins may be modified to accommodate individual anatomic or cosmetic considerations. The preferred treatment for lentigo maligna is complete surgical excision. However, the large size of many of these lesions coupled with their common occurrence on the face of elderly patients, warrants consideration of radiation therapy, cryotherapy, topical therapy, or observation in some cases (see Fig. 50.22).

For patients with stage IA disease (i.e. thin melanomas [<1.0 mm] without negative prognostic attributes such as ulceration, Clark's level IV–V, or extensive regression), wide local excision is sufficient treatment. For patients with stage IB–II disease (i.e. intermediate and thick lesions [>1.0 mm] without clinical evidence of nodal involvement), sentinel lymph node biopsy (SLNB) should be considered in conjunction with wide local excision.

SLN biopsy

Lymphatic mapping with SLN biopsy (SLNB) has become a common procedure performed at the time of wide local excision to identify regional nodal metastases for melanomas greater than 1 mm in thickness. Currently, SLNB is primarily a staging and prognostic tool with no proven therapeutic or survival benefit.

Before the development of SLNB, many patients underwent elective lymph node dissection (ELND) on the assumption that melanoma metastasized via the lymphatics and that removal of nodes with metastases prevented spread to distant sites. The advantage of SLNB over ELND is the relatively minimal invasiveness with which it identifies patients with clinically inapparent lymph node metastases. Another advantage of the current method of SLNB is the use of preoperative lymphoscintigraphy, a nuclear medicine study that permits identification of the specific draining nodal basin for a given melanoma. This technique is especially helpful when there is lymphatic drainage to more than one basin or if the drainage pattern is unpredictable, particularly with midline lesions and those on the head and neck. The selectivity of SLNB provides far fewer nodes to process and examine, making it more efficient and less likely for positive sections to be missed. Patients with metastatic melanoma found on SLNB typically undergo therapeutic 'completion' lymphadenectomy of the affected basin (Fig. 50.23). Those without evidence of melanoma in the SLNs are spared additional surgery.

Table 50.7 Surgical margins

Breslow thickness	Proposed surgical margins from the NCCN
In situ	0.5 cm
<1 mm	1.0 cm
1.01–4 mm	2.0 cm
>4 mm	≥ 2.0 cm

Preoperative lymphoscintigraphy identifies all draining nodal basins and helps to pinpoint the exact location of the SLN. At the time of surgery, the surgeon performs an intradermal injection of radioactive colloid and a blue dye around the site of the primary melanoma. The material then travels through the afferent lymph channels to identify the first draining or SLN. A gamma probe is then used intraoperatively to help map the most radioactive lymph node within a basin. After visualization of the blue dye, the SLN is located and removed. The hottest node and those with >10% radioactivity of the most radioactive node are removed. Histological analysis of the SLN(s) is then performed with H&E staining. Depending on the institution performing the procedure, additional tools used may include immunohistochemical staining for S-100, HMB-45 or MART-1 and possibly reverse transcriptase polymerase chain reaction (RT-PCR). Ideally, the procedure should be performed in conjunction with and before the wide local excision so the lymphatic drainage is not altered.

Sentinel lymph nodes are identified 87–100% of the time.[110–112] The yield depends on the technique and experience of the surgeon and institution. With improvements in technology and technique, the more recent rates approach 98% in most studies. Approximately 20% of SLNs are positive for melanoma, ranging from 12–36% in the literature.[110–114] Predictive factors for a positive SLN include primary melanomas with greater thickness, ulceration, high mitotic index (>5/high power field), axial location, and Clark level greater than III.[110,113,114] The mean thickness of the primary tumor in patients with a positive SLN is 2.5–3 mm, versus 1.5–2 mm when the SLN is negative. Positive nodes are exceedingly rare in those with melanomas less than 0.75 mm. The false negative rate ranges from less than 1 to 4%. This can be attributed to inability to locate the SLN or failure of histologic techniques to identify metastases. Again, with recent advances,

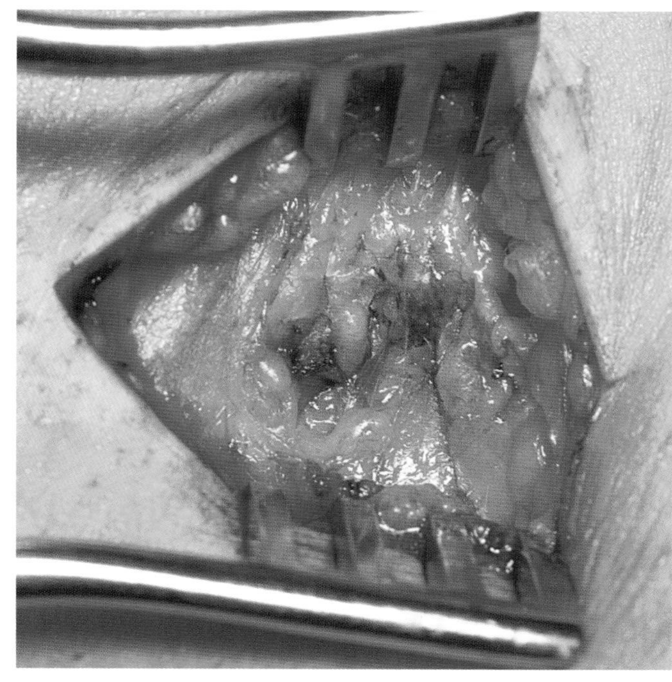

Figure 50.23 A blue node seen on sentinel lymph node biopsy.

the false negative rate is very low. False positives can occur with tests with high sensitivity, such as RT-PCR.

There are several advantages for performing SLNB. First is improved accuracy of staging. The new AJCC staging system takes into account pathologic staging information gained from SLNB. This provides the patient with valuable prognostic information because SLN status is the single most important predictor of survival. Second, patients with occult nodal metastases can be identified to undergo early therapeutic lymph node dissection and also adjuvant therapy. One study showed overall 5-year survival of 48% vs 27% in patients who had nodal micrometastases removed at ELND versus patients who waited for palpable nodes before undergoing therapeutic lymphadenectomy.[115] The current primary therapeutic implication of SLNB is that patients with positive SLNs are considered for adjuvant therapy with IFN or vaccines. Third, improved staging with SLNB will help define more homogeneous patient populations for participation in clinical trials. This will benefit studies of adjuvant therapies for patients with specific stages of disease. Previous trials that failed to demonstrate significant survival benefit may have combined patients of different stages who can now be stratified more clearly with the new AJCC clinical and pathologic staging.

The limitations of SLNB include cost, morbidity, and lack of proven therapeutic value. There are also potential complications of the surgical procedure, including lymphedema and retained blue dye. The procedure itself does not guarantee cure of nodal metastases or prevention of future spread of disease. It is possible to have skipped nodes when the melanoma spreads to a non-SLN. Distant metastases can also occur through nonlymphatic spread. There may be a false sense of security if the SLN is negative. Critics of the SLNB also point to the lack of proven benefit of adjuvant therapy as a reason not to pursue this costly procedure. There is significant disease-free survival benefit with some adjuvant therapy, but impact on overall survival remains inconclusive.

There are no proven survival benefits associated with SLNB at this time. It should not be used indiscriminately and the decision to undergo it should be individualized. The candidates who should be considered are those with melanomas >1 mm thickness and those with thin (<1 mm) melanomas demonstrating poor prognostic attributes (e.g. ulceration, extensive histologic regression, or Clark's level III+).

Adjuvant therapy

Adjuvant therapy should be considered for patients with thick primary tumors or positive lymph nodes who are at high risk for recurrence. Multiple approaches to adjuvant therapy including chemotherapy, immunotherapy, or vaccine therapy have been studied in this setting. Randomized studies of adjuvant treatment using bacillus Calmette–Guérin (BCG), *Corynebacterium parvum*, dacarbazine (DTIC), levamisole, vitamin A, or megestrol acetate alone or in combination have generally failed to show any benefit in disease-free or overall survival. Small subsets of isolated positive results have not been corroborated.

High-dose interferon-α is an FDA-approved adjuvant treatment for melanoma. It has shown increased disease-free survival and in one controlled study showed increased overall survival.[116] High-dose interferon alfa given for 1 full year in patients with stage IIB and III disease resulted in a median increase in overall survival from 2.8 to 3.8 years in treated patients.[116] There was significant toxicity associated with high-dose IFN therapy, but the treated group still had an increased quality of life adjusted survival time with a gain of 8.9 months without relapse and 7 months of overall survival time compared to the observation group.[117] Two other trials using high-dose IFN showed improvement only in disease-free survival in patients with positive nodal disease.[118,119] A trial comparing high-dose IFN and GM2-KLH/QS-21 vaccines revealed significant increases of disease-free and overall survival with IFN.[120] Low-dose IFN, although better tolerated, was ineffective in increasing overall survival in patients with positive or negative lymph nodes.[121,122] In summary, high-dose IFN results in prolonged relapse-free and overall survival in some patients with significant associated toxicity, but low-dose IFN has not been proven to be beneficial to overall survival.

Adjuvant vaccine therapy has been shown to be beneficial in a limited number of patients. To date, however, no vaccine has demonstrated significant survival benefit when compared to high-dose IFN or observation. Randomized, prospective studies have yet to show any significant increase in overall survival.[123–125] Vaccines are designed to stimulate an immune response. A variety of antigens have been tried,

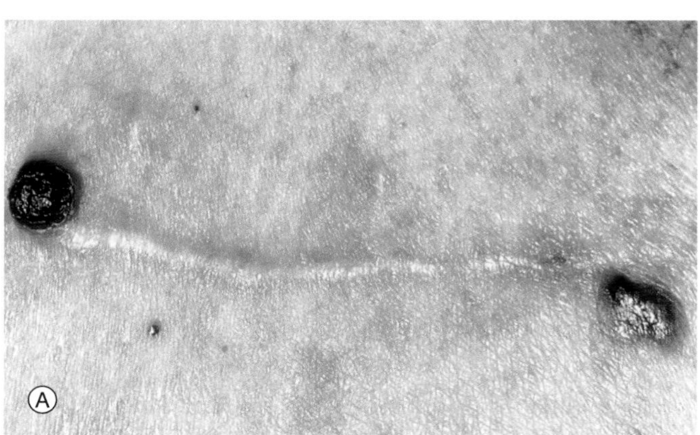

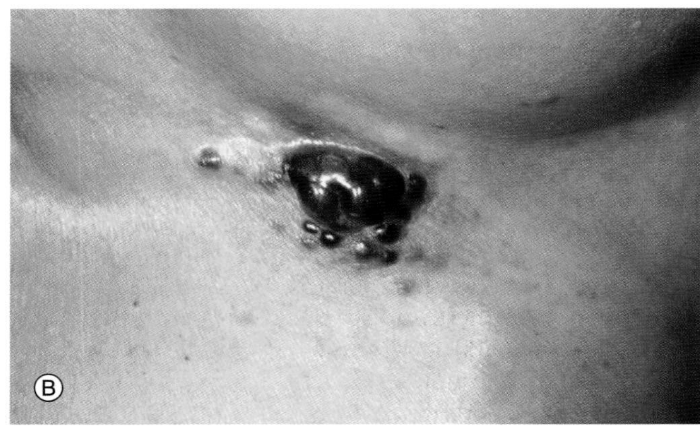

Figure 50.24 (A) Melanoma recurrence at the surgical site more then 1 year after initial excision. (B) Soft tissue and nodal metastases.

including whole cells, cell lysates, shed antigens, gangliosides, and peptides. In patients who develop an antitumor (humoral and/or cellular) response to a particular vaccine, disease-free and overall survival have been improved.[125] Patients not improving on one vaccine may have success with a different antigen. Additional ongoing trials are in progress to further evaluate the value of various vaccines.

Treatment of metastatic disease

In patients with metastatic melanoma distant to the local/regional site, curative resection of relatively stable remote nodal and soft tissue lesions, as well as isolated visceral lesions should be considered (Fig. 50.24). In symptomatic patients, palliative resection may also be appropriate. The lung is the most common visceral site of metastasis that is potentially curable with the resection of isolated lesions. Prolonged survival among some patients treated with surgical resection of limited liver, pulmonary, or brain metastases has been reported.[126–128] Palliative radiation therapy is an option in the setting of inoperable brain metastases, prolonging survival by 1–2 months.

Systemic chemotherapy with dacarbazine (DTIC) remains the mainstay of therapy for patients with extensive distant metastatic disease. Response rates are generally low (20%) and median duration of responses approaches 1 year. Complete responses are rare, usually less than 5%. Although several combination chemotherapy regimens have been evaluated over the years, none have demonstrated consistent improvements in survival compared to single-agent DTIC.[129,130]

Novel approaches to treatment of distant metastatic disease include the use of immuno 'biotherapies'—specifically IFN and IL-2—either alone or in combination with multidrug chemotherapy. Vaccine therapy is also well tolerated with low toxicity in advanced disease. Initial trials had promising results, with some patients having increased disease-free and overall survival when compared to historical controls. However, in a prospective trial comparing vaccine to chemotherapy there was no survival advantage, but there was significantly less toxicity.[131] The biologic agents and vaccines seem to benefit fewer people when compared to chemotherapy, but for the patients who do have complete responses, they are more likely to be durable. Large trials need to be conducted to evaluate the true benefits of the different agents.

■ POSTOPERATIVE CARE

Follow-up

Regular skin examinations are very important in patients with melanoma because these people are at significant risk of developing one or more subsequent new primary melanomas. Approximately 1–8% of patients with non-familial melanoma develop multiple primary melanomas.[132] Risk factors that increase the chance of developing new primary melanoma(s) in this population include older age and having atypical moles. A case–control study by Titus-Ernstoff et al. reported that patients with atypical moles have an increased risk for developing multiple primary melanomas (relative risk 8.8).[133]

The recommendation for the prevention of additional melanomas is sun protection, as discussed on page 830.

Patients with invasive primary malignant melanoma need regular follow-up for assessment of metastasis. A thorough review of systems and physical examination, including lymph node examination, should be performed on all follow-up visits. A focused review of systems aimed at patients with melanoma should include queries about weight loss, fatigue, headache, numbness, dizziness, shortness of breath, cough, abdominal pain, and bone pain. In addition to the complete cutaneous and lymph node examination, auscultation of the lungs, palpation of the liver and spleen, or a focused neurologic examination, may be warranted in selected patients.

Initially, patients with melanoma should be followed closely every 2–3 months. Although recurrences can occur at any time, even 10–20 years after the primary, the greatest risk is in the first years following diagnosis. Overall, 25% of all patients with melanoma develop recurrences. Most recur within 2–5 years. Therefore, surveillance is most important in the period immediately following treatment. After 1 or 2 years, if the patient remains free of disease, the interval between follow-up visits can be spaced out to between 6 months and 1 year, depending on individual risk factors. Time to recurrence for patients with node-negative disease varies inversely with the thickness of the primary tumor.[134] Thus, thin melanomas can potentially recur years after initial diagnosis. Every patient with a history of melanoma should be examined at least yearly.

Follow-up laboratory and imaging studies are guided by history, review of systems and symptoms, and findings on a complete skin examination and lymph node evaluation.[135] Most recurrences are found on physical examination or may produce symptoms that are revealed on a review of systems. A smaller percentage of metastases are found on chest radiography.[136] The first site of metastases is most commonly the skin and subcutaneous tissue, followed by lymph nodes, lung, liver, and brain.[137] In general, men and older patients have a worse prognosis than women and younger patients (Table 50.8).

The guidelines for treatment and follow-up from the National Comprehensive Cancer Network, American Academy of Dermatology, and the British Association of Dermatologists are summarized in Table 50.9.[109,138,139]

Table 50.8 Prognostic factors

Sex
Location
Age
Thickness
Ulceration
Regression
Mitotic index
Lymphocytic infiltrate
Angiogenesis
DNA ploidy
Nuclear volume
Microscopic satellitosis/in-transit metastases
Recurrent disease

Table 50.9 Published guidelines for managing patients with melanoma

		Margins	Workup	Followup
AAD	*In situ*	0.5 cm	H&P*; CXR, LDH (optional)	General recommendations not stage specific, should be based on individual risk. H&P 1–4×/year for 2 years then 1–2×/year
	<2 mm	1.0 cm		
	>2 mm	2.0 cm		Directed laboratory and imaging studies
	Stage III	Not discussed	Not discussed	Not discussed
	Stage IV	Not discussed	Not discussed	Not discussed
NCCN	*In situ*	0.5 cm	None	Not discussed
	<1 mm	1.0 cm	None	H&P every 6 months for 2 years, then yearly
	1–4 mm	1–2.0 cm	Consider SLNB; CXR, LFT (optional)	H&P 3–6 months for 3 years, then 6–12 months for 2 years. CXR, LFT every 6–12 months (optional)
	>4 mm	≥ 2.0 cm		
	Stage III	Excision and lymph node dissection	LFT, CXR; pelvic and other CT if indicated	H&P 3–6 months for 3 years then 4–12 months for 2 years, then yearly CXR, CBC, LFT every 3–12 months (optional), CT scans as indicated
	Stage IV	Excision of primary melanoma and focal resection of internal organs involved with metastatic melanoma (if feasible)	LFT, CXR; CT scans if indicated	Not discussed
BAD	*In situ*	0.2–0.5 cm	None	Self-examination, no follow-up required
	<1 mm	1 cm	None	H&P every 3 months for 3 years
	1–2 mm	1–2 cm	Stage II; Consider SLNB	H&P every 3 months for 3 years, then every 6 months for 2 years
	2.1–4 mm	2–3 cm	Stage IIB and up; LFT, LDH, CBC, CXR, liver ultrasound, CT chest, abdomen, pelvis	
	>4 mm	2–3 cm		
	Stage III	Excision and lymph node dissection		Not discussed
	Stage IV	Excision of primary melanoma and focal resection of internal organs involved with metastatic melanoma (if feasible)		Not discussed

**H&P includes review of systems, symptoms directed exam, full skin examination and lymph node examination*
AAD, American Academy of Dermatology; BAD, British Association of Dermatologists; CBC, complete blood count; CXR, chest X-ray; LDH, lactic dehydrogenase; LFT, liver function tests; NCCN, National Comprehensive Cancer Network; SLNB, sentinel lymph node biopsy.

Pitfalls and their management

- Not all patients with atypical mole syndrome are at equal risk for developing melanoma. The magnitude of the risk depends on factors such as the number of nevi, personal or family history of melanoma, and the presence of dysplastic nevi.
- Prophylactic removal of all atypical moles is not justified. The risk of any individual lesion turning malignant is low. Many melanomas develop de novo, not in association with a dysplastic nevus.
- The entire pigmented lesion should be removed in a biopsy to prevent sampling error and ensure that a small focus of melanoma is not missed.
- Sentinel lymph node biopsy is currently still a diagnostic procedure providing prognostic information—it has no proven therapeutic or survival benefits at this time.
- Most recurrences or metastases of melanoma are detected on physical examination or during a review of systems. Laboratory and imaging studies are of low yield and should be directed based on symptoms.
- Lifelong follow-up is crucial in patients with melanoma because recurrences can occur as long as 20 years after initial diagnosis and treatment. Patients also have an increased risk of developing a second primary melanoma.

SUMMARY

Compared to the general population, individuals with atypical moles are at increased risk for the development of malignant melanomas. Therefore, the management of these patients consists of strategies that could lower this risk and assist in the detection of early melanomas when they are most curable. Patients with atypical moles, or from families with atypical moles and/or melanomas should be educated about the hazards of sun exposure and methods of sun protection for themselves and their families. All patients with atypical melanocytic nevi, whether familial or sporadic, should have total cutaneous examinations at least once a year, beginning during adolescence. Total cutaneous photography creates an objective baseline that can help in lesion assessment during follow-up examinations. Teaching the techniques of cutaneous self-examinations may help in the identification of early melanomas, which can be treated with surgical excision. Thus, a combination of consistent follow-up and patient education is imperative for the most effective management of patients with atypical moles.

REFERENCES

1. Consensus Conference on precursors to malignant melanoma. J Dermatol Surg Oncol 1985; 11:537–542.
2. Friedman RJ, Rigel DS, Kopf AW. Early detection of malignant melanoma: the role of physician examination and self-examination of the skin. CA 1985; 35:130–151.
3. Consensus Development Panel on early melanoma. Diagnosis and treatment of early melanoma. JAMA 1992; 268:1314–1319.
4. Kraemer KH, Green MH. Dysplastic nevus syndrome: familial and sporadic precursors of cutaneous melanoma. Dermatol Clin 1985; 3:225–237.
5. Newton JA, Bataille V, Griffiths K, et al. How common is the atypical mole syndrome phenotype in apparently sporadic melanoma? J Am Acad Dermatol 1993; 29:989–996.
6. Newton JA. Familial melanoma. Clin Exp Dermatol 1993; 18:5–11.
7. Kraemer KH, Greene MH, Tarone R, Elder DE, Clark WH Jr, Guerry D 4th. Dysplastic naevi and cutaneous melanoma risk. Lancet 1983; 2:1076–1077.
8. Kopf AW, Friedman RJ, Rigel DS. Atypical mole syndrome. J Am Acad Dermatol 1990; 22:117–118.
9. Greene MH, Clark WH Jr, Tucker MA, et al. High risk of malignant melanoma in melanoma-prone families with dysplastic nevi. Ann Intern Med 1985; 102:458–465.
10. Lynch HT, Frichot BC III, Lynch JF. Familial atypical mole–melanoma syndrome. J Med Genet 1978; 15:352–356.
11. Clark WH Jr, Reimer RR, Greene M, et al. Origin of familial malignant melanomas from heritable melanocytic lesions. Arch Dermatol 1978; 114:732–738.
12. Huynh PM, Glusac EJ, Alvarez-Franco M, Berwick M, Bolognia JL. Numerous, small, darkly pigmented melanocytic nevi: the cheetah phenotype. J Am Acad Dermatol 2003; 48:707.
13. MacKie RM, English J, Aitchison TC, Fitzsimons CP, Wilson P. The number and distribution of benign pigmented moles (melanocytic nevi) in a healthy British population. Br J Dermatol 1985; 113:167–174.
14. Garbe C, Buttner P, Weiss J, et al. Risk factors for developing cutaneous melanoma and criteria for identifying persons at risk: multicenter case–control study of the central malignant melanoma registry of the German Dermatological Society. J Invest Dermatol 1994; 102:695–699.
15. Garbe C, Buttner P, Weiss J, et al. Associated factors in the prevalence of more than 50 common melanocytic nevi, atypical melanocytic nevi, and actinic lentigines: multicenter case–control study of the central malignant melanoma registry of the German Dermatological Society. J Invest Dermatol 1994; 102:700–705.
16. Harrison SL, MacLennan R, Speare R, et al. Sun exposure and melanocytic naevi in young Australian children. Lancet 1994; 344:1529–1532.
17. Stefanato CM, Romero JB, Kopf AW, Bart RS. Solar nevogenesis: a surrogate for predicting a rise in incidence of malignant melanoma because of ozone depletion. J Am Acad Dermatol 1993; 29:486–487.
18. Kopf AW, Lazar M, Bart RS, Dubin N, Bromberg J. Prevalence of nevocytic nevi on lateral and medial aspects of arms. J Dermatol Surg Oncol 1978; 4:153–158.
19. Kopf AW, Lindsay AC, Rogers GS, Friedman RJ, Rigel DS, Levenstein M. Relationship of nevocytic nevi to sun exposure in dysplastic nevus syndrome. J Am Acad Dermatol 1985; 12:656–662.
20. Kopf AW, Gold RS, Rogers GS, et al. Relationship of lumbosacral nevocytic nevi to sun exposure in dysplastic nevus syndrome. Arch Dermatol 1986; 122:1003–1006.
21. Stierner U. Melanocytes, moles, and melanoma. A study on UV effects. Acta Derm Venereol 1991; 168S:1–31.
22. Rivers JK, MacLennan R, Kelly JW, et al. The Eastern Australian childhood nevus study: prevalence of atypical nevi, congenital nevus-like nevi, and other pigmented lesions. J Am Acad Dermatol 1995; 32:957–963.
23. Abadir MC, Marghoob AA, Slade JS, Salopek TG, Yadav S, Kopf AW. Case–control study of melanocytic nevi on the buttocks in atypical mole syndrome: role of solar radiation in the pathogenesis of atypical moles. J Am Acad Dermatol 1995; 33:31–36.
24. Slade J, Marghoob AA, Salopek TG, et al. Atypical mole syndrome: risk factor for cutaneous malignant melanoma and implications for management. J Am Acad Dermatol 1995; 32:479–494.
25. Halpern AC, Guerry D 4th, Elder DE, et al. Natural history of dysplastic nevi. J Am Acad Dermat 1993; 29:51–57.
26. Tucker, MA, Fraser MC, Goldstein AM, et al. A natural history of melanomas and dysplastic nevi: an atlas of lesions in melanoma prone families. Cancer 2002; 94:3192–3209.
27. Swerdlow AJ, English J, MacKie RM, et al. Benign melanocytic naevi as a risk factor for malignant melanoma. Br Med J 1986; 292:1555–1559.
28. Holly EA, Kelly JW, Shpall SN, et al. Number of melanocytic nevi as a major risk factor for malignant melanoma. J Am Acad Dermatol 1987; 17:459–468.
29. Grob JJ, Gouvernet J, Aymar D, et al. Count of benign melanocytic nevi as a major indicator of risk for nonfamilial nodular and superficial spreading melanoma. Cancer 1990; 66:387–395.
30. Halpern AC, Guerry D 4th, Elder DE, et al. Dysplastic nevi as risk markers of sporadic (nonfamilial) melanoma: a case–control study. Arch Dermatol 1991; 127:995–999.
31. Roush GC, Nordlund JJ, Forget B, et al. Independence of dysplastic nevi from total nevi in determining risk for nonfamilial melanoma. Prev Med 1988; 17:273–279.
32. Garbe C, Kruger S, Stadler R, et al. Markers and relative risk in a German population for developing malignant melanoma. Int J Dermatol 1989; 28:517–523.
33. Augustsson A, Stierner U, Rosdahl I, et al. Common and dysplastic naevi as risk factors for cutaneous malignant melanoma in a Swedish population. Acta Derm Venereol (Stockh) 1991; 71:518–524.
34. Garbe C, Buttner P, Weiss J, et al. Risk factors for developing cutaneous melanoma and criteria for identifying persons at risk: multicenter case–control study of the central malignant melanoma registry of the German Dermatological Society. J Invest Dermatol 1994; 102:695–699.
35. Tucker MA, Halpern A, Holly EA, et al. Clinically recognized dysplastic nevi. A central risk factor for cutaneous melanoma. JAMA 1997; 277:1439–1444.
36. Marghoob AA. The dangers of the atypical mole (dysplastic nevus) syndrome. Teaching at risk patients to protect themselves from melanoma. Postgrad Med 1999; 105:147–148, 151–152, 154.
37. Rigel DS, Rivers JK, Kopf AW, et al. Dysplastic nevi: markers for increased risk for melanoma. Cancer 1989; 63:386–389.
38. Sagebiel, RW. Melanocytic nevi in histologic association with primary cutaneous melanoma of superficial spreading and nodular types: effect of tumor thickness. J Invest Dermatol 1993; 100:322S–325S.
39. Black WC. Residual dysplastic and other nevi in superficial spreading melanoma. Clinical correlations and association with sun damage. Cancer 1988; 62:163–173.
40. Novakovic B, Clark WH Jr, Fears TR, Fraser MC, Tucker MA. Melanocytic nevi, dysplastic nevi, and malignant melanoma in children from melanoma-prone families. J Am Acad Dermatol 1995; 33:631–636.
41. MacKie RM, McHenry P, Hole D, et al. Accelerated detection with prospective surveillance for cutaneous malignant melanoma in high-risk groups. Lancet 1993; 341:1618–1620.
42. Garbe C, Kruger S, Stadler R, Guggenmoos-Holzmann I, Orfanos CE. Markers and relative risk in a German population for developing malignant melanoma. Int J Dermatol 1989; 28:517–523.
43. Marghoob AA, Kopf AW, Rigel DS, et al. Risk of cutaneous malignant melanoma in patients with 'classic' atypical-mole syndrome: A case–control study. Arch Derm 1994; 130:993–998.
44. Marghoob AA, Slade J, Salopek TG, Rigel DS, Bart RS. Risk of developing multiple primary cutaneous melanomas in patients with the classic atypical-mole syndrome: a case–control study. Brit J Derm 1996; 135:704–711.
45. Tucker MA, Fraser MC, Goldstein AM, et al. Risk of melanoma and other cancers in melanoma-prone families. J Invest Dermatol 1993; 100:350S–355S.
46. Halpern, AC, Guerry D 4th, Elder DE, et al. A cohort study of melanoma in patients with dysplastic nevi. J Invest Dermatol 1993; 100:346S–349S.

47. Sober AJ, Burstein JM. Precursors to skin cancer. Cancer 1995; 75:645–650.

48. Rigel DS, Rivers JK, Friedman RJ, Kopf AW. Risk gradient for malignant melanoma in individuals with dysplastic nevi. Lancet 1988; 1:352–353.

49. MacKie RM, Freudenberger T, Aitchison TC. Personal risk-factor chart for cutaneous melanoma. Lancet 1989; 2:487–490.

50. Rhodes AR, Weinstock MA, Fitzpatrick TB, Mihm MC Jr, Sober AJ. Risk factors for cutaneous melanoma. A practical method of recognizing predisposed individuals. JAMA 1987; 258:3146–3154.

51. Tiersten AD, Grin CM, Kopf AW, et al. Prospective follow-up for malignant melanoma in patients with atypical-mole (dysplastic-nevus) syndrome. J Dermatol Surg Oncol 1991; 17:44–48.

52. Schneider JS, Moore II DH, Sagebiel RW. Risk factors for melanoma incidence in prospective follow-up: the importance of atypical (dysplastic) nevi. Arch Dermatol 1994; 130:1002–1007.

53. Halpern AC. The use of whole body photography in a pigmented lesion clinic. Dermatol Surg 2000; 26:1175–1180.

54. Kelly JW, Yeatman JM, Regalia C, Mason G, Henham AP. A high incidence of melanoma found in patients with multiple dysplastic nevi by photographic surveillance. Med J Aust 1997; 167:191–194.

55. Rigel DS, Friedman RJ, Kopf AW, et al. Importance of complete cutaneous examination for the detection of malignant melanoma. J Am Acad Dermatol 1986; 14:857–860.

56. Tucker MA, Greene MH, Clark WH Jr, Kraemer KH, Fraser MC, Elder DE. Dysplastic nevi on the scalp of prepubertal children from melanoma-prone families. J Pediatr 1983; 103:65–67.

57. Benmeir P, Baruchin A, Lusthaus S, et al. Melanoma of the scalp: the invisible killer. Plast Reconstr Surg 1995; 95:496–500.

58. Geller AC, Koh HK, Miller DR, Clapp RW, Mercer MB, Lew RA. Use of health services before the diagnosis of melanoma: implications for early detection and screening. J Gen Intern Med 1992; 7:2154–2157.

59. Romero JB, Stefanato CM, Kopf AW, Bart RS. Follow-up recommendations for patients with stage I malignant melanoma. J Dermatol Surg Oncol 1994; 20:175–178.

60. Marks R, Dorevitch AP, Mason G. Do all melanomas come from 'moles'? A study of the histological association between melanocytic nevi and melanoma. Aus J Dermatol 1990; 31:77–80.

61. Masri GD, Clark WH Jr, Guerry D IV, Halpern A, Thompson CJ, Elder DE. Screening and surveillance of patients at high risk for malignant melanoma result in detection of earlier disease. J Am Acad Dermatol 1990; 22:1042–1048.

62. Goldstein AM, Fraser MC, Clark WH, Tucker MA. Age at diagnosis and transmission of invasive melanoma in 23 families with cutaneous malignant melanoma/dysplastic nevi. J Natl Cancer Inst 1994; 86:1385–1390.

63. Crijns MB, Vink J, Van Hees CLM, Bergman W, Vermeer BJ. Dysplastic nevi. Occurrence in first- and second-degree relatives of patients with 'sporadic' dysplastic nevus syndrome. Arch Dermatol 1991; 127:1346–1351.

64. Albert LS, Rhodes AR, Sober AJ. Dysplastic melanocytic nevi and cutaneous melanoma: markers of increased melanoma risk for affected persons and blood relatives. J Am Acad Dermatol 1990; 22:69–75.

65. Bergman W, Palan A, Went LN. Clinical and genetic studies in six Dutch kindreds with the dysplastic nevus syndrome. Ann Hum Genet 1986; 50:249–258.

66. McCarthy JM, Rootman J, Horseman D, White VA. Conjunctival and uveal melanoma in the dysplastic nevus syndrome. Surv Ophthalmol 1993; 37:377–386.

67. Vink J, Crijns MB, Mooy CM, Bergman W, Oosterhuis JA, Went LN. Ocular melanoma in families with dysplastic nevus syndrome. J Am Acad Dermatol 1990; 23:858–862.

68. Friedman RJ, Rodriguez-Sains R, Jakobiec F. Ophthalmologic oncology: conjunctival malignant melanoma in association with sporadic dysplastic nevus syndrome. J Dermatol Surg Oncol 1987; 13:31–34.

69. Greene MH, Sanders RJ, Chu FC, Clark WH Jr, Elder DE, Cogan DG. The familial occurrence of cutaneous melanoma, intraocular melanoma, and the dysplastic nevus syndrome. Am J Ophthalmol 1983; 96:238–245.

70. Abramson DH, Rodriguez-Sains RS, Rubman R. B-K mole syndrome: cutaneous and ocular malignant melanoma. Arch Ophthalmol 1980; 98:1397–1399.

71. Bataille V, Bishop DT, Cuzick J, et al. Conjunctival melanoma in the atypical mole syndrome. Melanoma Res 1993; 3:61.

72. Rodriguez-Sains RS. Ocular findings in patients with dysplastic nevus syndrome. An update. Dermatol Clinics 1991; 9:723–728.

73. Leow YH, Tham SN. UV-protective sunglasses for UVA irradiation protection. Int J Dermatol 1995; 34:808–810.

74. Stoltz W, Braun-Falco O, Bilek P, Landthaler M, Cognetta AB. Basis of dermatoscopic and skin surface microscopy. In: Color atlas of dermoscopy. Cambridge: Blackwell 1994; 7–10.

75. Steiner A, Binder M, Schemper M, Wolff K, Pehamberger H. Statistical evaluation of epiluminescence microscopy criteria for melanocytic pigmented skin lesions. J Am Acad Dermatol 1993; 29:581–588.

76. Binder M, Schwarz M, Winkler A, et al. Epiluminescence microscopy. A useful tool for the diagnosis of pigmented skin lesions for formally trained dermatologists. Arch Dermatol 1995; 131:286–291.

77. Elwood JM, Willianson C, Stapleton PJ. Malignant melanoma in relation to moles, pigmentation, and exposure to fluorescent and other lighting sources. Br J Cancer 1986; 53:65–74.

78. Armstrong BK. Epidemiology of malignant melanoma: intermittent or total accumulated exposure to the sun? J Dermatol Surg Oncol 1988; 14:835–849.

79. Kopf AW, Bart RS, Rodriguez-Sains RS. Sunlight and malignant melanoma. J Dermatol Surg Oncol 1977; 3:45–48.

80. Jung EG, Bohnert E, Boonen H. Dysplastic nevus syndrome: ultraviolet hypermutability confirmed in vitro by elevated sister chromatid exchanges. Dermatologica 1986; 173:297–300.

81. Richard MA, Grob JJ, Gouvernet J, et al. Role of sun exposure on nevus. First study in age–sex phenotype-controlled populations. Arch Dermatol 1993; 129:1280–1285.

82. Kelly JW, Rivers JK, MacLennan R, Harrison S, Lewis AE, Tate BJ. Sunlight: a major factor associated with the development of melanocytic nevi in Australian school children. J Am Acad Dermatol 1994; 30:40–48.

83. Menter JM, Hollins TD, Sayre RM, Etemadi AA, Willis I, Hughs SN. Protection against UV photocarcinogenesis by fabric materials. J Am Acad Dermatol 1994; 31:711–716.

84. Naylor MF, Boyd A, Smith DW, Cameron GS, Hubbard D, Nelder KH. High sun protection factor sunscreens in the suppression of actinic neoplasia. Arch Dermatol 1995; 131:170–175.

85. Thompson SC, Jolley D, Marks R. Reduction of solar keratoses by regular sunscreen use. N Engl J Med 1993; 329:1147–1151.

86. Whitmore SE, Morison WL. Prevention of UV-B induced immunosuppression in humans by a high sun protection factor sunscreen. Arch Dermatol 1995; 131:1128–1133

87. Gallagher RP, Rivers JK, Lee TK, Bajdik CD, McLean DI, Coldman AJ. Broad-spectrum sunscreen use and development of new nevi in white children: a randomized controlled trial. JAMA 2000; 283: 2955–2960.

88. Pathak MA. Sunscreens: topical and systemic approaches for protection of human skin against harmful effects of solar radiation. J Am Acad Dermatol 1982; 7:285–312.

89. Westerdahl J, Olsson H, Masback A, Ingvar C, Jonsson N. Is the use of sunscreens a risk factor for malignant melanoma? Melanoma Res 1995; 5:59–65.

90. Garland CF, Garland FC, Gorham ED. Rising trends in melanoma. A hypothesis concerning sunscreen effectiveness. Ann Epidemiol 1993; 3:103–110.

91. Wolf P, Donawho CK, Kripke ML. Effect of sunscreens on UV radiation-induced enhancement of melanoma growth in mice. J Natl Cancer Inst 1994; 86:99–105.

92. Koh HK, Lew RA. Sunscreens and melanoma: implications for prevention. J Natl Cancer Inst 1994; 86:78–79.

93. Autier P, Dore JF, Lejeune F, et al. Cutaneous malignant melanoma and exposure to sunlamps or sunbeds: an EORTC multicenter case–control study in Belgium, France, and Germany. Int J Cancer 1994; 58:809–813.

94. Rossi JS, Blais LM, Redding CA, Weinstock MA. Preventing skin cancer through behavior change: implications for interventions. Dermatol Clin 1995; 13:613–622.

95. Grob JJ, Guglielmina C, Gouvernet J, Zarour H, Noe C, Bonerandi JJ. Study of sunbathing habits in children and adolescents: application to the prevention of melanoma. Dermatol 1993; 186:94–98.

96. Somach SC, Taira JW, Pitha JV, Everett MA. Pigmented lesions in actinically damaged skin. Histopathologic comparison of biopsy and excisional specimens. Arch Dermatol 1996; 132:1297–1302.

97. Ng PC, Barzilai DA, Ismail SA, et al. Evaluating invasive cutaneous melanoma: is the initial biopsy representative of the final depth? J Am Acad Dermatol 2003; 48:420–424.

98. Duray PH, Livolsi VA. Recurrent dysplastic nevus following shave excision. J Dermatol Surg Oncol 1984; 10:811–815.

99. Bondi EE, Clark WH Jr, Elder D, Guerry D, Greene MH. Topical chemotherapy of dysplastic melanocytic nevi with 5% fluorouracil. Arch Dermatol 1981; 117:89–92.

100. Halpern AC, Schuchter LM, Elder DE, et al. Effects of topical tretinoin on dysplastic nevi. J Clin Oncol 1994; 12:1028–1035.

101. Edwards L, Jaffe P. The effect of topical tretinoin on dysplastic nevi. A preliminary trial. Arch Dermatol 1990; 126:494–499.

102. Edwards L. Meyskens F, Levine N. Effect of oral isotretinoin on dysplastic nevi. J Am Acad Dermatol 1989; 20:257–260.

103. Dellavalle RP, Nicholas MK, Schilling LM. Melanoma chemoprevention: a role for statins or fibrates? Am J Ther 2003; 10:203–210.

104. Denkert C, Kobel M, Berger S, et al. Expression of cyclooxygenase 2 in human malignant melanoma. Cancer Res 2001; 61:303–308.

105. Wolf IH, Smolle J, Binder B, Cerroni L, Richtig E, Kerl H. Topical imiquimod in the treatment of metastatic melanoma to skin. Arch Dermatol 2003; 139:279–276.

106. Jemal A, Murray T, Samuels A, et al. Cancer statistics, 2003. CA Cancer J Clin 2003; 53:5–26.

107. Rigel DS, Carucci JA. Malignant melanoma: prevention, early detection, and treatment in the 21st century. CA Cancer J Clin 2000; 50:215–236.

108. Balch CM, Buzaid AC, Soong SJ, et al. Final version of the American Joint Committee on Cancer Staging System for cutaneous melanoma. J Clin Oncol 2001; 19:3635–3648.

109. Houghton A, Coit D, Bloomer W, et al. NCCN melanoma practice guidelines. National Comprehensive Cancer Network. Oncology (Huntingt) 1998; 12:153–177.

110. Gershenwald JE, Thompson W, Mansfield PF, et al. Multi-institutional melanoma lymphatic mapping experience: the prognostic value of sentinel lymph node status in 612 stage I or II melanoma patients. J Clin Oncol 1999; 17:976–983.

111. Cascinelli N, Belli F, Santinami M, et al. Sentinel lymph node biopsy in cutaneous melanoma: the WHO Melanoma Program experience. Ann Surg Oncol 2000; 7:469–474.

112. Clary BM, Brady MS, Lewis JJ, Coit, DG. Sentinel lymph node biopsy in the management of patients with primary cutaneous melanoma: review of a large single-institutional experience with an emphasis on recurrence. Ann Surg 2001; 233:250–258.

113. McMasters KM, Wong SL, Edwards MJ, et al. Factors that predict the presence of sentinel lymph node metastasis in patients with melanoma. Surgery 2001; 130:151–156.

114. Wagner JD, Gordon MS, Chuang TY, et al. Predicting sentinel and residual lymph node basin disease after sentinel lymph node biopsy for melanoma. Cancer 2000; 89:453–462.

115. Cascinelli N, Morabito A, Santinami M, Mackie RM, Belli F. Immediate or delayed dissection of regional nodes in patients with melanoma of the trunk: a randomized trial. Lancet 1998; 20; 351:793–796.

116. Kirkwood JM, Strawderman MH, Ernstoff MS, et al. Interferon alfa–2b adjuvant therapy of high-risk resected cutaneous melanoma: the Eastern Cooperative Oncology Group Trial EST 1684. J Clin Oncol 1996; 14:7–17.

117. Cole BF, Gelber RD, Kirkwood JM, et al. Quality-of-life-adjusted survival analysis of interferon alfa-2b adjuvant treatment of high-risk resected cutaneous melanoma: an Eastern Cooperative Oncology Group study. J Clin Oncol 1996; 14: 2666–2673.

118. Creagan ET, Dalton RJ, Ahmann DL, et al. Randomized, surgical adjuvant clinical trial of recombinant interferon alfa-2a in selected patients with malignant melanoma. J Clin Oncol 1995; 13:2776–2783.

119. Kirkwood JM, Ibrahim JG, Sondak VK, et al. High- and low-dose interferon alfa-2b in high-risk melanoma: first analysis of intergroup trial E1690/S9111/C9190. J Clin Oncol 2000; 18:2444–2458.

120. Kirkwood JM, Ibrahim JG, Sosman JA, et al. High-dose interferon alfa-2b significantly prolongs relapse-free and overall survival compared with the GM2-KLH/QS-21 vaccine in patients with resected stage IIB–III melanoma: results of intergroup trial E1694/S9512/C509801. J Clin Oncol 2001; 19:2370–2380.

121. Inman JL, Russell GB, Savage P, et al. Low-dose adjuvant interferon for stage III malignant melanoma. Am Surg 2003; 69:127–130.

122. Cascinelli N, Belli F, MacKie RM, et al. Effect of long-term adjuvant therapy with interferon alpha-2a in patients with regional node metastases from cutaneous melanoma: a randomized trial. Lancet 2001; 358:866–869.

123. Hersey P, Coates AS, McCarthy WH, et al. Adjuvant immunotherapy of patients with high-risk melanoma using vaccinia viral lysates of melanoma: results of a randomized trial. J Clin Oncol 2002; 20:4181–4190.

124. Wallack MK, Sivanandham M, Balch CM, et al. Surgical adjuvant active specific immunotherapy for patients with stage III melanoma: the final analysis of data from a phase III, randomized, double-blind, multicenter vaccinia melanoma oncolysate trial. J Am Coll Surg 1998; 187:69–77.

125. Bystryn JC, Zeleniuch-Jacquotte A, Oratz R, et al. Double-blind trial of a polyvalent, shed-antigen, melanoma vaccine. Clin Cancer Res 2001; 7:1882–1887.

126. Leo F, Cagini L, Rocmans P, et al. Lung metastases from melanoma: when is surgical treatment warranted? Br J Cancer 2000; 83:569–572.

127. Essner R. Surgical treatment of malignant melanoma. Surg Clin North Am 2003; 83:109–156.

128. Wronski M, Arbit E. Surgical treatment of brain metastases from melanoma: a retrospective study of 91 patients. J Neurosurg 2000; 93:9–18.

129. Falkson CI, Ibrahim J, Kirkwood JM, et al. Phase III trial of dacarbazine versus dacarbazine with interferon alpha-2b versus dacarbazine with tamoxifen versus dacarbazine with interferon alpha-2b and tamoxifen in patients with metastatic malignant melanoma: an Eastern Cooperative Oncology Group study. J Clin Oncol 1998; 16:1743–1751.

130. Young AM, Marsden J, Goodman A, et al. Prospective randomized comparison of dacarbazine (DTIC) versus DTIC plus interferon-alpha (IFN-alpha) in metastatic melanoma. Clin Oncol (R Coll Radiol) 2001; 13:458–465.

131. Mitchell MS. Perspective on allogeneic melanoma lysates in active specific immunotherapy. Semin Oncol 1998; 25:623–635.

132. Stam-Posthuma JJ, Van Duinen C, Scheffer E, et al. Multiple primary melanomas. J Am Acad Dermatol 2001; 44:22–27.

133. Titus-Ernstoff L, Duray PH, Ernstoff MS, Barnhill RL, Horn PL, Kirkwood JM. Dysplastic nevi in association with multiple primary melanoma. Cancer Res 1988; 15; 48:1016–1018.

134. Romero JB, Stefanato CM, Kopf AW, et al. Follow-up recommendations for patients with stage I malignant melanoma. J Dermatol Surg Oncol 1994; 20:175–178.

135. Huang CL, Provost N, Marghoob AA, et al. Laboratory tests and imaging studies in patients with cutaneous malignant melanoma. J Am Acad Dermatol 1998; 39:451–463.

136. Mooney MM, Kulas M, McKinley B, et al. Impact on survival by method of recurrence detection in stage I and II cutaneous melanoma. Ann Surg Oncol 1998; 5:54–63.

137. Balch CM, Soong SJ, Murad TM, et al. A multifactorial analysis of melanoma. IV. Prognostic factors in 200 melanoma patients with distant metastases (stage III). J Clin Oncol 1983; 1:126–134.

138. Sober AJ, Chuang TY, Duvic M, et al. Guidelines of care for primary cutaneous melanoma. J Am Acad Dermatol 2001; 45:579–586.

139. Roberts DL, Anstey AV, Barlow RJ, et al. UK guidelines for the management of cutaneous melanoma. Br J Dermatol 2002; 146:7–17.

Index

Notes
Page numbers in *italics* refer to figures: page numbers in **bold** refer to information in tables.
Abbreviations
BCC – basal cell carcinoma
BTX-A – botulinum toxin-A
Er:YAG laser – erbium:yttrium-aluminium-garnet laser
IPL – intense pulsed light
KTP laser – potassium-titanyl-phosphate laser
SCC – squamous cell carcinoma
SMAS – superficial musculoaponeurotic system

A
Abbe cross-lip flap, 348
perioral region reconstruction, 392–393
postoperative care, 361
technique, 359, *360*
ABCD features
dysplastic nevi, 821, *822*
melanoma, 828
abdomen, liposuction, 524–526, **525**, *527*
ablative laser skin resurfacing, 612–618
carbon dioxide laser, 431, 612–613, *613*
Er:YAG laser *vs.*, 616–617
history/development, 611–612
optimizing outcomes, 615–616
side effects, 615, **615**, *616*
contraindicated medications, 617
Er:YAG-carbon dioxide hybrid laser system, 614–615
Er:YAG laser, 613–615, *614*
ablation depth, 614
advantages, 614
carbon dioxide laser *vs.*, 616–617
disadvantages, 614
dyspigmentation, 614
history/development, 612
modulated, 614–615
optimizing outcomes, 616–617
photodamage, 614
preoperative preparation, 612
pulse duration, 614
short-pulsed, 613–614
side effects, 616, 617
superficial epidermal/dermal lesions, 614
optimizing outcomes, 615–617
patient compliance, 618
patient expectations, 618
patient selection, 617
pitfalls/management, 617–618
postoperative care, 617
preoperative preparation, 612
scar revision, 408
technical aspects, 612–615
abscesses
infected, 220–221
inflamed, *220*, 220–221
irrigation, 220
packing of wound, 220, *220*
postoperative care, 222
stab incision, 220, *220*
absorbable sutures, 63, 227–229, **228**
biopsies, 211
follicular unit hair transplantation donor closure, 561, *561*
monofilament, 63
absorption spectrum, chromophores, 579
absorptive dressings, 119
Accreditation Association of Ambulatory Health Care (AAAHC), 159, **159, 160**
healthcare standards, *161*
accreditation survey, 159–161, *160*, **161**
acetic acid, delayed grafts, 374
acitretin, skin cancer prevention, 811
acne
carbon dioxide laser skin resurfacing side effect, 615
cryosurgery, 196
deep (phenol) chemical peels, 476
dermabrasion, 592
pitfalls, 596, 597
keloids, 706, *715*, 716
prevalence, 617
Radiesse, 455
superficial chemical peels, 467
actinic keratoses. *see also* squamous cell carcinoma (SCC)
organ transplant recipients, 806
treatment, *814*
prevention, imiquimod, 811
as SCC precursor, 793
treatment
body chemical peels, 477, *478*
cryosurgery, 192, 197
deep (phenol) chemical peels, 476
5-fluorouracil, 793
imiquimod, 793
medium-depth chemical peels, 471, 472, *472*, *473*
photodynamic therapy, 793
tropical tretinoin, 811
actinomycin, 108
acute wounds. *see* wound(s)
Adaptic
composite grafts, 374
full-thickness grafts, 366, 368, *369*
adhesive tape, ellipse excision, 263
adrenaline. *see* epinephrine (adrenaline)
Adson forceps, 61
advancement flaps, 314–316. *see also* island pedicle flaps; rotation flaps
advantages, 314
bilateral, 314–315
bilateral T-plasty (A-T flap), 316
basis, *316*
bipedicle, 320
forehead wound, *321*
Burow's, 316, *318*
cheek, 286–287, *288*, 390
forehead and temple reconstruction, 385
H-plasty, 314–316
applications, 315–316
basis, *315*
eyebrow defects, 315
mucosal, 320
nose reconstruction, 387
O–T rotation flap, 316, *317*
perioral region reconstruction, 392
scalp reconstruction, 384
scar formation prevention, 402
unilateral, 314
basis, *315*
positioning, *315*
Advanta, **445**, 456–457
aesthetics
island pedicle flaps, 319–320
Mohs micrographic surgery, 790
random pattern cutaneous flaps, 335
age/aging, 425–435, *432*
artist's perception, 428
etiology
baseline elasticity, 430–431
craniofacial skeletal aging, 426, *426*
epidermal and dermal aging, 425
external aging, 425
facial shape changes, 428, *428*
gravitational aging myth, 428–429
internal aging, 425
lean aging face, sagging, 429, *430*
mimetic muscle aging, 425
oxidative damage, 425
skin/muscle interaction, 425–426
ultraviolet (UV) damage, 425
wound infection development, 138
facial animation, 426, *426*
facial atrophy pattern, 429, *430*
facial hypertrophy pattern, 429, *430*
fat distribution, 426–427, 427, *427*
atrophy, 427
autologous fat transfer, 431, *433*
body fat *vs.*, *429*, 429–430
hypertrophy, 427
redistribution, 426
sagging, 429
young *vs.*, 426–427, *427*
management
cosmetic management, 431, *432* (*see also specific problems and procedures*)
implants, 431
liposuction, 429
microsuction of fat hypertrophy, 431, *434*
mid-face lifting, 431
optimizing outcomes, 431, *432*
pitfalls/management, 428–431
practical applications, 431–432
sagging correction, 430, *431*

age/aging, (*cont'd*)
structural facial rejuvenation, 431–432
technical aspects, 425–428
photographic documentation of patient when younger, 432, *434*
AIDS. *see* HIV infection
Alabama, dermatology office accreditation, **170**
ala nasi, *8*
defect repair, 350
alar base nasolabial, *8*
alcohol abstention, follicular unit hair transplantation, 556
alcohol-based preparations
surgical hand scrub, 27–28, *28*, **28**
surgical site preparation, 31
alcohol, infection prevention, 139
alexandrite lasers
laser hair removal, 583, **584,** 586
long pulsed
hemangiomas, 634
vascular lesions, **629**
port-wine stain removal, 634
Q-switched lasers, 600, 601
wavelengths, 627
Alford's technique. *see* Z-plasty
alginate dressings, 119, **119,** *122*, 122–123, **133**
allergic contact dermatitis, ear piercing, 303
allergic reactions
anesthesia, 54
bovine collagen, 458
identification in preoperative assessment, 74
post-biopsies, 211–212
sutures, 227
Alloderm, **445,** 455
historical aspects, 439
preoperative preparation, 440
allografts, 125
wound dressing, 123
alpha hydroxy acids (AHAs)
chemical peels, 464
preoperative preparation, 465
superficial chemical peels, *469*, 469–470, **470**
Apligraf, *126*, 126–127
alternating current, electrosurgery, 178–179
aluminum chloride, 249, **252**
aluminum oxide crystals, 592–593
ambulatory phlebectomy, 649, 651
ambulatory surgery center (ASC) approval, 148
American Academy of Cosmetic Surgery, 592
American Academy of Dermatology, 835, **836**
American Academy of Dermatology (AAD)
chemical peels guidelines, 465
dermatology office accreditation, 171
liposuction surgical suite and set-up guidelines, 522
American Association for Accreditation of Ambulatory Surgical Facilities (AAAASF), 159
American Board of Hair Restoration Surgery (ABHRS), 550
American Health Information Management Association, 85
American Heart Association guidelines, 143–144
American Joint Committee on Cancer (AJCC), melanoma staging, 832, **832**
sentinel lymph node biopsy, 834
amides, anesthesia. *see* anesthesia, amides
aminocaproic acid (AMICAR), **253**
aminolevulinic acid (ALA), 580
amoxicillin, 141
amputation, lower limb, 745
Amstat (tranexamic acid), **253**
anagen hair growth, 576, *577*
analgesia
dressings, 132
laser surgery, 607
anaphylaxis, anesthesia, 54
androgenic alopecia, 551–553, **552**. *see also* follicular unit hair transplantation
diffuse patterned alopecia, 552
diffuse unpatterned alopecia, 552
hair pull test, 553
hair type changes, 576
Ludwig Classification, 552
miniaturization, 551, *551*
Norwood classification, 551–552, *552*, 553
telogen effluvium, 553
anesthesia, 39–58. *see also specific anesthetics*
additive substances, 41–43, **42**
adverse effects, 54–56
allergies, 789
medication interaction, 55, **55**
systemic toxicity, 55, **55**
amides, 40, **40**
pharmacological properties, 40, **41**
structure, *40*
applications, 56–57
benign subcutaneous lesions, 768, *769*
for biopsies, 205–206, 206
dermabrasion (*see* dermabrasion)
elliptical excision, 261
epidermal cysts, 217
fat pad extraction upper-eyelid blepharoplasty, 682
iontophoresis, 45
laser surgery, 601
lipomas, 214
nail surgery, 721, *722*
pulsed dye laser treatment of port-wine stains, 633
random pattern cutaneous flaps (*see* random pattern cutaneous flaps)
soft-tissue augmentation, 440–441
transconjunctival lower-eyelid blepharoplasty, 683
transcutaneous lower-eyelid blepharoplasty, 684–685
upper-eyelid blepharoplasty, 676
upper-eyelid blepharoplasty fat pad extraction, *682*
use in incision, draining and exteriorization, 213
vascular lesions laser/light treatment, 640
children, 56, **56**
classification, 40, **40**
esters, 40, **40**
pharmacological properties, 40, **41**
structure, *40*
field block, 46, *46*
practical applications, 56
history, 39
infiltrative techniques, 45–47
mechanism of action, 40–41
nerve fiber categories, 41, **42**
optimizing outcomes, 52
physiology, 40
pitfalls/management, 53–56
pregnancy, 40
bupivacaine, 55
epinephrine, 42
ring block, 46, *46*
practical applications, 56
structure, 39–40, *40*
techniques, 43–51
local (*see below*)
topical (*see below*)
tumescent (*see below*)
types, **41** (*see also specific types*)
benzyl alcohol, 54–55
combined, 42–43
diphenhydramine, 54–55
esters (*see above*)
general, 648
hemostatic (*see* hemostasis)
metoclopramide, 55
nerve block (*see* facial nerve (VIIth cranial); nerve blocks)
ophthalmic, 45
tramadol, 55
anesthesia, local, 45–46
allergy identification, 74
autologous collagen, 449
for biopsies, 205
elliptical excision, 261
follicular unit hair transplantation, 558, 559, **559**
hyaluronic acid gel injection, 452
laser surgery, 601
Mohs micrographic surgery, 782
random pattern cutaneous flaps, 336
anesthesia, topical, **43,** 43–45
benzocaine, 43, **43**
Betacaine-LA, 45
for biopsies, 205–206
cocaine, 43, **43**
cryoanesthesia, 43, **44**
EMLA, 44, **44**
hyaluronic acid gel injection, 452
laser hair removal, 585
lidocaine, **43,** 44, **44**
LMX, **44,** 44–45
practical application, 57
practical applications, 57
S-Caine patch, 45
S-Caine peel, 45
tetracaine, **44,** 45
topicaine, **44,** 45
anesthesia, tumescent, 46, **46**
autologous fat transfer, 535, 537
dermabrasion, 594
endovenous ablation, 655
radiofrequency closure of veins, 648, 649, *651*
radiofrequency with ambulatory phlebectomy, 649, 651
hemostasis, 248, 254–255
liposuction, 46, 513, 523–524, **524,** 528
minimum incision face lift, 657, 660–661, 662, *662*
neck liposuction, 693–694
practical applications, 57
random pattern cutaneous flaps, 336
angioedemas, **571**
angiofibromas, 592
angiogenesis, 108–109, *109*
acute wound dressings, 118
growth factors, 108–109, **109**
angiosarcomas, 796
angry patients, 415
angular artery, face, *15*

ankle nerve block, 51, *53*
ankle-to-brachial index (ABI), leg ulcers, 749, *750*
anterior button earlobe keloids, 711
anthropometric landmarks, 10, *12*. *see also specific landmarks*
antiandrogenic medications, 578
antibiotic(s), 137–146
  allergy identification, 74
  applications, 140–145
    endocarditis prophylaxis, 142–145, **144**
    epidermal cysts, 218
    hidradenitis suppurativa, 221
    indwelling device prophylaxis, 144–145
    leg ulcers, 753
    during pregnancy, 68
    soft tissue prostheses, 145
    vascular graft implantation, 145
  Centers for Disease Control and Prevention, 138
  National Nosocomial Infections Surveillance, 138
  optimizing outcomes, 145
  oral/systemic
    delayed grafts, 374
    follicular unit hair transplantation, 556
  personnel preparation, 139–140
  postoperative care, 142, 145, 339
  preoperative preparation, 139–140
  prophylaxis, 137–139, 140–142, **141**
    autologous fat transfer, 537, 546
    for biopsies, 205
    elliptical excision, 260, 269
    in patients with cardiovascular disease, 72
    surgical suite preparation, 139–140
    wound infection prevention, 140
  resistance, 137, 138
    leg ulcers, 753
  surgical site infection prevention, 137
  topical
    biopsies, 205
    wound infection prevention, 141–142
  wound classification, 140, **140**
anticoagulants
  cutaneous surgery risk, 73–74
  discontinuation
    blepharoplasty, 675, 687
    elliptical excision, 259–260
  Mohs micrographic surgery, 781
  random pattern cutaneous flap contraindication, 313
antilymphocyte antibodies, **804**
  immunosuppression induction, 802
antimicrobials
  dressings, 127
  leg ulcers, 753
  post-dermabrasion prophylaxis, 595
antiphospholipid syndrome (lupus anticoagulant syndrome), 746
antiseptic agents, 26
  dressings, 117
  leg ulcers, 753
  surgical hand scrub, 27–28, **28**
antiviral prophylaxis
  chemical peels, 465
  post-dermabrasion, 595
Apesos' technique, 293, *295*
Apligraf, 375
  leg ulcers, 761
  venous ulcers, 131
apocrine hidrocystoma, 219–220, *220*
  optimizing outcomes, 221–222
  postoperative care, 222
aponeurosis, 6
apoptosis, keloids, 707
appearance, psychiatric examination, 414
aprotinin (Trasylol), **253**
Aptos threads, facial soft tissue lifting, 670–671
  before and after photographs, *670, 671*
  results, *670*, 671, *671*
  technique, *670*, 670–671
Aquacel, 123
arachidonic acid, 104
Argamaso's technique, 298, *299*
argon laser, 599
Arizona, dermatology office accreditation, **165, 170**
arms
  liposuction, 526, 528
  reconstruction, 395–396
Arora's technique, 294, *296*
Artecoll, **444,** 453–454, *454, 455*
  allergic reaction, 458–459
  historical aspects, 438–439
  pitfalls, 458, 459
  polymethylmethacrylate, 453, *453*
Artefill. *see* Artecoll
arterial cutaneous flaps. *see* axial pattern flaps
arterial ulcers
  etiology, 744–745, *745*
  postoperative care/wound care, 131
  prevention, 751
artificial nails, 733
artificial skin equivalents, 282
aseptic technique, 25–37
  history, 25–26
  normal flora, 26
  pitfalls/management, 35
  preoperative preparation, 27–32 (*see also* patient preparation)
    environmental cleaning, 31–32
    patient, 30–31
    surgical instrument sterilization, 32
    surgical personnel (*see* personnel preparation)
  resources, online, 37
  surgical site infection, 26–27
  techniques and optimizing outcomes, 32–35
    draping, 33
    face mask, 33
    hair removal, 33
    instrument cleaning and sterilization, 33–34
    instrument packaging and quality assurance, 34, *34*
    sterile field maintenance, 34, *34*
    surgical gloves, 33
    surgical hand scrub, 32–33
    surgical site preparation, 33
    surgical technique, 34–35
    wound dressings, 35
aspiration pump, liposuction, 522
aspirin
  hemostasis impairment, **247,** 248, 259
  random pattern cutaneous flap contraindications, 313
  venous ulcers, 752
asymmetry
  chin implant complications, 496
  smile, BTX-A complications, 510
A-T flaps, hands, feet and digits reconstruction, 396
atrophic scarring
  1540 nm Erbium:glass laser skin resurfacing, 621
  pulsed dye laser treatment of port-wine stains, 631
atrophie blanche, inflammatory ulcers, 746
atypical fibroxanthomas, 796
  organ transplant recipients, 806
atypical moles. *see* dysplastic nevi
auriculotemporal nerve block, **47,** 48
autoclave sterilization, 32
autografts, 123, 125
  definitions, 365
  porcine xenograft viability, 375
  wound dressing, 123
autoimmune diseases, ablative laser skin resurfacing, 617
Autologen, **443,** 449–450
autologous collagen, 449–450
autologous fat transfer, 535–548
  complications, 546–547
    fat hypertrophy following weight gain, 546
    infection, 546
    intravascular penetration, 546
    overcorrection, 536, 546, *546*
  controversies in procedure, 536–537, **537**
  fat autograft muscle injection (*see* fat autograft muscle injection (FAMI))
  frozen fat use, 544–545, *545*
  harvesting, 537–538
    syringe aspiration, 537, *537*
  history/development, 438, 535–536
  indications for, 539–540
    age related facial atrophy, 536, *536*
    aging face, 431, *433*
    breast, calcification, 539
    facial rebalancing, 540, *540*
    full-face volume restoration, 536, 540
  Lipostructure™, 536, 540
  longevity, 542, 544
  new trends, 536
  optimizing outcomes, 542, 544–545
  pitfalls/management, 546–547
  preoperative preparation, 537
    prophylactic oral antibiotics, 537, 546
  processing, 538
    centrifugation, 538, *538*
    separation, 538, *538*
  technical aspects, 537–541
    injection techniques, 538–539, *539*
    sterile equipment, 546, *547*
  touch-up procedures, 544
    weight loss, 544, *545*
autologous grafts, dermal fillers, **446**
autolytic debridement
  dressing function in acute wounds, 118
  leg ulcers, 757
automatic external defibrillator (AED), 153
axial arteries, SMAS, 17
axial pattern flaps, 345–364
  Abbe cross-lip flap (*see* Abbe cross-lip flap)
  classification, 348
  dorsal nasal flap (*see* dorsal nasal flap)
  forehead flap, 346, *347* (*see also* paramedian forehead flap)
  history/development, 351
  median forehead flap, 348
  nasal reconstruction (*see* nasal reconstruction; *specific flap types*)

axial pattern flaps, (*cont'd*)
optimizing outcomes, 363
paramedian forehead flap (*see* paramedian forehead flap)
pitfalls/management, 363
postoperative care, 360–362
preoperative preparation, 351–352
skin cancer, 345–346
techniques, 352–360 (*see also specific techniques*)
azathioprine, **804**
immunosuppression maintenance, 803
skin cancer occurrence, 808

B

bacillus Calmette–Guérin, melanoma therapy, 834
bacteremia, 143
incidence, 140
bacterial endocarditis, 72
bacterial infections
dermabrasion pitfalls, *595*, 595–596, 597
leg ulcers, 753, 755–756
post-cryosurgery, 201
Baker's formula, 476, **476**
'banana rolls,' 526
banner transposition flaps, 330, *333*, *334*
Bard-Parker scalpels, *59*, 59–60, *60*
basal cell carcinoma (BCC), 791–792
clinical features, 791–792
contraindication to organ transplant, 815
cryosurgery, 197–198, *198*, *200*
hidrocystoma *vs.*, 772
histology, 791
leg ulcers, 750
metastases, 792
Mohs micrographic surgery, 780, 791, 812
specimen interpretation, 785–786
stains, 784
organ transplant recipients
incidence, 805
treatment, 812–813, *814*
recurrence, 792
treatment
cryotherapy, 791
electrodesiccation and curettage, 185–186, *186*, 812
ellipse excision, 262, *266*, *267*, *268*
Mohs micrographic surgery (*see above*)
pharmacological, 791
radiation therapy, 791
basal cell nevus syndrome, 216
baseline body photographs, 827, *828*
basement membrane zone (BMZ) restoration, 106, *106*
basiliximab, **804**
immunosuppression induction, 802
basophils, 102, **102**
histamine release, 103
basting sutures, 367
Beaver scalpels, 59, *59*, 60
Becker's nevus, laser surgery, *605*
Beer's law, pulse oximeter, 153
behavior modification, body dysmorphic disorder, 421–422
benign subcutaneous lesions, 767–776. *see also* cysts; lipomas
imaging, 767
pitfalls/management, 775
postoperative care, 775
preoperative preparation, 767–768
anesthesia, 768, *769*
excision within hairline, 768, *768*
Kraissl's lines, *768*
relaxed skin tension lines, 767, *768*
techniques, 768–773
benzocaine
combination, **43**
methemoglobinemia, 56
topical, 43, **43**
benzyl alcohol, 54–55
Ber-EP4 stain, 784
β-blockers (nonselective), 74
Betacaine-LA
topical anesthesia, 45
vascular lesions laser/light treatment, 640
Bier's block (intravenous regional anesthesia), 248–249
bilateral advancement flaps, 314–315
bilateral corrugator supercilii muscle, 14–15, **16**
bilateral flap from posterior and lateral portion of lobe (Buchan's technique), 297–298, *298*
bilateral partial nail avulsion, 733
bilateral T-plasty (A-T flap) advancement flaps. *see* advancement flaps
bilayered cellular matrix (BCM), 127
bilberry, hemostasis impairment, **247**
bilobed transposition flaps. *see* transposition flaps
Biobrane dermal replacement, 125
bioengineering skin equivalents, leg ulcers, 761, **761**
biofilms, 756
biologic dressings, 123–125
biometrics, digital imaging, 95, **95**
biopsies, 203–212. *see also* sentinel lymph node (SLN) biopsy
anesthesia, 205–206, 206
chemical hemostasis, 204
chlorhexidine gluconate, 205
complications, 211–212
bleeding following, 204, 212
hypertrophic scars, 203
contraindications, 211
hepatitis B vaccination, 203
indications
cutaneous tumors, 203
epidermal pathology lesions, 203
inflammatory conditions, 203–204
for lesions with epidermal pathology, 203
melanoma, 830–831
iodophors, 205
light microscopic examination, 204, **204**
nail surgery (*see* nail surgery, biopsies)
optimizing outcomes, 211
postoperative care, 211
antibiotics, 205
preoperative preparation, 204–206
anesthesia, 205–206
antibiotic prophylaxis, 205
biopsy site preparation, 205
informed consent, 204–205
medication allergies, 204, **204**
patient evaluation, 204
site choice, 203
site closure, 210–211
techniques, 206–211
curettage, 209, *210*
cutting needles, 211
diagnostic, 203
ellipse excision, 209, 210
excisional, 208–210, **209,** *210*
incisional, 210
nail biopsy (*see* nail surgery)
punch (*see* punch biopsies)
saucerization (*see* saucerization biopsy)
scissor, 206–207, *207*
shave, 206, **206,** *207*
superficial matrix, *723*, 723–724
therapeutic, 203
undermining, 210, **211**
ulcers, 203
biosurgical debridement, leg ulcers, 757
Biosyn sutures, **228,** 229
biosynthetic dressings, dermal replacements, 125–126
bipedicle advancement flaps. *see* advancement flaps
bipolar cautery
aseptic technique, 35
random pattern cutaneous flaps, 338
Bishop–Harmon forceps, 61
bleaching, hair removal, 578
bleeding. *see* hemorrhage
bleeding disorders, liposuction, 517, *518*
bleomycin
common warts (ungual), 734
keloids, 715
blepharoplasty, 673–689
anatomy, 673–675
canthal tendons, 673, *676*
cross-sectional structure, *675*
fat pads, 673, *676*
inferior oblique muscle, *675*
superficial periocular anatomy, *674*
anticoagulant discontinuation, 675, 687
complications, 675, 687–688
digital imaging, 88, *88*
examination template, 674, *679*–680
globe malposition, 674
levator function, 674–675
lid ptosis evaluation, 674, *681*
lower eyelids, 683–685
adjuvant procedures, 685
advanced considerations, 685
complications, 685
transconjunctival, 683–684, *684*
transcutaneous, 684–687
lower-lid laxity test, 674, *681*
patient questionnaire, *677*–678
pitfalls/management, 687–688
preoperative evaluation, 673–674
upper-eyelid, 673, *681*, *682*, 682–683, *683*
anesthesia, 676
skin and muscle excision, 676, *681*, 682
blindness, blepharoplasty complication, 687
blistering, laser hair removal, 587
blood clotting. *see* hemostasis
blood pressure cuffs, 153
blushing disorder, 637
body dysmorphic disorder, 416–422
clinical features, 418
complications/psychiatric comorbidity, 418–419
diagnosis, 416–417, **417**
epidemiology, 417
etiology/pathophysiology, 417–418
evaluation, 418
body dysmorphic disorder questionnaire, 418, *420*–421
muscle dysmorphia, **417**
treatment options, 419, 421–422
education, **419,** 421

selective serotonin reuptake inhibitors, 417, 422
body dysmorphic disorder questionnaire (BDDQ), 418, *420–421*
body peeling, chemical, 476–477, *477*, *478*
body, skin tension lines, *9*
body weight, aging face, 428
boilable rubber gloves, 26
bone chisels, 62
bone resorption, chin implants, 492, 494, 496
bony asymmetry, liposuction, 522
BOTOX. *see* botulinum toxin-A (BTX-A)
botulinum toxin, 431, 501–502. *see also* botulinum toxin-A (BTX-A)
aging face, 426
carbon dioxide laser skin resurfacing combination, 613
dose (*see specific procedures*)
medium-depth chemical peel combination, 474
MYOBLOC, 502
neck rejuvenation, 691
soft-tissue augmentation combination, 458
type A (*see* botulinum toxin-A (BTX-A))
botulinum toxin-A (BTX-A), 501–512
adverse effects/complications, 509–511
cervical complications, 510
infraorbital orbicularis injection complications, 509
periorbital complications, 510
upper face, 509, 510
applications
brow elevation, 504–505
brow shaping, 504–505
bunny lines, 506
crow's feet, *505*, 505–506, *506*
depressor anguli oris, 507, *507*, 510
eyebrow asymmetry, 505, *505*
facial asymmetry, 508
forehead lines, horizontal, 504, *504*
glabellar rhytidoses, *503*, 503–504, *504*
horizontal forehead lines, 504, *504*
hypertrophic orbicularis, 506
lower face, 506–507, 509, 510
masseteric hypertrophy, 508
melomental folds, 507
mental crease, 507
midface, 505–506
mouth frown, 507
nasalis, 506
nasolabial folds, 506
neck, 507–508
necklace lines, 507
'peau d'orange' chin, 507, *508*
perioral rhytides, 506, *506*
platysmal bands, 508
upper face, 503–504, 509, 510
as combination, 508–509
contraindications, 502–503
digital imaging, 88, *89*, *90*
history/development, 501
immunogenicity, 511
injection techniques, 503–508
pitfalls/management, 509–511
postoperative care, 509
preoperative preparation, 502–503
Bourneville–Pringle tuberous sclerosis, 734
bovine collagen, dermal fillers. *see* dermal fillers, bovine collagen
Bowenoid papulosis, 792
Bowen's disease (squamous cell carcinoma *in situ*), 736, 737, 792
Mohs micrographic surgery, 792
brachytherapy, keloids, 712–713
bradycardia, follicular unit hair transplantation, **571**
bradykinin, 103
'breadloaf' method, Mohs micrographic surgery, 778, *779*
breast enlargement, male, etiology, 529
breast liposuction (female), 530
breasts
calcification, autologous fat transfer, 539
sagging, 429–430
Breslow thickness, 833
British Association of Dermatologists, 835, **836**
broadband light therapy, BTX-A combination, 509
bromelain, hematoma resorption, 258
brow elevation
BTX-A, 504–505
forehead and temple reconstruction, 385
brow-forehead lift, 686
brow-lift surgery, 283–284, 673, 685–687
advanced considerations, 687
anatomy, 673
BTX-A combination, 508
complications, 687–688
digital imaging, 88, *92–93*
open *vs.* endoscopic surgery, 687
pitfalls/management, 687–688
preoperative evaluation, 676
Schirmer test, 676, 688
surgical technique, 686
traditional approaches, 686, *686*
transblepharoplasty browpexy, 687
Brown–Adson forceps, 61
brow ptosis, BTX-A complication, 510
brow shaping, BTX-A, 504–505
bruising, BTX-A complication, 510
buccal branches, facial nerve, *13*, *14*, 18
Buchan's technique, 297, 297–298, *298*
bulbar conjunctiva, *9*
bullae, leg ulcer grafting, 761
bulla repens, 733
bunny lines, BTX-A, 506
bupivacaine, **41**
lidocaine, combined with, 43
during pregnancy, 55
random pattern cutaneous flaps, 336
buried butterfly sutures, *240*, 240–241
buried vertical mattress sutures, 240, *240*, 278, *278*
ellipse excision, 263, *263*
Burow's advancement flaps, 316, *318*
Burow's graft (island graft), 369
Burow's triangle
forehead and temple reconstruction, 385
nose reconstruction, 387
buttocks
autologous fat transfer donor site, 537
liposuction, 526
button chin, 488, *489*, *494*
button keloids, 708
N-butyl-2-cyanoacrylate, 232–233
Byron closed neck dissector, 694, *695*

C

cabinets and storage, 151, *151*, 154
cadaveric dermal replacement, 125
cadexomer iodine preparations, 127, 753
café-au-lait macules, laser surgery, 601, 602, *602*
optimizing outcomes, 604–605
postoperative care, 607–608
treatment parameters, *605*
calcaneal (Achilles) tendon, *22*
calcaneus, *22*
calcineurin inhibitors, **804**
immunosuppression maintenance, 803
California, dermatology office accreditation, 164, **165**
camera selecting. *see* digital imaging, selecting a camera
candidiasis, chemical peels, 479–480, *480*
cannulae
fat autograft muscle injection, 540, *541*
liposuction, 522, *523*
neck and jowl liposuction, *661*
canthal tendons, 673, *676*
canthoplasty, 407
canthopexy, lateral, 284, *284*
capillarity, sutures, 226
capsulopalpebral fascia resuspension, 685
carbolic acid, 25–26
carbon dioxide lasers
common warts (ungual), 734
dermabrasion combination, 592
keloids, 712
matricectomy, 725
onychogryposis, 727
scar revision, 408
skin resurfacing (*see* ablative laser skin resurfacing, carbon dioxide laser)
steatocystoma, 219
carbon dioxide, solid, 470
carcinoembryonic antigen (CEA), 784
carcinoma cuniculatum, 736
carcinomas
epidermoid, 736, *736*
onycholemmal, 736
squamous cell, 736
cardiac pacemakers
electrosurgery, 181, 187, **189**, 189–190
prophylaxis, 144
cardiovascular disease, 68, 72
cardiovascular system, anesthesia toxicity, 55
cartilage grafts, 353, *353*
cartilage replacement, 374
caruncula lacrimalis, *9*
Casson's technique, 293, *295*
Castroviejo needle holders, 62
catagen hair growth, 576, *577*
cauterization
lipomas, bleeding, 214, *215*
pincer nails, 733
CEAP class symptoms, 648, **648**
cell membrane injury, arachidonic acid formation, 104
Center for Disease Control (CDC)
antibiotics, 138
surgical site infection definition, 26–27
central chin implants, 488, *489*, *494*
central local distant digital anesthesia, nail surgery, 721, *722*
central nervous system (CNS), anesthesia toxicity, 55
centrifugation
autologous fat transfer, 538, *538*
fat autograft muscle injection, 541
cephalexin, delayed grafts, 374
cephalosporin
allergy, 517
wound infection prevention, 141
certificate of need (CON), 163–164, **164**

cervical nerves, 18
cervicofacial rotation flaps, 281, *281*, 286, *286*
cervicomental esthetics, 692
chalazion clamp, 291, *292*
chamber cryosurgery technique, 193, *193*
Charcot foot, 745
cheeks
advancement flaps, 286–287, *288*
augmentation, autologous fat transfer, 539
as cosmetic units, *8*
melolabial interpolation flap, 350, *350*
reconstruction, 389–390, *390*, 397, **398**
preferred closure option, **398**
rotation flaps, *322*
undermining, 663–664
"cheetah" phenotype, dysplastic nevi, 821, *824*
chemical autoclave sterilization, 65
chemical burns, local anesthesia, 54
chemical hemostasis, post-biopsy, 204
chemical immersion sterilization, 32
chemical peels, 463–482
body peeling, 476–477, *478*
classification, **464**
complications, **478,** 478–480
candidiasis, 479–480, *480*
herpes simplex virus, 479, *479*
hyperpigmentation, 478, *478*
hypopigmentation, 477, 478
infection, *479*, 479–480
milia, 478
prolonged erythema, 478–479, *479*
scarring, 480, *480*
systemic, 480
consultation, 466, **466**
deep (phenol), 476, **476**
history, 463–465
leg ulcers, 757–758
medium-depth (*see below*)
penetration depth, 463, *464*
pitfalls/management, 477–478
preoperative preparation, 465–466
skin preparation, 463, **464,** 465
superficial (*see below*)
chemical peels, medium-depth, 471–475
adjunctive therapies, 474
agents, 471, **472**
definition, 471
healing time, 474, *475*
indications for, 471, 472, **472**
actinic keratoses, 471, 472, *472, 473*
trichodiscomas, 472, *473*
Jessner's solution, 472, 474
optimizing outcomes, 474
postoperative care, 474
appearance, 474, *475*
cleaning avoidance, 474, *475*
technical aspects, 472, 474
trichloroacetic acid, 471, 472, 474
chemical peels, superficial, 466–471
advantages of, 466, **466**
agents, 466, **466,** 468–470
alpha hydroxy acids, 469–470
glycolic acid peel, *469*, 469–470, **470**
Jessner's solution, 468–469, **469,** 470
salicylic acid, 470
solid carbon dioxide, 470
tretinoin, 467, 470
trichloroacetic acid, 468
application technique, 467
indications for, 466
acne scarring, 467
rhytides, 467
limitations of, 466, **467**
maintenance peeling, 471
neutralization, 468, 470
optimizing outcomes, 470–471
photoaging, 467
Glogau's classification, 467, **467**
postoperative care, 471
skin preparation, 467
technical aspects, 467–470
variables, 467–468, **468**
chemoprophylaxis
melanoma, 831
SCC treatment, 811
chest liposuction (male), 529
children, anesthesia, 56, **56**
chin
augmentation (*see* chin implants)
as cosmetic unit, *8*
fat autograft muscle injection, 541
muscles, 6
reconstruction, 393, 397, **398**
preferred closure option, **398**
rotation flaps, *322*
chin implants, 483–500
before and after pictures, *497*–499
anatomy, 485–486, *486*
autologous fat transfer, 539
complications, 492–496
asymmetry, 496
bone resorption, 492, 494, *495*, 496
extrusion, 495
hematoma, 495–496
implant removal, 494
infection, 495, *495*, 496
marginal mandibular nerve injury, 492–493, *493*, 496
mental nerve injury, 493, 496
migration/malposition, 494–495, 496
necrosis, 496
overcorrection, 493–494, 496
undercorrection, 494
visible/palpable projections, 494, *494*
digital imaging, 88, *91*–92
evaluation and examination, 487–488
dental occlusion, 488
head positioning, 487, *487*
hyoid bone position, 487–488
lip posture, 488
microgenia (small chin), 488
micrognathia, 488
pre-jowl sulcus, 488
history/development, 483
idealized profile, 483–485
implant selection, 488, **488**
intraoral surgery, 489
minimum incision face lift, 667
optimizing outcomes, 491–492
pitfalls/management, 492–496
postoperative care, 492
preexisting characteristic changes, 496
preoperative preparation, 487–489
profile analysis, 483–485, **484,** *485*
removal, 494
silastic, 488–489
silicone, 488–489, *489, 494*
strong chin, 483, *484*
submental surgery, 489–491, *490, 491*
implant insertion, *491*
mental nerve avoidance, 490
sizer implant insertion, 490, *492*
suturing, 491
supraperiosteal pocket, 492
surgical technique, 489–491
techniques, 489–491
weak chin, 483
Chin Implant Style 3, 489
chlorhexidine gluconate
biopsies, 205
follicular unit hair transplantation, 557
infection prevention, 139
surgical hand scrub, 27, **28**
surgical site preparation, 31
chloroprocaine, **41**
chloroxylenol. *see* parachlorometaxylenol (PCMX) (chloroxylenol)
chondroitin, hemostasis impairment, **247**
chromophores
absorption spectrum, 579
laser hair removal, 579–580, **580**
laser surgery, 599–600
chronic inflammation, 104–105
chronic wounds. *see* wound(s)
cicatricial ectropion, 386
ciprofloxacin, 141
circular defect, periorbital region reconstruction, 386
circumoral axial advancement flaps, 359–360, *360*
cleaning, instruments, 65
clindamycin
delayed grafts, 374
wound infection prevention, 141
Clinical picture, Etiology, Anatomic distribution and Pathophysiology (CEAP) classification system, 762, **763**
clonidine, 254
clopidogrel (Plavix), hemostasis impairment, **247**
closed cryosurgery technique, 193, *193*
closed wound care, random pattern cutaneous flaps, 339
Clostridium botulinum, 501
Closure catheter, 647, *647*
closure of wounds. *see* sutures/suturing; wound closure
coagulation, 101
coagulation factors, hemostasis, 245
coblation, 177
cocaine
anesthesia history, 39
tetracaine, 45
topical, 43, **43**
cocaine hydrochloride, hemostasis, **253**
cognitive-behavioral therapy (CBT), body dysmorphic disorder, 422
cold therapy
hemostasis, 255
liposuction postoperative care, 530
cold tolerance, cryosurgery, 192
collagen(s)
autologous, 449–450
basement membrane zone restoration, 106
biosynthesis of, 111, *111*
bovine (*see* dermal fillers, bovine collagen)
dermis, 5
dermoepidermal junction, 5
fibroplasia, 107
human (*see* human collagen)
synthesis, keloids, 707
tissue remodeling, 748
wound healing, 110–111

collagenase(s), **112**
leg ulcer debridement, 757
collagenase-1 (MMP-1), 105
collagen dressings, 123
collagenoses, proximal nail fold biopsy, 724
Colorado, dermatology office accreditation, **165**
Combes' formula. *see* Jessner's solution
common palmar digital branch ulnar nerve, *22*
compartment syndrome, arm liposuction, 526
complement system, 104
complete hair restoration, 556, **556**
composite grafts, 374
definition, 365
skin substitutes, 123, **124,** *126*, 126–127
wound dressing, 123
compound/deep hemangiomas, 635
comprehension level, psychiatric examination, 414
compression bandages
leg ulcers, 752
neck rejuvenation postoperative care, 699
venous ulcers, 130
compression garments
neck rejuvenation postoperative care, 699
venous ulcer prevention, 750
compression, hemostasis, 249, *249*
compression pump, venous ulcers, **129,** 130
compression stockings
hemostasis, 256
venous ulcers, **129,** 130
compression therapy
with Graftskin for leg ulcers, 762
keloids, 713
leg ulcers, 750, 751–752, **752**
venous ulcers (*see* venous ulcers, compression therapy)
computed tomography (CT), melanoma staging, 793, 832
conchal bowl, ear reconstruction, 393–394
condylomata, multiple, 195
congenital hypertrophic lip of the hallux, 728, *728*
congenital malalignment of the great toenail, *728*, 728–729, *729*
congenital vascular anomaly classification, **630**
conjunctival incision, 683, *684*
Connecticut, dermatology office accreditation, **165**–166
connective tissue, dermis, 5
consent. *see* informed consent
consultation area, 67
contact dermatitis
anesthesia, adverse effect, 54
carbon dioxide laser skin resurfacing side effect, 615
dressings, 131, *133*
leg ulcers, 748
continuous running sutures, 278–279, *279*
continuous wave lasers
carbon dioxide, hemostasis, 250
skin pigmentation removal, 599
continuous wave neodymium:yttrium aluminum garnet (Nd:YAG) laser, 250–251
contracted scar, V-to-Y repair, 405
conventional cutting needle, 231, *231*
Cook total body peel, 477, *477*
cooling, laser hair removal, 581–582, *582*, 585
copper vapor laser, 599
coronal forehead and brow lift, 686
corset platysma repair, 691, 696–697, *697*
corticosteroids, **804**
hidradenitis suppurativa, 221
immunosuppression
acute rejection, 803
induction, 802
maintenance, 803
keloids (*see* keloids)
prostaglandin synthesis inhibition, 104
suppression of wound healing, 112–113
topical, 471
venous ulcers, 753
cosmesis, electrodesiccation and curettage, 186
cosmetic management, aging face, 431, *432*
cosmetic units
elliptical excision evaluation, 260
scar formation prevention, 402
Cosmoderm, **442,** 450
historical aspects, 438
preoperative preparation, 440
Cosmoplast, **443,** 450
historical aspects, 438
preoperative preparation, 440
costs
dressings, 133–134
surgical suite design, 148, **150**
cotton swabs, cryosurgery use, 193
cover gowns, 29
cranial nerve V (trigeminal nerve), 18
cranial nerve IX (spinal accessory nerve), 19
lipomas, 774
neck reconstruction, 395
craniofacial skeletal aging, 426, *426*
crash carts, 150
credentialing
dermatology office accreditation, 161–162
inaccurate and incomplete, 171
crescent excision, 265, *266*
Crile–Wood needle holders, 62
crossfinger flap, 737, *738*
crown coverage, 556
crow's feet
bovine collagen injection, 449, *449*
BTX-A, *505*, 505–506, *506*
Zyderm I injection technique, *448*
crush injury, nail surgery, 726
crust formation, post-cryosurgery, 201
cryoanesthesia, 43, **44**
dermabrasion, 594
cryogens, 193–194
non-ablative radiofrequency skin resurfacing, 621
pulsed dye laser treatment of port-wine stains, 631
cryoglobulinemia, cryosurgery, 192
cryosurgery, 191–202
basic principle, 191
conductivity, 191
fractional, 199, *199*
golden rule, 191–192
halo thaw time, 191
history/development, 192
indications
acne, 196
actinic keratosis, 197
BCC, 197–198, *198, 200*, 791, 812
common warts (ungual), 734
condylomata, multiple, 195
cutaneous larva migrans, 195
hemangiomas, 196, *197*
hyperkeratotic growths, 474
Kaposi's sarcoma, 198
keloids, 196
molluscum contagiosum, 195
papillomavirus infection, 194–195
rhinophyma associated rosacea, 196
rosacea, 196
SCC, 198, 812
seborrheic keratosis, 195
solar lentigo, 195–196
vascular malformations, 196–197
verrucas, 194–195
interphase, 191
keloids (*see* keloids)
mechanism of action, 191
palliative treatment, 198–199, *199*
pitfalls/management, 200–201
postoperative care, 199–200
practical applications, 194–199, **195**
preoperative preparation, 192
techniques, 192–194
chamber technique, 193, *193*
closed technique, 193, *193*
cotton swab use, 193
cryogens, 193–194
large lesions, 194
open (spray) technique, 192–193
sticking, 193
storage, 194, *194*
tissue temperature, 194
total freeze time, 191
total thaw time, 191
treatment timeline, *200*
'cuff' hypothesis, venous ulcers, 744
curettes/curetting, 62, *62*
biopsies, 209, *210*
epidermal cysts, 217, *218*
hyperkeratotic growths, 474
curved island pedicle flaps, 320
curvilinear closure, regional reconstruction, 382
cutaneous flaps, 346–348. *see also specific types*
flap survival, 347
neovascularization, 347
random pattern flap, 348
risk factors, 347–348
tobacco exposure, 347
cutaneous larva migrans, cryosurgery, 195
cutaneous tumors, biopsies, 203
cyanoacrylate compounds, 232–233
cyclo-oxygenase-2 (COX2) inhibitors, melanoma prevention, 831
cyclosporine, **804**
immunosuppression maintenance, 803
skin cancer occurrence, 808
Cymetra, **445,** 455–456, *456*
historical aspects, 439
cysts, 213–214, 768–773. *see also* benign subcutaneous lesions
dermoid cyst, 771
digital myxoid cyst, 772
epidermal cyst (*see* epidermal cysts (epidermoid/infundibular cysts))
hidrocystoma, 772
infected, 220–221
inflamed, 220–221
milia (*see* milia)
mucous cyst (mucocele), 772
onycholemmal, 736
optimizing outcomes, 221–222
packing of wound, 220, *220*

cysts, (*cont'd*)
pilar (trichilemmal) cyst, 218, *219*, 770–771
pilonidal cyst/sinus, 772
pitfalls/management, 775
postoperative care, 222
proliferating trichilemmal cyst, 771
sac collapse, 217, *217*
scarred, removal difficulty, 223
stab incision, 220, *220*
steatocystoma multiplex, 772
cytokines, macrophage release, 103

D

dacarbazine, melanoma therapy, 834, 835
daclizumab, **804**
immunosuppression induction, 802
Dacron sutures, **229,** 230
Danna approach, 769, *769*
Deaver retractor
corset platysma repair, 696
midline platysma repair with transection, 695, *696*
debridement
autolytic facilitation, 118
leg ulcers (*see* leg ulcers)
optimizing outcomes, 132, *132*
debulking, Mohs micrographic surgery, 782–783
deep-brain stimulator implants, cutaneous surgery effect, 73
deep buccinator muscle, 17
deep cervical lymphatic nodes, *20*
deep (phenol) chemical peels, 476, **476**
deep fibular nerve block, 51, *53*
deep layer (dermal) sutures, 278
deep vein thrombosis risk, 648
defibrillators
implanted, 144
preoperative patient identification, 72
delayed grafts, 374–375
porcine xenografts, 375
delayed type hypersensitivity. *see* hypersensitivity
Deming circle, 162, *162*
Denecke's technique, 304, *305*
densitometer, follicular unit hair transplantation, 549, *551*
dental occlusion, 488
dentures, chin implants, 496
depilatories, chemical, 578
depressor anguli oris muscle, **16,** 17
BTX-A, 507, *507*, 510
chin implants, 485
depressor labii inferioris muscle, **16,** 17
chin implants, 485
Dermabond (octyl cyanoacrylate), 233
dermabrasion, 591–592, 593–597. *see also* microdermabrasion
acne scars, 592
anesthesia, 594
angiofibromas, 592
carbon dioxide laser combination, 592
epidermal nevi, 592
grafting, 378
optimizing outcomes, 596–597
pitfalls, 595–596, 597
bacterial infections, *595*, 595–596, 597
viral infections, 595, *595*, 597
postoperative care, 595–596
preoperative preparation, 593–594
test spot, 593–594, 597
rhinophyma, 592
rhytides, 592
scar removal, 592
scar revision, 407–408, *409*
seborrheic keratoses, 592
syringomas, 592
tattoo removal, 592
technique, *594*, 594–595
endpieces, *595*
trichoepitheliomas, 592
wart management, 811–812
Dermagraft, 126, *126*
dermal aging, 425
dermal fillers, **439, 440,** 441–449, **442–446**. *see also* dermal replacements; soft-tissue augmentation; *individual fillers/implants*
autologous grafts, **446**
bovine collagen, 441–449
allergic reaction, 458
contraindications, 448
historical aspects, 438
hypersensitivity, 447, *447*
injection technique, 448, *448*
serial punctures, 448, *448*
skin test, 447, *447*
threading injection technique, *448*, 449
injectable human collagen, 450
medium depth chemical peel combination, 474
placement sites, 441, *441*
repeated treatments, 441
DermLiteFOTO, 94–95
Dermalive, **444**
Dermalon sutures, **229,** 230
dermal pigmented lesions, laser surgery, 603, 606
dermal replacements, 123, **124,** 125–126. *see also* dermal fillers
Biobrane, 125
biosynthetic dressings, 125–126
cadaveric, 125
Dermagraft, 126, *126*
EZ Derm, 125
Integra, 125–126
Oasis, 125
Transcyte, 126
Dermaphot, 94, 95
dermatitis, contact. *see* contact dermatitis
dermatochalasis, 673
dermatofibrosarcoma protuberans, 795
Mohs micrographic surgery, 795
stains, 784
dermatology digital imaging software, **83,** 83–84
dermatology office accreditation, 159–173
accreditation survey process, 159–161, *160*, **161**
benefits, 172
certificate of need, 163–164, **164**
credentialing, 161–162
Medicare certification and reimbursement, 163
Office-Based Surgery Accreditation program, 161
Office of Inspector General, 163
optimizing outcomes, 171
organizations, 159
Accreditation Association of Ambulatory Health Care, 159, **159, 160**
American Association for Accreditation of Ambulatory Surgical Facilities, 159
Federation of Ambulatory Surgery Association, 163
Institute for Quality Improvement, 163
Joint Commission on Accreditation of Healthcare Organizations, 159
outdated/irrelevant policies/procedures, 171
pitfalls/management, 171–172
practical applications, 172
privileging, 161–162
quality assurance and improvement, *162*, 162–163
state legislation and regulation, 164–171, **165**–170
state licensing, 163–164
website addresses, **171**
dermatomes
grafting for leg ulcers, 760
harvesting in split-thickness grafts, 371, *371*
dermis. *see* skin
dermis reconstitution, 107
dermoid cyst, 771
dermoscopy
dysplastic nevi, 821, *821*, *822*, *829*, 829–830
melanoma, *829*, 829–830, *830*
Dexon II sutures, 227, **228**
Dexon S sutures, 227, **228**
diabetes mellitus
nail surgery, 721
wound infection development, 138
diabetic ulcers
etiology, 745, *745*
foot
biosurgical debridement, 757
postoperative care/wound care, 131
Graftskin, 762
prevention, 751
diazepam, dermabrasion, 594
dicloxacillin, delayed grafts, 374
diet, liposuction, 519
diffuse patterned alopecia (DPA), 552
diffuse unpatterned alopecia (DUPA), 552
digital dermoscopy, 95
digital exsanguination, matricectomy, 725
digital imaging, 77–96. *see also* photography
annotation, 84
archival storage, 83–84
biometrics, 95, **95**
blepharoplasty, 88, *88*
Botox documentation, 88, *89*, *90*
brow lift, 88, *92*–93
chin augmentation, 88, *91*–92
color correction, 84
dermatology software, **83,** 83–84
digital dermoscopy, 95
editing, 84
e-mail, 85
exposure correction, 84
facial photography for surgical procedures, 86–87, *87*
file compression, 83
file formats, 83, **83**
film photography *vs.*, 77, **78**
hair restoration, 88, *89*
hardware for capture, 77–79
camera memory systems, 78–79
liquid crystal displays (camera), 79
optical sensors, 77–78
resolution, print and display disparity, 78
storage media, 79, **79**

image databases, 85
medical imaging services management, 85–86
networked environments, 95
oral photography, 86
overexposure, 80
photomicroscopy, 77
practical applications, 86–95
presentations, 84–85
prints, 84, **84**
processing techniques, 86
resizing, 84
resources, online, 86
selecting a camera, 79–80
adapters, 80, **80**
ultra compact cameras, 79, **80**
skin surface microscopic photography, 94–95
specular reflection, 80
surgical specimen tracking, 88
techniques, 80–82
auto focus failure minimization, 80, *81*
basic digital photography, 80–82
bit depth, 81
color balance, 82
color imaging, 81
computer skills, prerequisite, 80
diagnostic indexing of patient images, 82
image labels, 81, *81*
macro photography, 80–81
multispectral imaging, 81
patient image labeling conventions, 82, **82**
photodynamic fluorescent photography, 81
proper exposure, 80
red-green-blue imaging, 81
sharpness (focus), 80
storage and retrieval software, 82
storing, retrieving, processing images, 82
ultraviolet photography, 81
view finders, 81
teledermatology, 85
total body photography (*see* total body photography)
total immersion photography, 82, **83,** 93
digital injury, anesthesia, 53
digital ischemia
digital block complication, 49
local anesthesia adverse effect, 54
digital myxoid cysts, 772
digital nerve blocks, 49, *50*
digit reconstruction, 396–397, **399**
dimpling, chin implant complication, 494
diode lasers
(810-nm), 652, 653, *653*, *654*
(940-nm), 652
(1450 nm)
non-ablative laser skin resurfacing, 620–621
skin resurfacing, *620*
compound/deep hemangiomas, 635
laser hair removal, 583, **584**
Q-switched lasers, 600
vascular lesions, **629**
wavelengths, 627
diphenhydramine, 54–55
diplopia
blepharoplasty complication, 687
BTX-A complication, 510
dipyridamole (Persantin), **247**
direct current, electrosurgery, 178
'dirty' anatomic areas, 140
dissecting table, follicular unit hair transplantation, 558, *558*
dissection, lipomas, 214
disseminated superficial actinic keratoses, 477, *478*
distal digital ring block, 721, *722*
distal flap necrosis, 341
distal interphalangeal crease, *22*
distal interphalangeal joint, 719
stiffness, 741
distal nail avulsion, 724, *724*
distal nail embedding, 731, *732*
distal nasal defects
bilobed transposition flaps, 330, *332*
repair, 350
distal phalanx, 719, *720*
distal subungual felon, 734
distal toenail embedding with normally directed nail, 727–728, *728*
distraction test, lower-lid laxity in blepharoplasty, 674, *681*
District of Columbia, dermatology office accreditation, **166**
dog-ear redundancy, **312**
repairs, 266–269, *269*, *270*
Dong Quai root, hemostasis impairment, **247**
donor sites
full-thickness grafts, 367
grafting, 376–377
selection, 367
split-thickness grafts, 372
Doppler ultrasound, endovenous ablation, 646
dorsal finger cysts, 735, *736*
dorsal nasal flap, 321, 322–323, *324*, 325, 348, 350
optimizing outcomes, 363
pitfalls/management, 363
technique, 356–358, *358*, *359*
dorsum
dorsal nasal flap repair, 356–358
nose, *8*
dorsum (hand) rejuvenation, 539
dorsum repair, 350
double-gloving, 30, 33
double imbricating suture, 253
double purse-string sutures, *255*
double rotation flap, 393
double transposition flaps (bilobed flaps), 389
drainage, 213–224
history, 213
liposuction postoperative care, 530
optimizing outcomes, 221
pitfall management, 223
placement, 270–271
postoperative care, 222
preoperative preparation, 213–214
drapes/draping, 31, 33
infection prevention, 139–140
dressings, 35, 117–135. *see also* wound care
acute wounds, 117–118
analgesia, 132
biopsies, 211
chronic wounds, 118
cost *vs.* cost-effectiveness, 133–134
definition, 117
elliptical excision, 269
functions, 117–118, **118**
hemostasis, 255–256
historical perspective, 117
leg ulcers, 753–754, **755**
optimizing outcomes, 132
pitfalls/management, 131
post-dermabrasion, 595
practical applications, 132–134
random pattern cutaneous flaps, 339
types, 118–127, **119**
absorptive, 119
alginates, 119, **119,** *122*, 122–123, **133**
antimicrobial, 127
biologic, 123–125
biosynthetic, 125–126
cadexomer iodine, 127
collagen, 123
contact layer, **133**
film (*see* film dressings)
foam (*see* foam dressings)
gauze, 119
hydrocolloids (*see* hydrocolloid dressings)
hydrofiber, 123, *123*
hydrogel, **119,** 121–122, *122*, **133**
nonadherent fabrics, 118
occlusive (*see* occlusive dressings)
relative performance, **133**
silver-impregnated, 127
drooling, BTX-A complication, 510
dry eye
blepharoplasty complication, 687
brow lift complications, 688
dry-heat sterilization, 65
surgical instruments, 32
dumbbell keloids, 708, 711–712, *712*
Duoderm, keloids, 714
Duplex ultrasound, endovenous ablation, 646, *647*
Dupuytren's contracture, wound healing, 110
Dynamic Cooling Device
epidermal protection from lasers, *628*
pulsed dye laser treatment of port-wine stains, 632
dyschromia, 431
dysmorphophobia. *see* body dysmorphic disorder
dysphagia, BTX-A complication, 510
dyspigmentation
Er:YAG laser resurfacing, 614
long-pulsed 532 nm KTP laser skin resurfacing, 619
dysplastic nevi, 821–839. *see also* melanoma
clinical features/presentation, 821, **822**
ABCD features, 821, *822*
appearance changes, 824, *825*, 826
"cheetah" phenotype, 821, *824*
dermoscopy, 821, *821*, *822*, *829*, 829–830
distribution, 821
increasing numbers, 824, *825*, 826
sun exposure, 824
distribution, *823*
melanoma risk, *826*, 826–827, *827*
melanoma *vs.*, 821
natural history/progression, 821, 824, 826
prophylactic excision *vs.* observation, 827, *827*
baseline body photographs, 827, *828*
total body photography, 90
dysplastic nevus syndrome, 821, *823*, *824*, **824**
Dysport (botulinum toxin-A), 502
dystrophic epidermolysis bullosa, grafting, 375

E
earlobes
keloids, *711*, 711–712, *712*
reduction, 303–307
elliptical excision, 304, *304*
lateral earlobe, 304, *305*
L-plasty with a superior based wedge (Fearson's technique), 307, *307*
medial portion of lobe, 305, *306*
optimizing outcomes, 307
postoperative care, 307
preoperative preparation, 303–304
techniques, 304–307
wedge excision, 304, *304*
split (*see* split earlobe repair)
ear piercing, 301–303
complications, 302–303, **303**
kits, 302
needle techniques, *301*, 301–302, *302*
optimizing outcomes, 302
pitfalls/management, 302–303
postoperative care, 302
preoperative preparation, 301
ear reconstruction, 393–394, 397, **398**
eccrine porocarcinomas, 796
ectropion
BTX-A, 510
carbon dioxide laser resurfacing, 616
lower-eyelid blepharoplasty, 685
Mohs micrographic surgery, 790
prevention, 407
repair, 406–407, *408*
V-to-Y repair, 405
eczematous dermatitis, 753
edema, postoperative
carbon dioxide laser skin resurfacing, 615
fat autograft muscle injection, 541, *544*
follicular unit hair transplantation, **571**
juvenile ingrown toenails, 729
laser surgery, 607
microdermabrasion, 591
post-cryosurgery, 199, 201
post-dermabrasion, 595
education
body dysmorphic disorder, **419,** 421
organ transplants, skin cancer in, 810
Effendi's technique, 294, *297*
eflornithine hydrochloride, 578
Eitner's technique, 305, *306*
ELA-Max. *see* LMX
elastic bandages, venous ulcers, **129,** 130
elastic fibers
dermis, 5
remodeling phase of wound healing, 111
elasticity
aging face, 430–431
sutures, 226
elastic recoil
aging face, 430
liposuction, 521
elastin, 111
elective lymph node dissection (ELND), 833
electrical burns, electrosurgery, 187, 188, *188*
electrical power, 179
electrical resistance, 179
electrical work, 179
electric-powered nylon screw operating room table, 150
electrocautery, 177, **182**
alcohol-based preparations caution, 27, *28*
aseptic technique, 34–35
ellipse excision, 262–263
sterile field maintenance, 34, *34*
electrocoagulation, 177, **182,** 183, 251–252
mechanism of action, *184*
optimizing outcomes, *184*, 186
random pattern cutaneous flaps, 338
electrocution, electrosurgery, 187, 188
electrodesiccation and curettage, 177, **182**
BCC treatment, 185–186, *186*, 812
indications, **185**
mechanism of action, *183*
optimizing outcomes, 185
SCC treatment, 812
electrodesiccation, 182–183
electrofulguration, 177, **182,** 182–183
mechanism of action, *183*
electrolysis, 177
hair removal, 578
electroradiosurgery, matricectomy, 725
electrosection, 177, **182,** 183–184
optimizing outcomes, 186–187
random clinical trials, 187
random pattern cutaneous flaps, 337
electrosurgery, 177–190
hemostasis (*see* hemostasis)
high-frequency, 177
indications, **185**
optimizing outcomes, 184–187
pitfalls, 187–190
cardiac pacemakers, 187, **189,** 189–190
electrical burns, 187, 188, *188*
electrocution/shocks, 187, 188
eye injuries, 187, 189
implantable cardiac defibrillators, 187, 189–190
infection transmission, 187, 188–189
postoperative care, 187
preoperative preparation, 181
principles, 177–179
alternating current, 178–179
area, 178, *178*
direct current, 178
techniques, 182–184
monopolar *vs.* bipolar, 182
monoterminal *vs.* biterminal, 182
transformers, 179, *180*
types, *182* (*see also specific techniques*)
units and waveforms, 179–181
waveforms, 179, *180*, 181, *181*
elevation, hemostasis, 255
ellipse excision, 259–272
earlobe reduction, 304, *304*
epidermal cysts, 218
excisional biopsy, 209, 210
indications
BCC, 262, *266*, *267*, *268*
melanoma, 262
SCC, 262
pitfalls, 270–271
postoperative care, 269–270
preoperative preparation, 259–261
anesthesia, 261
antibiotic prophylaxis, 260
anticoagulant cessation, 259–260
evaluation, 260
history taking, 259–260
implantable cardioverter–defibrillators, 260
informed consent, 260–261
pacemakers, 260
prepping and draping, 261
scar revision, 403, *403*
size/morphology, *261*
techniques, 261–269
crescent excision, 265, *266*
dog-ear repairs, 266–269, *269*, *270*
hemostasis, 262–263
incision, 262, *262*
M-plasty, 265–266, *267*
partial closure, 266
S-plasty (lazy S repair), 266, *268*
suturing, 263–264
undermining, 263
Elsahy's technique, 299, *299*
EMLA
laser hair removal, 585
methemoglobinemia, 56
topical anesthesia, 44, **44**
vascular lesions laser/light treatment, 640
Emmet's wedge excision, 730, *731*
endocarditis, antibiotic prophylaxis, 142–145, **144**
endoluminal laser ablation. *see* varicose veins, endovenous ablation
endoscopic brow lift, 686
open *vs.*, 687
endothelial cells, hemostasis, 245
endovenous laser treatment (EVLT™), 651–654. *see also* varicose veins, endovenous ablation
Enna and Delgado's technique, 304, *305*
Enterobacteriaceae, antibiotic resistance, 137
Enterococcus infections, 26
prevention, 141
environmental cleaning, 31–32
enzymatic debridement, leg ulcers, 757–758
eosinophils, 102, **102**
eosin stains, nail biopsy, 722
ephelides
cryosurgery, 195–196
laser surgery, 601, 602
epidermal aging, 425
epidermal cysts (epidermoid/infundibular cysts), 216–218, *769*, 769–770, *770*
anesthetic, 217
antibiotic use, 218
basal cell nevus syndrome association, 216
cyst sac collapse, 217, *217*
dissection of cyst wall, skin hook use, *217*
extrusion, 217, *217*
fibrosis, 218
fusiform excision, 218
Gardner syndrome association, 216
incision line, 217
irrigation, 217
preoperative preparation, 767
probing with a curette, 217, *218*
recurrent, 218
wound closure, 217
epidermal sutures, 278–280
epidermis, *4*
biopsies, 203
carcinoma, 736, *736*
cultured grafts, 123, **124,** 125
cysts (*see* epidermal cysts (epidermoid/infundibular cysts))
damage, laser hair removal, 586, *586*
pigmented lesions, laser surgery, 601–602, 604–606
protection, laser-tissue interaction principles, 627
epidermolysis bullosa
basement membrane zone (BMZ), 106
grafting for leg ulcers, 761
Graftskin, 762

epinephrine (adrenaline)
in anesthesia, 41–42, **42,** 45
adverse reactions, 54
with lidocaine (*see* lidocaine)
nonselective β-blockers reaction, 74
during pregnancy, 42
contraindications to use, 54
hemostasis, 248
random pattern cutaneous flaps, 336
sensitivity, liposuction, 517
epithelial cysts. *see* epidermis
eponychium, 720
equipment suppliers, 155–157
Erbium:glass laser (1540 nm), skin resurfacing, 621
erbium:yttrium-aluminium-garnet (Er:YAG) laser, 431
carbon dioxide hybrid laser system, 614–615
scar revision, 408
skin pigmentation removal, 599
skin resurfacing (*see* laser skin resurfacing)
Erb's point, 18, 19–20, *21,* 48, 49, *50*
lipomas, 774, *774*
neck reconstruction, 395
erosion wound, 98, *98,* **99**
erythema
chemical peels, 478–479, *479*
elliptical excision, 271
juvenile ingrown toenails, 729
laser surgery, 607
carbon dioxide laser skin resurfacing, 615
Er:YAG laser skin resurfacing, 616
hair removal, 586
post-dermabrasion, 596
therapy, 637–638
erythematous scars, pulsed dye laser, 639–640, *640*
erythromycin
endocarditis prophylaxis, 144
wound infection prevention, 141
erythroplasia of Queyrat, 792
eschar, post-cryosurgery, 199–200
Escherichia coli infections, 26
prevention, 141
Estlander flap, 393
Ethibond sutures, **229,** 230
hands, feet and digits reconstruction, 396
Ethicon needle abbreviations, 231, *232*
Ethilon sutures, **229,** 230
ethylene oxide gas sterilization, 65
etidocaine, **41**
eumelanin hair color, 577
examination glove allergy, 74
excessive granulation tissue, dressings, 131
excisional biopsy, 208–210, **209,** *210*
excision tray organization, *65,* 65–66
excision wounds, care, 127–128
exercise, liposuction, 519
exostoses, subungual, 734, *735*
expanded polytetrafluoroethylene (e-PTFE), 439
exposure keratopathy, 687–688
exsanguinating tourniquet, *251*
exteriorization, 213–224
history, 213
optimizing outcomes, 221
pitfall management, 223
postoperative care, 222
preoperative preparation, 213–214
external aging, 425
external carotid artery, *15*
external nasal nerve block, **47,** 48
extracellular matrix
angiogenesis, 109
remodeling phase of wound healing, 110
extramammary Paget's disease, 796
imiquimod therapy, 796
Mohs micrographic surgery, 784
extremities. *see also specific extremity*
reconstruction, 395–396, 397, **398**
skin tension lines, *10*
extremity nerve blocks, 49–51
extrusion
chin implants, 495
epidermal cysts, 217, *217*
exudation, post-cryosurgery, 201
eye(s)
as cosmetic units, *8, 9*
electrosurgery injuries, 187, 189
protection, laser hair removal, 585
eyebrows
asymmetry, BTX-A therapy, 505, *505*
as cosmetic units, *8, 9*
defects, H-plasty advancement flaps, 315
'Mr Spock,' BTX-A complication, 510
ptosis, facial soft tissue lifting using Aptos threads (*see* Aptos threads, facial soft tissue lifting)
eyelids
blepharoplasty (*see* blepharoplasty)
crease fixation, 682
ectropion, BTX-A combination, 509
excision, skin defect, 386
lower (*see* lower eyelid(s))
ptosis
blepharoplasty evaluation, 674
BTX-A complication, 510
retraction
blepharoplasty complication, 687
brow lift complication, 687–688
lower-eyelid blepharoplasty complication, 685
rotation flaps, *322*
EZ Derm, 125

F

face
age-related changes
animation, 426, *426*
atrophy, 429, *430,* 536, *536*
shape changes, 428, *428*
anatomy (*see below*)
anthropometric landmarks, 10, *12*
autologous fat transfer, 535, 540, *540*
BTX-A (*see* botulinum toxin-A)
chemical peels, 466
erythema, 637–638
pulsed KTP lasers, 641
fat *vs.* body fat, *429,* 429–430
hypertrophy pattern, 429, *430*
lower (*see* lower face, BTX-A)
minimally invasive brow lift, 687
non-ablative laser skin resurfacing (*see* non-ablative laser skin resurfacing)
parotid duct, *13*
photography for surgical procedures, 86–87, *87*
skin tension lines, 7, *9*
SMAS (*see* superficial musculoaponeurotic system (SMAS))
telangiectasias, 637
pulsed KTP lasers, 641
face, anatomy, 7, 10–17, 274–275
arterial supply, *15* (*see also specific arteries*)
facial artery, 12, *15, 16*
superficial temporal artery, 11, *13, 15*
temporal artery (*see below*)
bones (*see* face, bones)
cosmetic units (*see* face, cosmetic units)
facial nerve (*see* facial nerve (VIIth cranial))
facial vein, *15*
foramina, 10
infraorbital, 10, *11*
supraorbital, 10, *11*
frontal eminences, 10
glabella, 10
mastoid process, 10, *11*
mental foramen, *11*
muscles (*see* face, muscles)
parotid gland, 6, 10–11, *13, 15*
retaining ligaments, 658, *658*
superficial temporal vein, *15*
temporal artery
anterior branch, *15*
facial nerve relationship, *13*
frontal branch, *13*
temporal fossa, 11–12
zygomatic arch, 10, *11*
face, bones, *11*
frontal bone, 7, 10, *11*
mandible, 7, 10, *11*
maxillary bone, 7, *11*
nasal bone, *11*
parietal bone, *11*
temporal, 10, *11*
zygomatic bone, 7
face, cosmetic units, 6–7, *8,* 274, *274. see also specific components*
boundaries, 6
nasofacial sulcus, 6, *8*
wound closure effects, 274
cheeks, *8*
chin, *8*
eyes/eyebrows, *8, 9*
forehead, *8*
lips, *8*
nose, *8*
face lifts (rhytidectomy), 284, *284,* 431
followed by fat autograft muscle injection, 541
minimum incision face lift (*see* minimum incision face lift)
SMAS, 285, *285*
tissue thinning, *536*
face masks, 29–30, 33
face, muscles, 13–15, **16,** 17. *see also specific muscles*
chin, 6
ear muscles, 17
fat autograft injection, 541, **541,** *542*–543
dysfunction, 547
masseter muscle, 11, *13, 15*
nasal muscle, 17
perioral muscles, 6, 17
depressor anguli oris, **16,** 17
depressor labii inferioris, **16,** 17
levator anguli oris, **16,** 17
levator labii superioris, **16,** 17
levator labii superioris alaeque nasi, **16,** 17
mentalis, **16,** 17
orbicularis oris, **16,** 17
platysma, **16,** 17
risorius, **16**

face, muscles, (*cont'd*)
zygomaticus major, **16,** 17
zygomaticus minor, **16,** 17
periorbital muscles, 14–15, 17
bilateral corrugator supercilii, 14–15, **16**
levator palpebrae superioris, 14, **16**
orbicularis oculi, 14, **16,** 284
palpebral muscle, 14
procerus, 6, **16**
sternocleidomastoid muscle, 12–13
facial aging. *see* age/aging
facial artery, 12, *15, 16*
facial nerve (VIIth cranial), *13, 14*
buccal branches, *13, 14,* 18
cervical branch, *13, 14,* 18
forehead and temple reconstruction, 384–385
marginal mandibular branch, *13, 14,* 18, *19*
minimum incision face lift anatomy, 658, *659*
nerve blocks, 47–49, *48*
auriculotemporal, **47,** 48
external nasal, **47,** 48
greater auricular, **47,** 48–49, *50*
infraorbital, **47,** 48, *48, 49*
mental, **47,** 48, *48, 49*
random pattern cutaneous flaps, 336
supraorbital nerve, 47, **47,** *48*
supratrochlear nerve, 47, **47,** *48*
transverse cervical, **47,** 48–49
parotid nerve, *14*
temporal branches, *13, 14, 16,* 18, *19*
Whitnall's tubercle, *14*
zygomatic branches, *13, 14,* 18
facial plane (vertical line), chin implants, 484
facial vein, *15*
facial wrinkles, fine, deep (phenol) chemical peels, 476
far-far-near-near stitch. *see* vertical mattress sutures
Fascian, **444,** 450
fasciculation, chin implant complication, 494
Fatah's technique, 293–294, *296,* 299, *299*
fat atrophy, aging face, 427
fat augmentation, autologous. *see* autologous fat transfer; fat autograft muscle injection (FAMI)
fat autograft muscle injection (FAMI), 540–541, *544*
cannulae, 540, *541*
example protocol, 545, **545**
facial muscles, 541, **541,** *542*–543
full-face volume correction, 540
injection, 541, *543*
with liposuction of the neck, 541, *541*
weight gain, 546, *546*
fat hypertrophy
aging face, 427
autologous fat transfer, 546
microsuction of, 431, *434*
fat pads
blepharoplasty anatomy, 673, *676*
lower-eyelid blepharoplasty, 685
transconjunctival lower-eyelid blepharoplasty, 683–684, *684*
transcutaneous lower-eyelid blepharoplasty, 685
upper-eyelid blepharoplasty, 682, *682*
fat redistribution, aging face, 426
Fayman's technique, 300, *300*
Fearson's technique, 307, *307*
Federation of Ambulatory Surgery Association (FASA), 163
feet reconstruction, 396–397, 397, **399**
ferric sulfate (Monsel's solution), 249, **252**
feverfew, hemostasis impairment, **247**
Fibrel, 438
fibrin clots
development, 101
fibroplasia, 107
fibrin cuffs, venous ulcers, 744
fibrin sealant, 250, **252,** 438
fibroblasts
fibroplasia, 107
wound healing influence, 112
fibrokeratomas, ungual, 734, *734*
fibromas, periungual, 734
fibronectin
dermis, 5, 107
fibroplasia, 107
leg ulcer tissue remodeling, 748
macrophage release, 103
wound contraction, 108
fibroplasia, 107
fibrosis, epidermal cysts, 218
field block
anesthesia, 46, *46*
practical applications, 56
figure-of-eight suture, *256*
fillers. *see* dermal fillers
film dressings, **119,** *120,* 120–121, **133**
wound healing, 113
finasteride, 553, 556, 570, **570**
fingernails. *see* nail(s)
finger splinting, nail surgery, 721–722
fire safety, surgical suite design, 148
first metatarsal bone, *22*
fistula development
cheek reconstruction, 389
in hidradenitis suppurativa, 221
Fitzpatrick skin type, dermabrasion, 593
flaccid cheek, BTX-A complication, 510
flap(s). *see also specific types*
Abbe cross-lip flap (*see* Abbe cross-lip flap)
circumoral axial advancement flaps, 359–360, *360*
forehead and temple reconstruction, 385
full-thickness defect, *391,* 391–392
interpolation, 402
laser hair removal, 579
lower, SCC, 806, *806*
necrosis, minimum incision face lift, 668
optimizing outcomes, 363
perioral region reconstruction, 390, 392
regional reconstruction, 382
scar formation prevention, 402
technique, 359–360
upper, island pedicle flaps, *319*
wound healing, 99
flap creation from lateral portion of lobe (Pardue's technique), 297, *297*
flap creation from lateral portion of lobe and Z-plasty (Walike and Larrabee and Hamilton and La Rossa techniques), 297, *298*
flashlamp-pulsed dye laser, wavelengths, 627
flexor digitorum longus tendon, *22*
flexor hallucis longus tendon, *22*
flexor retinaculum, *22*
Florida, dermatology office accreditation, 164, **166**
Flowers Mandibular Glove, 489
fluence
laser hair removal, 581, **582**
laser-tissue interaction principles, 627
fluorescent pulsed light, laser hair removal, **584**
5-fluorouracil
actinic keratoses, 793
prevention, 811
keloids, 715
melanoma prevention, 831
SCC treatment, 813
flurazepam, dermabrasion, 594
flushing disorder, 637
foam dressings, 119, **119,** 120, *120,* **133**
wound healing, 113
fold, nail. *see* nail fold
follicular infundibulum rupture, 221
follicular neogenesis, 575
follicular unit composition, 549
follicular unit extraction (FUE), 549, 550, 559–560, **560**
follicular unit hair transplantation, 549–574
American Board of Hair Restoration Surgery, 550
densitometer, 549, *551*
digital imaging, 88, *89*
donor
closure, 561, *561,* **561**
harvest, 559
supply assessment, 554
follicular unit composition, 549
follicular unit extraction, 549, 550
history/development, 550–551
International Society of Hair Restoration Surgery, 550
local anesthesia, 558
mini-micrografting *vs.*, 550
operating room, 557–558, *558*
optimizing outcomes, 566–568
automation, 568
camouflage, 568, *569*
density, 568, *569*
finasteride, 570, **570**
forelock integration, 567–568, *569*
hair direction, 567, *567*
hairline placement, 567, *568*
minoxidil, **570**
recipient site influences, 566, *567*
transition zones, 566, *566*
visibility, 566, *566*
pitfalls/management, 568–573, **571, 572**
age, 570
angioedema, **571**
bleeding, **571**
bradycardia, **571**
donor problems, 570, 572
excessive coverage area, 573
graft problems, 568, 572–573, 573
hairline problems, 573
hypertension, **571**
medical therapy, lack of, 570
multiblade knife use, 572
postoperative edema, **571**
pruritus, **571**
tight scalp, 572
urticaria, **571**
postoperative care, 568, **570**
instructions, 565
medications, **565, 570**
preoperative preparation, 551–557
androgenic alopecia (*see* androgenic alopecia)
candidates for, **553,** 553–554

complete restoration, 556, **556**
contraindications, 554
expectations, 554
finasteride, 553
first transplant session planning, 555, **555**
instructions, 556, **557**
non-androgenetic hair loss, 552–553, **553**
patient evaluation and surgical planning, 551–553
patient preparation, 556–557, **557**
photographic documentation, 558–559
second transplant session planning, 555–556
subsequent transplant sessions, 556
recipient sites, 562–565
density, 563–564
distribution, *564*, 564–565
'forward weighting,' 564, *564*
hair direction, 563, *563*
insertion, 565, *565*
scalp regions, 564, *564*
'side weighting,' 564, *565*
size and orientation, 563
'stick and place,' 565
techniques, 558–565
follicular unit extraction, 559–560, **560**
graft dissection, 561–562, *562*, *563*
local anesthesia, 559, **559**
patient disposition, 565
strip excision, *560*, 560–561
vascular compromise, 555
Food and Drug Administration (FDA), microdermabrasion, 592
foot, anatomy, 20–21, *22*
footwear, 30
foramina, 10
forceps, 61, *61*
forehead, *8*
as cosmetic unit, *8*
flaps, 346, *347* (*see also* paramedian forehead flap)
axial pattern flaps, 351
bipedicle advancement flaps, *321*
horizontal lines, BTX-A, 504, *504*
lipomas, *216*
reconstruction, 384–386, *385*, 397, **398**
suspension sutures, 283–284
forelock integration, follicular unit hair transplantation, 567–568, *569*
'forward weighting,' follicular unit hair transplantation, 564, *564*
Fotofinder, 94
four-layer bandage, venous ulcers, **129,** 130
FOX test, 560
fractional cryosurgery, 199, *199*
FRAIL (For Recognition of Adult Immobilized Life), 748
frank exposure keratitis, 687
Frankfort horizontal plane, 484, *485*
frequent wound care, random pattern cutaneous flaps, 339
frontal bone, 7, 10, *11*
frontal eminences, 10
frontalis muscle, *14*, **16**
forehead lipomas, 215
frosting, chemical body peeling, 477, *477*
frozen fat, autologous fat transfer, 544–545, *545*
full-face volume correction
autologous fat transfer, 536, 540
fat autograft muscle injection, 540
full-thickness defect of the lips, *391*, 391–392
full-thickness skin grafts (FTSGs), 123, **124,** 366–370, *370*
Burow's graft (island graft), 369
definition, 365
equipment, 366
grafting for leg ulcers, 758
hair-bearing grafts, 369–370
procedure, 366–369, *368*, *369*
Adaptic, 368, *369*
basting sutures, 367
donor site selection, 367
Hypafix, 368
myocutaneous hinge flap, 369
subcutaneous hinge flap, 369
template formation, 367, *368*
tie-over bolster, 367–368, *369*
tie-over sutures, 368, *369*
Xeroform, 368
regional reconstruction, 382
trunk reconstruction, 395
wound dressing, 123, **124**
full-thickness wounds, 98, *98*, **99**
contraction, 108
postoperative care/wound care, 129
fungal infections, dermabrasion, 595–596, 597
fusiform excision. *see* ellipse excision

G

galea aponeurotica
forehead and temple reconstruction, 384
scalp reconstruction, 382
Gardner syndrome, 216
garlic, hemostasis impairment, **247,** 259
gas sterilization, 32
gauze dressings, 119
gelatinases, **112**
gelatin, hemostasis, **252**
gemfibrozil, 831
geometric broken-line closure, scar revision, 404, *404*
gigantomastia, liposuction, 530
ginger, hemostasis impairment, **247**
ginkgo, hemostasis impairment, **247,** 259
ginseng, hemostasis impairment, **247**
girdles, 530
glabella, *8*, 10
anthropometric landmarks, *12*
nose reconstruction, 388
rhytides, BTX-A, *503*, 503–504, *504*
tissue necrosis
soft-tissue augmentation, 459
Zyplast injection, 447, *447*
transposition flap, 388
glabellar frown line, Artecoll, 454, *454*
Glasgold Wafer, 489
chin implant repair, 494, 496
globe malposition, blepharoplasty, 674
Glogau's photoaging classification, 467, **467**
glomus tumors, subungual, 734–735, *735*
gloves, 30, 33
infection prevention, 139
Glu-stitch, 232–233
wound closure, 232–233
glycolic acid peel, *469*, 469–470, **470**
glycomer 631 (Biosyn) sutures, **228,** 229
glycoproteins, dermis, 5
glycosaminoglycans, dermis, 5
gnathion, *12*
gonion, *12*
Gore-Tex, **446,** 456
government accreditation inspections, 172
gowns, 30
infection prevention, 139–140
Gradle scissors, 60
grafts. *see* grafts/grafting
grafts/grafting, 123–125, 365–379. *see also* skin substitutes; *individual types*
applications
cheek reconstruction, 390
ectropion repair, 407
hands, feet and digits reconstruction, 396
keloids, 711
laser hair removal, 579
leg ulcers (*see* leg ulcers)
nose reconstruction, 388–389
perioral region reconstruction, 393
periorbital region reconstruction, 386
regional reconstruction, 382
scalp reconstruction, 384
definitions, 365
delayed grafts, 374–375
failure, 760
physiology, 365–366
pitfalls/management, 377–378
postoperative care, 375–377, *376*, *377*
preoperative preparation, 366
random pattern cutaneous flap combination, 281–282
size, ectropion prevention, 407
skin substitutes, 375
split-thickness graft (*see* split-thickness skin grafts (STSGs))
techniques, 366–375
types
allografts, 123, 125
autografts, 123, 125
composite grafts, 123, **124,** *126*, 126–127, 374
full-thickness skin graft (*see* full-thickness skin grafts (FTSGs))
porcine xenografts, 375, *376*
wound closure, 346, *346*
wound healing, 99, *100*
Graftskin, leg ulcers, 761–762
granulation phase, 100, *100*
dermis reconstitution, 107
extremities reconstruction, 396
fibroplasia, 107
juvenile ingrown toenails, 729
regional reconstruction, 382
scalp reconstruction, 383, *383*
trunk reconstruction, 395
granulocyte macrophage-colony stimulating factor (GM-CSF), 753
granulomas
in chronic inflammation, 105
foreign body, 458, 459, 460
gravitational aging, 428–429
minimum incision face lift (*see* minimum incision face lift)
great auricular nerve
minimum incision face lift, 662, *663*
nerve block, **47,** 48–49, *50*
great saphenous vein, 646
Duplex ultrasound, 646, *647*
grooves, nail. *see* nail grooves
ground substance
dermis, 5
remodeling phase of wound healing, 110

growth factors
angiogenic, 108–109, **109**
inflammatory response, 101, 104, **104**
keloids, 707
leg ulcer healing, 756
retention, 118
Guerrero-Santos' technique, 305, *306*
gutter treatment, ingrown toenails, 729

H

hair
anatomy, 575–576, *576*
follicle, 575
color, 577
excess, 577–578
removal (*see* laser hair removal)
follicular neogenesis, 575
growth, 576, *577*, **577**
following laser hair removal, 586
reduction, 578
telogen, 576, *577*
laser removal (*see* laser hair removal)
removal, 31, *31*, 33, 578
infection prevention, 139
restoration (*see* follicular unit hair transplantation)
types, 576–577
hair-bearing grafts, 369–370
hair bulb, 575–576
hair covers, *29*, 30
hair follicle, 575
thermal relaxation time, 580, **581**
hairline excision, benign subcutaneous lesions, 768, *768*
hairline placement, follicular unit hair transplantation, 567, *568*
hair pull test, androgenic alopecia, 553
hair systems, follicular unit hair transplantation, 556
hair thickeners, follicular unit hair transplantation, 556
half-buried horizontal mattress (tip) stitch, 236–237, *237*
half-buried mattress sutures, 280, *280*
half circle Ferguson needle, 665, *665*
halo thaw time, cryosurgery, 191
Hamilton and La Rossa technique, 297, *298*
hand
anatomy, 20–21, *22*
distal interphalangeal crease, *22*
hypothenar eminence, *22*
median nerve, *22*
metacarpophalangeal crease, *22*
proximal interphalangeal crease, *22*
proximal palmar crease, *22*
radial nerve, 20, *22*
thenar eminence, *22*
thumb interphalangeal crease, *22*
ulnar nerve, *22*
wrist crease, *22*
reconstruction, 396–397, 397, **398, 399**
wrist crease, *22*
hand scrub, 27–29, 32–33
antiseptic agents, 27–28, **28**
duration and method, 28–29
handwashing, infection prevention, 139
Hansen's disease, leg ulcers, 748
Harahap's technique, 294, *296*
head
lymphatics, 18–19, *20*
nerve supply, 18
head wrap, minimum incision face lift, 667, *667*
'healing secretion,' biosurgical debridement of leg ulcers, 757
healing time, cryosurgery, 200
Health Insurance Portability and Accountability Act (1996) (HIPPA)
digital imaging, 85
guidelines for patient privacy, 147
heated chemical vapor sterilization, surgical instruments, 32
helical chondrocutaneous advancement flap
conchal bowl, 394
ear reconstruction, *394*
hemangiomas, **630,** 634–635
children, cryosurgery, 192
compound/deep, treatment of, 635, *636*
cryosurgery, 196, *197*
involuting, treatment of, 635
long-pulsed alexandrite laser, 634
long-pulsed Nd:YAG laser, 634
proliferating hemangiomas, 634
pulsed dye laser, 634, *635*
pulsed dye lasers, 641
ulcerated, treatment of, 634–635, *635*
hematomas
chin implants, 495–496
development, 257–258
biopsies, following, 212
elliptical excision, 271
prevention, 113
random pattern cutaneous flaps, 341
minimum incision face lift, 668
hematoxylin/eosin staining
Mohs micrographic surgery, 784
nail biopsy, 722
hemophilia A, 73
hemophilia B, 73
hemorrhage(s)
biopsies, following, 204, 212
blepharoplasty complication, 675, 687
follicular unit hair transplantation, **571**
Mohs micrographic surgery, 789
nail surgery, 721
neck rejuvenation complication, 699, 700
transconjunctival lower-eyelid blepharoplasty, 684
hemostasis, 100, 101, **101,** 245–258
anatomic location, 254
compression, 249, *249*
tourniquets, 249, *250, 251*
definition, 245
electrosurgery, 251–253
electrocoagulation, 251–252
tissue damage, 252–253
wound necrosis, 253
elliptical excision, 262–263
hemostatic anesthesia, 248–249
epinephrine, 248
intravenous regional anesthesia (Bier's block), 248–249
topical lidocaine with epinephrine, 248
tumescent anesthesia, 248, 254–255 (*see also* anesthesia, tumescent)
hypertension, 254
laser surgery, 250–251
mast cell regulation of, 103
nail surgery, 721
physiological, 245–246
disorders, *246*, 246–247
postoperative care, 255–256
patient instructions, **257**
preoperative preparation, 245–248
evaluation, 246–247
history taking, 246, **246**
medications impairing hemostasis, **247,** 247–248
preparing surgical field, 248
procedures, 254–255
random pattern cutaneous flaps (*see* random pattern cutaneous flaps)
suture ligation, 253
double purse-string sutures, *255*
ex suture, *256*
figure-of-eight suture, *256*
mattress sutures, *254*
square/U suture, *256*
topical hemostatics, 249–250, **252, 253**
hemostatic anesthesia. *see* hemostasis
hemostats, 61
lipoma removal, 214, *215*
hepatitis, 72
hepatitis B
electrodesiccation and curettage, 189
vaccination for biopsies, 203
herbal supplements/medicines
hemostasis impairment, **247**
liposuction, avoidance for, 519, **520**
hereditary hemorrhagic telangiectasia, *638*
herpes labialis
ablative laser skin resurfacing, 617
non-ablative laser skin resurfacing, 622
herpes simplex virus infection, 72–73
chemical peels, 479, *479*
dermabrasion, 595, 597
heterografts. *see* xenografts (heterografts)
hidradenitis suppurativa, 221, *221*
optimizing outcomes, 221–222
pitfall management, 223
hidrocystoma, 772
hip liposuction, 526
hirsutism, 577
antiandrogenic medications, 578
histamine, 103
keloids, 707
Histoacryl, 232–233
histology, laser hair removal, 582, *583*
history taking, 68–73
cardiovascular disease, 68, 72
elliptical excision, 259–260
hemostasis, 246, **246**
hepatitis, 72
herpes simplex virus infection, 72–73
HIV infection, 72
hypertension, 68
implanted deep-brain stimulators, 73
inherited bleeding disorders, 73
Mohs micrographic surgery, 780–781, **781**
organ transplantation, 72
pregnancy, 68
prosthetic devices, 72
psychosocial issues, 416
questionnaire, 68, *70–71*
HIV infection
associated lipoatrophy, 454–455
cryosurgery for molluscum contagiosum, 195
cutaneous surgery effect, 72
dermabrasion, 593–594
SCC , organ transplant recipients, 809
wound infection development, 139
homograft, definition, 365
horizontal forehead lines, BTX-A, 504, *504*

horizontal mattress sutures, 236, *237*, 279–280
half-buried mattress suture, 280, *280*
'hospital gangrene,' 25–26
hostile patients, 415
H-plasty advancement flaps. *see* advancement flaps
human collagen
dermal filler, 450
historical aspects, 438
human papillomavirus (HPV)
electrodesiccation and curettage, 189
organ transplants, 809
SCC, 809
hyaluronic acid (hyaluronan)
biological function, 450
dressings, 123
gels, 450–453 (*see also individual types*)
historical aspects, 438
injection technique, 452
isovolemic degradation, 451–452
local anesthetic, 452
longevity of correction, 452–453
safety and efficacy, 451
threading injection technique, 452
topical anesthetic, 452
treatment reaction, 451
Tyndall effect, 452
remodeling phase of wound healing, 110
tissue remodeling in leg ulcers, 748
hyaluronidase, anesthesia additive, 42, **42**
hydraulic operating room tables, 149, 150
hydrocolloid dressings, **119,** 121, *121,* **133**
wound healing, 113, *113*
hydrofiber dressings, 123, *123*
hydrogel dressings, **119,** 121–122, *122,* **133**
hydrogen peroxide, wound care, 339
hydroquinone, chemical peels, 465
hydroxyzine hydrochloride, dermabrasion, 594
Hylaform, **442,** 450, 451
Hylaform Fine Line, 450, 451
Hylaform Fineline, **442**
Hylaform Plus, **443,** 450, 451
hylan gels, historical aspects, 438
Hylan Rofilan Gel, **445**
hyoid bone, 19
chin implant examination, 487–488
neck liposuction, 528
neck rejuvenation, 692
profile analysis, chin implants, 485
Hypafix, full-thickness grafts, 368
hyperandrogenic state, excess hair, 577
hyperkeratotic growths
cryofreezing with medium-depth chemical peels, 474
curetting with medium-depth chemical peels, 474
hyperpigmentation. *see also* pigmentary changes
chemical peels complication, 478, *478*
laser surgery, 604
carbon dioxide laser skin resurfacing, 616, *616*
Er:YAG laser skin resurfacing, 616
laser hair removal, 587, *587*
non-ablative laser skin resurfacing, 621, 622
pulsed dye laser of port-wine stains, 631
hypersensitivity
delayed-type, 54
ear piercing, 303
liposuction, 530
hypertension
cutaneous surgery effect, 68
follicular unit hair transplantation, **571**
hypertrichosis, 577
hypertrophic capillary (port-wine stain). *see* port-wine stains
hypertrophic orbicularis, BTX-A, 506
hypertrophic scars
ablative laser skin resurfacing, 617
biopsies, 203
carbon dioxide laser skin resurfacing side effect, 616
cryotherapy, 714–715
ear piercing, 303
intralesional steroids, 402
keloids *vs.*, 707
pulsed dye laser, 639–640, *640*
remodeling phase of wound healing, 110
split earlobes, 301
steatocystoma, 219
trunk reconstruction, 395
hyponychium, 720
hypopigmentation. *see also* pigmentary changes
chemical peels complication, 477, 478
keloid corticosteroid treatment, 710, *712*
keloid cryotherapy, 715
laser surgery, *605*
carbon dioxide laser skin resurfacing, 616
Er:YAG laser skin resurfacing, 617
laser hair removal, 587, *587*
pulsed dye laser, 631
post-cryosurgery, 201
tattoo removal, *606*
hypothenar eminence, *22*
hypoxia, wound healing, 112

I

idealized profile, chin implants, 483–485
Illinois, dermatology office accreditation, **166**
imaging. *see also specific techniques*
benign subcutaneous lesions, 767
melanoma staging, 832
imbibition, grafting, 365–366
imbrication, SMAS, 285
imiquimod, 777
actinic keratoses, 793
prevention, 811
BCC, 791
extramammary Paget's disease, 796
keloids, 714
melanoma therapy, 795, 831
immunogenicity, BTX-A, 511
immunohistochemical staining, *794*, 795, 833
immunosuppression, chemical peels, 466
immunosuppressive drugs, 802–804, **804**. *see also* organ transplants, skin cancer in
acute rejection, 803–804
change in use, **804**
induction, 802
maintenance, 802–803
mechanism of action, *803*
skin cancer occurrence, 808–809
implantable cardiac defibrillators (ICDs)
electrosurgery, 181, 187, 189–190
elliptical excision, 260
implanted deep-brain stimulators, 73
implants
aging face, 431
chin (*see* chin implants)
incision, 213–224
elliptical excision, 262, *262*
epidermal cysts, 217
history, 213
lipomas, 214
optimizing outcomes, 221
pitfall management, 223
postoperative care, 222
preoperative preparation, 213–214
incisional antibiotics, wound infection prevention, 141–142
incisional biopsies, 210
incision step-off, wound closure, **243**
incompetent mouth, BTX-A complication, 510
Indermil, 232–233
wound closure, 232–233
indwelling device prophylaxis, 144–145
infections, 26–27
abscesses, 220–221
autologous fat transfer, 546
biopsies, 212
carbon dioxide laser skin resurfacing, 615–616
chemical peels, *479*, 479–480
chin implant, 495, *495*, 496
cysts, 220–221
dressings, 131, *133*
ear piercing, 302–303
elliptical excision, 271
juvenile ingrown toenails, 729
keloids, 706
leg ulcers, 753
liposuction, 531
nail surgery (*see* nail surgery)
neck rejuvenation complication, 699
post-cryosurgery, 201
prevention, antibiotics, 137
random pattern cutaneous flaps, 341
transmission, 26
cryosurgery, 192
electrosurgery, 187, 188–189
infective endocarditis (IE), prophylaxis, 142
inferior labial artery, *15*
inferior oblique muscles, *675*
inferior segment, hair follicle, 575
infiltrating lipomas of the upper extremities, 216
infiltrative anesthesia, 45–47
inflammation
abscesses, *220*, 220–221
cysts, 220–221
leg ulcers, 746, *747*, **747**
ulcers, 746
inflammatory conditions, biopsies, 203–204
inflammatory response, 97, *97*, 99–105, *100*
cellular response, 101–103
chemical mediators, 103–104
chronic inflammation, 104–105
complement system, 104
granulation tissue formation, 100, *100*
growth factors, 101, 104, **104**
hemostasis, 100, 101, **101**
vascular response, 100–101
informed consent, 67, 75
axial pattern flaps, 351–352
biopsies, 204–205
chemical peels, 465–466
digital imaging, 85
elliptical excision, 260–261
form
follicular unit hair transplantation, 557, **557**

informed consent, (*cont'd*)
soft-tissue augmentation, 458
minimum incision face lift, 660
random pattern cutaneous flaps, 336
infraorbital area
autologous fat transfer overcorrection, 546, *546*
undermining, minimum incision face lift, 668
infraorbital crease, *9*
infraorbital foramen, 10, *11*
infraorbital nerve block, **47,** 48, *48, 49*
infraorbital orbicularis, 509
infundibular cysts, *769,* 769–770, *770*
infundibulum, 575
ingrown toenails, **727,** 727–730
in infancy, 727–729, *728*
congenital hypertrophic lip of the hallux, 728, *728*
congenital malalignment of the great toenail, *728,* 728–729, *729*
distal toenail embedding with normally directed nail, 727–728, *728*
juvenile, 729–730, *730, 731, 732*
pincer nails, 731, 733
trumpet nails, 731, 733
tubed nails, 731, 733
inherited bleeding disorders, 73
injectable paraffin, 437
inosculation, grafting, 366
Institute for Quality Improvement (IQI), 163
instruments, 59–66. *see also specific instruments*
bone chisels, 62
cleaning, 33–34
cleaning of, 65
curettes, 62, *62*
excision tray organization, *65,* 65–66
forceps, 61, *61*
injury prevention, 65
needle holders, 61–62, *62*
packaging and quality assurance, 34, *34*
periosteal elevators, 62
repair tray organization, 66, *66*
scalpels, 59–60, *60*
scissors, *60,* 60–61, *61*
sterilization, 32, 33–34, 65
technical aspects, 59–64
towel clips, 62
wound healing, 113
instrument tie knot, 233, *234*
integrin receptors, wound healing, 107–108, *108*
intelligence, psychiatric examination, 414
intense pulsed light (IPL). *see also* laser surgery
cooling, 605–606
laser hair removal, 583–584, **584**
poikiloderma, 638–639
skin pigmentation therapy, 601, 602
optimizing outcomes, 605–606
port-wine stains, *633,* 633–634
postoperative care, 608
telangiectasia, 637, *638*
skin resurfacing, 618
vascular lesions, 629–630, **630,** 642
wavelengths, 627
interferon-α (IFN-α)
BCC, 791
Kaposi's sarcoma therapy, 813
keloids, 710, 714
melanoma therapy, 795, 834
metastases, 835
organ transplant recipients, 813
interferon-γ (IFN-γ), keloids, 714
interferon(s), keloids, 707, 712, 714, 715
Integra dermal replacement, 125–126
interleukin-2 (IL-2)
antagonists, 802
melanoma metastases therapy, 835
intermittent claudication, arterial ulcers, 745
internal aging, 425
International Society of Hair Restoration Surgery (ISHRS), 550
International Transplant Skin Cancer Collaborative, 810, **811**
interphalangeal joint stiffness, distal, 741
interpolation flaps, 402
intralesional steroids
scar revision, 402
trapdoor deformity repair, 406
intraoral surgery, chin implants, 489
intravascular penetration, autologous fat transfer, 546
intravenous regional anesthesia (Bier's block), 248–249
involuting hemangiomas, 635
iodophors, biopsies, 205
iontophoresis anesthesia, 45
Iowa, dermatology office accreditation, **170**
iris scissors, 60, *60*
irrigation
abscesses, 220
epidermal cysts, 217
ischemic flap failure
Abbe cross-lip flap, 361
paramedian forehead flap repair, 360
island graft (Burow's graft), 369
island pedicle flaps, 316–320, *318. see also* advancement flaps
aesthetic repair, 319–320
basis, *318*
curved, 320
de-epithelialized, 320
mobility, 319
perinasal cheek defect, *319*
perioral region reconstruction, 392, *392*
underlying anatomy, 320
upper lip defect, *319*
V to Y advancement flap (*see* V to Y advancement flaps)
Isolagen, **445,** 449
isotretinoin
chemical peels, 466
dermabrasion, 593
keloids, 706
melanoma prevention, 831
organ transplant recipients, 811
SCC treatment, 813
isovolemic degradation, hyaluronic acid gels, 451–452
isthmus, 575

J

Jacobsen hemostat, 61
Jessner's solution
medium-depth chemical peels, 472, 474
superficial chemical peels, 468–469, **469,** 470
Jeweler's (splinter) forceps, 61
Joint Commission on Accreditation of Healthcare Organizations (JCAHO), 159
Joseph's technique, earlobe reduction, 304, *305*
jowl fat pad suspension, minimum incision face lift, 664, 666
jowl liposuction, 528–529
minimum incision face lift, 660, 661, *661,* 666
jugular veins, *20*
jugulodigastric lymphatic nodes, *20*
jugulo-omohyoid lymphatic node, *20*
Juvederm, **444**
juvenile ingrown toenails, 729–730, *730, 731, 732*
juxta-auricular S-form skin excision, 657, 662, *662*
preoperative marking, 667

K

Kalimuthu's technique, split earlobe repair, 294, *296*
Kalimuthu's technique (V-flap), split earlobe repair, 294, *296*
Kansas, dermatology office accreditation, **166**
Kaposi's sarcoma
contraindication to organ transplant, 815
cryosurgery, 198
organ transplant recipients, 806
interferon-α therapy, 813
pathogenesis, 809
treatment, 813
Karapandzic flap, perioral region reconstruction, 392
keloids, 705–718
clinical manifestations, 707–708
hypertrophic scars *vs.*, 707, **707**
limited mobility, 708, *708*
epidemiology, 705–706
ritual keloiding, 706, *706*
Yoruba tribe, 705, 706, *706*
etiology, **706,** 706–707
ablative laser skin resurfacing, 617
ear piercing, 303
split earlobes, 301
trunk reconstruction, 395
lobular, 708
mederma, 715
pathogenesis, 707
pedunculated (*see* pedunculated keloids)
prevention, 715–716
sessile (*see* sessile keloids)
spontaneous, 706
treatment (*see below*)
keloids, therapy, 708–715, **709**
bleomycin, 715
brachytherapy, 712–713
clinical trials, 708, **709**
compression therapy, 713
corticosteroids, 709–710, 716
combination, 710, 712, 715
hypopigmentation, 710, *712*
prevention, 715
cryotherapy, 196, 714–715
combination, 710, 715
Duoderm, 714
5-fluorouracil, 715
history, 705
interferon-a, 707, 710, 712, 714, 715
isotretinoin, 706
optimizing outcomes, 716
pitfalls/management, 716
radiation therapy, 712–713

Index

silicone gel sheeting, 709, 710, 712, 713–714
surgery, 710–712
earlobe keloids, *711*, 711–712, *712*
grafting, 711
laser surgery, 710, 712
techniques, 708–715
verapamil, 715
vitamin E, 715
keratinocyte growth factor-2, 753
keratinocytes
epidermis, 4
in re-epithelialization, 105–106
wound healing role, 98
keratinous cysts. *see* epidermal cysts
keratitis, blepharoplasty complication, 687
keratoconjunctivitis, blepharoplasty complication, 687
kinins, 103–104
Klippel–Trenaunay syndrome, 630
knee liposuction, 526
knot tying. *see* sutures/suturing
Koenen's tumor, 734
Kraissl's lines, *768*
krypton lasers, 599

L

labial artery, perioral region reconstruction, 391
labial incompetence, chin implant complication, 494, *495*
labrale inferius, *12*
labrale superius, *12*
lacrima puncta, eyes/eyebrows, *9*
lactate dehydrogenase (LDH) levels, melanoma staging, 832
lactomer (Polysorb) sutures, 227, **228**
lagophthalmos, 687
LaGrange scissors, 60
laminins, basement membrane zone restoration, 106, *107*
lanugo hair, 576
lap-joint technique (Argamaso's technique), 298, *299*
laser(s), 599–600, **600**. *see also individual types*
absorption spectra, *600*
tissue interaction principles, 625–630
electromagnetic radiation, 625
epidermal protection, 627, *627*, *628*
fluence, 627
pulse duration, 627
selective photothermolysis, 625–626
spot size, 627
thermal diffusivity, 627
thermal relaxation time, 627
wavelength, *626*, 626–627, **627**
wart management, organ transplant recipients, 811–812
laser hair removal, 575–588, *585*
adverse reactions, 586
blistering, 587
epidermal damage, 586, *586*
hair thinning, 586, 587
pigmentary changes, 586, 587, *587*
benefits, 579
chromophores, 579–580, *580*, **580**
contraindications, 578
cooling, 581–582, *582*
fluence, 581, **582**
histology, 582, *583*
laser systems, 582–585, **584**
alexandrite laser, 583, **584,** 586
diode laser, 583, **584**
fluorescent pulsed light, **584**
IPL, 583–584, **584**
Nd:YAG laser, 583, **584,** 586
ruby laser, 582–583, **584,** 586
leukotrichia, 586–587, 587
medical history, 578, **578**
microwave technology, 584–585
optical energy, **584**
optimal target, 580
optimizing outcomes, 585–586
parameters, 585, 586
photoprotection, 587
photothermal, **584**
pitfalls/management, 586–587
postoperative care, 586
preoperative preparation, 578–579
skin phototype classification, 578, **579**
pulse duration, 580–581, 586, *586*
risks, 579
skin types, 585–586
spot size, 581, *581*
techniques, 579–585
test spot, 586
treatment delivery, 585
treatment intervals, 586
vellus hair treatment avoidance, 586
wavelength, 580, *580*, **581**
laser skin resurfacing, 611–624
ablative (*see* ablative laser skin resurfacing)
BTX-A combination, 509
history/development, 611–612
lower-eyelid blepharoplasty, 685
medium-depth chemical peels combination, 474
non-ablative (*see* non-ablative laser skin resurfacing)
photorejuvenation, laser and light sources, 611, **611**
postoperative care/wound care, **128,** 128–129
wound infection prevention, 142
laser surgery
chemical peels combination, 471
chromophores, 599–600
ephilides, 601, 602
hemostasis, 250–251
hypopigmentation, 604
keloids, 710, 712
mechanism of action, 599–600
melanosome damage, 599–600
vascular lesions (*see* vascular lesions; *individual disorders*)
wavelength choice, 599–600, *600*
laser surgery, skin pigmentation, 599–609. *see also specific lesions*
café-au-lait macules (*see* café-au-lait macules, laser surgery)
complications, 607–608
history, 601
laser types, 599–601, **600**
optimizing outcomes, 604–607
dermal lesions, 606
endpoints, 604
epidermal lesions, 604–606
hyperpigmentation, 604
hypopigmentation, 604, *605*
postoperative care, 607–608
analgesia, 607
edema, 607
erythema, 607
sun protection, 607
preoperative preparation, 601
anesthesia, 601
patient evaluation, 601
safety, 601
tattoo removal (*see* tattoo removal)
techniques, 601–604
dermal lesions, 603
epidermal lesions, 601–602
treatment parameters, *605*
wavelength choice, 600
Lassus' technique, 305, *306*
lateral angle of eye, *9*
lateral canthopexy, 284, *284*
lateral canthus, *9*
lateral cheek/lateral neck skin flap, 662–663
lateral earlobe reduction, 304, *305*
lateral longitudinal nail biopsy, 722–723, *723*
lateral nail fold. *see* nail fold
lateral nail grooves, 720, 721
lateral neck/lateral cheek skin flap, 662–663
lateral palpebral commissure, *9*
lateral ridge, *8*
lateral side wall, *8*
latex allergy
identification in preoperative assessment, 74
liposuction, 517
layered closures, 275–277, *277*
'lazy S' excision, extremities reconstruction, 395
lean aging face sagging, 429, *430*
leg ulcers, 743–766
bioengineering skin equivalents, 761, **761**
compression therapy, 751–752, **752**
contraindicative medications, 749
debridement types, 754–758
autolytic, 757
biosurgical, 757
enzymatic and chemical, 757–758, *759*
mechanical, 757, *757*
surgical/sharp, 756, *757*
dressings, moist wound healing, 753–754, **755**
etiology, 743–746, **744**
arterial ulcers, 744–745, *745*
diabetic ulcers, 745, *745*
inflammatory ulcers, 746
pressure ulcers, *745*, 745–746
venous ulcers, 743–744, *745*
frequency, **744**
grafts/grafting, 758–762
bullae, 761
dermatome, 760
epidermolysis bullosa, 761
full-thickness skin graft, 758
graft failure, 760
meshing, 760, *760*
occlusive dressings, 761
optimizing outcomes, 760
'pinch grafting,' 760, *760*
pitfalls/management, 760
preoperative preparation, 758
split-thickness graft, 758
techniques, 760
infections, 753
diagnosis, 753, **754**
pharmacologic therapy, 752–753
pitfalls/management, 763
preoperative preparation, 748–751

leg ulcers, (*cont'd*)
diagnostic assessment, 749–750, *750*, **751**
medical history, 748–749
physical examination, 749, **749**
prevention, 750–751
For Recognition of Adult Immobilized Life, 748
shave therapy, 763
subfascial endoscopic perforator surgery, 762–763
Clinical picture, Etiology, Anatomic distribution and Pathophysiology classification system, 762, **763**
surgical techniques, 754–763
techniques, 751–763
types, **744**
wound preparation and debridement, 754–758
bacteria removal, 755–756
nonmigratory tissue removal, 756
senescent cell removal, 756
wound debridement, 755, *755*
wound repair physiology, 746–748
inflammation, 746, *747*, **747**
proliferation and tissue formation, 746
tissue remodeling, 746, 748
leiomyosarcomas, 806
lentigenes
cryosurgery, 195–196
laser surgery, 601
optimizing outcomes, 604
treatment parameters, *605*
lentigo simplex, cryosurgery, 195–196
leprosy, leg ulcers, 748
leukocytes, 101–103. *see also specific types*
leukoplakia, organ transplants, 806, *806*
leukotrichia, 586–587, 587
levamisole, 834
levator anguli oris muscle, **16,** 17
levator function, blepharoplasty, 674–675
levator labii superioris alaeque nasi muscle, **16,** 17
levator labii superioris muscle, **16,** 17
levator palpebrae superioris muscle, 14, **16**
levobupivacaine, **41**
Lewis' technique, 304, *305*
lidocaine, **41**
allergy
liposuction, 517
prevention, 53
autologous fat transfer, 537
bupivacaine, combined with, 43
dosage, **55**
EMLA (*see* EMLA)
with epinephrine
elliptical excision, 261
hemostasis, 248
post-dermabrasion, 595
history, 39
iontophoresis anesthesia, 45
liposuction, 523–524
LMX (*see* LMX)
random pattern cutaneous flaps, 336
tetracaine, 45
topical anesthesia, **43,** 44, **44**
toxicity, 55, **55**
lifting flaps, scar prevention, 402
lighting, 149, 151, *151*, 154
light microscopic examination, 204, **204**
Limberg transposition flap, *390*
Linton procedure, 762
lip(s)
augmentation
Alloderm, 455
Artecoll, 453, 454, *455*
Cymetra, 455–456, *456*
fat autograft muscle injection, 540
hyaluronic acid gels, 452, *453*
Isolagen, 449
Radiesse, 455
Restylane, 451
Softform implants, *457*
subdermal implant insertion procedure, 457
Zyplast, *447*
chin implants examination, 488
lipodermatosclerosis
leg ulcers, 749
shave therapy for venous ulcers, 763
stanozolol for venous ulcers, 752
venous ulcers, 744, *745*
lipomas, 213, 214–216, *773*, 773–775, *774*
anesthesia, 214
common sites, 214
dissection, 214
forehead, *216*
frontalis-associated, 215
hemostasis, 214, *215*
infiltrating, of the upper extremities, 216
optimizing outcomes, 221, 773–775
Erb's point, 774, *774*
liposuction, 774–775
spinal accessory nerve damage, 774
palpation of, 214, *214*
pitfall management, 222–223
incomplete removal, 222–223
pitfalls/management, 775
postoperative care, 222
preoperative preparation, 767
removal with hemostat, 214, *215*
skin incision, 214
wound closure, 215
running horizontal mattress suture, 215, *215*
Lipostructure™, 536, 540
liposuction, 513–533
abdomen, 524–526, **525,** *527*
aging face, 429
arms, 526, 528
breast, female, 530
buttocks, 526
cannulae, 522, *523*
chest, male, 529
consultation, 513, 517
contraindicated medications, 519, **520, 521**
diet, 519
dry technique, 513
exercise, 519
expectations, 519–521, 528
fat volume (maximum removal), 524
hips, 526
history, 513, 535
jowls, 528–529
knee, 526
lipomas, 774–775
long-term outcome, 531–532
neck (*see* neck rejuvenation, liposuction)
optimizing outcomes, 524–530
oversuction (*see specific anatomical areas*)
physical examination, 521–522
pitfalls/management, 530–532, **531**
postoperative care, 530
preoperative preparation, 513, 517, 519–521
contraindicated medications, 519, **520, 521**
medical and surgical history, 517, *518*, 519
medication history, 517, 519, **520**
preconsultation questionnaire, *514*–516, *518*
surgical risk, 517, **517**
preparatory procedure, 522–523
suboptimal results, 531
suction procedure, 524
surgical suite and set-up, 522
liposuction cannulae, 522, *523*
thighs, medial, 526
thighs, outer, 526, *528*
touch-up procedures, 531
tumescent anesthesia, 46, 513, 523–524, **524**
weight gain, 531
wet technique, 513
lips, as cosmetic units, *8*
'lip-switch' flap, 392
Liquid Bandage, 232–233
liquid nitrogen, cryosurgery, 192, 194
liquid silicone, 437–438
Listerism, 26
Lister, J
aseptic technique history, 25–26
dressings, 117
livedo reticularis, 746
LMX, 640
laser hair removal, 585
topical anesthesia, **44,** 44–45
lobular keloids, 708, 711, 712, *712*
local anesthesia. *see* anesthesia, local
Loeb's technique, 305, *306*
longitudinal melanonychia, *723*, 723–724
long-pulsed lasers
alexandrite (*see* alexandrite lasers)
dye, **629**
Louisiana, dermatology office accreditation, **170**
lovastatin, 831
lower cheeks, *8*
lower extremity lesions, 395
lower eyelid(s)
blepharoplasty (*see* blepharoplasty)
eyes/eyebrows, *9*
laxity, 687–688
laxity test, 674
Mohs defect, 386
suspension sutures, 284
lower face, BTX-A, 506–507
complications, 509, 510
lower lips, SCC, 806, *806*
lower nasal defects, 349
L-plasty (Fatah's technique), 293–294, *296*, 299, *299*
L-plasty with a superior based wedge (Fearson's technique), 307, *307*
Ludwig Classification, 552
lunula, 721
lupus anticoagulant syndrome, 746
lymphangiomas, 197
lymphomas, organ transplant recipients, 804–805
lymphoscintigraphy, melanoma, 793, *794*

Index

M
maceration prevention, dressings, 132, *132*
machine aspiration, autologous fat transfer, 537–538
macrophages, **102,** 102–103, **103**
cytokine release, 103
fibronectin release, 103
wound healing influence, 112
maggot therapy, leg ulcer debridement, 757
magnetic resonance imaging (MRI), melanoma staging, 793
maintenance peeling, 471
make-up application, post-dermabrasion, 596
malar area, *8*
autologous fat transfer, 535, 539
malar fat pad
facial soft tissue lifting using Aptos threads (*see* Aptos threads, facial soft tissue lifting)
minimum incision face lift, 657, 659, *660*, 664, *664*, 665–666
malignancy risk, keloid radiation therapy, 713
malignant fibrous histiocytomas, 796
malignant melanoma. *see* melanoma
malnutrition, wound infection, 138
mal perforans ulceration, 745
mammogram screen, 530
mandible, 7, 10, *11*
facial soft tissue lifting using Aptos threads (*see* Aptos threads, facial soft tissue lifting)
mandibular ligament, 658
mandibular nerve, 18
mandibular retaining ligament, partial release by periosteal elevator, 664, *664*
marginal mandibular nerve, *13*, *14*, 18, *19*
anatomy, chin implants, 485
avoidance in silicone chin implants, 489, *489*
injury, 485–486
chin implant complication, 492–493, *493*, 496
neck rejuvenation, 700
neck liposuction, 693, 694
marginal reflex distance (MRD), 674, *681*
marionette lines
Artecoll, 453, 454
autologous fat transfer, 539
bovine collagen injection, 449
Radiesse, 455
Softform implants, *456*
masks, infection prevention, 139
Massachusetts, dermatology office accreditation, **166**–167
masseteric hypertrophy, BTX-A, 508
masseter muscle, 11, *13*, *15*
mast cells, 102, **102,** 103
mastoid process, 10, *11*
matricectomy, 725, *725*
onychogryphosis, 727
matrilysins, **112**
matrix metalloproteinases (MMPs)
re-epithelialization, 105
remodeling phase of wound healing, 111–112, **112**
mattress sutures
buried vertical (*see* buried vertical mattress sutures)
half-buried, 280, *280*
hemostasis, *254*
horizontal (*see* horizontal mattress sutures)
running horizontal, 215, *215*
side-to-side complete split earlobe suture, 293, *294*
vertical (*see* vertical mattress sutures)
maxillary bone, 7, *11*
maxillary nerve, 18
Maxon sutures, **228,** 229
Mayo scissors, 60, *61*
Mayo surgical stand, 65–66, 152, *152*
McCollough's technique, 305, *306*
McCoy, Stark and Tipton technique, 304, *304*
McGregor's patch, 658
mechanical aspiration pump, liposuction, 522
mechanical creep, skin, 6, 275
mechanical debridement. *see also* dermabrasion; microdermabrasion
leg ulcers, 757
mederma, keloids, 715
medial angle of eye, *9*
medial canthus, *9*
medial malleolus, *22*
medial plantar artery, *22*
medial plantar nerve, *22*
median forehead flap, 348
median nerve. *see* hand, anatomy
median nerve block, 51, *52*
medical history. *see* history taking
Medicare Certificate, 161
reimbursement, 163
Medicare survey, 163
medication
allergies, 204, **204**
anesthesia interaction, 55
existing, cutaneous surgery effect, 68, 73–74
wound healing influence, 112
Mediskin 1, 375
medium-depth chemical peels. *see* chemical peels, medium-depth
megestrol acetate, melanoma therapy, 834
melanin
absorption peaks, 626, *626*
hair color, 577
laser hair removal, 579
melanocyte-stimulating hormone (MSH), 707
melanocytic nevi, laser surgery, 603
melanoma, 793–795, 821–839. *see also* dysplastic nevi
analysis algorithms, digital imaging, 86
clinical features/presentation, 793, **822**
detection/prevention, 793, **828,** 828–831, 832
ABCD, 828
biopsy, 830–831
chemoprevention, 831
dermoscopy, *829*, 829–830, *830*
immunostaining, 795
lymphoscintigraphy, 793, *794*
ophthalmologic examination, 829
routine dermatologic examination, 828, *829*
screening, 828–829
self examination, 828
sun protection, 830
ultraviolet precautions, 830, **830**
visual aids, 829–830
Wood's light, 829
development, *827*
dysplastic nevi *vs.*, 821
head/neck, 793
lifetime risk, 831
management, 777, 831–832
imiquimod, 795
interferon-α, 795
metastases, treatment, 835
organ transplant recipients, 806
incidence, 805
interferon-α therapy, 813
treatment, 813
postoperative follow-up, 835
guidelines, 835, **836**
prognostic factors, **835**
recurrence, 835
risk of, *826*, 826–827, *827*
sentinel lymph node biopsy, 793, *794*, *833*, 833–834
organ transplant recipients, 813
staging, 793, 832
survival data, **832**
surgery, 833–835
adjuvant therapy, 834–835
elective lymph node dissection, 833
ellipse excision, 262
Mohs micrographic surgery, 784, 794–795
sentinel lymph node biopsy, *833*, 833–834
surgical margins, 833, **833**
ungual, 736–737, *738*
melanophages, laser surgery, 603
melanosomes, laser surgery, 599–600
melasma, laser surgery, 603
melolabial flaps, cheek reconstruction, 389–390
melolabial folds, *8*
melomental folds, BTX-A, 507
membrane-type matrix metalloproteinases, **112**
memory of sutures, 226
mental crease, BTX-A, 507
mental foramen
age related changes, 486, *486*
anatomy, chin implants, 485, *486*
face, *11*
nerve block, 48, *49*
mental foramen, 10
mentalis muscle, **16,** 17
chin implants, 485
mental nerve
anatomy, chin implants, 485, *486*
avoidance, chin implants, 489, *489*, 490, 493, 496
nerve block, **47,** 48, *48*, *49*
mental protuberance, 485, *486*
mentolabial crease, 6
mentolabial sulcus, *12*
menton, *12*
meperidine hydrochloride, dermabrasion, 594
mepivacaine, **41**
Merkel cell carcinoma, 795
contraindication to organ transplant, 815
organ transplant recipients, 806
metastases, 807
Mohs micrographic surgery, 813
pathogenesis, 809
radiation therapy, 813
treatment, 813
radiation therapy, 795
Mersiline sutures, **229,** 230
meshing, grafting for leg ulcers, 760, *760*
metacarpal block, 721, *722*
metacarpophalangeal crease, *22*

metastases
melanoma, 835
Merkel cell carcinoma, 807
organ transplants, skin cancer in, 807–808, *808*
SCC, 792
organ transplant recipients, 807
methemoglobinemia
anesthesia, adverse effect, 56
prevention, 53
benzocaine, 56
EMLA, 56
prilocaine, 56
methicillin-resistant *Staphylococcus aureus* (MRSA), 137, 138
wound infection prevention, 141
methylene blue, laser hair removal, 580
methylparaben (lidocaine preservative) allergy, 517
metoclopramide, 55
Metzenbaum scissors, 60, *61*
microcystic adnexal carcinoma, 796
microdermabrasion, 589–591. *see also* dermabrasion
American Academy of Cosmetic Surgery, 592
clinical benefits, 593
edema, 591
Food and Drug Administration, 592
histologic changes, 590, *591*
history, 589–590
sebum levels, 590–591
technique, 592–593
transepidermal water loss, 591
microfibrillar collagen, hemostasis, **252**
microgenia (small chin), 488
micrognathia, chin implant, 488
microlipoinjection
autologous collagen, 449
historical aspects, 438
micro-marsupialization, mucous cyst, 772
microsphere targeting, laser hair removal, 579–580
microwave technology, laser hair removal, 584–585
midazolam, 254
mid-face
BTX-A, 505–506
suspension sutures, 284–285
mid-face lifting, 286
aging face, 431
mid forehead lift, 686
midline forehead flap, 351
midline platysma repair with transection, 695–696
migration of chin implant, 494–495, 496
milia, 218, 771
carbon dioxide laser skin resurfacing, 615
chemical peels complication, 478
dressings, 131
optimizing outcomes, 221–222
post-cryosurgery, 201
post-dermabrasion, 596, 597
Miller's technique, 305, *306*
mimetic muscle aging, 425
Mini-Mental Status Exam, 414–415
mini-micrografting, follicular unit hair transplantation *vs.*, 550
minimum incision face lift, 657–672
before and after photographs, *669*
anatomy, 657–658
facial nerve, 658, *659*
facial retaining ligaments, 658, *658*
great auricular nerve damage prevention, 662, *663*
optimizing outcomes, 666–667
photographic documentation, 660
pitfalls/management, 667–668
postoperative care, 667, *667*
preoperative preparation, 660
presurgical markings, 660, *661*
rhytidectomy variations, 658–660
deep-plane dissection, 658–659
malar fat pad, 659, *660*
mid-face, 659, *660*
SMAS lift, 659–660
subperiosteal, 658
sub-SMAS, 658
supra-SMAS (subcutaneous), 659
sensory nerves of the neck and head, *663*
SMAS, 657
plication, 657, 664–665, *665*
techniques, 660–666
cheek undermining, 663–664
facial soft tissue lifting using Aptos threads (*see* Aptos threads, facial soft tissue lifting)
instruments used, **668**
jowl fat pad suspension, 664, 666
juxta-auricular S-form skin excision, 657, 662, *662*, 667
malar fat pad suspension, 657, 664, *664*, 665–666
neck and jowl liposuction, 660, 661, *661*
periosteal elevator partial release of mandibular retaining ligament, 664, *664*
platysma plication (midline), 661–662
redundant skin, 666, *666*
skin closure, 666, *666*, 668
subcutaneous undermining of the lateral cheek/lateral neck skin flap, 662–663
tumescent anesthesia, 657, 660–661, 662, *662*
minoxidil, 556, **557**
follicular unit hair transplantation, **570**
Mississippi, dermatology office accreditation, **167**
mitral valve prolapse, endocarditis prophylaxis, 143
Mittelman Prejowl Implant, 488–489, *489*
mixed vascular malformations, cryosurgery, 197
Mohs defects of the lower eyelids, 386
Mohs micrographic surgery, 777–800
advantages, 778–779
axial pattern flaps, 345
cure rates, 312
ears, 780, *788*
history, 777–778
indications, **780,** 791–796
BCC (*see* basal cell carcinoma (BCC))
Bowenoid papulosis, 792
Bowen's disease (SCC *in situ*), 792
dermatofibroma sarcoma protuberans, 784, 795
eccrine porocarcinomas, 796
epidermoid carcinoma, 736
erythroplasia of Queyrat, 792
extramammary Paget's disease, 784
eyelid tumors, 779–780
facial malignancies, 779
genitals, 780
melanoma (*see* melanoma)
Merkel cell carcinoma, 813
primary eccrine adenocarcinomas, 796
primary mucinous carcinoma, 796
SCC (*see* squamous cell carcinoma (SCC))
sebaceous carcinoma, 796
verrucous carcinoma, 792
nose, 780
optimizing outcomes, 787–788
equipment, 787, *787*
pitfalls, 788–790
anesthetic allergies, 789
bleeding, 789
cosmetic results, 790
ectropion, 790
nerve injury, 789
periorbital areas, 789–790
postoperative care, 788
preoperative preparation, 780–781
history taking, 780–781, **781**
radiation therapy combination, 790
specimen interpretation, 785–787
technique, *779*, 781–787, *782*
'breadloaf' method, 778, *779*
debulking, 782–783
identification/delineation, *781*, 781–782
local anesthesia, 782
mapping/division, 783, *783*
reconstruction, 788
specimen numbering, *785*, 786
specimen processing, 783–784, *784*
specimen sectioning, 783–784
stage II excision, *786*
stage III excision, *786*
staining, 784, *785*
supplies, *788*
training programs, 777
moisture retentive dressings. *see* dressings; occlusive dressings
moisture vapor transmission rate (MVTR), 119
MoleMax system, 94
moles, atypical. *see* dysplastic nevi
molluscum contagiosum, cryosurgery, 195
Monocryl sutures. *see* poliglecaprone 25 (Monocryl) sutures
monocytes, 102, **102**
monofilament sutures, absorbable, 63
Monosof sutures, **229,** 230
Monsel's solution (ferric sulfate), 249, **252**
mood and affect, psychiatric examination, 414
morphing, digital imaging, 86
mouse lethality assay (MLA), 502
mouth frown, BTX-A, 507
M-plasty, 265–266, *267*
regional reconstruction, 382
MRSA. *see* methicillin-resistant *Staphylococcus aureus* (MRSA)
'Mr Spock' eyebrow, BTX-A complication, 510
mucocele, 772
mucosal advancement flaps, 320
mucous cyst (mucocele), 772
multiple condylomata, cryosurgery, 195
multiple Z-plasty, scar revision, 405, *405*
multispectral imaging, 81
mupirocin, 142
muscle dysmorphia, **417**
muscle resection, brow lift, 686
muscles, face. *see* face, muscles; *specific muscles*

muscle to periosteum suspension, 685
muscular asymmetry, liposuction, 522
Mustarde flaps
  cheek reconstruction, 390
  rotation flaps, 325–326
mycophenolate mofetil, **804**
  immunosuppression maintenance, 803
  skin cancer occurrence, 808
MYOBLOC (Botulinum toxin-B), 502
myocutaneous hinge flap, full-thickness grafts, 369
myofibroblasts, wound contraction, 108
myxoid pseudocysts, 735, *736*

N
nail(s)
  anatomy, 719–721, *720* (*see also individual features*)
  braces, 733
  clippings, 722, *723*
  hand scrub, 29
  surgery (*see below*)
  tumors (*see* nail tumors)
nail ablation (total), 725, *725*
nail avulsion, *724*, 724–725
  distal, *724*
  onychogryphosis, 727
  partial, 724–725
    foreign bodies, 726, *726*
    pincer nails, 733
  proximal, 724, *724*
nail bed, 720, 721
  biopsies, 723, *723*
  periosteal flap, 730
nail embedding, distal, 731, *732*
nail fold
  defects, 737, *739*
  lateral, 720
    biopsies, 724
    defects, 737
  proximal, 720, 721
    biopsies, 724
    defects, 737, *739*
nail grooves
  lateral, 720, 721
  proximal, 720, 721
nail matrix, 720, 721
  biopsies, 723, *723*
    superficial, *723*, 723–724
  defects, 737, 740–741
  graft, 737, 740
  horn, phenolization, 730, *731*, *732*
nail plate, 720, 721
nail surgery, 719–742
  biopsies, 208, *209*, 722–724, *723*
    ungual melanoma, 736
  distal interphalangeal joint stiffness, 741
  distal nail embedding, 731, *732*
  fold defects, 737, *739*
  foreign bodies, *726*, 726–727
  infection, 733–734, 741
  ingrown toenails (*see* ingrown toenails)
  instruments, 721
  lateral nail grooves, 721
  matricectomy, 725, *725*
  matrix defects, 737, *740*, 740–741
  nail ablation (total), 725, *725*
  nail avulsion (*see* nail avulsion)
  necrosis, 741
  onychogryphosis, 727
  optimizing outcomes, 741
  pachyonychia congenita, 727
  pincer nails, 731, 733
  pitfalls/management, 741
  preoperative preparation, 721–722, *722*
  racket fingers, 727, *728*
  reconstructive, 737, 740–741
  techniques, 722–741
  trauma, 726, *726*
nail tumors, 734–737
  benign, 734–735
    myxoid pseudocysts, 735, *736*
    subungual exostoses, 734, *735*
    subungual glomus tumors, 734–735, *735*
    ungual fibrokeratomas, 734, *734*
  malignant, 736–737
    epidermoid carcinoma, 736, *736*
    onycholemmal carcinoma, 736
    onycholemmal cyst, 736
    squamous cell carcinoma, 736
    ungual melanoma, 736–737, *738*
nail wall hypertrophy, 729
nasal alae
  defects, 374
  nose reconstruction, 386
nasal bone, *11*
nasalis, BTX-A, 506
nasal muscle, 17
nasal reconstruction, 348–350, 386–389, *388*, *389*, **398**
  ala defect repair, 350
  cheek melolabial interpolation flap, 350, *350*
  contour restoration, 349
  distal nasal defect repair, 350
  dorsal nasal flap, 350
  dorsum repair, 350
  full thickness defects, 349
    trilaminar reconstruction, 349, *349*
  function restoration, 349
  lower nasal defects, 349
  nasal tip repair, 350
  paramedian forehead flap, 350
  subunit replacement, 348, *348*, *362*
  supratip repair, 350
nasal root, nose reconstruction, 387
nasal symmetry, axial pattern flaps, 352
nasal tip
  dorsal nasal flap repair, 356–358
  repair, 350
nasion, *12*
nasofacial sulcus, 6, *8*
nasojugal folds, *9*
nasolabial folds, 6, 431
  Alloderm, 455
  Artecoll, 454
  autologous fat transfer, 539
  bovine collagen injection, 449
  BTX-A, 506
  Hylaform, 451, 452, *452*
  Radiesse, 455
  Restylane, Zyplast *vs.*, 452
  Softform implants, *457*
  subdermal implant insertion procedure, 457
  Zyplast, *441*
    Restylane *vs.*, 452
nasolabial junction, suspension sutures, 287
nasolabial transposition flaps, 330–331, 334, *335*
  nose reconstruction, 387, *389*
  suturing, 339
  trapdoor deformity, 334, *335*
National Comprehensive Cancer Network (NCCN)
  melanoma follow-up recommendations, 835, **836**
  melanoma surgery recommendations, 833
National Institute of Health, 830–831
National Nosocomial Infections Surveillance (NNIS), 138
N-duopropenide (NDP), 28
neck
  BTX-A, 507–508
    flexor weakness, 510
  ideal sculpture, chin implants, 485
  liposuction, 528–529, *529*
    with fat autograft muscle injection, 541, *541*
    minimum incision face lift, 660, 661, *661*, *666*
  reconstruction, 394–395, 397, **398**
  rejuvenation (*see* neck rejuvenation)
  undermining, 667–668
neck anatomy, 19–20
  Erb's pont, 19–20, *21*
  hyoid bone, 19
  jugular veins, *20*
  lymphatics, *20*
  nerve supply, 18
    spinal accessory nerve, 19
  omohyoid muscle, *20*
  posterior triangle, 19
  sternocleidomastoid muscle, 19
necklace lines, BTX-A, 507
neck lift, 431
neck rejuvenation, 691–701
  botulinum toxin, 691
  complications, 699, 700
  corset platysma repair, 691
  history, 692
  liposuction, 528–529, *529*, 691, 693–694, *695*
    instruments, **694**
    optimal candidate, *692*
    preoperative markings, 693, *693*
    sternocleidomastoid muscles, 694, *694*
  optimizing outcomes, 699–700
  patient evaluation, 692, 699
    poor skin quality, 692, *693*
    prominent platysmal banding, 692, *693*
  pitfalls/management, 700
  platysma repair, 691, 695–697
    corset platysma repair, *696*, 696–697, *697*
    midline platysma repair with transection, 695–696, *696*
    patient evaluation, 692
  postoperative care, 699
  radiofrequency tissue tightening, 692, 698–699, *700*
    ThermaCool TC, 692, 698–699, *699*
    treatment grid, 698, *699*
  SMAS plication, 691, 697–698, *698*
    patient evaluation, 692
  techniques, 693–699
necrosis
  chin implant complication, 496
  nail surgery, 741
needle holders, 61–62, *62*
needles, 64, *64*
  bending, wound closure, **243**
  cutting, biopsies, 211
  suturing (*see* sutures/suturing)

neodymium:yttrium aluminium garnet (Nd:YAG) laser
1064-nm, 653–654
1320 nm, 619–620, 653, 654, *654*
compound/deep hemangiomas, 635, *636*
endoluminal laser ablation, 653–654, 654, *654*
facial erythema, 638
keloids, 712
laser hair removal, 583, **584,** 586
long-pulsed
facial telangiectasia, 637, *637*
hemangiomas, 634
skin resurfacing, 619
vascular lesions, **629**
port-wine stains, 634
pulsed, 641–642
Q-switched, 600, 601
laser hair removal, 579
skin resurfacing, 618–619
skin pigmentation removal, 600–601
dermal lesions, 603
skin resurfacing, 619–620
telangiectases, 641
vascular lesions, 641–642
venulectases, 641
wavelengths, 627
neogenesis, follicular, 575
neomycin allergy, 74
neovascularization
angiogenesis, 108
grafting, 366
nerve blocks, 46–51. *see also individual nerve blocks*
ankle block, 51, *53*
digital block, 49, *50*
extremities, 49–51
peripheral, 47
practical applications, 56–57
regional, 601
wrist block, 51, *51*, *52*
nerve fibers, anesthesia, 41, **42**
nerve injury
local anesthesia adverse effect, 54
Mohs micrographic surgery, 789
nerve supply, 18
Neuro-smooth needle holders, 62
neurotrophic ulcer, 748
neutrophils, 102, **102**
nevi, dermabrasion, 592
nevus of Ota, laser surgery, 603, *603*
optimizing outcomes, 606
treatment parameters, *605*
nevus spilus, *605*
New Fill/Sculptra, **444,** 450
New Jersey, dermatology office accreditation, 164, **167**
New York State, dermatology office accreditation, 164, **167**–168
Nikolsky's sign, laser hair removal, 585
nipple ptosis, breast liposuction, 530
non-ablative laser skin resurfacing, 402–403, 618–622
cooling devices, 618
diode laser (1450 nm), *620*, 620–621
Erbium:glass laser (1540 nm), 621
IPL source, 618
long-pulsed 532 nm KTP laser, 619
Nd:YAG laser
1320 nm, 619–620
long-pulsed, 619
Q-switched, 618–619
optimizing outcomes, 621
patient expectations, 622
photodamage level, 621–622
pitfalls/management, 621–622
postoperative care, 621
preoperative preparation, 618
pulsed dye laser, 618
technical aspects, 618–621
non-ablative radiofrequency skin resurfacing, 621
nonabsorbable sutures, 63–64, **229,** 229–230
biopsies, 211
nonadherent fabric dressings, 118
non-androgenetic hair loss, 552–553, **553**
nonbiologic occlusive dressings, **119,** 119–123
non-steroidal anti-inflammatory drugs (NSAIDs), hemostasis impairment, **247**
North Carolina, dermatology office accreditation, **168**
Norwood classification, 551–552, *552*, 553
nose. *see under nasal*
as cosmetic unit, *8*
Novafil sutures, **229,** 230
Nurolon sutures, **229,** 230
nutritional supplements
cutaneous surgery risk, 73
hemostasis impairment, **247**
nylon sutures, 64, **229,** 230

O

Oasis dermal replacement, 125
grafting, 375
obsessive–compulsive disorder, 415
occipital lymphatic nodes, *20*
occipitofrontalis muscle, 384
occlusion, endoluminal lasers, 654
occlusive dressings, 119–127
alginates, **119,** *122*, 122–123, **133**
biologic, 123–125
biopsies, 211
collagen dressings, 123
films, **119,** *120*, 120–121, **133**
foams, **119,** 120, *120*, **133**
grafts, 123–125
leg ulcers, 761
hyaluronic acid dressings, 123
hydrocolloids, **119,** 121, *121*, **133**
hydrofibers, 123, *123*
hydrogels, **119,** 121–122, *122*, **133**
leg ulcers, 753–754, 757
moisture vapor transmission rate, 119
nonbiologic occlusive, **119,** 119–123
skin substitutes (*see* skin substitutes)
wound healing, 113, *113*
octyl cyanoacrylate (Dermabond), 233
oculocardiac reflex, blepharoplasty complication, 688
odor minimization, dressings, 132
Office-Based Surgery Accreditation program, 161
Office of Inspector General (OIG), 163
Quality Oversight of ASCs: A System in Neglect, 172
office space design, 147–148, *148*
Ohio, dermatology office accreditation, 164, **168,** 171
'Ohmic heating,' 179
Ohm's law, 179
Oklahoma, dermatology office accreditation, **168**
OKT3, **804**
immunosuppression induction, 802
omohyoid muscle, *20*
oncology, 790–797
one-needle ear piercing technique, 301, *301*
onychogryphosis, 727
matricectomy, 725, *725*
onycholemmal carcinoma, 736
onycholemmal cysts, 736
onychomycoses, partial nail avulsion, 724–725
open (spray) cryosurgery technique, 192–193
operating rooms
follicular unit hair transplantation, 557–558
tables, *150*, 150–151, 154
operating stools, adjustable, 150–151
ophthalmic anesthesia, 45
ophthalmic branch, facial nerve, 18
ophthalmologic examination, melanoma, 829
oral commissures
Artecoll, 454
Softform implants, *456*
Z-plasty, 405, *406*
oral contraceptive use, liposuction, 519
oral photography, digital imaging, 86
orbicularis, hypertrophic, 506
orbicularis oculi muscles, 14, **16,** 284
hypertrophy, 685
upper-eyelid blepharoplasty, 676
orbicularis oris muscles, **16,** 17
orbital septa plication, 685
OrCel, 127
Oregon, dermatology office accreditation, **168**
organ transplants
cutaneous surgery effect, 72
history, 801–802, **802**
immunosuppression (*see* immunosuppressive drugs)
incidence, **801,** 801–802
organ transplants, skin cancer in, 801–819. *see also* immunosuppressive drugs; *specific cancers*
aggressiveness, *807*, 807–808
epidemiology, 804–806
incidence, 805–806
hand, 806
histology, *806*, 806–807, *807*
leukoplakia, 806, *806*
management, 810–813
education, 810
follow-up guidelines, 810
sun protection, 810
metastases, 807–808, *808*
multiple hand lesions, 815–816, *816*
multiple scalp lesions, 815, *816*
pathogenesis, *808*, 808–809 (*see also* immunosuppressive drugs)
viral infections, **805**
risk factors, 809–810
scalp, 806
orientation, psychiatric examination, 414
orthonyx method, juvenile ingrown toenails, 729
ortho-phthalaldehyde (OPA) sterilization, 32
orthotic device, venous ulcers, **129,** 130, *130*
Osler-Rendu-Weber syndrome, *638*
osteomyelitis
leg ulcers, 750
scalp reconstruction, 383–384
osteonecrosis, scalp reconstruction, 384
O–T rotation flaps, 316, *317*
bilateral T-plasty advancement flaps *vs.*, 316

overlapping posterior-anterior flaps (Harahap's technique), 294, *296*
oxidative damage, aging face, 425
oxidized cellulose, hemostasis, **252**
oxyhemoglobin absorption peaks, 626, *626*
O–Z flaps (pinwheel flap)
chin reconstruction, 393
rotation flaps, 281, 326, *327*

P

pacemakers
elliptical excision, 260
preoperative identification, 72
pachyonychia congenita, 727
packing of wound
abscesses, 220, *220*
cysts, 220, *220*
Paget's disease. *see* extramammary Paget's disease
pain. *see also* analgesia; anesthesia
cryosurgery, 192
juvenile ingrown toenails, 729
nail surgery, 741
post-cryosurgery, 200
post-dermabrasion, 595
palliative treatment, cryosurgery, 198–199, *199*
palpation, of lipomas, 214, *214*
palpebral muscle, 14
pan-facial filler, 428
panniculitis, venous ulcers, 744
papain urea, 758, *759*
papillomavirus infection, 194–195
parachlorometaxylenol (PCMX) (chloroxylenol)
surgical hand scrub, 27, **28**
surgical site preparation, 31
parallel opposed flaps (Reiter and Alford's technique), 292, *293*
paramedian forehead flap, 348, 350, 351
optimizing outcomes, 363
pitfalls/management, 363
postoperative care, 360–361, *361*, *362*
preoperative preparation, 351–352, *352*
supratrochlear artery, 351
technique, *352*, 352–356, *353*, *354*, *355*, *356*, *357*
trapdoor deformity prevention, 354
paresthesias, 54
Pardue's technique, 297, *297*
parietal bone, *11*
paronychia, 733–734
parotid (Stenson's) duct, *13*
cheek reconstruction, 389
parotid gland, 6, 10–11, *13*, *15*
cheek reconstruction, 389
parotid lymphatic nodes, 19, *20*
parotid nerve, *14*
partial closure, elliptical excision, 266
partial nail avulsion. *see* nail avulsion
partial necrosis, staples, 232
partial-thickness skin graft. *see* split-thickness skin grafts (STSGs)
partial-thickness wounds, 98, *98*, **99**
contraction, 108
uncomplicated, 129
passive–aggressive patients, psychosocial issues, 415
patient counseling, random pattern cutaneous flaps, 314
patient education
hemostasis, **257**
Mohs micrographic surgery, 781
patient evaluation, 67–75. *see also specific disorders; specific techniques*
allergies, 74
for biopsies, 204
components, 67–68
consultation area, 67
laser surgery, 601
medical history (*see* history taking)
medication (existing), 68, 73–74
problem-focused physical examination, 68, *69*
procedure explanation, 68
smoking, 75
social history, 74–75
surgical history, 68, 74
wound closure, 225
patient expectations
follicular unit hair transplantation, 554
psychosocial issues, 416
patient preparation, 30–31
draping, 31
hair removal, 31, *31*
street clothes removal, 30–31
surgical site preparation, **28,** 31
patient privacy, 147
patient questionnaire, 68, *70–71*
patient safety, enhanced by accreditation, 172
PCMX. *see* parachlorometaxylenol (PCMX) (chloroxylenol)
'peau d'orange' chin, BTX-A, 507, *508*
pedicled nasolabial transposition flaps, 334
pedunculated keloids, 708, *708*
solo corticosteroid therapy, 709–710
surgery, 710–712
peeling agents, 431
peer-based quality improvement program, 171
peer-based reviews, 162
penicillin allergy, 74
liposuction, 517
Pennsylvania, dermatology office accreditation, **168**–169
Penrose drain tourniquet, *251*
pentoxifylline, venous ulcers, 752
periauricular zone, suspension sutures, 284–286
perifollicular crusting, laser hair removal, 586
perifollicular edema, laser hair removal, 586
perinasal cheek defect, island pedicle flaps, *319*
periocular tumor, skin defect, 386
periodic acid-Schiff (PAS), 722
perioral region
fat autograft muscle injection, 541
muscles (*see* face, muscles)
reconstruction, 390–393, 397, **398**
perioral rhytides, BTX-A, 506, *506*
periorbital region
BTX-A complications, 510
muscles (*see* face, muscles)
reconstruction, 386, 397, **398**
periorbital rhytidectomy, BTX-A combination, 509
periosteal elevators, 62
partial release of mandibular retaining ligament, 664, *664*
periosteal tacking sutures, 407
peripheral nerve blocks, 47
periungual fibromas, 734
Perlane, **443,** 451
Perma-Hand sutures, **229,** 229–230
personal digital assistant (PDA), 79
personnel preparation, 27–30
attire, *29*, 29–30
hand scrub (*see* hand scrub)
petrolatum
deep (phenol) chemical peels, 476
superficial chemical peels, 471
phenol chemical peels, 476, **476**
history, 463, 464
phenolization
ingrown toenails, 730, *731*, *732*
matrix horn, 730, *731*, *732*
of nail pocket, 725
onychogryphosis, 727
pheomelanin hair color, 577
philtral crest, *8*
philtrum, *8*
photoaging, 425
minimum incision face lift (*see* minimum incision face lift)
neck rejuvenation (*see* neck rejuvenation)
superficial chemical peels (*see* chemical peels, superficial)
photodynamic fluorescent photography, 81
photodynamic therapy (PDT)
actinic keratoses, 793
laser hair removal, 580
photographic dermography, 94–95
photography. *see also* digital imaging
aging face, 428, 432, *434*
autologous fat transfer, 544
BTX-A, 503
chemical peels, 465
dermabrasion, 593
follicular unit hair transplantation, 558–559
liposuction, 522
minimum incision face lift, 660
photomicroscopy, digital imaging, 77
photoprotection, laser hair removal, 586, 587
photorejuvenation, 611, **611**
photothermal laser hair removal, **584**
physician liability, digital imaging, 85
pigmentary changes. *see also* hyperpigmentation; hypopigmentation
dressings, 131
laser hair removal, 586
post-dermabrasion, 596, 597
pigmentary dyschromia, deep (phenol) chemical peels, 476
pilar (trichilemmal) cysts, 218, *219*, 770–771
pilonidal cyst/sinus, 772
pincer nails, 731, 733
'pinch grafting,' leg ulcers, 760, *760*
pin-cushioning, scar formation prevention, 402
pinwheel flaps. *see* O–Z flaps (pinwheel flap)
Pitanguy flap demarcator, 666, *666*
pivot point, random pattern cutaneous flaps, **312**
'pixie ear' deformity, 668
plane of elevation, random pattern cutaneous flaps, 337–338, *338*
Plan of Correction, Medicare certification and reimbursement, 163
plantar surface, 396, *396*
plasticity, sutures, 226
platelet(s)
function, 313
in hemostasis, 101
hemostasis, 245–246
histamine, 103
serotonin release, 103

platelet-derived growth factor (PDGF), 756
platelet gels, **252**
platysmal banding, prominent, 692, *693*
platysmal bands
BTX-A, 508
deformities following neck liposuction, 529
platysma muscle, **16,** 17
minimum incision face lift, 658, 661–662, 666–667
plication via corset platysmaplasty, 666–667
repair (*see* neck rejuvenation, platysma repair)
platysmaplasty, minimum incision face lift, 666–667
plication, SMAS, *286*
pogonion, *12*
poikiloderma, 431
of Civatte, 638–639, *639*
IPL, 638–639
poliglecaprone 25 (Monocryl) sutures, **228,** 229
follicular unit hair transplantation donor closure, 561, **561**
polybutester (Novafil) sutures, **229,** 230
polydioxanone sutures, 227–228, **228**
polyester coated sutures, 64, **229,** 230
sutures, **229**
polyester uncoated sutures, **229,** 230
polyfilament sutures, absorbable, 63
polyglactin 910 (Vicryl-rapide) sutures, 227, **228**
polyglycolic acid (Dexon II, Dexon S) sutures, 227, **228**
polyhexafluoropropylene-VDF (Pronova) sutures, **229,** 230
polymethylmethacrylate (PMMA), 453, *453*
foreign body granuloma, 459
historical aspects, 438
polypropylene (Prolene, Surgipro) sutures, 64, **229,** 230
Polysorb sutures, 227, **228**
polytrimethylene carbonate (Maxon) sutures, **228,** 229
porcine xenografts, 375, *376*
port-wine stains, 630–634
alexandrite laser treatment, 634
classification, **630**
cryosurgery, 196–197
IPL treatment, *633*, 633–634
Klippel–Trenaunay syndrome, 630
KTP laser treatment, 634
Nd:YAG laser treatment, 634
psychosocial morbidity, 631
pulsed dye lasers, *631*, 631–633, *632*, 641
Sturge–Weber syndrome, **630**
positron emission tomography (PET), melanoma staging, 793, 832
postauricular lymphatic nodes, 19, *20*
posterior button keloids, *711*
posterior tibial artery, *22*
posterior tibial nerve block, 51, *53*
posterior triangle, 19
postoperative care, 74–75. *see also* wound care; *specific conditions; specific techniques*
abscesses, 222
biopsies, 211
cryosurgery, 199–200
cysts, 222
exteriorization, 222
incision, 222
lipomas, 222
random pattern cutaneous flaps (*see* random pattern cutaneous flaps)
steatocystoma, 222
wound closure (*see* sutures/suturing; wound closure)
postoperative edema. *see* edema, postoperative
potassium-titanyl-phosphate (KTP) laser
facial erythema, 638
facial telangiectasia, 637
long-pulsed, 619
port-wine stains, 634
pulsed
facial erythema, 641
facial telangiectasias, 641
vascular lesions, 628, **628,** 641
wavelengths, 627
Q-switched, 600
skin cooling, *627*
skin pigmentation removal, 600
skin resurfacing, 619
povidone–iodine
elliptical excision, 261
surgical hand scrub, 27, **28**
surgical site preparation, 31
preauricular cheeks, *8*
preauricular sulcus, 6
prednisolone, **804**
skin cancer occurrence, 809
pregnancy
anesthesia (*see* anesthesia, pregnancy)
cutaneous surgery effect, 68
excisional biopsy, 210
laser hair removal, 578
Prejowl Chin Implant, 488, *489*
pre-jowl sulcus, chin implants, 488
preoperative patient assessment. *see* patient evaluation
preoperative preparation. *see also specific disorders; specific procedures*
aseptic technique (*see* aseptic technique, preoperative preparation)
biopsies, 204–206
cryosurgery, 192
draining, 213–214
exteriorization, 213–214
incision, 213–214
preoperative shaving, infection risk, 31, 35
pressure earrings, earlobe keloids, 711, 713
pressure ulcers
biosurgical debridement, 757
etiology, *745*, 745–746
postoperative care/wound care, 131
prilocaine
anesthesia, **41**
EMLA (*see* EMLA)
methemoglobinemia, 56
primary closure, regional reconstruction, 382
primary defects, definitions, **312**
primary eccrine adenocarcinomas, 796
primary face wound closure, 346
primary intention healing, 98–99
postexcision wounds, 127
primary lobe, random pattern cutaneous flaps, **312**
primary motion, random pattern cutaneous flaps, **312**
primary mucinous carcinoma, 796
privacy, digital imaging, 85
privileging
dermatology office accreditation, 161–162
inaccurate and incomplete, 171
probes, cryosurgery, 193, *193*
problem-focused physical examination, 68, *69*
procaine, 39
anesthesia, **41**
anesthesia history, 39
procedure explanation, 68
procerus muscle, 6, **16**
profile analysis, chin implants, 483–485, *485*
Prolene sutures, **229,** 230
proliferating hemangiomas, 634
proliferative phase (wound healing). *see* wound healing
proline hydroxylase, keloids, 707
Pronova sutures, **229,** 230
proparacaine, topical, **43**
prophylactic antibiotics. *see* antibiotic(s)
Propionibacterium acnes
normal flora, 26
resistance, 137
propoxyphene, post-dermabrasion, 595
prostaglandins
corticosteroid inhibition, 104
in inflammatory response, 104
prosthetic devices
cutaneous surgery effect, 72
implanted, prophylaxis, 144
prosthetic valve endocarditis (PVE), prophylaxis, 142–143
proteinases, remodeling phase of wound healing, 111–112
proteoglycans
remodeling phase of wound healing, 110
tissue remodeling in leg ulcers, 748
proximal interphalangeal crease, *22*
proximal nail avulsion, 724, *724*
proximal nail fold. *see* nail fold
proximal nail groove, 720, 721
proximal palmar crease, *22*
proximal subungual felon, 733
proximal toe block anesthesia, 729
pruritus, follicular unit hair transplantation, **571**
pseudoepitheliomatous hyperplasia, post-cryosurgery, 200
pseudohypopigmentation, post-dermabrasion, 596, 597
Pseudomonas aeruginosa infections
ear piercing infection, 303
elliptical excisions, 271
prevention, 140
resistance, 137
surgical site infection, 26
psychogenic attack, anesthesia, adverse effect, 54
psychosocial issues, 413–423. *see also* body dysmorphic disorder
angry patients, 415
hostile patients, 415
incidence, 413
obsessive–compulsive disorder, 415
passive–aggressive patients, 415
personality identification, 415
pitfalls, 415–416
psychiatric examination, 413–415
appearance, 414
comprehension level, 414
intelligence, 414
Mini-mental Status Exam, 414–415
mood and affect, 414
orientation, 414
thought processing, 414
sociopathic patients, 415

puberty, hair type changes, 576
pulley stitch, 241, *241*
elliptical excision, 266, *268*
functions, 275
pulp, 720
pulsed dye laser (PDL)
benign subcutaneous lesion removal, 767, *768*
facial erythema, 638
hemangiomas, 634, *635*, 641
hypertrophic and erythematous scars, 639–640, *640*
hypertrophic scars, 639–640, *640*
keloids, 712
5-fluorouracil combination, 715
laser skin resurfacing, 618
poikiloderma of Civatte, 638–639, *639*
port-wine stains, *631*, 631–633, *632*, 641
purpura, 628, 629, 641
rosacea-associated telangiectasia, 636, *637*
scar revision, 402
skin pigmentation removal, 600, 601
spider angiomas, 641
striae alba, 640
striae distensae, 640
striae rubra, 640
sunscreen protection, 641
telangiectases, 641
ulcerated hemangiomas, 635
vascular lesions, 627–628, **628,** 629, 641
warts, 640
pulse duration
laser hair removal, 580–581, 586, *586*
laser-tissue interaction principles, 627
pulse oximeter, 153, *153*, 154
punch biopsies, 207–208, *208*, **208**
closure, 211
melanoma biopsy recommendations, 830–831
punch technique (Tan's technique), 291–292, *293*
punctum, 769
puppet face lift, 286
purpura
laser hair removal, 586
pulsed dye lasers, 628, 629, 641
port-wine stains, 633
purse-string sutures, 241
double, *255*
pyoderma gangrenosum ulcer, leg ulcers, 748, *749*

Q

Q-switched lasers
alexandrite lasers, 600, 601
diode laser, 600
KTP laser, 600
Nd:YAG laser (*see* neodymium:yttrium aluminium garnet (Nd:YAG) laser)
pulse duration laser hair removal, 580
ruby lasers, 600, 601
quality assurance, dermatology office accreditation, 162–163
quality improvement programs, 162–163
inadequacy, 171–172
techniques, 162–163
Quality Oversight of ASCs: A System of Neglect, 172

R

racket fingers, nail surgery, 727, *728*
radial nerve
hand (*see* hand, anatomy)
nerve block, 51
radiation dermatitis, telangiectasia, 636, *636*
radiation therapy
BCC, 791
organ transplant recipients, 812
keloids, 712–713
Merkel cell carcinoma, 795
organ transplant recipients, 813
Mohs micrographic surgery combination, 790
SCC, 812
Radiesse filler, **445**, 454–455
historical aspects, 439
pitfalls, 459
preoperative preparation, 440
radiofrequency tissue tightening
neck rejuvenation (*see* neck rejuvenation)
varicose veins (*see* varicose veins, endovenous ablation)
radiotherapy. *see* radiation therapy
random pattern cutaneous flaps, 311–344, 348, 349. *see also specific types*
advantages, 312
anesthesia, 336
classification schemes, 311
complications, 341–342
contraindications, 313–314
definitions, 311, **312**
disadvantages, 312–313
dog-ear redundancy, **312**
graft combination, 281–282
hemostasis, 313, 338
history, 312
incision, 336–337
optimizing outcomes, 334–339
patient selection, 313–314
alternative surgery, 336
pivot point, **312**
plane of elevation, 337–338, *338*
postoperative care, 339–342
closed wound care, 339
dressings, 339
frequent wound care, 339
scar massage, 341
suture removal, 339–341
preoperative preparation, 312–314
aesthetic considerations, 335
informed consent, 336
patient counseling, 314
tumor removal confirmation, 312
primary lobe, **312**
primary motion, **312**
scalp reconstruction, 384
secondary lobe, **312**
secondary motion, **312**
surgical planning, 335–336
suturing, 338–339
tension vector, **312**
undermining, **337,** 337–338
vascular networks, 311
rapamycin, 808
Rassman handle, 560, *560*
razor blades, 60
recombinant human platelet-derived growth factor, 756
reconstructive nail surgery, 737, 740–741
rectangular flaps on anterior and posterior sides (Zolite's technique), 298, *299*
red-green-blue (RGB) imaging, 81
red hypertrophic scars, revision, 402
reduction mammoplasty, 530
re-epithelialization wound healing, 105–106
regeneration wound healing, 98
regional nerve blocks, 601
regional reconstruction, 381–399
cheeks (*see* cheeks)
chin (*see* chin)
closure options, preferred, **398**–399
digits, 396–397, **399**
ear, 393–394, *394*, **398**
extremities, 395–396, **398**
feet, 396–397, **399**
forehead/temple, 384–386, *385*, **398**
hands, 396–397, **398, 399**
healing, 381–382
secondary-intention healing, 381–382, **383**
neck, 394–395, **398**
nose (*see* nasal reconstruction)
perioral region, 390–393, *391*, *392*, **398**
periorbital region, 386, **398**
pitfalls/management, 397
scalp, 382–384, *383*, *384*, **398**
trunk, 395, **398**
wound closure, **381**
reinnervation, grafting, 366
Reiter and Alford's technique, 292, 293, *293*, *295*
Reiter technique. *see* Z-plasty
relaxed skin tension lines (RSTL)
scar formation prevention, 401
Z-plasty, 404
remodeling phase, wound healing. *see* wound healing
repair tray organization, 66, *66*
repair wound healing, 98
repetitive compulsive behavior, 418
resident flora, 26
rest, hemostasis, 255
Restylane, **443,** 451, *451*, 452
adverse events, 452
Restylane Fine Lines, **442,** 451
resurfacing, 431
resuscitative equipment, 153, 154
retinal transplant recipients, skin cancer prevention, 811
retinoids. *see also individual types*
organ transplant recipients, 811, 813
SCC treatment, 813
retroauricular island transposition flap, 393–394
retrobulbar hemorrhage, blepharoplasty, 687
retroplasmal fat, 696, *696*
reverse cutting needle, 231, *231*
reverse transcriptase polymerase chain reaction (RT-PCR), sentinel lymph node biopsy, 833
Reviderm Intra, **444,** 454
rhinion, *12*
rhinophyma
dermabrasion, 592
rosacea association, 196
Rhode Island, dermatology office accreditation, **169**
rhombic transposition flaps. *see* transposition flaps
rhytidectomy. *see* face lifts (rhytidectomy)
rhytides
aging face, 426
coarse, 431
dermabrasion, 592
Isolagen, 449

rhytides, (*cont'd*)
laser skin resurfacing (*see* laser skin resurfacing)
superficial chemical peels, 467
Riedel's profile analysis, 484, *485*
Rieger flap. *see* dorsal nasal flap
ring block, 46, *46*
applications, 56
risorius muscle, **16,** 17
root, forehead, *8*
ropivacaine, **41**
rosacea
cryosurgery, 196
facial erythema, 637
telangiectasia association, *637*
rotation flaps, 320–326. *see also* advancement flaps
basis, *321*
cervicofacial, 281, *281,* 286, *286*
cheek reconstruction, 390
chin, *322*
dorsal nasal rotation flap, 321, 322–323, *324,* 325
eyelid/cheek, *322*
mobility improvement, 321, *324*
Mustarde flaps, 325–326
nose reconstruction, 387
optimal rotation, 321, *323*
O–Z flaps (pinwheel flap), 281, 326, *327*
periorbital region reconstruction, 386
placement/creation, 321, *323*
scalp reconstruction, 384, *384*
scar formation prevention, 402
split earlobe repair, 294, *297*
suturing, 339, *340*
Tenzel flaps, *325,* 325–326, *326*
rounded needle, 231, *231*
'roundeye' repair, 509
rubber gloves, 26
Rubin's technique, 305, *306*
ruby lasers
hair removal, 582–583, **584,** 586
Q-switched, 600, 601
running horizontal mattress sutures, 215, *215*
running locked sutures, 238–239, *239*
ellipse excision, 263–264, *265*
running simple sutures, 238, *238*
running subcuticular sutures, 239, *240,* 280, *281*
running subdermal sutures, 241
running sutures, 238–239, 278–279. *see also specific types*
continuous, 278–279, *279*
ellipse excision, 263, *264*
horizontal mattress, 215, *215*
locked (*see* running locked sutures)
simple, 238, *238*
subcuticular, 239, *240,* 280, *281*
subdermal, 241

S
saddle bags, liposuction, 521, 522
sagging
aging face, 430, *431*
resulting from fat distribution, 429
salicylic acid, superficial chemical peels, 470
saphenous nerve block, 51, *53*
sarcopenia, 425
saucerization biopsies, 206
saucerization biopsy, 206
melanoma biopsy recommendations, 831
S-Caine patch, 45
S-Caine peel, 45
scalp
anatomy, 6
cyst, *770*
laxity, 554
organ transplants, skin cancer in, 806
reconstruction, 382–384, 397, **398**
regions, 564, *564*
scalpels, *59,* 59–60, *60*
scalp stains, follicular unit hair transplantation, 556
scars/scarring
biopsies, 212
chemical peels complication, 480, *480*
cysts, 223
elliptical excision, 271
follicular unit hair transplantation, 554
hypertrophic (*see* hypertrophic scars)
informed consent, 260
Isolagen, 449
massage, 341
post-dermabrasion, 597
prevention, 401–402
flap refinements, 402, *402*
revision (*see below*)
tissue formation, 111
wound healing, 98
scars/scarring, revision, 401–409
dermabrasion, 592
postoperative care, 408
techniques, 402–408
ablative lasers, 408
dermabrasion, 407–408, *409*
ectropion prevention, 407
ectropion repair, 406–407, *408*
fusiform elliptical excision, 403, *403*
geometric broken-line closure, 404, *404*
intralesional steroids, 402
non-ablative lasers, 402–403
oral commissure correction, 405, *406*
trapdoor deformity repair, 406, *407*
V-to-Y repair, 405–406, *406*
W-plasty, 403–404, *404*
Z-plasty, 404–405, *405, 406*
timing, 402
Schirmer test, 676, 688
scissor biopsy, 206–207, *207*
scissors, *60,* 60–61, *61*
scleral show
blepharoplasty complication, 687
lower-eyelid blepharoplasty complication, 685
screening, melanoma, 828–829
scrub suits, 29, *29*
sebaceous carcinoma, 796
sebaceous cysts. *see* epidermal cysts; steatocystoma
sebaceous skin, random pattern cutaneous flaps, 313
seborrheic keratoses
cryosurgery, 195
dermabrasion, 592
laser surgery, 602
sebum levels, microdermabrasion, 590–591
secondary defects, definitions, **312**
secondary-intention healing, 98–99, 345–346, *346*
follicular unit extraction, 560
perioral region reconstruction, 393
porcine xenografts, 375
postexcision wounds, 127–128
regional reconstruction, 381–382, **383**
surgical face wound closure, 345–346, *346*
secondary lobe, random pattern cutaneous flaps, **312**
secondary motion, random pattern cutaneous flaps, **312**
seizures, anesthesia, 56
selective lateral matrix excision, 730, *731*
selective photothermolysis
laser-tissue interaction principles, 625–626
vascular lesions, 627–630
selective serotonin reuptake inhibitors (SSRIs), body dysmorphic disorder, 417, 422
self-adherent wrap, venous ulcers, **129**
self examination
dysplastic nevi, 827
melanoma, 828
senescent cell removal, leg ulcers, 756
sentinel lymph node (SLN) biopsy
BCC treatment, 812–813
melanoma (*see* melanoma)
SCC treatment, 812–813
sepsis, 25
Septisol, deep (phenol) chemical peels, 476
septum incision, upper-eyelid blepharoplasty, 682, *682*
seroma formation
dressings, 131
neck rejuvenation complication, 699, 700
serotonin
in inflammatory response, 103
mast cell release, 103
platelet release, 103
sessile keloids, 708, *708*
solo corticosteroid therapy, 709–710
surgery, 710–712
shave biopsy, 206, **206,** *207*
shave therapy, venous ulcers, 130–131, 763
shaving, hair removal, 578
short-pulsed lasers, 599, 601
side-to-side closure, 291, *292,* 293, *294*
wound edge undermining (Apesos' technique), 293, *295*
Z-plasty at inferior margin (Casson's technique), 293, *295*
'side weighting,' follicular unit hair transplantation, 564, *565*
silastic chin implants, 488–489
silicone chin implants. *see* chin implants
silicone gel sheeting (SGS), 709, 710, 712, 713–714
silicone, liquid, 437–438
silk sutures, 63–64, **229,** 229–230
SilkTouch carbon dioxide laser, 612
silver-impregnated dressings, 127
silver nitrate, hemostasis, 249, **252**
simple sutures
ellipse excision, 263, *264*
interrupted, 278, *278*
single interrupted stitches, *235,* 235–236
sinks, surgical suite design, 151–152
sirolimus (rapamycin), **804**
immunosuppression maintenance, 803
site preparation, **28,** 31, 33
sizer implant insertion, 490, *492*
skeletal muscle wastage, 425
skin
atrophy, corticosteroid treatment, 710
biomechanical responses, 5–6, 275
mechanical creep, 6, 275
stress relaxation, 275
stress–strain curves, *5,* 5–6

cancer (*see also specific types*)
axial pattern flaps, 345–346
contraindication to organ transplant, 815
excision wounds, 761
metastasis, 198
primary tumors, 198
total body photography, 88, 90
closure (*see* sutures/suturing; wound closure)
cooling
epidermal protection from lasers, 627, *627*
pulsed dye laser treatment of port-wine stains, 631, 633
function, 3
head and neck, 6
intrinsic elasticity, 5
laser resurfacing (*see* ablative laser skin resurfacing; laser skin resurfacing; non-ablative laser skin resurfacing)
marking
transconjunctival lower-eyelid blepharoplasty, 683
transcutaneous lower-eyelid blepharoplasty, 684
upper-eyelid blepharoplasty, 676
muscle interaction, 425–426
phototype
ablative laser skin resurfacing, 617
classification, 578, **579**
non-ablative laser skin resurfacing, 622
redraping, 699
redundancy, liposuction, 522
structure, 3–5, *4*, 273–274
dermis, *4*, 5
dermoepidermal junction, 5
epidermis, 3–4, *4*
head, *7*
surface microscopic photography, 94–95
tension, keloids, 706, 715
types, laser hair removal, 585–586
skin closure tapes, 232
skin hooks, 61, 225
epidermal cysts wall dissection, 217, *217*
use, 34
skin preservation at apex (Boo-Chai's technique), 297, *297*
skin substitutes, 123–127. *see also* grafts/grafting
composite grafts, 123, **124,** *126*, 126–127
dermal replacements (*see* dermal replacements)
epidermal grafts, cultured, 123, **124,** 125
grafting, 375
skin tension lines
body, 9
elliptical excision evaluation, 260
extremities, *10*
face, 7, *9*
wound contraction, 108
sliding flaps, scar formation prevention, 402
slivering, follicular unit hair transplantation, 561–562, *562*
smile alterations, chin implants, 496
smoking
chemical peels, 466
cutaneous surgery risk, 75
follicular unit hair transplantation, 556, **557**
minimum incision face lift, 660, 667, 668
nail surgery, 741
random pattern cutaneous flaps, 313–314
wound infection development, 138
snap test
lower-lid laxity test in blepharoplasty, 674, *681*
neck rejuvenation, 692
social history, 74–75
social phobias, body dysmorphic disorder, 419
sociopathic patients, psychosocial issues, 415
sodium bicarbonate
anesthesia additive, 42, **42**
liposuction, 523–524
Sofsilk sutures, **229,** 229–230
Softform/Ultrasoft, **446,** 456, *456*, *457*
historical aspects, 439
soft-tissue augmentation, 437–462. *see also* dermal fillers; *individual fillers/implants*
BTX-A combination, 509
commonly used products, 441–457, **442–446**
autologous collagen, 449–450
hyaluronic acid gels (*see* hyaluronic acid (hyaluronan))
ideal properties, 437
subdermal fillers, 454–456
subdermal implants, 455, 456–457
expectations, 440
historical aspects, 437–439
optimizing outcomes, 458
patient preparation, 459
pitfalls/management, **440,** 458–460
extrusion, 459
implant palpation, 459
infection, 458, 459
tissue necrosis in glabellar region, 459
postinjection swelling/erythema, 459
postoperative care, 458
preoperative preparation, 439–441
skin test, 458
side effects, 459
technical aspects, 441–457
vasovagal episode, 459
soft tissue landmarks, profile analysis, **484**
soft tissue prostheses, antibiotics, 145
solar elastosis, soft-tissue augmentation, 458
solar lentigenes
cryosurgery, 195–196
laser surgery, *602*
solid carbon dioxide, cryosurgery, 194
SOOF (suborbicularis oculi fat) face lift, 286, *286*
South Carolina, dermatology office accreditation, **169**
speech alterations, chin implants, 496
spider angiomas, 636
pulsed dye lasers, 641
spinal accessory nerve. *see* cranial nerve IX (spinal accessory nerve)
S-plasty (lazy S repair), 266, *268*
excisional biopsy, 210
split earlobe repair, 291–301
complete split repair, 293–301
bilateral flap from posterior and lateral portion of lobe (Buchan's technique), 297–298, *298*
creation of flap from lateral portion of lobe (Pardue's technique), 297, *297*
creation of flap from lateral portion of lobe and Z-plasty (Walike and Larrabee and Hamilton and La Rossa techniques), 297, *298*
lap-joint technique (Argamaso's technique), 298, *299*
L-plasty (Fatah's technique), 293–294, *296*, 299, *299*
modifications, 300
overlapping posterior-anterior flaps (Harahap's technique), 294, *296*
partially incised T-plasty (Arora's technique), 294, *296*
pierced canal not preserved, 293–294
pierced canal preservation, 297–300
rectangular flaps on anterior and posterior sides (Zolite's technique), 298, *299*
rotational flap (Effendi's technique), 294, *297*
side-to-side closure, 293, *294*
with Z-plasty at inferior margin (Casson's technique), 293, 295
skin preservation at apex (Boo-Chai's technique), 297, *297*
superior based skin flaps (Elsahy's technique), 298, *299*
superior strip repair of tract and two Z-plasties (Fayman's technique), 300, *300*
undermining wound edges and side-to-side closure (Apesos' technique), 293, *295*
V-flap (Kalimuthu's technique), 294, *296*
Z-plasty (Tromovitch's, Reiter and Alford's techniques), 293, *295*
partial split repair, 291–292
parallel opposed flaps (Reiter and Alford's technique), 292, *293*
punch technique (Tan's technique), 291–292, *293*
side-to-side closure, 291, *292*
pitfalls and their management, 301
postoperative care, 301
preoperative preparation, 291
techniques, 291–301 (*see also individual techniques*)
split nail, 737, *740*
split-thickness skin grafts (STSGs), 123, **124,** 370–374
definition, 365
equipment, 370
extremities reconstruction, 395
fusiform elliptical excision, 403
grafting for leg ulcers, 758
hands, feet and digits reconstruction, 396
harvesting, 370–372
dermatomes, 371, *371*
mesher, 371–372, 372
Weck blade, 371, *371*
Zimmer electric dermatome, 371, *371*
Zimmer mesher, 372, *372*
postoperative care, 377, *377*
procedure, 372–374, *373*
regional reconstruction, 382
trunk reconstruction, 395
wound dressing, 123, **124**
spongiotic dermatitis, 631
spontaneous keloids, 706
spot size, laser principles, 627
spray cryosurgery technique, 192–193
spray refrigerants, dermabrasion, 594
squamous cell carcinoma (SCC), 736, 792–793. *see also* actinic keratoses
actinic keratoses precursors, 793
contraindication to organ transplant, 815
cryosurgery, 198

squamous cell carcinoma (SCC), (*cont'd*)
ellipse excision, 262
in situ (*see* Bowen's disease (squamous cell carcinoma *in situ*))
leg ulcers, 750
metastases, 792
Mohs micrographic surgery, 780, 812
specimen interpretation, 785–786
proliferating trichilemmal cyst differential diagnosis, 771
transplant recipients (*see below*)
squamous cell carcinoma (SCC), organ transplant recipients, 806
HIV infection, 809
human papillomavirus, 809
incidence, 805
lower lip, 806, *806*
metastases, 807
pathogenesis, 809
risk factors, 809–810
treatment, 810–813, *814*
adjuvant therapies, 813
chemoprophylaxis, 811
cryosurgery, 812
electrodesiccation and curettage, 812
isotretinoin, 813
Mohs micrographic surgery, 812
radiation therapy, 812
retinoids, 813
sentinel lymph node dissection, 812–813
surgery, 811–813
topical agents, 810–811
square knot, 233, **233**
square sutures, *256*
stab incision
abscesses, 220, *220*
cysts, 220, *220*
staff illness, infection prevention, 140
stainless steel sutures, 64
stanozolol, venous ulcers, 752
Staphylococcus aureus infection
ear piercing infection, 303
intranasal colonization, 138
resistance, 137
screen
dermabrasion, 593
electrodesiccation and curettage, 189
elliptical excisions, 271
surgical site infection, 26
wound infection prevention, 141
Staphylococcus epidermidis
normal flora, 26
wound infection prevention, 141
Staphylococcus viridans, 141
staples, 231–232
follicular unit hair transplantation donor closure, 561, *561*
wound closure, 231–232
state legislation and regulation, 164–171, **165**–170
state licensing, 163–164
steam autoclave sterilization, 65
surgical instrument sterilization, 32
steatocystoma, 219
optimizing outcomes, 221–222
postoperative care, 222
steatocystoma multiplex, 772
step-off correction, 235, 237–238, *238*, *241*
step-sectioning, melanoma biopsy recommendations, 831
stereomicroscopic dissection, follicular unit hair transplantation, 557–558, 561–562, *562*
sterile field maintenance, 34, *34*
sterile surgical gowns, 30
sterilization, instruments, 32, 33–34, 65
Steri-strips
ellipse excision, 263
scar formation prevention, 401
sternocleidomastoid muscles, 12–13, 19
neck liposuction, 694, *694*
steroids. *see* corticosteroids
'stick and place,' follicular unit hair transplantation, 565
stomion superius, *12*
stratum corneum, 4, *4*
stratum germinativum, epidermis, 4, *4*
stratum granulosum, 4, *4*
stratum spinosum, 4, *4*
street clothes removal, 30–31
stress relaxation, skin, 275
stress–strain curves, skin, 5, 5–6
striae alba, pulsed dye laser, 640
striae distensae, 640
pulsed dye laser, 640
striae rubra, 640
strip excision, follicular unit hair transplantation, *560*, 560–561
stromelysins, **112**
strong chin, 483, *484*
structural augmentation, 431
structural facial rejuvenation, 431–432
aging face, *433*
structural fat remodeling with age, 426–427, *427*
Sturge–Weber syndrome, **630**
subcutaneous fatty tissue, liposuction, 521
subcutaneous fibrosis, minimum incision face lift, 667–668
subcutaneous hinge flap, 369
subcutaneous lesions. *see specific types*
subcuticular sutures, running, 239, *240*, 280, *281*
subdermal fillers, 454–456
subdermal sutures, running, 241
subfascial endoscopic perforator surgery (SEPS), 762–763
submandibular lymphatic nodes, *20*
submandibular ptosis, facial soft tissue lifting using Aptos threads. *see* Aptos threads, facial soft tissue lifting
submental depressions, post-neck liposuction, 529
submental fat assessment, neck rejuvenation, 692
submental lymphatic nodes, 19, *20*
submental surgery. *see* chin implants, submental surgery
subnasale, *12*
suborbicularis oculi fat (SOOF) face lift, 286, *286*
subperiosteal minimum incision face lift, 658
subungual hematomas, 726, *726*
subungual hyperkeratoses, 724
subungual keratoses, 727
subungual exostoses, 734, *735*
subungual felon, 733, 734
subungual glomus tumors, 734–735, *735*
subungual infection, 734
suction machines, 149, 152
suicide attempts, body dysmorphic disorder, 419
sun avoidance, post-dermabrasion, 596
sun exposure, dysplastic nevi, 824
sun protection
laser surgery, 607
melanoma, 830, 835
organ transplants, skin cancer in, 810
sunscreens
chemical peels preparation, 465
pulsed dye lasers, 641
Supercut scissors, 60–61
superficial augmentation, 431
superficial branch radial nerve, *22*
superficial chemical peels. *see* chemical peels, superficial
superficial fibular nerve block, 51, *53*
superficial matrix biopsy, *723*, 723–724
superficial musculoaponeurotic system (SMAS), 6, 14, 17, *276*
axial arteries, 17
in face lifts, 285, *285*
identification, 273, 275
imbrication, 285
minimum incision face lift, 657, 664–665, *665*, 667
minimum incision face lifts, 657, 658, 659–660
plication, *286*
neck rejuvenation (*see* neck rejuvenation, SMAS plication)
wrinkles, 7
superficial temporal artery, 11, *13*, *15*
superficial temporal vein, *15*
superior based skin flaps (Elsahy's technique), 299, *299*
superior eyebrow, *8*
superior labial artery, *15*
superior palpebral sulcus, *9*
superior strip repair of tract and two Z-plasties (Fayman's technique), 300, *300*
supermedial cheeks, *8*
supraorbital foramen, 10, *11*
supraorbital nerve
forehead and temple reconstruction, 385
nerve block, 47, **47**, *48*
supraorbital transposition flaps, 282, *282*
supraperiosteal pocket, chin implants, 492
supra-SMAS (subcutaneous) minimum incision face lift, 658, 659
supratip, *12*
repair, 350, 356–358
supratrochlear artery, paramedian forehead flap, 351
supratrochlear nerve
forehead and temple reconstruction, 385
nerve block, 47, **47**, *48*
sural nerve block, 51, *53*
surgical attire, 29–30
surgical suite design, *147*, 147–148, 147–157, 149–153
ambulatory surgery center (ASC) approval, 148
arrangement of equipment, 152–153
cabinets and storage, 151, *151*, 154
carts, 151, *152*
ceilings, 149
consultant (architect) selection, 148
costs, 148, **150**
crash carts, 150
doors, 149, 154
equipment suppliers, 155–157
fire safety, 148

floors, 149, 154
Health Insurance Portability and Accountability Act of 1996 (HIPPA) guidelines for patient privacy, 147
hydraulic power tables, 149
lighting, 149, 151, *151*, 154
Mayo stand, 152, *152*
monitoring equipment, 153, *153*
office accreditation, 148
office space design, 147–148, *148*
operating room tables, *150*, 150–151, 154
operating stools, adjustable, 150–151
optimizing outcomes, 154
patient privacy, 147
pitfalls/management, 154
plumbing, 149
resuscitative equipment, 153, 154, *154*
room maintenance, 153
size, 148
suction machines, 149, 152
surgical sink, 151–152
walls, 149
waste disposal, 152, 154
wiring, 149
Surgilon sutures, **229,** 230
Surgipro sutures, **229,** 230
suspension (tacking) suture, 282–287
anchoring points, 283, *283*
forehead, 283–284
lower eyelid, 284
mid-face, 284–285
nasolabial junction, 287
periauricular zone, 284–286
placement, 283, *283*
random pattern cutaneous flaps, 339
technique, 283
suture-cutting scissors, 61, *61*
suture granuloma, dressings, 131
sutures/suturing, 62–64, **63,** 233–241
allergy to, 227
aseptic technique, 35
breakage during tying, **243**
capillarity, 226
chin implants submental surgery, 491
coating, 226
configuration, 225–226
elasticity, 226
elliptical excision, 263–264
follicular unit hair transplantation donor closure, 561, *561*
hands, feet and digits reconstruction, 396
hemostasis (*see* hemostasis)
knots, 226, 233–235
instrument tie, 233, *234*
slippage, **243**
square knot, 233, **233**
strength, 226
memory, 226
nasolabial transposition flaps, 339
needles, 64, *64*, 230–231, *231*
commonly used types, 231, *232*
Ethicon needle abbreviations, 231, *232*
optimizing outcomes, 241–242
placement, 242
plasticity, 226
properties, 225–227
random pattern cutaneous flaps (*see* random pattern cutaneous flaps)
removal, 242, *242*, **242**
biopsies, 211
elliptical excision, 269
random pattern cutaneous flaps, 339–341
rotation flaps, 339, *340*
scar formation prevention, 401
selection of, 242
size, 226
step-off correction, 235, 237–238, *238*, *241*
suture tracks, **243**
tensile strength, 226
tension, 241–242
tissue reaction, **226,** 226–227
types/materials, 62–64, **63,** 227–230 (*see also specific types*)
absorbable sutures (*see* absorbable sutures)
buried butterfly suture, *240*, 240–241
continuous running sutures, 278–279, *279*
deep layer (dermal) sutures, 278
double imbricating suture, 253
double purse-string sutures, *255*
epidermal sutures, 278–280
Ethibond sutures (*see* Ethibond sutures)
Ethilon sutures, **229,** 230
figure-of-eight suture, *256*
glycomer 631 (Biosyn), **228,** 229
half-buried horizontal mattress (tip) stitch, 236–237, *237*
half-buried mattress sutures, 280, *280*
lactomer (Polysorb), 227, **228**
Maxon sutures, **228,** 229
Mersiline sutures, **229,** 230
Monocryl sutures, **228,** 229
Monosof sutures, **229,** 230
nonabsorbable (*see* nonabsorbable sutures)
Novafil sutures, **229,** 230
Nurolon sutures, **229,** 230
nylon sutures, 64, **229,** 230
periosteal tacking sutures, 407
Perma-Hand sutures, **229,** 229–230
polybutester (Novafil), **229,** 230
polydioxanone, 227–228, **228**
polyester, uncoated (Dacron, Mersiline), **229,** 230
polyfilament absorbable, 63
polyglactin 910 (Vicryl-rapide), 227, **228**
polyglycolic acid (Dexon II, Dexon S), 227, **228**
polyhexafluoropropylene-VDF (Pronova), **229,** 230
polypropylene (Prolene, Surgipro), 64, **229,** 230
Polysorb, 227, **228**
polytrimethylene carbonate (Maxon), **228,** 229
Prolene, **229,** 230
Pronova, **229,** 230
pulley stitch, 241, *241*
running simple suture, 238, *238*
running subcuticular stitch, 239, *240*
running subdermal stitch, 241
silk, 63–64, **229,** 229–230
single interrupted stitches, *235*, 235–236
Sofsilk, **229,** 229–230
square, *256*
stainless steel, 64
surgical gut, 63, 227, **228**
Surgilon, **229,** 230
Surgipro, **229,** 230
suspension (*see* suspension (tacking) suture)
tacking (*see* suspension (tacking) suture)
Ticron, **229,** 230
tie-over, 368, *369*
traditional buried, 239–240, *240*, *241*
U sutures, *256*
Vicryl-rapide, 227, **228**
swelling, post-cryosurgery, 201
syringe aspiration, autologous fat transfer, 537, *537*
syringomas, dermabrasion, 592
systemic antibiotics. *see* antibiotic(s)
systemic lupus erythematosus (SLE), inflammatory ulcers, 746

T
tachycardia, following liposuction, 530–531
tacking sutures. *see* suspension (tacking) suture
tacrolimus, **804**
immunosuppression maintenance, 803
skin cancer occurrence, 808, 809
Tan's technique, split earlobe repair, 291–292, *293*
Tanzer's technique, earlobe reduction, 304, *305*
Targretin, 811
tattoo removal
dermabrasion, 592
laser surgery, 600, 603–604, *604*
amateur tattoos, 603–604, *604*
hypopigmentation, *606*
laser types, 606–607
optimizing outcomes, 606–607
treatment parameters, *605*
tattoos, pigments, 603–604
Tazarotene, 811
tear-through deformity, 540–541
Teflon (PTFE), historical aspects, 439
telangiectasias, 635–637
elliptical excision, 271
facial, 637, *637*
IPL, 637, *638*
Osler-Rendu-Weber syndrome, *638*
pulsed dye lasers, 641
KTP laser skin resurfacing, 619
radiation dermatitis, 636, *636*
rosacea-associated, 636, *637*
spider angiomas, 636
surrounding scars, 402
venulectasia, 637
teledermatology, 85
Telfa, full-thickness grafts, 366
telogen effluvium
androgenic alopecia, 553
follicular unit hair transplantation, 555
telogen hair growth, 576, *577*
temple reconstruction, 384–386, *385*
temporal bone, *8*, 10, *11*
temporal branches, facial nerve, *13*, *14*, *16*, 18, *19*
temporal fossa, 11–12
tenascin, post-dermabrasion, 596
tendon passers, Alloderm insertion, 455, *455*
Tennessee, dermatology office accreditation, **170**
tension vector, random pattern cutaneous flaps, **312**
Tenzel flaps, *325*, 325–326, *326*
terminal hair, 576
test spot, dermabrasion, 593–594, 597

tetracaine, **41**
cocaine, 45
history, 39
lidocaine, 45
topical anesthesia, **43, 44,** 45
Texas, dermatology office accreditation, **169,** 171
thenar eminence, *22*
therapeutic skin biopsies, 203
ThermaCool TC
neck rejuvenation, 692, 698–699, *699*
skin resurfacing, 621
thermal burns, local anesthesia adverse effect, 54
thermal damage time (TDT), 581
thermal diffusivity, laser-tissue interaction principles, 627
thermal relaxation time (TRT)
laser-tissue interaction principles, 627
pulse duration laser hair removal, 580, **581**
thermolysis, hair removal, 578
thighs
autologous fat transfer donor site, 537
liposuction
medial, 526
outer, 526, *528*
thought processing, psychiatric examination, 414
threading injection technique
bovine collagen, *448*, 449
hyaluronic acid gels, 452
thrombin, 245–246, **252**
thrombocytopenia, 247
thumb interphalangeal crease, *22*
tibialis posterior tendon, *22*
tibial nerve, *22*
Ticlid (ticlopidine), hemostasis impairment, **247**
ticlopidine (Ticlid), hemostasis impairment, **247**
Ticron sutures, **229,** 230
tie-over bolster, full-thickness grafts, 367–368, *369*
tie-over sutures, 368, *369*
tip stitch, 236–237, *237*
tissue adhesives
ellipse excision, 263
wound closure, 232–233
tissue damage
electrosurgery, 252–253
glabellar region, following soft-tissue augmentation, 459
tissue inhibitor metalloproteinases (TIMPs), 112
tissue reaction, sutures, **226,** 226–227
tissue remodeling, leg ulcers, 746, 748
tissue temperature, cryosurgery, 194
T lymphocytes, **102**
tobacco exposure, cutaneous flaps, 347
toenails. *see* nail(s)
toluidine blue, Mohs micrographic surgery, 784
tongue-in-groove technique, composite grafts, 374
topicaine, **44,** 45
topical anesthesia. *see* anesthesia, topical
topical antibiotics. *see* antibiotic(s)
total body photography, 77, 88, 90, 93–94, *94*
with digital dermoscopy, 95
total freeze time, cryosurgery, 191
total immersion photography, 82, **83,** 93
total thaw time, cryosurgery, 191
tourniquets, 249, *250, 251*
nail surgery, 721
towel clamps, suture tension, 242
towel clips, 62
T-plasty, partially incised (Arora's technique), 294, *296*
track marks, wound closure, 242
traditional buried stitches, 239–240, *240*
tramadol, 55
tranexamic acid (Amstat), **253**
transblepharoplasty browpexy, 687
transconjunctival lower-eyelid blepharoplasty, 683–684, *684*
transcutaneous lower-eyelid blepharoplasty, 684–687
Transcyte dermal replacement, 126
transepidermal water loss (TEWL), microdermabrasion, 591
transient flora, 26
transposition flaps, 326–334. *see also specific types*
applications
cheek reconstruction, 389, *390*
forehead and temple reconstruction, 385–386
perioral region reconstruction, 392
periorbital region reconstruction, 386
scalp reconstruction, 384
banner, 330, *333, 334*
bilobed, 281, 328, 330, *331*
cheek reconstruction, 389
distal nasal defects, 330, *332*
nose reconstruction, 387, *388*
scar formation prevention, 402
rhombic, 327–328, *329*
basis, *328*
hands, feet and digits reconstruction, 396
modified, *330*, 338
scar formation prevention, 402
supraorbital, 282, *282*
trapdoor deformity, 342
transthecal digital block, nail surgery, 721, *722*
transverse cervical nerve block, **47,** 48–49
trapdoor deformity
Abbe cross-lip flap, 361
nasolabial transposition flaps, 334, *335*
paramedian forehead flap repair, 354, 360
random pattern cutaneous flaps, 342
repair, 406, *407*
scar formation, 402, *402*
transposition flaps, 342
'trap' hypothesis, venous ulcers, 744
trauma
keloids, 706
nail surgery, 726
treatment timeline, cryosurgery, *200*
Trendelenburg position, operating room tables, 150
tretinoin
ablative laser skin resurfacing, 612
actinic keratoses management, 811
chemical peels preparation, 465
melanoma prevention, 831
post-dermabrasion, 596
SCC treatment, 813
superficial chemical peels, 467, 470
triamcinolone acetonide, 709–710
trichilemmal (pilar) cysts, 218, *219*, 770–771, 771
trichloroacetic acid (TCA) peels, 431
history, 463, 464
medium-depth, 471, 472, 474
superficial, 468
trichodiscomas, medium-depth chemical peels, 472, *473*
trichoepitheliomas, dermabrasion, 592
trichon, *12*
trimethoprim-sulfamethoxazole, 141
Triseptin, 27–28
Tromovitch's technique. *see* Z-plasty
trunk reconstruction, 395, 397, **398**
tumescent anesthesia. *see* anesthesia, tumescent
tumescent liposuction, 142
tweezing, hair removal, 578
two-needle ear piercing technique, 302, *302*
Tyndall effect, hyaluronic acid gels, 452

U

ulcers
arterial (*see* arterial ulcers)
biopsies, 203
diabetic foot ulcers (*see* diabetic ulcers)
hemangiomas, 634–635, *635*
pressure (*see* pressure ulcers)
venous ulcers (*see* venous ulcers)
wound, 98, *99*
ulnar nerve, *22*
nerve block, 51, *52*
Ultrapulse 5000 carbon dioxide laser, 612
Ultrasoft, 456
historical aspects, 439
ultrasound, Doppler, endovenous ablation, 646
ultraviolet (UV) light
melanoma precautions, 830, **830**
photography, 81
undermining
biopsies, 210, **211**
elliptical excision, 263
minimum incision face lift, 663–664, 667, 668
lateral cheek/lateral neck skin flap, 662–663
neck, 667–668
random pattern cutaneous flaps, **337,** 337–338
ungual melanomas, 736–737, *738*
ungual fibrokeratomas, 734, *734*
unilateral advancement flaps. *see* advancement flaps
Unna boot
leg ulcers, 752
venous ulcers, **129,** 130, *130*
upper eyelid blepharoplasty. *see* blepharoplasty
Urgent QR Powder, 249, **252**
urticaria, **571**
U sutures, *256*

V

vaccines, melanoma therapy, 834–835
Valsalva maneuver, 646
vancomycin
endocarditis prophylaxis, 142–143
wound infection prevention, 141
vapocoolants, topical anesthesia, 43, **44**
varicose veins
endovenous ablation (*see* varicose veins, endovenous ablation)
great saphenous vein ligation, 645

varicose veins, endovenous ablation, 645–655
ambulatory phlebectomy as combination, 645–646
Doppler ultrasound, 646
Duplex ultrasound, 646, *647*
endoluminal laser ablation, 645, 651–654
810-nm diode laser, 652, 653, *653*, *654*
940-nm diode laser, 652
1064-nm Nd:YAG laser, 653–654
1320-nm Nd:YAG laser, 653, 654, *654*
history/development, 645
occlusion with endoluminal laser, 654
pitfalls/management, 655
preoperative preparation, 646
radiofrequency closure, 645, 646–649, *648*
ambulatory phlebectomy combination, 649, 651
CEAP class symptoms, 648, **648**
clinical improvement time, 651, *652*
Closure catheter, 647, *647*
consent form, 649, *650*
ligation and/or ambulatory phlebectomy combination, 649
long-term effectiveness, 648
postoperative care, 651
postoperative instructions, 651, *653*
standard technique, 647–649
without phlebectomy, 649
reflux diagnosis, 646
techniques, 646–654
thermal sheath melting, 654, *654*
Valsalva maneuver, 646
vascular compromise, follicular unit hair transplantation, 555
vascular ectasia types, port-wine stain therapy, 632
vascular graft implantation, antibiotics, 145
vascular lesions, 625–644. *see also specific types*
hypertrophic and erythematous scars, 639–640
pulsed dye laser, 639–640, *640*
laser/light treatments, **627**
clinical applications, **630,** 630–640
IPL, 642
postoperative care, 640–642
preoperative preparation, 640
pulsed laser types, 641–642
safety procedures, 640–641
techniques, 640–642
poikiloderma, 638–639
poikiloderma of Civatte, 638–639, *639*
selective photothermolysis, 627–630
IPL, 629–630, **630**
long-pulsed dye lasers, **629**
pulsed dye laser, 627–628, **628,** 629
pulsed KTP lasers, 628, **628**
striae distensae, 640
warts, 640
wavelengths, 626
vascular malformations, cryosurgery, 196–197
vascular networks, random pattern cutaneous flaps, 311
vascular occlusion, autologous fat transfer, 546
vascular response, 100–101
vasculitis ulcers, 746
vasoconstrictors, in anesthesia, 41–42
vasovagal reaction
liposuction, 530
soft-tissue augmentation, 459
vellus hair, 576
laser hair removal avoidance, 586
venous ulcers, 129–131. *see also* arterial ulcers
compression therapy, **129,** 129–131
bandages, **129,** 130
orthotic device, **129,** 130, *130*
pumps, **129,** 130
self-adherent wrap, **129**
stockings, **129,** 130
Unna boot, **129,** 130, *130*
etiology, 743–744, *745*
Graftskin, 762
pharmacologic therapy, 752–753
prevention, 750
shave therapy, 130–131
subfascial endoscopic perforator surgery, 762
wound dressings, 130–131
ventricular ectopy, liposuction, 530
venulectases, pulsed Nd:YAG lasers, 641
venulectasia, 637
verapamil, keloid therapy, 715
vermilion border
lips, *8*
perioral region reconstruction, 390
verrucae, cryosurgery, 192, 194–195
verrucous carcinoma, 792. *see also* squamous cell carcinoma (SCC)
vertical band formation, neck rejuvenation complication, 700
vertical line (facial plane), chin implants, 484, *485*
vertical mattress sutures, 236, *236*, 279, *279*
ellipse excision, 263–264, *265*
scar formation prevention, 401
V-flap (Kalimuthu's technique), split earlobe repair, 294, *296*
Vicryl-rapide sutures, 227, **228**
viral infections, post-dermabrasion, 595, *595*, 597
Virginia, dermatology office accreditation, **169**
vitamin A, melanoma therapy, 834
vitamin E
hemostasis impairment, **247,** 259
keloids, 715
voltage, 179
volumetric aging. *see* minimum incision face lift
von Willebrand disease (vWD), 246–247
cutaneous surgery effect, 73
von Willebrand factor (vWF), 245
V to Y advancement flaps, 317, *318*
ectropion repair, 407
regional reconstruction, 382
scar revision, 405–406, *406*

W

Walike and Larrabee technique, 297, *298*
warfarin
hemostasis impairment, **247,** 248
random pattern cutaneous flap contraindications, 313
warts, 640
nail tumors, 734
organ transplant recipients
pathogenesis, 811
treatment, 811–812, **812,** *814*
pulsed dye laser, 640
Washington, dermatology office accreditation, **169**
waveforms, electrosurgery, 179, *180*, 181, *181*
wavelength, laser-tissue interaction principles, *626*, 626–627, **627**
waxing, hair removal, 578
website addresses, dermatology office accreditation, **171**
Webster needle holders, 62
Weck blade, 371, *371*
wedge excision, earlobe reduction, 304, *304*
weeping, post-cryosurgery, 199
weight gain
autologous fat transfer, 546
fat autograft muscle injection, 546, *546*
following liposuction, 531
weight loss, autologous fat transfer touch-up procedures, 544, *545*
Westcott scissors, 60
whirlpool baths, leg ulcers, 757, *757*
white roll, perioral region reconstruction, 392
Whitnall's tubercle, *14*
wire brush dermabrasion, 431
Wood's light, melanoma staging, 829, 832
wound(s)
acute, 97–98, 99
dressing functions, 117–118
Graftskin, 762
postoperative care/wound care, 127–129
antibiotic therapy/prophylaxis, 137–139, 140–142, **141**
care (*see* wound care)
chronic, 97–98
dressing functions, 118
postoperative care/wound care, 129–131
classification, 140
antibiotics, 140, **140**
closure (*see* wound closure)
contraction, 108
culturing, leg ulcers, **754**
debridement
leg ulcers, 755, *755*
optimizing outcomes, 132, *132*
post-cryosurgery, 200
dehiscence, random pattern cutaneous flaps, 341
dressings (*see* dressings)
healing (*see* wound healing)
necrosis, electrosurgery, 253
wound adhesive strips, 242
wound care, 127–131. *see also* postoperative care
acute wounds, 127–129
arterial ulcers, 131
chronic wounds, 129–131
diabetic foot ulcers, 131
dressings, 145
elliptical excision, 269
full-thickness, uncomplicated, 129
grafting, 376–377
laser resurfacing, **128,** 128–129
Mohs micrographic surgery, 788
partial-thickness, uncomplicated, 129
postexcision wounds, 127–128
pressure ulcers, 131
venous ulcers (*see* venous ulcers)
wound closure, 225–244, 242, *242*, **242,** 273–290. *see also* sutures/suturing; *specific techniques*
cutaneous flaps, 346–348
axial pattern flaps (*see* axial pattern flaps)
blood supply, 347

wound closure, (*cont'd*)
flap survival, 347
neovascularization, 347
random pattern flap, 348
risk factors, 347–348
tobacco exposure, 347
direct, 99, 113
edge inversion, **243**
epidermal cysts, 217
eversion, scar formation prevention, 401
factors influencing choice, **381**
grafts, 346, *346*
keloids, 711
leg ulcers, 746–748
lipomas, 215
materials, 62–64, 225–233
skin closure tapes, 232
staples, 231–232
tissue adhesives, 232–233
minimum incision face lift, 666, *666*, 668
pitfalls, 242–243, **243,** 289
postoperative care, 242, *242*, **242,** 287
preoperative evaluation, 225
preoperative preparation, 273–277
leg ulcers, 754–758
primary closure, 346
staples (*see* staples)
suturing (*see* sutures/suturing)
techniques, 277–287
artificial skin equivalents, 282
complex closure, 280–282
transcutaneous lower-eyelid blepharoplasty, 685
upper-eyelid blepharoplasty, 683, *683*
wound healing, 97–115
acute wound creation, 99
cellular response, 101–103
direct closure, 99
factors influencing, 112–113
flaps, 99
grafts, 99, *100*
keratinocytes role, 98
optimizing outcomes, 113, *113*
phases, 97, *97*, 99–112 (*see also specific phases*)
proliferative phase, 97, *97*, 105–109
angiogenesis, 108–109, *109*, **109**
basement membrane zone restoration, 106, *106*, *107*
dermis reconstitution, 107
fibroplasia, 107
integrin receptors, 107–108, *108*
leg ulcers, 746
re-epithelialization, 105–106
wound contraction, 108
remodeling phase, 97, *97*, 109–112, *110*
collagen, 110–111, *111*
elastic fibers, 111
extracellular matrix, 110
proteinases, 111–112, **112**
repair types, 98, **99**
secondary intention (*see* secondary-intention healing)
wound types, 97–99
acute, 97–98
chronic, 97–98
erosion, 98, *98*, **99**
full-thickness, 98, *98*, **99**
partial-thickness, 98, *98*, **99**
primary intention healing, 98–99
secondary intention healing, 98–99
ulcer, 98, *99*
wounding, keloids, 707
W-plasty
regional reconstruction, 382
scar revision, 403–404, *404*
wraparound keloids, 711, *711*, 712
wrinkles, 431
SMAS, 7
wrist nerve block, 51, *51*, *52*

X

xenografts (heterografts)
definition, 365
porcine, 375, *376*
wound dressing, 123
Xeroform
composite grafts, 374
full-thickness grafts, 366, 368

Y

Yoruba tribe, keloids, 705, 706, *706*

Z

zaleplon, dermabrasion, 594
Zimmer electric dermatome, 371, *371*
Zimmer mesher, 372, *372*
zinc chloride paste, 249, **252**
Zolite's technique, 298, *299*
zolpidem tartrate, 594
Z-plasty
random pattern cutaneous flaps, 342
scar revision, 404–405, *405*
split earlobe repair, 293, *295*
flap creation from lateral portion of lobe, 297, *298*
with superior strip repair of tract, 300, *300*
Zyderm, 441, **442**
allergy rate, 459
historical aspects, 438
preoperative preparation, 440
skin test, 458
zygomatic arch, 10, *11*
zygomatic bone, 7
zygomatic branches, facial nerve, *13*, *14*, 18
zygomatic ligament (McGregor's patch), 658
zygomaticus major muscles, **16,** 17
zygomaticus minor muscles, **16,** 17
Zyplast, 441, *441*, **443,** 447, *447*
allergy rate, 459
historical aspects, 438
preoperative preparation, 440
skin test, 458